Procedures Content

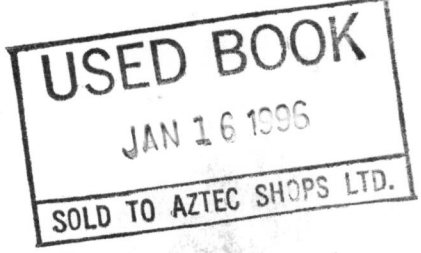

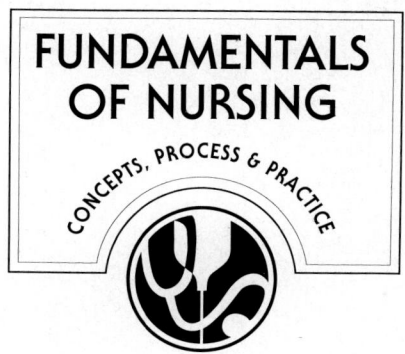

FUNDAMENTALS OF NURSING

CONCEPTS, PROCESS & PRACTICE

FUNDAMENTALS OF NURSING

CONCEPTS, PROCESS & PRACTICE

PATRICIA A. POTTER, RN, MSN

Director of Nursing Practice
Barnes Hospital
St. Louis, Missouri

ANNE G. PERRY, RN, MSN, EdD

Associate Professor
Saint Louis University School of Nursing
St. Louis, Missouri

THIRD EDITION

*with over 632 illustrations,
including 560 in color*

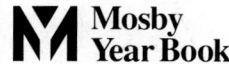

St. Louis Baltimore Boston Chicago London Philadelphia Sydney Toronto

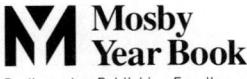
Mosby
Year Book
Dedicated to Publishing Excellence

Managing Editor: Susan R. Epstein
Developmental Editor: Beverly J. Copland
Project Manager: Carol Sullivan Wiseman
Senior Production Editor: Pat Joiner
Designer: David Zielinski

THIRD EDITION

Printed in the United States of America

Mosby–Year Book, Inc.
11830 Westline Industrial Drive
St. Louis, Missouri 63146

Library of Congress Cataloging in Publication Data
Potter, Patricia Ann.
    Fundamentals of nursing : concepts, process, and practice/
Patricia A. Potter, Anne G. Perry.–3rd ed.
        p.   cm.
    Includes bibliographical references and index.
    ISBN 0-8016-6667-8
    1. Nursing.   I. Perry, Anne Griffin.   II. Title.
    [DNLM: 1. Nurse-Patient Relations.   2. Nursing Care.   3. Nursing
Process.   WY 100 868f]
RT41.P844   1992
610.73—dc20
DNLM/DLC
for Library of Congress   92-49926
                                                                            CIP

94 95 96 97 CL/VH/CL 9 8 7 6 5 4 3 2

Contributors

Della Aridge, RN, MSN
Clinical Nurse Specialist, General Surgery Division
Saint Louis University Hospital
St. Louis, Missouri

Susan Cole, RN, MSN, CCRN
Clinical Resource Nurse, Department of Surgery
Saint Francis Medical Center
Cape Girardeau, Missouri

Dorothy McDonnell Cooke, RN, PhD
Assistant Professor, School of Nursing
Saint Louis University
St. Louis, Missouri

Sharon H. Cox, MSN, CNAA
Consultant
Creative Nursing Management, Inc.
Minneapolis, Minnesota

Catherine Doerrer, RN, MSN
Director of Medicine
Barnes Hospital
St. Louis, Missouri

Sally M. Featherstone, RN, MN, CS
Director of Psychiatric Nursing Services
Barnes Hospital
Washington University Medical Center
St. Louis, Missouri

Lois K. Hess, RN, JD
Assistant In-House Counsel
Jewish Hospital Healthcare Systems, Inc.
Louisville, Kentucky

Nancy C. Jackson, RN, BSN, MSN, CCRN
Pulmonary Clinical Nurse Specialist
St. Mary's Health Center
St. Louis, Missouri

†Sister Kathleen Krekeler, RN, PhD
Professor of Nursing, School of Nursing
Saint Louis University
St. Louis, Missouri

Pamela A. Lesser, RN, MS
Women's Services Coordinator
Women and Infants Service
Barnes Hospital
St. Louis, Missouri

Gail B. Lewis, RN, MSN
Associate Professor
Barnes College
St. Louis, Missouri

Annette Lueckenotte, RN, MS, CS
Director of Nursing
Barnes Extended Care — Clayton
St. Louis, Missouri

Mary Kay Knight Macheca, RN, MSN(R), CDE
Diabetes Clinical Nurse Specialist
Barnes Hospital
St. Louis, Missouri

Sharon L. Merritt, RN, EdD
Assistant Professor, Medical-Surgical Nursing
College of Nursing;
Interim Director, Center for Narcolepsy Research
University of Illinois at Chicago
Chicago, Illinois

Ann M. Popkess, RN, BSN
Manager, Barnes Home Health Services
St. Louis, Missouri

Susan A. Reed, RNCS, MSN
Clinical Nurse Specialist
Substance Abuse Programs/Psychiatry
Fort Howard VA Medical Center
Baltimore, Maryland

Janet Robuck, MS, RD
Associate Professor of Nutrition
School of Nursing
University of Alabama
Birmingham, Alabama

Judith A. Roos, RN, MSN
Faculty
Jewish Hospital College of Nursing and Allied Health
St. Louis, Missouri

Janice Rumfelt, RNC, MSN(R), EdD
Assistant Professor, School of Nursing
Southern Illinois University at Edwardsville
Edwardsville, Illinois

Rachel E. Spector, RN, PhD, CTN
Associate Professor, Boston School of Nursing
Chestnut Hill, Massachusetts

Martha Spies, RN, MSN
Assistant Professor, Deaconess College of Nursing
St. Louis, Missouri

Joetta A. Vernon, RN, MS
Doctoral Candidate, University of Nebraska
Lincoln, Nebraska

Mary Walker, RN, MA
Psychiatric Clinical Nurse Specialist
VA Medical Center
Knoxville, Iowa

Valerie Yancey, BA, AD, BSN, MSN
Assistant Professor
Barnes College
St. Louis, Missouri

v

†Deceased

Consultants

Cynthia Hoppe Allen, BSN, MN, MPH
School of Nursing
Southeastern Louisiana University
Hammond, Louisiana

Charlene A. Allred, RN, PhD
Assistant Professor
College of Nursing
Medical University of South Carolina
Charleston, South Carolina

Genevieve Bahrt, RN, MN
Lecturer
School of Nursing
University of California-Los Angeles
Los Angeles, California

Karen Bailey, RN, MSN
Instructor
School of Nursing
Marshall University
Huntington, West Virginia

Billie J. Bodo, RN, MSN
Assistant Professor
Lakeland Community College
Mentor, Ohio

Eleanor Lee Brown, RNC, MSN
Assistant Professor
Department of Nursing
Macon College
Macon, Georgia

Victoria Brown, RN, PhD
Associate Professor
School of Nursing
Georgia College
Milledgeville, Georgia

Mary Coppola, RN, MSN
Assistant Professor
Salem State College
Salem, Massachusetts

Amy Deutschendorf, RN, MSN
Clinical Nurse Specialist
Sinai Hospital of Baltimore;
Faculty Associate
University of Maryland
Baltimore, Maryland

Susan Dicke, BSN, BA, MS
School of Nursing
Mansfield General Hospital
Mansfield, Ohio

Cathy Franklin, RN, BSN, MA
Professor of Nursing
Researcher
Director of Weekend Evening Program
Caldwell Community College
Hudson, North Carolina

Brenda Goodner, RN, MSN, CS
Psychotherapist
Santa Teresa, New Mexico

Renee Harrison, RN, MSN
Assistant Professor
Tulsa Junior College
Tulsa, Oklahoma

Susan Herman, RN, MSN
Assistant Professor of Nursing
Chaffey College
Alta Loma, California

Wendy F. Higden, BN
Teacher and Clinical Instructor
Nursing Department
Vanier College
St. Laurent, Quebec, Canada

Karen Hill, RN, MN
Assistant Professor
School of Nursing
Southeastern Louisiana University
Hammond, Louisiana

Judith Hupcey, CRNP, EdD
Assistant Professor
School of Nursing
Pennsylvania State University
Hershey, Pennsylvania

Susan S. Johnson, RN, MSN
Lead Instructor
Nursing Education Options Program
Guilford Tech Community College
Jamestown, North Carolina

Donna M. Kauffman, RN, MSN
Associate Professor
School of Nursing
Purdue University
West Lafayette, Indiana

Patricia T. Ketcham, RN, MSN, PhDc
Assistant Professor
Undergraduate Program Director
Oakland University
Rochester, Michigan

Marjorie Knox, RN, MA, MPA
Professor of Nursing
Community College of Rhode Island
Warwick, Rhode Island

Jan L. Lee, CS, RN, PhD
Assistant Professor
Medical-Surgical/Physiological Section
School of Nursing
University of California-Los Angeles
Los Angeles, California

Martha Long, RN, MSN, CIC
Infection Control Practitioner
University of Alabama Hospital
Birmingham, Alabama

Ruth Ludwick, RNC, MSN, PhDc
Assistant Professor
School of Nursing
Kent State University
Kent, Ohio

Janet Morgan, RN, MS
Associate Professor of Nursing
Tompkins-Cortland Community College
Dryden, New York

Kathleen Nuwayhid, RN, BSN, MN
Instructor of Nursing
Vanier College
St. Laurent, Quebec, Canada

Susan Opas, RNC, MSN, CNS, CHES
Lecturer
School of Nursing
University of California-Los Angeles
Los Angeles, California

Victoria L. Poole, RN, DSN
Assistant Professor
School of Nursing
University of Alabama at Birmingham
Birmingham, Alabama

Cheryl A. Prandoni, RN, MSN
Director of Learning Resources
School of Nursing
Catholic University of America
Washington, D.C.

Caroline Pritchard, RN, MSN, ND
Instructor and Clinical Director
BSN Program
Case Western Reserve University
Cleveland, Ohio

Peg Reiter, RN, MS
Assistant Professor
Galveston College
Galveston, Texas

Susan Schaffer, RN, MS, CFNP
Assistant Professor of Nursing
Old Dominion University
Norfolk, Virginia

Patti Pond Scott, RN, BS
Instructor
Kilgore College
Longview, Texas

Margaret Souders, RNC, MSN
Instructor
Department of Nursing
Phoenix College
Phoenix, Arizona

Ruth Stephens, RN, PhD
Professor of Nursing
Florida Community College at Jacksonville
Jacksonville, Florida

Jean Urick, RN, MN
Assistant Professor
School of Nursing
Southeastern Louisiana University
Hammond, Louisiana

Flora Weirich, RN, MSN, CEN
Instructor
School of Nursing
Pennsylvania State University
University Park, Pennsylvania

Joyce Williams, RN, MSN
Assistant Professor
School of Nursing
George Mason University
Fairfax, Virginia

Diane M. Wink, RN, MSN, MA, EdD
Assistant Professor
University of Central Florida
Orlando, Florida

Toni Wortham, RNC, MSN
Associate Professor
Nursing Program
Madisonville Community College
Madisonville, Kentucky

To the professional nurses of Barnes Hospital for their excellence in client care.

Pat Potter

To the nurses at Saint Louis University Hospital and the School of Nursing for their commitment to excellence in nursing practice, education, administration, and research.

In Loving Memory of
Sr. Kathleen Krekeler, RN, PhD, CCVI
1928-1992
Teacher, mentor, friend
Her knowledge, compassion, humor,
and gentle demands for excellence
were cherished gifts to all of us.

Anne Perry

Preface

The art and science of professional nursing practice continue to evolve and expand. The growing body of nursing research and the explosion of technological advances challenge and stimulate nurses to acquire knowledge and refine critical-thinking skills. The goal of nursing education is to prepare today's student to meet tomorrow's challenge.

More than ever, the nurse of tomorrow will need a broad knowledge base from which to provide the expert care needed in a rapidly developing profession. The student must first master the basic theories and skills and then develop and refine the ability to apply analytical thinking to each clinical situation. Finally, the nurse must combine competency and critical thinking with caring and an awareness of the uniqueness of each client's specialized needs.

Fundamentals of Nursing: Concepts, Process, and Practice has been developed to provide today's students with a solid foundation of nursing principles to prepare them to meet the challenges of tomorrow. This textbook is designed for beginning students in all levels of professional nursing programs. The comprehensive coverage provides fundamental nursing concepts, skills, and techniques of nursing practice and a firm foundation for more advanced areas of nursing study.

The text presents the theoretical and practical information necessary to make sound clinical judgments while emphasizing cognitive, interpersonal, and psychomotor skills needed to carry out fundamental nursing activities. Each aspect of the educational approach is organized to guide the student to interrelate principles and skills while developing a critical-thinking approach to each clinical situation.

 FEATURES

This third edition has been revised and expanded to reflect the realities of current nursing practice and the learning needs of today's students. The content and presentation have been designed to ensure that students can readily master the theoretical and practical knowledge needed to make sound clinical judgments and carry out fundamental nursing activities.

ORGANIZATION. The content is presented in a logical building-block approach. Realistic clinical examples are presented throughout to clearly illustrate the application of theoretical concepts in practice. Chapter by chapter, the student builds on and reinforces knowledge already mastered to understand additional principles and clinical skills.

NURSING PROCESS FRAMEWORK. The five-step nursing process serves as the organizing framework for narrative discussions of clinical content. In each clinical chapter nursing process is discussed in narrative accompanied by a series of boxes illustrating the application of the nursing process to client care. These boxes provide pertinent examples of possible NANDA diagnoses, samples of the diagnostic process, related sample nursing care plans, and sample evaluations of interventions against expected outcomes. A distinct logo alerts students to nursing process content. This logo precedes each step in the narrative and is repeated in each box, visually linking the narrative discussion to the boxed displays for quick recognition. As the discussion guides students through the process, the boxes demonstrate *how* to apply it. For example, sample diagnostic process boxes contain assessment activities and corresponding defining characteristics that form nursing diagnoses.

The sample nursing care plans clearly demonstrate the development of individualized care plans. Based on NANDA-approved nursing diagnoses through the Tenth Conference in 1992, the sample care plans feature client goals, expected outcomes, and interventions with rationales.

LEARNING AIDS. Each chapter in *Fundamentals of Nursing* begins with a chapter outline and learning objectives to focus students' attention on important content. Key terms are boldfaced and defined within the chapter to ensure comprehension. A list of key terms in each chapter appears in the chapter review.

Nearly 100 step-by-step procedures with research-based rationales detail how, and why, nursing skills are performed. Large, full-color photos and drawings clarify and support the narrative to visually prepare students for clinical experience.

Boxed research highlights emphasize the relevance of nursing research to practice. A new feature, client teaching boxes, stresses the growing importance of the nurse's role in preparing clients for self-care. Whereas the narrative instructs students *how* to teach, the boxes highlight *what* to teach. Numerous tables, boxes, and illustrations emphasize and support important content.

Each chapter closes with a brief summary followed by a new feature, the chapter review, including key concepts, key terms with reference to the page where the definition can be found, and critical thinking exercises. This review assists students to evaluate learning and test their ability to apply what they have learned. References and additional readings guide students desiring further exploration.

NEW AND EXPANDED CONTENT. A completely rewritten nursing process unit expands coverage of the diagnostic process and planning phase. The assessment chapter includes Gordon's Functional Health Patterns. Total quality improvement has been incorporated to provide a basis for evaluation to ensure quality client care.

The chapter on health care delivery expands coverage of financial issues and their impact on health care. The home health care chapter has been expanded to include discussions of admission and discharge to address these key areas of client care.

The culture and ethnicity chapter adds consideration of the nurse's and client's cultures in planning care. The teaching-learning chapter has been expanded to prepare students for increased responsibility in preparing clients for self-care. Body substance isolation (BSI) precautions are incorporated and stressed throughout the text to reflect their increasing inclusion in agency protocols. The oxygenation chapter now includes cardiovascular factors and basic content on interpretation of ECGs.

This edition also features two new chapters. The skin integrity chapter focuses on prevention and care of pressure ulcers and incorporates the latest AHCPR and NPUAP guidelines for risk identification, prevention, and treatment. The mobility and immobility chapter presents mobility on a continuum of health care needs to address the impact of varying levels of mobility on the client.

VISUAL APPEAL. A contemporary, attractive design features an easy-to-read typeface and bold headings. Special logo visually highlight content on nursing process, teaching, and research boxes to help students locate these important elements. Other key content is highlighted in tables and boxed displays. The addition of hundreds of new, large, full-color illustrations enhances learning and understanding.

 ORGANIZATION

The textbook is organized into nine units that emphasize a logical progression in the learning process.

Unit 1, The Nurse, Client, and Health Care Environment, introduces the student to the profession of nursing by presenting a historical overview, discussing nursing theories, and addressing the health care system, client, and environment. Cultural considerations of the nurse and client are presented with discussions of financial issues in health care, current regulatory standards, admission and discharge, and home health care.

Unit 2, The Nursing Process, discusses the use of the nursing process as a whole and considers each component in detail. Five separate chapters emphasize the importance of each step of the process.

Unit 3, Professional Nursing Concepts and Issues, discusses the importance and relevance of basic nursing concepts. A chapter on research emphasizes the importance of conducting research and integrating new findings into practice. A comprehensive overview of the principles of values, ethics, legal issues, communication skills, client teaching, and leadership related to nursing practice is provided.

Unit 4, Professional Nursing Skills, details nursing actions and skills applicable to all health care settings for a wide variety of clients. The unit progresses from simple skills of measuring vital signs to more complicated techniques of physical assessment and medication administration. The importance of observing BSI precautions and accurately reporting and recording are stressed throughout.

Unit 5, Growth and Development for the Individual and Family, presents the differing health care needs of specific age groups. It begins with a discussion of the family and proceeds from conception through older adulthood. The last chapter discusses nursing measures regarding death, loss, and grieving.

Unit 6, Human Needs in Health and Illness, explores the psychosocial needs of clients and explains how to assess these needs and incorporate interventions into nursing care. The student learns about the influence of a client's emotional, sexual, and spiritual needs on health beliefs and practice.

Unit 7, Basic Physiological Needs, details nursing care for clients with problems in hygiene, nutrition, sleep, comfort, oxygenation, fluid balances, and urinary and bowel elimination. Each chapter discusses normal physiological structure, alterations, assessment criteria, and the use of the nursing process.

Unit 8, Providing a Safe Environment, stresses the importance of maintaining a safe environment for the client. The chapter on mobility and immobility addresses body mechanics on a continuum of needs to emphasize the importance of individualized care. The new chapter on skin integrity focuses on prevention and care of pressure ulcers. Discussions of sensory alterations and substance abuse address the special needs of clients with these problems.

Unit 9, Caring for the Perioperative Client, presents care for inpatient and outpatient surgical clients. Preoperative and postoperative care are discussed, with a separate chapter on nursing interventions to promote wound healing.

The text concludes with an appendix of normal laboratory values, an extensive glossary of important terms introduced in the text, and a detailed, cross-referenced index. Common abbreviations have been listed inside the back cover for quick referral.

In organizing the text, every attempt was made to ensure a logical progression of concepts and skills and a meaningful grouping of related subjects. We recognize that instructors may assign chapters in different sequences and therefore have made each chapter as independently understandable as possible with extensive cross-references throughout the text.

The clinical examples in the text depict men and women practicing nursing in a variety of health care settings. We have attempted to delete sexist language and cumbersome terms such as *he/she* and *his/her* as much as possible when referring to clients and nurses in the text.

We acknowledge the differences in opinion related to use of the terms *client* and *patient*. We have chosen to use the term *client* because it suggests a more active, participatory role for the person who has entered the health care delivery system. In its broadest sense, *client* refers to the client-family unit and the client-significant other unit, as well as the individual.

TEACHING AND LEARNING PACKAGE

A number of ancillaries have been developed to assist instructors and students in the teaching and learning process. These include an instructor's resource manual and test bank, *Computest* (a computerized test bank), a set of overhead transparency acetates, a student study guide, and procedure performance checklists for students.

The *Instructor's Resource Manual and Test Bank* includes learning objectives, key terms, topical out-

lines, sample nursing care plan exercises, suggestions for classroom and clinical activities, and procedure performance checklists for all chapters of the textbook. These performance checklists are formatted for convenient duplication for class use. The questions in the test bank are formulated to parallel the type of questions students will encounter on the NCLEX examination. The answer key provides coding of responses according to the NCLEX blueprint categories of nursing process and client needs. The manual is perforated so that pages can be easily removed for lesson planning and test construction.

A Study Guide to Accompany Fundamentals of Nursing, by Kathleen Hoover, has been developed to furnish a meaningful self-instructional tool focusing on the essential concepts, principles, and skills presented in the text. Each chapter parallels the chapters in the text and includes prerequisite readings, objectives, review of key concepts, critical-thinking and experiential exercises, additional readings, and answers for the review of key concept exercises.

Computest, a computerized test bank of over 500 multiple choice questions related to content in the text, aids instructors using computers in test construction. All questions on the disks are also printed in the *Instructor's Resource Manual.*

The *Overhead Transparency Acetates* set includes 100 illustrations from the text, selected for effective use in classroom discussions and for instructional value. Many of these are full-color; the remaining transparencies are two-color.

The *Procedure Performance Checklists* provided in the *Instructor's Resource Manual* are also available for student purchase. These checklists are bound and perforated and are offered individually or packaged with the text.

In addition, schools adopting this text will receive a video from the new Mosby's Nursing Skills Video Series.

ACKNOWLEDGMENTS

To Susan Epstein, a multi-talented editor whose knowledge, experience, good humor, and patience nurtured our creativity while she demanded excellence in developing this edition.

Our development editor, Beverly Copland, for her attention to detail, motivation, commitment to excellence, and magical skills for tracking contributors, manuscript, illustrations, and at times the authors.

The professional nursing staffs of Barnes Hospital and the Saint Louis University Hospital. Their commitment to excellence in nursing care has instilled many ideas for this text. A special thanks to members of the administrative staffs for their support and belief in this project.

Saint Louis University School of Nursing for providing an environment in which faculty and students can achieve their highest potential. Thanks to faculty members and students who lent their time and expertise for many of the photographic sessions.

Patrick Watson, a highly creative individual whose photographs are visually realistic. Through Pat's patience and a determination to achieve visual perfection, his photographs make each chapter very special.

Our illustrators, Vicki M. Freidman and Marcy H. Hartstein, for their meticulous line and full-color drawings.

Our family and friends for their patience, understanding, and support during times that were often difficult at best. They provided an emotional strength that made all our efforts worthwhile.

Our reviewers and nursing advisory panel, whose expertise and astute recommendations helped develop a text of high standards to meet the needs of beginning nursing students.

The book production editing, design, and manufacturing staff at Mosby–Year Book, whose talents and commitment to quality resulted in a visually appealing and readable textbook.

We also wish to acknowledge a friendship that continues to grow, protect, and nurture each of us in our personal and professional challenges.

Patricia A. Potter
Anne G. Perry

Detailed Contents

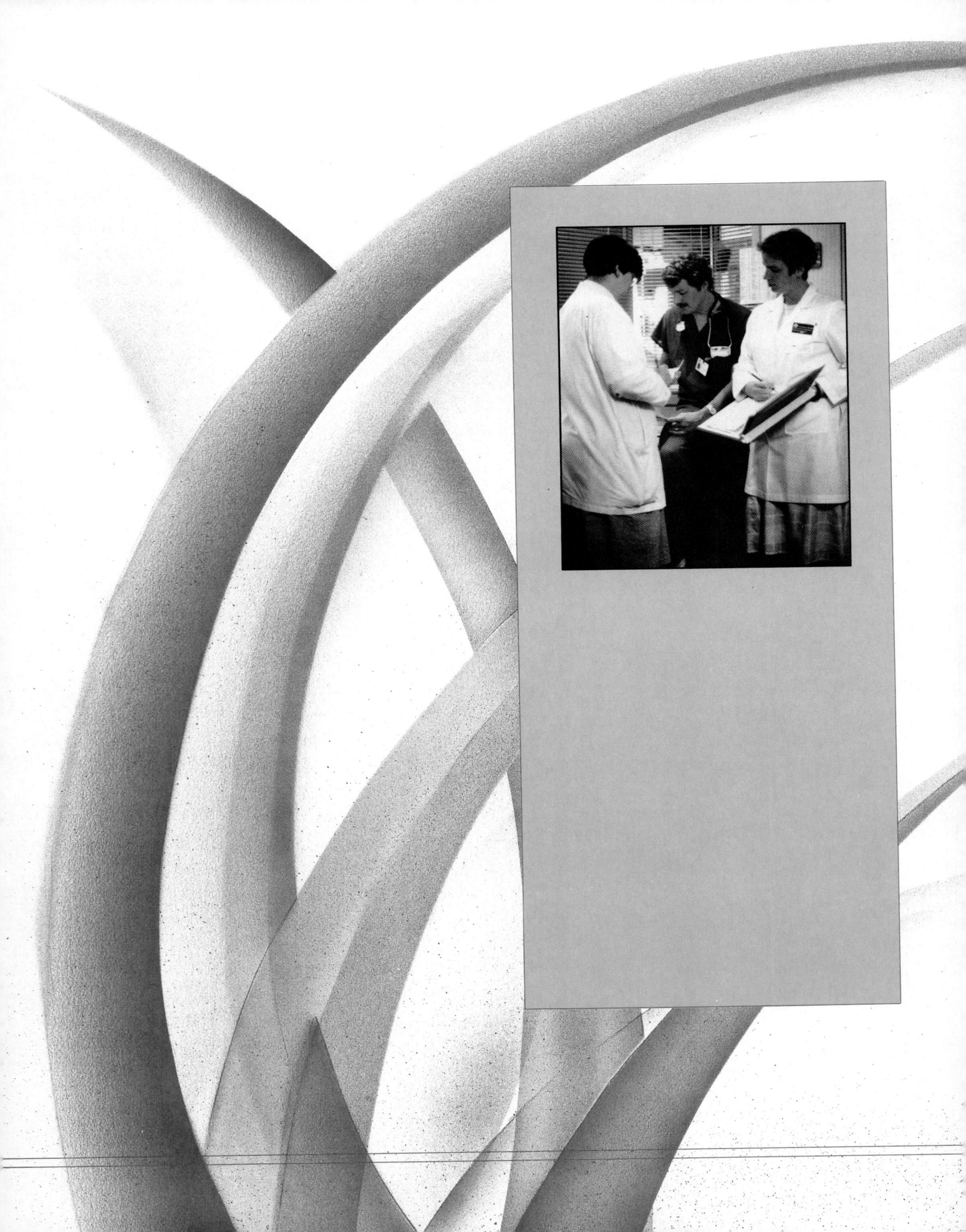

UNIT 1

The Nurse, Client, and Health Care Environment

CHAPTER 1

The Profession of Nursing

OBJECTIVES

Mastery of content in this chapter will enable the student to:
- Define the key terms listed.
- Discuss the historical development of professional nursing.
- Discuss the modern definitions, philosophies, and theories of nursing practice.
- Describe educational programs for becoming a registered nurse.
- Describe practice settings for nurses.
- Describe the roles and function of a nurse.
- List the five characteristics of a profession and discuss how nursing demonstrates these characteristics.
- Discuss the influence of social and economic changes on nursing practice.
- Discuss the influence of nursing on political issues and health care policy.

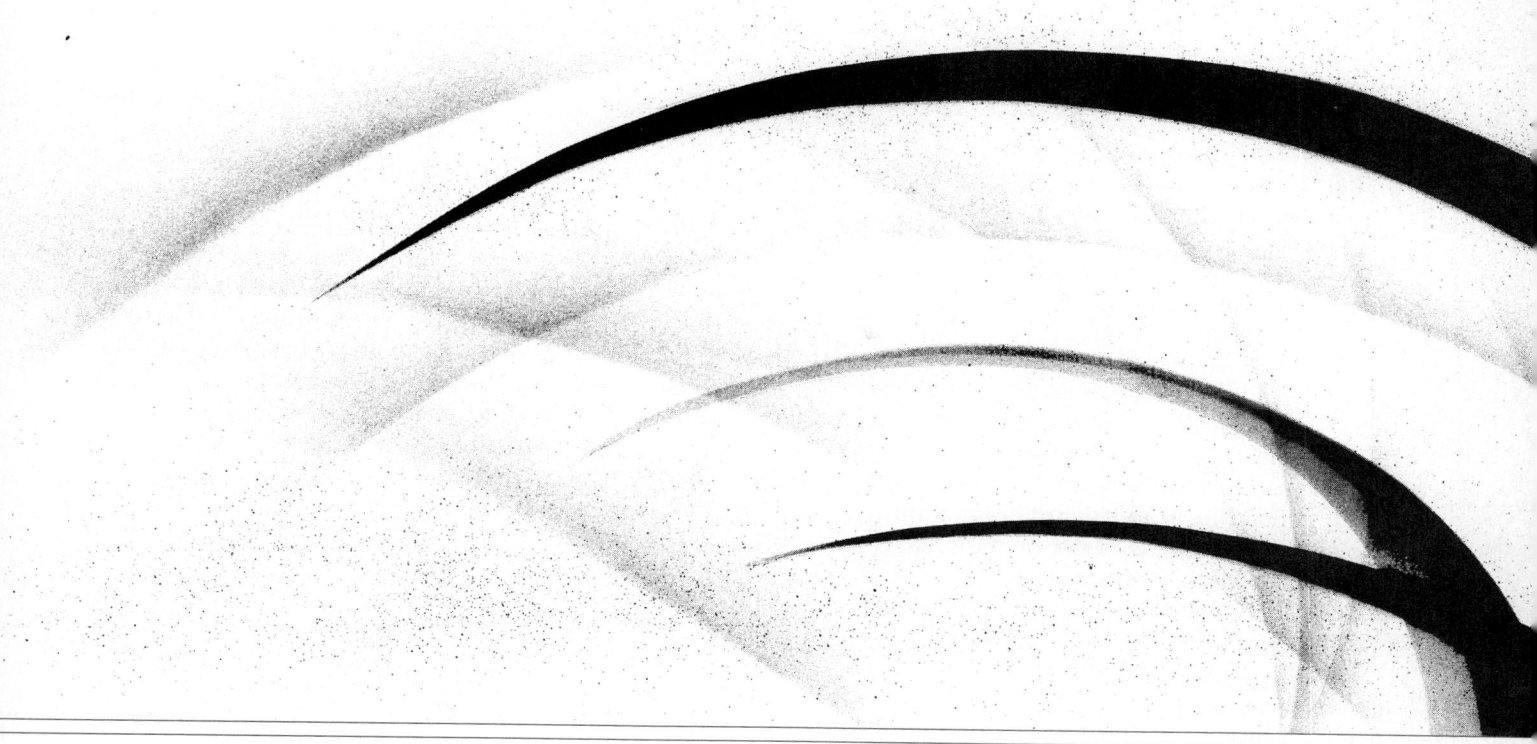

CHAPTER OUTLINE

Modern nursing involves many activities, concepts, and skills related to basic sciences, social sciences, growth and development, contemporary issues, and other areas. Nursing as a profession is unique because it addresses the responses of individuals and families to actual and potential health problems in a humanistic and holistic manner. Nurses have many roles, such as care givers, decision makers, advocates, and teachers, and they must often assume several roles at the same time. Because of the diversity of nursing roles, nurses need a philosophy of nursing to guide their practice. Over the years, nurses have developed many philosophies and definitions of nursing. The following definition, written by Virginia Henderson and adopted by the **International Council of Nurses (ICN)** (1973), is a concise statement with which most nursing theorists would agree:

The unique function of the nurse is to assist the individual, sick or well, in the performance of those activities contributing to health, its recovery, or to a peaceful death that the client would perform unaided if he had the necessary strength, will, or knowledge. And to do this in such a way as to help the client gain independence as rapidly as possible.

The profession of nursing is complex and multifaceted. Nurses practice in many settings that emphasize different aspects of nursing care and nursing roles. In addition, individuals can become registered nurses through a variety of educational programs, and a variety of career opportunities become available as nurses gain experience and continue their education.

Expertise in nursing is the result of knowledge and clinical experience. The expertise required to interpret clinical situations and make complex decisions is the basis for the advancement of nursing practice and the development of nursing science (Benner, 1984; Benner, Tanner, 1987). To deliver nursing care, the nurse must be able to make relevant observations, recognize health problems, and develop appropriate plans to address those problems (Tanner et al, 1987). Expertise is gained through this continual process.

The profession of nursing evolves as society and health care needs and policies change. Nursing responds and adapts to changes, meeting new challenges as they arise.

 HISTORICAL PERSPECTIVE

Nursing was distinguished in its early history as a form of community service and was originally related to a strong instinct to preserve and protect the family (Donahue, 1985). Nursing began as the desire to keep people healthy and provide comfort, care, and assurance to the sick. Although the general goals of nursing have remained relatively the same over the centuries, the practice of nursing has been influenced by society's changing needs, and thus nursing has gradually evolved into a modern profession.

Nursing is as old as medicine. Throughout history, nursing and medicine have been interdependent. During the era of Hippocrates, medicine was practiced without nursing, and during the Middle Ages, nursing was practiced without medicine (Donahue, 1985).

In ancient cultures, religious beliefs and myths were the bases for health care and medical practice. Religious leaders assumed the responsibility for diagnosis and treatment, and many cultures believed that illness was caused by the gods' displeasure. In these cultures, nurses usually had a role subservient to religious leaders.

Many ancient societies did not value human life in the same way we do today, so the care takers of life were less respected. Nurses delivered custodial care and depended on physicians or priests for direction (Kelly, 1981). Under the direct supervision of a physician the nurse tended to the hygiene of clients in the home. Nurses did not participate in activities to promote health or teach families how to care for the ill.

One consistent role of the nurse from early civilization is that of the midwife. Throughout medical and nursing histories the midwife has been accepted in the role of assisting women during childbirth.

Under the influence of Christianity, nurses began to gain respect, and the practice of nursing expanded. One of the earliest records of Christian nursing detailed the formation of the Order of the Deaconesses, a group somewhat like today's public health or visiting nurses. The Order's goals included meeting the following basic needs of the society (Dolan et al, 1983; Donahue, 1985):

1. To feed the hungry
2. To give water to the thirsty
3. To clothe the naked
4. To visit the imprisoned
5. To shelter the homeless
6. To care for the sick
7. To bury the dead

Historically, men and women have held the role of nurse. The entry of women into nursing can be traced to approximately AD 300 (Shryock, 1959; Donahue, 1985). Women entered nursing because the social position of Roman women improved (Shryock, 1959), Christians taught that men and women are equal before God (Shryock, 1959; Dolan et al, 1983), and Christians appealed to women "to carry on His work in behalf of all who were in distress" (Shryock, 1959).

The Benedictine order, founded in the sixth century, increased the number of men entering nursing. Although the Benedictines were scholars, librarians, teachers, and agriculturalists, nursing the sick eventually became the chief function and duty of their community life (Donahue, 1985).

During the Middle Ages, the Crusades became a stimulus for expanded nursing and health care. Military nursing orders for men were formed, and hospitals were established. After the Crusades, large cities began to develop and grow with the decline of feudalism. The extensive population growth in cities led to certain health problems (see box) and an increased need for health care. Some of these problems still exist in urban areas today, although the mortality rates associated with them have greatly declined.

Secular groups were also formed to meet specific health care needs during the Middle Ages. The Hospital Brothers of St. Anthony cared for victims of the disease called *St. Anthony's fire*, the Brothers of Misericordia in Italy provided transportation services for the ill (Fig. 1-1), and the Alexian Brothers (a group still active today) cared for victims of bubonic plague.

The lack of hygiene and sanitation and the increasing poverty in urban centers resulted in serious health problems in the fifteenth to seventeenth centuries. Societal factors, such as laws punishing the poor and the Window Tax (which led to decreased ventilation because landlords bricked in windows to avoid paying the tax), created conditions and health needs to which nursing responded.

The Sisters of Charity was founded in 1633 by St. Vincent de Paul. The sisters cared for people in hospitals, asylums, and poorhouses. In addition, the sisters became widely known as visiting nurses because they cared for sick people in their homes. The first supervisor of the Sisters of Charity was Louise de Gras, a widow of high social standing. de Gras, who entered the order and was later known as St. Louise de Marillac, established perhaps the first educational program to be associated with a nursing order. She recruited intelligent, refined, and compassionate women (Donahue, 1985). The program included experience in the care of the sick in the hospital, as well as home visits. The Sisters of Charity were introduced in America by Mother Elizabeth Seton in 1809, and later their name was changed to the Daughters of Charity (Donahue, 1985).

In the eighteenth century, the further growth of cities brought an increase in the number of hospitals and a larger role for nurses. Smallpox epidemics in the French colonies and during the Revolutionary War in the English colonies increased the need for nursing services. Nursing skills and knowledge were

---

Health Problems Associated with the Growth of Cities

- Overcrowding
- Poor ventilation
- Poor heating and cooling
- Poor sanitation, garbage collection, and plumbing
- Poor water supply
- Inadequate methods of preserving foods
- Ignorance of elementary hygiene practices

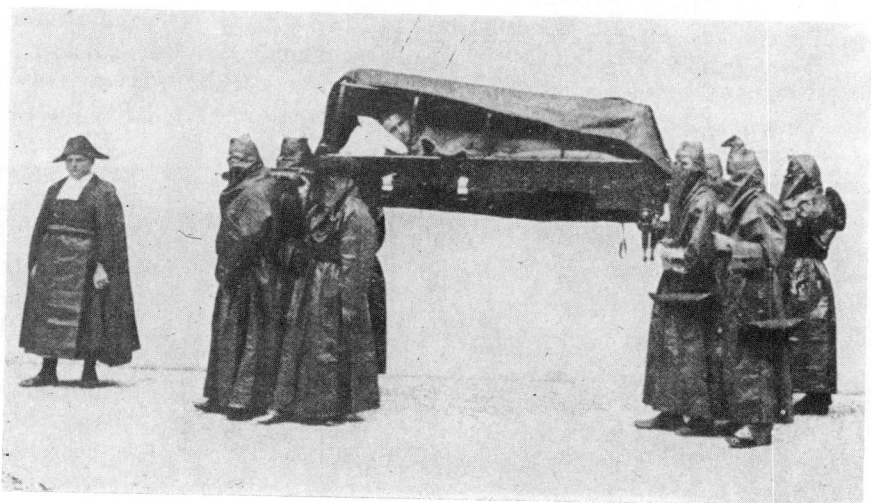

Fig. 1-1   The Brothers of Misericordia taking a patient to the hospital in Florence.
From Dolan JA et al: *Nursing in society,* ed 15, Philadelphia, 1983, Saunders.

generally passed on by experienced nurses because there was still little formal education for them.

During the nineteenth century, the Deaconess Order was revived by Protestant churches. The Deaconess Institute at Kaiserswerth, Germany, was established in 1836 by Pastor Theodore Fliedner (Woodham-Smith, 1983; Donahue, 1985). The regeneration of this nursing order was stimulated by the recognition of the need for the services of nurses.

In October 1846, Florence Nightingale received the *Yearbook of the Institution of Deaconesses at Kaiserswerth* (Woodham-Smith, 1983). In 1847, she went to Kaiserswerth to work with the Deaconesses (Woodham-Smith, 1983; Donahue, 1985).

In 1853, Nightingale went to Paris to study with the Sisters of Charity and was later appointed superintendent of the English General Hospitals in Turkey. During this period, she brought about major reforms in hygiene, sanitation, and nursing practice and reduced the mortality rate at the Barracks Hospital in Scutari, Turkey, from 42.7% to 2.2% in 6 months (Cohen, 1984; Woodham-Smith, 1983; Donahue, 1985).

In 1860, Nightingale wrote *Notes on Nursing: What It Is and What It Is Not* for the lay person. Her philosophy of nursing practice reflected the changing needs of society. She saw the role of nursing as having "charge of somebody's health" based on the knowledge of "how to put the body in such a state to be free of disease or to recover from disease" (Nightingale, 1860). During the same year, she developed the first organized program of training for nurses, the Nightingale Training School for Nurses at St. Thomas' Hospital in London (Fig. 1-2).

The Civil War stimulated the growth of nursing in the United States. Clara Barton, founder of the American Red Cross, tended soldiers on the battlefields, cleansing their wounds, meeting their basic needs, and comforting them in death. The American Red Cross was ratified by the United States Congress in 1882 after 10 years of lobbying by Barton. Dorothea Lynde Dix, Mary Ann Ball (Mother Bickerdyke), and Harriet Tubman also influenced nursing during the Civil War (Donahue, 1985). As superintendent of the female nurses of the Union Army, Dix organized hospitals, appointed nurses, and oversaw and regulated supplies to the troops. Mother Bickerdyke organized ambulance services, supervised nurses, and walked abandoned battlefields at night looking for wounded soldiers. Harriet Tubman was active in the Underground Railroad movement and assisted in leading over 300 slaves to freedom (Donahue, 1985).

After the Civil War, nursing schools in the United States and Canada began to pattern their curricula after the Nightingale School. In Canada the first training school, St. Catherine's in Ontario, was founded in 1874 (Donahue, 1985; Raab, 1985). In 1884, Mary Agnes Snively took over the directorship of the Toronto General Hospital. She helped form the Canadian National Association of Trained Nurses in 1908 (Donahue, 1985; Raab, 1985). The name was later changed to the **Canadian Nurses Association (CNA)** in 1924 (Donahue, 1985).

Isabel Hampton (later Isabel Hampton Robb), a graduate of St. Catherine's in Ontario, was the first superintendent of the Johns Hopkins Training School in Baltimore, Maryland. She authored the following textbooks: *Nursing: Its Principles and Practice for Hospital and Private Use* (1894), *Nursing Ethics* (1900), and *Educational Standards for Nurses* (1907) (Donahue, 1985). She helped found the Nurses' Associated Alumnae of the United States and Canada in 1896. The Canadian affiliation was removed in 1899, and the organization became the **American Nurses Association (ANA)** in 1911. Hampton was also one of the original founders of the *American Journal of Nursing* (Wheeler, 1985; Donahue, 1985).

Nursing in hospitals expanded in the late nineteenth century, but nursing in the community did not increase significantly until 1893 when Lillian Wald and Mary Brewster opened the Henry Street Settlement, which focused on the health needs of poor people who lived in tenements in New York (Silverstein, 1985; Donahue, 1985). Nurses working in this settlement had greater responsibility for their clients than nurses working in hospitals because they frequently encountered situations requiring action independent of a physician's orders. In addition to the treatment of illness, poor people needed nursing

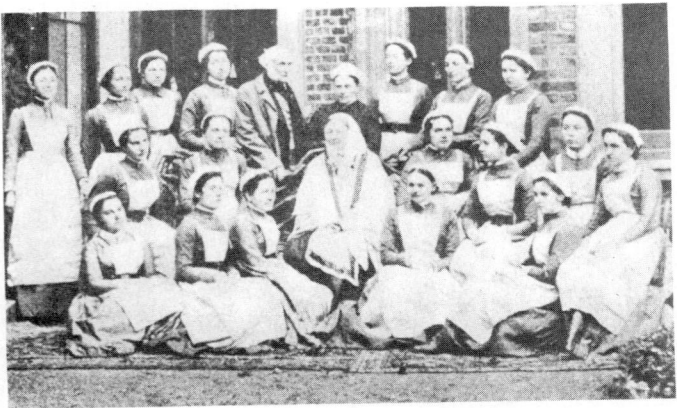

Fig. 1-2 Florence Nightingale (*center*) and students at St Thomas' Hospital in London in 1887.
From Dolan JA et al: *Nursing in society*, ed 15, Philadelphia, 1983, Saunders.

therapies aimed at restoring nutrition, providing shelter, and maintaining hygiene. Wald authored the following books describing her activities with the Henry Street Settlement: *The House on Henry Street* (1915) and *Windows on Henry Street* (1934).

Advances were made in hospital care, public health, and nursing education in the early twentieth century. Mary Adelaide Nutting, a member of the first graduating class at Johns Hopkins Hospital and successor to Isabel Hampton Robb as superintendent of the Johns Hopkins Training School, was instrumental in the affiliation of nursing education with universities. She became the first professor of nursing at Columbia University Teachers College in 1907 (Donahue, 1985).

In 1923 the Rockefeller Foundation funded a survey of nursing education, the Goldmark Report. The report concluded that nursing education needed increased financial support and suggested that the money be given to university schools of nursing. As a result the Rockefeller Foundation funded the expansion of nursing programs at Yale University, Vanderbilt University, and the University of Toronto. Frances Payne Bolton provided financial support for the nursing school at Western Reserve University.

As nursing education developed, nursing practice also expanded. In 1901 the Army Nurse Corps was established, followed in 1908 by the Navy Nurse Corps. Nursing specialization was also developing. In the 1920s, graduate nurse-midwifery programs were initiated, and beginning in the 1950s, specialty nursing organizations such as the Association of Operating Room Nurses (1949), American Association of Critical-Care Nurses (1969), and Oncology Nursing Society (1975) were formed.

In 1965 the National Commission on Nursing and Nursing Education explored issues that included the supply of and demand for nurses, clarification of nursing roles and functions, education of nurses, and career opportunities available to nurses. Their report, often called the *Lysaught report* after Jerome P. Lysaught, the director of the study, called for clarification of nursing roles and responsibilities in relation to those of other health care professionals. It also advocated greater financial support for nurses and more career opportunities to attract nurses and retain them in the profession (Lysaught, 1970).

As nursing practice and education evolved to meet the needs of society, nursing's code of ethics, which was initially discussed in 1897, also evolved (Viens, 1989). The first written ANA Code of Ethics was proposed in 1926 at the organization's annual convention. The purpose of this code was to "create a sensitiveness to ethical situations and to formulate general principles which result in the formation of conscious

and critical judgment resulting in action in specific situations" (ANA, 1926). Again as technology and the needs of society changed, the Code underwent multiple revisions, the most recent being the 1985 Code for Nurses with Interpretive Statements (Sward, 1978; ANA, 1985) (see Chapter 13).

Nurses and nurse educators are revising nursing practice and curricula to meet the ever-changing needs of society. Advances in high technology, rising acuity of clients, and early discharge of clients from health care institutions require nurses to have a strong and current knowledge base from which to practice.

CONCEPTUAL AND THEORETICAL MODELS OF NURSING PRACTICE

The development of nursing science and theory is a scholarly activity. Developing this science involves generating knowledge; although this knowledge can be used with knowledge from other disciplines, it is designed to advance and support nursing practice and health care (Hinshaw, 1989). One method for creating nursing's scientific knowledge base is through the development and use of **nursing theory**.

Historically, nursing theories were studied in an isolated academic environment independent of nursing practice. There is, however, a contemporary move toward theory-based practice. Nurses now and in the future need to have models of care from which their practice is based (Parse, 1990).

As nursing continues to evolve, nurses theorize about the nature of nursing practice, the principles on which practice is based, and the proper goals and functions of nursing in society. Conceptual and theoretical nursing models are used to provide knowledge to improve practice, guide research and curricula, and identify the domain and goals of nursing practice. Nursing theories provide the nurse with goals for assessment, nursing diagnosis, and intervention; common ground for communication; and professional autonomy and accountability. They also guide future directions for nursing research, practice, education, and administration (Marriner-Tomey, 1989; Chinn, Jacobs, 1987; Fawcett, 1989; Meleis, 1985; Torres, 1986; Parse, 1987) (see box on p. 8).

A historical review of the last 120 years demonstrates that nursing has developed a growing body of knowledge. Nursing concepts and theories have evolved since Nightingale, who, in establishing the discipline of nursing, spoke with firm conviction about the "nature of nursing as a profession that required knowledge distinct from medical knowledge" (Nightingale, 1860). The overall goal of this knowl-

---

Goals of Theoretical Nursing Models

- Guide research to establish empirical knowledge base for nursing
- Identify area to be studied
- Identify research techniques and tools that will be used to validate nursing interventions
- Identify nature of contribution that research will make to advancement of knowledge
- Formulate legislation governing nursing practice, research, and education
- Formulate regulations interpreting nurse practice acts so that nurses and others better understand laws
- Develop curriculum plans for nursing education
- Establish criteria for measuring quality of nursing care, education, and research
- Prepare job descriptions used by employers of nurses
- Guide development of nursing care delivery systems
- Provide knowledge to improve nursing administration, practice, education, and research
- Provide systematic structure and rationale for nursing activities
- Identify domain and goals of nursing

---

edge has been to explain the practice of nursing as different and distinct from the practice of medicine, psychology, and social work (Torres, 1986; Chinn, Jacobs, 1987; Fawcett, 1989).

A significant milestone influencing the development of nursing concepts and theory was the establishment of the journal, *Nursing Research,* in 1952. This journal reports on the scientific investigations being conducted by nurses and other professionals. The journal has encouraged scientific productivity and has helped to provide the framework for a questioning attitude that has set the stage for further inquiries into theoretical nursing (Meleis, 1985).

In the mid-1950s, nursing leaders began to formulate theoretical views of nursing and concerns about subjects to include or exclude from nursing curricula. Teachers College Columbia University offered masters and doctoral programs in nursing education and administration (Meleis, 1985). Several prominent nurse theorists graduated from this institution; these include Peplau, Henderson, Hall, Abdellah, King, Wiedenbach, and Rogers.

During the 1960s, Yale University School of Nursing defined nursing even further. "Nursing was considered a process rather than an end, an interaction rather than content, and a relationship between two human beings rather than an interaction between unrelated nurse and patient" (Meleis, 1985). In addition, the ANA's 1965 position paper defined nursing and concluded that one of the most significant goals for nursing was theory development. The ANA supported and lobbied for the need for continuing efforts to develop the body of nursing knowledge (ANA, 1965; Meleis, 1985). As a result, federal support was also provided to nurses pursuing masters and doctoral degrees.

Theory development was emphasized from the mid-1960s to 1970. A series of symposia, sponsored by Case Western Reserve University, was held to assist in the development of nursing theory. During the mid-1970s the **National League for Nursing (NLN)**, the accrediting institution for nursing education programs, made theory-based curriculum a requirement for accreditation. Thus schools of nursing were expected to use a conceptual framework in the development and implementation of their curricula (Meleis, 1985).

Definitions and theories of nursing can help the nursing student understand how the roles and actions of nurses fit together in nursing. The following sections describe, in chronological order, concepts basic to selected nursing theories (Table 1-1).

Nightingale's Theory

Contemporary authors are beginning to explore Florence Nightingale's work as a potential theoretical and conceptual model for nursing (Chinn, Jacobs, 1987; Marriner-Tomey, 1989; Meleis, 1985; Torres, 1986). Meleis (1985) notes that Nightingale's concept of environment as the focus of nursing care and her admonition that nurses need not know all about the disease process are early attempts to differentiate between nursing and medicine.

Nightingale did not view nursing as limited merely to the administration of medications and treatments but rather as oriented toward providing fresh air, light, warmth, cleanliness, quiet, and adequate nutrition (Nightingale, 1860; Torres, 1986). Through observation and data collection, she linked the client's health status with environmental factors and, as a result, initiated improved hygiene and sanitary conditions during the Crimean war.

Torres (1986) notes that Nightingale provided basic concepts and propositions that could be validated and used for practice in nursing. Nightingale's "descriptive theory" provides nurses with a way to think about nursing or a frame of reference that focuses on patients and the environment (Torres, 1986). Nightingale's letters and writings direct the nurse to act on

TABLE 1-1   Summary of Nursing Theories

Theorist	Goal of Nursing	Framework for Practice
Nightingale (1860)	To facilitate "the body's reparative processes" by manipulating client's environment (Torres, 1986)	Client's environment is manipulated to include appropriate noise, nutrition, hygiene, light, comfort, socialization, and hope.
Peplau (1952)	To develop interaction between nurse and client (Peplau, 1952)	Nursing is significant, therapeutic, interpersonal process (Peplau, 1952). Nurses participate in structuring health care systems to facilitate natural ongoing tendency of humans to develop interpersonal relationships (Marriner-Tomey, 1989).
Henderson (1955)	To work interdependently with other health care workers (Marriner-Tomey, 1989), assisting client to gain independence as quickly as possible (Henderson, 1964). To help client gain lacking strength (Torres, 1986)	Nurses help client to perform Henderson's 14 basic needs (Henderson, 1966) (see p. 11).
Abdellah (1960)	To provide service to individuals, families, and society. To be kind and caring but also intelligent, competent, and technically well prepared to provide this service (Marriner-Tomey, 1989)	This theory involves Abdellah's 21 nursing problems (Abdellah et al 1960) (see p. 11).
Orlando (1961)	To respond to client's behavior in terms of immediate needs. To interact with client to meet immediate needs by identifying client behavior, reaction of nurse, and nursing action to be taken (Torres, 1986; Chinn, Jacobs, 1987)	Three elements, including client behavior, nurse reaction, and nurse action, compose nursing situation (Orlando, 1961).
Hall (1962)	To provide care and comfort to client during disease process (Torres, 1986)	The client is composed of the following overlapping parts: person (core), pathologic state and treatment (cure), and body (care). Nurse is care giver (Chinn, Jacobs, 1987; Marriner-Tomey, 1989).
Wiedenbach (1964)	To assist individuals in overcoming obstacles that interfere with the ability to meet demands or needs brought about by condition, environment, situation, or time (Torres, 1986)	Nursing as practice is related to individuals who need help because of behavioral stimulus. Clinical nursing has the following components: philosophy, purpose, practice, and art (Chinn, Jacobs, 1987).
Levine (1966)	To use conservation activities aimed at optimal use of client's resources	This adaptation model of human as integral whole is based on "four conservation principles of nursing" (Levine, 1973).
Johnson (1968)	To reduce stress so that client can move more easily through recovery process	This basic needs framework focuses on seven categories of behavior (see p.12). Individual's goal is to achieve behavioral balance and steady state by adjustment and adaptation to certain forces (Johnson, 1980; Torres, 1986).
Rogers (1970)	To maintain and promote health, prevent illness, and care for and rehabilitate ill and disabled client through "humanistic science of nursing" (Rogers, 1970)	"Unitary man" evolves along life process. Client continuously changes and coexists with environment
Orem (1971)	To care for and help client attain total self-care	This is self-care deficit theory. Nursing care becomes necessary when client is unable to fulfill biological, psychological, developmental, or social needs (Orem, 1985).

Continued.

TABLE 1-1 Summary of Nursing Theories—cont'd		
Theorist	Goal of Nursing	Framework for Practice
King (1971)	To use communication to help client reestablish positive adaptation to environment	Nursing process is defined as dynamic interpersonal process between nurse, client, and health care system.
Travelbee (1971)	To assist individual or family to prevent or cope with illness, regain health, find meaning in illness, or maintain maximal degree of health (Marriner-Tomey, 1989)	Interpersonal process is viewed as human-to-human relationship formed during illness and "experience of suffering."
Neuman (1972)	To assist individuals, families, and groups to attain and maintain maximal level of total wellness by purposeful interventions	Stress reduction is goal of systems model of nursing practice (Torres, 1986). Nursing actions are in primary, secondary, or tertiary level of prevention.
Roy (1979)	To identify types of demands placed on client, assess adaptation to demands, and help client adapt	This adaptation model is based on the physiological, psychological, sociological, and dependence-independence adaptive modes (Roy, 1980).
Patterson and Zderad (1976)	To respond to human needs and build humanistic nursing science (Patterson, Zderad, 1976; Chinn, Jacobs, 1987)	Humanistic nursing requires participants to be aware of their "uniqueness" and "commonality" with others (Chinn, Jacobs, 1987).
Leininger (1978)	To provide care consistent with nursing's emerging science and knowledge with caring as central focus (Chinn, Jacobs, 1987)	With this transcultural care theory, caring is central and unifying domain for nursing knowledge and practice (Leininger, 1980).
Watson (1979)	To promote health, restore client to health, and prevent illness (Marriner-Tomey, 1989)	This theory involves philosophy and science of caring; caring is interpersonal process comprising interventions that result in meeting human needs (Torres, 1986).
Parse (1981)	To focus on man as living unity and man's qualitative participation with health experience (Parse, 1981) (Nursing as science and art [Marriner-Tomey, 1989])	Man continually interacts with environment and participates in maintenance of health (Marriner-Tomey, 1989). Health is continual, open process rather than state of well-being or absence of disease (Parse, 1981; Marriner-Tomey, 1989; Chinn, Jacobs, 1987).

the behalf of the client. Her principles encompass the areas of practice, research, and education. Most important, her concepts and principles shaped and delineated nursing practice (Marriner-Tomey, 1989). Nightingale taught and used the nursing process, noting that "vital observation [assessment] . . . is not for the sake of piling up miscellaneous information or curious facts, but for the sake of saving life and increasing health and comfort."

Peplau's Theory

Hildegard Peplau's theory (1952) focuses on the individual, nurse, and interactive process (Peplau, 1952); the result is the nurse-client relationship (Torres, 1986; Marriner-Tomey, 1989). According to this theory the client is an individual with a felt need, and nursing is an interpersonal and therapeutic process. Nursing's goal is to educate the client and family and to help the client reach mature personality development (Chinn, Jacobs, 1987). Therefore the nurse strives to develop a nurse-client relationship in which the nurse serves as a resource person, counselor, and surrogate.

When the client seeks help, the nurse first discusses the nature of the problem and explains the services available. As the nurse-client relationship develops, the nurse and client mutually define the problem and potential solutions. The client gains from this relationship by using available services to meet needs, and nurses assist the client in reducing anxiety related to the health care problem. Peplau's theory is unique in that the collaborative nurse-client relationship creates a "maturing force" through which interpersonal effectiveness assists in meeting the client's needs (Beeber, Anderson, Sills, 1990). When the original needs have been resolved, new needs may emerge. The nurse-client interpersonal relationship is characterized by the following overlapping phases: orientation, identification, explanation, and resolution (Chinn, Jacobs, 1987).

Peplau's theory and ideas were developed to provide a design for the practice of psychiatric nursing. Nursing research on anxiety, empathy, behavioral tools, and tools to evaluate verbal responses resulted from Peplau's conceptual model (Marriner-Tomey, 1989).

Henderson's Theory

Virginia Henderson's nursing theory (1955) involves basic needs of the whole person. Henderson (1964) defines nursing as

assisting the individual sick or well in the performance of those activities contributing to health or its recovery . . . that he would perform unaided if he had the necessary strength, will, or knowledge. And to do this in such a way as to help him gain independence as rapidly as possible.

The following needs, often called *Henderson's 14 basic needs,* provide a framework for nursing care (Henderson, 1966):

1. Breathe normally.
2. Eat and drink adequately.
3. Eliminate by all avenues of elimination.
4. Move and maintain a desirable position.
5. Sleep and rest.
6. Select suitable clothing; dress and undress.
7. Maintain body temperature within normal range.
8. Keep the body clean and well groomed.
9. Avoid dangers in the environment.
10. Communicate with others.
11. Worship according to faith.
12. Work at something that provides a sense of accomplishment.
13. Play or participate in various forms of recreation.
14. Learn, discover, or satisfy the curiosity that leads to normal development and health.

Abdellah's Theory

The nursing theory developed by Faye Abdellah et al (1960) emphasizes delivering nursing care for the whole person to meet the physical, emotional, intellectual, social, and spiritual needs of the client and family. When using this approach, the nurse needs knowledge and skills in interpersonal relations, psychology, growth and development, communication, and sociology, as well as a knowledge of the basic sciences and specific nursing skills. The nurse is a problem solver and decision maker. The nurse formulates an individualized view of the client's needs, which may occur in the following areas:

1. Comfort, hygiene, and safety
2. Physiological balance
3. Psychological and social factors
4. Sociological and community factors

In these four areas, Abdellah et al (1960) identified the following specific client needs, which are often referred to as *Abdellah's 21 nursing problems:*

1. To maintain good hygiene and physical comfort
2. To achieve optimal activity, exercise, rest, and sleep
3. To prevent accident, injury, or other trauma and prevent the spread of infection
4. To maintain good body mechanics and prevent and correct deformities
5. To facilitate the supply of oxygen to all body cells
6. To facilitate the maintenance of nutrition to all body cells
7. To facilitate the maintenance of elimination
8. To facilitate the maintenance of fluid and electrolyte balance
9. To recognize the physiological responses of the body to disease conditions—pathological, physiological, and compensatory
10. To facilitate the maintenance of regulatory mechanisms and functions
11. To facilitate the maintenance of sensory function
12. To identify and accept positive and negative expressions, feelings, and reactions
13. To identify and accept the interrelatedness of emotions and organic illness
14. To facilitate the maintenance of effective verbal and nonverbal communication
15. To facilitate the development of productive interpersonal relationships
16. To facilitate progress toward achievement of personal spiritual goals
17. To create and/or maintain a therapeutic environment
18. To facilitate awareness of the self as an individual with varying physical, emotional, and developmental needs
19. To accept the optimum possible goals in light of limitations—physical and emotional
20. To use community resources as an aid in resolving problems arising from illness
21. To understand the role of social problems as influencing factors in the cause of illness

Orlando's Theory

To Ida Orlando (1961), the client is an individual with a need that, when met, diminishes distress, increases adequacy, or enhances well-being (Chinn, Jacobs, 1987). Orlando's theory focuses on nurses' reactions to client behavior in terms of the client's immediate need (Torres, 1986). Orlando's theory contains a conceptual framework for professional nursing. Three elements—client behavior, nurse reaction, and nurse actions—compose the nursing situation (Marriner-Tomey, 1989). After nurses thoroughly assess the client's needs, they recognize the impact of that need on the client's level of health and then act automatically or deliberately to meet the need, ultimately reducing the client's distress (Chinn, Jacobs, 1987).

Levine's Theory

Myra Levine's nursing theory, formulated in 1966 and published in 1973, views the client as an integrated being who interacts with and adapts to the environment. Levine believes that nursing intervention is a conservation activity, with conservation of energy as a primary concern (Fawcett, 1989). Health is viewed in terms of the conservation of energy in the following areas, which Levine calls the *four conservation principles of nursing:*
  1. Conservation of client energy
  2. Conservation of structural integrity
  3. Conservation of personal integrity
  4. Conservation of social integrity
With this approach, nursing care involves conservation activities aimed at the optimal use of the client's resources.

Johnson's Theory

Dorothy Johnson's theory of nursing (1968) focuses on how the client adapts to illness and how actual or potential stress can affect the ability to adapt. The goal of nursing is to reduce stress so that the client can move more easily through recovery (Johnson, 1968). Johnson's theory focuses on basic needs in terms of the following categories of behavior:
  1. Security-seeking behavior
  2. Nurturance-seeking behavior
  3. Master of oneself and one's environment according to internalized standards of excellence
  4. Taking in nourishment in socially and culturally acceptable ways
  5. Ridding the body of waste in socially and culturally acceptable ways
  6. Sexual and role-identity behavior
  7. Self-protective behavior

According to Johnson, the nurse assesses the client's needs in these categories of behavior, called *behavioral subsystems.* Under normal conditions the client functions effectively in the environment. When stress disrupts normal adaptation, however, behavior becomes erratic and less purposeful. The nurse identifies this inability to adapt and provides nursing care to resolve problems in meeting the client's needs.

Rogers' Theory

In her theory, Martha Rogers (1979) considers man (unitary human being) as an energy field coexisting within the universe. Man is in continuous interaction with the environment. In addition, man is a unified whole, possessing personal integrity and manifesting characteristics that are more than the sum of the parts (Rogers, 1979). Unitary man is a "four dimensional energy field identified by pattern and manifesting characteristics that are specific to the whole and which cannot be predicted from the knowledge of parts" (Marriner-Tomey, 1989). The four dimensions used in Rogers' theory—energy fields, openness, pattern and organization, and four dimensionality—are used to derive principles about how human beings develop.

Rogers views nursing primarily as a science and is committed to nursing research. Nursing therefore incorporates knowledge of the basic sciences and physiology, as well as nursing knowledge:

The science of nursing aims to provide a body of abstract knowledge growing out of scientific research and logical analysis and capable of being translated into nursing practice. Nursing's body of scientific knowledge is a new product specific to nursing . . . . Nursing is a humanistic science.

Orem's Theory

Dorothea Orem (1971) developed a definition of nursing that emphasizes the client's self-care needs. Orem describes her philosophy of nursing in this way:

Nursing has as a special concern man's needs for self-care action and the provision and management of it on a continuous basis in order to sustain life and health, recover from disease or injury, and cope with their effects. Self-care is a requirement of every person—man, woman, and child. When self-care is not maintained, illness, disease, or death will occur. Nurses sometimes manage and maintain required self-care continually for persons who are totally incapacitated. In other instances, nurses help persons to maintain required self-care by performing some but not all care measures, by supervising others who assist patients, and by instructing and guiding individuals as they gradually move toward self-care.

Thus the goal of Orem's theory is helping the client perform self-care. According to Orem, nursing care is necessary when the client is unable to fulfill biological, psychological, developmental, or social needs. The nurse determines why a client is unable to meet these needs, what must be done to enable the client to meet them, and how much self-care the client is able to perform.

King's Theory

Imogene King's theory (1971) focuses on the interpersonal relationship between client and nurse. The nurse-client relationship is the vehicle for the nursing process, which is a dynamic interpersonal process in which the nurse and client are affected by each other's behavior, as well as by the health care system (King, 1971). The nurse's goal is to use communication to assist the client in reestablishing or maintaining a positive adaptation to the environment.

Neuman's Theory

Betty Neuman (1972) defines a total-person model incorporating the holistic concept and an open-systems approach (Marriner-Tomey, 1989). To Neuman, the person is a dynamic composite of physiological, sociocultural, and developmental variables that function as an open system. As an open system, the person interacts with, adjusts to, and is adjusted by the environment, which is viewed as a stressor (Chinn, Jacobs, 1987). Stressors disrupt the system. Neuman's model includes intrapersonal, interpersonal, and extrapersonal stressors. Intrapersonal stressors are forces occurring within the person; interpersonal stressors such as role expectations occur between persons, and extrapersonal stressor such as financial circumstances occur outside the person (Neuman, 1982; Marriner-Tomey, 1989).

Neuman believes that nursing is concerned with the whole person. The goal of nursing is to assist individuals, families, and groups in attaining and maintaining a maximal level of total wellness (Neuman, Young, 1972). The nurse assesses, manages, and evaluates client systems. Nursing focuses on the variables affecting the client's response to the stressor (Chinn, Jacobs, 1987). Nursing actions are in the primary, secondary, and tertiary levels of prevention. Primary prevention focuses on strengthening a line of defense through the identification of actual or potential risk factors associated with stressors. Secondary prevention strengthens internal defenses and resources by establishing priorities and treatment plans for identified symptoms, and tertiary prevention focuses on readaptation. The principal goal in tertiary prevention is to strengthen resistance to stressors

through client education and to assist in preventing a recurrence of the stress response (Chinn, Jacobs, 1987; Marriner-Tomey, 1989; Torres, 1986; Neuman, 1982).

Roy's Theory

Sister Callista Roy's adaptation theory (Roy, Obloy 1979; Roy, 1980) views the client as an adaptive system. According to Roy's model, the goal of nursing is to help the person adapt to changes in physiological needs, self-concept, role function, and interdependent relations during health and illness (Marriner-Tomey, 1989). The need for nursing care arises when the client cannot adapt to internal and external environmental demands. All individuals must adapt to the following demands:

1. Meeting basic physiological needs
2. Developing a positive self-concept
3. Performing social roles
4. Achieving a balance between dependence and independence

The nurse determines what demands are causing problems for a client and assesses how well the client is adapting to them. Nursing care is then directed at helping the client adapt.

Watson's Theory

Watson's philosophy of caring (1979) attempts to define the outcome of nursing activity in regard to the humanistic aspects of life (Watson, 1979; Marriner-Tomey, 1989). The action of nursing is directed at understanding the interrelationship of health, illness, and human behavior. Nursing is concerned with promoting and restoring health and preventing illness.

Watson's model is designed around the caring process, which she defines as 10 "carative" factors. Each factor describes the caring process of how a client attains or maintains health or dies peacefully. Caring represents all of the factors the nurse uses to deliver health care to the client (Watson, 1987).

 ## ANA DEFINITION OF NURSING PRACTICE

In 1955 the ANA published the following official definition of nursing practice*:

The practice of professional nursing means the performance for compensation of any act in the observation, care, and counsel of the ill, injured, or infirm or in the mainte-

---

*From ANA: *Am J Nurs* 55:1474, 1955.

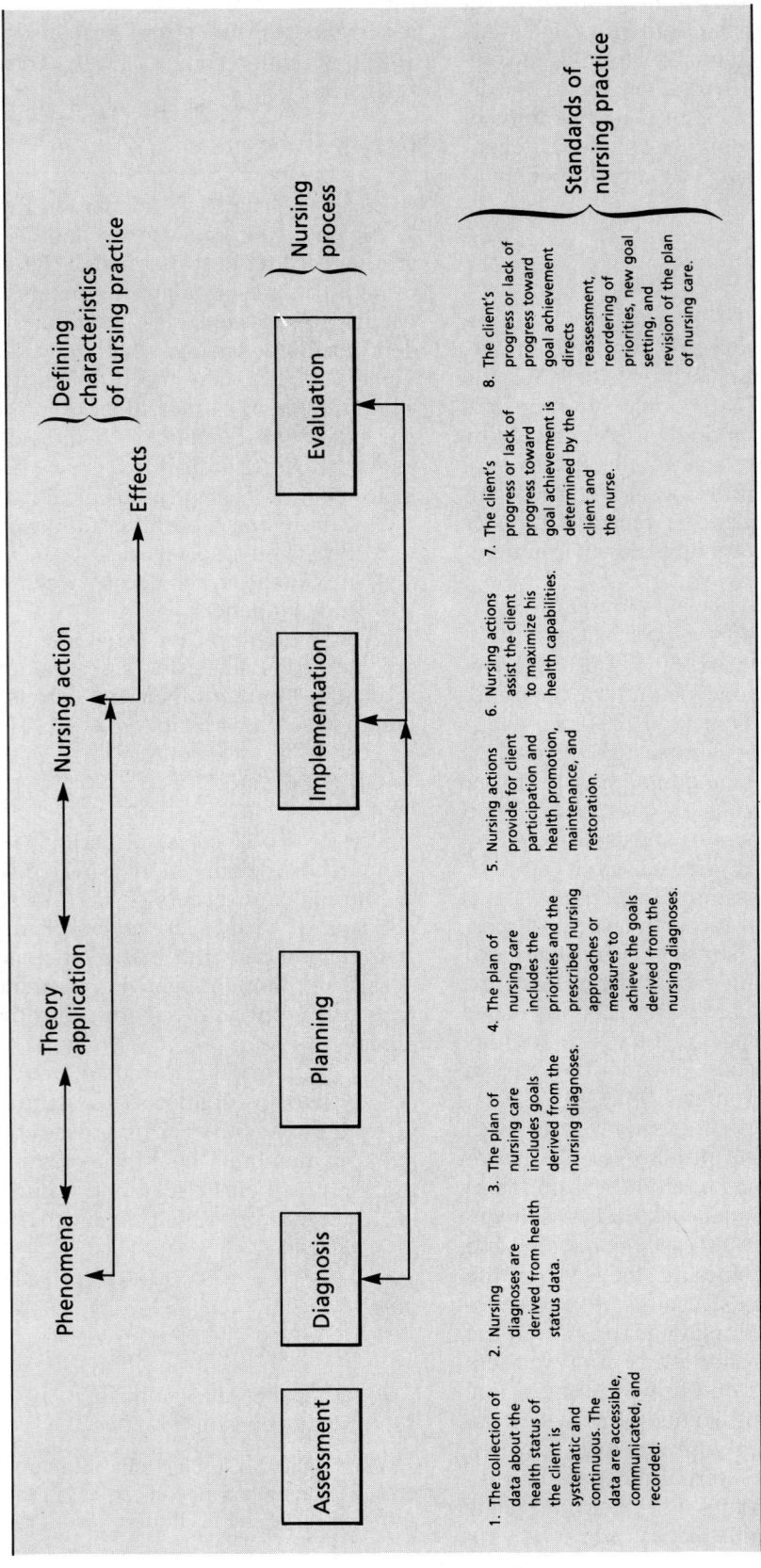

Fig. 1-3 Defining characteristics of nursing practice: relationship to the nursing process and the standards of nursing practice.
Modified from the American Nurses Association: *Nursing and social policy statement*, Kansas City, Mo, 1980, The Association.

nance of health or prevention of illness of others, or in the supervision and teaching of other personnel, or the administration of medications and treatments as prescribed by licensed physician or dentist, requiring substantial specialized judgment and skill and based on knowledge and application of the principles of biological, physical, and social sciences. The foregoing shall not be deemed to include acts of diagnosis or prescription of therapeutic or corrective measures.

This early definition by the ANA is significant in its attempt to define nursing practice in a fairly specific manner. Nonetheless, it tends to stress nursing's dependent role, an emphasis no longer accepted. In 1965 the ANA Committee on Education issued a position paper that presents a fuller definition of nursing and emphasizes nursing as an independent profession*:

Nursing is a helping profession and, as such, provides services which contribute to the health and well-being of people.

Nursing is a vital consequence to the individual receiving services; it fills needs that cannot be met by the person, family, or other persons in the community.

Three essential components of professional nursing are care, cure, and coordination. The care aspect is more than "to take care of"; it is also "caring for" and "caring about." It is dealing with human beings under stress, frequently over long periods of time. It is providing comfort and support in times of anxiety, loneliness, and helplessness. It is listening, evaluating, and intervening appropriately.

The promotion of health and healing is the cure aspect of professional nursing. It is assisting clients to understand their health problems and helping them cope. It is the administration of medications and treatments. It is also the use of clinical nursing judgment in determining, on the basis of patient outcomes, whether the plan of care needs to be maintained or changed. It is knowing when and how to use existing and potential resources to help patients toward recovery and adjustment by mobilizing their own resources.

Professional nursing practice is this and more. It is sharing responsibility for the health and welfare of all people in the community, and it is participating in programs designed to prevent illness and maintain health. It is coordinating and synchronizing medical and other professional and technical services that affect patient care. It is supervising, teaching, and directing all those involved in nursing care.

In 1979 the Committee of Chairpersons of the ANA determined that the **Congress for Nursing Practice** should define the nature and scope of nursing practice. The Congress is the part of the ANA concerned with legal aspects of nursing practice, public recognition of the significance of nursing

---

*From ANA: *Am J Nurs* 65:106, 1965.

practice to health care, and implications for nursing practice of trends in health care.

In 1980 the Congress defined nursing as the diagnosis and treatment of human responses to actual or potential health problems (ANA, 1980). This definition involves the following characteristics of nursing: phenomena, theory application, nursing action, and evaluation of the effects of action (Fig. 1-3). *Phenomena* are the human responses to actual or potential health problems. The nurse identifies the client's responses by assessing health status and obtaining data. The nurse applies nursing *theory* to understand these responses. The nurse takes *actions* to resolve actual or potential health care problems. The nurse then evaluates the *effects* of the actions on the client's responses. These four characteristics are related to the nursing process, which is described in Unit 2.

 ## CNA DEFINITION OF NURSING PRACTICE

The CNA in the 1980 *Definition of Nursing and Standards of Practice* defined nursing as follows*:

The nursing profession exists in response to a need of society and holds ideals related to man's health throughout his life span. Nurses direct their energies toward the promotion, maintenance, and restoration of health; the prevention of illness; the alleviation of suffering, and the ensurance of a peaceful death when life can no longer be sustained. Nurses value a holistic view and regard an individual as a biopsychosocial being who has the capacity to set goals and make decisions and who has the right and responsibility to make informed choices congruent with personal beliefs and values. Nursing, a dynamic and supportive profession guided by its code of ethics, is rooted in caring, a concept evident throughout its four fields of activity: practice, education, administration, and research.

Founded in 1908, the CNA provides leadership to practicing nurses in the Canadian provinces. Through the actions and activities of the CNA, nurses can meet the health care demands of the changing Canadian society (Meilicke, Larsen, 1988).

 ## EDUCATIONAL PREPARATION

Registered Nurse Education

As the profession of nursing grew, various educational routes for becoming a **registered nurse (RN)** were developed. Initially, schools were usually associated with a specific hospital. The primary purpose of

---

*From CNA: *Definition of nursing standards and practice*, Ottawa, 1980, The Association.

such a school was to educate nurses who would work within that institution.

As nursing increasingly defined its own body of knowledge, formalized educational processes developed to ensure a consistent level of education in institutions. Such consistency was also necessary for RN licensure.

Currently in the United States, an individual can become an RN through an associate degree, diploma, or baccalaureate degree program. In Canada, there are diploma and baccalaureate degree programs.

Associate Degree Education

The associate degree program in the United States is a 2-year program usually offered by a college or junior college. This program focuses on the basic sciences and on theoretical and clinical courses related to the practice of nursing. Graduates of this type of program take the state board examination for RN licensure.

Diploma Education

The diploma program in the United States is a 2- or 3-year program usually associated with a hospital. Diploma programs also focus on the basic sciences and on theoretical and clinical courses related to nursing practice. Some diploma programs are affiliated with a colleges or universities, which grant college credit for nonnursing courses. Graduates of a diploma program receive a diploma from the hospital and take the state board examination for RN licensure. In the United States, diploma programs are declining in numbers. In Canada, diploma programs are offered in community colleges or hospitals and are 2-year programs (or 3 years in some hospital-based programs) compared with associate degree programs in the United States.

Baccalaureate Education

The baccalaureate degree program usually encompasses 4 years of study in a college or university. The program focuses on the basic sciences and on theoretical and clinical courses, as well as courses in the social sciences, arts, and humanities to support nursing theory. In Canada, a Bachelor of Science in Nursing (BScN) or a Bachelor in Nursing (BN) is the equivalent to the Bachelor of Science in Nursing (BSN) in the United States.

The American Association of Colleges of Nursing (AACN) published the *Essentials of College and University Education for Professional Nursing* (1986). This document delineated essential knowledge, practice and values, attitudes, personal qualities, and professional behaviors for the baccalaureate-prepared nurse. The goal of this document was to provide standards by which "faculty can measure the content of the curriculum and the performance of the graduate" (AACN, 1986).

Two other types of degree programs offer eligibility to take the state board examinations for RN licensure. First, some programs offer a master's degree in nursing as the first professional degree. At present, these programs exist at Yale University and Massachusetts General Hospital. The second type of program, the nursing doctorate (ND) at Case Western Reserve University, offers the doctorate as the first professional degree.

Accreditation and Licensure

To be accredited, nursing programs must meet certain criteria established by the NLN. This voluntary accreditation is available for basic nursing education programs and master's degree programs in nursing (National Commission on Nursing, 1983).

RN licensure for practice in most states and provinces requires that the student complete a prescribed course of study from an approved program. In the United States the program must be approved by the State Board of Nursing in the state in which the student is seeking licensure. In Canada the program must be approved by a Provincial Board of Nursing in the province in which the student is seeking licensure.

In the United States, RN candidates must pass the National Council Licensure Examination for Registered Nurses (NCLEX-RN), which is administered by each state's board of nursing. In Canada the CNA Testing Service (CNATS) administers the test to qualified candidates in each province. Whether nurses can practice in a state or province other than their own depends on the agreement between the states or provinces involved. In some instances, reciprocity is considered on an individual basis.

Graduate Nursing Education

As expressed by the ANA (1969), the purpose of a graduate program in nursing is to prepare nurse clinicians capable of improving nursing care through the advancement of nursing theory and sciences. A person completing a graduate program can receive the degree of Master of Arts in Nursing (MA), Master in Nursing (MN), or Master of Science in Nursing (MSN). The NLN has described the characteristics of and standards for accredited master's degree nursing programs (see box).

A master's degree in nursing can be valuable for nurses seeking expanded roles such as that of nurse educator, clinical nurse specialist, nurse administrator, or practitioner. These roles are described later in this chapter.

Characteristics of Graduate Education in Nursing Leading to the Master's Degree

The master's program in nursing is offered by an educational institution of higher learning and is built on a baccalaureate curriculum, including an upper-division major in nursing. It provides students with an opportunity to:

- Acquire advanced knowledge from the sciences and the humanities to support advanced nursing practice and role development
- Expand knowledge of nursing theory as a basis for advanced nursing practice
- Develop expertise in a specialized area of clinical nursing practice
- Acquire the knowledge and skills related to a specific functional role in nursing
- Acquire initial competence in conducting research
- Plan and initiate change in the health care system and in the practice and delivery of health care
- Further develop and implement leadership strategies for the betterment of health care
- Actively engage in collaborative relationships with others to improve health care
- Acquire a foundation for doctoral study

Modified from NLN: *Characteristics of graduate education in nursing leading to the master's degree,* New York, 1978, The League.

States that Require Mandatory Continuing Education

STATE

- Alabama
- California
- Colorado
- Florida
- Iowa
- Kansas
- Kentucky
- Massachusetts
- Minnesota
- Nebraska
- Nevada
- New Mexico
- Texas

From American Nurses Association: Oct 1991, Washington, DC The Association.

The first nursing doctorate program opened in 1953 at the University of Pittsburgh. The need for nurses with doctorate degrees is rising (Institute of Medicine, 1983). It was estimated that over 13,000 doctorally prepared nurses would be needed by 1990 (Holzemer, 1987). Professional doctoral programs in nursing (DSN or DNSc) emphasize the application of research findings to clinical nursing. Other programs emphasize more basic research and theory and award the Doctor of Philosophy (PhD) in nursing (Holzemer, 1987).

Continuing Education

Because nursing is a dynamic profession, **continuing education** programs help nurses remain current in nursing skills, knowledge, and theory. Continuing education involves formal, organized, and educational programs offered by educational and health care institutions. As expressed by the ANA (1975), the goals of continuing education in nursing are to improve and maintain nursing practice, promote and exercise leadership in effecting change in health care delivery systems, and fulfill professional learning needs. Other goals include helping nurses become specialized in a particular area of practice and teaching nurses new skills and techniques.

In general, continuing education programs are short term and are designed for all nurses. The ANA or the state board of nursing is the accrediting agency for these programs. The ANA awards continuing education units on completion of specific courses. Some states require nurses to take continuing education courses for license renewal (Table 1-2).

In-Service Education

An **in-service education** program is instruction or training provided by a health care agency or institution. An in-service program is held in the institution and is designed to increase the knowledge, skills, and competencies of nurses and other health care professionals employed by the institution. For example, a hospital might offer an in-service program to inform nurses about primary nursing before it is implemented at the hospital.

All nurses have access to continuing education and in-service programs organized and conducted by a university, private hospital, private continuing education service, or the employing institution or agency. Such programs assist the practicing nurse in acquiring new knowledge and skills necessary for today's highly technical and fast-changing health care delivery system.

Licensed Practical Nurse Education

A licensed practical or vocational nurse is trained in basic nursing techniques and direct client care. The **licensed practical nurse (LPN)** practices under the supervision of a registered nurse in a hospital or community health practice setting. A licensed practical nurse, **licensed vocational nurse (LVN)**, or in Canada a registered nurse's assistant (RNA) generally receives 1 year of education and training in a hospital, community college, or other agency. The LPN is licensed by the state board of nursing after completing the educational program and passing the licensure examination.

Career Mobility and Clinical Ladder

Education continues to be important after the nurse begins practice, whether the practice setting focuses on the adult or child, the chronically or acutely ill, or the home or hospital. Nursing encompasses an ever-widening range of roles. Multiple career paths and goals are open to new and experienced practitioners (Hefferin, Kleinknecht, 1986).

In the past, career mobility for nurses was somewhat limited. However, with expanding roles in nursing practice, this situation has changed. The clinical-ladder approach to advancement has been discussed in many nursing journals and put into practice in various settings (Anderson, Denyes, 1975; Colavecchio, Tescher, Scalgi, 1974; Zimmer, 1974). The clinical ladder unifies clinical practice and nursing administration, fosters collaboration between nursing education and service, and is a professional advancement system.

The clinical ladder contains structure, criteria for clinical competencies, promotional procedures, and incentives for advancement (Huey, 1982). The structure is individualized for a specific institution and may include multiple levels on the clinical, administration, research, and education pathways (ANA, 1984). There are specific objective, measurable criteria for each level within the structure. Within a clinical-ladder system, nurses are no longer promoted strictly on the basis of education and seniority within the institution. Promotional procedures within the clinical ladder are clearly delineated, thereby promoting self-appraisal and peer appraisal for career mobility within the system. The incentive for advancement may include increased autonomy of practice, raise in salary or promotion within the organizational structure itself, increased expertise, and personal self-fulfillment.

The clinical ladder is a method for career mobility by which one program can encourage and motivate nurses to remain in the health care setting. Career

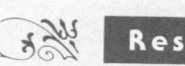

Research Highlight

Hefferin and Kleinknecht developed the Nursing Career Preference Inventory (NCPI), which assists a nurse in identifying work interests or preferences and in determining the primary nursing practice areas and hospital-based nursing role positions that most often reflect the interest patterns. The NCPI was developed from the response of 2735 nurses. The researchers noted that the NCPI filled a void in career counseling for nurses and assisted nurses in identifying and achieving career goals.

Hefferin EA, Kleinknecht MK: Development of the nursing career preference inventory, *Nurs Res* 35(1):44, 1986.

counseling is another method for retention and promoting within the settings.

Hefferin and Kleinknecht (1986) developed the Nursing Career Preference Inventory to assist nurses in determining which of the four primary nursing practice areas—clinical, administration, research, or education—reflects their personal work activity interests or preferences (see research highlight). Career inventories are valuable in retaining bright, talented nurses within an institution and decreasing the risk of experienced nurses leaving the profession.

Research has demonstrated that the early years of clinical practice are critical. During this period, job satisfaction, commitment to the employing institution, and professionalism decrease. New graduates and experienced nurses entering a new work environment are at risk. As the nurse gains graduate education, the decline in satisfaction is significantly reduced (McCloskey, McCain, 1987).

 NURSING PRACTICE

Nurses practice in a variety of settings, in many roles within those settings, and with other care givers in the allied health professions. The practice of nursing is guided only in part by administrators in hospitals and other health care agencies and institutions. State and provincial nurse practice acts establish specific legal regulations for practice, and professional organizations establish standards of practice as criteria for nursing care.

Standards of Nursing Practice

As nursing has gained independence as a profession, it has increasingly set its own standards for

---

TABLE 1-2   ANA Standards of Nursing Practice

Standard	Element
ASSESSMENT	
The nurse collects client health data.	The priority of data collection is determined by the client's immediate condition of needs.
	Pertinent data are collected using appropriate assessment techniques.
	Data Collection involves the client, significant others, and health care providers when appropriate.
	The data collection process is systematic and ongoing.
	Relevant data are documented in a retrievable form.
DIAGNOSES	
The nurse analyzes the assessment data in determining diagnoses.	Diagnoses are derived from the assessment data.
	Diagnoses are validated with the client, significant others, and health care providers, when possible.
	Diagnoses are documented in a manner that facilitates the determination of expected outcomes and plan of care.
The nurse identifies expected outcomes individualized to the client.	Outcomes are derived from the diagnoses.
	Outcomes are documented as measurable goals.
	Outcomes are mutually formulated with the client and health care providers, when possible.
	Outcomes are realistic in relation to client's present and potential capabilities.
	Outcomes are attainable in relation to resources available to the client.
	Outcomes include a time estimate for attainment.
	Outcomes provide direction for continuity of care.
PLANNING	
The nurse develops a plan of care that prescribes interventions to attain expected outcomes.	The plan is individualized to the client's condition or needs.
	The plan is developed with the client, significant others, and health care providers, when appropriate.
	The plan reflects current nursing practice.
	The plan is documented.
	The plan provides for continuity of care.
IMPLEMENTATION	
The nurse implements the interventions identified in the plan of care.	Interventions are consistent with the established plan of care.
	Interventions are implemented in a safe and appropriate manner.
	Interventions are documented.
EVALUATION	
The nurse evaluates the client's progress toward attainment of outcomes.	Evaluation is systematic and ongoing
	The client's responses to interventions are documented.
	The effectiveness of interventions is evaluated in relations to outcomes.
	Revisions in diagnoses, outcomes, and the plan of care are documented.
	The client, significant others, and health care providers are involved in the evaluation process, when appropriate.

From ANA: *Standards of clinical practice,* Washington, DC, 1991, The Association.

practice. Standards for practice are important as objective guidelines for nurses to provide care and as criteria for evaluating care. When standards are clearly defined, clients can be assured they are receiving high-quality care, nurses know exactly what is necessary to give nursing care, and administrators can determine that care meets acceptable standards.

Moreover, standards of practice are important if a legal dispute arises over whether a nurse practiced appropriately in a particular case (see Chapter 14). The ANA and the CNA have published standards of nursing practice (Tables 1-2 and 1-3). In addition, the ANA has published standards for professional performance (see box on p. 21).

TABLE 1-3 Summary of CNA Standards for Nursing Practice	
Standard	Elements
Nursing practice requires that a conceptual model for nursing be the basis for the independent part of that practice.	Nurses are required to have a clear idea or conception of the distinct goal of nursing. Nurses are required to have a clear idea or conception of the client. Nurses are required to have a clear idea or conception of their roles in response to the health needs of society. Nurses are required to have a clear idea or conception of the source of client difficulty. Nurses are required to have a clear idea or conception of the focus and modes of nursing intervention. Nurses are required to have a clear idea or conception of the expected consequences of nursing activities.
Nursing practice requires the effective use of the nursing process.	Nurses are required to collect data in accordance with their conception of the client. Nurses are required to analyze data collected in accordance with their conception of the goal of nursing, their role, and the source of client difficulty. Nurses are required to plan their nursing actions based on the identified actual and potential client problems and in accordance with their conception of the focus and modes of intervention. Nurses are required to perform nursing actions that implement the plan. Nurses are required to evaluate all steps of the nursing process in accordance with their conceptual models for nursing.
Nursing practice requires that the helping relationship be the nature of the client-nurse interaction.	Nurses are required to increase the likelihood that the client will perceive the health service experience as understandable, manageable, and meaningful at the outset. Nurses are required to set mutually agreed on expectations as a means of increasing the likelihood that the client will perceive the health service experience as understandable, manageable, and meaningful. Nurses are required to ensure a successful termination of the helping relationship.
Nursing practice requires nurses to fulfill professional responsibilities.	Nurses are required to respect statuses and policies relevant to the profession and the practice setting. Nurses are required to comply with the Code of Ethics of their profession. Nurses are required to function as members of a health team.

Modified from CNA: *A definition of nursing practice standards for nursing practice*, Ottawa, 1980, (rev 1987), The Association.

Nurse Practice Acts

In all states in the United States and all provinces in Canada, nurse practice acts regulate the licensure and practice of nursing. Each state or province defines for itself the scope of nursing practice, but most have similar practice acts. The definition of nursing practice published by the ANA in 1955 (see p.13) is in some ways representative of the scope of nursing practice as defined in most states and provinces. In the last decade, however, many states have revised their nurse practice acts to reflect nursing's growing autonomy and the expanded roles of nurses in practice. The 1955 ANA prohibition against diagnosis and treatment, for example, has been removed from nurse practice acts in many states or rephrased to differentiate between nursing diagnosis and treatment and medical diagnosis and treatment. Nurse

---

Standards of Professional Performance

- The nurse systematically evaluates the quality and effectiveness of nursing practice.
- The nurse evaluates his/her own nursing practice in relation to professional practice standards and relevant statues and regulations.
- The nurse acquires and maintains current knowledge in nursing practice.
- The nurse contributes to the professional developement of peers, colleagues, and others.
- The nurse's decisions and actions on behalf of clients are determined in an ethical manner.
- The nurse collaborates with the client, significant others, and health care providers in providing client care.
- The nurse uses research findings in practice.
- The nurse considers factors related to safety, effectiveness, and cost in planning and delivering client care.

From ANA: *Standards of clinical practice*, Washington, DC, 1991, The Association.

TABLE 1-4 Employment Settings of Registered Nurses

Setting	United States*	Canada†
Hospital	68%	74%
Nursing homes	8%	7%
Community health	7%	9%
Physician and dentist offices	6%	2.5%
Schools	4%	—
Nursing education	4%	3%
Occupational health	4%	—
Other	4%	3%
Unknown	—	3%

*Data from American Nurses Association: *Facts about nursing 86-87*, Kansas City, Mo, 1987, The Association.
†Data from Statistics Canada and Canadian Nurses Association: *Nursing in Canada, 1987*, Ottawa, 1988, Canadian Nurses Association.

practice acts are discussed in more detail in Chapter 14.

Practice Settings

As nursing's role in the health care system has expanded, the settings in which nurses practice have also increased. Table 1-4 gives statistics on the numbers of nurses in practice settings.

Hospitals and Other Institutions

The largest group of practicing nurses are those working in hospitals or other health care agencies. Two other groups are the nurse practitioners and clinical nurse specialists (Gordin, 1991). Current reimbursement practices of private and federal or state insurance groups have resulted in shorter hospital stays (see Chapter 3). Thus clients are being discharged from hospitals sooner, frequently requiring continued nursing care in the home. Today's hospital-based professional nurse is not only adept in providing nursing care but is also able, through early discharge planning, to meet the home care needs of clients.

The increased older adult population and rising acuity rates have resulted in part from new disease entities and new forms of supportive therapy. Infections associated with acquired immunodeficiency syndrome (AIDS), organ transplantation, and techno-

logical equipment used in the critical care setting are a few factors contributing to a higher percentage of critically ill clients in hospitals.

In addition to the rising acuity rate, there has been a sharp upward spiraling of health care costs. To adjust for this increase, hospitals are reducing the number of people on staff without decreasing the workload. Professional nurses are caught in this dilemma (McClure, 1991). Today's professional nurses are challenged to meet the multiple health care needs of clients with reduced resources.

In hospitals, nursing services operate 24 hours a day. Hospitals use different staffing patterns to meet the need for nursing care. Some hospitals have three 8-hour shifts, whereas other hospitals use two 12-hour shifts or three 10-hour shifts that overlap during the early morning, late afternoon, and night. The roles and responsibilities of nurses employed in hospitals vary because hospitals differ widely in size and organizational structure (see Chapter 3).

Regardless of the practice environment, nurses are challenged to deliver quality care. Nursing research linking quality patient outcome studies with cost effectiveness provides documentation that nurses are meeting the challenge. Nurses are active in speaking out about health care issues at all levels of government (Holzemer, 1990).

Clients in hospitals generally require 24-hour nursing care. Hospitals may be acute, long-term, and rehabilitation care facilities. Nurses employed in an acute-care setting care for clients with severe illnesses and complex problems. Today these clients are usually more dependent and more seriously ill than patients in the past because of shorter periods of hospitalization. As a result, nursing practice in acute-care settings has become more specialized and complex. The skills and knowledge needed to practice in this setting are determined by the clinical area of practice.

The rapid rise in the number of older adults, clients with chronic illnesses, and clients with functional impairments has resulted in the growth of long-term care facilities. Long-term care is provided in institutions such as chronic disease hospitals, psychiatric hospitals, and nursing homes. Nursing homes are the most common agencies providing inhouse, long-term care.

Rehabilitation facilities generally employ many types of health care professionals. The goal of these institutions is to teach disabled clients to achieve a maximal level of function and to teach families to help them reach that level.

Community Settings

Since 1974 the number of nurses employed in community-based practice settings has increased substantially. The rising costs of institutional care have created the need for community-based nursing services aimed at health promotion and disease prevention.

Nursing in community-based settings is concerned primarily with health promotion and maintenance, education and management, and coordination and continuity of care within the community. Community-based nurses assess the health needs of individuals, families, and communities and help clients cope with threats to health and problems of illness. Whereas institutional health care focuses on the individual and family, community-based nursing is directed toward the health of the community and the interaction of individuals within that community. A community can be a particular location such as an urban or rural area or a group of people related by occupation, school, or another common interest or characteristic. Thus community-based nurses are employed in a variety of practice settings, including community and occupational health centers, schools, home health care agencies, and private practices.

COMMUNITY HEALTH CENTERS. Community health centers offer comprehensive programs for health maintenance and promotion, education and management, and coordination of care within the community. Community health centers provide ambulatory care (care sought by clients able to come to the centers), as well as care within the home. Persons seeking health care at a community health center usually live near the center.

Nurses employed in these centers often work more independently than nurses working in institutional settings. Community health centers also employ other health professionals, but nurses generally provide most of the care. In some settings, physicians are called in only when specific needs arise. Examples of community health centers are planned parenthood clinics and family care and mental health centers.

SCHOOLS. Community-based health services are common in schools and on college campuses. Nursing services include health education in disease prevention, health promotion, and sex education. In addition, nurses working in schools may provide care for students with nonemergency acute illnesses such as upper respiratory tract infections, influenza, and viruses. School nurses also make referrals for students and their families when additional, more specialized health care is needed.

OCCUPATIONAL HEALTH SETTINGS. Many companies in large office buildings and factories provide health services to employees in occupational health centers located on the premises. Nursing care in these settings involves five areas. The nurse may develop programs aimed at increasing health and safety in the workplace by reducing the number of occupational accidents, the risk of occupational disease, or the transmission of a contagious disease among the workers. The nurse may provide programs for health promotion, disease prevention, and health education. The nurse also treats nonemergency acute illnesses and provides first aid. In emergency situations such as heart attacks or trauma, the nurse gives emergency care and arranges transportation to a hospital. The nurse also refers employees to additional health resources when necessary.

HOME HEALTH CARE AGENCIES. A client often needs specific nursing care that can be given efficiently in the home. Some hospital-based nursing services have initiated their own institutional-based home health care services (see Chapter 5). Nurses in these agencies provide home-based nursing care to clients discharged from that particular institution. Other agencies providing home health care include visiting nurse associations, public health nursing agencies, hospices, and private home care agencies.

The nurse who functions in the home must also be skilled at teaching. Rising health care costs have limited the duration and frequency of visits. As a result the home health care nurse often teaches the client or family to competently perform nursing activities and self-care. Caring for the client in the home environment requires the nurse to be flexible, resourceful, creative, and self-confident, as well as clinically competent (see Chapter 5).

Other Settings

These are the most common areas in which nurses are employed, but there are a number of other settings in which nurses' roles and responsibilities vary widely. A nurse employed in a physician's office, for example, may have little independent responsibility, but a nurse in solo practice or joint practice with other nurses or other health care professionals may provide care with much independence. Nurses are also employed in educational and research positions.

 # ROLES AND FUNCTIONS OF THE NURSE

Contemporary nursing requires that the nurse possess knowledge and skills in a variety of areas. In the past the principal role of nurses was to provide care and comfort as they carried out specific nursing functions, but changes in nursing have expanded the role to include increased emphasis on health promotion and illness prevention, as well as concern for the client as a whole. The contemporary nurse functions in the interrelated roles of care giver, decision maker, protector and client advocate, manager, rehabilitator, comforter, communicator, and teacher.

Care Giver

As care giver, the nurse helps the client regain health through the healing process. Healing is more than just curing a specific disease, although treatment skills that promote physical healing are important to care givers. The nurse addresses the holistic health care needs of the client, including measures to restore emotional and social well-being. The care giver helps the client and family set goals and meet those goals with a minimal cost of time and energy.

Decision Maker

To provide effective care, the nurse uses decision-making skills throughout the nursing process. Before undertaking any nursing action, whether it is assessing the client's condition, giving care, or evaluating the results of care, the nurse plans the action by deciding the best approach for each client. In some situations the nurse makes these decisions alone or with the client and family, and in other cases the nurse works with other health care professionals.

Protector and Client Advocate

As protector the nurse helps maintain a safe environment for the client and takes steps to prevent in-jury and protect the client from possible adverse effects of diagnostic or treatment measures. Confirming that a client does not have an allergy to a medication and providing immunization against disease in a community-based practice are examples of the nurse's protective role.

In the role of client advocate, the nurse protects the client's human and legal rights and provides assistance in asserting those rights if the need arises. For example, the nurse may provide additional information for a client who is trying to decide whether to accept treatment. The nurse may also defend clients' rights in a general way by speaking out against policies or actions that might endanger clients' well-being or conflict with their rights.

Manager

Nurses coordinate the activities of other members of the health care team, such as nutritionists and physical therapists, when managing the client's total care. Nurses must also manage their own time and the resources of the practice setting when concurrently providing care to several clients. Differentiated practice models offer nurses opportunities to make decisions about their career paths. In a differentiated practice setting, nurses can choose between roles as managers of patient care or as associate nurses who carry out the care manager's decisions (Manthey, 1990). As managers, nurses coordinate and delegate care responsibilities and supervise other health care workers.

Rehabilitator

Rehabilitation is the process by which individuals return to maximal levels of functioning after illness, accidents, or other disabling events. Frequently clients experience physical or emotional impairments that change their lives, and the nurse helps them adapt as fully as possible. Rehabilitative activities range from teaching clients to walk with crutches to helping clients cope with lifestyle changes often associated with chronic illness.

Comforter

The role of comforter, caring for the client as a person, is a traditional and historical one in nursing and has continued to be important as nurses have assumed new roles. Because nursing care must be directed to the whole person rather than simply the body, comfort and emotional support often help give the client strength to recover. While carrying out nursing activities, nurses can provide comfort by demonstrating care for the client as an individual with unique feelings and needs. As comforter, nurses should help the client reach therapeutic goals rather than encourage emotional or physical dependence.

Communicator

The role of communicator is central to all other nursing roles. Nursing involves communication with clients and families, other nurses and health care professionals, resource persons, and the community. Without clear communication, it is impossible to give care effectively, make decisions with clients and families, protect clients from threats to well-being, coordinate and manage client care, assist the client in rehabilitation, offer comfort, or teach. The quality of communication is a critical factor in meeting the needs of individuals, families, and communities.

Teacher

As teacher, the nurse explains to clients concepts and facts about health, demonstrates procedures such as self-care activities, determines that the client fully understands, reinforces learning or client behavior, and evaluates progress in learning. Some teaching can be unplanned and informal, such as when a nurse responds to a question about a health issue in casual conversation. Other teaching activities may be planned and more formal, such as when the nurse teaches a client with diabetes to self-administer injections. The nurse uses teaching methods that match the client's capabilities and needs and incorporates other resources, such as the family, in teaching plans.

Career Roles

The preceding roles and functions apply to all nurses in most practice settings. Career roles, on the other hand, are specific employment positions. Because of increasing educational opportunities for nurses, the growth of nursing as a profession, and a greater concern for job enrichment, the nursing profession offers expanded roles and different kinds of career opportunities. Examples of career roles include nurse educators, clinical nurse specialists, nurse practitioners, certified nurse-midwives, anesthetists, administrators, and researchers. Additional nonclinical roles include risk managers, quality assurance nurses, and product consultants.

Nurse Educator

A **nurse educator** works primarily in schools of nursing, staff development departments of health care agencies, and client education departments. Nursing educators generally have a background in clinical nursing, which provides them with practical skills and theoretical knowledge. A faculty member in a school of nursing prepares students to function as nurses. Nursing faculty members are responsible for teaching current nursing practice theory and necessary skills in laboratories or clinical settings. Nurse educators in nursing schools are usually required to have graduate degrees in nursing education. In addition, they generally have a specific clinical specialty and advanced clinical experience.

Nurse educators in staff development departments of health care institutions provide educational programs for nurses within their institution. These programs include orientation of new personnel, critical care nursing courses, and instruction about new equipment or procedures.

The primary focus of the nurse educator in an agency's department of client education is to teach ill or disabled clients and families to provide care in the home. In most health care agencies, however, the budget does not permit a separate client education department. Therefore staff nurses usually incorporate education into a client's plan of care.

Clinical Nurse Specialist

The **clinical nurse specialist (CNS)** has a master's degree in nursing and expertise in a specialized area of practice. A CNS works in a critical, acute, long-term, or community health care agency. In addition, a CNS may specialize in the management of a disease such as cancer, diabetes, or cardiovascular or pulmonary disease or in a specific field such as pediatrics or gerontology. The CNS functions as a clinician, educator, manager, consultant, and researcher within the area of practice to plan or improve the quality of nursing care for the client and family.

Nurse Practitioner

The **nurse practitioner** provides health care to clients, usually in an outpatient, ambulatory care, or community-based setting (Roy, Obloy, 1978; Molde, Diers, 1986). Molde and Diers noted that nurse practitioners care for clients with complex problems and attend more to symptoms of nonpathological conditions, comfort, and comprehensiveness of care.

A significant percentage of primary care encounters extend beyond the boundaries of medicine and demand the expertise of the nurse. The nurse practitioner is able to establish a collaborative provider-client relationship (Kasch, 1986).

A nurse practitioner may work with a specific group of clients or clients of all ages and health care needs. The major practitioner categories are adult, family, pediatric, obstetrics-gynecology, and geriatric nurse practitioner. A nurse practitioner has the knowledge and skills necessary to detect and manage limited acute and chronic stable conditions. The nurse practitioner's educational preparation includes a practitioner program or a master's degree in nursing.

An adult nurse practitioner (ANP) provides primary, ambulatory care to adults with a nonemergency acute or chronic illness. ANPs are usually employed in ambulatory care centers or outpatient clinics and work in collaboration with a primary physician.

A family nurse practitioner (FNP) provides primary ambulatory care for families, usually in collaboration with a family care physician. The FNP meets the family's general health care needs, manages some illnesses by providing direct care, and guides or counsels the family as needed.

A pediatric nurse practitioner (PNP) provides health care to infants and children. An obstetrics-gynecology nurse practitioner (OB-GYN), provides primary ambulatory care to women seeking obstetrical or gynecological health care. The nurse practitioner who is also a certified nurse-midwife may independently deliver infants. A geriatric nurse practitioner (GNP) provides ambulatory or inpatient care to older adults. The GNP's activities include interventions for health maintenance, illness prevention, or health restoration.

Certified Nurse-Midwife

A **certified nurse-midwife (CNM)** is educated in nursing and midwifery and is certified by the American College of Nurse-Midwives. The practice of nurse-midwifery involves providing independent care for women during normal pregnancy, labor, and delivery, as well as care for the newborn. It may include some gynecological services such as routine Papanicolaou (Pap) smears, family planning, and treatment for minor vaginal infections. A CNM practices with a health care agency that provides medical consultation, collaborative management, and referral.

Nurse Anesthetist

A **nurse anesthetist** is an RN who has received advanced training in an accredited program in anesthesiology. Nurse anesthetists provide surgical anesthesia under the guidance and supervision of an anesthesiologist, who is a physician with advanced knowledge of surgical anesthesia.

Nurse Administrator

A **nurse administrator** manages client care and the delivery of specific nursing services within a health care agency. This administrator may hold a middle management position, such as head nurse or supervisor, or an upper-level management position, such as assistant or associate director or director of nursing services. Functions of administrators include budgeting, staffing, strategic planning of programs and services, employee evaluation, and employee development. Middle-management positions usually require at least a baccalaureate degree in nursing, and upper-level positions generally require a master's degree.

Nurse Researcher

The **nurse researcher** investigates problems to improve nursing care and to further define and expand the scope of nursing practice (see Chapter 11). The nurse researcher may be employed in an academic setting, hospital, or independent professional or community-service agency. The minimum educational requirement is a graduate degree in nursing.

Health Care Team

In most practice settings the nurse works with other health care professionals to provide total care for clients. The health care team comprises four general types of professionals, including nurses, physicians, allied health professionals such as therapists and technicians, and other specialists such as social workers and chaplains. The involvement of many different persons in the client's health care, however, may cause a fragmenting of care. Because nurses have the greatest opportunity to interact with all of the other professionals in the health care team, they often have the role of coordinating and integrating services within the plan of care.

Physician

A **physician** is a professional who has earned a degree of Doctor of Medicine (MD) or Doctor of Osteopathy (DO). The physician has completed a required curriculum, has had a specific period of postgraduate training, and has passed a licensing examination. A physician is licensed for the medical diagnosis and treatment of clients.

Most physicians specialize in diseases involving one body system (for example, a cardiologist specializes in heart diseases) or in one specific disease (for example, an oncologist specializes in cancer). Physicians may also specialize in surgery or in treating a certain age group.

Nurses work with physicians in many capacities. One nurse may work in a setting in which most nursing care depends on the physician's orders. An intensive care nurse may follow written guidelines that permit more independent nursing actions. A clinical nurse specialist or nurse practitioner may function in a collaborative capacity with a physician; for example, when preparing a client with newly diagnosed diabetes for discharge, the nurse and physician work together to teach the client and family about home care.

Physician Assistant

A **physician assistant** (**PA**) is trained in certain aspects of the practice of medicine to provide support to physicians. PAs practice in the United States but not in Canada and must work under the direction and supervision of a physician. PAs practice in hospitals, clinics, or private physicians' offices.

Allied and Other Health Care Professionals

THERAPIST. A **physical therapist** (**PT**) is licensed to assist in the examination, testing, and treatment of physically disabled or handicapped people through the use of special exercises, the application of heat and cold, the use of sonar waves, and other techniques. A PT usually receives training in a 4-year college program leading to a bachelor of science degree in physical therapy. A PT practices in hospitals, clinics, rehabilitation centers, and community-based agencies.

An **occupational therapist** (**OT**) is licensed or certified to develop and use adaptive devices that help chronically ill or handicapped clients carry out activities of daily living. OTs usually receive education and training in 4-year college programs, and like a PT, work in a variety of settings.

A **respiratory therapist** (**RT**) is licensed to deliver treatment designed to improve clients' ventilatory function or oxygenation. Educational and training programs vary. They range from 6-month training programs to educational programs in 4-year colleges. An RT is usually employed in an institutional health care setting.

Nurses work with therapists in a collaborative capacity. Care initiated by therapists is frequently continued and evaluated by nurses. Nurses and therapists together consider the client's progress and develop goals and discharge plans that include the client and family. In addition, nurses refer clients to therapists for further care. For example, a nurse caring for a person with severe pulmonary disease may refer the client to a PT to learn exercises for strengthening the upper arm muscles, to an OT to learn energy-saving techniques for activities of daily living, and to an RT for techniques to promote airway clearance.

PHARMACIST. A **pharmacist** is a licensed professional who formulates and dispenses medications. The pharmacist may practice only within a pharmacy or may be involved in client care conferences or in the development of medication administration systems (see Chapter 21). The pharmacist's education ranges from a bachelor of science degree to a doctorate in pharmacology. A pharmacist practices in an institutional or outpatient setting.

The pharmacist is a valuable resource for nurses. For example, the nurse can request information about new drugs from the pharmacist. The nurse must know the action, desired effect, correct dosage, and side effects of all drugs administered. If this information is unavailable in standard reference books such as textbooks or hospital formularies, the nurse should consult the pharmacist.

Pharmacists also provide information about which drugs are compatible and which can be mixed or administered together. In addition, pharmacists can tell the nurse which over-the-counter drugs may interact adversely with prescribed drugs so that this information can be incorporated into the discharge teaching plan.

SOCIAL WORKER. A **social worker** is trained to counsel clients and families. Counseling services may include providing emotional support for clients and families during severe or terminal illnesses, arranging placement in extended care facilities, and locating financial resources. The social worker generally has a baccalaureate or master's degree in social work and is employed in every type of agency in the health care system. A nurse frequently refers clients to a social worker, and they work together to identify resources for meeting clients' present and future health care needs.

SPIRITUAL ADVISORS. **Spiritual advisors** offer spiritual support and guidance to clients and families and may be employed by an agency or institution or be provided by a religious affiliation within the community. Spiritual advisors are ministers, priests, nuns, rabbis, or lay members of religious congregations. A client may request to see a spiritual advisor, or the nurse may initiate a referral.

 ## NURSING AS A PROFESSION

Professionalism

Nursing is not simply a collection of specific skills, and the nurse is not simply a person trained to perform specific tasks. Nursing is a profession.

No one factor absolutely differentiates a job from a profession, but the difference is important in terms of how nurses practice. When we say a person acts "professionally," for example, we imply that the person is conscientious in actions, knowledgeable in the subject, and responsible to self and others. Etzioni (1961) describes professions in terms of the following primary characteristics:

1. A profession requires an extended education of its members, as well as a basic liberal foundation.
2. A profession has a theoretical body of knowledge leading to defined skills, abilities, and norms.
3. A profession provides a specific service.
4. Members of a profession have autonomy in decision making and practice.
5. The profession as a whole has a code of ethics for practice.

Nursing clearly shares, to some extent, each of these characteristics. Nursing is still evolving as a profession, however, and faces controversial issues as nurses strive for greater professionalism.

Education

As a profession, nursing requires that its members possess a significant amount of education. The issue of standardization of nursing education is a major controversy today. Most nurses agree that nursing education is important to practice and that it must respond to changes in health care created by scientific and technological advances. The ANA's 1965 position paper on nursing education emphasizes the role of education in the profession (see box).

In 1984 the ANA described two levels of practice, the associate nurse and the professional nurse, which require the bachelors of science in nursing. The NLN also supports a proposal that associate and diploma graduates take one licensing examination. North Dakota was the first state to implement such a policy. In January 1987, North Dakota's Supreme Court ruled that the state board "has the authority . . . to direct that only associate and baccalaureate degree graduates may sit for practical and registered nursing license examinations respectively" (News, 1987).

Theory

As nursing has emerged as a profession, nursing knowledge has been developed through nursing theories. Theoretical models serve as frameworks for nursing curricula and clinical practice. Nursing theories also lead to further research that increases the scientific basis of nursing practice.

A theory is a way of understanding a reality, and in this general sense, all practicing nurses use the theories they have learned. Several of the approaches described in the section on definitions and philosophies are parts of fully developed nursing theories.

Premises for ANA's First Position Paper on Education for Nursing

- Nursing is a helping profession and, as such, provides services which contribute to the health and well-being of people.
- Nursing is of vital consequence to the individual receiving services; it fills needs which cannot be met by the person, by the family, or by other persons in the community.
- The demand for services of nurses will continue to increase.
- The professional practitioner is responsible for the nature and quality of all nursing care that patients receive.
- The services of professional practitioners of nursing will continue to be supplemented and complemented by the services of nurse practitioners who will be licensed.
- Education for those in the health professions must increase in depth and breadth as scientific knowledge expands.
- In addition to those licensed as nurses, the health care of the public, in the amount and to the extent needed and demanded, requires the services of large numbers of health occupation workers to function as assistants to nurses. These workers are presently designated: nurses' aids, orderlies, assistants, attendants, etc.
- The professional association must concern itself with the nature of nursing practice, the means for improving nursing practice, the education necessary for such practice, and the standards for membership in the professional association.

From ANA: *A position paper: educational preparation for nurse practitioners and assistants to nurses,* Kansas City, Mo, 1965, The Association.

Service

Nursing has always been a service profession, although in the past the service was usually viewed as a charitable one. Today, nursing is a vital and indispensable component of the health care delivery system.

Autonomy

Autonomy means that a person is reasonably independent and self-governing in decision making and practice. It has been difficult for nurses to attain the degree of autonomy enjoyed by other professionals. In the past, physicians, hospital administrators, and others in the health care delivery system have found nursing autonomy difficult to understand and support. Through clinical competence and greater educational preparation, however, nurses are increasingly taking on independent roles in nurse-run clinics, collaborative practice, and advanced nursing careers.

With increased autonomy come greater responsibility and accountability. *Accountability* means that the nurse is responsible, professionally and legally, for the type and quality of nursing care provided. The nurse is accountable for keeping abreast of technical skills and knowledge needed to perform nursing care. The nursing profession itself regulates accountability through nursing audits and standards of practice.

Code of Ethics

Nursing has a code of ethics, which defines the principles by which nurses function. In addition, nurses incorporate their own values and ethics into practice. Chapter 13 gives several examples of specific statements of nursing's code of ethics.

Professional Organizations

A **professional organization** is created to deal with issues of concern to those practicing in the profession. In North America the major professional nursing organizations are the ANA, CNA, and NLN. The CNA and the ANA were formed in the late nineteenth century to improve standards of health and availability of health care, to foster high standards for nursing, and to promote the professional development and general and economic welfare of nurses. The ANA and CNA are part of the ICN. The objectives of the ICN parallel those of the CNA and ANA; the ICN promotes national associations of nurses, improves standards of nursing practice, seeks a higher status for nurses, and provides an international power base for nurses.

The NLN is concerned with the improvement of nursing education, nursing service, and health care delivery in the United States. In Canada the Canadian Association of University Schools of Nursing and the Canadian Association of Practical and Nursing Assistants perform similar functions.

Nursing students also take part in organizations such as the National Student Nurses Association (NSNA) in the United States and the Canadian Student Nurses Association (CSNA) in Canada. These organizations consider issues of importance to nursing students and often cooperate in activities and programs with the professional organizations.

Some professional organizations are special-interest groups focusing on specific areas such as critical care, nursing administration or research, or nurse-midwifery. These organizations seek to improve the standards of practice, expand nursing roles, and foster the welfare of nurses within the specialty areas. In addition, professional organizations present education programs and publish journals. Some representative specialty organizations are discussed in the following paragraphs.

The Association of Operating Room Nurses (AORN) in the United States and the National Conference of Operating Room Nurses in Canada are concerned with continuing education for operating room nurses, higher standards for operating room care, and increased research activities.

The Nurses Association of the American College of Obstetricians and Gynecologists (NAACOG) includes Canadian and American nurses and promotes standards of practice in obstetrical and gynecological nursing, encourages professional growth for its members, and is an accrediting body for advanced programs in obstetrical and gynecological nursing.

The National Association of Pediatric Nurse Associates/Practitioners (NAPNAP) is a national organization for nurses prepared by training or experience to give primary care to children. NAPNAP works in conjunction with the American Academy of Pediatrics.

The American Association of Critical Care Nurses (AACN) is a national organization of nurses working in critical care areas. It is concerned with nursing education, practice, and research as they involve critical care nursing.

 ## SOCIETY'S INFLUENCE ON NURSING

Throughout history, nursing has responded to society's needs. Contemporary nursing education, practice, and research are an outgrowth of economic, technological, demographic, sociological, and political issues.

Technological Advances

In recent years, scientific and technological advances have affected almost every aspect of life. Health care has changed in many ways, including the use of new equipment, new diagnostic tests and treatment measures, and new drugs. Nursing has adapted and will continue to respond to these changes with continuing education, in-service programs, and other educational approaches. Nursing is also uniquely concerned with the *human* side of technological advances. Society as a whole seems to accept technological advances in health care, but clients often experience problems related to them. For example, dialysis machines have been used for many years to treat clients with kidney problems, but that fact does not lessen the emotional conflict a client may experience after learning that dialysis is needed. As health care technology becomes increasingly complex and sophisticated, nurses must help clients adjust to the use of technology in care.

Demographic Changes

Demographic changes affect the population as a whole. Changes that have influenced health care in recent decades include the population shift from rural areas to urban centers; increasing life span; the higher incidence of chronic, long-term illness; and the increased incidence of diseases such as alcoholism and lung cancer. Nursing as a profession responds to such changes by exploring new methods for providing care, by changing educational emphases, and by establishing practice standards in new areas. To better meet the changing health care needs of clients, the nurse also responds to demographic changes in the population served by the practice setting.

Consumer Movement

The consumer movement is a heightened awareness of the value and costs of products and services; in short, consumers want their money's worth. Health care in general has been influenced by the consumer movement in ways as diverse as new kinds of health care agencies such as health maintenance organizations, new forms of health insurance, and concern about the rising costs of health care (see Chapter 5). Also, consumers are more knowledgeable about health and illness and are becoming more vocal in their desire for high-quality care. Because nurses generally interact with clients more than other health care professionals, they must often answer questions about the quality and costs of health care. Health care consumers are also more aware of their rights as clients, and the nurse supports these rights in the role of client advocate.

Health Promotion

Related to the consumer movement is a greater emphasis in society on health promotion and illness prevention. Exercise and nutrition are subjects that interest many people. Nursing has responded to this greater concern for health promotion in many ways, from programs in the community to specific health promotion and teaching activities for clients in hospitals and other health care settings. Health promotion activities are a part of many of the roles of a nurse, including care giver, client advocate, rehabilitator, communicator, and teacher.

Women's Movement

The women's movement has brought about many changes in society as women have increasingly sought economic, political, occupational, and educational equality. Nursing is responding in two ways. Because most nurses are women, they are increasingly asserting their equal rights as human beings, employees, and health care professionals. The women's movement has encouraged nurses to seek greater autonomy and responsibility in providing care in an environment that has been and continues to be patrician (Bunning, Campbell, 1990). The women's movement has caused female clients to seek more responsibility for and control over their bodies, health, and lives in general. As women become more aware of their own needs and unique qualities, they seek health care that can help them meet those needs.

Human Rights Movement

Like the women's movement, the human rights movement is changing the way society views the rights of *all* of its members, including minorities, clients with terminal illness, pregnant women, and older adults. Many groups have special health care needs, and nursing has responded by respecting all clients as individuals with a right to good care and with basic human rights. Nurses advocate the rights of all clients, but they have also recognized the special needs of some groups and thus have created bills of rights for dying, hospitalized, and pregnant clients, as well as other groups, to ensure that quality care is provided without sacrificing these rights.

 ## TRENDS IN NURSING

This chapter has emphasized that nursing is not a static, unchanging profession but is continuously growing and evolving as society changes, as health care emphases and methods change, as lifestyles change—and as nurses themselves change. To speak of nursing at all is to speak of nursing as it is at a given time, and in this sense, this chapter is about trends in nursing.

The current philosophies and definitions of nursing demonstrate the holistic trend in nursing—to address the whole person in all dimensions, in health and illness, and in interaction with the family and community. Nursing continues to draw on the social sciences and other fields as the focus of nursing care expands.

One trend in nursing education is the growing number of students receiving basic nursing education in community colleges and universities. Professional nursing organizations continue to stress the importance of education for nurses seeking new and expanded roles.

Nursing practice trends include a growing variety of settings in which nurses have greater independence. Nurses continue to gain autonomy and respect as members of the health care team. Nursing roles continue to expand with the broadening focus of nursing care. The clinical ladder and new career roles also represent current trends in nursing practice.

Trends in nursing as a profession include the growing emphasis on the aspects of nursing that characterize it as a profession, including education, theory, service, autonomy, and ethical codes. The activities of nursing's professional organizations reflect all the trends in nursing education and practice. Finally, all the influences of society on nursing also reflect trends in contemporary nursing.

Two other trends need to be discussed: the increasing political influence of nursing and nursing's influence on health care policy and practice.

Political Influence of Professional Nursing

Historically, nurses' involvement in politics has been limited. Although individual nurses such as Florence Nightingale, Lillian Wald, and Margaret Sanger have influenced decision making in areas such as sanitation, nutrition, and birth control, nurses have accomplished less as a group. The recent women's movement, however, has inspired nurses to address health care issues. In addition, as more college-educated people enter the profession, they bring to nursing the activism and involvement of the university campuses.

In 1974, the ANA formed the Nurses Coalition in Politics (N-CAP), which was the first political action committee (PAC) for nurses. This organization, which was later renamed ANA-PAC, is a major PAC that is sought for support for candidates seeking federal offices (Mason, 1990).

Political power is the ability to influence or persuade an individual holding a government office to exert the power of that office to affect a desired outcome (Rogge, 1987). Traditionally, nurses have been uncomfortable with politics because the majority of nurses are women and politics has been male dominated. Nurses are also unaware of historical precedents established by nurses in the political arena, and because they are not politically astute, nurses lack the political education to successfully compete in politics (Mason, Talbott, 1985; Mason, 1990).

Nurses' involvement in politics is receiving greater emphasis in nursing curricula, professional organizations, and health care settings (Stanhope, Belcher, 1982). Professional nursing organizations have employed lobbyists to urge state legislatures and the U.S. Congress to improve the quality of health care. Kalisch and Kalisch (1982) note that the ANA

works for the improvement of health standards and the availability of health care services for all people; fosters high standards of nursing, stimulates and promotes the professional development of nurses, and advances their economic and general welfare. The purposes are unrestricted by considerations of nationality, race, creed, lifestyle, color, sex, or age.

The ANA employs RNs as lobbyists at the federal level, and state nursing organizations also hire lobbyists and legislative specialists to work on state nursing issues and assist with federal efforts. Finally, lobbyists working on behalf of nursing are employed in Washington, D.C., by professional interest groups such as the American Federation of Teachers, NLN, American College of Nurse Midwives, American Public Health Association, and AACN. These groups aim to remove financial barriers to health care, increase the quality of nursing care available, increase economic rewards to nurses, and expand professional nursing roles (Aiken, 1982).

In addition, individual nurses work to effect change in the health care system. According to Mullane (1975), if nurses become serious students of social needs, activists in influencing policy to meet those needs, and generous contributors of time and money to nursing and their organizations and to candidates working for universal good health care, then the future is bright indeed.

Nursing's Influence on Health Care Policy and Practice

Nurses are becoming more involved in changes in health care reform. *Nursing's Agenda for Health Care Reform* supports the creation of a health care system that ensures access, quality, and services at affordable costs (ANA, 1991). The plan for reform focuses on primary health care services and the promotion, restoration, and maintenance of health (ANA, 1991) (see Chapter 3).

Political activism and commitment are a part of professionalism, however, and politics are an important aspect of the delivery of health care. Therefore nurses should not view politics as "dirty business" but as a reality that includes the arts of influence, compromise, and social interaction.

Nurses have been involved in a different sort of politics in schools of nursing and in health care settings when seeking additional resources, more self-direction, and accountability with authority. The skills gained in such experiences can be transferred to the politics of health care policy-making.

As long as nurses maintain involvement in health care policy and practice, misinformed outsiders cannot attempt to impose their will on nursing and nursing practice. Nonnursing groups, often led by other health care providers, have made attempts to impose institutional licensure, mandatory continuing education, curtailment of advanced nursing practice, and other constraints on a profession that should have its own voice in decisions made in these and numerous other areas affecting the quality of nursing care. Although nurses have often successfully prevented infringement on the profession's self-governance, the future of nursing requires that nurses individually and collectively seek a greater influence on health care policies affecting nursing practice.

 SUMMARY

Nursing as a profession is complex and multifaceted. The nurse's role includes that of care giver, teacher, counselor, advocate, and researcher. The nurse needs a theoretical or conceptual model from which to practice in a variety of settings. The professional growth and development of today's nurse requires information on research and on ways to perform a research study, as well as on the use of findings in a clinical practice setting. The standards of practice set forth by professional nursing associations provide guidelines for competent, safe, and professional practice. Historical origins of nursing have assisted today's professionals in their development and future needs.

CHAPTER 1 REVIEW

Key Concepts

- Nursing is an essential part of society; it has grown out of society and has evolved with it.

- Nursing has responded to the health care needs of society, which were influenced by economic, social, and cultural variables of a specific era.

- Formalized education programs for professional nursing were established in the nineteenth century by Florence Nightingale.

- The growth of nursing and nursing education in the United States was stimulated by the Civil War.

- The Canadian Nurses Association and the American Nurses Association were established in the late nineteenth century.

- The opening of the Henry Street Settlement by Lillian Wald and Mary Brewster marked the expansion of nursing into the community setting.

- Nursing education became affiliated with universities early in the twentieth century.

- Expansion of nursing into the military occurred in the early twentieth century, and the development of specialty nursing organizations began in the 1950s and has continued to the present.

- The Lysaught Report (1970) emphasized the need for clarification of nursing roles and responsibilities, greater financial support for nurses, and more career opportunities.

- Nursing definitions reflect changes in the practice of nursing and help bring about changes by identifying the domain of nursing practice and guiding research, practice, and education.

- Conceptual and theoretical nursing models provide knowledge to improve practice, guide research and nursing curricula, and identify the domain and goals of nursing practice.

- Conceptual and theoretical nursing models provide a basis for clinical nursing practice.

- Educational preparation of the registered nurse can be through one of three programs in the United States or two programs in Canada.

- A license for a registered nurse in each state or province is granted after a candidate has completed a prescribed course of study in an accredited program and passed a licensing examination.

- Graduate nursing programs prepare nurse clinicians to improve nursing care through the advancement of nursing theory and sciences.

- Continuing education programs can be accredited by the American Nurses Association or the state board of nursing.

- The clinical ladder incorporates opportunities for advancement in nursing through an administrative or clinical track.

- Nursing standards provide the guidelines for implementing and evaluating nursing care.

- The rapid rise in the number of older adults and rate of chronic illnesses and functional impairments has resulted in an increased number of long-term care facilities.

- Community-based agencies focus primarily on health promotion, maintenance, education, and management, as well as coordination and continuity of care within the community.

- The multiple roles and functions of the nurse include care giver, decision maker, protector, client advocate, manager, rehabilitator, comforter, communicator, and teacher.

- Specific employment positions include nurse educator, clinical nurse specialist, nurse practitioner, certified nurse-midwife, nurse anesthetist, administrator, and researcher.

- The health care team is multidisciplinary and may include a physician, physician assistant, physical therapist, occupational therapist, respiratory therapist, pharmacist, social worker, and spiritual advisor.

- Nursing is a profession encompassing educational preparation for the nurse, nursing theory, a provided service, autonomy, and a code of ethics.

- Professional nursing organizations deal with issues of concern to specialist groups within the nursing profession.

- Changes in society, such as increased technology, new demographic patterns, consumerism, health promotion, and the women's and human rights movements, have led to changes in nursing.

- Nurses are becoming more politically sophisticated and, as a result, are able to increase nursing's influence on health care policy and practice.

Key Terms

American Nurses Association (ANA), p. 6

Canadian Nurses Association (CNA), p. 6

Certified nurse-midwife (CNM), p. 25

Clinical nurse specialist (CNS), p. 24

Congress for Nursing Practice, p. 15

Continuing education, p. 17

In-service education, p. 17

International Council of Nurses (ICN), p. 4

Licensed practical nurse (LPN), p. 18

Licensed vocational nurse (LVN), p. 18

National League for Nursing (NLN), p. 8

Nurse administrator, p. 25

Nurse anesthetist, p. 25

Nurse educator, p. 24

Nurse practitioner, p. 24

Nurse researcher, p. 25

Nursing theory, p. 7

Occupational therapist (OT), p. 26

Pharmacist, p. 26

Physical therapist (PT), p. 26

Physician, p. 25

Physician assistant (PA), p. 26

Professional organization, p. 28

Registered nurse (RN), p. 15

Respiratory therapist (RT), p. 26

Social worker, p. 26

Spiritual advisors, p. 26

Critical Thinking Exercises

1. You are assigned to care for a client who needs to learn how to manage cardiac medication. Describe the criteria you would use to select a nursing theory for a basis for clinical practice.

2. You are assigned to interview a nurse in an expanded role. What information would you need about the role before conducting your interview?

3. Part of your education includes experiences in different types of health care settings. What differences would you expect between nurses who practice in hospitals, skilled care facilities, and home care agencies? Would you expect any commonalities?

REFERENCES

Abdellah FG et al: *Patient-centered approaches to nursing,* New York, 1960, Macmillan.

Aiken LH: The impact of federal health policy on nursing. In Aiken LH, editor: *Nursing in the 80's: crises, opportunities, challenges,* Philadelphia, 1982, Lippincott.

American Association of Colleges of Nursing: *Essentials of college and university education for professional nursing: a final report,* Washington, DC, 1986, The Association.

American Nurses Association: A code of ethics, *Am J Nurs* 26:621, 1926.

American Nurses Association: Educational preparation for nurse practitioners, *Am J Nurs* 65(12):106, 1965.

American Nurses Association: *Statement on graduate education in nursing,* New York, 1969, The Association.

American Nurses Association: *Nursing and social policy statement,* Kansas City, Mo, 1980, The Association.

American Nurses Association: *Career ladders: an approach to professional productivity and job satisfaction,* ANA Pub No N5-27, Kansas City, Mo, 1984, The Association.

American Nurses Association: *Code for nurses with interpretive statements,* ANA Publ No G-56, Kansas City, Mo, 1985, The Association.

American Nurses Association: *Standards for continuing education in nursing,* Washington, DC, 1991, The Association.

American Nurses Association: *Nursing's agenda for health care reform,* Washington, DC, 1991, The Association.

Anderson MI Denyes MJ: A ladder for clinical advancement in nursing practice, *J Nurs Adm* 5(2):16, 1975.

Beeber L, Anderson CA, Sills GM: Peplau's theory in practice, *Nurs Sci Q* 3(1):6, 1990.

Benner P: *From novice to expert: excellence and power in clinical nursing practice,* Menlo Park, Calif, 1984, Addison-Wesley.

Benner P, Tanner C: How expert nurses use intuition, *Am J Nurs* 87(1):23, 1987.

Bunning S, Campbell JC: Feminism and nursing: historical perspectives, *ANS* 12(4):11, 1990.

Chinn PL, Jacobs MK: *Theory and nursing: a systematic approach,* ed 2, St Louis, 1987, Mosby–Year Book.

Cohen IB: Florence Nightingale, *Sci Am* 250(128):137, 1984.

Colavecchio R, Tescher B, Scalgi C: A clinical ladder for nursing practice, *J Nurs Adm* 5:54, 1974.

Dolan JA et al: *Nursing in society: a historical perspective,* ed 15, Philadelphia, 1983, Saunders.

Donahue MP: *Nursing: the finest art, an illustrated history,* St Louis, 1985, Mosby–Year Book.

Etzioni A: *The semi-professionals and their organizations,* New York, 1961, Free Press.

Fawcett J: *Analysis and evaluation of conceptual models of nursing,* ed 2, Philadelphia, 1989, Davis.

Gordin P: Launching a leadership role, *MCN* 16(1):24-26, 1991.

Hefferin EA, Kleinknecht MK: Development of the nursing career preference inventory, *Nurs Res* 35(1):44, 1986.

Henderson V: The nature of nursing, *Am J Nurs* 64:62, 1964.

Henderson V: *The nature of nursing,* New York, 1966, Macmillan.

Hinshaw AS: Nursing science: the challenge to develop knowledge, *Nurs Sci Q* 2(4):162, 1989.

Holzemer W: Doctoral education in nursing: an assessment of quality: 1979-1984, *Nurs Res* 36(2):110, 1987.

Holzemer WL: Quality and cost of nursing care: is anybody out there listening, *Nurs Health Care* 11(8):412, 1990.

Huey FL: Looking at ladders, *Am J Nurs* 82:1520, 1982.

Institute of Medicine, Division of Health Care Services: *Nursing and nursing education: public policies and private actions,* Washington, DC, 1983, National Academy Press.

International Council of Nurses: *Code for nurses,* Geneva, 1973, The Council.

Johnson DE: Theory in nursing: borrowed and unique, *Nurs Res* 11:206, 1968.

Johnson DE: The behavioral system for nursing. In Riehl JP, Roy C, editors: *Conceptual models for nursing practice,* ed 2, New York, 1980, Appleton-Century-Crofts.

Kalisch BJ, Kalisch PA: *Politics of nursing,* Philadelphia, 1982, Lippincott.

Kasch CR: Establishing a collaborative nurse-patient relationship: a distinct focus of nursing action of primary care, *Image J Nurs Sch* 18:44, 1986.

Kelly LY: *Dimensions of professional nursing,* New York, 1981, Macmillan.

King IM: *Toward a theory for nursing,* New York, 1971, Wiley.

Leininger MM: Caring: a central focus of nursing and health care services, *Nurs Health Care* 1(3):135, 1980.

Levine MC: *An introduction to clinical nursing,* ed 2, Philadelphia, 1973, Davis.

Lysaught JP: *An abstract for action,* New York, 1970, McGraw-Hill.

Manthey M: 1990 nursing: a profession of choice, *Nurs Manage* 21(9):17, 1990.

Marriner-Tomey A: *Nursing theorists and their work,* ed 2, St Louis, 1989, Mosby–Year Book.

Mason DJ: Nursing and politics: a profession comes of age, *Orthop Nurs* 9(5):11, 1990.

Mason DJ, Talbott SW: *The political action handbook for nurses,* Menlo Park, Calif, 1985, Addison-Wesley.

McCloskey JC, McCain BE: Satisfaction, commitment, and professionalism of newly employed nurses, *Image: J Nurs Sch* 19(1):20, 1987.

McClure ML: Nursing and hospital cost containment, *J Prof Nurs* 7(1):4, 1991.

Meilicke D, Larsen, J: Leadership and the leadership of the Canadian Nurses Association. In Baumgart AJ, Larsen J, eidtors: *Ca-*

nadian nursing faces the future: development and change, St Louis, 1988, Mosby–Year Book.

Meleis AI: *Theoretical nursing: development and progress,* Philadelphia, 1985, Lippincott.

Molde S, Diers D: Nurse practitioner research: selected literature review and research agenda, *Nurs Res* 34(6):362, 1986.

Mullane MK: Nursing care and the political arena, *Nurs Outlook* 23:699, 1975.

National Commission on Nursing: *Source book: National Commission on Nursing,* Chicago, 1983, American Hospital Association.

Neuman B: *The Neuman systems model: application to nursing education and practice,* New York, 1982, Appleton-Century-Crofts.

Neuman BM, Young RJ: A model for teaching total person approach to patient problems, *Nurs Res* 21:264, 1972.

News: North Dakota's High Court frees nursing board to enforce its BSN requirement for RN licensure, *Am J Nurs* 87(3):372, 1987.

Nightingale F: *Notes on nursing: what it is and what it is not,* London, 1860, Harrison & Sons.

Orlando IJ: *The dynamic nurse-patient relationship: function, process, and principles,* New York, 1961, Putnam.

Orem DE: *Nursing: concepts of practice,* New York, 1971, McGraw-Hill.

Orem DE: *Nursing: concepts of practice,* ed 3, New York, 1985, McGraw-Hill.

Parse RR: *Man-living-health: theory of nursing,* New York, 1981, Wiley.

Parse RR: *Nursing science: major paradigms, theories, and critiques,* Philadelphia, 1987, Saunders.

Parse RR: Nursing theory-based practice: a challenge for the 90s, *Nurs Sci Q* 3(2):53, 1990.

Patterson JG, Zderad LT: *Humanistic nursing,* New York, 1976, Wiley.

Peplau HE: *Interpersonal relations in nursing,* New York, 1952, Putnam.

Raab DM: Nursing in Canada: perseverance in practice, *Health Care* September 1985, p 27.

Rogers ME: *An introduction to the theoretical basis of nursing,* Philadelphia, 1970, Davis.

Rogge MM: Nursing and politics: a forgotten legacy, *Nurs Res* 36(1):26, 1987.

Roy C: The Roy adaptation model. In Riehl JP, Roy C, editors: *Conceptual models for nursing practice,* New York, 1980, Appleton-Century-Crofts.

Roy C, Obloy SM: The practitioner movement: toward a science of nursing, *Am J Nurs* 79:1698, 1979.

Shryock RH: *The history of nursing: an interpretation of the social and medical factors involved,* Philadelphia, 1959, Saunders.

Silverstein NG: Lillian Wald at Henry Street 1893-1895, *ANS* 7(2):1, 1985.

Stanhope M, Belcher AE: Political imperatives for nursing practice. In Lancaster J, Lancaster W, editors: *Concepts for advanced nursing practice,* St Louis, 1982, Mosby–Year Book.

Sward, K: The code for nurses: an historical perspective. In American Nurses Association: *Perspectives on the code for nurses,* Publ No G-132, Kansas City, Mo, 1978, The Association.

Tanner CA et al: Diagnostic reasoning strategies of nursing and nursing students, *Nurs Res* 36(6):358, 1987.

Torres G: *Theoretical foundations of nursing,* Norwalk, Conn, 1986, Appleton-Century-Crofts.

Viens DC: A history of nursing's code of ethics, *Nurs Outlook* 37(1):45, 1989.

Watson J: *Nursing: the philosophy and science of caring,* Boston, 1979, Little, Brown.

Watson J: Nursing on the caring edge: metaphorical vignettes, *ANS* 10(1):10, 1987.

Wheeler CE: *The American Journal of Nursing* and the socialization of a profession: 1900-1920, *ANS* 7(2):20, 1985.

Woodham-Smith C: *Florence Nightingale,* New York, 1983, McGraw-Hill.

Zimmer MJ: Rationale for a ladder for clinical advancement, *J Nurs Adm* 5:18, 1975.

Zimmer MJ: A suggested code, *Am J Nurs* 26:599, 1926.

ADDITIONAL READINGS

American Nurses Association Committee on Education: *A position paper,* New York, 1965, The Association.

Canadian Nurses Association: *Definition of nursing standards and practice,* Ottawa, 1980, The Association.

Canadian Nurses Association: *Nursing in Canada: 1985,* Ontario, Canada, 1986, The Association.

Crosby LJ, Facteau LM, Donley R: Priorities for nurse training act legislation: a national survey of nursing deans, *Image: J Nurs Sch* 15(4):107, 1983.

Curran CR, Minnick G, Moss J: Who needs nurses? *Am J Nurs* 87:444, 1987.

Dennis KE, Prescott PA: Florence Nightingale: yesterday, today, and tomorrow, *ANS* 7(2):66, 1985.

Dickoff J, James P: A theory of theories: a position paper, *Nurs Res* 17(3):197, 1968.

Diers D, Hamman A, Molde S: Complexity of ambulatory care: nurse practitioner and physician caseloads, *Nurs Res* 35(5):310, 1986.

Fairman JA: Sources and references for research in nursing history, *Nurs Res* 36(1):56, 1987.

King IM: *A theory for nursing: system, concepts, process,* New York, 1971, Wiley.

Knox SL: A clinical advancement program, *J Nurs Adm* 10(7):29, 1980.

Leininger MM: *Transcultural nursing: concepts, theories and practices,* New York, 1978, Wiley.

Leininger MM: *Transcultural care, diversity and universality: a theory of nursing,* Thorofore, NJ, 1985, Slack.

Newman MA: Nursing's theoretical evolution, *Nurs Outlook* 20(7):449, 1972.

Parse RR, Cogne AB, Smith MJ: *Nursing research: qualitative methods,* Bowie, Md, 1985, Brady.

Roy C: Adaptation: a conceptual framework for nursing, *Nurs Outlook* 18(3):42, 1970.

Roy C: *Introduction to nursing: an adaptation model,* ed 2, Englewood Cliffs, NJ, 1984, Prentice Hall.

Roy C, Roberts S: Theory construction in nursing: an adaptation model, Englewood Cliffs, NJ, 1981, Prentice Hall.

Shamansky SL, Schilling LS, Holbrook TL: Determining the market for nurse practitioner services: the New Haven experience, *Nurs Res* 34(4):242, 1985.

Silva MC, Rothbart D: An analysis of changing trends in philosophies of science on nursing theory development and testing, *ANS* 6(2):1, 1984.

Stevens BJ: *Nursing theory: analysis, application, evaluation,* ed 2, Boston, 1984, Little, Brown.

Taylor MS, Covaleski MA: Predicting nurse's turnover and internal transfer behavior, *Nurs Res* 34(4):237, 1985.

Travelbee J: *Interpersonal agents of nursing,* ed 2, Philadelphia, 1971, Davis.

Walker LO: Toward a clearer understanding of the concept of nursing theory, *Nurs Res* 20(5):428, 1971.

Watson J: *Nursing: human science and human care,* New York, 1985, Appleton-Century-Crofts.

Watson J et al: *A model of caring: an alternative health care model for nursing practice and research,* ANA Pub No NP-59-3M 8179 190, Kansas City, Mo, 1979, American Nurses Association.

White S: The expanded role for nurses, *Nurs* 77 7:90, 1977.

Wiedenbach E: *Clinical nursing: a helping art,* New York, 1964, Springer.

CHAPTER 2

Health and Illness

OBJECTIVES

Mastery of concepts in this chapter will enable the student to:

- Define the key terms listed.
- Discuss the definition of health and related concepts.
- Discuss the health-illness continuum, high-level wellness, agent-host-environment, health-belief, evolutionary-based, and health-promotion models.
- Describe health-promotion and illness-prevention activities.
- List and discuss the three levels of preventive care.
- List and explain four kinds of risk factors.
- Describe variables influencing health beliefs and practices.
- Describe variables influencing illness behavior.
- List and discuss the stages of illness behavior.
- Describe the impact of illness on the client and family.
- Discuss the nurse's role for the client in health and illness.

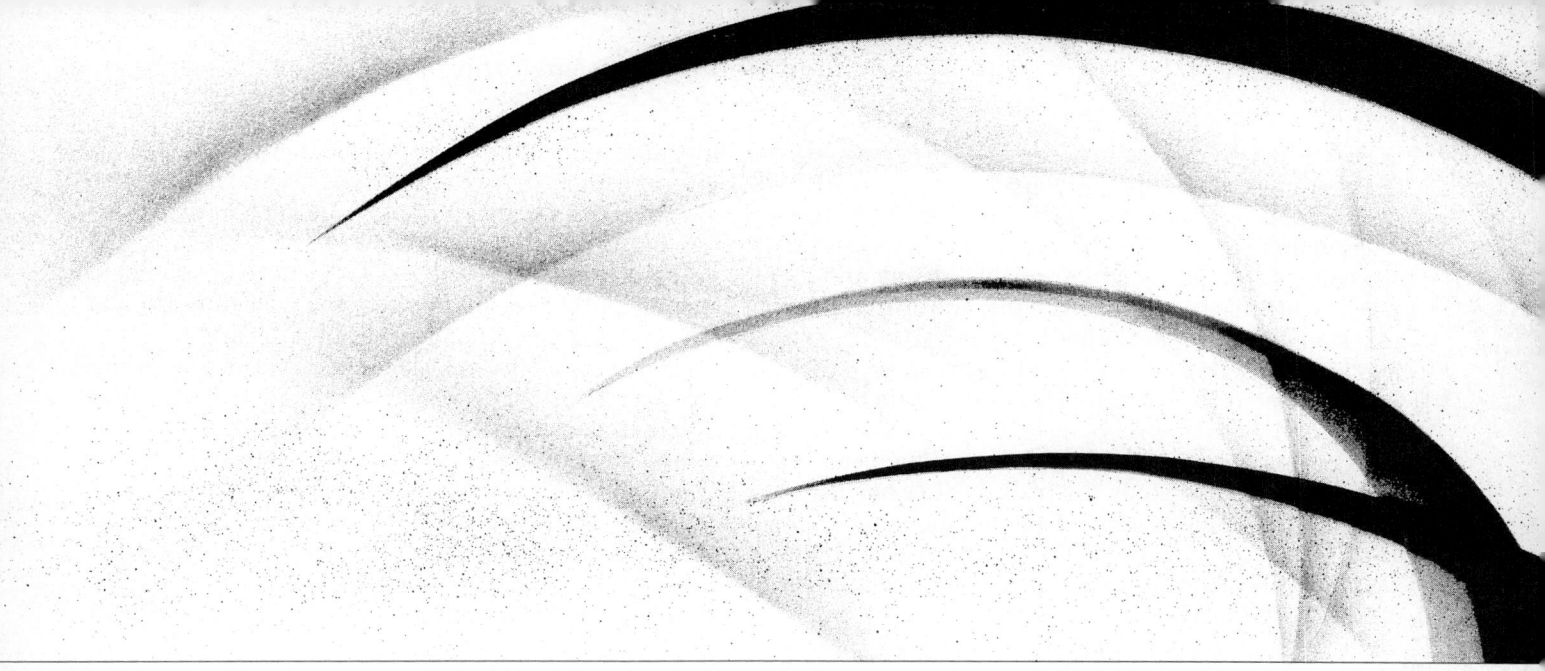

CHAPTER OUTLINE

Definition of Health

Models of Health and Illness

Health-illness continuum
High-level wellness model
Agent-host-environment model
Health-belief model
Evolutionary-based model
Health-promotion model

Variables Influencing Health Beliefs and Practices

Internal variables
External variables

Health Promotion and Illness Prevention

Levels of preventive care
Acute and chronic illness

Risk Factors

Genetic and physiological factors
Age
Environment
Lifestyle

Illness and Illness Behavior

Variables influencing illness behavior
Stages of illness behavior

Impact of Illness on Client and Family

Behavioral and emotional changes
Impact on family roles
Impact on body image
Impact on self-concept
Impact on family dynamics

In the past, most individuals and societies have viewed good health or wellness as the opposite or absence of disease. This attitude toward health remains popular with many health professionals. It assumes that people are normally healthy and that people with disease are unhealthy and in an abnormal state. This simple, either-or attitude can be easily applied; a person is considered healthy or ill, with no range in between. Nevertheless, this attitude ignores states of health between disease and good health. Also, it emphasizes the physiological dimension of a person, considering only the body as ill or healthy. In addition, this limited view overlooks the complex interrelationships between the physiological, emotional, intellectual, sociocultural, developmental, and spiritual dimensions.

Since Nightingale's time, there has been an association between the practice of nursing and the concept of health (Tripp-Reimer, 1984). Today's health and medical care services are shaped largely by the way health professionals and consumers define *health* and *illness* (Weitzel, 1989; Balog, 1982).

Health care professionals' definitions serve as bases for determinations about the types and quality of health care services that should be provided. Not all health care professionals, however, agree on the definition of these concepts. Consumers of health care frequently view their health as an absence of disease, and the better people believe their health to be, the more active they are in maintaining those levels of health (Yarcheski, Mahon, 1989; Weitzel, 1989).

However, the definition of good health or wellness from a health care worker's perspective may not always correspond with a client's concept. Each client's concept of health and health care practices is unique and based on lifestyle, cultural background, spiritual beliefs, and economic and psychosocial status. Therefore to provide individualized care for the client, the nurse needs to be aware of variables influencing health beliefs and practices.

People also have different attitudes about illness and react to it in different ways. Medical sociologists call the reaction to illness, *illness behavior.* The nurse needs to understand the way that clients react to illness and the way that illness affects clients and families. Illness can have an enormous impact on them. The nurse who recognizes this impact and the factors involved can take steps to minimize the effects of illness and assist the client and family in maintaining or returning to the highest level of functioning.

The nurse also identifies actual and potential risk factors that predispose a person or group of people to illness. Risk factors are genetic, behavioral, environ-

mental, gender, and age-related items that predispose an individual to an increased risk for disease. Types of risk factors are discussed later in this chapter. Nursing actions involving health promotion and illness prevention assist the client not only in maintaining and increasing the existing level of health but also in achieving an optimal level of health.

The nurse assesses all dimensions of the whole person, including the physical, intellectual, emotional, developmental, and spiritual aspects. The nurse also observes interactions with family and community. To best assist the client in health maintenance and promotion, illness prevention, and adaptation to the changes that illness produces in every dimension of functioning, the nurse must understand all these dimensions (Edelman, Mandle, 1990).

 ## DEFINITION OF HEALTH

Good **health** or wellness is not merely the absence of **illness.** Defining good health is difficult because each person has a personal concept of health. Health is not an acquired piece of scientific knowledge; nor is it a thing, a part of the body, or a function of the body such as hearing, seeing, or breathing. Health is a state of being that people define in relation to their own values.

No current definition of health is acceptable to all health care workers. The World Health Organization (WHO) defines health as a "state of complete physical, mental and social well-being, not merely the absence of disease or infirmity" (WHO, 1947). Yet this definition of health has not been universally accepted. Those opposed to it believe that it is unrealistic because people from underdeveloped countries and many persons of low economic status would not be considered healthy (Fuchs, 1974). In addition, the WHO definition is difficult to use when trying to scientifically determine who is or is not healthy or to determine the point at which a person becomes ill rather than healthy (Breslow, 1972).

The WHO definition, however, has the following characteristics that promote a more positive concept of health (Edelman, Mandle, 1990):

1. A concern for the individual as a total system
2. A view of health that identifies internal and external environments
3. An acknowledgment of the importance of an individual's role in life

Another issue related to defining health is the unique attitude of each client toward health, which involves much more than the absence of illness or disability. To help clients identify and reach health goals, the nurse must discover and use information about their concepts of health. As a result, health goals may be different for each client.

Nurses also differ on their definitions of health. They plan care based on a definition of health and accepted standards of health care. Neuman's system model (1989, 1990) focused on health as the totality of life processes, and disease was included as a process. In addition, health is measured on a graded scale or continuum (see Chapter 1).

Health in its broadest sense is a dynamic state in which the individual adapts to changes in internal and external environments to maintain a state of well-being. The internal environment includes many factors that influence health, including genetic and psychological variables, intellectual and spiritual dimensions, and disease processes. The external environment includes factors outside the person that may influence health, including the physical environment, social relationships, and economic variables. Because both environments continuously change, the person must adapt to maintain a state of well-being.

Health and *illness* therefore must be defined in terms of the individual. Health can include conditions that the client or nurse may have previously considered to be illness. For example, a person with epilepsy who has learned to control seizures with medication and who functions at home and at work may now not consider himself ill. Health is also closely related to an individual's lifestyle, and some illnesses can be considered to be the result of that lifestyle. A client who experiences constant stress may have frequent gastrointestinal upsets. In such a case, treating the condition may have no effect on the pattern of behavior, and the person may not even consider a gastrointestinal upset an illness at all if it seems a "normal" or usual aspect of life. A health professional's rigid attitude toward health and illness, in which the whole person is not considered, may have little meaning for such a person's future health.

Therefore because the attitudes of client and nurse toward health may not coincide exactly, the nurse uses the nursing process as a tool to work with the client and family to mutually establish goals of care and plan individualized care.

MODELS OF HEALTH AND ILLNESS

A model is a theoretical way of understanding a concept or idea. Because health and illness are complex concepts, models are used to understand the relationships between these concepts and the client's attitudes toward health and health practices.

Health beliefs are a person's ideas, convictions, and attitudes about health and illness. Health beliefs may be based on factual information or misinformation, common sense or myths, or reality or false expectations. Because **health behaviors** usually result from health beliefs, they can positively or negatively affect health. Positive health behaviors are activities related to maintaining, attaining, or regaining good health and preventing illness. Common positive health behaviors include immunizations, proper sleep patterns, and adequate exercise, diet, and nutrition. Negative health behaviors include practices actually or potentially harmful to health, such as smoking, drug or alcohol abuse, poor diet, and refusal to take necessary medications.

Nurses have developed health models to understand clients' health behaviors and beliefs so that effective health care can be provided. These models allow nurses to understand and predict clients' health behaviors, including how they use health services and adhere to recommended therapies.

A client's health beliefs depend on many factors, including perception of the level of health, modifying factors such as demographics, personality, and perception of benefits resulting from positive health behaviors. Health models usually incorporate these components.

The health-illness continuum, the high-level wellness, and agent-host-environment models describe the relationships between health and illness. The health-belief model explains and predicts a client's health behavior; the evolutionary-based and health-promotion models were developed by nurses and focus on health promotion. These models are not meant to conflict theories but represent ways of approaching complex issues and understanding clients' attitudes toward health and illness differ.

Health-Illness Continuum

According to Neuman (1990), "health on a continuum is the degree of client wellness that exists at any point in time, ranging from an optimal wellness condition, with available energy at its maximum, to death, which represents total energy depletion." According to this **health-illness continuum** model, health is a dynamic state that continuously alters as a person adapts to changes in the internal and external environments to maintain a state of physical, emotional, intellectual, social, developmental, and spiritual well-being. Illness is a process in which the functioning of a person is diminished or impaired in one or more dimensions, when compared with the person's previous condition. Because health and illness are relative qualities, existing in varying degrees, it is more accurate to consider

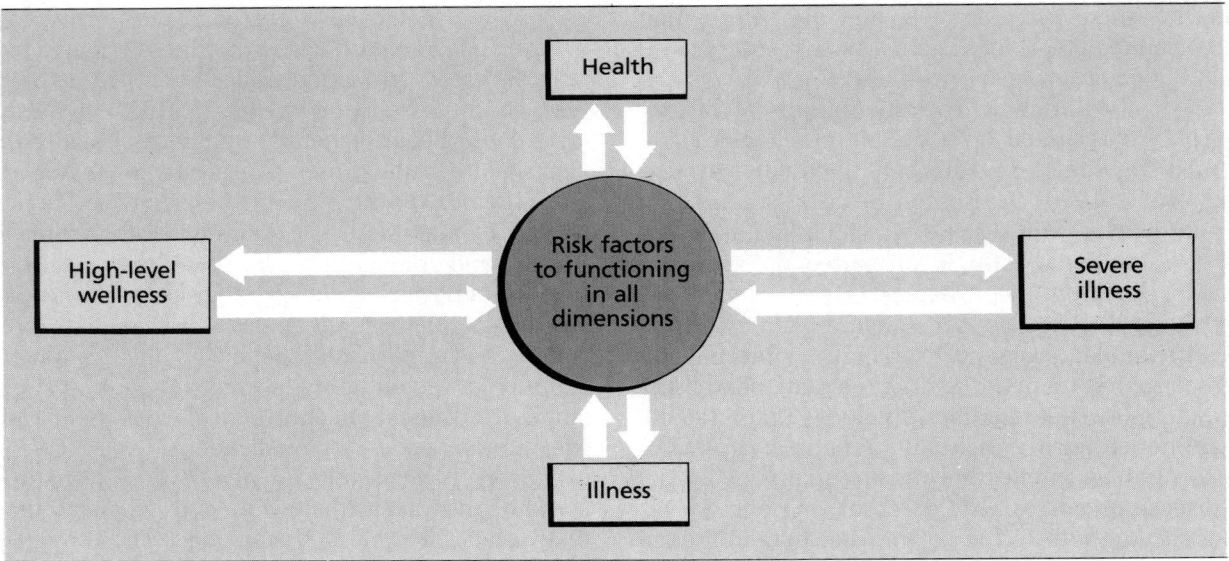

Fig. 2-1   The health-illness continuum, ranging from high-level wellness to severe illness, provides a method of identifying a client's level of health. Level of health is a reflection of the client's level of functioning in all dimensions.

health and illness in terms of a point on a scale or continuum rather than an either-or, absolute state (Fig. 2-1).

The literature supports the view that health and the attainment of it is a central concept and a goal of nursing practice (Meleis, 1990; Pender, 1975, 1986, 1987, 1990; Parse, 1981, 1990; Neuman, 1989, 1990). A nurse can determine a client's level of health at any point on the health-illness continuum. High-level wellness and severe illness are the opposite ends of the continuum, with a full range of states in between. A client's risk factors (variables that make illness more likely in any dimension) are important in identifying level of health. Risk factors include genetic and physiological variables such as age, lifestyle, and environment (see later sections). As a person progresses through the developmental stages, certain risk factors are more common than others. An adolescent, for example, is more likely than an adult to experience stressors related to body image and self-concept, and an older adult is more likely than a child to develop cardiac illness.

The way clients view their levels of health depends on their attitudes toward health and their values, beliefs, and perceptions of their physical, emotional, intellectual, social, developmental, and spiritual well-being. To help clients set goals to reach an optimal level of health, the nurse helps them identify their positions on the health-illness continuum (Meleis, 1990).

The drawback of the health-illness continuum is that it is not always easy to describe a client's level of health in terms of one point between two extremes. For example, is a man who has a broken leg but who has adapted to limited mobility more or less healthy than a physically healthy man experiencing severe depression after the death of his spouse? The model is effective when it is used to compare a client's present level of health with previous levels of health. Subsequently it is useful as the nurse helps the client set goals to attain a future level of health.

High-Level Wellness Model

First developed in the late 1950s and revised by Dunn (1977), the high-level wellness model is oriented toward maximizing the health potential of an individual. This model requires the individual to maintain a continuum of balance and purposeful direction within the environment. It involves progress toward a higher level of functioning, an open-ended and ever-expanding challenge to live at the fullest potential. Last, there is continued integration of health practices by the individual at increasingly higher levels throughout life (Dunn, 1959, 1977; Pender, 1987).

Nursing models of wellness are directed at behavioral change and have been successful in nurse-managed centers for older adults (Gilpatrick, 1989; Smith, Sorrell, 1989). In the behavioral change approach to wellness, nurses implement nursing interventions that help clients modify selected high-risk behaviors. These interventions are in broad categories and are based on principles of adult learning (Gilpatrick, 1989).

Health care directed at helping a client achieve high-level wellness emphasizes health-promotion and illness-prevention activities rather than treatment for illness. Such were the goals in the successfully nurse-managed Stay Well Center for older adults (Smith, Sorrell, 1989). High-level wellness is a dynamic process, not a passive, static state.

The high-level wellness model can also be applied to family and community health. Families and communities have many functions, and high-level wellness involves successful functioning in an integrated manner.

Agent-Host-Environment Model

The agent-host-environment model of health and illness originated in the community health work of Leavell et al (1965) and has since been expanded as a model for describing the cause of illness in other health areas. According to this approach, the level of health or illness of an individual or group depends on the dynamic relationship of the agent, host, and environment.

The **agent** is any internal or external factor that by its presence or absence can lead to disease or illness. Agents can be biological, chemical, physical, mechanical, or psychosocial. The presence of these agents does not mean a person will become ill, but an agent must be present (or absent, as in a lack of adequate nutrition) for a particular illness to occur.

The **host** is the person or persons who may be susceptible to a particular illness or disease. Host factors are physical or psychosocial situations or conditions putting an individual or group at risk for becoming ill. Examples of such factors are the host's family history, age, or lifestyle.

The **environment** consists of all factors outside of the host. Physical environment includes economic level, climate, living conditions, and elements such as light and sound levels. Social environment consists of factors involving a person's or group's interaction with others, including stress, conflicts with others, economic hardships, and life crises such as the death of a spouse.

The agent-host-environment model emphasizes that health and illness depend on the dynamic interaction of all three variables. Community health nursing has further developed the interaction between agent-host-environment into a causal model for addressing the health needs for homeless families (Fig 2-2). This model, first developed by Pesznecker (1984) and recently reported by Berne et al (1990), proposes that health-promoting or health-damaging responses are shaped by interaction between the individual or group and the environment and that the responses are further mediated by public policy. For example, homeless persons are faced with a variety of stressors or agents that can affect their levels of health; exposure to inadequate shelter, crime, and exposure to nature's elements increase the homeless client's risk for illness.

The agent-host-environment model has been expanded into a general theory of the multiple causes of disease. Until recent decades, it was commonly believed that single causes of a disease could be identified. Infectious diseases in particular were thought to have single causes; the agents (for example the bacteria or viruses) were considered solely responsible. It is now recognized that most diseases have multiple causes, as the agent-host-environment model demonstrates. The theory of the multiple causes of disease is important to nurses because nursing emphasizes holistic care of the client, which is based on knowledge of environmental, psychosocial, and lifestyle factors.

Health-Belief Model

Rosenstoch's (1974) and Becker and Maiman's (1975) **health-belief model** (Fig. 2-3) addresses the relationship between a person's belief and behaviors. It provides a way of understanding and predicting how clients will behave in relation to their health and how they will comply with health care therapies (see Chapter 16).

The first component in this model involves the individual's perception of susceptibility to an illness. For example, a client needs to recognize the familial link for coronary artery disease. After this link is recognized, particularly when one parent and two siblings have died in their fourth decade from myocardial infarction, the client may perceive the personal risk of heart disease. The second component is the individual's perception of the seriousness of the illness. This perception is influenced and modified by demographic and sociopsychological variables, perceived threats of the illness, and cues to action (for example, mass media campaigns and advice from family, friends, and medical professionals).

The third component—the likelihood that a person will take preventive action—is the person's perception of the benefits of taking action. Preventive action may include lifestyle changes, increased adherence to medical therapies, or a search for medical advice or treatment.

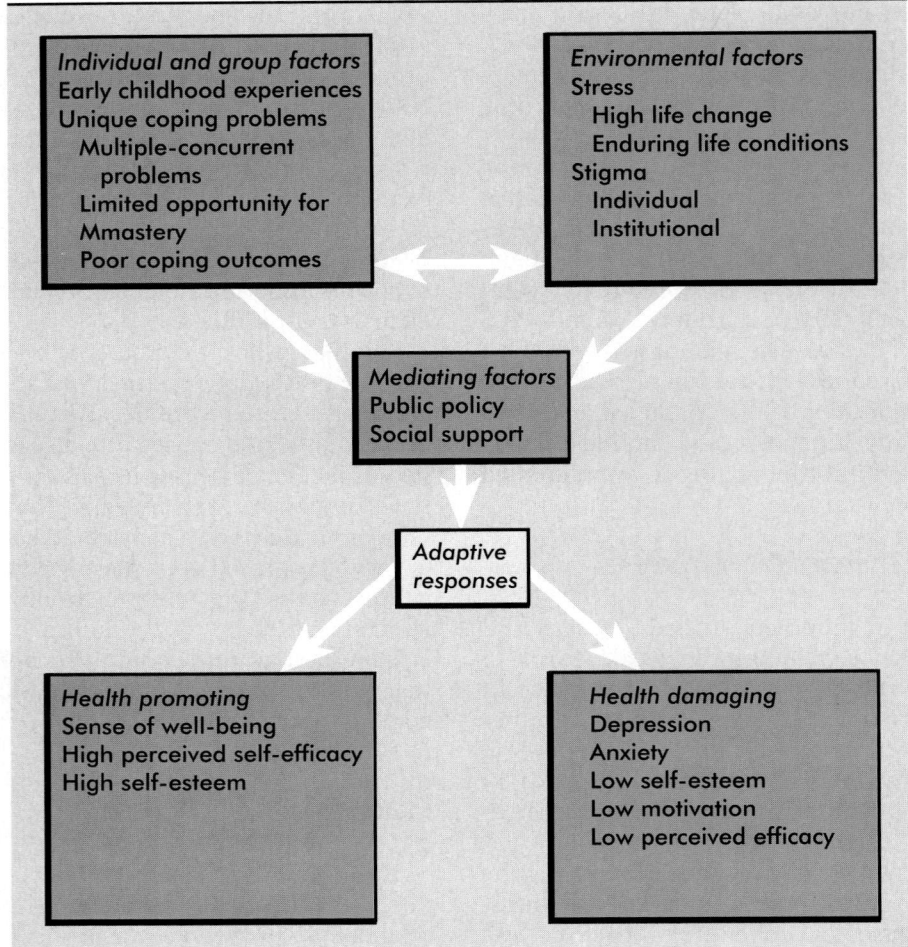

Fig. 2-2 Adaptational model of poverty.
Adapted from Pesznecker BL: *Public Health Nurs* 1(4):237, 1984.

The health-belief model helps nurses understand factors influencing clients' perceptions, beliefs, and behavior and plan care that will most effectively assist clients in maintaining or regaining health and preventing illness. A research study by Prewitt (1989) investigated the correlation between health beliefs and preventive health behaviors and educational materials dealing with acquired immunodeficiency syndrome (AIDS) (see research highlight).

Evolutionary-Based Model

The evolutionary-based model of health and viability is supported by the principle that illness and death sometime serve an evolutionary function (Dixon, Dixon, 1984). The model (Fig. 2-4) interrelates the following elements:

1. Life events, which reflect developmental variables and variables associated with chance, such as accidents or relocation
2. Life-style determinants, which are personal and learned adaptive strategies that an individual uses to make lifestyle changes
3. Evolutionary viability within the social context, which reflects the extent to which individuals function to promote survival and well-being (Dixon, Dixon, 1984)
4. Control perceptions, which reflect the extent to which a person can influence the circumstances of life
5. Viability emotions, which are "affective reactions" developed from life events or lifestyle determinants
6. Health outcomes, which are the physiological, behavioral, and psychological states resulting

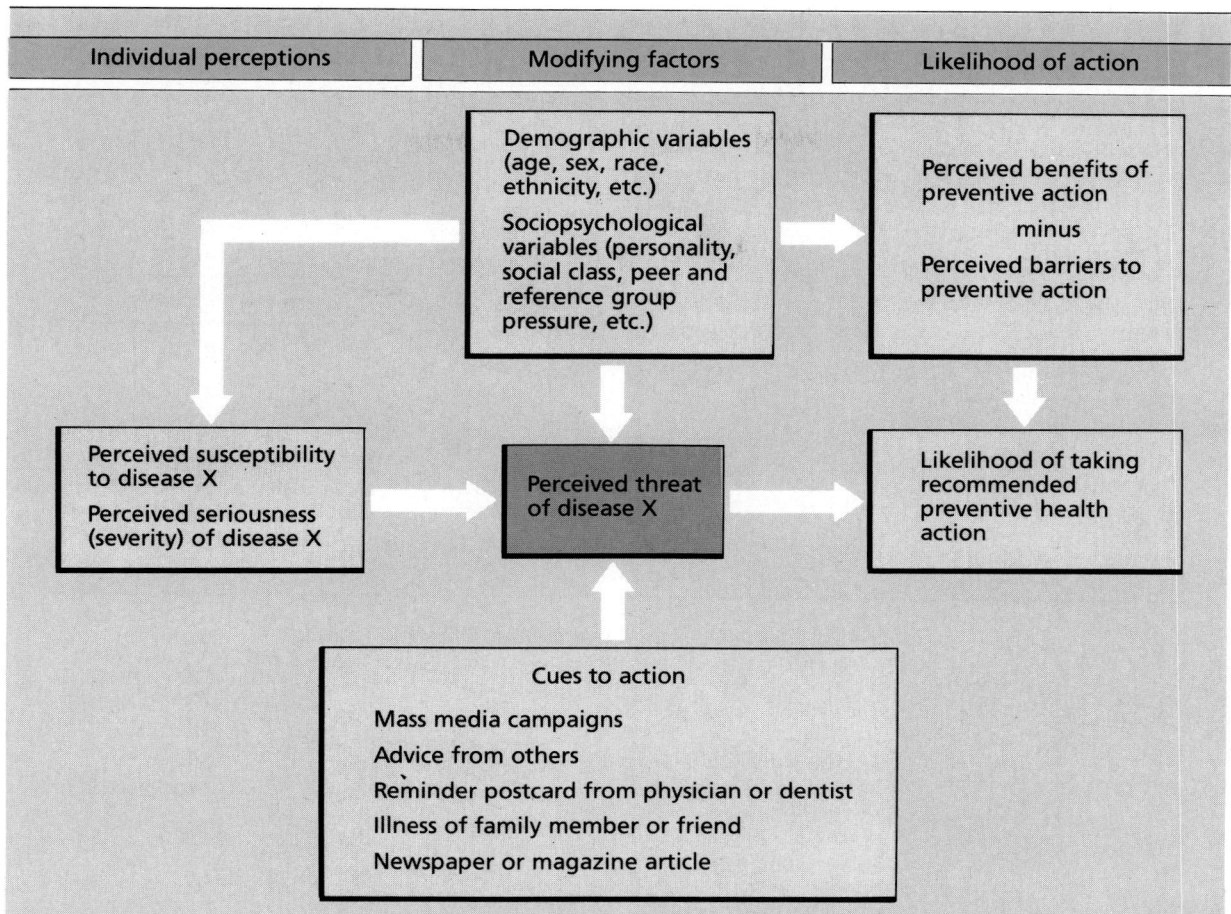

Fig. 2-3   Health belief model.
From Becker MH, Maiman LA: *Med Care* 13(1):12, 1975.

Research Highlight

One of the most explosive health threats of the 1990s is the AIDS epidemic; professional and trade literature describe this syndrome as one of America's most urgent medical problems. The research objective of Prewitt's was to identify the effectiveness of the educational materials for AIDS and the correlation between health beliefs and preventive health behavior. The researcher reviewed English-language educational pamphlets targeting African Americans, intravenous drug users, homosexual and heterosexual men and women, college students, and teenagers. These pamphlets were ob-

tained from a wide geographical selection. There was a high correlation between the content of the pamphlet and the health-belief model. The messages in the educational material focused on susceptibility; if the individual perceives a risk, then a behavior is modified. There was a correlation between the content of the pamphlet and the preventive health behavior. Thus the researcher was able to conclude that the perceived threat to health provided a reason for changing behavior in the case of AIDS prevention.

Prewitt VR: Health beliefs and AIDS educational materials, *Fam Community Health* 12:65, 1989.

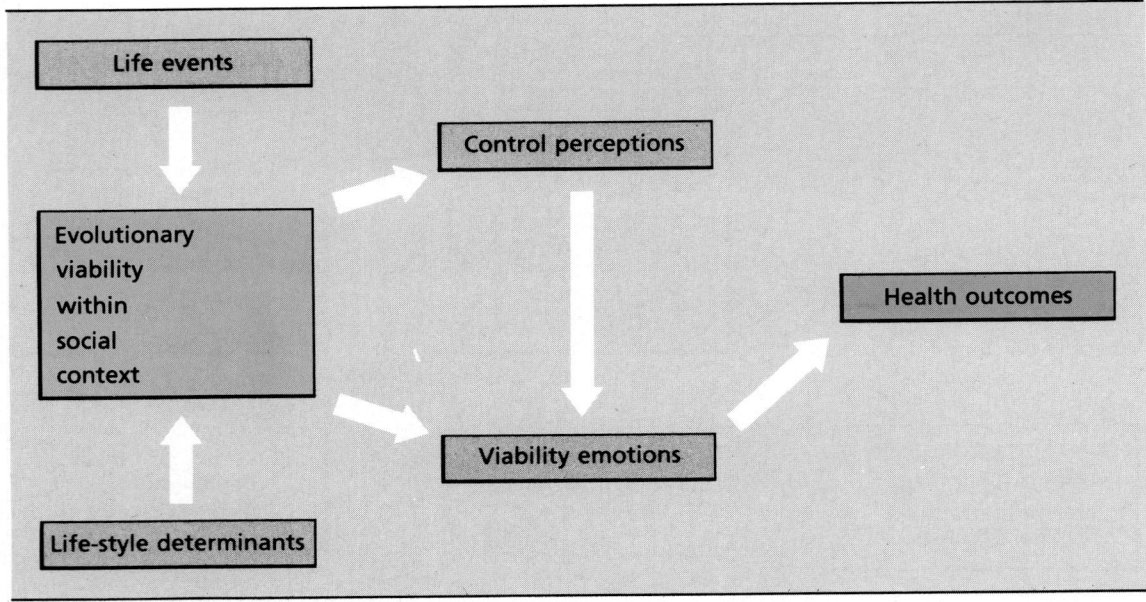

Fig. 2-4   Evolutionary-based model of viability and health.
Redrawn from Dixon JK, Dixon JP: *ANS* 6(3):1, 1984.

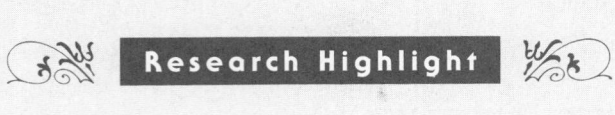

Pender's health-promotion model was tested with 179 blue-collar workers. The most powerful predictors of health-promotion behaviors were perceptions of health status and self-efficacy. Thus the better that persons perceive their health, the more likely that they will act in ways to maintain it. In addition, believing in the ability to accomplish a behavior (for example, increasing exercise and decreasing fat intake) acts as a motivation to perform that behavior. This study suggested that blue-collar workers were interested and involved in health promotion and work-site health-promotion programs would benefit workers and employers in reducing absenteeism related to illness.

Weitzel MH: A test of the health-promotion model with blue-collar workers, *Nurs Res* 38:99, 1989.

from viability emotions and the other factors within the model

With this model, nursing interventions can be developed for all six client dimensions. The full scope of clinical experience may require assisting clients to regain a sense of viability. This is particularly important in nursing because of the opportunity for long-term contact with the client and family (Dixon, Dixon, 1984).

Health-Promotion Model

The health-promotion model proposed by Pender (1982, 1984) was designed to be a "complimentary counterpart to models of health protection." Health promotion is directed at increasing a client's level of well-being (Pender, 1987). The model focuses on three functions (Fig. 2-5). It identifies factors (for example, demographic and social) that enhance or decrease participation in health promotion. The model also organizes cues into a pattern to explain the likelihood of a client's participation in health-promotion behaviors (Pender, 1987). The focus of this model is to explain the reasons that individuals engage in health activities. It is not designed for use with families or communities. This model has been tested with a variety of populations because it is a reliable indicator of health promotion (see research highlight).

■ VARIABLES INFLUENCING HEALTH BELIEFS AND PRACTICES

Nurses need to understand the variables that can influence clients' health beliefs and practices. Internal and external variables can influence how a person thinks and acts. Understanding the way in

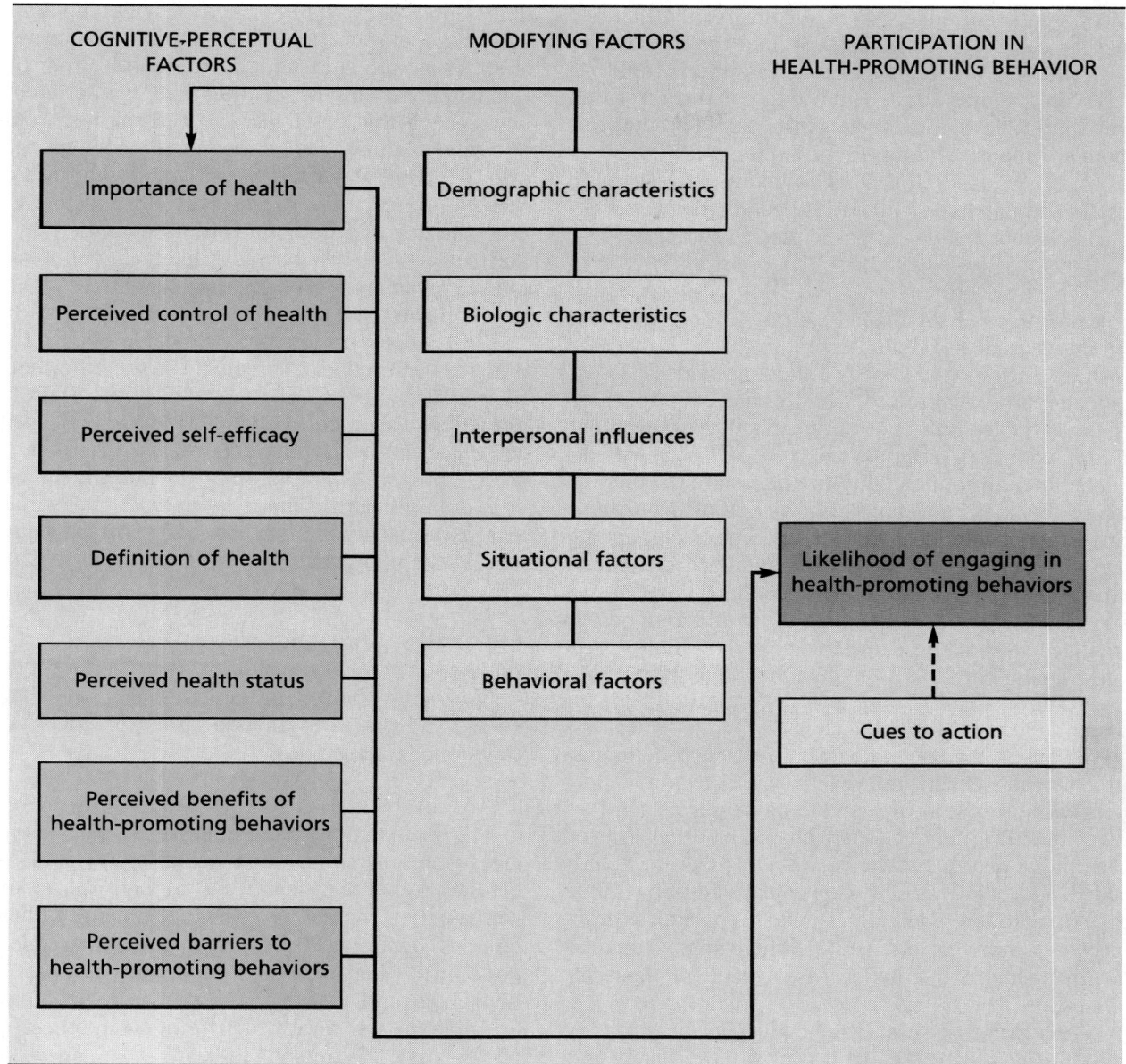

Fig. 2-5 Health promotion model.
From Pender NJ: *Health promotion in nursing practice,* ed 2, Norwalk, Conn, 1987, Appleton & Lange.

which these variables affect a client allows the nurse to plan and deliver individualized care for that client.

Internal Variables

Internal variables include a person's developmental stage, intellectual background, perception of personal functioning, and emotional and spiritual factors.

Developmental Stage

A person's thought and behavior patterns change throughout life. The nurse must consider level of growth and development when using the client's health beliefs and practices as a basis for planning care. For example, a young child is not generally able to recognize the potential seriousness of illnesses and needs to be motivated to act in ways beneficial to a treatment plan or to develop habits for illness prevention. An adolescent's emotional development may influence personal beliefs about health-related matters such as the use of contraception, and the nurse thus uses different techniques of teaching than would be used for a young adult. Knowledge of the stages of growth and development helps the nurse predict the client's response to the present illness or the threat of future illness (see Unit 5). The planning of nursing care is then adapted to these expectations, as well as to the client's abilities to participate in self-care.

Intellectual Background

A person's beliefs about health are shaped in part by intellectual variables, including knowledge (or misinformation) about body functions and illnesses, educational background, and past experiences. These variables influence a person's thoughts. In addition, cognitive abilities shape the *way* a person thinks, including the ability to understand factors involved in illness and apply knowledge of health and illness to personal health practices. Cognitive abilities also relate to a person's developmental stage. A nurse considers intellectual background when trying to understand a client's beliefs about health and health practices so that these variables can be incorporated into nursing care.

Perception of Functioning

The way a person perceives physical functioning affects health beliefs and practices. For example, persons with chronic heart conditions perceive their levels of health differently than people who have never had major health problems. As a result, the health beliefs and practices of these people tend to be different. In addition, individuals who have successfully recovered from severe acute illnesses may change health beliefs and practices as a result of those illnesses.

When nurses assess a client's level of health, they gather subjective data about the way the client perceives physical functioning, such as level of fatigue, shortness of breath, or pain. They also obtain objective data about actual functioning such as blood pressure and height measurements and lung sound assessment. This information allows nurses to more successfully plan and implement individualized care.

Emotional and Spiritual Factors

Emotional and spiritual factors also influence health beliefs and practices. A person experiencing a stress response with each change in life tends to respond to any sign of illness (see Chapters 30 and 33), such as worrying that the illness is life threatening. A person who generally is very calm may have little emotional response during illness, whereas an individual unable to cope emotionally with the threat of

illness may deny the presence of symptoms and not take therapeutic actions. For example, a man who is short of breath and coughs frequently may blame this condition on cold weather if he cannot emotionally accept the possibility of a respiratory illness. Many people have strong emotional reactions against even thinking about the risk of cancer and will deny symptoms and refuse to take preventive action. Other illnesses are more emotionally acceptable, however, and the person will be more likely to acknowledge the symptoms and seek appropriate care.

If religious beliefs include the belief that physical health is necessary for spiritual health, clients' health practices will reflect that belief. On the other hand, if their religious beliefs require refusal of certain kinds of medical treatment, health care may be avoided. In some cases, clients may believe that illness is a deserved punishment and thus do nothing to regain or maintain health. Thus as with emotional variables, a nurse must understand clients' spiritual values to involve them effectively in nursing care (see Chapter 33).

External Variables

External variables influencing a person's health beliefs and practices include family practices, socioeconomic factors, and cultural variables.

Family Practices

The way that clients' families use health care services generally affects their health practices. Healthy families generally seek ways to help all members achieve their highest potential . Flexibility in healthy families encourages members to change role resposibilities. For example, men can assume some household and child-care responsibilities. Members are able to temporarily perform each others tasks (deChesnay, Magnuson, 1988).

If a child's parents treated every virus and illness as a potentially severe disease and immediately sought health care, the child generally does the same in adulthood. A person with this type of family background would be more likely to stay home from school or work with a cold, whereas others would attempt to carry on as usual. Likewise, the adult clients are also more likely to practice prevention if their families did so. For example, people whose parents took them for annual checkups as children are more likely to take their own children for regular checkups.

Socioeconomic Factors

Social and psychosocial factors can increase the risk for illness and influence the way that a person defines and reacts to illness. Psychosocial variables include the stability of the person's marital or intimate relationship, lifestyle habits, and occupational environment.

A person's social network is also related to health behavior (Steele, 1982; Parsons, 1958). Neighbors, peers, and co-workers are usually aware of a person's level of health, and if the person is unexpectedly absent from work or a planned activity or is experiencing a symptom of illness, a member of the social network may encourage medical attention. A person generally seeks approval and support from social groups, and this desire for approval and support affects health beliefs and practices. For example, if it is socially acceptable in a particular peer group for teenage girls to smoke, the pressure to conform may be stronger than the concern about smoking being harmful to health.

Social variables partly determine how the health care delivery system provides medical care. Because the health care system is organized in certain ways, it determines how clients can obtain care. The system provides care for clients with health problems that society considers "legitimate" and "acceptable." In addition, the system defines the treatment method, the economic cost to the client, and potential reimbursement to the health care agency or client. The health care system is a complex structure on which clients depend for care. Chapter 3 describes this system in detail.

Economic factors, like social factors, can affect a client's level of health by increasing the risk for disease, by influencing how or at what point the client enters the health care system, or by limiting compliance with a prescribed treatment plan.

Epidemiological studies have shown that persons at low economic levels have a greater risk for pulmonary disease, cancer, and diabetes mellitus than persons at higher levels (Goldsmith, 1975; Davidson, 1971). In addition, a large number of people at low economic levels live in urban areas and therefore have a greater risk for disease because of their environment.

Economic factors also influence the way a client enters the health care system. A worker who has health insurance is more likely to seek care and treatment for a chronic cough than an individual who is out of work and has no insurance.

A person's compliance with the treatment that is designed to maintain or improve health is also affected by economic status. A person who has high utility bills, a large family, and a low income tends to give a higher priority to food and shelter than to costly drugs or treatment or expensive foods for special diets.

Cultural Background

Cultural background influences individual beliefs, values, and customs. It influences entry into the health care system and personal health practices. For example, a study of health education practices for African Americans showed that most individuals did not have access to health education as a means for primary prevention (Airhihenbuwa, 1989).

Sociocultural differences between clients and nurses can affect the nurse-client relationship and the quality of nursing care delivered (Anderson, 1987). If nurses are not aware of their own and other cultural patterns of behavior and language, they may not be able to recognize and understand a client's behavior and beliefs and may have difficulty with interacting with the client. For example, a client from a culture that strongly values and expects close, warm, and supportive family relationships may experience cultural conflict with a nurse who does not value or has not experienced close kinship ties (Leininger, 1977). The nurse must identify and incorporate cultural factors into a client's care plan to avoid conflict between goals and methods of care and the client's cultural background (see Chapter 4).

◼ HEALTH PROMOTION AND ILLNESS PREVENTION

Nurses emphasize health promotion and illness-prevention activities as important forms of health care. Nurses assist clients in maintaining good health and improving their levels of health instead of merely providing care after illness occurs. Health promotion and illness prevention are closely related concepts and, in practice, overlap to some extent. Activities involving **health promotion** help clients maintain or enhance their present levels of health. Activities for **illness prevention** protect clients from actual or potential threats to health. Both types of activities are future oriented. The difference between them involves motivations and goals. Health-promotion activities motivate people to act positively to reach the goals of more stable levels of health. Illness-prevention activities motivate people to avoid declines in health or functional levels.

Health-promotion activities can be passive or active. With **passive strategies of health promotion,** individuals gain from the activities of others without doing anything themselves. The fluoridation of municipal drinking water and the fortification of homogenized milk with vitamin D are two examples of passive health-promotion strategies.

With **active strategies of health promotion,** individuals are motivated to adopt specific health programs. Weight reduction and smoking cessation programs require clients to be actively involved in measures to improve their present and future levels of wellness while decreasing the risk of disease.

Health-promotion and illness-prevention activities have become an important focus of health care. Although scientific and medical advances since the 1940s have resulted in cures for many infectious diseases, there are still no cures for many chronic diseases. Thus there is greater motivation for preventing the occurrence of these diseases. In addition, the rapid rise of health care costs has motivated consumers to seek ways of decreasing the incidence and minimizing the results of illness or disability. Last, society as a whole has become increasingly conscious of health and the value of maintaining or increasing the level of health.

Pender (1987) has developed the Lifestyle and Health Habits Assessment (LHHA), which is divided into 10 sections (see box). The assessment tool uses *yes* and *no* responses. The rating in each section, as well as the total score, provides the information necessary to design an individualized health-protection and health-promotion program for the client. Use of the LHHA may increase the client's awareness of living patterns and assist in motivating behavior changes (Pender, 1987).

The LHHA provided a starting point for the Health-Promoting Lifestyle Profile (HPLP) (Walker, Sechrist, Pender, 1987). This instrument focuses on health-promotion behaviors and is being, the research findings validate (see research highlight).

The HPLP focuses on health-promoting behaviors. Health-damaging behaviors (for example, smoking and alcohol) did not conceptually fit with health-promotion activities and were deleted from the profile, further supporting the idea that health promotion and illness prevention are different activities (Pender, 1987).

The goal of a total health program is to improve a client's level of well-being in all dimensions, not just physical health. Total programs are based on the belief that many factors can affect level of health. Health can be influenced by individual practices such as poor eating habits and little or no exercise. It can also be affected by physical stressors, a poor living environment, exposure to air pollutants, and an unsafe environment. Psychological stressors and hereditary factors can also influence level of health. Total health-promotion programs are directed at changing lifestyle by developing habits that can improve level of health. The following categories are identified as important determinants of health status (Edelman, Mandle, 1990):

1. Smoking
2. Nutrition
3. Alcohol use
4. Habituating drug use
5. Driving
6. Exercise
7. Sexuality and contraceptive or barrier use
8. Family relationships
9. Risk-factor modification
10. Coping and adaptation

Other programs are aimed at specific health care problems. For example, the American Lung Association has developed smoking cessation clinics that include group support (Fig. 2-6). Exercise programs

---

Categories of Lifestyle and Health Habits Assessment*

- General competencies of self-care
- Nutritional practices
- Physical or recreational activities
- Sleep patterns
- Stress management
- Self-actualization
- Sense of purpose
- Relationships with others
- Environmental control
- Use of health care system

*The complete LHHA and the rating scale are described in detail in Pender NJ: *Health promotion in nursing practice*, ed 2, Norwalk, Conn, 1987, Appleton & Lange.

 **Research Highlight**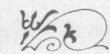

Walker, Sechrist, and Pender developed an instrument focusing on health-promotion behaviors. The 48-item HPLP was used with 952 adults and was evaluated and statistically analyzed. As a result, each of the 48 items on the inventory was placed into one of the following categories: self-actualization, health responsibility, exercise, nutrition, interpersonal support, and stress management. The researchers noted that their results were similar to other findings on health practice and high-level wellness. These data help support the validity of the HPLP for health-promotion behaviors.

Walker SN, Sechrist KR, Pender NJ: The health-promoting life-style profile: development and psychometric characteristics, *Nurs Res* 36:76, 1987.

encourage participants to regularly schedule exercise. Stress-reduction programs teach participants to cope with stressors.

Some health-promotion and-illness prevention programs are operated by health care agencies. Others are independently operated. Many corporations have developed health-promotion activities for employees. Likewise, colleges and community centers offer health-promotion and illness-prevention programs. Nurses may be actively involved in these programs or may serve as consultants or give referrals. The goal of these activities is to improve level of health through preventive health services, environmental protection, and health education.

Health-promotion and illness-prevention activities are important to the consumer and the health care provider. Whether an activity uses the active or passive strategy, the goal is to maintain or improve the level of physical, emotional, intellectual, social, developmental, and spiritual well-being. Although activities are often organized in specific programs, nurses in all areas of practice often have opportunities to assist clients in adopting activities to promote health and decrease risks of illness.

Levels of Preventive Care

Nursing care oriented to health promotion and illness prevention can be understood in terms of health activities on the primary, secondary, and tertiary levels (Table 2-1).

Primary Prevention

Primary prevention is true prevention; it precedes disease or dysfunction and is applied to clients considered physically and emotionally healthy. It is not

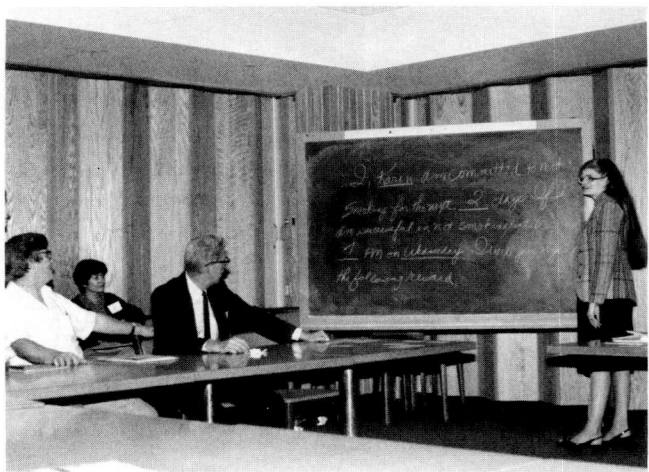

Fig. 2-6 The American Lung Association has developed client-centered smoking cessation clinics that include group support.
Courtesy American Lung Association of Eastern Missouri.

TABLE 2-1   The Three Levels of Prevention

Primary Prevention		Secondary Prevention		Tertiary Prevention
Health Promotion	Specific Protection	Early Diagnosis and Prompt Treatment	Disability Limitations	Restoration and Rehabilitation
Health education Good standard of nutrition adjusted to developmental phases of life Attention to personality development Provision of adequate housing and recreation and agreeable working conditions Marriage counseling and sex education Genetic screening Periodic selective examinations	Use of specific immunizations Attention to personal hygiene Use of environmental sanitation Protection against occupational hazards Protection from accidents Use of specific nutrients Protection from carcinogens Avoidance of allergens	Case-finding measures: individual and mass Screening surveys Selective examinations Cure and prevention of disease process to prevent spread of communicable disease, prevent complications, and shorten period of disability	Adequate treatment to arrest disease process and prevent further complications Provision of facilities to limit disability and prevent death	Provision of hospital and community facilities for retraining and education to maximize use of remaining capacities Education of the public and industries to use rehabilitated persons to the fullest possible extent Selective placement Work therapy in hospitals Use of sheltered colony

Modified from Leavell H, Clark AE: *Preventive medicine for doctors in the community,* New York, 1965, McGraw-Hill.

therapeutic, does not use therapeutic treatments, and does not involve symptom identification (Edelman, Mandle, 1990). Activities are directed at decreasing the probability of specific illnesses or dysfunctions. In addition, primary prevention includes health education programs, immunization, or physical and nutritional fitness activities. Primary prevention can be provided to an individual or to a general population, or it can focus on individuals at risk for developing specific diseases.

Secondary Prevention

Secondary prevention focuses on individuals who are experiencing health problems or illnesses and who are at risk for developing complications or worsening conditions. Activities are directed at diagnosis and prompt intervention, thereby reducing severity and enabling the client to return to normal health at the earliest possible point (Pender, 1987; Edelman, Mandle, 1990). A large portion of secondary level nursing care is delivered in the home, hospital, or skilled nursing facility to prevent complications. Secondary prevention includes screening techniques and treatment of early stages of disease to limit disability by averting or delaying the consequences of advanced disease.

Tertiary Prevention

Tertiary prevention occurs when a defect or disability is permanent and irreversible. It involves minimizing the effects of the disease or disability by interventions directed at preventing complication and deterioration (Edelman, Mandle, 1990). Activities are directed at rehabilitation rather than diagnosis and treatment (Pender, 1987). Care at this level aims to help clients achieve as high a level of functioning as possible, despite the limitations caused by illness or impaired functioning. This level of care is called *preventive care* because it involves prevention of further disability or reduced functioning. A nurse who provides tertiary care to a recently blinded client, for example, not only assists the client in adapting to the disability through activities such as teaching techniques to perform personal hygiene, but also directs attention to the goal of preventing future problems such as accidents in the home or potential problems with child rearing.

Acute and Chronic Illness

There are a variety of ways to classify illnesses and their impact on the clients. For the purposes of this chapter, two general classifications of illness are presented: acute and chronic illness.

Acute Illness

An **acute illness** is characterized by a relatively short duration of symptoms that are usually severe. The symptoms appear abruptly, are intense, and subside after a relatively short period. An episode of acute illness results in a state of recovery comparable to the client's previous level of wellness and activity. In some cases the acute episode results in death or passage into a chronic disease process.

Chronic Illness

A **chronic illness** lasts more than 3 months. Presently, 13% of the population report limitations caused by chronic illness. Also, there is a significant increase in chronic limitations experienced between the ages of 45 and 64; 25% to 30% of the population experience symptoms of chronic disease (Edelman, Mandle, 1990).

Because of this rise in chronicity, nurses are challenged to provide chronically ill clients with client-centered goals designed to optimize their levels of functioning and their ability to live with the illness (Cooper, 1990). In addition to planning interventions directed at the physical limitations of the illness, nurses must deal with the impact of chronic illness in all components of their clients' lives. Social supports and psychosocial resources are identified and individualized for the clients and families (Burckhardt, 1987; Leidy, 1990; Tilden, Weinert, 1987).

 ## RISK FACTORS

A **risk factor** is any situation, habit, environmental condition, physiological condition, or another variable that increases the vulnerability of an individual or group to an illness or accident. For example, a person whose father and paternal grandfather died of acute myocardial infarctions in their forties is at risk for coronary disease. Likewise, members of a community exposed to industrial air pollution are at risk for developing pulmonary disease. Risk factors include variables other than physical conditions. For example, a person who has experienced emotional stressors over a long period risks developing many kinds of illness.

The presence of risk factors does not mean that a disease state will develop, but risk factors increase the chances that the individual will experience a particular disease. Risk factors can occur in different aspects of a person's internal or external environment. Nurses and other health care professionals are concerned with them for several reasons. Risk factors play a major role in how a nurse identifies a client's health status. They can also influence health beliefs and practices if a person is aware of their presence. Identifying risk factors is also important for health-promotion and illness-prevention activities; such identificaton allows modification or elimination of the risk factors.

Risk factors can be placed in the following interrelated categories: genetic and physiological factors, age, physical environment, and lifestyle.

Genetic and Physiological Factors

Physiological risk factors involve the physical functioning of the body. Certain physical conditions, such as being pregnant or overweight, place increased stress on a person's physiological systems (for example, the circulatory system), increasing susceptibility to illness in these areas. Heredity, or genetic predisposition to specific illness, is a major physical risk factor. For example, a person with a family history of diabetes mellitus is at risk for developing the disease later in life. Other documented genetic risk factors include family histories of cancer, coronary disease, and renal disease.

Age

Age increases susceptibility to certain illnesses. For example, the risk of cardiovascular disease increases with age for both sexes. The risks of birth defects and complications of pregnancy increase after age 35. Many kinds of cancer pose a greater risk for persons over age 45 than for younger persons. Age risk factors are often closely associated with other risk factors such as family history and personal habits. For example, a man at age 60 who has smoked 40 years is at a greater risk for developing lung cancer than a man at age 30 who has smoked 10 years.

Environment

The physical environment in which a person works or lives can increase the likelihood that certain illnesses will occur. For example, some kinds of cancer and other diseases are more likely to develop when industrial workers are exposed to certain chemicals or when people live near toxic waste disposal sites. Screening for these environmentally based risk factors are directed at the short-term effects of the exposure and the potential for long-term effects (Edelman, Mandle, 1990).

Air, water, and noise pollution increase the risk of illness. High crime rates or overcrowding can also lead to stresses that make individuals more susceptible to disease.

In the home the physical environment may include conditions that pose risks to an individual or family. Unclean, poorly heated or cooled, or overcrowded dwellings increase the likelihood that infections and other diseases will be contracted and spread. Within the family, conflicts or other problems may create stressors that put individual members or the family as a whole at increased risk of illness.

Lifestyle

Many activities, habits, and practices involve risk factors; the stresses of life crises and frequent lifestyle changes also are risk factors. Health practices and behaviors can have positive or negative effects on health. Practices with potential negative effects are risk factors; these include overeating or poor nutrition, insufficient rest and sleep, and poor personal hygiene. Other habits that put a person at risk for illness include smoking, alcohol or drug abuse, and activities involving a threat of injury such as skydiving or mountain climbing. Some habits are risk factors for specific diseases. For example, excessive sunbathing increases the risk of skin cancer, and being overweight increases the risk of cardiovascular disease.

Any emotional stress can be a risk factor if it is severe or prolonged or the person is unable to cope adequately with it. In such a case, emotional stress may increase the chance of illness. Emotional stressors may occur with events such as divorce, pregnancy, and arguments. Any area of life that leads to long-term emotional stress can be a risk factor. Job-related stresses, for example, may overtax a person's cognitive skills and decision-making ability, leading to "mental overload" or "burnout."

Holmes and Rahe (1967) developed a classic social readjustment rating scale that correlates life changes with the risk of illness. Their research has shown that there is a greater risk for illness when a person has encountered a major life event change or multiple changes.

Adjustments that clients must make in hospitals and other health care settings also involve a risk for further illness. Volicer (1974) developed a hospital stress rating scale (Table 2-2) that closely parallels the Holmes and Rahe scale. The objective of this scale is to predict the risk of a long hospital stay, complications, and pain; all of these factors may be linked to further disability or prolonged illness. The hospital stress rating scale assigns a numerical value to actual or potential stressors experienced during

TABLE 2-2 Hospital Stress Rating Scale

Rank	Event	Mean Score
1	Possibility of loss of function of senses (e.g., eyesight, hearing)	116.8
2	Admission for life-threatening illness	107.1
3	Possibility of loss of an organ	92.1
4	Anticipated bad experience with medications	80.3
5	Inadequate insurance to cover hospitalization	78.5
6	Possibility of disfigurement	75.8
7	Anticipated future loss of income as a result of illness	75.5
8	Admission for surgery	73.7
9	Inadequate explanation of diagnosis	71.8
10	Undiagnosed ailment at time of admission	71.1
11	Inadequate finances for family during hospital stay	71.0
12	Being away from home	60.4
13	Inadequate explanation of treatment	58.0
14	Presence of severely ill roommate	57.8
15	Isolation for contagious condition	57.5
16	Anticipated improvement in functioning	56.8
17	Unconcerned attitude of hospital staff	56.4
18	Spouse at home	55.7
19	Anticipated pain or discomfort as a result of treatment	54.6
20	Dependent children at home	53.9
21	Hospitalization at considerable distance from home	53.2
22	Hospitalization as the result of an accident	50.7
23	Anticipated relief of pain or discomfort	50.2
24	Emergency admission	50.0
25	Experience of esthetically unpleasant surroundings	47.7
26	Admission for diagnostic tests only	46.2
27	Not having visitors	44.5
28	Prior hospitalization experience	43.3
29	Anticipated improved appearance	43.0
30	Change in amount of physical activity	41.6
31	Holiday or special family occasion during hospitalization	41.3
32	Change in amount of independent behavior	41.0
33	Major change in eating habits	40.1
34	Cared for by unfamiliar physician	39.6
35	Major change in sleeping habits	38.8
36	Being away from job	38.0
37	Language problem in communication with staff	36.2
38	Presence of unfamiliar machines or mechanical devices	35.1
39	Isolation from friends	34.5
40	Acquaintance with someone else with the same medical problem	34.3
41	Change in amount of personal privacy	33.6
42	Change in amount of interaction with other people	32.2
43	Extensive medical knowledge	30.7
44	Change in awareness of world or local events	27.2
45	Being away from school	26.3

From Volicer BJ: *Nurs Res* 23(3):235, 1974.

hospitalization. The higher the total score, the greater the risk that complications will develop, that pain medications will be necessary, and that the hospital stay will be prolonged. A high score on the scale does not mean that a client will experience complications or a long hospital stay. However, it does predict general risks and therefore helps a nurse identify risks so that nursing interventions can be developed to reduce hospital stress and the incidence of complications (Volicer, 1974).

 ## ILLNESS AND ILLNESS BEHAVIOR

Illness is not merely the presence of a disease process. Illness is a state in which a person's physical, emotional, intellectual, social, developmental, or spiritual functioning is diminished or impaired compared with that person's previous experience. Cancer is a disease process, but one client with leukemia who is responding to treatment may not perceive himself as ill and may continue to function as usual, whereas another client with breast cancer who is preparing for surgery may perceive herself as ill and be affected in dimensions other than the physical.

Illness therefore is not synonymous with disease. Although nurses must be familiar with different kinds of diseases and their treatments, they are concerned more with illness, which may include disease but also the effects on functioning and well-being in all dimensions.

People who are ill generally act in a way that medical sociologists call *illness behavior.* Illness behavior involves the ways persons monitor their bodies, define and interpret their symptoms, take remedial actions, and use the health care system (Mechanic, 1982). If individuals perceive themselves to be ill, illness behaviors can serve as coping mechanisms. For example, illness behavior may be a means of obtaining reassurance. A person who has been off work for a week because of illness may need to be reassured that his employer missed his contribution and that others care about him (Lambert, Lambert, 1987). The health team can also be a source of support and reassurance for clients. This support is particularly important for clients with chronic diseases. Clients with severe cardiac impairments who are unable to care for themselves look to the health team for support. Clients may need reassurance that the inability to care for themselves is due to the physical disease and not to a lack of motivation or desire. In addition, illness behavior can result in clients being released from roles, social expectations, or responsibilities. For

a housewife, for example, the "flu" may be a temporary release from child care and household responsibilities.

Variables Influencing Illness Behavior

Just as health behavior is affected by internal and external variables, so is illness behavior. To understand the client's behavior and plan individualized care, the nurse needs to understand the influences of these variables. They are complex in their origins and effects.

Internal Variables

Important internal variables influencing the way clients behave when they are ill are their perceptions of symptoms and the nature of the illness itself. If clients believe that the symptoms of their illnesses disrupt their normal routine, they are more likely to seek health care assistance than if they do not perceive the symptoms to be disruptive. If clients believe that the symptoms are serious or perhaps life threatening, they are also more likely to seek assistance. Persons awakened by crushing chest pains in the middle of the night generally view this event as a symptom of a potentially serious and life-threatening illness and will probably be motivated to seek assistance. However, such a perception can also have the opposite effect. Individuals may fear serious illness, react by denying it, and not seek medical assistance.

Cox (1985) investigated the reliability of the Health Self-Determination Index (HSDI) and noted that, although further testing is needed, the tool could assist nurses in determining and predicting client responses to health problems and needs. Therefore knowing how clients react to health problems enables the nurse to anticipate their needs, questions, and concerns and, ultimately, assist them in adopting positive health practices.

A client's illness behavior can also be affected by the nature of the illness. Acute illnesses involve symptoms of relatively short duration that are usually severe and that may affect functioning in any dimension. Chronic illnesses persist over a long period, usually longer than 6 months, and can affect functioning in any dimension. Several variables influence the illness behavior of a client with a chronic illness. The client may fluctuate between a state of maximal functioning and serious recurrences that may be life threatening.

If a chronic illness cannot be cured and the symptoms are only partially relieved by therapy, the client may not be highly motivated to comply with the therapy plan. In addition, in the present system, health care professionals are sometimes not highly motivated to remain involved in a client's care, and the client's own motivation may also lessen. The present system is geared to short, intensive client interactions. Continuity is often lacking, and health care services and community support systems vital for management of chronic illness do not always maintain adequate communication with one another (Aiken, 1976).

Clients with acute illnesses are more likely to seek health care and comply readily with therapy. Chronically ill clients may become less actively involved in their care, may experience greater frustration, and may comply less readily with care. Because nurses generally spend more time with chronically ill clients than other health care professionals, they are in the unique position of being able to assist these clients in overcoming problems related to illness behavior.

External Variables

External variables influencing a client's illness behavior include the visibility of symptoms, social group, cultural background, economic variables, accessibility of the health care system, and social support.

The visibility of the symptoms of an illness can affect body image and illness behavior. For example, a person who has a draining sore on the lip may seek assistance sooner than a person with a sore throat because people may comment on the sore, the sore changes the person's appearance, and the drainage requires continual care.

Clients' social groups may assist them in recognizing the threat of illness or support the denial of potential illness. For example, two 35-year-old women in two different social groups have identified breast masses while performing breast self-examination; both discuss the finding with their friends. The first woman's friends might encourage her to seek medical attention to determine whether a biopsy is necessary, whereas the second woman's friends might tell her that the lump probably represents only fibrocystic disease and that she does not need to rush to a doctor. These examples show the influence that friends may have on a client. The client's interaction with family members, peers, and others may have similar results.

Illness behavior can be interpreted and explained in terms of personal experiences and expectations. Cultural and ethnic background teaches an individual how to be healthy, recognize illness, and be ill. Meanings attached to health and illness are related to the basic culture-bound values by which a person defines a given experience and perception (Spector, 1991).

Western culture has emphasized a specific, systematic, causal explanation for trying to understand disease. In addition, the effects of disease and its interpretation also vary according to cultural circumstances. For example, there is a higher mortality rate from measles in underdeveloped countries, than in Western cultures (Moore et al, 1980). Therefore to develop individualized therapy, a nurse needs to understand a client's cultural background. For example, two studies of the way that cultural groups respond to pain (Leininger, 1977; Zborowski, 1952) demonstrated several cultural variations. Older New Englanders, for instance, avoided responding to pain and tended to suffer in silence and not seek relief. Members of the Irish cultural group tended to deny pain. Members of the Italian and Jewish cultural groups sought relief for pain, but Italians were more concerned about the implications of pain for their future levels of wellness and functioning.

Economic variables also influence the way that a client reacts to illness. Because of economic constraints, an individual may delay treatment and in many cases continue to work, rear children, or go to school. In addition, there are economic constraints within the health care system, and a client with inadequate health insurance cannot gain access to the health care system (Larkin, 1987).

Clients' access to the health care system is closely related to the influence of economic factors. The health care system is a socioeconomic system that clients must enter, interact within, and exit. For many clients, entry into the system is complex or confusing, and some clients may seek nonemergency medical care in an emergency room because they do not otherwise know how to obtain health services. The physical proximity of clients to a hospital, clinic, or health care agency often influences how soon they enter the system after deciding to seek care. In addition, some clients are reluctant to seek care from a large, complex medical center and will more readily visit a community agency. Clients frequently feel that a large medical center is impersonal, that care is provided in a mechanized, assembly-line approach, and that health care personnel are always looking for the worst. Some clients, however, may seek care only from a large medical center because they believe diagnosis and treatment procedures are more modern.

Social support has been linked to health practices such as seat belt use, exercise, nutrition, smoking cessation, and health screening practices (Muhlenkamp, Sayles, 1986). Research notes that clients react positively to social support during participation in positive health practices (Hubbard, Muhlenkamp, Brown, 1984). Thus persons who view themselves as being part of a social group and having emotional and personal resources on which they can rely are more likely to practice positive health behaviors.

These internal and external factors can interact in various ways to influence how persons behave when ill and how and when they seek health care. Mechanic (1982) summarized the influences on illness behavior in a list of 10 primary determinants (see box). A nurse who knows the variables that affect illness behavior can better understand such behavior. Nursing care can then be planned and delivered in a way that involves clients' resources so they are restored to maximal levels of health.

Stages of Illness Behavior

Although the behavior of ill individuals is influenced by internal and external variables, people generally pass through five stages of illness behavior (Fig. 2-7). This pattern involves how a person seeks, finds, and completes health care.

A nurse encounters clients in various stages of illness behavior. Knowledge of these stages enables the nurse to assess client behavior, determine the stage of illness behavior, and develop interventions to promote optimal physical, emotional, intellectual, social, and spiritual functioning throughout the illness.

Stage 1: Symptom Experience

During the initial stage, a person is aware that "something is wrong." A person usually recognizes a physical sensation or a limitation in functioning but does not suspect a specific diagnosis.

Ten Determinants of Illness Behavior

- The visibility and recognizability of the illness's symptoms
- The extent to which the person perceives the symptoms as serious (the person's estimate of the present and future risks)
- The person's information, knowledge, and cultural assumptions and understanding related to the perceived symptoms
- The extent to which symptoms disrupt family, work, and social activities
- The frequency of the appearance of the symptoms and their persistence
- The extent to which others exposed to the person tolerate the symptoms
- The extent to which basic needs are denied because of the illness
- The extent to which meeting other needs competes with illness responses
- The extent to which the person gives other possible interpretations to the symptoms
- The availability and physical proximity of treatment resources and the psychological and monetary costs of taking action (including costs in time and effort, as well as costs such as stigma, social distance, and feelings of humiliation)

Modified from Mechanic D: The epidemiology of illness behavior and its relationship to physical and psychological distress. In Mechanic D: *Symptoms, illness behavior, and help seeking*, New York, 1982, Prodist.

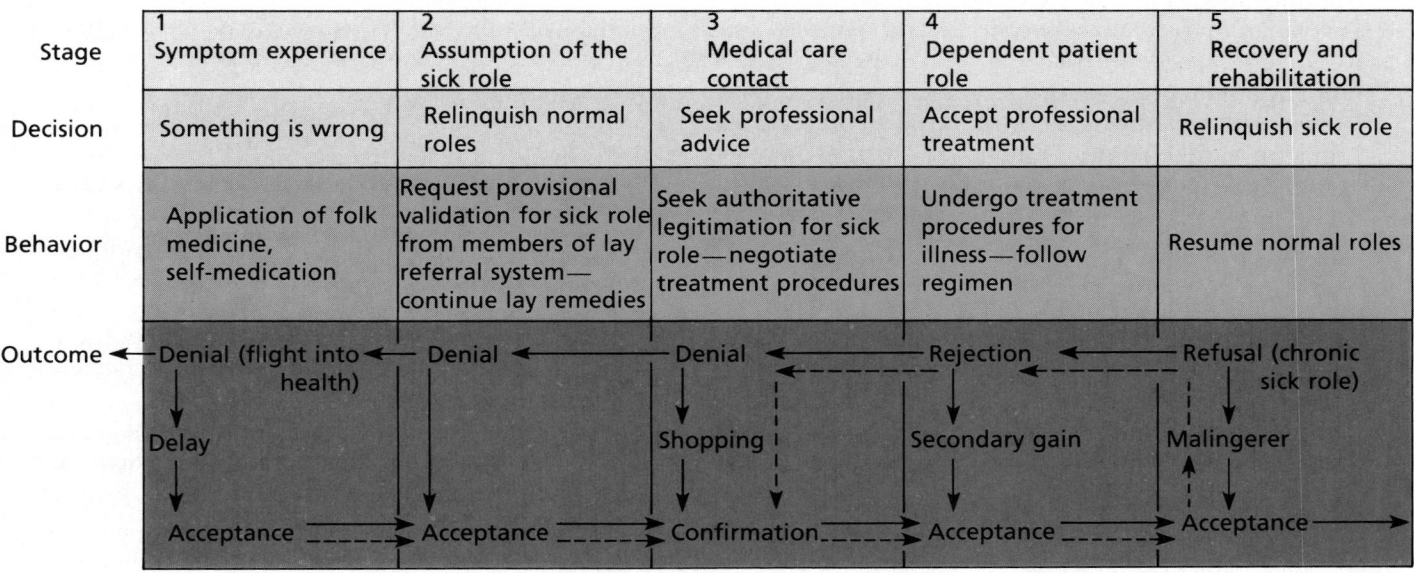

Fig. 2-7   Stages of illness behavior.
From Suchman EA: *J Health Hum Behav* 6:114, 1965.

The person's perception of a symptom includes awareness of a physical change such as pain, a rash, or a lump; evaluation of this change and a decision that it is a symptom of an illness; and an emotional response.

For example, a 38-year-old woman detects a lump during monthly breast self-examination. She knows the lump is not related to hormonal changes because she recently completed her menstrual period. She decides that the lump means that something is wrong and that it may be a symptom of cancer. She becomes anxious and fearful about this diagnosis.

After acknowledging the presence of a symptom or symptoms, a person may behave in many ways. One person may decide that the symptoms are mild or are not life threatening, such as in the case of a cold, so this person attempts self-medication strategies rather than seeks health care. Frequently, the individual uses over-the-counter drugs and home remedies.

If the symptoms are regarded as severe or life threatening, immediate care may be sought or the symptoms' presence or implications may be denied. If a person denies the symptoms or their meaning for future wellness, advice or treatment may be delayed. Before progressing to the next stage of illness behavior, the person must first acknowledge the presence of a health problem.

Stage 2: Assumption of the Sick Role

If symptoms persist and become severe, clients assume the sick role. At this point the illness becomes a social phenomenon, and sick people seek confirmation from their families and social groups that they are indeed ill and that they should be excused from normal duties and role expectations (Coe, 1978). The social group recognizes the illness and may also support continued self-medication.

The assumption of the sick role results in emotional changes, such as withdrawal or depression, and physical changes. Emotional changes may be simple or complex, depending on the severity of the illness, the degree of disability, and the anticipated length of the illness.

In the case of an illness requiring intervention from health professionals, the person may deny that such intervention is necessary and thus delay contact with the health care system. After accepting the persistent nature of the symptoms or the potential threat to present and future levels of wellness, the person seeks contact with the health care system and becomes a client.

Stage 3: Medical Care Contact

If symptoms persist despite the home remedies, become severe, or require emergency care, the person is motivated to seek professional health services. In this stage the client seeks expert acknowledgment of the illness, as well as treatment. In addition, the client seeks an explanation of the symptoms, the cause of the symptoms, the course of the illness, and the implications of the illness for future health.

The severity of the illness influences the amount of time the person waits before making contact with health care professionals. A person with a life-threatening illness or trauma may seek immediate contact, whereas a person with a persistent skin rash may delay contact for several weeks or months. In addition, the psychosocial and cultural variables that affect illness behavior may influence the length of the delay.

Clients' illnesses can be validated at any point on the health-illness continuum. A health professional may determine that they do not have an illness or that illnesses are present and may be life threatening. Clients then accept or deny this diagnosis, depending on several factors. The variables that affect illness behavior influence client reaction. If clients accept the diagnoses, they usually follow with the prescribed treatment plan. If they deny the diagnoses, they may begin "shopping" within the health care system. In such a case, clients consult several health care providers until they find one who makes the desired diagnosis or until they accept the initial diagnoses. Clients who consider themselves ill, even if health professionals regard them as healthy, may "shop" with a variety of doctors and therapists to obtain the desired diagnoses of illness. Conversely, clients initially diagnosed as ill, particularly with life-threatening illnesses, may seek another expert to tell them that their health or lives are not threatened. Clients with diagnosed cancer may seek opinions from several physicians in an attempt to avoid facing the diagnosis.

Stage 4: Dependent Client Role

After accepting the illness and seeking treatment, the client enters the fourth stage of illness behavior. In this stage, the client depends on health care professionals for the relief of symptoms. The client accepts care, sympathy, and protection from the demands and stresses of life. A client can adopt the dependent role in a health care institution, at home, or in a community setting.

It is socially permissible for clients in the dependent role to be relieved of normal obligations and tasks. The more ill the clients, the more they are excused from responsibilities.

After entering the dependent stage, the client must also adjust to the disruption of a daily schedule. This disruption affects the client's role in occupation, family, and community and may lead to stress in the emotional, intellectual, social, developmental, and spiritual dimensions.

Stage 5: Recovery and Rehabilitation

The final stage of illness behavior—recovery and rehabilitation—can arrive suddenly, such as when a fever subsides. If recovery is not prompt, long-term care may be required before the client is able to resume an optimal level of functioning (for example, the case of a fractured leg). In the case of chronic illness, the final stage may involve an adjustment to a prolonged reduction in health and functioning.

■ ■ ■

Not all clients go through each stage, nor do they all move through them at the same rate or in the same manner. People who have been in good health but suddenly suffer heart attacks and are taken to the emergency room, for example, are put immediately into the dependent client role, even though they have not progressed emotionally through the earlier stages. Nonetheless, the described pattern of illness behavior occurs in many cases, and an understanding of these stages helps a nurse identify clients' changing illness behaviors and plan effective nursing care with clients.

IMPACT OF ILLNESS ON CLIENT AND FAMILY

Illness is never an isolated life event. The client and family must deal with changes resulting from illness and treatment. Each client responds uniquely to illness, and therefore nursing interventions must be individualized. The client and family commonly experience behavioral and emotional changes, as well as changes in roles, body image, self-concept, and family dynamics.

Environment, personal behaviors, and psychosocial factors play an interactive role in illness and health. The health care professional can no longer focus only on physical functioning. Diagnostic assessment from a biopsychosocial perspective is more comprehensive and results in more specific diagnoses and interventions (Shaver, 1985).

Behavioral and Emotional Changes

People react differently to illness or the threat of illness. Individual behavioral and emotional reactions depend on the nature of the illness, the client's attitude toward it, the reaction of others to it, and the variables of illness behavior.

Short-term, non-life-threatening illnesses evoke few behavioral changes in the functioning of the client or family. A husband and father who has a cold, for example, may lack the energy and patience to spend time in family activities and may be irritable and prefer not to interact with his family. This is a behavioral change, but the change is subtle and does not last long. Some may even consider such a change a normal response to illness.

Severe illness, particularly one that is life threatening, can lead to more extensive emotional and behavioral changes, such as anxiety, shock, denial, anger, and withdrawal. These are common responses to the stress of illness. The nurse develops interventions to assist the client and family in coping with this stress because the stressor itself cannot usually be changed (see Chapter 30).

Anxiety

Anxiety is a feeling of apprehension, uneasiness, agitation, uncertainty, and fear that occurs when individuals anticipate threats. The symptoms of an illness may not create as much anxiety as the anticipation of the way the illness may affect future health. For some, the anxiety is a fear of a possible diagnosis, particularly a diagnosis of cancer. Others may become more anxious over impending surgery and anticipated pain. Anxiety responses vary from client to client, family to family, and stage to stage in illness behavior, but the nurse who knows their signs develops appropriate interventions (see Chapter 30).

Shock

When clients or families are informed of a severe or life-threatening illness, shock responses may occur. The shock response is a powerful emotional state. For some, the state may be an adaptive mechanism that allows them time to absorb what they have been told. Some people describe themselves as "numb" or "immobilized." People hearing that they have cancer or a severely debilitating disease such as parkinsonism may react with shock. They hear what has been said to them but fail to respond or respond in a totally inappropriate manner.

Denial

Denial is a mechanism by which the client or family avoids emotional conflict and anxiety by refusing to acknowledge difficult facts. A family learning that a loved one has cancer may deny the diagnosis and attempt to continue as though nothing were wrong. Short-term denial, however, can be an effective way of coping with an illness. The nurse must determine when denial is no longer productive and may be a hindrance to therapy.

Anger

The client or family may experience anger because of the illness. The anger of family members might be directed at the client because the illness has disrupted their routine, their plans, and, in some cases, their economic and emotional support. This anger might also be directed toward themselves. For example, a 50-year-old man has a heart attack while cleaning the garage; throughout hospitalization and recovery, his teenage son is very angry and makes no attempt to hide his anger. The nurse might discover that the son has been angry at himself for not cleaning the garage because he thinks that his father would not have suffered the heart attack if he had. In addition, the client or family might become angry with the health care team for making the diagnosis.

Anger, like other emotions, may take irrational forms. The client who suffered the heart attack may be angry at the disease process itself, as if it had singled him out. Anger also may have effects on a client's social or spiritual dimensions. For example, a client may become unsociable or blame a supreme being for the illness (see Chapter 33). Regardless of the kind of anger, the nurse helps the client and family work through their emotions and cope with the associated stresses.

Withdrawal

Illness, particularly long-term or severe illness, may cause clients to withdraw. Regardless of whether clients are in a hospital or at home, they may avoid interaction, remain in their rooms, or resort to solitary activities such as continuously watching television. Withdrawal is a symptom of depression and may be an effect of the illness or diagnosis. Family members may also withdraw from contact with ill persons because of anger or depression. When such withdrawal occurs, the nurse needs to work with clients and families to plan activities that promote the continuation of family functioning and support.

Impact on Family Roles

People have many roles in life such as wage earner, decision maker, professional, and parent. When an illness occurs, the roles of client and family may change. Such a change may be subtle and short term or drastic and long term. An individual and family generally adjust more easily to subtle, short-term changes. In most cases they know that the role change is only temporary. For example, the mother of two preschool children has a viral infection, and her illness continues for a week; during this time, she gives up her roles of housewife and child care provider. Initially, she may welcome giving up these

roles to be able to care for herself. As she gets better, however, she begins to look forward to resuming her roles.

With short-term role changes, a client does not go through prolonged adjustment phases. Long-term changes, however, require an adjustment process similar to the grief process (see Chapter 28). The client and family often require specific counseling and guidance to assist them in coping with the role changes. The following case study illustrates the way that such changes can occur.

Mr. Lampe is a married 40-year-old construction worker with three sons. The family is very active in outdoor activities and goes hiking and camping every 2 weeks during the summer and fall. Mr. Lampe is injured while hiking, and his injury necessitates the amputation of one leg. Because of the injury, Mr. Lampe has to change jobs and as a result receives a lower salary. The family activities change from active outdoor ones to passive indoor ones. Mrs. Lampe becomes angry because the reduction in income makes it difficult for the family to maintain its previous standard of living. The three sons become angry because their dad no longer takes them camping and hiking. Mr. Lampe becomes angry because he feels that his wife and children should be grateful that he is alive and should not worry about material things. The anger in the family gradually increases to the point that Mr. Lampe becomes unable to function at his highest level. The visiting nurse notices these changes in the family and observes angry outbursts. She refers the family for counseling sessions with a family therapist to help them cope with the anger resulting from the changes in Mr. Lampe's roles.

In some cases, family members may mistakenly assume that the ill person needs to be free of decisions and responsibilities. Family members take over all the roles of the client, including wage earner and decision maker. For instance, although Mr. Lampe does need to recover physically from his illness, he does not have to relinquish all of his roles in the family. If the family attempts to relieve him of all responsibility, he may feel isolated and withdraw from them. Because changes in a client's role affect family, nurses must incorporate the family into the plan of care (deChesnay, Magnuson, 1988).

Impact on Body Image

Body image is the subjective concept of physical appearance (see Chapter 31). Some illnesses result in changes in physical appearance, and clients and families react differently to these changes. The reactions of clients and families to changes in body image depend on the following:

1. The types of changes (for example, loss of a limb, a special sense, or an organ)

2. Their adaptive capacity
3. The rate at which changes take place
4. Supportive services available

When a change in body image occurs, such as that resulting from a leg amputation, the client generally adjusts in the following phases: shock, withdrawal, acknowledgment, acceptance, and rehabilitation. Initially the client may be shocked by the change or impending change and may depersonalize it and talk about it as though it were happening to someone else. As the client and family recognize the reality of the change, they become anxious and may withdraw, refusing to discuss it. Withdrawal is an adaptive coping mechanism that can assist the client in making the adjustment. As the client and family acknowledge the change, they move through a period of grieving. At the end of the acknowledgment phase, they accept the loss. During rehabilitation, the client is ready to learn how to adapt to the change in body image through use of a prosthesis or changes in lifestyle and goals.

Impact on Self-Concept

Self-concept is the individuals' mental image of themselves, including how they view their strengths and weaknesses in all aspects of their personalities. Self-concept depends in part on body image and roles but also includes other aspects of psychological and spiritual self (see Chapters 31 and 33). The impact of illness on the self-concept of clients and family members may be more complex and less readily observed than role changes.

Self-concept is important in a person's relationships with other family members. A client whose self-concept changes because of illness may no longer meet the expectations of the family, leading to tension or conflict. As a result, family members may change their interactions with the client. For example, the client may no longer be part of the family's decision-making process or may not be perceived as being able to provide emotional support to other family members or friends. Finally, the client may be left out of social functions. In the course of providing care, a nurse is able to observe changes in the client's self-concept—or in the self-concepts of family members—and develop a care plan to help them adjust to the impact of illness.

Impact on Family Dynamics

Because of the effects of illness on the client and family, family dynamics often change. Nursing interventions need to be directed toward the family and client (Reeder, 1991). Family dynamics is the process by which the family functions, makes decisions, gives support to individual members, and copes with everyday changes and challenges. If a parent in a family becomes ill, family activities and decision making often come to a halt as the other family members wait for the illness to pass, or they delay action because they are reluctant to assume the ill person's roles or responsibilities. In some cases of prolonged illness, the family often has to shift to a new pattern of functioning, a change that can lead to emotional stress. Young children, for example, may experience a strong sense of loss if either parent is hospitalized or is unable to provide affection and a sense of security. Emotional difficulty may continue even when the other parent or family members are successful in assuming the roles and responsibilities of the hospitalized parent. If a parent of an adult becomes ill and cannot carry out usual activities, the adult child often assumes many of the parent's responsibilities and in essence becomes a parent to the parent. Such a reversal of the usual situation can lead to stress, conflicting responsibilities for the adult child, or direct conflict over decision making.

Chapter 23 discusses family dynamics and the impact of illness on family functioning. Illness can disrupt a family's patterns of living, just as it can disrupt the functioning of the client in all dimensions. A nurse must view the whole family as a client and plan care to meet the same goal that must be met for the ill person—to regain the maximal level of functioning and well-being.

 ## SUMMARY

The concepts of health and illness continuously change. Health is not merely the absence of illness or disability. It is a dynamic state in which individuals adapt to internal and external environments to maintain well-being. To provide effective nursing care and assist clients in regaining and maintaining high levels of wellness, nurses must understand clients' concepts of health and their health beliefs and practices.

Health care professionals and consumers are emphasizing health-promotion and illness-prevention activities, which are designed to help clients reduce the risks of illness and maintain maximal health.

When persons become ill, they progress through stages of illness behavior. If the illnesses are serious enough for people to enter the health care system and receive nursing care, a nurse should be able to identify the factors influencing behavior and the impact of illnesses on clients and families. Nursing care is thus directed at preventing illness and promoting health, helping clients adjust to illnesses and their impact, and helping regain maximal functioning.

CHAPTER 2 REVIEW

Key Concepts

- A healthy individual adapts to changes in the internal and external environment and thus maintains a state of well-being in all dimensions.

- An illness may be a disease, but it also includes reduced functioning in any human dimension.

- A person's state of health or illness should be considered in relation to individual values, personality, and lifestyle rather than measured by any absolute standard.

- According to the health-illness continuum model, health and illness are in a dynamic, relative relationship. This model allows a nurse to compare a client's state of health with past states.

- The high-level wellness model describes health as an integrated method of functioning oriented at maximizing an individual's potential.

- The agent-host-environment model describes disease or illness as the result of the dynamic interaction of factors related to the agent, host, and environment. No one factor is the cause of disease or illness.

- The health-belief model considers factors influencing health beliefs. This model helps nurses understand and predict the behaviors of clients in seeking or complying with health care.

- The evolutionary-based model of health and viability is based on the principle that illness and death sometimes serve as evolutionary functions.

- The health-promotion model is directed at increasing an individual's level of well-being and self-actualization.

- Health beliefs and practices are influenced by internal variables, including developmental stage, intellectual background, perception of functioning, and emotional and spiritual factors, and by external variables, including family practices and socioeconomic and cultural factors.

- To individualize care and ensure maximal participation in it, the nurse considers the client's health beliefs and practices when planning care.

- Health-promotion activities maintain or enhance a person's health.

- Illness-prevention activities protect against risk factors and thus maintain a person's level of health.

- Nursing incorporates health-promotion and illness-prevention activities rather than simply treating illness after it occurs.

- Primary preventive care helps healthy people maintain and increase their levels of health.

- Secondary preventive care helps ill persons avoid complications or further health problems.

- Tertiary preventive care helps clients adapt to or overcome disability or reduced functioning caused by illness.
- Risk factors threaten a person's health, influence health practices, and are important considerations in illness-prevention activities.
- Risk factors are commonly associated with genetic or physiological variables, age, environment, and lifestyle.
- Illness behavior, like health practices, is influenced by many variables and must be considered by the nurse when planning care.
- Although no two ill individuals behave in exactly the same way, most pass through the following stages of illness behavior: symptom experience, assumption of the sick role, medical care contact, the dependent role, and recovery and rehabilitation.
- Illness can have many effects on the client and family, including behavioral and emotional changes and changes in roles, body image, self-concept, and family dynamics.
- To plan and implement holistic nursing care that assists in attaining states of maximal functioning and well-being, a nurse must consider all of the effects of an illness on a client and family.

Key Terms

Active strategies of health promotion, p. 47
Acute illness, p. 50
Agent, p. 41
Chronic illness, p. 50
Environment, p. 41
Health, p. 38
Health behaviors, p. 39
Health-belief model, p. 41
Health promotion, p. 47
Health-illness continuum, p. 39

Host, p. 41
Illness, p. 38
Illness behavior, p. 53
Illness prevention, p. 47
Passive strategies of health promotion, p. 47
Primary prevention, p. 49
Risk factor, p. 50
Secondary prevention, p. 50
Tertiary prevention, p. 50

Critical Thinking Exercises

1. You are working in a day-care setting. You're asked to design an early education health promotion program for the 4-year-old group. You initially focus on diet and exercise. How do you begin to design the program? What resources do you need?

2. One of the students in your school seeks your advice for smoking cessation programs. How do you identify appropriate resources? Which programs would be suitable for this person? What information does the client need about the potential programs?

3. Assess your own lifestyle. Identify three areas for change. Select one area, determine what needs to change, how to identify resources to promote change, how to select and implement the resources, and how to evaluate the effectiveness of the change.

REFERENCES

Aiken LH: Chronic illness and responsive ambulatory care. In Mechanic D: *The growth of bureaucratic medicine*, New York, 1976, Wiley.

Airhihenbuwa CO: Health education for African Americans: a neglected task, *Health Educ* 20:9, 1989.

Allinger RL: Study of illness referral in a Spanish speaking community, *Nurs Res* 26:53, 1977.

Anderson JM: The cultural context of caring, *Can Crit Care Nurs J* 4(4):7, 1987.

Balog JE: The concepts of health and disease: a relativistic perspective, *Health Values* 6:7, 1982.

Becker MH, Maiman LA: Sociobehavioral determinants of compliance with health and medical care recommendations, *Med Care* 33(1):1021, 1975.

Berne AS et al: A nursing model for addressing the health needs of homeless families, *Image J Nurs Sch* 22:8, 1990.

Breslow L: A quantitative approach to the World Health Organization definition of health: physical, mental and social well-being, *Int J Epidemiol* 1:347, 1972.

Burckhardt CS: Coping strategies of the chronically ill, *Nurs Clin North Am* 22: 534, 1987.

Coe R: *Sociology of medicine*, ed 2, New York, 1978, McGraw-Hill.

Cooper MC: Chronic illness and nursing's ethical challenge, *Holistic Nurs Pract* 5(1): 19, 1990.

Cox CL: The health self-determination index, *Nurs Res* 34:177, 1985.

Davidson JK: Diabetes in socio-economically deprived neighborhoods. In American Diabetes Association: *Diabetes mellitus: diagnosis and treatment*, New York, 1971, The Association.

deChesnay M, Magnuson N: How healthy families cope with stress, *AAOHN J* 36:361, 1988.

Dixon JK, Dixon JP: An evolutionary-based model of health and viability, *ANS* 6(3):1, 1984.

Dunn H: What high level wellness means, *Health Values* 1:9, 1977.

Dunn HL: High-level wellness for man and society, *Am J Public Health* 49:789, 1959.

Edelman CL, Mandle CL: *Health promotion throughout the life span*, ed 2, St Louis, 1990, Mosby–Year Book, Inc.

Fuchs VR: *Who shall live? Health, economics, and social choice*, New York, 1974, Basic Books.

Gilpatrick DM: Moving clients toward wellness: behavioral change, *Clin Nurse Spec* 3(1):25, 1989.

Goldsmith JR: Health effects of air pollution, *Basics RD* 4(2):4, 1975.

Holmes TH, Rahe RH: Social readjustment rating scale, *J Psychosom Res* 11:213, 1967.

Hubbard P, Muhlenkamp AF, Brown N: The relationship between social support and self-care practices, *Nurs Res* 33:266, 1984.

Lambert CE, Lambert VA: Psychosocial impacts created by chronic illness, *Nurs Clin North Am* 22:527, 1987.

Larkin J: Factors influencing one's ability to adapt to chronic illness, *Nurs Clin North Am* 22:535, 1987.

Leavell HR et al: *Preventive medicine for the doctor in his community*, ed 3, New York, 1965, McGraw-Hill.

Leidy NK: A structural model of stress, psychosocial resources, and symptomatic experience in chronic physical illness, *Nurs Res* 39:230, 1990.

Leininger M: Cultural diversities of health and nursing care, *Nurs Clin North Am* 12(1):5, 1977.

Mechanic D: The epidemiology of illness behavior and its relationship to physical and psychological distress. In Mechanic D: *Symptoms, illness behavior, and help seeking*, New York, 1982, Prodist.

Meleis AI: Being and becoming healthy: the core of nursing knowledge, *Nurs Sci Q* 3:107, 1990.

Moore LG et al: *The biocultural basis of health: expanding views of medicine anthropology*, Prospect Heights, Ill, 1980, Waveland Press.

Muhlenkamp AF, Sayles JA: Self-esteem, social support and positive health practices, *Nurs Res* 35:334, 1986.

Neuman B: *The Neuman Systems Model*, ed 2, Norwalk, Conn, 1989, Appleton & Lange.

Neuman B: Health as a continuum based on the Neuman Systems Model, *Nurs Sci Q* 3:129, 1990.

Parse RR: *Man-living-health: a theory of nursing*, New York, 1981, Wiley.

Parse RR: Health: a personal commitment, *Nurs Sci Q* 3:136, 1990.

Parsons T: Definitions of health and illness in light of American values and social structures. In Joco EG, editor: *Patients, physicians, and illness*, New York, 1958, Free Press.

Pender NJ: A conceptual model for preventive health behavior, *Nurs Outlook* 23:385, 1975.

Pender NJ: *Health promotion and nursing practice*, Norwalk, Conn, 1982, Appleton-Century-Crofts.

Pender NJ: Health promotion and illness prevention. In Werley HH and Fitzpatrick JJ, editors: *Annual review of nursing research*, New York, 1984, Springer.

Pender NJ, Pender AR: Attitudes, subjective norms, and intentions to engage in health behaviors, *Nurs Res* 35(1):15, 1986.

Pender NJ: *Health promotion in nursing practice*, ed 2, Norwalk, Conn, 1987, Appleton & Lange.

Pender NJ: Expressing Health through lifestyle patterns, *Nurs Sci Q* 3:115, 1990.

Pesznecker E: The poor: a population at risk, *Public Health Nurs* 1:237, 1984.

Prewitt VR: Health beliefs and AIDS educational materials, *Fam Community Health* 12:65, 1989.

Reeder JM: Family perception: a key to intervention. In American Association of Critical-Care Nurses: *AACN clinical issues in critical care nurse,* 1991, The Association.

Rosenstoch I: Historical origin of the health belief model, *Health Educ Monogr* 2:334, 1974.

Shaver JF: A biopsychosocial view of human health, *Nurs Outlook* 33:186, 1985.

Smith JM, Sorrell V: Developing wellness programs: a nurse-managed stay-well center for senior citizens, *Clin Nurse Spec* 3(1): 198,1989.

Spector RE: *Cultural diversity in health and illness,* ed 3, Norwalk, Conn, 1991, Appleton & Lange.

Steele RL: Social networks as a means of health maintenance, *Health Values* 6(6):6, 1982.

Tilden VP, Weinert, C: Social support and the chronically ill individual, *Nurs Clin North Am* 22:613, 1987.

Tripp-Reimer T: Reconceptualizing the construct of health: integrating emic and itic perspectives, *Res Nurs Health* 7:101, 1984.

Volicer BJ: Patient's perceptions of stressful events associated with hospitalization, *Nurs Res* 2(3):235, 1974.

Walker SN, Sechrist KR, Pender NJ: The health-promoting lifestyle profile: development and psychometric characteristics, *Nurs Res* 36:76, 1987.

Weitzel MH: A test of the health promotion model with blue-collar workers, *Nurs Res* 38:99, 1989.

World Health Organization Interim Commission: *Chronicle of WHO,* Geneva, 1947, The Organization.

Yarcheski A, Mahon N: A causal model of positive health practices: the relationship between approach and replication, *Nurs Res* 38:88, 1989.

Zborowski M: Cultural components in response to pain, *J Soc Issues* 8:16, 1952.

ADDITIONAL READINGS

Alexy B: Goal setting and health risk reduction, *Nurs Res* 34(5):283, 1985.

Brown BJ: Reorganizing hospital-based nursing practice: an analysis of patient outcomes, provider satisfaction and costs. In Aiken LH, editor: *Health policy and nursing practice,* New York, 1981, McGraw-Hill, Inc.

Collier JAH: Developmental and systems perspectives on chronic illness, *Holistic Nurs Pract* 5(1):1, 1990.

Dunn H: *High level wellness,* Arlington, Va, 1961, Beatty.

Dunn HL: What high-level wellness means, *Can J Public Health* 50:447, 1959.

Ferrans CE, Powers MJ: Quality of life index: development and psychometric properties, *ANS* 8(1):15, 1985.

Fries JF: The future of disease and treatment: changing health conditions, changing behaviors, and new medical technology, *J Prof Nurs* 2(1):10, 1986.

Hyman RB, Woog P: Stressful life events and illness onset: a review of crucial variables, *Res Nurs Health* 5:155, 1982.

Mechanic D: *Medical sociology,* ed. 2, New York, 1978, Free Press.

Milsum JH: Health, risk factor reduction and life-style changes, *Fam Community Health* 3:1, 1980.

Parsons T: *The social system,* New York, 1951, Free Press.

Pollock SE: Human responses to chronic illness: physiologic and psychosocial adaptation, *Nurs Res* 35:90, 1986.

Steinfels P: The concept of health: an introduction, *Hastings Cent Rep* 1(3):3, 1973.

Rotter J: Generalized expectancies for internal versus external control of reinforcement, *Psychol Monogr* 80:1, 1966.

Suchman EA: Stages of illness and medical care, *J Health Human Behav* 6:114, 1965.

Volicer BJ: Perceived stress levels of events associated with the experience of hospitalization: development and testing of a measurement tool, *Nurs Res* 22:491, 1973.

Volicer BJ, Bahannon MW: A hospital stress rating scale, *Nurs Res* 24:354, 1975.

Wolinsky FD: *The sociology of health: principles, professionals and issues,* Boston, 1980, Little, Brown.

The Health Care Delivery System

OBJECTIVES

Mastery of content in this chapter will enable the student to:

- Define the key terms listed.
- Discuss major events in the evolution of the health care system.
- Describe society's influence on the health care delivery system.
- Discuss factors influencing entry into the system.
- Describe the six types of health care agencies.
- Discuss the client's right to health care and describe client rights within the health care delivery system.
- Compare the various methods for financing health care.
- Explain the advantages and disadvantages of a prospective reimbursement system.
- Describe the problems of the health care delivery system.
- Explain solutions for each problem of the health care delivery system.

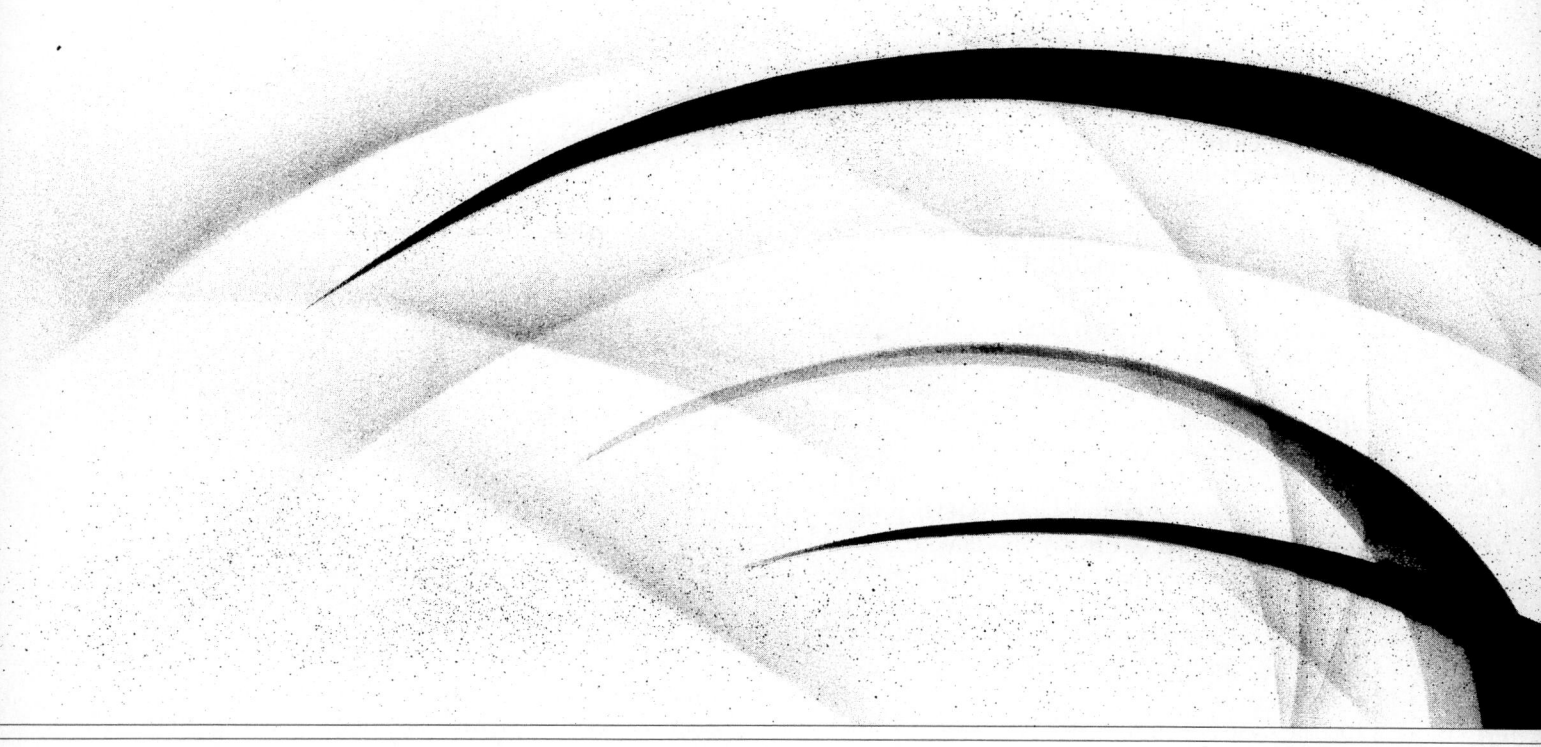

CHAPTER OUTLINE

Evolution of the Health Care Delivery System

Types of Health Care Services
Health promotion
Illness prevention
Diagnosis and treatment
Rehabilitation

Types of Agencies
Outpatient agencies
Institutions
Community-based agencies
Support groups
Volunteer agencies
Hospices
Government agencies

Factors Influencing Health Care Delivery
Society and the consumer's movement
New knowledge and technology
Legal issues and ethics
Economics
Politics

The Client and the Health Care Delivery System
Right to health care
Rights within the system
Entry into the system

Financing Health Care Services
Private insurance plans
Health maintenance organizations
Preferred provider organizations
Long-term insurance
U.S. government insurance plans
Canadian government health insurance

Problems With the System
Issues for the 1990s
Solutions for the 1990s

The health care system is experiencing a period of revolutionary change. Health care institutions are no longer thriving economically. The cost of health care services continues to skyrocket. Because business, industry, and the government are paying the majority of health care bills, they are demanding greater controls, regulations, and evidence that quality health care is being received by clients (Sovie, 1990). Health care insitutions are scrambling to find better ways to provide health care at a lower cost. At the same time, they are being evaluated very closely by regulatory agencies such as the Joint Commission on Accreditation of Healthcare Organizations (JCAHO), professional review organizations (PROs), and state health departments. The reviews focus on the outcomes of health care and whether clients leave health care institutions in an improved state of health with the capacity to manage their continued health care needs.

Rising costs of and restrictions placed on health care services by private and government third-party payers (insurers) lower the frequency and quality of the care of people from varying socioeconomic backgrounds. Many clients do not have access to health care. A two-tiered health care system exists in which clients with private insurance often receive a different quality of care than those with public insurance. Income, social class, and place of residence frequently dictate accessibility to and type of health care received. Small hospitals that provide illness care to rural areas are becoming less financially viable. There is a crisis in the United States in regards to eligibility for health care dollars. In many parts of the country a family of three with an income of more than $5000 per year is too well off to qualify for Medicaid (Rooks, 1990).

Nursing is a major component of the health care delivery system, and nurses make up the largest employment group within the system. Nursing services are necessary for virtually every client seeking care of any type, including health promotion, diagnosis and treatment, and rehabilitation. Because nursing is such an important part of the health care delivery system and because the delivery of nursing services is tied to other components of the health care delivery system, the nurse needs to understand the system to effectively deliver quality care within it. Every nurse practicing today needs to appreciate that health care is a business. The success of any health care business depends on nursing's participation in changing the systems for delivering cost-effective care and creating strategies to ensure that clients receive quality care.

 ## EVOLUTION OF THE HEALTH CARE DELIVERY SYSTEM

It is important to understand the developments leading to the American health care delivery system. At the turn of the century, only a few urban hospitals existed in the United States. These institutions served the poor, whereas the affluent and middle-class members of the population were treated at home (McMahon, 1987). The early hospitals were primarily financed by voluntary donations and supported by groups such as churches. By the late 1920s, because of the very high losses faced by hospitals (many clients were unable to pay), a new system of payment was introduced—third-party payment (Smith, 1990). Hospital insurance plans quickly developed, and the cost of health care has grown ever since.

From the mid-1920s to mid-1930s, there was much discussion at the government level regarding costs of medical care. President Franklin Roosevelt attempted to fight the effects of the Great Depression by developing an extensive system of long-range social insurance and short-term public assistance (Smith, 1990). Controversy over the program ran high, and no immediate legislation was proposed. Finally in 1935, passage of the Social Security Act facilitated public assistance to blind persons, older adults, and dependent children. A major national health care conference in 1938 resulted in the first national discussion of a national health care program in the United States. A general consensus emerged from the conference about principles for improving the nation's health, but there was no agreement about how the costs of health care would be divided beteen federal and state governments (Smith, 1990). That problem still exists.

Before 1945 the U.S. government was not involved in the health care industry. The Hill-Burton Act of 1945 was passed, providing money for hospital construction, expansion, or improvement (Beck, 1985). As a result, new hospitals were built in suburban and rural settings. Large urban medical centers were expanded for scientific research and technological advances.

With the passage of the Medicare and Medicaid amendments to the Social Security Act in 1965, the U.S. government established national and state health insurance programs for certain segments of the population. The Medicare program provides medical and hospital insurance for persons who are over 65 years of age or disabled. The Medicaid program provides a joint federal and state health insurance program for low-income persons in specific groups, including families with dependent children, older adults, blind or disabled persons, and persons who cannot afford medical care. In Canada, similar but more inclusive medical services are provided by provincial medical care plans. The Social Security Amendments Act of 1972 changed the Medicare and Medicaid program, largely to control costs. From 1974 to 1981, succeeding amendments were made to control costs and improve cost-effectiveness strategies. In 1977 a new Federal Health Care Financing Administration (HCFA) was created to administer the Medicare and Medicaid programs.

The National Health Planning and Resources Development Act of 1974 (PL 93-641) introduced a comprehensive system of health care planning. The purpose of the law was to bring together the work of new Health Systems Agencies (HSA) with that of the state planning agencies. Previously fragmented federal programs for health planning, such as Hill-Burton programs for health care facility construction and regional medical programs for health care delivery programs, were combined into one system. Consumers would shape local health plans and cut medical costs. A purpose of the Act was to improve planning and health care accessibility. For example, the construction of any new facility or the addition of beds to a hospital would be reviewed by planning groups. Unfortunately the HSA was not provided with authority over federal health facilities (such as Veterans Administration [VA] hospitals). Local governments, private health care providers and community groups failed to support the local and state planning agencies. Marmor (1983) notes that the HSA's authority was restricted and insufficient to reshape the local politics of medicine.

Although legislation was designed to provide for the expansion of hospitals and payment of services and to develop a system of health care planning, some legislation did affect certain professionals. The Rural Health Clinics Act of 1978 represented the U.S. government's willingness to allow nurse practitioners to deliver primary health care. This act provides for the development of rural health clinics in medically underserved areas, for the use of nurse practitioners as clinic staff, and for direct reimbursement to clinics for services provided by nurse practitioners to Medicare and Medicaid recipients. This law demonstrates the trend toward involving nurses in primary health care delivery.

During the 1970s, research was underway to understand the hospital industry, particularly to identify similarities and differences between hospitals. Much attention was paid to the resources used by hospitals. Resource use depended on the severity and types of

patients for whom a hospital cared, as well as usual treatments and procedures used. Yale University collaborated with the Federal Social Security Administration and the State of New Jersey to determine whether the concept of defining groups of similar patients for resource **utilization review** could be used as a system for payment (Smith, 1990). In other words, if research showed that patients with similar diagnoses could be cared for at similiar costs and with favorable results, diagnostic categories might be used as a system for establishing payment of hospital costs nationally. The outcome of the research was the 1983 Medicare prospective pricing plan approved by Congress for most inpatient services as part of the Social Security Amendments of 1983. Hospitals would no longer be reimbursed for all costs incurred in the care of a client. The prospective payment system has been one of the most significant factors affecting the health care industry. Payment for hospital services to Medicare clients is based largely on flat rates per admission based on diagnostic categories.

Health care is a business; as a result, central issues are escalating costs and the availability of quality health care services. Financial pressures have forced hospitals and other health care institutions to shift organizational priorities. There is a concern that institutions will make financial incentives a priority over quality humane care. Nursing professionals are in a position to restructure care delivery systems while maintaining a level of excellence in health care. More than ever, the role of nursing in client advocacy will be critical to ensure that the health care needs of all populations are served.

 ## TYPES OF HEALTH CARE SERVICES

A broad variety of health care services (see box on p. 68) are available to clients and families, depending on the nature and extent of a health problem. The types of services offered often depend on the site in which clients seek health care (for example, a hospital or mental health clinic). Nurses play an active role in all forms of health care service. The types of services can best be categorized as health promotion, illness prevention, diagnosis and treatment, and rehabilitation.

Health Promotion

Health-promotion services have developed rapidly within the health care delivery system. By keeping people healthy, the overall costs of health care de-

Examples of Health Care Services

HEALTH PROMOTION

- Prenatal classes
- Classes on care of elderly parents
- Nutrition counseling
- Exercise classes
- Stress management
- Specific disease–management classes (e.g., diabetes, arthritis)
- Smoking cessation classes

ILLNESS PREVENTION

- Screening programs (e.g., hypertension, high cholesterol levels, breast cancer [mammography])
- Routine check-ups or physical examinations
- Mental health counseling and crisis prevention
- Immunizations
- Occupational health and safety measures (e.g., workplace ventilation, protective eye wear, noise control)
- Public legislation (e.g., seat belts, air bags, school bus codes)

DIAGNOSIS

- Radiological procedures (e.g., magnetic resonance imaging and computed tomography scans, x-ray studies)
- Physical examinations
- Blood testing

TREATMENT

- Client education
- Surgical intervention
- Laser therapies
- Pharmacological therapies

REHABILITATION

- Cardiovascular programs
- Pulmonary programs
- Sports medicine
- Alcohol- and drug-dependence programs
- Mental illness programs
- Stroke and spinal-cord–injury programs

cline. Health-promotion activities, including specific health education programs, are designed to help clients reduce the risk of illness, maintain maximal function, and promote habits related to good health. Health-promotion activities take place in many settings. For example, hospitals offer programs such as prenatal nutrition classes in which the essentials of good nutrition during pregnancy, after childbirth, and for the infant are taught. These classes promote the general health of the woman, fetus, and infant.

Illness Prevention

Illness prevention is another type of service provided by the health care delivery system. The nurse helps prevent illness by assisting the client and family in reducing risk factors and avoiding the need for primary, secondary, or tertiary health care. Usually prevention activities involve the client directly and include measures such as periodical physical examinations and identification of familial risk factors for illnesses such as cardiovascular disease. After risk factors are identified, the client can engage in positive health practices such as changing the diet to prevent illness.

Illness-prevention activities also include environmental programs to reduce the threat of illness or disability. For example, public health departments control the breeding of mosquitoes with insecticides during hot, humid weather to reduce the risk of encephalitis.

Occupational safety measures and educational programs are also illness-prevention activities. In the painting and construction industry, for example, the use of respirators by employees exposed to dust and paint fumes reduces the risk of lung disease.

Public education programs and legislation are also involved in illness and injury prevention. Laws requiring the use of approved infant or toddler restraint seats in automobiles, for example, are directed at preventing severe injury or death.

Preventive health education and practices are generally very effective in reducing the risk of disease and disability, and prevention activities help improve the client's and community's level of health. Furthermore, it is becoming evident that preventive measures reduce the costs of health care.

Diagnosis and Treatment

The diagnosis and treatment of illness have traditionally been the most commonly used services of the health care delivery system. Advances in technology and computers have resulted in more sophisticated diagnostic procedures and greater chances for early diagnosis. Many new diagnostic tests are noninvasive and painless. Furthermore, diagnostic services can now be brought to a client; hospitals have equipped motorized vans with diagnostic x-ray equipment and offer services at sites such as shopping malls and public libraries.

Nurses' activities in the community can be directed at early diagnosis and education. For example, nurses can teach women about breast self-examination (see Chapter 20), enabling them to discover a breast mass at an early stage and to know the importance of seeking early treatment. In other community settings, such as schools, special programs have been organized to detect health problems, such as hypertension, elevated cholesterol, or visual or hearing impairments, at an early stage.

Treatment methods have also expanded because of advances in technology and knowledge. Clients are receiving newer, more innovative health care treatments based on the most recent research. Treatment of illnesses has also expanded outside hospitals and other institutions, even to the home. When treatment is initiated within an institution, nurses teach the client and family to complete the treatment plan at home and in the outpatient setting.

Rehabilitation

Rehabilitation is the restoration of a person to normal or near-normal function after a physical or mental illness, injury, or chemical addiction. Rehabilitation was once available primarily for clients with illnesses or injury to the nervous system, but the health care delivery system has expanded its scope of such services. Today, specialized rehabilitation services, such as cardiovascular rehabilitation programs, help clients and families adjust to necessary changes in lifestyle after heart attacks. Pulmonary rehabilitation programs aim to increase the exercise tolerance of clients with chronic pulmonary diseases.

Rehabilitation services begin the moment a client enters the health care system with an illness or injury. Initially, rehabilitation may focus on the prevention of complications related to the illness or injury. As the condition stabilizes, rehabilitation is directed at maximizing the client's functioning and level of independence.

These programs take place in many health care settings, including specific rehabilitation institutions, outpatient settings, and the home. Frequently, clients needing long-term rehabilitation have severe disabilities affecting their ability to carry out the activities of daily living. When rehabilitation services are provided in outpatient settings, clients receive treatment at specified times during the week but remain at home the rest of the time. Specific rehabilitation strategies are applied to the home environment so that maximal levels of function and independence can be achieved. Nurses and other members of the health care team visit homes and help clients and families learn to adapt to illness or injury.

 TYPES OF AGENCIES

As a result of the expansion of the health care system and increasing specialization, the variety and number of health care agencies have increased. Services once delivered primarily by hospitals are now provided in many other types of settings through agencies that include outpatient, institutional, community-based, volunteer, hospice, and government programs.

Outpatient Agencies

Clients who do not require hospitalization can receive health care in an alternative site such as a physician's office, clinic, or another ambulatory care facility. **Outpatient services** are generally directed at the diagnosis and treatment of acute and chronic illnesses. An outpatient setting is designed to be convenient and easily accessible to clients.

Physicians' Offices

Physicians' offices provide primary care for a large segment of the population. Physicians in office practice tend to focus on the diagnosis and treatment of specific illnesses rather than on health promotion and other services. With more competition in health care, physicians' offices now offer a wider range of diagnostic and therapeutic services. Some offices have complete laboratory facilities for analyzing blood specimens and urine samples and obtaining electrocardiograms and radiographs (x-ray films). Diagnostic procedures such as sigmoidoscopy and ultrasound can also be performed. Simple surgical procedures such as biopsies and removal of skin lesions are offered.

Nurses employed in physicians' offices can assume many roles. Some nurses have the traditional role of registering clients, taking vital signs, preparing the client for examination or laboratory studies, and providing basic information. Other nurses working with physicians have the expanded role of conducting physical examinations and histories, offering health education, and recommending therapies for clients in stable health states.

Clinics

Clinics traditionally involve a department in a hospital where clients not requiring hospitalization receive medical care, a group practice of physicians, or a community agency that delivers a particular type of health service such as immunizations. Frequently, clients who use clinics are from a lower socioeconomic level because the costs for services are lower. Often a client cannot assume that the same primary care provider will be available during each clinic visit. The roles of nurses in a clinic are very similar to those of nurses in a physician's office.

Ambulatory Care Centers

Ambulatory care centers, like clinics, provide health services on an outpatient basis. The centers may be affiliated with hospitals or function independently under a corporation or a single physician or group of physicians. An ambulatory care center may be located within an inpatient facility, however, most are located away from a major inpatient institution. An urgent-care center is an example of an ambulatory care center that provides 24-hour service to clients for minor injuries or illnesses such as lacerations and influenza. The urgent care center offers an alternative to a hospital emergency room.

Nurses providing primary care in an ambulatory setting work in a more expanded role as a nurse practitioner or clinical nurse specialist (see Chapter 1). These nurses have a specific caseload of clients and provide follow-up care when the clients visit the care center.

Institutions

Institutional agencies include hospitals, extended care facilities, psychiatric facilities, and rehabilitation centers offering health care services to **inpatients** (clients admitted to a stay within an institution for diagnosis, treatment, or rehabilitative services).

Hospitals

Hospitals traditionally have been the major agency of the health care system. Typically a client would come to a hospital for diagnosis and treatment. The client would remain hospitalized until almost fully recovered. However, prospective reimbursement has changed how patients are cared for in hospitals. A client within a certain **diagnostic-related group (DRG)** is expected to be cared for and discharged within a projected time period. For example, a woman who delivers a baby by natural childbirth is expected to be discharged home within 23 hours in many hospitals. If the client is not fully recovered, al-

ternative care sites are found, including extended care facilities, nursing homes, and home care. Many insurers even deny hospitalization for clients with "minor" conditions.

Today, clients who enter hospitals are usually acutely ill and need comprehensive and specialized health care. The services provided by hospitals vary considerably. Small rural hospitals with only 40 beds may only offer limited emergency and diagnostic services, as well as general inpatient services. In comparison, large urban medical centers offer comprehensive, state-of-the-art diagnostic services, emergency care, surgical intervention, intensive care units, inpatient services, and rehabilitation facilities. Larger hospitals also offer professional staff from a variety of specialties such as social service, respiratory therapy, physical and occupational therapy, and speech therapy. The focus in hospitals is to provide the highest quality of care possible so that clients can be discharged early but safely to the home or a facility that can adequately manage remaining health care needs.

Hospitals are classified as *public* and *private*. Public and private hospitals exist throughout Canada and the United States. A public hospital is financed and operated by a government agency at the local, state, provincial, or national level. Many clients in public hospitals cannot afford to pay for care. The hospitals provide services at a not-for-profit rate. Private hospitals are owned and operated by groups such as churches, corporations, businesses, and charitable organizations. The majority of clients who enter private hospitals have some type of insurance or medical assistance to pay for care. Private hospitals are operated on a for-profit or not-for-profit basis. The profit status influences how revenue can be used for services and taxation purposes. Many large corporations such as Humana and the Hospital Corporation of America (HCA) operate groups of for-profit hospitals across the United States.

Two other types of hospitals include military and VA hospitals. Military hospitals are located throughout the United States and in countries around the world to provide medical care for members of the armed forces and their families. VA hospitals provide health care to veterans with service-related and non-service-related illnesses or disabilities.

A nurse who works within a hospital has the opportunity to work in a variety of roles and different departments. The care of clients on an inpatient nursing unit or within an intensive care unit requires the nurse to have the knowledge and skills for applying the nursing process (see Unit 2), providing client education, coordinating health care services and discharge planning, and delivering a variety of therapies. As the depth of nursing knowledge increases, many nurses specialize their practice. This allows them to become expert in the care of select patient populations. Many hospitals have, for example, specialized units for the care of clients with oncological, orthopedic, pulmonary, or cardiac problems. Other opportunities within a hospital setting may include the role of patient educator, nurse manager, clinical nurse specialist, and infection control coordinator.

Extended Care Facilities

An **extended care facility** is an institution providing intermediate and long-term medical, nursing, or custodial care for clients recovering from acute illness or clients with chronic illnesses or disabilities. Extended care facilities include intermediate care and skilled nursing facilities, long-term care and nursing homes, and some retirement community institutions. At one point, extended care facilities primarily cared for older adults. However, as hospitals manage clients toward early discharge, there is a greater need for intermediate care settings for clients of all ages. For example, a young client who has experienced a stroke or traumatic accident may be transferred to an extended care facility for rehabilitative or supportive care until discharge to the home becomes a safe option.

The growth of extended care facilities increases as the number of older adults grows. The average life expectancy of the U.S. urban population in 1988 was 75 years. The percentage of persons over the age of 65 is likewise increasing (U.S. Bureau of the Census, 1988). With a "graying" population on the rise, more extended care facilities are needed. Namazi (1988) estimated that, of the 28 million older adults living in the United States during 1988, 6 million were in need of some form of long-term care.

An intermediate care or skilled nursing facility offers skilled care from a licensed nursing staff. This may include administration of intravenous fluids, wound care, long-term ventilator management, and physical rehabilitation. Extensive supportive care is provided until clients can move back into the community or into residential care. Third-party payers cover skilled nursing care. Extended care facilities provide around-the-clock nursing coverage. Nurses employed in such a setting have expertise similiar to that of nurses working in acute-care inpatient settings. In addition, the nurse should have a background in gerontologic nursing principles.

A long-term care facility or nursing home provides 24-hour intermediate and custodial care such as bathing, dressing, feeding and exercise therapy for clients of any age with chronic or debilitating illnesses. The majority of clients in long-term care facilities are older adults. Custodial care is not reimbursed by most insurers. Long-term care has been under attack for years because of claims regarding inadequate care and abuses. Many of the claims have been justified. However, much of the negative public opinion about nursing homes is based on misconceptions about the level of care provided. The box on p. 72 compares nursing functions in long-term and acute care institutions. It is important for a nurse working in a long-term care facility to accept the philosophy that long-term care is not the end for the older adult, that life continues with meaning and value, and that the nurse is an important person in the older adult's life. The nurse can assist the individual to move in a positive direction to attain or retain that meaning and value (Gensberg, 1981).

A third type of extended care facility is a residential or retirement community. Clients live in separate apartments or condominiums that compose a residential center. The clients remain relatively independent within a partially protective setting. Usually people keep all personal possessions in their residences. Services available within retirement communities include 24-hour nursing care, emergency medical care, housekeeping, laundry, transportation, social activities, and food service. The residential community bridges the gap between independent living and placement in a nursing home.

Psychiatric Facilities

Clients who suffer emotional and behavioral problems such as depression, violent behavior, and eating disorders often require special counseling and treatment in **psychiatric facilities.** Located in hospitals, independent clinics, or private mental health hospitals, psychiatric facilities offer inpatient and outpatient services, depending on the seriousness of the problem. Clients may enter these facilities voluntarily or involuntarily, if there is concern that these clients will harm themselves or others. A comprehensive multidisciplinary treatment plan involving clients and families is established for clients with psychiatric illness. Medicine, nursing, social work, and activity therapy collaborate to develop a plan of care that will enable clients to return to functional states within the community. At discharge, clients are usually referred for follow-up care at clinics or with counselors.

Rehabilitation Center

A **rehabilitation center** is a residential institution providing therapy and training to restore clients to optimal levels of functioning and independence. Re-

Nursing Functions in Caring for Older Adults in Institutions

LONG-TERM CARE

- Provide a milieu for living rather than illness and dying.
- Teach clients and families.
- Counsel clients and family.
- Learn about and use community resources, advise family and client of same.
- Establish short-term and long-term goals; evaluate progress toward both periodically.
- Secure and maintain health, recreation, and social history.
- Plan and coordinate care.
- Teach ancillary personnel.
- Communicate clients' needs in written and verbal form.
- Give treatments, medications, and rehabilitative exercises.
- Observe and evaluate client response to treatment, medications, and care plan.
- Teach health care maintenance to staff and clients.
- Keep physician aware of changes in clients' condition.
- Institute life-saving measures in the absence of a physician.
- Perform physical assessment of clients.
- Ensure adequate medical, dental, and podiatric care for clients.
- Maintain hydration, nutrition, aertion, and comfort.

ACUTE CARE

- Support client in achieving highest level of autonomy possible in situation.
- Provide appropriate information to client and family about treatment plan, medications, and diagnosis in collaboration with physician.
- Collaborate with multiprofessionals, client, and family to develop a comprehensive care plan.
- Supervise ancillary personnel.
- Recognize implications of syndromes for client care (e.g., renal failure, coronary disease, emphysema).
- Protect clients from injury or iatrogenic disease.
- Perform physical and psychosocial assessments and integrate in nursing care plan.
- Initiate action as outlined in nursing protocols regarding various conditions.
- Provide emergency treatment as needed (e.g., cardiopulmonary resuscitation, amelioration of shock, hemorrhage, convulsions, poisoning).
- Alert physician to changes in client status and abnormal findings of tests.
- Maintain hydration, nutrition, aeration, and comfort.

From Ebersole P, Hess P: *Toward healthy aging: human needs and nursing response*, ed 3, St Louis, 1990, Mosby–Year Book.

habilitation centers actively involve clients and families in providing health care. The goal of rehabilitation is to decrease the clients' dependence on the care provided so that they assume responsibility for personal care.

Rehabilitation centers employ persons from nursing, medicine, and the allied health fields such as physical therapy. Many rehabilitation centers focus on physical rehabilitation programs to teach the client and family to achieve maximal physical function after a stroke, head or spinal cord injury, or other physical impairment. **Drug rehabilitation centers** help the client become free from drug dependence and return to the community. Nurses employed in rehabilitation centers are committed to long-term continuity of nursing services and must be knowledgeable in their specialized area.

Community-Based Agencies

Community-based health care agencies focus on providing health care to clients within their neighborhoods. Examples of such agencies are adult daycare centers, home health care agencies, rural primary care hospitals, crisis intervention centers, and specialized support groups such as Alcoholics Anonymous. Nurses may have a variety of roles within these agencies.

Adult Day-Care Centers

Adult day-care centers provide health care to specific client populations during the day. They may be associated with a hospital or nursing home or exist as independent centers. Frequently the clients of such centers do not require hospitalization but need continuous health care services while their families or support persons work. These clients include elderly individuals needing daily physical rehabilitation, individuals with emotional illnesses needing daily counseling, and individuals with chemical dependence problems who are involved in rehabilitation programs. Adult day-care centers reduce the cost of health care and allow clients to retain more independence by living at home.

Nurses working in day-care centers provide continuity between care delivered in the home and in the center. For instance, nurses can ensure that the client continues to take prescribed medication and administer specific treatments; the nurse can also assist the client through counseling sessions. Knowledge of community needs and resources is essential in providing adequate support of clients who often spend only a few hours a week in the day-care setting (Ebersole, Hess, 1990).

Home Health Care Agencies

A **home health care agency** is an organization providing professional and nonprofessional health care services in the home (see Chapter 5). It is one of the fastest growing areas of health care due to the emphasis on early discharge by hospitals. Many hospitals now operate home health care agencies. Other corporations, such as the Visiting Nurses Association and community health centers, provide home care. The range of home health care services is growing from skilled nursing to home intravenous therapy. Home health care nurses employed by agencies deliver continuing and comprehensive care that is preventive, curative, and rehabilitative. Home health care agencies, like community health care agencies in general, provide care based on the belief that care directed at the individual, family, and group contributes to the health of the population as a whole.

Rural Primary Care Hospitals

In 1989 the Omnibus Budget Reconciliation Act (OBRA) directed the Department of Health and Human Services to create a new health care entity, rural primary care hospitals (RPCH). A RPCH provides 24-hour emergency care, with no more than six inpatient beds for providing temporary care for 72 hours or less to clients needing stabilization before transfer to a larger hospital. Physicians, nurse practitioners, or physician assistants staff the RPCH (Sharp, 1991). Access to health care in rural areas has been a serious problem. Numerous rural hospitals have been forced to close because of economic failure. The RPCH can provide inpatient care to acutely ill or in-

jured persons before they are transferred to better equipped facilities. Basic radiological and laboratory services are also available.

Nurses who work in an RPCH function independently in the absence of a physician. Competence in physical assessment, clinical decision making, and emergency care are essential. Nurse practitioners use medical protocols under the guidance of a staff physician.

Crisis Intervention Centers

Crisis intervention centers provide emergency psychiatric care and counseling to clients experiencing extreme stress or conflict, often involving suicide attempts or drug or alcohol abuse. These centers, which are usually self-contained units within a hospital or community health care center, provide services 24 hours a day. The services may be delivered directly on the premises, or counseling may be provided over the telephone. The primary objectives of crisis intervention centers are to help the person cope with the immediate problem and to offer guidance and support for long-term therapy (see Chapter 30).

Support Groups

Support groups provide self-help services for clients with select health problems. Participants receive emotional support and information on ways to adjust to personal and health problems. For example, Alcoholics Anonymous is an international nonprofit organization of recovering alcoholic persons whose purpose is to help alcoholics stop drinking and remain sober through group support, shared experiences, and faith in a higher power. Meetings are held in a central community location such as a church, school, or hospital. Al-Anon assists families in helping alcoholic family members, and Alateen helps teenagers cope with alcoholism in their families.

Support groups are usually organized by groups of clients who have experienced common health problems. Reach to Recovery is an example of a support group comprising clients who have undergone mastectomy or breast reconstruction surgery. Through support groups, clients can discuss problems and learn that other people share those problems. Participants also learn to problem solve and offer each other the emotional support needed to deal with crises.

Volunteer Agencies

Volunteer agencies are not-for-profit health care agencies established nationally or within a community to meet a specific need. Examples are the American Lung Association and the American Cancer Society and, in Canada, the Canadian Lung Association and the Canadian Heart Foundation. Most volunteer agencies do not provide treatment but have programs for the prevention and detection of specific illnesses; public education is a major focus. In addition, some volunteer agencies provide financial support for training of physicians and nurses, as well as for biomedical research directed at the prevention, detection, or treatment of certain diseases.

Volunteer agencies depend heavily on professional and lay volunteers to perform many of its activities. Financial support is generally derived from fund-raising activities, federal grants, and donations from individuals. Many health professionals donate time and resources to agencies within their specialty.

Hospices

The trend of seeking care outside of institutions has led to the development of hospices to meet the needs of the terminally ill. A **hospice** is a system of family-centered care designed to make the terminally ill person comfortable and ensure a satisfactory lifestyle through the terminal phase of illness (see Chapter 28). Hospice care can benefit a client in the terminal phases of any disease, such as cardiomyopathy, multiple sclerosis, acquired immunodeficiency syndrome (AIDS), cancer, emphysema, or renal disease.

A client entering a hospice has reached the terminal phase of illness, and the client, family, and physician have agreed that no further treatment could reverse the disease process. The client and family must accept the fact that the hospice will not use emergency measures such as cardiopulmonary resuscitation to prolong life. Instead, the hospice provides pain control and comfort measures to maintain the quality of life. Hospices do not have rigid visiting policies or other prescribed limits, and the environment for the client and health care workers is very relaxed.

Hospices are operated in many settings. Independent hospices provide only hospice care and are not affiliated with a hospital or medical center. Other hospices operate within a hospital setting, and many hospitals are now developing hospice units in a separate area of the institution. Many home care agencies also offer these services and involve neighborhood and community resources in providing care and emotional support for terminally ill clients and their families.

Nurses who work in hospices are employed in institutional and community settings. Hospice nurses are committed to the philosophy and objectives of the facilities for which they work. They provide care and support for the client and family during the terminal phase and continue to give the family emotional support throughout the grieving period.

Some organizations affiliated with hospices also offer **respite care**. Caring for a terminally ill spouse or relative can be emotionally and physically draining. Respite care provides a primary care provider such as a spouse or family member the opportunity to have some time alone. A nurse or specially trained volunteer comes to the home so that the primary care provider can run errands or have a break from the responsibility of direct care. The respite care service is important in maintaining the health of the care giver and family.

Government Agencies

Government agencies are clinics, hospitals, and other health services supported by local, state, provincial, or national taxes. Local government agencies include city hospitals and public health clinics. Agencies at the state or provincial level include state psychiatric hospitals and hospitals for clients with pulmonary disease. National agencies include primary research institutions such as the National Institutes of Health (NIH) and agencies administering health and welfare programs for a country such as the Canadian Department of Health and Welfare.

The types of local and state or provincial agencies and the allocation of resources for these agencies vary from one city, state, or province to another. Usually, agency funds originate in the tax base and are controlled by elected or appointed officials.

Health departments at the city or county level are generally concerned with specific health needs of the community and may receive additional support from the state or provincial health organization. Federal agencies provide specific kinds of health services on a national level. Of the many health-related national agencies in the United States and Canada, two are described in the following paragraphs: VA hospitals and the Canadian health care system.

VA Hospitals

VA hospitals were established after World War II to provide care for injured and disabled veterans. They are generally near medical schools and major medical centers with teaching and training functions. Many of the medical staff members in a VA hospital are supplied by the medical school.

Nursing services in VA hospitals are provided around the clock. Nursing services and nursing roles in these hospitals are similar to those in nongovernment hospitals.

Canadian Health Care System

The Canadian health care system includes a Department of National Health and Welfare, which is responsible for enforcing federal laws about harmful foods and drugs, providing health care services for certain categories of people, promoting fitness and amateur sports, administrating social welfare programs, and overseeing financial and technical programs (Stewart, 1985).

Most general and specialized hospital costs are financed by provincial hospital insurance plans. Each province organizes and administers its own plan, but plans have many common features, and each plan must meet certain federal standards (Soderstrom, 1981). In all provincial plans, insured services must be available to all residents. Members of the military and the Royal Canadian Mounted Police and inmates of federal prisons are excluded because their insurance is financed through other federal agencies.

 ## FACTORS INFLUENCING HEALTH CARE DELIVERY

Changes in the health care delivery system have increased rapidly during the last decade. The present system is the result of changes associated with social and consumer influences, new knowledge and technology, legal and ethical trends, and economic and political factors. An understanding of the factors influencing the health care system will enable nurses to adjust to changes, create better ways of providing nursing care, and develop new nursing roles.

Society and the Consumer's Movement

Consumers of health care delivery services have increased their knowledge and awareness of health promotion, illness prevention, and treatment practices. As a result, these consumers are exerting influence on health care and its delivery. No longer do consumers simply accept a health care professional's recommendations. Consumers are curious. They expect that information will be provided so that they might gain an understanding of health problems and their implications.

As consumers have become more knowledgeable about health in general, they have gained a greater awareness of the impact of lifestyle on health. As a result, consumers have expressed a greater need for

knowledge and services related to illness prevention and health promotion (see Chapter 2). Similarly, businesses and corporations have instituted programs to promote wellness and fitness. The costs of health care has a direct impact on businesses. Increased sick time and disability of employees cause significant financial loss. The interest society holds for more information about health care is growing. Consumers seek diagnosis and treatment of illness, but this is no longer the exclusive or even primary focus of health care. More people wish to learn about self-care so that they may remain as independent as possible.

Another major influence on societal trends has been the "baby-boomers," people born during the decade after World War II. That segment of the population is now middle-age and is beginning to express concerns about the availability and quality of health care. As this group approaches old age, significant changes will probably occur in health care delivery systems. For example, health maintenance services, which allow persons with chronic disease to achieve a high level of wellness and functioning, will become more important.

The health care beliefs and practices of society are as complex as those of an individual, depending on continuously evolving values, ethics, concepts of health, and other factors. In general, however, consumers' desire for health promotion, health maintenance, and new cures and treatments has led to changes in the health care delivery system. Many institutions and community-based agencies provide a wide range of outpatient health-promotion and health-maintenance programs on a regular basis. Volunteer agencies have arisen to meet specific needs in health maintenance and promotion, and consumers have become more active in fund raising to support research in these areas.

New Knowledge and Technology

Scientific knowledge continues to rapidly increase. Research has led to new treatments and cures for life-threatening conditions such as cancer, cardiovascular diseases, and diabetes mellitus. Clients have the opportunity to receive the most advanced treatment in the form of organ transplantation, laser surgery, and even gene-alteration therapies.

The disadvantages of this knowledge explosion are related to three factors. First, it is increasingly difficult for health care professionals to remain well informed about advances in their field. With the volume of knowledge available, it is difficult to stay a generalist. For example, a practicing nurse has trouble staying competent in all areas of general nursing practice. More care givers are becoming specialized so that they can focus on exclusive areas of knowledge and skills. Nurses may choose oncology or critical care as a specialty. Institutions bear the costs of keeping professional staff educated and updated on advances in health care.

A second disadvantage is the costs related to technology. New third-generation antibiotics, diagnostic imaging equipment, and specialized beds or support surfaces are just a few examples of technologies that are introduced daily into health care settings. Consumers must ask about whether these new technologies improve the quality of care and are cost effective. Nurses play a key role in evaluating new products and determining whether they help improve nursing practice. The costs of technologies are eventually transferred to clients. The ultimate factors in the use of technologies may be the economic resources available and the wants and needs of society as a whole.

The third disadvantage of advanced technology relates to its impact on health care delivery. Because technology causes greater specialization in health care, there is a risk of more fragmentation in care. It is important to have a single care giver who coordinates a client's health management. For example, one physician directs the course of therapy, using advice from radiologists, surgeons, and perhaps rehabilitation experts. However, diverse specialization usually introduces multiple care givers who do not always communicate clearly to ensure well-coordinated client care. Increased fragmentation of care also adds to health care costs.

Legal Issues and Ethics

As people become more aware of their rights to health care and humane treatment, legal and ethical issues arise when care becomes compromised. Health care providers are under increased scrutiny as consumers gain a better understanding of their health problems. Safe, efficacious, and humane health care is an expectation of society. When this expectation is unmet, legal actions can be taken against care givers, and the ethical dilemmas that arise are enormous.

A legal right is that to which a person is entitled by law. For example, a person has a legal right to competent licensed professionals and safe practices within a medical treatment center (see Chapter 14). In contrast, an ethical right, such as a person's desire to refuse life-saving therapies, has no legal guarantees (see Chapter 13). Ethics is the principles or

standards governing proper conduct. The legal and ethical concerns raised by consumers have changed the health care system. Standards have been implemented by various regulatory agencies to ensure that health care staff are competently educated. Policies within an institution dictate proper procedures for obtaining client consent to treatment. Institutions have created ethics committees to review professional practices and offer guidance when client rights are threatened. More attention is being given to client advocacy. Health care institutions are more intent on keeping clients and families informed and ensuring that staff members are responsible for their practice.

Economics

Ultimately, someone must pay for all health care services. Clients with private resources or insurance policies are generally able to seek health-promotion and health-maintenance services, but, too often, those with lower economic status or inadequate health insurance must defer seeking health services until they are very ill. As the total economy of a community or a country declines, its overall use of health care services also declines. During recent years, physicians have avoided hospitalization for clients whenever possible. More individuals are being treated on an outpatient basis.

During inflationary times and periods of high unemployment, more people avoid seeking diagnosis and treatment. The use of health care services declines because of the high cost of services and because of loss of insurance by the unemployed. Only the acutely ill seek health care. In some situations the health care delivery system responds to the declining use of in-hospital services by expanding less costly services such as health-promotion activities. Frequently, institutions react to economic pressures rather than proact to find creative solutions to problems. For example, many hospitals facing financial difficulty have reduced the number of employed registered nurses and added less educated care givers. This reduction in staff can have serious consequences on the quality and safety of nursing care.

Politics

The health care delivery system is also influenced by political decisions and factors. Through health care legislation, government at all levels affects how health care is provided and who pays for it. For example, a federal administration that makes health care a high priority can benefit the health care delivery system by introducing legislation that increases funding for health education and research.

Although politics influences the system, the client must adjust to changes caused by health care legislation. The poor frequently must delay seeking preventive or tertiary care because of economic restraints resulting from government policies such as increasing Medicare copayments.

 ## THE CLIENT AND THE HEALTH CARE DELIVERY SYSTEM

People usually have little or no interaction with the health care delivery system while experiencing good health. However, if they become ill, feel ill, or are motivated for other reasons to seek health care, they must enter the health care delivery system. Some clients enter the system easily by walking into a clinic or hospital emergency room or by making an appointment with a physician in private practice. Other clients experience difficulties in entering the system because of confusion or unfamiliarity with the agencies or because of inadequate health insurance.

Clients entering the system have rights. Society generally believes that all people have a right to health care. However, after persons enter the health care delivery system, they become clients and thus have certain rights *within* the system. People as health care consumers have a general right to determine *what* kind of health care should be available for present and future needs. Each of these rights affects how health care is delivered, but practices ensured by these rights are also influenced by society's attitudes and the system itself.

Right to Health Care

Society has generally come to believe that all people have a right to health care, regardless of cultural, economic, or other factors. In the 1960s, this belief led to the development of the federal Medicare and Medicaid programs. These two programs seek to meet the health care needs of older adults and the poor, the groups generally least able to afford health care on their own. However, the Medicare and Medicaid programs do not cover all health care costs. Therefore rising overall costs require clients to assume more and more of the cost.

Nursing services have also been affected. Discharge planning has a high priority and must be implemented the first day of hospital admission. In some institutions, a high ratio of nurses to patients is viewed as too expensive, so there has been a reanaly-

sis of the appropriate methods for delivering care with fewer nurses. In addition, in an attempt to further reduce nursing costs, lower-salaried, nonprofessional health care workers may be hired (Smith, 1985).

Rising costs, nursing shortages, and changing demographics have forced smaller, rural hospitals to close or consolidate with larger medical centers. In addition, smaller, rural hospitals are unable to diversify services (for example, same-day surgery centers, home health care, and fitness programs) to compete with larger centers.

Health care costs continue to rise for three reasons. First, rising poverty levels reduce the percentage of low-income mothers receiving prenatal care. Hence, premature births, low-birth-weight infants, and infant mortality and morbidity rates increase in the indigent population. Second, the increase in the number of clients with AIDS or AIDS-related illness is costly to the health care system, as well as to public and private insurance carriers. Third, modern technology provides physicians and nurses with skills and treatments to care for victims of trauma and disease who, 10 years ago, would have died from the same problems.

Rights Within the System

In 1973 the American Hospital Association developed a Patient's Bill of Rights (see Chapter 14), which lists 12 specific rights of hospitalized clients. The bill offers some guidance and protection to clients by stating the responsibilities of the hospital and staff to clients and families. However, it is not a legally binding document. The Patient's Bill of Rights supports consumer activities for clients in the health care system. Clients have the right to information pertaining to diagnosis and treatment, fees for services, and continuity of care. Clients have the right to refuse any diagnostic or treatment procedures. Above all, the Patient's Bill of Rights reaffirms clients' rights to information and privacy while receiving health care.

One of the client's specific legal rights in any health care facility is **informed consent,** which is obtaining permission from the client to perform certain kinds of actions. Informed consent must be obtained before beginning any invasive procedure, administering an experimental drug, or placing a client in a research study. Informed consent must meet the following criteria:

1. The consent document must be written in language that the client or guardian can understand.

2. The consent document must delineate all possible risks and actions of the physician or researcher to minimize the risks.
3. The consent document must list the benefit of the procedure to the client; if there is no known benefit at present, the consent document must state that fact.
4. Any alternatives to the procedure must be specified, even if the only alternative is nonparticipation.
5. The document must state that participation is voluntary and that the client can refuse to participate or withdraw from participation without having further health care withheld.
6. A client who gives informed consent must be rational and competent or represented by a competent guardian and must be told how to reach the physician or researcher performing the procedure.

Clients' rights and informed consent affect the way the health care system delivers care. Most agencies now have committees to evaluate client suggestions and complaints about the delivery of health care. In many institutions, this committee is called a *patient care committee.* Another committee, an institutional review board, ensures that elements of informed consent are consistent with federal guidelines. Although the need to protect clients' rights sometimes results in increased work and paperwork, this protection is necessary to ensure that all clients maintain their rights within the health care delivery system.

Entry into the System

The three most common ways that clients enter the health care system are entry by referral from a health team member, entry when the client has a specific health need, and entry related to financial resources. Other methods of entry are self-referral, employer referral, and social referral.

A client may enter the system by referral from a health team member in the case of an acute, potentially life-threatening problem, such as severe chest pain, or in the case of a less threatening problem such as a rash of unknown cause. In an emergent situation a client typically calls a physician who refers the client directly to emergency services. In less acute situations the nurse is frequently the professional in a position to refer the client to the system. Such referrals may be given to a neighbor seeking advice, a child and family at a school where the nurse practices or does volunteer work, and the family of a client to whom the nurse has previously provided care.

Clients also enter the system on their own because of a specific need. For example, a college student may seek health care for treatment of a sore throat or gastrointestinal upset and thus may enter the health care system at the primary care level through the student health center. Another student may be involved in a severe automobile accident and enter the health care system through a hospital emergency room.

Finally, entry into the health care system may be influenced by financial situations. People who are employed and have insurance may readily enter hospitals for elective surgical or diagnostic procedures because they have the financial resources to seek and pay for primary health care. However, employers may only offer certain health care plans, thus restricting employees' choices of physicians and agencies. Unemployed persons with limited resources may seek care only if the illness becomes acute and may then go to hospital emergency rooms. Frequently the only type of care some clients can obtain is that supported by local, state, provincial, or federal programs.

Regardless of the manner of entry into the system, all clients encounter nurses and nursing services. The first impression that the client has of the care delivered by a nurse may form a significant and lasting impression about nursing and health care in general. Nurses therefore have the opportunity to increase client awareness of such services and the types of quality care they can and should expect.

 ## FINANCING HEALTH CARE SERVICES

The rapid rise in health care costs has been the subject of discussion by government officials, the media, health care professionals, and consumers. The United States spends more on health than any other country. In 1987, 11.2% of the gross national product (GNP) was spent on health care. In contrast, only 8.6% of Canada's GNP was spent on health care (Harrington, 1990). It has become increasingly difficult, if not impossible, for people to meet health care costs with their own resources. In fact, many Americans have no means to pay for health care. Approximately 60% of insured Americans are underinsured, and 33 million Americans have no insurance at all. Government agencies and private companies have developed a variety of prepaid health care, insurance, and social service programs to subsidize the cost of health care. A topic frequently discussed as a solution to the financial crisis in health care is the creation of a national health care plan.

Private Insurance Plans

Traditionally, health care systems operated on a fee-for-service basis. Basically, health care providers were encouraged to use health care resources with little reservation. The philosophy was the more you do, the more you get paid (Hillman, 1989). The traditional "private-pay" insurance policy supported fee-for-service activities. Such an insurance policy can be obtained by an individual or through a group plan offered by employers. This type of plan is a retrospective fee-for-service option. Health insurance programs pay for some, most, or all of the expenses of health care for the client. Such payments are called *third-party reimbursements* because the costs of health care services are met, not by the health care agency or the client, but by the third party, the insurer. Ultimately, of course, consumers bear the costs through insurance premiums. The United States had 1000 for-profit commercial health insurers and 85 Blue Cross and Blue Shield plans in 1990 (U.S. Department of Commerce, 1990).

Health Maintenance Organizations

After the enactment of the Medicare and Medicaid amendments to the Social Security Act in 1965, considerable public attention was directed at finding ways to control health care costs. By the end of 1969 the federal government supported the formation of comprehensive prepaid, group practice corporations to stimulate competition, improve health system efficiency, raise the quality of care, and increase access to health services (Drew, 1989). The **Health Maintenance Organization (HMO)** Act of 1973 instituted the establishment of HMOs to provide comprehensive, preventive, and treatment services to a specific group of voluntary enrolled persons under a fixed, prepaid plan. Members of an HMO pay periodic payments in advance for expected costs of benefits for a population group. The HMO's promise to deliver specifically defined services within a fixed, prepaid system offers an incentive to contain costs and unnecessary use of services. If the HMO cannot provide services using the dollars paid by participants, the organization will not succeed financially.

Philosophically an HMO provides clients with all health care needed to maintain wellness and prevent illness. When clients are hospitalized, the HMO monitors their progress carefully to be sure that hospital care is managed efficiently. It is predicted that up to 80% of the insured population will be enrolled in HMOs or some form of group health plan in the next 10 years (Smith, 1990). Hospitals have the incentive to provide care for specific conditions or diagnoses while guaranteeing quality at a low cost. The focus on health maintenance is a significant shift away from the illness orientation of private insurers, whose plans pay little for preventive health care.

There are four types of HMO models (see box). Each is organized to provide members with comprehensive services. When clients join HMOs, they are required to use only the HMO member physicians and facilities (except in an emergency). Most HMOs have a large group of participating physicians from a variety of specialties. The inability to choose a preferred physician who routinely manages care is one disadvantage of an HMO. However, more HMOs are contracting directly with independent practicing physicians. This **independent practice association (IPA)** model adds more physicians to the HMO's approved medical provider list and thus adds clients to the system.

An HMO operates under a managed care system. Specific guidelines are established for levels of health

---

Health Maintenance Organization Models

INDEPENT PRACTICE ASSOCIATION (IPA)

- An HMO contracts with physicians who agree to care for HMO plan members. Physicians practice out of their own offices. It is the most common HMO model.

GROUP PRACTICES

- Health care services are provided by groups of participating physicians at one or more sites.

STAFF

- HMO employs its own physicians, who deliver services at one or more central locations.

NETWORK

- HMO contracts with one or more medical groups or IPAs to deliver care to plan members in different geographic locations.

care service, length of hospitalization, and medical specialist access. Clients with select diagnoses may be required to seek care only on an outpatient basis. Before clients qualify for hospitalization, a second opinion from a different physician is often required to prevent unnecessary hospitalization. The use of specialists or consultants in a case must be approved by the HMO physician, further controlling health care costs.

Preferred Provider Organizations

Consumers' confusion about health care insurance options is easily understandable. **Preferred provider organizations (PPOs)** are an example of a group health plan that frequently becomes confused with an HMO. A PPO is a contractual arrangement between a set of providers (usually physicians and hospitals) and one or more purchasers (usually self-insured employers or insurance plans) (Ermann, 1987). In a PPO plan, physicians or hospitals agree to provide comprehensive health services at a discount to companies under contract. These plans are also called *industry-based health plans*. They may be for-profit or not-for-profit.

A client who is insured through a group insurance plan by an employer may have a PPO option. The client can then obtain services from any provider, whether associated with the PPO or not. However, there are incentives to use a PPO, including expanded benefits, reduced deductibles on initial medical care, and reduced copayments.

PPO providers agree to accept utilization review as a way of controlling unnecessary expenses in providing health care. For example, clients may not be able to enter hospitals without meeting preadmission certification. This screening process eliminates unnecessary hospitalization and directs clients to appropriate outpatient treatment options. PPOs reimburse providers on a fee-for-service basis and exact a discount (Ermann, 1987). The hospital or physician may accept 80% of the usual charge as payment in full from the PPO client. In exchange for the discounted service, the provider recieves an increased number of clients and rapid payment of claims. The client receives care at a reduced rate, and the hospital gains because it can provide services at lower costs when its services are used by more clients.

Long-Term Insurance

About 75% of the elderly in the United States are covered by some type of private health insurance; however, most plans cover the same as Medicare (Ebersole, Hess, 1990). As a result, there is little if any coverage for long-term care. Most persons who are 50 years or older will need some form of long-term care for themselves or parents. As much as $22,000 to $50,000 per year can be spent for nursing home care for a spouse or parent (Ebersole, Hess, 1990). The unavailability of long-term care insurance is a national concern.

Private insurance companies have begun to add long-term care policies. The policy will provide an insured person $24 to $100 daily for an unlimited period of time or for as little as 2 years (Ebersole, Hess, 1990). There is also discussion to expand Medicare long-term care benefits.

Perhaps the most promising plan is to offer long-term care benefits through a national health care plan. Several proposals including the Physicians for a National Health Program (PNHP), the Pepper Commission, the Heritage Foundation, and the Health Security Partnership have been submitted to various committees in the U.S. Congress for consideration (Harrington, 1990; Curtin, 1991).

U.S. Government Insurance Plans

The Social Security Act of 1965 provided two plans for a national health insurance program. Beneficiaries include older adults and impoverished or disabled persons. Medicare and Medicaid were designed to improve access of health care to those most in financial need.

Medicare

Persons entitled to **Medicare** coverage include adults who are 65 years of age or older, persons of any age with permanent kidney failure, and select individuals with disabling illnesses. The program is administered by the Health Care Finacing Administration (HCFA) and is funded in part through Social Security (FICA) taxes. The original Medicare program (Title XVIII) has undergone numerous changes since its inception. There are still two parts to the program, however. Part A is basically acute-care hospital insurance; Part B covers physician and certain outpatient services (see box). Most persons do not pay monthly premiums directly for Medicare because of deductions of premiums from monthly social security checks.

Medicare does not pay for the full cost of certain services. For example, a diagnostic test such as a mammogram will only be reimbursed for a flat amount of $50. If a radiological center charges more than the flat rate, the client must pay the remainder. Hospitals and physicians voluntarily choose to partic-

---

Health Care Services Covered and Not Covered by Medicare

EXAMPLES OF COVERED SERVICES

- Acute hospital care
- Selected skilled nursing care
- Home health care within defined limits
- Diagnostic laboratory testing
- Diagnostic radiologic testing
- Physical therapy
- Speech pathology services
- Ambulance (when health is at risk)
- Kidney dialysis or transplant
- Medications given in the hospital or skilled nursing facility
- Selected outpatient medications
- Physician care for medical and surgical services, treatments, tests, and procedures
- Outpatient and emergency care for illness or accidents
- Prosthetic devices
- Durable medical equipment (e.g., oxygen, wheelchairs, home dialysis)
- Medical supplies (e.g., syringes, dressings)
- Hospice benefits
- Respite care under specific conditions
- Mental health services (only 180 days paid for a lifetime)

EXAMPLES OF SERVICES NOT COVERED

- Long-term care
- Preventive health services (e.g., immunizations, physical examinations)
- Hearing examinations and hearing aids
- Dental care (nonserious)
- Eye examinations and eye glasses

---

jor diagnostic categories (for example, diseases of the respiratory system or diseases of the circulatory system). Most of the categories contain a medical and surgical division. Each division is then further broken down into DRGs, totaling 492 (Lorenz, 1992). The specific DRG assigned depends primarily on a client's principal medical diagnosis. However, secondary diagnoses, operating room procedures, age, discharge status, complications, and comorbidities (preexisting conditions) are also considered. A hospital receives one payment for each Medicare discharge based on the DRG classification, regardless of actual cost for caring for a client. The formula for determining payment is weighted, depending on the intensity and changes in resource consumption. Each DRG is assigned an average length of stay.

CASE STUDY OF CALCULATING DRG PAYMENT

Case description: Mr. Truman was admitted to the hospital on Nov. 1 after experiencing chest pain and shortness of breath. He had undergone cardiac surgery almost 10 years before but was beginning to again have symptoms of problems. He was scheduled for a cardiac catheterization, but it was delayed until Nov. 3. The physician also referred Mr. Truman for diet counseling for a low-cholesterol diet. The cardiac catheterization proceeded without complications, and surgery was unnecessary. Mr. Truman remained hospitalized overnight to ensure that no problems developed. He was discharged on Nov. 4.

- *Principal diagnosis:* Ischemia, heart
- *Secondary diagnosis:* Disturbances, heart, functional, long-term effect of cardiac surgery
- *DRG assigned:* DRG 125: circulatory disorders except acute myocardial infarction with cardiac catheterization without complex diagnosis
- *Assigned or allowed length of stay:* 2.2 days
- *Actual length of stay:* 3.1 days
- *Payment calculation (based on 2.2 days):* Payment per discharge × DRG weight = $3400 × 0.7015 = $2385
- *Actual hospital costs for Mr. Truman:* $2960
- *Loss for hospital:* $575

---

ipate in Medicare, although many states are considering making it mandatory for licensure. If a physician accepts assignment (that is, the Medicare payment), there is a percentage of the fee (for example, 20%) is paid by the client. Participants in the program are encouraged to purchase supplemental insurance plans through private insurers. Coverage by Medicare can be confusing to a client. The Social Security Administration offers pamphlets explaining all benefits.

Payment by the government for services offered under Medicare is based on the DRG classification system. This classification system is based on 23 ma-

A significant change in Medicare arose with passage of OBRA in 1990. To meet the federal government's deficit reduction target for 1991, OBRA caused a reduction in Medicare payments for physician and other part-B services by 2%. The bill prohibits physicians who accept Medicare as payment-in-full from recovering the reduction by billing clients. Payment rates for other health care providers such as nurse practitioners, nurse midwives, and nurse anesthetists were also reduced (Grimaldi, 1991). There is a growing concern that Medicare benefits will continue to drop.

Medicaid

Medicaid is the government insurance program for persons of very low income. Coverage is regulated by states. Nationally, the average income eligibility requirement for Medicaid is less than half of the 1990 federal poverty level (nationally defined income level below which a family is considered "poor") (Rooks, 1990). Specifically, a family of three with an income of more than $5000 per year was too well off to qualify for Medicaid.

Medicaid has financed a large portion of maternal and child care for the poor. Since 1963 the Medicaid program has helped improve child health and reduce infant mortality rates through prenatal care. However, in 1981, major cuts in Medicaid programs were instituted by the Reagan administration. A financial crisis threatened most government-funded social and health programs.

With demands exceeding resources, many states toughened Medicaid eligibility rules. A study in 1988 showed that the United States had the nineteenth lowest infant mortality rate among industrialized nations (Cohen, 1990). This embarassing statistic prompted Congress to take steps to restore Medicaid funding. As of 1989, all states must provide Medicaid coverage for pregnant women and for children up to the age of 6 if family income is less than 133% of the federal poverty level.

An increased number of impoverished people who fail to qualify for Medicaid do not have access to health care. With the growing number of poor, the funds for Medicaid are dwindling. Many hospitals and other agencies are taking measures to minimize treatment of medicaid clients because they are not reimbursed for their costs. Obvious reforms to the Medicaid system are needed. Many Medicaid-eligible citizens are being asked to enter HMO plans for better managed medical care.

DRGs

In 1983, the Medicare health insurance part A plan converted to prospective reimbursement using the DRG system. Originally, 383 DRGs were used to establish fixed payments for select medical conditions regardless of actual hospital costs (see box). Today there are 492 DRGs. In theory the objective of the **prospective payment** system is to provide incentives for hospitals to lower costs. For example, the DRG fee for gallbladder removal requiring hospital stay of 5 days might be set at $2500, a figure set on the basis of services that should be required over a projected length of stay. In hospital X, however, these services might typically cost $3000 and the hospital charged $3500. Because Medicare reim-

burses the hospital only $2500, regardless of actual costs, the hospital operates at a loss. The hospital is given the incentive to find other methods of providing quality care to recover costs and make a profit. The hospital is also motivated not to keep the client hospitalized longer than necessary because the reimbursement is the same regardless of the client's actual length of stay.

In theory, prospective payments should help contain costs and even be an incentive for improved quality. Hospitals know the projected length of stay for each DRG and the anticipated payment. Opportunities to reduce system delays and inefficiencies, find better diagnostic measures, coordinate care more efficiently, and reduce unnecessary procedures should improve quality care. The longer clients are hospitalized, the greater risk for complications. On the other hand, there is public concern that prospective payments might reduce the quality of care in certain cases. For example, the hospital might be tempted to discharge the client who had gallbladder surgery after 5 days, even though, by its past standards, the client would have remained in the hospital another day or two.

Regulatory mechanisms within the Medicare system protect clients from premature discharge and reduced standards of care. Protection of clients is ensured by audits of records by federal authorities. If these audits identify a trend to prematurely discharge clients, resulting in readmission to the hospital within 7 days, the hospital risks losing reimbursement funds.

Catastrophic Health Insurance

The advanced technology of medical care in the United States has created challenging problems. More people are surviving illness and are living longer. Conditions that in the past would have proved fatal can now be treated successfully. The high costs associated with major and chronic illness are not covered by most insurance programs. In July 1988 the Medicare Catastrophic Coverage Act was passed to provide protection against the overwhelming out-of-pocket costs of major lengthy illnesses. Medicare recipients must pay flat premiums for the coverage. In addition, Medicare recipients who file income tax returns pay an additional fee based on taxable income.

The catastrophic coverage includes benefits for clients hospitalized over 60 days. There is also a limit on the amount that clients will be required to pay for physician fees. Expanded coverage for medications has also been added. Despite the revisions, it is estimated that only 17% of Medicare enrollees will benefit from the change (Ebersole, Hess, 1990).

Canadian Government Health Insurance

The Canadian government has an integrated health care system with national health insurance. All citizens of Canada are covered by the mandatory program financed with tax dollars. Benefits are comprehensive, including short- and long-term care, and involve use of private-sector providers of services. The plan bypasses middlemen. Thus the government negotiates directly with providers to establish reasonable health care rates. Canada has substantially lower health care costs than the United States (8.6% of the GNP compared with 11.2%) (Harrington, 1990). The Canadian health care plan is more cost effective in that it has fewer expenditures on insurance, prepayment, and administration costs, and the costs to hospitals and physicians are also lower.

 PROBLEMS WITH THE SYSTEM

The health care system in the United States is one of the largest and most extensive in the world. However, it has many problems. The problems that plague health care are not new but have been aggravated by societal changes and system mismanagement. Because nurses make up the largest segment of health care professionals and because they care for clients 24 hours a day, they have an opportunity to work for solutions to the problems. Ironically, during a time of turmoil, nursing has one of its best opportunities as a profession to show its unique contributions to health care.

Issues for the 1990s

Cost Control

As health care costs rise (see box) and reimbursement for services declines, institutions are being asked to exercise cost containment. The challenge is to reduce costs without sacrificing the quality of care. If measures to reduce costs are not well planned, clients may suffer. For example, there is an ongoing effort to reduce resource utilization in the delivery of care to hospitalized clients. Physicians and nurses are being asked to use fewer resources such as laboratory or radiological tests, types of equipment, and even medications. If these resources are reduced without appropriate clinical analysis of possible client outcomes, serious problems can arise. Clients may suffer more complications and ultimately remain hospitalized longer. Similarly, there is considerable effort

---

Common Causes for High Costs of Medical Care

- Increased population and demand for services
- Increased number of people with chronic illnesses
- Increased cost of new technology and equipment
- Inflation
- Increased specialization of care
- Increased number of people over 65 years of age
- Increased number of clients surviving traumatic, disabling injuries or life-threatening illnesses
- Increased survival rates of infants with low birth weight and neonates who are ill
- Increase in the acuity of hospitalized clients using more resources
- Increased need for more professional staff members to care for acutely ill clients
- Use of unnecessary diagnostic and therapeutic services

---

to discharge clients from hospitals as soon as possible. Shorter hospitalizations can reduce complications and overall costs. However, if a client's length of stay is shortened without proper consideration of resources needed for health care in the home, the system may not serve a client properly. Coordination of care must remain an essential part of care delivery.

Specialization

Advanced scientific knowledge and technology have resulted in the increasing specialization of health care in areas such as cardiac disease, kidney disease, and cancer. Although specialization allows each professional to provide clients with highly advanced care, the delivery of total care is often fragmented. The number of primary physicians and care givers has gradually declined, and many families might have a different physician for each family member or illness. As a result, care is not provided for the family as a unit or for the whole person. The care giver is therefore unable to assess family or personal dynamics and its impact on level of health. With so many specialists involved, the client can be lost to follow-up simply because it is too difficult to cope with so many specialists. Furthermore, as the client goes from one specialist to another, the cost of care increases, the client can be overmedicated or undermedicated, and quality of life is changed because of the time involved in obtaining care.

Older Adult Population

Older adults comprise a significant portion of clients within the health care system. Chronic illnesses affect older adults more often than children or young adults. Because people live longer, the number of clients with chronic disease grows. Quality of life versus length of time that one is able to remain alive also becomes an issue as physicians develop treatments that prolong life. The health care system must address the special care requirements of the chronically ill by providing proper health care facilities and ensuring that professionals are prepared to care for the needs of older adults.

Access

Even though a large percentage of the GNP goes to health care, a significant portion of the population has limited access to the health care delivery system. Access is restricted by geographic, financial, and attitudinal barriers. Many people living in rural areas are simply not close to a source for health care. Low-income communities do not often have the fiscal resources necessary to establish or maintain major health care services. As competition for hospital cost containment increases, small hospitals that provide illness care to rural areas become less financially viable (Mitchell et al, 1990).

A person who does not have a source of funds to pay for personal health care is a victim of financial barriers. The number of people covered by private hospital insurance is shrinking because the number of part-time and service industry jobs, which provide limited or no health insurance, is growing. Meanwhile, the number of manufacturing and transportation jobs that usually provide full insurance coverage is shrinking (Hudson Institute, 1987).

Governmental health insurance plans were designed to help older adults and needy people access health care. However, federal budget cuts have reduced the number of indigent persons receiving help. Basically a person must be very poor to receive available funds. Estimates from a variety of resources reveal that the number of uninsured and underinsured continues to grow. To further aggravate accessibility, the number of institutions that once cared for the indigent is declining. To collect a reserve of money to be used for care of indigent clients, a hospital at one time could increase the price for an insured client above the actual costs. Prospective reimbursement through the DRG system prevents this practice. The costs of uncompensated care are now borne directly by institutions and providers, threatening their existence.

A true health care delivery system should include activities that promote health and prevent, treat, and rehabilitate from disease (Mitchell et al, 1990). Unfortunately, the U.S. health care system has traditionally focused on treatment or care of disease. In contrast, the Canadian health care system is more comprehensive. To have an adequate health care policy, there must be an integration of social factors such as housing, nutrition, and long-term care for chronic ailments. The present attitude of the U.S. health care system excludes the promotion of community and societal health.

Quality

As public awareness about health care improves and as the statistics for performance of the health care system become available, quality of care will become a serious issue. For example, the United States has one of the worst infant mortality rates for the poor. Hospital mortality and morbidity rates are now available for public review and raise questions about the efficacy of certain therapies. To determine the quality of health care, a person must ask about the outcomes of care. Outcomes are the result (desirable or undesirable) of care delivered (Williams, 1991). For example, nosocomial (hospital-acquired) infection rates, surgical wound healing, and ability to perform self-care are all outcomes. The JCAHO has created an *Agenda for Change* with objectives for the 1990s. Health care facilities will have to demonstrate a commitment to quality of care for all clients. Unless quality can be proved, institutions will not remain accredited, and government funding will be withdrawn.

Solutions for the 1990s

Nursing's Agenda for Change (ANA, 1991) is supported by numerous health care organizations such as the ANA and NLN. The document presents nursing's recommendations for steps to achieve immediate health care reform (see box). Successful achievement of this agenda will shift the focus of health care from illness and cure to wellness and care (ANA, 1991). A variety of solutions are needed to create excellence in health care.

Managed Care and Case Management

In the past, care givers from all disciplines such as nursing, medicine, and social work managed a client's care within a hospital by contributing their own plans of care. There has always been an objective to coordinate the work of all care givers so that a single plan was followed with favorable outcomes. This was not always easy to accomplish, depending on the nursing delivery-of-care model (see Chapter 1) or the collaboration of all care givers. For example, team

Nursing's Agenda for Health Care Reform

The basic components of nursing's "core of care" include:

- A restructured health care system that:
  - Enhances consumer access to services by delivering primary health care in community settings
  - Fosters consumer responsibility for personal health, self-care, and informed decision making in selecting health care services
  - Facilitates the use of the most cost-effective providers and therapeutic options
- A federally-defined standard package of essential health care services available to all citizens and residents of the United States, provided and financed through an integration of public and private plans and sources:
- A phase-in of essential services, so that the health care delivery system can be fiscally responsible in the:
  - Coverage of pregnant women and children, which is critical
  - Design of services that specifically assist vulnerable popuations who have had limited access to the health care delivery system. (A "Healthstart Plan" is proposed to improve the health status of these individuals.)
- Planned change to anticipate health care service needs that correlate with changing national demographics
- Steps to reduce health care costs, including:
  - Required use of managed care in a public health plan and encouraged in private plans
  - Incentives for consumers and providers to use managed-care arrangements

- Controlled growth of the health care delivery system through planning and prudent resource allocation
- Incentives for consumers and providers to be more cost efficient in exercising health care options
- Development of health care policies based on effectiveness and outcomes research
- Ensurance of direct access to a full range of qualified providers
- Elimination of unnecessary bureaucratic controls and administrative procedures
- Case management required for clients with continuing health care needs
- Provisions for long-term care, including:
  - Public and private funding for services of short duration to prevent personal impoverishment
  - Public funding for extended care
  - Emphasis on the consumers' responsibility to financially plan for long-term care needs
- Insurance reforms to ensure improved access to coverage
- Access to services ensured by no payment at the point of service and elimination of balance billing in public and private plans
- Establishment of public or private-sector review—operating under federal guidelines and including payers, providers, and consumers—to determine resource allocation, cost reduction approaches, allowable insurance premiums, and fair and consistent reimbursement levels (This review would progress in a climate sensitive to ethical issues.)

Adapted from ANA: *Nursing's agenda for health care reform*, Kansas City, Mo, 1991, The Association.

nursing was so focused on the tasks of nursing care that little effort was given to ensure continuity of discharge planning and participation by all care givers. Managed-care and case-management systems are improving collaboration of care givers and the ability to deliver quality services. The "product" of most health care agencies is the provision of services by health care professionals in an efficient and effective manner with expected outcomes (Pierog, 1991). With managed care and case management, typically one care giver coordinates care from admission through discharge from an acute-care setting into an outpatient or home health care environment. A multidisciplinary plan is implemented so that all care givers work with one plan to achieve the same client outcomes.

A popular tool used in managed care and case management is a **critical pathway.** These pathways are multidisciplinary treatment plans that sequence interventions over a projected length of stay for specific case types. Initially developed by Zander (1988) at the New England Medical Center in Boston, a critical path tells care givers what care needs to be given and when so that a client is discharged on time and in as healthy a condition as possible. Ideally, critical pathways incorporate expected outcomes throughout hospitalization and at the time of discharge (Fig 3-1). Typically a primary nurse, often called a *case manager,* coordinates a client's progress through a pathway. The nurse is responsible for communicating with other care givers so that a client's progress is uninterrupted. In some settings, the nurse case man-

BARNES		**CARE PATH** **560 RENAL TRANSPLANT**				
SERVICE						
PHYSICIAN		PRIMARY NURSE				
DC DATE	ADM DATE	DATE OF SURGERY	**A-8**			

PROBLEM NUMBER	**PATIENT PROBLEMS / NURSING DIAGNOSES**
#1	POTENTIAL FOR INFECTION
#2	ALTERATION IN FLUID VOLUME
#3	LACK OF KNOWLEDGE
#4	DECREASED ACTIVITY TOLERANCE
#5	ADJUSTMENT TO ILLNESS / TREATMENT
#6	INCREASED RISK FOR NUTRITIONAL ALTERATION

PROBLEM NUMBER		**PRE - ADMIT**	**DAY 1 PRE-OP / DOS**	**DAY 2 POD 1**	**DAY 3 POD 2**	**DAY 4 POD 3**	**DAY 5**
#1 **#2**	**ASSESSMENT / MONITORING**		ADM Weight / VS I & O q 1 Hr Wgt. immed. post-op VS q 30 min x 4 hr q 1hr x 24 BGM q 30 min - 1hr Foley	I & O q 1 Hr Wgt q AM VS q 2hr x 24 hr BGM q 2hr Daily Care Foley	I & O q 1 Hr Wgt q AM VS q 4hr if stable x1 x2 x3 x4 x5 x6 BGM q 2hr Daily Care Foley	I & O q Shift Wgt q AM VS q 4hr if stable x1 x2 x3 x4 x5 x6 BGM qid x1 x2 x3 x4 Daily Care Foley **UO ≥ 50 cc/hr. Absence of inflammation at surgical site** **No peripheral edema**	I & O q Shift Wgt q AM VS q 4hr if stable x1 x2 x3 x4 x5 x6 BGM qid x1 x2 x3 x4 Daily Care Foley
	CONSULTS		Renal Service Metabolism TXP. Coord	Dietary Referral P.T. O.T. Social Work DM CNS referral if indicated			
#1 **#2**	**PROCEDURE / TEST**		On Admission: Labs EXG CXR	Daily CBC SMA6 CSA	Daily CBC SMA6 If glucose ≥200 inititate bld glucose monitoring CSA	Daily CBC SMA6 If glucose ≥200 inititate bld glucose monitoring CSA	Daily CBC SMA6 If glucose ≥200 inititate bld glucose monitoring CSA
#1 **#2**	**TREATMENT**		TCDB q 2 hr IS q 2 hr 40% HHM	TCDB q 2 hr IS q 2 hr D/C O₂	TCDB q 2 hr IS q 2 hr	D/C TCDB D/C IS **Lungs clear to ausculation**	
#4	**ACTIVITY**		Bedrest	Up walking with assist qid P.T. x1 x2 Nursing x3 x4	P.T.: Increase amb distance until up ad lib TID P.T. x1 x2 Nursing x3	P.T.: Increase amb distance until up ad lib TID P.T. x1 x2 Nursing x3 **Independence with bathing at sink**	P.T.: Increase amb distance until up ad lib TID P.T. x1 x2 Nursing x3

Fig. 3-1   Example of a section of a care path.
Courtesy Barnes Hospital, St Louis.

ager may even coordinate care on a pathway when the client is transferred to a different unit. There are also institutions that assign case managers only to high-risk clients.

If pathways are developed correctly, fewer resources (for example, laboratory or radiological tests) are used; yet the clinical outcomes of care (for example, avoidance of complications or successful achievement of rehabilitation) are realized in a desired time frame. By reducing costs and ensuring quality outcomes, critical pathways are a solution to major health care delivery problems. Critical pathways may also be developed for home health or skilled nursing facilities.

National Health Care Plan

Because of the problems of access and rising health care costs, there is growing public interest in a national health care plan. The goal of such a plan would be to provide all Americans with health insurance coverage. The task of nursing as a profession is to understand and select the best option for a health care plan. Harrington (1990) summarizes the types of plans under debate:

1. Incremental expansion of existing public programs (that is, Medicare and Medicaid)
2. Mandatory requirements on employers to offer private health insurance to employees
3. A comprehensive national health plan inclusive of all medically necessary care (acute, long term, rehabilitation, dental, and occupational health) financed through progressive taxes

The expansion of existing public programs would greatly benefit the poor. Several groups who have made health care reform proposals (Table 3-1) have also recommended adding long-term care benefits. This is popular among the elderly and disabled because only 52% of nursing home services as of 1990 were covered by public or private insurance (Harrington, 1990). A problem with Medicare expansion proposals is that a part-C voluntary program would be added. Persons with low incomes and the greatest need for services would likely not contribute. Another problem is the administrative inefficiency of incremental expansion programs. Medicaid and Medicare are regulated through different eligibility requirements and benefits across states. A single, integrated program is needed to ensure fair distribution to all.

TABLE 3-1 Health Care Reform Proposals	
Coverage	Benefits
KENNEDY/WAXMAN	**BENEFITS**
Employers would cover full-time workers; Medicaid covers low-income and uninsured workers.	Plan would provide hospital, physician, all prenatal and well-baby examinations, diagnostic test, and some mental health benefits. Maximum, out-of-pocket expenses are $3000 per family.
PHYSICIANS FOR A NATIONAL HEALTH PROGRAM	
National health program would cover everyone under public insurance program.	Plan would include all medically necessary care, including acute, long-term, rehabilitation, dental, and occupational health care and prescriptions; there is no cost sharing.
ENTHOVEN/KRONICK	
Employers would provide insurance to employees and their dependents; Medicare and Medicaid would continue with states offering subsidized voluntary insurance for all others.	Plan would include basic benefits packages of HMO Act subject to tighter definitions and restrictions. Physician, inpatient, and outpatient hospital services; medically needed emergency services; alcohol, drug, and medical referral services; laboratory and radiology services; home health care and preventative services. Out-of-pocket costs cannot exceed 100% of insurance premium.
PEPPER COMMISSION	
This is combined employment-based and public plan. Businesses with more than 100 employees would be required to provide private health insurance or contribute to public plan for all employees and dependents.	Plan would include basic hospital and physician services, limited mental health benefits, and preventative services. Maximum out-of-pocket expense per person is $3000

The employer-based financing programs combine public and private financing mechanisms. Employers offer private insurance plans or pay taxes for public insurance coverage (Harrington, 1990). In addition, employers can buy insurance directly through public sponsors, and individuals would be encouraged to join managed care plans such as HMOs. Medicaid and Medicare would continue with most of these plans; however, there could be some restructuring to shift resources from acute to chronic and long-term care.

The problem with this category of plan is that many people would not be covered because small businesses, the self-employed, and part-time workers would be exempt.

The comprehensive national health plan is modeled like the Canadian health plan. The plan would be mandatory and cover all individuals for comprehensive health services. Private-sector providers would provide services. Costly copayments and deductibles common with traditional insurance would be eliminated. It is believed that a single well-administered health plan would save millions of dollars. Hospitals and nursing homes would receive annual lump sum payments for all expenses ("global budgets"), based on past expenses, clinical performance, volume services, wages, and costs (Himmelstein, Woolhandler, 1989). Physicians would be paid on a fee-for-service plan. The concerns over the national health plan comes from the proposed progressive tax system needed to fund the plan.

Nursing Services

The problems of the health care system raise the question as to the worth of the medical model, which focuses primarily on illness. Nursing has always supported a holistic model for health care, integrating the person, care givers, society, environment, and health. However, the present health care system continues to emphasize curing rather than caring for an individual. Nursing can make a significant contribution by becoming more involved in all levels of health care. Nurses can provide services at a more cost-effective and qualitative level than other providers (Maraldo, 1989). Fagin and Maraldo (1989) note that, if nurses were willing to take a percentage of physician charges rather than an equal fee-for-service charge, it would be possible to have a more cost-effective delivery of services. Consumers must learn what nurses can offer in preventive and **primary care** services. Primary care is the first contact in a given episode of illness that leads to a decision regarding a course of action to resolve the health care problem. In addition, nurses should take an active lead in reorganizing and coordinating health care systems.

Gerontological Care

As the number of older adults within our population increases, it becomes critical for nursing and other professions to understand the unique science of gerontology. For a long time, physicians and nurses have accepted pediatrics as a branch of medicine concerned with the development and care of children. Only during the last two decades has a specific body of knowledge been established pertaining to the physiologic characteristics of aging, diseases of aging, and the psychologic, economic, and sociologic problems of the older adults. An older adult has different health concerns than a middle-age adult. Gunter (1987) defines *gerontologic nursing* as

a health service that incorporates gerontic nursing methods and specialized knowledge about the aged to establish conditions within the client and/or environment that will increase health-conducive behaviors, minimize health losses and disability, provide comfort and sustenance and facilitate diagnosis, palliation, and treatment of disease in the aged.

The rapidly growing specialty of gerontologic nursing prepares nurses to design strategies aimed at helping older adults maintain functioning and independence. The collaboration of all health care disciplines is needed for improved care. More long-term care facilities designed to provide safe, functional, and stimulating environments for older adults are needed. Finally, gerontologic nurses can administer the type of care needed to support chronically ill and disabled older adults.

Quality Improvement

Efforts in ensuring and improving the quality of health care have never been as important as they are today. The health care agencies that survive in the 1990s will be able to guarantee a superior level of quality of care. Third-party payors will likely contract with successful organizations. For example, if a hospital uses managed care to successfully lower complications and improve clients' functional states after treatment for cancer, the hospital will receive payer support.

Health care is behind industry in regards to quality management. The terms most frequently discussed in the health care literature have been *quality assurance* and *quality improvement*. Quality assurance (QA) is the ongoing systematic monitoring or evaluation of nursing practice, medical practice, or practice of other disciplines. Traditionally, QA has focused on clinical practice, providing information on the appropriateness of nursing care processes and activities. QA programs direct staff to inspect and repair rather than prevent, innovate, and develop personnel (Schroeder, 1988). Deming is the American businessman responsible for creating the now famous management strategies that have elevated the Japanese in the world market. Deming's work (1986) has created the quality-improvement movement in American business. Quality improvement (QI) has become the new focus in health care. It is a more integrated,

coordinated approach to find ways to continually improve practices and services. A focus is the elimination of barriers that impede clients' use of the health care system at a nursing unit or agency. The JCAHO agenda for the 1990s will be to have health care disciplines collaborate more to identify the best possible clinical practice that can gurantee repeated favorable outcomes for clients.

SUMMARY

The health care industry is the most rapidly growing and changing in North America. Because of its rapid expansion and increased costs, patterns of use by clients have changed, and new emphases are emerging. Consumers of health care now demand health-promotion and health-maintenance services that are affordable and accessible. The growing population of needy persons and older adults in the United States require an aggressive look at solutions needed to improve the quality and availability of health care.

Today's health care delivery system is much better than in the past, but it still has problems. Financing health care has placed a burden on private and government resources. Technological advances have resulted in high-quality specialized care, but specialization has led to fragmentation of care. Finally, health care services are still unevenly distributed.

Nursing is in a position to influence the future of health care. The traditional medical model for health care is no longer responsive to the holistic needs of clients. Cost-effectiveness, expansion of nursing services, and QI are just some examples of nursing activities that will help solve health care system problems.

CHAPTER 3 REVIEW

Key Concepts

- Health care services are provided in a large number of settings, across all age groups, and for the chronically and acutely ill.
- The growth of the health care industry has resulted in specialization of health care professionals.
- Consumers are requesting more information, especially on services related to illness prevention and health promotion.
- Chronically ill and disabled clients are seeking knowledge and skills to maximize their levels of wellness and independence.
- Needy persons in the United States have reduced accessibility to health care services.
- Increased technology and new biomedical equipment increase the risk of health care professionals giving greater attention to the machine than to the client.
- A nation's economy directly affects the fiscal resources of the health care delivery system.
- The Medicare prospective reimbursement system is based on payment calculated on the basis of DRG assignment.
- Health-promotion activities are designed to help clients reduce the risk of illness, maintain maximal function, and promote lifestyle habits related to good health.
- Illness-prevention activities are directed at helping the client and family reduce risk factors.
- Diagnosis and treatment activities are usually disease-specific, with the goal of curing the client.
- Rehabilitation allows an individual to return to a level of normal or near-normal function after a physical or mental illness, injury, or chemical dependency.
- Community-based agencies focus on providing health care to clients within their neighborhoods.
- Crisis intervention centers provide emergency psychiatric treatment and counseling to clients experiencing extreme stress or conflict.
- A rehabilitation center uses a multidisciplinary health care team to restore the client to a maximal level of physical, emotional, or mental wellness.
- Psychiatric mental health agencies provide inpatient and outpatient counseling services to clients with behavioral or emotional illnesses.
- A hospice provides family-centered care to help clients maintain satisfactory levels of comfort and lifestyles through the terminal phases of illness.
- Government agencies can be local, regional, or national and are supported by revenues obtained through taxes.
- Prepaid health care can be obtained through health maintenance organizations, preferred provider organizations, or individual practice associations.

- Clients may enter the health care system through referral and because of specific health needs.
- Financing of health care services is primarily through private and managed health care plans or government support.
- Nursing is able to reduce health care costs by implementing cost-containment measures, such as primary care, and expanding nursing activities into low-income and rural regions.

Key Terms

Adult day-care centers, p. 72

Crisis intervention centers, p. 73

Critical pathway, p. 85

Diagnostic-related group (DRG), p. 70

Drug rehabilitation centers, p. 72

Extended care facility, p. 71

Government agencies, p. 74

Health Maintenance Organization (HMO), p. 79

Home health care agency, p. 73

Hospice, p. 74

Independent practice association (IPA), p. 79

Informed consent, p. 77

Inpatients, p. 70

Medicaid, p. 82

Medicare, p. 80

Outpatient services, p. 69

Preferred provider organizations (PPOs), p. 80

Primary care, p. 88

Prospective payment, p. 82

Psychiatric facilities, p. 71

Rehabilitation, p. 69

Rehabilitation center, p. 71

Respite care, p. 74

Third-party reimbursements, p. 79

Utilization review, p. 67

Volunteer agencies, p. 73

Critical Thinking Exercises

1. Trinity hospital is a 300-bed acute-care hospital that provides outpatient and inpatient services. Recently the percentage of clients cared for under Medicare has risen from 35% to 42%. In addition, another 36% of the clients belong to PPOs. Approximately 10% have Medicaid and the remainder have private insurance. What can be done to improve the hospital's ability to be profitable? What would the role of the nurse be in those improvements?

2. Consider Mr. Wilson, a 68-year-old client who will have major surgery to replace the joint in his hip. Afterward, extensive therapy will be needed for him to again walk normally. Describe the type of health care agencies that might become involved in the care of Mr. Wilson.

3. Explain the different problems faced by a client living in a large urban area versus a small rural community with respect to accessibility to health care services.

4. Nurse managers are responsible for ensuring that the nursing staffs under their supervision provide quality and cost-effective care to clients. What might the managers study before deciding to recommend a new type of bed for clients?

REFERENCES

American Nurses Association: *Nursing's agenda for health care reform,* Kansas City, Mo, 1991, The Association.

Beck DF: The hospital's financial future: DRGs and beyond, *Health Care Superv* 3:1, 1985.

Cohen S: The politics of Medicaid: 1980-1989, *Nurs Outlook* 38(5):229, 1990.

Curtin L: Rube Goldberg and the great American healthcare system, *Nurs Manage* 22(5):9, 1991 (editorial).

Deming WE: *Out of the crisis,* Cambridge, Mass 1986, MIT Center for Advanced Engineering.

Drew JC: Health maintenance organizations: history, evolution and survival, *Nurs Health Care* 11(3):145, 1989.

Ebersole P, Hess P: *Toward healthy aging: human needs and nursing response,* ed 3, St Louis, 1990, Mosby–Year Book.

Ermann D: Preferred provider organizations: implications of the fatest growing health care options, *Consultant* 27(4):102, 1987.

Fagin CM and Maraldo P: An interview with Claire M. Fagin: perspectives on Nursing in today's health care envirnoment, *Nurs Econ* 7(4):186, 1989.

Gensberg F: Long-term care nursing. In Ebersole P, Hess P: *Toward healthy aging: human needs and nursing response,* St Louis, 1981, Mosby–Year Book.

Grimaldi PL: Congress slices Medicare physician fees, *Nurs Manage,* 22(1):22, 1991.

Gunter LM: Nomenclature: what is in the name "gerontic nursing"? *J Gerontol Nurs* 13:7, 1987 (editorial).

Harrington C: Policy options for a national health care plan, *Nurs Outlook* 38(5):223, 1990.

Hillman AL: Cost containment incentives in HMOs: what's known, what's not known, *Consultant* 29:84, 1989.

Himmelstein DU and Woolhandler S: A national health program for the United States, *N Engl J Med* 320:102, 1989.

Hudson Institute: *Workforce 2000: work and workers for the 21st century,* Indianapolis, 1987, The Institute.

Lorenz E: *DRG working guidebook,* St. Anthony's Publishing, 1992, Alexandria, Va.

Maraldo PJ: The nursing solution, *Health Manage Q* 11(4):18, 1989.

Marmor TR: *Political analysis and american medical Care,* Cambridge, Mass, 1983, Cambridge University Press.

McMahon LF: The development of diagnosis-related groups. In Burdsley M, Coles J, Jenkins L, editors: *DRGs and health care,* London, 1987, King Edward Hospital Fund for London.

Mitchell PH et al: The crisis of the healthcare nonsystem, *Nurs Outlook* 38(5):214, 1990.

Namazi K: *Summary of environmental design issues,* Chardon, Ohio, 1988, Corinne Dolan Alzheimer Center (unpublished manuscript).

Pierog LJ: Case management: a product line, *Nurs Adm Q* 15(2):16, 1991.

Rooks JP: Let's admit we ration health care—then set priorities, *Am J Nurs* 90:39, 1990.

Schroeder P: Directions and dilemmas in nursing quality assurance, *Nurs Clin North Am* 23(3):657, 1988.

Sharp N: Rural healthcare: new opportunities for nurses, *Nurs Manage* 22(3):22, 1991.

Smith CE: DRGs: making them work for you, *Nurs 85* 15:1, 1985.

Smith JP: The politics of American healthcare, *J Adv Nurs* 15:487, 1990.

Soderstrom L: *The Canadian health care system,* London, 1981, Croom Helm.

Soderstrom L.: Soaring hospital costs: the brewing revolt, *U.S. News & World Report,* Aug 22, 1983.

Sovie M: Redesigning our future: whose responsibility is it? *Nurs Econ* 8(1):21, 1990.

Stewart M et al: Community health nursing in Canada, Toronto, 1985, Gage.

US Bureau of the Census: 1988.

US Department of Commerce: 1990.

Williams AD: Development and application of clinical indicators for nursing, *J Nurs Care Qual* 6(1):1, 1991.

Zander K: Managed care within acute care settings: design and implementation via nursing care management, *Health Care Superv* 6(2):27, 1988.

ADDITIONAL READINGS

American Hospital Association: *AHA Medicare payment: special report 3*, Chicago, 1983, The Association.

Canadian Hospital Association: *Introduction to nursing management: a Canadian perspective to nursing management*, Ottawa, 1985, The Association.

Dunston J: How managed care can work for you, *Nurs 90* 90:56, 1990.

Fagin CM: Nursing as an alternative to high-cost care, *Am J Nurs* 82:56, 1982.

Flomann MP, Shaffer FA: DRGs as one of nine approaches to case mix in transition, *Nurs Health Care* 4(8):438, 1983.

Fox RT: DRGs: a management control tool in hospitals and multi-institutional systems, *Hosp Prog* 62:52, 1981.

Fromer MJ: *What's fair?* Paper presented at the Forum of the Health Care Financing Administration, Washington, DC, April 16-21, 1985.

Griffith H: Who will become the preferred providers? *Am J Nurs* 85:538, 1985.

Halloran E, Halloran DC: Exploring the DRG/nursing equation, *Am J Nurs* 85:1093, 1985.

Hunt K: DRG: what it is, how it works, and why it will hurt, *Med Econ* 60:262, 1983.

Maraldo PJ, Solomon SB: Nursing's window of opportunity, *Image J Nurs Sch* 19:83, 1987.

Moccia P: 1989: Shaping a human agenda for the nineties, *Nurs Health Care* January, 1989.

Moccia P, Pfordresner K: If nurses had their way, *Ms* 146:104, 1983.

Shukla RK, Tuner WE: Patient's perception of care under primary nursing and team nursing, *Res Nurs Health* 7:93, 1984.

Waters S: What happens if your hospital bills separately for nursing? *RN* 48(7):18, 1985.

White CH: Redefining professional nursing: solution to the chronic shortage? *Hosp Prog* 62:40, 1981.

Yano-Fong D: Advantages and disadvantages of product-line management, *Nurs Manage* 19(5):27, 1988.

CHAPTER 4

Culture, Ethnicity, and Nursing

OBJECTIVES

Mastery of the content in this chapter will enable the student to:

- Define the key terms listed.
- Explain the need for a nurse's self-evaluation when providing care to clients from other sociocultural backgrounds.
- Describe heritage-consistent and heritage-inconsistent attributes.
- Describe the relationship of sociocultural background to health and illness beliefs and practices.
- Describe cultural phenomena—environmental control, biological variations, social organization, communication, space, and time—that apply to culturally sensitive nursing practice.
- Compare concepts of traditional and modern health and illness beliefs and practices.
- List general health and illness beliefs and practices of Asian, African, Native, Spanish, and European Americans.
- Perform a cultural assessment using the heritage-consistency assessment tool.
- Discuss several ways in which planning and implementation of nursing interventions can be adapted to a client's ethnicity.

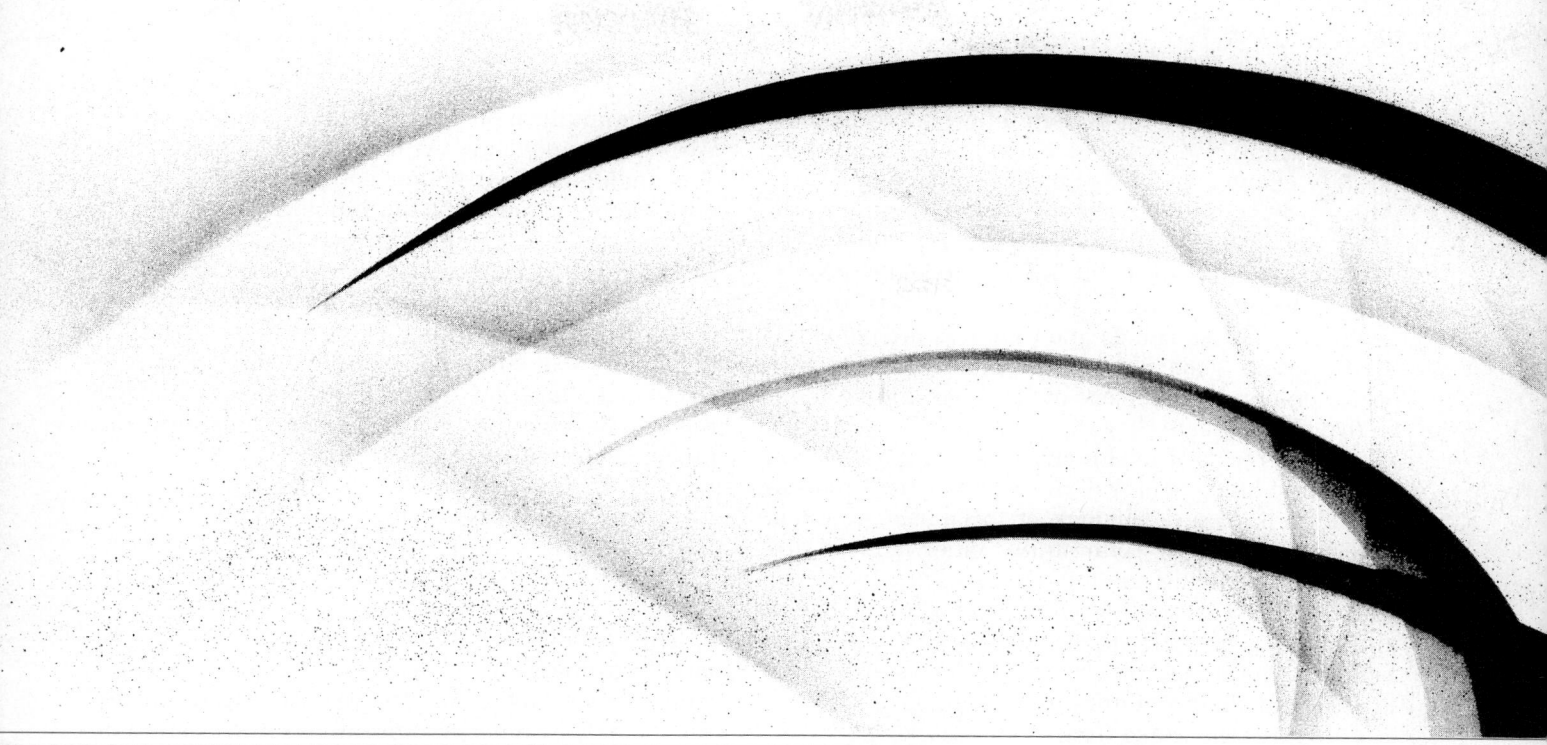

CHAPTER OUTLINE

Nurses often come from different ethnic, cultural, and religious backgrounds than their clients. At the same time, nurses must understand that clients have differing world views and interpretations about health and illness that are based on sociocultural and religious beliefs. When awareness of and sensitivity to clients' unique health and illness beliefs and practices are conveyed by the nurse, good rapport is established. This rapport promotes the delivery of safe and culturally effective nursing care.

A broad range of health and illness beliefs exist in the United States. Many of these beliefs have roots in the cultural, ethnic, religious, or social background of a person, family, or community. When anticipating fear or experiencing an illness or crisis, a person may use a **modern** or **traditional** approach to prevention and healing, or both approaches may be used. The following questions must be asked in respect to the nurse's and client's cultural backgrounds.

1. Who is the nurse from a cultural perspective?
   Who is the client from a cultural perspective?
2. What is the nurse's heritage?
   What is the client's heritage?
3. What are the health traditions of the nurse's heritage?
   What are the health traditions of the client's heritage?
4. What cultural phenomena interact with the nurse's health care needs?
   What cultural phenomena interact with the client's health care needs?

The answers to these questions will help the nurse successfully provide care for a client of a different cultural or ethnic background. It will also allow effective transcultural communication. **Transcultural communication** occurs when each person attempts to understand the other's point of view from that person's cultural frame of reference. Effective transcul-tural communication is facilitated by identification of areas of commonalities. After reaching a cultural understanding, the nurse must consider the client's cultural factors throughout the nursing process. In the last decade, major nursing organizations have emphasized the importance of considering cultural factors when delivering nursing care. The subspecialty of **transcultural nursing** represents an effort by nurses from all cultural backgrounds and clinical areas to come together and define concepts that enable them to develop the knowledge and skills needed to provide culturally sensitive care.

IMMIGRATION AND DEMOGRAPHY

The population of the United States consists largely of the descendants of immigrants. The only truly native Americans are the American Indians, Aleuts, and Eskimos because they settled here thousands of years before the Europeans, Asians, and Africans. People have come to this land from every nation of the world and continue to legally and illegally immigrate. The passage of Public Law 99-603, The Immigration Reform and Control Act of 1986, made it possible for several million people to become legal aliens in this country if they have lived here since 1982 and have proof of employment.

The **demographics** of the United States' population is changing. The European majority has been shrinking (Fig. 4-1); the African, Spanish, Asian, and Native American populations are growing. If current immigration and birth trends continue, it is predicted that the Spanish population will increase by 21%, the Asian by 22%, African by 12%, and European by 2%. (Henry, 1990). Furthermore, it is predicted that by the year 2065 the "average" American resident will be of African, Asian, Spanish, Arabian, or Pacific-Is-

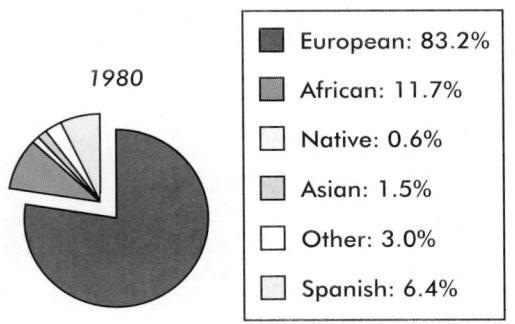

1980

- European: 83.2%
- African: 11.7%
- Native: 0.6%
- Asian: 1.5%
- Other: 3.0%
- Spanish: 6.4%

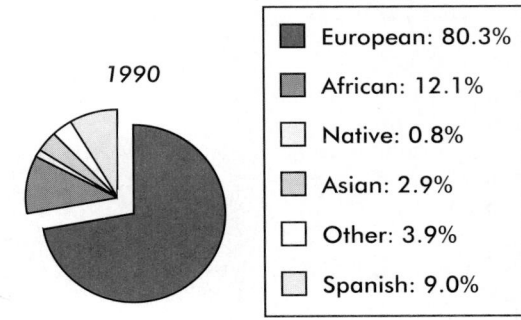

1990

- European: 80.3%
- African: 12.1%
- Native: 0.8%
- Asian: 2.9%
- Other: 3.9%
- Spanish: 9.0%

Fig. 4-1   United States population comparison: 1980-1990 census.
From *New York Times*, March 11, 1991, p 1.

lands descent—not European. (Fuller, 1989) The terms *European, African, Asian, Native,* and *Spanish American* will be used to address the major cultural groups because they indicate each group's country of origin.

The social explosion in the United States in the mid-1960s resulted in a surge of group consciousness. African, Spanish, Asian, Native and European Americans have asserted their cultural group identities. The rebirth of ethnic identity eroded both the **melting pot** myth and the belief that an American culture would decrease group awareness (Giordano, Giordano, 1977).

Every immigrant group has its own cultural attitudes about health and illness. Each group also has widely ranging beliefs and practices regarding these areas. Health and illness can be interpreted in terms of personal experience and expectations. There are countless ways to explain health and illness, and people base their responses on cultural, religious, and ethnic backgrounds. The responses are culture specific, based on clients' experiences and perceptions.

HERITAGE CONSISTENCY

One way of analyzing belief systems is through the melting-pot theory in which people assume the characteristics of the dominant culture (acculturation) via schools, television, radio, and motion pictures. Another theory is **heritage consistency,** which looks at **acculturation** on a continuum (Table 4-1). Using this theory, the degree to which people identify with the dominant and traditional cultures is assessed. It is possible to assess health beliefs by determining people's ties to traditional beliefs and their stage of acculturation. A relationship exists between strong personal identities and heritage or level of acculturation and health beliefs.

Heritage consistency was originally developed by Estes and Zitzow (1980) to assess and counsel alcoholic Native Americans within a cultural context. It describes the degree to which lifestyle reflects tribal culture. The theory has been expanded in an attempt to study the degree to which lifestyle reflects the tra-

TABLE 4-1 Heritage Continuum	
Heritage Consistency Factors	Heritage Inconsistency Factors
Childhood development occurred in the individual's country of origin or in a U.S. neighborhood of like ethnic group.	Childhood development did not occur in the individual's country of origin or in an immigrant neighborhood of like ethnic group.
Extended family members encouraged participation in traditional religious or cultural activities.	Extended family members did not encourage participation in traditional religious or cultural activities.
Individual engaged in frequent visits home to the country of origin or to the "old neighborhood" in the United States.	Individual does not engage in visits home to the country of origin or the "old neighborhood" in the United States.
Family homes are within the ethnic community.	Family was not in the ethnic community.
Individual participates in ethnic cultural events such as religious festivals, "national holidays," singing, dancing, and costumes.	Individual does not participate in ethnic cultural events.
Individual was raised in an extended family setting.	Individual was not raised in an extended family setting.
Individual maintains regular contact with the extended family.	Individual does not maintain contact with the extended family.
Individual's name has not been Americanized.	Individual's name has been Americanized.
Individual was educated in a parochial (nonpublic) school with a religious or ethnic philosophy similar to personal background.	Individual was educated in public schools.
Individual engages primarily in social activities with others of the same ethnic background.	Individual does not engage primarily in social activities with others of the same ethnic background.
Individual has knowledge about the ethnic culture and language.	Individual does not have knowledge about ethnic culture and language.
Individual possesses elements of personal pride about the national and ethnic origin.	Individual does not possess elements of personal pride about the national and ethnic origin.
Individual incorporates elements of historical beliefs and practices into personal philosophies.	Individual does not incorporate elements of historical beliefs and practices into personal philosophies.

Modified from Spector RE: *Cultural diversity in health and illness,* ed 3, Norwalk, Conn, 1991, Appleton & Lange.

ditional culture, whether it is Asian, African, European, Native, or Spanish.

Culture

Culture represents nonphysical traits, such as values, beliefs, attitudes, and customs, shared by a group of people and passed from one generation to the next. Culture is also the sum of beliefs, practices, habits, likes, dislikes, norms, customs, and rituals learned from the family during the years of socialization. Many people's beliefs, thoughts, and actions, both conscious and unconscious, are determined by cultural background (Spector, 1991).

Ethnicity

Ethnicity is a sense of identification associated with a cultural group's common social and cultural heritage. Ethnicity is "complex, ambivalent, paradoxical, and elusive" (Senior, 1965). A person is born into an ethnic group but may also adopt characteristics of another ethnic group. The characteristics of an ethnic group include common language and dialect, migra-

tory status, race, and religious faith and practices. People share traditions, values, symbols, literature, folklore, music, and food preferences. Settlement and employment patterns and special political interests are often similar. People from the same ethnic group often have a sense of uniqueness. These characteristics extend from family to neighborhood to communities. There are at least 106 different ethnic groups in North America and more than 170 Native American tribes (Thernstrom, 1980).

Religion

Religion is a belief in a divine or superhuman power (or powers) to be obeyed and worshipped as the creator and ruler of the universe. Ethical values and religious beliefs and practices further clarify ethnicity by providing a frame of reference and a perspective within which to organize information (Abramson, 1980). Religious teachings help formulate a meaningful philosophy and system of practices through a system of beliefs, practices, and social controls having specific values, norms, and ethics that vary between religious groups. Some religious prac-

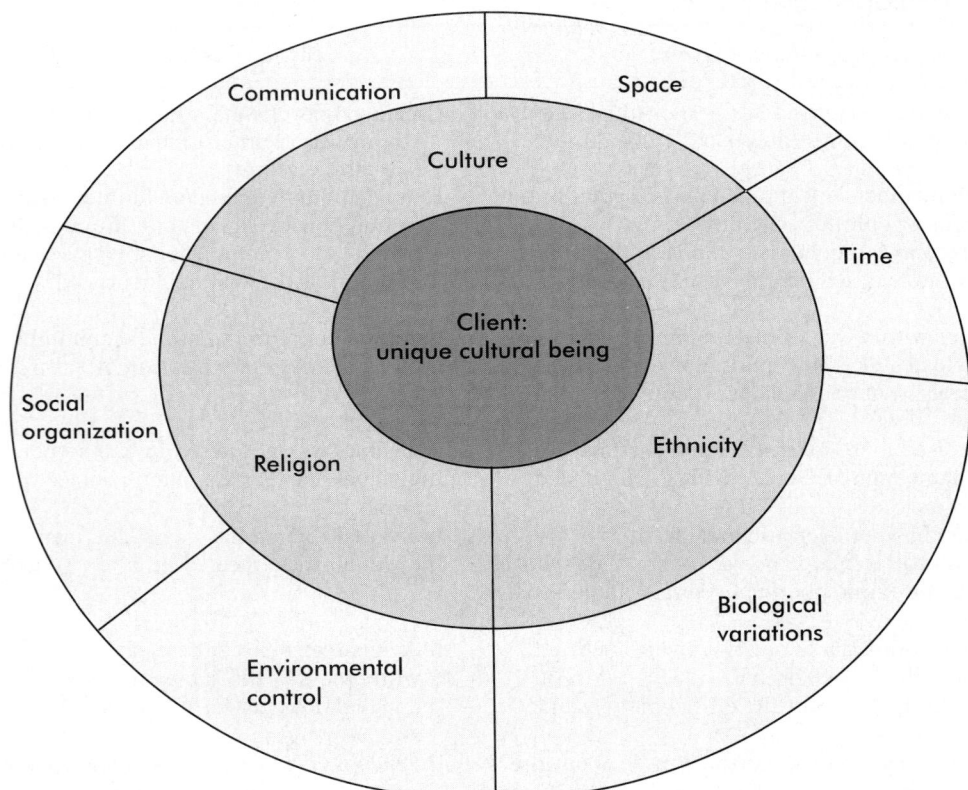

Fig. 4-2   Model of the client within a culturally unique heritage and the cultural phenomena that have an impact on nursing care.
Adapted from Spector RE: *Cultural diversity in health and illness,* ed 3, Norwalk, Conn, 1991, Appleton-Lange; and Giger JN, Davidhizar RE: *Transcultural nursing,* St Louis, 1991, Mosby–Year Book.

tices are health related. For example, some religions teach that adherence to a code or mandate is conducive to harmony and health and that breaking it may cause disharmony or illness (Thernstrom, 1980).

The degree of heritage consistency is evaluated by determining the importance of culture, ethnicity, and religion to a person, although it is difficult to isolate the specific aspects of culture, ethnicity, and religion that shape a person's world view. Fig. 4-2 illustrates the way that culture, ethnicity, and religion relate to the socialization of a person. When religion is discussed, culture and ethnicity must also be included. However, within the diverse U.S. society, descriptions and comparisons of ethnic, religious, and cultural behavior in health and illness may be made.

The client comes from a distinct heritage involving ethnic, cultural, and religious background. Heritage consistency is ever-changing . It is not designed to ste-

reotype or diagnose. Rather, it is a way of understanding whether a person interprets a health or illness event in a modern or traditional way. The factors constituting **heritage inconsistency** and consistency are presented in Fig. 4-9.

 CULTURAL PHENOMENA

In addition to heritage consistency, there are six cultural phenomena that Giger and Davidhizar (1991) have identified as varying between cultural groups. These are environmental control, biological variations, social organization, communication, space, and time. Fig. 4-3 illustrates how ethnicity, religion, and culture are affected by cultural phenomena, thus further defining heritage consistency.

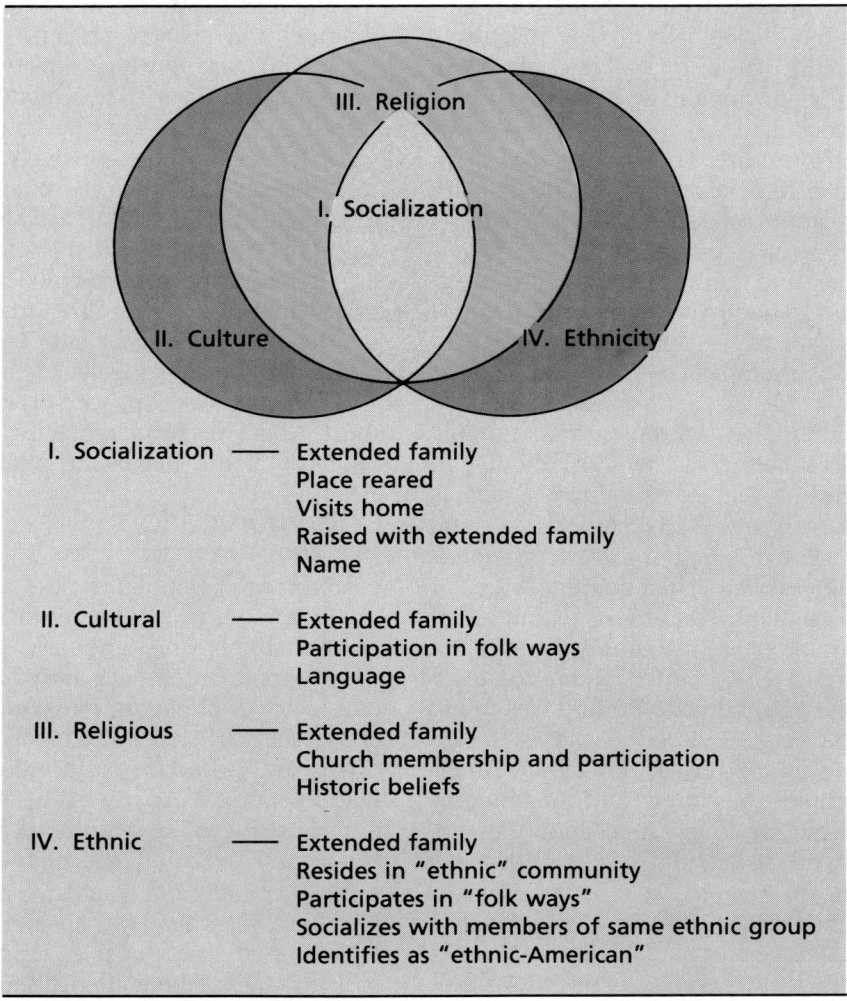

Fig. 4-3 Model of heritage consistency.
From Spector R: *Cultural diversity in health and illness,* ed 3, Norwalk Conn, 1991, Appleton & Lange.

Environmental Control

Environmental control refers to the ability of members of a particular cultural group to plan activities that control nature or direct environmental factors. (Giger, Davidhizar, 1991). Included are the complex systems of traditional health and illness beliefs, the practice of folk medicine, and the use of traditional healers. This particular cultural phenomenon plays an extremely important role in the way clients respond to health-related experiences, including the ways in which they define health and illness and seek and use health and nursing care resources and social supports. Table 4-2 presents a summary of data related to environmental control and other cultural phenomena that have an impact on nursing care.

Biological Variations

There are several ways in which people from one cultural group differ biologically (that is, physically and genetically) from members of other cultural groups. The following are a few of the significant examples to consider:

1. Body build and structure. There are specific bone and structural differences between groups, such as the smaller stature of Asians.
2. Skin color. There are variations in tone, texture, healing abilities, and hair follicles.
3. Enzymatic and genetic variations. These variations include the way a client may respond to drug and dietary therapies.
4. Susceptibility to disease. Many diseases have higher morbidity rates within certain groups. These include tuberculosis, which is higher in Native Americans; diabetes mellitus, which is higher in Spanish and Native Americans; and hypertension, which is higher in African Americans. Other illnesses are listed in Table 4-2.
5. Nutritional Variations. Countless examples of nutritional preferences, ranging from the hot and cold preferences found among Spanish Americans, the *yin* and *yang* preferences found among Asian Americans, and the rules of the kosher diet found among Jewish and Islamic Americans are examples. A common nutritional disorder is that of lactose intolerance, found among Mexican, African, Asian, and Eastern European Jewish Americans. (Giger, Davidhizar, 1991).

The high incidence of acquired immunodeficiency syndrome in the African and Spanish communities is an emerging public health concern. As of April 1, 1991, there was a total of 171,876 cases reported in the United States; 28% of these cases are among African Americans, who compose 12.1% of the population. About 16% are among Spanish Americans, or 9% of the population (Carr, 1991)

Social Organization

The social environment in which people grow up and live plays an essential role in their cultural development and identification. Children learn the responses of life events from the family and its ethnoreligious group (Table 4-2). This **socialization** process is an inherent part of heritage—cultural, religious and ethnic background. *Social organization* refers to the family unit, (nuclear, single-parent or extended family) and the social group organizations (religious or ethnic) with which clients and families may identify.

Social Barriers to Health Care

Several social barriers, such as unemployment, underemployment, homelessness, lack of health insurance, and poverty prevent people from entering the health care system. Poverty is by far the most critical factor. *Poverty* is a relative term and changes from time and place. In the United States, poverty is pervasive and found extensively among people in certain geographical areas (for example Appalacia, other rural areas, and urban areas) and certain groups (for example, African, Spanish, and Native Americans; rural populations; older adults; migrant workers; and illegal aliens). Poor health, crippling diseases, drug and alcohol abuse, poor education, and inferior education are contributing social causes of poverty.

Government and private programs aid people with short- and long-term problems. The nurse must be aware of clients' needs and financial resources.

Communication

Communication differences are presented in many ways, including language differences, verbal and nonverbal behaviors, and silence (Table 4-2).

Language differences are possibly the most important factor in providing transcultural nursing care because they affect all stages of the nursing process. Clear and effective communication is important when dealing with any client, especially if language differences create a cultural barrier between the nurse and client. If the client does not speak the nurse's language, a translator is necessary. More often, however, the client speaks the nurse's language with limited ability or uses language with denotative or connotative meanings different from the nurse's meanings. For example, a client with limited language ability might know customary greetings such

TABLE 4-2 Cross-Cultural Examples of Cultural Phenomena Impacting on Nursing Care

Nations of Origin	Environmental Control	Biological Variations*	Social Organization	Communication	Space	Time Orientation
Asian China Hawaii Philippines Korea Japan Southeast Asia (Laos, Cambodia, Vietnam)	Traditional health and illness beliefs Use of traditional medicines Traditional practitioners: Chinese doctors and herbalists	Liver cancer Stomach cancer Coccidioidomycosis Hypertension Lactose intolerance	Family: hierarchical structure, loyalty Devotion to tradition Many religions, including Taoism, Buddhism, Islam, and Christianity Community social organizations	National language preference Dialects, written characters Use of silence Nonverbal and contextual cuing	Noncontact people	Present
African West Coast (as slaves) Many African countries West Indian Islands Dominican Republic Haiti Jamaica	Traditional health and illness beliefs Folk medicine tradition Traditional healer: rootworker	Sickle cell anemia Hypertension Cancer of the esophagus Stomach cancer Coccidioidomycosis Lactose intolerance	Family: many female, single parent Large, extended family networks Strong church affiliation within community Community social organizations	National languages Dialect: Pidgen, Creole, Spanish, and French	Close personal space	Present over future
Europe Germany England Italy Ireland Other European countries	Primary reliance on modern health care system Traditional health and illness beliefs Some remaining folk medicine tradition	Breast cancer Heart disease Diabetes mellitus Thalassemia	Nuclear families Extended families Judeo-Christian Religions Community social organizations	National languages Many learn English immediately	Noncontact people Aloof Distant Southern countries: closer contact and touch	Future over present
Native American 170 Native American Tribes Aluets Eskimos	Traditional health and illness beliefs Folk medicine tradition Traditional healer: medicine man	Accidents Heart disease Cirrhosis of the liver Diabetes mellitus	Extremely family oriented Biological and extended families Children taught to respect traditions Community social organizations	Tribal languages Use of silence and body language	Space very important and has no boundaries	Present
Hispanic countries Spain Cuba Mexico Central and South America	Traditional health and illness beliefs Folk medicine tradition Traditional healers: *Curandero, Espiritista, Partera, Senora*	Diabetes mellitus Parasites Coccidioidomycosis Lactose intolerance	Nuclear family Extended families Compadrazzo: godparents Community social organizations	Spanish or Portuges primary language	Tactile relationships Touch Handshakes Embracing Value physical presence	Present

*Indicates a high morbidity incidence.
From Giger JN, Davidhizar RE: *Transcultural nursing*, St Louis, 1991, Mosby–Year Book.

as "How are you?" or "Hello" but not understand health terms such as "pain" or "temperature" that are usually understood by lay persons in the dominant cultural group. Failure to communicate effectively with the client not only may cause delays in diagnosis and treatment but may also lead to tragic results. In one incident, for example, an English-speaking nurse failed to determine that the client truly understood preoperative instructions about washing the surgical site with povidone-iodine (Betadine). The non-English-speaking Asian client, throughout the instruction period, kept nodding and smiling when the nurse asked her, "Do you understand what I told you?" The nurse judged that the client understood the instructions. Much to the nurse's dismay, the client drank the whole bottle of povidone-iodine solution instead of washing with it. Appropriate medical measures were instituted to save the client's life.

The nurse should not assume that the client understands communication. A more appropriate nursing intervention would be a demonstration of *how* to wash the area with povidone-iodine. Then the client returns the demonstration. No words have to be spoken; yet by doing this procedure or any other procedure in pantomime, the client grasps what the nurse is teaching and is then able to follow directions.

When deprived of the most common medium of interaction with clients—the spoken word—nurses often become frustrated and ineffective. As a result, nurses need to communicate with clients limited in the use of the dominant language. Some nurses tend to avoid clients with whom they cannot communicate. This creates a vicious circle of cultural misunderstandings. According to Muecke (1970), the nurse might behave toward clients in the following ways that could be misconstrued:

1. The nurse shouts the same words louder. Raising the voice will not make the words more understandable, and such actions could also suggest hostility to clients.
2. The nurse focuses on tasks rather than on clients. This suggests that the nurse is more interested in the tasks than in the clients.
3. The nurse stops talking with clients and starts doing things for them instead of with them, possibly implying clients' inferiority.

The effect of the nurse's actions is the painful isolation of clients who do not speak the dominant language and who are in an unfamiliar environment. Consequently, clients experience cultural shock and may react by withdrawing, becoming hostile or belligerent, or being uncooperative.

Language differences can be bridged, however. The nurse can ask family members who speak in the dominant language to interpret. The family can also provide information about the client's background that could be valuable in holistic care. The health care institution can also facilitate the search for an interpreter. For example, a list of bilingual or multilingual staff members and volunteers in a hospital might be kept in a central place such as the information desk.

Medical terms must be clearly explained to all clients, especially those with limited skills in the dominant language. Jargon presents problems even for alert, oriented, adult clients who speak the dominant language. For example, there may be many clients who think that *force fluids* means "force urination" or "force elimination of fluids."

Differences in denotative meanings may exist between members of two cultures, causing miscommunication. For instance, when African American youths say "That's bad" and mean "That's good," European adults might be confused. The youths are speaking in an argot, or a special linguistic code of their cultural group. Another linguistic block to communication between ethnic groups comes from differences in connotative meanings for certain words, even when the denotative meanings are the same. For example, to a European American, *hospital* may mean a facility where modern health care is provided. Navajos, however, associate hospitals with death, because they believe the ground and the building where any person dies become contaminated for an indeterminate period with evil spirits that will infect anyone who steps on this ground (Hall, 1963). Thus they avoid hospitals.

By giving special attention to the communication process, nurses can work to overcome language differences with clients who do not speak the dominant language. Observing nonverbal behaviors, for example, can help clarify communication, although nonverbal communication is also influenced by culture. Nurses can also learn to phrase questions and statements to elicit information from clients whose ethnic background shapes their response. For example, when a Mexican American man is asked if he feels pain, he may simply say *no* if he believes that admitting pain is a sign he is not manly. The nurse might ask instead whether he feels pain with a change in position, while coughing, or at night.

Finally, the nurse who practices in an area where many members of an ethnic group live should attempt to learn the clients' language. No nurse can learn all the languages that may be encountered in practice, but it is possible for a nurse to learn one other language. With more difficult languages, such as Vietnamese, the nurse can learn some basic terms. Many community health nurses have learned the languages of their clients.

Space

Personal space involves people's behaviors and attitudes toward the space around themselves. **Territoriality** is an attitude toward an area people have claimed and defend or react emotionally about when others encroach on it. Both are influenced by culture, and thus different ethnic groups have varying norms related to the use of space (Table 4-2).

Staff members and other clients frequently encroach on clients' territory in hospitals, which includes their rooms, beds, closets, and belongings. The nurse should try to respect their territory as much as possible, especially when performing nursing procedures. The nurse should also welcome visiting members of the family and extended family. This can remind clients of home, lessening the effects of isolation and shock from hospitalization.

Personal space is involved in many nursing activities, and the nurse should be sensitive about the client's attitudes toward personal space. For example, providing nursing care often involves touching the client, an action that has different meanings in different cultures and for different individuals. Actions comforting to one client may be threatening to another. Standards of behavior vary also in terms of who, male or female, can touch the client, and where. The meaning of personal space also varies among cultures. Hall (1963) has studied the meaning of space and has identified behaviors common in the following zones:

1. *Intimate zone* extends up to 1½ feet. Because this distance allows adults to have the most bodily contacts for perception of breath and odor, they do not find this acceptable in public places. Visual distortions are also present.
2. *Personal distance* extends from 1½ to 4 feet. This is an extension of the self that is like having a "bubble" of space surrounding the body. At this distance the voice may be moderate, body odor may not be apparent, and visual distortion may have disappeared.
3. *Social distance* extends from 4 to 12 feet. This is reserved for impersonal business transactions. Perceptual information in much less detailed.
4. *Public distance* extends 12 feet or more. Individuals interact only impersonally. Communicators' voices must be projected, and subtle facial expressions may be lost.

These generalizations about the use of personal space are based on studies of the behavior of European North Americans. Use of personal space varies between individuals and ethnic groups. The extreme modesty practiced by members of some cultural groups and lower socioeconomic groups may prevent members from seeking preventive health care.

Time

Certain cultures in the United States and Canada tend to be future oriented. The members of these cultures are concerned with long-range goals and with health care measures in the present to prevent the occurrence of illness in the future. They prefer to plan ahead in making schedules, setting appointments, and organizing activities. **Time orientation** varies among different cultural groups, however, and a nurse who has one attitude toward time may find it difficult to understand and plan care for clients with a different time orientation. Some African, Spanish, and Southern European Americans are oriented more to the present than the future. These clients may not share the nurse's attitude toward matters related to time. Clients may be late for appointments, not because of reluctance or lack of respect for the nurse but because they are less concerned about planning ahead to be on time than with the activity in which they are currently engaged. This time orientation difference may become important in health care measures such as long-term planning and explanations of medications schedules. For example, if clients have not been regularly taking medications prescribed to lower blood pressure, teaching about the potential effects of hypertension should emphasize short-term problems rather than only long-term problems, which may be less important to them.

 ## TRADITIONAL HEALTH AND ILLNESS BELIEFS

When health beliefs and practices are discussed as they relate to culture, ethnicity, and religion, the word *may* should be used to prevent stereotyping. The range of health and illness definitions, beliefs, and practices is infinite, and there are differences within and between groups. However, some discernible commonalities exist. The nurse must remember that it is important to constantly assess and communicate with clients to clarify their beliefs about health and illness.

Traditional Beliefs

Culturally based folk beliefs often determine the definitions of health and illness for people who have traditional belief systems. The prevention and treatment of an illness depend on understanding its cause. Traditional health beliefs about the cause of illness may differ vastly from the Western model of epidemiology. It is therefore important to understand traditional epidemiology, or the causes of illness within a belief system. Cultural, ethnic, and religious backgrounds often reflect the beliefs held about this phenomena. In the modern epidemiological model, the causes of an illness may be stress and maladaptation, viruses, bacteria, or carcinogens (agents causing cancer). In the traditional epidemiological model, there are vastly different causative agents, including soul loss, spirit possession, spells, evil eyes, and hexes. Illness may be due to people who have the ability to make others ill (for example, witches). People who believe in these forces must exercise great care to protect themselves. Envy, hate, and jealousy are also forces to be avoided. A person may practice prevention by avoiding situations that could provoke the envy, hate, or jealousy of another. If health is viewed as the reward for good behavior, every effort is made to avoid situations in which social or religious behavior is compromised (Spector, 1991).

Traditional Practices

Many traditional practices are used to prevent and treat illness; these include the use of objects, substances, and religious practices, also known as *folk medicine*. Indeed, folk medicine is related to other types of medicine practiced in society. It has coexisted, with increasing tensions, with modern medicine and was derived from academic medicine of earlier generations. Folk practices of ancient times have only in part been abandoned by modern health care belief systems. Many of these beliefs and practices continue to be observed today. Today's "popular medicine" is in a sense commercial folk medicine. The following are varieties of folk medicine (Yoder, 1972):

1. **Natural folk medicine** is one of human's earliest uses of the natural environment and is the use of herbs, plants, minerals and animal substances to prevent and treat illnesses.
2. **Magicoreligious folk medicine** represents a human's use of charms, holy words, and holy actions to prevent and cure illnesses.

Natural Folk Medicine

Natural folk medicine is widely practiced in the United States and the world. In general, this form of prevention and treatment is found in old-fashioned remedies and household medicines. These remedies have been passed down for generations, and many are in common use today. Much of this field is herbal in nature, and the customs and rituals related to the use of these herbs vary among ethnic groups. The common aspects of the use of herbs is the knowledge that they are present in nature to be used as a source of therapy. The way that these medicines are gathered and the specific uses may vary by group and region. In general, folk-medicine traditions prescribe the time of year in which the herb was to be picked; the way it is dried and prepared; and the method, amount, and frequency for consumption (Yoder, 1972).

Magicoreligious Folk Medicine

Magicoreligious folk-medicine, too, has existed for as long as humans have sought to cure their ailments. It is now labeled by some as "superstition"; yet for believers, it may take the form of religious practices related to healing. One example of this is a form of unofficial religious healing known as *pow-wowing, charming,* or *conjuring.* In these practices charms, amulets, and physical manipulations are used in the attempt to heal illness (Yoder, 1972).

Use of Protective Objects

Protective objects can be worn, carried, or hung in the home. Amulets are objects with magical powers (for example, charms worn on a string or chain around the neck, wrist, or waist to protect the wearer from the evil eye or evil spirits). Amulets exist in societies all over the world and are associated with protection from trouble (Budge, 1978). People may also use talismans or "consecrated religious objects" (Budge, 1978). Talismans are believed to possess extraordinary powers and may be worn on a rope around the waist or carried in a pocket or purse. People who wear amulets or carry a talisman should be allowed to do so in a health care institution.

Use of Substances

Substances are ingested in certain ways or amounts or are worn or hung in the home. This practice uses diet and consists of many different observances. In many belief systems, the body is kept in balance or harmony by the type of food eaten, so many food taboos and combinations exist. For example, it is believed that some food substances can be ingested to prevent illness. To prevent illness, people from many ethnic backgrounds eat raw garlic or onion, wear them on the body, or hang them in the home. The rules of kosher practiced among Jewish people mandate the elimination of pork and shellfish from the diet. They are allowed fish with scales and fins and only certain cuts of beef from animals with cleft hooves that chew cud (cattle and lambs). Jews also believe that milk and meat must never be mixed or eaten at the same meal (Steinberg, 1947). Moslems also adhere to many dietary practices.

Religious Practices

Another traditional approach to illness prevention centers around religion and includes practices such as the burning of candles, rituals of redemption, and prayer. Religion strongly affects the way people attempt to prevent illness, and it plays a strong role in rituals associated with health protection. Religion dictates social, moral, and dietary practices designed to keep a people healthy and in balance. Religion also plays a vital role in those persons' perceptions of illness prevention. Many people believe illness can be prevented by strictly following religious codes, morals, and practices and view illness as punishment for violating a religious code. Religious practices such as the Catholic custom of blessing of the throats on St. Blaise Day are performed to prevent sore throats and choking.

Traditional Remedies

The use of folk or traditional medicine is increasing, and the practice is seen among people from all walks of life and cultural and ethnic backgrounds. Use of folk medicine is not a new practice among heritage-consistent people, so many of the remedies have been used and passed on for generations. The pharmaceutical properties of vegetation—plants, roots, stems, flowers, seeds, and herbs—have been studied, tested, cataloged, and used for countless centuries. Many of these plants are used by specific communities. Others cross ethnic and community lines and are used in certain geographic areas. These remedies are purchased in special stores or market

places in the United States and may also be purchased in the person's country of origin.

When clients do not take the medications that have been prescribed, the nurse must make an effort to determine whether they are taking traditional remedies. Frequently, the active ingredients of traditional remedies are unknown. If clients are taking them, the nurse must determine the remedy and its active ingredients. Often, these ingredients can be antagonistic or synergistic to prescribed medications. If this is the situation, the medication may have no effect, or a severe overdose may occur. The richness of this pharmacopoeia far exceeds the limits of this chapter; thus only a limited sample of the remedies of each population will be highlighted.

Healers

In the traditional context, healing is the restoration of the person to a state of harmony between the body, mind, and spirit, or the restoration of holistic health. Within a given community, specific people are known to have the power to heal. The healer is thought to have received the gift of healing from a divine source.

In many instances a heritage-consistent person may consult a traditional healer before, instead of, or along with a modern health care provider. Many differences exist between the Western physician and the traditional healer (Kaptchuk, Croucher, 1987) (Table 4-3). The relationship between the person and the healer, for example, is often much closer than that between the person and the health care profes-

TABLE 4-3   Comparisons: Traditional Healer Versus Physician

Healer	Physician
Maintains an informal, friendly, affective relationship with the entire family	Is business-like and formal, dealing primarily with the client
Comes to the house day or night	Stays in a physician's office or *clinic* where the client must go for services. Rarely, if ever, makes home visits
For diagnosis, consults with head of house, creates a mood of awe, talks to all family members, is not authoritarian, has social rapport, builds expectation of cure	Deals primarily with the ill person, may address only that person's illness (authoritarian manner can create fear)
Is generally less expensive than the physician	Is generally more expensive than the healer
Has ties to the "world of the sacred," has rapport with the symbolic, spiritual, creative, or holy force	Is primarily secular, pays little attention to the religious beliefs of a client or meanings of an illness.
Shares the world view of the client (i.e., speaks the same language, lives in the same neighborhood or in the same similar socioeconomic conditions, may know the same people, understands the lifestyle of the client)	Generally does not share the world view of the client (i.e., may not speak the same language, live in the same neighborhood or in the same socioeconomic conditions, may not understand the lifestyle of the client)

Modified from Spector RE: *Cultural diversity in health and illness*, ed 3, Norwalk, Conn, 1991, Appleton & Lange.

sional. The person sees the healer as one who understands the problem within the cultural context, speaks the same language, and shares a similar world view. Examples of traditional healers follow:

1. Medicine man: the traditional healer of the Native Americans
2. *Senora:* a Puerto Rican woman knowledgeable in the treatment of illness
3. *Espiritista:* a person possessing more sophisticated skills than the *Senora*
4. *Curandero:* a person of Mexican heritage with the God-given ability to heal using a religious-psychiatric approach
5. *Partera:* a Mexican-American midwife
6. Root-worker: a African person able to determine the cause of an illness and the treatment

Traditional healers have always been a part of cultures. The methods used by these healers were developed over generations by trial and error and are often based on religious beliefs and social circumstances. Effective methods have been preserved and adapted to meet the needs of the present time. The traditional healer is aware of the cultural and personal needs of the client and is able to understand this problem in today's world.

CULTURAL ASPECTS OF HEALTH AND ILLNESS

Many cultures exist in the United States today (Table 4-1 and Fig. 4-1). Nurses must be aware of these groups and be familiar with the basic characteristics of each. The following "culture capsules" provide a general overview of Asian, African, Native, Spanish, and European American cultures. Each capsule includes a synopsis of the culture's background, traditional definitions of health and illness, and traditional beliefs about the causes of illness, methods of prevention, and remedies.

These capsules illustrate the dynamic similarities and differences between groups of people. However, clients must be assessed as individuals. Characteristic beliefs of a cultural group are not necessarily shared by each individual in that group. However, this background may be used as a framework for providing culturally sensitive nursing care.

Asian Americans

Asian Americans originated in China, Hawaii, the Philippines, Korea, Japan, Laos, Cambodia, and Vietnam. Many Asian Americans have lived in the United States for several generations. Others arrived more recently, and still others are still entering the country, especially in California.

Within the Asian community, Chinese medicine provides an overall framework for Asian cultures and teaches that health is a state of spiritual and physical harmony between a body, mind, and spirit in harmony with nature. In addition, the forces of *yin* (female, negative energy) and *yang* (male, positive energy) must be in balance. Illness is the result of imbalance between *yin* and *yang*. The body is viewed as a gift from parents and ancestors. It is not the person's personal property and must be cared for and maintained. The primary role of the physician in ancient China was to help safeguard the body and to prevent illness. If a person became ill despite preventive measures, it was not necessary to pay the physician for treatment.

Illness Cause and Prevention

Illness may be caused by an upset in the balance of *yin* and *yang*. The weather, overexertion, and prolonged sitting may also cause illness, which may be prevented by adhering to a proper diet to maintain the body's balance, exercising, avoiding temperature changes, and taking certain remedies.

Remedies

The following examples are a few traditional remedies used to prevent and treat ailments among Asian Americans (Fig. 4-4):

Jen Shen Lu Jung Wan is a brown-colored, thick liquid used as a general tonic to brace up the whole system and improve digestion. It may be taken before elective surgery. *Thousand year eggs* are uncooked eggs covered with carbon or straw and stored in large vases for a long time. They are eaten daily with rice for good health. *Huo Li Jian Mei Su* are small, brown, coated pills taken twice a day to counteract senility, for the relief of fatigue, and for the maintenance of youth, health, and beauty. *Tiger balm* is a salve used for temporary relief of minor aches and pains. *Ginseng root* is the most famous Chinese medicine. It has universal medicinal usage in "building the blood," especially after childbirth. Chinese legend states that the more the root looks like a man, the more effective it is. Ginseng is native to the United States and is used in this country as a restorative tonic. *White flower* is a liquid used to treat colds, influenza, headaches, and coughs. Other methods of treatment include the use of *acupuncture,* a method of treating disease by puncturing the skin at certain points of the body with metal needles, and moxibustion, the application of heat to these same points (Spector, 1991).

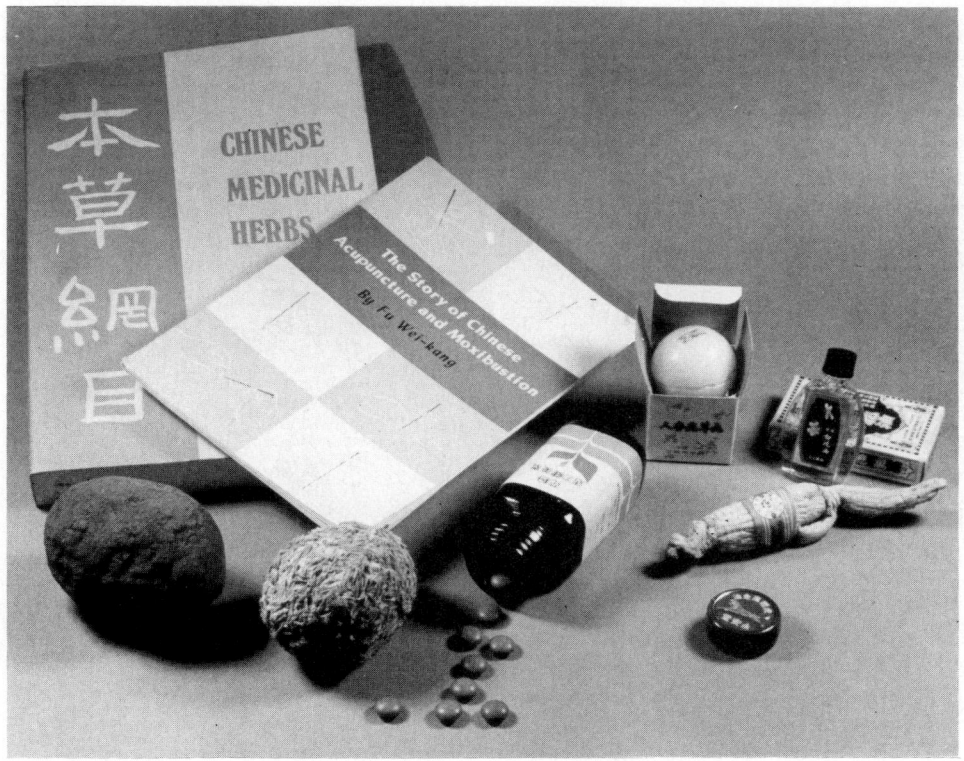

Fig. 4-4   Asian American remedies include *Jen Shen Lu Jung Wan*, thousand year eggs, *Huo Li Jian Mei Su*, Tiger Balm, ginseng root, and white flower.
Photograph by Lucy Rozier, Boston College Audio Visual Services, Boston College, Chestnut Hill, Mass, from the author's private collection.

African Americans

Most African Americans were brought to the United States as slaves between 1619 and 1860 from the west coast of Africa. Today, many have also immigrated to the United States from African countries, the West Indies, the Dominican Republic, Haiti, and Jamaica.

The traditional definition of health stems from the African belief about life and the nature of being. To Africans, life is a process rather than a state, and the nature of a person is viewed in terms of an energy force rather than matter. When healthy, a person is in harmony with nature. Illness is seen as a disharmony of the mind, body, and spirit or as a disharmony between man and nature. Researchers and epidemiologists have noted chronic illnesses and illness patterns that are associated with cultural and ethnic groups. Berg and Berg (1989) describe the correlation between psychological stress and hypertension found in African Americans (see research highlight).

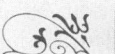 **Research Highlight**

In this study, Berg and Berg addressed dietary adherance among 23 African Americans with end-stage renal disease (ESRD). They observed that health care providers have difficulty in convincing these clients to adhere to their diets because the providers may lack awareness of culturally related dietary habits. The researchers collected data by interviewing persons in the sample group and monitoring the laboratory analyses of their blood. Although these persons claimed to be adhering to the necessary dietary restrictions, their blood analysis suggested the opposite. Berg and Berg attempted to explain their findings by speculating that the renal dietary restrictions were too rigid and alien in the context of African American cultural eating patterns.

Berg J, Berg BL: Compliance, diet, and cultural factors among black Americans with end-stage renal disease, *J Nat Black Nurses Assoc* 3(2):18, 1989.

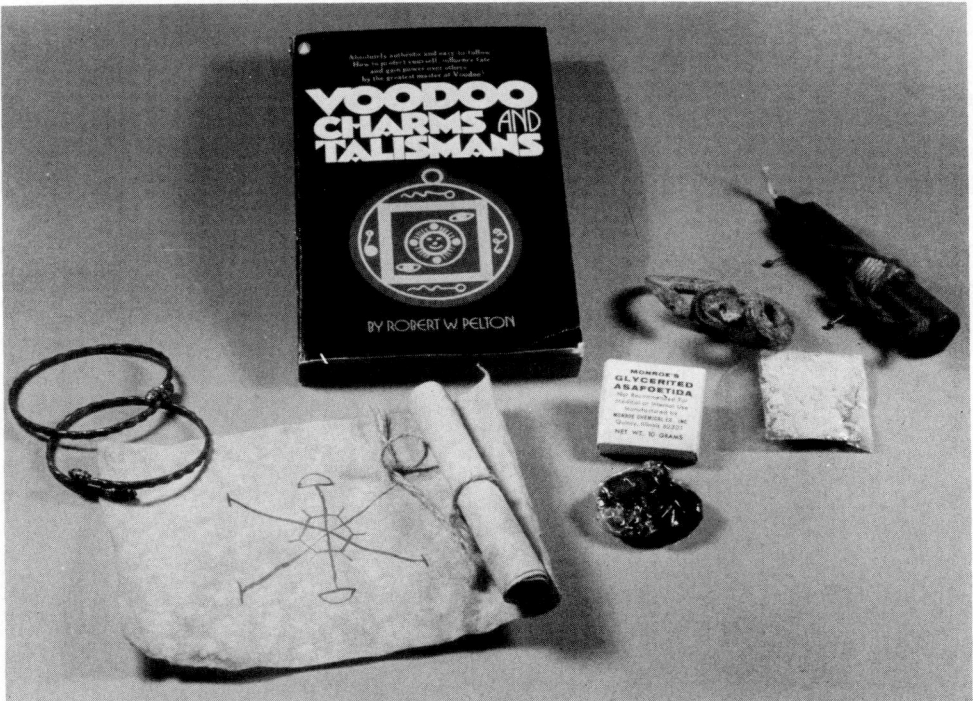

Fig. 4-5 African American remedies include bangles, talisman, *Asafoetida*, snake, and Voo Doo candle.
Photograph by Lucy Rozier, Boston College Audio Visual Services, Boston College, Chestnut Hill, Mass, from the author's private collection.

Illness Cause and Prevention

Illness (disharmony) is often attributed to demons and evil spirits. Several methods are used as protection from these forces, including the ancient belief and practice of voodoo. Voodoo is believed to cause, as well as prevent, the action of malevolent forces. "White" magic protects against these forces, and "black" magic directs their energy to a specific person or body area. The extent of the belief in this magic is unknown. Traditional beliefs about prevention of illness focus on avoiding people believed to carry evil spirits. Prayer and a well-balanced diet are considered helpful.

Remedies

The following examples are a few traditional remedies used to prevent or treat ailments among African Americans (Fig. 4-5).

Bangles are silver bracelets worn by people originating from the West Indies. They overlap but are open to let out evil and closed to prevent evil from entering the body. They are worn from infancy and are replaced as the person grows. These bracelets tarnish and leave a black ring on the skin when a person is becoming ill. The black ring serves as a signal to rest, improve the diet, and take any other needed precautions. Some people wear many bangles, believing that their sound frightens away evil spirits. Many people believe that they are extremely vulnerable to evil, even to death, when the bangles are removed, so removal of these bracelets can cause a great deal of anxiety.

Talismans protect the wearer from all sickness and are worn on a string around the waist or carried in a pocket or in a purse. *Asafoetida* is a foul-smelling, gummy substance worn to ward off colds and evil. It is known as the incense of the devil. A dehydrated garden *snake* is ground into a powder and dissolved in water. The liquid is applied to skin lesions such as poison ivy. *Voodoo candles* have a peculiar spiritualistic character and are used for sacred rituals and rites. Colors also have significance. For example, pink means love; white means peace, and blue means success and protection from harm (Spector, 1991).

Native Americans

There are approximately 170 Native American tribes in the United States, predominantly in the

Western states. Although many Native Americans remain on reservations, many also live off of them.

Health reflects the ability to live in total harmony with nature and the ability to survive under extremely difficult circumstances. People are believed to have an intimate spiritual relationship with nature. The earth is considered a living organism, the body of a higher individual, with a will and a desire to be well and experience health and illness. The body and earth must be treated with respect. Because the earth provides food, shelter, and medicine to man, it must be protected. According to Basque (1975), "The land belongs to life, life belongs to the land, and the land belongs to itself." Thus to stay healthy a person must maintain a positive, balanced relationship with nature.

Another explanation of the Native American view of health is that the body is divided into two halves, plus and minus. There are also, in every whole, two energy poles, positive and negative. People have the power to control themselves, and with this potency, spiritual power (control of the body's energy) is derived. Health is described as the harmony or balance between the two halves or the two energy poles. Illness is the disharmony of the body, mind, and spirit (Boyd, 1974).

Illness Cause and Prevention

Sources causing illness vary from nation to nation or tribe to tribe. Hopi Indians associate illness with evil spirits and therefore strive to avoid or ward off these spirits. Navahos see illness as the result of displeasing the holy people, annoying the elements, disturbing animal and plant life, neglecting the celestial bodies, misusing a sacred Indian ceremony, or tampering with witches or witchcraft. Hawk Littlejohn (1979), an Eastern Band Cherokee medicine man, describes illness as the imbalance of the body, mind, or spirit caused by an excess in one domain and the neglect of the other two. For example, a student who spends too much time studying—developing the mind—may neglect the body and spirit and will therefore be vulnerable to disharmony and illness. The main principle for the prevention of illness is the maintenance of harmony with the body, mind, and spirit and the avoidance of factors that cause disharmony.

Remedies

The following examples are remedies used by Native Americans to prevent or treat illness (Fig. 4-6):

Sand painting is the creation of a sand painting by the Navaho medicine man while diagnosing an ailment. The painting is created by the medicine man in an elaborate diagnostic ceremony of motion of the

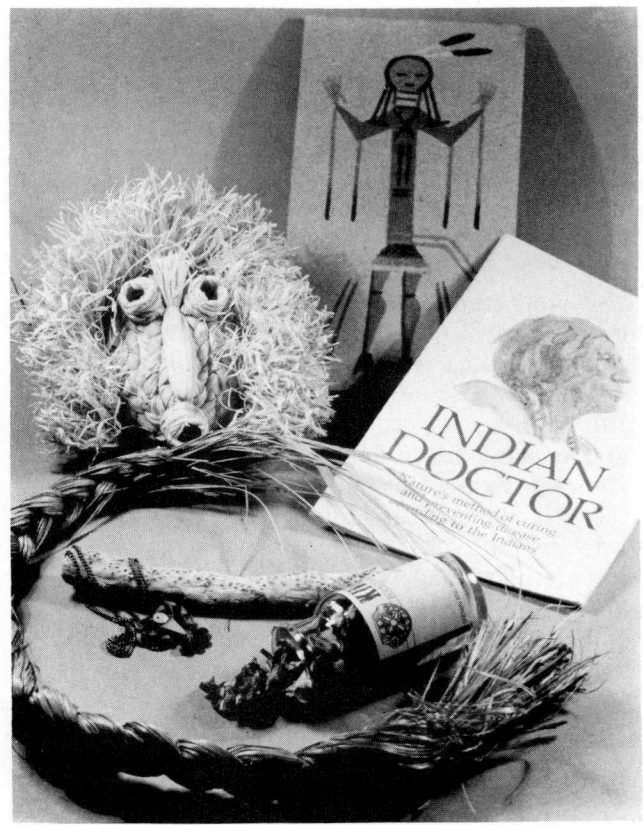

Fig. 4-6   Native American remedies include sand painting, mask, sweet grass, thunderbird, and *Estafiate*.
Photography by Lucy Rozier, Boston College Audio Visual Services, Boston College, Chestnut Hill, Mass., from the author's private collection.

hand. When the hand moves in a certain way, the medicine man knows that it is indicative of a specific illness and is able to prescribe the correct treatment.

A *mask* is worn to hide the self from the devil or evil spirits. *Sweet grass* is burned as a rite of purification by the medicine man. A *thunderbird* is an amulet worn for good luck and protection. *Estafiate* are dried leaves used in a tea to treat stomach problems (Spector, 1991).

Spanish Americans

Members of the Spanish community originate in Spain, Cuba, Mexico, Puerto Rico, and other Spanish-speaking countries. Health is often believed to be the result of good luck or a reward from God for good behavior. Health represents a state of equilibrium within the universe where the forces of hot, cold, wet, and dry are balanced. Blood is hot and wet, and yellow bile is hot and dry; phlegm is cold and wet, and black bile is cold and dry. The concept originated with the early Hippocratic theory of health and the four humors. Health exists when the four humors are in a balanced state. Health is maintained by the diet and other practices that keep the humors balanced. Illness is viewed as misfortune or bad luck, punishment from God for evil thoughts or actions, or the imbalance of hot and cold.

Illness Cause and Prevention

Several factors cause illness. A hot-cold imbalance, for example, is primarily-caused by improper diet. Food substances are classified as *hot* or *cold* without regard to their actual temperature. This classification can vary from person to person, but essentially, certain foods are known to be hot, and others are known to be cold. Examples of cold food are chicken, honey, avocados, bananas, and lima beans. Examples of hot foods are chocolate, coffee, corn meal, garlic, kidney beans, onions, and peas. Illness can occur if these foods are eaten in improper combinations or amounts. For example, *friadad del estomago* (cold stomach) is caused by eating too many cold foods. There are several conditions in which a person maintains health by adhering to this hot-cold system. A pregnant woman avoids hot foods. During menstruation and after childbirth, she avoids cold foods. An infant who requires formula that contains a hot food such as evaporated milk may be fed a cold food such as whole milk.

Other factors believed to cause illness are the "dislocation of body parts" and magic or supernatural causes outside the body such as *mal ojo* (bad eye). *Envidia* (envy) is also a cause of illness and bad luck, and many means are used to prevent it. Many people of Spanish origin believe that to succeed is to fail (that is, when a person's success provokes the envy of friends and neighbors, misfortune or illness may follow). Illness may be prevented by proper diet, avoidance of "harmful" people, the wearing of amulets for protection, the use of candles, and prayer.

Remedies

The following remedies are used among people of Spanish Americans (Fig. 4-7) for the prevention or treatment of illness:

All kinds of novena *candles* may be burned to ward off evil. *Jabon de la Mano Milagrosa* (soap of the miraculous hand) is used to cleanse and protect a person. *Amulets* such as *Milagros* (Mexican) are worn as protection from evil. The *Mano Negro* (Blackhand) amulet of Puerto Rico may be placed on a baby at birth and is believed to protect it from the evil eye.

Manzanilla is a herb made into tea and used to treat stomach and intestinal pain, uterine cramps, anxiety, and insomnia. *Anis* are star-shaped seeds

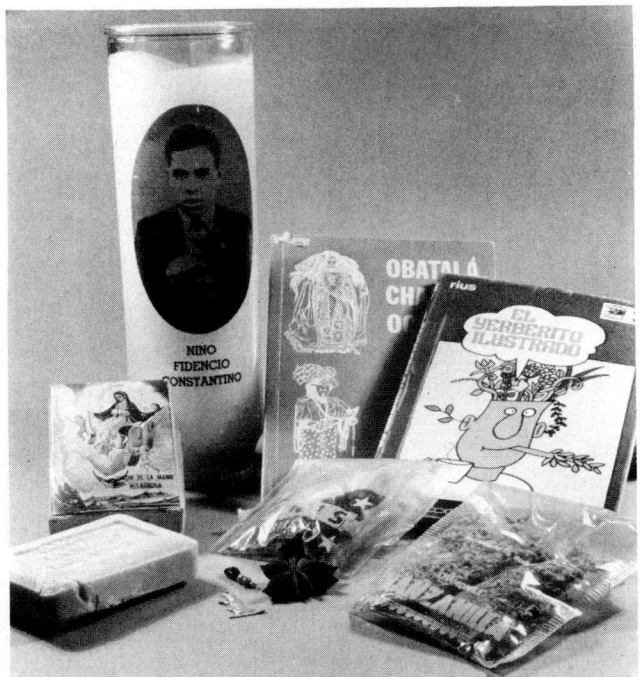

Fig. 4-7 Spanish American remedies include candles, *Jabon de la Mano Milagrosa*, and amulets—*Milagros* (Mexican), *Mano Negro* (Puerto Rican), and *Manzanilla, Anis*. Photograph by Lucy Rozier, Boston College Audio Visual Services, Boston College, Chestnut Hill, Mass, from the author's private collection.

used to treat painful gases, upset stomach, colic, and anorexia and to increase breast milk (Spector, 1991).

European Americans

Members of most European American communities originated in Europe and have been migrating to this country since 1620. This population is a diverse mixture of people from many countries, speaking numerous languages and observing a wide variety of health beliefs and practices. The 1980 census was the first to attempt to break down the population by country of origin. The largest groups were from Germany, England, Ireland, and France.

Health and illness are defined in many ways, including the ability to perform activities of daily living, a state of physical and emotional well-being, and a state free of illness. Illness is described as the inability to perform activities of daily living, the presence of disease symptoms and pain, and the malformation of body organs.

Illness Cause and Prevention

To Europan Americans, traditional beliefs about the causes of illness are many and varied. Examp-

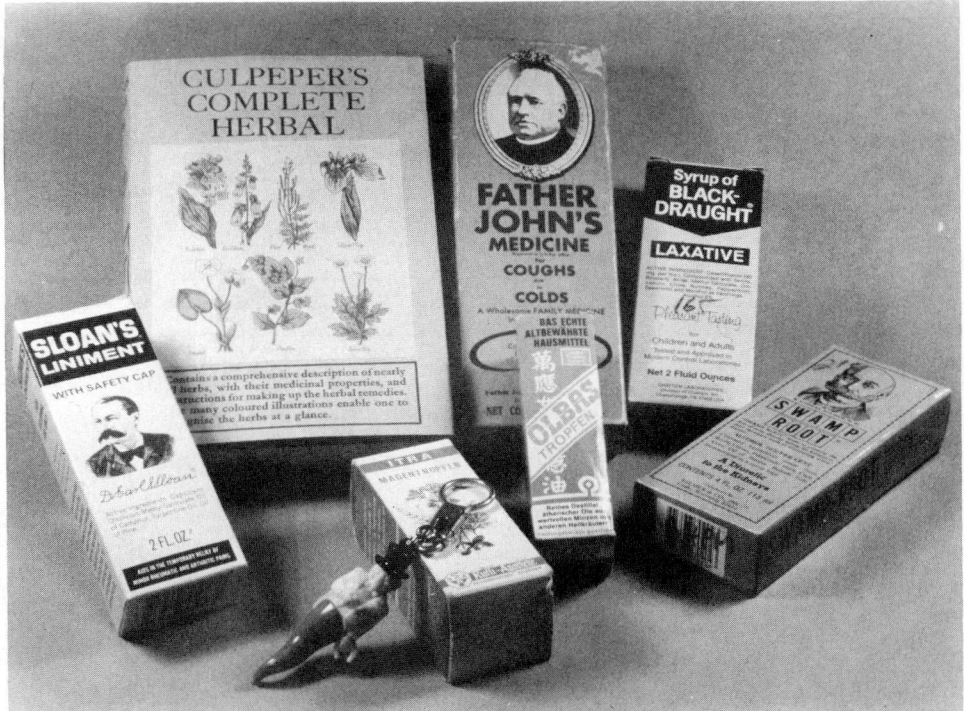

Fig. 4-8   European American remedies include Sloan's Liniment, *Malocchio, Olbas* and *Magentropfen,* swamp root, Syrup of Black Draught, and Father John's Medicine. Photograph by Lucy Rozier, Boston College Audio Visual Services, Boston College, Chestnut Hill, Mass, from the author's private collection.

les of these causes include breaking of religious rules, exposure to causative agents, punishment from God, drafts, climatic changes, and the abuse of the body. A wide variety of methods for preventing illness may be found among European Americans, including diet, exercise, religious rituals, and the wearing of amulets.

Remedies

The following are a few examples of remedies reported among European Americans (Fig 4-8).

Sloan's Liniment aids in the temporary relief of minor pains resulting from arthritis and other ailments. *Malocchio* is an Italian horn worn to prevent the evil eye. The hunchbacked man *Gobo* worn on a horn offers extra protection; he holds a horseshoe for luck in his left hand and points the index and baby finger of his right hand to ward off the evil spirit.

Olbas and *magentropfen* are medicines sold in Germany to treat sore throats and lack of appetite. *Swamp root* is an over-the-counter liquid used as a diuretic. *Syrup of Black Draught* is used as an over-the-counter laxative. *Father John's Medicine* is a family medicine that has been used for colds and coughs since 1855 (Spector, 1991).

 ## CULTURAL FACTORS AND THE NURSING PROCESS

When nurses provide care to clients from other backgrounds, they must be aware of and sensitive to their own unique heritage and health traditions and then to the clients' sociocultural background. They must assess and listen carefully to health and illness beliefs and practices and respect and not challenge cultural, ethnic, or religious values and health care beliefs (Fig. 4-9 on pp. 112 and 113). The nursing process enables the nurse to provide individualized care (see Unit 2) and can be adapted to provide culturally sensitive care (Table 4-4 on p. 113).

The nurse should begin assessment by determining the client's cultural heritage, social organization background (Fig. 4-9 and Table 4-4), and language skills. The client should be asked about the cause of the illness or problem. The nurse should then determine whether the person is taking any home remedies to treat the symptoms and whether social support services are available.

When clients are cared for outside of the hospital, the assessment process of transcultural nursing

Heritage Assessment Tool

1. Where was your mother born? _____
2. Where was your father born? _____
3. Where were your grandparents born?:
   a. Your mother's mother? _____
   b. Your mother's father? _____
   c. Your father's mother? _____
   d. Your father's father? _____
4. How many brothers _____ and sisters _____ do you have?
5. What setting did you grow up in? Urban _____ Rural _____ Suburban _____
6. What country did you parents grow up in?
   Father _____
   Mother _____
7. How old were you when you came to the United States? _____
8. How old were your parents when they came to the United States?
   Mother _____
   Father _____
9. When you were growing up, who lived with you?
   Nuclear _____ or Extended _____ Family
10. Have you maintained contact with:
    a. Aunts, uncles, cousins?   (1) Yes _____ (2) No _____
    b. Brothers and sisters?   (1) Yes _____ (2) No _____
    c. Parents   (1) Yes _____ (2) No _____
    d. Your own children?   (1) Yes _____ (2) No _____
11. Did most of your aunts, uncles, cousins live near to your home?
    (1) Yes _____ (2) No _____
12. Approximately how often did you visit your family members who lived outside of your home?
    (1) Daily _____ (2) Weekly _____ (3) Monthly _____
    (4) Once a year of less _____ (5) Never _____
13. Was your original family name changed?
    (1) Yes _____ (2) No _____
14. What is your religious preference?
    (1) Catholic _____ (2) Jewish _____
    (3) Protestant _____ Denomination _____ (4) Other _____ (5) None _____
15. Is your spouse the same religion as you?
    (1) Yes _____ (2) No _____
16. Is your spouse the same ethnic background as you?
    (1) Yes _____ (2) No _____
17. What kind of school did you go to?
    (1) Public _____ (2) Private _____ (3) Parochial _____
18. As an adult, do you live in a neighborhood where the neighbors are the same religion and ethnic background as yourself?
    (1) Yes _____ (2) No _____
19. Do you belong to a religious institution?
    (1) Yes _____ (2) No _____
20. Would you describe yourself as an active member?
    (1) Yes _____ (2) No _____
21. How often do you attend your religious institution?
    (1) More than once a week _____ (2) Weekly _____ (3) Monthly _____
    (4) Special holidays only _____ (5) Never _____
22. Do you practice your religion in your home?
    (1) Yes _____ (2) No _____ (if yes, please specify)
    (3) Praying _____ (4) Bible reading _____ (5) Diet _____
    (6) Celebrating religious holidays _____

Fig. 4-9   Heritage assessment tool.
From Spector RE: *Cultural diversity in health and illness,* ed 3, Norwalk, Conn, 1991, Appleton-Lange.

Heritage Assessment Tool—cont'd

23. Do you prepare foods of your ethnic background?
    (1) Yes _____ (2) No _____
24. Do you participate in ethnic activities?
    (1) Yes _____ (2) No _____ (if yes, please specify)
    (3) Singing _____ (4) Holiday celebrations _____
    (5) Dancing _____ (6) Festivals _____
    (7) Costumes _____ (8) Other _____
25. Are your friends from the same religious background as you?
    (1) Yes _____ (2) No _____
26. Are your friends from the same ethnic background as you?
    (1) Yes _____ (2) No _____
27. What is your native language? _____
28. Do you speak this language?
    (1) Prefer _____ (2) Occasionally _____ (3) Rarely _____
29. Do you read your native language?
    (1) Yes _____ (2) No _____

The greater the number of *yes* answers, the more likely the client is to strongly identify with a traditional heritage. (The one *no* answer that indicates heritage identity is "Was your name changed?")

Fig. 4-9, cont'd   Heritage assessment tool.

TABLE 4-4   Cultural Adaptation of the Nursing Process

Process	Action
Assessment	
Heritage consistency	Perform heritage-consistency assessment (Fig. 4-9) on self and client.
Environmental control	Ask about the client's beliefs of the nature of the health problem and actions being taken at home or in the community to treat and resolve it.
	Ask about other health care resources being used.
Biological variations	Ask about nutritional preferences.
	Observe body structure, skin tone, and color.
	Be aware of health problems that may be more common in that client's background.
Social organizations	Conduct community activities.
Communication skills	Determine the needs of the client who does not speak the dominant language and provide competent interpreters.
Space	Be aware of territoriality; seek permission before intruding in the client's territory.
	Be aware of touch and eye-contact expectations.
Time	Understand the differences in time orientation
Nursing diagnosis	
Development of problem list	Ask about the client's interpretation of the problem and possible effective interventions.
Planning	Include client, family, and community in plans as needed.
Implementation	Alter usual ways of interacting to adjust to client's social interaction and etiquette.
	Incorporate interventions agreeing with client's cultural heritage, educational level, and language skills.
Evaluation	With client, determine whether nursing care has met expectations and needs.

Ethnocultural Social Organization Assessment Tool

- Demographic data that includes:
  - Total population size of city or town
  - Breakdown by areas: residential concentrations of target group
  - Breakdown by ages
  - Education
  - Occupations
  - Income
- Traditional health and illness beliefs found within target group
- Traditional health and illness practices within target group
- Use and sources of home remedies
- Identity of traditional healers

---

comes alive the moment the confines of the institutional setting are left and the nurse delves into the community. One way that sensitivity and appreciation for a given ethnoreligious community can be developed is for the nurse to go out and witness the daily life of that community. The box lists various social organizational factors that the nurse may want to explore as a way of acquiring this awareness. The "answers" to the various areas raised are generally found in libraries or through interviews with people from the community. A second approach to this activity is to walk through the community and view the churches, social organizations, and health-related services available. If possible, the nurse can visit a community health care provider or clinic, a church or community center that serves the target group, or grocery stores and pharmacies to observe differences in foods and over-the-counter remedies. If possible, the nurse should eat a meal in a neighborhood restaurant.

Assessment enables the nurse to cluster relevant data and develop actual or potential nursing diagnoses related to the cultural or ethnic need of the client. In addition, the nursing diagnosis should state the probable cause. The identification of the cause of the problem further individualizes the nursing care plan and encourages selection of appropriate interventions.

When establishing the goals of care and planning specific interventions, the nurse again considers cultural variables as they relate to the client. The extended family should be involved in care, for example, if the family is the client's strongest support group. Cultural beliefs and practices can be implemented into therapy (Berg, Berg, 1989) (see research highlight). The client's cultural heritage, educational level, and language skills should be considered when planning teaching activities. To avoid confusion, misunderstanding, or cultural conflict, explanations of aspects of care usually not questioned by acculturated clients may be required for clients who do not speak the dominant language or who are not acculturated (De Santis, Thomas, 1990) (see research highlight). The nurse may have to alter usual ways of interacting to avoid offending or alienating a client with different attitudes toward social interaction and etiquette. A client who is modest and self-conscious about the body may need psychological preparation before some procedures and tests that are usually viewed as routine (for example, obtaining a chest x-ray film or electrocardiogram [ECG]).

The nurse can find out what care clients consider appropriate by involving them and families in planning it and by asking about their expectations. This should be done in every case, even if the nursing care cannot be modified. Because the nurse and clients are likely to take many aspects of their cultures

Research Highlight

The planning of culture-specific health teaching of immigrant groups has proved to be a challenge to nurses. DeSantis and Thomas assessed 30 immigrant Haitian mothers regarding their health beliefs and practices. The mothers used preventive methods from the Western health care system and traditional Haitian systems. About 97% used magicoreligious measures; 47% administered home remedies, and 35% used a variety of measures to ensure that cold air did not enter the neonates and cause illness or pain. They found that these methods were successful because the children did not get sick. The mothers consulted with a variety of individuals and established their own health care networks.

DeSantis L, Thomas J: The immigrant Haitian mother: transcultural nursing perspective on preventive health care for children, *J Transcult Nurs* 2:2, 1990.

for granted, questions should be clear, and explanations should be explicit. Discussing cultural variables with clients and families during planning helps the nurse implement clients' personal health beliefs and practices so that interventions can be individualized.

The nurse evaluates the results of nursing care by determining the extent to which the individualized goals of care have been met. Evaluation continues throughout the nursing process and should include feedback from the client and family. Self-evaluation is crucial as the nurse increases skills for interaction. The nurse should consider the following questions:

1. Are nurses open to understanding ways in which the client's values differ from theirs?
2. Have nurses given sufficient attention to communicating with the client with limited skills in the dominant language?

3. Have nurses successfully involved the client's family in the nursing process?
4. Are nurses incorporating the client's beliefs and practices into nursing therapies?
5. Are nurses therapeutic relationships with the client grounded on respect for the client, regardless of cultural differences?

Nurses should evaluate their attitudes toward providing transcultural nursing care. Some nurses may believe they should treat all clients the same and simply "act naturally." However, this attitude fails to acknowledge that cultural differences exist and that there is no one natural human behavior. The nurse cannot act the same with all clients and still hope to deliver effective, individualized, holistic care. Sometimes, inexperienced nurses are so self-conscious about cultural differences and so afraid of making a mistake that they impede the nursing process by not asking questions about areas of difference or by asking so many questions that they seem to pry into the client's personal life. The process of self-evaluation can help the nurse become more comfortable when providing care to clients from diverse backgrounds.

 SUMMARY

Nurses need to be aware of and sensitive to the cultural needs of clients. The body of knowledge relevant to transcultural nursing is rapidly growing, and it is imperative that nurses from all cultural backgrounds be aware of nursing implications in this area. The practice of nursing today demands that the nurse identify and meet the cultural needs of diverse groups; understand the social and cultural reality of the client, family, and community; develop expertise to implement culturally acceptable strategies to provide nursing care; and identify and use resources available and acceptable to the client (Boyle, 1987).

CHAPTER 4 REVIEW

Key Concepts

- Cultural background affects all dimensions of health; it is vital that the nurse consider cultural background when planning care.
- Many ethnic and cultural groups in North America retain their cultural heritage.
- The way that culture influences behaviors, attitudes, and values depends on many factors and thus may not be the same for individual members of a cultural group.
- Although basic human needs are the same for all people, the way a person seeks to meet those needs is influenced by culture.
- Ethnocentrism can impede the delivery of care to ethnic minority clients.
- Stereotyping ethnic group members can lead to mistaken assumptions about a client.
- The nurse should have an understanding of the prevalant characteristics of the five major groups in North America—Asian, African, Native, Spanish, and European Americans—but should always individualize care rather than generalize about all clients in these groups.
- Before assessing the cultural background of a client, nurses should assess how they are influenced by their own cultures.
- Nursing diagnoses for clients should include potential problems in interaction with the health care system and problems involving the effects of culture.
- The planning and implementation of nursing interventions should be adapted as much as possible to the client's cultural background.
- Evaluation should include the nurse's self-evaluation of attitudes and emotions toward providing nursing care to clients from diverse sociocultural backgrounds.

Key Terms

Critical Thinking Exercises

1. Ms. Sanchez, a recent immigrant from South America, has been admitted to the hospital for the first time in her life. She appears apprehensive. What are two activities that you may undertake to help her adjust to this strange environment.

2. Mr. Jabar is a practicing Muslim and on a clear liquid diet. He refuses to eat the Jello that he is served. What intervention would be helpful in respect to his diet?

3. When a client is often late for a clinic appointment, what interventions may prevent this from becoming a problem?

4. Mrs. Chan, a 57-year-old Asian immigrant, is going home and is refusing to accept follow-up nursing care. What assessment questions may be helpful in determining who and what will be helpful for her?

REFERENCES

Abramson HJ: Religion. In Thermstrom S, editor: *The Harvard encyclopedia of American ethnic groups,* Cambridge, Mass, 1980, Harvard University Press.

Basque W: Lecture notes, Boston, 1975, Boston College.

Berg J, Berg BL: Compliance, diet, and cultural factors among black Americans with end-stage renal disease. *J Nat Black Nurses Assoc* 3(2):18, 1989.

Boyd D: *Rolling thunder,* New York, 1974, Random House.

Boyle JS: The practice of transcultural nursing, *Transcultural Nursing Society Newsletter* 7:2, 1987.

Budge EAW: *Amulets and superstitions,* New York, 1978, Dover Publications. (Originally published in London, 1930, by Oxford University Press).

Carr E et al: AIDS surveillance summary: state and national comparisons, *AIDS Newsl* 7(4), 3, 1991.

DeSantis L, Thomas J: The immigrant Haitian mother: transcultural nursing perspective on preventive health care for children, *J Transcult Nurs* 2:2, 1990.

Estes G, Zitzow D: Heritage consistency as a consideration in counseling Native Americans. Paper presented at the convention of the National Indian Education Association, Dallas, 1980.

Fuller WP: Recent trends in U.S. refugee policy, *America* 161:238, 1989.

Giger JN, Davidhizar RE: *Transcultural nursing assessment and intervention,* St Louis, 1991, Mosby–Year Book.

Giordano J, Giordano GP: *The ethno-cultural factor in mental health,* New York, 1977, Institute of Pluralism and Group Identity.

Hall ET: Proxemics: the study of man's spatial relations. In Goldstein I, editor: *Man's image in medicine and anthropology,* New York, 1963, International Universities Press.

Henry WA III: Beyond the Melting Pot, *Time* 135:28, April 9, 1990.

Kaptchuk T, Croucher M: *The healing arts,* New York, 1987, Summit Books.

Littlejohn H: Interview, Boston, 1979.

Muecke MA: Overcoming the language barrier, *Nurs Outlook* 18:53, 1970.

Senior C: *The Puerto Ricans: strangers then neighbors,* Chicago, 1965, Quadrangle.

Spector RE: *Cultural diversity in health and illness,* ed 3, Norwalk, Conn, 1991, Appleton & Lange.

Steinberg M: *Basic Judaism,* New York, 1947, Harcourt, Brace, & World.

Thernstrom S, editor: *The Harvard encyclopedia of American ethnic groups,* Cambridge, Mass, 1980, Harvard University Press.

Yoder D: Folk medicine. In Dorson RH, editor: *Folklore and folk-life,* Chicago, 1972, University of Chicago Press.

ADDITIONAL READINGS

Airhihenbuwa CO: Health education for African Americans: a neglected task, *Health Educ* 20:9, 1989.

Anderson JM: The cultural context of caring, *Can Crit Care Nurs J* 4(4):7, 1987.

Becerra, RM, Shaw D: *The elderly Hispanic: a research and reference guide,* Lanham, Md, 1984, University Press of America.

Bienvenue RM, Goldstein JE: *Ethnicity and ethnic relations in Canada,* ed 2, Toronto, 1985, Butterworths.

Boyle JS, Andrews MM: *Transcultural concepts in nursing care,* Glenview, Ill, 1989, Scott, Foresman.

Braithwaite RL et al: Community organization and development for health promotion within an urban black community: a conceptual model, *Health Educ* 20:56, 1989.

Bryant CA: *The cultural feast: an introduction to food and society,* St Paul, 1985, West.

Carnegie ME: *The path we tread: blacks in nursing:* 1854-1984, Philadelphia 1987, Lippincott.

Carson VB: *Spiritual dimensions of nursing practice,* Philadelphia, 1989, Saunders.

Conway FJ, Carmona PE: Cultural complexity: the hidden stressors, *J Adv Med Surg Nurs* 1(4):65, 1989.

Curry MA: *Access to prenatal care: key to preventing low birthweight,* Kansas City, Mo, 1987, American Nurses Association.

Delaney J, Lupton MJ, Toth E: *The curse: a cultural history of menstruation,* Chicago, 1988, University of Chicago Press.

DeSantis L: A profile of cultural diversity in nursing practice, *Fla Nurse* 37:15, 1989.

Dinnerstein L, Reimers DM: *Ethnic Americans,* ed 3, New York, 1988, Harper & Row.

Flaskerud JH, Rush CE: AIDS and traditional health beliefs and practices of black women, *Nurs Res* 38(4):210, 1989.

Fuentes C: *The old gringa* New York, 1985, Farrar, Straus, Giroux.

Gibbs JT et al: *Children of color,* San Francisco, 1988, Jossey-Bass.

Gonzalez-Wippler M: *Tales of the Orishes,* New York, 1985, Original Books.

Gonzalez-Wippler M: *Santeria-African magic in Latin America,* Bronz, NY, 1987, Original Books.

Hammerschlag CA: *The dancing healers: a doctor's journey of healing with Native Americans,* San Francisco, 1988, Harper & Row.

Hirsch ED: *Cultural literacy: what every American needs to know,* Boston, 1987, Houghton Mifflin.

Huttlinger K, Wiebe P: Transcultural nursing care: achieving understanding in a practice setting, *J Transcult Nurs* 1:17, 1989.

Kleinman A: *Patients and healers in the context of culture,* Berkeley, 1980, University of California Press.

Lawless EJ: *God's peculiar people,* Lexington, KY, 1988, University of Kentucky Press.

Leininger M: Importance and use of ethnomethods: ethnography and ethnonursing research, *Recent Adv Nurs* 17:12, 1987.

Leininger M: Leininger's theory of nursing: cultural care diversity and universality, *Nurs Sci Q* 1(4):152, 1988.

Leininger M: Transcultural eating patterns and nutrition: transcultural nursing and anthropological perspectives, *Holistic Nurs Pract* 3(1):16, 1988.

Leininger M: The transcultural nurse specialist: imperative in today's world, *Nurs Health Care* 10(5)250, 1989.

Leininger M: Transcultural nurse specialists and generalists: new practitioners in nursing, *J Transcult Nurs* 1:4, 1989.

Leininger M: Transcultural nursing: quo vadis (where goeth the field? *J Transcult Nurs* 1:33, 1989.

Leininger M: Issues, questions, and concerns related to the nursing diagnosis cultural movement from a transcultural nursing perspective, *J Transcult Nurs* 2:23, 1990.

Leininger M: The significance of cultural concepts in nursing, *J Transcult Nurs* 2:52, 1990.

Lesnoff-Caravaglia G, editor: *Realistic expectations for long life,* New York, 1987, Human Sciences Press.

McNall MCC, Benner P: Healing we cannot explain, *Am J Nurs* 89(9):1162, 1989.

Meyer CE: *American folk medicine,* Glenwood, Ill, 1985, Meyerbooks.

Morrison T: *Tar baby,* New York, 1981, Knopf.

Morrison T: *Beloved,* New York, 1987, Knopf.

Murray P: *Song in a weary throat: an American pilgrimage,* New York, 1987, Harper & Row.

Stoll RI: *Concepts in nursing: a Christian perspective,* Madison, Wisc, 1990, InterVaristy Christian Fellowship.

Strange H et al: *Aging and cultural diversity,* South Hadley, Mass, 1987, Bergin & Garvey.

Sullivan LW: Guest editorial: issues on health care, *J Nat Black Nurse Assoc* 3:3, 1989.

Tripp-Reimer T: Cross-cultural perspectives on patient teaching, *Nurs Clin North Am* 24(3), 613 1989.

Walker A: *The temple of my familiar,* New York, 1989, Harcourt, Brace, Jovanovich.

Zahler D, Zahler KA: *Test Your cultural literacy,* New York, 1988, Arco.

Zambrana RE, editor: *Work, family, and health: Latina women in transition,* New York, 1982, Fordham University Press.

NURSING RESOURCES

American Nurses Association
600 Maryland Avenue SW
Suite 100 West
Washington, DC 20024
Council on Cultural Diversity in Nursing Practice
Publishes *Cultural Connections* and council membership is available to members of the ANA

Transcultural Nursing Society
Official Journal—*Journal of Transcultural Nursing*
Membership information is available from
M. Germain
3132 South Calumet Ave.
Chicago, IL 60616
Transcultural Nursing Certification information is available from:
Dr. G. Roessler
8401 Munster Drive
Huntington Beach, CA 92646

Council on Nursing and Anthropology
c/o Millie Roberson
Nursing and health Sciences
Salisbury State University
Salisbury, MD 21801

CULTURAL GROUP SPECIFIC NURSING ORGANIZATIONS AND RESOURCES

National Black Nurses Association, Inc.
P.O. Box 1823
Washington, D.C. 20013
(202) 393-6870
Publishes *The Journal of the National Black Nurses Association*

National Association of Hispanic Nurses
2300 W. Commerce, Suite 304
San Antonio, TX 78207
(512) 226-9743

Indian Health Service
The IHS Primary Care Provider—a monthly publication of the IHS Clinical Support Center. It can be obtained from Department of Health and Human Services
Indian Health Service/PHS
4212 North 16th Street
Phoenix, AZ 85016
(602) 263-1581

The NIHB Health Reporter—a monthly newsletter. It can be obtained from
National Indian Health Board
50 S. Steele, Suite 500
Denver, CO 80209
(303) 394-3500

University Microfilms International
300 North Zeeb Road
P.O. Box 1764
Ann Arbor, MI 48106
Publishes *Black Studies* a catalog of selected doctoral dissertation research

Letteria Dalton Sigma Omega Foundation, Inc.
P.O. Box 6479
Cincinnati, OH 45206-0479
This organization is a public foundation founded on the principle that the empowerment of the black family is necessary for a strong, viable community.

Federal Government
U.S. Department of Health and Human Services
U.S. Public Health Service
Office of the Assistant Secretary for Health
Office of Minority health
200 Independence Avenue S.W., Room 118F
Washington, D.C. 20201
This agency provides countless resources, including a listing of selected Minority and Disadvantaged Support Programs in Science and Research.

Admission, Discharge, and Home Health Care

OBJECTIVES

Mastery of content in this chapter will enable the student to:
- Define the key terms listed.
- Describe the nurse's role in maintaining continuity of care from admission, transfer, and discharge from an acute-care facility.
- Identify purposes of health care referrals.
- Identify clients in need of comprehensive discharge planning.
- Identify types of home health care agencies and reimbursement mechanisms.
- Identify recent social, economic, technological, and government forces that have influenced the development of home health nursing.
- Describe roles and responsibilities of nurses in home health care.
- Describe how regulatory standards and quality assurance guidelines affect the clinical practice of home health nursing.
- Identify at least two areas of specialized nursing care in the home.
- Identify future trends in home health care and the way they affect clinical practice.

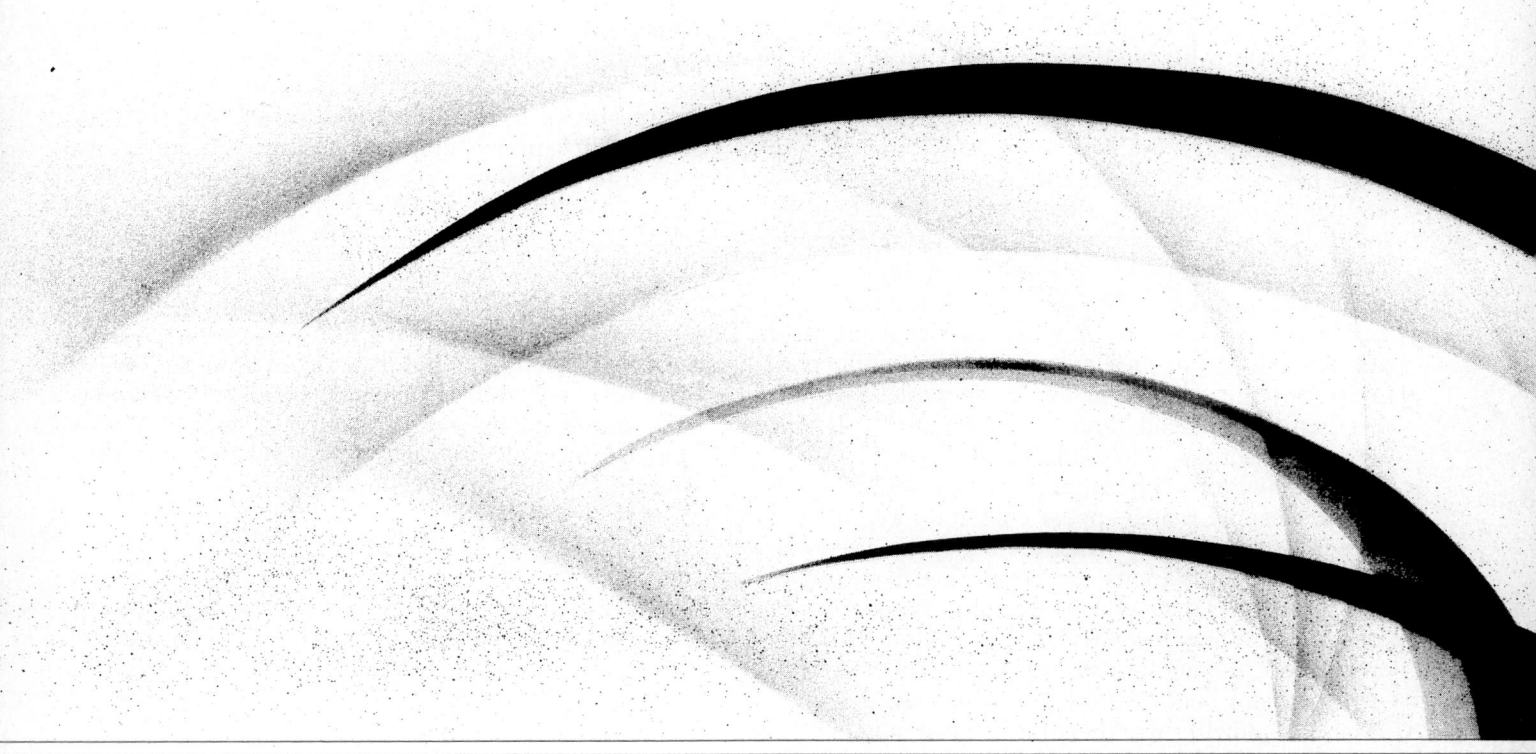

CHAPTER OUTLINE

Continuum of Care
    Regulatory agencies

Admission Process
    Initial admitting procedures
    Admission to a nursing division

Multidisciplinary Discharge Planning
    Nursing's role
    Referrals for health care services
    Transfers within an agency
    Discharge from the hospital

Home Health in the Continuum of Care

Types of Home Health Care Services and Reimbursement
    Home health care agencies
    Private duty agencies
    Durable medical equipment companies

Increased Demand for Home Health Care

Nursing Roles and Responsibilities
    Clinical practice
    Home health care management
    Teaching and research activities
    Legal and ethical responsibilities
    Discharge planning

Delivery of Home Health Nursing Care
    Assessment
    Nursing diagnosis
    Planning
    Implementation
    Evaluation

Clinical Aspects of Quality Assurance

Specialty Nursing Areas
    Hospice
    Home IV therapy
    Home respiratory care

Future Trends

The health care delivery system is an array of services with professional staff that offers a variety of ways to assist clients toward an improved level of health. Entrance into and movement through the system is not always simple, however, because of a complexity of issues. There is the challenge of providing clients with the appropriate services to meet their needs, as well as the challenge of doing this as quickly as possible. Reimbursement guidelines (see Chapter 3) now result in clients leaving hospitals earlier. As a result, clients require continued care within the home. The ability of clients to move through the health care system and have their needs met holistically and comprehensively depends on a well-coordinated continuum of care.

Admission into a hospital is an extremely stressful event. Hospital rooms appear cold and foreign. Often it seems unclear as to which care giver is directing a treatment plan. Various procedures are depersonalizing, uncomfortable, and frightening. Once hospitalized, a client may move to various locations within an institution, depending on the nature of the health care problem being treated. A client can feel powerless, not knowing whether the hospital stay will lead to an improvement in health. It is common for a client to question whether life will ever be the same after hospitalization. To be a partner in the plan of care, a client must have a clear sense of what to expect once admitted to a hospital. Similarly, it is crucial that a client knows what to expect in regard to continuing health care at home.

Nurses play a key role in coordinating care from admission through discharge. Unlike other care givers, nurses spend the most time with clients. Therefore they have the best perspective of the holistic approach needed in a client's care. Nurses coordinate the many resources required to ensure a smooth transition from the hospital to the home.

To separate the processes of admission and discharge is a critical error. The two processes should be well integrated into one. The nurse identifies the client's health care needs, anticipates physical and psychological deficits that have implications for resumption of normal activities, involves family members in the plan of care, and assists in having health care resources made available in the hospital and home. Ultimately the client and family should be prepared to understand the implications of health problems and the responsibilities for care in the home.

 ## CONTINUUM OF CARE

The concept of a continuum of care has become more important with the arrival of prospective reim-

bursement for hospitals (see Chapter 3). When a client enters the hospital, the cost for hospitalization in most cases is a predetermined amount, regardless of the resources used by care givers. As a result, for hospitals to survive financially, there is pressure to discharge clients as soon as possible. Given a client's usual limited length of stay in a hospital, the timely and accurate determination of health care needs and their prioritization are critical. To ensure a continuum of care, all care givers must know the client's prioritized needs so that a thoroughly integrated plan of care can be administered. Fragmentation of care— a client receiving a variety of services that may be repetitious, unrelated, or inappropriate—is unacceptable. A well-coordinated, multidisciplinary approach ensures a continuum of care from admission to discharge.

Regulatory Agencies

Any agency involved in the regulation of health care requires that health care institutions coordinate the admission and discharge process. The U.S. gov-

---

Examples of JCAHO Standards*
for Admission and Discharge

NURSING

- Each client's need for nursing care related to admission is assessed by a registered nurse.
- Each client's assessment includes consideration of biophysical, psychosocial, environmental, self-care, educational, and discharge planning factors.
- The client and family are involved in care as appropriate.
- Nursing staff members collaborate, as appropriate, with physicians and members of other clinical disciplines to make decisions regarding the client's need for nursing care.
- In preparation for discharge, continuing care needs are assessed and referrals for such care are documented in the client's medical record.

ADMINISTRATION

- Each hospital provides policies and procedures on discharge planning. These will include mechanisms to identify a client who requires discharge planning to foster continuity of medical or other care to meet the identified needs.
- There are mechanisms to initiate discharge planning on a timely basis.

*From Joint Commission on Accreditation of Healthcare Organizations: *Manual of hospital accreditation: 1992 standards*, Chicago, 1992, The Commission.

ernment through Medicare and the health departments of all 50 states have created specific standards addressing the importance of **discharge planning** and a continuum of care from hospital to the home. The Joint Commission on Accreditation of Healthcare Organizations (JCAHO) conducts regular accreditation visits of hospitals throughout the United States. The JCAHO seeks to improve the quality of health care provided to the public and stimulate health care organizations to meet or exceed standards of practice (JCAHO, 1992). Specific standards pertaining to making a client's admission and discharge a well-coordinated process can be found in the box on p. 122.

Regulatory standards regarding the admission-discharge process aim to provide a clear direction for all health care providers. It is assumed that a client will recieve the best quality of care within shorter time frames if health care is well coordinated from the moment the client enters a hospital. Success in meeting these standards requires collaboration from all professional care givers.

 ADMISSION PROCESS

A client can access the health care system in a variety of ways (for example, hospital, emergent care center, clinic, or physician's office) (see chapter 3). This section focuses primarily on admission into a hospital system. Commonalities exist for all settings (see box at right).

Initial Admitting Procedures

Each institution follows a different set of policies and procedures for admitting a client. A client's condition determines the extent of the admitting procedure. For example, a client entering through the emergency room may not be in a condition to undergo the same interview process that takes place in a hospital admitting office. In the case of an emergency admission, family members provide pertinent information for the hospital's records while the client is transported directly to a nursing division. In contrast, an elderly client who can no longer attend to daily chores but who is still independent enough to perform some self-care will undergo extensive screening before being accepted as a nursing home resident.

Admitting officers, secretaries, and technicians are the personnel primarily involved with the preliminary procedures for admitting clients into an agency. Some hospitals have a small satellite admitting office within the emergency room. Clients experience con-

---

Common Procedures for Admission to a Health Care Agency

- Placement of client in appropriate receiving area
- Assessment of client's health care problems and needs
- Determination of client's payment source for health care
- Explanation of client's rights
- Orientation to the health care agency's policies and procedures
- Preliminary testing and screening (specific for each agency)
- Development of an individualized plan of care

---

siderable anxiety about the admission process so all personnel should treat them courteously and professionally. If one person shows an uncaring attitude, clients may assume that all personnel are unprofessional. By making clients and families feel welcome, nurses and other staff members begin to establish a therapeutic relationship with the client.

The first step in admitting a client is to acquire identifying information, including full legal name, age, birth date, address, next of kin, admitting physician, religion, occupation, and type of insurance. This information ensures correct legal identification of the client. Data may be entered into a computer that provides a printout of an admission sheet that is placed within the client's permanent medical record. Each client receives a permanent identification number for the hospital record.

After this identifying information is gathered, the client receives an identification bracelet used when therapies or procedures such as medication administration or x-ray examinations are performed. The bracelet should be secure so that it remains in place throughout hospitalization. It is especially important for children or confused or comatose clients to have identification bracelets.

The hospital is responsible for ensuring the clients' legal rights at admission. The admitting officer will instruct clients or legal guardians on the general consent form for treatment. The signature on the consent form gives the hospital permission to perform routine procedures and selected therapies. In addition, the hospital must give clients written information about their rights under state law to make decisions about medical care, including the right to accept or refuse medical or surgical treatment. Clients must receive information about their rights to formulate advance directives such as living wills. The Patient Self-Determination Act, passed as a part of the Omnibus Budget Reconciliation Act (OBRA) of 1990, became effective in December 1991. Each state determines how the law concerning advance directives is to be stated. Finally, it is important for the client to also receive information regarding the *Patient's Bill of Rights* from the American Hospital Association (AHA) (AHA, 1972). This document must be posted within an admitting office for all clients to see. In addition, most institutions give clients copies of the *Patient's Bill of Rights* in their admission booklets. The bill describes clients' rights to be well informed and receive respectful, competent, continuous, and confidential health care.

Each hospital has policies and procedures that the client should know. Usually the client or family receives a brochure explaining available services (for example, pastoral care and social work), visiting hours, meal time schedules, smoking policies, and any other policies or rules that affect the person's conduct as a client. At admission, a client is usually quite anxious and unable to remember a great deal of information. A booklet gives the client a resource to be used at any time.

In some cases, clients may undergo laboratory and x-ray testing in the admitting office. However, the majority of testing is now done on an outpatient preadmission basis to control the costs of inpatient care. Such tests can be performed safely and more cheaply before the client is hospitalized.

After all necessary information has been collected and the client is thoroughly informed, the next step is transportation of the client to the nursing division. To begin ensuring continuity of care, the admitting office notifies the nursing division of the client's admission, current status, and room assignment. The formal admission of the client to the nursing divison begins (Procedure 5-1) This allows nursing staff to prepare a room and obtain necessary equipment for the arrival. In some hospitals the nursing department determines room assignments. This ensures that the client who requires frequent observation and therapy is placed in a room accessible to the nursing staff.

Admission to a Nursing Division

Members of the admitting office or emergency room transport the client to the nursing division under an escort. The client's condition determines whether ambulation or use of a wheelchair or stretcher is most appropriate. On arrival on the division the client and family are introduced to the nurse assuming the client's care. The initial moments spent with a client begins the orientation phase of the nurse-client relationship (see Chapter 6).

The nurse completes a number of procedures during the admission process, including orientation of the client to the room and unit procedures, collection of a nursing history (see Chapter 6) and physical assessment (see Chapter 20), collection of specimens, and a clarification of client questions and expectations. The nurse must always be conscious of the client's level of fatigue and comfort. The admission process can be exhausting, especially if there is a delay in the admitting office for a room assignment. When the client is experiencing physical or psychological symptoms, the nurse determines whether any portion of the admission process can be completed later.

 MULTIDISCIPLINARY DISCHARGE PLANNING

As soon as a client is admitted to a hospital, all members of the health care team begin preparations for discharge. Successful discharge planning is a centralized, coordinated, multidisciplinary process that ensures that the client has a plan for continuing care after leaving the hospital (AHA, 1983). Discharge planning facilitates the transition of the client from one environment to another (see box). The following levels of outcomes must be ensured for a client's successful disharge plan:

1. Client and family understand the diagnosis, anticipated level of functioning, discharge medications, and anticipated medical follow-up.
2. Specialized instruction or training is provided to the client and family to ensure proper care after discharge.

Client Risk Factors for Discharge Planning

- Lack of knowledge of treatment plan
- Newly diagnosed chronic disease
- Major surgery
- Radical surgery
- Prolonged recuperation from major surgery or illness
- Social isolation
- Emotional or mental instability
- Complex home care regimen
- Lack of financial resources
- Lack of available or approximate referral sources
- Terminal illness

Adapted from Burgess W, Ragland EC: *Community health nursing: philosophy, process, practice,* Norwalk, Conn, 1983, Appleton-Century-Crofts.

STEPS	RATIONALE
ROOM PREPARATION	
1. Wash hands.	Reduces spread of microorganisms.
2. Prepare assigned room with necessary equipment and personal care items: a. Bedpan and urinal b. Wash basin c. Bath towel and washcloth d. Toiletry items (e.g., soap, toothpaste, hand lotion) e. Tissue paper f. Water pitcher and drinking glass g. Kidney or emesis basin h. Thermometer i. Sphygmomanometer	Promotes comfort by preventing unnecessary delays during care. (Clients often prefer to bring personal care items from home into health care agency.)
3. Prepare bed by adjusting it to lowest horizontal position. Turn down top sheet and spread.	Makes getting into bed easier and safer. If client is to be transferred to bed from stretcher, place bed in high position.
4. Arrange room furniture for easy access to the bed.	
5. Assemble special equipment such as suction equipment, oxygen supplies, and pole for intravenous line. Be sure that it is in working order.	Prevents delays in case immediate treatment is necessary.
ADMISSION PROCESS	
6. Greet client and family cordially. Introduce yourself by name and job title; state that you are responsible for client's care. (Primary nurse may be assigned at this time.)	Reduces anxiety about admission and expedites client requests.
7. Escort client and family to assigned room. Introduce them to roommate if semiprivate room is assigned.	Orientation begins with introduction to roommate.
8. Assess client's general appearance, noting signs or symptoms of physical distress.	Provides baseline assessment. (If client is experiencing acute physical problems, postpone routine admission procedures until client's immediate needs are met.)
9. Assess client's and family's psychological status by noting nonverbal behaviors and verbal responses to greetings and explanations.	Anxiety influences ability to adapt to health care environment and amount of instructions that will be retained.
10. Check physician's orders for treatment measures that should be initiated immediately.	Delay can cause worsening of condition
11. Orient client to nursing division. a. Introduce staff members who enter room. Always introduce client by last name.	Promotes ability to recognize care givers.
b. Tell client name of head nurse or charge nurse of division and role in solving problems.	Provides means for client to communicate problems.
c. Explain visiting hours and their purpose.	Willingness to observe visiting hour policy ensures client will receive adequate rest. .
d. Discuss smoking policy. e. Demonstrate equipment use (e.g., bed, overbed table, lighting).	Client's safety depends on understanding correct use of equipment.
f. Show client how to use nurse call light and position it in a convenient place. Have client demonstrate use of light.	Ensures client knows how to call for assistance.
g. Escort client to bathroom (if able to ambulate). h. Explain hours for mealtime and nourishments	

Admitting a Client to a Nursing Division

STEPS	RATIONALE
i. Describe services available (e.g., chaplain visitation, gift shop, activity therapy).	Offers client options for making decisions.
12. Assess vital signs (see Chapter 19).	Provide baseline measurement to compare future findings. Determines alterations from normal expected range.
13. Have family leave room unless they choose to assist client with undressing. Close door and curtains. Help client undress and assist into comfortable position.	Provides for privacy. Prepares client for care.
14. Obtain nursing history to include the following assessment categories (see Chapter 6): a. Client's perceptions of illness b. Past medical history c. Presenting signs and symptoms d. Risk factors for illness	Provides data necessary to develop individualized plan of care based on client's identified health problems.
e. History of allergies (Provide client with allergy band, similar to size of identification band, listing allergies of foods, drugs, or substances).	Alerts nurses to substances to which client is allergic.
f. Medication history (If medications are brought to agency, have client or family take drugs home; otherwise, medications are stored on division for safekeeping. (Follow individual hospital policy.)	Therapeutic drug administration depends on correct dosages, proper timing of dosages, and avoidance of drug incompatibilities.
g. Alterations in activities of daily living	Helps identify client and family needs on discharge to the home.
h. Family resources and support i. Client's knowledge of health problems and implications for long-term care	Allows nurse to plan necessary instruction to prepare client for discharge.
15. Conduct physical assessment of appropriate body systems (see Chapter 20).	Provides objective data for identifying health problems.
16. If not obtained in admitting, instruct client on acquiring urine specimen. Inform client about technicians who will obtain blood specimens and perform tests.	Urinalysis, complete blood count, electrocardiogram, and chest x-ray study are basic screening tests.
17. Inform client about procedures or treatments scheduled for the next shift or day (e.g., visits by physician or dietitian).	Client has right to be informed of any scheduled procedures or treatments. Being able to anticipate planned therapies minimizes anxiety.
18. Give client chance to ask questions about procedures or therapies.	Provides opportunity to clarify expectations and misconceptions.
19. Collect valuables client chooses to keep. Complete listing sheet (see agency policy) and have client or family member sign it. Place valuables in safe.	Accounts for placement of valuables and prevents loss.
20. Allow client and family time together to spend alone, if desired.	Admission procedure can be stressful and fatiguing. Allows time for decision making.
21. Be sure call light is within easy reach, bed is in low position, and side rails are raised.	Provides for client's safety.
22. Wash hands.	Reduces spread of microorganism.
23. Record history and assessment findings on appropriate forms.	Prompt and thorough documentation prevents deletion of data.
24. Notify physician of client's arrival; report any unusual findings.	Client's condition may require immediate attention.
25. Begin to develop nursing plan of care. Confer again with client as needed.	Provides for continuity of care.

3. Community support systems are coordinated to enable the client to return home.
4. Relocation of the client and coordination of support systems or transfer to another health care facility are performed.

Every client in a hospital requires discharge planning. There are conditions, however, that place a client at greater risk for being unable to meet continuing health care needs after discharge (see box). When a client has one of these conditions, it is especially important to coordinate referrals to appropriate outside agencies such as a home health care agency or a rehabilitation center.

All care givers who care for a client with a specific health problem must participate in discharge planning. Development of a plan with mutually accepted outcomes and ongoing communication about its progress is essential. For example, a client admitted to the hospital for a major surgical procedure involving the lung will probably require the collaboration of the physician, nurses, respiratory therapists, physical therapists, social workers, and home health care staff. The client will need pain control, early physical ambulation, aggressive pulmonary therapy, and training for improved exercise tolerance. The client's smooth transition from hospital to home may not be accomplished if, for example, the nurse's pain control measures are not used before physical therapy, the physician chooses to prescribe bed rest an extra day, or the social worker is not informed of the lack of family support. All care givers must work together for a discharge plan to be successful.

Nursing's Role

The nursing process (see Unit 2) is a systematic, purposeful method of helping clients regain, maintain, or promote health. Often the first health care provider to encounter a client, the nurse must ensure that an organized approach to care begins immediately. Application of the nursing process ensures effective discharge planning. Assessment of a client's health care problems and responses to those problems, identification of specific problems requiring intervention, development of a plan to eliminate or modify problems, provision of appropriate interventions, and evaluation of interventions is the nursing process. If any step is incorrectly performed, discharge will not go smoothly.

Nurses in different hospitals conduct the discharge planning process differently. When the delivery-of-care system is primary nursing, a single nurse is responsible for coordinating care from admission to discharge. Even though the primary nurse is unable to be with the client every day, it is that nurse's responsibility to identify the client's discharge planning

needs and then be sure that all members of the health care team are aware of these needs. Clear communication of discharge planning information in the client's medical record is essential. Many hospitals also have discharge planning rounds on nursing divisions. During rounds, various members of the health care team discuss the status of each client with respect to potential discharge. Rounds allow members of all disciplines to interact and discuss the best treatment options for each client.

In some hospitals, nurses assume the role of case manager. The role builds on the accountability practiced in primary nursing (Zander, 1988). The case manager is responsible for specific client outcomes. Care expected to be delivered by various disciplines throughout a hospital is planned and managed through formal **case management** plans, sometimes called *critical paths* (Zander, 1988). The critical paths are multidisiciplinary treatment plans that predict certain interventions and clinical outcomes over a projected length of stay. The plan of care from each discipline, such as nursing, medicine, social work, and dietary, is integrated into a single plan, the critical path. The case manager uses the critical path as a blueprint for a client's treatment and management. The discharge plan is the critical path, because it provides clear direction for the care to be delivered to a client. The case manager can always individualize a plan of care, but the critical pathway provides a useful standard of practice for a particular health problem.

Referrals for Health Care Services

Often a client will require the services of various disciplines within a hospital, such as dietary, social work, and/or physical therapy. The nurse is often the first to recognize the client's needs. For example, a client may have had a poor appetite for several days and reveals to the nurse a dislike for many of the food choices on the menu. A referral to a dietitian could result in identifying food preferences appropriate to the client's diet. It is important to remember that other health professionals specialize in skills and knowledge that give a client services that the nurse cannot offer. Referrals should be made as soon as possible after the client's need is identified.

In many agencies a physician's order is needed for a referral, especially when specific therapies are planned (for example, physical therapy). It is ideal to have clients participate in referral processes so that they are involved in decision making. If clients fail to understand the purpose of referrals, they may refuse proposed treatment measures. The box on p. 128 summarizes the role that various disciplines can play in a treatment plan.

Health Disciplines Used in Referrals

DIETITIAN

- Provides proper nutrient and food source requirements in clients' diets
- Instructs clients on meal planning and diet restrictions

SOCIAL WORKER

- Provides counseling for major life crises such as terminal illness and family problems
- Assists in finding community resources such as equipment for home health care or an agency that will accept clients after discharge from a hospital
- Assists in finding financial resources to cover medical costs

PHYSICAL THERAPIST

- Assists in the examination and treatment of physically disabled or handicapped persons
- Assists in rehabilitating clients and restoring normal musculoskeletal function

OCCUPATIONAL THERAPIST

- Trains clients to adapt to physical handicaps by learning new vocational skills or activities of daily living

SPEECH THERAPIST

- Assists clients with disorders affecting normal oral communication

CLINICAL NURSE SPECIALIST

- Consults with nursing staff on appropriate interventions for complex nursing diagnoses
- Provides instruction to clients and family members who will assume self-care

HOME HEALTH CARE NURSE

- Provides follow-up discharge visits to a client's home for the delivery of nursing services

When multiple referrals are made for a client's plan of care, the nurse coordinates referral activities. Often it is necessary to have different therapists collaborate so that a client's care is uninterrupted. For example, there may be certain times in the day when a client can better tolerate physical therapy or is most receptive to instruction. The nurse attempts to plan referral activities at these times.

Transfers within an Agency

Discharge planning can become more complicated when a client transfers from one nursing division to another. This often occurs when the client requires a different type of medical service. For example, a client may be admitted to a medical nursing division for diagnosis of chest pain but is eventually transferred to a surgical nursing division for an open-heart procedure. Transfers to different divisions require considerable preparation. Nurses on the sending division coordinate activities with nurses on the receiving division; these activities include preparing the client's medical record, transporting medications and personal supplies, orienting the client and family to the transfer procedure, and transporting the client to the new division. Before a transfer is initiated, it is criti-

Elements of Reporting a Client Transfer

- Review of client's current condition
- Review of current nursing diagnoses
- Review of nursing plan of care
- Review of client's medications and medical therapies, clarification of treatments ordered for the day
- Acquisitions of special equipment for client care

cal to determine a client's physical condition. A client who is not stable may require special equipment such as oxygen, a cardiac monitor, or intravenous fluids during transfer to a new division. Regardless of where a client is transferred, the discharge care plan must remain current and appropriate for all team members to follow. Nurses on a receiving area must acquire complete information about the client's medical needs and nursing care so that continuity of care is not sacrificed. Nurses from the sending division provide a complete report (see box) to nurses on the receiving area. The client's discharge plan may stay the same regardless of a transfer to a new area, but it is important for the client, family, nurses, and other health care providers to validate it. Nurses must have a clear understanding of the client's progress and the interventions planned.

After a client arrives on a new division, the nursing staff is responsible for assessing the client's condition and determining whether revisions to the plan of care are needed. Throughout the transfer process, the client and family are kept informed to minimize anxiety and fear.

Discharge from the Hospital

If discharge planning is successful, the discharge of a client from a hospital should be uneventful. The nurse monitors the client's progress on an ongoing basis (see Unit 2). As a client successfully meets the expected outcomes of care, goals of care are met, and the client achieves an improved level of health or maintenance of a preexisting health state. At the same time the nurse assists in coordinating the care of other disciplines. Procedure 5-2 outlines the steps taken in the successful discharge of a client.

At discharge, clients must have the necessary knowledge, skill, and resources to meet self-care needs. Most clients are able to return home. The nurse and health care team determine whether resources are available to assist clients at home or whether home health care services are required. Clients who require more extensive care may enter skilled nursing facilities or rehabilitation programs or become residents of nursing homes. When health care continues after discharge, health care providers must receive a thorough review of client needs. The hospital nurse may talk directly with care givers in other agencies or provide a detailed summary of the care plan on a discharge document. Care should continue in the new setting with little interruption.

Discharge Against Medical Advice

Occasionally a client chooses to leave a hospital against medical advice (AMA). In this situation, there is a risk that the client will suffer complications from leaving the hospital prematurely. The client must sign a form that releases the physicians and hospital from any legal responsibility for the client's health. Before an AMA form is completed, the nurse and/or physician discusses with the client the possible outcomes of the decision. The client must clearly understand all risks. The AMA form is signed by the client and is witnessed by the physician or nurse (depending on agency policy). Usually staff inform the risk-management department of any AMAs.

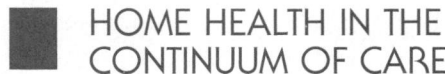

HOME HEALTH IN THE CONTINUUM OF CARE

Home health care is the provision of medically related professional and paraprofessional services and equipment to clients and families in their places of residence for health maintenance, education, illness prevention, diagnosis and treatment of disease, palliation, and rehabilitation. The most common services include nursing; medical and social work; physical, occupational, speech, and respiratory therapy; nutrition therapy; and physician care. Of these services, nursing is used most often as a result of client needs.

Paraprofessional services include home health aides, housekeepers, and companions. Many of these care givers provide personal care and household support services that prevent the need for costly hospitalization or care in a skilled nursing facility.

Home health care equipment is any medically related product adapted for home use, including highly technical items such as mechanical ventilators and intravenous (IV) infusion pumps and nontechnical items such as hospital beds and walkers.

Home health care agencies have extended almost every type of health care service into the client's residence. Health promotion and education are traditionally the primary objectives of home care. The focus is encouragement of client and family independence through teaching of self-care. Recovery and stabilization of illness must be addressed in the home, where problems related to lifestyle, safety, environment, family dynamics, and health care practices can be readily identified.

Clients needing home health care have a variety of physical, socioeconomic, and psychological problems. Most of these clients are medically unstable and have an acute problem such as wound infection or an exacerbation of a chronic condition such as lung disease. They usually require home treatment, professional assessment, education, and frequent changes in therapy. Some clients may be medically stable (for example, persons with chronic insulin-dependent diabetes), but they require long-term care to prevent exacerbations and hospitalization. Insurance reimbursement for medically unstable clients has improved, but most policies and government funds do not reimburse clients for long-term care.

TYPES OF HOME HEALTH CARE SERVICES AND REIMBURSEMENT

To meet client needs for home health care services and equipment and to ensure adequate reimburse-

Discharging a Client

STEPS

RATIONALE

DISCHARGE PLANNING

1. From time of admission, assess client's health care needs for discharge, using nursing history, care plan, and ongoing assessments of physical abilities and cognitive function (see Unit 2).

Plan for discharge begins at admission and continues throughout client's stay in agency.

2. Assess client's and family's need for health teaching related to home therapies, restrictions resulting from health alterations, and possible complications.

Will improve understanding of health care needs and ability to achieve self-care at home. Inclusion of family member in teaching sessions provides client with available resource.

3. Assess with client and family environmental factors within home that might interfere with self-care (e.g., size of rooms, doorway clearances, steps, bathroom facilities). (A home health care nurse may be available on referral to assist with assessment.)

May pose risks to safety as a result of limitation created by illness or need for certain therapies.

4. Collaborate with physician and other disciplines (e.g., physical therapy) in assessing need for referral for skilled home health care services or an extended care facility.

Clients eligible for home health care are confined to home as result of illness, are under physician's care, and require skilled nursing care on intermittent basis. A multidisciplinary assessment ensures a comprehensive discharge plan.

5. Assess acceptance of health problems and related restrictions.

Acceptance of health status can affect willingness to adhere to therapies and restrictions after discharge.

6. Consult other health team members about needs after discharge) (e.g., dietitian, social worker, home health care nurse). Make appropriate referrals.

Members of all health care disciplines should collaborate to determine client's needs and functional abilities.

7. Develop appropriate nursing diagnoses (see Chapter 7) and care plan (see Chapter 8). Implement plan of care (see Chapter 9). Evaluate progress on an ongoing basis (see Chapter 10). Develop relevant goals for client's discharge:

Well-coordinated plan of care ensures that client will meet desired clinical outcomes by discharge.

   a. Client will understand health care problems and related implications.

Client and family teaching will better prepare client to care for individual needs.

   b. Client will be able to care for individual needs.

Planned discussion periods will give client opportunity to ask questions and clarify information.

   c. Home environment will be safe.

Family members can make changes before client's arrival to make home safer. A home health care nurse may be able to assess home.

   d. Health care resources in the home will be available.

Early referral to home health care services will allow nurses to assess client's needs more thoroughly.

PREPARATION BEFORE DAY OF DISCHARGE

8. Suggest ways to change physical arrangement of home to meet client's needs.

Client's level of independence and ability to retain function can be maintained within safe environment.

9. Provide client and family with information about community health care resources.

Communities resources often offer services client or family cannot provide.

STEPS	RATIONALE
10. Conduct teaching sessions with client and family as soon as possible during hospitalization (e.g., signs and symptoms of complications; information regarding medications, use of medical equipment follow-up care, diet, exercise; restrictions imposed by illness or surgery). Pamphlets or books may be given to client.	Gives opportunities to practice new skills, ask questions, and obtain necessary feedback to ensure learning.

DAY OF DISCHARGE

STEPS	RATIONALE
11. Let client and family ask questions or discuss issues related to home health care (optional).	Allows for final clarification of information previously discussed. Helps relieve anxiety.
12. Check physician's discharge orders for prescriptions, change in treatments, or need for special appliances. (Orders should be written as early as possible.)	Discharge is authorized only by physician. Early check of orders permits you to attend to any last-minute treatments or procedures well before discharge.
13. Determine whether client or family has arranged for transport home.	Client's condition at discharge will determine method for transport.
14. Offer assistance as client dresses and packs all personal belongings. Provide privacy as needed.	Promotes comfort.
15. Check all closets and drawers for belongings. Obtain copy of valuables list signed by client and have security or appropriate administrator deliver valuables to client. Account for all valuables.	Prevents loss of personal items. Client's signature will verify receipt of items. Removes nursing department of liability for losses.
16. Provide client with prescriptions or medications ordered by physician. Review previous instruction.	Review of drug information provides feedback to determine success in learning about medications.
17. Contact agency's business office to determine whether client needs to finalize arrangements for payment of bill. Arrange for client or family to visit office.	Source of concern for many clients is whether agency has accepted insurance or other payment forms.
18. Acquire utility cart to move client's belongings. Obtain wheelchair for clients unable to ambulate. Clients leaving by ambulance will be transported on ambulance stretchers.	Provides for safe transport of client.
19. Assisting client to wheelchair or stretcher using proper body mechanics and transfer techniques. Escort client to entrance of agency where source of transportation is waiting (see agency policy).	Prevents injury to you and client. Agency policy requires escort to ensure client's safe exit.
20. Lock wheelchair wheels. Assist client in transferring into automobile or transport vehicle. Help family place personal belongings in vehicle.	Agency's liability ends once client is safely in vehicle.
21. Return to division and notify admitting or appropriate department of time of discharge.	Allows agency to prepare for admission of next client.
22. Document discharge on discharge summary form (see Chapter 22). In many institutions, client receives signed copy of form (see Step 10).	Discharge summary is essential for documenting client's status when leaving health care agency. Signed copy demonstrates plan was communicated to and agreed to by client.
23. Document status of health problems at discharge.	Allows final evaluation of plan of care.

CONTINUED

ment, nurses must understand the services available and the way clients are reimbursed. Home health care services are reimbursed by three mechanisms, including government funds, private insurance, and private pay.

Home Health Care Agencies

Home health care agencies provide skilled, intermittent professional and home health aide services, usually once or twice a day up to 7 days a week. Visits usually last 1 hour. Professional services include the implementation of a plan of treatment and skilled assessment and instruction. Home health aides provide personal care such as bathing, feeding, and bed making. Use of these services allows clients to live independently, usually with the help of family members.

Approved agencies that provide these services usually receive reimbursement from the government (such as Medicare and Medicaid in the United States), private insurance, and private pay. The Medicare and Medicaid programs have strict, and elaborate regulations governing reimbursement for home health care services. An agency cannot simply charge for a service and expect to receive full reimbursement. Most professional services provided through a Medicare-licensed agency are reimbursed at the costs for providing the service by government programs. Commercial payers, such as Blue Cross, often negotiate contract rates or provide reimbursement for billed charges. Because of the increasing costs of health care, all reimbursement mechanisms are closely evaluated.

Private Duty Agencies

Private duty agencies provide professional and paraprofessional home health care services on a more continuous basis, usually by registered nurses, licensed practical nurses, housekeepers, companions, or home health aides. These agencies provide nursing coverage for 4 to 24 hours a day.

The cost of 24-hour, private-duty nursing care ranges from $7000 to $12,000 (U.S.) a month, depending on the level of the professional providing the care. Government funds will not pay for private-duty nursing care, so reimbursement is provided primarily by private insurance and private pay. Some government programs are available for homemaker services. As expected, these services are generally affordable only to people for whom commercial insurance provides reimbursement or to those who can afford to pay privately.

Durable Medical Equipment Companies

Most **durable medical equipment (DME)** companies provide medical equipment, such as hospital beds, wheelchairs, commodes, and ventilators, as well as disposable supplies. Home oxygen is also available from most DME companies. Reimbursement is through government and private insurance. Fairly stringent guidelines exist for determining reimbursement for equipment. Many DME companies are now encouraged to seek JCAHO accreditation to ensure quality of equipment and services.

The DME industry is one of the most rapidly growing areas in the health care field. Nurses and therapists are frequently employed by these companies to provide client education and assist with sales and marketing activities. Referrals can be made to DME companies by any health care professional. The physician must certify medical necessity by signing a prescription for the equipment.

 ## INCREASED DEMAND FOR HOME HEALTH CARE

Home health care has evolved into a challenging and rapidly growing field. Because of recent economic, social, government, and technological developments, home health professionals are caring for clients who are more ill, who go home from the hospital sooner, and who have more needs for highly technical care and complex equipment than ever before.

Other forces causing more demand for home health care services include increases in the number of older adults and chronically ill persons, advances in home care technology, and the breakdown of the extended family. Most households require two incomes, which leaves fewer family members at home to care for the older adults and disabled persons. Clients are more acutely ill when discharged from the hospital and require more intensive services.

The U.S. government's health care payment system has resulted in major cutbacks that have made an impact on the home health care industry. Funding for hospital care has been drastically cut, especially for older adults, resulting in a tremendous increase in the need for home health care services by clients who would have previously been hospitalized. As a result, many of these clients require more highly skilled and technical services.

Many agencies are able to provide many highly technical services in the home; these include IV therapy, mechanical ventilation, infant apnea monitoring, and preterm labor monitoring. Because of the nature of these services, the agency is required to provide 24-hour staff availability and services 7 days a week. Although the cost for providing many of these services at home is much less than in an institutional setting, less government funding of the health care system has forced home health agencies to operate efficiently or fail.

 ## NURSING ROLES AND RESPONSIBILITIES

Nurses assume many roles in home health care, from nurse to agency owner and director. Home health care provides a great deal of autonomy and flexibility and offers opportunities for independent clinical practice, management, marketing, teaching, clinical specialization, and research.

Clinical Practice

Home health nurses provide creative and adaptive care to clients in the home. A holistic, nonjudgmental, and family-centered philosophy is essential for the nurse in the home. The nurse must understand another's value systems and beliefs. The nurse helps clients grow and develop independence and usually has an interest in health promotion and maintenance. Most of all, home health nurses must take the initiative to assess and diagnose client problems, implement appropriate therapies, and evaluate outcomes. Some agencies use the nurse as a case manager, who is the person responsible for initiating the plan of care and ensuring continuous follow-up with progress toward discharge.

Home health care nurses provide individualized care and have one-on-one contact with clients and families. They are independent and have their own caseloads, and they help clients adapt to the plan of care and disease processes. For example, a terminally ill client receiving daily heparin injections is helped by the nurse to establish a medication schedule that compliments daily home routines. Nurses also help clients adjust to the influences of cultural and environmental factors and have the opportunity to develop the nurse-client relationship more fully than nurses in hospitals.

Home health nursing requires clinical assessment and judgment, teaching skills, and the ability to coordinate and document care provided. A home health care nurse needs a broad knowledge of community resources, cultural and socioeconomic factors, family

dynamics, and psychology. Writing skills that include demonstrated knowledge and application of regulatory and reimbursement guidelines are essential abilities. In most settings, the home health care nurse is a generalist, one who applies nursing care skills and knowledge for clients of all ages and a wide range of health problems.

Home Health Care Management

Most home health agency directors, managers, and field supervisors are nurses possessing advanced training in administration and experience in home health care practice. They provide a vital link among care givers, clients, physicians, community resources, advisory board members, and regulatory and reimbursement agencies. In addition to clinical and personnel management, they are responsible for financial management, quality assurance, and program development. Home health nursing management requires a strong ability to promote staff excellence while containing costs and complying with reimbursement and regulatory guidelines.

Teaching and Research Activities

Most nurses in home health care agencies are involved in many educational activities. In fact, the primary focus of home health care nursing is client and family education to establish self-care and independence. Nurses determine client and family learning abilities and needs, develop and implement individualized teaching plans, and evaluate the success of the client in meeting learning objectives. Frequent visits to homes allow the nurse to evaluate whether clients are successfully applying new knowledge to health care practices.

Most home health care agencies coordinate staff educational activities, including orientation, case conferences, monthly in-service workshops, and physical assessment courses. Workshops about specialty services are also important as home care becomes more technical and intensive.

The home health care nurse must also know how to solve problems. Frequently the nurse enters a client's home to find an absence of resources. Managers and field staff must refine problem-solving skills and further develop them into more formalized research activities. Many agencies are engaged in formalized studies to document the following:

1. Cost effectiveness of clinical problems
2. Staffing needs
3. Consumer satisfaction
4. Quality assurance and improvement activities

These research activities will become important as competition and regulations increase and funding sources decrease.

Legal and Ethical Responsibilities

Nurses are legally able to perform independent nursing activities based on educational preparation and experience. Nurses can evaluate clients for home health care services without a medical order but must provide care under the direction of a written plan of treatment signed by a physician. Home health care nurses often establish the plan of care and then collaborate with the physician for medical treatment plans. The most controversial legal issues in home health clinical practice include the following:

1. Risks associated with providing highly technical procedures, such as administration of IV medication and blood products, in the home
2. Legal aspects of client teaching such as liability for errors made by family care givers based on misuse of information provided by the nurse
3. Compliance with Medicare or other government home health care regulations

Because of limited and highly fragmented funding for home care, home health care nurses must determine whether to continue providing services when there is risk of inadequate reimbursement for services. Often Medicare coverage expires, but clients need ongoing care but are unwilling or unable to pay privately for it. Many nurses face ethical dilemmas when torn between complying with regulations and caring for the needs of older adults and indigent and chronically ill clients. The nurse must be very knowledgeable about home health care policies to provide clinical documentation that will result in optimal reimbursement for the client. Nursing managers must also be very knowledgeable about regulations and follow the legal steps necessary to overturn coverage denials when appropriate.

Discharge Planning

Discharge planning is a major function of most home health care agencies, especially those affiliated with hospitals (see Procedure 5-2). Agencies hire experienced nurses to function as home health coordinators or discharge planners. Nurses attend discharge planning rounds and consult with medical, nursing, and social work staffs in hospitals and clinics. They facilitate access to all home health equipment and services during a client's discharge from the hospital or clinic. The coordinator screens all referrals to see whether the client is eligible for home health services in terms of insurance coverage, health care needs, and family and home situation. After determining that a client is eligible for home health care services, the coordinator completes a referral form based on information obtained from the following:

1. Client and family interviews
2. Consultation with physicians, other nurses, and staff members
3. The client's medical records

Thorough assessment and data collection by the coordinator before hospital discharge facilitates continuity of care and, in many cases, can speed the discharge process. To promote independence, initial teaching begins before the client leaves the acute-care facility. A complete discharge assessment allows home health care nurses to better understand the client's medical problems. It provides more information for making decisions about home health care planning.

Another aspect of discharge planning occurs when the client is discharged from home health care. The home health nurse (case manager) usually collaborates with the client and family and other home health care staff (such as nurses, therapists, and social workers) to plan the discharge. All necessary referrals are made to community resources for follow-up care. For example, a client with chronic lung disease may be referred to breathing clubs, support groups, or outpatient rehabilitation programs. The home health care staff follows up on these referrals to assess client satisfaction and evaluate effectiveness.

DELIVERY OF HOME HEALTH NURSING CARE

Assessment

Client and family assessment begins at referral. The coordinator submits written referral forms to the home health nurses. These forms usually include demographic data, physician's orders, medications, treatments, nursing and medical diagnoses, goals and prognoses, and functional limitations and activities.

Special problems and concerns at discharge should be communicated to the home health care staff. In complicated specialty cases (for example, IV therapy, mechanical ventilation, and hospice care), home health nurses may also visit the client in the hospital before discharge to identify needs, initiate discharge teaching, and prepare the client and family for care.

Before the nurse can thoroughly assess the client and family, a preassessment phase must take place. This phase involves incorporating information about the client's environment and gradually establishing a nurse-client relationship. The preassessment phase is based on acceptance of individuals and families (Stuart-Siddall, 1986). The nurse combines information from the referral with an assessment of the client and family in the home; the nurse uses interviews, physical assessments, and histories to do this. For this reason, the assessment is complex and time consuming. An assessment usually includes data about the following areas:

1. Physical assessment and history of all body systems, with emphasis on the present illness
2. Psychosocial assessment (education, ethnicity, and social relations)
3. Family dynamics (decision making and rituals)
4. Community resources (need for financial assistance and follow-up care)
5. Environmental factors (housing, transportation, and neighborhood)
6. Functional limitations (problems resulting in inabilities related to activities of daily living)
7. Client and family knowledge and attitudes toward illness and health behaviors and the impact on their lifestyle

 ## Nursing Diagnosis

After collecting data about the client and the home, the home health care nurse selects nursing diagnoses. Any nursing diagnosis may apply to a client in the home; however, some health problems are seen routinely (see diagnoses box). If the nurse has assessed an insufficient number of defining characteristics for a diagnosis, additional information from family or friends may help confirm a diagnosis. The diagnostic process (see box) requires the correct use of assessment skills in revealing defining characteristics for client problems.

 ## Planning

The plan of care identifies nursing diagnoses and establishes long- and short-term goals. The nursing diagnoses and goals should be related to the primary disease processes, treatment plan, functional limitations, and psychosocial, financial, and environmental problems.

The planning process in home health care requires involvement of the client and family. All care is given in the home. The client and family are accustomed to having control, and the nurse must not

---

 Examples of Nursing Diagnoses Routinely Identified for Clients Requiring Home Health Care

NANDA-APPROVED NURSING DIAGNOSES

Altered skin integrity related to:
- Physical immobility
- Radiation
- Pressure

Altered nutrition related to:
- Inability to ingest or digest food
- Inability to absorb nutrients

Bathing/hygiene self-care deficit related to:
- Pain
- Musculoskeletal impairment
- Decreased endurance

Pain related to:
- Chronic disability

Knowledge deficit related to:
- Lack of experience
- Cognitive limitation

High risk for infection related to:
- Inadequate primary or secondary defenses
- Inadequate acquired immunity
- Malnutrition

 Sample Nursing Diagnostic Process for Home Health Care

Assessment Activities	Defining Characteristics	Nursing Diagnosis
Ask if client has had experience with self-administering IV medications.	Client communicates never having given IV medications in past and requests information.	
Instruct client to read written instructions and note level of reading comprehension.	Client reads written words but demonstrates poor retention (e.g., why catheter is flushed).	*Knowledge deficit* regarding home IV antibiotic administration related to lack of previous experience
Observe client's behavior when receiving instruction of how to flush catheter.	Client hesitates to hold syringe and defers all teaching to significant other.	

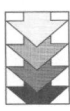

Sample Nursing Care Plan for Knowledge Deficit

Nursing diagnosis: *Knowledge deficit regarding home IV antibiotic administration* related to lack of previous experience.
Definition: Knowledge deficit is the state in which specific information is lacking (Kim, McFarland, McLane, 1991).

Goal	Expected Outcomes	Nursing Interventions	Rationale
Client will acquire knowledge and skill of basic IV therapy by 7/16.	Client will demonstrate correct handwashing and aseptic technique by second visit.	Demonstrate and watch client return demonstration of proper handwashing and aseptic technique.	Learning that is applied immediately is retained longer and is more subject to immediate use than that which is not.
	Client will demonstrate correct preparation and administration of IV fluids and medication by third visit.	Demonstrate and watch client return demonstration of inspection of bag label for date and name, inspection of solution, priming of tubing with fluid, and insertion of needle into cap.	
	Client will explain knowledge of effects of medication by second visit.	Instruct client on three side effects of medication. Praise client for correct answer.	Learning is facilitated when learner receives feedback.
	Client will safely dispose of used equipment by third visit.	Demonstrate proper disposal of IV equipment and explain safety issues.	Relating skill to home improves retention of information.

lose sight of this fact. Home health care professionals have minimal control over the environment, unlike hospital nurses who work in a very controlled environment. Client involvement in planning and teaching leads to better compliance with care. The client is urged to take an active role. The following factors must be considered when planning home care:

1. Socioeconomic, cultural, and environmental factors
2. Family and community resources
3. Client teaching
4. Interdisciplinary collaboration between home health care and hospital professionals
5. The client's physician and other health care providers, who must be consulted and informed on a regular basis

Short- and long-term goals must be realistic and measurable. They are planned with involvement of the client and family, who are also involved in discharge planning. Home health staff must foster independence to prepare the client for discharge from home health care services.

Implementation

Implementation of the plan of care (see care plan) requires close collaboration among clients, family members, home health care personnel, and physicians. Skilled interventions include assessments, teaching, consultation with physicians about changes in therapy, and initiation of complex procedures such as dialysis, IV therapy, phototherapy, and mechanical ventilation. Most procedures can be taught to the client and family. Government and private insurers pay for visits only until the client and family have had time to learn procedures. Some interventions such as prenatal assessments and the administration of blood products require the skill of a registered nurse. These interventions would not be taught to the family. Thorough documentation of the visit would support reimbursement resulting from the necessity of skilled care.

Planned interventions are not always easily achieved in many home. Nurses in home care must adapt interventions to all types of environmental, social, financial, and cultural constraints. Family and community resources must be used to assist with implementation.

Evaluation

Evaluation of outcomes of care is an ongoing process, which is the key to the success of home health care (see evaluation box). Outcomes of care must be

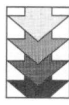

Sample Evaluation of Interventions for Knowledge Deficit

Goal	Evaluative Measures	Expected Outcomes
Client will acquire knowledge and skill of basic IV therapy by 7/16.	Have client demonstrate appropriate use of aseptic technique.	Client will demonstrate correct hand-washing and aseptic technique by second visit.
	Observe IV sites routinely.	Signs/symptoms of infection will be absent from catheter site.
		There will be no evidence of unresolved infection or lack of healing.
	Have client demonstrate preparation and administration of IV fluids.	Client will demonstrate correct preparation and administration of IV fluids and medication by third visit.
		Correct number of doses will be administered.
		No unused, expired medication will be found in home.
		There will be no side effects of medication from improper administration.
	Ask client to describe side effects of medication.	Client will list three side effects of medication by second visit.
	Observe client disposing of equipment. Check disposal containers.	Needle container will be filled with appropriate waste. Client will have no incidence of needlesticks or exposures in home. There will be no improperly disposed of needles, bags, or tubing in home by third visit.

documented for continuity of care, reimbursement, accreditation, and research. Evaluation of client response to teaching, treatments, and medications results in identification of changes needed in therapy. It also helps identify obstacles that may interfere with the effectiveness of the care plan. Effective, ongoing evaluation of outcomes and thorough follow-up for necessary changes are the most important functions of home health care personnel.

 ## CLINICAL ASPECTS OF QUALITY ASSURANCE

Many government and private regulatory agencies have established standards and guidelines for the operation and reimbursement of home health care agencies. All regulations directly or indirectly have an impact on the clinical and administrative practice of home health care nurses.

The United States and Canadian governments have established specific reimbursement guidelines for coverage of home health care services. Government agencies, specifically the Health Care Financing Administration (HCFA), distribute funds for all claims and monitor for compliance with guidelines.

Two independent organizations have established comprehensive standards for home health care. They are the JCAHO and the Community Health Accreditation Program (CHAP). To receive accreditation, all hospital-based home health care agencies must meet the standards of the JCAHO. Other organizations elect to achieve JCAHO or CHAP accreditation for quality assurance and reimbursement purposes. Most states also require licensure of home health care agencies. State guidelines follow those of Medicare but may also include additional regulations. Accreditation standards focus on documentation and case management because they affect the day-to-day practice of home health nurses.

The client's clinical record must contain comprehensive, updated care plans and detailed nursing notes from each visit. Visit reports must contain evidence that a visit was necessary and that skilled care was given (for example, assessments, which reflect medical instability, and client teaching and consultation with physicians). Homebound status, safety measures, progress toward discharge, client comprehension of instruction, and functional limitations must also be well documented.

Each client must be assigned a case manager who coordinates all aspects of care, including planning and collaboration with all home health care disciplines, community resources, and physicians. The case manager plans the client's discharge from a home health care program and implements follow-up as needed. A monthly case conference must be held on each client and followed by written documentation.

The goal of case management is to ensure the quality of interdisciplinary planning and coordination of care. The purpose of quality assurance is to ensure delivery and documentation of quality care and agency compliance with regulatory and reimbursement guidelines. Even though direct client care must be the primary consideration of the home health nurse, these regulatory procedures must also be performed. Failure to comply with these guidelines can result in considerable damage to clients and possibly the lifetime loss of their home health care benefits.

 SPECIALTY NURSING AREAS

Home health care clients increasingly need more specialized and technically advanced services. Most agencies realize that general home health care nurses are not trained to provide this level of care. As a result, agencies have developed specialty nursing teams in areas such as hospice care, IV and pulmo-

nary therapy, obstetrics, psychiatry, pediatrics, oncology, and diabetes care. Many larger agencies employ clinical nurse specialists to develop and manage specialty nursing programs.

Hospice

Hospice is a philosophy of care. It exists to provide support and care for persons in the last months of an incurable illness so that life can be lived as fully and comfortably as possible.

Hospice care has evolved into a specialization. Nurses working in this area require highly technical skills related to pain control and other palliative therapies. They also need to know the psychology of dealing with dying clients and their families (see Chapter 28). This specialized philosophy of care is applied to clients and families in the comfort of their own homes. In the United States, about 80% of certified hospice care is provided in the homes. Most programs are managed by home health care agencies. Home hospice care is preferred over inpatient hospice care for clients whose family members provide home care.

Home IV Therapy

Clients are now receiving **home IV therapies,** including hydration, antibiotic medications, parenteral nutrition, blood products, and analgesic and chemotherapeutic agents (see research highlights).

In the United States, many agencies require national IV therapy certification offered through the Intravenous Nurses Society (INS) for nurses administering home IV therapy. These nurses are usually

  Research Highlight

Nieweg et al performed a study of continuous IV administration of 4-epidoxorubin (4-ED) over 21 days. The purpose of this study was to achieve optimal patient instruction to make continuous IV infusion via an Infuse-a-Port (implanted venous access device) possible on an outpatient basis. The nurse explained the treatment to clients. They were taught to mix the medication and manage the pump. The clients were instructed on emergency measures and contacting the outpatient unit. They were seen once a week in an outpatient setting. At the end of the study, 22 clients had been given a total of 57 completed cycles over 1197 infusion days. Serious complications were not observed. Several advantages of outpatient therapy were discussed. The authors concluded that clients could successfully be treated safely and effectively on an outpatient basis when they had proper instruction and support systems.

Nieweg R et al: A patient education program for a continuous regimen on an outpatient basis, *Cancer Nurs* 10(7):177, 1987.

 Research Highlight

Niederpruem identifies compliance as a major factor affecting the success of a client on home IV therapy. The author uses the health-belief model to predict outcomes of health behaviors affecting the success or failure of a client on home IV antibiotic therapy. The following key factors in determining compliance were identified: physiological, psychosocial, and nursing and medical support. The author also discusses the use of teaching and learning principles to promote compliance and identifies possible solutions to problems that can occur.

Niederpruem MS: Factors affecting compliance in the home IV antibiotic therapy client, *J Intravenous Nurs* 12(3):136, 1989.

certified in chemotherapy, as well. IV therapy nurses must have good teaching and assessment skills (see teaching box. A multidisciplinary approach is often used to offer the client a complete range of IV services. A pharmacist, dietitian, nurse, and physician are part of many home health care agency's infusion therapy team. Comprehensive discharge planning is needed to ensure safe and effective home care.

Home Respiratory Care

Clients with chronic lung and other debilitating diseases are discharged sooner, are more ill, and need more complicated and technical care and equipment. They may require oxygen, mechanical ventilation, and tracheostomies (see Chapter 38).

Respiratory care technology has responded to the needs of these clients. Small, portable ventilators are now as efficient and effective as most hospital ventilators. Nurses caring for these clients not only need to know procedures for operating this equipment but must also have advanced knowledge and skills in respiratory nursing care and client and family teaching.

 ## FUTURE TRENDS

In 1991, the home care industry grew to $10 billion. Industry experts anticipate continued growth to the next century (Powells, 1989). This growth is accompanied by many challenges. The following list presents trends in the field of home care (Griffith, 1987):

1. The focus of home care will change to preventive care and the individual's responsibility for health. These shifts in perspectives will provide new roles and responsibilities for home care nurses, as client educators and case managers.
2. Emergence of managed health care systems and government pressure to respond to the needs of the poor and catastrophically ill will affect reimbursement and the development of future home health care programs. Home care agencies will be asked to define and defend pricing systems.
3. Hospital-based agencies will grow as the move to divest health services from conglomerates continues. Commitment and strong marketing efforts will be required of hospital administrators to ensure the future of these agencies.
4. Computers and new technology will continue to revolutionize the home care industry. Computerized documentation systems and improved financial software will increase the productivity of home health care agencies.

Home health care agencies will be challenged by a focus on preventative health care delivery, cost containment through managed care, industry competition, and growth of technology in the next decade.

 ## SUMMARY

The challenge in health care today is to provide clients with appropriate services as quickly as possible. A hospital is a foreign and threatening place. There, the nurse plays a key role in helping a client adjust and know what to expect from various health care providers. From admission through discharge, the nurse coordinates client care so that a smooth transition from hospital to the home or alternative health care facility occurs. A multidisciplinary approach is needed to ensure that clients receive all available resources. Discharge planning ensures a continuum of care after the client leaves the hospital.

As more clients leave hospitals with continuing health care needs, increasing numbers receive health care in the home. Nurses assume many roles in home health care through different types of agencies. Although some aspects of nursing care in the home are the same as practiced in other health care settings, home health care nurses pay particular attention to collaboration among family members, the client, and other members of the health care team. Quality assurance of safe and effective care in the home is also particularly important.

Client Teaching for Home IV Therapy

OBJECTIVE

- Client will demonstrate, with assistance of caregiver, the correct technique for administering home IV antibiotic therapy.

TEACHING STRATEGIES

- Discuss the importance of infection control and safe IV administration.
- Demonstrate and client will return demonstration of mixture, administration, and discontinuance of IV solution.
- Have family member or significant other observe administration procedure.

EVALUATION

- Client will correctly administer first dose of medication.

CHAPTER 5 REVIEW

Key Concepts

- Admission into a hospital begins with ensuring that a client knows what to expect during the hospital stay.
- Prospective reimbursement has created pressure to discharge clients as soon as possible.
- Discharge planning begins when a client is admitted to a hospital.
- Regulatory agencies have created standards for discharge planning.
- During admission, clients are given information about their rights in making decisions about medical care, including the right to refuse treatment.
- A medical condition may place a client at risk for needing thorough discharge planning.
- A nurse should refer clients to other health care providers when it becomes apparent that the expertise of other disciplines is needed.
- The ultimate outcome of discharge planning is to give clients the knowledge, skills, and resources needed to assume self-care after discharge.
- Home health care is a rapidly changing field affected by many forces and trends in society.
- Nursing is the essential and predominant component of home health care. Nurses hold many roles from top management to bedside clinician.
- Delivery of home health nursing care involves assessment, nursing diagnosis, planning, implementation, and evaluation, as well as accurate documentation.
- Home health care is closely regulated by government and accreditation agencies, which have a tremendous impact on the clinical practice of home health nurses.
- The future of home health care nursing will be marked by rapid growth, specialization, high technology, reimbursement reform, and a change in focus to preventive care.
- Discharge planning is an integral part of home health nursing.

Key Terms

Critical Thinking Exercises

1. Mr. Simon is a 60-year-old client, newly diagnosed with cancer, who enters the hospital for removal of a portion of his colon. Until this time, he has been very healthy. He lives alone in a small rural community, with family residing in a town about 300 miles away. He belongs to the local Catholic church. As the nurse assigned to Mr. Simon, consider his risks for needing comprehensive discharge planning. Develop a discharge plan.

2. When a client transfers from one nursing division to another, there is information that must be reported to the receiving division. Give examples of this information.

3. Mrs. Jones, age 46, is diagnosed with end-stage cancer of the cervix. She lives at home with her husband and two teenage sons. You are the home health care nurse making the initial visit. Identify at least three assessment areas you will need to gather data about to prepare a care plan.

4. Mr. Oaks is a 70-year-old man with a neurgenic bladder requiring self-catheterization. His vision is poor. He lives alone and is very independent. He has received some instruction in the technique of self-catheterization. Describe your approach to teaching this client.

5. Mrs. Phillips is a 55-year-old woman with high blood pressure. You visit her twice a week to instruct about medication side effects and administration, and you measure her blood pressure. Today, her blood pressure is high, and she tells you she cannot afford her medicine. She has just enough income to cover living expenses. Identify a nursing diagnosis and one goal of care for Mrs. Phillips.

REFERENCES

American Hospital Association: Patients' bill of rights, *Nurs Outlook* 24:29, 1972.

American Hospital Association: *Introduction to discharge planning for hospitals,* Chicago, 1983 American Hospital Publishing.

Griffith E: Homecare prophecies and predictions, I. *Home Healthc Nurse* 5(6):10, 1987.

Joint Commission on Accreditation of Healthcare Organizations: *Manual of hospital accreditation: 1992 standards,* Chicago, 1992, The Commission.

Kim MJ, McFarland GK, McLane AM: *Pocket guide to nursing diagnoses,* ed 4, St Louis, 1991, Mosby–Year Book.

Powells S: Home care's future, *Hospitals,* 63(1):42, 1989.

Stuart-Siddall S: *Home health care nursing: administrative and clinical perspectives,* Rockville, Md, 1986, Aspen.

Zander K: Managed care within acute care settings: design and implementation via nursing care management, *Health Care Superv* 6(2):27, 1988.

ADDITIONAL READINGS

American Nurses Association: *Standards of nursing care for home health care practice,* Kansas City, Mo, 1986, The Association.

Benefield LE, editor: *Home health care management,* Englewood Cliffs, NJ, 1988, Prentice Hall.

Fortinsby RH, Granger CV, Seltzer GB: The use of functional assessment in understanding home care needs, *Med Care* 19(5):489, 1981.

Gorski LA: Effective teaching of home IV therapy, *Home Healthc Nurse* 5(5):10, 1987.

Handy CM: Home care of patients with technically complex nursing needs, *Nurs Clin North Am* 23(2):315, 1988.

Jennings ME, editor: *Nursing care planning guides for home health care,* Baltimore, Md, 1989, Aspen.

Keating SB, Kelmer GB: *Home health care nursing: concepts and practice,* Philadelphia, 1988, Lippincott.

Martinson IM, Widmer A: *Home health care nursing,* Philadelphia, 1989, Saunders.

Meisenheimer CG: *Quality assurance for home health care,* Rockville, Md, 1989, Aspen.

Mitchell MK, Storfield JL, editors: *Standards of excellence for home care organizations: Community Health Accreditation Program (CHAP),* New York, 1989, National League for Nursing.

National Health Publishing: *Home health and hospice manual regulations and guidelines,* Owings Mills, Md, 1985, Rynd.

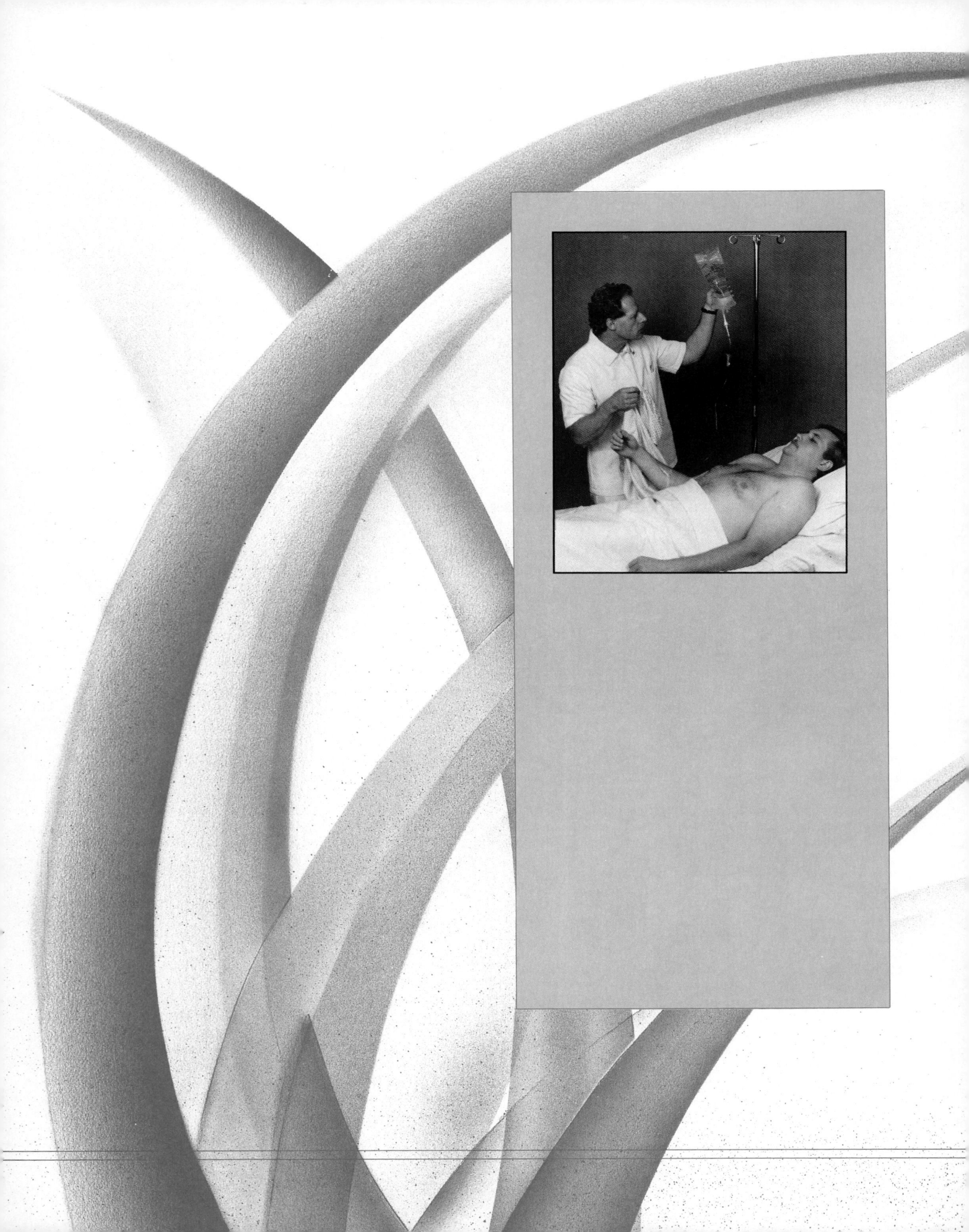

UNIT 2

The Nursing Process

CHAPTER 6

Assessment

OBJECTIVES

Mastery of content in this chapter will enable the student to:
- Define the key terms listed.
- State the five components of the nursing process.
- Describe the three components of nursing assessment.
- Discuss the purposes of nursing assessment.
- Differentiate between objective and subjective data.
- State the sources of data for a nursing assessment.
- Describe the four interviewing techniques.
- State the purpose of a nursing history.
- State the purpose of a physical examination.
- Demonstrate the four skills of physical examination.
- Conduct and record a nursing assessment.

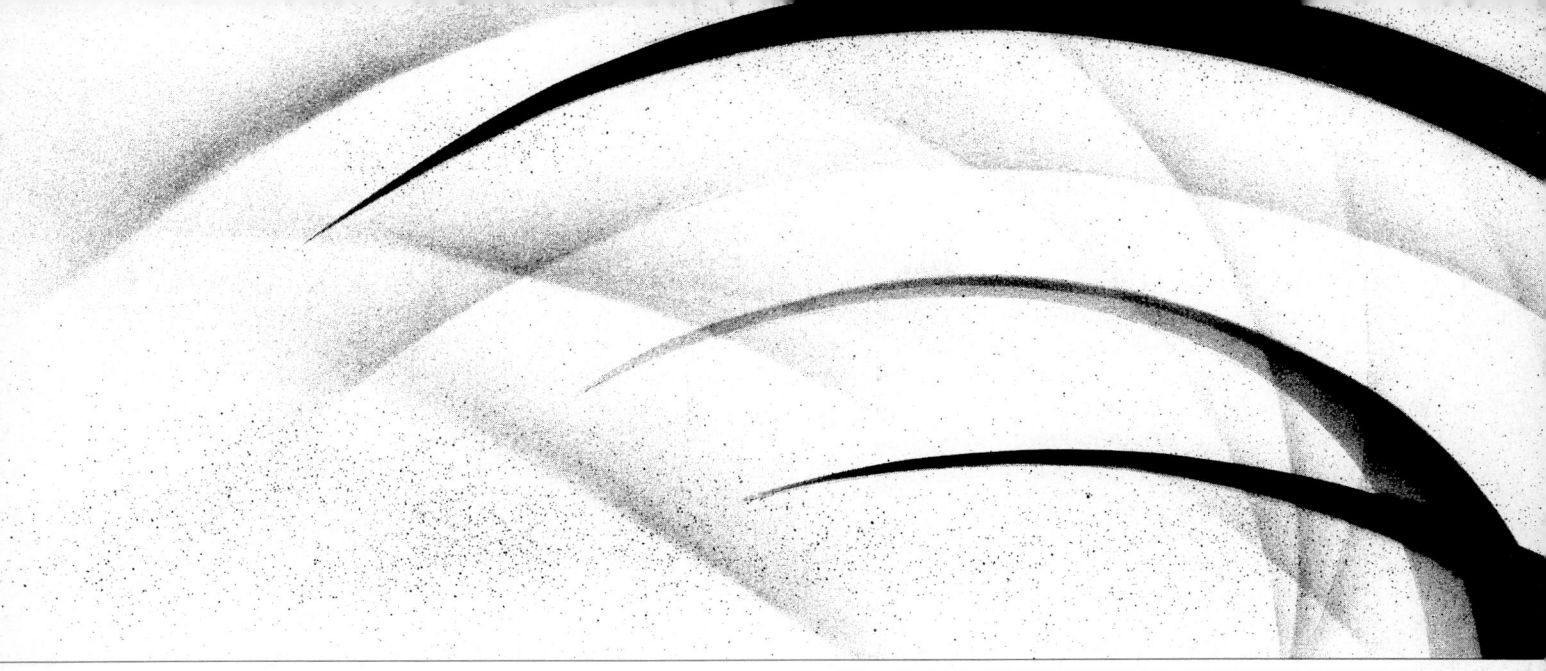

CHAPTER OUTLINE

The **nursing process** is a method for organizing and delivering nursing care. To understand its functions, components, and interactions, the nurse should have a working knowledge of the nature of a process. A process is a series of steps or components leading to achievement of a goal. The three characteristics of a process are purpose, organization, and creativity (Bevis, 1978). Purpose is the goal or specific aim of the process. Organization is the series of steps or components needed to achieve the goal. Creativity is the continual development of the process itself. In summary, a process is a continuous progression from one point to another to achieve a specific goal.

The nursing process provides the creative and organizational structure and framework for nursing care; yet it is flexible enough to be used in all settings. The purposes of the nursing process are to identify the client's health care needs, determine priorities of care goals and expected outcomes, establish a nursing care plan to meet client-centered needs, provide nursing interventions designed to meet these needs, and evaluate the effectiveness of nursing care in achieving client goals (Table 6-1).

The components of the nursing process—assessment, nursing diagnosis, planning, implementation, and evaluation—provide the organizational structure for achieving the purpose of the process (Fig. 6-1). Throughout the process, the nurse collects and analyzes data to identify clients' actual or potential health care needs and determine priorities of care goals. The nurse then develops and implements individualized care plans and evaluates clients' responses to the plans, determining whether the goals have been achieved or changed. If they have changed, the nurse modifies the original plan of care.

Evaluation and modification bring creativity to the nursing process. In addition, the evaluation and modification of the existing care plan allow continual growth of the nursing process. With this process, the nurse can meet the client's health care needs as they arise or change. The creativity of the nursing process is also demonstrated by its application in a wide variety of settings. For example, the nursing process is readily applicable for the neonate or the geriatric client and for the client in a critical care or general medical-surgical unit or inpatient or community-based setting.

TABLE 6-1 Summary of Nursing Process

Component	Purpose	Steps
Assessment	To gather, verify, and communicate data about client so data base is established	1. Collecting nursing health history 2. Performing physical examination 3. Collecting laboratory data 4. Validating data 5. Clustering data 6. Documenting data
Nursing diagnosis	To identify health care needs of client, to formulate nursing diagnoses	1. Analyzing and interpreting data 2. Identifying client problems 3. Formulating nursing diagnoses 4. Documenting nursing diagnosis
Planning	To identify client's goals; to determine priorities of care, to determine expected outcomes, to design nursing strategies to achieve goals of care	1. Identifying client goals 2. Establishing expected outcomes 3. Selecting nursing actions 4. Delegating actions 5. Writing nursing care plan 6. Consulting
Implementation	To complete nursing actions necessary for accomplishing plan	1. Reassessing client 2. Reviewing and modifying existing care plan 3. Performing nursing actions
Evaluation	To determine extent to which goals of care have been achieved	1. Comparing client response to criteria 2. Analyzing reasons for results and conclusions 3. Modifying care plan

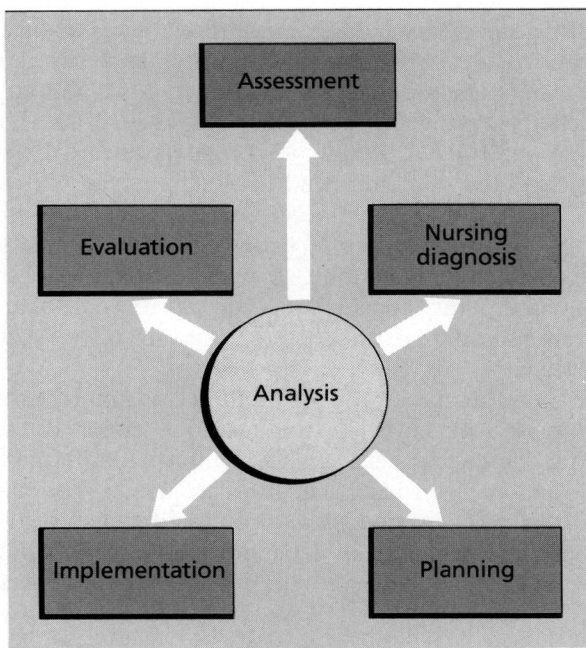

Fig. 6-1 Five-step nursing process model.

■ HISTORICAL PERSPECTIVE

The nursing process has traditionally been defined as a systematic method for assessing health status, diagnosing health care needs, formulating a plan of care, initiating the plan, and evaluating the effectiveness of the plan. The use of the nursing process in providing individualized care requires the nurse to rely on scientific knowledge to make clinical nursing judgments and set priorities.

The term *nursing process* was first introduced by Lydia Hall in 1955. Although this term has been used in education and practice for 30 years, its definition has evolved and been modified (Table 6-2). Hall described the following types of relationships between nursing and the client: nursing at, to, for, and with the client (Hall, 1955, 1963).

Dorothy Johnson (1959), Ida Orlando (1961), and Ernestine Wiedenbach (1963) introduced a three-step nursing process model into nursing education and practice. With all of these models, the nurse had to first identify or assess client needs. However, steps two and three differed. Only Wiedenbach included an evaluation component within her model.

In 1967, Lois Knowles presented a process model that she called the *five D's:* discover, delve, decide, do, and discriminate. During the first two phases (discover and delve), the nurse collects data on the health status of the client and then selects a plan of action (decide) and carries it out (do). During the last phase (discriminate), the nurse establishes health care priorities and assesses the client's reaction to the nursing actions (Knowles, 1967).

In 1967 the Western Interstate Commission of Higher Education (WICHE) defined the nursing process as "the interrelationship between a patient and a nurse in a given setting; it incorporates the behaviors of patient and nurse and the resulting interaction." They listed the steps in the process as perception, communication, interpretation, intervention, and evaluation (WICHE, 1967). The faculty at the Catholic University of America (1967) divided the nursing process into the following phases: assessment, planning, intervention, and evaluation (Yura, Walsh, 1988).

In 1969 Dolores Little and Doris Carnevali used a four-step process in the development of written nursing care plans; they combined health assessment and designation of the problem into the first step.

In 1973, Kristine Gebbie and Mary Ann Lavin at St. Louis University School of Nursing initiated national conferences on the classification of nursing diagnoses (Gebbie, Lavin, 1975). In addition, nursing educators and practicing nurses began to use the five-step nursing process model on a regular basis. Since 1973, conferences on the classification of nursing diagnoses have been held every 2 years.

Also in 1973 the American Nurses Association (ANA) published the *Standards of Nursing Practice,* which describes the five step nursing process model (ANA, 1973). Further commitment by the ANA to the five-step nursing process model was documented in the *1980 Nursing and Social Policy Statement* (ANA, 1980), which made this model the standard for professional nursing practice. The 1991 revision of the ANA's *Standards of Clinical Nursing Practice* continues to use the five-step model (ANA, 1991).

In 1992, the Joint Commission on Accreditation of Healthcare Organizations (JCAHO) continues to require the nursing process as a means for documenting the planning of client care. Thus to receive accreditation, hospitals were required to incorporate the nursing process into their policies and practices.

In 1981, Ruth Freeman and Janet Heinrich introduced a six-step nursing process for community health nursing. The first step of their process is the establishment of a working relationship. Second is the assessment of the situation as it relates to health and nursing care, as well as to the balance between health conditions and the reinforcing or counteracting forces that mediate them. The third and fourth steps are the development and negotiation of action goals with the client and the collaboration between nurse and client to decide possible courses of action. The fifth step is the implementation phase in which the step-by-step course of action is taken. The sixth and final step is validation of the effectiveness of the action taken. With this model the decisions and actions of multiple health care professionals are continually coordinated.

 ## OVERVIEW OF THE NURSING PROCESS

Purpose

The purposes of the five-step process are to establish a client data base; identify the client's health care needs; determine priorities of care, goals, and expected outcomes; establish a nursing care plan; provide nursing interventions to meet client needs; and determine the effectiveness of nursing care in meeting expected outcomes and achieving client goals.

Relationship of the Nursing Process Steps

Each step of the nursing process is essential to the problem-solving technique and is closely interrelated with the other four steps. During assessment, the nurse collects data about the client from a variety of sources. This information is used for problem identification so that planning and implementation are appropriate to the client's needs. It is also the basis for accurate evaluation.

The nursing diagnosis step involves formulating diagnostic statements that identify the client's health-related problems. The accuracy of these statements depends on the thoroughness of data collection, sorting, clustering, and validation. The identified nursing diagnoses form the framework for the nursing care plan. Thus the nursing diagnoses provide the nurse with an individualized, client-centered focus.

During the planning step of the process, a care plan is formulated. It is individualized based on the assessment data base and nursing diagnoses. The nursing care plan contains expected client outcomes and goals, appropriate nursing interventions, and criteria for evaluation.

Implementation is the action step of the nursing process. During this step, problem-oriented individualized client care is delivered according to the care plan. Interventions are continually modified as deemed necessary by ongoing nursing assessment of the client's response and diagnostic analysis. The success of this step is examined during evaluation.

The last step of the process is evaluation. The nurse determines the client's progress toward meeting expected outcomes and achieving goals and the success of nursing interventions. The success of implemented interventions, achievement of expected outcomes, and resolution of nursing diagnoses are evaluated. This step provides for the revision of the nursing care plan as necessary to resolve health problems.

The entire process is sequential and interrelated. Each step depends on the previous one. The sequence is logical because client information is gathered before determining health care needs. The plan is based on client needs, and nursing care is provided according to that plan. Last, nursing care is evaluated in terms of achievement of expected outcomes.

The nursing process is dynamic because any step may be reviewed and revised during evaluation. This dynamic flexibility allows the nurse to respond to changing client needs.

Theoretical Comparison

The focus of the nursing process is problem identification and resolution (McHugh, 1986). Problem solving and the scientific method are theoretical approaches used to identify and resolve problems in nursing and other professions (Table 6-2).

TABLE 6-2   Steps in Problem Solving, the Scientific Method, and the Nursing Process

Problem Solving	Scientific Method	Nursing Process
Encountering problem	Recognizing problem	Assessing
Collecting data	Collecting data	
Identifying exact nature of problem	Formulating hypothesis	Formulating nursing diagnosis
Determining plan of action	Selecting plan for testing hypothesis	Planning
Carrying out plan	Testing hypothesis	Implementing
Evaluating plan in new situation	Interpreting results	Evaluating
	Evaluating hypothesis	

Problem-Solving Method

In nursing, a problem arises when a client is unable to meet health care needs. Problem solving is a specific method for obtaining a solution, and it is used by nurses to assist clients in meeting health care needs. The problem-solving method used in clinical nursing practice is a six-step model that enables the nurse to make judgments and be held accountable for these judgments.

Scientific Method

The scientific method is a testable, systematic process for solving problems. There are seven steps to this method, which is used in clinical practice when the nurse wants to investigate or research a specific nursing intervention or phenomena. The use of the scientific method enables nurses to do clinical research to expand the scientific basis for nursing practice (see Chapter 11).

Benefits

When the nursing process is used to organize and deliver nursing care, the client becomes an active participant in an individualized health care process. The client receives comprehensive and consistent care. The evaluation of successful achievement of expected outcomes and quality assurance and improvement studies document the quality of care provided. The process model also assists in cost containment because nursing care is based on client needs.

Nursing also benefits from the nursing process model. The systematic approach encourages efficient use of nursing time and resources. This organized method is used to document delivery of professional nursing care. Complete and accurate documentation of each step demonstrates professional competence, responsibility, and accountability in meeting client health care needs.

 ASSESSMENT

Nursing **assessment** is the process of gathering, verifying, and communicating data about a client. The purpose of the assessment is to establish a data base about the client's level of wellness, health practices, past illnesses and related experiences, and health care goals. The information contained in the **data base** is the basis for an individualized plan of nursing care developed throughout the nursing process.

Collection of data includes the nursing health history, physical examination, results of laboratory and diagnostic tests, and information from health care team members and the client's family. Data gathered during the health history are obtained when the nurse interviews the client. To collect data from an interview, the nurse initiates the nurse-client relationship (see Chapter 15), uses various interview techniques, and progresses through the orientation, working, and termination phases of an interview. The skills of inspection, palpation, percussion, and auscultation permit the nurse to collect data from the physical examination (see Chapter 20). Laboratory and diagnostic tests validate the findings of the history and examination and can lead to identification of problems not previously noted.

In 1982, Marjory Gordon introduced a typology (analysis based on types) of functional health patterns (see box). This framework is not conceptually linked to one nursing theoretical model. Thus it is adaptable to all models (Gordon, 1987). The functional health pattern model can be used with individuals, families, or communities, and it evolves from the relationship of the client and the environment.

For each of the 11 patterns the nurse assesses clients by organizing patterns of behavior and physiological responses that pertain to a functional health category. The nurse then compares assessment data with the client's baseline (for example, usual blood pressure, weight, and nutritional intake); established norms based on age, gender, height, and weight; and cultural, social, or other norms, such as religious practices, ethnic dietary guidelines, and health care practices (Gordon, 1987).

The assessment of each of the 11 patterns represents the interaction of the client and the environ-

---

Typology of 11 Functional Health Patterns

- Health perception–health management pattern
- Nutritional-metabolic pattern
- Elimination pattern
- Activity-exercise pattern
- Cognitive-perceptual pattern
- Sleep-rest pattern
- Self-perception–self-concept pattern
- Role-relationship pattern
- Sexuality-reproductive pattern
- Coping-stress-tolerance pattern
- Value-belief pattern

From Gordon M: *Manual of nursing diagnosis: 1991-1992*, St Louis, 1991, Mosby–Year Book.

ment, which Gordon calls "biopsychosocial integration." No one health pattern can be understood without knowledge of the other patterns (Gordon, 1991). Description and evaluation of health patterns assist the nurse in identifying functional patterns (client strengths) and dysfunctional patterns (nursing diagnoses), which assist in developing the nursing care plan (Gordon, 1987, 1991). For example, the sleep-rest pattern focuses the nursing assessment on the patterns of sleep, rest, and relaxation. It includes patterns of sleep and rest-relaxation periods during the 24-hour day, as well as the individual's perception of the quality and quantity of sleep and rest and perception of energy level. Also included are aids to sleep (for example, medications, meditation, nighttime routines) (Gordon, 1991). The assessment of Mr. Roberts' sleep-rest pattern reveals that the client has difficulty falling and remaining asleep. He describes the quality of his sleep as "poor" and states that he averages about "3 hours of sleep per night." He reports that, at times, he feels he is awake throughout the whole night. Further assessment reveals that the client uses over-the-counter sleeping aids, drinks caffeinated beverages, vigorously exercises, and snacks heavily before retiring. The assessment data support a dysfunctional sleep-rest pattern that results in the nursing diagnosis *sleep pattern disturbance*.

 ## DATA COLLECTION

Data collected during assessment should be descriptive, concise, and complete and should not include interpretative statements. Descriptive data originate in the client's perception of a symptom, the perceptions and observations of the family, the nurse's observations, or reports from other members of the health team. For example, a client may describe pain as a "sharp, throbbing pain in the abdomen." The nurse's observation may be, "The client lies on the side holding the abdomen. Facial grimacing present throughout assessment." The nurse records only observations and does not interpret behavior (for example, "The client tolerates pain poorly"). Concise data briefly describe the information obtained. The information is summarized in a short format using correct medical terms (for example, "Patient describes a constant, sharp, throbbing pain in the upper right quadrant of the abdomen. Pain began 48 hours before hospitalization, 2 hours after a high-fat meal. Pain was not relieved by antacids"). Complete data collection results when the nurse obtains all information relevant to the actual or potential health problem. To confirm that complete data have

been collected, the nurse might ask, "Do I have the information to answer the questions when, where, and what are the duration and influencing factors?" For example, a nurse in an outpatient clinic uses these questions to write clear, concise, descriptive, and accurate information on the assessment form of a client seeking treatment for recurrent headaches.

Mrs. Cooper is seeking treatment for recurrent headaches. She describes the headaches as occurring every morning after she rises from bed. The pain is localized over the left front maxillary sinus and is described by Mrs. Cooper as "pulsating." The headaches last anywhere from 1 hour to "all day." In the past the pain has been relieved with 10 grains of aspirin, but the client states that the aspirin has not been effective during the past 10 days. Mrs. Cooper notices an increase in the intensity of the headache during cold, damp weather.

The collection of inaccurate, incomplete, or inappropriate data leads to incorrect identification of the client's health care needs and subsequent inaccurate, incomplete, or inappropriate nursing diagnoses. Inaccurate data result if the nurse fails to collect information relevant to a specific area or if the nurse is disorganized or unskilled in assessment techniques. Data are incomplete if the nurse neglects to obtain all information about a specific area, jumps to conclusions about a potential problem, or makes assumptions without validation. Inappropriate data are those unrelated to the area being assessed.

 ## TYPES OF DATA

During assessment, the nurse obtains two types of data, subjective and objective. **Subjective data** are clients' perceptions about their health problems. Only clients can provide this kind of information. For example, the presence of pain is a subjective finding. Only clients can provide information about its frequency, duration, location, and intensity. Subjective data usually include feelings of anxiety, physical discomfort, or mental stress. Although only clients can provide subjective data relevant to these feelings, the nurse must be aware that these problems can result in physiological changes, which are identified through objective data collection.

Objective data are observations or measurements made by the data collector. Identifying the presence of a total body rash is an example of observed objective data. The measurement of objective data is based on an accepted standard, such as a thermometer, on which the Fahrenheit or centigrade scale is the standard of measure, or a unit of measure. An elevated body temperature and measurement of head circumference are examples of measured objective data.

Ms. Johnson is taking care of Mr. Woods 1 day after an appendectomy. Ms. Johnson asks Mr. Woods about any pain or discomfort. He replies, "I have an occasional twinge in my right side, but I'm fine." Ms. Johnson observes that he is diaphoretic and has tachycardia and that his blood pressure is elevated.

Mr. Woods' description of his pain is subjective, but the physiological changes of elevated blood pressure, tachycardia, and diaphoresis are the bases for additional objective data.

SOURCES OF DATA

Data are obtained from the client, family, health care team members, health record, other records, physical examination, results of diagnostic and laboratory tests, and pertinent nursing and medical literature. Each source provides information about the client's level of wellness, risk factors, health practices and goals, and patterns of illness, as well as information relevant to the client's health care needs.

Client

In most situations the client is the best source of information. The client who is oriented and answers questions appropriately can provide the most accurate information about health care needs, lifestyle patterns, present and past illnesses, perception of symptoms, and changes in activities of daily living.

Family

Families can be interviewed as primary sources of information about infants or children and critically ill, mentally handicapped, disoriented, or unconscious clients. In cases of severe illness or emergency situations, families may be the only available sources of data about clients' health-illness patterns, current medications, allergies, onset of illness, and other information needed by nurses and physicians.

The family can supply additional data about the client's health status and may be able to indicate how the client reacts to changes in level of wellness and functioning. Finally, the family can make pertinent observations about the client's needs that can affect the delivery of care.

Health Care Team Members

The health team consists of physicians, nurses, allied health professionals, and nonprofessional employees working in a health care setting (see Chapter 3). Because assessment is an ongoing process, the nurse must communicate with other health care team members, including physical therapists, social workers, community health workers, and spiritual advisers. Health care team members can provide data about the way the client interacts within the health care environment, reacts to information about diagnostic tests, and responds to visitors. Every member of the health care team is a potential source of information, and the team can identify and communicate data and verify information from other sources.

Medical Records

The present and past medical records of the client can verify information about past health patterns and treatments or can provide new information. By reviewing medical records, the nurse can identify patterns of illness and past methods of coping.

Other Records

Other records such as educational, military, and employment records may contain pertinent health care information. If the client received services at a community health center or day-care clinic, the nurse should obtain data from these records but must first obtain written permission from the client or guardian to see them. Any information obtained is confidential and is treated as part of the client's legal medical record (see Chapter 14).

Literature Review

Reviewing nursing and medical literature about an illness help the nurse complete the data base. The review increases the nurse's knowledge about the symptoms, treatment, prognosis of specific illnesses, and established standards of therapeutic practice. The knowledgeable nurse is able to obtain pertinent, accurate, and complete information for the assessment data base.

METHODS OF DATA COLLECTION

The nurse uses the interview, the nursing health history, the physical examination, and results of laboratory and diagnostic tests to establish the data base. Each method allows the nurse to collect complete information about past and present level of wellness.

Interview

The first step in establishing the data base is to collect subjective information by interviewing the client. The interview is a pattern of communication initiated for a specific purpose and focused on a specific content area. In nursing, the major purposes of the interview are to obtain a nursing health history, identify health needs and risk factors, and determine specific changes in level of wellness and pattern of living. The interviewer obtains information about the client's health state, lifestyle, support systems, patterns of illness, patterns of adaptation, strengths and limitations, and resources.

When conducting the interview, the nurse uses specific communication skills to focus attention on the client's level of wellness. The nurse also helps the client understand changes that are occurring or will occur in pattern of living. This chapter describes communication skills and the interview, whereas Chapter 15 discusses the total communication process and details the various communication techniques necessary for nursing practice.

The nursing interview achieves several objectives (see box). First, the nurse-client relationship is initiated. A **nurse-client relationship** is the association between the nurse and the client that has a mutual concern, the client's well-being. This relationship encourages the sharing of information, ideas, and emotions.

During the interview, the nurse obtains information about a client's physical, developmental, emotional, intellectual, social, and spiritual dimensions.

Objectives of the Nursing Interview

- Establish a therapeutic relationship with the client.
- Introduce the client to the facility in a manner that is not threatening.
- Gain insight about the client's concerns and worries.
- Determine the client's expectations of the health care delivery system.
- Obtain cues about parts of the data collection phase that require in-depth investigation (branching).

Physical and developmental information reflects normal functioning and the pathological changes in a person's pattern of living induced by illness, trauma, or developmental crisis. Emotional information includes the behavioral responses to changes in health and pattern of living. Relevant emotional information includes mood, perceptions, body image, self-concept, and attitudes about sexuality. Intellectual information includes intellectual performance, problem-solving ability, educational level, communication patterns, and attention span. Social information involves environmental, cultural, ethnic, or social patterns that can affect the present or future level of wellness. The nurse also collects information about values, beliefs, and religious practices, which are part of the spiritual dimension.

The interview also provides the nurse with the opportunity to observe the client. The nurse observes interactions between the client and family and between the client and the health care environment; the nurse also observes the use of eye contact, nonverbal communication, and other body language. While observing this behavior, appearance, and interaction with the environment, the nurse determines whether the data obtained by observation are consistent with those obtained by verbal communication. For example, if the client states no concern about an upcoming diagnostic test but appears anxious and irritable, the data conflict. The observation provides additional data for the health history.

The interview is a mechanism by which the client can obtain information, as well. If a positive nurse-client relationship has been established, the client will feel comfortable enough to ask the nurse questions about the health care environment, treatments, diagnostic testing, and available resources. The client needs this information to participate in establishing goals and planning care. In addition, the interview is a first step toward establishing a therapeutic relationship between the nurse and client so that health interventions such as education or counseling can occur. To interview a client successfully and achieve the purpose and objectives of the interview, the nurse needs skills in initiating the nurse-client relationship, using the various types of interviews, and moving from one phase of the interview to the next.

Types of Interview Techniques

The client's personality and health care needs and the health care setting affect the **interview** process. An emergency situation may require one type of interview technique, whereas a chronic illness requires another. The interview in an emergency room usually centers on the present illness or trauma, precipitating factors, medications, and allergies. By contrast, an interview with a client undergoing extensive rehabilitation may focus on past and present illnesses and coping strategies, family and community resources, and present limitations and goals for rehabilitation. The nurse can use many interview techniques to elicit the necessary information from the client or another source.

PROBLEM-SEEKING TECHNIQUE. The **problem-seeking interview** identifies the client's potential problems, and subsequent data collection focuses on those problems. For example, the nurse may ask the client about changes in digestion such as lack of appetite, nausea, vomiting, or diarrhea. If the client says that some of these symptoms have occurred, the nurse may proceed with problem-solving questions that focus on the specific change in digestion.

PROBLEM-SOLVING TECHNIQUE. The **problem-solving interview** technique focuses on gathering in-depth data on specific problems identified by the client or nurse (Ivey, 1988). For example, if the client has experienced nausea, the interviewer gathers information about the onset, aggravating factors, associated symptoms, relief measures that the client has tried, and the effectiveness of these measures.

DIRECT-QUESTION TECHNIQUE. The **direct-question interview** is a structured format requiring one- or two-word answers and is frequently used to clarify previous information or provide additional information (Ivey, 1988). With this technique, the questions do not encourage the client to volunteer more information than is directly requested. This type of questioning is useful in obtaining biographical data and specific information about health problems such as symptoms, precipitating factors, and relief measures.

OPEN-ENDED QUESTION TECHNIQUE. The **open-ended question interview** is aimed at obtaining a response of more than one or two words. This technique leads to a discussion in which clients actively describe their health status. This method strengthens the nurse-client relationship because it demonstrates that the nurse wants to invest time in hearing clients' thoughts. Examples of open-ended questions follow:

1. "What are your health care needs?"
2. "How have you been feeling?"
3. "What can you tell me about your problem?"

Phases of the Interview

The interview involves the orientation, working, and termination phases. Before interviewing the client, the nurse prepares by reading the past medical record, obtaining information about the present illness, reviewing literature on the health problem, and creating an environment conducive to an interview. An interview with a hospitalized client should be scheduled for a time when interruptions by other health care professionals or families will be minimal and the client will not be receiving visitors. An environment in which the client is comfortable and relaxed is also conducive to a good interview. A client interviewed at home may prefer that the interview take place in a bedroom away from other family members. Finally, the nurse selects a place private enough to allow the client to be comfortable when providing personal information (Hickey, 1990).

ORIENTATION PHASE. Before beginning, the nurse reviews the purposes for the interview, the types of data to be obtained, and the methods most appropriate for conducting the interview. The review encourages the nurse to consider the reason for the interview, specific data needed from the client, and interview techniques to use. The interview helps establish the nurse-client relationship. While conducting the interview, the nurse remains aware that the client is forming an impression about nursing.

The nurse opens the interview by explaining the purposes of the interview. The nurse also discusses the types of questions that will be asked and the client's role in the process. Then the nurse spends a few minutes becoming acquainted with the client.

Mr. Coffey is preparing an admission history on Mr. Rose, a 21-year-old man hospitalized for the first time.

Mr. Coffey: Good afternoon, Mr. Rose. I'm Bill Coffey, and I'm the nurse who will be managing your care during your hospital stay and through discharge to your home.

Mr. Rose: Hi, Bill. Please call me Jim. What do you mean by managing my care?

Mr. Coffey: That means I'm totally responsible for all your nursing care while you're hospitalized and planning for your discharge back to your home. Although other nurses will sometimes take care of you when I'm off, I'm the nurse who plans your care. Once you're discharged, I'll call you at home to see how you are doing and if you have any questions.

Mr. Rose: I guess that's a lot like being a coach. You may not play the game, but you're responsible for winning or losing.

Mr. Coffey: I suppose that's one way of looking at it. Sometime this afternoon I'd like to ask you some questions about your health. We call this a *health interview*. The interview is done so I can best plan your care, and any information you give me is confidential. The total interview should take about 20 to 30 minutes. When could I interview you?

Mr. Rose: Could I do it now? My girlfriend is coming to visit later this afternoon. We coach a Little League team in the evenings, so she'll have to be at the game tonight.

Mr. Coffey: That's fine. Since you're in a private room, is it OK if we stay here? (Mr. Rose nods.) Good, let me close the door. Before we start, do you have any questions about anything in your room?

Mr. Rose: Yes. Why is there an outlet for oxygen on the wall above my bed? Does that mean that I'm really sick—did they put me in a special room?

Mr. Coffey: No, that's not it. Every bed in this hospital has an oxygen outlet located on the wall above the head of the bed. The reason is that this hospital has a central oxygen delivery system, and when a patient needs oxygen, we're able to supply it quickly, easily, and safely.

Mr. Rose: OK. I wasn't actually worried. I was basically just curious. That was the only piece of equipment I couldn't explain.

Mr. Coffey: (pause) Jim, you mentioned that you and your girlfriend are coaches for a Little League team. What's that like?

In this example, Mr. Coffey introduced his role to the client. He reviewed the interview process, and its objectives, confidentiality, and length. The nurse and client agreed mutually on an interview time. Before beginning the interview, Mr. Coffey asked his client if he had any questions. Mr. Coffey's answer about the oxygen allowed Mr. Rose to clarify his concern so that he would not be distracted during the interview. Mr. Coffey used the client's experience with coaching as a means of becoming acquainted before proceeding to the health interview. He chose coaching because Mr. Rose had made reference to his coaching experience. Mr. Coffey asked an open-ended question about coaching to encourage Mr. Rose to talk.

WORKING PHASE. As the interview progresses, the nurse asks questions to form a data base from which the nursing care plan will be developed. The four techniques of interviewing are implemented as needed. In addition, the nurse uses 10 communication strategies (see box) to facilitate communication and ensure that nurse and client clearly understand what the other is saying (see Chapter 15).

TERMINATION PHASE. As in the other phases of the interview, termination requires skill on the part of the interviewer. Ideally the client should be given a clue that the interview is coming to an end. For example, the nurse may say, "There are just two more questions," or "We'll be finished in 5 to 6 minutes." With this method the client can maintain attention without being distracted by wondering how much longer the interview will last. Also, the client may ask any final questions before the interview ends.

The nurse should be as organized during this phase as during the opening. The interview is terminated in a friendly manner, with the nurse indicating specifically when there will be additional contact. For example, an appropriate way to end an interview would be, "Thank you for answering these questions. They'll be helpful in planning your care. Another nurse will be caring for you this evening, but I'll be back on duty tomorrow morning. Do you have any other questions? Is there anything I can do for you now?"

The nurse's interviewing skills and techniques are essential in developing a data base. The skillful inter-

---

Strategies for Effective Communication

- *Silence* is helpful for making observations and provides the client with time to organize thoughts and present complete information to the interviewer.
- *Attentive listening* demonstrates interest in the client's needs, concerns, and problems. Listening can be facilitated by maintaining eye contact, remaining relaxed, and using appropriate touch techniques.
- *Conveying acceptance* demonstrates the interviewer's willingness to listen to the client's beliefs, values, and practices without being judgmental.
- *Related questions* are planned. When asking these questions, the nurse uses words and word patterns in the client's normal sociocultural context.
- *Paraphrasing* provides an opportunity for the interviewer to validate information from the client without changing the meaning of the statement. Paraphrasing is the interviewer's formulation of what the client has said in more specific words.
- *Clarifying* facilitates correct communication of information. It is achieved by asking the client to restate the information or by providing an example.
- *Focusing* eliminates vagueness in communication, limits the area of discussion, and helps the interviewer direct attention to the pertinent aspects of a client's message.
- *Stating observations* provides the client with feedback about how the interviewer observes behavior, action, facial expression or activities.
- *Offering information* allows the interviewer to clarify treatments, initiate health teaching, and identify and correct misconceptions.
- *Summarizing* condenses the data into an organized review. It validates data because the client has the opportunity to confirm that they are correct. Summarizing indicates the end to a particular part of the interview.

viewer is able to adapt interview strategies to different clients and health care environments. Pertinent health data are obtained when the nurse is prepared for the interview and is able to carry out each interview phase.

Initiating the Nurse-Client Relationship

Perhaps the most difficult client interview for a nurse to conduct is the first. For some clients, being interviewed by a nurse is a new experience. Therefore the nurse must establish an effective nurse-client relationship before proceeding to the nursing health history.

The first step in initiating the relationship is for nurses to introduce themselves as interviewers, stating their names, positions, and the purposes of the interview.

Good afternoon, Mr. Carney. I am Miss West, the student nurse who will be taking care of you tomorrow. I would like to talk to you for 30 to 40 minutes about your health and answer any questions you may have about your care. The reason for the interview is so I can plan your nursing care. Do you have any questions at this time? May I talk to you now?

In this example the nurse introduced herself as the interviewer, gave an estimate of the time needed for the interview, and told Mr. Carney the reason for the interview. Indicating the interview length is important because it helps ensure cooperation. A client, even one in a hospital, should not be considered a captive audience, and the nurse should take steps to ensure that a client's time is not used inappropriately. Stating the length of the interview demonstrates that time will not be abused. In the example, the nurse also gave Mr. Carney an opportunity to ask questions. It is important to determine whether the client has any pressing questions before beginning the interview. By answering these questions, the nurse can meet some of the client's immediate needs, and the client may feel more comfortable about answering questions. For example, a client who is unsure about how the hospital bed operates may be thinking about the bed instead of the interviewer's questions and therefore may not provide complete information for the data base. Finally, the nurse asked whether it was all right to conduct the interview at that time, thereby giving the client a choice.

The next step in initiating the nurse-client relationship is to communicate trust and confidentiality to clients. Illnesses that cause people to seek help are often accompanied by anxiety, helplessness, disrup-

tion of family relationships, and changes in self-image. Frequently, clients are asked to provide very personal information about themselves and their families. Generally, people share such information only with close friends, and there is a certain amount of trust that this information will not be shared with others. The nurse assures clients that interviews are confidential before asking them to share personal information concerning past or present levels of wellness or family relationships.

Finally, the nurse-client relationship is enhanced by the professionalism and competence conveyed by the nurse. The nurse's attitude of professionalism and professional manner and appearance encourages a supportive therapeutic relationship with the client so that they can communicate freely, thereby allowing identification of health care needs and objectives. The nurse is involved with the client and family and becomes an advocate for the client. The nurse as a client advocate intercedes for the client and encourages others to put the client's needs high on their list of priorities.

Nursing Health History

The **nursing health history** is data collected about the client's level of wellness, changes in life patterns, sociocultural role, and mental and emotional reactions to illness. The nursing history is obtained during the interview, and it is the first step in performing assessment. The objective is to identify patterns of health and illness, risk factors for physical and behavioral health problems, deviations from normal, and available resources for adaptation (Perry, 1982).

Patterns of health and illness are identified by collecting data about the physical, developmental, intellectual, emotional, social, and spiritual dimensions (Fig. 6-2 on p. 156). Incorporating data from all dimensions enables the nurse to develop a complete plan of care. Although many formats for the nursing health history have been given in the literature, all contain similar basic components (see box on p. 157).

Biographical Information

Biographical information is factual, demographic data about the client. The client's age, address, working status, marital status, and types of insurance coverage should be included.

Reason for Seeking Health Care

The nurse asks why the client sought health care because the information contained on the admission form may differ greatly from the subjective reason for seeking health care, as in the following example:

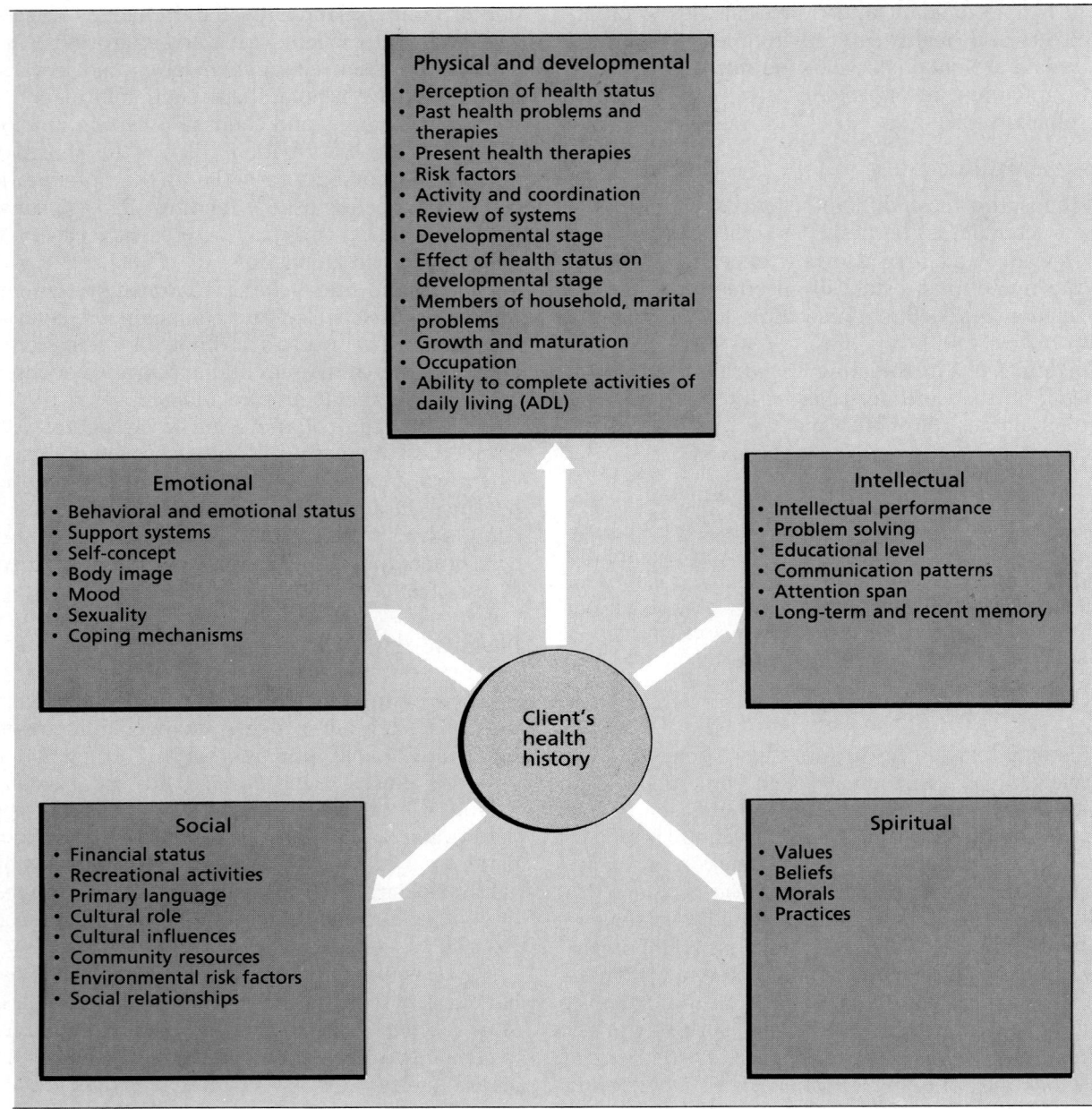

Physical and developmental
- Perception of health status
- Past health problems and therapies
- Present health therapies
- Risk factors
- Activity and coordination
- Review of systems
- Developmental stage
- Effect of health status on developmental stage
- Members of household, marital problems
- Growth and maturation
- Occupation
- Ability to complete activities of daily living (ADL)

Emotional
- Behavioral and emotional status
- Support systems
- Self-concept
- Body image
- Mood
- Sexuality
- Coping mechanisms

Intellectual
- Intellectual performance
- Problem solving
- Educational level
- Communication patterns
- Attention span
- Long-term and recent memory

Client's health history

Social
- Financial status
- Recreational activities
- Primary language
- Cultural role
- Cultural influences
- Community resources
- Environmental risk factors
- Social relationships

Spiritual
- Values
- Beliefs
- Morals
- Practices

Fig. 6-2 Dimensions for gathering data for a health history.

Mr. Brown has been seen in the outpatient clinic for chronic diarrhea and is scheduled for a series of gastrointestinal diagnostic tests. During the nursing health history the nurse asks Mr. Brown his reason for seeking health care. "To find out why I have this pain in my stomach," the client replies. The information can make the nurse aware of any discomfort that may be related to chronic diarrhea.

The statement made by the client is not a diagnostic statement but is the client's perception of reasons for seeking health care. Clarification of the client's perception identifies potential areas for education, counseling, or community resources required throughout all phases of diagnoses and recovery. When recorded, the statement is enclosed in quotation marks to indicate the client's words.

Present Illness

If an illness is present, nurses gather essential and relevant data about the onset of symptoms. The nurse determines whether the symptoms began sud-

Basic Components for a Nursing Health History

- *Biographical information:* date of birth, sex, address, family members' names and addresses, marital status, religious preference and practices, occupation, source of health care, and insurance
- *Reasons for seeking health care:* goals of care, expectation of the services and care delivered, and expectations of the health care system
- *Present illness or health concern:* onset, symptoms, nature of symptoms (e.g., sudden or gradual), duration, precipitating factors, relief measures, and weight loss or gain
- *Past health history:* prior illnesses throughout development, injuries and hospitalizations, surgeries, blood transfusions, allergies, immunizations, habits (e.g., smoking, caffeine intake, alcohol or drug abuse), prescribed and self-prescribed medications, work habits, relaxation activities, and sleep, exercise, and eating or nutritional patterns
- *Family history:* health status of the immediate family and living relatives, cause of death of relatives, and risk factor analyses for cancer, heart disease, diabetes mellitus, kidney disease, hypertension, or mental disorders
- *Environmental history:* hazards, pollutants, and physical safety
- *Psychosocial and cultural history:* primary language, cultural group, community resources, mood, attention span, and developmental stage
- *Review of systems (ROS):* head-to-toe review of all major body systems, as well as the client's knowledge of and compliance with health care (e.g., frequency of breast or testicular self-examination or last visual acuity examination)
- *Functional health patterns*

denly or gradually and whether they are always present or come and go. The nurse also asks about the duration of symptoms. In the section of the history on present illness, the nurse records specific information such as location, intensity, and quality of a symptom. The nurse needs to know whether any action precipitates the symptoms, makes them worse, or provides relief.

It is also appropriate to learn clients' expectations of the health care providers. The nurse determines whether clients expect to be "cured," "free of pain," or "able to care for themselves." This information assists in establishing the goals of nursing care, as well as in determining whether clients' expectations of

themselves and the health care providers are realistic. In addition, such expectations provide the nurse with information on client perceptions about patterns of illness or changes in lifestyle.

Past Health History

The information collected about past history provides data on the client's health care experiences. The nurse determines whether the client has ever been hospitalized or has undergone surgery. Also essential in planning nursing care are descriptions of allergies, including allergic reactions to food, drugs, or pollutants. If an allergy is present, the specific reaction and treatment are noted on the assessment form.

The nurse also identifies habits and lifestyle patterns. Use of alcohol, tobacco, caffeine, or drugs or routinely taken medications can place the client at risk for diseases involving the liver, lungs, heart, nervous system, or thought processes. Noting the type of habit, as well as the frequency and duration of use, provides essential data.

Assessing patterns of sleep, exercise, and nutrition is important when planning nursing care. The nursing care plan within a health care setting should be correlated with a client's lifestyle patterns. Frequently, variations in sleep, activity, and nutritional patterns can be accommodated.

Family History

The purpose of the family history is to obtain data about immediate and blood relatives. The objectives are to determine whether the client is at risk for illnesses of a genetic or familial nature and to identify areas of health promotion and illness prevention. The family history also provides information about family structure, interaction, and function that may be useful in planning care (see Chapter 23). For example, a cohesive, supportive family can be a resource in helping a client adjust to an illness or disability and should be incorporated into the plan of care. On the other hand, if the client's family is not supportive, it may be better to not involve them in care, particularly if the family history reveals that the client is experiencing stress related to familial relationships.

Environmental History

The environmental and psychosocial histories provide data about clients' home environments and any support systems that they or family members may need to use. The environmental history, for example, identifies exposure to pollutants that can affect health, high crime that prevents clients from walking around their neighborhoods, and resources that can assist clients in the return to the community.

Psychosocial History

The psychosocial history includes information about ways that the client and family cope with stressors. The nurse asks about resolved stressors to determine the types of stressors encountered and available coping resources (see Chapter 29).

Review of Systems

The **review of systems (ROS)** is a systematic method for collecting data on all body systems. During the ROS, the nurse asks the client about the normal functioning of each system and any noted changes. Such changes are usually subjective data because they are described as perceived by the client.

As the nurse proceeds through the nursing health history, the data obtained are recorded in a clear, concise manner using appropriate terminology. A clear, concise record is necessary because other health care professionals may use the nursing health history when delivering health care. The sample in Fig. 6-3 shows the correct way to record such information. Chapters in this unit and the clinical chapters present nursing process boxes and examples of nursing care plans to illustrate how each component of the nursing process is integrated into practice.

The **functional health patterns** serve as a focus or organizing framework for the nursing assessment (see box on p. 149). Information in the nursing health history permits a systematic description of the 11 functional health patterns and the client's perception, evaluation, and explanation of any particular problems. The 11 patterns assist in establishing the nursing data base because the historical and current information about all health patterns is collected and the information is used as base-line criteria against which any future changes are evaluated (Gordon 1987, 1991). Assessment of functional health patterns and biomedical systems are easily integrated and aid in completing the client's physical and behavioral assessment data base.

Physical Examination

The **physical examination** and collection of diagnostic and laboratory data involves the gathering of objective, observable information undistorted by client perceptions (see Chapter 20). The physical examination is the taking of vital signs and other measurements and the examination of all body parts using the techniques of inspection, palpation, percussion, and auscultation. The examiner looks for abnormalities that may yield information about past, present, and future health problems. The physical examination is conducted after the nursing health history so that data gathered can be verified. In addition, new data are obtained during the examination.

Throughout the examination, data are measured against a **standard,** which is an established rule or basis of comparison in measuring or judging capacity, quantity, content, and value of objects in the same category. The term *norm* is frequently used synonymously with *standard* in the literature. Selected standards are reliable and relevant for the category being compared. For example, established standards for ideal height and weight are used to determine whether an individual is taller or shorter than the standard or is overweight or underweight. The nurse conducting the physical examination uses inspection, palpation, percussion, and auscultation to verify information and collect further data, which are compared with the standards to determine whether the findings are normal or abnormal. Chapter 20 discusses these skills in more detail, but they are presented as an overview of physical examination.

Before conducting the physical examination, the nurse prepares the client, environment, and necessary equipment. The nurse informs the client about the process of the physical examination, specifically its purposes, the nurse's role, the client's role, and the approximate duration.

Order of Examination

The physical examination is carried out in a systematic manner similar to the ROS (see Chapter 20). This component of assessment usually begins with data on the client's height, weight, and vital signs (see Chapter 19).

Next the examiner writes a general statement about perceptions of the client and the client's level of health. This statement, called the *general survey*, includes information about mental status, body development, nutritional status, sex and race, chronological versus apparent age, appearance, and speech.

Last is a head-to-toe examination of the body systems. The examiner records objective data obtained , using clear, concise, and appropriate language in describing each system examined.

Inspection

The nurse inspects clients' bodies and observes moods, including all responses and nonverbal behaviors. This **inspection** begins with the nurse's first contact with clients and continues throughout the nursing history. Inspection is used to systematically collect data about significant behaviors or physical features. It is important to be accurate and thorough, using a systematic approach such as head-to-toe.

Palpation

With **palpation,** the examiner uses the hands and sense of touch to gather data. Palpation is used to detect tenderness, temperature, texture, vibration, pul-

Date *April 10, 19--*

Biographical information

Name *William Brown* _____ Date of birth *06/20/19* _____ Sex *M*

Address *4511 Front Street*

Family member or significant other name *Hannah — 40 years*

Address *same*

Marital status S (M) D W   Religious preference *Methodist*

Religious practices *Attends church weekly*

Occupation (present) *carpenter*

Length of occupation *32 years client has owned his own remodeling firm for the past 20 years*

Source of health care *private doctor, Dr. Kelly*

Insurance *Blue Cross — Blue Shield*

Client's reason for seeking health care *"To find out why I've had diarrhea for 3 weeks"*

Present illness

Onset *3 weeks ago* _____ , Sudden or gradual *sudden*

Duration *continued to present*

Symptoms *watery diarrhea, no cramping or GI pain noted*

Precipitating factors *occurs following a meal, diarrhea is sudden*

Relief measures *some relief noted when client eats small meals*

Expectations of health care providers *"To stop diarrhea" and "to tell me I don't have stomach cancer"*

Past history

Illnesses: Childhood *measles, mumps, and chickenpox*

Injuries & hospitalizations *(1) age 12 - tonsillectomy, (2) age 46 - broken leg*

Operations *see above*

Major illnesses *none*

Allergies: Type *roses, no drugs or food allergies stated*

Reaction *sneezing, runny nose*

Treatment *Allerest tablets*

Immunizations: *current*

Habits: ETHANOL *6-pack/day* SMOKING *2 packs/day for 20 years* _____ DRUGS *none*

Duration of each _____

Medications: Prescribed *none*

Self-medicated *Allerest*

Sleep patterns *usually retires at 11pm and rises at 6 AM*

Exercise patterns *plays tennis or racquetball 3 times a week*

Nutritional patterns *large breakfast-lunch, salad for evening meal*

Work patterns *works 50-60 hours a week*

Fig. 6-3   Nursing health history.

Continued.

Family history

Health of parents, siblings, spouse, children _____

Risk factor analysis: cancer, heart disease, diabetes mellitus, kidney disease, hypertension, mental disorders

mother died at 58 from stomach cancer; father died at 75 from heart attack; brother died at 42 from stomach cancer; 2 sisters, 50 and 48, alive and well; 1 son, 35, alive and well

Environmental history

    Cleanliness *lives in rehabilitated city home*

    Hazards *some street crime*

    Pollutants *auto fumes*

Psychosocial/cultural history

    Primary language *English*

    Cultural group *neighbors*   Community resources *his church*

    Mood *sociable, talkative, asked if symptoms were cancer related.*

Developmental stage *an adult male who appears to assume the responsibilities of an adult role.*

Review of systems (ROS) _____

Head, eyes, ears, nose, and throat (HEENT)

    Head: Headaches *occasional*   Dizziness *no*

    Vision: Last eye exam *2 months ago*

         Glasses *yes, bifocals* Contacts _____ (Hard _____ Soft _____ Long wearing _____)

         Blurring *no*

         Diplopia *no*   Pain *no*   Inflammation *yes, during allergy season*

         Surgery *no*

    Hearing: Impaired *no*   Type of hearing aid _____

         Date of new batteries _____

         Pain *no*   Drainage *no*   Tinnitus *occasionally*

    Nose: Allergic rhinitis *yes*   Type allergen *roses*

         Relief measures *Allerest tablets*

         Frequency of colds per year *1*

         History of polyps *no*

         Sinuses *no problems*

         Nose bleeds *none*

    Throat & mouth: Last dental exam *6 months ago*

         Dentures *no*

         Speech disorders _____

         Swallowing problem *no*

    Respiratory: Cough *yes*   Sputum *yes on rising in the morning*

         Dyspnea *no*   Dyspnea on exertion *no*

         Activity tolerance *plays racquetball 3 times per week*

         Last chest x-ray *this hospitalization*

         Pain *no*   Hemoptysis *no*

Fig. 6-3 cont'd   Nursing health history.

Circulatory: Pain _no_   Palpitations _no_

Edema _no_   Numbness _no_   Tingling _no_

Changes in color _no_   Changes in hair _no_

Distribution on extremities _no_

Syncope _no_   Dizziness _no_

PND _no_

Nutritional: Appetite _good until 3 weeks ago_

Nausea _____   Vomiting _____

Elimination (bowel):

Routine pattern _every other day_ Use of laxatives _none_

Colostomy _____   Ileostomy _____

Constipation _____   Diarrhea _began 3 weeks ago_

Melena _____

(Urine) incontinence _no_   Infections _once — 10 years ago_

Hematuria _no_   Catheter _no_

Reproductive:

Pregnancies _N/A_   Children _____

Last Pap test _____   Results _____ LMP_____

Excessive bleeding _____   Vaginal discharge _____

Self breast exam

Prostate problems

Neurological:

Confusion _no_   Convulsions _no_

Paralysis _no_   Paresthesia _no_   Weakness _no_

Incoordination _no_   Headaches _relieved with ASA 10 gr_

Musculoskeletal:

Pain _no_   Stiffness _no_

Exercise patterns _racquetball 3 times a week_

Adaptive responses _no_

Skin: Rashes _no_   Lesions _no_   Color _white_

Texture _smooth_   Turgor _good_

Fig. 6-3 cont'd   Nursing health history.

sations, masses, and other changes in structural integrity. Each body part is palpated, usually after a systematic assessment pattern. Palpation rules out or confirms suspicions raised during interview and inspection. Because touching may elicit fear, embarrassment, pain, or other strong emotions, the nurse should explain the actions and reasons for them. In addition, the client should be instructed to let the nurse know whether palpation produces tenderness, pressure, or pain. The two palpation techniques, light and deep, are described in detail in Chapter 20.

Percussion

Percussion is the tapping of the body's surface to produce vibration and sound. The sounds indicate the density of the underlying tissue and thus detect the location of body organs and structures. For example, percussion over a hollow organ such as the stomach produces a high-pitched, drumlike sound called *tympany*. Percussion over a dense organ such as the liver produces a low-pitched, thudlike sound called *dullness*. Percussion requires the examiner to place the palmar surface of one hand against the client's body while tapping with the other.

Auscultation

Auscultation is the process of listening to sounds produced by the body. Three systems produce sounds for the examiner to auscultate, including the cardiovascular system, the respiratory system, and the gastrointestinal system. For auscultation of these systems the nurse uses a stethoscope, an instrument that amplifies sounds produced by internal organs.

Diagnostic and Laboratory Data

The final source of assessment data is the results of diagnostic and laboratory tests. These data verify alterations identified in the nursing health history and physical examination. They include baseline information about the response to illness and information about the effects of later treatment measures.

Laboratory data are compared with the established norms for a particular test, age group, and sex. The nurse identifies variations from the normal and interprets findings according to the disease process and treatments. In addition, laboratory data can be used to evaluate the success or failure of nursing and medical interventions.

Laboratory tests are selected according to the symptoms or disease. However, common tests may be used for a large number of clients (see box). Specific laboratory tests and the nursing responsibilities associated with them are detailed in Unit 7.

Laboratory data are one more source of information the nurse uses in completing a data base. In ad-

---

Common Laboratory and Diagnostic Tests

BLOOD ANALYSIS

- Complete blood count (CBC)
- Electrolyte tests: sequential multiple analysis—6 (SMA_6), SMA_{12}
- Arterial blood gas (ABG) analysis
- Fasting blood sugar (FBS) test
- Glucose tolerance test (GTT)

URINE ANALYSIS

- Urinalysis (UA)
- Urine culture and sensitivity test

RADIOLOGICAL EXAMINATIONS

- Chest roentgenogram (CXR)
- Upper gastrointestinal (UGI) test
- Lower gastrointestinal (LGI) test
- Scans of the body, head, chest, and bone

STOOL ANALYSIS

- Guaiac tests
- Ova and parasite tests

SPUTUM ANALYSIS

- Culture and sensitivity test
- Acid-fast bacilli (AFB) test
- Cytology tests

OTHER

- Electrocardiogram (ECG)
- Stress test
- Tuberculosis (TB) skin test

---

dition to verifying abnormal findings noted in the history and examination, laboratory data can identify actual or potential health care problems not previously noted by the client or examiner.

 DATA VALIDATION

After gathering the subjective and objective data, the data must be validated to ensure its accuracy. Validation of each source of assessment data is obtained by comparing the data with another source. The client should validate the interview and health history when the nurse summarizes pertinent areas of the interview and asks about its accuracy. Any addition or corrections should be added to the historical information. Findings concerning physical examination and observation of client behavior can be validated by comparing data in the medical record with consultation from another health team member or family member. A literature review can confirm that the data are consistent with the medical diagnosis.

 ## DATA CLUSTERING

After collecting and validating the subjective and objective data, the nurse organizes the information into meaningful clusters. The nurse bases the sorting of data on professional knowledge. During data clustering, the nurse organizes data and focuses attention on functions needing support and assistance for recovery. The box demonstrates focused data clustering using system-oriented assessment and functional health pattern assessment.

 ## DATA DOCUMENTATION

Data documentation is the last part of a complete assessment. Thoroughness and accuracy are necessary when recording data. If an item is not recorded, it is lost and unavailable as part of the data base.

Thoroughness in data documentation is essential for two reasons. First, all data pertinent to client status are included. Even information that does not seem to indicate an abnormality should be recorded. It may become pertinent later, serving as a baseline for a change in status. A general rule of thumb is that if it is assessed it should be recorded.

Second, observation and recording of client status is a legal and professional responsibility. The nurse practice acts in all states and the ANA *Policy Statement* (1980) and ANA *Standards of Clinical Nursing Practice* (1991) mandate accurate data collection and recording as independent functions essential to the role of the professional nurse.

Being factual is easy after it becomes a habit. The basic rule is to record all observations. When recording data, a nurse should pay attention to facts and should make an effort to be as descriptive as possible. Anything heard, seen, felt, or smelled should be reported exactly. Conclusions about such data become nursing diagnoses. Because assessment includes the collection and documentation of subjective and objective data, the nurse should make certain that the data base is complete and factual before data clustering. Premature clustering can lead to inaccurate nursing diagnoses. In situations in which the client has just been admitted or when the client's status is changing rapidly, it is better to continually collect and document the new data and delay clustering.

Focused Data Clustering

SYSTEM-ORIENTED FORMAT
Integumentary System

- Intact, flushed skin, which is hot and dry to touch
- Dry oral mucosa, coated tongue and cracked lips

Gastrointestinal System

- Distended, firm abdomen, which is tender to palpation in lower quadrants
- Hyperactive bowel sounds in all quadrants
- History of anorexia, nausea, vomiting, and diarrhea for 2 days

Medical Record

- Laboratory tests indicating elevated white blood cell (WBC) count and hematocrit level: hypernatremia
- Abdominal x-ray examination showing gas-filled loops of bowel
- Admitting diagnosis of gastroenteritis

FUNCTIONAL HEALTH PATTERN FORMAT
Activity and Exercise Pattern

- Statement of increased fatigue when walking
- Demonstration of ability to perform activities of daily living (ADLs)
- Fatigued, dyspneic, and diaphoretic appearance when performing ADLs
- Increased pulse from 90 to 126 beats per minute during ADLs

Sleep and Rest Pattern

- Report of difficulty in falling and remaining asleep
- Denial of use of sleeping aids

Medical Record

- Previous history of decreased activity tolerance and poor sleeping 2 weeks before hospital admission for congestive heart failure
- Chest x-ray film showing pulmonary congestion

 ## SUMMARY

Nursing assessment is the gathering and verification of data about a client to establish a data base. The health history, physical examination, and collection of laboratory data are components of assessment.

After collecting data, the nurse validates and sorts data so that they are clustered into related groups. Validation, sorting, and clustering are the preparatory steps to formulation of nursing diagnoses.

CHAPTER 6 REVIEW

Key Concepts

- The nursing process is a method for organizing and delivering nursing care.
- The purpose of the nursing process is to identify the client's health care needs, establish a nursing care plan, and complete nursing interventions designed to meet these needs.
- Organization of the nursing process is based on five components, including assessment, nursing diagnosis, planning, implementation, and evaluation.
- During assessment, the nurse gathers, verifies, and communicates data about a client by interview, nursing health history, physical examination, and laboratory and diagnostic tests.
- Written data statements should be descriptive, concise, and complete and should not include interpretative statements.
- Collection of inaccurate, incomplete, or inappropriate data may result in incorrect identification of the client's health care needs.
- Objective data can be measured by the data collector, but subjective data are the client's or family's perceptions.
- The client is the principal source of data.
- Families can be a primary source of information about the client's health status.
- Every member of the health care team is a potential source of information.
- Other data sources include the health record, other records, and pertinent literature.
- Review of the pertinent literature increases the nurse's knowledge about the symptoms, treatment, and prognosis of a specific illness.
- The interviewer identifies the client's needs, risk factors, and specific changes in level of wellness and pattern of living.
- Use of effective communication skills enables the nurse to initiate the nurse-client relationship and complete the interview.
- The interview has three phases: orientation, working, and termination.
- During the interview, information is obtained about the physical, developmental, intellectual, emotional, social, and spiritual dimensions of the client.
- The interview allows the nurse to observe the client and interaction between the client and family.
- The four primary interview techniques include problem solving, problem seeking, direct question, and open-ended question.
- The nursing health history involves data about level of wellness, past medical history, family history, environmental history, psychosocial and cultural history, and a review of the body systems.
- Physical examination requires the skills of inspection, palpation, auscultation, and percussion.
- Laboratory and diagnostic tests add to the data base and verify data gathered through the nursing health history and physical examination.

Key Terms

Assessment, p. 149

Auscultation, p. 162

Data base, p. 149

Direct-question interview, p. 153

Functional health patterns, p. 158

Inspection, p. 158

Interview, p. 152

Norm, p. 158

Nurse-client relationship, p. 152

Nursing health history, p. 155

Nursing process, p. 146

Objective data, p. 150

Open-ended question interview, p. 153

Palpation, p. 158

Percussion, p. 162

Physical examination, p. 158

Problem-seeking interview, p. 153

Problem-solving interview, p. 153

Review of systems (ROS), p. 158

Standard, p. 158

Subjective data, p. 150

Critical Thinking Exercises

1. During the initial phase of assessment, you observe that your client seems reluctant to answer your questions. What information do you need to understand this reluctance? What can you do to increase the client's comfort? What changes might you make in the interview style?

2. You are going to assess two clients: one client for a physical examination and behavioral assessment and the other client for a follow-up after a hospital admission for pneumonia and congestive heart failure. What types of changes will you make in your assessment technique, length of assessment, types of questions you ask, and interview techniques between these two clients?

3. You are assigned to provide health care to a three-generation family in your school's community. How do you modify your assessment tool to obtain all data for each developmental level and to assess for environmental factors that influence health promotion?

REFERENCES

American Nurses Association: *Standards of nursing practice,* Kansas City, Mo, 1973, The Association.

American Nurses Association: *Nursing: a social policy statement,* Kansas City, Mo, 1980, The Association.

American Nurses Association: *Standards of clinical nursing practice,* Kansas City, Mo, 1991, The Association.

Bevis EM: *Curriculum building in nursing: a process,* St Louis, 1978, Mosby–Year Book.

Freeman RB, Heinrich J: *Community health nursing practice,* ed 2, Philadelphia, 1981, Saunders.

Gebbie K, Lavin MA: *Classification of nursing diagnoses,* St Louis, 1975, Mosby–Year Book.

Gordon M: *Nursing diagnosis process and application,* ed 2, New York, 1987, McGraw-Hill.

Gordon M: *Manual of nursing diagnoses: 1991-1992,* St Louis, 1991, Mosby–Year Book.

Hall LE: *Quality of nursing care.* Address given at the meeting of the Department of Baccalaureate and Higher Degree programs of the New Jersey League for Nursing, Public Health News, New Jersey Department of Health, 1955.

Hall LE: A center for nursing, *Nurs Outlook* 11:805, 1963.

Hickey PW: *Nursing process handbook,* St Louis, 1990, Mosby–Year Book.

Ivey AE: *Intentional interviewing and counseling: facilitating client development,* ed 2, Pacific Grove, Calif, 1988, Brooks/Cole.

Johnson D: A philosophy of nursing, *Nurs Outlook* 7:198, 1959.

Joint Commission on Accreditation of Healthcare Organizations: *Manual of hospital accreditation: 1992 standards,* Chicago, 1992, The Commission.

Knowles L: *Decision making in nursing: a necessity for doing, 1966 ANA clinical sessions,* New York, 1967, Appleton-Century-Crofts.

Little DE, Carnevali DV: *Nursing care planning,* Philadelphia, 1969, Lippincott.

McHugh M: Nursing process: musings on the method, *Holistic Nurs Pract* 1(1):21, 1986.

Orlando I: *The dynamic nurse-patient relationship,* New York, 1961, Putnam.

Perry AG: Analysis of the components of the nursing process. In Carlson JH, Craft CA, McGuire AD, editors: *Nursing diagnosis,* Philadelphia, 1982, Saunders.

Western Interstate Commission of Higher Education: *Defining clinical content: Graduate Nursing Programs, Medical and Surgical Nursing Programs,* Seattle, 1967, The Commission.

Wiedenback E: The helping art of nursing, *Am J Nurs* 63:64, 1963.

Yura H, Walsh M: *The nursing process: assessing, planning, implementing, and evaluating,* ed 5, Nowalk, Conn, 1988, Appleton & Lange.

ADDITIONAL READINGS

Brown MD: Functional assessment of the elderly, *J Gerontol Nurs* 14:13, 1988.

Bellack JP, Bamford DA: *Nursing assessment: a multidimensional approach*, 1984, Belmont, Calif, Wadsworth.

Bermost LS: Interviewing: a key to therapeutic communication in nursing practice, *Nurs Clin North Am* 1:205, 1966.

Bowers AC, Thompson JM: *Clinical manual of health assessment*, ed 3, St Louis, 1988, Mosby–Year Book.

Edelman C, Mandle CC: *Health promotion throughout the lifespan,* ed 2, St Louis, 1990, Mosby–Year Book.

Eggland ET: How to take a meaningful nursing history, *Nurs 77* 7:22, 1977.

Fields WL, McGinn-Campbell KM: *Introduction to health assessment*, Reston, Va, 1983, Reston.

Fraser C, Filler MJ: The assessment factor most nurses forget, *RN* March 1989, p 32.

Gordon M: *Manual of nursing diagnosis: 1991-1992,* St Louis, 1991, Mosby-Year Book.

Jones DA: *Health assessment manual,* New York, 1984, McGraw-Hill.

Jones DA, Lepley MK, Baker BA: *Health assessment across the life span,* New York, 1984, McGraw-Hill.

Kesler AR: Pitfalls to avoid in interviewing outpatients, *Nurs 77* 7:70, 1977.

Levin RF, Crosley JM: Focused data collection for the generation of nursing diagnoses, *J Staff Development* 2 (2):56, 1986.

Loveridge CE, Heinkeken J: Confirming interactions, *J Gerontol Nurs* 14:27, 1988.

Luekenotte AG: *Pocket guide to gerontologic assessment*, St Louis, 1990, Mosby–Year Book.

Malasanos L et al: *Health assessment,* ed 4, St Louis, 1989, Mosby–Year Book.

Marriner A: *The nursing process: a scientific approach to nursing care,* ed 4, St Louis, 1987, Mosby–Year Book.

McCain RF: Nursing by assessment, not intuition, *Am J Nurs* 65:82, 1965.

Mengel A: Getting the most from patient interviews, *Nurs 82,* 12(11):46, 1982.

Moss AR: Determinants of patient care: Nursing Process or nursing attitudes? *J Adv Nurs* 13: 615, 1988.

Norris L: Coaching the question, *Nurs 86* 16(5):100, 1986.

CHAPTER 7

Nursing Diagnosis

OBJECTIVES

Mastery of content in this chapter will enable the student to:

- Define the key terms listed.
- Describe the way defining characteristics and the etiological process individualizes a nursing diagnosis.
- List and discuss the steps of the nursing diagnostic process.
- Demonstrate the nursing diagnostic process.
- Differentiate between a nursing diagnosis and a medical diagnosis.
- Explain what makes a nursing diagnosis correct.
- Discuss the advantages of nursing diagnoses for the client and the nursing profession.
- Discuss the limitations of nursing diagnoses.
- Formulate nursing diagnoses from a nursing assessment.

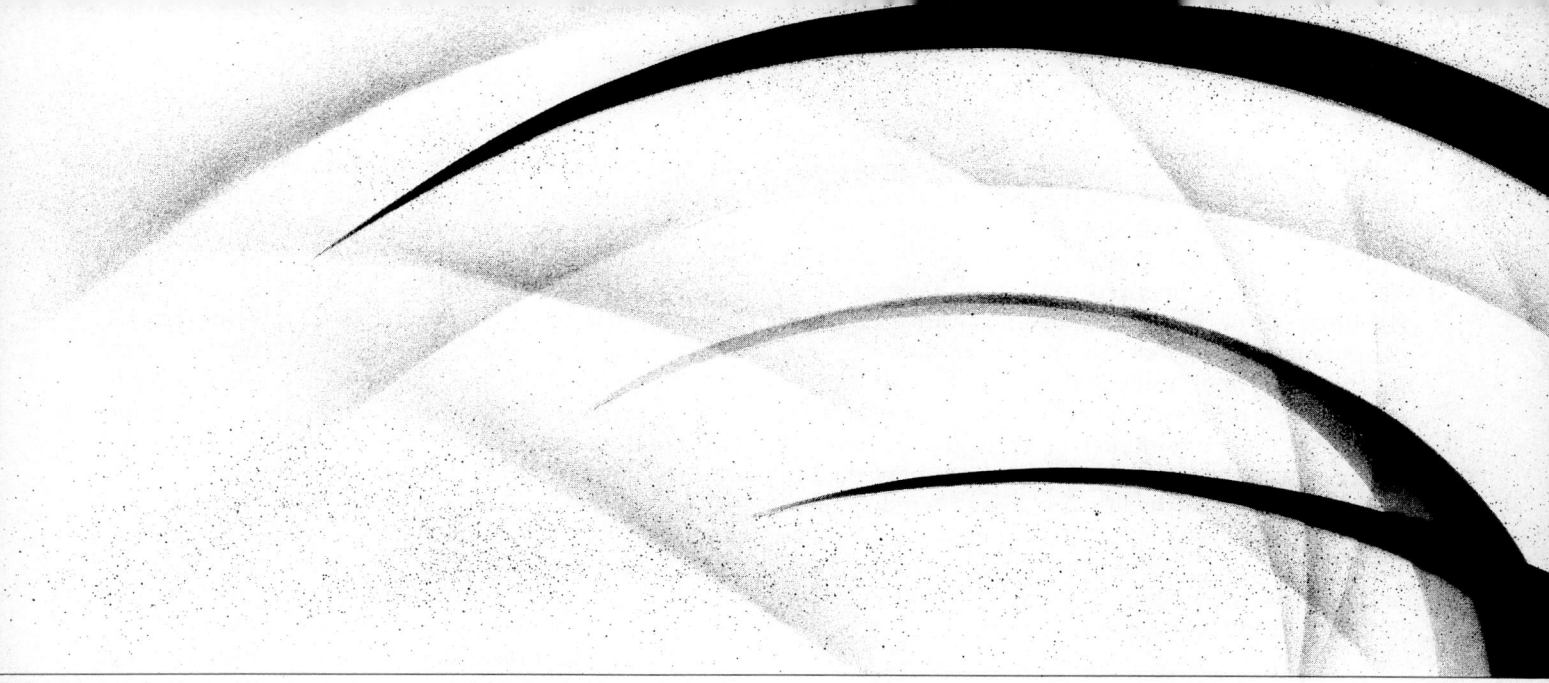

CHAPTER OUTLINE

After completing the nursing assessment, the nurse proceeds to the nursing diagnosis, a statement that describes the client's actual or potential response to a health problem that the nurse is licensed and competent to treat. The purposes of the nursing diagnosis are to analyze assessment data and identify health problems involving the client and family and to provide direction for the nursing care plan. The statement of a nursing diagnosis is the culmination of a diagnostic process during which the nurse analyzes assessment data to identify the client's health problems. Nursing diagnoses are developed for a client, family, or community and take into account the physical, developmental, intellectual, emotional, social, and spiritual data obtained during assessment.

EVOLUTION OF NURSING DIAGNOSIS

Nursing has attempted to define itself professionally and functionally since the writings of Nightingale, who stated that the purpose of nursing care was "to put the patient in the best condition for nature to act upon him" (Nightingale, 1860).

Initially, nursing curricula were organized around disease entities or medical models. However, in the mid-1950s and early 1960s, nursing leaders and educators started to revise curricula around **client-centered problems** (Carpenito, 1989). According to McFarland and McFarlane (1989), the term was first introduced in the nursing literature in 1950. Fry (1953) proposed that nursing could enhance its creativity by the formulation of nursing diagnosis and an individualized nursing care plan. This was not supported by professional nursing, and in 1955 the Model Nurse Practice Act of the American Nurses Association (ANA) excluded diagnosis or prescriptive therapies (ANA, 1955). As a result, nurses were hesitant to use the nursing diagnostic label.

However, the works of Henderson, Abdellah, and other theorists encouraged defining nursing in terms of patient problems. These early theorists, by defining nursing action in terms of client-centered problems, paved the road for the interest and eventual use of nursing diagnosis in contemporary nursing education, practice, administration, and research.

Nursing literature in the 1960s included articles for and against the use of nursing diagnoses. In fact, other health care professions, in particular the medical profession, debated the issue. In an article in the *Journal of the American Medical Association*, King (1967) refuted the argument that only physicians diagnose. His article listed the following criteria necessary for a diagnosis: a preexisting series of categories that provide a reference for the diagnosis, a particular entity that is to be diagnosed, and a deliberate judgment that the assessed data belongs to a particular category (McFarland, McFarlane, 1989; King, 1967).

During the 1970s and 1980s, activities concerning nursing diagnosis increased. There was an increase in the number of articles about and support for nursing diagnosis in the nursing literature. Nursing diagnosis was first incorporated into ANA's 1973 *Standards of Nursing Practice* (ANA, 1973) and revised in 1991 *Standards of Clinical Nursing Practice* (ANA, 1991). In 1980, the ANA went a step farther in its support of nursing diagnosis. *Nursing: A Social Policy Statement* (see Chapter 1) defined nursing as "the diagnosis and treatment of human responses to actual or potential health problems" (ANA, 1980).

In 1973, the first conference for the Classification of Nursing Diagnosis was held to identify nursing functions and establish a classification system. To date, participants of 10 conferences have developed the current list of nursing diagnostic categories (see box). As a result of the initial conferences, an international association was developed. In 1982 a professional association, the **North American Nursing Diagnosis Association (NANDA)** was established. The purpose of NANDA was "to develop, refine, and promote a taxonomy of nursing diagnostic terminology of general use for professional nurses" (Kim, McFarland, McLane, 1984). The ANA has officially sanctioned NANDA as the organization to govern the development of a classification system of nursing diagnosis (Carpenito, 1989).

As nursing curricula continue to incorporate nursing diagnosis into the educational preparation of nurses, the research in this field will continue to grow. As a result, new diagnostic labels are developed, researched, and added to the NANDA listing, which is by no means complete. Continued evolution of nursing diagnosis draws from the collective wealth of nursing knowledge. Through the ongoing collaboration of nursing educators, administrators, researchers, and practitioners, nursing diagnosis has the potential to enrich the nursing profession as a whole.

DEFINITION

Nursing literature contains many definitions for *nursing diagnosis*. These definitions have evolved as the profession's acceptance of nursing diagnosis strengthened. Table 7-1 on p. 172 lists some definitions and their sources. However, some common components of these definitions include nursing, client, and health problems. In addition, each definition implies clinical judgment or decision making.

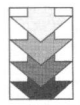

Activity intolerance
Altered family processes
Altered growth and development
Altered health maintenance
Altered nutrition: less than body requirements
Altered nutrition: more than body requirements
Altered nutrition: high risk for more than body requirements
Altered oral mucous membrane
Altered parenting
Altered patterns of urinary elimination
Altered protection*
Altered role performance
Altered sexuality patterns
Altered thought processes
Altered (specify type) tissue perfusion (cerebral, cardiopulmonary, renal, gastrointestinal, peripheral)
Anticipatory grieving
Anxiety
Bathing/hygiene self-care deficit
Body-image disturbance
Bowel incontinence
Care giver role strain†
Chronic low self-esteem
Chronic pain
Colonic constipation
Constipation
Decisional conflict (specify)
Decreased cardiac output
Defensive coping
Diarrhea
Diversional activity deficit
Dressing/grooming self-care deficit
Dysfunctional grieving
Dysfunctional ventilatory weaning response (DVWR)†
Dysreflexia
Effective breastfeeding*
Family coping: potential for growth
Fatigue
Fear
Feeding self-care deficit
Fluid volume deficit (1)
Fluid volume deficit (2)
Fluid volume excess
Functional incontinence
Health seeking behaviors (specify) or desire for high-level wellness (specify)
High risk for activity intolerance
High risk for altered body temperature
High risk for altered parenting
High risk for care giver role strain†
High risk for fluid volume deficit
High risk for aspiration
High risk for disuse syndrome
High risk for impaired skin integrity
High risk for infection
High risk for injury
High risk for peripheral neurovascular function†

High risk for poisoning
High risk for self-mutilation†
High risk for suffocating
High risk for trauma
High risk for violence: self-directed or directed at others
Hopelessness
Hyperthermia
Hypothermia
Impaired adjustment
Impaired gas exchange
Impaired home maintenance management
Impaired physical mobility
Impaired skin integrity
Impaired social interaction
Impaired swallowing
Impaired tissue integrity
Impaired verbal communication
Inability to sustain spontaneous ventilation†
Ineffective airway clearance
Ineffective breastfeeding
Ineffective breathing pattern
Ineffective denial
Ineffective family coping: compromised
Ineffective family coping: disabled
Ineffective individual coping
Ineffective infant feeding pattern†
Ineffective management of therapeutic regimen (individual)†
Ineffective thermoregulation
Interrupted breastfeeding†
Knowledge deficit (specify)
Noncompliance (specify)
Pain
Parental role conflict
Perceived constipation
Personal identity disturbance
Post trauma response
Powerlessness
Rape-trauma syndrome
Rape trauma syndrome: compound reaction
Rape-trauma syndrome: silent reaction
Reflex incontinence
Relocation stress syndrome†
Self-esteem disturbance
Sensory/perceptual alterations (specify) (auditory, gustatory, kinesthetic, olfactory, tactile, visual)
Sexual dysfunction
Situational low self-esteem
Sleep pattern disturbance
Social isolation
Spiritual distress (distress of the human spirit)
Stress incontinence
Toileting self-care deficit
Total incontinence
Unilateral neglect
Urge incontinence
Urinary retention

*Diagnoses accepted in 1990. †Diagnoses accepted in 1992.

TABLE 7-1 Definitions of Nursing Diagnosis	
Author	Definition
Abdellah (1957)	"The determination of the nature and extent of nursing problems presented by the individual patients or families receiving nursing care."
Durand, Prince (1966)	"A statement of a conclusion resulting from a recognition of a pattern derived from a nursing investigation of the patient."
Gebbie, Lavin (1975)	"The judgment or conclusion that occurs as a result of nursing assessment."
Bircher (1975)	"An independent nursing function. . . . An evaluation of a client's personal responses to his human experience throughout the life cycle, be they developmental or accidental crises, illness, hardship, or other stresses."
Aspinall (1976)	"A process of clinical inference from observed changes in patient's physical or psychological condition; if it is arrived at accurately and intelligently, it will lead to identification of the possible causes of symptomatology."
Gordon (1976)	"Actual or potential health problems which nurses, by virtue of their education and experience, are capable and licensed to treat."
Roy (1982)	"Nursing diagnosis is a concise phrase or term summarizing a cluster of empirical indicators representing patterns of unitary man."
Shoemaker (1984)	"A nursing diagnosis is a clinical judgment about an individual, family, or community which is derived through a deliberate, systematic process of data collection and analysis. It provides the basis for prescriptions for definitive therapy for which the nurse is accountable. It is expressed concisely and includes the etiology of the condition when known."
Carpenito (1987)	"A nursing diagnosis is a statement that describes the human response (health state or actual/potential altered interaction pattern) of an individual or group which the nurse can legally identify and for which the nurse can order the definitive interventions to maintain the health state or to reduce, eliminate, or prevent alteration."
NANDA (1990)	"A nursing diagnosis is a clinical judgment about individual, family, or community responses to actual and potential health problems and life processes. Nursing diagnoses provide the basis for selection of nursing interventions to achieve outcomes for which the nurse is accountable."
Carlson et al (1991)	"Nursing diagnosis is a summary statement about the health status of a client(s) derived through the assessment process and requiring intervention from the domain of nursing."

Modified from Carlson JH et al: *Nursing diagnosis: a case-study approach*, Philadelphia, 1991, Saunders.

TABLE 7-2 NANDA Nursing Diagnosis Format	
Diagnostic Statement	Related Factors
Constipation	Less than adequate diet
	Medications
	Lack of privacy
	Pregnancy
Fatigue	Discomfort
	Excessive emotional demands
	Increased energy requirement
Impaired skin integrity	Edema
	Excessive secretions
	Immobilization
	Diaphoresis (sweating)

It is not the purpose of this chapter or text to create a new definition of nursing diagnosis or to critique the present definitions. Rather, the definition used in this text is to assist the student in using nursing diagnoses as a framework for delivering nursing care. This component, like all components of the nursing process, enables the student to plan individualized nursing care.

A **nursing diagnosis** then is a statement that describes the client's actual or potential response to a health problem that the nurse is licensed and competent to treat. The client's actual and potential responses are obtained from the assessment data base and a review of literature, client's past medical records, and consultation with other professionals, all of which were collected during assessment. Last, the client's actual or potential responses require interventions from the domain of nursing (Carlson et al, 1991).

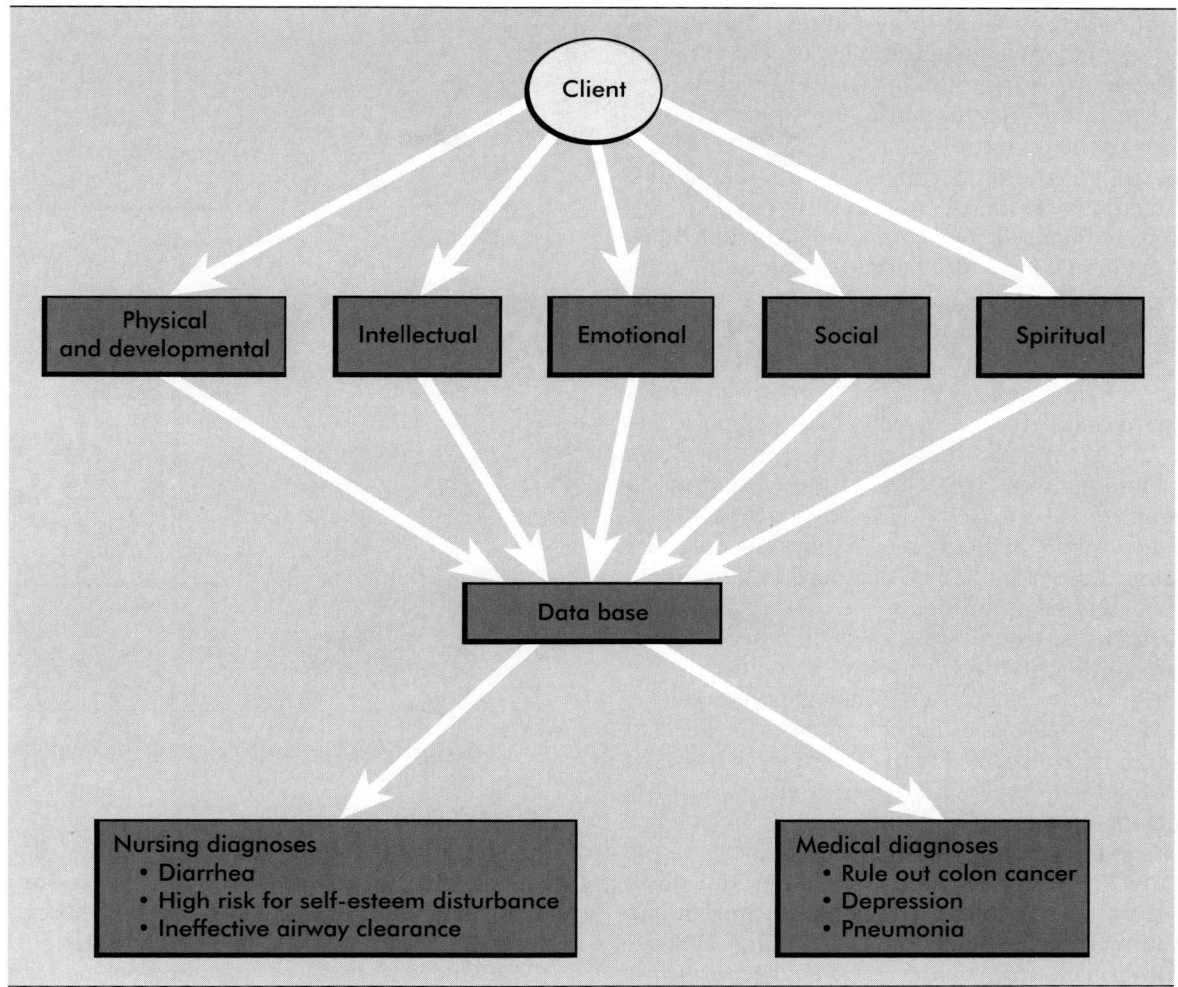

Fig. 7-1   Comparison of nursing and medical diagnoses using the same data base.

Nursing Diagnosis Format

The nursing diagnosis format (that is, how the actual diagnosis is stated) flows from the diagnostic process, which is discussed in a later section. However, the format is presented here to provide the beginning nurse with familiarity and rationale for the structure of a nursing diagnostic statement.

Throughout this text, nursing diagnoses are stated in a two-part format accepted by NANDA (McLane, 1987): the diagnostic statement followed by a statement of related factors (see Table 7-2). The diagnostic labels are categories approved by NANDA (see box on p. 171). The related-factor statement refers to the contributing or etiological factors that affect the client's actual or potential response to the health problem and that the nurse is licensed and competent to treat.

This two-part format is accepted by the majority of nursing leaders (Carlson et al, 1991; Soares O'Hearn, 1990; Carpenito, 1989; Gordon, 1987). It assists the nurse in individualizing a client's nursing diagnoses and provides direction for selection of appropriate interventions. This format supports the delivery of individualized nursing care for one client or a group of clients.

Nursing Diagnosis and Medical Diagnosis

Until recent years the term *diagnosis* was almost exclusive to the medical profession. A **medical diagnosis** is the identification of a disease condition based on a specific evaluation of physical signs, symptoms, history, laboratory tests, and procedures (Fig. 7-1). Physicians are licensed to treat these diseases or pathological processes by performing surgery, prescribing medication, and ordering specific invasive and noninvasive therapies. During the last three decades, however, the term *nursing diagnosis* has appeared more frequently in the literature.

A nursing diagnosis is a statement of a client's actual or potential response to a health problem that the nurse is licensed and competent to treat. It reflects the client's level of health or response to a disease or pathological process. Medical and nursing diagnoses are derived from the physiological, psychological, sociocultural, developmental, and spiritual dimensions of the client (Fig. 7-1). Nursing diagnosis is a nursing activity and responsibility supported by the ANA, first in 1973 and reaffirmed in the Social Policy Statement in 1980 and 1991 *Standards of Clinical Nursing Practice* (ANA, 1973, 1980, 1991).

The goals and objectives of a nursing diagnosis differ from those of a medical diagnosis. The goal of a nursing diagnosis is to identify actual and potential client responses, whereas the goals of a medical diagnosis are to identify and to design a treatment plan for curing the disease or the pathological process.

The objective of a nursing diagnosis is development of an individualized plan of care so that the client and family are able to adapt to changes resulting from health problems. The objective of the medical diagnosis is to prescribe treatment. A medical diagnosis of appendicitis, for example, requires the physician to remove the infected appendix. After the appendectomy the client may have a nursing diagnosis of *impaired physical mobility related to painful incision.* The nursing care would be directed at gradually increasing the client's mobility to preoperative levels.

 ## NURSING DIAGNOSTIC PROCESS

The **diagnostic process** is the decision-making steps the nurse uses to develop a diagnostic statement (Carnevali et al, 1984). This process includes analysis and interpretation of data, identification of problems, and formulation of nursing diagnoses (Fig. 7-2). Data validation and clustering follow assessment (see Chapter 6) and lead to analysis and interpretation of data.

Analysis and Interpretation of Data

In the assessment phase, data were collected from a variety of sources, validated, and sorted into clusters. The data base is continually revised to include changes in the client's physical and emotional status, as well as the results of laboratory and diagnostic

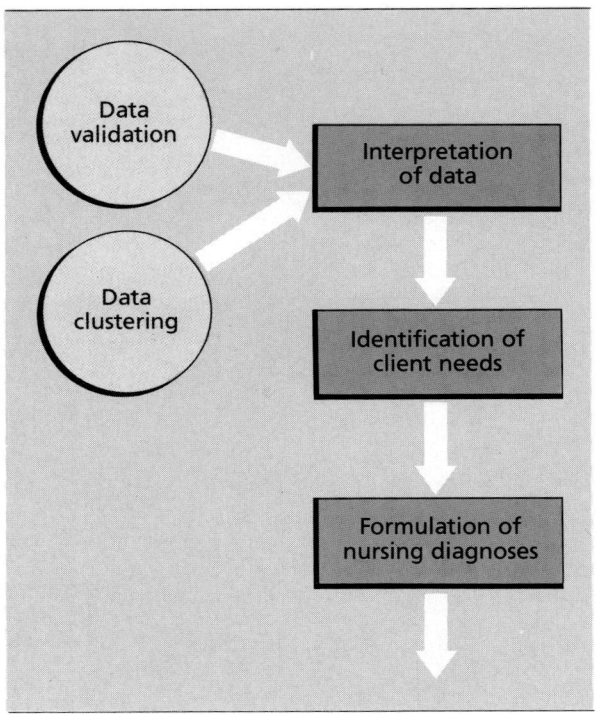

Fig. 7-2 Nursing diagnostic process.

tests. During this step, the nurse using knowledge and experience, analyzes and interprets, or draws conclusions from the data clusters (Benner, 1984; Carnevali, et al, 1984; Carlson et al, 1991).

The analysis involves recognizing patterns and trends, comparing these patterns with normal health patterns, and drawing conclusions about the client's response (see box). When looking for patterns or trends in the data, the nurse examines the clusters in the data base. When a relationship among these patterns is identified, a list of client-centered problems or needs begins to emerge. The nurse may group together these clusters and patterns. This grouping consists of defining characteristics. *Defining characteristics* are the clinical criteria that support (validate) the presence of the diagnostic catergory. Clinical criteria are objective or subjective signs and symptoms, clusters of signs and symptoms, or risk factors (Carpenito, 1989). Multiple defining characteristics resulting from assessment data support the nursing diagnosis (Carpenito, 1987). The presence of one sign or symptom does not support the nursing diagnostic label. Instead, the clustering of multiple defining characteristics supports the diagnosis. Absence of these characteristics suggests that the diagnosis should be rejected. Diagnostic categories and their defining characteristics provide structure for the cognitive process in the identification of client

---

Example of Data Analysis

Recognize pattern (possible defining characteristics).

- No bowel movement for 4 days
- Painful defecation with straining
- Last stool small and hard
- Abdomen firm and distended

Compare with normal standards.

- Soft, formed stool daily
- Defecation not painful
- Abdomen soft, nondistended

Make a reasoned conclusion.

- Bowel elimination problem

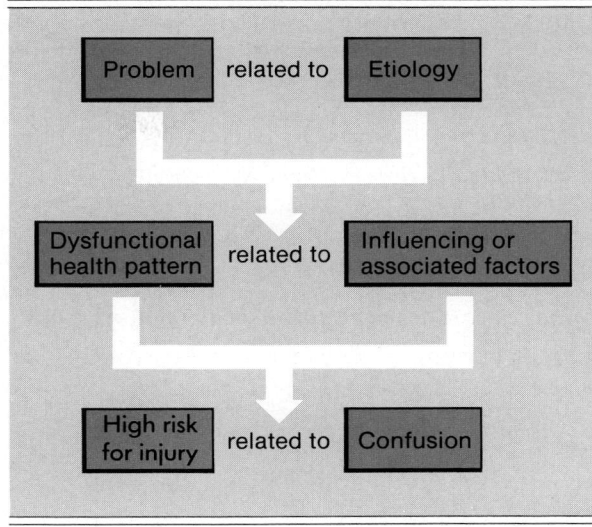

Fig. 7-3   Relationship between diagnostic statement and format.
Redrawn from Hickey P: *Nursing process handbook*, St Louis, 1990, Mosby–Year Book.

needs and actual formulation of the nursing diagnoses (Hurley, 1986).

Identification of patterns is perhaps demonstrated through the following example. Gray hair does not necessarily indicate that a person is an older adult. However, if gray hair is clustered with wrinkled skin, age spots, and slowed gait, then these characteristics probably indicate that the person is an older adult.

The identified pattern is compared with normal healthful standards. The nurse uses widely accepted norms, such as normal laboratory and diagnostic test values, and professional knowledge as the basis for comparison and judgment. When comparing the patterns, the nurse decides whether the grouped signs and symptoms are normal and within healthful standards. Defining characteristics that are beyond healthful norms form the basis for problem identification.

Identification of Client Problems

Before formulating the nursing diagnosis, the nurse identifies the client's problems. When identifying these problems, the nurse considers all assessment data and focuses on pertinent and abnormal data. It may help the inexperienced nurse to think of this identification phase as the general health care problem and the formulation of the nursing diagnosis as the specific health care problem. Thus in describing health care problems, the nurse moves from general to specific.

To identify the client's need, the nurse first determines what the client's health problems are and whether they are actual or potential problems. An **actual health problem** is one that is perceived or experienced by the client, such as a *sleep pattern disturbance related to a noisy environment.* A **potential health problem** is one for which the client is at risk, such as an overweight smoker at risk for *ineffective airway clearance related to incisional pain.*

The problem-identification step brings the nurse closer to forming a nursing diagnosis and making general analyses of the clustered data; thus this step assists the nurse in making a nursing diagnosis.

Formulation of Nursing Diagnoses

Formulation of the nursing diagnosis is based on identification of client needs. The diagnostic label should include the problem (for example, *potential for injury*) and its etiology (for example, *related to confusion*). The problem is actual or potential, and the etiology is a condition or situation that can be affected by nursing interventions.

The connecting phrase between the diagnostic label and the etiology establishes a relationship between the two parts of the statement. This is not a cause-and-effect statement, but rather it indicates that the etiology can contribute to or be associated with the problem (Fig. 7-3).

The **etiology** identifies the cause of the problem. It may be a direct or contributing factor in the development of the client need and subsequent nursing diagnosis. The etiology is represented in the nursing

TABLE 7-3   Comparison of Interventions for Nursing Diagnoses with Different Etiologies

Nursing Diagnoses	Interventions
CLIENT A	
Ineffective airway clearance related to obesity	Place client in high Fowler's position.
	Have client cough and deep breathe every 2 hours while awake.
	Start weight-reduction diet (1200 calories) to decrease obesity.
Feeding self-care deficit related to bilateral arm casts	Encourage family to visit during meals.
	Be certain staff or family members are available to feed client.
	Provide high-calorie milkshakes with straw at 3 and 8 PM.
Social isolation related to protective isolation	Plan staffing patterns to include visits to client's room 4 times a day.
	Relax visiting hours for family.
CLIENT B	
Ineffective airway clearance related to poor coughing	Teach client deep breathing and coughing.
	Splint client's abdominal incision during coughing.
Feeding self-care deficit related to inability to grasp feeding utensils	Provide large-handled eating utensils.
	Offer finger foods cut in large pieces for between-meal snacks: 10-2-8.
Social isolation related to recent move into neighborhood	Provide client with phone numbers and location of local senior citizens' center.
	Draw client a map of neighborhood stores, restaurants, and libraries.

Summary of Relevant Assessment Data

PHYSICAL AND DEVELOPMENTAL DATA

- Diarrhea for 3 weeks
- Productive cough on rising each morning
- 15-pound weight loss 2 weeks before hospitalization
- Hemoglobin level of 10 g
- Slight change of emphysema shown on chest x-ray film
- Crackles in bilateral lung bases
- Distended abdomen
- Squamous cell cancer
- 20-year history of smoking, 2 packs a day (40 pack-years)
- Family history of stomach cancer
- Family history of heart attacks
- 40-year marriage
- 20-year self-employment
- One adult son, 35 years old
- Two sisters, 50 and 48, with no major health problems
- Temporary colostomy
- Abdominal incision

INTELLECTUAL DATA

- Talkative affect
- Frequent questions about whether he has cancer
- Good attention span

EMOTIONAL DATA

- Anxiety
- Withdrawal after biopsy report of squamous cell cancer
- Avoidance of viewing of abdomen

SOCIAL DATA

- Tennis three times a week
- Active role in his neighborhood

SPIRITUAL DATA

- Methodist
- Weekly church attendance
- Daily Bible reading

TABLE 7-4 Formulation of Nursing Diagnoses		
Clustering Data	Identification of Client Need	Nursing Diagnosis Formulation
Diarrhea for 3 weeks Distended abdomen Family history of stomach cancer	Alteration in elimination patterns	*Diarrhea related to unknown cause*
Weight loss: 15 pounds Diarrhea Anemia, hemoglobin level of 10 g	Excessive weight loss	*Altered nutrition: high risk for less than body requirements related to chronic diarrhea for 3 weeks*
40 pack-year history of smoking Slight change of emphysema shown on chest x-ray film Crackles auscultated in lung fields	Risk for postoperative respiratory complications	*High risk for ineffective airway clearance after surgery related to incisional pain*
Temporary colostomy Abdominal incision Client resistance to viewing of abdomen	Change in body image	*High risk for self-esteem disturbance related to change in body image*
Client verbalization of fear of stomach cancer Client withdrawal after biopsy report	Changes in interpersonal interactions	*High risk for ineffective individual coping related to unknown prognosis*

diagnostic statement after the phrase *related to*. Inclusion of the etiology individualizes the nursing diagnosis and subsequent interventions (Table 7-3).

Etiological factors are difficult to validate. In some settings, medical diagnoses are recorded as the etiology of the nursing diagnosis. This is incorrect. Nursing interventions cannot change the medical diagnosis. However, nursing interventions can be directed at etiological factors and the diagnostic label. For example, the nursing diagnosis, *pain related to breast cancer,* is incorrect. Nursing actions cannot affect the medical diagnosis of breast cancer. Rewording the diagnosis to read, *pain related to mastectomy incision* results in nursing interventions directed at improving comfort and pain control.

As the client's needs change, nursing diagnoses are modified. For example, a client's pertinent assessment data includes decreased dietary fiber and limited fluid intake, no bowel movement for 3 days, decreased bowel sounds, distention of the lower abdomen, hard fecal material extracted during digital rectal examination, and a guaiac-negative stool specimen. The nursing diagnosis was, *constipation related to limited fiber intake.* After appropriate nursing intervention, the constipation was resolved, and the nursing diagnosis was modified to read, *high risk for constipation related to limited fiber intake.* The risk exists based on the client's past history of constipation and decreased fiber intake.

After the health problem has been resolved, the nursing diagnosis for that problem is no longer relevant. In addition, as the client's physiological and emotional status change, the health problem may remain relevant, but the cause may change. Therefore the nursing diagnosis must be modified, or new nursing diagnoses are developed as the client's needs and status change.

The modification of nursing diagnoses is ongoing. As the level of nursing care and level of wellness change, these changes are reflected in the statement of nursing diagnoses. Outdated nursing diagnoses do not accurately reflect the client's current needs and result in a lower quality of nursing care.

Assessment Data and the Diagnostic Statement

As nurses begin to develop nursing diagnoses, they need to be sure that assessment data support the diagnostic label and etiology. It may help to identify assessment activities that produce specific kinds of data. For example, asking the client about the quality and perception of pain results in subjective data. However, palpating an area and eliciting a painful grimace provides objective information. Likewise, asking a client to describe the perception of an irregular heartbeat elicits subjective information, and using auscultation to obtain a pulse produces an objective measurement for heart rate and rhythm.

The box contains a summary of the pertinent assessment data that may lead to the identification of an actual or potential health care problem. Table 7-4 demonstrates data clustering, identification of client need, and formulation of nursing diagnoses from the pertinent assessment data that are presented in the box.

TABLE 7-5	Defining Characteristics and Etiologies to Support Nursing Diagnoses		
Assessment Activities	Defining Characteristics	Nursing Diagnoses	Etiologies ("Related to")
Auscultate lungs. Observe respiration. Observe cough. Inspect skin color. Ask client about shortness of breath and observe for it. Ask client about smoking.	Abnormal breath sounds Changes in rate or depth of respiration Cough Cyanosis Dyspnea Smoking history	*Actual or high risk for ineffective airway clearance*	■ Decreased energy or fatigue ■ Tracheobronchial infection, obstruction, or secretion ■ Pain
Observe client's grooming. Observe client's willingness to participate in rehabilitation. Review history of traumatic injury.	Verbal or nonverbal response to actual or perceived change in structure of function Missing or impaired body part, not looking or touching body or body part Trauma to body Refusal to acknowledge change	*Actual or high risk for self-esteem disturbance*	■ Biophysical factors (e.g., amputation or loss of function of extremity) ■ Cognitive or perceptual factors (e.g., expressions of worthlessness and sorrow) ■ Psychosocial factors (e.g., withdrawal behavior or excessive crying)

Measures for Avoiding Diagnostic Errors

■ Identify client's response to illness.
■ State a NANDA diagnostic statement.
■ Identify an etiology treatable by nursing.
■ Identify a client need associated with a treatment or test.
■ Identify client's response to equipment.
■ Identify client's, not nurse's, problem.
■ Identify client's problem, not interventions.
■ Identify client's problem, not goals.
■ Avoid prejudicial statements.
■ State the etiology legally.
■ Identify a problem and an etiology.
■ Identify only one client problem in a diagnostic statement.

Table 7-5 uses the three nursing diagnoses, *high risk for ineffective airway clearance, high risk for self-esteem disturbance,* and *high risk for ineffective individual coping,* to demonstrate the way that the defining characteristics and probable etiologies assist in the development of the total diagnostic label. The

defining characteristics and relevant etiologies are from the text *Pocket Guide to Nursing Diagnosis* by Kim, McFarland, and McLane (1991) and are derived from the NANDA classification. A complete list of the current NANDA classification of nursing diagnostic labels is in the box on p. 171).

 SOURCES OF ERROR

The diagnostic process has potential for errors. One type of error is the incorrect identification of a client need or no identification at all. A second type of error occurs when the nurse identifies a need important to the nurse and not the client. With the third type of error, the identification of the need is correct, but the diagnostic statement is worded incorrectly. Errors in the diagnostic process result in the development of an incomplete or inappropriate nursing care plan.

Gordon (1982, 1987) groups errors into the following categories: errors of omission and errors of commission. An **error of omission** occurs when the nurse fails to identify a health care problem, which can occur when incomplete data are collected from the client, when data are clustered incorrectly in the analysis process, or when data are interpreted im-

TABLE 7-6 Examples of Errors in Formulating the Nursing Diagnostic Statement

Correct Statement	Stated as Medical Diagnosis	Stated in Medical Terminology	Stated as a Nursing Intervention
Diarrhea related to unknown cause	Diarrhea	Alteration in bowel elimination related to lesion in descending colon	Offer bedpan frequently because of diarrhea.
Altered nutrition: high risk for less than body requirements related to chronic diarrhea for 3 weeks	Potential malnutrition	High risk for alteration in nutrition: less than body requirements owing to malnutrition	Provide high-protein diet due to high risk for altered nutrition.
High risk for ineffective airway clearance after surgery related to abdominal incisional pain	Potential pneumonia	High risk for ineffective airway clearance owing to emphysema	Have client cough frequently because of ineffective airway clearance.
High risk for self-esteem disturbance related to change in body image	Avoidance reaction to colostomy	High risk for disturbance in self-concept owing to colostomy	Encourage client to interact with others.
High risk for ineffective coping related to terminal prognosis	Fear of cancer	High risk for ineffective coping owing to squamous cell cancer	Encourage client to verbalize fear.

properly. An **error of commission** occurs from overdiagnosing or diagnosing nonexistent health care problems. For example, a client who enters a hospital for a diagnostic test may be prematurely diagnosed as having *knowledge deficit related to unfamiliarity with procedure.* However, after further assessment, the nurse may learn that the client has undergone the test before and has no questions.

Errors in data clustering can lead to errors of commission because data are clustered prematurely, incorrectly, or not at all (Gordon, 1982). Premature closure of clustering occurs when the nurse makes the nursing diagnosis before all data have been grouped. Incorrect clustering occurs when the nurse tries to make the nursing diagnosis fit the signs and symptoms obtained. The nursing diagnosis should be derived from the data, not the other way around. An incorrect nursing diagnosis affects quality of care.

The last type of error that can occur is the manner in which the nursing diagnosis is stated. There are some common guidelines to reduce errors in the diagnostic statement itself (see box). The statement should be worded in appropriate, concise, and precise language, which involves using correct terminology reflecting the *nursing* needs of the client. Concise wording ensures that the nursing need can be easily communicated to other nurses and health care professions. The diagnostic statement should also be precise, identifying unique nursing needs, and

should be stated in the problem-etiology format. A diagnostic statement such as, *unhappy and worried about health,* can lead to errors. The language needs to be more precise and appropriate, such as, *high risk for ineffective individual coping related to fear of medical diagnosis.*

In addition, there are three incorrect ways to state the diagnostic label, including nursing diagnoses stated as medical diagnoses, use of medical terminology to describe the cause, and statement of the nursing diagnosis as an intervention. These are errors because they shift the focus of the statement from nursing to medicine or shift the focus from the cause to the intervention. Table 7-6 states the correct nursing diagnoses formulated from assessment data from Chapter 6 and compares them with the three errors of medical diagnosis, medical terminology, and nursing intervention. As expertise with the diagnostic process is gained, the likelihood of errors is reduced, and the nurse is able to develop the nursing diagnoses based on the actual or potential nursing needs of the client.

NURSING DIAGNOSES: APPLICATION TO CARE PLANNING

The use of nursing diagnoses is a mechanism for identifying the domain of nursing. The formulated nursing diagnoses provide direction for the planning process and the selection of nursing interventions to achieve the desired outcomes. Thus the expected outcomes are developed for each nursing diagnosis (McFarland, McFarlane, 1989). The care plan (see Chapter 8) is a mechanism for demonstrating accountability (Carlson et al, 1991; Carpenito, 1987, 1989). In addition, the nursing diagnoses and subsequent care plan assist in communicating to other professionals the client-centered problems through the nursing care plan, consultations, discharge planning, and client care conferences.

Advantages of Nursing Diagnoses

The nursing diagnosis is advantageous for nurses and clients. It facilitates communication among nurses about a client's level of wellness and discharge planning. The health care delivery system today requires greater numbers of health care professionals. As more people become responsible for the care of a client, it is essential that these professionals be able to clearly communicate with one another about the client's problems. Nursing diagnoses facilitate communication in several ways. The initial list of nursing diagnoses is an easily obtainable reference to the client's current health care needs. Nursing diagnoses also encourage the nurse to develop organizational skills because they help prioritize the client's needs. As the nurse communicates with other professionals, the use of nursing diagnoses encourages organized communication relevant to the client's goals and priorities.

Nursing diagnoses are also used for charting in the nurse's progress notes, writing referrals, and providing effective transition of care from one unit to another, from one clinic to another, or from the hospital to the community. Discharge planning is the set of decisions and activities involved in giving continuity and coordination to nursing care (McKeehan, 1979). Discharge planning is necessary when a client is discharged from one hospital to another or from the hospital to the community. In discharge planning, nursing diagnoses are the mechanism for communicating and delineating care the client still requires (Carpenito, 1987)(see Chapter 5).

Nursing diagnoses can also serve as a focus for quality assurance and improvement and peer review. Quality assurance is the monitoring and evaluation of the quality and appropriateness of client care compared with accepted standards. Quality improvement is an appraisal, by professional co-workers of equal status, of the way a nurse conducts practice, education, or research. Quality assurance and peer review use accepted standards as measures against which performance is weighed. The nursing diagnosis is a method of identifying the focus of nursing activity. When focusing on the nursing diagnosis, the reviewer can determine whether nursing care was correct and delivered according to standards of practice.

The benefits of nursing diagnosis for the profession are also important for the client and family. Better communication among health care professionals helps eliminate potential problems in giving care and maintains a focus on meeting the client's health care goals. Similarly, the ultimate reason for quality assurance and improvement and peer review is to ensure that high-quality care is given to clients and families. Furthermore, the client benefits from the individualization of nursing care resulting from appropriate goal setting, correct selection of priorities, selection of appropriate interventions, and establishment of outcome criteria.

Limitations of Nursing Diagnoses

Nursing diagnoses have limitations, and the beginning practitioner should be aware of their existence. Because of the continuous evolution of the term and use of nursing diagnoses, the language can occasionally be verbose and contain jargon. This may limit the use of nursing diagnoses to only nursing professionals and result in confusion among other members of the health care team (Shamansky, Yanni, 1985).

Imprecise language of the diagnostic label may incorrectly "label" a client. One such diagnostic label is *noncompliance*. The term is value laden and incomplete (Edel, 1985; Stantis, Ryan, 1982).

In addition, the evolution of a standardized terminology in the form of a taxonomy has resulted in confusion about the language of the diagnostic label (Lunney, 1986; Porter, 1986). The 1986 National Conference for the Classification of Nursing Diagno-

sis first proposed a taxonomic structure for an organizational framework of current and future diagnostic labels (McLane, 1987). To date, the revised taxonomic structure serves as a classification system for nursing diagnosis (Carlson et al, 1991).

The evolving taxonomy can limit nursing practice. Nursing diagnoses, developed by the Task Force of the National Group for the Classification of Nursing Diagnoses, are only the beginning of a total classification system. Through formulation and use of other nursing diagnoses, the taxonomy will grow and expand the focus of professional nursing.

 ## SUMMARY

The analysis of data obtained during nursing assessment results in the formulation of nursing diagnoses. Nursing diagnoses are developed through a process in which data are validated and clustered, the client's needs are identified, and the specific nursing diagnoses are formulated. The stated nursing diagnoses reflect the client's individual responses to a disease or pathological process.

Formulation of the nursing diagnosis is a cognitive activity focusing on the client's health care needs and expectations. The formulation of nursing diagnoses enables the nurse and client to determine client goals, priorities, and projected outcomes of nursing care in the planning component of the nursing process.

CHAPTER 7 REVIEW

Key Concepts

- The statement of nursing diagnosis is the result of the diagnostic process.
- The diagnostic process includes analysis and interpretation of data, identification of client problems, and formulation of nursing diagnoses.
- The interpretation of data requires the nurse to validate and cluster data.
- Nursing diagnoses state the actual or potential problems in the client's health status.
- Nursing diagnoses are written for the physical, developmental, intellectual, emotional, social, and spiritual dimensions of the client.
- Nursing diagnoses are necessary to develop a plan of care that will help the client and family adapt to changes resulting from an illness or change in lifestyle.
- Nursing diagnostic errors can occur by omission or commission.
- Errors of omission occur when the nurse has failed to identify a health problem.
- Causes of errors of omission are incomplete data collection, incorrect data clustering, or improper interpretation of data.
- Errors of commission occur when the nurse over-diagnoses or diagnoses nonexistent health problems.
- Causes of errors of commission are incomplete data collection and incorrect data clustering.
- Diagnostic statement errors include using inappropriate or imprecise language, stating a medical diagnosis as a nursing diagnosis, using medical terminology to describe the cause, and stating the nursing diagnosis as an intervention.
- Nursing diagnoses improve communication between nurses and other health professionals.
- Nursing diagnoses can serve as a focus for quality assurance and improvement and peer review.

Key Terms

Actual health problem, p. 175

Client-centered problems, p. 170

Defining characteristics p. 174

Diagnosis, p. 173

Diagnostic process, p. 174

Error of commission, p. 179

Error of omission, p. 178

Etiology, p. 175

Medical diagnosis, p. 173

North American Nursing Diagnosis Association (NANDA), p. 170

Nursing diagnosis, p. 172

Potential health problem, p. 175

Critical Thinking Exercises

1. Your client's nursing Kardex contains a care plan for *bathing/hygiene* and *toileting self-care deficit: related to decreased mobility of right arm.* What data do you need from the assessment data base to determine whether the nursing diagnosis is current?

2. How do you organize assessment data to derive nursing diagnosis that reflect client response to illness, hospitalization, and lifestyle changes?

3. How can you organize assessment data to avoid errors in data clustering, which can lead to errors in nursing diagnosis?

REFERENCES

American Nurses Association: *Model nurse practice act,* Kansas City, Mo, 1955, The Association.

American Nurses Association: *Standards of nursing practice,* Kansas City, Mo, 1973, The Association.

American Nurses Association: *Nursing: a social policy statement,* Kansas City, Mo, 1980, The Association.

American Nursing Association: *Standards of clinical nursing practice,* Kansas City, Mo, 1991, The Association.

Benner P: *From novice to expert,* Menlo Park, Calif, 1984, Addison-Wesley.

Carlson JH et al: *Nursing diagnosis: a case-study approach,* Philadelphia, 1991, Saunders.

Carnevali DL et al: *Diagnostic reasoning in nursing,* Philadephia, 1984, Lippincott.

Carpenito LJ: *Nursing diagnoses: application to clinical practice,* ed 2, Philadelphia, 1987, Lippincott.

Carpenito LJ: *Nursing diagnoses: application to clinical practice,* ed 3, Philadelphia, 1989, Lippincott.

Edel MK: Noncompliance: an appropriate nursing diagnosis? *Nurs Outlook* 33:183, 1985.

Fry VS: The creative approach to nursing, *Am J Nurs* 53:301, 1953.

Gordon M: *Nursing diagnoses: process and practice,* New York, 1982, McGraw-Hill.

Gordon M: *Nursing diagnosis: process and application,* ed 2, New York, 1987, McGraw-Hill.

Hurley ME: *Classification of nursing diagnoses,* St Louis, 1986, Mosby–Year Book.

Kim MJ, McFarland GR, McLane AM, editors: *Classification of nursing diagnoses: proceedings of the Fifth Conference (NANDA),* St Louis, 1984, Mosby–Year Book.

Kim MJ, McFarland GK, McLane AM: *Pocket guide to nursing diagnoses,* ed 4, St Louis, 1991, Mosby–Year Book.

King LS: What is a diagnosis? *JAMA* 202:154, 1967.

Lunney M: Nursing diagnoses: refining the system, *Am J Nurs* 82:456, 1986.

McFarland GK, McFarlane EA: *Nursing diagnosis and intervention: planning for patient care,* St Louis, 1989, Mosby–Year Book.

McKeehan KM: Nursing diagnosis in a discharge planning program, *Nurs Clin North Am* 14:517, 1979.

McLane AM, editor: *Classification of nursing diagnoses: proceedings from the Seventh Conference (NANDA),* St Louis, 1987, Mosby–Year Book.

Nightengale F: *Notes on nursing: what it is and is not,* London, 1860, Harrison & Sons.

Porter EJ: Critical analysis of NANDA nursing diagnoses taxonomy. I. *Image J Nurs Sch* 18:137, 1986.

Shamansky SL, Yanni CR: In opposition to nursing diagnosis: a minority opinion, *Image J Nurs Sch* 17:47, 1985.

Soares O'Hearn CA: Nursing diagnosis: a phenomenological structural description and multidimensional taxonomy or typological redefinition. In Chaska N: *The nursing profession: turning points,* St Louis, 1990, Mosby–Year Book.

Stantis MA, Ryan J: Noncompliance, an unacceptable diagnosis, *Am J Nurs* 82:941, 1982.

ADDITIONAL READINGS

Aspinall MJ: Nursing diagnosis: the weak link, *Nurs Outlook* 24:433, 1976.

Aspinall MJ: Use of a decision tree to improve diagnostic accuracy, *Nurs Res* 28:182, 1979.

Benner P, Tanner C: How expert nurses use intuition, *Am J Nurs* 87:23, 1987.

Dalton J: A descriptive study: defining characteristics of the nursing diagnosis: cardiac output, alterations in, decreased, *Image J Nurs Sch* 17:113, 1985.

Fehring RJ: Validating diagnositic labels: standardized methodology. In Hurley M, editor: *Classification of nursing diagnoses: proceedings of the Sixth Conference (NANDA)*, St Louis, 1986, Mosby–Year Book.

Gebbie KM, Lavin MA: Classifying nursing diagnoses, *Am J Nurs* 74:250, 1974.

Gleit CJ, Tatro S: Nursing diagnoses for healthy individuals, *Nurs Health Care* 8:456, 1981.

Gordon M: Nursing diagnoses and the diagnostic process, *Am J Nurs* 76:1298, 1976.

Gordon M: Classification of nursing diagnoses, *J NY State Nurses Assoc* 9:5, 1978.

Gordon M: The concept of nursing diagnoses, *Nurs Clin North Am* 14:487, 1979.

Halloran EJ: Nursing workload, medical diagnosis related groups and nursing diagnoses, *Res Nurs Health* 8:421, 1985.

Hickey P: *Nursing process handbook,* St Louis, 1990, Mosby–Year Book.

Iyer PW, Taptich BJ, Bernocchi-Losey D: *Nursing process and nursing diagnoses,* Philadelphia, 1986, Saunders.

Jacoby MK: The dilemma of physiological problems: eliminating the double standard, *Am J Nurs* 85:281, 1985.

Kim MJ: Nursing diagnoses in critical care, *Dimens Crit Care Nurs* 2:5, 1983.

Kim MJ: Without collaboration, what's left? *Am J Nurs* 85:281, 1985.

Levin RF, Crosley JM: Focused data collection for the generation of nursing diagnoses, *Nurs Staff Dev* 2(2):56, 1986.

Martens K: Let's diagnose strengths, not just problems, *Am J Nurs* 86:192, 1986.

Nettle C et al: Community nursing diagnosis, *J Community Health* 6(3):135, 1989.

Popkess SA: Diagnosing your patient's strengths, *Nurs 81* 11:34, 1981.

Shoemaker JK: Essential features of a nursing diagnosis. In Kim MJ et al, editors: *Classification of nursing diagnoses: proceedings of the Fifth Conference (NANDA)*, St Louis, 1984, Mosby–Year Book.

Walker L: Nursing diagnoses and interventions: new tools to define nursing's unique role, *Nurs Health Care* 7(6):323, 1986.

CHAPTER 8

Planning

OBJECTIVES

Mastery of content in this chapter will enable the student to:
- Define the key terms listed.
- Discuss the process of priority setting.
- Describe goal setting.
- List the seven guidelines of a written outcome statement.
- Discuss the difference between a goal and an expected outcome.
- Discuss the process of selecting nursing interventions.
- Define the three types of interventions.
- Discuss the differences between dependent, independent, and interdependent interventions.
- List the purposes of the nursing care plans. and community health settings.
- Describe the differences between care plans used in hospital and community health settings.
- Develop a care plan from a nursing assessment.
- List the six steps involved in consultation.
- Discuss the consultant process.

CHAPTER OUTLINE

ursing assessment and the formulation of nursing diagnoses initiate the planning step of the nursing process. **Planning** is a category of nursing behaviors in which client-centered goals are established and strategies are designed to achieve the goals. During planning, priorities are set, goals are determined, expected outcomes are developed, and a nursing care plan is formulated. In addition to collaborating with the client and family, the nurse consults with other members of the health care team, reviews pertinent literature, modifies care, and records relevant information about the client's health care needs and clinical management.

ESTABLISHING PRIORITIES

After formulating specific nursing diagnoses, the nurse establishes the priorities of the diagnoses by ranking them in order of importance. Priorities of care are established to identify the order in which nursing interventions will be provided when an individual has multiple problems or alterations (Carpenito, 1989).

Establishing priorities is not merely a matter of numbering the nursing diagnosis on the basis of severity or physiological importance. Rather, it is a method by which the nurse and the client mutually rank the diagnoses in order of importance based on the client's desires, needs, and safety.

Maslow's hierarchy of needs can be useful in designating priorities (see Chapter 29). Basic physiological needs are given priority over safety needs. The needs for love, esteem, and self-actualization may have a lower priority. The nurse may encounter situations in which there are no emergency physical needs but in which high priority must be given to the psychological, sociocultural, developmental, or spiritual needs of the client.

Because clients have multiple diagnoses, the nurse is not able to treat all of them when they are identified. The nurse selects mutually agreed on priorities based on the urgency of the problem, the nature of the treatment indicated, and the interaction among the diagnoses (Gordon, 1987).

Priorities are classified as *high, intermediate,* or *low.* Nursing diagnoses that, if untreated, could result in harm to the client or others have the highest priorities (Gordon, 1987). High priorities occur in the psychological and physiological dimensions, and the nurse should avoid classifying only physiological nursing diagnoses as high priority.

Intermediate-priority nursing diagnoses involve the nonemergency, non-life-threatening needs of the client. Low-priority nursing diagnoses are client needs that may not be directly related to a specific illness or prognosis.

Whenever possible, the client should be involved in priority setting. In some situations the client and nurse assign different priority rankings to the nursing diagnoses. If both place a different value on health care needs and treatments, these differences can be resolved through open communication. However, when the client's physiological and emotional needs are at stake, the nurse needs to assume primary responsibility for setting priorities.

When the nurse assigns priorities to nursing diagnoses, the needs of the client, resources of the health care system, and limitations of time are considered. Table 8-1 displays priority settings and rationales. These priorities involve client needs and resources and limitations of the health care system.

TABLE 8-1   Priority Setting

Nursing Diagnoses	Rationale
HIGH PRIORITY	
Diarrhea related to unknown cause	Prompt resolution of diarrhea and cause prevents further decline in physiological and emotional status.
High risk for ineffective individual coping related to unknown medical diagnosis	Prompt intervention for ineffective coping will help client prepare for a diagnostic test, treatment, or diagnosis.
High risk for ineffective airway clearance after surgery related to abdominal incisional pain	Because of the risk of post-operative pulmonary complications, nurse will institute preventive client education early in nursing care.
INTERMEDIATE PRIORITY	
High risk for altered nutrition: less than body requirements related to chronic diarrhea for 3 weeks	This nursing diagnosis does not affect client's immediate physiological or emotional status. Possible surgery will also assist nurse in resolving diagnosis.
LOW PRIORITY	
High risk for chronic infections related to history of smoking for 20 years	This nursing diagnosis reflects client's long-term needs.

Development of client goals may occur with the establishment of priorities. However, for clarity and explanation, determining goals is presented in the next section.

 ## ESTABLISHING GOALS AND EXPECTED OUTCOMES

Goals and expected outcomes are specific statements of client behaviors or responses that the nurse anticipates from nursing care. After assessing, diagnosing, and establishing priorities about the client's health care needs, the nurse formulates goals and expected outcomes with the client for each diagnoses (Hickey, 1990).

The purposes for writing goals and expected outcomes are twofold. First, goals and expected outcomes provide direction for the individualized nursing interventions. Second, the goals and outcomes are used to determine the effectiveness of the interventions.

A variety of terms are used interchangeably in the nursing literature when addressing goals and outcomes. These terms include *objectives, goals, outcome criteria,* and *outcomes.* Regardless of the terms, the purpose of this step is to identify a specific means to evaluate the client's response to nursing care (Hickey, 1990). In this text, the terms *goals* and *expected outcomes* are used to indicate anticipated client responses. Fig. 8-1 illustrates the relationships between nursing diagnoses, goals, and expected outcomes.

Each goal and expected outcome statement must have a time frame for evaluation. The time element depends on the nature of the problem, etiology, overall condition of the client, and treatment setting.

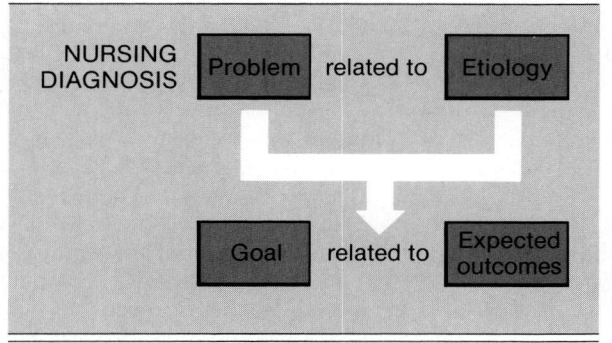

Fig. 8-1 Relationship of parts of the nursing diagnosis to the goals and expected outcomes.
Redrawn from Hickey P: *Nursing process handbook,* St Louis, 1991, Mosby–Year Book.

Goals of Care

Nursing care is planned according to nursing diagnoses, and priority setting reflects the goals of care established by the client and nurse. The nursing diagnoses formulated are based on the client's response and perception of changes in level of wellness, activities of daily living, lifestyle patterns, and role performance. Because each person responds uniquely to a situation, the nursing diagnoses and client goals of health care are also unique.

Individual nursing diagnoses and priority setting helps determine the goals of care. Bulechek and McCloskey (1985), define **goals** as "guideposts to the selection of nursing interventions and criteria in the evaluation of nursing interventions." Setting goals is an activity that includes the client and family.

Role of the Client in Goal Setting

A **client-centered goal** is a specific and measurable objective designed to reflect the client's highest level of wellness and independence in function. Client-centered goals require active involvement by the client in goal setting and the development of expected outcomes and the care plan.

Because clients participate in goal setting, they should be alert and have some degree of independence in completing activities of daily living, problem solving, and decision making. When developing goals, the nurse can act as an advocate for the client to prevent further deterioration in the level of wellness or cognitive and physical functioning.

When clients' cognitive and physical impairments are so severe that they are unable to actively participate in goal setting, the nursing team acts in their behalf to develop client-centered goals. These clients may include comatose individuals, totally disoriented individuals, individuals unable to participate in decision making, and abandoned infants or infants removed by the courts from parental custody.

Goals should not only meet the immediate needs of the client but should also include prevention and rehabilitation. Two types of goals are developed for the client; they are short-term goals and long-term goals.

Short-Term Goals

A short-term goal is an objective that is expected to be achieved in a short period of time, usually less than a week (Alfaro, 1986; Carpenito, 1989). With the present health care system and shorter hospital stays, short-term goals are the direction for the immediate care plan. (Long-term goals may be more appropriate for problem resolution after discharge [Carpenito, 1989]). A short-term goal for a client with ineffective airway clearance, for example, may be "absence of abnormal lung sounds within 2 days."

Long-Term Goals

A long-term goal is an objective that is expected to be achieved over a longer period of time, usually over weeks or months (Alfaro, 1986; Carpenito, 1989). Long-term goals may be carried over into discharge to skilled nursing facilities, rehabilitation settings, or return to the home. For example, a long-term goal for a client with an ineffective airway clearance may be to "remain free of upper respiratory infection for 6 months." These goals often focus on prevention, rehabilitation, discharge, and health education. Failure to set long-term goals may prevent the client from receiving continuity of care for discharge planning.

Goal setting establishes the framework for the nursing care plan. Table 8-2 shows the progression from nursing diagnoses to goals, which are individualized to meet client needs. Through goals, the nurse is able to provide continuity of care and promote opti-

mal use of time and resources. Ultimately the goal leads to the development of expected outcomes.

Expected Outcomes

An **expected outcome** is the specific, step-by-step objective that leads to attainment of the goal and the resolution of the etiology for the nursing diagnosis (Table 8-2). An outcome is the measurable behavior change of the client in response to nursing care (Alfaro, 1986; Hickey, 1990). Outcomes are the desired response of client condition in the physiological, social, emotional, developmental, or spiritual dimensions. This change in condition is documented through observable or measurable client responses. The expected outcomes determine when a specific, client-centered goal has been met and later assist in evaluating the response to nursing care and resolution of the nursing diagnosis.

Expected outcomes have several functions. Projected before nursing actions are formulated, ex-

TABLE 8-2 Examples of Goal Setting with Expected Outcomes		
Nursing Diagnosis	Goals	Expected Outcomes
Ineffective individual coping related to fear of negative prognosis	Client will openly discuss diagnosis.	Client will ask pertinent questions about diagnosis by 6/1. Client will express fears of unfavorable outcome by 6/2. Client will identify at least two strategies for dealing with fear by 6/4.
High risk for ineffective airway clearance related to incisional pain	Client's lungs will remain clear throughout postoperative period.	Client will turn, cough, and deep breath every hour. Client will use incentive spirometer every hour. Client will request pain medication as needed before breathing exercises.
Knowledge deficit regarding postoperative care at home related to inexperience	Client will state four postoperative risks before discharge.	Client will identify need to drink 2 to 3 L of fluid every day by 6/2. Client will name three signs of infection by 6/3. Client will demonstrate aseptic wound care by 6/4. Client will state home activity restrictions by 6/5.
High risk for altered peripheral tissue perfusion related to potential thrombophlebitis secondary to postperative venous status	Client will maintain adequate tissue perfusion by discharge.	Client will perform active range of movement exercises every 2 hours while restricted to bed. Client will continuously wear antiembolic stockings. Client will progressively increase ambulation by 50 feet every day.

pected outcomes provide a direction for nursing activities (Gordon, 1987). They also include observable client behaviors and measurable criteria for each goal. They also provide a projected time span for goal attainment and an opportunity to state any additional resources that may be required to achieve the goal, including additional equipment, personnel, or knowledge. Finally, the nurse uses expected outcomes as criteria to evaluate the effectiveness of nursing activities.

Expected outcomes are derived from short- and long-term client-centered goals and are based on nursing diagnoses developed during the second component of the nursing process (Table 8-2). When writing expected outcomes, the nurse should ensure that the outcome statement is written in measurable behavior terms. This allows the nurse to note specifically the behavior and the type of behavioral response expected for resolution of the problem. The expected outcome statements should be written sequentially, with given time frames. This provides the nurse with an order for the interventions, as well as a time reference for resolution of the problem.

Multiple expected outcomes are developed for each goal and nursing diagnosis. The rationale for the multiple expected outcomes is that few client problems can be resolved by one nursing action. In addition, the listing of the step-by-step expected outcomes gives the nurse practical guidance in planning interventions.

Guidelines for Writing Goals and Expected Outcomes

There are seven guidelines for writing goals and expected outcomes. These seven guidelines involve client-centered, singular, observable, measurable, time-limited, mutual, and realistic factors.

Client-Centered Factors

Because nursing care is directed from nursing diagnoses, the goals and expected outcomes focus on the client. These statements reflect expected client behaviors and responses as a result of nursing interventions.

A common error in writing goals and expected outcomes is to write the statement as an intervention. The correct statement is, "client will ambulate in the hall three times a day." A common error is to write, "nursing assistant will ambulate client in the hall three times a day."

Singular Factors

Each goal or expected outcome statement should only address *one* behavioral response. This singular-

ity provides a more precise method to evaluate client response to the nursing action. If the statement reads, "client's lungs will be clear to auscultation and respiratory rate will be 22/min by 8/22" and the lungs are clear but the respiratory rate is 28/min after nursing actions, it is difficult to determine whether the expected outcome has been achieved. By splitting the statement into two parts, "lungs will be clear to auscultation by 8/22" and "respiratory rate will be 22/min by 8/22," the nurse can determine specifically the outcome that has been achieved. In addition, singularity assists the nurse in modification of the care plan.

Observable Factors

The desired outcome of nursing care must be observable. Through observation, the nurse notes that the change has taken place. Observable changes can occur with changes in physiological findings and the client's level of knowledge, comfort, or anxiety. The measurable results can be obtained by directly asking the client about the condition or can be measured by using assessment skills. Examples of outcomes involving assessment skills are, "lungs will be clear on auscultation by 8/22" and "nonpurulent wound drainage will occur by 9/12."

Measurable Factors

Goals and expected outcomes contain outcome criteria and are written to give the nurse a standard against which to measure the client's response to nursing care. Examples are "body temperature will remain 98.6" and "apical pulse will remain between 60 and 100 beats per min." A goal or an outcome that is stated in measurable terms allows the nurse to objectively quantify changes in the client's status.

Common mistakes are made when the nurse uses vague qualifiers such as *"normal, acceptable, or sufficient"* in the expected outcome statement. Vague qualifiers have different meanings to different people. Using such terms results in guesswork in determining the client's response to care. Terms specifically describing quality, quantity, frequency, and weight allow the nurse to evaluate that the expected outcome was or was not achieved.

Time-Limited Factors

The time frame for each goal and expected outcome indicates when the expected response should occur. Time frames assist the nurse and client in determining that progress is being made at a reasonable rate.

Time limits assist the nurse in keeping expected outcomes in order. When the date of evaluation arrives, the nurse assesses the client to determine whether that particular expected outcome has been reached. If the expected outcome is still appropriate for the client's care, another future evaluation date is set.

Mutual Factors

Mutual setting of goals and expected outcomes ensures that the client and nurse agree on the direction and time limits of care. Mutual goal setting can increase the client's motivation and cooperation.

During this mutual setting of goals and outcomes, the nurse does not impose personal values on the client. However, the nurse must also be aware of client safety and basic human needs. Using experience and acquired knowledge, the nurse may need to direct some of the goals and expected outcomes to keep the client physically and emotionally stable and safe in the environment.

Realistic Factors

Short, realistic goals and expected outcomes can quickly provide the client and nurse with a sense of accomplishment. In turn, this sense of accomplishment can increase the client's motivation and cooperation. When establishing realistic goals, the nurse, through assessment, must know the resources of the health care facility, family, and client; the client's physiological, emotional, cognitive, and sociocultural potential; and the economical cost and resources available to reach expected outcomes in a timely manner. Establishing goals and expected outcomes without assessment of client, environment, or resources can be frustrating to the client and nurse because the plan then contains unrealistic goals.

 ## DESIGNING NURSING INTERVENTIONS

Nursing interventions, strategies, or actions are selected after goals and expected outcomes are established. However, implementation of these strategies occurs during the implementation phase of the nursing process (see Chapter 9).

Choosing suitable nursing strategies is a decision-making process. The nurse uses assessment data, priority setting, knowledge, and experience to select actions that will successfully meet the established goals and expected outcomes (Prescott, Dennis, Jacox, 1987).

Each expected outcome has interventions. The method of intervention selection is always the same, but the types of interventions are individualized to the client's needs. Fig. 8-2 illustrates the relationship of interventions to goals and expected outcomes.

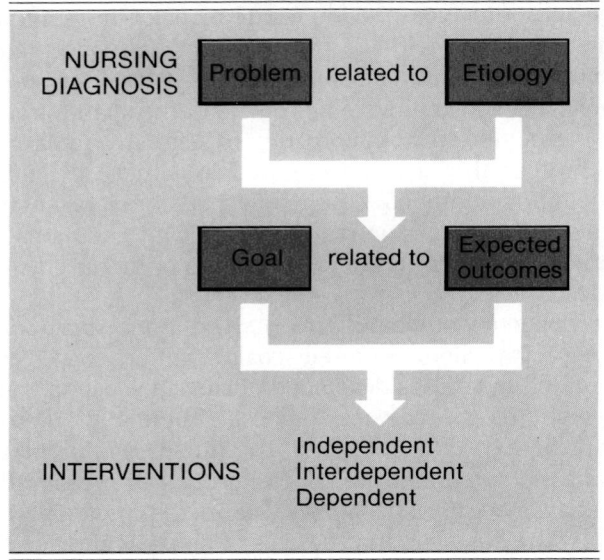

Fig. 8-2 Relationship of interventions to goals and expected outcomes.
Redrawn from Hickey P: *Nursing process handbook,* St Louis, 1991, Mosby–Year Book.

Types of Interventions

There are three categories of nursing interventions: independent, interdependent, and dependent. The category selection is based on client needs. One client may have all three categories on the care plan, whereas another client may have only independent and interdependent categories on the care plan.

Independent Factors

Independent interventions involve aspects of professional nursing practice encompassed by applicable licensure and law. These interventions require no supervision or direction from others. For example, designing interventions for increasing a client's knowledge about adequate nutrition or activities of daily living related to hygiene is an independent nursing action.

Independent interventions can solve the client's problems without consultation or collaboration with physicians or other health care professionals (Kim, 1986). Additional examples of independent nursing interventions include progressive relaxation and guided imagery techniques and therapeutic touch and massage (Snyder, 1985).

In delineating the scope of nursing practice, the ANA (1980) listed 10 areas in nursing's domain (see box). This list, with the continuing work of NANDA and nurse researchers, clarifies and elaborates the realm of independent nursing practice.

Delineation of Nursing Practice

- Self-care limitations
- Impaired functioning in areas such as rest, sleep, ventilation, circulation, activity, nutrition, elimination, skin, or sexuality
- Pain and discomfort
- Emotional problems related to illness and treatment, life-threatening events, or daily experiences such as anxiety, loss, loneliness, or grief
- Distortion of symbolic function, reflected in interpersonal and intellectual processes such as hallucinations
- Deficiencies in decision making and the ability to make personal choices
- Self-image changes required by health status
- Dysfunctional perceptual orientations to health
- Strains related to life processes such as birth, growth and development, and death
- Problematic affiliative relationships

From American Nurses Association: *Nursing: a social policy statement,* Kansas City, Mo, 1980, The Association.

Independent nursing interventions do not require a physician's order or an order from another professional. Physicians frequently include in their written orders the specifics of independent nursing interventions. However, according to the nurse practice acts in a majority of states, nursing actions pertaining to activities of daily living, health education, health promotion, and counseling are in the domain of nursing practice. These acts delineate the legal scope of the practice of nursing within the geographical boundaries of the jurisdiction (see Chapter 14).

Interdependent Factors

Interdependent interventions are carried out by the nurse with another health care professional. An example of an interdependent action is implementation of a hypertension protocol, in which the nurse has criteria to change drug and diet therapies.

Interdependent interventions also provide a solution to a client's problem in a collaborative manner through judgment and recommendations of the interdisciplinary health care team. The ANA (1980) defines **collaboration** as a

partnership in which the power on both sides is valued by both, with recognition and acceptance of separate and combined spheres of activity and responsibility, mutual safeguarding of legitimate interests of each party, and a commonality of goals that is recognized by both parties.

Dependent Factors

Dependent interventions are based on the instruction or written orders or another professional. Administering a medication, implementing an invasive procedure, changing a dressing, and preparing a client for diagnostic tests are dependent nursing interventions. It it is not within the legal practice of nursing for the nurse to prescribe and order these treatments, but it is within the practice of nursing for the nurse to complete such orders.

Each dependent nursing intervention requires specific nursing responsibilities and technical nursing knowledge. When administering medications, the nurse is responsible for knowing the classification of the drug, its physiological action, normal dosage, side effects, and nursing interventions related to its action or side effects (see Chapter 21). Nursing interventions associated with administering medication depend on the physician's written order.

Ms. Kline is caring for a preoperative client, Mrs. Wells, who has the following medication order: "Atropine sulfate, 0.4 mg intramuscularly at 8 AM today." Ms. Kline recalls that atropine is an anticholinergic medication and that the desired preoperative effect is to control salivation, bronchial secretions, and rhinorrhea during surgical anesthesia. She consults a resource to determine that 0.4 mg is a normal preoperative dose. Ms. Kline prepares Mrs. Wells for the injection and tells Mrs. Wells to expect an increase in thirst caused by medication. After administration of the drug, she observes the client for any side effects such as flushing, tachycardia, restlessness, or disorientation, and she records in the client's medical record that the drug has been administered.

With an invasive procedure or dressing changes, the nurse is responsible for knowing when the procedure is necessary, the clinical skills necessary to complete it, and its expected outcome and possible side effects; the nurse is also responsible for adequate preparation of the client and proper communication of the results.

When a specific diagnostic or laboratory test is ordered by a physician, the nurse is responsible for scheduling the test, preparing the client, and knowing the normal findings and nursing implications associated with it.

All of these interventions require nursing judgment and decision making. When encountering an order for a dependent intervention, the nurse does not automatically implement the order but stops to determine whether the requested order is appropriate for the client. Every nurse encounters an inappropriate or incorrect order at some time. The nurse with a strong knowledge base will recognize the error and seek clarification of it. The ability to recognize incorrect orders is particularly important when administering medications or implementing procedures. An error can occur in writing the order or transcribing it to the Kardex or medication card. Clarifying an order is competent nursing practice, and it protects the client and members of the health care delivery system. The nurse carrying out an incorrect or inappropriate order is as much in error as the person who wrote or transcribed the original order and is liable for any complications resulting from the error. Chapter 14 explains legal issues affecting nursing practice.

Selection of Interventions

When selecting interventions, the nurse deliberates about all possible interventions to achieve the expected outcomes; researches standardized care plans, textbooks, and nursing and related health care literature; and collaborates with other health care professionals. During deliberation, the nurse reviews client needs, priorities, and previous experiences to select nursing interventions that have the best potential for achieving the expected outcomes. As the nurse gains experience, this deliberation process becomes more efficient and experienced based (Benner, 1984).

Research of standardized care plans, textbooks, and nursing and related literature addresses usual problems and nursing actions for given conditions. Although they are written in general terms, the nurse uses these resources to acquire new client care knowledge. This knowledge then assists in the individualization of the intervention.

Collaboration completes the selection of interventions. Through collaboration the nurse is able to tap the best resources to individualize the nursing actions to meet the expected outcomes. During collaboration, the nurse also collaborates with the client to select suitable interventions that are congruent with the client's hopes, belief, values, resources, and expectations. The collaboration process is discussed in a later section of the chapter.

Usually the nurse will have more interventions than are necessary to meet the desired outcome. Some are discarded as inappropriate, and some are adapted to the client's needs and abilities. As a result, the list of possible interventions is narrowed down to those suitable to the client (Redman, 1988). These interventions are then written on the nursing care plan.

NURSING CARE PLAN

One product of the planning component is the nursing care plan, which is based on assessment data and the nursing diagnoses, priorities, and goals and expected outcomes. Generally, nursing care plans involve the following areas: nursing diagnoses, goals, specific nursing activities and strategies, and expected outcomes.

Purpose of Care Plans

The **nursing care plan** is a written guideline for client care. Written care plans document the client's health care needs, which are determined by assessment and the nursing diagnoses, priorities, and goals and expected outcomes formulated during planning.

The care plan also coordinates nursing care, promotes continuity of care, and lists outcome criteria to be used in the evaluation of nursing care (Little, Carnevali, 1983). In addition, the written care plan communicates to other nurses and health care professionals pertinent assessment data, a list of problems, and therapies. A written care plan decreases the risk of incomplete, incorrect, or inaccurate care.

The care plan is organized so that any nurse can quickly identify the nursing actions to be delivered. In hospitals and outpatient and community-based settings, the client often receives care from more than one nurse, physician, allied health professional, and health technician. The written nursing care plan makes possible the coordination of nursing care, subspecialty consultations, and scheduling of diagnostic tests.

The care plan can also identify and coordinate resources used to deliver nursing care. The listing of specific equipment and supplies necessary for nursing actions is an economically efficient mechanism for selecting equipment. If all equipment and supplies are included in the care plan, the nurse's time is used more effectively in providing care as opposed to locating supplies.

The nursing care plan enhances the continuity of nursing care by listing specific nursing actions necessary to achieve the goals of care. These nursing activities can be carried out throughout the day and from day to day. A correctly formulated nursing care plan facilitates the continuity of care from one nurse to another. As a result, all nurses have the opportunity to deliver the same quality of care.

Written nursing care plans organize information exchanged by nurses in change-of-shift reports.

Nurses focus these reports on nursing care and treatments delineated in care plans. At the end of shifts, nurses discuss care plans with the next care givers. Thus all nurses are able to discuss current and pertinent information about the client's care plan.

The written care plan can also be adapted to the discharge needs of the client. Incorporating the goals of the care plan into discharge planning is particularly important for a client who will be undergoing long-term rehabilitation in the community. The adaptation of the care plan enhances the continuity of nursing care between nurses in the hospital and community.

Same-day surgeries and earlier discharges from hospitals require the nurse to plan discharge needs on the care plan the moment the client enters a health care agency. Mortensen and McMullin (1986) note that incomplete assessments and the absence of measurable outcome criteria extend client stays in short-term, one-day surgical centers. Client stays were lengthened because there were no documented, measurable criteria for discharge readiness on the postoperative nursing care plan, resulting in confusion among all the health care professionals as to when the client could safely be discharged from the setting.

When developing an individualized care plan, the nurse involves the family and client. The family is a resource that can be used to help the client meet health goals. In addition, meeting some of the family's needs can improve the client's level of wellness.

The last item documented on the nursing care plan is the expected outcome criteria used in evaluation of care. Proper listing of the criteria provides the nurse with objective statements that help determine whether the goals of care have been achieved.

The complete care plan is the blueprint for nursing action. It provides direction for implementation of the plan and a framework for evaluation of the client's response to nursing actions.

Care Plans in Various Settings

The structure of the nursing care plan varies from one health care setting to another. For example, the care plan used in a hospital is different from one used in a community health setting. The nursing care plan developed for the client returning home is usually based solely on long-term health needs. In addition, the client and family are more involved and assume more responsibility for care because the client is receiving nursing care in the home. Although the structure of the care plan varies depending on the setting, its overall purpose is to provide a written guideline for care so that the health care needs of the client and subsequent therapies are communicated among the health care team.

Institutional Care Plans

Institutional (staff) care plans are concise documents that become part of the client's medical record. Many hospitals use the Kardex nursing care plan. **Kardex** is a trade name for a card-filing system that allows quick reference to the particular needs of the client for certain aspects of nursing care. Each card is folded once. Information about medications, activity levels, level of self-care, diet, treatments, and procedures is usually included on the outside of the card. The nursing care plan is commonly placed on the inside (Fig. 8-3 on p. 196). Each institution has its own format for the Kardex, but the basic information contained on it is universal. The care plan section of the Kardex also has institutional variations. One institution might use a three-column nursing care plan, which includes the problem, goal, and nursing action. Another institution may incorporate a four-column nursing care plan, which includes the nursing diagnosis, goal, nursing action, and evaluation. As the five-step nursing process has gained popularity, the nursing care plan on the Kardex in many hospitals has been revised to include the following components of the nursing process: assessment, nursing diagnosis, goal, implementation, and evaluation (Fig. 8-4 on p. 196).

STANDARDIZED CARE PLANS. The use of computers and the need to efficiently organize the nurse's time have resulted in standardized care plans, which are forms created for a specific clinical area (for example, coronary care, abdominal surgery, postpartum, and same-day surgery units). Each care plan lists generalized nursing diagnoses, goals, outcome criteria, and interventions for specific clients (Fig. 8-5 on p. 197).

After completing a nursing assessment, the nurse, using a standardized format, determines whether it should be used for that particular client. Even if the care plan is generally appropriate for a client, the nurse must add or delete information on the standardized form to individualize it for the client's needs. Failure to do so can result in incomplete and inaccurate care.

Standardized nursing care plans are a method to streamline and augment care planning. They are not intended to replace the nursing care plan process but to avoid a situation in which the nurse must write the same generalized plan again.

Medical Diagnosis and other pertinent medical information:

10/25 LBP c̄ RLE Sciatica
10/26 Laminectomy L4-L5 c̄ Bone Graft

Condition Satis   PMH:
Allergies (Drugs, food, other) PCN, ASA, Codeine   DM

Adm. Date 10/23 | Age 64 | Religion Cath | Mode of Travel
Service Ortho | Doctor Ford | Resident Kowalski | Intern

FREQUENTLY ORDERED ITEMS		Date	Specimens/Daily Lab	Date	Treatments		
Temp. Pulse & Resp.	> q4°	10/25	Adm. Blood work	10/24	BR and Logroll q2°		
BP		10/25	UA c̄ Micro				
		10/25	BS				
I & O	q8°						
Weights							
Spot Checks							
Chest P.T.							
Incentive Spirometer							
P.T.							

ACTIVITIES		NUTRITION	Date	Diagnostic Procedures			
Ad lib		Diet Regular	10/25	Myelogram			
Ambulate	X2			CT Scan			
Chair							
BRP			Date				
Bedrest		Feedings	10/25	CXR			
Self	Bath		10/25	ECG			
Tub		Assist c̄ meals					
Shower		FLUID BALANCE					
Bed	✓	Force					
Assist.		D E N					
		Restrict					
		D E N					

Orderlies Needed
Family:

NURSING CARE PLAN

Date	Nursing Diagnosis	Expected Outcomes	Nursing Plan/Orders
10/26	Pain related to incisional Swelling	1. Client requests for pain med. decreases by 10/28. 2. Client respiratory expansion ↑ by 10/27.	1. Encourage client to Log Roll when Turning. 2. Instruct client in relaxation exercizes.
10/27	Impaired physical mobility related to pain	1. Client increases ambulation from BID to QID or greater by 10/28. 2. Client assumes ADL by 10/29.	1. Ambulate in Hall c̄ client 20 min. after administration of analgesic. 2. Encourage family to walk client. 1. Allow client extra time to do self-care for hygiene needs.

Discharge Planning: Destination: | Transportation: | Probable Date: | Referral Agencies: | Appointment:
Supplies:

Patient Name

Fig. 8-3 Nursing care plan on a nursing Kardex.

Assessment	Nursing diagnosis	Goal	Implementation	Evaluation
Weight loss: 15 lbs. in 10 days. Eats only portion of meal due to full feeling immediately after beginning a meal.	High risk for altered nutrition: less than body requirements related to sensation of fullness c̄ meals.	Weight will remain 185 lbs for next 6 months.	1. Weigh daily. 2. Small frequent high calorie feedings: 8-10-12-2-4-6	Weight is 185 lbs. Client consumes all food delivered on meal tray.

Fig. 8-4 Five-column nursing care plan.

NURSING STANDARD CARE PLAN

Nursing Diagnosis: INEFFECTIVE BREATHING PATTERN

Related to: _____

(respiratory muscle fatigue, anxiety, pain, impaired respiratory
mechanics such as chest tubes, incisions, anatomy)

Date Initiated / Initials	Expected Outcomes	Date to be Met / Initials	Date Met / Initials
_____	Patient will verbalize understanding of _____ .	_____	_____
_____	Patient will demonstrate ability to perform _____ .	_____	_____
_____	Patient will pace and schedule activities.	_____	_____
_____	Patient will use relaxation techniques for breathing control.	_____	_____
_____	Patient will maintain respiratory rate of _____ with PaCO2 of _____ .	_____	_____
_____	Other: _____	_____	_____

Relevant baseline data: _____

_____

Referrals: (date contacted)

☐ Nurse Specialist: _____   ☐ Home Care: _____   ☐ Social Work: _____

☐ Other: _____   ☐ Other: _____

Date Initiated / Initials	Nursing Interventions	Date Inactivated / Initials
	1. Assess respiratory function for rapid, shallow, irregular, or slow breathing, dyspnea, use of accessory muscles, breath sounds, restlessness, confusion, and cyanosis every _____ .	
	2. Monitor patient's mental status/LOC every _____ .	
_____ _____ _____	3. Maintain adequate airway by: ☐ a. cough/splinting every _____ ☐ b. suction every _____ ☐ c. incentive spirometry every _____	_____ _____ _____
	4. Pace and schedule activity to avoid dyspnea resulting from fatique. Schedule is _____	
	5. Provide physical and emotional support during episodes of respiratory distress by: _____	
_____ _____ _____ _____ _____	6. Provide teaching specific to patient or support person's needs. Initiate individual plan: ☐ a. pursed lip breathing ☐ b. coughing/splinting techniques (specify) _____ ☐ c. relaxation techniques (specify) _____ ☐ d. diaphragmatic breathing _____ ☐ e. other: _____	_____ _____ _____ _____ _____
_____ _____ _____ _____	7. Other interventions specific to patient: a _____ b _____ c _____ d _____	_____ _____ _____ _____
	Signature/Initials: _____	

☐ **PLAN OF CARE MUTUALLY SET WITH PATIENT AND/OR FAMILY.**

Fig. 8-5 Standardized nursing care plan.

TABLE 8-3 Scientific Rationale for the Student Care Plan

Assessment	Goals	Implementation	Rationale	Expected Outcomes
Nursing diagnosis: *High risk for impaired of skin integrity* related to immobility resulting from coma				
Definition: High risk for impaired skin integrity is the state in which an individual's skin is at risk of being adversely altered.*				
Fever: higher than 102°F for 72 hours Diaphoresis Incontinence of urine	Absence of break in skin Absence of redness Absence of decreased muscle mass over bony prominences	Turn client every 2 hours in following sequence: 8 AM—supine 10 AM—left side Noon—prone Repeat, beginning with supine position.	Critical time for skin tissue breakdown is between 1 and 2 hours of constant pressure.†	No skin breakdown is noted. Skin color, temperature, and capillary return are normal. Client is afebrile.
Decreased skin turgor No skin breakdown noted		Keep client's skin dry at all times.	Moisture increases maceration of skin and promotes bacterial growth‡	Skin remains dry and intact. Skin turgor is improved.

*Data from Kim MJ, McFarland GK, McLane AM: *Pocket guide to nursing diagnoses*, ed 4, St Louis, 1991, Mosby–Year Book.
†Data from Bereck KH: *Nurs Clin North Am* 10(1):160, 1975; Braden: 1988.
‡Data from Kavchack-Keys MA: *Nurs* 77 7:60, 1977; Braden: 1988; Bergstrom: 1987; Greenleaf: 1984.

Student Care Plans

Nursing students learn to write and use a nursing care plan as part of their education. The student care plan is essential for learning the problem-solving technique, the nursing process, skills of written and verbal communication, and organizational skills needed for nursing care. Most important, by using the nursing care plan, students can apply the knowledge gained from nursing and medical literature and the classroom to a practice situation.

The student care plan is more elaborate than a care plan in a hospital or community health care agency because its purpose is to teach the process of planning care. To learn the care-planning process, the student must progress in a step-by-step manner, beginning with assessment and ending with evaluation. Student care plans vary from one educational program to another and between beginning and more advanced students. Some educational institutions model the student care plan on the care plan used in the affiliated health care agency. The only modification may be that the instructor requires the beginning student to include the scientific rationale for the nursing actions selected (Table 8-3). A **scientific rationale** is the reason that, based on supporting literature, a specific nursing action was chosen.

 ## WRITING THE NURSING CARE PLAN

As an initial step in planning, the nurse assigns a priority to each nursing diagnosis; priority can be based on Maslow's hierarchy of needs, urgent client physiological and safety needs, and important needs perceived by the client. The nursing diagnosis with the highest priority is the beginning point for the nursing care plan and is followed by other nursing diagnoses in order of assigned priority.

When using the five-column plan, in the assessment column (column 1), the nurse includes all data relevant to the corresponding nursing diagnosis (column 2). The nurse includes the previously developed goals in the next column (column 3). At this point, the nurse begins to translate the short- and long-term goals into action plans that anticipate the needs of the client, coordinate nursing care, and select appropriate nursing measures.

The nurse writes the action plan in the implementation column (column 4) of the care plan. Each nursing action is written to include information necessary to implement nursing care. It may help the beginning nurse to ask whether the stated interventions answer the following questions:

TABLE 8-4 Frequent Errors in Writing Nursing Interventions

Type of Error	Incorrectly Stated Nursing Intervention	Correctly Stated Nursing Intervention
Failure to precisely or completely indicate nursing actions	Primary nurse will turn client every 2 hours.	Primary nurse will turn client every 2 hours, using the following schedule: 2 PM—right side 8 AM—supine Repeat 10 AM—left side at 4 PM and 2AM Noon—prone
Failure to indicate frequency	Primary nurse will observe client cough and deep breathe.	Primary nurse will observe client cough and deep breath at 10 AM—2 PM—6 PM—10 PM.
Failure to indicate quantity	Primary nurse will provide hydrogen peroxide (H_2O_2) mouthwash to client every 2 hours while awake: 8-10-12-2-4-6-8-10.	Primary nurse will provide 50 ml of H_2O_2 mouthwash to client every 2 hours while awake: 8-10-12-2-4-6-8-10.
Failure to indicate method	Primary nurse will change client's dressing once a shift: 6 AM—2 PM—10 PM.	Primary nurse will replace client's dressing, with Neosporin ointment to wound and two dry 4 × 4 dressings secured with hypoallergenic tape, once a shift: 2 PM—10 PM—6 AM.
Failure to indicate person to perform the action	Irrigate nasogastric (NG) tube every 2 hours (even) round the clock with 30 ml of normal saline (NS).	Primary nurse will irrigate NG tube every 2 hours (even) around the clock with 30 ml NS.

1. *What* is the intervention?
2. *When* should each intervention be implemented?
3. *How* should the intervention be performed?
4. *Who* should be involved in each aspect of intervention?

In addition, the nurse should understand the reason for a specific intervention. Nonspecific nursing interventions result in incomplete or inaccurate nursing care, lack of continuity among care givers, and poor use of resources.

Common omissions in writing nursing interventions include action, frequency, quantity, method, or person to perform them. These errors can occur if the nurse is unfamiliar with the planning process. Table 8-4 illustrates these types of errors by showing incorrect and correct statements of nursing interventions.

Column 5 of the nursing care plan contains the projected outcome criteria previously identified. Listing the criteria on the care plan gives a written estimation of when the goal of care has been achieved, thus indicating when a particular nursing diagnosis is no longer relevant to the client's plan of care.

 ## CONSULTING OTHER HEALTH CARE PROFESSIONALS

Planning nursing care involves consultation with other members of the health care team. Consultation may occur at any step in the nursing process but is needed most often in the planning and intervention steps because the nurse is more likely to identify a problem requiring additional knowledge or skills or a need to obtain community or agency resources. **Consultation** is a process in which the help of a specialist is sought to identify ways to handle problems in client management or the planning and implementation of programs. Consultation is based on the problem-solving approach, and the consultant is the stimulus for change.

In clinical nursing, consultation is used to solve problems in the delivery of nursing care or the use of resources. Nurse consultants are most frequently approached for advice about difficult clinical problems. Nurses are consulted for their clinical expertise, client education skills, or staff education skills.

Nurses also consult with other members of the health care team, such as physical therapists, nutritionists, and social workers. Again, the consultant focuses on problems in nursing.

When to Consult

The need for consultation in nursing occurs when the nurse has identified a problem that cannot be solved using personal knowledge, skills, and resources. Consultation increases the nurse's knowledge about the problem and helps in learning skills and obtaining the resources needed to solve the problem. After the consultation, the nurse may be able to resolve similar problems in the future. For example, a nurse encountering a patient with a recent colostomy might request a consultation from an enterostomal therapist to determine the materials needed to clean the colostomy site and the specific techniques to use during the procedure.

Consultation is also used when the exact problem remains unclear. A consultant who is objectively entering a situation can more clearly assess and identify the exact nature of the problem, whether it is client, personnel, or equipment oriented. An unbiased consultant can often objectively identify the problem and outline a method for resolving it.

How to Consult

The first step in the consultation process is identification of the general problem area, which will give the consultant a starting point for identifying the problem. Second, the consultation should be directed to the appropriate professional, who may be another nurse or another member of the health care team. A consultation requested of the wrong individual delays problem solving and diminishes the quality of care delivered to the client.

Third, the nurse provides the consultant with pertinent information and resources about the problem area. Pertinent information includes a brief summary of the problem, methods used to resolve the problem, and outcome of those methods. Other resources can include the client's medical record, nurses and other members of the health team, and the client's family.

Fourth, the nurse should not bias consultants. Consultants are in the clinical setting to identify and resolve a nursing problem, and biasing them can hinder problem resolution. Bias can be avoided by not overloading consultants with subjective and emotional conclusions about the client and problem.

Fifth, the nurse requesting consultation should be available to discuss the findings and recommendations. When a consultation is requested, the nurse provides a private, comfortable atmosphere in which the consultant and client can meet. However, this does not mean that the nurse leaves the environment. A common mistake is turning the whole problem over to the consultant. The consultant is not there to take over the problem but to assist the nurse in resolving it. The nurse requesting assistance should request the consultation for a day when both are scheduled to work and a time when distractions are minimal. Thus the consultant is available to the nurse, and the nurse is also available to the consultant.

Finally, the nurse incorporates the consultant's recommendations into the care plan. The success of the advice depends on the implementation of the problem-solving techniques suggested.

The use of consultants is a valuable adjunct to nursing care. In clinical nursing practice, competent and experienced nurses encounter problems beyond their knowledge or experience. Professional and competent nurses recognize their limitations, seek appropriate consultation, and learn from the findings and recommendations.

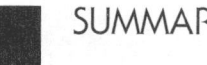 ## SUMMARY

The planning component of the nursing process results in the development of the nursing care plan, which details the selected nursing interventions and the appropriate evaluation criteria for each client. The nursing student learns the process of planning care in the educational and the clinical settings. Although the format of the care plan varies from one educational institution to another and from one health care setting to another, the student nurse will encounter the student care plan and the institutional care plan throughout the educational process.

Planning nursing care involves a cognitive and written process. The student learns to solve a client's health care problems by selecting appropriate nursing interventions. In addition, the student learns to communicate the client's health care needs through the written care plan. Individual care plans are the result of the nurse's knowledge and expertise, as well as the knowledge and expertise gained through the use of consultants.

Complete and accurate planning of nursing care results in individualization, coordination, and continuity of nursing care. Planning establishes the framework of nursing care to be delivered during implementation.

Key Concepts

- During the planning component, client goals are determined, priorities are established, expected outcomes of nursing care are developed, and a nursing care plan is written.

- Nursing care is planned and organized around specific nursing diagnoses, resulting in an individualized care plan.

- When establishing priorities, the nurse ranks nursing diagnoses and goals in order of importance.

- The nurse begins the nursing care plan with the nursing diagnoses that have the highest priority.

- Goals include prevention, rehabilitation, and the crisis or urgent needs of the client.

- Goal setting establishes a framework for the care plan.

- Using expected outcomes, the nurse evaluates the effectiveness of the care plan.

- In general, care plans include the nursing diagnosis, goals, specific actions by the nurse, and expected outcomes.

- The care plan is a written guideline for client care so that the care given can be quickly understood by all members of the health care team.

- The care plan increases communication among nurses and facilitates the continuity of care from one nurse to another and from one health care setting to another.

- The development of an individualized care plan requires involvement of the client and family during the planning phase.

- Care plans become part of a client's medical record.

- The care plan is a method for teaching students to transfer knowledge gained from nursing and medical literature and the classroom into practical experience.

- Poorly written nursing care plans result in incomplete or inaccurate nursing care, lack of continuity among care givers, and poor use of resources.

- Correctly written nursing interventions include actions, frequency, quantity, method, and the person to perform them.

- Independent nursing interventions can solve the client's problems without consultation or collaboration with physicians or other health care professionals.

- Interdependent nursing interventions are completed with or without a physician's order or are written at a nurse's suggestion and can provide the solution to the client's problem in a collaborative manner with judgment and recommendations of the interdisciplinary health team.

- Dependent nursing interventions are completed with a physician's order but require nursing judgment or decision making.

- Planning nursing care often involves consultation with other members of the health care team.

- The need for consultation in nursing occurs when a a problem that cannot be solved using the nurse's knowledge, skills, and resources is identified.

Key Terms

Client-centered goal, 189

Collaboration, p. 193

Consultation, p. 199

Dependent interventions, p. 193

Expected outcome, p. 190

Goals, p. 189

Independent interventions, p. 192

Interdependent interventions, p. 193

Kardex, p. 195

Nursing care plan, p. 194

Planning, p. 188

Scientific rationale, p. 198

Critical Thinking Exercies

1. How do you derive goals of nursing care from nursing diagnoses?

2. What criteria do you use to determine expected outcomes for a given set of client-centered goals?

3. What information do you need to plan nursing interventions for your clients? If you had nursing assistants, how would you plan those nursing strategies that could be delegated to these persons?

REFERENCES

Alfaro R: *Application of nursing process: a step by step guide,* Philadelphia, 1986, Lippincott.

American Nurses Association: *Nursing: a social policy statement,* Kansas City, Mo, 1980, The Association.

Benner P: *From novice to expert: excellence and power in clinical nursing practice,* Menlo Park, Calif, 1984, Addison-Wesley.

Bulechek G, McCloskey J: *Nursing interventions: treatments for nursing diagnoses,* Philadelphia, 1985, Saunders.

Carpenito LJ: *Nursing diagnosis application to clinical practice,* ed 3, Philadelphia, 1989, Lippincott.

Gordon M: *Nursing diagnosis: process and application,* ed 2, New York, 1987, McGraw-Hill.

Hickey PW: *Nursing process handbook,* St Louis, 1990, Mosby–Year Book.

Kim MJ: In Hurley MA, editor: *Classification of nursing diagnoses: proceedings of the Sixth Conference (NANDA),* St Louis, 1986, Mosby–Year Book.

Little DE, Carnevali DC: *Nursing care planning,* ed 3, Philadelphia, 1983, Lippincott.

Mortensen M, McMullin C: Discharge score for surgical outpatients, *Am J Nurs* 86:1347, 1986.

Prescott PA, Dennis KE, Jacox AK: Clinical decision-making of staff nurses, *Image* 19:56, 1987.

Redman BK: *The process of patient education,* ed 6, St Louis, 1988, Mosby–Year book.

Snyder M: *Independent nursing interventions,* New York, 1985, Wiley.

ADDITIONAL READINGS

Bower FL: *The process of planning nursing care,* St Louis, 1983, Mosby–Year Book.

Caplan G: *The theory and practice of mental health consultation,* New York, 1970, Basic Books.

Hendrix MJ, LaGodna GE: Consultation: a political process aimed at change. In Lancaster J, Lancaster W, editors: *Concepts for advanced clinical nursing practice,* St Louis, 1982, Mosby–Year Book.

Iyer PW, Taptich BJ, Bernocchi-Losey D: *Nursing process and nursing diagnosis,* Philadelphia, 1986, Saunders.

Kissinger JF, Munjas BA: Nursing process: student attributes and teaching methodologies, *Nurs Res* 30:242, 1981.

Mayers MG: *A systematic approach to the nursing care plan,* ed 2, New York, 1978, Appleton-Century-Crofts.

McHugh M: Nursing process: musings on the method, *Holistic Nurs Pract* 1:21, 1986.

Pilcher MW: Post-discharge care: how to follow-up, *Nurs 86,* 16:50, 1986.

Sanborn CW, Blount M: Standard plans for care and discharge, *Am J Nurs* 84:1394, 1984.

Westfall UE: Outcome criteria generation: a process and product. In Harley MA, editor: *Classification of nursing diagnoses: proceedings of the Sixth Conference (NANDA),* St Louis, 1986, Mosby–Year Book.

Yura H, Walsh MB: *The nursing process: assessment, planning, implementing, evaluation,* ed 4, New York, 1983, Appleton-Century-Crofts.

CHAPTER 9

Implementation

OBJECTIVES

Mastery of content in this chapter will enable the student to:
- Define the key terms listed.
- Discuss the differences between protocols and standing orders.
- Describe the information-processing model for selecting nursing interventions.
- List and discuss the five steps of the implementation process.
- Describe the five different implementation methods.
- Select appropriate implementation methods for an assigned client.

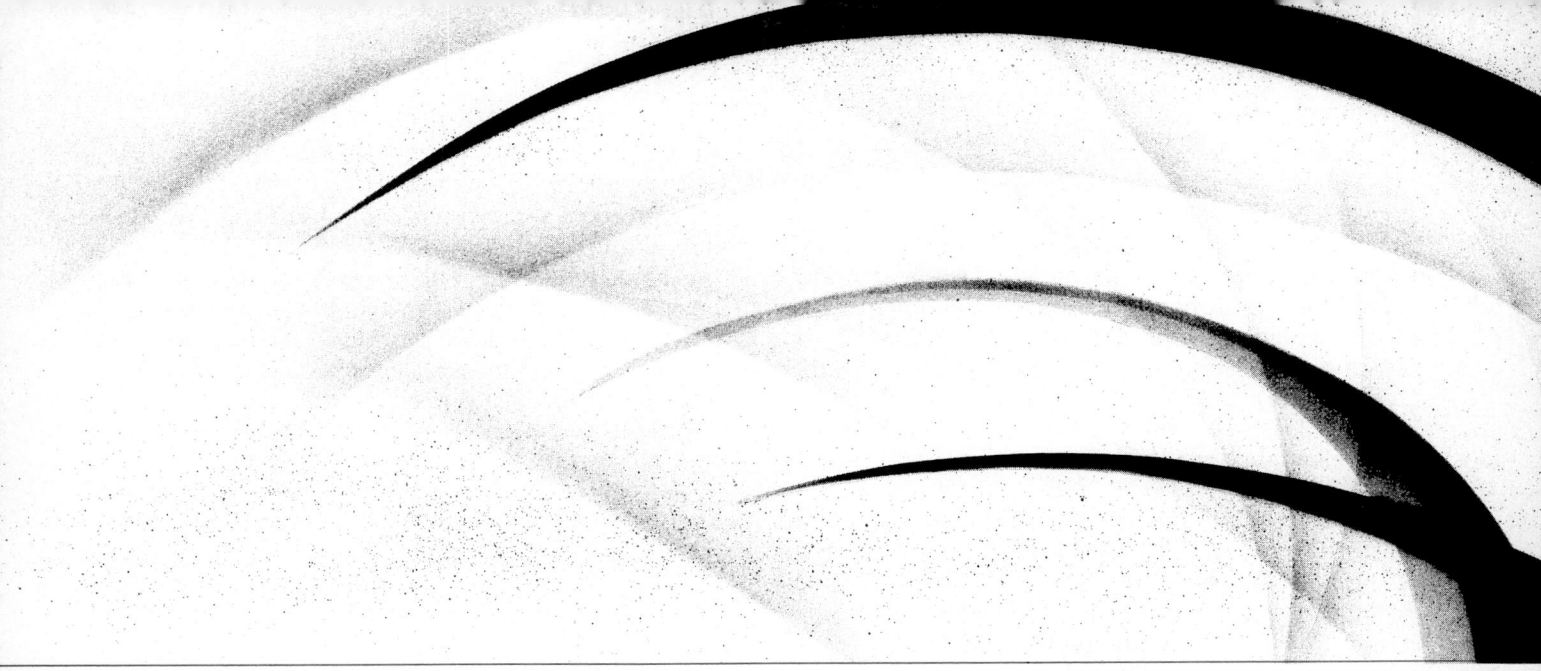

CHAPTER OUTLINE

Types of Nursing Interventions
Protocols and standing orders

Decision-Making Strategies for Choosing Nursing Interventions

Implementation Process
Reassessing the client
Reviewing and modifying the existing nursing care plan
Identifying areas of assistance
Implementing nursing interventions
Communicating nursing interventions

Implementation Methods
Assisting with activities of daily living
Counseling
Teaching
Giving care to achieve client goals
Giving care to achieve attainment of goals
Supervising and evaluating the work of other staff members

n theory, implementation of the nursing care plan follows the planning component of the nursing process. However, in practice settings, implementation may begin directly after assessment. Immediate implementation is necessary when the nurse identifies urgent needs of the client, such as a threat to physiological status (for example, a cardiac arrest), psychological status (for example, a sudden death of a loved one), socioeconomic status (for example, the sudden loss of a home in a fire), or spiritual status (for example, an illness viewed as God's punishment).

Implementation is a category of nursing behavior in which the actions necessary for achieving the expected outcomes of nursing care are initiated and completed. Implementation includes performing, assisting, or directing the performance of activities of daily living, counseling and teaching the client or family, giving direct care to achieve client-centered goals, supervising and evaluating the work of staff members, and recording and exchanging information relevant to the client's continued health care.

Implementation begins after the care plan has been developed and focuses on the initiation of nursing interventions to achieve the goals and expected outcomes of care. A **nursing intervention** is any act by a nurse that implements the nursing care plan or any specific objective of the plan. The client may require intervention in the form of support, medication, treatment for the current condition, client-family education, or treatment to prevent future health problems.

Implementation is continuous and interacts with the other components of the nursing process. During implementation, the nurse reassesses the client, modifies the care plan, and rewrites expected outcomes as necessary. To complete implementation effectively, the nurse is knowledgeable about types of interventions, the implementation process, and specific implementation methods.

■ TYPES OF NURSING INTERVENTIONS

Implementation puts the care plan into action. After the plan has been developed according to client needs and priorities, the nurse performs specific nursing interventions, which can be dependent, independent, or interdependent (see Chapter 8). In addition, nursing interventions may be entirely based on protocols or standing orders. Although these types of interventions may be viewed by some as a form of a dependent or interdependent order, a clear description of each is necessary.

Protocols and Standing Orders

A **protocol** is a written plan specifying the procedures to be followed during an assessment or when providing treatment. For example, nurses providing primary care for clients in an outpatient setting follow a protocol. In such a setting, nurses assess the client and identify abnormalities. The established protocol delineates the conditions that nurses are permitted to treat and the types of treatment that they are permitted to administer.

A protocol can also be strictly within the framework of nursing such as a protocol for admission and discharge, relaxation training, or pain management. Protocols are also used in interdisciplinary settings for diagnostic testing and physical, occupational, and speech therapies.

A **standing order** is a written document containing rules, policies, procedures, regulations, and orders for the conduct of client care in various stipulated clinical settings. Standing orders are approved and signed by the physician in charge of care before their implementation. They are commonly found in critical care settings, where clients' needs can change rapidly and require immediate attention. An example of such a standing order is one that specifies a certain drug for an irregular heart rhythm. After assessing the client and identifying the irregular rhythm, the critical care nurse gives the appropriate medication without first notifying the physician. Standing orders are also common in the community health setting, in which the nurse encounters situations that do not permit immediate contact with a physician. Thus standing orders and protocols give the nurse the legal protection to intervene appropriately in the client's best interest.

Nursing interventions implemented during the nursing process include dependent, independent, and interdependent interventions. Before implementing any therapy, including those included in protocols and standing orders, the nurse must use sound judgment in determining whether the intervention is correct and appropriate. Second, the nurse implementing any intervention has the responsibility to obtain correct theoretical knowledge and develop the clinical competency necessary to perform the intervention. Nursing responsibility is equally great for all types of interventions.

■ DECISION-MAKING STRATEGIES FOR CHOOSING NURSING INTERVENTIONS

Nurses using the nursing process make two major types of decisions. The diagnostic process defines the client's strengths and problems at the conclusion of the assessment and throughout the diagnostic stage (Hickey, 1991; McFarland, McFarlane, 1989). Specific nursing interventions are also selected during the planning stage (Grier, 1981; Gordon, 1987).

The student must carefully select the interventions designed to achieve expected outcomes and know the way that dependent, independent, and interdependent interventions differ. Several factors make decision making more difficult when choosing among independent nursing interventions (Snyder, 1985). One factor is the absence of objective data concerning the probable consequences of the interventions. Another factor is that independent nursing interventions are often not mutually exclusive from medical therapies. For example, the nurse may need to augment relaxation, massage, and guided imagery techniques with prescribed analgesics for pain management (see Chapter 37).

Snyder (1985) proposes an information-processing model of decision making (Table 9-1). The objective of this model is to characterize the sequence of the thought process used by problem solvers. In addition, Snyder incorporates a behavioral decision model for decision making; this model focuses on decisions that will be made rather than the ways that they are made. Therefore the information-processing model identifies how decisions are made, and the behavioral decision model denotes the decisions made. Because

of the information-processing model, a student uses the following components of decision making when determining nursing interventions (Snyder, 1985):

1. The set of all possible nursing actions
2. A listing of all possible consequences associated with each possible nursing action
3. The determination of the probability that each of the consequences will occur
4. A judgment based on the value of that consequence to the client

This model is effective in teaching the student clinical decision making. However, the beginning student or practitioner still needs supervision from an instructor or experienced nurse.

 ## IMPLEMENTATION PROCESS

The implementation component of the nursing process has five steps: reassessing the client, reviewing and modifying the existing nursing care plan, identifying areas of assistance, implementing nursing strategies, and communicating interventions.

Reassessing the Client

Assessment is a continuous process. Each time a nurse interacts with a client, additional data are gath-

TABLE 9-1   Information-Processing Model for Pain Related to Abdominal Incision Healing

Possible Actions	Possible Consequences Associated with Action	Probability of Consequence	Value of Consequence to Client
Teach relaxation exercises.	Client is able to control perception of pain.	Moderate	Ability to control perception and response to pain
	Pain is unrelieved.	Moderate	
	Pain increases.	Low	
Teach client use of controlled analgesia.	Client is able to control administration of analgesia within preset limits.	High	Ability of client to use analgesia to continuously relieve pain
	Pain is relieved.	High	
	Pain is unrelieved.	Moderate	
	Pain increases.	Low	
Administer narcotic analgesia every 4 hours.	Client is unable to control administration of analgesia.	High	Inability to control administration of analgesia
	Pain increases in intensity before nurse administers narcotic analgesia.	Moderate to high	Increase or decrease of pain perception based on blood levels of narcotic analgesia
	Pain is relieved.	Moderate to high	
	Client is confused after administration of narcotic analgesia.	Low to moderate	

ered to reflect physical, developmental, intellectual, emotional, social, and spiritual needs. The student nurse begins to reassess such needs each time the client and student interact. When new data are assessed and a new need is identified, the nurse modifies nursing care.

During the initial phase of implementation, the nurse reassesses the client. This is a partial assessment and may only focus on one dimension or system. The purpose of the reassessment is to gather new data that can affect the implementation or outcome of care.

A nursing care plan has been developed for Mrs. Coyle (Table 9-2). The nursing diagnosis, *Altered patterns of urinary elimination related to perineal swelling after vaginal delivery*, provided the focus for the plan. Before inserting the straight catheter, the nurse conducts reassessment to determine that Mrs. Coyle has not voided spontaneously; if Mrs. Coyle has, the catheterization procedure would no longer be appropriate.

The reassessment phase of the implementation component thus provides a mechanism for the nurse to determine whether the proposed nursing action is appropriate for the client's level of wellness.

Reviewing and Modifying the Existing Nursing Care Plan

Although the nursing care plan was developed according to the nursing diagnoses identified during assessment, changes in the client's status can neces-

sitate modification of planned nursing care. Before beginning care, the nurse reviews the care plan and compares it with assessment data to validate the stated nursing diagnoses and determine whether the nursing interventions are the most appropriate for the clinical situation. If the client's status has changed and the nursing diagnosis and related nursing interventions are no longer appropriate, the nursing care plan needs to be modified (see Chapter 10).

Modification of the existing care plan includes several steps. First, data in the assessment column are revised to reflect the client's current status. New data entered in the care plan should be dated to inform other members of the health care team of the time that the change occurred. Whenever possible, new data should be recorded in a different color to alert other care givers to changes.

Second, nursing diagnoses are revised. Nursing diagnoses that are no longer relevant are deleted, and new nursing diagnoses are added and dated. Because the client's status and health care needs have changed, the priorities, goals, and expected outcomes also must be revised. The revisions are also dated on the care plan.

Third, specific implementation methods are revised to correspond to the new nursing diagnoses and client goals. This revision reflects the client's present status. The new implementation methods indicate the client's greater independence from or dependence on nursing. In addition, revised implementation can include the client's specific needs for health care resources.

Finally, the nurse evaluates the client response to the nursing actions. If client response is not consis-

---

TABLE 9-2 Sample Nursing Care Plan

Assessment	Goal	Implementation	Evaluation
Nursing diagnosis: *altered patterns of urinary elimination* related to perineal swelling after vaginal delivery			
Definition: Altered patterns of urinary elimination is the state in which an individual experiences a disturbance in urine elimination.*			
Client has not voided in 8 hours.	Facilitate emptying of bladder	Insert straight catheter, using sterile technique, if patient has not voided in 8 hr and bladder is palpable.	1000 ml of clear yellow urine is returned via straight catheter.
Fluid intake for last 8 hr is 2400 ml.			Bladder is not palpable.
Client states that she "feels the urge to void" and experiences bladder discomfort.			Client no longer has sensation to void.
Bladder is palpable to 2 cm below umbilicus.			Client no longer complains of bladder discomfort.

*Data from Kim MJ, McFarland GK, McLane AM: *Pocket guide to nursing diagnoses*, ed 4, St Louis, 1991, Mosby–Year Book.

tent with the established expected outcomes, further revisions for the plan of care are needed. For example, a preoperative care plan was developed for Mr. Brown. As he progressed through the postoperative period, his nursing needs changed. New data were noted in blue ink and dated. The nurse made modifications in the care plan for one nursing diagnosis: *high risk for ineffective airway clearance after surgery related to abdominal incisional pain* (Table 9-3). On the second postoperative day, the nurse assessed Mr. Brown and noted decreased chest wall movements, crackles that were auscultated in the right lower lobes, and an elevated temperature (39° C). Mr. Brown had a standing order for a chest x-ray examination, which was taken immediately and revealed the collapse of alveoli in the right lower lobe. The nursing diagnosis was revised to read *Ineffective airway clearance related to abdominal incision.* The goal of "maintaining a patent airway" was still appropriate. Specific nursing interventions were developed to assist in achieving a patent airway. Finally, the projected evaluation criteria were rewritten to reflect the desired level of wellness and indicate when the need had been resolved.

The astute nurse is sensitive to changes in the client's status and readily incorporates these changes into the care plan. The health status of the client is dynamic and changes continuously. Therefore the care plan needs to be flexible to incorporate necessary changes. An out-of-date or incorrect care plan compromises the quality of nursing care, whereas review and modification enable the nurse to provide nursing care that meets the client's needs.

Identifying Areas of Assistance

Some nursing situations require the nurse to seek assistance. The assistance can fall in the following categories: additional personnel, knowledge, or nursing skills. Before implementing care, the nurse evaluates the plan to determine the need for assistance and the type required.

TABLE 9-3   Modified Nursing Care Plan for Mr. Brown

Assessment	Goals	Implementation	Evaluation
Nursing diagnosis: *High risk for ineffective airway clearance after surgery* related to abdominal incision			
Definition: High risk for ineffective airway clearance after surgery is the state in which an individual is unable to clear secretions or obstructions from the respiratory tract to maintain airway patency.[*]			
Smoked two packs/day 20 years; chest x-ray film showing slight change of emphysema; crackles auscultated in lung field; scheduled for abdominal surgery	Maintain a patent airway.	Demonstrate turn, cough, and deep breathing to client.	Productive cough produced. Airway clear to auscultation.
		Client demonstrates turning, coughing, and deep breathing exercises.	
MODIFIED 24 HOURS AFTER SURGERY			
Decreased chest wall movements; crackles in base that do not clear with coughing	Promote airway clearance.	Administer chest physiotherapy to all lobes of the lung: 8-12-4-8-12-4.	Lung fields are clear on auscultation. Client becomes afebrile.
		Ensure that Mr. Brown coughs and deep breathes every 2 hours around the clock.	Chest x-ray film demonstrates atelectasis resolving.
		Suction nasotracheal area every 2 hours if client is unable to cough productively.	
		Teach client to splint incision with pillow before and during coughing.	Client does not report increased pain during coughing.

[*]Data from Kim MJ, McFarland GK, McLane AM: *Pocket guide to nursing diagnoses,* ed 4, St Louis, 1991, Mosby–Year Book.

Situations requiring additional personnel vary. For example, a nurse assigned to care for an overweight, immobilized client may need additional personnel to help turn, transfer, and position the client because of the physical work involved. The nurse also needs to determine when the personnel are needed. If the client needs to be turned and repositioned every 2 hours, additional personnel will be needed every 2 hours. The nurse then must determine the number of persons needed and must discuss the need for assistance with potential resources. Finally, the nurse needs to take time to plan care so that the additional personnel do not become overburdened.

Additional personnel are also required when a client's health status declines or when the number of clients on a nursing division increases. In both situations the required level of nursing care is too much for one nurse to deliver safely.

Mr. Douglas is assigned to care for two postoperative clients, Mr. West and Mrs. Jade. Two hours into the shift, Mr. West begins to hemorrhage and goes into shock. Mr. Douglas spends the next hour stabilizing Mr. West's condition. At this point, he reviews the care plan for Mrs. Jade and the new care plan for Mr. West. The nurse's assessment of the situation is that for the next 2 hours he will need to spend all of his time with Mr. West. He approaches his supervisor with this assessment and requests additional help for the next 2 hours.

Some nursing situations require additional knowledge and skills. A nurse needs additional knowledge when administering a new medication or implementing a new procedure. Such information can be obtained from a hospital's formulary or procedure book. If the nurse still is uncertain about the new medication or procedure, other members of the health care team can be consulted.

Because of the continual growth of health care professions and related technology, a nurse may lack the skills needed to carry out a procedure. When this occurs, information about the procedure is obtained from the literature and the agency's procedure book. Next, all equipment necessary for the procedure is collected. Finally, another nurse who has completed the procedure correctly and safely provides assistance. The assistance can come from another staff nurse, a supervisor, an educator, or a nurse specialist.

Requesting assistance occurs frequently in all types of nursing practice and is a learning process that continues throughout educational experiences and into professional development.

Implementing Nursing Interventions

The nurse uses nursing interventions to achieve the goals of care and selects from the following methods to achieve the goals of nursing care:

1. Assisting in the performance of activities of daily living
2. Counseling and educating the client and family
3. Giving care to achieve therapeutic goals
4. Giving care to facilitate attainment of therapeutic goals by the client
5. Supervising and evaluating the work of other staff members

Nursing practice is composed of cognitive, interpersonal, and psychomotor (technical) skills. Each type of skill is needed to implement interventions. The nurse is responsible for knowing when one of these methods is preferred over another and for having the necessary theoretical knowledge and psychomotor skills to implement each. A later section introduces the general theoretical information for each method and refers to subsequent chapters that detail the necessary theoretical and psychomotor skills.

Cognitive Skills

Cognitive skills involve nursing knowledge. The nurse must know the rationale for each therapeutic intervention, understand normal and abnormal physiological and psychological responses, be able to identify client learning and discharge needs, and recognize the need for preventive and compensatory nursing actions.

Interpersonal Skills

Interpersonal skills are essential to effective nursing action. The nurse must communicate clearly with the client, family, and other members of the health care team. Client teaching and counseling must be done to the level of the client's understanding. The nurse must also be sensitive to the client's emotional response to the illness and treatment. Use of interpersonal skills enable the nurse to be perceptive to the client's verbal and nonverbal communication (see Chapter 15).

Psychomotor Skills

Psychomotor skills involve the direct care needs of clients such as changing a dressing, giving an injection, or suctioning a tracheostomy. The nurse has a professional responsibility to correctly complete these skills. Some of these skills may be new. If that is the case, the nurse must assess the present level of competency and obtain the necessary resources to ensure that the client receives the treatment safely.

Communicating Nursing Interventions

Nursing interventions are written or communicated orally. When written, nursing interventions are incorporated into the nursing care plan and client's medical record. The care plan usually reflects proposed nursing interventions. After the interventions are implemented, pertinent information is written in the client's record. This information usually includes a brief description of the nursing assessment, the specific procedure, and the client's response to nursing care.

A brief description of pertinent assessment findings in the client's medical record validates the need for a specific nursing intervention. Writing the time and the details of the intervention document that the procedure was completed. A summary of the client's response to the procedure evaluates its effectiveness.

Nursing interventions are also communicated orally from one nurse to another or to other health professionals. Nurses commonly communicate orally when changing shifts, transferring a client to another unit, or discharging a client to another health agency. Whether the nursing intervention is written or communicated orally, the language should be clear, concise, and to the point. Chapter 15 discusses the communication skills necessary in nursing practice, and Chapter 22 describes the skills needed to record pertinent information in the client's medical record.

 IMPLEMENTATION METHODS

The nurse carries out the nursing care plan by using several implementation methods. For example, the client with the nursing diagnosis, *impaired physical mobility related to bilateral arm casts,* may require assistance in performing activities of daily living. The client coping inadequately because of fear of a medical diagnosis requires counseling as a method of nursing intervention. The client with a diagnosed knowledge deficit needs interventions through health education. The totally immobilized or disoriented client requires nursing interventions providing total client care. Another method of implementation involves the supervision and evaluation of other members of the health care team.

For each nursing diagnosis the nurse is able to identify the need for one specific implementation method rather than another. Each method of implementation includes specific theoretical knowledge and clinical skills.

Assisting with Activities of Daily Living

Activities of daily living (ADLs) are activities usually performed in the course of a normal day; they include eating, dressing, bathing, brushing the teeth, and grooming. Conditions resulting in the need for assistance with ADLs can be acute, chronic, temporary, permanent, or rehabilitative. An acute disease is characterized by symptoms that are usually severe and that are present for a relatively short period of time, usually less than 6 months. An episode of acute disease results in recovery to a state of health and activity comparable to the state before the disease, passage into a chronic phase of the disease, or death. For example, the postoperative client is unable to complete ADLs independently because of the acute health problem, surgery. While progressing through the postoperative period, the client gradually depends less on nurses for completing ADLs.

A chronic disease persists longer. Although the symptoms are usually less severe than those of the acute phase of the same disease, chronic disease may result in complete or partial disability. A client with partial paralysis after a cerebrovascular accident has a chronic impairment requiring long-term assistance with ADLs.

The client's need for assistance with ADLs may be temporary, permanent, or rehabilitative. In the case of temporary assistance with ADLs, the client needs assistance during a specific time period. A client with impaired mobility because of bilateral arm casts has a temporary need for assistance. After the casts are removed, the client will gradually assume responsibility for ADLs. A client with a total self-care deficit related to an injury high in the cervical spinal cord has a permanent need for assistance. It is unrealistic for the nurse to plan a rehabilitation program with the goal that the client will be able to independently complete all ADLs. This client may have a rehabilitative need for assistance with ADLs. Through rehabilitation, the client will learn new ways to perform ADLs, thus becoming more independent and better able to perform self-care.

Through assessment, the nurse collects data that verify the need for assistance with ADLs. As the nurse analyzes this data, nursing diagnoses are formed in relation to such assistance.

Counseling

Counseling is an implementation method that helps the client use a problem-solving process to recognize and manage stress and that facilitates interpersonal relationships among the client, family and health care team. Nurses provide counseling to help the client accept actual or impending changes resulting from stress. Counseling is emotional, intellectual, spiritual, and psychological support. A client and family who need nursing counseling have "normal" adjustment difficulties and are upset or frustrated but are not psychologically disabled. Psychologically disabled clients require counseling by nurses specializing in psychiatric nursing, social workers, psychiatrists, or psychologists.

Many counseling techniques are used to foster cognitive, behavioral, developmental, experiential, and emotional growth in clients (see box). Counseling encourages individuals to examine available alternatives and to decide which choices are useful and appropriate. When clients are able to examine alternatives, they can develop a sense of control and are able to better manage stress. To assist clients in need of counseling techniques, the nurse must be able to identify the need for counseling and possess communication skills to develop a therapeutic relationship (Sundeen et al, 1989).

Clients or families needing counseling include persons who must adjust lifestyle patterns, such as stopping smoking, reducing weight, or decreasing activity levels. Clients coping with chronic or disabling diseases require counseling to help them accept changes in lifestyle or body image as the disease progresses. During life-threatening illnesses, clients and families need counseling to cope with the possibility of death.

Teaching

Counseling is closely aligned to teaching. Both involve using communication skills to effect a change in the client. However, with counseling the change results in the development of new attitudes and feelings, whereas in teaching the focus of change is intellectual growth or the acquisition of new knowledge or psychomotor skills (Redman, 1988).

Teaching is an implementation method used to present correct principles, procedures, and techniques of health care to clients and to inform clients about their health status (see Chapter 16). As a nursing responsibility, teaching is implemented in all health care settings. The nurse is responsible for assessing the learning needs of clients and is accountable for the quality of education delivered.

The **teaching-learning process** is an interaction between the teacher and learner in which specific learning objectives are presented (Redman, 1988). This process provides the organizational structure and framework for client education. The teaching-learning process is much like the basic nursing process and has the following components: assessment, nursing diagnosis, planning, implementation, and evaluation.

During assessment, the nurse determines the client's learning needs and readiness to learn. The nurse then interprets the data to formulate nursing diagnoses reflecting these learning needs. When planning, the nurse and client establish goals for learning. Implementation is the initiation of the teaching strategies designed to achieve the learning goal. Finally, evaluation measures the learning that has occurred. The purpose of the teaching-learning process is to develop and implement a teaching plan individualized for the client's needs, level of knowledge, and learning resources.

Giving Care to Achieve Client Goals

To achieve the therapeutic goals for the client, the nurse initiates interventions to compensate for adverse reactions, uses precautionary and preventive measures in providing care, applies correct techniques in administering care and preparing the client for special procedures, and initiates lifesaving measures in emergency situations. The following sections briefly discuss the nursing interventions in these areas. The specific knowledge and skills needed to carry out these nursing procedures are detailed in subsequent chapters.

Compensation for Adverse Reactions

An **adverse reaction** is a harmful or unintended effect of a medication, diagnostic test, or therapeutic intervention. Adverse reactions can follow independent, dependent, or interdependent nursing interventions. Nursing actions that compensate for adverse reactions reduce or counteract the reaction. To inter-

---

Examples of Counseling Strategies Used by Nurses

- Behavior modification
- Bereavement counseling
- Biofeedback
- Relaxation training
- Reality orientation
- Crisis intervention
- Guided imagery
- Play therapy

vene, the nurse must have knowledge of the potential undesired effects. For example, when administering a medication, the nurse understands the known and potential side effects of the drug. After administration of the medication the nurse assesses the client for any side effects. The nurse should be aware of drugs that can counteract the side effects. For example, a client may have an unknown hypersensitivity to penicillin, and hives develop after three doses. The nurse records the reaction and stops administration of the drug. The nurse also consults the physician's standing orders and administers an antipruritic medication to relieve the itching and an antihistamine to reduce the allergic response.

When caring for a client who is undergoing or who has undergone a particular diagnostic test, the nurse uses an understanding of the test and its potential adverse effects. For example, a client has not had a bowel movement in 24 hours after a barium enema. Because a bowel impaction is a potential side effect of a barium enema, the nurse administers increased fluids, gives a stool-softening medication, and instructs the client to let the nursing personnel know when a bowel movement occurs.

Therapeutic interventions may also have potential adverse effects.

Ms. Rice, the nurse, assesses a stage 1 pressure ulcer on Mr. Allen's sacrum. She develops interventions designed to prevent further skin breakdown and promote wound healing. She obtains an order for an alternating air mattress and Tegaderm (film dressing). Ms. Rice also changes Mr. Allen's turning schedule from every 2 hours to every hour while awake, and every 2 hours while asleep (2200-0700 hrs). After the second day of treatment, Ms. Rice reassesses Mr. Allen's skin and notes stage I pressure ulcers on both heels; the sacral ulcer has also progressed to a stage III ulcer. To counteract the continued skin breakdown, the nurse discontinues the air matress and obtains an order for the Clinitron bed, Tegaderm for the heel ulcers, and a hydrogel dressing for the sacral ulcer.

Although adverse effects are not common, they do occur. The nurse learns potential side effects, is able to recognize the presence of an adverse reaction, and is able to intervene accordingly.

Preventive Measures

Preventive nursing actions are directed at preventing illness and promoting health to avoid the need for secondary or tertiary health care. Prevention includes assessment and promotion of the client's health potential, application of prescribed measures such as immunizations, health teaching, early diagnosis and treatment, and development of rehabilitation potential.

In the case of a client who has a hypersensitivity to penicillin, the nurse can implement several preventive measures. The nurse indicates the penicillin allergy in the client's medical record, informs the client and family of the need for a Medic-Alert bracelet, and teaches them actions they should take if the client is given penicillin again. The nurse also teaches the client and family about the allergy and specific drugs to avoid.

Preventive nursing actions are used to meet the therapeutic goals of the client. Through preventive actions the nurse is able to help the client attain the highest level of wellness.

Correct Techniques in Administering Care and Preparing a Client for Procedures

The administration of nursing care requires the nurse to be experienced in many **techniques,** which are methods followed in performing specific procedures such as administering medications, changing clients' dressings, or inserting Foley catheters. Client care, particularly in the hospital, involves many techniques. Every procedure the nurse does for the client is carried out by a specific method.

To carry out a procedure, the nurse must be knowledgeable about the procedure itself, times it is needed, its steps, and its expected outcome. In a hospital the nurse is required to complete many procedures each day. Some of these procedures might be new, so before entering into a new procedure the nurse assesses personal competencies and determines the need for assistance, new knowledge, or new skills.

Lifesaving Measures

A **lifesaving measure** is an independent, dependent, or interdependent nursing intervention implemented when a client's physiological or psychological state is threatened. The purpose of the lifesaving measure is to restore physiological or psychological equilibrium. Such measures include administering emergency medications, instituting cardiopulmonary resuscitation, restraining a confused or violent client, and obtaining immediate counseling from a crisis center for a severely anxious client.

The initiation of lifesaving measures is an essential component of nursing practice. As with any procedure, the nurse must be knowledgeable about the lifesaving procedure itself, times it is necessary, its steps, and its expected outcome. If an inexperienced nurse happens on a situation requiring emergency measures, the proper nursing action is to get an experienced professional.

Giving Care to Achieve Attainment of Goals

The nurse achieves the attainment of health care goals by providing an environment conducive to meeting such goals; adjusting care in accordance with clients' expressed or implied needs; stimulating and motivating clients, thereby enabling them to achieve self-care and independence; and encouraging them to accept care or adhere to the treatment regimen. For each nursing intervention, the nurse and clients work together to meet the goals they developed. With some interventions, the nurse assumes a more active role, and with others, the nurse assumes a more passive role.

Nurses can create a health care environment conducive to achieving clients' goals. Ideally the nurse develops an environment that provides clients with adequate privacy for meeting basic needs and that allows them to feel safe and free to interact with the health care team. An early step in creating an appropriate environment is to orient clients and families to the health care agency. If it is a hospital, clients need to be oriented to their rooms, the health care team, and other clients. Clients in clinics should be oriented to clinic policies and procedures, the location of restrooms and cafeterias, and the health care team. When clients receive care in the home, the nurse should take time to acquaint them and their families with the purposes and expectations of the home visits.

Whether clients are in the hospital, outpatient clinic, or a community setting, the nurse takes measures to provide privacy. Obviously, clients need privacy to carry out activities of hygiene, grooming, and elimination. In addition, they need privacy to talk with families, friends, or members of the health care team. In an environment of privacy, clients feel free to share concerns, ask questions about diagnosis and treatment, and resolve personal problems.

Nursing care and other therapeutic measures are designed to meet the client's needs. As a further aid in the attainment of health care goals, the nursing care plan includes some flexibility so that the client is not placed into a fixed routine. Obviously the degree of flexibility depends on the nature of the need, the severity of the client's disability or illness, and the client's dependence on nursing care. However, even the smallest degree of flexibility, giving the client an opportunity to have some choice about the type or timing of nursing care, is valuable.

Clients with severe and chronic diseases should be encouraged to increase their levels of self-care and independence, a difficult task often disheartening for them and the nurse. To avoid discouraging clients, it is best to attempt to achieve this nursing goal gradually. The care plan is implemented so that clients successfully achieve one level of independence before attempting the next.

Mr. Porter is a 50-year-old executive, husband, and father of three teenagers. He is recovering from a severe myocardial infarction (heart attack) and cardiac arrest. For the past 10 days, all of Mr. Porter's hygiene and grooming needs have been met by the nursing staff. One day, Mr. Porter expresses doubts of ever getting his energy back and being able to care for himself. That evening Mr. Martin, a student nurse, assesses Mr. Porter and develops a nursing care plan. One of the goals is complete self-care by Mr. Porter within 1 week. With the help of his instructor, Mr. Martin implements the following nursing care plan, which is designed to achieve the overall goal of independence in various phases:

Day 1   Wash face and comb hair
Day 2   Wash face, shave, and comb hair
Day 3   Feed himself breakfast, wash face, shave, and comb hair
Day 4   Feed himself meals, wash face, shave, and comb hair
Day 5   Perform grooming activities and feed himself
Day 6   Perform grooming activities and feed himself
Day 7   Shower

Each day included achievable tasks for Mr. Porter. Placing the tasks in sequential order served the following purposes: (1) each task was developed with the knowledge that Mr. Porter could indeed successfully complete the activity, (2) a sequence of successes motivated Mr. Porter to continue with the plan, and (3) the sequence was designed to gradually increase Mr. Porter's activity tolerance.

Clients with chronic diseases are frequently on a regimen that requires strict adherence to treatment modalities. **Client adherence** means that clients and families must invest time in carrying out the required home treatments. For example, a client with chronic obstructive pulmonary disease must spend several hours a day performing respiratory therapies designed to keep the airway open and maintain an acceptable level of wellness.

Some treatment plans include the need for the client and family to adjust to functional changes as a result of medications. For example, a client with high blood pressure treated with atenolol (Tenormin) occasionally feels increasingly fatigued during the early stages of treatment, or a client with cancer who is undergoing chemotherapy has changes in energy level and body image as a result of the medication.

Finally, adherence to treatment plans can require an increased financial investment by the client and family. For example, for a client who has cardiac disease, a two-story house may no longer be suitable because the client is unable to climb stairs without feeling short of breath. Thus the client and family must invest in a new house.

Investments of time, money, and personal resources for a long period of time can be discouraging. The discouraged client may neglect the treatment regimen. After the client begins to reduce adherence to treatment, level of wellness declines.

Nurses are able to intervene and assist the client in adhering to a treatment plan. Adequate discharge planning and education of the client and family help promote a smooth transition from one health care setting to another or to the home. They also help increase the client's level of knowledge about the treatment plan. Counseling helps the client and family adapt to change resulting from the disease process or treatment. Continuity of care also provides a supportive professional who is familiar with the client's pattern of living, pattern of wellness, and treatment. In addition, reinforcing successes with the treatment plan encourages the client to adhere to the regimen.

Supervising and Evaluating the Work of Other Staff Members

The nurse who develops the care plan frequently does not perform all of the nursing interventions. Some may be delegated to another member of the health care team. Noninvasive interventions such as skin care, range of joint motion exercises, ambulation, grooming, and hygiene measures can be assigned to another staff nurse, a nursing assistant, or a licensed practical nurse. The nurse assigning tasks is responsible for ensuring that each task is assigned to an individual skilled in it. The nurse is also responsible for ensuring that the delegated task was completed according to the standard of care.

SUMMARY

In the fourth component of the nursing process, implementation, the nurse initiates and carries out the objectives of the nursing care plan. During implementation, the nurse completes dependent, independent, and interdependent nursing interventions.

As with the other components of the nursing process, implementation itself is a process. It comprises the following steps: reassessing the client, reviewing and modifying the existing care plan, identifying areas of assistance, implementing nursing interventions, and communicating nursing interventions. During reassessment the nurse focuses on one part of the total nursing assessment to determine the presence of changes affecting nursing interventions. The nurse gathers and analyzes data from the reassessment and reviews or modifies the care plan as needed. The review and modification of the plan reflect the client's current health care needs and appropriate nursing actions. Before implementing nursing interventions, the nurse identifies areas of assistance that require additional personnel, knowledge, or nursing skills. After implementing of nursing interventions, the nurse writes or orally communicates the specific nursing intervention and client responses.

Nursing interventions are selected from five methods, including assisting with ADLs, counseling and teaching, giving care to achieve the therapeutic goals for the client, giving care to facilitate the attainment of health care goals by the client, and supervising and evaluating the work of other staff members. Each implementation method requires the nurse to use theoretical knowledge and clinical skills.

Knowledge of the implementation process and the selection of appropriate nursing strategies enable the nurse to provide individualized and competent care. Through implementation, strategies are designed to accomplish the goals delineated in the nursing care plan.

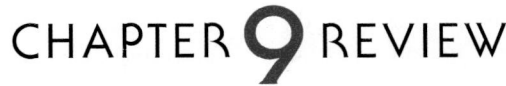

Key Concepts

- The purpose of implementation is to carry out the nursing care plan developed in the planning component.

- Implementation requires the nurse to reassess the client, review and modify the existing care plan, identify areas in which assistance is needed, implement nursing interventions, and communicate nursing interventions.

- The care plan is modified as a client's level of wellness and health care needs change.

- The implementation of nursing care may require additional knowledge, nursing skills, and personnel.

- After implementation, the nurse writes in the client's record a brief description of the nursing assessment, specific procedures, and client's response to nursing care.

- Implementation methods fall into the following categories: assisting with activities of daily living, counseling and teaching, giving care to achieve therapeutic goals, giving care to facilitate attainment of health goals, and supervising other personnel.

- Counseling helps the client use problem solving to recognize and manage stress and facilitates interpersonal relationships among the client, family, and health care team.

- Teaching is used to present correct principles, procedures, and techniques of health care to clients; inform clients about their health status; and refer clients and families to appropriate resources.

- Nursing actions to achieve therapeutic goals include compensation for adverse reactions, preventive measures, correct techniques for administering care and preparing the client for procedures, and lifesaving measures.

- Nursing actions that achieve the attainment of health care goals include providing a conducive environment, adjusting care to fit the client's needs, and stimulating and motivating the client.

- Delegating care to other personnel involves ensuring that the individuals are skilled in the tasks and evaluating that each task was completed according to the standard of care.

- To complete any nursing procedure, the nurse must be knowledgeable about the procedure, times it is needed, its steps, and its expected outcome.

Key Terms

Activities of daily living (ADLs), p. 211
Adverse reaction, p. 212
Client adherence, p. 214
Counseling, p. 211
Implementation, p. 206
Lifesaving measure, p. 213
Nursing intervention, p. 206

Preventive nursing actions, p. 213
Protocol, p. 206
Standing order, p. 206
Teaching, p. 212
Teaching-learning process, p. 212
Techniques, p. 213

Critical Thinking Exercises

1. You are preparing to carry out the following nursing intervention: If the client is voiding infrequently and producing small amounts of urine, insert a straight catheter at 1200 to relieve bladder distension. What additional data must you obtain from the client to determine whether this is an appropriate intervention?

2. You are assigned to ambulate with Mr. Clay who had abdominal surgery 24 hours before. Mr. Clay weighs 270 lbs and is 6 feet tall. What questions do you need to answer before you attempt to ambulate with this client?

3. Your client needs a complicated wound irrigation and dressing change. What measures will you take to reduce the risk of an adverse reaction to this intervention?

REFERENCES

Brown JJ, Fanner CA, Padrick KP: Nursing's search for scientific knowledge, *Nurs Res* 33:26, 1984.

Gordon M: *Nursing diagnosis: process and application,* ed 2, New York, 1987, McGraw-Hill.

Grier M: The need for data in making nursing decisions. In Werley H, Grier M, editors: *Nursing information systems,* New York, 1981, Springer.

Hickey P: *Nursing process handbook,* St Louis, 1991, Mosby–Year Book.

McFarland GK, McFarlane EA: *Nursing diagnosis and intervention: planning for patient care,* St Louis, 1989, Mosby–Year Book.

Redman BK: *The process of patient education,* ed 6, St Louis, 1988, Mosby–Year Book.

Snyder M: *Independent nursing interventions,* New York, 1985, Wiley.

Sundeen SJ et al: *Nurse-client interaction: implementing the nursing process,* St Louis, ed 4, 1989, Mosby–Year Book.

ADDITIONAL READINGS

American Nurses Association: *Nursing: a social policy statement,* Kansas City, Mo, 1980, The Association.

Carpenito LJ: *Nursing diagnosis application to clinical practice,* ed 3, Philadelphia, 1989, Lippincott.

Chesney MA: Behavior modification and health enhancement. In Matarazzo JD et al: *Behavioral health,* New York, 1984, Wiley.

Halloran E, Kiley M: Case mix management for nurses, *Nurs Manage* 15(2):39, 1984.

Iyer PW, Taptich BJ, Bernocchi-Losey D: *Nursing process and nursing diagnosis,* Philadelphia, 1986, Saunders.

Kim MJ: Degree of independence of nursing interventions for nursing diagnoses. In Hurley MA, editor: *Classification of nursing diagnoses: proceedings of the Sixth Conference (NANDA),* St Louis, 1986, Mosby–Year Book.

Kim MJ: Nursing diagnoses: a Janus view. In Hurley ME, editor: *Classification of nursing diagnoses: proceedings of the Sixth Conference (NANDA),* St Louis, 1986, Mosby–Year Book.

Marriner A: *The nursing process: a scientific approach to nursing care,* ed 4, St Louis, 1987, Mosby–Year Book.

McMurrey PH: Toward a unique knowledge base in nursing, *Image J Nurs Sch* 14:12, 1982.

CHAPTER 10

Evaluation

OBJECTIVES

Mastery of content in this chapter will enable the student to:
- Define the key terms listed.
- Explain the relationship between expected outcomes and goals of care.
- Describe the interaction of the components of the nursing process.
- Give examples of evaluation measures used to determine progress toward outcomes.
- Evaluate nursing actions selected for a client.
- Explain the differences and similarities between quality assurance and quality improvement.
- Give examples of the 10 steps to quality improvement.

CHAPTER OUTLINE

The **evaluation** component of the nursing process measures the client's response to nursing actions and the client's progress toward achieving goals. Evaluation is ongoing and occurs when the nurse has contact with a client. The emphasis is on client outcomes. The nurse evaluates whether the client's behaviors or responses reflect a reversal or improvement in a nursing diagnosis or maintenance of a healthy state. During evaluation, the nurse judges the success of the previous steps of the nursing process by examining the client's responses and comparing them with the behaviors stated in the expected outcomes.

Another aspect of evaluation involves measurement of the quality of nursing care provided in a health care setting and the quality of nursing care for a client. The quality, effectiveness, and appropriateness of nursing care has been the focus of the Joint Commission on Accreditation of Health Care Organizations (JCAHO) and **professional standards review organizations (PSROs)**. Quality assurance is an ongoing, systematic, comprehensive evaluation of health care services and the impact of those services on health care consumers. The emphasis is on client outcomes and the care givers and the systems in which they practice. Legal criteria and professional standards are often used to evaluate the quality of care. Evaluation of nursing activities determine the types of nursing actions performed and the level of success in achieving client goals. It ensures quality professional nursing practice.

DYNAMICS OF EVALUATING THE NURSING PROCESS

While caring for clients, the nurse compares observed results (for example, reversal of pain symptoms, improved knowledge of illness, and proper use of equipment by the client) with expected outcomes. Critical thinking is required when the nurse analyzes the findings of evaluative measures. For example, when evaluating a client for a change in vital signs, the nurse must apply knowledge of disease processes and physiological responses to interpret whether a change has indeed occurred. Positive evaluations occur when desired results are met, leading the nurse to conclude that the care plan effectively met client goals. Negative evaluations or undesired results indicate that the problem was not resolved or that potential problems were not avoided. As a result, the nurse must change the care plan, and the entire nursing process sequence is repeated.

This sequence continues until problems are resolved. The nurse must realize that evaluation is dynamic and ever changing, depending on the client's nursing diagnoses and condition. A client whose health status continuously changes requires more frequent evaluation. In addition, priority diagnoses are often evaluated first. For example, a nurse evaluates a client's acute pain before evaluating the status of knowledge deficit.

EVALUATION OF GOAL ACHIEVEMENT

The purpose of nursing care is to assist the client in resolving actual health problems, preventing the occurrence of potential problems, and maintaining a healthy state. Evaluation of goals determines whether this purpose was accomplished. The nurse matches the client's behavior (for example, self-administration of insulin or relief of anxiety) or physiological response (for example, decrease in size of pressure ulcer or fall in body temperature) with the behavior or response specified in the goal. The initial assessment of a client provides the baseline data to determine whether the desired changes occurred. For example, during assessment, a client may report acute abdominal pain, rate the pain 8 on a scale of 10 (see Chapter 37), and grimace or hold the abdomen during attempts to move in bed. This baseline is used by the nurse to identify the nursing diagnosis of *Pain* and establish the goal, "client will be able to perform self-care measures without discomfort in 3 days." One outcome may include, "client will verbalize pain at 3 on a scale of 10." After nursing actions are performed, the nurse reassesses the client by measuring the subjective report of pain and observing facial expressions. The new data are compared with outcome criteria to determine whether predicted changes have occurred (Table 10-1). To objectively evaluate the degree of success in achieving a goal, the nurse should use the following steps:

1. Examine the goal statement to identify the exact desired client behavior or response.
2. Assess the client for the presence of that behavior or response.
3. Compare the established outcome criteria with the behavior or response.
4. Judge the degree of agreement between outcome criteria and the behavior or response.

There are different degrees of goal attainment. If the client's response matches or exceeds the outcome criteria, the goal is met. If the client's behavior begins to show changes but does not yet meet specified criteria, the goal is partially met. If there is no progress, the goal is not met (Table 10-2). A clearly defined goal with specific outcomes is easily measured.

Evaluative Measures and Sources

Evaluative measures are simply the assessment skills and techniques used to collect data for evaluation. For example, auscultation of lung sounds, observation of a client's skill performance, inspection of the skin, and inquiry regarding the severity of pain are all evaluative measures. The new data collected from evaluation measures are critically analyzed and compared with expected outcomes to determine whether changes occurred (Table 10-3 on p. 222). After caring for a client over a long period, the nurse is able to make subtle comparisons of responses and behaviors. The accuracy of any evaluation improves when the nurse is familiar with the client's behavior and physiological status.

The primary source of data for evaluation is the client. However, the nurse also uses the family and other care givers. The importance of documentation and reporting in the evaluation process is critical. The written nursing progress notes and information shared between nurses during change-of-shift reports (see Chapter 22) should communicate a client's progress toward meeting expected outcomes and

---

TABLE 10-1   Examples of Objective Evaluation of Goal Achievement

Goals	Outcome Criteria	Client Responses	Evaluation
Client will self-administer insulin by 12/18.	Client prepares insulin dosage in syringe by 12/17. Client demonstrates self-injection by 12/18.	Client prepared accurate dosage in syringe on 12/17. Client administered morning insulin dosage; self-injection was correctly performed on 12/18.	Outcome criteria and client response agree; goal was met.
Client's lungs will be free of secretions by 11/30.	Lungs will be clear to auscultation by 11/30. Coughing will be nonproductive by 11/29. Respirations will be 20 per minute by 11/30.	Lungs were clear to auscultation on 11/30. Client coughed frequently but nonproductively on 11/29. Respirations were 18 per minute on 11/29.	Outcome criteria and client response agree; goal was met.
Client will be able to perform self-care measures without discomfort in 3 days.	Client will verbalize pain at 3 on a scale of 10 within 3 days.	Client reports severe right sided abdominal pain at 5 on a scale of 10 while attempting bathing on day 3.	Outcome criteria and client response disagree; goal was not met.

TABLE 10-2   Comparison of Client Goal and Response in Goal Evaluation

Client Goals	Client Responses	Evaluation
Client will self-administer prepared insulin dosage by 12/18.	Client prepared dosage correctly using proper infection-control technique and self-administered insulin on 12/18.	Client met all criteria of goal statement; goal was met.
Client will have a soft, formed bowel movement every other day by 4/22.	Client had no bowel movement for 3 days.	Client has made no progress toward goal achievement; goal was not met.
Client will identify four signs of infection by 2/4.	Client discussed teaching booklet and information related to signs of infection on 2/3. Client identified two signs of infection on 2/4.	Client is making progress toward goal achievement; goal was partially met.

TABLE 10-3   Evaluation Measures to Determine the Success of Goals and Expected Outcomes

Goals	Evaluation Measures	Expected Outcomes
Client's pressure ulcer will heal within 7 days.	Inspect color, condition, and location of pressure ulcer. Measure diameter of ulcer daily. Note odor and color of drainage from ulcer.	Erythema will be reduced in 2 days. Diameter of ulcer will decrease in 5 days. Ulcer will have no drainage in 2 days. Skin overlying ulcer will be closed in 7 days.
Client will tolerate ambulation to end of hall by 11/20.	Palpate client's radial pulse before exercise. Palpate client's radial pulse 10 minutes after exercise. Observe client for dyspnea or breathlessness during exercise. Assess respiratory rate during exercise.	Pulse will remain below 110 beats per minute during exercise. Pulse rate will return to resting baseline within 10 minutes after exercise. Respiratory rate will remain within 2 breaths of client's baseline rate. Client will deny feeling of breathlessness by 11/20.
Client will self-administer prescribed insulin dosage correctly by 12/18.	Observe client preparing insulin dosage. Have client explain how to prevent infection while preparing a syringe. Observe client administering self-injection.	Client will correctly prepare prescribed dosage of insulin on 12/17. Client will describe 3 ways to prevent infection while preparing syringe and administering injection. Client will perform return demonstration of self-injection on 12/18.

goals. All members of the health care team should have a sense of the client's progress. Each nurse summarizes data on an ongoing basis to ensure that the client is progressing to a better level of health.

Expected Outcomes

Expected outcomes are statements of progressive, step-by-step responses or behaviors that the client needs to accomplish to remove or modify the etiology of the nursing diagnosis. Expected outcomes are established during the planning phase of the nursing process (see Chapter 8). For example, for a nursing diagnosis of, *anxiety related to fear of hospitalization,* the client must understand the reason for hospitalization and the procedures to expect during hospitalization. In addition, the client must have a sense of relief after understanding this information. To determine whether anxiety has been resolved, the nurse establishes outcomes measuring the client's improved knowledge level and acknowledgement of anxiety relief. Expected outcomes have short time frames (depending on the health care setting) and include as few as one or two intervention sessions (Hickey, 1991). To provide truly objective measurements, the outcomes are stated behaviorally and have time frames for evaluation.

After a specified time interval or when all interventions for an expected outcome have been completed, the nurse evaluates the client's ability to demonstrate the behavior or response stated in the outcome criteria. Evaluation of each expected outcome and its place in the sequence is essential. Failure to evaluate each expected outcome results in an inability to determine the place in which the sequence faltered.

If the client achieves the expected outcome, the nurse continues with the care plan. If evaluation determines that the expected outcome was not met or only partially met, the nurse begins reassessment and revision.

Goals

A goal specifies the behavior or response that indicates resolution of a nursing diagnosis or maintenance of a healthy state. It is a summary statement of what is to be accomplished when all outcomes have been met. Each nursing diagnosis in the client's care plan has a goal, and every goal has a time frame for evaluation. The nurse evaluates goals after comparing evaluative findings with all expected outcomes. When a goal has been accomplished, the nurse knows that interventions have been successful and that the client is progressing.

As hospital stays become shorter, many clients are discharged before all goals are met and all nursing diagnoses are resolved. When preparing a client for discharge, the nurse evaluates the status of each nursing diagnosis and writes an evaluative statement identifying the client's progress toward goal achievement and problem resolution. Appropriate revisions to the care plan are made for home or follow-up care (for example, an extended-care facility). The nurse must clearly distinguish between goals that have been met and goals that require continued intervention. A home health nurse will probably revise interventions to adapt them to the client's home.

 ## CARE PLAN REVISION

After goals have been evaluated, adjustments to the care plan are made as indicated. If a goal was successfully met, that portion of the care plan is discontinued. Unmet and partially met goals require the nurse to reactivate the nursing process sequence. After reassessment, modification or addition of nursing diagnoses, goals, expected outcomes, and interventions is made as needed. The nurse also reestablishes priorities. At this point, evaluation is again performed to review client progress.

Discontinuing a Care Plan

After determining that expected outcomes and goals have been achieved, the nurse confirms this evaluation with the client. If both agree that the expected outcome have been met, the nurse discontinues that portion of the care plan. For example, a client has the nursing diagnosis, *knowledge deficit regarding insulin therapy related to inexperience;* to achieve the goal of accurate client administration of insulin, the nurse establishes outomes such as, "client will describe the purpose of insulin and the side effects of hypoglycemia." The nurse discusses the information with the client and learns whether the client understands explanations and is comfortable with the information provided. It is unnecessary to teach additional information about insulin.

A nurse must promptly document and report on goal achievement. This ensures that other nurses will not unnecessarily continue a care plan. Continuity of care assumes that care provided is relevant to client needs. Significant time is wasted when achieved goals are not communicated.

Modifying a Care Plan

When goals are not met, evaluation involves identifying the variables or factors that interferred with goal achievement. Usually a change in the client's condition, needs, or abilities makes alteration of the care plan necessary. For example, when teaching

self-administration of insulin, the nurse discovers that the client has a literacy problem or a visual impairment that prevents the reading of insulin dosages on the syringe. As a result, original outcomes cannot be met. Thus the nurse uses new interventions and revises outcomes to meet the goal of care.

Lack of goal achievement may also result from an error in nursing judgment or failure to follow each step of the nursing process. Clients frequently have very complex problems. The nurse should always remember the possibility of overlooking or misjudging something. When there is failure to achieve a goal, no matter what the reason, the entire nursing process sequence is repeated to discover changes that need to be made to promote, maintain, or restore the client's health.

Reassessment

A complete reassessment of all client factors relating to the nursing diagnosis and etiology is the first step in reactivating the nursing process. Reassessment requires critical thinking when the nurse compares new data about the client's condition with previously assessed information. Often a nurse applies intuitive knowledge from previous experience to direct the reassessment process. In this case, a nurse compares the actual data with knowledge of client expectations. As in the original assessment, data are collected from all available sources. Depending on the nurse's findings, it may be necessary to assess variables that were not covered on the initial assessment.

Reassessment ensures that the data base is accurate and current. It may also reveal the missing link; that is, a critical piece of new information was previously overlooked and thus interferred with goal achievement. All new data are sorted, validated, and clustered to analyze and interpret differences from the original data base. The nurse documents reassessment data to alert other nursing staff to the client's status.

Nursing Diagnoses

After reassessment, the nurse reevaluates all nursing diagnoses and determines whether the diagnostic statement was accurately formulated for the situation. The nurse asks whether the correct diagnosis was selected and whether it and the etiologic factor are current. The problem list should then be revised to reflect the client's changed status. A new diagnosis may be made. If a previous diagnosis no longer accurately reflects the problem, it should be discontinued, and a modified statement is entered. For example, if the nurse finds that a client with diabetes has a serious visual impairment, it may be unlikely that the client will be able to self-administer insulin.

The nurse's assessment reveals that a family member is available as a resource. To develop a plan designed to educate an alternate care giver about the administration of insulin, the nurse then establishes a new diagnosis, *Altered health maintenance related to visual impairment.*

A nurse's care is based on an accurate list of nursing diagnoses. Accuracy is more important than the number of diagnoses selected. As the client's condition changes, the diagnoses do too.

Goals and Expected Outcomes

Every goal and expected outcome should be evaluated for needed changes. Even the goals for unchanged nursing diagnoses should be examined for appropriateness. Determining that each goal and expected outcome is realistic for the problem, etiology, and time frame is particularly important. Unrealistic expected outcomes and time frames make goal achievement difficult.

The nurse clearly documents goals and expected outcomes for new or revised nursing diagnoses so that all team members are aware of the revised care plan. When the goal is still appropriate but has not yet been met, the nurse may change the evaluation date to allow more time. All goals and expected outcomes should be client centered, with realistic expectations for client achievement.

Interventions

The evaluation of interventions examines two factors: the appropriateness of the interventions selected and the correct application of the implementation process. The appropriateness of an intervention may be based on the **standard of care** for a client's health problem. If the client has a specific nursing diagnosis such as, *ineffective airway clearance,* the standard of care established by a nursing department for this problem may include pain control measures with coughing or deep breathing exercises to help a client breathe more easily with a clear airway. The nurse reviews the standard of care to determine whether the right interventions have been chosen or if additional ones are required.

It may only be necessary to increase or decrease the frequency of interventions. The nurse uses judgment based on previous experience, as well as the client's actual response to therapy. For example, if a client continues to have congested lung sounds, the nurse increases the frequency of coughing exercises to remove secretions.

During evaluation, the nurse may determine that some planned interventions are designed for an inappropriate level of nursing care. If the level of care needs to be changed, a different action verb, such as

assist in place of *provide,* may be substituted. Sometimes the level of care is appropriate, but the interventions are unsuitable because of a change in the expected outcome. In this case, the interventions should be discontinued, and new ones are planned.

During implementation, the nurse evaluates the client's response during and immediately after intervention. This is the beginning of the evaluation process. Evaluation must be integrated with ongoing nursing care activity. If the response is favorable, implementation continues. Reevaluation occurs when the intervention proves unsuccessful. The nurse then examines the other components of implementation such as client and environment preparation, anticipated complications, or use of personal or technical skills during care delivery (Hickey, 1991).

Changes in implementation should be guided by the nature of the client's unfavorable response. Consulting with other nurses may yield suggestions for improving the approach to care delivery. Senior nurses are often excellent resources because of their experience. Simply changing the care plan is not enough. The nurse must implement the new plan and reevaluate the client's response to the nursing actions. Evaluation is continuous.

Occasionally an error during care planning and delivery is discovered during evaluation. This should be anticipated. The nursing process is designed to be a systematic, problem-solving approach to individualized client care, but there is a wide array of variables for each client with a health care problem. Clients with the same health care problem are not treated the same. As a result, sometimes, the nurse makes errors in judgment. The systematic use of evaluation provides a way for nurses to catch these errors in judgment. The nurse consistently incorporates evaluation into practice to minimize error and ensure that the most appropriate interventions are used.

Evaluation is the final step of the nursing process, a systematic method for organizing and delivering nursing care. The exclusion of evaluation from the nursing process prevents the nurse from evaluating nursing practice and determining whether the outcomes of client care are beneficial. The regular application of evaluation ensures that a client's care plan is current and appropriate. The case study box summarizes each step of the nursery process:

■ QUALITY ASSURANCE AND QUALITY IMPROVEMENT

The evaluation of health care is a process used to determine the quality of service provided to clients. The process is receiving more attention than ever be-

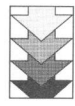

Nursing Process Case Study

Ms. Jenner is a 39-year-old woman entering the orthopedic clinic with acute lower back pain.

Nursing History: Client has had continuous "mild backaches" for almost a year. Three days ago she began exercising for back strengthening and noticed a "pull in my lower back, so I stopped exercising." Acute back pain developed the next morning. Ms. Jenner went to work but was only able to stay a few hours. After driving home, "the pain worsened and it traveled down my right leg." Ms. Jenner is normally very active, walking 2 miles daily. She enjoys gardening and dancing. She lives alone and has a large golden retriever. "The dog is playful and causes me to bend over a lot." She has a close friend who lives 15 minutes away. Ms. Jenner is employed as a nurse and states "I'm worried about missing work."

Physical Assessment: Acute lumbar pain is graded as a 9 on a scale of 10. Pain radiates down right leg while client stands, disappears while she is lying supine. Client limps noticeably and holds lower back when asked to walk. Range of motiton decreased when client bends forward. Reduced sensation exists along distribution of peroneal nerve from just above the right knee and down to the outer 3 toes of the right foot. During assessment, Ms. Jenner asked many questions about the possible cause of her back pain. Because she is a nurse, she knows that symptoms could indicate a ruptured intravertibral disk. Her facial expression and tone of voice is tense.

Medical Findings: Radiological examination revealed no ruptured disk. Client has malalignment of L5 to S1 vertebrae, which will be treated conservatively.

DIAGNOSTIC PROCESS

Assessment activities	Defining characteristics	Nursing diagnoses
Questione client about character of symptoms.	Acute lower back pain, radiates down right leg, worsens with standing, relieved while lying supine	*Pain* related to musculoskeletal injury
Observe client's facial expression.	Tense expression, grimaces	
Observe for changes in body function	Unable to walk without limping, range of motion of lower back reduced	
Interview client about perception of back problem.	Asks questions about cause of pain and effects on work	*Anxiety* related to threat to health status
Review nursing history.	Had acute pain for first time, 2 days ago	
	As a nurse, knows potential implications of back injury (fears consequences)	
Observe facial expression.	Tense expression	

NURSING CARE PLAN

Nursing diagnosis: *Pain* related to musculoskeletal injury

Definition: Pain is the state in which an individual experiences and reports the presence of severe discomfort or an uncomfortable sensation.

Goal	Expected outcomes	Interventions	Rationale
Client will gain freedom of back movement without pain within 4 weeks.	Client will report reduction in pain severity (less than 9) after nursing theraphies.	Instruct client on use of patient controlled analgesia (PCA).	PCA device allows client to self-administer analgesia as needed for acute pain.
	Client will exhibit fewer signs and symptoms of pain within 5 days.	Keep client properly positioned in pelvic traction with hips and knees flexed 30 degrees and head of bed slightly elevated.	Position relieves pressure from lower back by reducing lumbar curve.*
		Reduce activities requiring client to get out of bed to sit or stand.	Sitting or standing during an acute bakc injury can increase back pain.
Client will initiate good body mechanics during daily activities without fear of injury within 1 week.	Client will discuss fears related to back injury within 2 days.	Plan periods during routine care for client to discuss fears about back injury.	Provides opportunity for client to clarify misconceptions about extent of back injury.

Continued.

Nursing Process Case Study—cont'd

NURSING CARE PLAN-CONT'D

Nursing diagnosis: *Anxiety* related to threat to health status
Definition: Anxiety is a vague, uneasy feeling, the source of which is often nonspecific or unknown to the individual.

Goal	Expected outcomes	Interventions	Rationale
Client participates in care without undue anxiety within.	Client will initiate self-care activities independently within 1 week.	Educate client regarding body mechanics to be used during daily activities: using straight-backed chairs, keeping knees higher than hips during sitting, avoiding prone position, and for work activities, lifting, techniques.	Gives client control over minimizing further back injury.

EVALUATION OF INTERVENTIONS

Goals	Evaluative measures	Expected outcomes
Client will gain freedom in back movement without pain within 4 weeks.	Observe client's facial expression and body positioning during movement. Have client rate pain severity on scale of 1 to 10 after care activities (e.g., repositioning, walking to bathroom).	Client will exhibit fewer signs and symptoms of back pain within 5 days. Client will report a reduction in pain severity (less than 9) after nursing therapies.
Client will initiate good body mechanics during daily activities without fear of injury within 2 weeks.	Observe client's affect and tone of voice for signs of anxiety. Question client about fears relating to ability to resume normal activities. Have client describe body mechanic techniques to use during daily activities at home and work.	Client will discuss fears related to back injury within 2 days. Client will initiate self-care activities independently within 1 week.

Ms. Jenner responded well to pain-control measures. By the third day of hospitalization, she reported less severe pain. The news that her treatment would be conservative and the reduction in pain severity led to a noticeable reduction in her anxiety. She was attentive to discussions about body mechanics. At the time of discharge, she was able to walk with less discomfort.

Data from Beare PG, Myers JL: *Principles and practice of adult health nursing*, St Louis, 1990, Mosby–Year Book.

fore because of the increasing costs of health care. A health care organization faced with economic pressures must identify the factors that differentiate it from other organizations. Quality of care is the answer. Nursing has participated in the monitoring of quality for many years. For nurses to be accountable for their practice, they must discriminate between effective and ineffective aspects of care. They must determine what activities favorably influence a client's recovery. Quality assurance and quality improvement are two methods used to measure the quality of care. The JCAHO has defined **quality assurance (QA)** as a planned and systematic process for the monitoring and evaluation of the quality and appropriateness of client care and for resolving identified problems

(JCAH, 1986). Early QA programs were centralized; nursing units throughout a hospital or home health agency monitored using the same clinical criteria. Measurement was often performed with agency surveys or by QA staff members who collected data about nursing units. The problem with this approach was that care activities differ from one unit to another. Often, QA evaluation failed to provide meaningful information about the delivery of quality care on a specific unit. As a result, few nurses felt that the problems were defined, and thus nursing practice infrequently changed.

The development of unit-based QA programs places the responsibility and authority for monitoring on professional staff nurses. In a unit-based program,

TABLE 10-4 Characteristics of Quality Assurance and Quality Improvement	
Quality Assurance	Quality Improvement
Focuses on Clinical care	Focuses on all system activities
Organizes structure by department	Crosses department systems
Focuses on process of care	Focuses on outcomes of care
Focuses on problem	Focuses on continuous improvement
Divides analysis of effectiveness and efficiency	Integrates analysis of quality and cost

---

JCAHO's Ten Steps for QI

- Establish responsibility and accountability for a QI program.
- Define the scope of service for a clinical area.
- Define the key aspects of service for the clinical area.
- Develop quality indicators to monitor the outcomes and appropriateness of care delivered.
- Establish thresholds for evaluation of indicators.
- Collect and analyze data from monitoring activities.
- Evaluate results of monitoring activities to determine the need for change in practice.
- Resolve problems through development of action plans.
- Reevaluate to determine if the action plan was successful.
- Communicate results of QI to members of the organization.

---

each unit has a QA committee whose members identify clinical priorities for a unit, monitor quality indicators, evaluate monitoring results, and recommend changes in nursing practice. Unit-based committees are participative, decentralizing decision making and accountability for practice and placing it on the level of the staff nurse.

As health care organizations become more attuned to business trends (see Chapter 3), QA activities are being replaced with **quality improvement (QI)** programs. QA activities have often been very crisis focused (Table 10-4). Staff members monitored a specific practice issue such as client education, identified and resolved the problem, and then moved to a new practice issue. This problem-focused approach often missed opportunities for improvement in other areas. For example, a nursing staff choose to monitor success in the clients' ability to explain the purpose of discharge medications. A review of clients for a month indicates that most clients are unable to explain their medications. With a QA approach, nurses offer clients more information to "fix" the problem and then remonitor to see whether there was improvement. With a QI approach, prevention is the focus. In this example, nurses monitor not only the clients' ability to discuss medications, but also the system being used in client education. Monitoring and evaluation are designed to objectively and systematically pursue opportunities for continuous improvement in client's care. Often, this involves participation from various health care departments such as nursing, clinical specialists, and nursing educators.

The JCAHO's "Agenda for Change" has established objectives for health care organizations to develop more comprehensive QA and QI programs (JCAHO, 1987). This will give data to QI participants so that they can evaluate clinical practice and the management of their facilities (Schroeder, 1988). Ultimately an effective QA and QI program will lead to improved clinical practice, better participation by professional staff members, and increased sophistication of evaluation. It will also achieve better outcomes for clients.

Components of a QI Program

A well-organized QI program clearly distinguishes between the measurement and evaluation of quality. The JCAHO's 10 steps to QI (see box) are incorporated within most health care organizations' QI programs. These steps ensure a systematic approach for identifying opportunities to improve quality of health care services and to take appropriate action in resolving problems.

Responsibility for Program

The vice president or director of nursing is usually responsible and accountable for ensuring that nursing service has a QA or QI program. A nurse manager such as a head nurse of a unit or practice area often is responsible for supporting a unit-based program. Individual staff nurses on unit-based committees are responsible for monitoring quality, making decisions about practice, and ensuring that quality care is administered.

Scope of Service

Each nursing unit or practice area is involved in the care of a select group of clients, providing a well-defined set of services to them. An analysis of a unit's scope of service reveals the types of clients who receive nursing care. An example might be an orthopedic unit that cares for young, middle, and older adults undergoing major joint replacements, back surgery, and trauma. An understanding of the scope of service allows nurses to focus on quality issues related to typical client groups.

Key Aspects of Service

The unit-based committee reviews activities or services considered most important in providing quality service to clients. Examples of key aspects of service on the orthopedic unit might include client education, rehabilitation, postoperative monitoring, and administration of blood products. To identify the greatest opportunity for measuring quality, nurses categorize the key aspects of service by high volume, high risk, and problem areas. They are then able to focus on the most important care activities.

Developing Quality Indicators

A **quality indicator** is a quantitative measure of an important aspect of care that determines whether quality of service conforms to requirements. There are three types of indicators: structure, process, and outcome.

Structure indicators evaluate the structure or systems for delivering care. For example, an emergency cart contains all necessary equipment for cardiac resuscitation, or a nurse working in a coronary care unit completes a critical care course. **Process indicators** evaluate the manner in which care is delivered (Williams, 1991). For example, the nurse turns an immobilized client every 2 hours, or the nurse has a postoperative client use an incentive spirometer every 2 hours. **Outcome indicators** evaluate the results of nursing interventions and the effectiveness of care. They represent measurable changes in a client's status related to the receipt of nursing care (Marek, 1989). For example, the client's skin remains intact after bed rest, or the client's lungs are clear on auscultation by the third postoperative day.

Most organizations stress the use of quality indicators for quality monitoring because the indicators focus on the client. Quality is best evaluated when nurses test standards of care for desired outcomes. If a standard of care for maintenance of skin integrity involves a turning schedule and use of special support surfaces, the evaluation of the incidence of skin breakdown will reveal outcomes of care. This should be a natural step for nurses because outcome evaluation is a part of the nursing process.

Establishing Thresholds for Evaluation

After selecting a quality indicator, nurses must determine ways to quantitatively measure the indicator. The occurrence of an indicator, or the percentage of times the indicator is observed (for example, the number of clients who can successively explain self-care instructions compared with the number instructed), are common measures. After the measurement is determined, nurses then establish a threshold that they choose to reach. The **threshold** is a standard for determining whether a problem with quality exists. A measurement that falls below a threshold indicates a problem. For example, nurses may set a threshold of 85% of clients explaining self-care instructions. If the threshold is not met, nurses must thoroughly review the factors interfering with successful client education. When QI is an ongoing process, nurses will continuously work to improve outcomes or performances by raising thresholds.

Data Collection and Analysis

On unit-based committees, nurses monitor criteria for each quality indicator for a predetermined number of clients or cases. Nurses must collect meaningful information that allows accurate analysis of the appropriateness of care. An example of an indicator is the incidence of skin breakdown on all clients who have had total hip replacements. In this case, nurses observe potential pressure areas for skin breakdown. In addition, nurses may monitor the nursing interventions used, age of clients, and their mobility status. Collection of relevant data allows accurate analysis of potential problems with quality and their possible causes.

Evaluation of Care

Using assessment data, nurses evaluate their nursing care. If results exceed or meet the threshold, no problem has been identified. When thresholds for satisfactory care have not been met, nurses must attempt to determine the cause of problems. For example, nurses may set a threshold of 100% of clients having intact skin after total hip procedures. When only 90% of clients meet that goal, nurses must determine the reasons for this. This step requires nurses to honestly review practice activities and look for opportunities to reinforce nursing care standards or improve practice.

Resolution of Problems

After evaluating the success in meeting established quality indicators, nurses develop action plans to resolve any problems. It is important to establish actions that will result in success. For example, the action of merely notifying staff that a problem exists is unlikely to change practice or improve outcomes. An action plan should be more direct. In-service seminars, revision of assessment tools, or creation of standard nursing protocols are examples of specific action steps that nurses can recommend.

Evaluation of Improvement

After implementing an action plan to improve quality of care, nurses must reevaluate the success of the plan. Remonitoring of quality indicators will reveal whether change has occurred. The change may be positive or negative. For example, if the incidence of skin breakdown for clients who have had total hip replacements decreases from previous measures, nurses have successfully improved outcomes. Similarly, if the incidence worsens during the next monitoring period, a new plan of action is needed. As is the case with the nursing process, when desired outcomes (QI criteria) are not met, nurses reinstitute the QI process.

Communication of Results

The results of QI activities must be communicated to nurses and appropriate organizational departments. If findings and results are not communicated, it is unlikely that practice changes will be incorporated by all staff members. Regular discussion of QI activities in staff meetings, distribution of QI newsletters or memos, and a mechanism for QI committee members to personally report to other nurses are examples of communication strategies. Often a QI study reveals information that applies to other units or departments. In this case the organization must be responsible for responding to the problem with quality. Revision of policies and procedures, modification of standards of care, or implementation of system changes are examples of the ways that an organization may respond to quality issues.

The incorporation of a QI program within a health care setting benefits the client, professional staff, and institution. With a focus on client outcomes, QI activities will lead to a selection of interventions that result in improved client care. Professional staff members learn from their own practice, identify opportunities to change practice, and gain greater satisfaction from improved client outcomes. An institution will benefit from an improved level of care delivery that reduces excessive use of resources and improved client satisfaction with services.

 SUMMARY

The evaluation process determines the effectiveness of the nursing care plan, offering nurses the information needed to ensure optimum client outcomes. A systematic process of evaluation requires the nurse to use critical thinking when comparing expected outcomes with actual results. When client goals are achieved, the client has reached an improved level of health. If goals are unmet, the nurse analyzes the cause and reestablishes a more appropriate care plan.

QA and QI are processes that evaluate the quality of nursing care delivered on a unit. Active participation ensures that relevant practice issues are monitored as they influence client outcomes. QI activities provide opportunities for all health care professionals to elevate the level of care delivered to clients.

CHAPTER 10 REVIEW

Key Concepts

- Evaluation determines a client's response to nursing actions and the extent to which goals of care have been met.
- The nurse compares the client's response to nursing actions with expected outcomes established during planning.
- Evaluation may reveal new health care needs.
- Evaluation measures are assessment skills used to collect data for evaluation.
- The nursing care plan is modified based on data obtained during evaluation.
- As a result of evaluation, client priorities may change.
- Expected outcomes are stated in behavioral terms to describe the desired effect of nursing actions.
- Assessment data gathered during evaluation determine the need to revise and modify the care plan.
- Evaluation enables the nurse to determine the reason that the care plan was successful or unsuccessful.
- For nurses to be accountable for their practice, they must know the outcomes of care.
- Evaluation involves critical thinking because the nurse determines the optimal way to deliver nursing care.
- Prevention is the focus for quality improvement activities.
- The three types of quality indicators are structure, process, and outcome.
- After monitoring a quality indicator, professional nurses analyze the findings and establish an action plan when problems are identified.

Key Terms

Evaluation, p. 220

Outcome indicators, p. 228

Process indicators, p. 228

Professional standards review organizations (PSROs), p. 220

Quality assurance (QA), p. 226

Quality improvement (QI), p. 227

Quality indicator, p. 228

Standard of care, p. 224

Structure indicators, p. 228

Threshold, p. 228

Critical Thinking Exercises

1. The nurse enters Mr. Myers room at 8 AM to begin his morning care. Vital signs are scheduled to be measured at this time. After the vital signs are measured the nurse begins the bath and inspects the condition of the client's skin. The night shift reported that Mr. Myers received a pain medication at 7 AM for surgical incision pain. The nurse looks at Mr. Myer's incisional dressing and asks if the pain has been relieved. In this situation, determine which nursing activities are assessment measures and which are evaluation measures. Explain the difference.

2. Mr Ross's care plan includes the goal of "achieving self-care independence by the third day after surgery." How might the nurse evaluate the success in achieving this goal?

3. A nurse's responsibility is to plan for a client's discharge from a health care setting. Other care givers such as social workers and physical therapists participate in a discharge plan. Describe how goals and expected outcomes facilitate discharge planning.

4. As a nurse on a neurological unit you care for a number of clients with parkinsonism, a disorder that causes an unsteady gait, muscle weakness, and muscular rigidity. Over the last month five clients with parkinsonism have fallen. Develop a quality indicator and monitoring criteria to measure this practice problem.

REFERENCES

Hickey PW: *Nursing process handbook,* St Louis, 1991, Mosby.

Joint Commission on Accreditation of Health Care Organizations: Agenda for change, *News from the Joint Commission* 1(1):1, 1987.

Joint Commission on Accreditation of Hospitals: *Accreditation manual for hospitals,* Chicago, 1986, The Commission.

Marek KD: Outcome measurement in nursing, *J Nurs Qual Assur* 4(1):1, 1989.

Schroeder P: Directions and dilemmas in nursing quality assurance, *Nurs Clin North Am* 23(3):657, 1988.

Williams AD: Development and application of clinical indicators for nursing, *J Nurs Care Qual* 6(1):1, 1991.

ADDITIONAL READINGS

Arikian VL et al: Education and QA: a model for continuous improvement in skin integrity, *J Nurs Qual Assur* 5(1):1, 1990.

Anderson PA, Davis SE: Nursing peer review: a developmental process, *Nurs Manage* 18(1):46, 1987.

Beckman JS: What is a standard of practice: *J Nurs Qual Assur* 1(2):1, 1987.

Beyers J: Quality: the banner of the 1980s, *Nurs Clin North Am* 23(3):617, 1988.

Cobb MD: Evaluating medication errors, *J Nurs Adm* 16(4):41, 1986.

Coyne C, Killien M: A system for unit-based monitors of quality of nursing care, *JONA* 17(1)26, 1987.

Crockett D, Sutcliffe S: Staff participation in nursing quality assurance, *Nurs Manage* 17(10):25, 1986.

Davis-Martin S: Outcome and accountability: getting into the consumer dimension, *Nurs Manage* 17(10):25, 1986.

Driever MJ: Interpretation: a critical component of the quality assurance process, *J Nurs Qual Assur* 2(2):55, 1988.

Foglesong D: Standards promote effective production, *Nurs Manage* 18(1):24, 1987.

Given B et al: Relationships of processes of care to patient outcomes, *Nurs Res* 28(2):85, 1979.

Greaves PE, and Loquist RS: Impact evaluation: a competency-based approach, *Nurs Adm Q* 7(3):81, 1983.

Grohar ME, Myers J, McSweeney M: A comparison of patient acuity and nursing resource use, *J Nurs Adm* 16(6):19, 1986.

Hegyvary ST: Issues in outcomes research, *J Nurs Qual Assur* 5(2):1, 1991.

Iyer PW, Taptich BJ, Bernocchi-Losey D: *Nursing process and nursing diagnosis,* Philadelphia, 1986, Saunders.

Kunkle V: Accountability standards balance quality and efficiency, *Nurs Manage* 18(1):34, 1987.

Lillesand KM, Korff S: Nursing process evaluation: a quality assurance tool, *Nurs Adm Q* 7(3):9, 1983.

Lunde KF, Durbin-Lafferty E: Evaluating clinical competency in nursing, *Nurs Manage* 17(8):47, 1986.

Maciorowski LF, Larson E, Keane A: Quality assurance evaluate thyself, *J Nurs Adm* 15(6):38, 1985.

Standards of nursing practice, *Am Nurse* 6:11, 1974.

Marringer A: *The nursing process; a scientific approach to nursing care,* St Louis, 1983, Mosby–Year Book.

Meisenheimer CG: Incorporating JCAH standards into a quality assurance program, *Nurs Adm Q* 7(3):1, 1983.

Peters DA, Pearlson J: Clinical evaluation: research for quality assurance, *J Nurs Qual Assur* 3(3)1, 1989.

Potter PA: An assessment tool for developing quality indicators, *J Nurs Care Qual* 6(1):30, 1991.

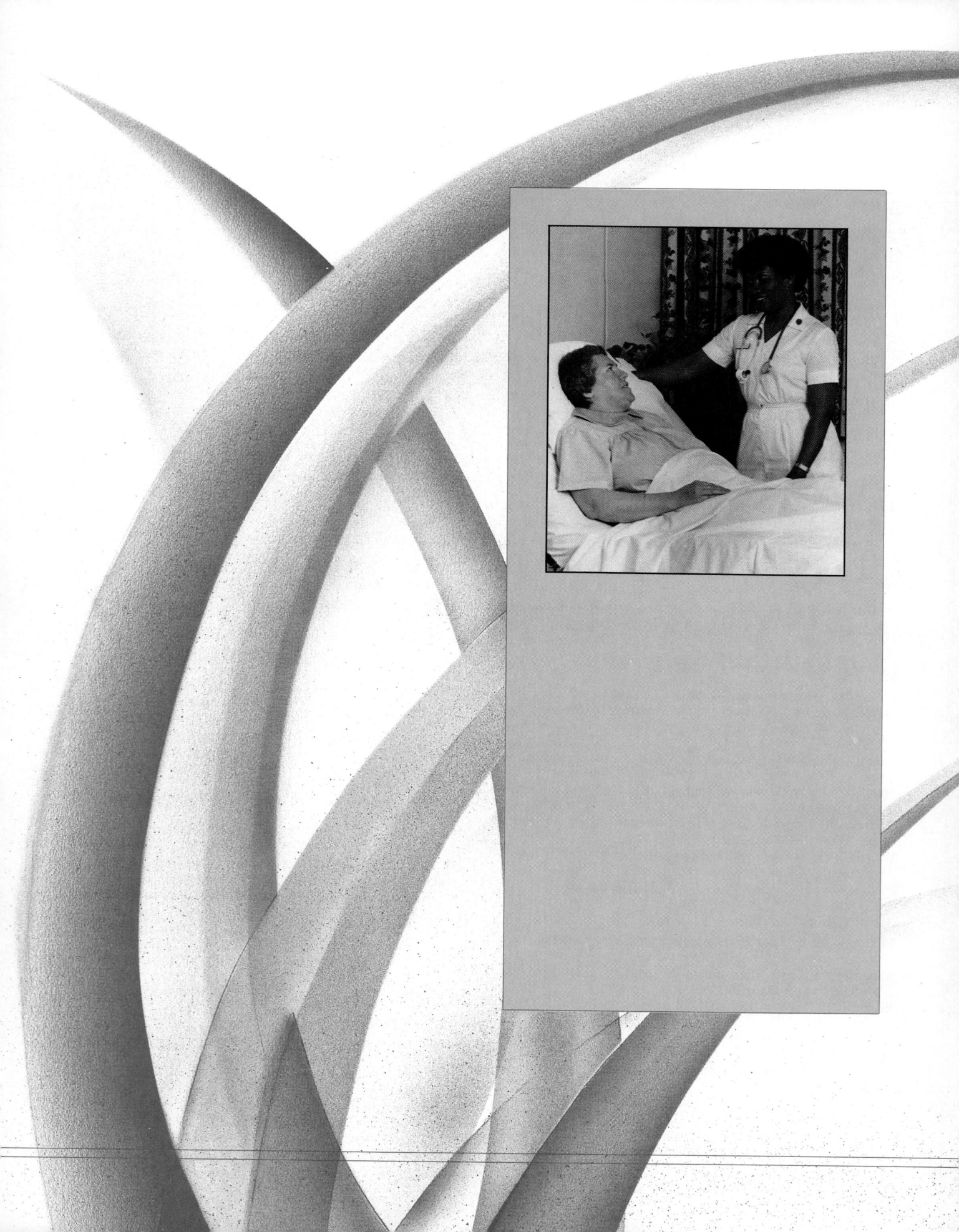

UNIT 3

Professional Nursing Concepts and Practices

CHAPTER **11**

Research

OBJECTIVES

Mastery of content in this chapter will enable the student to:
- Define the key terms listed.
- Compare the various ways to acquire knowledge.
- List the characteristics of scientific investigation.
- Compare methods for developing new nursing knowledge.
- Define scientific and nursing research.
- Compare the research process with the nursing process.
- List ANA's priorities for nursing research.
- Explain the rights of human research subjects.
- Explain the rights of others who assist in human research studies.
- Describe a typical research report.
- Discuss methods of locating research reports in nursing and related areas.
- Explain how to organize information from a research report.
- List the characteristics of a clinical nursing problem that can be researched.
- List the criteria for using research findings in nursing practice.

CHAPTER OUTLINE

Scientific Research in Nursing

Acquiring knowledge
Nursing and the scientific method
Definitions of scientific and nursing research
Nursing research and the nursing process
Nurse researchers

Ethical Issues in Research

Rights of human subjects
Rights of other research participants

Nursing Research in Nursing Practice

Identifying research studies
Locating research studies
Organizing information from a research study
Identifying clinical nursing problems
Using findings in nursing practice

For about 30 years, many nursing leaders and organizations have made considerable efforts to increase nurses' awareness of the importance of conducting nursing studies and using research as a foundation for practice. In 1974 the American Nurses Association (ANA) House of Delegates passed a resolution calling for more nursing research to focus on clinical problems that nurses face in professional practice. Until the 1970s, nursing studies tended to focus on the roles and characteristics of nurses rather than on problems in delivering professional care to clients (Gortner, 1980). In 1981 the ANA published specific recommendations for studying research at the different nursing education levels (ANA, 1981a). A study of nursing by the Institute of Medicine (1983) recommended that the federal government increase funds for scientific research in nursing and that steps be taken to establish a national organization to place nursing research "in the mainstream of scientific investigation." Acting on this recommendation in 1985, the U.S. Congress overrode two presidential vetoes to establish the National Center for Nursing Research under the National Institutes of Health. According to Merritt (1986), this National Center was established

for the purpose of conducting a program of grants and awards supporting nursing research and research training related to patient care, the promotion of health, and the prevention of disease and the mitigation of the effects of acute and chronic illnesses and disabilities.

In 1991 the ANA revised the *Standards of Clinical Nursing Practice.* Within this document are the *Standards of Professional Performance* (see Table 1-5). Standard 7 mandates that the professional nurse use "research finding in practice" (ANA, 1991). Thus the ANA requires nurses to incorporate research findings in clinical practice to restore health, prevent illness, and minimize the effects of acute and chronic disease and disability.

 ## SCIENTIFIC RESEARCH IN NURSING

Acquiring Knowledge

Human beings acquire knowledge in many ways. A person continuously takes in and processes numerous pieces of information to understand experiences. The scientific researcher also seeks to explain or understand reality, but the scientist's process of acquiring knowledge is systematic and logical. This process, or scientific method, is the foundation of research. Scientific research is the most reliable and objective of all methods of gaining knowledge.

One way of learning is by tradition. One generation passes knowledge to the next. For example, children often learn about traditional holidays such as Christmas and Passover through traditional or customary family practices. In nursing, certain traditional methods of practice such as the change-of-shift report and other daily hospital work practices are passed from one practitioner to the next. Tradition is an efficient way of learning, although it can also limit the ability to seek new ways of doing things. If tradition becomes so ingrained that a person does not question the custom, other, more appropriate or efficient ways may be overlooked.

Knowledge is also acquired by seeking information from experts in a particular field. Experts are often asked to solve problems or answer questions. For example, at income tax time an accountant's help is sought to fill out tax forms. Similarly, nursing students often seek the advice of instructors and practicing nurses when assessing and caring for clients. Authority, like tradition, is not infallible, although it is commonly treated as absolute truth.

A person also learns through experience. Without this process, a person would have to relearn a procedure every time it was performed. Practice leads to the development of routines that help build skills. For example, a student nurse taking a blood pressure measurement for the first time may feel awkward and unsure of hearing the sounds, but with pratice the student's technique and confidence improve. Although experience is an important way of learning, it has limitations. A person may continue to do something simply because it was learned that way and may overlook improved or other ways of doing the same thing. If experience causes a person to learn something incorrectly, the person uses knowledge inappropriately.

Learning by trial and error is yet another way of gaining knowledge. Making mistakes or repeatedly trying various ways of accomplishing something will eventually result in problem solving. This method of learning is practical, but it is unsystematic and often a haphazard way of learning. In nursing, because clients' health status depends on nursing actions, trial and error is not an appropriate way of acquiring new knowledge.

The scientific method is the most advanced, objective means of acquiring knowledge. It is characterized by systematic, orderly procedures that, although not without fault, seek to limit the possibility for error and minimize the likelihood that any bias or opinion by the researcher might influence the results of research and thus the knowledge gained. Polit and Hungler (1991) describe the characteristics of scientific investigation as follows:

1. The steps of planning and conducting an investigation are undertaken in a systematic, orderly fashion.
2. Scientists attempt to control external factors that are not under direct investigation but that can influence a relationship between phenomena they are studying. For example, if a scientist were studying the relationship between diet and heart disease, other characteristics such as stress would have to be eliminated as contributing factors to this disease.
3. Evidence that is part of reality (**empirical data**) is gathered directly or indirectly through use of the human senses and is the basis for discovering new knowledge.
4. The goal is to understand phenomena in such a way that the knowledge gained can be applied generally, not just to isolated cases or circumstances.
5. Scientists strive to conduct investigations that contribute to testing or developing theories, thereby advancing the knowledge that can be applied toward increasing understanding of people, places, or life events.

Nursing and the Scientific Method

Compared with other ways of acquiring knowledge, the scientific method is more orderly and objective in its approach. Nurses use this approach to develop knowledge. In the past, much of the information used in nursing practice was borrowed from biology, physiology, psychology, and sociology. Often, this information was applied to nursing without testing or comparing ways for caring for clients. For example, nurses use several methods to help clients sleep. Interventions such as giving a client a backrub, making sure that the bed is clean and comfortable, preparing the environment by dimming the lights, and talking to a worried or anxious client are frequently used nursing measures and, in general, are logical, commonsense approaches. However, when these measures are considered in greater depth, questions may arise about their applications for different clients in different situations.

Research provides a way for nursing questions and problems to be studied in greater depth. Frequently, nurses generally rely on personal experience or the statements of nursing experts. If an intervention works for most clients, the nurse may be satisfied with this success without questioning whether there might be a better way. If the intervention is not successful, the nurse might use an approach practiced by a colleague or try a different sequence of accepted measures. Even if an intervention discovered with this approach is effective for one or more clients, it may not be appropriate for other clients in other settings. Approaches need to be tested to determine the measures that work best with specific clients.

Definitions of Scientific and Nursing Research

According to Kerlinger (1986), **scientific research** is a "systematic, controlled, empirical, and critical investigation of natural phenomena guided by theory and hypotheses about the presumed relations among such phenomena." Several factors affect scientific research. When scientists use systematic, controlled methods for studying events or problems, they have more confidence that the results are accurate and are not influenced by opinion or belief. These studies are well organized and follow a specific procedure. For a study to be empirical, the evidence collected must come from objective findings. In addition, other researchers should be able to examine the evidence and see the same **phenomena** (results). To guide the design of a research study, scientists create a hypothetical proposition (**hypothesis**) about what they expect to see before conducting the study. Finally, scientists generally study the way that characteristics or events are different or the way that one event causes another.

When reading research studies, nurses should avoid interpreting results in terms of cause and effect because there is a difference between cause-and-effect and other kinds of relationships. For example, as people get older, they tend to lose their hair, and their skin becomes wrinkled. These factors are related to each other as part of the aging process, but neither causes the other. Researchers often study such relationships without being able to determine why or how these changes take place.

Biomedical research is concerned mainly with discovering the causes and treatments of disease. In contrast, **nursing research** is directed toward helping well people improve their health status and stay healthy, as well as assisting clients who are sick or disabled by an illness to maintain or improve their health. Nursing also focuses on the full range of human responses, which sometimes do not lend themselves to scientific methodology rather than the biological or physical ones.

The Commission on Nursing Research of the ANA (1981b) has defined nursing research as follows:

Nursing research develops knowledge about health and the promotion of health over the full life span, care of persons with health problems and disabilities, and nursing actions to enhance the ability of individuals to respond effectively to actual or potential health problems.

The International Council of Nurses (1986) supports the need for nursing research as a means for improving the health and welfare of people. Nursing research is a way to identify new knowledge, improve professional education and practice, and use resources effectively.

The effects of preoperative teaching on postoperative recovery is an area that has been studied extensively. Some studies (Schmidt, Wooldridge, 1973; Wolfer, Davis, 1970) have examined the emotional responses (for example, postoperative anxiety and fear) and physiological responses (for example, the return to usual oral intake and urinary retention) of clients to a surgical experience. Teaching clients what they can expect on the day of surgery and in the immediate postoperative period is now a widely accepted and implemented nursing measure. Such teaching often includes, for example, information about when vital signs will be monitored after surgery and the deep breathing and coughing techniques they will be asked to perform. This information is provided to relieve fear and anxiety and to help clients recover from surgery.

Because nurses are interested in acquiring knowledge about a wide range of human needs and responses to health problems, nursing research uses many methods to study clinical problems (see box). The hallmark of scientific research is the **experiment.** In a true experimental study, the conditions under which a measure is investigated are tightly controlled. The study usually includes a control or **comparison group,** which does not receive the nursing measure being investigated. The results for this group are compared with those of a study or **experimental group,** the group that receives some form of treatment or intervention. The **subjects,** persons selected for the comparison and experimental groups, are chosen at random from among those eligible for the study. Designing an experiment to study physical causes of disease is less difficult than designing an experiment that also includes psychological or social aspects of health. For example, to study the relationship between postoperative anxiety and preoperative teaching, the researcher can control one psychological factor by using only subjects having surgery for the first time. However, the researcher cannot control other experiences that the clients may have had, such as hearing a friend's "horror" stories about surgery or reading about surgical experiences in the newspapers. These psychological factors that cannot be controlled may influence the subject's level of anxiety.

Nursing studies use many methods for investigating clinical problems; some may be similar to the experimental approach. Other methods may be similar to those used in the social sciences such as anthropology and sociology. The amount of knowledge known about the problem and the type of problem being investigated are some factors that determine the methods used. Nursing is a practice discipline that deals with unique physical, emotional, and social problems that people experience in regaining, maintaining, and promoting health. Carper (1978) describes the following patterns of knowing in nursing:

1. Empirics: the science of nursing
2. Esthetics: knowledge about the art of nursing
3. Personal knowledge: concrete, experiential knowing
4. Ethics: moral nursing knowledge

Types of Research

HISTORICAL RESEARCH

Systematic collection and critical evaluation of data relating to past events*

EXPLORATORY RESEARCH

Initial study designed to develop or refine research questions or to test and refine data-collection methods*

EVALUATION RESEARCH

Study that tests how well a program, practice, or policy is working

DESCRIPTIVE RESEARCH

Study in which the objective is to accurately identify characteristics of persons, situations, or groups and the frequency with which certain events or characteristics occur

EXPERIMENTAL RESEARCH

Study in which the investigator controls the independent variable and randomly assigns subjects to different conditions

QUASI EXPERIMENTAL RESEARCH

Study in which subjects cannot be randomly assigned to treatment conditions, although the researcher controls the independent variables

CORRELATIONAL RESEARCH

Study that explores the interrelationships among variables of interest without any active intervention by the researcher

*Data from Polit D, Hungler B: *Nursing research: principles and methods,* ed 4, Philadelphia, 1991, Lippincott.

Each pattern represents a necessary but incomplete approach to the problems that nurses face in clinical practice.

Experimental approaches to studying a problem require that the information about human subjects be collected and quantified in a prescribed manner. **Quantitative research** is concerned with information as statistics. **Qualitative research** is concerned with the nature of something. Knowledge collected through qualitative research methods do not involve the statistical organization and interpretation of information; rather it involves the discovery of important characteristics and the way that they might be related. For example, a qualitative research study might involve a survey measuring clients" perceptions of a teaching program. Findings would not prove that one method of teaching is better than another. Yet data would reveal perceived characteristics of the program. When qualitative methods are used, the investigator uses first-hand strategies such as open-ended interviews and case histories to study people under natural conditions as they are dealing with the reality of their health situation. Personal and ethical knowing are particularly relevant when qualitative methods of studying a problem are used.

Nursing Research and the Nursing Process

The research process (Seaman, 1987; Abdellah, Levine, 1986) consists of phases or steps that can be compared and contrasted with those of the nursing process. Both are problem-solving processes used by nurses in practice (Table 11-1), but they are very different. The nursing process is used to determine health needs and plan nursing care for clients. It is used as a basis for gaining and using information about clients to help them restore, maintain, or promote health. Depending on the nursing diagnosis, knowledge from a number of disciplines may be used in the nursing process to help clients solve particular health problems.

In contrast, the **research process** is used to gain knowledge that can be used in other, similar situations. Nurses may want to gain knowledge about the reason a particular event happens or the best way to provide care for clients with a certain health problem. The research process is used to gain knowledge that can be applied to a whole group or class of clients.

During assessment, the nurse caring for a client with sleeping difficulties determines factors that might interfere with the ability to sleep. These may include the client's concern about health status, pain, a noisy environment, or a messy or uncomfortable bed. After assessing these aspects, the nurse for-

TABLE 11-1 Comparison of Phases of the Nursing Process and the Research Process

Nursing Process	Research Process
Assessment	Select the topic and identify the research problem.
	Formulate a summary of the proposed research.
	Review the literature for theory and other related studies.
	Define concepts and variables to be studied.
Nursing diagnosis	State hypotheses about expected observation or questions to be studied.
	Determine ethical implications of the proposed study.
	Identify assumptions and limitations.
Planning	Describe the research design and methods for data collection.
	Define the study population and sample.
	Determine how to process, analyze, and summarize data.
	Plan for communicating findings.
Implementation	Collect data from subjects.
Evaluation	Analyze and interpret data.
	Communicate findings in written and other forms.

Data from Seaman CH, : *Research methods: principles, practice and theory for nursing,* Norwalk, Conn, 1987, Appleton-Century-Crofts; Abdellah FG, Levine E: *Better patient care through nursing research,* ed 3, New York, 1986, Macmillan.

mulates a nursing diagnosis, plans interventions, implements these interventions, and evaluates the subjective and objective evidence that indicates whether the client is able to sleep.

In contrast, a researcher studying sleeping difficulties seeks new information that can be applied to more than one client. For example, a nurse notices that many clients seem to have a difficult time sleeping the night before a particular diagnostic procedure. Based on work with these clients, the nurse determines that most of them express concerns about the results of the test. In this situation the nurse might design a research study in which some of the clients receive the usual nursing care and others receive care based on relieving anxiety. After collecting information about the effects of the usual care for one group and the new approach for the other, the nurse researcher compares the results to determine whether clients who received the new care had less difficulty sleeping than those who received the normal care. If the clients receiving the new care slept better, the nurse has acquired new knowledge about how generally to help clients.

Nurse Researchers

In 1981 the ANA published the following list of priorities for nursing research*:
1. Promoting health, well-being, and competency for personal care among all age groups
2. Preventing health problems throughout the life span that have the potential to reduce productivity and satisfaction
3. Decreasing the negative impact of health problems on coping abilities, productivity, and life satisfaction of individuals and families
4. Ensuring that the care needs of particularly vulnerable groups are met through appropriate strategies
5. Designing and developing health care systems that are cost effective in meeting the nursing needs of the population

In 1985 the Cabinet on Nursing Research of the ANA outlined predictions about consumers of nursing services, health care systems, and nursing for the year 2000 (ANA, 1985a). On the basis of these predictions, priorities for nursing research were further specified (see box).

With these priorities, the profession demonstrates to nurses, other health care professionals, and the general public the areas in which nurses need further knowledge to improve their services. Nurses can use these priorities to guide policy makers and decisions about participation in a research project.

Nurses conduct research in a variety of settings. Student nurses and practitioners may be asked to participate in studies that investigate client outcomes and the effectiveness of nursing care. These types of research projects are commonly called *quality assurance* or *improvement studies* (see Chapter 10). Data are collected to determine the impact that nurses have on achievement of client care objectives in a particular clinical setting. Because the results of such research are usually applicable only in one institution, this is not scientific research as discussed earlier. However, such research is important to the institution because the nursing department can use it to demonstrate the contributions made by nurses to client care. For example, an editorial in the *American Journal of Nursing* (Mallison, 1987) urged nurses to

participate in client outcome studies to determine how staffing levels affect the quality of care. Mallison sees these types of studies as important in light of a growing nursing shortage and the understaffing experienced in many clinical agencies.

Clinical nursing research should be undertaken by nurses trained to conduct scientific investigations.

ANA Nursing Research Priorities

GENERATION OF KNOWLEDGE ENABLING NURSES TO:

- Promote health, well-being, and the ability to care for oneself among all age, social, and cultural groups.
- Minimize and prevent behaviorally and environmentally induced health problems that compromise the quality of life and reduce productivity.
- Minimize the negative effects of new health technologies on the adaptive abilities of individuals and families experiencing acute or chronic health problems.
- Ensure that the care needs of particularly vulnerable groups, such as the elderly, children with congenital health problems, individuals from diverse cultures, the mentally ill, and the poor, are met in effective and acceptable ways.
- Classify nursing practice pheonomena.
- Ensure that principles of ethics guide nursing research.
- Develop instruments to measure nursing outcomes.
- Develop integrative methodologies for the holistic study of human beings as they relate to their families and lifestyles.
- Design and evaluate alternative models for delivering health care and for administering health care systems so that nurses will be able to balance high quality and cost-effectiveness in meeting the nursing needs of identified populations.
- Evaluate the effectiveness of alternative approaches to nursing education for the kind of practice that requires broad knowledge and a wide repertoire of skills, and for the kind of practice that requires specialized knowledge and a focused set of skills.
- Identify and analyze historical and contemporary factors that influence the shaping of nursing professionals' involvement in national health policy development.

From American Nurses Association: *Directions for nursing research: toward the twenty-first century,* Kansas City, Mo, 1985, The Association.

---

*American Nurses Association, Commission on Nursing Research: *Research priorities for the 1980s: generating a scientific basis for nursing practice,* Kansas City, Mo, 1981, The Association.

Generally, nurse researchers hold master's and doctoral degrees. A student nurse asked to participate in a nursing study as a subject or by collecting data is entitled to receive information about the qualifications of the person conducting the study. The researcher's educational background and biographical sketch give some information about the person's qualifications. An experienced researcher is usually more qualified to undertake a complex, long-term project than a beginning researcher. Nurses new to research may, however, make important contributions by assisting with data collection, conducting replicated studies (studies previously performed elsewhere), or by conducting less complex studies.

Nurses with a master's degree in nursing are prepared to collaborate in the design and conduct of research and provide expertise for reviewing studies and integrating studies into practice (ANA, 1989). At the baccalaureate level, nurses are prepared to read research critically and determine the readiness of research for use in practice, promote understanding of ethical research principles, identify clinical problems needing research, and assist experienced investigators in conducting research studies. Nurses with associate degrees are expected to use research findings in practice sometimes under the guidance of nurses prepared at higher levels of education, identify clinical problems needing study, and assist in the conduct of nursing studies.

ETHICAL ISSUES IN RESEARCH

Rights of Human Subjects

To refine existing knowledge and develop new knowledge, clinical research is sometimes directed at trying new procedures whose outcome is doubtful or unknown (ANA, 1975). This kind of research may conflict with the purpose of nursing practice, which is to meet specific clients' needs. In such cases the researcher is responsible for structuring the investigation to avoid or minimize harm to the subjects. Although it is not always possible to anticipate all potential undesirable effects, researchers are obligated to inform everyone involved about the known potential risks. Other basic human rights must also be observed. These principles, as set forth by the Canadian Nurses Association (CNA) (1983), are outlined in the box on p. 242.

Informed consent means that research subjects are (1) given full and complete information about the purpose of the study, procedures, data collection, potential harm and benefits, and alternative methods of treatment; (2) capable of fully understanding the re-

search and the implications of participation; and (3) assured of free choice in giving consent, including the right to withdraw from the study at any time. Procedures for obtaining informed consent must be outlined in the study protocol.

Confidentiality means that the privacy of subjects will be respected. **Anonymity** (refusal to disclose one's name) is often used to ensure privacy and, if promised, must be respected.

In addition, the researcher planning to conduct a study must possess the knowledge and skills necessary to undertake the research. Generally, a nurse planning to conduct a study involving psychiatric clients should be familiar with psychiatric nursing principles and theory. Current ANA (1985b) and CNA (1983) guidelines state that qualified nurse researchers have a right to engage in research and have a right of access to resources needed to conduct studies.

In the United States, any agency receiving federal funds must have an institutional review board (Armiger, 1977). This group reviews all studies conducted in the institution to ensure that ethical principles (see Chapter 13) are observed. Not all research undertaken in clinical areas involves experimentation with human subjects. Research not using a new treatment with subjects may involve minimal or no risk to clients. For example, a survey designed to measure clients' perceptions of stress in intensive care units holds little risk for participants. Nonetheless, a major responsibility of the institutional board is to determine the risk status of all research projects. The nurse's responsibility is to protect the clients' rights at all times.

Rights of Other Research Participants

Student and practicing nurses may be asked to participate in research as data collectors or may be involved in the care of clients participating in a study. All participants, including health care professionals caring for clients, have the right to be fully informed about the study, its procedures (including informed consent and risk factors), and any physical or emotional injury that clients could experience as a result of participation. Often the physical risks are more obvious than emotional risks. Depending on the problem being studied, clients may be asked to give highly personal and intrusive information. Because this type of research can lead to anxiety or stress for some clients, the researcher should prepare all participants, including nurses delivering care, for this possibility and assist them in coping with the effects. Participants also have the right to see review forms from the institutional review board that certify ap-

---

Ethical Guidelines for Conducting Nursing Research with Human Subjects

I. Scientific merit of the research
   A. Study of the problem or question(s) under study must be ethical.
   B. The problem or question(s) must be worthwhile (e.g., significant ones for nursing).
   C. The design and methods of the study must meet established scientific criteria, (e.g., meet reliability and validity criteria, make optimal use of time and resources).
   D. The study must be designed with accepted ethical boundaries.
II. Consent and human subject protection and confidentiality
   A. Informed consent
      1. Information must be provided so that subjects can make an informed and educated decision about participation, including the following:
         a. Nature/purpose of study
         b. Purpose, extent and duration of participation
         c. Type of information that is requested
         d. Use of records
         e. Use of information during and after study
         f. Inconvenience, potential risks, and potential benefits
         g. Standard treatment that may be withheld
         h. Freedom to withdraw at any time without recrimination
         i. How anonymity and confidentiality will be maintained
      2. Persons who are competent to consent must be free to do so without threat that they must participate to maintain benefits (e.g., high-quality care). If not competent to give consent, it must be sought from an individual who can act as an advocate for the noncompetent person.

      3. Verbal or written consent may be obtained, provided ethical considerations are observed. Who consented, under what circumstances, the information provided to subjects, and assurance of the right to withdraw and that no coercion was used must be documented by the investigator.
      4. Other persons affected by the subject's participation must be informed of the study and consent obtained if necessary (e.g., staff nurse, spouse).
   B. Confidentiality
      1. Information must be handled so that confidentiality and anonymity are maintained.
      2. Information may not be used or released outside the terms of the agreement.
   C. Protection of subjects
      1. Subjects must be protected from all types of harm.
      2. Potential benefits must outweigh potential risks.
      3. When the well-being of the subject conflicts with the integrity of the research, a decision must be made that favors the subject.
III. The research setting
   A. The investigator must make a specific request to the agency where the research is to be conducted and provide the agency with the knowledge needed to make an informed consent about approval.
   B. The agency has an obligation to provide a valid system for review.
   C. All nurses have an obligation to collaborate in the research process with the investigator.
   D. Investigators have a responsibility to provide adequate information to the staff members involved in or affected by the study.
   E. Staff members have the right to participate or not, and should be informed if this is a condition of employment in a particular agency.

From Canadian Nurses Association: *Ethical guidelines for nursing research involving human subjects*, Ottawa, 1983, The Association.

---

proval of the study. Any student, nurse, or other participant has the right to refuse to carry out any research procedures if concerned about their ethical aspects.

Besides dealing with the harmful effects of a research project, nurses may be faced with other ethical dilemmas (Brink, Wood, 1988). For example,

some clients may feel they have to participate in an investigation to please the health care professionals on whom they depend for care. They may feel that they will receive inferior care if they refuse to participate. Research ethics require that clients not be made to feel that they are obliged to participate in a study. The ultimate decision rests with the client.

Withholding proper care or in any way implying that care will be withheld from clients who refuse to participate is unethical.

Another ethical dilemma in research involves withholding a new intervention from clients who might benefit from its use. In an experiment investigating a new intervention, for example, the experimental group may receive the new intervention while the comparison group receives the usual care. In such cases, clients in the comparison group are deprived of a new treatment that could be beneficial to them. One way of managing this dilemma is to offer the new nursing care to the comparison group after data necessary to the experimental study have been collected.

 ## NURSING RESEARCH IN NURSING PRACTICE

Identifying Research Studies

When reading nursing literature, the practicing or student nurse must be able to differentiate a research report or article from other types of writing. This may not be as simple as it seems. Even if the title has the word *research* in it, the article does not necessarily report the results of a research study. The nurse can determine whether an article reports a research study only by examining its contents.

Sometimes, however, an article's title can give a clue to its contents. Phrases such as *a study of* or *comparison of* suggest a research report. The abstract and the introductory paragraphs of an article can also indicate whether the article is based on research. An **abstract** is a short summary of the purpose of a study, the subjects included in the research, the way the study was conducted, and the results obtained in the investigation. An abstract is often very brief and does not contain all essential information from the article. The first few paragraphs of the article should provide further clues about whether it describes a research study. Phrases such as *the purpose of this study was* and *this research was carried out to determine* are indications that the article is a research report. If the article describes only the author's experience with a particular aspect of nursing care, it probably is not a research article. In addition to the abstract, a typical research report has the following parts:

1. *Introduction* section: an introductory section presenting the purpose, a summary of literature used to formulate the study, and the hypotheses tested

2. *Methods* section: description of the methods used to conduct the study, including the sample (what or who was studied), and to collect data, including the device or instrument used to measure empirical information

3. *Results* section: description of the results obtained in the study, including statistical tests used to analyze data

4. *Discussion* section: presentation of the author's interpretation of the results, including conclusions and implications that can be drawn from the study

5. *Reference* list (articles used to support the study's methodology)

If the report is written by one of the researchers in the study, it is a **primary source.** Any other article about the study is considered a **secondary source** (for example, an article in which the author was not directly involved in conducting the study but collected the information from a primary or another secondary source). Most nursing textbooks are secondary sources of information. Authors of these texts incorporate knowledge and information gathered from nursing and related literature, including research written by original investigators.

The fact that a report is a primary source does not guarantee its accuracy, which depends on the ability of researchers to be scientific, impersonal, and impartial in conducting studies. However, a primary source does report firsthand knowledge, whereas a secondary source may include another person's interpretation of the original work.

Locating Research Studies

Students and practicing nurses often need to find research articles on subjects that interest them. In the health care field, a number of resources are useful when searching the literature for research articles.

To locate primary research sources related to a particular subject, the first source is the journals where original research reports are usually published. The most efficient way to locate research articles is to consult an index of journal articles. The *Cumulative Index to Nursing and Allied Health Literature (CINAHL)*, published bimonthly, contains listings from over 300 English-language nursing and allied health journals, as well as publications of the ANA and National League for Nursing. The *International Nursing Index*, published four times a year, contains listings from over 200 nursing journals from around the world. *Index Medicus,* an international index published monthly, includes listings from approximately 2900 biomedical journals, including about 60 nursing journals. The *Hospital Literature Index*, published quarterly, contains listings from journals dealing with planning and providing health care programs and services. These indexes are generally found in reference sections of medical and nursing libraries.

These indexes can save time in locating articles. Each index uses a list of key words that form subject headings and subheadings: article listings are grouped or organized under these headings. For example, a person might find subject headings such as *pain* or *primary nursing*, whereas subheadings might include *physiology* or *history* respectively. An author listing is also available, making it possible to find articles published during a certain time period by a particular person. Articles on a particular subject are found by first checking the subject headings to see whether the key term listed in the index matches the subject. The key term listing may also lead to other subject groupings that contain articles similar in content. Using an index may at first seem time consuming, but it saves time because the alternative is looking through many journals trying to find articles pertinent to the subject.

Many nursing and medical libraries provide computerized searches for articles. MEDLINE, a data base available through the Medical Literature Analysis and Retrieval System (MEDLARS), is a system available in many libraries for locating research materials. Information in this system is retrieved from *Index Medicus* and the *International Nursing Index*. In addition, the CINAHL is available as a computerized data base. A list of articles and abstracts is transmitted over telephone lines within hours of being requested. Computer searches generally involve a user's fee. Reference librarians have information about this type of resource.

Nurses having access to microcomputers and modems may subscribe individually to bibliographic services available through a data base vendor. Some of the more popular services include *Knowledge Index* available through DIALOG Information Services, *GRATEFUL MED* available through the National Library of Medicine, and *BRS Colleague* available through W.B. Saunders Co. Most of these vendors charge an initial subscription fee and an hourly fee for time connected to the central computer. There are also charges for telephone time. These services often provide access to data bases in other disciplines (for example, psychology and sociology).

Major nursing journals publishing research studies include *Advances in Nursing Science, Applied Nursing Research, International Journal of Nursing Studies, Nursing Research, Research in Nursing and Health,* and *Western Journal of Nursing Research.* Although not all articles published in these journals are research reports, most issues are devoted to primary reports of nursing studies. Other nursing journals also publish original reports of research studies.

For example, *Heart and Lung,* a specialty journal, often includes research reports. Recently, more specialty practice journals appear to be publishing research articles.

Secondary literature sources such as books can be helpful in finding primary research sources. Nursing students seeking research articles should use reference lists or bibliographies at the end of textbook chapters. To document the scientific basis for their writing, authors frequently cite primary sources as references, and these references are a valuable resource for nursing students who want more information.

Other secondary resources helpful in finding primary nursing research articles are research reviews such as the *Annual Review of Nursing Research* and the *Review of Research in Nursing Education*. Each volume is devoted to certain topics. For example, the 1990 edition of the *Annual Review of Nursing Research* (Fitzpatrick, Tauton, Benoliel, 1990) contains a chapter on cardiovascular research in nursing written by Marie Cowan who is a prominent nurse researcher in this area. A review can help determine the status of research on a topic and can direct the reader toward other primary research sources. Research reviews are relatively new in nursing.

Organizing Information from a Research Study

Articles listed in a bibliography or reference section are called **citations**. A citation provides the author's name and information about where "ideas" or "quotations" were originally published. Writers are ethically obligated to give credit to others whose thoughts are used, even if the original author's exact words are not quoted.

There are many ways to list a citation. The style recommended by the American Psychological Association (1983) is widely used. This format avoids footnotes. All citations are arranged alphabetically at the end of the report. Schools of nursing use many formats, however, and nursing students should ask about the citation format used at their own schools. Listing citations according to the recommended guidelines prevents students from listing incomplete citations.

A book citation includes author names, date of publication, title, edition if appropriate, place of publication, and publisher. Journal citations include author names, date of publication, title of article, name of the journal in which the article appeared, volume and issue numbers, and the exact page numbers of the article. The page numbers of direct quotations should be noted. The order of information in citations, the punctuation used, and the use of underlining and quotation marks depend on the particular citation format.

The use of index cards for recording information helps maintain consistency and accuracy in record keeping. One card is used for notations about each article. Other categories of information should be noted for future use of the research study as a foundation for nursing practice. These categories include *when* the study was conducted, *what* problem area was studied, *how* information and data were collected and compared, *who* was included in the study, *where* the study was conducted (including type of setting and geographical region), a brief summary of the *results* (including major findings and conclusions of the study), and how many *citations* or references were used in the report. Any direct quotation from the report should be noted on the index card with quotation marks and the exact page number on which the quotation appears (see box).

The date of publication gives the approximate time the study was conducted. Sometimes, researchers define the exact time period in the article because a considerable time (as long as 2 years) may pass between the time a study was completed and the time the article was published. Noting when a study was conducted allows the reader to track the development of knowledge in a particular area.

In nursing, many kinds of clinical problems can be studied. The subject of the study provides information about the topics been investigated by nurse researchers. Studies undertaken in a particular problem area can then be collected and evaluated.

There are often many ways to investigate a particular research problem. Knowing the way that researchers studied a question helps students evaluate the thoroughness of the investigation.

A major purpose of scientific research is to increase knowledge about general classes of people or events. Knowledge about the subjects in a research study gives the nurse information about clients to whom the conclusions may be applied. When similar results are obtained with different groups of clients, nurses can be more confident when using the new methods with other clients.

Because nursing care is provided for clients in varying circumstances, the location of research can influence whether the results might apply in a different setting or region. This information is particularly relevant for research involving psychological aspects of nursing care. Different regions of the country have unique traditions and customs. Nursing interventions appropriate for people with certain attitudes and beliefs may not be relevant in regions or settings where attitudes and beliefs differ substantially.

A summary of the results concerns what was demonstrated in a particular problem area. When the

---

Sample Bibliography Card

WHEN

Walike, B.C. and Walike, J.W. (1977). Relative lactose intolerance: A clinical study of tube-fed patients. *Journal of American Medical Association, 238*, 948-951.

WHAT

Lactose intolerance of tube-fed patients

HOW

Consistency, frequency and composition of stools; body weight; selected blood studies, including electrolyte, protein, glucose, cholesterol, total bilirubin, and blood urea nitrogen levels; 24-hour urine studies; glucose tolerance test; lactose tolerance test; symptoms of gastrointestinal distress

WHO

20 white patients between the ages of 46 and 74 receiving both lactose and lactose-free nasogastric tube feedings after head or neck surgery for cancer; 4 patients dropped from the study due to complications unrelated to tube feeding

WHERE

Inpatient hospital clinical research unit (14 patients) in Seattle, Wash, location of 6 patients not stated

RESULTS

Significant differences in stool frequency and consistency were found for patients on tube feeding diets that contained lactose (milk sugar) when compared to how these same patients tolerated lactose-free diets. Nine patients also experienced at least one other symptom of gastrointestinal distress. Lactose intolerance is relative and should be viewed in relation to both increased amount and ability of the intestines to break down milk sugar. "The results indicate that lactose should be reduced or eliminated from tube-feeding diets to improve patient tolerance and comfort and to reduce diarrhea." (p. 948)

CITATIONS

18 references

---

findings and conclusions are similar in a number of research studies, the conclusions are considered more significant than in the case of an isolated research project. The effects of preoperative teaching on the postoperative recovery of clients is an example of a problem area in which collective evidence provides a reasonable scientific foundation for nursing practice.

Many books and journal articles in nursing and related disciplines provide more detailed information about reading and evaluating research studies. Learning to find and read nursing research studies is not a simple task, but nursing research is based on principles of logic, and with a thoughtful approach, the nursing student can learn to understand and evaluate nursing research studies.

Identifying Clinical Nursing Problems

Diers (1979) defined a **clinical nursing problem** as "a difference between two state of affairs, a discrepancy between the way things are and the way they ought to be, or between what one knows and what one needs to know to eliminate the problem." The following questions are raised by this definition:

1. Given the nursing interventions recommended for clients with a particular health care problem, how might the suggested care be improved so that the results or outcomes of care are better?
2. Given the knowledge about how to provide nursing care, what additional information would be needed to plan new interventions for clients with a particular health care problem?

Unanswered questions and the desire to improve nursing practice can provide the stimulus for conducting a research study.

Experience can make it possible to identify a researchable clinical nursing problem, but a nurse does not need to have years of clinical practice to identify a nursing problem. Sometimes a person who is relatively new in a situation can more easily see how things could be improved than those who have more experience and who take present conditions for granted. The nurse also considers whether the problem frequently occurs in a particular client group, whether it can be consistently and accurately measured, and whether a possible nursing solution might change the way care is delivered (Fuller, 1982).

Sometimes nursing students or practicing nurses think their ideas about nursing problems for study are not worthwhile unless they are certain that the proposed clinical study would make a radical change in client care. However, research efforts also may have to refine ideas about a clinical problem before the investigator can test alternative nursing interventions. In fact, some nurse researchers think that more investigative work needs to be done to describe the client response before research is designed to test an alternative intervention. In addition, the researcher may have to devise correct ways for measuring results before the study can proceed. All these factors may discourage a nurse from undertaking a nursing research project. On the other hand, such projects can be viewed as stimulating challenges because much information has yet to be scientifically tested for its relevance to nursing practice.

Studies by Barbara Walike Hansen et al (Walike et al, 1975) illustrate how research can progress from the phase of clinical problem refinement to the testing of new nursing measures. This early study documented the need for further research into tube-feeding procedures and the way clients are affected by this method of meeting nutritional needs. Flynn et al (1987) found that tube-fed patients experience problems similar to those identified by Walike. A number of factors associated with clients' responses to tube feedings have been studied, including tube location for proper formula administration; temperature, volume, and rate of formula administration; attitudes and adjustments of clients toward tube feeding; and responses to the formula contents and other complications. Some of the studies dealing with these aspects of care are outlined in Table 11-2.

Determining the proper insertion length for a nasogastric tube so that it is located properly in the stomach is a topic frequently covered in nursing texts. Hanson (1979, 1980) described an improved method for determining the proper insertion length that increased from 72% to 91% the likelihood that the tube would be properly located in the body or fundus of the stomach. Metheny, Spies, and Eisenberg investigated risk factors associated with tube displacement (1986) and the accuracy of methods used to monitor tube location (1988). Metheny (1988) also reviewed research about testing the placement of nasogastric and nasointestinal feeding tubes at the bedside and concluded that little research exists to support the effectiveness of commonly recommended clinical measures.

The temperature, volume, and rate of administration of tube-feeding formula are regulated and monitored by nurses. The effects of cold, room-temperature, and warm (body-temperature) feedings on gastrointestinal function have been reported by Kagawa-Busby et al (1980), who found that healthy volunteers tolerated room-temperature feedings as well as they did warm formula. Some subjects experienced cramping and diarrhea 6 to 9 hours after receiving cold feedings. Heitkemper et al (1981) found that the volume and rate of administration for volunteer subjects are related to subjective symptoms of gastrointestinal distress; the recommended rate for tube feeding in this study was less than 60 ml/min for the usual volume feeding of 250 ml. When larger volumes (up to 750 ml per feeding) were needed to meet nutritional needs, subjects were able to tolerate them when administered at a rate of 30 ml/min. Six

TABLE 11-2 Summaries of Selected Tube Feeding Studies

Author and Purposes	Subjects and Procedures	Major Findings

GENERAL EXPLORATORY AND DESCRIPTIVE STUDY

Author and Purposes	Subjects and Procedures	Major Findings
*Walike et al (1974): Assess and describe problems associated with tube feeding, develop hypotheses about methods for reducing eliminating problems	121 adults: 48 female, 73 male (ages, 14-90). Survey (145 variables) reviews factors influencing incidence and causes of problems: demographic and health status data; feeding method, diet, intake and output, vital signs; physical and emotional status, drug therapy, attitudes and reactions to diet; blood chemistry; hematological and urine data. Data collection tools were developed by investigators.	Various types and tube sizes were used. Variations in procedure were found for client position during feeding; use of gastric aspiration; rate, temperature and volume of administration; number of feedings per day; and contents of solutions. Adverse responses included diarrhea, gastrointestinal complications, weight loss, and elevated blood urea nitrogen levels. Scant information about attitudes and adjustments to feedings was found.

TUBE LOCATION AND PLACEMENT

Author and Purposes	Subjects and Procedures	Major Findings
*Hanson (1979): Identify noninvasive techniques and criteria for predicting proper length of stomach tube placement and clinical means for determining appropriate tube length	104 adults: 99 cadavers, 5 normal volunteers. Comparison of external body measurements to actual distance from tip of nose to lower esophageal sphincter.	New formula for predicting length was found to accurately predict length 91% of the time, compared with a 72% accuracy rate using traditional nose-to-ear-to-ziphoid measurement.
Metheny, Spies, Eisenberg (1986): Describe frequency with which nurses reported being able to aspirate fluid and measure gastric retention, predict accurate tube placement by client's ability to speak, and predict accurate placement by auscultation of air	Staff nurses supplied data for 20 clients fed by nasogastric tubes (128 tube days) and 55 clients fed by nasointestinal tubes (247 tube days). Data included results of withdrawing 5 ml of fluid, air auscultation, speaking ability and gastric retention.	This study measured the ability to aspirate fluid varied from 79% (large-bore tubes) to 33% (small-bore tubes) and check for gastric retention (90% large and 45% small). All clients could speak. 47% of time, nurses reported hearing epigastric air when tube was located anywhere besides stomach. New methods for checking placement need to be developed, and tubes that will allow proper monitoring need to be identified.

RATE, VOLUME, AND TEMPERATURE OF ADMINISTRATION

Author and Purposes	Subjects and Procedures	Major Findings
*Heitkemper et al (1981): Determine effects of volume and rate of administration of enteral tube feedings on client tolerance and gastric pressure changes	14 healthy volunteers: 9 females, 5 males (ages, 21-35). Studied for 10-12 trials on separate days. Feedings were administered at various volumes and rates after 10 hr of fasting.	Firsttime feedings are more likely to be associated with discomfort, which subside with subsequent feedings. Rate of infusion should be no greater than 60 ml/min. Volume of feeding does not affect sbjective tolerance as long as rate per minute is within suggested guidelines.
*Kagawa-Busby et al (1980): Determine effects of nasogastric feedings at various temperatures on gastric motility, total gastrointestinal transit time and diarrhea, and subjective distress symptoms	6 healthy volunteers: 4 female, 2 male. Nine trials per subject, for a total of 54 at 3 different temperatures for infusion. Rate was 50 ml/min for all administrations.	All three temperatures resulted in similar gastric motility pattern after feeding. All showed similar decrease in gastric contraction and return of gastric activity during and after feeding. Two subjects reported diarrhea after cold feedings; no gastrointestinal disturbances were found after warm feeding.

---

*Tube Feeding Consortium Group study.

Continued.

TABLE 11-2 Summaries of Selected Tube Feeding Studies — cont'd

Author and Purposes	Subjects and Procedures	Major Findings
ATTITUDES AND ADJUSTMENTS		
*Padilla et al (1979): Determine type, incidence and subjective level of distress experienced by clients experiencing tube feedings	30 alert adult clients. Interviewed via 47-item tube-feeding and hospital experience checklist, tool developed by investigators to measure distress associated with tube feedings and hospitalization.	Clients identified sore nose or throat, having nothing by mouth, limited mobility, and dry mouth and runny nose as some uncomfortable aspects of having feeding tube. Interventions to reduce unpleasant experiences were identified by health care professionals familiar with these problems
FORMULA CONTENTS AND/OR COMPLICATIONS		
Cataldi-Betcher et al (1983): Evaluate incidence of complications for patients receiving enteral nutrition support	253 subjects: 53% male (mean age 62.8), 47% female (mean age, 63.8). Standardized protocols for enteral feedings were followed by majority of physicians ordering enteral feedings. Most clients had weighted nasogastric tubes. 30 (11.7%) experienced gastrointestinal (6.2%), mechanical (3.5%), or metabolic (2%) complications.	For clients with functioning gastrointestinal tract, enteral feedings are preferred method of support. Diarrhea is most frequent complication; cause is multifactorial. Correct tube selection is important to prevent mechanical-complications; small- and large-bore tubes have strengths and limitations. Metabolic complications are often less severe than those associated with parenteral nutrition. Recommendations for preventing all complications were discussed.
Taylor (1982): Compare incidence of diarrhea and/or aspiration pneumonia in neurosurgical clients receiving continuous versus intermittent infusion tube feedings	13 clients (5 on intermittent, 7 on continuous, and 1 on both) (ages, 19 to 64). Investigator developed instruments to measure vital signs, relevant laboratory data, medications, and incidence of diarrhea and/or aspiration.	Descriptive study documented that diarrhea and aspiration occur with continuous and intermittent feedings. Procedure used in both protocols may reduce incidence of apiration. Further research needs to be done on use of tube feedings with clients with neurological problems.
*Walike and Walike (1973): Determine the proportion of diarrhea that could be accounted for in clients by lactose content of diet and other factors that contribute to remaining gastrointestinal symptoms.	11 clients (9 males, 2 females) studied for a mean of 9.4 days on lactose and lactose-free nasogastric diets. Data collected included relevant laboratory data, frequency and consistency of stools, and lactose tolerance tests.	Lactose content of diets commonly used for patients fed by nasogastric tube is major cause of diarrhea. Intolerance to lactose cannot be determined by traditional test with patients. Relative lactose intolerance may be present in majority of adults; this becomes important when size of lactose load is beyond client's ability to hydrolyze it. Elimination of lactose from tube feeding diets will reduce gastrointestinal side effects.
*Walike and Walike (1977)	(See box on p. 245 for summary of results.)	

of the fourteen subjects experienced nausea or abdominal discomfort with the first feeding. Tolerance improved with subsequent formula administrations.

Other studies investigated the distressful objective and subjective symptoms experienced by clients. The first study (Padilla et al, 1979) described the psychosensory irritations and deprivations commonly experienced by 30 clients. Sensory irritations included dry mouth, sore throat, and thirst. Deprivation of taste when chewing and swallowing food were reported by these clients. A follow-up study (Padilla et al, 1981) explored the effects of four different ways of providing information to clients about tube-feeding procedures to reduce distress. The teaching intervention most effective for subjects in this study provided sensory information about the procedure and coping behaviors to increase comfort during and after tube insertion. In addition, clients who perceived that they had control over their environment and behavior did not express less distress than clients perceived that they had no control.

Results of the Walike and Walike study (1977) dealing with the effects of lactose (milk sugar) on stool frequency and consistency are shown in the box. As a result of this research, commercially prepared tube-feeding formulas that do not contain lactose are now available. One problem in this study was the difficulty experienced by the researcher in finding a reliable and uniform way to measure stool consistency (Hansen, 1984). The investigators found that the nurses used "very creative and imaginative descriptions" to describe the characteristics of stool, and these descriptions differed among nurses participating in data collection. A stool consistency diagram (Fig. 11-1) was developed to group descriptions into nine categories. The actual water content of stools in each category was analyzed to confirm these categories objectively. At the time of the study, only one rating form for stool consistency of meconium (material in a newborn's stool) existed in the research literature. The experience of these investigators in having to develop a reliable, valid way of measuring a human phenomenon is common among nursing researchers. Much of nursing practice deals with identifying and describing human responses to health care problems that are insufficiently defined and classified to permit general agreement about observations. Other studies dealing with complications associated with tube feedings are outlined in Table 11-2.

These articles represent a sample of tube-feeding research. Through collaborative efforts, the Tube Feeding Consortium Group (Bergstrom et al, 1984) was able to study a large number of subjects in many locations to make the findings more generalized. The clinical nursing problems addressed in these studies

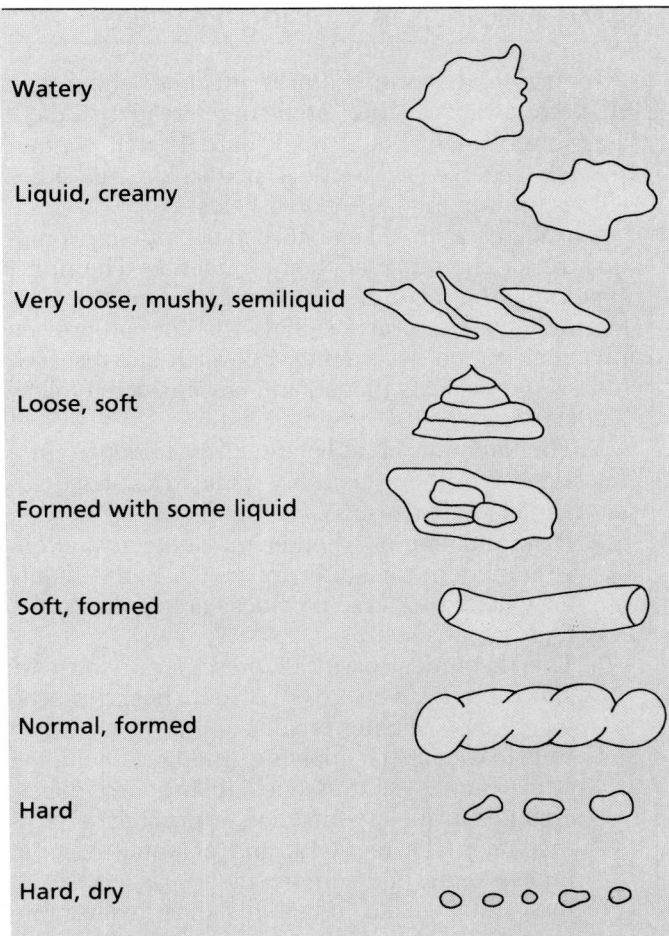

Watery

Liquid, creamy

Very loose, mushy, semiliquid

Loose, soft

Formed with some liquid

Soft, formed

Normal, formed

Hard

Hard, dry

Fig. 11-1   Stool consistency diagram.

involve aspects of care with which nurses must deal in everyday practice. Client safety might be improved, for example, if the new method for determining length of inserting a feeding tube were widely used in professional nursing practice. The problem of diarrhea in clients receiving tube feedings can be minimized by changing the contents of the formula. This has been a significant nursing problem, especially with clients who are immobilized or who have decreased levels of consciousness. The scientific foundation on which decisions about the nursing care of such clients can be based has been strengthened by the work of researchers who are investigating tube feeding. These studies originated in questions about procedures for and clients' responses to a common nursing measure. The results of these studies did not lead to the invention of a completely new nursing intervention, but a substantial scientific basis has been established for improving nursing care for clients.

Using Findings in Nursing Practice

To use findings in clinical practice, the nurse must be aware of the problems already studied. Therefore nurses should read journals that contain research reports, as well as textbooks and other sources, in nursing and related fields.

Not all research related to clinical nursing problems can or should be applied in practice. The nurse must judge the scientific worth of a study before considering its use in practice. This chapter can provide only a foundation for judging the worth of a research study. Other aspects that should be considered follow (Stetler, Marram, 1976; Stetler, 1985):

1. The amount of substantiating evidence provided by other scientific studies that have obtained similar results
2. Determination of whether the subjects and environment in the study are similar to the clients for whom the nurse provides care in the particular practice setting
3. The theoretical basis for present nursing care and the effectiveness of current theory in solving clinical nursing problems
4. The feasibility of applying findings, including ethical and legal limitations, institutional policy, changes in the organization of nursing services that might be required, and potential costs in time, money, and equipment

The nurse must make judgments that involve validating the scientific soundness of a study, comparatively evaluating whether any use can be made of the findings, and deciding type of application that would be appropriate (Stetler, 1985).

Haller, Reynolds, and Horsley (1979) note that **research utilization** (using research findings in day-to-day practice) begins with the identification of a clinical nursing problem that has been investigated through conceptually related studies; the results of these studies can be used in clnical practice. The problem area chosen must have an establisehd research base, be relevant to practice, and be reliably evluated by nurses in clinical settings. When selecting the problem area, the nurse is concerned with whether a solid research base exists for changing practice, the scientific merit of the studies that constitute the research base, and the potential risk to the client in implementing the practice change. The final phases include developing a clinical protocol that can be used to implement the change and clinically evaluating the outcomes of the new nursing care to determine its effectiveness.

Nurses often participate in quality assurance (QA) or quality improvement (QI) studies that evaluate the processes and outcomes (results) of nursing care (see Chapter 10). These studies measure how well nursing interventions are being implemented with specific clients by examining expected outcomes related to the nursing process protocols and procedures of a specific setting. Some questions about nursing care provided for tube-fed clients that might be examined in a QA study include the following:

1. Regarding tube obstruction, how frequently do tubes becomes obstructed and need replacement? What are the causes of the obstruction?

2. Related to tube placement and respiratory complications, are the methods being used to check placement correctly determining tube position? How frequently do clients with poor cough or gag reflex experience tube malposition and pulmonary complications?

3. Regarding gastrointestinal complications, how frequently are clients experiencing diarrhea, and what are the etiologies among the clients studied?

The knowledge base developed by investigators (see Table 11-2) provides a means for examining nursing measures and outcomes. Kohn and Keithley (1989) suggest research-based nursing interventions that can be implemented to minimize these complications. By examining the quality of care provided for clients in their own setting and changing care as needed based on knowledge developed in studies, nurses can use resesarch to improve the quality of care.

Nurses should not change from accepted to unproven ways of providing client care without careful deliberation and consultation with colleagues. Experimenting with new nursing measures is inappropriate, especially if an increased risk to the clients' health is possible.

Some people estimate that the half-life of knowledge in the health care field is about 5 years. This means that half of what nurses learn today may be out of date in 5 years. By developing skills necessary to read and understand nursing research studies, nurses can remain current throughout their careers.

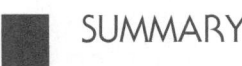 ## SUMMARY

Research is an essential part of the nursing process because it is an advanced, objective method of gaining new knowledge about human needs and people's responses to illness, treatments, therapies, and other health-related factors. The research process, a problem-solving method, involves a number of phases from the identification of a problem to the development and testing of hypotheses to the analysis, interpretation, and communication of findings. To gain new knowledge in a variety of nursing areas, nurses conduct clinical research in many settings, involving many kinds of research subjects whose rights must carefully be protected.

Nurses indirectly involved in conducting research also gain from nursing research findings. Nurses therefore must develop skills for locating and identifying research studies and for organizing research information for clinical application. The successful use of research findings in practice depends on the skills of the nurse to judge the scientific worth of a study, determine whether findings can be applied to a particular clinical setting and group of clients, and consider other practical issues such as ethical implications, institutional policies, and implementation costs. These skills are important for all nurses because of the continuously evolving nursing knowledge base needed to practice professional nursing in all settings.

CHAPTER 11 REVIEW

Key Concepts

- People acquire knowledge through tradition, from authorities in a field, through experience, by trial and error, and through application of the scientific method.
- The scientific method is the most objective method of gaining new knowledge.
- A scientific investigation is an orderly, planned, and controlled way of studying reality that can be applied to general situations and contributes to the testing of theories about people, places, or life events.
- Nursing research is conducted to study the physical or psychosocial responses of people of all ages in health and illness.
- An experimental research study controls factors that could influence the results, includes comparison and experimental treatment groups of subjects, and uses random means for selecting study subjects.
- A qualitative research study organizes information in narrative format so that phenomena can be described and patterns of relationships can be discovered.
- Participation of human subjects in research studies requires the researcher to obtain informed consent of study subjects, maintain the confidentiality of subjects, and protect subjects from undue risk or injury.
- The researcher conducting a study is required to inform all persons assisting in the study about the purposes of the research and to prepare them for any adverse effects the subjects could experience.
- Research reports are most commonly found in specialized journals.
- A number of indexes for the health care field are available for finding research articles.
- When sumamrizing data reported in a research study, the nurse should note when, how, where, and by whom the investigation was conducted and who and what was studied.
- A researchable clinical nursing problem is one that is not satisfactorily resolved by present nursing interventions, occurs frequently in a particular group, can be consistently and accurately measured, and has a possible solution within the realm of nursing practice.
- To determine whether research findings can be used as a basis for nursing practice, the nurse should consider the scientific worth of the study, the substantiating evidence provided in other studies, the similarity of the research setting to the nurse's own clinical practice setting, the status of current nursing theory, and factors affecting the feasibility of application.

Key Terms

Abstract, p. 243
Anonymity, p. 241
Biomedical research, p. 237
Citations, p. 244
Clinical nursing problem, p. 246
Comparison group, p. 238
Confidentiality, p. 241
Empirical data, p. 237
Experiment, p. 238
Experimental group, p. 238
Hypothesis, p. 237

Nursing research, p. 237
Phenomena, p. 237
Primary source, p. 243
Qualitative research, p. 239
Quantitative research, p. 239
Research process, p. 239
Research utilization, p. 250
Scientific research, p. 237
Secondary source, p. 243
Subjects, p. 238

Critical Thinking Exercises

1. The nurse is concerned about learning to properly clean a pressure ulcer. Explain the benefits to the client if the nurse learns how to clean the sore by the scientific method versus trial and error.

2. If you wished to determine the best method for cleaning a pressure ulcer, what type of research method would you use for study?

3. The nurses working on an orthopedic unit decided to study the factors that commonly result in client falls on their unit. Explain why this QI study is not scientific research. How could it be made into a scientific research study?

4. If you were participating in a study that tested a new drug, what do you believe should be included in a client's informed consent?

REFERENCES

Abdellah FG, Levine E: *Better patient care through nursing research*, ed 3, New York, 1986, Macmillan.

American Nurses Association: *Human rights guidelines for nurses in clinical and other research*, Kansas City, Mo, 1975, The Association.

American Nurses Association, Commision on Nursing Research: *Guidelines for the investigative function of nurses*, Kansas City, Mo, 1981a, The Association.

American Nurses Association, Commission on Nursing Research: *Research priorities for the 1980s: generating a scientific basis for nursing practice*, Kansas City, Mo, 1981b, The Association.

American Nurses Association: *Directions for nursing research: toward the twenty-first century*, Kansas City, Mo, 1985a, The Association.

American Nurses Association: *Human rights guidelines for nurses in clinical and other research*, Kansas City, Mo, 1985b, The Association.

American Nurses Association: *Education for participating in nursing research*, Kansas City, Mo, 1989, The Association.

American Nurses Association: *Standards of clinical practice*, Washington, DC, 1991, The Association.

American Psychological Association: *Publication manual of the American Psychological Association*, ed 3, Washington DC, 1983, The Association.

Armiger B: Ethics of nursing research: profile, principles, perspective, *Nurs Res* 26:330, 1977.

Bergstrom N et al: Collaborative nursing research: anatomy of a successful consortium, *Nurs Res* 33:20, 1984.

Brink PJ, Wood MJ: *Basic steps in planning nursing research: from question to proposal*, ed 3, North Scituate, Mass, 1988, Duxbury Press.

Canadian Nurses Association: *Ethical guidelines for nursing research involving human subjects*, Ottawa, 1983, The Association.

Carper BA: Fundamental patterns of knowing in nursing, *ANS* 1:13, 1978.

American Nurses Association, Commission on Nursing Research: *Guidelines for the investigative function of nurses*, Kansas City, Mo, 1981a, The Association.

Diers D: *Research in nursing practice*, Philadelphia, 1979, Lippincott.

Fitzpatrick JJ, Tauton RL, Benoliel JQ: *Annual review of nursing research*, vol 8, New York, 1990, Springer.

Flynn KT et al: Enteral tube feedings: indications, practices and outcomes, *Image* 19:16, 1987.

Fuller ED: Selecting a clinical nursing problem, *Image* 14:60, 1982.

Gortner SR: Nursing research: out of the past and into the future, *Nurs Ress* 29:204, 1980.

Haller KB, Reynolds MA, Horsley, JA: Developing research-based innovation protocols: process, criteria, and issues, *Res Nurs Health* 2:45, 1979.

Hansen BW: Personal communication, Feb 14, 1984.

Hanson RL: New approach to measuring adult nasogastric tubes for insertion, *Am J Nurs* 80:1334, 1980.

Hanson RL: Predictive criteria for length of nasogastric tube insertion for tube feeding, *J Parenter Enter Nutr* 3:160, 1979.

Heitkemper ME et al: Rate and volume of intermittent enteral feeding, *J Parenter Enter Nutr* 5:125, 1981.

Institute of Medicine, Division of Health Care Services: *Nursing and nursing education: public policies and private actions*, Washington DC, 1983, National Academy Press.

International Council of Nurses: *Nursing research: ICN position statement*, Geneva, 1986, The Council.

Kagawa-Busby KS et al: Effects of diet temperature on tolerance of enteral feedings, *Nurs Res* 29:276, 1980.

Kerlinger FN: *Foundations of behavioral research*, ed 3, New York, 1986, Holt, Rinehart & Winston.

Kohn CL, Keithley JK: Enteral nutrition: potential complications and patient monitoring, *Nurs Clin North Am* 24:330, 1989.

Mallison MB: The shortage that destroys, *Am J Nurs* 87:899, 1987.

Merritt DH: The National Center for Nursing Research, *Image* 18:84, 1986.

Metheny N: Measures to test placement of nasogastric and nasointestinal feeing tubes: a review, *Nurs Res* 37:324, 1988.

Metheny NA, Spies MA, Eisenberg P: Frequency of nasoenteral tube displacement and associated risk factors, *Res Nurs Health* 9:241, 1986.

Metheny NA, Spies MA, Eisenberg P: Measures to test placement of nasoenteral feeding tubes, *West J Nurs Res* 10:367, 1988.

Padilla GV et al: Subjective distresses of nasogastric tube feeding, *J Parenter Enter Nutr* 3:53, 1979.

Padilla GV et al: Distress reduction and the effects of preparatory teaching films and patient control, *Res Nurs Health* 4:375, 1981.

Polit DV, Hungler BP: Nursing research: principles and practice, ed 4, Philadelphia, 1991, Lippincott.

Schmidt FE, Woolridge PJ: Psychological preparation of surgical patients, *Nurs Res* 22:108, 1973.

Seaman CH: *Research methods: principles, practice and theory for nursing,* Norwalk, Conn, 1987, Appleton-Century-Crofts.

Stetler C: Research utilization: defining the concept, *Image* 17:40, 1985.

Stetler CB, Marram G: Evaluating research findings for applicability in practice, *Nurs Outlook* 25:559, 1976.

Walike BC, Walike JW: Relative lactose intolerance: a clinical study of tube-fed patients, *JAMA* 238:948, 1977.

Walike BC et al: Patient problems related to tube feeding. In Batey MV, editor: *Communicating nursing research,* vol 7, Boulder, Colo, 1975, Western Interstate Commission for Higher Education.

Wolfer JA, Davis CE: Assessment of surgical patients: preoperative emotional condition and postoperative welfare, *Nurs Res* 19:402, 1970.

ADDITIONAL READINGS

American Nurses Association, Cabinet on Nursing Research: *Establishment of a National Institute of Nursing: a statement of rationale (mimeographed),* Kansas City, Mo, 1983, The Association.

Binger JL, Jensen LM: *Lippincott's guide to nursing literature: a handbook for students, writers, and researchers,* Philadelphia, 1980, Lippincott.

Byers PH, Wiggins CL, Morelli, CC: Effect of enteral alimentation and antibiotic usage on diarrhea, *Nut Supl Serv* 8:14, 1988.

Cataldi-Betcher EL et al: Complications occurring during enteral nutrition support: a prospective study, *J Parenter Enter Nutr* 7:546, 1983.

Edes TE, Wlk BE, Austin JL: Diarrhea in tube-fed patients: feeding formula not necessarily the cause, *Am J Med* 88:91, 1990.

Eisenberg P, Metheny N, McSweeney M: Nasoenteral feeding tube properties and the ability to withdraw fluid via syringe, *Appl Nurs Res* 2:168-172, 1989.

Eisenberg P et al: Characteristics of patients who remove their nasal feeding tube, *Clin Nurse Spec* 1:94, 1987.

Fox DA: *Fundamentals of research in nursing,* Norwalk, Conn, 1983, Appleton-Century-Crofts.

Hermann ME et al: Subjective distress during continuous enteral alimentation: superiority of silicone rubber to polyurethane, *J Parenter Enter Nutr* 13:281, 1989.

Horsley JA, Crane J, Haller KB: *Reducing diarrhea in tube-fed patients: CURN project,* New York, 1981, Grune & Stratton.

Keohane PP et al: Relation between osmolality of diet and gastrointestinal side effects in enteral nutrition, *Br Med J* 288:678, 1984.

Metheny N, Eisenberg P, McSweeney M: Effect of feeding tube properties and three irrigants on clogging rates, *Nurs Res* 37:165, 1988.

Metheny NA, Eisenberg P, Spies MA: Aspiration pneumonia in patients fed through nasoenteral tubes, *Heart Lung,* 15:256, 1986.

Metheny N et al: Effectiveness of pH measurements in predicting feeding tube placement, *Nurs Res* 38:280, 1989.

Metheny N et al: Effectiveness of the auscultatory method in predicting feeding tube location, *Nurs Res* 39:262, 1990.

Sarter B: *Paths to knowledge: innovative research methods for nursing,* New York, 1988, National League for Nursing.

Smith CE et al: Diarrhea associated with tube feeding in mechanically ventilated, critically ill patients, *Nurs Res* 39:148, 1990.

Taylor TT: A comparison of two methods of nasogastric tube feedings, *J Neurosurg Nurs* 14:49, 1982.

Trussell P, Brandt A, Kanpp S: *Using nursing research: discovery, analysis, and interpretation,* Wakefield, Mass, 1981, Nursing Resources.

Walike BC, Walike JW: Lactose content of tube feeding diets as a cause of diarrhea, *Laryngoscope* 83:1109, 1973.

Werley HH, Fitzpatrick J: *Annual review of nursing research,* vol 4, New York, 1986, Springer.

Williams KR: Effect of the temperature of tube feeding on gastric motility in monkeys, *Nurs Res* 24:4, 1975.

Wilson HS: *Research in nursing care,* ed 2, Redwood City, Calif, 1989, Addison-Wesley.

Woods NF, Catanzaro M: *Nursing research: theory and practice,* St Louis, 1987, Mosby–Year Book.

CHAPTER 12

Values

CHAPTER OUTLINE

Nurses are concerned with each client's basic human needs (see Chapter 29) and the ultimate well-being of the client. While performing the "work" of nursing, professional nurses are faced with a variety of decisions about a client's care and whether the client's well-being can be assured as a result of that care. In clinical practice, nurses act as interfaces between the client and physician (Stenberg, 1979). There is an expectation that nurses thus play a key role in making decisions about therapies that will lead to the best outcomes. Nurses control and are accountable for independent nursing interventions. Interdependent interventions are initiated after collaboration between the nurse and some other care giver. The nurse makes decisions that often influence the way that such interventions are delivered. In the case of medical interventions prescribed by physicians, nurses implement therapies chosen by others and are accountable for implementing these therapies correctly. Nurses must judge the appropriateness of any therapy; however, in the case of dependent therapies the physician is the primary decision maker.

Facing decisions with a clear perspective and purpose is no simple task. Every day brings situations that require thought, critical decision making, and action. Frequently the person deciding is confused over the many options involved in a decision, including the way a decision is made, persons affected by it, and its implications. Decisions are based in part on a person's conscious or unconscious values. A **value** is a personal belief about the worth of a given idea or behavior upon which a person acts. Values are standards that influence behavior. An individual's needs, the culture and society in which a person lives, and the significant others to whom the individual relates are a reflection of personal values. Values vary from person to person, developing and changing as a person grows and matures.

A value is not the same as an attitude. An **attitude** is a feeling toward a person, object, or idea (Steele, 1986). A person's attitudes are relatively constant. With any attitude a person evaluates whether the person, object, or idea is good or bad, positive or negative. A person may have an attitude about certain ideas without valuing them. Values have a strong motivational component that directs conduct. Attitudes can also influence behavior. However, values are the beliefs that a person acts on and thus become the standards for guiding actions, developing and maintaining attitudes toward relevant objects, morally judging self and others, and comparing self and others (Rokeach, 1973).

Nurses practice under a personal and professional set of values. As persons, nurses have the right to express and act on their values (Bernal, 1985). Each client also has a value system of unique personal needs and preferences. Many values that nurses hold (for example, beliefs in the importance of human dignity, independence, or positive human relationships) can influence a client's care. Conflict between nurses' and clients' values may lead to ethical dilemmas (see Chapter 13). Nurses must understand their own values and those of their clients. Nurses try to minimize the effect of personal values on the client's recovery. For example, a nurse may personally value the importance of the family in providing support regarding decisions. If a client fails to hold the same value, a nurse may inappropriately try to persuade the client to pursue family involvement in care decisions. A systematic analysis of value systems helps nurses to act in a more professional and knowledgeable way.

The threats posed by illness cause individuals to reassess their health-related values. The frequency and intensity with which people practice health-promoting behaviors depend on the value placed on reducing the threat of illness and promoting health. The nurse helps clients clarify personal values, reorder value priorities, minimize conflict, and achieve consistency among values and behaviors related to illness prevention and health promotion. The nurse helps clients understand themselves and the impact of certain behaviors on their well-being.

 ## NATURE AND FUNCTION OF VALUES

The values a person chooses to exercise are a part of that person's identity. Values represent a way of life. They are expressed as behaviors that a person tries to maintain (Omery, 1989). Rokeach (1973) has observed that the total number of values a person possesses is relatively small and that values are organized into value systems. The values that influence behavior may be conscious or unconscious. An individual may express values openly or demonstrate them through verbal and nonverbal behaviors.

There are only a few values (for example, friendship, quality of health, religious freedom, or material gain) that a person consciously acknowledges as important and most significant in influencing life. Only a few values consistently and predictably have an impact on behavior. No two individuals give equal importance to the same values. The values that hold the greatest importance in shaping thoughts and actions are a part of a person's unique identity.

Values related to one another form a **value system.** Examples of value systems are those related to religion and health. Rokeach (1973) describes value systems as learned principles and rules to allow choice and guide decisions. Zuzich (1978) described the internalized value system that a person uses repeatedly in making judgments as standards of conduct. A person's values about health determines the choices made about health promotion and the use of health care resources during a time of illness. For example, eating a balanced diet, exercising, and seeking early medical attention during illness are the result of a person's value of health. The behaviors that a person assumes as a result of personal values should be realistic. A young man with severe heart disease cannot set unrealistic expectations for the maintenance of physical strength and endurance, for example. A realistic value system allows the person to be flexible and attain greater satisfaction from the attitudes, behaviors, and feelings influenced by personal values.

Values may be classified as intrinsic or extrinsic (Steele, 1986). Intrinsic values are related to the maintenance of life such as the value of food or love. Values categorized as extrinsic originate from outside a person and are not essential to the maintenance of life. For example, values associated with the choice of an occupation are extrinsic. Some values appear less important than others, depending on the type of choices a person must make or the priority of the values held.

A person's perceptions of other individuals are influenced by personal values. When meeting someone for the first time, for example, a person notes the other person's behavior. Values direct a person's responses toward another. The nurse who grasps the outstretched hand of a dying client values caring and compassion. The client knows this by the nurse's actions: speaking softly, offering comfort measures, or staying at the client's side. The nurse may perceive the dying client's value of being able to maintain courage during a time of suffering. The client expresses a need to stay strong in the presence of family members. The nurse respects the client's values by making the client as comfortable as possible and having basic needs met before family members visit. Values shape reactions to others and form a basis for evaluating human interaction and relationships.

 FORMATION OF VALUES

Values are learned through observation and experience. An individual observes not only behavior but also the setting in which it occurs and the response it creates. For example, a beginning nursing student closely observes a clinical instructor's actions at the client's bedside and the client's reactions. If the client remains relaxed and accepting as the instructor administers care, the student learns to value being a competent and caring nurse. The instructor's competence and caring as a professional nurse are incorporated into the student's value system.

Values are also acquired through experience. After repeatedly experiencing the same situations, a person looks back on personal successes and failures to determine what behaviors led to the desirable effects and how other people responded to those behaviors. The nursing student who receives an instructor's praise after performing a task well will probably continue to value high standards of achievement. Repeated reinforcement results in the student becoming a skilled clinician.

Brill (1973) has summarized the following manner in which values are learned or acquired:

1. A particular circumstance demands a reaction from an individual.
2. The individual responds on a trial-and-error basis or on the basis of principle.
3. The individual selects an effective response.
4. The individual comes to believe that this is the "right" response because it works for him or her.
5. The individual believes that people who respond differently in the same situation are "wrong."

People learn values by observing and interacting with others. Persons have values that they believe to be important for a satisfying life. People often transmit their values to others in an effort to influence their attitudes and behaviors.

Modes of Value Transmission

Values are learned over a lifetime. This is not a deliberate process whereby individuals consciously choose the values they wish to have. Values become a part of an individual during socialization in the family, school, work, church, and other social groups. When children observe parents, family, and friends, they internalize behaviors that become the foundation of their value system.

The people who influence a child are generally unaware of the way they transmit their values. For example, if a mother consistently demonstrates honesty in dealings with others, her child will likely see the value of telling the truth. The child becomes honest without the mother's insistence or threat. However, the process of imposing values can be deliberate, as when a parent says to a child who has lied, "You should be ashamed of yourself. Good girls don't lie." There are five traditional modes of value transmission. Table 12-1 on p. 260 demonstrates the way these modes may lead to widely varying effects.

TABLE 12-1 Modes of Value Transmission	
Descriptions	Implications
MODELING	
Persons act in way to show others preferred way to behave. People acquire values from variety of role models.	Children initially wish to be like their parents, and thus parents can model values they perceive as significant. Modeling may not lead to socially acceptable behavior (e.g., viewing another's aggressive behavior). Unless parents point out the most desirable values, children can follow any role model.
MORALIZING	
Parents and teachers hold standards for right and wrong and rigidly enforce children to conform to their sets of values.	This approach can be very authoritarian. Moralizing parents may be unwilling to consider alternative values for children. With this approach, one way is often the only way. Young persons reared by moralizing adults often have difficulty with making independent choices.
LAISSEZ-FAIRE	
At times, people aquire values by behaving informally without restrictions or limitations. No one value system is right for everyone, and children form values without parents' rigid guidelines.	Parents want children to be free to explore a variety of life experiences. Children are encouraged to be inquisitive and learn from experiences. Parents may refrain from discipline. Limitation is that no one assumes responsibility for children's behavior. Conflict and confusion may arise if children have no direction.
RESPONSIBLE CHOICE	
Balance of freedom and restriction allows children to select values that lead to personal satisfaction and parental support. Children's choices are more limited as compared with laissez-faire approach.	Values are not strictly imposed by parents. As children choose values, parents, other family members, and teachers allow them to explore within boundaries new behaviors and their consequences. Children who can freely discuss their behavior and its effects will learn to understand their own values.
REWARD AND PUNISHMENT	
Offering rewards for certain valued behaviors serves to control behavior. When children fail to assume certain behaviors, parents administer punishment.	Parents may choose to use either form of value transmission more frequently. Using rewards can be positive approach to strengthen preferred values. Punishment may teach that violence is acceptable.

Influence of Development

Value formation, modification, and reaffirmation occur throughout a person's life. Cognitive and emotional level of development influence the way values are learned.

Infant

Infants rely on their parents for physical and emotional care. Although infants possess no real ability to

reason, they acutely sense the emotions and behaviors of people around them. The manner in which parents react to their children is often a function of their values. Infants begin to grow in emotional security through prompt and consistent responses of the parents to their needs.

Toddler

A toddler learns acceptable behavior by imitating others and seeking approval. As the child strives for a sense of autonomy, an identity forms, shaped by the values of the people with whom the child associates. The parents balance the child's need for independence against the need for safety and protection. The setting of appropriate limits allows the toddler to continue identity development.

Preschool Child

The preschool child is at the stage of cognitive development when concept formation begins. Concepts are objects, events, and experiences that have acquired meaningful labels: dogs bark, trees have leaves, a mother holds and comforts. The child can understand the terms *right* or *wrong* as applied to single acts. If repeatedly told not to hit or push playmates, the child learns that this act is wrong but does not yet have an abstract understanding of all "wrong" behaviors. Parents must provide kind, fair, and consistent limits for behavior and help direct the child toward behaviors that they value.

School-Age Child

The school-age child is exposed to diverse groups of people with a variety of values. Parents usually encourage the child to be involved in activities at home and outside the home. Goal setting and achievement are incorporated, promoting values related to doing good, avoiding harm, and choosing between activities. Important behaviors are being involved in problem solving and living by choices.

Adolescent

Adolescence is a critical developmental period that provides rapid and varied learning experiences. Adolescents' primary concerns are to achieve a balance between personal identity and the identity established with peers. Because of rapid physical and psychosocial development, adolescents frequently doubt themselves and the values they have been taught. As adolescents mature and the physical and emotional changes stabilize, they examine and incorporate values that frequently resemble their parents'. However, because their social contacts expand greatly, adolescents are no longer limited by parental values.

Adult

The mature adult is able to examine, maintain, or change values based on continuing life experiences and the acquisition of new knowledge. Marrying, rearing children, and choosing a career often require young adults to redefine their values.

Middle-age adults begin to redefine self-concept to suit the needs of later life. Middle-age adults whose values have been reinforced have a growing sense of security. However, the onset of aging may pose a threat to adults who value youth and vitality.

During late adulthood, an individual faces significant changes in life, including retirement from work, the physical alterations of aging, and the loss of close friends and family. It is important for the older adult to remain active and independent so that life continues to be enriching. The older adult may see many personal values threatened as it becomes more difficult to stay active and maintain meaningful interpersonal relationships. It is therefore essential for the adult to remain open to new ideas and values so that the opportunity for growth and satisfaction exists despite advancing age.

Sociocultural Influences

Values are formed in social settings where the educational, socioeconomic, spiritual, and cultural backgrounds of people vary. Leininger (1978) describes culture as "a way of life belonging to a designated group of people." A culture can have subcultures—small groups that assume an identity of their own—that have similarities to the larger culture (Steele, 1986). In the United States, there are many subcultures (for example, Native, Italian, or German Americans) that share some values with the larger culture while adopting some values unique to their subculture (see Chapter 4).

It is difficult to establish norms for any subculture because no absolute agreement about acceptable values exists within a particular subculture. Nurses are expected to respect the values of the client, even when their cultural backgrounds differ.

A particular culture's value orientation influences the way in which members pursue health care. Individuals as social groups face a certain number of problems, and there are a finite number of solutions to those problems. Persons in certain cultural groups may seek health care for the slightest problems, whereas those in other groups seek care only when their conditions are serious.

To give effective care, nurses must understand the influence of cultural traditions on health behaviors, response to stress, use of health care services, and adjustment to illness. Professional care givers' value systems may differ from those of clients. However, nurses must also realize that no single culture agrees on what is "right" or "wrong." Nurses must respect cultural orientation but also look further into and understand clients' uniqueness.

 ## VALUES IN PROFESSIONAL NURSING

Nurses assist clients in various life situations. Virginia Henderson (1964) defined nursing as assisting an individual sick or well in the performance of those activities that contribute to health or its recovery, that he or she would perform unaided if they had the necessary will, strength, or knowledge. And to do this in such a way as to help them gain independence as rapidly as possible.

Because nursing care involves people, it is important for nurses to understand the human values that facilitate the giving of help (Raatikainen, 1989). Nurses have their own set of values that are the result of personal choice or learning. Society's values regarding how persons should be cared for also influence nurses. Finally, the values of the institutions in which nurses are employed also influence practice. When nurses' personal and professional values are similar, they readily assume a professional role. When personal and professional values differ, nurses can become dissatisfied. The central values that direct nurses in clinical decision making and support of clients may not always be clear. However, many authors identify one value involved in the nurse-client relationship: caring (Table 12-2).

The Value of Caring

There is an important link between the value of caring and nurses' views on persons and their human dignity (Fry, 1989). **Caring** involves a sense of dedication to another person. When unable to exhibit caring to clients, nurses can no longer deliver the nurturing activities designed to assist people. Such a situation creates a dilemma for nurses and can be a serious source of dissatisfaction. Changes within the health care delivery system (see Chapter 3) have created situations that threaten nurses' ability to exercise caring toward clients. Specialization in health care has led to a subdivision of tasks by care givers; this often leads to depersonalization. Health care institutions and even society expect nurses to do more with fewer resources; yet nurses often lack the autonomy and authority to decide how care will be provided (Kurtz, Warry, 1991).

Advanced technology often endangers a humane approach to nursing care when the nurse gives more importance to monitoring of equipment than to sustaining the nurse-client relationship. Caring benefits the nurse and client. Kurtz and Warry (1991) argue that caring makes curing possible. However, caring is more than simply having concern for another person. For caring to influence a nurse's practice, it must be integrated as a standard of performance in all care activities. Fry (1988) and Veatch (1987) identify four criteria that define caring as a moral value that serves as an ethical standard for nursing practice:

1. Caring must be viewed as an ultimate or overriding value to guide one's actions.
2. Caring must be considered a universal value and, hence, must be applied to all persons in similar circumstances.
3. Caring must be considered prescriptive in that certain behaviors (for example, empathy, support, compassion, and protection) are preferred.
4. Caring must be other-regarding in that it must consider the human flourishing of others and not just one's own welfare.

Caring is an all encompassing part of nursing. Specific professional behaviors demonstrate a nurse's commitment to caring and excellence in practice. The American Association of Colleges of Nursing (1986) recommends seven values essential for the professional nurse (Table 12-3). The professional

---

TABLE 12-2 Caring as a Foundational Value of Nursing

Definition	Central Concepts
WATSON	
Caring is foundation of nursing as human science. It requires commitment on part of nurse to protect human dignity and preserve humanity.	Nurse-client relationship (caring as value of central importance) Caring as mode of being, natural state of human existence Caring as required for one to care for self or others Caring occurring in society to serve human needs
NODDING	
To care may mean to be charged with protection, welfare, or maintenance of something or someone. Person-to-person encounter results in joy as basic human affect.	Receptively (acceptance by care giver of person cared for) Relatedness (relation of care giver to one cared for as fact of human existence) Responsiveness (commitment of care giver to one cared for)
FRANKENA	
Caring involves respect for persons. It is basis of normative human judgments in general.	Respect (caring requiring identifiable form of response on part of care giver to person cared for)

Adapted from Kurtz RJ, Warry J: *Nurs Forum* 26(1):4, 1991.

TABLE 12-3   Essential Nursing Values and Behaviors*

Essential Values	Attitudes and Personal Qualities	Professional Behaviors
ALTRUISM Concern for the welfare of others	Caring Commitment Compassion Generosity Perseverance	Gives full attention to the patient/client when giving care. Assists other personnel in providing care when they are unable to do so. Expresses concern about social trends and issues that have implications for health care.
EQUALITY Having the same rights, privileges, or status	Acceptance Assertiveness Fairness Self-esteem Tolerance	Provides nursing care based on the individual's needs irrespective of personal characteristics. Interacts with other providers in a nondiscriminatory manner. Expresses ideas about the improvement of access to nursing and health care.
ESTHETICS Qualities of objects, events, and persons that provide satisfaction	Appreciation Creativity Imagination Sensitivity	Adapts the environment so that it is pleasing to the patient/client. Creates a pleasant work environment for self and others. Presents self in a manner that promotes a positive image of nursing.
FREEDOM Capacity to exercise choice	Confidence Hope Independence Openness Self-direction Self-discipline	Honors individual's right to refuse treatment. Supports the rights of other providers to suggest alternatives to the plan of care. Encourages open discussion of controversial issues in the profession.
HUMAN DIGNITY Inherent worth and uniqueness of an individual	Consideration Empathy Humaneness Kindness Respectfulness Trust	Safeguards the individual's right to privacy. Addresses individuals as they prefer to be addressed. Maintains confidentiality of patients/clients and staff. Treats others with respect regardless of background.
JUSTICE Upholding moral and legal principles	Courage Integrity Morality Objectivity	Acts as a health care advocate. Allocates resources fairly. Reports incompetent, unethical, and illegal practice objectively and factually.
TRUTH Faithfulness to fact or reality	Accountability Authenticity Honesty Inquisitiveness Rationality Reflectiveness	Documents nursing care accurately and honestly. Obtains sufficient data to make sound judgments before reporting infractions of organizational policies. Participates in professional efforts to protect the public from misinformation about nursing.

*The values are listed in alphabetical rather than priority order.
From American Association of Colleges of Nursing: *Essentials of college and univesity education for professional nursing,* Washington, DC, 1986, The Association; reprinted from American Nurses Association: *Code for nurses,* Kansas City, Mo, 1976, The Association.

nurse assigns priorities to these values when making decisions. Incorporation of these values into the personal and professional value system enables the nurse to be more humane and authentically caring.

 ## VALUES AND CLINICAL DECISION MAKING

Nurses identify diagnoses and make clinical judgments on the basis of subjective and objective information that they collect about the client. The decision-making process involves critical thinking and is an important nursing responsibility. Each client's needs are analyzed so that correct decisions are made about care.

A nurse's values influence clinical decision making. When a nurse values equality, the care delivered to a client will be based on the person's needs and provided in a nondiscriminatory way. When facing life-and-death decisions regarding a client's care, the nurse consistently applies a set of values in decision making (Taylor, 1985). Persons who believe in the sanctity of life support the concept that life is a paramount right that must be protected at all costs. A nurse who values sanctity of life may not be able to easily assist with an abortion. In contrast, persons supporting the value of quality of life believe that no life at all is better than a life with suffering or deficits (Taylor, 1985). A nurse may be better able to withhold treatment from a terminally ill client if quality of life is part of the personal value system. Taylor (1985) warns that decision making can become biased when quality of life becomes a criterion in health care. Differences in social and economic class can define quality of life in a variety of ways. For example, an intelligent, socially accomplished and technically skilled person may become biased as to the type of care that an uneducated, illiterate, or physically handicapped person would seek.

Nurses care for clients who possess unique values about life and the human experience. Clients' values must be respected. Therefore nurses must know their own values and the ways that they interact with the values of clients. To make intelligent and thoughtful decisions about care, nurses must be aware of the influence that values have in decisions.

 ## VALUES CLARIFICATION

Because individuals are not always consciously aware of their values, they can have difficulty when they have to make choices or when they feel forced

---

> ### Three Steps of Values Clarification
>
> **Choosing one's beliefs and behaviors**
> - Choosing from alternatives
> - Choosing freely
> - Considering all consequences
>
> **Prizing one's beliefs and behaviors**
> - Prizing and cherishing the choice
> - Publicly affirming the choice
>
> **Acting on one's beliefs**
> - Making the choice part of one's behavior
> - Acting with a pattern of consistency and repetition

Modified from Raths LE, Harmin M, Simon SB: *Values and teaching,* ed 2, Columbus, Ohio, 1979, Merrill.

---

to change their values. In addition, individuals must realize the implications that their values have for their own behavior. Yet people do not suddenly become aware of their values, and many people are unable to define their values clearly and meaningfully. To achieve an awareness of personal values, individuals use cognitive processes of values clarification.

Values clarification, or valuing, is a process of self-discovery that helps people gain clearer insights into their values. It is not a set of rules that interferes with conscientious decision making. Values clarification does not imply that a specific set of values should be accepted by all persons. It is also not a method of indoctrination to religious, moral, or cultural standards. When clarifying values in given situations, people learn what choices to make when alternatives are presented and how to determine whether choices are rationally made. The result of valuing is greater self-awareness and personal insight.

Raths, Harmin, and Simon (1979) pioneered values clarification as an approach to appraisal of values. Valuing involves three steps: choosing, prizing, and acting (see box). Using values clarification, the person ranks personal values in hierarchical order. The resultant hierarchy reveals to the individual a personal value system that provides a guide for personal conduct, lifestyle, and interpersonal interactions. First, the person must choose personal values freely. The freedom to select among alternatives allows a person to cherish the final choice. However, the individual must understand the alternatives. For example, an older woman may experience the sudden loss of her husband. As she shares her concerns with a community health nurse, it is clear that she has several choices. She can continue to live alone and grieve for her husband, move in with her daughter and away from friends, or live at home and begin to regularly socialize with male and female companions. The nurse helps the woman examine her choices without passing judgment or offering advice. A clear understanding of all alternatives and their consequences will ensure that the woman's final choice is the right one for her.

Prizing is showing private and public satisfaction with the value chosen. A person holds a value in esteem by feeling good about a choice. A nurse helps a client use values clarification so that the person is able to affirm personal values in the presence of significant others. When the widow decides to begin socializing again after her husband's death, she prizes her decision by being able to share it with her daughter. By announcing personal values, a person reaffirms their importance or relevance.

Acting on a chosen value solidifies its acceptance. Acting requires a translation of values into behavior. The widow begins to attend church socials and volunteers at a local hospital. Raths, Harmin, and Simon (1979) suggest that persons should act consistently and regularly on chosen values. It would be important for the widow to regularly pursue opportunities to spend time with friends and acquaintances. It may, however, be difficult to act consistently on a chosen value. For example, a client who values independence may be too disabled by illness to safely function alone. However, the client may be able to make personal decisions about self-care activities. The nurse carefully clarifies alternatives for clients so that they can act on the best possible choices.

Values Clarification Versus Ethical Decision Making

Values clarification is inadequate as a guide for solving ethical dilemmas (Bernal, 1985). There are often conflicts in values among health care professionals and clients that lead to ethical dilemmas (see Chapter 13). For example, a client may decide not to have surgery for lung cancer. The physician believes that surgery is the client's only choice. The nurse may believe in a client's autonomy but is unsure whether this client has made a rational decision.

When many different values are expressed in a situation, values clarification will probably not resolve the dilemma. Each person may benefit from knowing the other's values; yet they may not agree on the final decision. Ethical decisions require a clear analysis of all facts, with the nurse assuming a client-advocate role. It must be assumed that some values are better than others. Until health care professionals and clients can jointly agree on one value, such as client autonomy or freedom, ethical decisions cannot be easily made.

Strategies for Values Clarification

A system of strategies can help make valuing more insightful, practical, and meaningful for the person whose values are unclear. These **values clarification strategies** are exercises to help an individual clarify personal values using the three steps of valuing. The nurse can use the strategies with clients or for personal values clarification. For example, the strategy of completing unfinished sentences (see box) helps nurses determine and explore their own attitudes, beliefs, interests, and goals, which are indicators of their professional values. The finished sentences can be shared with a group to give nurses an opportunity to affirm their choices. The strategy of rank ordering (see box on p. 266 [left]) requires the selection of priorities among different values. The nurse can develop a similar exercise to help clients order their values in specific situations. This strategy demonstrates that many issues require more consideration of values than is usually given in decision making.

The health value scale (see box on p. 266 [right]) is an exercise for setting value priorities. It consists of 10 values that a client ranks in order of importance. The client ranks items in a way that accu-

---

Sentence Completion

Complete the following sentences. Use them to examine your feelings and values.
- I believe I succeed as a nurse when . . .
- A patient has a right to . . .
- I wish the director of nursing would . . .
- Physicians and nurses work together best when . . .
- I fail as a nurse if I cannot . . .
- The most difficult patient is one who . . .

Modified from Simon SB et al: *Values clarification: a handbook of practical strategies for teachers and students*, New York, 1978, Hart.

Rank Ordering

Choose 3 things from the 14 choices below that give you the most satisfaction in your work.
1. To be excited by what you're doing
2. To help others solve problems
3. To contribute to society with worthwhile work
4. To be recognized as an authority
5. To motivate yourself
6. To figure things out
7. To work within a structured situation
8. To think though new solutions
9. To have choice about time
10. To make a lot of money
11. To work in a team
12. To work out-of-doors
13. To be respected for your work
14. Other _____

From Ross R: *Prospering woman*, San Rafeal, Calif, 1982, Whatever Publishing.

Health Value Scale

Below you will find 10 values listed in alphabetical order. Arrange the values in order of their importance as guiding principles in your life. Study the list carefully and choose the one value that is most important to you. Write the number *1* in the space to the left of that value. Write the number 2 for the value that ranks second in importance. Continue in the same manner for the remaining values until you have included all ranks from *1* to *10*. Each value will have a different rank.
____ A comfortable life (a prosperous life)
____ An exciting life (a stimulating, active life)
____ A sense of accomplishment (lasting contribution)
____ Freedom (independence, free choice)
____ Happiness (contentedness)
____ Health (physical and mental well-being)
____ Inner harmony (freedom from inner conflict)
____ Pleasure (an enjoyable, leisurely life)
____ Self-respect (self-esteem)
____ Social recognition (respect, admiration)

Modified from Uustal DB: *Am J Nurs* 78:2058, 1978.

rately reflects a personal value hierarchy. If health is ranked in one of the top four positions, the client places a high value on health. The value placed on health is moderate if ranked *5, 6,* or *7* and low if ranked *8, 9,* or *10*. Information obtained from this exercise can help the nurse plan health care teaching methods. Another way to complete this exercise is by having the client freely name 10 values and to then establish a priority for them.

Nurses' Values Clarification

When values clarification is used for personal benefit, personal growth and professional satisfaction can be gained. During contacts with clients, peers, physicians, and other health care professionals, the nurse's values are challenged and tested. Examples of challenges follow:
1. How does the nurse show a willingness to be accountable for actions as a professional?
2. How do the nurse's attitudes about clients influence the care provided?
3. When another nurse performs some action unsafely, what should be done?
The nurse has difficulty assuming the role of a professional when personal values are poorly con-

ceived and unclear. Values clarification helps a nurse explore values and decide whether to act on beliefs (see box on p. 264). The nurse is able to establish more effective relationships with clients and better meet their needs after clearly defining personal values. Thus values clarification facilitates decision making and problem solving.

Values clarification can be used by nurses and other health care workers who face similar value conflicts daily. Sharing values about clients, their families, and colleagues assists nurses in recognizing their commonly held values. This sharing helps nurses understand the behavior of colleagues. Communication lines also become more open when dealing with controversial issues.

Clients' Values Clarification

Valuing is a useful tool in helping clients and families adapt to the stress of illness and other health-related problems. The nurse helps clients sort out emotions to clarify their meaning and significance. Values clarification helps clients gain awareness of personal priorities, identify ambiguities in values, and resolve major conflicts between values and behavior. Communication with clients becomes more effective because the nurse is able to focus attention on clients' comments and the reasons for them. Clients becomes more willing to express problems and true feelings, and thus the nurse is able to establish an individualized care plan.

A nurse is responsible for educating clients about health-promoting behaviors. The nurse's goal is to help clients establish health-protecting or health-promoting behaviors. Frequently clients are taught facts and concepts about their conditions, but their health behaviors remain unchanged. The nurse who learns about clients' values is able to devise a more successful teaching program. Giving clients meaningful and practical information increases the likelihood that they will assume behaviors that promote well-being.

Values Clarification as a Tool in Client Care

Merely encouraging the client to express feelings may provide inadequate information if the real problem is a conflict in values. For example, a middle-age man has just been diagnosed with a terminal disease. His values of health, economic security, and family unity are threatened. When encouraged to discuss his feelings, he may be unable to clearly describe how he feels. The nurse who is familiar with values clarification can help the client define values, clarify goals, and seek solutions.

Helping clients clarify values is not an attempt at psychoanalysis. The nurse's role is to shape responses to the client's questions or statements to stimulate introspection. Clarification of verbal response comes from the awareness that the valuing process will motivate a client to examine personal thoughts and actions. Such responses can help the client choose a value freely, consider alternatives, prize the choice, affirm the choice with others, act on the choice, and incorporate into life the behaviors that reflect the value selected.

When the nurse makes a clarifying response, it should be brief, selective, nonjudgmental, thought provoking, and spontaneous. A good clarifying exchange between nurse and client lasts only a short time. The nurse's response makes the client think about values after the exchange. Clarifying responses are used only when values conflict is the issue. For example, when the nurse explains a medical procedure, an attempt at values clarification is not needed. A nurse makes a clarifying response only for situations in which no right or wrong answer exists. Situations lacking answers are those involving beliefs, aspirations, feelings, and attitudes.

The nurse's response does not judge the client's values. A client will be unable to find comfort in personal values if the nurse moralizes or advises about choices. The nurse's response must evoke the client's creative thinking. For example, a client might be undecided about whether to seek another physician's opinion about a medical problem. It would be simple (although unethical) for the nurse to inform the client about the most skillful physicians in a given area. Likewise, the nurse could easily explain the hazards of proposed surgery. However, it is the client who must live with the choice of physicians; the focus must be on the client and the possible outcomes of the decision.

A nurse's spontaneity helps a client think creatively. The nurse often has little warning when the client seeks solutions to a values dilemma. With experience, a nurse can learn to make clarifying responses without advanced planning. For example, a client has been encouraged by doctors to undergo experimental surgery but has been unable to make a decision. The client asks the nurse, "What would you do?" The nurse should respond, "This is obviously a difficult decision for you. Have you weighed the pros and cons?" Although the response is consciously and deliberately designed to stimulate thought, it should not appear contrived.

Values clarification can occur in any setting. The bedside, a clinic office, or the home is a suitable place for clients to express feelings. Valuing is often more successful when the nurse has the opportunity for repeated contact with clients. It is difficult for the nurse to help clients meaningfully achieve each step of the valuing process when little time is spent giving care to them.

Ultimately the client perceves that valuing provides personal satisfaction. Values clarification promotes effective reasoning and decision making. The client becomes more aware of the way that values influence actions, and this awareness is an essential component of problem solving.

CASE STUDY

Mrs. James is a 73-year-old woman who fractured her ankle in a fall at home. Mrs. James' daughter is concerned about her mother's welfare and wants Mrs. James to live with her family. The daughter has voiced concern to the nurse that Mrs. James is incapable of caring for herself. Mrs. James' rehabilitation has progressed well. One day, Mrs. James asks the nurse, Ms. Fryer, "What should I do? I know my daughter worries about me, but I don't want to be cared for like a child."

Ms. Fryer realizes that Mrs. James is experiencing a conflict in her values for her independence, love for her daughter, and health. The nurse thinks the values clarification process would help Mrs. James make her choice. Ms. Fryer begins by helping Mrs. James choose from the alternatives available.

Choosing from Alternatives. The nurse's response depends partly on Mrs. James' age, education, and level of maturity. Mrs. James is an alert woman, knowledgeable about her needs, and capable of making decisions for herself. She has demonstrated motivation in her rehabilitation.

Examining All Consequences. Mrs. James loves her daughter and knows that the offer to join the daughter's family is genuine. Mrs. James says that she has many friends in her apartment building and that moving to her daughter's home would make it very difficult for her to socialize with her friends. Mrs. James' apartment is on the second floor, which requires her to climb one flight of stairs. A downstairs apartment will soon be vacant.

The nurse says, "Perhaps it would be helpful to weigh the advantages and disadvantages of joining your daughter against moving into the downstairs apartment." When making this suggestion, the nurse carefully avoids letting her own values influence Mrs. James' thinking, even though she has a close relationship with her own daughter and has been very happy when they shared her house on extended visits.

Choosing Freely. The next day, Ms. Fryer enters Mrs. James' room during breakfast. Her goal is to determine whether Mrs. James was able to make a decision of her own. Mrs. James says, "I've decided to move into the downstairs apartment," Ms. Fryer asks, "Was this a difficult choice to make?"

Prizing the Choice. Mrs. James acknowledges that she does not want to hurt her daughter's feelings; however, she knows her decision was the best one. "I still have many friends and they have encouraged me to stay in the apartment. I still feel spry and able to take care of myself." The nurse recognizes that it is important for Mrs. James to be satisfied with her choice.

Affirming the Choice. It is important that Mrs. James be able to speak out in support of her decision. She may need assistance from the nurse in thinking of ways to affirm the choice. An appropriate response by Ms. Fryer is, "What will be the best way to share your decision with your daughter?" Mrs. James replies, "My daughter and son-in-law are coming by to visit this evening. I've decided to let them know tonight."

Acting on the Choice. Mrs. James has made the decision to retain her independence. She is able to share her choice and the rationale for it with her daughter. The nurse using values clarification recognizes Mrs. James' need to act on her decision. She asks, "What can you do to begin planning for your move?"

Mrs. James calls the apartment manager to arrange for her new home. She is going to stay with her daughter for a week after discharge from the hospital. Meanwhile, she will have the opportunity to select new paint and wallpaper for the apartment. Mrs. James' value of independence remains alive in the measures she has taken to accomplish her move.

Acting with a Pattern. A month after discharge, Mrs. James returns to her physician's office for a checkup. She stops by the nursing division to visit with Ms. Fryer. Ms. Fryer is interested in learning whether Mrs. James has continued to retain her independence; for independence to be meaningful to Mrs. James, it must become integrated into her lifestyle. Ms. Fryer asks, "Was your choice to remain in the apartment the right one?" Mrs. James responds, "For now, yes. I am feeling much better and there are many friends to help me. My daughter visits every week. You know, though, I do have to be cautious in the way I walk around. I know someday I may have to live with my daughter."

As Mrs. James becomes more physically dependent, a conflict will arise between the independence she prizes and her ability to act on that value. The value of the genuine love and concern expressed by Mrs. James' daughter may become a higher priority than the value of independence. Mrs. James' maturity will be reflected in her eventual ability to modify her values. As she becomes more physically dependent, she must adapt her values accordingly. Mrs. James will still be alert and capable of making decisions. The daughter's ability to provide a safe environment for her mother without compromising Mrs. James' ability to make her own decisions should prove to be mutually satisfying.

As in the preceding case study, it takes time for nurses to develop values clarification as a tool for a client's care. Nurses cannot attempt to help a client explore values unless they have insight into their own. Values clarification can be a valuable means of helping a client sort out true feelings and beliefs and gain a better awareness of goals in life.

 ## SUMMARY

A person's unique set of values influences personal decisions and actions. Although values may be acquired and held unconsciously, a person's conscious awareness of values helps in reaching decisions and avoiding conflicts. A client who is conscious of personal values related to health and health behaviors is able to participate fully in health care, and nurses conscious of their own values are better able to help a client clarify values and make decisions.

People form values through observation and experience, noting the responses evoked by their own and others' behaviors. Values are acquired from parents and other family members in a continuous process that begins in infancy. Values are transmitted through various modes: modeling, moralizing, laissez-faire, responsible choice, and reward and punishment. While maturing and recognizing that life poses a variety of changes, a person must remain open to new ideas and their influence on personal values.

Nursing involves caring for human beings. The values of caring, respect for others, equality, and human dignity are important in enabling a nurse to assist clients most effectively. An individual who enters the profession of nursing possesses a personal set of values. If these values complement those of professional nursing, the role of a nurse is more easily ensured. However, societal, institutional, and even client values can create conflicts for a nurse, making decisions about client care difficult. Having a clear understanding of personal and professional values helps a nurse become more committed to excellence in nursing practice. Values clarification is the use of various strategies to explore the meaning of values and behaviors. The valuing process involves choosing, prizing, and acting on one's beliefs. When values are clearly detailed and positively affirmed, the client and nurse are more able to make objective decisions about health care.

CHAPTER 12 REVIEW

Key Concepts

- When nurses can clearly differentiate their personal values from their professional values, they are better able to help clients understand their values.
- Values provide a standard for acceptable behavior.
- A person acquires values after observing behaviors that prove successful for others.
- A child acquires values from parents, other family members, school, church, and other social institutions.
- Value formation begins in the early developmental stages and continues throughout life.
- Sociocultural background influences a person's values toward health and health care.
- The value of caring facilitates the giving of help to another human being.
- Values clarification is not an indoctrination method but a process that promotes an understanding of personal values.
- A person must be able to choose values freely from available alternatives and understand the consequences of choosing.
- A person may have an attitude about a certain idea, without valuing it.
- A nurse's values influence decisions made about a client's care.
- When making clinical decisions, the nurse establishes priorities for values inherent to professionalism.
- Values clarification helps a nurse explore personal values and feelings and decide whether to act on personal beliefs.
- The nurse who learns about a client's values is better prepared to help the client assume health-protecting or health-promoting behaviors.
- Values clarification strategies are useful tools that help clients and nurses understand their own values.
- Nurses who use values clarification with clients offer clarifying responses that stimulate introspection about values and behavior.
- Values clarification promotes effective reasoning and decision making.
- A nurse who assists a client in clarifying values and making decisions does so nonjudgmentally.
- Changes within the health care delivery system may threaten a nurse's ability to exercise caring.
- Caring serves as an ethical standard for nursing practice.

Key Terms

Attitude, p. 258

Caring, p. 262

Value, p. 258

Value system, p. 258

Values clarification, p. 264

Values clarification strategies, p. 265

Critical Thinking Exercises

1. It has been very difficult to care for Mr. Jones, a 26-year-old client who was shot in the head after leaving the scene of a robbery. He has been unconscious since reaching the hospital. Although Mr. Jones is still alive on a ventilator, the physicians offer no hope of survival. The nurse from the day shift reports that the family has been complaining about the care Mr. Jones is receiving, she notes, "They are just so ungrateful." Ms. Wells is the nurse caring for Mr. Jones during the evening shift. She spends extra time positioning her client and making sure his airway is clear. The above situation describes an attitude, value, and potential ethical dilemma. Identify each.

2. Ms. Russo is considering having a tubal ligation. She is 38 years old and has never had children. Her clinic nurse, Ms. Morris is 28 years old and married and has been unable to have children despite trying for 2 years. Ms. Russo asks the nurse to explain the tubal ligation procedure and its risks. Describe how Ms. Morris's personal values might influence this interaction.

3. Mr. Liles has been told he has cancer and that chemotherapy is his only choice of treatment. The client's brother died 2 years earlier after receiving extensive chemotherapy. The side effects of the medication caused Mr. Liles' brother to be very uncomfortable. A nurse assists Mr. Liles in values clarification. What are his choices and how might he be able to prize and act on each?

REFERENCES

American Association of Colleges of Nursing: *Essentials of college and university education for professional nursing,* Washington, DC, 1986, The Association.

Bernal EW: Values clarification: a critique, *J Nurs Educ* 24:174, 1985.

Brill NI: *Working with people, the helping process,* Philadelphia, 1973, Lippincott.

Fry ST: The ethic of caring: can it survive in nursing? *Nurs Outlook* 36(1):48, 1988.

Fry ST: Toward a theory of nursing ethics, *ANS* 11(4):9, 1989.

Henderson V: The nature of nursing, *Am J Nurs* 64:62, 1964.

Kurtz RJ, Warry J: Caring ethic: more human kindness, the care of nursing science, *Nurs Forum* 26(1):4, 1991.

Leininger M: *Transcultural nursing: concepts, theories, and practices,* New York, 1978, Wiley.

Omery A: Values, moral reasoning, and ethics, *Nurs Clin North Am* 24(2):499, 1989.

Raatikainen R: Values and ethical principles in nursing, *J Adv Nurs* 14:92, 1989.

Raths LE, Harmin M, Simon SB: *Values and teaching,* ed 2, Columbus, Ohio, 1979, Merrill.

Rokeach M: *The nature of human values,* New York, 1973, Free Press.

Steele SM: AIDS: clarifying values to close in on ethical questions, *Nurs Health Care* 7(5):246, 1986.

Stenberg MJ: Ethics as a component of nursing education, *ANS* 1(3):53, 1979.

Taylor SG: The effect of quality of life and sanctity of life on clinical decision making, *AORN J* 41:924, 1985.

Veatch RM, Fry ST: *Case studies of nursing ethics,* Philadelphia, 1987, Lippincott.

Zuzich A: Some frameworks for ethical development. In Reilly DE, editor: *Teaching and evaluating the affective domain in nursing programs,* Thorofare, NJ, 1978, Slack.

ADDITIONAL READINGS

Brink PJ: Value orientation as an assessment tool in cultural diversity, *Nurs Res* 33:198, 1984.

Cannon RB et al: A values clarification approach to cultural diversity, *Nurs Health Care* 5:161, 1984.

Gortner SR et al: Appraisal of values in the choice of treatment, *Nurs Res* 33:319, 1984.

Kurtz RJ, Warry J: The caring ethic; more than kindness, the core of nursing science, *Nurs Forum* 26(1):4, 1991.

Leininger M: Caring: a central focus of nursing and health care services. *Nurs Health Care* 1:135, 1980.

McNally JM: Values. I. *Superv Nurse* 11:27, 1980.

Syby CA: Ethical dilemmas: a need for values clarification education *CCQ* 7(1):1, 1984.

Ross R: *Prospering woman,* San Rafael, Calif, 1982, Whatever Publishing.

Steele SM, Harmon VM: *Values clarification in nursing,* Norwalk, Conn, 1983, Appleton-Century-Crofts.

Uustal DB: Values clarification in nursing: application to practice, *Am J Nurs* 78:2058, 1978.

CHAPTER 13

Ethics

OBJECTIVES

Mastery of content in this chapter will enable the student to:

- Define the key terms listed.
- Discuss the influence of ethics on nursing practice.
- Discuss the influence of personal and professional values on ethical decisions.
- Compare responsibility and accountability in nursing practice.
- Identify the purposes of a professional code of ethics.
- Identify and apply the primary and secondary principles of ethics to clinical situations.
- Discuss the types of ethical conflicts confronted by nurses.
- Discuss and apply to a clinical situation the process used to resolve ethical problems.
- Identify and analyze the ethical dilemma of any clinical situation for presentation to an ethics committee.

CHAPTER OUTLINE

Definition of Ethics

Foundations of Ethical Decision Making
    Values
    Morals
    Ethics in nursing

Nurses' Codes of Ethics

Accountability and Responsibility
    Ethical Principles

    Respect for persons
    Respect for autonomy
    Beneficence and nonmaleficence
    Justice
    Veracity, confidentiality, and fidelity

Process for Resolving Ethical Problems

Methodology for Decision Making

Bioethics Committees

Ethics is the study of standards for professional behavior related to "right" and "wrong" professional conduct. **Ethics** arises in situations that are complex and involve many different factors. It is possible to arrive at different ethical views by analyzing different aspects of the same problem. For example, there is a situation involving a client who has been declared to be brain dead, and the client's family is considering organ donation. The nurse supports the client by providing complete physical and psychological care to allow time for family members to agree on organ donation. The nurse may question whether the expensive measures provided to prolong the client's life are justifiable. However, fidelity to the client requires the nurse to support both the client and family until a final determination is made.

Ethical principles help the nurse choose the quality of care provided in situations involving profound life issues. Decision making concerning appropriate care is further complicated when knowledge is incomplete and requires further study (Ashley, 1978). In some cases, the client's choice or values may conflict with the nurse's. An example of this situation for nurses is the controversy related to abortion. In one case, a nurse who does not believe in abortion may find it difficult to care for a woman who has had an abortion. On the other hand, a nurses who believes in choice may find it difficult to care for a client who plans to give birth to a baby with multiple malformations.

The health care system has undergone dramatic changes in recent years (see Chapter 3). As a result, nurses work in health care settings that generate a variety of ethical situations. Many factors contribute to the complexity of today's health care environment. Advances in technology are the primary reasons for the changing scope of nursing activities. As a result, conflicts arise as nurses provide care within these environments. Situations involving **euthanasia**, informed consent, and quality of life can present ethical dilemmas. Other ethical dilemmas challenge today's nurses because of changes in nursing practice. For example, nurses are more independent and more willing to exercise responsibility for making clinical decisions.

Nurses maintain their primary commitment to clients; however, they are also accountable to physicians, other health team members, and the institutions for which they work. Clients are also more aware of their rights within the health care system and make additional demands on health care workers. The nurse acts as the liaison between clients and other health care team members to ensure that clients' rights are honored and that clients know and understand their options. Clients seek information from nurses to understand their choices; nurses are asked to assist them in decision making. Daily and frequent personal contact with clients places nurses in a unique position compared with other health care professionals. The nurse is present during the most basic of human activities such as bathing, eating, ambulating, and elimination. The nurse performs specific treatment activities such as medication administration, complex dressing changes, and ongoing physical assessments. The establishment of this relationship is the foundation of nursing ethics.

The nurse provides psychological support to clients experiencing pain, fear, joy, or grief. For example, the nurse remains with the mother of the stillborn infant until other family members can be present. The nurse provides comfort, using touch and empathy to encourage the mother to express her grief. Experiences such as this place the nurse in a special relationship with the client. The situation allows the nurse to show care for the client, and this caring is the foundation of the nurse-client relationship.

 DEFINITION OF ETHICS

Ethics reflects the principles or standards that govern proper conduct related to professional behaviors. The values of the client, nurse, and society interact to set the environment for ethical behavior. If the value systems of all involved are not cohesive, ethical dilemmas can occur. A dilemma is a choice between equally unsatisfactory alternatives (Syby, 1984). Ethical dilemmas require the nurse to make challenging and often difficult decisions about the best way to care for clients.

For example, the nurse is obligated to act for the benefit of the client and to prevent harm. An ethical dilemma can arise from conflict between these two values. The nurse can do good for the client with terminal lung cancer by providing the prescribed narcotic to reduce pain and provide comfort, but that same action may also cause harm by hastening death from respiratory depression. In this example, the situation is further complicated by the client's need for comfort and understanding of the potential side effects of the narcotic. Family members have expressed their concerns related to the side effects of the narcotic and request the nurse to withhold the drug or administer a less effective medication. In this example, a dilemma remains, even if the family and client agree on the administration of the narcotic. That dilemma still requires the nurse to choose between doing good by providing the benefit of a narcotic and avoiding harm as a result of side effects of the narcotic.

An understanding of ethical decision making will assist nurses in making proper clinical decisions that will benefit the client and themselves. As nurses develop these decision-making skills, they can help and support clients to manage their own decisions related to health care.

FOUNDATIONS OF ETHICAL DECISION MAKING

The primary moral imperative of nursing is to improve the quality of the lives of those who seek or receive nursing services (Curtin, 1986). To gain the knowledge to make ethical decisions for the benefit of clients or to support clients in making decisions for themselves, nurses must understand the relationship between values, morals, and ethics.

Values

Values (see Chapter 12) are principles or standards that influence behavior and decision making. Values are based on experience, religion, education, and culture. Additional sources of values for nurses are the professional peer group (other nurses) and employing institutions. Values underlie all decision making and influence beliefs about the worth of ideas or behavior. Values are associated with the emotional and conceptual aspects of life and influence behavior. When people value something, they choose it over other alternatives and freely make that choice. They also prize their choice and are proud and happy with it; they are also willing to publicly share it with others. In addition, people act, using the choice as a part of their behaviors, and they repeat that behavior.

Values are the building blocks for the development of morals (personal conduct) and ethics (professional conduct). Values are not the same all the time; they can develop and change over time. Changes in values produce changes in attitude and behaviors. Values can be identified in everyday experiences and are expressed as behaviors or verbalized standards of conduct that a person endorses and tries to maintain (Omery, 1989).

Morals

A moral belief is the personal conviction that something is absolutely right or wrong in all situations. A person is generally unwilling to change personal opinions on issues of a moral nature. To one person, for example, abortion may be an absolute moral wrong; in other words, there are no acceptable reasons for a woman to end a pregnancy prematurely. If this person holds consistent moral views, capital punishment is also a moral wrong. Not all persons hold the same moral views. A moral issue becomes an ethical one when the choice is no longer clear between right and wrong.

Ethics in Nursing

Nursing ethics provides the standards for professional behavior and is the study of principles of right and wrong conduct for nurses. Nursing ethics states the duties and obligations of nurses to their clients, other health professionals, the profession, and the community. Ethics promotes the philosophical and theological study of morality, moral judgments, and moral problems. There are three types of ethics. Descriptive ethics presents a factual narrative of moral behaviors. Descriptive studies do not produce moral judgments on these behaviors. Metaethics is concerned with theoretical issues of meaning and justification. It is the portion of ethics that centers on the extent to which judgments are reasonable or otherwise justifiable. Normative ethics raises questions about what is right or what ought to be done in a situation that calls for an ethical decision (for example, deciding whether to prolong life in a terminally ill client). Discussions regarding ethics in this chapter refer to normative ethics.

NURSES' CODE OF ETHICS

Nursing has developed codes of ethics that determine the profession's standards of conduct. These codes of ethics describe the goals and values of the nursing profession. Students must make a commitment to uphold these obligations when they become nurses.

A code is a set of ethical principles generally accepted by members of the profession. These principles assist nurses in deciding on the proper conduct for a specific situation. There are several codes for professional nurses (see boxes on pp. 276 and 277). These codes differ in their language and specific emphasis, but all reflect the same underlying principles of respect for autonomy (self-determination), beneficence (doing good), nonmaleficence (avoiding harm), justice (treating people fairly), veracity (truth-telling), fidelity (keeping promises), and confidentiality (respecting privileged information).

American Nurses Association Code of Ethics

- The nurse provides services with respect for human dignity and the uniqueness of the client unrestricted by considerations of social or economic status, personal attributes, or the nature of health problems.
- The nurse safeguards the client's right to privacy by judiciously protecting information of a confidential nature.
- The nurse acts to safeguard the client and the public when health care and safety are affected by the incompetent, unethical, or illegal practice of any person.
- The nurse assumes responsibility and accountability for individual nursing judgments and actions.
- The nurse maintains competence in nursing.
- The nurse exercises informed judgment and uses individual competence and qualifications as criteria in seeking consultation, accepting responsibilities, and delegating nursing activities to others.
- The nurse participates in activities that contribute to the ongoing development of the profession's body of knowledge.
- The nurse participates in the profession's efforts to implement and improve standards of nursing.
- The nurse participates in the profession's efforts to establish and maintain conditions of employment conducive to high-quality nursing care.
- The nurse participates in the profession's effort to protect the public from misinformation and misrepresentation and to maintain the integrity of nursing.
- The nurse collaborates with members of the health professions and other citizens in promoting community and national efforts to meet the health needs of the public.

From American Nurses Association: *Code for nurses with interpretive statements*, Kansas City, Mo, 1985, The Association.

International Council of Nurses Code for Nurses

- The fundamental responsibility of the nurse is fourfold: to promote health, to prevent illness, to restore health, and to alleviate suffering.
- The need for nursing is universal. Inherent in nursing is respect for life, dignity, and rights of man. It is unrestricted by considerations of nationality, race, creed, color, age, sex, politics, or social status.
- Nurses render health services to the individual, the family, and the community and coordinate their services with those of related groups.

NURSES AND PEOPLE

- The nurse's primary responsibility is to those people who require nursing care.
- The nurse, in providing care, promotes an environment in which the values, customs, and spiritual beliefs of the individual are respected.
- The nurse holds in confidence personal information and uses judgment in sharing this information.

NURSES AND PRACTICE

- The nurse carries personal responsibility for nursing practice and for maintaining competence by continual learning. The nurse maintains the highest standards of nursing care possible within the reality of a specific situation.
- The nurse uses judgment in relation to individual competence when accepting and delegating responsibilities.
- The nurse when acting in a professional capacity should at all times maintain standards of personal conduct which reflect credit upon the profession.

NURSES AND SOCIETY

- The nurse shares with other citizens the responsibility for initiating and supporting action to meet the health and social needs of the public.

NURSES AND CO-WORKERS

- The nurse sustains a cooperative relationship with co-workers in nursing and other fields. The nurse takes appropriate action to safeguard the individual when his care is endangered by a co-worker or any other person.

NURSES AND THE PROFESSION

- The nurse plays the major role in determining and implementing desirable standards of nursing practice and nursing education.
- The nurse is active in developing a core of professional knowledge.
- The nurse, acting through the professional organization, participates in establishing and maintaining equitable social and economic working conditions in nursing.

From International Council of Nurses: *ICN code for nurses: ethical concepts applied to nursing*, Geneva, 1973, Imprimeries Populaires.

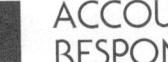

ACCOUNTABILITY AND RESPONSIBILITY

A nurse assumes responsibility and accountability for nursing care provided. **Responsibility** refers to the execution of duties associated with the nurse's particular role (ANA, 1985). When administering medications, the nurse is responsible for assessing clients' need for the drugs, giving them safely and correctly, and evaluating the responses. A nurse who acts in a responsible manner gains the trust of clients and other professionals. A responsible nurse remains competent in knowledge and skills and demonstrates a willingness to perform within the ethical guidelines of the profession.

Accountability means being answerable for one's own actions. A nurse is accountable to self, the client, the profession, the employer, and society (see box). If a wrong dose of medication is given, the nurse is accountable to the client who received it, the physician who ordered it, the nursing service that set standards of expected performance, and society, which demands professional excellence. To be ac-

---

Canadian Nurses Association Code of Ethics

The body of the code is divided into the following sources of nursing obligations:

CLIENTS

- A nurse is obliged to treat clients with respect for their individual needs and values.
- Based on respect for clients and regard for their rights to control their own care, nursing care should reflect respect for the clients' right of choice.
- The nurse is obliged to hold confidential all information about a client learned in the health care setting.
- The nurse has an obligation to be guided by consideration for the dignity of clients.
- The nurse is obliged to represent the ethics of nursing before colleagues and others.
- The nurse is obliged to advocate all clients' interests.
- In all professional settings, including education, research, and administration, the nurse retains a commitment to the welfare of clients. The nurse has an obligation to act in a fashion that will maintain trust in nurses and nursing.

HEALTH TEAM

- Client care should represent a cooperative effort, drawing on the expertise of nursing and other health professions. By acknowledging personal or professional limitations, the nurse recognizes the perspective and expertise of colleagues from other disciplines.
- The nurse, as a member of the client's health care team, is obliged to take steps to ensure that the client receives competent and ethical medical and nursing care.

SOCIAL CONTEXT OF NURSING

- Conditions of employment should contribute to client care and to the professional satisfaction of nurses. Nurses are obliged to work toward securing and maintaining conditions of employment that satisfy these goals.

RESPONSIBILITIES OF THE PROFESSION

- Professional nurses' organizations recognize a responsibility to clarify, secure, and sustain ethical nursing conduct. The fulfillment of these tasks requires professional organizations to remain responsive to the rights, needs, and interests of clients and nurses.

From Canadian Nurses Association: *Code of ethics for nursing*, Ottawa, 1985, The Association.

Maintaining Professional Accountability

SELF
- Report any personal conduct that endangers clients.
- Stay informed of current nursing practice theory and issues.
- Make judgments based on facts.

CLIENT
- Provide clients with accurate information about care.
- Conduct nursing care in a manner that ensures client safety and well-being.

PROFESSION
- Maintain ethical standards in practice.
- Encourage peers to follow the same.
- Report a colleague's unethical behavior.

EMPLOYING INSTITUTION
- Follow policy and procedures defined by the institution.

SOCIETY
- Maintain ethical conduct in the care of all clients in all settings.

countable, the nurse acts according to the professional code of ethics. Thus when an error is made, the nurse reports it and initiates care to prevent further injury. Accountability calls for an evaluation of a nurse's effectiveness in practice. Professional accountability serves the following purposes:

1. To evaluate new professional practices and reassess existing ones
2. To maintain standards of health care
3. To facilitate personal reflection, ethical thought, and personal growth on the part of health care professionals
4. To provide a basis for ethical decision making

To be accountable, the nurse practices within the codes of the profession. Accountability requires an evaluation of the nurse's performance in providing nursing care. The Joint Commission on Accreditation of Healthcare Organizations (JCAHO) has recommended the establishment of standards for the delivery of nursing care. The standards are developed by clinical experts within the department of nursing. These standards provide a basic structure against which nursing care is objectively measured. These standards do not eliminate the need for individualized care plans. Instead, the nurse incorporates the standards into care plans. Accountability is better ensured because the quality of care can be measured.

 ## ETHICAL PRINCIPLES

The code of ethics from the American Nurses Association (ANA) assists nurses in defining their ethical duties and actions. Thus the code allows the nurse to practice and act in a responsible and accountable manner. In the preamble of the *Code for Nurses with Interpretive Statements* (ANA, 1985), the following ethical principles are defined:

When making clinical judgements, nurses base their decisions on consideration of consequences and of universal moral principles, both of which direct and justify nursing actions. The most fundamental of these principles is respect for persons. Other principles stemming from this basic principle are respect for autonomy, beneficence, nonmaleficence, veracity, confidentiality, fidelity, and justice.

The ethical principles within the ANA code provide a foundation for nursing practice. Beauchamp and Childress (Fowler, 1989) also identify respect for autonomy, nonmaleficence, beneficence, and justice as the basic ethical principles (Table 13-1). The secondary principles include veracity, confidentiality, and fidelity. These secondary principles can be incorporated into the primary principles when interpreting ethical issues and making clinical decisions.

TABLE 13-1 Ethical Principles

Definitions	Nursing Implications
AUTONOMY	
Personal liberty of action, self-determination	Promote client decision making. Support client's right to informed consent. Make decisions when client's choice poses harm. Exercise autonomy when members of the health care team agree to importance of autonomy.
NONMALEFICENCE	
Duty to do no harm	Avoid deliberate harm, risk of harm, and harm that occurs during performance of nursing actions. Consider degree of risk permissible. Determine whether use of technological advances provides benefits that outweigh risks.
BENEFICENCE	
Doing or active promotion of good	Provide health benefits to clients. Balance benefit and risks of harm. Consider how client is best helped.
JUSTICE	
Fairness or equity	Ensure fair allocation of resources, such as appropriate staffing or mix of staff to all clients. Determine order in which clients should be treated (e.g., priority treatment for clients in pain).

According to the ANA code, respect for persons is the fundamental principle of professional behavior. Nurses are obligated to respect human existence and the individuality of persons to whom they provide nursing care. Nurses must take all reasonable means to protect and sustain human life where there is hope of recovery or when clients can benefit from life-prolonging treatment (ANA, 1985).

Respect for Persons

The principle of respect for persons does not only apply to clinical situations, but it applies to all of life's situations. This principle directs individuals to treat themselves and others with a respect inherent to man's humanness. It requires recognition in a sense that all mankind shares a common human destiny

(Fowler, 1989). The principle of respect for persons needs to be simplified as it affects nursing practice. A nurse's respect for persons generally means respect for autonomy.

Respect for Autonomy

Autonomy means that individuals are able to act for themselves to the level of their capacity (Fowler, 1989). Part of the shared human destiny includes the recognition of autonomy.

The concept of people as autonomous individuals leads nurses to respect their values and choices. It is important to remember that persons are not fully autonomous and cannot act solely for their own purposes; consideration and respect for the rights of others is included in the principle of respect for autonomy.

The principle of respect for autonomy has received special recognition in today's health care setting because of the long tradition of emphasis on the principle of beneficence. When the principle of beneficence (the duty to do good) overrides the client's autonomy, the result is paternalism. **Paternalism** is doing what the health professional believes is in the client's best interests regardless of the client's own determinations. Frequently the principles of respect for autonomy and beneficence conflict. An example of this situation is the elderly woman who is alert but forgetful and unsteady on her feet. In the past, she has fallen, and the nurses are concerned for her safety. The client does not remember to call for assistance; therefore the nurses have suggested that she wear a restraint. The client is embarrassed by the restraint and refuses to wear it. In this situation, the nurse plans the client's care to include specific times for the client to move about with assistance as needed. In addition, the nurse gains the client's cooperation by placing the restraint under her clothing and explaining the importance of safety when the client is alone.

Informed consent is a method that promotes and respects a person's autonomy. To make autonomous decisions and actions, clients must be offered enough information to make decisions and must be free of internal or external influences so that they can act. Properly administered, informed consent helps clients understand all of their options.

The client must have all the information a reasonable person, in a comparable situation, would need. Additional information that is relevant to a client because of age, gender, occupation, and risk should also be provided. The information must be communicated in a manner that the client can understand (Fowler, 1989). Clients who have retarded or delayed development, are legally incompetent, are minors, or are psychiatrically disturbed have the right to participate in health care decisions to the extent their condition or ability allows.

Free consent is a willingness to participate in situations related to informed consent. There are internal and external constraints to voluntariness (willingness). Internal constraints include pathophysiological conditions that alter the ability to process information. Examples of internal constraints include significant trauma, neurological damage, hypoxia, and other compromised physiological states. Psychological factors such as grief, suffering, or anxiety can also limit willingness to participate. The external constraints that can influence voluntariness include coercion, duress, fraud, deceit, or undue influence.

Respect for autonomy must be acknowledged when the client disagrees with health care professionals, as well as when the client agrees with the recommendations of the health care team. The health care team, for example, must respect the decision of a client to stop renal dialysis. The nurse provides ongoing comfort measures to assist the client in preparing for death.

Respect for autonomy does not apply when clients are unconscious. Clients must be able to participate in decision making. If clients cannot speak for themselves, during emergencies, there is presumed consent based on the following (Fowler, 1989):

1. It is reasonable to assume that injured or ill clients would want treatment.
2. Health care providers have a social contract based on social trust that requires that clients be treated and not abandoned if they cannot speak for themselves.

The situation changes if unconscious or seriously ill clients have made their wishes known to family members or has written advance directives. Respect for autonomy requires that members of the health care team follow these directives.

In 1990, the Patient Self Determination Act (Advance Directives Act) became law and was implemented in all health care institutions effective December 1, 1991. The law requires that all persons receiving medical care in an institution recognized by Medicare and Medicaid be given written information about their rights under the state law to make decisions about medical care, including the right to accept or refuse medical or surgical treatment. The information must be provided at admission. Clients must be provided with information about their rights to formulate advance directives such as a living will or to appoint someone to speak for them through a durable power of attorney for health care (Flarey, 1991). In addition, a client's treatment wishes must be documented and periodically reviewed with the client.

A **living will** lists the medical treatment a person chooses to omit or refuse if the person is unable to make decisions and is terminally ill. A durable power of attorney for health care appoints a person (relative or trusted friend) to make medical decisions on a client's behalf when the client can no longer make decisions. Under the law, institutions are required to provide written information at admission to allow clients to exercise these rights. Failure to comply could cause agencies to lose their reimbursement.

The wishes of clients must be documented in medical records. Advance directives make it possible for clients to receive the treatment and care they desire when they are unconscious or incompetent. For example, the client with end-stage pulmonary disease, who does not wish to be placed on a ventilator, will be made comfortable and treated medically with other support therapies. This client will not be resuscitated when respiratory failure occurs. The challenge for the nurse is to provide the comfort and support that the client requires, help the client discuss the decision openly, provide necessary medications for comfort, and minimize activities that cause respiratory distress. Nursing obligations related to respect for autonomy include the following:

1. Assist and promote client decision making.
2. Support clients' rights to informed consent.
3. Follow the advance directives that clients provide.
4. Support competent clients' decisions.

Nonmaleficence and Beneficence

The principles of beneficence and nonmaleficence are viewed on a continuum ranging from not inflicting harm (**nonmaleficence**) to benefitting others (**beneficence**). The continuum has the following dimensions:

1. Noninflection of harm (nonmaleficence)
2. Removing harmful conditions (beneficence)
3. Preventing harm (beneficence)
4. Doing good or benefiting others (beneficence)

Generally, nonmaleficence takes precedent over beneficence. In clinical situations, however, it is often difficult to draw the line between not inflicting harm and preventing or removing harmful situations. For example, the nurse at the well-baby clinic who immunizes children for diptheria, whooping cough, and tetanus inflicts some degree of harm or pain; however, the benefit of being protected against whooping cough is more important. Another example

of these principles is the case of the client who must receive surgical treatment. Surgery for cancer of the bowel can be seen as inflicting harm; however, the benefit of removing the tumor for the client generally outweighs the harm related to the risk of surgery.

The beneficence principle requires the balancing of harms and benefits. Benefits promote the client's welfare and health, whereas harms or risks detract from the client's health or welfare. Clients, nurses, and physicians must consider the risks and benefits when making decisions related to treatment and research. The principle of beneficence requires assessment and balancing of risks and benefits in clinical settings. For example, the client with cancer must weigh the benefits and risks of experimental cancer drugs before choosing to receive the treatments. The nurse must provide the information that the client requests by discussing it with the client or keeping the physician informed of the client's need for information.

The principles of beneficence and nonmaleficence direct nurses to promote good and avoid causing harm. However, these principles do not give direction for distribution of resources when they may be insufficient for the number of clients who would benefit from them. In the health care system today, resources are limited. Examples related to limited resources are the insufficient number of available beds in the intensive care unit, the imbalance in nurse-client ratios on some nursing units, and the limited number of organs available for transplantation. Decisions about who should receive available resources require further consideration and direction from the principles of justice. The principle of beneficence requires the nurse to provide health benefits to clients, balance the benefits against the harm in situations in which a choice must be made, and determine the best way to assist the client. The principles of nonmaleficence requires the nurse to avoid harming clients during delivery of nursing care and weigh the benefits against the harms for the use of advanced technologies in specific clinical situations.

Justice

The principle of **justice** requires treating others fairly and giving persons their due. When there are resources to distribute in health care, nurses should allocate them in such a way that equal shares go to equal recipients. The following problems complicate the application of distributive justice:

1. Not everyone is equal in every way. Sometimes there are situations in which it seems that one

person should receive a greater or lesser share than another.

2. Resources are limited. There is not always enough for each person to receive an equal share.

Some of the suggestions that have been made to aid equal distribution include contracts, individual need, individual effort, ability to pay, social contribution, and merit. In daily life, different bases for distribution are used for different settings. Welfare payments are made based on individual need, but jobs and promotions are usually distributed for achievement and merit (Davis, Aroskar, 1983). The distribution of nursing care is determined by the individual needs of clients and by nurses who establish priorities for client needs. Certain clients require skilled nursing care more than others. To live and avoid permanent disability, these clients are usually more seriously ill and require immediate intervention. For example, the client who is admitted to the neurological unit after suffering head trauma usually requires immediate assessment and surgical intervention to prevent brain damage associated with edema or hemorrhage. Other clients who are more physically stable are cared for as the nurse makes time for other necessary nursing activities such as discharge teaching and routine care. Some clients die despite any help that the nurse can provide. The criteria of need, added with the client's prognosis, is basic to the practice of **triage**, which is used by nurses and other health care professionals when resources are in short supply.

In contrast to cases of urgent need are clients who require long-term needs created by handicaps. Examples are mentally retarded children or a client who has an injured spinal cord. Justice for these clients may mean providing additional assistance because they might be able to achieve their best results only with additional health care resources.

Unequal treatment to clients always requires justification. For example, should a client who does everything possible to improve health be cared for differently from a client who refuses to follow medical restrictions? The principle of justice supports the argument that there should be at least equal initial access to health care for assessment of the client's needs. This view has limitations, but it supports a more critical evaluation of distribution of scarce health care resources. Continued support to a client who repeatedly refuses health care advice may not seem to be the best way to use resources. However, the principle of justice requires the nurse to ensure fair allocation of resources to all clients.

Veracity, Confidentiality, and Fidelity

The secondary principles of ethical conduct outlined in the ANA Code of Nurses include the following.

1. **Veracity,** or the duty to tell the truth
2. **Confidentiality,** or the duty to respect privileged information
3. **Fidelity,** or the duty to keep promises

The secondary ethical principles of veracity, confidentiality, and fidelity are frequently meshed into the context of primary principles. An example is truth-telling (veracity) as it relates to informed consent. A young man requests information related to kidney transplantation and the drugs that he will be required to take for the rest of his life. The nurse explains the side effects of the medications, including their effect on being able to have children. The client must weigh the benefits of transplantation against the risk of becoming sterile as a result of drug therapy. The nurse must answer the client's questions with honesty even though the client may choose to remove himself from the transplant list.

Confidentiality is a basic ethical principle that ensures a client's privacy. Nurses avoid discussing the condition of a client with anyone who is not involved in the client's care. Often a dilemma arises when a client chooses to keep confidential information that places the client or others at risk. An example, is the client who is suffering from acquired immunodeficiency syndrome (AIDS) and chooses not to reveal the diagnosis to family members. If family members will assume the health care of the client, the nurse may believe that they have the right to be properly informed. The principle of veracity guides the nurse in encouraging the client to share information about illness. However, in the end it is the client's decision. The principle of fidelity requires that nurses keep promises made to clients and is based in relationships that continue over time.

Frequently, ethical dilemmas can develop when the principles of fidelity and justice conflict. For example, the nurse promises to stay with an assigned primary client, who suffers terminal cancer, during the next work shift. Because of the familiarity with the client's needs, the primary nurse is best suited to care for the client. However, several clients are admitted to the unit on an emergency basis during the shift. The same primary nurse is also the most experienced nurse in the unit and is needed in the emergent situation. The principle of justice related to the allocation of resources (nurse's time) places this nurse in conflict. Fidelity can be preserved in this situation by having the primary nurse talk with the client, delegate care to a competent colleague, and monitor the cancer client's progress during the shift.

PROCESS FOR RESOLVING ETHICAL PROBLEMS

Ethical reasoning is similar to the nursing process in that it requires critical thinking skills. A nurse can best solve ethical dilemmas by systematically considering all options for solving the dilemma. An ethical dilemma occurs as a result of conflict between moral principles that support different courses of action. Uustal (1991) has outlined the following characteristics of ethical dilemmas.

1. The choice is between equally undesirable alternatives.
2. Real choice exists between possible courses of action.
3. The persons involved place a significant value judgment on possible actions or on the consequences of actions.
4. Data also will not help resolve the dilemma.
5. "Resolutions" to the ethical dilemmas come from different resources (that is, psychology, sociology, and theology).
6. Actions taken in an ethical dilemma will result in unfavorable outcomes and/or will constitute a breach of a person's duty to another.
7. The choices made in an ethical dilemma have far-reaching effects on the perceptions of human beings and definition of personhood, relationships with others, and people and society as a whole.
8. Any ethical decision involves the allocation and expenditure of resources that are finite or limited.
9. Ethical dilemmas are not solvable but rather, resolvable.
10. There is no "right" or "wrong" when dealing with two equally unfavorable actions.

Curtin and Flaherty (1982) used similar characteristics to assist nurses in distinguishing ethical problems from other problems in the health care setting. These characteristics follow:

1. The problem cannot be resolved solely through a review of scientific data.
2. The problem is perplexing. A person cannot easily think logically or make a decision about the problem.
3. The answer to the problem will have great relevance for several areas of human concern.

An example of the interrelatedness of these problems occurs for nurses caring for the premature infant who has several major malformations that require extensive surgeries with poor prognoses. The choices for the parents are to make the infant comfortable and not perform the surgeries or have the surgeries performed and risk causing increased pain for the infant. In addition to other problems, the newborn cannot digest formula; she vomits after every feeding. After a nasogastric tube is inserted, the infant digests the formula. However, the tube seems to cause discomfort for the newborn, and she cries. The nurses face the dilemma of whether to bottle-feed the infant or feed her through the nasogastric tube, which causes pain.

The nurses are doing good and avoiding harm but are causing pain. This is an example of the dilemmas that may arise when nurses care for clients. In the end, the nurse must deal with such problems, and after reviewing a situation and recognizing that an ethical problem does indeed exist, the nurse uses a consistent methodology to determine a plan for action.

METHODOLOGY FOR DECISION MAKING

Each ethical dilemma will be different. However, the nurse in any setting can follow a model for ethical decision making to increase the probability that all factors are weighed equally. The previous example of the premature infant will be used in applying the decision-making model, which includes the following steps:

1. *Identify the important factors.* List everyone involved in the decision-making process, including physicians and nurses. (In the previous example, the parents, physician, and nurses should be included.)
2. *Presume good will.* Everyone involved is concerned with providing comfort and care to the infant.
3. *Gather relevant and factual information,* which should include preferences of the client (or family if the client is unable to express preferences), family systems, social considerations, daily life, planned medical intervention, community surroundings, care givers' input, and the "ideal picture" that the care giver perceives in solving the dilemma (see box). (For example, some nurses believe that the feeding and holding of infants is the care that they provide under most circumstances and, since the outcome

will be death, it is important to maximize this routine care.)

4. *State values (principles).* (Related to beneficence and nonmaleficence, the nurses in the example provide nourishment, which is doing good. The nurse will not do harm by causing pain or by allowing starvation. Related to fidelity, the nurses care for the comfort of the infant as promised to the parents).

5. *Rank values* The nurse and parents rank the value of comfort over nutrition. The burden faced by nurses is the risk of causing vomiting or possible starvation.

6. *Take action.* The nurse follows the action of bottle feeding, which can be physically satisfying, by stimulating the infant's sucking reflex.

No two ethical dilemmas are the same. Using a systematic model for ethical decision making increases the probability that all ethical principles and values involved are reviewed. The nurse acts after evaluating all alternative courses of action. It is also essential that the nurse does not act alone. Communication of the plan for resolving ethical dilemmas must be shared with all health care team members. A systematic approach to ethical decision making allows the nurse to practice in a professional manner and to increase the ability to deal with complex, ethical situations.

 BIOETHICS COMMITTEES

Health care workers recognize that scientific and technological advances and increased public awareness and participation in health care issues have raised complex ethical, legal, and social questions about clients and the care activities provided to them. In the past 15 years, health care institutions have focused on the development of ethics committees. Other titles for these committees include *human values committees*, *medical-moral committees*, or *bioethics committees*. The committees serve several purposes (see box). All members of the health care team

---

Data Collection Sheet for Ethical Care Plan

CLIENT PREFERENCES
- Parents are unsure of best way to feed infant.
- Parents express concern over infant's comfort.

FAMILY SYSTEMS
- Other family members have same concern for infant's comfort.

SOCIAL CONSIDERATIONS
- Health care team respects parents' wishes.

DAILY LIFE
- Parents are involved in death of their child.

MEDICAL INTERVENTION
- Physician has ordered amount and kind of formula.
- Physician treating the infant believes nutrition is basic care.

COMMUNITY SURROUNDINGS
- Infant's hospitalization is paid through private-insurance. Minimal financial expense is on public funds or parents.

STAFF INPUT
- Nurses are divided. Some believe they should bottle-feed infant because of pain related to nasogastric tube feedings. Other nurses are concerned that infant is not retaining formula and thus might starve.

IDEAL PICTURE
- Nurses want to provide comfort and not have infant suffer.

Primary Functions of Ethics Committees

- To direct educational programs that provide knowledge regarding ethical principles and issues for the medical and professional community
- To assist the hospital and medical staff in the development and review of policies related to ethical responsibilities. Two examples include the "do not resuscitate" policy and the advance directives policy
- To serve in an advisory capacity and/or as a resource for persons involved with a specific client to resolve ethical situations or make decisions related to the client's care
- To evaluate institutional experiences related to reviewing decisions having ethical implications

can bring issues to an ethics committee for formal review. Ethics committees contribute to the management of clients without disruption or interference with research and practice.

The establishment of ethics committees is an additional resource for clients and health care professionals. Nurses should not view ethics committees as the new "quick fix" to the many ethical dilemmas in the health care setting. It is still necessary for nurses to deal with ethical issues in an objective and systematic way. All options should be tried before seeking formal help from an ethics committee. The ethics committee holds promise for assisting clients, families, and health care professionals to make decisions related to health care. Bioethics committees should not be viewed as the answer for all problems, and they do not remove the hospital's responsibility for the care provided. In addition, ethics committees do not replace the client-physician decision making for health care provided.

The composition of an ethics committee should be multidisciplinary and include physicians, nurses, administrators, social workers, spiritual advisors, attorneys, and lay representatives. To be most effective, ethics committees should be a standing hospital and medical staff committee. Members appointed to it should be approved by the hospital's authority. When an ethical issue is presented to the committee the client's privacy and confidentiality must be respected and maintained. Names are eliminated from discussion. The committee uses a formal process for analyzing the ethical dilemma and making recommendations. The chairperson should report the activities of the committee to the president of the hospital and the president of the medical board on an annual basis. The JCAHO standards released for 1991 emphasize the importance of ethics committees in all health care institutions (JCAHO, 1991). Nurses have the responsibility to be knowledgeable about the existence of an ethics committee within the health care environment and about how to access committee members for assistance in ethical situations.

 ## SUMMARY

Ethics is the study of the standards for professional behavior related to "right" and "wrong" conduct. The nurse works in situations that have complex and sometimes conflicting problems related to client care. Ethical behavior develops from the values that nurses hold throughout their lives. Values are formed from observation and experience occurring from infancy through adulthood. Values are personal (morals) and professional (ethics).

Nurses practice ethically by following the codes of their profession. Nurses study and integrate the pri-

mary principles of respect for autonomy, beneficence, nonmaleficence and justice into their practice. The secondary principles of truth-telling (veracity), fidelity, and confidentiality are also studied and incorporated into practice. The responsible nurse maintains competency when practicing. The nurse is responsible to the client, physician, peer group, and employing institution.

In their daily work, nurses are placed in a variety of situations in which ethical questions arise. The nurse uses a systematic method to identify and attempt to resolve these problems. Ethical dilemmas are not easily resolved, and the decisions are difficult to make. When available, the nurse uses the ethics committee and other professionals as resources.

Key Concepts

- Technological advances in health care have created many types of ethical dilemmas.
- The nurse's role has become multifaceted, a situation that has increased the number and diversity of ethical dilemmas that a nurse encounters in practice.
- The special relationship between nurse and client is the foundation for nursing ethics.
- An ethical dilemma results from conflicts in values, causing uncertainty in decision making.
- Clients have the right to safe and effective nursing care.
- Experiences in nursing practice adapt personal values to professional values.
- The integration of personal and professional values assists the nurse in practicing nursing.
- A professional nursing code of ethics directs nurses' activities to champion clients assigned to their care.
- Professional nurses have a commitment to client, profession, employing institution, and society to provide high-quality care.
- An ethical nurse maintains skill competency and assumes responsibility for nursing care.
- Responsibility refers to the scope of function and duties a nurse is required to perform.
- A nurse is accountable when demonstrating a willingness to assume responsibility for nursing care.
- When nurses witness acts that may endanger clients, they are obligated to report them.
- The nurse establishes a methodical approach to resolving ethical dilemmas.
- The nurse evaluates all sides of the ethical dilemma before acting.
- The ethics committee is an excellent resource to help the nurse understand and support the care of the client.
- Advance directives are important to the ethical care of the client.

Key Terms

Accountability, p. 277

Autonomy, p. 279

Beneficence, p. 280

Confidentiality, p. 281

Ethics, p. 274

Euthanasia, p. 274

Fidelity, p. 281

Justice, p. 280

Living will, p. 280

Nonmaleficence, p. 280

Paternalism, p. 279

Responsibility, p.277

Triage, p. 281

Veracity, p. 281

Critical Thinking Exercises

1. Your basic or governing values influence your behavior. To determine your governing values, ask, "What do I really want?" Imagine your ideal self. How do you want to act, feel, and think? Examples of governing values include integrity, sincerity, and love of family. Identify three or four of your governing values and explain briefly what each means to you.

2. Compare and contrast a nurse's "accountability" with a nurse's "responsibility."

3. A woman with a husband, grown children, and grandchildren and who was a nurse at a local hospital indicates to other nurses and her husband that she did not want life-prolonging procedures administered unless she would be able to function as a relatively "normal" person. The woman has a stroke and is admitted to the hospital where she was employed. Routine treatment procedures did not produce the desired results. The family authorized treatment, which required use of a respirator and a feeding tube for a time after the procedure. The family was aware that without the treatment she had no hope of living; with the treatment the probabilities of recovery were fifty-fifty. The procedure was initiated. After several days it was clear that the procedure was not effective and the client would remain comatose. Some on the hospital staff believe once a treatment is initiated, it cannot be withdrawn. For this situation:
   a. State the ethical dilemma.
   b. Identify the elements that are not relevant to the resolution of the dilemma.
   c. Identify individuals who should participate in the resolution of the dilemma.
   d. State who should have the power to decide how this dilemma is resolved. List the reasons.
   e. State which ethical principles are involved. Explain. If there are more than one, contrast the relationships among them.

4. A 20-year-old person begins studies and training to become a registered nurse. The student plans marriage and a family. The student's training includes clinical practice rotations on each nursing division of a teaching hospital. The medicine division has a number of patients being treated for acquired immuno deficiency syndrome (AIDS). The student cares about people, including self and the family to be. The student wants to provide the best nursing care possible; yet this person is hesitant to care for patients with AIDS. For the preceding situation:
   a. State the ethical dilemma.
   b. Identify the elements that are not relevant to the resolution of the dilemma.
   c. Identify the individuals who should participate in the resolution of the dilemma.
   d. State who should have the power to decide how this dilemma is resolved. List the reasons.
   e. Identify which ethical principles are involved. Explain. If there are more than one, contrast the relationships among them.
   f. Determine what would you would say when asked to summarize the situation and present a recommendation; list the rationale for that position.

5. Based on your knowledge, describe a realistic situation that involves an ethical dilemma related to nursing practice. Then using the information in Table 13–1, critically assess the various aspects of the dilemma.

6. Give an example of a situation that you would refer to your ethics committee. Describe the assistance you expect from the committee.

REFERENCES

American Nurses Association: *Code for nurses with interpretive statements*, Kansas City, Mo, 1985, The Association.

Ashley B, O'Rourke K: *Health care ethics*, St Louis, 1978, The Catholic Hospital Association.

Curtin LL: The nurse as advocate: a philosophical foundation for nursing. In Chinn P, editor: *Ethical issues in nursing*, Rockville, Md, 1986, Brady.

Curtin LL, Flaherty MJ: *Nursing ethics: theories and pragmatics*, Norwalk, Conn, 1982, Appleton & Lange.

Davis A, Aroskar M. Perspectives on ethical-moral principles. In Davis A, Aroskar M, editors: *Ethical dilemmas in nursing practice*, ed 2, Norwalk, Conn, 1983, Appleton & Lange.

Flarey DL: Advanced directives: in search of self-determination, *JONA* 21(11):16, 1991.

Fowler M: Ethical decision making in clinical practice, *Nurs Clin North Am* 24(4):956, 1989.

Joint Commission on the Accreditation of Healthcare Organizations: *Accreditation manual for health care organizations*, Oakbrook Terrace, Ill, 1991, The Comission.

Omery A: Values, moral reasoning and ethics, *Nurs Clin North Am* 24(2):499, 1989.

Syby CA: Ethical dilemmas: a need for values clarification education, *CCQ* 7(1):1, 1984.

Uustal DB: *A consultant review of bioethical principles and theories*, presentation at a workshop, 1991.

ADDITIONAL READINGS

American Nurses Association: Code for nurses, *Am J Nurs* 50:196, 1950.

American Nurses Association: *Position statement on nursing and the patient self-determination act,* Kansas City, Mo, 1991, The Association.

Annas GJ: Rules for research in nursing homes, *N Engl J Med* 315:1157, 1986.

Applegate ML, Entrekin NM: *Teaching ethics in nursing,* New York, 1984, The National League for Nursing.

Aroskar MA: Anatomy of an ethical dilemma: the theory, *Am J Nurs* 80:658, 1980.

Aroskar MA: Anatomy of an ethical dilemma: the practice, *Am J Nurs* 80:661, 1980.

Aroskar MA: Nurses as decision makers: ethical dimensions, *Imprint* 32:29, 1985.

Bandman B: Option rights and subsistence rights. In Bandman EL, Bandman B, editors: *Bioethics and human rights,* Boston, 1978, Little, Brown.

Creighton H: *Law every nurse should know,* ed 5, Philadelphia, 1986, Saunders.

Creighton H: The maintenance of life: 1983-1985. II. *Nurs Manage* 17: 12, 1986.

Curtin LL: Ethical issues in nursing practice and nursing education. In National League for Nursing: *Ethical issues in nursing and nursing education,* New York, 1980, The League.

Edwards BJ, Haddad AM: How we help nurses handle questions of ethics, *RN* 50(9):14, 1987.

French DG: Ethics: nurse, am I going to live? *Nurs Manage* 15:43, 1984.

Fry S: Toward a theory of nursing ethics, *Adv Nurs Sci* 11(4):9, 1989.

Gilbert DA: The ethics of mandatory elder abuse reporting statutes, *ANS* 8:51, 1986.

Grady C: Ethical issues in providing nursing care to human immunodeficiency virus–infected populations, *Nurs Clin North Am* 24(2):523, 1989.

International Council of Nurses: *ICN code for nurses: ethical concepts applied to nursing,* Geneva, 1973, Imprimeries Populaires.

Kloosterman N et al: Statement on ethics in critical care research. I. *Focus Crit Care* 12(3):47, 1985.

Kloosterman N et al: Statement on ethics in critical care research. II. *Focus Crit Care* 12(4):58, 1985.

Lanik G, Webb AA: Ethical decision making for community health nurses, *J Community Health Nurs* 6(2):95, 1989.

MacMillan-Scattergood D: Ethical conflicts in a prospective payment home health environment, *Nurs Econ* 4(4):165, 1986.

O'Rourke KD: Ethics of research on human subjects, *Parameters* (publication of Saint Louis University) Spring-Summer 1986, p 16.

Parent BL: Moral, ethical, and legal aspects of infection control, *Am J Infect Control* 13:278, 1985.

Robinson A: Genetic screening's medical progress prompts ethical questions, *AORN J* 43(5):1137, 1986.

Scott RS: When it isn't life or death, *Am J Nurs* 85:19, 1985.

Smith SJ, Davis AJ: Ethical dilemmas: conflicts among rights, duties, and obligations, *Am J Nurs* 80:1463, 1980.

Steele SM: AIDS: clarifying values to close in on ethical questions, *Nurs Health Care* 7(5): 247, 1986.

Thompson JE, Thompson HO: Teaching ethics to nursing students, *Nurs Outlook* 37(2):84, 1989.

Viens DC: A history of nursing's code of ethics, *Nurs Outlook* 37(1):45, 1989.

Weeks LC et al: How can a hospital ethics committee help? *Am J Nurs* 89:651, 1989.

Yarling RR, McElmurry BJ: The moral foundation of nursing, *ANS* 8:63, 1986.

Younger SJ et al: Psychosocial and ethical implications of organ retrieval, *N Engl J Med* 313:321, 1985.

CHAPTER 14

Legal Issues

OBJECTIVES

Mastery of content in this chapter will enable the student to:
- Define the key terms listed.
- Explain legal concepts that apply to nurses.
- Describe the legal responsibilities and obligations of nurses.
- List sources for standards of care for nurses.
- Define legal aspects of nurse-client, nurse-physician, nurse-nurse, and nurse-employer relationships.
- Give examples of legal issues that arise in nursing practice.

CHAPTER OUTLINE

Legal Limits of Nursing
  Standards of care
  Licensure
  Student nurses

Legal Liability in Nursing
  Torts
  Malpractice

Legal Concepts and the Nurse-Client Relationship
  Assault
  Battery
  Invasion of privacy
  Informed consent
  Death and dying

Legal Safeguards and Nursing Practice
  Physician orders
  Short staffing
  "Floating"
  Incident reports
  Reporting obligations
  Good Samaritan laws
  Contracts
  Controlled substances

Legal Issues in Specialty Practice Areas
  Perinatal nursing
  Pediatric nursing
  Medical-surgical nursing
  Critical care units
  Psychiatric nursing
  Home health nursing
  Acquired immunodeficiency syndrome

Contemporary law is a composite of all of the rules and regulations by which society governs itself. Without law, society could not deal with disputes and problems in an orderly fashion. The laws of any society are flexible and ever changing through either legislative process or judicial decisions.

The law has many valuable functions when applied to nursing practice. It differentiates nursing practice from the practice of other health care professions. It also describes and protects the rights of clients and nurses. For these reasons, nurses should understand basic legal concepts as they relate to nursing practice.

Many nurses view the law with apprehension because they fear being named in a malpractice lawsuit. With increased emphasis on clients' rights, nurses today must understand their legal obligations and responsibilities to clients. Nurses who give competent care based on their education will seldom need to worry about a malpractice lawsuit.

The public is better informed than in the past about health and illness. Through reports in newspapers and magazines and on television, more information is available to consumers of health services. Many clients are knowledgeable about their rights, and nurses are challenged to become advocates for clients. In 1972 the American Hospital Association (AHA) developed and adopted a Patient's Bill of Rights. In 1974 the Dying Person's Bill of Rights was completed, and in 1975 the Pregnant Patient's Bill of Rights was written. Although these documents are not considered legally binding, many hospitals use them to provide guidelines for care.

 LEGAL LIMITS OF NURSING

Standards of Care

One of the functions of law, as applied to nursing practice, is to define the standards of care that nurses must provide. All U.S. state legislatures and Canadian provincial parliaments have passed nursing practice acts that define the scope of nursing practice in their particular state or province. These **nursing practice acts** set educational requirements for nurses, distinguish between nursing and medical practice, and generally define nursing practice. All nurses are responsible for knowing the provisions of the act for the state or province in which they work.

Professional organizations are another source for defining the scope of care. The American Nurses Association (ANA) and Canadian Nurses Association (CNA) have developed standards for nursing practice, policy statements, and similar resolutions. These standards are general and include recommendations such as the obligation of nursing service departments to provide continuing education programs.

The written policies and procedures of the employing institution detail how nurses are to perform their duties. Such policies are usually quite specific and are set down in procedure manuals in most nursing units. For example, a procedure policy outlining the steps that should be taken when changing a dressing or administering medication gives specific information about how nurses are to perform these tasks. These policies provide another definition of standards of care.

Standards of care concern nurses' accountability or obligations to account for their actions. General duty nurses are legally responsible for meeting the same standards as other general duty nurses in similar settings. However, specialized nurses such as nurse anesthetists, intensive care nurses, certified nurse-midwives, or operating room nurses are held to standards of care and skill exercised by those in the same specialty as defined by applicable standards. All nurses should know the standards of care they are expected to meet.

Standards of care are very important. **Standards of care** are guidelines by which nurses should practice. If nurses do not perform duties within accepted standards of care, they may place themselves in jeopardy of legal action. In a malpractice lawsuit, these standards are used to determine whether the nurse has acted as any reasonably prudent nurse with the same level of education and experience would act. Standards of care are thus guidelines for determining whether nurses performed duties in an appropriate manner. If nurses are named as defendants in a malpractice lawsuit and it is shown that neither the accepted standards of care outlined by the state or province nursing practice act nor the policies of the employing institution were followed, the nurses' legal liability is clear.

One of the first and most important cases to discuss a nurse's liability was *Darling v Charleston Community Memorial Hospital*. The case was decided by the Illinois Supreme Court in 1966, and it has been adopted in almost every state. It involved an 18-year-old man with a fractured leg. When the cast was applied to his leg, the physician placed insufficient padding under the plaster. The man's toes became swollen and discolored, and he had decreased sensation in them. He complained to the nursing staff many times. Although nurses recognized his symptoms as signs of impaired circulation, they failed to tell their supervisor that the physician did not respond to their calls or the client's needs. During the next 4 days, gangrene developed, and the man's leg had to be amputated. The physician in the emergency room was liable for incorrectly applying the cast. The nursing staff was also liable because they had not adhered to the standards of care appropriate to the client's symptoms.

Licensure

All registered nurses are licensed by the board of nursing of the state or province in which they practice. The requirements for licensure vary among states in the United States and provinces in Canada, but in most nurse licensing acts, requirements exist for education, and nurses must pass examinations. Licensure permits persons to offer special skills to the public, but it also provides legal guidelines for protection of the public. All states use the National Council Licensure Examinations (NCLEX) for registered nurse and licensed practical nurse examinations. Nurse licensing statutes usually require that nurses be 21 years of age, be citizens or have work permits, and exhibit good moral character.

A license can be suspended or revoked by the board of nursing if nurses' conduct violates provisions contained in the licensing statute. For example, nurses who perform illegal acts such as selling or taking controlled substances jeopardize their license status. Before licenses are revoked, nurses must be notified of the charges and permitted to attend hearings in which evidence can be presented on their behalf. These hearings are not court proceedings but are usually conducted by the state or provincial board of nursing. Some states and provinces provide for judicial review of such cases if nurses have exhausted all other forms of appeal.

Student Nurses

If a client suffers harm as a direct result of nursing students' actions or lack of action, the liability for the incorrect action is generally shared by the students, instructor, hospital or health care facility, and university or educational institution. Student nurses should never be assigned to tasks for which they are unprepared and should be carefully supervised by instructors as they learn new procedures. Although student nurses are not considered employees of the hospital, the institution has a responsibility to monitor the acts of nursing students. Student nurses are expected to perform as professional nurses would at that point in their experience. Faculty members are usually responsible for instructing and observing students, but in some situations, staff nurses may share these responsibilities. Every nursing school should provide clear definitions of responsibility.

Sometimes student nurses are employed as nursing assistants or nurse's aides when not attending classes. If student nurses are employed in this capacity, they should not perform tasks that do not appear in a job description for a nurse's aide or assistant. For example, even if a student has learned to administer intramuscular medications in class, this task may not be performed as a nurse's aide.

 LEGAL LIABILITY IN NURSING

Two basic sources exist for contemporary law. **Statutory law** is created by elected legislative bodies such as state or provincial legislatures, the U.S. Congress, administrative bodies such as state boards of nursing, or the Parliament of Canada. **Common law** is created by judicial decisions made in courts when cases are decided.

Civil law is concerned with relationships among people and the protection of a person's rights. Although violations of civil law might cause harm to an individual or property, no grave threat to society as a whole usually exists. For example, defamatory statements made about a person might lead to personal problems, but they do not threaten society in general.

Criminal law is concerned with relationships between individuals and governments and with acts that threaten society and its order. Misuse of controlled substances is an example of criminal conduct for nurses.

A **crime** is an offense against society that violates a law. Criminal acts are prosecuted in the criminal justice system. There are two classifications of crimes. A **felony** is a crime of a serious nature that carries a penalty of imprisonment for greater than 1 year or death. A **misdemeanor** is a crime of a less serious nature, and the penalty is usually a fine or imprisonment for less than a year. In nursing there are few crimes nurses would commit if they practiced within accepted standards of care. For the purpose of this chapter, flagrant criminal activity such as murder and illegally dispensing controlled substances will not be discussed. Laws pertaining to such offenses apply to nurses and all individuals.

Torts

A **tort** is a civil wrong committed against a person or property. Torts may be subtle. They may be classified as unintentional or intentional. Unintentional torts include negligence. An example of an unintentional tort, or negligence, is malpractice. Intentional torts are willful acts that violate another's rights. Examples are assault, battery, defamation, invasion of privacy, false imprisonment, and fraud.

Negligence

Negligence is conduct that falls below the standard of care. It is established by law for the protection of others against unreasonable risk of harm. It is characterized chiefly by inadvertence, thoughtlessness, or inattention.

If nurses give care that does not meet appropriate standards, they may be held liable for negligence. Negligence may involve carelessness such as not checking an armband and consequently administering the wrong medication. However, carelessness is not always the cause. If nurses perform procedures for which they have not been trained and do it carefully but still harm the client, a claim of negligence could be made.

Nurses have been involved in several common negligent acts. Such acts are also known as *malpractice*. Examples follow:
1. Intravenous therapy errors resulting in infiltrations or phlebitis
2. Burns to clients
3. Falls resulting in injuries to clients
4. Failure to use aseptic technique where required
5. Errors in sponge, instrument, or needle counts in surgical cases

Nurses are responsible for performing all procedures correctly and exercising professional judgment as they carry out physicians' orders and duties not ordered but for which they have authority. Any nurse who does not meet accepted standards of practice or care or who performs duties in a careless fashion runs a risk of being found negligent.

Malpractice

Malpractice is professional misconduct, unreasonable lack of skill or fidelity in professional duties, evil practice, or illegal or immoral conduct. In a malpractice lawsuit against a nurse, the following criteria must be established:
1. The nurse (defendant) owed a duty to the client (the plaintiff)
2. The nurse did not carry out that duty
3. The client was injured
4. The client's injury was a result of the nurse's failure to carry out the duty.

The best way for nurses to avoid being named in lawsuits is to follow standards of care, give competent health care, and develop empathetic rapport with clients. In addition, careful, complete, and objective documentation are keys to avoiding malpractice. Nurses must also keep current with the practice. They should know and follow the policies and procedures of the institution in which they work. Finally, nurses should be sensitive to the common sources of client injury, such as falls. Poor client relations is a leading cause of lawsuits. Clients who believe that nurses performed duties correctly and were concerned with their welfare are unlikely to initiate a lawsuit.

Malpractice Insurance

All nurses should consider purchasing insurance, even if the employing institution has coverage. Such insurance ensures that nurses are adequately protected in all aspects of professional practice because nurses employed by institutions may also practice in a noninstitutional setting (for example, assisting a neighbor or doing volunteer work). Because nurses are professionals, it is difficult, if not impossible, to separate the private person from the professional for purposes of limiting their exposure to suits for malpractice.

 ## LEGAL CONCEPTS AND THE NURSE-CLIENT RELATIONSHIP

The nurse deals with many people, including the client and family, physicians, other nurses, and other health care professionals, as well as the employing institution. In nurse-client interactions, several legal issues may arise. The Patient's Bill of Rights, adopted by the AHA, is a statement of guidelines related to nurse-client interaction (see box).

Assault

Assault is any willful attempt or threat to harm another, coupled with the ability to actually harm the other person. The victim believes harm will come as a result of the threat. Assault may be subtle; for example, a nurse might attempt to coerce a client into taking a drug. A more obvious example might involve a nurse handling an uncooperative client in the emergency room. If the exasperated nurse yells, "If you don't take off those filthy clothes, I'm going to rip them off you!" and moves toward the client, a claim of assault could be made.

Battery

Battery is any intentional touching of another's body or anything the person is touching or holding without consent. Injury is not a requirement. There have been instances of battery of confined clients in mental institutions. In a less drastic case, if a nurse attaches fetal electrodes during labor without the consent of the mother, a claim of battery could be made. The important issue is informed consent. In some situations consent is implied. For example, if a nurse says, "I have your injection for you, Mr. Jones," and he holds out his arm, he is giving implied consent to the injection.

It is unimportant whether the procedure that constitutes battery helps the client. In a classic case in 1905, *Mohr v Williams,* the client gave written consent for surgery on his right ear. After the client was anesthetized, the physician discovered that the left ear was more seriously affected, and he operated on the left ear. The client sued because surgery was performed on the "wrong" ear. Within the context of battery is the issue of informed consent, which will be discussed later.

Invasion of Privacy

Clients have claims for **invasion of privacy** when their private affairs, with which the public has no concern, have been publicized. Clients are entitled to confidential health care. All aspects of care should be free from unwanted publicity or exposure to public scrutiny. An example of invasion of privacy occurs when clients are unnecessarily exposed in the room or in corridors.

Another form of invasion of privacy is the release of information to an unauthorized person such as a member of the press or the client's employer. Gossiping about a client's activities is another form of invasion of privacy and could lead to a charge of slander against the nurse. Another example is a nurse's unwanted intrusion in private family matters. A nurse has no right to intrude in matters not directly related to the client's well-being. For example, a nurse should respect a wish not to inform the client's family of a terminal illness.

An individual's right to privacy may conflict with the public's right to information. For example, a threat or benefit to public health may override the individual's right to privacy. Disclosures of private information were made about individuals who had toxic shock syndrome and who were involved in the Tylenol poisoning cases. Sometimes the client is a public figure whose physical condition is considered newsworthy. There are also cases in which information is given out about a scientific discovery or a major medical breakthrough, as with the first heart transplant cases or the first artificial heart recipient. If an event falls into any of these categories, information should be channeled through the public relations department of the institution to ensure that invasion of privacy does not occur. The nurse should not attempt personally to decide the legality of disclosing information.

Defamation of Character

Defamation of character is the act of holding up of a person to ridicule, scorn, or contempt within the

Patient's Bill of Rights

1. The patient has the right to considerate and respectful care.
2. The patient has the right to obtain from his physician complete current information concerning his diagnosis, treatment, and prognosis in terms the patient can be reasonably expected to understand.
3. The patient has the right to receive from his physician information necessary to give informed consent prior to the start of any procedure and/or treatment. . . . Where medically significant alternatives for care or treatment exist, or when the patient requests information concerning medical alternatives, the patient has the right to such information (and) to know the name of the person responsible for the procedures and/or treatment.
4. The patient has the right to refuse treatment to the extent permitted by law, and to be informed of the medical consequences of his action.
5. The patient has the right to every consideration of his privacy concerning his own medical care program.
6. The patient has the right to expect that all communications and records pertaining to his care should be treated as confidential.
7. The patient has the right to expect that within its capacity a hospital must make reasonable response to the request of a patient for services.
8. The patient has the right to obtain information as to any relationship of his hospital to other health care and educational institutions insofar as his care is concerned (and) any professional relationships among individuals, by name, who are treating him.
9. The patient has the right to be advised if the hospital proposes to engage in or perform human experimentation affecting his care or treatment (and) has the right to refuse to participate.
10. The patient has the right to expect reasonable continuity of care.
11. The patient has the right to examine and receive an explanation of his bill regardless of source of payment.
12. The patient has the right to know what hospital rules and regulations apply to his conduct as a patient.

From American Hospital Association: *A patient's bill of rights,* Chicago, 1972, The Association.

community. There are two types of defamation: slander and libel. For example, if a nurse tells a client that his physician is incompetent, the nurse could be held liable for **slander** (defamation in the form of spoken words). The nurse who writes such a comment could be sued for **libel** (defamation in the form of written words). The important issue in a claim of defamation of character is whether harm is done to the reputation of the plaintiff.

Informed Consent

Informed consent is a person's agreement to allow something to happen (for example, surgery) based on a full disclosure of facts needed to make an intelligent decision (that is, knowledge of risks involved, benefits, alternatives, or consequences of refusal). The law has long recognized that individuals have the right to be free from bodily intrusion. In *Schloendorff v Society of New York Hospital,* decided in 1914, the court observed that "every human being of adult years and sound mind has a right to determine what shall be done with his body." The doctrine of informed consent not only requires that a person be given all relevant information required to reach a decision regarding treatment but also that the person be capable of understanding the relevant information and does in fact give consent. One who performs a procedure on a client without informed consent may be found civilly liable for committing battery.

A signed consent form is required for all routine treatment, hazardous procedures such as surgery, some treatment programs such as chemotherapy, and research. A client signs general consent forms when admitted. Separate, special consent forms must be signed by the client or a representative before specialized procedures are performed. The following factors must be verified for a consent to be valid:

1. The person must be mentally and physically competent and be legally an adult.
2. The consent must be given voluntarily. No forceful measures may be used to obtain it
3. The person giving consent must thoroughly understand the procedure, its risks and benefits, and alternative procedures.
4. The person giving consent must have the opportunity to have all questions answered satisfactorily.

If a client is deaf or has some other impediment in communication (such as speaking a foreign language), an interpreter should be available to explain the terms of consent. Fig. 14-1 is an example of a consent form for admission to the hospital.

THE CHILDREN'S MERCY HOSPITAL
Kansas City, Missouri

TERMS AND CONDITIONS OF ADMISSION

NECESSARY MEDICAL TREATMENT:
Recognizing the need for hospital care for the child whose name appears herein, consent is hereby given to The Children's Mercy Hospital for hospital services rendered under the general and specific instructions of the attending physician and treatment to be necessary for the safety, welfare and health of the child.

PROFESSIONAL CARE:
The patient is under the professional care of an attending physician who arranges for services for the care and treatment of the patient. The attending physician is usually selected by the patient's parent or guardian, but may when not designated or under emergency circumstances be otherwise selected.

RELEASE OF INFORMATION:
The Hospital is authorized to furnish information from the patient's medical record to any insurer, compensation carrier or welfare agency who may be providing financial assistance for hospital care.

PHOTOGRAPHS:
Photographs of the patient may be taken under the supervision of The Children's Mercy Hospital by members of the Staff or other persons for teaching, medical research purposes or for publicity as deemed proper by the Hospital and the taking of pictures, unless specifically denied in writing, shall not be deemed an invasion of privacy.

PERSONAL VALUABLES:
The Hospital shall not be liable for loss or damage to any personal property of the patient brought into The Children's Mercy Hospital.

PAYMENT FOR HOSPITAL CARE:
I/We do hereby assume financial responsibility for and agree to make payment in full to The Children's Mercy Hospital for all charges for services or medical supplies furnished the above patient. Payment is to be made within 30 days as bills are presented with settlement in full, or arrangements for same to be made in the Financial Counseling Department before departure of the patient.

I/We do certify that the financial information given is true, accurate and complete to the best of my/our knowledge, and further authorize The Children's Mercy Hospital to investigate any and all financial information given on this admission under their normal investigative procedures.

I/We do hereby assign and authorize payment directly to the above named Hospital and physician(s) of all hospitalization or insurance benefits and physician fee benefits and guarantee to pay any balance, with the understanding that the account is not settled or closed until after the insurance benefits are received by the Hospital and if there is a remaining balance I/we agree to pay the same. I/We are aware of the above contents.

I/We hereby certify that I/we have read all parts of this Admission Form and agree and accept all terms and conditions hereon and state that all representations made by me are true.

I am aware of the above contents.

A photocopy of this agreement shall be considered as valid and effective as the original.

SIGNED ADDRESS PHONE

RELATION TO PATIENT DATE

WITNESS DATE

SECOND WITNESS (TELEPHONE CONSENTS) DATE

Fig. 14-1 Sample consent form for admission to the hospital.
Courtesy The Children's Mercy Hospital, Kansas City, Mo.

Because nurses do not perform surgery or direct the medical procedure, obtaining client consent does not fall within the nursing duty. However, in many institutions the nurse assumes responsibility for confirming consent. When a nurse takes consent forms for clients to sign, the nurse should ask if they understand the procedures for which consent is being given. If clients deny understanding or the nurse suspects that they do not, the nurse is obligated to notify the physician or nursing supervisor and to make certain that clients are informed before signing. The court says that clients' right to self-determination gives them the right to clear information with which to make decisions for informed consent. Fig. 14-2 is a sample consent form for a special procedure that is similar to some consent forms for surgery. Possible complications are listed to make certain that the client understands them.

If a client participates in an experimental treatment program or submits to the use of experimental drugs or treatments, an even more detailed and stringently regulated informed consent form is used. The Federal Food and Drug Administration and the institutional review board review the information in the consent form for research involving human subjects. The client is always given the option of withdrawing from the experiment at any time.

A client refusing surgery or other medical treatment must be informed about any harmful consequences. If the client persists in refusing, the rejection should be written, signed, and witnessed.

Parents are usually the legal guardians of pediatric clients and therefore are the persons who must sign consent forms. Occasionally a parent or guardian refuses treatment for a child. In these cases the court may intervene on the child's behalf. The practice of making a child a ward of the court, administering necessary treatment, and then returning legal guardianship to the parents is relatively common in such cases. A nurse involved in such a case should inform the nursing supervisor, who will enlist the aid of the appropriate hospital administrator.

In some instances, obtaining informed consent is difficult. If the client is unconscious, for example, consent must be obtained from a person legally authorized to give consent on the client's behalf. If a person has been declared legally incompetent in a judicial proceeding, consent must be obtained from the person's legal guardian. In emergency situations, if it is impossible to obtain consent from the client or an authorized person, the procedure required to benefit the client (or perhaps save a life) may be undertaken without liability for failure to obtain consent. In those instances, the law presumes the client would wish to be treated.

Death and Dying

Many legal issues surround the events of death, including a basic definition of the actual point at which a person is considered dead. The literature agrees that death occurs when there is an absence of brain function, despite function of other body organs. One reason for the development of this definition is to facilitate recovery of organs for transplantation. This definition is also useful when there is a question of whether to continue life support. Nurses must be aware of legal definitions of death because they must document all events that occur when the client is in their care.

Ethical (see Chapter 13) and legal questions are raised by the issue of **euthanasia.** Active euthanasia (intentionally administering a lethal dose of morphine to a client to cause death, for example) is defined as intentional homicide. The less well-defined area of passive euthanasia, such as removing breathing support or withholding a blood transfusion from a terminally ill client with irreversible brain damage, raises legal questions that are being dealt with by the courts.

In other situations involving death, nurses have specific legal duties. For example, nurses have the legal obligation to treat a deceased person's remains with dignity. Consent for an autopsy must be given by the decedent (before death) or a close family member. Laws in many states and provinces give an order of priority for family members who may give consent for autopsy. Autopsies are required in circumstances, such as death resulting from an accident or suspected child abuse or other criminal activity.

Handling of Bodies

Nurses are legally obligated to treat a deceased person's remains with dignity and care (see Chapter 28). Wrongful handling could cause emotional harm to the survivors. In one case, for example, survivors sued when a mislabeling of bodies led to an Orthodox Jew's body being prepared for a Roman Catholic funeral and a Roman Catholic's body being prepared for a Jewish burial.

Autopsy

Consent for autopsy must be given by the decedent (before death) or a close family member. Laws in many states and provinces give an order of priority for family members who may give consent. For an adult male, for example, his wife, then his children, and then any other family member may give consent.

INFORMED CONSENT FOR AMNIOCENTESIS

I. I hereby request and authorize Doctor ______________ to perform a diagnostic amniocentesis (pass a needle through the abdominal wall and withdraw some of the amniotic fluid). I further request that an attempt be made to perform the following test(s) on my unborn child:

A. Chromosome analysis ________ (Initial)
B. Alpha-fetoprotein ________ (Initial)
C. Acetylcholinesterase (If indicated) ________ (Initial)
D. ______________ ________ (Initial)

II. I consent to the performance of an ultrasound examination for the purpose of dating the pregnancy, locating the placenta and selecting a site for placement of the needle.

III. I understand that:

A. the procedure of amniocentesis involves a small risk to both mother and fetus and that these risks include; discomfort at the site where the needle was inserted, cramping, bloody spotting, leakage of amniotic fluid, intrauterine infection and miscarriage.

B. there is a possibility that growing the fetal cells may not be successful and that repeat amniocentesis would then be required.

C. although the liklihood of an error is considered to be extremely small, a complete and correct diagnosis of the condition of the fetus based on the test(s) performed cannot be guaranteed.

D. the results provided of normal chromosomes or normal biochemical status of the fetus does not eliminate the possibility that the child may have birth defects and/or mental retardation because of other disorders.

E. in the case of twins, the results may apply to only one of the pair.

F. in some Rh negative mothers Rh sensitization has occurred following amniocentesis.

IV. I have had my questions answered and understand and accept the risks and limitations of this test.

Signed: ______________________ (Patient)
______________________ (Spouse)
______________________ (Witness)
Date: ______________

Fig. 14-2 Sample consent form for a special procedure.
Courtesy The Children's Mercy Hospital, Kansas City, Mo.

Autopsies may resolve legal and medical questions and are required in certain circumstances such as death resulting from suspected child abuse or other criminal activity. Sometimes an autopsy consent stipulates exclusions (such as no studies involving the brain). As with any consent, the physician should not use coercion to obtain consent for autopsy.

Organ Donation

Legally competent persons are free to donate their bodies or organs for medical use. Consent forms are available for this purpose. In many states, adults may sign the back of their driver's licenses. A nurse may serve as a witness when individuals wish to give consent for the donation of organs or the body.

In most states, required request laws stipulate that, at the time of a person's death, a qualified health care giver must ask family members to consider organ or tissue donation. In the past, this option has not been offered to the family. Required request laws came about because of the shortage of suitable organs for transplantation.

The Uniform Anatomical Gift Acts address many problems of organ donation and stipulates that the physician who certifies death shall not be involved in removal or transplant of organs. The National Organ Transplantation Act prohibits selling or purchasing organs and facilitates this area of medical and nursing practice. Organ and tissue donation remains voluntary. Consent forms are available for this purpose. A nurse may serve as a witness when a person wishes to give consent for a donation.

Living Wills and Health Care Surrogates

In light of the attention being given to the rights of the terminally ill and people in a persistently vegetative (permanently comatose) state, the nurse may find that many clients have living wills or health care surrogates. If they do not, they may ask the nurse to provide information about them. The federal government has recently passed the Patient Determination Act. This act requires health care institutions to provide information about advance directives such as living wills. The nurse should be familiar with the institution's policies complying with the Act.

Living wills are documents instructing physicians to withhold or withdraw life-sustaining procedures in clients whose death is imminent. The procedures are considered to prolong the dying process rather than promote life.

Each state providing for living wills has its own requirements for executing them, but generally two witnesses, neither of whom can be a relative or doctor, are needed when the client signs the document. Many states are passing such laws.

Health care surrogate statutes are sometimes also referred to as *durable powers of attorney*. Clients execute these documents to appoint someone to make health care decisions if and when the time comes when they are no longer able to make decisions on their own behalf.

 ## LEGAL SAFEGUARDS AND NURSING PRACTICE

In addition to encountering legal problems in the care of clients, nurses may share liability for errors made by physicians and other health care personnel or for inadequate care provided by the employing institution.

Physician Orders

The physician is responsible for directing medical treatment. Nurses are obligated to follow physicians' orders unless they believe the orders are in error or would be detrimental to clients. Therefore all orders must be assessed, and if one is determined to be erroneous or harmful, further clarification from the physician is necessary. If the physician confirms the order and the nurse still believes that it is inappropriate, the supervising nurse should be informed. A written memorandum to the supervisor detailing the events in chronological order and the reasons for refusing to carry out the order should protect the nurse from any disciplinary action. The supervising nurse should help resolve the questionable order. A nurse carrying out an inaccurate order may be legally responsible for any harm suffered by the client.

The physician should write all orders, and the nurse must make sure that they are transcribed correctly. Verbal orders are not recommended because they leave possibilities for error. If a verbal order is necessary (during an emergency, for example), it should be written and signed by the physician as soon as possible, usually within 24 hours.

A difficult area regarding physician orders involves an order of "no code" or "do not resuscitate" (DNR) for a terminally ill client. Many physicians are reluctant to write such orders because they fear legal repercussions for "abandoning" a client. If a physician has documented in progress notes that the client's condition is deteriorating and that the decison not to administer cardiopulmonary resuscitation has been made, the physician is perfectly justified in writing a no code order. Unless the physician decides that such a discussion would be detrimental to the client's condition, the order should be discussed with the client. In such cases, the physician should also discuss the order with the family. A no code order should be written, not given verbally. Physicians should regularly review DNR orders in case the client's condition warrants a change.

According to guidelines adopted by the American Heart Association, cardiopulmonary resuscitation is not intended for use when a client has an irreversible illness in which death is expected (Cushing, 1981). Partial code or "slow code" verbal instructions have occasionally been suggested as a way for a physician to avoid writing a no code order. *Slow code* may be defined differently by various institutions but usually means resuscitative procedures should be performed more slowly than recommended by the American Heart Association. These codes are not recommended, however, because they may be interpreted as not performing resuscitative procedures as a competent person would and may therefore be the basis for a lawsuit.

Short Staffing

During nursing shortages, the issue of inadequate staffing may arise. The Joint Commission for the Accreditation of Healthcare Organizations (JCAHO) requires institutions to have guidelines for determining the number (staffing ratios) of nurses required to give care to a specific number of clients. Legal problems may arise if there are not enough nurses to provide competent care. If assigned to care for more clients than is reasonable, nurses should attempt to reject assignments by informing the nursing supervisor that they are inappropriate. If nurse are required to accept assignments, they should make written protests to nursing administrators. Although these protests would not relieve nurses of responsibility if a client suffered because of inattention, it would show that they were attempting to act in good faith. Nurses should not walk out when staffing is inadequate because charges of abandonment could be made.

"Floating"

Nurses are sometimes required to "float" from the area in which they normally practice to other nursing units. In one case, a nurse in obstetrics was assigned to an emergency room. A client entered the emergency room and complained of chest pain. The client was given a markedly increased dosage of lidocaine by the obstetrical nurse and died after suffering irreversible brain damage and cardiac arrest. The nurse lost the malpractice lawsuit against her.

Nurses who float should inform the supervisor of any lack of experience in caring for the types of clients on the new nursing unit. They should also request and be given orientation to the unit.

Incident Reports

An **incident report** is filed when something arises that could or did cause injury and that was not consistent with good care. For example, if a nurse administers an incorrect dose of medication, a client falls out of bed, or an intravenous solution infiltrates the skin causing sloughing and scar formation, the nurse should complete an incident report. Most institutions provide specific forms for this purpose. The nurse records all of the details of the incident, and the physician examines the client and indicates adverse effects caused by the error (Fig. 14-3 on p. 300).

Many nurses are reluctant to file incident reports because they believe these reports harm their employment records. Actually, incident reports are used by institutions' administrations for quality assurance and risk management. By reviewing incident reports, administrators can determine areas of client risk. For example, if a certain kind of problem has occurred repeatedly such as pressure ulcers, educational methods can be used to prevent the problem in the future. In addition, the insurance carrier for a hospital or other institution relies on incident reports to assess liability and possible future claims. Incident reports supplement quality assurance programs to ensure provision of high-quality care. With this system, several steps are taken to identify and correct problems that could compromise care. Incident reports are not mentioned in the chart because they cannot be used in a court of law. However, the nurse is advised to check the appropriate state law.

Incident reports are the tools used by risk managers. Risk management is a system of ensuring appropriate nursing care. Steps involved in risk management include identifying possible risks, analyzing them, acting to reduce them, and evaluating steps taken. One tool used in risk management is an incident report.

For nurses in practice, the underlying rationale for quality assurance and risk management programs is the highest possible quality of care. Some insurance companies, medical and nursing organizations, and the JCAHO require the use of quality assurance and risk management procedures.

Reporting Obligations

In some situations, nurses are required to report certain communicable diseases or criminal activities, such as abuse, gunshot wounds, attempted suicide, or rape, to the appropriate authority. For example, most states require health care professionals to report suspicions of child abuse. Because cases that must be reported vary among states and provinces, the nurse should be familiar with appropriate statutes.

The Children's Mercy Hospital
INCIDENT REPORT
An incident is any happening which is not consistent with routine operation of the hospital or care of a particular patient. It may be an accident or a situation which might result in an accident.

Person(s) involved ______

Complete as applicable if possible injury:

- ☐ Patient → ☐ Inpatient ☐ Outpatient — Diagnosis ______ Age ______ Who was supervising patient? ______
- ☐ Employee → Department ______ Job title ______ Length of time on job ______ Age ______ Home phone ______
- ☐ Other → Home address & phone ______ Reason for being at hospital ______

Exact location of incident ______ Date of incident ______ Time ______

Names & addresses of witnesses ______

INCIDENT FACTS ______

(Use reverse side if necessary.)

Was person involved seen by CMH physician because of incident?
☐ No ☐ Yes Date ______ Time ______

Signature of person reporting ______ Date written ______

PHYSICIAN'S STATEMENT (Clinical information on patients must ALSO be charted.)
Description of any injury ______
Treatment given or recommended ______
If employee involved, when is return to work permitted? ______
Signature of physician ______ Date ______ Time ______

If patient, parent, or nursing personnel involved, send to Nursing Supervisor. Send all others to Administration.

The Children's Mercy Hospital
INCIDENT REPORT

INCIDENT FACTS (continued from reverse side) ______

DO NOT WRITE BELOW THIS LINE

Incident report number ______
Reviewers and dates of review
______ / / ______ / /
______ / / ______ / /
______ / / ______ / /

Fig. 14-3 Sample incident report.
Courtesy The Children's Mercy Hospital, Kansas City, Mo.

Good Samaritan Laws

Good Samaritan laws have been enacted in almost every state and province to encourage health care professionals to assist in emergency situations. These laws limit liability and offer legal immunity for people helping in an emergency, providing they give reasonable care. If a nurse stops at the scene of an automobile accident and gives appropriate emergency care (for example, using caution when moving the injured person in case there is a spinal injury or applying pressure to stop hemorrhage), the nurse is acting within accepted standards, even though proper equipment was not available.

Contracts

A contract is a written or oral agreement between two people in which goods or services are exchanged. An oral contract is as legally binding as a written one but may be more difficult to prove. A breach of contract occurs if either party fails to carry out agreed obligations.

By accepting a job, a nurse enters into an agreement with an employer. The nurse will perform professional duties competently, adhering to the policies and procedures of the institution. In return, the employer not only pays for the nurse's services but also furnishes facilities and equipment in proper working order to enable the nurse to provide efficient and competent care.

Nurses also enter into contractural agreements with clients. Nurses agree to give competent care, and clients agree to pay for the services. When clients sign admission forms when entering the hospital or agree to nursing care in any health care agency, they initiated the contract. Private duty nurses have specific written contracts with their clients. It is from such contracts that the duty to perform competently arises and the failure for which leads to the concept of negligence.

Controlled Substances

Another legal issue that might arise for nurses involves the use of controlled substances. In 1970 the

Comprehensive Drug Abuse Prevention and Control Act was passed in the United States. It covers substances such as narcotics, depressants, stimulants, and hallucinogens. The act regulates hospital distribution systems, rehabilitation programs for drug abuse, and research into the medical treatment of addiction. Canadian law similarly regulates controlled substances. Nurses may administer controlled substances only under the direction of a licensed physician.

Controlled substances should be kept securely locked, and only authorized personnel should have access to them. Criminal penalties exist for misuse of controlled substances. There have been cases in which physicians illegally prescribed and dispensed controlled substances, and if nurses employed by such physicians fail to report these activities, they are legally accountable for aiding and abetting the physicians.

 ## LEGAL ISSUES IN SPECIALTY PRACTICE AREAS

Many possible legal liabilities exist in all areas of nursing practice. Any nurse working in a specialized field should study the legal issues pertaining to that area of practice. Space does not permit a complete discussion of all legal liabilities, but a few issues involved in some practice areas are discussed in the following sections.

Perinatal Nursing

Perinatal nursing involves care of women before, during, and immediately after pregnancy, as well as care of newborn. Many legal issues are involved in the care of a mother and her infant.

Some of the ethical issues involved in contraceptive counseling are discussed in Chapter 13. From a legal standpoint, persons receiving sexual counseling or treatment for venereal disease have a right to privacy and confidentiality. However, some states have passed laws requiring that parents of minors be informed if a minor seeks contraceptive information or treatment for venereal disease or if a minor girl becomes pregnant.

Infertility of couples desiring to have children may pose legal questions that usually arise from the solution that they choose. One solution is the artificial insemination of a woman with sperm from a donor other than her husband. Because of the potential legal problems, the mother, her husband, and the donor must give written consent to the procedure. Preferably the husband and wife are not told the identity of the donor and vice versa.

Another solution to the problem of infertility is the use of a "surrogate mother." The husband donates sperm to be artificially inseminated into a woman who is not his wife. The woman bears the child and then relinquishes it to the husband and wife. Legal questions arise if the surrogate mother receives monetary compensation because this might be defined as illegal "baby selling". Kentucky has equated mother-surrogate arrangements to the sale of infants and has made the practice illegal in that state. Legal problems may also occur if the surrogate mother changes her mind and wants to keep the baby. The highly publicized Stern-Whitehead Baby M case in New Jersey illustrates some of the legal problems inherent in the practice of using surrogate mothers. Some philosophers describe the use of commercial mother surrogates (in which the woman is paid for her services) as exploitative of women and dehumanizing to infants.

Abortion is one of the most emotionally charged issues confronting perinatal nurses. After the U.S. Supreme Court ruling on *Roe v Wade* in 1973, which legalized abortion, two conflicting groups formed, those who support the woman's right to make decisions about her own body and those who support the fetus' right to life. Legal decisions, including other Supreme Court cases, continue the debate. For example, in *Webster v Reproductive Health Services* in 1989, the Supreme Court declared as unconstitutional the provision in a Missouri statute that required that all second-trimester abortions be performed in a hospital. In the *City of Akron v Akron Center for Reproductive Health, Inc.,* a similar provision was declared unconstitutional. Provisions dealing with parental consent, 24-hour waiting periods for informed consent, and disposal of fetal remains were also declared unconstitutional in this case. More recent cases have held the requirement of parental notification to be constitutional. Spousal notification remains unconstitutional.

In most states and provinces, laws concerning abortion include provisions known as *conscience clauses*. These clauses allow nurses, physicians, and institutions to refuse to assist in abortions without fear of reprisal if abortion is against their ethical, moral, or religious principles. If nurses are ethically or morally opposed to assisting in abortions, they should exercise the right provided by conscience clauses. However, the nurses should never impose their values on clients (see Chapter 12).

Nurses have legal responsibilities regarding fetal monitoring during labor (Wiley, 1976). A claim of battery may be made if nurses do not obtain consent before attaching monitor leads. They are also responsible for recognizing abnormal monitor patterns. If they note signs of fetal distress, they must notify the physician and nursing supervisor and prepare for emergency treatment such as a cesarean section.

There are legal requirements in providing nursing care for newborns, such as properly identifying the infant-mother pair as soon as possible with fingerprints, footprints, and wrist bands, or obtaining a blood sample for phenylketonuria (PKU) testing when required by law. Standards of practice include providing a clear airway, clamping the umbilical cord, applying antibiotics or silver nitrate to the eyes, and minimizing stress by drying and keeping the infant warm. Resuscitation equipment must be in the delivery room. When a stillborn infant is delivered, the nurse must record all events about the delivery. Although the atmosphere in a delivery room is disquieting, the nurse must complete legal requirements by careful documentation.

When an infant requiring intensive care is born, the nurse has many legal responsibilities similar to those in other intensive care settings. Ethical problems involved in removing infants from ventilatory support are discussed in Chapter 13.

An important legal issue that has surfaced in neonatal practice has surrounded "Baby Doe Regulations." The original 1982 case involved an infant born in Indiana with Down syndrome complicated by esophageal atresia. The infant's parents refused permission for surgical repair of the defect, and the infant died. An ongoing debate began, with court decisions and federal statutes regulating the treatment of handicapped infants. Most authorities agree that a compromise supporting the rights of disabled infants yet not imposing governmental interference on parents and physician decisions is necessary. In a 1986 Supreme Court ruling, *Bowen v American Hospital Association,* the court ruled that the Rehabilitation Act did not apply to Baby Doe situations.

The most recent Baby Doe legislation, The Child Abuse and Neglect Amendment of 1984, was passed by the U.S. Congress. This legislation requires states to establish programs that would respond to any reports of medical neglect, including possible withholding of medical treatment from handicapped infants with life-threatening conditions. This law does not mandate that all disabled infants be treated but promotes parent and physician decision making in these cases. Many medical centers use "ethics committees" to help the decision-making process.

Iatrogenic disease in a critically ill infant in a neonatal intensive care unit (NICU) may have legal consequences for those involved in the infant's care. An iatrogenic disease results from treatment administered. For example, retrolental fibroplasia, a form of blindness caused by too much oxygen, is an iatrogenic disease. Frequent monitoring of the inspired oxygen concentration and frequent blood gas deter-

minations are standards of care that must be met by nurses working in an NICU.

Pediatric Nursing

Every state and province with child abuse legislation requires that suspected child abuse or neglect be reported. Health care professionals such as nurses are mandated to report suspected cases. To encourage reports of suspected cases, states and provinces provide legal immunity for the reporter if the report is made in good faith and without malice. Health care professionals who do *not* report suspected child abuse or neglect may be liable for civil or criminal legal action.

As in all areas of nursing practice, negligence involving pediatric clients is possible. A $450,000 settlement was awarded in a New York case, *Beardsley v Wyoming County Community Hospital,* in 1981; a 6-year-old boy was taken to the hospital after a sledding accident. Although his prognosis was good after a splenectomy, the nurses administered D_5W as his only intravenous fluid instead of alternating it with isotonic saline solution as ordered. Brain damage occurred, and although the boy's condition improved during the next 10 mo, he had permanent residual damage. The monetary award was large because the boy had lost future earnings because of the negligent acts, which did not meet appropriate standards of care.

Pediatric nurses are responsible for preventing children in their care from accidentally harming themselves. Cribs, which sometimes have a restraining device over the top, are designed to keep infants and toddlers from climbing out of bed and injuring themselves. All poisonous substances and sharp objects should be kept out of the reach of children. Children should be kept under constant surveillance to minimize opportunities for accidental harm.

Medical-Surgical Nursing

As in the case of pediatric clients, disoriented adults may require some form of restraint to prevent accidental self-injury. Standards of care, laws, and regulations about the use of restraints and supervision apply to nursing practice with medical-surgical and other clients. Side rails are available on most hospital beds for adult clients. Some disoriented older adults may also require belt restraints to prevent them from falling out of bed. If clients fall out of bed and injure themselves, they may bring a lawsuit against the nurses and institution.

Critical Care Units

Nurses working in critical care settings are also legally accountable for performing their duties. Critical care nurses require additional training and ongoing in-service education to provide them with information about advances in care methods.

The staffing ratio in an intensive care setting should be one nurse for each client or at most 1:2½, depending on the severity of clients' conditions. The JCAHO recommends these ratios because of the intensity of care required by such clients. These clients usually require careful observation and assessment of their conditions and many treatment procedures and medications. If a nurse is assigned to three or four intensive care clients and is unable to give appropriate care and a client suffers harm, the nurse is liable for accepting the client assignment.

Possible legal problems for critical care nurses are associated with the use of electronic monitoring devices. No monitor can be considered totally reliable, and the nurse must not completely depend on it. There may also be electrical hazards. The equipment should be checked routinely by engineers to ensure that a client will not receive an electrical shock.

Psychiatric Nursing

The primary purpose for hospitalizing clients with mental illnesses is rehabilitation so that they may return to society as useful and healthy citizens. Current principles of treatment suggest that mentally ill clients should be given as much freedom as possible. One problem arising from this freedom is the possibility that clients will slip away, or elope. If the nurse fails to prevent client elopement, the nurse and employer would be held liable for any injuries that clients sustain or inflict as a result of the elopement.

Another concern is the possibility of client suicide. If history and medical records indicate suicidal tendencies, the client must be kept under supervision.

Home Health Nursing

An evolving trend in nursing is an increased provision of nursing services in the home. Although community nursing programs have existed for years, the model of nursing care in the home has expanded to include more hours per day, up to full-time, 24-hour care. Many hospitals are dismissing clients with more complex problems requiring sophisticated physical care such as those who need continuous intravenous therapy or those with increased oxygen requirements, including ventilatory support.

Nurses functioning in this area of practice must provide reasonable care within guidelines and standards of care governing home health care (see Chapter 5). Legal exposure exists in this area of practice, as in more traditional settings, and nurses should review their need for malpractice insurance.

Acquired Immunodeficiency Syndrome

The mention of acquired immunodeficiency syndrome (AIDS) causes fear and panic in many members of society. This lethal disease is found in clients in virtually every segment of nursing practice, from AIDS victims on medical-surgical units, to mothers and infants in perinatal units, to young children with hemophilia in pediatric settings.

Legal questions surround this disease in relation to the civil liberties of the victim. An example is whether clients with AIDS have the right to withhold information about the diagnosis from the family members who will care for them. Rights of the individual versus protection of public health are debated. In the future, new laws enacted by the legislature and many court cases addressing this problem will arise. The nurse should treat all clients as if they could be infected. Thus gloves must to be worn when handling blood and other bodily fluids (see Chapter 18). Gowns, masks, and protective eyewear should also be worn when appropriate.

Currently, the federal government is considering whether health care workers should disclose to clients that they are HIV positive. At least two court cases have found a compelling need for physicians to disclose their HIV status to the hospitals in which they work and to their clients.

 SUMMARY

There are many legal issues confronting practicing nurses today, but nurses should view the law not with apprehension but as a helpful adjunct to defining nursing practice. Nurses aware of legal rights and obligations are better prepared to care for clients.

Nursing standards of care delineate and define appropriate nursing care. Some standards are stated in general terms such as those enacted in nursing practice acts and those provided by professional nursing organizations. More specific standards are defined by the employing institution. If nurses act within the accepted standards of care, their chances of being involved in a malpractice lawsuit are reduced.

Some legal issues, such as the necessity for informed consent and avoiding negligence, are involved in almost every branch of nursing. Issues are confined to specific areas, such as conscience clauses for perinatal nurses asked to assist in abortions. However, regardless of the situation, nurses are responsible for knowing the laws that apply to their areas of nursing practice.

Key Concepts

- With increased emphasis on client rights, nurses in practice today must understand their legal obligations and responsibilities to clients.

- The civil law system is concerned with the protection of a person's private rights, and the criminal law system deals with the rights of individuals and society as defined by legislative statutes.

- Under the law, practicing nurses must follow standards of care, which originate in nurse practice acts, the guidelines of professional organizations, and the written policies and procedures of employing institutions.

- Registered nurses and licensed practical nurses are licensed by the state or province in which they practice; licensing is based on educational requirements, the passing of an examination, and other criteria.

- Student nurses are expected to perform as professional nurses, should be assigned only to tasks for which they are prepared, and should be carefully supervised.

- Nurses are responsible for performing all procedures correctly and exercising professional judgment as they carry out physician orders. Otherwise they may be liable for negligence.

- All clients are entitled to confidential health care and freedom from unauthorized release of information. Otherwise nurses may be liable for invasion of privacy, slander, or libel.

- Nurses should act and speak carefully to avoid frightening, coercing, or physically intimidating clients (assault).

- Informed consent allows physical procedures to be carried out in a lawful manner, without fear of battery.

- A nurse can be found liable for malpractice if the following criteria are established: the nurse (defendant) owed a duty to the client (plaintiff), the nurse did not carry out that duty, the client was injured, and the nurse's failure to carry out the duty caused the client's injury.

- Nurses are responsible for confirming that informed consent has been given for any surgery or other medical procedure before the procedure is performed.

- In emergency situations, informed consent is not necessary if it is impossible to obtain consent from the client or an authorized person.

- Legal issues involving death include documenting all events surrounding the death, treating a deceased person with dignity (wrongful handling is grounds for a lawsuit), and obtaining consent for an autopsy from the decedent (before death) or a close family member (after death).

- A competent adult can legally give consent to donate specific organs, and nurses may serve as witnesses to this decision.
- Nurses are obligated to follow physicians' orders unless they believe the orders are in error or could be detrimental to clients.
- Staffing standards have been set for the ratio of nurses to clients, and if the nurse is required to care for more clients than is reasonable, a formal protest should be made to the nursing administration.
- Nurses must file incident reports in all situations when someone could or did get hurt. These reports are also used for quality assurance and risk management.
- Depending on state and province laws, nurses are required to report possible criminal activities such as child abuse, gunshot wounds, attempted suicide, rape, and certain communicable diseases.
- Conscience clauses in most states and provinces allow any health care professional or institution to refuse to assist in abortions without fear of reprisal if it is against ethical, moral, or religious principles.
- Nurses practicing in specialized areas such as critical care are legally accountable for performing specialized duties and therefore require additional training and ongoing in-service education.
- All nurses should know the laws that apply to their area of practice.

Key Terms

Assault, p. 294

Battery, p. 294

Civil law, p. 293

Common law, p. 293

Crime, p. 293

Criminal law, p. 295

Defamation of character, p. 295

Euthanasia, p. 297

Felony, p. 293

Incident report, p. 299

Informed concent, p. 296

Invasion of privacy, p. 295

Libel, p. 296

Living wills, p. 298

Malpractice, p. 294

Misdemeanor, p. 293

Negligence, p. 294

Nursing practice acts, p. 292

Slander, p. 296

Standards of care, p. 292

Statutory law, p. 293

Tort, p. 293

Critical Thinking Exercises

1. Nurse Smith is enroute to the hospital to begin his shift. On the way, he is flagged down by his next door neighbor. The woman stated that her 2-year-old son was in the bathtub, during which time she ran down the street to get a carton of cigarettes. When she returned from the store, he was floating face down in the tub. She pulled him out, but he did not begin breathing. She asked Nurse Smith to help her. Nurse Smith told her to call the ambulance, and he began CPR, when he realized he did not carry private malpractice insurance. He continued CPR until the ambulance arrived. The ambulance transported the child to the nearest emergency department, where he was pronounced dead on arrival. The childs mother sued Nurse Smith for malpractice after the child welfare workers cited her for neglect, due to Nurse Smith's "hotline" call to the State Department of Children and Family Services.
   a. Was Nurse Smith obligated to stop and render assistance?
   b. Did Nurse Smith have a legal obligation to report the woman to the State Department of Children and Family Services? What was that legal obligation?
   c. Does Nurse Smith have any legal protection from the lawsuit, since he carried no private malpractice insurance? Explain.

2. Mrs. Lee has leukemia and has been hospitalized for acute and extreme anemia. She is married and has two young daughters. The physician has ordered blood transfusions to assist Mrs. Lee over her crisis. Unfortunately, Mrs. Lee's religion prohibits her from receiving blood transfusions. The husband has stated that, although he does not share her religion, he will concur with her wishes. Without the transfusion, Mrs. Lee will die. The physician has told you that he will declare a medical emergency and order you to initiate the transfusions as soon as Mrs. Lee slips into a coma from lack of oxygen. He has told you that if you do not comply, he will report you to the nursing supervisor and make sure that you are fired.
   a. What risks do you face if you administer the transfusion?
   b. What should you do?
   c. Would your answer change if this woman was admitted in a coma and there was no information regarding her wishes concerning blood transfusions?

3. Mr. Andrews is an 80-year-old man, was admitted for gallbladder surgery. He is recuperating. On the day that the physician allows him to walk down the hall with assistance, he asks you to help him do so. Mr. Andrews has on antiembolism hose, and he has slippers in the closet in his room. You get Mr. Andrews out of bed and assist him in his walking down the hall, which has newly-buffed linoleum floor. You forget to put on his slippers, although you knew about them. While walking down the hall, you turn to look at a very good-looking resident who has just begun to make rounds for the morning. As you are looking around, Mr. Andrew's foot slips out from under him, and he falls to the floor, breaking his hip. Identify the elements of negligence and use this scenario to apply those elements.

4. Mr. Jones is a 30-year-old man who has just been admitted with a suspicious pneumonia. He and his wife are in the hospital room while you and the physician are taking the history. The physician asks the client if he has engaged in any risky behavior that may have contributed to his pneumonia. He says "No." After the physician leaves the room, the wife asks you to step outside. She tells you that her husband is an intravenous drug abuser and that he was diagnosed as having the AIDS virus 2 weeks earlier at a different hospital in another city. You are asked not to reveal this information to anyone in the hospital—not even the physician (the client's symptoms are all consistent with AIDS). You tell the wife that you must tell this information to the physician, and you do so. The husband learns of this, and he checks himself out of the hospital against medical advice. He tells you that he is going to the Medical Center across town and that none of his clients information should be given to the Medical Center. The

physician tells you to call the Medical Center and tell them that Mr. Jones is on his way. Ten minutes later, the admitting physician at the Medical Center calls to ask you about Mr. Jones (The physician who saw the client at your hospital has left for a medical conference and cannot be reached.) You tell the physician the client's history.

   a. Has there been a breach of patient confidentiality?

   b. Are there any exceptions to the rule that would provide protection for the nurse?

   c. Should the nurse have divulged this confidential information, or should someone else have done this? Who?

REFERENCES

Beardsley v Wyoming County Community Hospital, 435 NYS 2d 862, 1981.

Bowen v American Hospital Association, 106 S Ct 2101, 1986.

City of Akron v Akron Reproductive Health, 462 U.S. 416 (1983).

Cushing M: Verbal no-code orders, *Am J Nurs* 81:1215, 1981.

Darling v Charleston Community Memorial Hospital, 33 Ill2d 326, 1966.

Mohr v Williams, 95 Minn 261, 1905.

National Organ Transplant Act, Public Law 98-507, Oct 19, 1984.

Roe v Wade, 410, U.S. 113 (1973).

Schloendorff v Society of New York Hospital, 211 NY 125, 1914.

Webster v Reproductive Health Services, U.S.L.W. 5023, July 3, 1989.

Wiley J: The nurse's legal responsibility in obstetric monitoring, *JOGNN* 5(suppl):77s, 1976.

ADDITIONAL READINGS

AIDS symposium, *J Hosp Law* 21(10):249, 1988.

American Hospital Association: *Required request legislation: a guide for hospitals in organ and tissue donation,* Chicago, 1988, The Association.

Anderson GC et al: Living wills: do nurses and physicians have them? *Am J Nurs* 86:271, 1986.

Annas GJ: Contracts to bear a child: compassion or commercialism? *Harvey Lect* 11(2):23, 1981.

Annas GJ: The baby broker boom, *Hastings Cent Rep* 16(3):30, 1986.

Arbeiter J: A buyer's guide to malpractice insurance, *RN* 49:22, 1986.

The basis for the right of committed patients to refuse psychotropic medication, *J Health Hosp Law* 22(6):176, 1989.

Black HC: *Black's law dictionary,* ed 5, St Paul, Minn, 1979, West.

Callahan D: How technology is reframing the abortion debate, *Hastings Cent Rep* 16(1):33, 1986.

Creighton H: *Law every nurse should know,* ed 5, Philadelphia, 1986, Saunders.

Cruzan et al v Director, Missouri Department of Health, III L ed 2 224,1990.

Cushing M: *Nursing jurisprudence,* Norwalk, Conn, 1988, Appleton & Lange.

Estate of William Beringer, M.D. v Medical Center of Princeton, docket no. L88-2550 (Sup Ct NJ), 1991.

Fenner K: *Ethics and law in nursing: professional perspectives,* New York, 1980, Van Nostrand Reinhold.

Feutz SA: Professional liability insurance. In Northrop CE, Kelly ME: *Legal issues in nursing,* St Louis, 1987, Mosby–Year Book.

Fiesta J: *The law and liability for nurses,* ed 2, New York, 1988, Wiley.

Fost N: Putting hospitals on notice, *Hasting Cent Rep* 12(4):5, 1982.

Goff v St. Luke's Hospital in Kansas City, Mo, MO 748 SW 2d 557, 1989.

Harris C: Legal and ethical issues. In Bobak IM, Jensen MD, Zolar MK, editors: *Maternity and gynecologic care: the nurse and the family,* ed 4, St Louis, 1989, Mosby–Year Book.

Hemelt MD, Mackert ME: *Dynamics of law in nursing and health care,* ed 2, Reston, Va, 1982, Reston.

Horsley JE: Short-staffing means increased liability for you, *RN* 44:73, 1981.

In Re Application of the Milton S. Hershey Medical Center, PA Super Ct No 361, Harrisburg, 1991.

In Re Schiller, 148 NJ Super 168, 1977.

Kreitzer M: Legal aspects of child abuse: guidelines for the nurse, *Nurs Clin North Am* 16(1):149, 1981.

Levine C et al: AIDS: public health and civil liberties, *Hastings Cent Rep* 16(6):9, 1986.

Moskop JC, Saldanha RL: The Baby Doe rule: still a threat, *Hastings Cent Rep* 16(2):8, 1986.

Ney CA: Living wills: the ethical dimemmas, *Crit Care Nurse* 9(8):20, 1989.

Northrop CE, Kelly ME: *Legal issues in nursing* St Louis, 1987, Mosby–Year Book.

Orlikoff J, Vanagunas AM: *Malpractice prevention and liability control for hospitals,* ed 2, Chicago, 1988, American Hospital Publishing.

Prosser W, Keeton W: *Prosser and Keeton on the law of torts,* ed 5, St Paul, Minn, 1988, West.

Regan WA: Nursing malpractice: a giant leap in damages, *RN* 44:69, 1981.

Rhodes A: *Nursing and the law,* ed 3, Rockville, Md, 1984, Aspen.

Rocereto LR, Maleski CM: *The legal dimensions of nursing practice,* New York, 1982, Springer.

Rothman DA, Rothman NL: *The professional nurse and the law,* Boston, 1977, Little, Brown.

Scott DJ: Withholding consent for medical care of a child: the ultimate parental decision, *J Health Hosp Law* 23:3, 1990.

Stark JL et al: Attitudes affecting organ donation in the intensive care unit, *Heart Lung* 13:400, 1984.

Weil WB: The Baby Doe regulations: another view of change, *Hastings Cent Rep* 16(2):12, 1986.

Whalen ER: Informed consent: the opinions of critical care nurses, *Heart Lung* 13:662, 1984.

Withdrawal of nutrition and hydration symposium, I. *J Health Hosp Law* 23(8):225, 1990.

Younger SJ: Do-not-resuscitate orders: no longer secret, but still a problem, *Hastings Cent Rep* 17(1):17, 1987.

CHAPTER 15

Communication

OBJECTIVES

Mastery of content in this chapter will enable the student to:
- Define the key terms listed.
- Describe differences between the three levels of communication.
- Identify characteristics of verbal and nonverbal communication.
- Discuss the functions of communication in the nurse-client relationship.
- Explain the role of communication in the nursing process.
- Describe each element of the communication process.
- Identify factors that promote and inhibit communication.
- Give examples of techniques that promote therapeutic communication.
- List and discuss the phases of a therapeutic helping relationship.
- Explain the dimensions of a helping relationship.
- Discuss nursing care measures for clients with communication alterations.

CHAPTER OUTLINE

Levels of Communication

Elements of the Communication Process
Referent or stimulus
Sender
Message
Channels
Receiver
Feedback

Modes of Communication
Verbal communication
Nonverbal communication

Factors Influencing Communication
Development
Perceptions
Values
Emotions
Sociocultural background
Gender

Knowledge
Roles and relationships
Environment
Space and territoriality

Therapeutic Communication
Social interaction
Caring and methods of effective communication
Barriers to effective communication

Helping Relationships
Dimensions of helping relationships
Phases of a helping relationship

Communication and the Nursing Process
Assessment
Nursing diagnosis
Planning
Implementation
Evaluation

Communication is the basic element of human interactions that allows people to establish, maintain, and improve contacts with others. Because communicating is something persons do every day, they often mistakenly think it is simple. However, communication is a complex and multifaceted process that involves behaviors and relationships and allows individuals to associate with others and the world around them. It is an ongoing, dynamic series of events in which meaning is generated and transmitted.

Communication refers to nonverbal and verbal behavior within a social context and includes all symbols and clues used by persons in giving and receiving meaning (Satir, 1983). An instructor's descriptions, a student's question, or a nurse's gestures create responses in those who observe, listen, and interact. Communication refers not only to content but also to feelings and emotions that people may convey in a relationship. A nurse listening to an anguished husband whose wife has died is an example of communication. Therefore not only does communication convey information but it also influences a relationship; it is an act of sharing.

Nursing is based on establishing a caring and helping relationship. Many theoretical systems for nursing are based on this interpersonal process. Nursing theorists emphasize communication as an integral part of the unique function of nursing (Severtsen, 1990; Lindberg, Hunter, Kruszewski, 1990). Sarvimaki (1988) describes nursing as communicative interaction and believes that the foundation of nursing lies in the "communicative attitude." This attitude is manifested in the striving for mutual understanding, coordination, and coaction. Instead of striving for control over clients by manipulating them to behave in specific ways or by defining success as setting and meeting predetermined, definite goals, communicative interaction emphasizes clients as cosubjects and is oriented at reaching a shared understanding.

A critical component of nursing practice is the ability to communicate effectively. A nurse uses a wide range of communication techniques with clients. Fritz et al (1984) point out several advantages to nurses who use effective communication skills. They help generate trust between the nurse and clients, prevent legal problems in practice, and provide the nurse with professional satisfaction. Communication is also a means for bringing about change. The nurse listens, speaks, and acts to negotiate change that promotes clients' well-being. Communication is also the foundation of the relationship between the nurse and other members of the health team. For example, the quality of the communication between the nurse and physician influences the outcome of client care. Knaus et al (1986) discovered that the lowest death rates in hospitals were related to interaction between the nurse and physician and the resulting coordinated response to the clients' needs rather than to administrative structure, specialization, or teaching status. Therefore poor working relationships and failure to communicate can lead to serious problems for the nurse and clients and can threaten the nurse's professional credibility. The process of communication cannot be simply memorized and put into practice. It is complex and requires a persistent and conscious application of principles.

LEVELS OF COMMUNICATION

Communication occurs at the intrapersonal, interpersonal, and public levels. **Intrapersonal communication** occurs within an individual. It is self-talk or an internal dialogue that occurs constantly and consciously. The goal of intrapersonal communication is self-awareness, which is influenced by self-concept and feelings of self-worth. Positive self-concept and self-awareness that come through internal dialogue can help nurses express themselves appropriately to others. For example, when a nurse walks into the client's room and thinks, "He looks uncomfortable. I'd better turn him on his side," the communication is intrapersonal.

Interpersonal communication is the interaction that occurs between two people or in a small group. It is often face-to-face and is the type most frequently used in nursing situations. Individuals communicating are continuously aware of one another. Healthy interpersonal communication allows problem solving, sharing of ideas, decision making, and personal growth. In nursing, there are many situations that challenge interpersonal communication skills. Each encounter with a client, such as collecting a blood specimen or taking a medical history, requires exchange of information. Meetings with staff members, physicians, social workers, and therapists test the nurse's communication skills with people who may have different opinions and experiences. Being a member of a nursing committee challenges the nurse's ability to express ideas clearly and decisively. Interpersonal communication is the heart of nursing practice. A nurse can help a client by communicating at a meaningful interpersonal level.

Public communication is interaction with large groups of people. Giving a lecture to a roomful of students and speaking to a consumer group on health education are examples of public communication.

Being a competent communicator with an audience requires the ability to envision oneself speaking to a group. Special platform skills such as use of posture, body movements, and tone of voice help a person express a point.

ELEMENTS OF THE COMMUNICATION PROCESS

Examination of the components of the communication process helps a person understand communication. A model can simply and graphically demonstrate complex processes, but it can also oversimplify. A model provides the nursing student with a framework for observing, understanding, and predicting what occurs as two people communicate.

A communication model must incorporate several principles. Communication is complex, involving many verbal and nonverbal symbols and messages exchanged between persons. Communication is a process. After a client and nurse begin to communicate, each subsequent message or thought has its base in what was said before (Fritz et al, 1984). Messages may be sent intentionally or unintentionally. Often, a person conveys messages about personality or attitude without being aware of it. Communication is a response between two or more persons as they send and receive stimuli or messages.

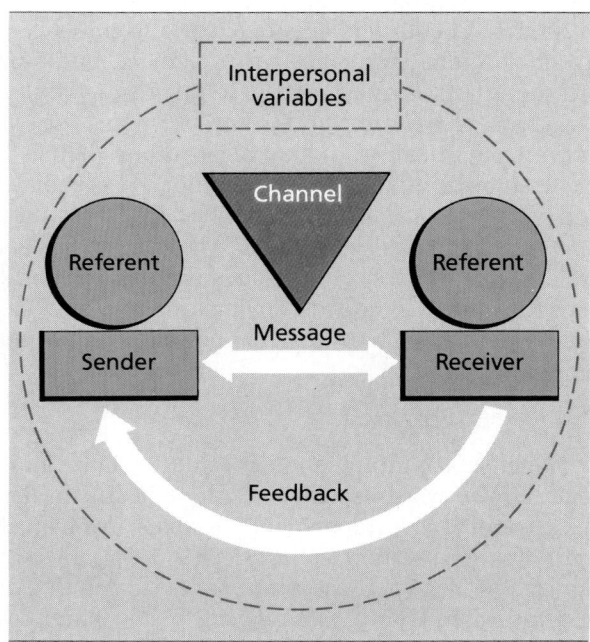

Fig. 15-1 Communication as an active process between sender and receiver.

Communication occurs on a social level, with participants engaged in intrapersonal and interpersonal contact. The process is dynamic, with the meaning of messages negotiated by participants. During communication, the person may or may not be aware of each element of communication (Fig. 15-1). During casual conversation participants do not bother to analyze the meaning of every gesture or word. For example, a person may become quite animated, using hands to express an idea without consciously thinking, "I'll wave my hand to stress this point." The nurse, however, learns to be conscious of each element of the communication process. In this way, the nurse can interact effectively with clients and remain aware of communication's effect on them. Because of the of the interaction between sender and receiver involved in communication, the model tends to oversimplify a complex process. However, each element is crucial. Information and meaning can be gained or lost if any element is altered.

Referent

The **referent** or stimulus motivates a person to communicate with another. It may be an object, experience, emotion, idea, or act. Individuals who consciously consider the referent during intrapersonal interaction can carefully develop and organize messages.

Sender

The **sender,** also called the *encoder,* is the person who initiates the interpersonal communication or message. The sender puts the referent such as an idea into a form that can be transmitted and assumes responsibility for the accuracy of the content and the emotional tone of the message. The role of sender may switch back and forth between participants at any time when information is transmitted.

Message

The **message** is the information that is sent or expressed by the sender. The most effective message is clear and organized and is expressed in a manner familiar to the person receiving it. An appropriate amount of information must be given, and the receiver must be ready to hear the message. For example, professional jargon (technical terminology used by health care providers) needs to be reserved for interactions between professionals and not between nurses and clients. Likewise, teaching would be inappropriate if nurses tried to teach the client everything in one sitting or teach the client to manage a colostomy when the client is not willing to look at the stoma. The message may comprise verbal and nonverbal language symbols (for example, spoken words, facial expressions, or gestures). Unfortunately, not all symbols have universal meaning; therefore difficulties in communication may occur with the message if the sender is not aware of this factor and does not seek clarification.

Channels

The message is sent along a channel of communication. **Channels** are means of conveying messages, such as through visual, auditory, and tactile senses. The sender's facial expression visually conveys a message. The spoken word travels via auditory channels. Placing a hand on an individual while communicating uses the channel of touch. Generally, the more channels the nurse uses to send a message, the better the client will understand it. For example, when attempting to relieve pain, the nurse verbalizes concern, expresses a sense of compassion, and repositions the client gently to lessen the pain.

Receiver

The **receiver,** also called the *decoder,* is the person to whom the message is sent. For communication to be effective, the receiver must perceive or become aware of the message. The message from the sender then acts as one of the receiver's referents. It prompts the receiver to decode and respond to the sender's message. The nurse learns to engage in intrapersonal communication to analyze and interpret the client's comments. Ideally, the sender's intention is perceived by the receiver. There is no guarantee that this will occur because words and symbols have multiple meanings. However, the more that the sender and receiver have in common, the more likely that the sender's meaning will be communicated.

Feedback

Communication is an ongoing process. The receiver returns a message to the sender. This **feedback** helps to reveal whether the meaning of the message is received. Mere intent to communicate is insufficient to ensure that a message is accurately received. The receiver's verbal and nonverbal response sends feedback to the sender to reveal the receiver's understanding of the message. To be effective, the two must be sensitive and open to each other's message, clarify the message, and modify behavior accordingly. In a social relationship, both persons involved assume equal responsibility for seeking openness and clarification, whereas the nurse assumes major responsibility in the nurse-client relationship.

 MODES OF COMMUNICATION

People send messages in the verbal and nonverbal modes, which are closely bound together during interpersonal interaction. As we speak, we express ourselves through movements, tone of voice, facial expressions, and general appearance. These modes can convey the same or different messages. The nurse who learns skills of communication masters techniques of each mode.

Verbal Communication

Verbal communication involves spoken or written words. Words are tools or symbols used to express ideas or feelings, arouse emotional responses, or describe objects, observations, memories, or inferences. They may also be used to convey hidden meanings, test the other's interest or degree of concern, or express hostility, or fear. *Language* is defined as the words, their pronounciation, and the method of combining them that is used and understood by a community (Boyle, Andrews, 1989). Language is a code that conveys meaning. A single word can change the meaning of a phrase or sentence. Language is effective only when each person communicating understands the message clearly.

A nurse encounters clients of various cultures who speak different languages. Also, some clients speak the same language as the nurse but use subcultural variations of certain words. For example, the word *dinner* may mean a midday meal to one person and the last meal of the day to another. These dialects and subdialects confuse meaning. Consequently, a nurse often works with clients who speak the same language but interpret messages differently from the way the nurse intended. To make a message clear, the nurse uses effective verbal communication techniques.

Clarity and Brevity

Effective communication is simple, short, and direct. Fewer words spoken result in less confusion. Because of the intrapersonal variables involved, human communication is imprecise in many ways. Vague phrases such as *you know* add little to clarity of a message. Clarity is achieved by speaking slowly and enunciating clearly. Using examples can make an explanation easier to understand. For instance, instructing a client with arthritis about self-care measures at home is more meaningful when the nurse provides specific examples, including demonstrations to reinforce the verbal message.

Repeating important parts of a message also makes communication clearer. The receiver should know the what, why, how, when, who, and where of ideas communicated.

Brevity is best achieved by using words that express an idea simply. "Tell me where your pain is" is better than "I would like you to describe for me the location of your discomfort." A simple, clear phrase communicates more effectively.

Vocabulary

Communication is unsuccessful if the receiver is unable to translate the sender's words and phrases. In nursing and medicine, there are many technical terms and jargon. If the nurse uses these terms, the client may become confused and unable to follow instructions or learn important information. Rather than telling the client, "Sit up while your lungs are auscultated," it might be better to say, "Sit up while I listen to your lungs." The first statement might make the client feel anxious. A message spoken in terms the client understands makes communication more effective.

Denotative and Connotative Meaning

A single word can have several meanings. A **denotative** meaning is one shared by individuals who use a common language. For example, the word *baseball* has the same meaning for all individuals who speak English, and the word *code* denotes cardiac arrest to nurses. The denotative meaning is used to define a word so that it means the same to everyone.

The **connotative** meaning of a word is the thoughts, feelings, or ideas that people have about the word (Duldt et al, 1984). Using the word *serious* to describe conditions may suggest to families that clients are close to death, but nurses may not consider them to be near death unless the word *critical* is used. Connotations are shades or interpretations of a word's meaning rather than different definitions.

When nurses communicate with clients, they carefully select words that cannot be easily misinterpreted. This is important when explaining conditions, therapies, or purposes of therapies.

Pacing

Verbal communication is more successful when expressed at an appropriate speed or pace. Talking rapidly, using awkward pauses, or speaking too slowly and deliberately can convey an unintended message. In the following example, the nurse uses awkward pauses during an explanation to a client:

Client: Do you know if the doctor found anything wrong?
Nurse: No (pause), but I'm sure if he did (longer pause) he would have come to explain things to you. (then very rapidly) Now let's get back to where we were.

Long pauses and rapid shifts to another subject may give the client the impression that the truth is being hidden. Also, speed and pace of speech varies, depending on geographical location.

The speed with which a message is verbalized, in addition to the presence, absence, and length of pauses, can determine the degree to which communication satisfies the listener. The nurse should not talk so quickly that words are unclear. Pauses should be used to accentuate or stress a particular point, giving the listener time to hear and comprehend the meaning of words. Proper pacing is achieved by thinking about what to say before saying it. Looking for nonverbal cues from the listener that might suggest confusion or misunderstanding is also useful. A person can also ask a listener if the pace is too fast or too slow or if the message needs repeating.

Timing and Relevance

Timing is critical to reception of a message. If the boss is in a bad mood, the time is wrong to ask for a raise. If a client is crying in pain, the time is wrong to explain the risks of surgery. Even though a message is clearly and concisely stated, poor timing can prevent it from being accurately received. Therefore the nurse must be sensitive to the appropriate time for discussions. Often the best time for interaction is when a client expresses an interest in communicating. By asking a simple question such as, "Would you like to talk about your surgery?" the nurse can avoid wasting time and energy if the client does not.

A person is more likely to communicate when a message is important. For example, when a client is facing open-heart surgery the next day, a discussion of the risks of cigarette smoking has less relevance than a review of preoperative procedures. An explanation of the side effects of birth control pills is relevant to the young woman who has received her first prescription for the medication. Verbal communication is more likely to have an impact when messages pertain to an individual's interests and needs.

Humor

Humor can be a powerful tool in promoting well-being. The phrase, "laughter is the best medicine," applies when nurses use humor to help clients adjust to stress imposed by illness. Dugan (1989) notes that laughter helps relieve stress-related tension and pain, increases the nurse's effectiveness in providing emotional support to clients, and humanizes the experience of illness. Laughter serves as a psychological and physical release. Studies have shown that humor stimulates the production of catecholamines and hormones that enhance feelings of well-being, improve pain tolerance, reduce anxiety, facilitate respiratory relaxation, and enhance metabolism (Sullivan, Deane, 1988; Williams, 1986).

Nurses can appropriately use humor in conversations with clients by telling jokes, sharing humorous incidents or situations, and using puns. A client who has become fearful or tense over events related to hospitalization can relax and become more open to interaction as a result of humor. When withdrawn because of emotional grief, the client can release emotional tensions through humor. Sullivan and Deane (1988) have found clients to be more self-disclosing and willing to share concerns of deeper significance.

Humor, is not always appropriate, however (for example, after the death of a loved one). Nurses need to be cautious in using humor to mask their own fears and discomforts or their inability to communicate with clients. Humor therefore should not become the only means of communication, but it can be an effective approach in helping clients to interact more openly and honestly.

Nonverbal Communication

Actions often speak louder than words. **Nonverbal communication** is transmission of messages without the use of words. It is one of the most powerful ways people convey messages to others. We continuously communicate nonverbally in every face-to-face encounter. Gestures impart meanings that are more significant than words. Ekman (1965) describes the ways in which nonverbal communication and verbal communication are interrelated. Nonverbal cues add meaning to the verbal message (Table 15-1).

A nurse needs to be aware of verbal and nonverbal messages sent to clients. Even the phrase, "Good morning, how are you?" can convey a number of meanings. A verbal message should be reinforced or complemented by nonverbal cues. Clients may sense a lack of trust or anxiety when a mismatch exists between a nurse's verbal and nonverbal messages.

During assessment, the nurse observes clients' verbal and nonverbal messages. Clients who say that they feel fine but grimace with movement are communicating two different messages. Becoming a good observer of nonverbal behavior requires time and practice. The nurse who perceives nonverbal messages is better able to understand clients, detect changes in conditions, and determine nursing care needs.

TABLE 15-1 Relationships Between Verbal and Nonverbal Communication	
Relationship	Example
Repeating—verbal and nonverbal cues saying the same thing but in different ways	When a mother describes how tall her son is, she also holds her hands at a distance above the floor equal to the child's height.
Contradicting—verbal and nonverbal cues conveying different messages	The nurse tells the client that obtaining a blood specimen "won't hurt a bit," but her sarcastic grin delivers a different message.
Complementing—nonverbal messages adding to verbal messages.	A client says she is afraid to be admitted to the hospital, and her anxious expression and trembling hands leave little doubt of her fear.
Accenting—nonverbal cues emphasizing verbal messages	A wave of the hand while saying hellow accentuates the word spoken.
Relating and regulating—nonverbal cues indicating when to begin or stop talking	A client who continually opens and closes her mouth briefly as her physician is talking is seeking an opportunity to speak.
Substituting—a nonverbal cue being used instead of words	A person nods vigorously to show approval of another's decision.

Metacommunication

Communication depends not only on the message but also on the relationship of the speaker to the other person. This is **metacommunication**. Satir (1983) defined *metacommunication* as "a comment on the literal content and nature of the relationship between the person involved." It is a message within a message that conveys the sender's attitude toward the self and the message and the attitudes, feelings, and intentions toward the listener. Metacommunication can be verbal or nonverbal. Verbal metacommunication is usually an explicit statement on how to decode a message (for example, "That's an order" or "I was only kidding"). Nonverbal metacommunication is more implicit and therefore may show genuine feelings or may be an attempt to hide feelings (for example, smiling when angry).

Personal Appearance

The general impression formed of another person influences the response to that person (Zunin, 1988).

A person's appearance is one of the first things noticed during an interpersonal encounter. People form an impression about another person within 20 seconds to 4 minutes. This impression is based 84% on appearance (Lalli-Ascosi, 1990). Physical characteristics, dress, grooming, and the presence of jewelry and adornment provide clues to the person's physical well-being, personality, social status, occupation, religion, culture, and self-concept. Paying attention to one's appearance can contribute to positive self-image and professional image.

Clothing, cosmetics, and jewelry that are not part of a professional uniform represent a personal choice and are taken as clues to the way people want others to respond to them. The way that a person dresses can also influence behavior. Knapp (1978) notes that clothes fulfill functions of decoration, protection (psychological and physical), sexual attraction, self-assertion, group identity, and role display.

Nurses can help clients maintain a sense of worth by allowing them to wear their own clothes if possible or if not contraindicated by treatment regimens. Hospital gowns are drab and ill fitting. Personal clothes give a sense of physical recovery and mental alertness.

Physical characteristics, such as the condition of hair, color of skin, weight, energy level, and presence of a physical deformity, also communicate information about the level of health. There are no established standards for physical characteristics that demonstrate good health. Each individual displays combinations of physical characteristics. The nurse remains alert for changes in physical appearance because they can be significant signs of disease.

Physical appearance often leads to impressions about personality and self-concept. Unfortunately, stereotyped views regarding the "perfect body" also influence the image of a person's body. Nurses should assess the importance of physical appearance to a client threatened with loss of body parts or function. They also need to consider their own views and values about body image.

The nurse's physical appearance influences the client's perception of care received. Each client has a preconceived image of a nurse. The traditional white uniform can be a symbol of purity and cleanliness. Although the uniform is not a reflection of abilities, it may become more difficult to establish a sense of trust and reliability if the nurse fails to meet the client's image. A professional nurse today wears uniforms, scrubsuits, and laboratory coats, as well as street clothes, to perform duties. A neat, well-tailored look conveys the message of a competent professional. Conversely, a nurse who has bad breath or cigarette breath, "messy" hair, poorly manicured nails, or dirty shoes, for example, will be considered unprofessional and may be taken less seriously than a nurse who has paid attention to these details of personal appearance.

Intonation

The tone of a speaker's voice can have a dramatic impact on a message's meaning. Depending on intonation, the simple question, "How are you?" can express enthusiasm, concern, indifference, and even annoyance. A person's emotions can directly influence tone of voice. Often this effect is unconscious, and the words send one message while the tone conveys the opposite. The nurse must be aware of emotions when interacting with clients. Intention to convey sincere interest in a client's welfare can be blocked if the nurse's tone of voice gives a different mood or meaning. Clients may question credibility if a nurse's voice is not sincere and pleasing. Voice tone can be a cue to a client's emotional state. Fear, anger, and grief can be expressed through intonation and pitch. Similarly, tone may indicate a client's energy level. A rested, alert person usually has a voice full of variations and inflections in tone and rapidity, whereas a fatigued person tends to talk in a mumbled monotone with incomplete sentences (Duldt et al, 1984).

Facial Expression

The face is rich in communication potential. A mutual glance or meeting of eyes between two people set the tone for an interpersonal encounter. The face and eyes send overt and subtle cues that assist in interpretation of messages. Studies show that the face reveals six primary emotions: surprise, fear, anger, disgust, happiness, and sadness (Knapp, 1978). Facial expressions often become the basis for important interpersonal judgments. Because of diversity in facial expressions, their meanings may be difficult to judge. The face may reveal genuine emotions or contradict true emotions, or facial expressions may be suppressed. Often people are unaware of the messages that their expressions convey. Providing clear feedback helps lessen confusion created by conflicting messages and expressions. When facial expressions fail to reveal clear messages, the receiver should seek verbal feedback to be sure of the speaker's intent.

For example, nurses are frequently watched by clients. Consider the impact of a nurse's facial expression on a client who asks, "Am I going to die?" The slightest change of expression can reveal the nurse's true feelings. It is difficult to control all facial expressions, but the nurse learns to be aware of what they can reveal. For example, when caring for a debilitated or deformed client, the nurse should avoid expressions of disgust.

Eye contact is an important facial expression. Wide eyes are associated with frankness, terror, and naiveté; downward glances reflect modesty or shyness. Raised upper eyelids reveal displeasure, and a stare is often associated with hatred and coldness. When two people confront each other, eye contact often prefaces a message. Initiating eye contact shows a willingness to communicate. Persons who maintain eye contact during a conversation are perceived as believable. Maintaining eye contact allows a person to become a good observer. It has been suggested that the level at which eye contact occurs significantly influences communication. The nurse should avoid looking down at a client during a discussion. One way this can be avoided is to sit down. The nurse appears less dominant and threatening sitting near the client at the same eye level (Fig 15-2).

Posture and Gait

The way that people stand and move is a visible form of self-expression. Posture and gait reflect attitudes, emotions, self-concept, and physical wellness. Leaning forward or toward a person conveys attention to that person. Leaning backward in a more relaxed manner shows less interest and caution.

An erect posture and a quick, purposeful gait communicate a sense of well-being and assuredness. A slumped posture and a slow, shuffling gait may indicate depression or discomfort. A bent-over posture may be a protective response to physical disease and injury. Nurses can collect useful information by observing clients' posture and gait. Specific illnesses cause identifiable gaits such as the shuffle of parkin-

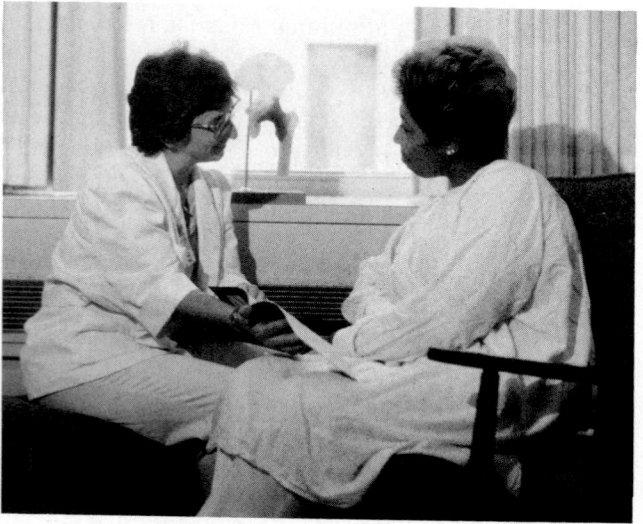

Fig. 15-2 Holding a client's hand or gently touching a client is useful in therapeutic communication.

sonism. Gait may be altered by many physical factors such as pain, drugs, or fractures.

Gestures

A wave of the hand, a salute, and shifting of feet are gestures. They are visual italics, which emphasize, punctuate, and clarify the spoken word. Duldt et al (1984) identify three functions of gestures: illustrating an idea, expressing an emotional state, and signaling by use of a sign. Gestures alone may reveal specific meanings, or with other communication cues, they may send messages.

Gestures are used to illustrate an idea that is difficult or inconvenient to describe in words. Pointing to an area of pain may be more accurate than describing the pain's location. Gestures may be used to convey emotions about the self or others. Covering the eyes, touching a part of the face, or pointing an accusing finger can reveal inner feelings.

Touch

Touch is a personal form of nonverbal communication. Persons engaged in communication must be close to each other when touch is used. Because touch is more spontaneous than verbal communication, it generally seems more authentic. Various messages, such as affection, emotional support, encouragement, tenderness, and personal attention, are conveyed through touch (Fig. 15-3). Touch is an important part of the nurse-client relationship, but it must be used with discrimination because strong social norms govern its use. Who, when, why, and where people touch are determined by unwritten sociocultural guidelines. Many persons mistakenly perceive touch as having only sexual implications.

Nurses rely on touch when carrying out interventions. Nurses can touch clients while performing physical assessments, giving baths, providing backrubs, and assisting with dressing. The nurse who is unaccustomed to touching or being touched may feel uncomfortable when performing interventions.

Similarly, persons who are ill must permit closer physical contact than they normally tolerate. Illness places people in dependent roles that call for the nurse to initiate and maintain closer interpersonal contact. It is important to remain sensitive to clients' dispositions toward touching. If clients shy away from the nurse's touch or refuse to hold the nurse's hand during pain, they are probably uncomfortable with being touched. Finally, touch can be a useful therapeutic tool. Holding the hand of grieving clients can often convey understanding better than words or other gestures. A nurse must be sure to use touch purposefully during interactions. Although touch can be helpful to clients, its use must be clearly understood and accepted (Vortherms, 1991).

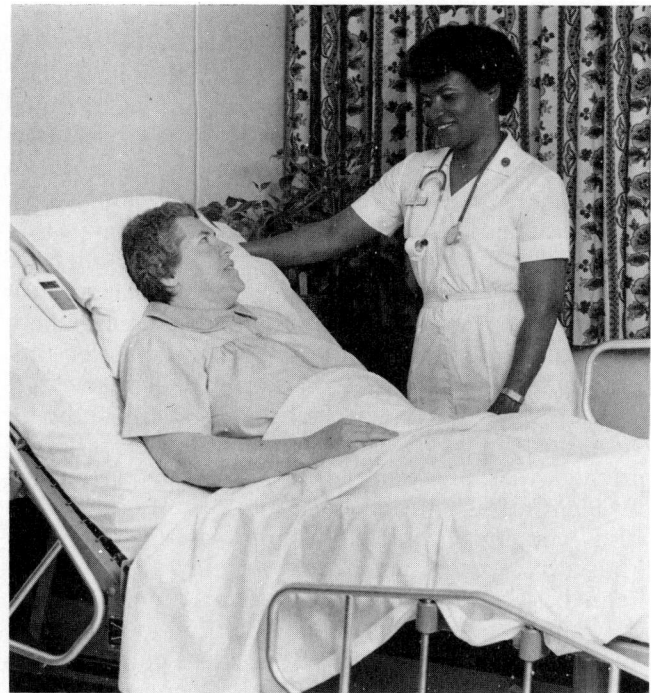

Fig. 15-3 Gently touching the client's hand conveys encouragement and support.

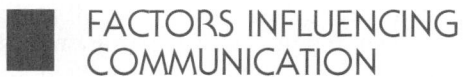

FACTORS INFLUENCING COMMUNICATION

Perceptions, values, cultural background, knowledge, roles, and the setting of interaction influence the content of a message and the manner in which it is shared. Interpersonal communication is made more complex because each person is influenced differently by these intrapersonal variables. Intrapersonal variables make each interpersonal communication unique. Each person makes different associations and interpretes messages differently. An understanding of these factors helps a nurse know the reasons that a client may have difficulty communicating and the strategies needed to help.

Development

Children are born with the physical mechanisms and capacity to develop speech and language skills. The rate of speech development varies and is directly related to neurological competence and intellectual development (Whaley, Wong, 1991). A child's environment must also offer stimulation for normal development. The environment provided by parents also affects the ability to communicate. The nurse uses special techniques to communicate with children of different developmental stages (see p. 358).

To communicate effectively with children, the nurse must understand the influence of development on language and thought processes. Both affect the way children communicate and the manner in which the nurse can successfully interact with them.

Perceptions

Each person senses, interprets, and understands events differently. **Perception** is the personal view of events. A nurse might state, "I've noticed you have been quiet since your family left. Would you like to talk about it?" The client's perception of the nurse's intent will affect the willingness to talk. Perceptions are formed by expectations and experiences. Differences in perceptions between people who are interacting can be a barrier to communication.

Values

Values are standards that influence behavior (see Chapter 12). They are what a person considers important in life and thus influence expression of thoughts and ideas. Values also affect interpretation of messages. Because values are a general guide to behavior, it is important for a nurse to develop awareness of them. Some values may be identified easily and without conflict (for example, confidentiality or good skin care for an immobile client); others may lead to a high level of conflict and be difficult to articulate (for example, values about death or the right to die). Knowing and clarifying values is important to decision making and interaction. A nurse does not allow personal values to interfere with professional relationships. Judgmental attitudes destroy trust and can be detrimental to effective communication.

Emotions

Emotions are a person's subjective feelings about events. The way a person relates or communicates with others is influenced by emotions. A client who is angry may react to nurses' instructions differently than one who is frightened. Emotions influence the ability to successfully receive a message. Emotions can also cause a person to misinterpret or not hear a message. Nurses should not take it personally if clients ventilate their emotions on them. Nurses can assess clients' emotions by observing them interact with family, physicians, or other nurses.

When nurses care for clients, they must be aware of their own emotions. It is difficult to hide emotions. Clients are perceptive and can sense anger, frustration, or sadness. It is usually inappropriate to discuss personal emotions with clients. A social support system of colleagues allows nurses to express emotions.

Sociocultural Background

Culture is the sum total of the learned ways of doing, feeling, and thinking; it is a form of conditioning that shows itself through behavior (see Chapter 4). Language, gestures, values, and attitudes reflect cultural origin. Often nurses care for clients who speak different languages. Culture, however, influences more than language or accent. Winkler and Doherty (1983) believe that communication style is highly dependent on cultural factors. For example, their research shows that American couples tend to be more calm and reasonable in communicating with one another than Israeli couples, who are verbally more aggressive. The influence of culture sets limits for the way people act and communicate.

Culture also influences methods of communicating symptoms or distress to others (Boyle, Andrews, 1989). Differences exist in self-disclosure or the willingness to convey emotions and psychological information to others. For example, European Americans are more open and willing to discuss private family matters, whereas Spanish, African, and Asian Americans are reluctant to reveal personal or family information to strangers, such as nurses or physicians. Some groups (for example, Spanish and Asian Americans) value a quiet demeanor and self-restraint; to be open or argumentative is thought to reflect negatively on family honor. In other groups, talking about oneself is considered bragging; Native Americans, for example, value silence and are comfortable with it. For a number of ethnic or racial groups, an inhibited silence occurs only in the presence of strangers or professionals of the dominant culture; sometimes this is due to historical distrust based on discrimination. At other times, it can be attributed to family loyalties and an agreement not to share problems outside of the family.

Language differences can also hamper communication and relationships. When a nurse cares for a client who speaks another language, an interpreter may be necessary. Except on a social basis or for care activities, a hospital interpreter is preferrable to a family member. Hospital interpreters generally understand medical terminology and can convey hospital policies and procedures. If a family member serves as an interpreter, it may be easier for the nurse to devise ways to communicate with the client. The nurse learns key words such as *water, pain,* or *bathroom* to ensure that the client's basic needs are assessed and understood.

Gender

Lakoff (1975) pioneered linguistic research on language and gender that focused on sex differences in communication behaviors and the way that they influence interaction. Sayers (1988) surveyed studies that revealed that certain speaker and listener behaviors support sex-linked deference and dominance patterns (that is, behaviors that show men dominating conversations by controlling the opportunity to speak and women providing support for this pattern of interaction). Tannen (1990), however, shows that women and men have different communication styles. From age 3, girls play with a best friend or in a small group and use language to seek confirmation, minimize differences, and establish or reinforce intimacy. Boys, on the other hand, use language to establish independence and negotiate status activities in large groups; even when they want to make friends, they are likely to do it by playfully butting heads. Carrying these styles into adulthood, women and men have completely different impressions of the same conversation. Tannen claims that the frictions between the sexes arise because girls and boys grow up in essentially different cultures, so conversation between them is, in effect, cross-cultural. This approach differs from the deference-dominance theories and focuses instead on a predominate female pattern of seeking relationships and connection with others and a predominate male pattern of accomplishing tasks and seeking independence and status. Although such an approach does not explain all problems that arise in relationships between women and men, it makes it possible to explain dissatisfactions without blame and without discarding the relationship.

Certainly nurses need to be aware of these differences when working with clients or other health team members of the opposite sex. Active listening and seeking clarification will help prevent misperceptions and misunderstandings.

Knowledge

Communication can be difficult when the persons communicating have different levels of knowledge. A message will not be clear if the words or phrases are not part of the listener's vocabulary. "The incision is well approximated without drainage" means the same as "The incision is clean and healing fine," but the latter is more easily understood by a client.

Nurses communicate with clients and professionals who have different levels of knowledge. A common language is essential when communicating across different knowledge levels. Nurses assess clients' knowledge by noting their responses to questions, abilities to discuss health problems, and questions that they ask. After assessment, nurses use terms and phrases that clients understand to promote attention and interest.

Roles and Relationships

People communicate in a style appropriate to their roles and relationships. Students talk with friends in different ways than with instructors, physicians, or ministers. Words, facial expressions, tone of voice, and gestures depend on the person receiving the communication.

Nurses may feel comfortable communicating with colleagues, joking about daily events, and sharing amusing stories. However, communicating with a client entering a clinic for the first time requires a different role. Anticipating apprehension, nurses convey respect by using the client's last name and avoid humor until they can determine the client's reaction to them. The client is probably looking for support rather than funny stories. Later, when the relationship between nurse and client is stronger, casual conversation and addressing the client on a first-name basis may be appropriate.

The better people know an individual, the more liberty they can take in expressing ideas. People feel more comfortable when expressing ideas to individuals with whom they have developed positive, satisfying relationships. As a nurse-client relationship develops, the nurse and client gain confidence in relating ideas and feelings. Communication is more effective when the participants remain aware of their roles in a relationship.

Environment

People tend to communicate better in a comfortable environment. A warm room, free of noise and distractions, is best. Noise and lack of privacy or space may create confusion, tension, or discomfort. For example, a client fearful of the diagnosis of cancer would hesitate to discuss the illness in a busy, crowded waiting room. Environmental distractions can distort the messages sent between two people.

The nurse has some control when selecting the setting for communicating with clients. A quiet office or lounge is ideal. When the client is visited at home, a bedroom or den may be best. The nurse's efforts to convey information must not be blocked by environmental distractions.

Space and Territoriality

Territoriality is the drive to gain, maintain, and defend an exclusive right to an area of space (Pluckhan, 1978). Territory is important because it provides people with a sense of identity, security, and control. In other words, individuals feel threatened when others invade their territory because it disrupts psychological homeostasis, creates anxiety, and produces feelings of loss of control. Hall (1969) coined the term *proxemics,* which means the use of space in interpersonal relationships or the distance between communicators. During social interaction, people consciously maintain a distance between themselves. Personal space is an invisible "bubble," and it is mobile—it goes with a person. Territory can be separated and made visible to others, such as a fenced-in yard, towel on the beach, or hospital bed. When personal space is threatened by intrusion, a defensive response occurs, preventing effective communication. Nurses often work with clients in situations in which space and territory are important. As with touch, the distance separating nurses from clients must be judged by the situation and culture. Physically restraining clients in danger of self-injury, giving mouth-to-mouth resuscitation, holding crying infants, and facilitating the excretory functions of incontinent clients require invasion of intimate space. Intimate distance or space includes an area in which people are able to touch one another or make physical contact to an area of 18 inches. Clients are sensitive about how nurses use distance. Nurses must convey confidence and gentleness.

As the distance becomes greater, the client and nurse feel more at ease. Greater flexibility is afforded when intimate contact is not required. Sitting with a client to conduct an interview, discuss personal feelings or thoughts, or teach are examples of personal distance (18 inches to 4 feet). Increasing the physical distance makes it easier for the client and nurse to communicate because the nurse becomes less imposing. Social distance (4 to 12 feet) is needed when dealing with groups. Making rounds with physicians is an example of group interaction. Communication at a social distance is less threatening than communication in an intimate or personal space because intimate sharing of thoughts and feelings is less likely to occur. Public distance (greater than 4 feet) is the distance maintained for formal speaking. A community health nurse presenting a seminar on hypertension to older adults or a professor lecturing to a class are examples.

 THERAPEUTIC COMMUNICATION

Beginning nursing students are often told to "get to know your clients" as they establish interpersonal relationships with clients. This is not easy, and sometimes it becomes the only barrier to an effective relationship. Nurses cannot get to know clients without being able to appreciate their uniqueness. Without knowing this, nurses are unable to help clients cope with health problems. Therapeutic communication helps nurses form working relationships with clients and fulfills the purposes of the nursing process.

Therapeutic communication is not casual. Instead, it is a planned, deliberate, professional act. However, preoccupation with the techniques of communication can cause the nurse to forget the client as a person. When theraputic communication techniques are first used, the communication process may seem artificial and contrived. It is more helpful to perceive each client interaction as an opportunity to achieve a positive relationship and shared understanding that results in attainment of mutual care goals.

Social Interaction

The first attempt at communicating with a client usually consists of a brief social interaction. The messages conveyed are superficial in that neither the nurse nor client discusses deeply personal matters of concern. Interpersonal exchange tends to be based on intuitive, unthinking, and automatic responses. Superficial interaction makes participants feel safe because the discussion has no hidden intent for personal disclosures.

A nurse often uses superficial social interaction at the beginning of a conversation with a client to lay a foundation for a closer relationship. For example, the nurse might greet a client by saying, "Good morning, Mrs. Sears, it's nice to see you today," or "Hi, Mr. Simpson, how do you like the great weather we're having?"

The skillful nurse does not allow social interaction to dominate a conversation but does maintain a congenial and warm style to build the client's trust. The goal is to help the client feel comfortable in sharing attitudes and feelings.

Caring and Methods of Effective Communication

The nurse uses communication skills while establishing a therapeutic relationship. There is no formula for forming a relationship with a client. Each person communicates uniquely, and each client requires different communication techniques. The nurse should be flexible in techniques used to foster communication with each client.

Listening Attentively

Listening is one of the most effective therapeutic communication techniques. It conveys a nonverbal, interest in the client's needs, concerns, and problems. It requires complete attention. Attentive listening involves an attempt to understand the entire verbal and nonverbal message that a person is commu-

nicating. Although hearing is a passive, neurological process of receiving information, listening is an active, learned process.

Listening effectively may at first seem awkward and time consuming, but like any skill, it requires practice. An effective listener, however, gains satisfaction from working with people and understanding their deeper health concerns. To be an attentive listener, the nurse uses the following skills:

1. Face clients while they speak.
2. Maintain natural eye contact to show willingness to listen.
3. Assume an attentive posture. Avoid crossing the legs and arms because this conveys a defensive posture.
4. Avoid distracting body movements, such as wringing hands, tapping feet, or fidgeting with an object in the hands.
5. Nod in acknowledgment when clients talk about important points or look for feedback.
6. Lean toward speakers to communicate involvement.

The nurse must appear natural while listening to clients. Nonverbal cues, such as leaning toward the speaker, should not become overbearing or threaten intimate space. Listening skillfully during a nursing procedure is beneficial and is an efficient use of time. For example, much can be learned and conveyed by the nurse who listens while giving clients baths. Clients, not the bath procedures, become the center of attention.

Conveying Acceptance

Showing acceptance means not judging another person and demonstrates the interviewer's willingness to listen to the client's beliefs, values, and practices. This is difficult at times because a nurse meets clients of diverse backgrounds. Acceptance is not the same as agreement. Acceptance is a willingness to hear the person without conveying doubt or disagreement.

Certainly a nurse does not accept all aspects of a client's behavior or illness. The nurse works to bring about change that improves a client's level of health. Acceptance is tolerance toward others that fosters a relationship between nurse and client.

To show acceptance the nurse remains aware of personal nonverbal expressions. The nurse avoids facial expressions and gestures that suggest disapproval, such as frowning, rolling the eyes upward, or shaking the head in disbelief. The following show that the nurse accepts what a client has to say:

1. Listening without interrupting
2. Providing verbal feedback that demonstrates understanding

3. Being sure that nonverbal cues match verbal communication
4. Avoiding arguing, expressing doubts, or attempting to change the client's mind

Asking Related Questions

Questioning is a direct method of communicating. The nurse's aim is to gain specific information about the client. Questions used during a conversation set the tone of the verbal interaction and control its direction. Questions are most effective when they relate to the topic or subject being discussed and use words and word patterns in the client's normal sociocultural context. During assessment of the client's health status, questions follow a logical sequence. The following example demonstrates this technique:

Nurse: Mr. James, can you tell me where you are having pain?
Client: Well, it seems to be in my back.
Nurse: What part of your back?
Client: Here, in the lower part.
Nurse: How would you describe the pain?
Client: It feels like a knife went through me.

The nurse's line of questioning helps the client tell a story. Each question focuses on a specific aspect of the story. The nurse is careful not to ask more than one question at a time or move on to another subject until the current topic is adequately explored. The nurse selects a question on the basis of the client's previous response so that information flows logically.

If the nurse wants the client to elaborate, open-ended questions are most effective. They give a client a chance to talk more completely about problems or concerns. Such questions cannot be answered with *yes* or *no*. Examples of open-ended questions include the following:

1. "Would you describe the pain you have been feeling?"
2. "What seems to be the problem?"
3. "Could you explain how your family feels about your illness?"

Asking the client open-ended questions allows the nurse to assess a number of factors. The client's verbal and nonverbal responses can reveal emotions. The nurse may be able to judge the level of the client's vocabulary and understanding of health by the response. Often the nurse seeks details of physical signs and symptoms, and the open-ended question elicits more accurate and detailed descriptions. Because an open-ended question prompts a lengthy response, the nurse can assess gaps or discrepancies.

Paraphrasing

Paraphrasing is restating clients' messages in the nurse's own words. Usually a paraphrased statement uses fewer words than the Through paraphrasing, the nur that lets clients know whether th understood and prompts further c following example illustrates this

Client: I've had it. My doctor won't on. He doesn't seem to care what I
Nurse: You're frustrated because y haven't talked about your diagnosis?
Client: Yes, he obviously doesn't know what it's like to be sick.

Practice is required to paraphrase accurately. If the meaning of a message is changed or distorted through paraphrasing, communication may become ineffective. For example, a client may say, "I've been overweight all my life and never had any problems. I can't understand why I need to be on a diet." Paraphrasing this statement by saying, "You mean you don't care if you're overweight or not?" is incorrect. "It seems that you're not convinced you need a diet because you've remained healthy," is a proper way of paraphrasing the statement.

Clarifying

Despite efforts at paraphrasing, the nurse may not understand the client's message. When a misunderstanding occurs, the nurse momentarily stops the discussion to clarify meaning. Without clarification, valuable information can be lost. Information critical to the client's care plan can be incomplete unless confusing or conflicting data are clarified. The nurse can attempt to repeat the message or admit confusion and ask the client to restate the message. In the following example, a client has come to the clinic for a checkup:

Client: I knew I might have a problem. It seems to be in my family. The last time I was here, though, it wasn't bad, so I didn't mention it.
Nurse: Excuse me, Mr. Brewer, can you tell me what type of problem you're having?

The nurse must also clarify messages. Examples can be used to clarify a vague, abstract idea. When using examples, the nurse describes ideas or situations to which the client can easily relate. In the following dialog, a nurse is explaining activity restrictions to a client who has had eye surgery:

Nurse: Now, Mr. Lee, once you go home you are not supposed to place stress on your eye.
Client: I'm not sure I know what you mean.
Nurse: Well, you're not allowed to stoop or bend over with your head down. For example, if you want to pick up your slippers off the floor or pick up a basket of laundry, don't bend over. Instead, bend your knees and keep your head up.

I have a dog at home. I guess I can't bend over to
pick him up?
Nurse: That's right. Bend your knees to lower yourself
down if you want to pick up your dog.

The more specific a clarifying message, the more
likely it will be understood. Clients who are easily
confused by the complex terms and jargon of medicine appreciate a simple, down-to-earth explanation
that uses familiar examples.

Focusing

Focusing eliminates vagueness in communication
by limiting the area of discussion. As clients discuss
topics related to health, their messages often become
vague. For example, a client may say to the nurse,
"Well, I've just been feeling funny lately. It doesn't
really bother me that much. It's just this feeling I'm
having in my head." This description tells little except that the client does not feel well. If the nurse
does not help focus specifically on the physical complaint, the client will likely continue to use vague descriptions.

To focus the discussion, the nurse might respond
to the client by saying, "You said you've been feeling
funny lately. Tell me when this feeling first started,"
or "Describe the feeling in your head." As in clarifying, the nurse seeks meaning in the client's message.
In the case of focusing, however, the nurse understands the client's message but realizes that it is nonspecific or vague.

The nurse does not use focusing if it interrupts clients while discussing an important issue. If conversations continue without new information or clients
begin to repeat themselves, focusing is useful.

Stating Observations

When communicating, people are often unaware
of the way that their messages are received. Feedback from others tells them whether they communicated the intended message. One way the nurse can
provide feedback is by sharing with clients observations of their behavior during communication. The
nurse describes the impressions created by the nonverbal cues. The following example illustrates this
point:

Miss Tucker is sitting in the waiting room of her physician's office. She is slumped in the chair, her body movements are slow, and she yawns while speaking with the
nurse. The nurse says, "Miss Tucker, you appear to be
quite tired."

If the client's verbal message conflicts with nonverbal cues, the nurse's observation may help convey

a clearer message. Stating observations often leads
the client to communicate more clearly without the
need for extensive questioning, focusing, or clarification.

The nurse does not state observations that might
embarrass or anger the client. The nurse in the preceding example would not say, "Miss Tucker, you
look a mess." Even if such an observation is made
with humor, the client can become resentful.

Offering Information

When two people communicate, the process is
rarely one sided. In an interaction with a client, the
nurse frequently offers information that gives the client additional data or insight. The client in the following dialog is scheduled to have surgery the next
day for an abdominal tumor removal:

Client: My doctor has told me I'm first on the schedule for
surgery tomorrow.
Nurse: Yes, we'll be awakening you about 6 AM.
Client: My family would like to be here then.
Nurse: That's no problem. They are free to come at 6, and
we'll show them where to wait for you once you've left
for the operating room.

Providing the client with additional information
encourages further response. Offering information
on an ongoing, timely basis not only facilitates communication but also promotes health teaching.

It is usually not helpful to withhold information
from clients, particularly when they seek it. If the
nurse avoids sharing information or gives only partial
information, clients may lose trust in the nurse. If
physicians chose to withhold information, the nurse
will need to clarify the reasons with them. However,
there is a wide range of information the nurse can
share (see Chapter 16). The nurse must avoid advising a client when giving information. Information
can facilitate a client's decision making, but the
nurse does not make the decision.

Maintaining Silence

Silence allows the nurse and client to organize
thoughts. The use of silence can be effective but is
difficult because pauses in conversation that last several seconds or minutes can cause unease. Beginning nurses may need to practice this technique before feeling comfortable.

The use of silence requires skill and timing. Silence allows the client an opportunity to communicate intrapersonally, organize thoughts, and process
information. It gives clients time to search for words
or feelings. Silence is particularly useful when clients
are confronted with difficult decisions that they are
not sure how to share with the nurse. For example,
silence may help clients gain the confidence needed
to share the decision to refuse medical treatment.

Silence also allows the nurse to observe clients. The nurse pays particular attention to nonverbal messages, such as worried expressions or loss of eye contact. Remaining silent demonstrates the nurse's willingness to wait for a response. Often the nurse has many questions, but some, especially older adults, are unable to reply quickly. Impatience expressed by the nurse frustrates clients' efforts at communication. Silence shows that the nurse is interested and will accept any response clients can express.

When clients become emotionally upset, silence helps them gather thoughts. A quiet period may diffuse an emotionally tense situation. A nurse's silence acknowledges clients' needs for a few moments of privacy. After clients are ready to talk again, they will more likely express feelings clearly.

Using Assertiveness

Assertiveness is standing up for one's rights without violating those of others (Stanhope, Lancaster, 1992). Through assertive techniques, people express feelings and emotions confidently, spontaneously, and honestly. Assertive persons make choices and decisions and are able to control their lives more effectively than nonassertive individuals. Nurses can teach clients assertiveness skills and use them to promote their own health.

Examples of assertiveness skills include speaking clearly, dealing with manipulation, and protecting against criticism. A clear message is complete and specific and includes all information a client needs to understand. The following example illustrates the incorrect technique for communicating a message:

Nurse: Your recovery depends on your ability to exercise right.
Client: Does that mean I can begin running?

The nurse should have been more specific when transmitting the message and should have given the client more information, as shown in the following example:

Nurse: Your recovery will include walking daily, progressing to about a mile a day within a month. Your therapist should be consulted before you begin to run.

To avoid being manipulated, nurses acquire skills to protect themselves from others who consciously or unconsciously use them. Learning to say *no* and resisting guilt imposed intentionally by others are two helpful techniques. Learning to say *no* is illustrated in the following case study:

Staff member: Listen, I'm really in a rush. Can you help me get this report completed?
Nurse: I've planned a home visit this morning. Perhaps my schedule will permit it tomorrow. I'll let you know.

Constructive criticism can promote growth, but manipulative criticism makes people vulnerable (Stanhope, Lancaster, 1992). The following example illustrates a method of protecting against criticism:

Supervisor: Nancy, I've been concerned about your performance lately.
Nurse: What have your concerns been?
Supervisor: I see you've been involved in two separate incidents with medication errors.
Nurse: Can you suggest ways I might avoid errors next time?

Negative inquiry is a skill that involves asking for more information when a criticism has been made. The person remains unemotional and low-key when asking for information and avoids sounding angry or sarcastic. Using criticism for growth helps nurses feel good about themselves.

Summarizing

Summarization is a concise review of main ideas that have been discussed. It sets the tone for further interactions between the nurse and client. Beginning a new interaction by summarizing a previous one helps the client recall topics discussed and shows the client that the nurse has analyzed their communication. In the folowing example, the nurse, Ms. Spier, has been working for several days to help the client, Mrs. Ramos, learn about diabetes:

Ms. Spier enters the client's room and says, "Good morning, Mrs. Ramos. I've come to talk with you more about your diabetes. If you recall, yesterday we discussed the purpose of insulin, its side effects, and how to give an injection."

Summarizing helps the nurse review key aspects of an interaction. Further communication can then focus on relevant issues. Clients will be able to sense whether the nurse understood their part of the message. With a summary the client is able to review information and make additions or corrections.

Barriers to Effective Communication

Some communication techniques or styles result in interpersonal interactions that are not therapeutic. These barriers can be damaging when a nurse is building a client relationship. Many techniques that normally promote effective communication can be harmful if used improperly.

Giving an Opinion

Giving an opinion takes decision making away from the client. It inhibits spontaneity, stalls problem solving, and creates doubt. The following example demonstrates how giving an opinion can be harmful:

Nurse: Mr. Jones, you look like you're deep in thought.

Client: Oh, no, not really. I was just thinking about whether my daughter is coming to see me.

Nurse: Well, if you ask me, she should have been here before now. It would mean so much to you.

Often the client simply needs an opportunity to express feelings. Giving an opinion prevents the client from developing solutions to problems.

At times, clients may require suggestions. For example, when a client is selecting a special diet, the nurse's help may be needed to choose the right food choice. Suggestions are presented to clients as options because the final decision rests with the client.

Offering False Reassurance

When a client is seriously ill, the nurse is tempted to offer hope to the client with statements such as "You'll be fine" or "There's nothing to worry about." When a client is reaching out for understanding, false reassurance from the nurse may discourage open communication. The following example illustrates this point:

Client: I'm so afraid of becoming dependent on my wife. I feel I'm never going to get any better.

Nurse: There's no reason to be so afraid. Things will get better.

Genuine, truthful reassurance, however, is important and helps validate a client's self-worth and sense of hope. Bradley and Edinberg (1990) have identified six basic conditions in which verbal reassurance can be given; a client can be reassured:

1. That there is hope
2. That the nurse is listening
3. That care is available
4. That certain undesirable changes can be expected (for example, loss of hair from chemotherapy)
5. That the client will be treated like a person
6. That the client's problem is understood

The following dialog shows how the nurse conveys a willingness to understand a client's concerns without falsely reassuring her that the illness or symptoms are minor:

Mrs. Stevens is a 58-year-old woman with terminal cancer. Her nurse, Ms. Fry, is sitting by her side.

Mrs. Stevens: I sometimes think this isn't happening to me. It seems so unfair. . . . Oh, I'm sorry. You don't want to hear my problems.

Ms. Fry: No, please, Mrs. Stevens, I do want to hear how you feel.

Being Defensive

Defensiveness in response to criticism suggests that the client has no right to an opinion. When a nurse becomes defensive the client's concerns are often ignored. The following example illustrates their point:

Mr. Locke has been a regular visitor to the health clinic for several years. The last time he visited the clinic, he had symptoms that resulted in his hospitalization. He now is returning to the clinic for a checkup 1 week after discharge from the hospital.

Mr. Locke: Well, I hope I don't have to see Dr. Warren today.

Nurse: I don't understand, Mr. Locke, is something wrong? Dr. Warren has been your doctor here for some time.

Mr. Locke: I don't care. He was the one who put me in the hospital, and that was a waste of time.

Nurse: That's silly. Dr. Warren is an excellent physician.

Mr. Locke: You think so, huh? He hasn't put you in the hospital for no reason.

Nurse: You were very ill, Mr. Locke. I know Dr. Warren made the right decision.

The nurse has threatened the relationship with Mr. Locke. He will probably not trust the nurse to keep his concerns confidential. The nurse is ignoring the client's feelings and will probably not take any action to remedy the problem. After this conversation, the nurse will have difficulty continuing a rapport that will prompt the client to discuss additional problems.

When clients express criticism, the nurse should listen to what they have to say. Listening does not imply agreement. To learn the reasons behind the client's criticism, the nurse avoids becoming defensive. There are two sides to any story, and the nurse attempts to learn why clients have become angry or dissatisfied. The following dialog demonstrates this technique:

Mr. Locke: Well, I hope I don't have to see Dr. Warren today.

Nurse: You seem upset, would you like to talk about it?

Mr. Locke: I just don't think he should have put me in the hospital.

Nurse: You believe hospitalization was unnecessary?

Mr. Locke: Yes, they really didn't do much of anything. They took a few tests and did some x-rays.

Nurse: Mr. Locke, did your doctors tell you what the tests showed?

Mr. Locke: No, not really. That's why I'm, so angry.

The nurse's patience led to an identification of the client's real concern, not knowing the results of his diagnostic tests. By avoiding defensiveness the nurse defused Mr. Locke's anger so that he could describe his concerns.

Showing Approval or Disapproval

Expressing excessive approval can be as harmful to a nurse-client relationship as stating disapproval. Offering excessive praise implies that the behavior being praised is the only acceptable one. Often the client shares a decision with the nurse, not in an effort to seek approval but to provide a means to discuss feelings. The following example illustrates this point:

Client: I've decided that when I leave the hospital I'll stay with my son. He doesn't want me to go home and be alone.
Nurse: Oh, I'm so glad to hear that. I think you definitely made the right decision. It's best for you to be with your son.

This nurse's comment will likely end further discussion of the topic. The client may perceive that the nurse agrees with the son. Perhaps the client would be better off with his or her son. On the other hand, the client may have a strong desire to remain independent, and now that has been discouraged. The nurse's excessive approval did not allow the client to think or act freely and inhibited the potential for decision making. A better response by the nurse might be, "You seem concerned about losing your independence."

On the other hand, disapproval implies that the client must meet the nurse's expectations or standards. In the following example, the nurse's response may hinder the client's positive attitude and recovery:

Client: Oh, I feel good, I was able to get up in the chair once today.
Nurse: Only once? You're going to have to get up more often than that!

It would have been better for the nurse to say, "You're making fine progress. Your doctor would like you to try to be up at least three times today. Do you think you'd like to sit up just before going to bed?" A disapproving statement causes the client to feel rejected. The client may avoid further interaction with the nurse, thus potentially slowing recovery.

Stereotyping

Everyone is unique. However, stereotyped responses inhibit uniqueness and oversimplify the situation. **Stereotypes** are generalized beliefs held about people. The use of stereotypes inhibits communication and can threaten a nurse-client relationship. Stereotyping statements, such as "Older adults are always confused" or "Clients with back problems cannot tolerate pain," seriously impair interpersonal communication.

Another nontherapeutic communication is the use of meaningless, stereotyped responses. Their use minimizes the importance of a person's message. The following example illustrates this point:

Client: I slept poorly last night. My incision seemed to be pulling.
Nurse: You can't win them all. At least the incision is healing well.

Asking Why

When people disagree with or fail to understand others, they are tempted to ask why the others believe or have acted in such a way. Clients frequently interpret "why" questions as accusations. They may also think that the nurse knows the reasons and is simply testing them. Regardless of clients' perceptions of the nurse's motivation, "why" questions can cause resentment, insecurity, and mistrust.

If the nurse wants additional information, there are more effective ways of phrasing questions. For example, rather than asking, "Why didn't you do your exercises?" the nurse could say, "You didn't do your exercises. Is something wrong?" Rather than asking, "Why are you anxious?" the nurse could say, "You appear upset. Would you like to talk?"

Changing the Subject Inappropriately

A nurse might inadvertently stop a client from discussing a subject of importance by changing the subject. Abruptly interrupting conversation is rude and shows a lack of empathy, as the following example shows:

Nurse: Good morning, Mr. Jones. How are you feeling?
Mr. Jones: (facial expression shows discomfort) Oh, not so good. My incision is rather sore.
Nurse: Well, let's get you up in a chair. We need to discuss your exercises.

The nurse's comment shows an unwillingness to discuss Mr. Jones' discomfort. The chance for a therapeutic assessment of his discomfort is lost. In this example, changing the subject was not therapeutic because the nurse ignored a potentially serious problem.

Changing the subject stalls progress of a therapeutic communication. The client's thoughts and spontaneity are interrupted, ideas become tangled, and as a result, the information provided may be inadequate. It is particularly important to avoid changing the subject during assessment. If the client has the opportunity to complete a message, the information shared will be more thorough and useful.

 ## HELPING RELATIONSHIPS

The nurse-client relationship is more than a mutual partnership. It is a process in which the helper is asked to intervene in the life of the client to help the client engage in more effective behavior. Travelbee (1971) calls it a *human-to-human relationship*. King (1971) says that the nurse-client relationship is a "learning experience whereby two people interact to face an immediate health problem, to share, if possible, in resolving it and to discover ways to adapt to the situation."

The nurse uses skills of interpersonal communication to develop a relationship with clients that allows understanding of them as total persons. This helping relationship is therapeutic, promoting a psychological climate that brings positive client change and growth. The relationship also focuses on meeting the clients' needs. Although the nurse may gain much satisfaction from the relationship, clients should be the primary recipients and determiners of benefits.

Creation of a therapeutic environment rests on the nurse's ability to provide physical and psychosocial comfort to the client. The nurse ensures that the client's physiological needs are satisfied. For example, the nurse positions the client so that breathing is normal for comfortable sleep. The nurse's actions consider the client's preferences. The nurse and client mutually determine how needs are met. In the following example, the nurse involves the client in her own care:

Mrs. Greer is a 63-year-old widow who is hospitalized for lung cancer. She makes frequent requests for pain medication before a dose is due. When a nurse delivers the medication, Mrs. Greer criticizes her for being late. Nothing the nurses do seems to satisfy Mrs. Greer.

Ms. Edwards has cared for Mrs. Greer for the past 2 days. She could easily be tired of her but chooses to be assigned to her for another day. Ms. Edwards enters her client's room and begins to straighten out the bed linen. Ms. Edwards asks, "Are you comfortable in that position, Mrs. Greer? Would you like a pain shot now?" Mrs. Greer accepts the offer and begins to relax in Ms. Edwards' presence. The nurse helps Mrs. Greer assume a more comfortable position on her side.

Once the client's pain has diminished, Ms. Edwards sits by her bed and says, "I know you've been experiencing much discomfort. Over the past few days we have not always been able to help you feel better. Can you help me to know the best way to make you feel comfortable?"

Efforts at improving Mrs. Greer's comfort make her more willing to discuss problems. The nurse soon learns of Mrs. Greer's great fear of death. The client has made frequent requests of the nurses to avoid feeling lonely. By discussing Mrs. Greer's fears, the nurse and client are able to find ways to minimize loneliness. The nurse's concern leads to solutions to the client's problems.

A helping relationship between the nurse and client does not just happen. It is built with care as the nurse uses therapeutic communication techniques.

Dimensions of Helping Relationships

Characteristics of any helping relationship are trust, empathy, caring, autonomy, and mutuality (Sundeen et al, 1989). They are essential if the nurse wants to establish positive and supportive relationships with clients.

Trust

With respect to helping relationships, Travelbee (1971) defines trust as "the assured belief that other individuals are capable of assisting in times of distress and will probably do so." Unless clients believe that a nurse wishes to care for their needs, a trusting relationship cannot develop. Trust fosters open, therapeutic communication. Previous experiences may affect clients' willingness to trust a nurse. Lack of previous health care experience or traumatic experiences causes clients to hesitate in trusting care givers. To foster trust, the nurse acts consistently, reliably, and competently. Honesty in sharing information with clients also builds trust. Without trust, a nurse-client relationship does not progress beyond social interaction and tending only to superficial needs.

Empathy and Sympathy

Empathy is widely accepted as a clinical component of the helping relationship, and within nursing it is considered an essential part of the nurse-client relationship. Definitions of empathy reflect the influence of psychotherapist Carl Rogers, who is well known for his work in identifying and describing the characteristics of a helping relationship. Empathy is the ability to enter into the life of another and accurately perceive feelings and meaning (Sundeen et al, 1989). Empathy is sensing, comprehending, and sharing the client's frame of reference, beginning with the problem the client recognizes. It is a fair, sensitive, and objective look at what another person experiences.

Empathy helps clients explain and explore their feelings so that problem solving might occur. It takes time for empathy to develop in a relationship. A nurse cannot automatically understand a client's feelings or experiences. In the following case study, being open and receptive helps the nurse learn to be empathetic:

Ms. Vincent has been caring for Mr. Pierce since his admission to the hospital 2 days before. Mr. Pierce is scheduled to have open-heart surgery the next day. Ms. Vincent enters the client's room, makes eye contact with him, and sits in the chair beside his bed. The following conversation occurs:

Ms. Vincent: Hello, Mr. Pierce. You look as though you're rather deep in thought.
Mr. Pierce: Oh, I suppose I do. It's just that I can't help but think about what tomorrow will bring.
Ms. Vincent: Would you like to talk about your surgery? I imagine you have a lot of questions.
Mr. Pierce: Yes, I would like to know more.

The nurse could easily have avoided Mr. Pierce's true concerns and even attempted to change the subject. An unhelpful remark would have been, "Don't worry about tomorrow, Mr. Pierce. Would you like me to get you something to read?" Such a comment would ignore Mr. Pierce's fears about surgery and prevent development of a meaningful relationship between the nurse and client. The skillful nurse moves the conversation forward to learn more about the client.

In contrast to empathy, sympathy is the expression of one's own feelings about another's predicament. It is the concern, sorrow, or pity shown by the nurse for the client in which the needs of the client are seen as the nurse's needs. Sympathy has a place in human relationships; sharing with another feels good, creates an alliance, and minimizes differences. Sundeen et al (1989) claim that this poses a difficulty in the helping relationship, however; helpers who share the needs of the client may be unable to help the client identify realistic alternatives and problem solve.

Social scientists and nurse researchers are rethinking, reviewing, and reinvestigating the role of empathy in the nurse-client relationship and the way that it is operationalized in nursing practice. The concept of empathy is not without controversy (see research highlight).

Caring

Caring is having a positive regard for another person. It is basic to a helping relationship. Most clients directly or indirectly express a need to be cared for at some time. Nurses show caring by accepting clients for who they are and respecting them as individuals. When clients feel cared for, they feel secure in threatening or anxiety-producing situations. Caring also promotes trust and decreases anxiety. Diminished anxiety and stress increase the body's defense and helps promote healing. Touching is an effective way for nurses to communicate care.

 Research Highlight

Pike reviews the literature on empathy to help clarify the concept and analyzes the relationship of empathy to recent findings on expert caring in nursing. Although they agree about the definition and process of empathy, authors disagree about the goals of empathic relationships. Two differing viewpoints generally emerge. Some authors (Rogers, Rawnsley, Zderad, Ehmann) hold that the goal is to objectively analyze another's experience and thereby bring about a therapeutic personality change. Others (Tyner, Travelbee) maintain that the end point of empathy is to share another person's pain or distress to relieve the person of carrying it alone.

Still others, particularly Benner and Wrubel, who examined actual practices of expert nurses, do not describe caring behavior as empathy. In their data, there are no accounts of nurses sensing a client's experience as if it were their own or vicariously experiencing the client's world. Instead, expert nurses have a storehouse of experiences that allows them to understand the client's "lived experience" without necessarily experiencing it themselves. Considering this data on caring practice, it appears that expert nurses do not routinely use empathy as it has been described in previous nursing literature.

According to Pike, determining whether empathy is a valid concept for practice, whether it is a crucial component of the nurse-client relationship, and whether it can be used by practicing nurses will be important for the future understanding of professional nursing.

Pike AW: On the nature and place of empathy in clinical nursing practice, *J Prof Nurs* 9(4):235, 1990.

Autonomy and Mutuality

Autonomy is an ability to be self-directed. Mutuality involves sharing with another. These are important in any helping relationship. The nurse and client work as a team, participating in care. The nurse offers opportunities to make decisions, even if it is as simple as choosing a bath time. As a client becomes more independent, the nurse offers more opportunities for decision making. The nurse also acts as an advocate to keep the client informed of health care alternatives and give support in decision making.

Phases of a Helping Relationship

The helping relationship is established and maintained by the professional nurse and consists of the preinteraction, orientation, working, and termination phases. The relationship is reciprocal; nurse and client relate to each other as they progress to therapeutic rapport. A helping relationship progresses over time as the nurse and client interact, but the helping relationship is not the same as the nursing process. The nursing process is a series of steps taken to manage a client's health problems. A helping relationship is a bond that allows the nurse to be more effective in carrying out the nursing process. The nurse is responsible for directing the client through the helping relationship to ensure that the client's needs are met.

Chapter 6 discusses the interview as a method for obtaining a nursing health history and identifying changes in the client's level of wellness and living patterns. Although the phases of an interview and of a helping relationship are the same, communication patterns are different. The interview can initiate a nurse-client relationship because it may be the first encounter. However, the interview is not the mechanism for maintaining a long-term therapeutic relationship. A helping relationship goes beyond the scope of an interview to establish rapport that is the basis for an ongoing resolution of the client's health problems.

Preinteraction Phase

Before a first meeting with a client, the nurse reviews information pertaining to the client. Such information may include the medical or nursing history, an entry in the nurse's notes of the medical record, or a discussion with another nurse who cared for the client. During this review, the nurse thinks about concerns that may develop. For example, before entering a relationship with a young cancer client, the nurse considers how the client is adjusting and whether death may be discussed. The preinteraction phase is a time when the nurse plans an approach. This process helps avoid stereotyping clients and allows the nurse to think about personal values or feelings. Although the nurse may feel anxious about a client, this sharpens mental processes and helps planning. The beginning nursing student should seek assistance from instructors if anxiety becomes intense.

A final step of the preinteraction phase is to choose a location and setting for the first meeting with a client. A comfortable, private, and attractive setting fosters interpersonal interaction. The nurse also plans sufficient time for discussion.

Orientation

The orientation phase begins when the nurse and the client first meet. It sets the tone for the rest of the nurse-client relationship. The orientation phase is superficial and is often marked by uncertainty and exploration.

During any initial encounter, both participants closely observe each other. The nurse and client make inferences and form judgments about each other's behaviors. Therapeutic communication will be more effective if the nurse is genuine, emphatic, and caring.

The nurse and client meet and identify each other by name. It is wise to address the client formally by using last names; for example, the nurse might say, "Good morning, Mr. Spencer. My name is Ms. Tucker. I am a student nurse assigned to take care of you today." As the therapeutic relationship develops, a client may ask the nurse to be more informal. Failure to identify oneself can create uncertainty because the client often encounters many personnel when seeking health care.

At the beginning of the relationship, neither individual is able to perceive the other's uniqueness. The nurse perceives a person who has a health-related problem. The client perceives the nurse as one of many health care professionals whose job is to help. Engaging in a social interaction initially helps the nurse and client become relaxed. The following dialog demonstrates communication to place a client at ease:

Nurse: It certainly is a lovely day, Mrs. Spier.
Client: Yes, isn't it? If I were home and feeling better, I'd be planting my garden.
Nurse: You're a gardener? What types of plants do you enjoy growing?
Client: Oh, a little of everything. I like some tomatoes, lettuce, radishes, and maybe some squash.

The nurse directs the conversation so that she and Mrs. Spier feel at ease. Rushing into a therapeutically oriented discussion when the client feels uncomfortable serves no purpose. The nurse and Mrs. Spier can come to know each other better and begin to develop a meaningful relationship if the social interaction is properly directed.

TESTING. The client often tests the nurse during the orientation phase. This is caused by the client's difficulty in acknowledging a need for help, fear of expressing true feelings, and anxiety over the need to change. The nurse who is aware of the client's concerns attempts to display confidence and competence. The nurse should not be defensive during testing but should be open and interested in the client's concerns. The client may use silence to avoid communicating. The nurse can show a desire to help by explaining the actions taken and performing care smoothly. The following case study shows communication involving testing:

Mr. Miles is a 52-year-old businessman who has been hospitalized for treatment of a bleeding stomach ulcer. He is very independent, and he is accustomed to making decisions for himself. Ms. Rains, the nurse, enters the client's room.

Ms. Rains: Good morning, Mr. Miles. My name is Ms. Rains, and I will be caring for you today.

Mr. Miles: You will, huh? Tell me, how long have you been a nurse?

Ms. Rains: About 2 years. I have worked in this hospital since graduating from nursing school.

Mr. Miles: Well, you won't have to worry about me. I can take care of myself.

Ms. Rains: I can imagine it's frustrating to be very independent one minute and then suddenly become ill and feel as though everyone is telling you what to do.

Mr. Miles: You can say that again. I'm just not used to needing help.

Ms. Rains: Mr. Miles, I'm not here to take away your independence. There are a number of things I need to do for you, but there are also many things I want you to be able to do for yourself. Let me explain some of the procedures I will be doing.

Mr. Miles: OK, I appreciate that.

Ms. Rains recognizes Mr. Miles' attempt to test her competence. Mr. Miles is fearful of losing his independence. If Ms. Rains has had minimal experience in developing relationships with clients, she may have felt the need to remain superficial and nondirective. The client will sense the nurse's superficiality during testing and avoid meaningful discussion. In this case, Ms. Rains acknowledges concerns and acts to eliminate Mr. Miles' fears.

BUILDING TRUST. Trust is relying on someone without doubt or question. Confidence, dependability, confidentiality, and credibility result in a trusting relationship. It is not easy for a client to perceive the need for help or to ask for it. Often a client trusts the nurse but is incapable of asking for assistance. Trust provides the foundation for effective communication as an individual becomes more open in expressing feelings and thoughts.

Trusting another person involves risk. As clients begin to share feelings and attitudes with the nurse, they become vulnerable. Clients must become comfortable in revealing personal information. The nurse who is insecure with clients may choose superficial methods to build trust: sharing secrets, telling private jokes, or encouraging clients to establish the relationship on a first-name basis. Some clients accept such behaviors, but others may resent being treated differently. Instead of enjoying the nurse's extra attention, they become distrustful.

Genuine caring is a powerful method for acquiring trust. The nurse shows sensitivity and understanding of the client's needs. Expressing concern is one way to establish trust. By showing concern, the nurse encourages the client's growth and progress. The following dialog demonstrates communication to build trust:

Mr. Squires: I've been home now for 4 days, and I just don't know what to do.

Ms. Ramsey: You're obviously upset. Tell me what the problem is. I'd like to help.

Mr. Squires: The doctor put me on that new diet. It seemed easy in the hospital, but I'm afraid I'm not eating right.

Ms. Ramsey: You've improved so much since your hospitalization. Let's sit down together and see what kinds of foods you should eat. Then we'll look at the types of foods you like that are allowed in your new diet.

Mr. Squires begins to trust Ms. Ramsey, who shows a willingness to help, not out of duty but out of a desire to meet his needs.

Mr. Squires: You shouldn't have to go to so much trouble for me.

Mr. Ramsey: You're not causing me trouble at all. An important part of my job is to help you stay healthy. Helping you to understand your diet better is part of my job.

Mr. Squires: Well, if I can learn to fix and eat the right foods, my doctor says I may stay out of the hospital longer this time.

Ms. Ramsey: Your doctor is right. Now let's go over what you know so far.

Another element that aids establishment of trust is recognizing Mr. Squires' individuality. He realizes that Ms. Ramsey respects him as a unique person.

Mr. Squires: The doctor said I should eat more vegetables and fruits. I really don't like many vegetables.

Ms. Ramsey: Well, let's make a list of what you do like. You know there are different ways to prepare the same kinds of foods. If you're able to eat the things you like, you'll be able to follow the diet more easily.

Mr. Squires: That sounds good. Before I left the hospital, I didn't think I would have much choice in what I ate.

Ms. Ramsey: Sure you do. I'll show you that you can have a lot of variety in your diet and even enjoy it. It's important that the diet be planned for you and not someone else.

Trust develops on a foundation of caring. Ms. Ramsey's time, patience, and conscientiousness show her concern for Mr. Squires' welfare.

IDENTIFYING PROBLEMS AND GOALS. During the initial encounter, the nurse begins to assess the client's health status. Through observations and interaction the nurse begins to make diagnostic conclusions. The client's health problems may be simple, such as moving without discomfort, choosing foods that will be easily tolerated, or getting out of bed safely. The relationship with the client is strengthened if the nurse identifies important client problems. Also, the client may not be able to recognize problems. During the orientation phase, the nurse uses communication techniques to direct the client to an awareness of problems, focus on the nature of the problems, and explore potential solutions. As problems are identified, the nurse and client mutually set goals. When the client is able to participate in goal setting and see the desired benefits, nursing interventions are more effective.

Sometimes the aim of the interaction is a mutual sharing of information, thoughts, and feelings rather than identification or addressing of problems. The nurse may find that the client is recovering without difficulty or coping well with the situation.

Identification of problems uses attentive listening, open-ended questioning, paraphrasing, and clarifying. Initially the nurse avoids identifying a large number of actual or potential problems. Bombarding the client with too many questions can result in emotional and physical fatigue. Also, it makes the client less trusting and more suspicious of the nurse's intentions. Limiting problem identification facilitates the client's understanding of the client's and nurse's roles. The following case study demonstrates communication to identify problems and goals:

Mr. Sachs is a 58-year-old man who has suffered a partial paralysis of his right side. Mr. Sachs needs to regain function in his right hand to retain his job as a telephone repairman. He is also fearful of damage to his self-image. He feels deformed and unable to live normally again.

Mr. Sachs: So much has happened to me. I know I may never again be able to do the things I once enjoyed.
Nurse: I know it's a difficult time for you now, but there are many things we can do to help you regain normal function.
Mr. Sachs: But there are so many things wrong with me.
Nurse: Let's take one at a time. What is most important to you?
Mr. Sachs: If only I could use my hand.
Nurse: Your doctor has ordered some exercises to increase the strength in your hand. I'll show you how to do each one. Are you willing to try them?
Mr. Sachs: You bet I am. If only I could use my hand again to work.

Nurse: Let's start with some simple goals. First we'll help you gain strength in your fingers so you can grasp eating utensils, a comb, or a razor. After that we'll try some more strenuous exercises.
Mr. Sachs: OK, that sounds reasonable. Show me what I need to do.

CLARIFYING ROLES. After a helping relationship is initiated, roles must be clarified. This occurs through a sharing of information, including the client's immediate needs, the client's perception of those needs, nursing care measures to be instituted, and steps for ensuring client participation in care. The helping relationship requires participation from both parties, but the nurse assumes the leadership role. Leadership does not mean control in the manipulative sense. Instead, the nurse takes the initiative in determining the client's point of view. The client assumes a role as receiver of care but also assumes an ongoing role as a participant in care.

FORMING CONTRACTS. After goals and roles are clearly defined, the nurse may establish a contract with the client. Generally, this involves a brief verbal interchange. Elements of the contract include location, frequency, and length of contacts with the client and duration of the relationship. The nurse should not present the contract in an overly formal way, but should outline an agreement in a way that clarifies expectations and summarizes steps for facilitating progress toward health. The following example demonstrates communication to form a contract:

Nurse: Mr. Reed, I'll be seeing you each morning for the next 4 days. After we practice your exercises together, I'd like you to do them on your own. Practice the exercises as often as you can without feeling pain or fatigue. On Friday, I'll introduce you to the nurse who will work with you next week. I'll be sure she knows the types of exercises you're doing.

It is important to let the client know when the relationship will be terminated. If the relationship is successful, the nurse and client frequently share respect and concern. The closer the nurse and client become in working together, the more difficult it is to end the relationship. If the client can anticipate the length of the relationship, termination will be less stressful. A student nurse often spends time with only one or two clients, often resulting in close relationships. Clients must be prepared for the end of the student's clinical experience; otherwise the client may become angered or disappointed.

Working Phase

During the working phase of a helping relationship, the nurse strives to meet goals set during the orientation phase. The nurse and client work together. The relationship broadens and becomes more flexible as the nurse and client are more willing to share feelings and discuss problems.

The nurse encourages the client's open expression of feelings. This may best be achieved by listening. If a client is unaccustomed to sharing feelings, the nurse is patient and understanding. The nurse's empathy and respect helps explore the client's true thoughts and feelings.

As the relationship progresses, clients participate in more self-exploration and are better able to discuss relevant issues. The nurse helps clients understand their feelings so that change can occur when necessary. Sundeen et al (1989) describe confrontation, immediacy, and self-disclosure as communication skills that will help clients gain self-understanding.

If the working phase is successful, clients are able to act on ideas and feelings. This often requires risk, and the nurse must remain supportive. Clients must deal with success and failure as they make decisions and resolve problems. Any attempt at change should be within clients' abilities. Change becomes less of a threat when clients express feelings about change and accept temporary setbacks. The nurse should encourage even the slightest progress.

CONFRONTATION. The nurse makes clients aware of inconsistencies in behavior or thoughts that interfere with self-understanding. The technique helps clients recognize growth or deal with important issues. The following case study demonstrates confrontation:

Ms. Perkins is a 60-year-old client with a history of obesity and high blood pressure. She has been returning to the clinic monthly for checkups.

Ms. Perkins: I feel frustrated, and I'm tired of being fat.
Nurse: When I saw you last month you told me you had lost 10 pounds and your clothes fit better. I can tell the difference.
Ms. Perkins: You're right, but it takes so much time to lose weight. I just get down on myself.

IMMEDIACY. The nurse focuses interaction on the present situation between nurse and client. Clients learn to understand how they interact with others. This involves drawing attention to clients' behaviors or statements. The following example demonstrates immediacy.

Nurse: As we've talked, you've seemed distant.
Client: Um-hm.
Nurse: Perhaps you are upset since I was not able to come talk with you as soon as I had promised.

SELF-DISCLOSURE. The nurse reveals personal experiences, thoughts, ideas, values, or feelings in context of the relationship. This is not therapy for the nurse. It shows clients that their experiences can be understood. The following dialog illustrates self-disclosure:

Ms. Wells' mother died just a month before. Since then, she has had difficulty with following her diet.

Nurse: This has been a difficult time for you.
Ms. Wells: It seems as though my world's collapsed.
Nurse: Three years ago I lost my mother. It was a very difficult time. I came to realize though that her death was a part of life and that she would want me to continue living life to its fullest.

INTEGRATING COMMUNICATION WITH NURSING ACTIONS. Nursing actions can generally be divided into four groups: physiological, psychological, spiritual, and socioeconomic. Bradley and Edinberg (1990) categorize the groups by their visibility. Physiological actions that attend to a client's physical needs, such as nutrition, elimination, and comfort, have high visibility. Most physiological actions are nonverbal and routinely performed. Traditionally, emphasis has been placed on a nurse's ability to perform physiological actions. Their high visibility allows the client to recognize the nurse as a good practitioner.

In contrast, psychological, socioeconomic, and spiritual nursing actions have low visibility. Psychological actions serve emotional needs. Socioeconomic actions, such as referring clients to community health agencies, assist clients in adapting to an environment. Spiritual actions help clients gain support for their belief systems. Low-visibility tasks are not readily observed or measured by others. Psychological, socioeconomic, and spiritual actions require cognitive and affective skills that are not routine and have traditionally led to less reward for the nurse.

Communication is important in performing both high- and low-visibility tasks (Fig. 15-4 on p. 352). Giving emotional support or educating the client's family obviously require effective communication, but basic nursing care procedures do too. The following case study shows how the nurse can integrate communication with nursing actions.

The nurse, Ms. Thomas, silently enters Mr. Richards' room. She tells him, "It's time for your pain shot." He is mildly startled and grimaces as he turns to see Ms. Thomas. As Mr. Richards starts to ask a question, she quickly reaches for his arm and prepares to inject the needle.

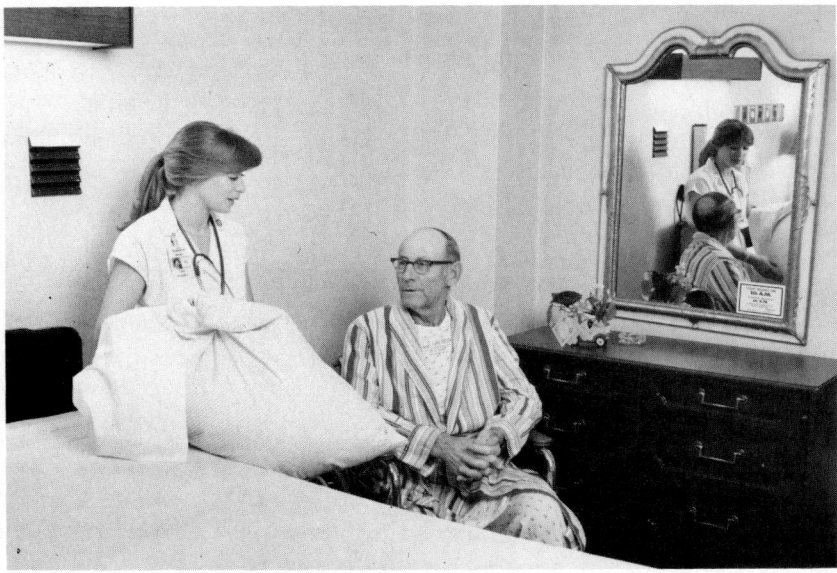

Fig. 15-4   The nurse integrates therapeutic communication skills into all aspects of care.

In contrast, a second nurse, Mr. Ives, enters Mr. Richards' room and says, "I have that pain medication you requested. Are you still feeling uncomfortable?" He turns and replies, "Yes, my back feels like a knife went through it. Will the pain ever go away?" Mr. Ives lays the syringe on the table, sits down next to Mr. Richards, and says, "It's normal to have pain the first few days after surgery. Let me give you that shot, and then I can show you how to move more carefully in bed to avoid worsening the pain."

Through communication, a nurse can convey the confidence, credibility, and knowledge that clients expect. In this example a few words of concern and reassurance (low-visibility communication skills) make receiving an injection more acceptable and encourage Mr. Richards to express his feelings.

Communication facilitates all nursing care measures. Integrating high- and low-visibility tasks allows Mr. Ives to accomplish several goals simultaneously. He quickly and efficiently assesses Mr. Richards' pain, provides a reassuring explanation, and demonstrates an alternative way of relieving pain. Therapeutic communication during high-visibility tasks increases the client's acceptance and understanding of procedures, lessens anxiety, and improves the client's willingness to cooperate.

Termination

During the orientation phase, the nurse tells the client when to expect the relationship to end. When termination occurs, the client should not be surprised. By remaining aware of goals of the relationship, the client should be prepared to function effectively without the nurse's support. Termination can nonetheless be difficult and painful for the client. The primary objective at the end of any helping relationship is termination in a planned and satisfying manner. Summarizing accomplishments and reviewing any unmet needs or follow-up care are helpful.

EVALUATION OF GOAL ACHIEVEMENT. Vital to termination is evaluation of goals. The nurse encourages assessment of the appropriateness and outcome of goals established. The following case study shows communication to evaluate goals.

Ms. Garner has worked with the client, Mr. Adams, during his 4-week stay in the hospital. Mr. Adams had surgery for repair of a fractured leg. Together, Ms. Garner and Mr. Adams set goals for his physical rehabilitation and return home.

Ms. Garner: Well, Mr. Adams, your doctor has discharged you for tomorrow morning. How do you feel about going home?

Mr. Adams: Oh, I'll be glad to get out of here. My leg feels pretty good.

Ms. Garner: Do you feel comfortable walking with the crutches?

Mr. Adams: Yes, I do. As you suggested, I practiced climbing stairs quite a bit in physical therapy. As you know, I have five stairs to climb up to my front door. I can climb them now without losing my balance.

Ms. Garner: You've also worked hard on learning to transfer from the bed and chair to a standing position with the crutches.

Mr. Adams: It's a lot easier now. All the practice you suggested helped. Since you've explained all of the right ways to hold the crutches, they feel like a natural part of me. I do hope I can get rid of them soon though.

Ms. Garner: Well, it sounds like you're ready to leave. Continue your leg exercises as you've done them here, and soon you won't need those crutches.

Mr. Adams: Thanks again for your help. I didn't think I'd ever be able to walk with these things, but now the crutches are no problem.

Both Ms. Garner and Mr. Adams experience satisfaction in meeting goals, particularly because the goals are mutually set. If goals are left unaccomplished, the reasons are examined, and plans are made for attainment in the future. Mr. Adams has not achieved the ability to walk without his crutches. Ms. Garner encourages him to continue his exercise regimen so that he will become strong enough to walk independently.

SEPARATION. Depending on the relationship between nurse and client, the client may have feelings of anxiety or ambivalence as termination nears. Ideally the client expresses feelings regarding termination. The nurse plans time to allow the client to share concerns or fears.

If the client remains in the health care setting and the nurse is the one leaving as a result of a scheduled day off or vacation, the client may feel abandoned. The nurse makes sure the client's care is uninterrupted by introducing the new nurse or communicating the client's needs with a written care plan. The nurse shares information that might foster the development of a helping relationship between other nurses and the client.

 ## COMMUNICATION AND THE NURSING PROCESS

Communication is important to the nursing process. A nurse uses communication skills during each step of the process (see box at right). Assessment, nursing diagnosis, planning, implementation, and evaluation of a client's care depends on effective communication between the nurse, client, family, and health care team. Through communication a

---

Communication Through the Nursing Process

ASSESSMENT

- Interviewing and history taking
- Physical examination (use of visual, auditory, and tactile channels)
- Observation of nonverbal behavior
- Review of medical records, literature, diagnostic tests

NURSING DIAGNOSIS

- Written analysis of assessment findings
- Discussion of health care needs and priorities with client and family

PLANNING

- Written care plans
- Health team planning sessions
- Discussions with client and family to determine methods of implementation

IMPLEMENTATION

- Discussion with other health professionals
- Health teaching
- Provision of therapeutic support
- Contact with other health resources
- Record of client's progress in care plan and nurse's notes

EVALUATION

- Acquisition of verbal and nonverbal feedback
- Written results of expected outcomes
- Update of written care plan
- Explanation of revisions to client

---

nurse and client come to an agreement about how to successfully meet the goals of care. According to Kasch (1986), the nurse functions as a communication strategist who strives to meet a client's communicative functions (see box on p. 354). These functions are part of the ongoing nursing process.

Communication is also important when caring for clients with communication problems. If clients are unable to interact with people because of illness, developmental delays, physical limitations imposed by therapy, or emotional reasons, the nurse encourages communication. The nurse uses the nursing process to ensure that clients communicate in a meaningful and effective way.

Communication Functions in Nursing

INFORMATION

- Gathering assessment information on which to base diagnosis and decision making
- Using methods to provide information that promotes client understanding, retention, and comprehension

INFLUENCE

- Using communication techniques when helping clients to change attitudes, beliefs, and actions

COMFORTING

- Interacting with clients to provide reassurance, support, and comfort
- Reducing a client's uncertainty during stressful times to alleviate or moderate emotional distress

RELATIONS

- Interacting to define, control, and modify the relationship between nurse and client
- Establishing, maintaining, repairing, and ending relationships
- Establishing a collaborative provider-client relationship*

IDENTITY

- Establishing self-identities to present oneself in ways that build credibility and produce friendliness, respect, and nurturing
- Presenting oneself in way that reflects competency

*Data from Barsky AH et al: *Soc Sci Med* 14a:653, 1980; Kim HS: Collaborative decision making in nursing practice: a theoretical framework. In Chinn PL, editor: *Advances in nursing theory development*, London, 1983, Aspen.

Assessment

Assessment can begin with a review of factors that influence communication. The client's developmental level, perceptions, emotions, cultural orientation, and knowledge are just a few items that the nurse must understand before planning ways to promote communication. It may be difficult to assess all of these factors if a client has physical barriers to communication. Family or friends then may become important for the nurse's assessment.

TABLE 15-2 Assessment of Physical Communication Barriers

Speech and Language Mechanisms	Alterations Affecting Speech
Respiratory system	Extreme dyspnea (shortness of breath)
	Artificial airways: endotracheal tube or tracheostomy
	Laryngectomy (surgical removal of larynx)
Oral and nasal cavities	Cleft palate
	Loose-fitting dentures
	Neurological disease affecting articulation (e.g., parkinsonism)
Speech center	Aphasia related to cerebrovascular accident (stroke) or brain tumor
Auditory system	Conduction or nerve deafness

Physical and Psychological Barriers to Communication

A client may suffer physical or psychological alterations that impair communication. To speak spontaneously and clearly, a person must have an intact respiratory system, normal oral and nasal cavities, and a functioning speech center in the cerebral cortex. Normal reception of language requires an intact auditory system. In the case of a child, the nurse assesses a child's ability to communicate, including the observation of sounds, gestures, and vocabulary expressed. When an adult develops hearing problems later in life, the ability to receive and understand messages is impaired. Review of medical history and physical assessment provide clues to the client's physical ability to communicate (Table 15-2). Physical barriers cause loss of speech, impaired articulation, or inability to find or name words.

The nurse should also consider whether clients are taking medication that impairs speech. Some medications, such as antidepressants, neuroleptics, or sedatives, may cause a client to slur words or use incomplete sentences. The nurse should be familiar with common side effects of such medications.

Some psychological illnesses such as psychosis or depression influence the ability to communicate. The client may demonstrate flight of ideas, constant verbalization of the same words or phrases, or a loose association of ideas. The nurse must isolate psychological causes of speech problems from possible neurological causes.

Nursing Diagnosis

The inability to communicate effectively influences a client's ability to express needs or react to the environment. After collecting assessment data the nurse clusters pertinent signs and symptoms or defining characteristics. The nurse's success in identifying the client's communication problem will ensure the formulation of an accurate nursing diagnosis (see diagnoses box). The diagnosis should focus on the cause of the communication disorder so that appropriate interventions are chosen (see diagnostic process box).

The nurse may also diagnose problems in clients who have difficulty with interacting with other persons. In these situations the client's difficulty of expression or a change in communication patterns leads the nurse to make a diagnosis.

Planning

Effective communication takes practice and concentration. The nurse makes a conscious effort at considering ways to help clients and families communicate thoughts and feelings more effectively. Planning an appropriate place and organizing care to allow sufficient time are essential. Consideration must also be given to interventions and communication techniques appropriate for the client's age and culture. Communication aids, such as a writing board for a client with a tracheostomy or a special

call light for a client who is paralyzed, may be useful. The nurse also needs to identify family members and other members of the health care team to whom communication problems can be referred or from whom the nurse can seek assistance in designing appropriate communication strategies. Some referrals might include the speech therapist for the client experiencing **aphasia** (neurological condition in which language function is defective or absent), an interpreter for a client who speaks a foreign language, or a psychiatric liaison nurse for the angry or highly anxious client.

It is especially important to have the client make decisions about the care plan. A person must feel

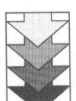

Examples of Nursing Diagnoses Related to Communication Alterations

NANDA-APPROVED NURSING DIAGNOSES

Impaired verbal communication related to:
- Physical barrier or artificial airway
- Neurological deficit
- Cultural difference
- Developmental deficit

Ineffective individual coping related to:
- Situational crises
- Maturational crises

Impaired social interaction related to:
- Communication barriers

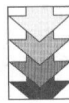

Sample Nursing Diagnostic Process for Communication Alterations

Assessment Activities	Defining Characteristics	Nursing Diagnosis
Ask whether client can speak or write English.	Unable to speak English language	*Impaired verbal communication* related to cultural difference
Ask whether client can read or understand English.	Lacks ability to answer question	
Determine the language that client speaks.	Communicates verbally in foreign language	
Observe whether nonverbal language is client's only means of communication (e.g., nods or uses hand gestures).	Able to express pain through use of facial gestures and pointing to affected body part	
Ask client to perform turning and deep-breathing exercises.	Lacks ability to follow instructions	

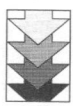

Sample Nursing Care Plan for Impaired Verbal Communication

Nursing diagnosis: *Impaired verbal communication* related to cultural differences
Definition: Impaired verbal communication is the state in which an individual experiences a decreased or absent ability to use or understand language in human interaction (Kim et al, 1991).

Goals	Expected Outcomes	Interventions	Rationale
Client will express basic needs clearly by 10/1.	Client will use simple English phrases.	Talk clearly and somewhat slower than normal in simple, short sentences.	Client will have difficulty following rapid speech. These techniques will promote communication when language barrier exists and no interpreter is present.
Client will express needs with minimal frustration by 10/1.	When unable to speak English, client will speak in Spanish or use an alternate method of communication.	Use attentive listening.	Listening wil help nurse understand meaning client is trying to convey and help build trusting relationship (Sundeen et al, 1989).
		Use alternative methods of communication, including: Communication board with key words spelled in English and client's language (Spanish)	When client does not speak English well enough to express needs or understand comments, client may become highly stressed and anxious. In these circumstances, nurse may need to use alternative communication methods (Boyle, Andrews, 1989).
		Use expressive nonverbal or body language	Body language is excellent nonconventional tool when spoken language is barrier. Nurse must be sensitive to variations across languages and cultures.
		Encourage client and family to teach staff some words or greeting in Spanish.	Language is viewed as source of communication power. Willingness to learn other's language helps promote feelings of acceptance and shows respect (Boyle, Andrews, 1989).
		Use an interpreter (Mrs. Santiago, Lab Dept, ext. 5444) as needed.	It is impossible to teach client or family if common language cannot be found or if literature in client's language is not available. In this situation, interpreter will be necessary. It is important to find an interpreter who will literally interpret comments made by client and nurse and who will be sensitive to client's culture and rephrase questions in acceptable way as needed.

comfortable and willing to communicate if effective interaction is to occur.

Success in promoting a client's ability to communicate depends not only on the client's participation in goal setting but also on the nurse's style of communication and the ability to establish a helping relationship. The use of therapeutic communication skills allows the nurse to perceive, react to, and respect the client's uniqueness. Successful interpersonal interaction meets the following goals of care for a client:

1. It transmits clear, concise, and understandable messages.
2. The client gains a sense of trust in the nurse as a care giver.
3. The nurse and client send and receive feedback.

After goals are mutually determined, expected outcomes are designated, and specific interventions are planned (see care plan).

 ## Implementation

With all clients the nurse tries to develop a helping therapeutic relationship. Clients will then feel more comfortable in interaction despite communication alterations.

Developing Social Skills

If ineffective coping or impaired social interaction is present, the nurse's interventions focus on helping clients do the following:

1. Express feelings and needs.
2. Develop conversational skills.
3. Communicate thoughts and feelings clearly (verbally and nonverbally).
4. Demonstrate assertiveness.
5. Solve problems.
6. Facilitate conversation with peers and staff.

A nurse who has more exerience with communication skills and interpersonal dynamics may assist clients through role playing. This allows clients to practice situations in which they have difficulty communicating. The following simple interventions can also be used to reinforce attempts at interaction:

1. Encourage participation in normal social activities.
2. Discuss neutral topics or subjects in which clients have interests.
3. Give positive reinforcement for acceptable social interactions.
4. Help clients identify persons with whom they feel comfortable and encourage activities with them.

5. Change bed or room assignments (in hospital) to encourage friendships or associates with same interests.
6. Minimize clients' idle time.

Controlling the Environment

If an environment is uncomfortable or distracting, a client will have difficulty with communicating, regardless of the problem. The nurse can control the environment so that it is conducive to interpersonal interactions. Methods of environmental control include the following:

1. Regulating room temperature to a comfortable level
2. Eliminating or reducing loud noises in the room (for example, radio or equipment alarm)
3. Making the client comfortable
4. Asking other staff members or family (if appropriate) not to enter room during interaction
5. Reducing bright or glaring light

Communicating with Clients with Special Needs

At times, it is necessary for nurses to use special communication techniques for successful nurse-client interactions. Clients with sensory and motor impairments, as well as children and older adults, require individualized approaches to communication.

PROVIDING ALTERNATE COMMUNICATION METHODS. Clients with physical communication barriers (for example, a client with a laryngectomy or endotracheal tube) may be unable to speak, or clarity of speech is so poor that alternate methods of communication are needed (see box). For these clients the

---

Communication Aids

- Pad and felt-tipped pen or magic slate
- Communication board with words, letters, or pictures denoting basic needs (e.g., water, bedpan, pain medication)
- Call bells or alarms
- Sign language
- Use of eye blinks or movement of fingers for simple responses (e.g., *yes* or *no*)
- Flash cards with common words or phrases the client may use
- Language cards for clients who do not speak the dominant language

---

Techniques for Communicating with Children

INFANT

- The child communicates primarily nonverbally (e.g., coos, smiles, cries) and seeks comfort.
- The nurse should avoid loud, harsh sounds and sudden movements.
- Gentle, close physical contact helps a child to become quiet.
- The nurse keeps the mother in view while holding and interacting with the child.

TODDLER OR PRESCHOOLER

- The child communicates verbally and nonverbally.
- The child is egocentric with all activities focused on the *self*.
- Speech and thought processes are concrete.
- The nurse should focus discussion on the child's personal needs and concerns.
- The child is told specifically what he or she can do and how he or she will feel.
- The child should be allowed to explore the environment (e.g., handle a stethoscope, play with a tongue blade).
- The nurse uses simple, short sentences, familiar words, and concrete explanations and avoids ambiguous phrases that the child can not interpret (e.g., "the shot will just feel like a bee sting" or "take this medicine for your tummy ache").

SCHOOL-AGE CHILD

- Speech is primarily verbal.
- The child seeks explanations of the world and is interested in functional aspects of objects and events.
- The child is concerned about body integrity.
- The nurse should give simple explanations, demonstrate how equipment works, and allow the child to manipulate equipment (e.g., hold a percussion hammer, wear a stethoscope).
- The child should be allowed to express fears or concerns.

ADOLESCENT

- An adolescent thinks more abstractly, fluctuates between childish and adult thinking behavior, and likes talking with adults outside of the family.
- The nurse should avoid imposing values or judgments.
- The nurse allows the adolescent to talk, is attentive, and avoids interrupting or showing gestures of disapproval.
- The nurse avoids embarrassing questions or the impulse to give advice.
- Adolescents frequently use a language of their own; the nurse should clarify unfamiliar terms.

---

nurse provides methods that are simple to use. Anything complicated can be frustrating and make communication more difficult. The nurse is patient as the client tries to communicate. The client must be able to physically use the method that the nurse provides. Clients must have the communication board or pencil and pad nearby. A client who is unable to speak can be at risk for injury unless personal needs can be quickly communicated.

COMMUNICATING WITH A CHILD. Communication with a child requires special considerations so that the nurse can develop a working relationship with both the child and family. The nurse receives much information from parents. Because contact between parent and child is usually close, information communicated by parents can be assumed to be reliable. However, some parents may exaggerate. If the client is a young child, it helps to offer toys or materials for play so that the parent can give full attention to the nurse. The nurse gives periodic attention to infants and younger children as they play to make them participants. An older child can be actively involved in communication.

Children, particularly the young, are especially responsive to nonverbal messages. Sudden movements or threatening gestures can frighten them. The nurse walking into an examination room with a broad grin and animated hand movements might inhibit formation of a relationship. The nurse should remain calm and gentle. It helps to let children make the first moves in interpersonal contacts. A quiet, friendly, confident tone of voice is best.

Children dislike being stared at. Adults looking down on them make them feel vulnerable. While communicating with young children, the nurse should meet them at eye level. Children feel helpless in most situations involving health care personnel.

When it is necessary to give explanations or directions, the nurse uses simple, direct language. The nurse must be honest with children. Deceiving children into thinking painful procedures are painless will only make them angry. To minimize fear and anxiety, the nurse should always tell children what to expect immediately before a procedure.

Drawing and play are two effective ways to communicate with young children. Drawing provides an opportunity for them to communicate nonverbally (by making drawings) and verbally (by explaining pictures). The nurse can use children's drawings as bases for initiating conversation. Techniques for communicating with children also vary with age (see box at left).

COMMUNICATING WITH OLDER ADULTS. Communication is more than talking and listening or reading and writing; it is a tool for social interaction that can aid understanding. This is often particularly evident in older adults who often suffer a "silence barrier" on three levels: social, emotional, and physical (Dreher, 1987). Social barriers include the loss of spouse or friends through death or separation and a restrictive living location when they change residence or children move away. For some older adults, the cost of transportation or a telephone may further restrict social interaction.

Fear of rejection or lowered self-esteem result in emotional barriers. Using good communication skills, particularly active listening and friendly therapeutic touch, can help relieve or diminish feelings of isolation and vulnerability. For older adults not inhibited by cost, telephoning can be a good method for maintaining contact with family and friends if travel and distance are barriers to communication.

Physical barriers can also occur; gradual changes in the body's muscles and nerves that affect voice, articulation, and hearing may result in slower and less precise speech. Sensory alterations such as a decreasing hearing acuity and an increasing threshold for intensity or loudness may prevent the older adult from receiving messages clearly. This can be complicated by ill-fitting hearing aids and poorly fitting dentures. Particular illnesses that are more common in older adults than in other age groups, such as can-

cer, stroke, and degenerative neurological diseases, can also distort speech and language. Motor disturbances such as **dysarthria** interfere with clarity of pronunciation. Many elderly adapt to the sensory losses (see Chapter 27) and can learn to communicate effectively. When obvious deficits exist, the nurse maximizes existing motor and sensory function so that the client can communicate more effectively (see box below).

COMMUNICATING WITH THE UNCONSCIOUS CLIENT. Even when persons are unconscious or nonresponsive, they may be able to receive stimuli. Hearing is thought to be the last sensation lost with unconsciousness and the first to be regained with consciousness. Therefore nurses need to be careful not to say anything to unconscious clients or within their hearing range that they would not say to fully conscious clients. Other important nursing interventions

---

Communicating with Sensorially or Motor-Impaired Clients

CLIENT WHO IS HEARING IMPAIRED

- Be sure hearing aid is clean, inserted properly, and has functioning battery.
- Adjust volume of hearing aid to comfortable level.
- Speak slowly and articulate clearly.
- Stand in front of client to provide opportunity for lip reading.
- Talk toward client's best ear.
- Reduce background noise.

CLIENT WHO IS VISUALLY IMPAIRED

- Keep eyeglasses clean and intact (allows client to see nonverbal communication).

CLIENT WHO HAS APHASIA

- Ask simple questions that require *yes* or *no* answers.
- Allow time for understanding and a response.
- Use visual cues (e.g., for example, words, pictures, objects) when possible.
- Talk one at a time.
- Do not shout or speak too loudly.

CLIENT WHO HAS DYSARTHRIA

- Listen attentively, be patient, and do not interrupt.
- Encourage client to converse.
- Refer to speech therapist as needed.

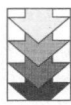

Sample Evaluation of Interventions for Impaired Verbal Communication

Goals	Evaluative Measures	Expected Outcomes
Cli nt will express basic needs clearly by 10/1.	Observe client use communication board. Ask family to question client about whether needs have been met.	Client will use alternate method of communication by 9/29.
Client sends clear, concise, and understandable messages by discharge from intensive care unit.	Observe client's interactions with nurse and family.	Client uses effective sign language by day after surgery.
	Confirm meaning of client's message by paraphrasing it.	Client makes appropriate requests by second day after surgery.
Client gains a sense of trust in the nurse as care giver by third home visit.	Observe client's openness and willingness to discuss personal thoughts or feelings.	Client voluntarily discusses thoughts or feelings with the nurse by second visit. Client expresses accomplishment of goals of relationship by third visit. Client shares feelings about termination of helping relationship by third visit.

include talking with the client while providing care; explaining procedures; providing orientation information, such as the nurse's name, place, date, and time of day; and avoiding bedside conversations with others about the client.

Evaluation

Evaluating whether or not communication has been therapeutic aids a client in improving communication, and it improves the nurse-client relationship. The nurse evaluates nursing interventions based on the previously established client goals to determine whether strategies or interventions were effective and what client changes resulted because of the interventions.

Successful communication is evaluated by the nurse's observations of client interactions. The nurse not only determines that communication exists, but also that the client appears satisfied that the message was received. For example, the nurse might ask the following questions:

1. Does the client appear more physically comfortable?
2. Does the client talk about feelings, reactions, and thoughts, or was conversation superficial?
3. Were the appropriate team members consulted?

Nurses compare actual outcomes with expected outcomes when determining the success or effect of interventions (see evaluation box). It is also useful for nurses to frequently evaluate the effectiveness of their own unique communication styles and techniques and to make periodic written "process recordings" of the verbal and nonverbal interactions between them and the client. Interactions and responses can then be examined by nurses, other designated nurses, or communication specialists. Some questions that could be asked during such examinations follow:

1. Did nurses encourage openness and allow the client to express thoughts and tell the story?
2. Did responses block the client's efforts? If so, how?
3. Were responses supportive or critical, opinionated, or trite?
4. Were open-ended or closed-ended questions used? Were they used appropriately?
5. How could communication be more effective?

If expected outcomes are not met or progress is not satisfactory according to the client, the nurse needs to reassess and modify the plan of care.

 SUMMARY

Communication is one of the most important nursing skills. It allows nurses to better understand clients' needs and develop relationships that will help clients attain healthy behaviors. Nurses' competence depends on their ability to send timely and intelligent messages as clients' needs dictate and on their ability to understand the client's communications. Communication is affected by many factors and is a complex process that includes verbal and nonverbal communication.

Therapeutic communication with the client involves planned, deliberate interactions that foster a helping relationship. Throughout the relationship the nurse uses skills that promote communication and avoids words and actions that inhibit communication. Through effective communication the nurse helps the client adapt to changes resulting from health alterations. The nurse acts to help clients with special communication problems communicate effectively in spite of physical, emotional, or developmental limitations.

CHAPTER 15 REVIEW

Key Concepts

- Effective communication is the process that allows nurses to establish working relationships with clients.

- Successful communication requires the message intended by the speaker to be similar or identical to the meaning acquired by the receiver.

- The way a person receives a message depends on past experiences, sensory function, and personal expectations.

- Words that have different connotative meanings can be easily misinterpreted by the person receiving the message.

- Effective verbal communication requires clear and concise phrasing of words, a proper pacing of statements, and an understandable vocabulary.

- When the sender's verbal and nonverbal communications complement each other, a receiver is unlikely to misinterpret a message.

- Communication aids the nurse in effectively and efficiently performing nursing care measures.

- Communication is the means by which the nurse helps clients adjust to changes imposed by illness.

- A nurse uses selective communication skills when interacting with clients.

- Skills that normally promote positive communication can also be detrimental to nurse-client relationships if they are used improperly.

- Ineffective communication skills inhibit the client's willingness to openly express ideas or concerns.

- Trust, empathy, caring, autonomy, and mutuality are basic dimensions of a helping nurse-client relationship.

- The working phase of a helping relationship involves the nurse and client working together so that the client can express thoughts and feelings freely and constructively.

- Clients with physical communication barriers may be able to express themselves more effectively with communication aids.

- Clients with ineffective social skills may benefit from positive reinforcement and encouragement to participate in interactions.

Key Terms

Aphasia, p. 355
Assertiveness, p. 323
Channels, p. 312
Communication, p. 310
Connotative, p. 313
Denotative, p. 313
Dysarthria, p. 359
Feedback, p. 312
Interpersonal communication, p. 310
Intrapersonal communication, p. 310
Message, p. 311

Metacommunication, p. 314
Nonverbal communication, p. 314
Paraphrasing, p. 321
Perception, p. 317
Proxemics, p. 319
Public communication, p. 310
Receiver, p. 312
Referent, p. 311
Sender, p. 311
Stereotypes, p. 325
Verbal communication, p. 312

Critical Thinking Exercises

1. You are working in the ICU and assigned to care for Tony, an 8-year-old boy who was hit by a car while riding his bicycle. He is unconscious as a result of a head injury. His mother, a 32-year-old engineer, is at the bedside. As you enter the room you notice her holding Tony's hand and crying.
   a. Identify at least two ways you might respond to Tony's mother.
   b. What factors that influence communication would you need to consider before developing a plan to help you respond to Tony's mother as she deals with this traumatic event? What additional information would you need?

2. Identify a habit you have of using a particular sort of obstructive message. (Pick one [e.g., such as holding arms across the chest] that you would sincerely like to break!)
   a. Sensitize youself to this habit by developing an exercise in which you use this message to excess.
   b. Now pick alternative messages from the list of caring or confirming techniques identified in the chapter, substitute it for the obstructive message in the exercise above, and practice using it over and over.

REFERENCES

Benner P, Wrubel J: *The primacy of caring,* Reading, Mass, 1989, Addison-Wesley.

Boyle JS, Andrews MA: *Transcultural concepts in nursing care,* Glenview, Ill, 1989, Scott, Foresman.

Bradley J, Edinberg MA: *Communication in the nursing context,* ed 3, Norwalk, Conn, 1990, Appleton & Lange.

Dreher BB: *Communication skills for working with elders,* New York, 1987, Springer.

Dugan DO: Laughter and tears: best medicine for stress, *Nurs Forum* 24(1): 18, 1989.

Duldt BW et al: *Interpersonal communication in nursing,* Philadelphia, 1984, Davis.

Ehmann VE: Empathy: its origin, characteristics, and process, *The Lamp* 28:25, 1971.

Ekman P: Communication through nonverbal behavior: a source of information about an interpersonal relationship. In Tomkins SS, Izard CE, editors: *Affect, cognition, and personality,* New York, 1965, Springer.

Fritz P et al: *Intrapersonal communication in nursing: an interactionist approach,* East Norwalk, Conn, 1984, Appleton & Lange.

Hall ET: *The hidden Dimension,* New York, 1969, Doubleday.

Kasch CR: Toward a theory of nursing action: skills and competency in the delivery of nursing care, *Nurs Res* 35(4):226, 1986.

Kim MJ, McFarland GK, McLane AM: *Pocket guide to nursing diagnoses,* ed 4, St Louis, 1989, Mosby–Year Book.

King I: *Toward a theory for nursing,* New York, 1971, Wiley.

Knapp M: *Nonverbal communication in human interaction,* New York, 1978, Holt, Rinehart & Winston.

Knaus WA et al: An evaluation of outcome from intensive care in major medical centers, *Ann Intern Med* 104(3):410, 1986.

Lakoff R: *Language and woman's place,* New York, 1975, Harper & Row.

Lalli-Ascosi S: Polishing your self-image, *Healthc Trends Transition* 1(2):15, 1990.

Lindberg JB, Hunter ML, Kruszewski AZ: *Introduction to nursing: concepts, issues, and opportunities,* Philadelphia, 1990, Lippincott.

Pluckhan ML: *Human communication: the matrix of nursing,* New York, 1978, McGraw-Hill.

Rawnsley MM: Toward a conceptual base for affective nursing, *Nurs Outlook* 28:244, 1980.

Rogers CR: The characteristics of a helping relationship, *Personnel Guid J* 37:6, 1958.

Sarvimaki A: Nursing care as moral, practical, communicative and creative activity, *J Adv Nurs* 13:462, 1988.

Satir V: *Conjoint family therapy,* ed 3, rev, Palo Alto, Calif, 1983, Science & Behavior Books.

Sayers F: Sex, sex-role and conversation: review of the literature and rationale. In Valentine CA, Hoar N, editors: *Women and communication power: theory, research, and practice,* Annandale, Va, 1988, Speech Communication Association.

Severtsen BM: Therapeutic communication demystified, *J Nurs Educ* 29(4): 190, 1990.

Stanhope M, Lancaster J: *Community health nursing: process and practice for promoting health,* ed 3, St Louis, 1992, Mosby–Year Book.

Sullivan JL, Deane DM: Humor and health, *J Gerontol Nurs* 14(1):20, 1988.

Sundeen SJ et al: *Nurse-client interaction: implementing the nursing process,* ed 4, St Louis, 1989, Mosby–Year Book.

Tannen D: *You just don't understand: women and men in conversation,* New York, 1990, Morrow.

Travelbee J: *Interpersonal aspects of nursing,* ed 2, Philadelphia, 1971, Davis.

Tyner R: Elements of empathetic care for dying patinets and their families, *Nurs Clin North Am* 20:393, 1985.

Vortherms RC: Clinically improving communication through touch, *J Gerontol Nurs* 17(5):6, 1991.

Whaley LF, Wong DL: *Nursing care of infants and children,* ed 4, St Louis, 1991, Mosby–Year Book.

Williams H: Humor and healing: therapeutic effects in geriatrics, *Gerontologist* 1(3):14, 1986.

Winkler I, Doherty WJ: Communication styles and marital satisfaction in Isreali and American couples, *Fam Process* 22:221, 1983.

Zderad C: Empathetic nursing, *Nurs Clin North Am* 4:655, 1965.

Zunin L: *Contact: the first four minutes,* New York, 1988, Ballantine.

ADDITIONAL READINGS

Beck C, Rawlins R, Williams S: *Mental health–psychiatric nursing: a holistic life-cycle approach,* ed 2, St Louis, 1988, Mosby–Year Book.

Bermosk LS: Interviewing: a key to therapeutic communication in nursing practice, *Nurs Clin North Am* 1(2):205, 1966.

Bird B: *Talking with patients,* Philadelphia, 1973, Lippincott.

Cameron JE: Giant leap forward begins with the nursing interview, *Aust Nurses J* 12(2):47, 1982.

Carpenito LJ: *Nursing Diagnosis: application to clinical practice,* ed 3, Philadelphia, 1989, Lippincott.

Chenevert M: *STAT: special techniques in assertiveness training for women in the health processions,* ed 3, St Louis, 1988, Mosby–Year Book.

Coad-Denton A: Therapeutic superficiality and intimacy. In Longo D, Williams R: *Clinical practice in psychosocial nursing: assessment and intervention,* ed 2, New York, 1986, Appleton & Lange.

Doona ME: *Traveller's interventions in psychiatric nursing,* ed 2, Philadelphia, 1979, Davis.

Ebersole P, Hess P: *Toward healthy aging,* ed 3, St Louis, 1990, Mosby–Year Book.

Egan G: *The skilled helper: a systematic approach to effective helping,* ed 4, Pacific Grove, Calif, 1990, Brooks/Cole.

Enelow A, Swisher SS, editors: *Interviewing and patient care,* ed 3, New York, 1985, Oxford University Press.

Flynn JM, Heffron PB: *Nursing from concept to practice,* ed 2, Norwalk, Conn, 1988, Appleton & Lange.

Goda S: Speech development in children, *Am J Nurs* 70:276, 1970.

Hein EC: *Communication in nursing practice,* ed 2, Boston, 1980, Little, Brown.

Kemp CG: *Perspectives on the group process,* Boston, 1964, Houghton Mifflin.

Kennedy CS, Garvin BJ: Nurse-physician communication, *Appl Nurs Res,* 1(3):122, 1988.

Knowles RD: Building rapport through neuro-linguistic programming, *Am J Nurs* 83:1011, 1983.

Loweree F et al: Admitting an intoxicated patient, *Am J Nurs* 84:617, 1984.

Marchione J, Stearns SJ: Ethnic power perspectives for nursing, *Nurs Health Care* 11(6):229, 1989.

Marsden, C: Ethics of the "doctor-nurse game," *Heart Lung* 19:422, 1990.

McKay M, Davis M, Fanning P: *Messages: the communication book,* Oakland, Calif, 1983, New Harbinger.

Morath J: Empathy training: development of sensitivity and caring in hospitals, *Nurs Manage* 20(3):60, 1989.

Murray RB: Therapeutic communication for emotional care. In Murray RB, Huelskoetter MM: *Psychiatric and mental health nursing: giving emotional care,* Englewood Cliffs, NJ, 1987, Appleton & Lange.

Olson JK, Iwasiw CL: Effects of a training model on active listening skills of post-RN students, *J Nurs Educ* 26(3):104, 1987.

Pike AW: On the nature and place of empathy in clinical nursing practice, *J Prof Nurs* 6:235, 1990.

Podrasky DL, Sexton DL: Nurses' reaction to difficult patients, *Image J Nurs Sch* 20(1):16, 1988.

Purtilo R: *Health professional and patient interaction,* ed 4, Philadelphia, 1990, Saunders.

Raudseff E: 7 ways to cure communication breakdowns, *Nurs 90,* 20(4):132, 1990.

Rogers CR: *On becoming a person,* Boston, 1972, Houghton Mifflin.

Rothenberger RL: Transcultural nursing: overcoming obstacles to effective communication, *AORN J* 51:1357, 1990.

Satir V: *The new peoplemaking,* Palo Alto, Calif, 1988, Science & Behavior Books.

Walker R: Effective listening, *Am J Med Technol* 35:8, 1969.

CHAPTER 16

Teaching-Learning Process

OBJECTIVES

Mastery of content in this chapter will enable the student to:
- Define the key terms listed.
- Describe the similarities and differences between teaching and learning.
- Identify the purposes of client education.
- Describe how to incorporate communication principles into the teaching-learning process.
- Describe the domains of learning.
- Differentiate factors that determine the motivation to learn from those that determine the ability to learn.
- Compare the nursing process with the teaching process.
- Write learning objectives for a teaching plan.
- Describe characteristics of a good learning environment.
- Identify different teaching approaches to use for clients with specific learning needs.
- Describe the instructional method best suited for a client with a specific learning need.
- Describe ways to incorporate teaching with routine nursing care.
- Identify methods for evaluating learning.

CHAPTER OUTLINE

Standards for Client Education

Purposes for Client Education
Maintenance of health and illness prevention
Restoration of health
Coping with impaired functioning

Teaching and Learning
Role of the nurse in teaching and learning
Teaching as a form of communication

Domains of Learning
Cognitive learning
Affective learning
Psychomotor learning

Basic Learning Principles
Motivation to learn
Ability to learn
Learning environment

Integrating the Nursing and Teaching Processes
Assessment
Nursing diagnosis
Planning
Implementation
Evaluation

Client education has become one of the more important roles for nurses working in every type of health care setting. Teaching healthy mothers in a physician's office about prenatal care, instructing clients visiting a clinic about immunization of children, and teaching heart attack victims about newly prescribed medications are examples of client education. Clients and family members have the right to health education so that they can make intelligent, informed decisions about their health and lifestyle. Many clients who previously received treatments in hospitals now receive them on an outpatient basis, or if they are hospitalized, they are discharged earlier (Kruger, 1991). Effective health education is essential if nurses are to care for increasing numbers of clients in the community and if the effects of preventable disease are to be minimized (Noble, 1991).

Increased demands on nurses' time and the need to give seriously ill clients concise and meaningful information as soon as possible emphasizes the importance of quality client education. As nurses try to find the best way to educate clients, the general public has become more assertive in seeking knowledge and understanding of personal health and the resources available within the health care system (Kruger, 1991). Providing clients with needed information about health care is necessary to ensure continuity of care from the hospital to the home. A well-designed, comprehensive teaching plan that fits clients' learning needs can reduce health care costs, improve the quality of care, and help clients gain more independence.

The significance of client education is enhanced because of clients' rights to know and be informed about their diagnoses, prognoses, treatments, and risks. Information provided should be readily understandable. It is negligent to assume that clients will learn on their own. Accurate and timely information is needed for clients to make decisions about their health. More attention is being paid in courts of law as to whether clients are adequately informed about ways to manage their health. Competent professional nursing practice includes client education. The nurse can provide adequate education only by identifying clients' learning needs and by using the most appropriate teaching strategies.

 ## STANDARDS FOR CLIENT EDUCATION

Client education has been a standard for professional nursing practice. According to Virginia Henderson (1966), part of a nurse's role is to "improve the

patient's level of understanding and therefore promote health." Accrediting agencies in the United States and Canada set guidelines for provision of client education within health care institutions. The guidelines ensure that the client and family receive the information necessary to maintain the client's optimal level of health. In the United States, the Joint Commission on Accreditation of Healthcare Organizations (JCAHO) (1992) has established standards for client education within hospitals:

> Throughout the client's stay, the client and, as appropriate, his/her significant other(s) receive education specific to the client's health care needs. This includes information regarding proper administration of medications, proper use of medical equipment, and instructions on how to obtain follow-up care after discharge.

The successful accomplishment of this standard is based on the nurse's accurate assessment of the client's educational needs, inclusion of the client and family in teaching plans, and evaluation of learning. The JCAHO standards ensure that the client will be taught information about procedures in acute care settings and the assumption of self-care activities.

In 1986, the Alberta Association of Registered Nurses developed a set of client education standards (see box). These standards address the educational process related to adults. The usefulness of the standards helps direct nurses in client education.

 ## PURPOSES FOR CLIENT EDUCATION

Nursing's Agenda for Health Care Reform by the American Nurses Association (ANA) (1991) recommends a restructuring of the health care system and focuses on wellness and care rather than illness and cure. With this plan, client and family education emphasizes the promotion, restoration, and maintenance of health. Clients are becoming more knowledgeable about health and thus seek involvement in their health maintenance. Nursing is pursuing opportunities to provide education as a part of primary health care delivery so that clients receive information about their care in more convenient and familiar places (ANA, 1991). Comprehensive client education includes three important purposes, each involving a separate phase of health care (see box on p. 350).

Maintenance of Health and Illness Prevention

The public has become more health conscious in recent years. Participation in fitness clubs, diet pro-

Client Education Standards

STRUCTURE

Standards in regard to structure relate to human and material resources, including administration and management of the health care agency. Nurses in both staff and administrative roles should contribute to their development and implementation.

Standard 1

The health care agency has a philosophy, goals, and objectives that reflect its mandate and provide direction for client education.

Standard 2

Client education is integrated into all areas of nursing practice in the health care system.

Standard 3

The nursing department of the health care agency is active in developing a comprehensive plan for client education.

Standard 4

An individual/department is responsible for facilitating and coordinating matters of client education.

PROCESS

Process standards outline criteria by which client education is delivered. The educational process includes the same steps as the nursing process.

Standard 1

The primary focus of the educational process is the client.

Standard 2

An educational assessment is done by the nurse in collaboration with the client.

Standard 3

The nurse demonstrates planning in the educational process.

Standard 4

The nurse applies principles of the educational process in implementation of client education.

Standard 5

A written outline of the educational process is available as a communication tool, a resource to health professionals, and as a record.

OUTCOME

Outcome standards are the criteria to meaure results of the educational process.

Standard 1

The nurse evaluates the educational process.

Standard 2

The client participates in evaluating the educational process.

From the Alberta Association of Registered Nurses: *Client education: position statement and guidelines,* 1985, Edmonton, Alberta, Canada, 1986, The Association.

Topics for Health Education

HEALTH PROMOTION AND ILLNESS PREVENTION

- First aid
- Avoidance of risk factors (e.g., smoking, alcohol)
- Stress management
- Growth and development
- Hygiene
- Immunizations
- Prenatal care and normal childbearing
- Nutrition
- Exercise
- Safety (in home and hospital)
- Screening (e.g., blood pressure, vision, cholesterol level)

RESTORATION OF HEALTH

- Client's disease or condition
  - Anatomic structure and physiologic condition of body system affected
  - Cause of disease
  - Origin of symptoms
  - Expected effects on other body systems
  - Prognosis
  - Limitations on function
  - Rationale for treatment
  - Medications

- Tests and therapies
- Nursing measures
- Surgical intervention
- Expected duration of care
- Hospital or clinic environment
- Hospital or clinic staff
- Long-term care
- Methods for client participation in care
- Limitations posed by disease or surgery

COPING WITH IMPAIRED FUNCTIONS

- Home care
  - Medications
  - Intravenous Therapy
  - Diet
  - Activity
  - Self-help devices
- Rehabilitation of remaining function
  - Physical therapy
  - Occupational therapy
  - Speech therapy
- Prevention of complications
  - Knowledge of risk factors
  - Implications of noncompliance with therapy
  - Environmental alterations

---

grams, regular exercise activities, and health-screening programs are examples of ways that people pay more attention to their health.

The nurse is a convenient resource for clients who want to improve their physical and psychological well-being. In the school, home, clinic, or workplace, the nurse provides information and skills that will allow clients to assume healthier behaviors (see box above). For example, in childbearing classes, nurses teach expectant parents what to anticipate and do during pregnancy. The expectant parents learn about the stages of fetal (unborn child) development and factors that can alter normal growth. Information about the physical and psychological changes that the woman undergoes during pregnancy is also a part of the class. After learning about normal childbearing the mother is more likely to eat healthy foods, get physical exercise, and avoid drugs or other substances that might harm the fetus. Promoting healthy behavior through education increases clients' self-esteem by allowing them to assume more responsibility for their health. With greater knowledge

persons can maintain better health habits. When clients become more health conscious, they are more likely to seek early diagnosis of health problems.

Restoration of Health

Clients who are injured or ill need information and skills that will help them regain improved levels of health (see box above). Clients recovering from illness or injury and adapting to the associated limitations often seek information about their conditions. However, clients who find it difficult to adapt to illness may become uninterested in learning. The nurse learns to identify clients' willingness to acquire knowledge and institutes methods to motivate interest.

The family is often a vital part of a client's return to health and needs to know as much as the client. If the nurse excludes the family from a teaching plan, conflicts may arise. For example, if the family does not understand a client's need to regain independent function, their efforts may cause the client to become unnecessarily dependent and retard progress.

Coping with Impaired Functioning

Not all clients fully recover from illness or injury. Many must learn to cope with permanent health alterations. Knowledge and skills are often necessary for clients to continue activities of daily living (see box on p. 350). For example, the client whose ability to speak is lost after surgery of the larynx learns new ways of communicating, and the client with severe heart disease learns to avoid physical activities that might cause further heart damage.

In the case of serious disability the client's role within the family may change, making understanding and acceptance by family members necessary. The family's ability to provide support is a result of education. Education begins as soon as the client's needs are identified and the family displays a willingness to help. The nurse teaches family members to assist the client with health care management. This includes, for example, giving medications and baths and applying dressings. Families of clients with other kinds of alterations, such as alcoholism, mental retardation, or drug dependence, learn to adapt to the emotional effects.

A nurse learns to recognize the information to teach to clients at different levels of wellness. To do this, the nurse must consider clients' needs in relation to their ability to meet them. Learning occurs when information is practical and useful. Comparing clients' desired levels of health with the actual states enables the nurse to plan meaningful teaching programs.

 ## TEACHING AND LEARNING

It is impossible to separate teaching from learning. **Teaching** is an interactive process between a teacher and one or more learners (Redman, 1988). It consists of a deliberate set of actions that help individuals gain knowledge or perform new skills. A teacher provides information that prompts the learner to participate in or initiate activities that lead to desired cognitive or behavioral change.

Learning is dynamic and fluid and is a shared, lifelong event (Rendon et al, 1986). To learn is to acquire knowledge or skills through reinforced practice and experience. For example, a diabetic client demonstrates to a nurse the technique for preparing insulin in a syringe. An arthritic client learns the best ways to perform self-care activities at home. Generally teaching and learning begin when a person identifies a need for knowing or acquiring an ability to do something. According to Knowles (1970), adults can learn, learning is an internal process, and there are superior conditions of learning and principles of teaching. Teaching is most effective when it responds to a learner's needs. The teacher identifies these needs by asking questions and determining the learner's interests. Teaching relies on principles of interpersonal communication. In other words, the teacher must send messages of significance to the learner and receive the learner's feedback.

Role of the Nurse in Teaching and Learning

Clients often ask nurses for information about their health. A client may request information about what will happen during an x-ray procedure. Family members may question the reason for their father's pain. A school may ask for information about childhood immunization. Identification of the need for teaching is easy when clients request information. Often, however, a client's need for teaching may be less obvious.

The nurse is frequently able to anticipate clients' needs for information. Client's physical conditions or treatment plans established by physicians often require that clients acquire new knowledge or skills. It is the nurse's responsibility to teach information that clients and their families need. Although the physician is ultimately responsible for providing information about a diagnosis, treatment, and prognosis, the nurse must help clients understand their responses to illness. A nurse clarifies information provided by physicians and becomes the primary source of information that assists clients' adjustment to their health problems.

To be an effective educator, a nurse must do more than just pass on facts; the nurse must engage the client in learning (Spicer, 1982). Nurses have numerous opportunities to pass on facts. However, there is no assurance that the client learns from these facts. As an educator, a nurse must carefully determine what clients need to know and find the time when they are ready to learn.

It is critical for nurses to perceive the role of educator as important (see research highlight on p. 352). More research is needed to demonstrate the relationship between client education and favorable client outcomes. A goal of client education is to change client behavior and to maintain or improve the client's health. When nurses value client education and are able to implement it into practice, clients will be better prepared for assuming their own health care responsibilities.

Research Highlight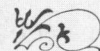

Kruger surveyed a sample of staff nurses, nurse administrators, and nurse educators, asking how nurses perceive their role as client educator and how well they believe that they are meeting client education needs. Staff nurses presented their views from actual practice. Nurse administrators provided the leadership for nursing practice and were selected because of their broad perspective of trends related to client education. Nurse educators presented the educational perspective of client education by nurses.

Of 1230 surveys mailed, 756, or 61.4%, were returned. Respondents represented each of the three professional groups and included all educational levels and specialty areas.

The survey included two items regarding the nurse's responsibility for education and three subsets of items:

preparation of clients receiving care, preparation of clients being discharged from a health care facility, and documentation of client education activities. There were significant differences when comparing responses on these three areas. Preparing clients to receive care (e.g., instructions, explanations of procedures) rated the highest, followed by preparing clients for discharge (e.g., self-care, disease prevention). Documenting client education activities received the lowest rating.

All three nurse groups believed that nurses should hold a high level of responsibility for client education; the majority of all nurses believed that the nurse providing nursing care should have primary responsibility for client education. The findings from this study support the nurse's role as client educator and emphasize the importance of role development.

Kruger S: The patient educator role in nursing, *Appl Nurs Res* 4 (1):19, 1991.

TABLE 16-1 Comparison of Terms Used in Teaching and Communication

Communication	Teaching	Communication	Teaching
REFERENT		**CHANNELS**	
Idea that initiates reason for communication	Perceived need to provide person with information, establishment of relevant learning objectives by teacher	Methods used to transmit message (e.g., visual, auditory, touch)	Methods used to present content (e.g., visual and auditory materials, touch, taste, smell)
SENDER		**RECEIVER**	
Person who conveys message to another	Teacher who performs activities aimed at assisting other person to learn	Person to whom message is transmitted	Learner
INTRAPERSONAL VARIABLES (SENDER)		**INTRAPERSONAL VARIABLES (RECEIVER)**	
Knowledge, values, emotions, and sociocultural influences that affect sender's thoughts	Teacher's philosophy of education (based on learning theory); knowledge of teaching content; teaching approach; experiences in teaching; teacher's emotions and values	Knowledge, values, emotions, and sociocultural influences that affect receiver's thoughts	Willingness and ability to learn (i.e., physical and emotional health, education, experience, developmental level)
MESSAGE		**FEEDBACK**	
Information expressed or transmitted by sender	Content or information taught	Information revealing that true meaning of message was received	Determination of whether learning objectives were achieved

Teaching as a Form of Communication

The teaching process closely parallels the communication process (see Chapter 15). Effective teaching depends in part on effective interpersonal communication. A teacher applies each element of the communication process while imparting information to students. Thus the teacher and student become involved in a teaching process that increases the student's knowledge and skills.

The steps of the teaching process can be compared with those of the communication process (Table 16-1). In teaching, the referent represents the need to provide the client with information. The client may request information, or the nurse may perceive a need for it. The nurse then identifies specific learning objectives. A learning objective describes what the learner will be able to do after successful instruction.

The nurse as teacher is the sender, whose aim is to convey a message to the client. The nurse promotes learning by communicating in a language recognizable to the learner. Many intrapersonal variables influence the nurse's style and approach. The nurse's attitudes, values, emotions, and knowledge influence the way that messages are sent. Past experiences with teaching help the nurse choose the best way to present information.

The message or content to be taught is delivered clearly and precisely. The nurse organizes information to be taught in a logical sequence so that the client will more easily understand skills or ideas. Each lesson is presented in a meaningful progression from simple to more complex skills or ideas.

The nurse may use several channels to present teaching content. All of the senses are channels for presenting information. The auditory channel is the simplest, as in a lecture or discussion. However, the learning process becomes more stimulating when several sensory channels are used. For example, a client with newly diagnosed heart disease will learn how to measure a pulse best by actually feeling the pulsation of an artery.

The receiver in the teaching-learning process is the learner. A number of intrapersonal variables affect motivation and ability to learn. Clients are ready to learn when they express a desire to do so and are more likely to receive the message when they understand the content. Attitudes, anxiety, and values are a few factors that influence the ability to comprehend a message. The ability to learn depends on factors such as emotional and physical health, education, stage of development, and previous knowledge.

An effective teacher provides a mechanism for evaluating the success of a teaching plan. Having a client demonstrate a newly learned skill and asking the client to describe the correct dosage schedule for a medication are ways to gather feedback. Feedback must show the success of the learner in achieving objectives; that is, the learner restates information or provides a return demonstration of skills learned.

 ## DOMAINS OF LEARNING

Learning occurs in three areas or domains: cognitive (understandings), affective (attitudes), and psychomotor (motor skills). Any topic to be learned may involve all domains or only one. For example, clients learn to understand about diabetes, the way that it affects the body, and ways to control blood sugar levels for healthier lifestyles (cognitive domain). In addition clients learn to accept the long-term nature of the disease (affective domain). Many diabetic clients must also learn to administer insulin injections on a daily basis (psychomotor domain). The characteristics of learning within each domain affect the teaching and evaluation methods used. Understanding each learning domain prepares the nurse to select proper teaching techniques. However, the nurse needs to also be able to apply the basic principles of learning to any teaching method (see later section).

Cognitive Learning

The **cognitive learning** domain involves intellectual behaviors. Bloom (1956) classifies cognitive behaviors in an ordered hierarchy. The simplest behavior is acquiring knowledge, whereas the most complex is evaluation.

Knowledge

Using knowledge is acquiring new facts or information and being able to recall them. For example, a client learns about a prescribed medication and is able to describe its purpose and potential side effects.

Comprehension

Comprehension is the ability to understand the meaning of learned material. For example, the client is able to explain specifically how the new medication will improve physical condition.

Application

Application involves using abstract, newly learned ideas in concrete situations. For example, the client learns to self-administer the medication according to a meal schedule to minimize side effects.

Analysis

Analysis involves relating ideas in an organized way. It allows a person to distinguish important from unimportant information. For example, the client is able to distinguish which side effects are more likely to be experienced from the medication and to compare them with the effects experienced by another person.

Synthesis

Synthesis is the ability to recognize parts of information as a whole. For example, the client experiences side effects from a medication and is able to take preventive steps.

Evaluation

Evaluation is a judgment of the worth of a body of information for a given purpose. For example, a client is able to recognize a symptom associated with the medication.

Affective Learning

Affective learning deals with expression of feelings and acceptance of attitudes, opinions, or values. Values clarification (see Chapter 12) is an example of affective learning. The simplest behavior in the hierarchy is receiving, and the most complex is characterizing (Krathwohl et al, 1964).

Receiving

Receiving is being willing to attend to another person's words. For example, a woman shows a willingness to listen to a nurse explain the surgical procedure for removal of a breast.

Responding

Responding involves active participation through listening and reacting verbally and nonverbally. The person feels satisfied from the response. For example, the client asks the nurse about the appearance of the incision that she will have.

Valuing

Valuing means attaching worth to an object or behavior. This is shown through the learner's behavior. The person is motivated to act out the behavior. For example, the client expresses a concern about the effect of surgery on her appearance. After surgery, the client refuses to look at the incision and wears a gown with a high neck.

Organizing

Organizing is developing a value system by identifying and organizing values and resolving conflicts.

For example, the client learns to accept changes created by surgery and is willing to participate in social activities.

Characterizing

Characterizing involves acting and responding with a consistent value system. The person behaves consistently when values are tested or challenged. For example, the client assumes a normal lifestyle after having breast surgery. She is able to discuss with others her positive feelings about herself.

Psychomotor Learning

The **psychomotor learning** domain involves acquiring skills that require the integration of mental and muscular activity such as the ability to walk or to use an eating utensil. The simplest behavior in the hierarchy is perception, whereas the most complex is origination (Simpson, 1972).

Perception

Perception is being aware of objects or qualities through the use of sense organs. A person associates a sensory cue with the task to perform. For example, after hearing the siren of an ambulance a person considers driving to the curb to avoid a collision.

Set

A set is a readiness to take a particular action. There are three sets: mental, physical, and emotional. For example, a person uses judgment to determine the best way to perform a motor act (mental readiness). Before performing the act, such as rising from a wheelchair, the person aligns and postures properly (physical readiness). A client might make the commitment (emotional set) to regularly perform exercises.

Guided Response

A guided response is the performance of an act under the guidance of an instructor. This involves imitation of a demonstrated act. For example, a client prepares an insulin injection after watching a nurse's demonstration. The nurse provides immediate reinforcement after the client correctly performs the act.

Mechanism

A mechanism is a higher level of behavior whereby a person has gained confidence and skill in performing the behavior. Usually the skill is more complex or involves several more steps than a guided response. For example, a client is able to fill the insulin syringe for different insulin doses.

Complex Overt Response

A complex overt response involves performing a motor skill involving a complex movement pattern. The person performs the skill smoothly and accurately without hesitation. For example, a client is able to self-administer an insulin injection using several sites.

Adaptation

Adaptation occurs when a person is able to change a motor response when unexpected problems arise. For example, as a nurse administers an injection, the appearance of blood during aspiration results in changing the way that the syringe is handled.

Origination

Origination is a highly complex motor act that involves creating new movement patterns. A person acts on the basis of existing psychomotor skills and abilities. For example, a nurse uses a different method of venipuncture on a client whose arm is swollen.

 ## BASIC LEARNING PRINCIPLES

To teach effectively the nurse must first understand the ways that people learn. Learning depends on three conditions: the willingness or motivation to learn, the ability to learn, and the learning environment. Motivation addresses a person's willingness to put effort into learning (Redman, 1988). The client's willingness to become involved in learning influences a nurse's teaching approach. Previous knowledge, attitudes, and sociocultural factors influence motivation.

The ability to learn depends on physical and cognitive attributes. Developmental level, physical wellness, and intellectual thought processes determine a person's ability to learn. If a person's learning ability is impaired, a teacher may postpone teaching activities or modify strategies to better meet the learner's needs.

The environment has a significant impact on the ability to learn. One of the teacher's major tasks is to manipulate environmental conditions to facilitate learning. This can be particularly challenging for a nurse in a busy health care setting.

Motivation to Learn

Attentional Set

People's minds generally function with mental pictures. For example, as a teacher explains how to give support to a dying client, students might envision grasping the fragile hand of a person taking a last breath. Before individuals can learn, they must give attention to, or concentrate on, information to be learned. An attentional set is the mental state that allows the learner to focus and comprehend the material. A number of factors influence this ability to attend, including physical discomfort, anxiety, and environmental distractions.

Any physical condition that impairs the ability to concentrate interferes with learning. Pain, fatigue, hunger, thirst, and even the urge to urinate or defecate create barriers to learning.

Anxiety may increase or decrease the ability of a person to learn. Anxiety is uneasiness from anticipation of threat or danger. When faced with change or the need to act differently, a person feels anxiety. Learning requires a change in behavior and thus produces anxiety. A mild level of anxiety may motivate learning. However, a high level of anxiety prevents learning; it incapacitates a person, creating an inability to attend to anything other than its immediate relief.

Environmental distractions (discussed in a later section) interfere with the ability to attend to a teacher and learning activities. Unplanned interruptions or an uncomfortable environment are not conducive to learning.

Motivation

Motivation is an internal impulse that causes a person to take action; it is the desire to learn. It implies that at some point in time a person is receptive to learning. A person may become motivated to learn by an idea, emotion, or physical need. If a person does not want to learn, it is unlikely that learning will occur.

The social, task mastery, and physical motives stimulate a person to learn. Social motives are a need for affiliation, social approval, or self-esteem. People normally seek out others with whom to compare opinions, abilities, and emotions. For example, a student often works hard to win praise from a teacher or the admiration of peers.

Task mastery motives are based on needs such as achievement and competence. A nursing student repeatedly works in a laboratory to learn the technique for giving an injection because of the motivation to master the task or skill. After a success, there is usually greater motivation to achieve more.

Often the motives of a client are physical. If a client suffers a physical change in function, that change may become a motivator for learning. According to Tanner (1989), knowledge that is necessary for survival creates a stronger stimulus for learning than knowledge that merely promotes health. For example, when a client experiences a loss in strength of a body part, there is motivation to learn exercises that will rehabilitate and restore normal strength.

Not everyone is interested in maintaining health. A person with lung disease may continue to smoke. A woman whose obesity worsens her heart condition may refuse to follow her diet. No therapy will have an effect unless a person is motivated by the belief that health is important. The trend in health care is to treat clients in their homes after they recover from the acute phase of illness. Such treatment is successful only if clients follow the recommendations of their physicians and health care team. Clients must believe that they will benefit from changing behaviors that do not contribute to healthier lifestyles. **Compliance** is clients' fulfillment of the prescribed course of therapy. The goal of a nurse's teaching plan is to help clients improve their levels of health and quality of life.

Clients' health beliefs and behaviors are major targets of teaching, and at the same time they affect the probability that change will occur (Redman, 1988). Health beliefs can be powerful motivators, and they are influenced by a number of variables (see Chapter 2). The following health beliefs are critical to people taking a health action (Rosenstock, 1960):

1. They believe that they are susceptible to the disease in question.
2. They believe that the disease would have serious effects on their lives if they contracted it.
3. They believe that actions can be taken to reduce the likelihood of contracting the disease or lessen its severity.
4. They believe that the threat of taking these actions is not as great as the threat of the disease itself.

The health-belief model (see Chapter 2) was originally designed to explain the reasons that persons attempt health actions. Later the model was used to predict compliance with therapies. Motivation now appears to play a role in the application of the health-belief model. Motivation is a cue for preventive health action. Further research is still needed on the usefulness of the model in predicting changes in client behavior. However, proven examples of motivational triggers are interpersonal crisis, interference of symptoms with valued social activity, and the nature and quality of symptoms (Redman, 1988).

Nurses can use the health-belief model in health education. If a nurse can modify clients' perceptions of their susceptibility to a disease or its severity, they may be more receptive to learning. When the perceived threat of a disease and the benefit of professional intervention are recognized, educational measures can lead to predictable changes in health behavior. The model does not prescribe strategies for changing health behavior. There is no standard method for motivating a person with a given health belief. However, the model can be useful in the assessment of a client's educational needs and willingness to learn.

Health education often involves changing attitudes and values that are not altered by simple teaching of facts. Therefore the nurse gives attention to ideas or beliefs that motivate a person to learn and applies the motivating factor to the teaching plan. The following example illustrates this point:

Mr. James is a 42-year-old businessman with high blood pressure. The nurse recognizes that Mr. James needs to learn about his condition, the type of treatment, and implications of his illness for his busy lifestyle. Mr. James is a highly motivated man who works hard for success. He admits that he has always felt himself invincible to any physical malady. Now he tells the nurse that he knows he cannot continue his hectic work pace unless he regains his health.

The nurse's teaching plan will integrate two principal motivators that Mr. James has acknowledged: the desire to succeed and the concern that high blood pressure will seriously affect his work life. The nurse will use Mr. James' motivation for success as the means to help him acquire better health habits. Mr. James will learn the ways that high blood pressure impairs physical function and the ways in which he can avoid factors that can aggravate blood pressure problems.

Psychosocial Adaptation to Illness

Loss of health, whether temporary or permanent, is difficult for people to accept. The process of grieving gives them time to adapt psychologically to the emotional and physical implications of illness. The stages of grieving (see Chapter 28) are a series of responses that clients experience during illness. People experience these stages at different rates and sequences, depending on their self-concepts before illness, the severity of illness, and the changes in lifestyle that the illness creates. Effective supportive care guides clients through the grieving process.

Readiness to learn is significantly related to the stage of grieving (Table 16-2). When unwilling or unable to accept the reality of illness, clients cannot learn. However, properly timed, teaching can facilitate adjustment to illness or disability.

The nurse identifies the client's stage of grieving on the basis of typical behaviors. When the client enters the stage of acceptance, during which learning can occur, the nurse presents a teaching plan. Continuous assessment of the client's behaviors deter-

TABLE 16-2   Relationship Between Psychosocial Adaptation to Illness and Learning

Stage	Client's Behavior	Learning Implications	Rationale
Denial or disbelief	Client avoids discussion of illness ("There's nothing wrong with me"), withdraws from others, and disregards physical restrictions. Client suppresses and distorts information that has not been presented clearly.	Provide support, empathy, and careful explanations of all procedures while they are being done. Let client know you are available for discussion. Explain situation to family. Teach in present tense (e.g., explain current therapy).	Any attempt to convince or tell client about illness will result in further anger or withdrawal. (Client is not prepared to deal with problem.) Provide only information client pursues or absolutely requires.
Anger	Client blames and complains and often directs anger toward nurse.	Do not argue with client, but listen to concerns. Teach in present tense. Reassure family of client's normality.	Client needs opportunity to express feelings and anger; client is still not prepared to face future.
Bargaining	Client offers to live better life in exchange for promise of better health ("if God lets me live, I promise to be more careful").	Continue to introduce only reality. Teach only in present tense.	Client is still unwilling to accept limitations.
Resolution	Client begins to express emotions openly, realizes that illness has created changes, and begins to ask questions.	Encourage expression of feelings. Begin to share information needed for future, and set aside formal times for discussion.	Client begins to perceive need for assistance and is ready to accept responsibility for learning.
Acceptance	Client recognizes reality of condition, actively pursues information, and strives for independence.	Focus teaching on future skills and knowledge required. Continue to teach about present occurrences. Involve family in teaching information for discharge.	Client is more easily motivated to learn. Acceptance of illness reflects willingness to deal with its implications.

mines the stage of grieving. Teaching continues as long as the client remains in a stage wherein learning can occur.

Active Participation

A client's involvement in learning implies an eagerness to acquire knowledge or skills. It also improves the opportunity for the client to make decisions during teaching sessions. For example, a client diagnosed with diabetes learns to monitor blood glucose levels to gain control of the disease. Through participation with the nurse, the client learns to adapt a monitoring system and schedule to personal lifestyle (Fig. 16-1). The client helps decide the type of glucose meter that will be easiest to use.

Roter (1987) describes a partnership model for health education; the partnership is between nurse and client. The model stresses the value of client collaboration with nurses during any educational activ-

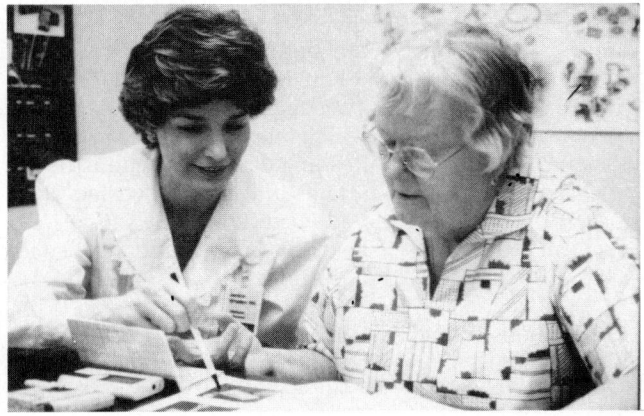

Fig. 16-1   Nurse instructing client with glucose meters. Courtesy Barnes Hospital, St. Louis.

ity. There is a greater transfer of knowledge when a client learns by participating. In addition, the learner gains confidence in the ability to solve problems. The client also gains knowledge and skills that will be useful and meaningful in day-to-day experiences.

Ability to Learn

Developmental Capability

Cognitive level of development influences a person's ability to learn. A nurse can be a competent teacher, but teaching will be unsuccessful if the client's intellectual abilities are not considered. For example, a teaching booklet is not useful if a client is illiterate, and a client who is unable to perform simple mathematical calculations will have difficulty learning to calculate medication doses.

Learning, like developmental growth, is an evolving process. A required level of maturation and cognitive development is needed before an individual becomes capable of learning. The nurse must know clients' levels of knowledge and intellectual skills before beginning teaching plans. In addition, learning occurs more readily when new information complements existing knowledge. Table 16-3 shows the types of learning problems that clients may have when their intellectual skills are not fully developed.

AGE GROUP. Age reflects the developmental capability for learning and the type of learning behavior that can be acquired (Table 16-4). Without proper biological, motor, language, and personal-social develop-

ment, many types of learning cannot take place. Learning occurs when behavior changes as a result of experience or growth (Whaley, Wong, 1991).

Physical Capability

The ability to learn often depends on the level of physical development and overall physical health. To learn psychomotor skills, a client must possess the necessary level of strength, coordination, and sensory acuity. For example, it is useless to teach a client to transfer from a bed to a wheelchair if the client has insufficient upper body strength. An older client cannot learn to apply an elastic bandage if eyesight is poor and if the fingers cannot grasp the bandage tightly. Therefore the nurse should not overestimate the client's physical development or status. The following physical attributes are required to learn psychomotor skills:

1. Size, or the height and weight to match the task to perform or the equipment to use (for example, crutch walking)
2. Strength, or the ability to follow a strenuous exercise program
3. Coordination, or the dexterity needed for complicated motor skills (for example, using utensils or changing a bandage)
4. Sensory acuity, or the sensory modalities needed to receive and respond to messages taught (for example, vision, hearing, touch, taste, and smell)

Any condition (for example, pain) that depletes a person's energy will also impair the ability to learn. A client who spends a morning undergoing diagnostic studies will possibly not be capable of a learning discussion. When an illness becomes aggravated by complications, such as a high fever or respiratory difficulty, teaching should be postponed. The nurse assesses energy level by noting a client's willingness to communicate, amount of activity initiated, and responsiveness toward questions. The nurse may halt teaching temporarily if a client needs rest. The nurse achieves greater teaching success when the client is an active participant in learning.

Learning Environment

The physical environment where teaching takes place makes learning pleasant or difficult. The nurse chooses a setting that helps the client focus on the learning task. The following factors are important when choosing the setting:

1. Number of persons being taught
2. Need for privacy
3. Temperature

TABLE 16-3 Cognitive Skills and Learning Implications

Intellectual Skill	Examples of Potential Problems
Math calculation	Computing drug doses, measuring liquid or solid food allotments, reading thermometer or syringe calibrations
Reading	Reading directions and instructions in teaching booklets and on medication labels
Problem solving	Learning how to regulate insulin doses on basis of signs and symptoms
Comprehension and application	Understanding physical restrictions imposed by illness; following directions when performing self-care in accordance with limitations

TABLE 16-4 Developmental Capacities for Learning

Learning Capacity	Teaching Methods
INFANT	
Infant relies on parents for basic needs.	Keep routines (e.g., feeding, bathing) consistent.
Infant learns to trust adults when they convey love and compassion.	Hold infant firmly while smiling and speaking softly to convey sense of trust.
Infant explores environment through senses.	
TODDLER	
Toddler learns to understand words and express feelings verbally.	Use play to teach procedure or activity (e.g., handling examination equipment, applying bandage to doll).
Toddler learns by associating words with objects.	Offer picture books that describe story of children in hospital or clinic.
Toddler likes to explore environment through play.	Use simple words such as *cut* instead of *laceration* to promote understanding.
PRESCHOOLER	
Vocabulary grows.	Use role playing, imitation, and play to make it fun for preschoolers to learn.
Preschooler uses language without comprehending meaning of words, especially concepts (e.g., right or left, time).	Encourage questions and offer explanations. Use simple explanations and demonstrations.
During play, child expresses feelings more through actions than words.	Encourage children to learn together through pictures and short stories of how to perform hygiene.
Preschooler asks questions and imitates adults.	
SCHOOL-AGE CHILD	
Child interacts with adults and peers outside immediate family.	Teach psychomotor skills needed to maintain health. (Complicated skills, such as learning to use a syringe, may take considerable practice.)
Child begins to acquire ability to relate series of events and actions to mental representations that can be expressed verbally and symbolically.	Offer opportunities to discuss health problems and answer questions.
Child is able to make judgments.	
Child matures physically.	
Play becomes more formal and imaginative.	
Child is inquisitive and asks many questions about health.	
ADOLESCENT	
Adolescent struggles between childlike feelings of dependence and independence of adults.	Help adolescent learn about feelings and need for self-expression.
Teenager wants to be in control but, during illness, fears loss of self-concept or body image.	Use teaching as collaborative activity.
Adolescent is able to solve abstract problems.	Allow adolescents to make decisions about health and health promotion (e.g., safety, sex education, substance abuse).
Teenager learns best when immediate benefit is gained.	Use problem solving to help adolescents make choices.
YOUNG OR MIDDLE ADULT	
Adult complies with health teaching because client fears the results, is trying to gain approval, is responding to nurse's attitude, or knows it is in best interest.*	Encourage participation in teaching plan by setting mutual goals.
Learning occurs when adult values information being taught.	Encourage independent learning.
	Offer information so that adult can understand effects of health problem.

*Data from Woodward S: *Preoperative patient education seminar presentation*, Denver, 1983, Resource Applications.

Continued.

TABLE 16-4 Developmental Capacities for Learning—cont'd	
Learning Capacity	Teaching Methods
OLDER ADULT	
Often, there is decline in visual and auditory acuity, which impairs perception of stimuli.	Teach when client is alert and rested.
Sensory alterations, mobility limitations, and physical coordination problems affect capacity to learn.	Involve adult in discussion or activity.
	Focus on wellness and the person's strength.
Sleep-wake cycles are more fragmented.	Use approaches that enhance sensorially impaired client's reception of stimuli (see Chapter 45).
Older adult takes pride in being independent and caring for self.	Keep teaching sessions short.
There is no decline in intelligence with age.	

4. Lighting
5. Noise
6. Ventilation
7. Furniture

The ideal environment for learning is a room with good lighting, good ventilation, appropriate furniture, and a comfortable temperature. A darkened room interferes with the client's ability to see, especially during demonstrations and use of visual aids. A room that is cold, hot, or humid and stuffy makes the client too uncomfortable to pay attention to the nurse's activities. Comfortable furniture helps eliminate distractions, such as the need to continually change position or shift body weight. A businesslike yet warm and accepting atmosphere promotes learning in children and adults (Klausmeier, 1985; Redman, 1988). Posters, displays, or equipment for practicing skills motivates a learner by stimulating curiosity. It is also important to choose a quiet setting to minimize distractions.

When a nurse works with only one client, the best setting for learning is one that is quiet and offers privacy. The nurse can provide privacy even in a busy hospital by closing cubicle curtains or taking the client to a quiet spot. In a home a bedroom might separate the client from household activities. If the client desires, family members might share in discussions. However, some clients are reluctant to discuss their illnesses when others, even close family members, are in the room.

Teaching a group of clients requires a room that allows everyone to be seated comfortably and within hearing distance of the teacher. The size of the room should not overwhelm the group, tempting participants to sit outside the group along the room's perimeter. Arranging the group to allow participants to observe one another further enhances learning. More effective communication occurs as learners observe others' verbal and nonverbal interactions.

 ## INTEGRATING THE NURSING AND TEACHING PROCESSES

A relationship exists between the nursing and teaching processes. With the nursing process, a thorough assessment reveals the client's health care needs. The nursing diagnoses identified are unique to the client's situation. A care plan is individualized, prescribing nursing therapies designed to improve or maintain the client's level of health. Evaluation determines the level of success in meeting goals.

While diagnosing a client's health care problems, the nurse may also identify the need for education. When education becomes a part of the care plan, the teaching process begins. Like the nursing process, the teaching process requires a thorough assessment, in this case analyzing the client's need, motivation, and ability to learn (Table 16-5). A diagnostic statement specifies the information or skills required by the client. When establishing a teaching plan, the nurse sets specific learning objectives. The implementation of a teaching plan involves the use of learning and teaching principles to ensure that the client acquires knowledge and skills. Finally, the teaching process requires an evaluation of learning based on learning objectives. If objectives are unmet, additional teaching is provided.

The nursing and teaching processes are not the same. The nursing process requires an assessment of all sources of data to determine a client's total health care needs. The teaching process focuses primarily on the client's learning needs and the willingness and capability to learn.

TABLE 16-5 Comparison of the Nursing and Teaching Processes

Basic Steps	Nursing Process	Teaching Process
Assessment	Collect data about client's physical, psychological, social, cultural, developmental, and spiritual needs from client, family, diagnostic tests, medical record, nursing history, and literature.	Gather data about client's learning needs, motivation, ability to learn, and teaching resources from client, family, learning environment, medical record, nursing history, and literature.
Nursing diagnosis	Identify appropriate nursing diagnoses.	Identify client's learning needs on basis of three domains of learning.
Planning	Develop individualized care plan. Set diagnosis priorities based on client's immediate needs. Collaborate with client on care plan.	Establish learning objectives, stated in behavioral terms. Identify priorities regarding learning needs. Collaborate with client on teaching plan. Identify type of teaching method to use.
Implementation	Perform nursing care therapies. Include client as active participant in care. Involve family in care as appropriate.	Implement teaching methods. Actively involve client in learning activities. Include family participation as appropriate.
Evaluation	Identify success in meeting desired outcomes and goals of nursing care.	Determine outcomes of teaching-learning process. Measure client's ability to achieve learning objectives. Reteach as needed.

 ## Assessment

The nurse must assess the skills and knowledge that the client may require, the client's motivation and ability to learn, and methods and resources for instruction. The client, family members, and the health care team are resources for this assessment.

Learning Needs

The nurse determines the information that is critical for the client to learn. The client's learning needs determine the choice of teaching content. Learning needs can change from the time a client enters a health care agency to the time of discharge from the agency and after the client resumes self-care at home. The nurse must therefore conduct an ongoing assessment of potential learning needs. All individuals do not have common learning needs. An effective assessment should be the basis by which instruction can be individualized to a client's lifestyle and perceived needs (Redman, 1988). The nurse assesses the following:

1. Questions raised by the client or family about health issues. When a client feels a need to know something, the nurse recognizes that the client will likely be receptive to learn.
2. Client's level of understanding of current health status, implications of illness, types of therapy, and prognosis. This information helps to determine a client's perception of the threat of illness and its effect on lifestyle.
3. Information or skills needed by the client to perform self-care and to understand the implications of a health problem. Health care members anticipate learning needs related to specific health problems. For example, a newly diagnosed diabetic client will obviously need to learn about dietary control. A client who has had major surgery must learn the physical restrictions imposed by the procedure.
4. Client's experiences that influence the need to learn. For example, a client who has had previous surgery is more likely to be familiar with preoperative procedures.
5. Information that family members require to support the client's needs. The extent of information depends on the extent of the family's role in helping the client.

Motivation to Learn

Nurses can use several assessment tools to assess the client's motivation to learn. In the absence of such tools the nurse can ask questions that will help define motivation. These questions focus on determining whether the client is prepared and willing to learn. Even though a client may have a variety of learning needs, a lack of motivation seriously threatens the success of the teaching plan. The nurse assesses the following motivational factors:

1. Client behavior (for example, attention span, tendency to ask questions, memory, and ability to concentrate during questioning). In acute care settings a client's physical condition can easily detract from learning.
2. Client's health beliefs and perception of the severity of a health problem, efficacy of current treatment, and extent of possible bodily harm.
3. Client's attitudes about health care providers (for example, role of client and nurse in making decisions). Mutually set goals are more likely to be valued by the client.
4. Client's description of information to learn. The client must play an active role in seeking health-based information.
5. Pain, fatigue, anxiety, or other symptoms that can interfere with the ability to attend and participate.
6. Client's sociocultural background. A client's beliefs and values about health and various therapies may be influenced by sociocultural norms or tradition (see Chapter 4).
7. Client's learning-style preference. When various options are available for learning (for example, brochures, videotape, and discussion), a client may perceive one approach as being more interesting. Merritt (1991) studied learning-style preferences of clients who underwent cardiac surgery and found that they preferred organized, detailed instruction using oral and pictorial-graphic modes of presentation over independent instruction modes.

Ability to Learn

The nurse determines the client's physical and cognitive capabilities to learn. Health care providers often underestimate the client's cognitive deficits. A variety of factors can impair cognition, including body temperature, electrolyte levels, oxygenation status, and blood glucose level. In an acute care setting, several of these factors may influence a client at one time. The nurse assesses the following factors related to the ability to learn:

1. Physical strength, movement, and coordination. The nurse determines the extent to which the client can perform skills.
2. Sensory deficits (see Chapter 45) that may affect the client's ability to understand or follow instruction. The following example illustrates this point:

Mrs. Lyon is a 68-year-old woman who received a prescription from her physician for a heart medication that slows the heart's rate. Mrs. Lyon must learn to check her pulse to be sure that her heart does not beat too slowly. Assessment reveals that Mrs. Lyon is unable to feel an arterial pulse because her fingers are stiff and callused. No one who lives nearby is consistently available to check her pulse. However, Mrs. Lyon's hearing is still good. The nurse chooses instead to teach Mrs. Lyon to listen to her heart beat with a stethoscope.

---

3. Client's reading level. This can be difficult to assess because a functionally illiterate client is often able to conceal it. The nurse asks a client to read instructions from a teaching brochure and then explain its meaning.
4. Client's developmental level. This influences the approaches chosen by the nurse during teaching (see Table 16-4).
5. Client's cognitive function, including memory, knowledge, association, and judgment (see Chapter 20). Fig. 16-2 is an example of a tool that can be used to screen cognitive function.

Teaching Environment

The environment for a teaching session must be conducive to learning. The nurse assesses the following factors when seeking a place to teach clients:

1. Distractions or persistent noise. A quiet area should be set aside for teaching.
2. Comfort of the room, including ventilation, temperature, lighting, and furniture.
3. Room facilities and available equipment.

Resources for Learning

A client may require the support of family members or significant others. In this case the nurse assesses the readiness and ability of family and friends to learn the information necessary for the care of the client. The nurse also needs to understand the home environment. Assessment of resources also includes a review of any teaching tools available. The nurse assesses the following resources for learning:

1. Family members' perceptions and understanding of the client's illness and its implications. Family perceptions should match those of the client; otherwise, conflicts may arise in the teaching plan.
2. Client's willingness to have family members involved in the teaching plan and to provide health care. Information about the client's health care is confidential unless the client chooses to share it. Sometimes, it is difficult for the client to accept the help of family members, especially when bodily functions are involved.
3. Family's willingness to participate in care.
4. Resources within the home. These include persons willing to assist the client with procedures

Examiner _____ Date _____   Addressograph Plate

Instructions: Check items answered correctly. Write incorrect or unusual answers
in space provided. If necessary, urge patient once to complete task.

Introduction to patient: "I would like to ask
you a few questions. Some you will find
very easy and others may be very hard.
Just do your best."

1) What day of the week is this? ___
2) What month? ___
3) What day of the month? ___
4) What year? ___
5) What place is this? ___
6) Repeat the numbers 8 7 2. ___
7) Say them backwards. ___
8) Repeat these numbers 6 3 7 1. ___
9) Listen to these numbers 6 9 4.
   Count 1 through 10 out loud, then
   repeat 6 9 4. (Help if needed. Then
   use numbers 5 7 3.) ___
10) Listen to these numbers 8 1 4 3.
    Count 1 through 10 out loud, then
    repeat 8 1 4 3. ___
11) Beginning with Sunday, say the
    days of the week backwards. ___
12) 9 +3 is ___
13) Add 6 (to the previous answer
    to "to 12"). ___
14) Take away 5 ("from 18"). ___
    Repeat these words after me
    and remember them; I will ask for
    them later: HAT, CAR, TREE,
    TWENTY-SIX.

15) The opposite of fast is slow. The
    opposite of up is ___
16) The opposite of large is ___
17) The opposite of hard is ___
18) An orange and a banana are both
    fruits. Red and blue are
    both ___
19) A penny and a dime are both ___
20) What were those words I asked
    you to remember? (HAT) ___
21) (CAR) ___
22) (TREE) ___
23) (TWENTY-SIX) ___
24) Take away 7 from 100, then take
    away 7 from what is left and
    keep going: 100 − 7 is ___
25) Minus 7 ___
26) Minus 7 (write down answers;
    check correct subtraction of 7) ___
27) Minus 7 ___
28) Minus 7 ___
29) Minus 7 ___
30) Minus 7 ___
TOTAL CORRECT
(maximum score = 30) ___

Patient's occupation (previous, if not employed) _____ Education _____ Age _____

Estimated intelligence (based on education, occupation, and history, not on test score):

    Below average, Average, Above average _____

Patient was: Cooperative ___ Uncooperative ___ Depressed ___ Lethargic ___ Other ___

Medical diagnosis: _____

IF PATIENT'S SCORE IS LESS THAN 20, THE DIMINISHED COGNITIVE CAPACITY IS PRESENT.
THEREFORE, AN ORGANIC MENTAL SYNDROME SHOULD BE SUSPECTED AND THE FOL-
LOWING INFORMATION SHOULD BE OBTAINED.

Temp. ___   BUN ___   Endocrine dysfunction? _____

BP   ___   Glu ___ T_3, T_4,   Ca,   P,   etc.

Hct ___ Po_2 ___   History of previous psychiatric difficulty _____

Na   ___ Pco_2 ___   Drugs: _____

K   ___   Steroids?L-Dopa?Amphetamines?Tranquilizers?Digitalis?

Cl   ___   Focal neurological signs: _____

CO_2 ___

EEG _____   DIAGNOSIS: _____

ECG _____

Fig. 16-2 Cognitive
capacity screening
examination.
From Gehi M et al:
Gen Hosp Psychiatry
3:186, 1980.

such as bathing or taking medications, financial or material resources such as obtaining health care equipment, and architectural resources such as arrangement of rooms or stairways.

5. Teaching tools, including printed materials, audiovisual aids, or charts. Printed material should match the client's reading level and present subject material clearly and logically. Brochures or booklets must be current.

Nursing Diagnosis

After assessing information related to the client's need, motivation, and ability to learn, the nurse uses data to analyze and select nursing diagnoses that reflect specific learning needs (see diagnoses box). This ensures that teaching will be goal directed and individualized. If a client has several learning needs, the nurse specifies nursing diagnoses so that teaching priorities are set (see diagnostic process box).

Each diagnostic statement describes the client's specific learning need and its related cause. Classifying diagnoses by the three learning domains can help the nurse focus on what and how to teach.

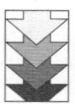

Examples of Nursing Diagnoses Related to Learning Needs

NANDA-APPROVED NURSING DIAGNOSES

Altered health maintenance related to:
- Lack of knowledge about health practices
- Lack of fine motor skills

Knowledge deficit (affective) related to:
- Misunderstanding of prognosis

Knowledge deficit (cognitive) related to:
- Newly diagnosed disease
- Newly prescribed therapy

Knowledge deficit (psychomotor) related to:
- Inexperience with skill
- Lack of interest in learning

Noncompliance with medications related to:
- Poor understanding of therapies
- Disbelief of health risk

Bathing/hygiene self-care deficit related to:
- Neuromuscular impairment
- Unfamiliarity with preventive care measures

Impaired social interaction related to:
- Poor communication skills

Some health care problems can be managed or eliminated through education. In these situations the etiology may be a knowledge deficit. For example, a client may have difficulty interacting socially because of a lack of effective communication skills, or a self care deficit may exist because of an inadequate knowledge base. Some nursing diagnoses may indicate barriers to effective learning (for example, pain or activity intolerance). In these cases the nurse delays teaching until the nursing diagnosis is resolved or the health problem is controlled.

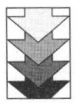

Sample Nursing Diagnostic Process Related to Learning Needs

Assessment Activities	Defining Characteristics	Nursing Diagnoses
Ask client to describe understanding of planned surgery.	States that physician has not yet provided explanation.	*Knowledge deficit (cognitive) regarding impending surgery* related to inexperience
Observe response to discussion about surgery.	Unable to describe purpose of surgery. Asks numerous questions and requests further information.	
Review medical record for history.	No previous surgical experience. Surgery is elective.	
Observe client attempt exercise program.	Unable to follow through with all exercise steps.	*Knowledge deficit (psychomotor) regarding ambulation training* related to impaired cognition
Ask client to describe steps to follow in exercises.	Cannot describe proper steps in sequence.	
Assess body temperature.	Fever of 38.8° C (102° F).	
Ask client to preform simple memory tests.	Unable to repeat sequence of numbers backward. Short-term memory of events is reduced.	

Planning

After determining the nursing diagnoses that indicate a client's learning needs, the nurse develops a teaching plan to promote cognitive, affective, and psychomotor learning (see care plan). The teaching plan incorporates the information learned about the client into individualized educational strategies. The client should be an active participant in the teaching plan. For example, the cient should agree to the plan, help choose instructional methods, and recommend times for instruction.

Developing Learning Objectives

The first step in forming a teaching plan is developing learning objectives. The **learning objectives** of health teaching are the behaviors desired as a result of the learning process (Redman, 1988). A learning objective identifies the expected outcome of a planned learning experience and helps establish priorities for learning. Despite all planning, a particular instructional session often leads to unanticipated learning. It may be difficult to anticipate all objectives for a teaching session. However, objectives cause a teacher to plan teaching sessions so that time is maximized and the best resources are available for learning.

Objectives are either short or long term. Short-term objectives relate to the client's immediate learning needs, such as knowing the nature of gallbladder disease to understand an upcoming test. Long-term objectives relate to acquisition of the knowledge and skills that are needed to permanently adapt to a health problem (for example, learning to plan a diet within restrictions caused by gallbladder disease). Like a goal of care, a long-term objective is usually all encompassing. Short-term objectives can be compared with the steps taken to achieve long-term goals.

Sample Nursing Care Plan for Knowledge Deficit

Nursing Diagnosis: *Knowledge deficit (cognitive) regarding impending surgery* related to inexperience
Definition: Knowledge deficit is the state in which specific information is lacking (Kim, McFarland, McLane).

Goals	Expected Outcomes*	Interventions	Rationale
Client will describe preoperative surgical care experience by 7/8.	Client will describe preoperative routines planned on morning before surgery (7/8), including monitoring and treatments, visit by anesthesiologist, and surgery time.	Five days before surgery, send client brochure on preoperative care.	Early timing and reinforcement of preoperative teaching may improve knowledge of surgery routines (Cupples, 1989).
		Make follow-up phone call 48 hours before surgery to discuss information.	Discusson helps client understand implications of surgery.
Client will participate in preoperative and postoperative surgical care procedures (7/8 and 7/9).	Client will demonstrate breathing and range of motion exercises by 7/8.	Demonstrate and have client return demonstration of breathing and exercise routines, including coughing, deep breathing, turning, and leg exercises.	Return demonstration effectively reveals success in learning motor skill.
	Client will describe postopertive routines and related rationale for recovery by 7/9.	Discuss benefits exercises have in preventing complications.	Cognitive learning is needed to give learners understanding of importance of motor skills.
		Discuss procedures to anticipate after surgery.	Discussion is appropriate teaching method for cognitive learning (Redman, 1988).
		Have client view videotape of postoperative surgical experience.	Videotape can be stimulus for follow-up discussion on points of interest.

*Teaching objectives.

The objectives established by the nurse and client guide the teaching plan. Poorly determined objectives can create confusion throughout the teaching-learning process. Thus a learning objective includes the same criteria as goals or outcomes in a nursing care plan (see Chapter 8), including the following:

1. Singular behaviors
2. Observable or measurable content
3. Timing or conditions under which the objective is measured
4. Goals mutually set between the nurse and client

Each objective is a statement of a singular behavior that identifies the learner's ability to do something after a learning experience. A behavioral objective contains an active verb describing what the learner will do after the objective is met, such as *to perform* a crutch gait, *to administer* an injection, or *to identify* drug dosages (Bloom, 1956). The verb should have few interpretations and be stated in terms of what the learner is to learn rather than what the teacher is to teach (Redman, 1988) (see box). Singular behaviors are easier to evaluate at the end of instruction.

Behavioral objectives are measurable and observable, indicating content to be learned (for example, "to perform *the three-point crutch gait*" or "to prepare *foods without using salt*"). The objective describes precise behaviors and content. An example of a vague or nonspecific objective might be "to be familiar with knowledge about diabetes." This example does not explain what the learner is to do, and it raises questions about how the behavior can be mea-

sured. The nurse observes for measurable behavioral changes in the client after instruction. Thus objectives should specify singular areas of content.

An objective is more precise when it describes the conditions or timing under which the behavior occurs. Conditions or time frames should be realistic and designed for the learner's needs (for example "to identify the side effects of Ritalin by discharge"). It also helps to consider conditions under which the client or family will typically perform the learning behavior (for example, "to walk from bedroom to bath using crutches"). The conditions for acceptable performance set a standard by which achievement of objectives is measured. A teacher sets conditions on the basis of a desired level of accuracy, success, or satisfaction. For example, a client undergoing therapy for a fractured leg will walk on crutches *to the end of the hall within 3 days*. Conditions are more acceptable when established by the teacher and learner. However, the nurse serves as a resource in setting the minimal conditions for success. Mutually agreed on conditions help define expected behaviors and quality of performance. The client uses the conditions as a form of self-evaluation, which is a powerful motivator of behavior.

Integrating Basic Teaching Principles

Teaching is the process of leading someone to learn. When developing a teaching plan, the nurse considers the principles that improve its effectiveness. The realm of teaching deals with teachers' behavior, reasons that they behave the way they do, and effects of their behavior on students. There is no single way to teach correctly. The best way to teach is determined by each learning situation. The principles of teaching are basically techniques for supporting the principles of learning.

SETTING PRIORITIES. Priorities for instruction are based on nursing diagnoses and the learning objectives established for the client. A client's learning needs must be set in order of priority to conserve the time and energy of the client and nurse. For example, a client who suffers a permanent leg injury has a knowledge deficit regarding the nature of the injury, its implications, and the types of skills needed to resume a normal life. The client will benefit most from first learning about the injury and the resultant physical changes before learning how to cope with the disability.

TIMING. The nurse determines the right time to teach, whether it is before clients enter clinics or hospitals, during admission to health care agencies, or at discharge. Each of these times may be appropri-

---

Terms Used for Objectives

TERMS WITH MANY INTERPRETATIONS

- To know
- To understand
- To realize
- To value
- To feel

TERMS WITH FEW INTERPRETATIONS

- To identify
- To describe
- To label
- To classify
- To demonstrate
- To select

ate because clients need to learn as long as they stay in the health care system. Teaching must be timed to coincide with readiness to learn.

Timing can be difficult in acute care settings because emphasis is placed on early discharge. For example, after surgery, it may take several days for a client to become free of discomfort. A variety of medications can cause the client to be drowsy and unable to attend to learning. By the time the client feels ready to learn, discharge may already be scheduled. The nurse should plan teaching activities for a time when the client is most attentive, receptive, and alert. Many hospitals are providing information to clients before their admission and after they return home. The client's activities should be organized to provide time for rest teaching-learning interactions.

The length of teaching sessions also influences learning ability. Prolonged sessions cause decreased concentration and attentiveness. Frequent sessions lasting 20 to 30 minutes are more easily tolerated and retain the client's interest. The nurse can assess for decreased concentration by observing for nonverbal cues, such as poor eye contact or slumped posture. After decreased concentration is noted, the session should be stopped. However, teaching sessions should not be too brief. The client needs time during each session to comprehend the information and to give feedback.

Teaching sessions should be planned frequently enough to document learning. The frequency of sessions depends on the learner's abilities and the complexity of the material. Intervals between teaching sessions should not be so long that the client might forget information. For a client discharged early, home health nurses must reinforce learning.

ORGANIZING TEACHING MATERIAL. A good teacher carefully plans the order in which to present information. An outline helps organize information into a logical sequence. Material should progress from simple to complex ideas because a person must learn the basics before making associations or complex interpretations of ideas. For example, to teach a client to calculate a 1200-calorie diet, the nurse first teaches the definitions of calories, proteins, and carbohydrates and then uses simple math to help the client learn to calculate amounts.

The nurse begins any instructional session with essential content. Clients are more likely to remember information that is taught during the first third of a teaching session (Miller, 1985). For example, after removal of a cancerous lung tumor, the client's risk for recurrence makes learning the warning signs of cancer crucial. The nurse starts with essential information and then completes a teaching session with informative but less critical content. Finally, a summary of the most important points covered during instruction is very useful. Repetition reinforces learning. A concise summary of key topics helps the learner know the most important information.

PROMOTING LEARNER ATTENTION AND PARTICIPATION. Active participation is a key learning principle. However, it is the teacher's responsibility to find ways to keep learners interested and involved. Learning is improved when more than one of the body's senses are stimulated. Audiovisual aids, drawings, and group participation are ways to stimulate learner attention. Several approaches can be used to promote participation, particularly when teaching sessions are lengthy.

A teacher's actions can also increase learner attention and interest. When conducting a discussion with a client, the teacher should stay active by changing tone and intensity of voice, making eye contact, and using gestures that accentuate key points. An effective teacher often uses as much energy as the learner, talking and moving among a group rather than remaining stationary behind a lectern or table. A client remains interested when the teacher is enthusiastic.

BUILDING ON EXISTING KNOWLEDGE. A client learns best on the basis of preexisting cognitive abilities and knowledge. Thus a teacher can be more effective by building on a learner's knowledge. To successfully build on a knowledge base, the nurse must conduct a thorough assessment of the learner's knowledge about the topic. A teaching plan must be individualized based on the client's learning needs. A client quickly loses interest if a nurse begins with familiar information.

SELECTION OF TEACHING METHODS. During planning the nurse chooses appropriate teaching methods and encourages the client to offer suggestions. A teaching method is the way that the teacher delivers information and is based on the client's learning needs (see box on p. 388). For example, a client with a psychomotor deficit learns best through demonstrations and supervised practice. The client masters skills by manipulating equipment and practicing manual skills. Discussions, question-and-answer sessions, and formal lectures are effective for promoting cognitive learning. Clients with intellectual deficits are given the opportunity to explore new ideas, recognize new relationships, and apply knowledge to their unique needs. More than one method may be used for instruction.

Teaching Methods

COGNITIVE

Discussion (one-on-one or group)

- May involve nurse and client or nurse with several clients
- Promotes active participation and focuses on topics of interest to client
- Allows peer support
- Enhances application and analysis of new information

Lecture

- Is more formal method of instruction because it is controlled by teacher
- Helps learner acquire new knowledge and gain comprehension

Question-and-answer session

- Is designed specifically to address client's concerns
- Assists client in applying knowledge

Role play, discovery

- Allow client to actively apply knowledge in controlled situation
- Promote synthesis of information and problem solving

Independent project (computer-assisted instruction), field experience

- Allow client to assume responsibility for completing learning activities at own pace
- Promote analysis, synthesis, and evaluation of new information and skills

AFFECTIVE

Role play

- Allows expression of values, feelings, and attitudes

Discussion (group)

- Allows client to acquire support from others in group
- Permits client to learn from other experiences
- Promotes responding, valuing and organization

Discussion (one-on-one)

- Allows discussion of personal, sensitive topics of interest or concern

PSYCHOMOTOR

Demonstration

- Provides presentation of procedures or skills by nurse
- Permits client to incorporate modeling of nurse's behavior
- Allows nurse to control questioning during demonstration

Practice

- Gives client opportunity to perform skills using equipment
- Provides repetition

Return demonstration

- Permits client to perform skill as nurse observes
- Is excellent source of feedback and reinforcement

Independent projects, games

- Require teaching method that promotes adaptation and origination of psychomotor learning
- Permit learner to use new skills

Writing Teaching Plans

In all health care settings, nurses develop written teaching plans for use by colleagues. When one nurse, such as a primary nurse, is responsible for developing the initial teaching plan, all information about the client is incorporated appropriately.

The teaching plan includes topics for instruction, optional resources (for example, equipment or teaching booklets), recommendations for involving family, and objectives of the teaching plan. A plan may be lengthy or in outline form.

The setting influences the complexity of any teaching plan. In an acute care setting, plans are concise and focused on the primary learning needs of the client because there is limited time for teaching. A home health care teaching plan may be more involved because nurses often have more time to instruct clients.

A plan should provide continuity of instruction, particularly when several nurses are involved in caring for the client. The more specific the plan, the easier it is for nurses to follow through. A step-by-step description of content areas to be covered (Fig. 16-3) is useful if several teaching sessions are needed. To avoid duplication, the nurse should know the point at which the last teaching session ended.

BARNES

C-33

DIABETIC INSTRUCTION RECORD

TI = TEACHING INITIATED
D/V = DEMONSTRATES/VERBALIZES UNDERSTANDING
FI = FAMILY INCLUDED

ADDRESSOGRAPH PLATE

ASSESSMENT

1. HIGHEST LEVEL OF FORMALIZED
   EDUCATION ATTAINED *High School*
2. VISION *Glasses required for reading*
3. LITERACY *Able to read and explain information in teaching booklet*
4. IDENTIFIED BARRIERS TO
   LEARNING

	DATE & INITIAL			
	TI	D/V	FI	COMMENTS
A) DISEASE OVERVIEW	P.L.	R.K.	P.L.	*Wife included in teaching*
1. DEFINITION OF DIABETES	3/28	3/29	3/28	*session*
2. LONGTERM COMPLICATIONS (MICROVASCULAR/MACROVAS-CULAR/NEUROPATHY)	P.L. 3/28	R.K. 3/29	P.L. 3/28	
3. 3 FACTORS OF CONTROL (DIET, EXERCISE, MEDICATION)	P.L. 3/28	R.K. 3/29	P.L. 3/28	
B) DIET	R.K. 3/29			
1. TYPE *1800 Cal. ADA*				
SNACK TIMES *8:00 PM*	3/29 R.K.			
2. MEAL TIMING *8am 12N 6pm*	3/29 R.K.			
3. FOOD TYPES TO AVOID (FRIED FATTY FOODS, SIMPLE SUGARS)				
4. IMPORTANCE OF WEIGHT CONTROL				
C) EXERCISE				
1. TYPE				
2. FREQUENCY				
3. DURATION				
4. EFFECTS ON BLOOD SUGAR CONTROL & INSULIN UTILIZATION				
D) MEDICATION				
1. NAME/DOSAGE				
2. ORAL AGENT				
a. WHEN TO TAKE				
b. ACTION OF MEDICATION				
3. INSULIN				
a. ACTION, KINDS, STORAGE				
b. PREPARATION, ADMINISTRATION				
c. SITE SELECTION/ROTATION				

Fig. 16-3 Documentation tool for client teaching.
Courtesy Barnes Hospital, St Louis.

Implementation

Implementation of a teaching plan involves application of all teaching and learning principles, including the following:

1. Know the client's learning needs.
2. Select a time that coincides with the client's readiness and ability to learn.
3. Know the client's ability to comprehend (Streiff, 1986) (see research highlight).
4. Select a teaching method that fits the learning domain for the client's learning need.
5. Select and establish priorities for content.
6. Actively involve the client and family in the teaching plan.
7. Be aware of personal teaching abilities (know content, be interested in the learner, and be aware of personal motives).
8. Use appropriate teaching aids and resources.
9. Control the environment so that it is conducive to learning.
10. Use repetition and reinforcement appropriately.
11. Give the client feedback.

Implementation involves viewing each interaction with a client as an opportunity to teach. The nurse

 Research Highlight

The problem of functional illiteracy is growing in the United States. Nurses often rely on educational pamphlets or brochures as teaching aids for clients. However, most are written at well above the eighth-grade level. A reading level below fifth grade is considered functional illiteracy.

Streiff conducted a study to determine whether clients in an ambulatory care setting read at a level allowing them to comprehend educational material. Streiff interviewed 106 adults, and their reported and actual reading levels were compared. Reported reading levels, indicated by the client's last grade completed in school, were significantly higher (mean = 3.1 grades) than actual reading level. The majority of clients (54.7%) read at levels that did not allow them to comprehend any educational materials available at their site of primary care.

Streiff LD: Can clients understand our instructions? *Image J Nurs Sch* 18(2):48, 1986.

maximizes opportunities for effective learning and uses a diversified approach to create an active learner-teacher exchange of ideas.

Teaching Approaches

A nurse's approach in teaching is different from teaching methodologies. Approach involves the nurse's task and relationship behaviors (Paulish, 1987). Some situations require a teacher to be directive, whereas others require a nondirective approach. An effective teacher concentrates on the task and recognizes that the approach may change based on the learner's response and the relationship with the client. A client's needs and motives can change over time. Thus the nurse must always be aware of the need to modify teaching approaches. Paulish (1987) suggests a model for teaching approaches based on situational leadership theory (see Chapter 17).

TELLING. This approach (high task–low relationship behavior) is appropriate when limited information or instructions must be taught. For example, preparing a client for an emergency diagnostic procedure. If a client is highly anxious but it is vital for information to be given, telling can be effective. Paulish (1987) warns that telling may not be effective, especially when client participation is desirable. When using telling, the nurse outlines the task (cognitive or psychomotor) to be done by the client and gives explicit instructions. There is no opportunity for feedback from the client.

SELLING. Although the nurse still provides structure and instruction in this approach (high task–high relationship), two-way communication is used. The nurse paces instruction on the basis of client response. Specific feedback is given to the client who shows success at learning. For example, a client learns the step-by-step procedure for a dressing change. The nurse uses the client's feelings about performing the procedure to adapt the teaching approach.

PARTICIPATING. This approach (high relationship–low task behaviors) involves the nurse and client setting objectives and participating in the learning process together. The client helps decide content, and the nurse guides and counsels the client with pertinent information. For example, a client with diabetes must learn about diet, exercise, and possible complications of the disease. Learning activities must be adapted to incorporate elements of the home environment. There is opportunity for discussion, feedback, and revision of the teaching plan during participation.

ENTRUSTING. With this approach (low relationship–low task behaviors) the client shows the ability to manage self-care. Responsibilities are accepted, and tasks are performed well. The nurse observes the client's progress and remains available to assist without introducing a lot of new information. For example, a diabetic client has been self-administering insulin for over 3 months. Injections are performed correctly, and the client can explain signs and symptoms of low blood glucose levels. The nurse instructs the client about a new prescribed dose of medication.

REINFORCING. The principle of reinforcement applies to the process of learning; however, the teacher must often be the source of reinforcement. **Reinforcement** is using a stimulus that increases the probability of a response. A learner who receives reinforcement before or after a desired learning behavior will likely repeat the behavior. Feedback is a common form of reinforcement.

Reinforcers are positive or negative. Positive reinforcement, such as a smile or approval, produces desired responses. A reinforcement is negative if its removal after a learner's response produces the desired behavior. Threatening, complaining, and criticizing are examples of negative reinforcers. People usually respond better to positive reinforcement. The effects of negative reinforcement are less predictable and often undesirable.

There are three types of reinforcers: social, material, and activity. When a nurse works with clients, most reinforcers are social (for example, smiles, compliments, words of encouragement, or physical contact). A nurse uses verbal and nonverbal communication when acknowledging that a skill has been learned well. Examples of material reinforcers are food, toys, and music. These work best with young children. Activity reinforcers rely on the principal that people are motivated to engage in activities if promised that, after its completion, they will be able to do something else they like better. Clients are more likely to perform painful exercises if given the chance to take naps afterwards.

Choosing an appropriate reinforcer involves careful thought and attention to preferences. Observing behavior often helps reveal the best reinforcer to use. Reinforcers should never be used as threats, and reinforcement is not always effective with every client. A young child responds more to social reinforcers than older children or adults. An adult with whom

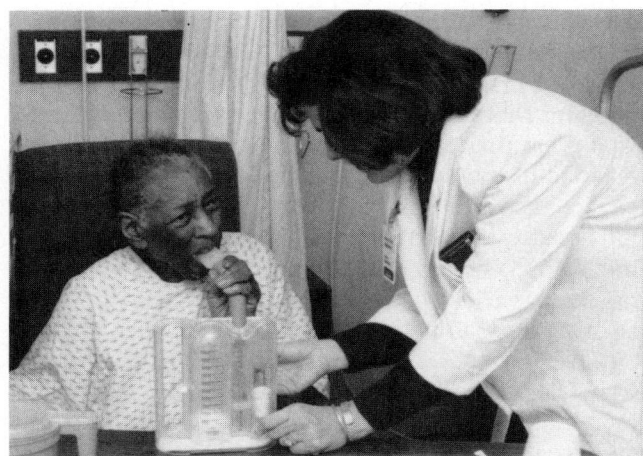

Fig. 16-4   Nurse teaching client at the bedside.

the nurse has a good relationship is more effectively reinforced than an adult with whom the nurse has a poor relationship.

Incorporating Teaching with Nursing Care

Many nurses find that they can teach more effectively while delivering nursing care. For example, while bathing a diabetic client the nurse discusses foot care, or while administering drugs the nurse may explain a medication's side effects. An informal, unstructured style relies on the positive therapeutic relationship between nurse and client, which fosters spontaneity in the teaching-learning process. This does not suggest that teaching should occur without a formal plan. When the nurse follows a teaching plan in an informal way, the client feels less pressure to perform, and learning becomes more of a shared activity. In addition, teaching during routine care is very efficient and cost effective (Fig. 16-4).

Instructional Methods

The methods chosen by a nurse in teaching depend on the client's learning needs (domain of learning), the time available for teaching, the setting, the resources available, and the nurse's own comfort level with teaching. Redman (1988) notes that teachers who are less knowledgeable and skilled in teaching often give information that they think is needed. More skilled teachers are flexible in altering teaching methods according to the learner's responses. An experienced teacher uses more techniques and teaching aids. A nurse cannot expect to be an expert educator when first entering nursing practice. Learning to become an effective educator takes time and practice.

When first starting to teach clients, it helps to remember that clients perceive the nurse as an expert. However, this does not mean that the nurse must have all of the answers. It simply means that clients expect that the nurse will keep them appropriately informed. The nurse can provide an effective teaching plan, keeping it simple and focused on clients' needs. A variety of teaching methods can be used, and a variety of teaching aids is usually available.

ONE-ON-ONE DISCUSSION. Perhaps the most common method of instruction used by a nurse is one-on-one discussion. By teaching clients at the bedside, in a physician's office, or in the home, the nurse shares information directly with them. Various teaching aids can be used during discussions, depending on clients' learning needs. Information is usually given in an informal manner, allowing clients to ask questions or share concerns. The nurse uses unstructured and informal discussion when helping clients understand the implications of illness and ways to cope with health stressors.

GROUP INSTRUCTION. A nurse uses group instruction with clients or families for one of the following reasons (Redman, 1988):
1. Groups are an economical way to teach a number of clients at one time.
2. The experience of being part of a group may be the most likely way for clients to meet learning objectives.

Group instruction often involves lecture and discussion. Lectures are highly structured and are efficient in helping groups of clients learn standard content about a subject. For example, a nurse might teach groups of clients about the warning signs of breast cancer, the health risks of smoking, or the normal development of a fetus. A lecture does not ensure that learners are actively thinking about the material presented, and thus discussion and practice sessions are essential (Redman, 1988).

After hearing information from a lecture, learners need the opportunity to share ideas and seek clarification. Group discussions allow clients and families to learn from each other as they review common experiences. A productive group discussion helps participants solve problems and arrive at solutions toward improving each member's health. To be an effective group leader, the nurse must be able to guide participation. Acknowledging a look of interest, asking questions, and summarizing key issues foster group involvement. However, not all clients benefit from group discussions, and sometimes physical or emotional level of wellness may prohibit participation.

PREPARATORY INSTRUCTION. Frequently, clients face unfamiliar tests or procedures that create significant anxiety. Providing information about procedures helps clients form realistic images of what to anticipate. This is a common expectation of clients in acute care settings because information helps to give them a sense of control. When an experience matches expectations, the client is more likely to attend to the nurse's future explanations. A nurse gains authority and respect when preparatory explanations prove useful. The nurses use the following guidelines for preparatory explanations:
1. Physical sensations during the procedure are described but not evaluated. For example, Mr. Reynolds is to have blood drawn as a routine admission test. The nurse explains that he will feel a sticking sensation as the needle punctures the skin. The nurse does *not* say, "It won't hurt very much."
2. The cause of the sensation is described, preventing misinterpretation of the experience. For example, the nurse tells Mr. Reynolds that often a needle insertion burns because alcohol used to clean the skin enters the puncture site.
3. Clients are prepared only for aspects of the experience that have commonly been noticed by other clients. For example, the nurse explains that, while blood is being drawn, the tight tourniquet often causes the hand to tingle and feel numb.

The client finds comfort in knowing what to expect. When the nurse's descriptions are accurate, the client copes more effectively with stress of procedures and therapies. The known is less threatening than the unknown.

DEMONSTRATIONS. A demonstration is an acting out for a learner and includes the teacher showing an intellectual skill or attitude or even a motor skill (see box). The client is able to observe a skill before practicing it. Demonstrations are most effective when learners first observe the teacher and then practice the skill in mock or real situations (**return demonstrations**). Nurses commonly use demonstrations for teaching motor skills; however motor skills are not learned separately from attitudes and factual knowledge (Redman, 1988). A demonstration should be combined with discussion to clarify concepts and

---

Examples of Skills Taught Using Demonstration

- Preparation of a syringe and self-injection
- Bathing an infant
- Crutch walking
- Transferring a client from wheelchair to bed
- Measuring a pulse
- Changing a dressing and cleaning a wound
- Range of motion exercises
- Deep-breathing exercises
- Stress-reduction techniques
- Communication techniques
- Conflict resolution

---

feelings. Before a demonstration of a motor skill the nurse follows these steps:

1. Be sure that the learner can easily see the demonstration. Position the learner to provide a clear view of the skill being performed.
2. Review the rationale and steps of the procedure.
3. Assemble and organize equipment. Be sure that all equipment works.
4. Prepare to perform each step in sequence while analyzing knowledge and skills involved.
5. Determine at what step explanations are to be given, considering the client's learning needs.
6. Judge proper speed and timing of the demonstration, based on the client's cognitive abilities and anxiety level.

The nurse demonstrates a skill in the same order in which the client will perform it. The demonstration involves the following:

1. Performing each step slowly and accurately
2. Encouraging the client to ask questions so that each step is understood
3. Explaining the rationale for each step
4. Allowing the client to observe each step
5. Avoiding a hurried approach
6. Allowing the client to handle equipment and practice the skill under supervision

The client demonstrates the procedure to ensure that learning has occurred. The independent demonstration should occur under the same conditions found at home or place where the skill is to be performed. For example, if a client is learning to walk with crutches, the nurse simulates the home envi-

ronment. If short, narrow steps lead to the client's bedroom, the client should learn to climb similar stairs in the hospital.

ANALOGIES. Learning occurs when a teacher translates complex language or ideas into words or concepts that the client understands. In addition, the client benefits by integrating new information into daily routines. **Analogies** supplement verbal instruction with familiar images that make complex information more real and understandable (Elsberry, Sorensen, 1986). For example, when explaining intestinal peristalsis to a client, an analogy would be the movement of an earthworm as the wave moves down the length of the worm. Another is comparing arterial blood pressure to the flow of water through a hose. To use analogies the nurse follows the following general principles:

1. Be familiar with the concept.
2. Know the client's background, experience, and culture.
3. Keep the analogy simple and clear.

ROLE PLAYING. A nurse uses role play for teaching ideas and attitudes. For example, a nurse may teach parents to respond to a child's behavior, help spouses to react to one another's anger, and assist families in communicating with dying relatives. During role play, people are asked to play themselves or someone else. The technique involves rehearsing a desired behavior. As a result of role play, clients are taught the skills required and feel more confident in being able to perform independently.

DISCOVERY. Discovery is a useful technique for teaching clients problem solving, application, and independent thinking. During individual or group discussion a nurse may pose a problem or situation for clients to solve. The problem pertains to the clients' learning needs. For example, clients with heart disease may be asked to plan a meal low in cholesterol. The clients in the group work together to decide which foods would be appropriate in the diet. The nurse asks the group members to present their diet, providing an opportunity to identify mistakes and reinforce correct information.

Speaking the Client's Language

It is important to use words that clients can understand. The nurse defines unfamiliar medical or nursing terms and uses them consistently throughout a teaching session. Medical jargon can be confusing. Byrne and Edeani (1984) found that clients under-

TABLE 16-6 Teaching Tools for Instruction	
Description	Learning Implications
PRINTED MATERIAL	
Written teaching tools available as pamphlets, booklets, brochures	Material must be easily readable for learner. Information must be accurate and current. Method is ideal for understanding complex concepts and relationships.
PROGRAMMED INSTRUCTION	
Written sequential presentation of learning steps requiring that learners answer questions and that teachers tell them whether they are right or wrong	Instruction is primarily verbal, but teacher may use pictures or diagrams. Method requires active learning, giving immediate feedback, correcting wrong answers, and reinforcing right answers. Learner works at own pace.
COMPUTER INSTRUCTION	
Use of programmed instruction format in which computers store response patterns for learners and select further lessons on basis of these patterns (Programs can be individualized.)	There is limited availability for health care clients. Method requires reading comprehension, psychomotor skills, and familiarity with computer.
NONPRINT MATERIALS **Diagrams**	
Illustrations that show interrelationships by means of lines and symbols	Method demonstrates key ideas, summarizes, and clarifies key concept.
Graphs (bar, circle, or line)	
Visual presentations of numerical data	Graphs help learner to grasp information quickly about single concept.
Charts	
Highly condensed visual summary of ideas and facts that may highlight series of ideas, steps, or events	Charts demonstrate relationship of several ideas or concepts. Method helps learners know what to do.
Physical objects	
Use of actual equipment, objects, or models to teach concepts or skills	Models are useful when real objects are too small, large, or complicated or are unavailable. Learners can manipulate objects that are to be used later in skill.
Other audiovisual materials	
Slides, audiotapes, television, and videotapes used with printed material or discussion	Materials are useful for clients with reading comprehension problems and visual deficits.

stand fewer medical words than health professionals predict. The problem of functional illiteracy is also real and growing. The nurse uses simple terminology to enhance clients' understanding. Frequently asking clients for feedback determines whether they comprehend terms used.

Using Teaching Tools

Many teaching tools are available for nurses to use when instructing a client. Selection of the right tool depends on the instructional method chosen, the client's learning needs, and the client's ability to learn (Table 16-6). For example, a printed pamphlet may

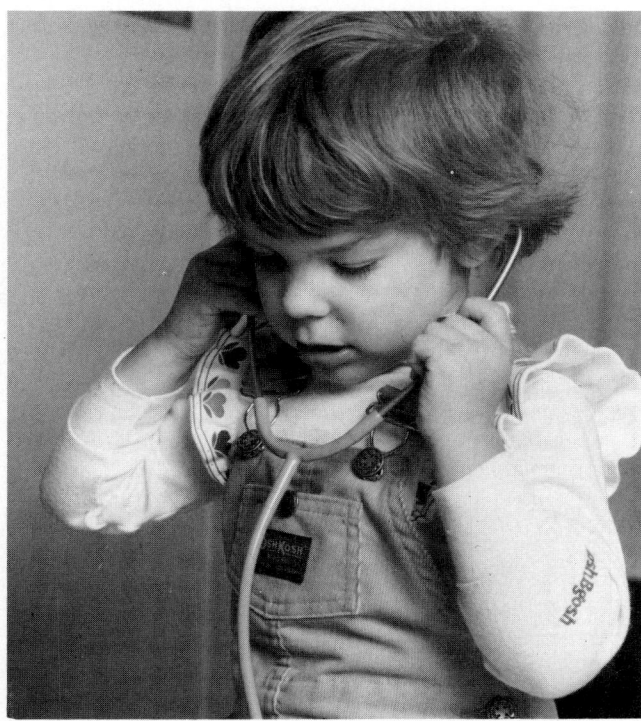

Fig. 16-5 The preschool child learns not to be afraid of medical equipment by being allowed to handle the stethoscope and imitating its use.

Teaching Strategies for Older Clients

- Use a slow pace of presentation.
- Give smaller amounts of information.
- Repeat information frequently.
- Reinforce oral teaching with audiovisual material, written exercises, and practice.
- Use analogies and examples.
- Reduce interruptions.
- Allow more time for learners to express themselves.
- Establish reachable short-term goals.
- Apply teaching to present situations.
- Base new information on what patients already know.

Adapted from Weinrich SP et al: *J Gerontol Nurs* 15(11):17, 1989

---

not be the best tool to use for a client with poor reading comprehension and, an audiotape may be the best choice for a client with visual impairment.

Special Needs of Children and Older Adults

A nurse's selection of instructional methods and application of teaching-learning principles may be based on a client's age. Children, adults, and older adults learn in different ways because of developmental differences. The nurse uses teaching strategies that maximize strengths and minimize the deficits that children and older adults bring to a learning experience.

Children pass through several developmental stages before adolescence (see Unit 5). In each developmental stage, children acquire new cognitive abilities that foster different types of learning (Fig. 16-5). For example, a nurse can teach school-age children about health as they acquire the ability to see things through the point of view of others. Dental hygiene, nutrition, safety measures, and sex education are examples of topics that may be presented to school children of varying ages. Parental input is incorporated in planning health education for children.

Older adults experience numerous physical and psychological changes as a result of aging (see Chapter 27). These changes can create barriers to learning unless adjustments are made in nursing interventions. Sensory changes such as visual and hearing deficits require techniques that enhance older adults' functioning senses (see Chapter 45). For example, the nurse sits to face clients with hearing problems and speaks in a low tone of voice during discussions. Clients with visual problems can benefit from the use of printed materials containing large print. Research shows that the ability of older adults to learn and remember is virtually as good as ever, especially if specific care is taken with the pace, the relevance of material, and the appropriateness of feedback (Hesse, 1984; Whitman, 1986). Although older adults have slower cognitive function and reduced short-term memory, nurses can facilitate learning in several ways (see box). When teaching older clients, the nurse should include family members who may be assuming partial care for the client.

 ### Evaluation

Client education is not complete until the nurse evaluates outcomes of the teaching-learning process (see evaluation box). The nurse determines whether clients have learned the material. Evaluation reinforces learners' correct behavior, helps learners realize how they should change incorrect behavior, and helps the teacher determine adequacy of teaching (Cronbach, 1977). The nurse evaluates clients' success at meeting each learning objective by measuring performance of each expected behavior under the desired conditions (see evaluation box). Success depends on clients' abilities to meet established performance criteria within the time frames identified within each objective.

Direct observation of behavior is useful when determining how a person will act in the future. Watching a client demonstrate a skill helps the nurse to know if the correct technique is being used. However, a client may choose to behave differently later. The most difficult measurement of behavior occurs with the affective domain because an individual can easily control the expression of feelings (Redman, 1988). Observation works best in a situation when a client is unaware of being watched.

Oral and written questioning are other useful evaluation methods. A client's success in cognitive learning can be measured verbally by answering questions about a specific topic that was taught. Questions measure behaviors that are not easily observed. The nurse should carefully phrase questions to be sure that the learner understands them and that objectives are truly measured.

Another form of evaluation includes self-reports (oral and written) and self-monitoring (written). This involves clients' or family members' providing information independently. An example might include a client's report of the foods eaten during a specific week, matched against a newly prescribed diet. The nurse relies on the client's honesty and memory in self-reporting.

During evaluation the nurse has the client demonstrate the behaviors described in the learning objec-

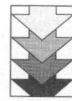

Sample Evaluation of Interventions for Knowledge Deficit

Goal	Evaluative Measures	Expected Outcomes
Client will describe preoperative surgical care experience by 7/8.	Ask client to identify procedures anticipated before surgery.	Client will describe preoperative routines planned on morning before surgery.
Client will participate in preoperative surgical care procedures by 7/8.	Have client demonstrate breathing exercises.	Client will demonstrate deep breathing exercises.
	Ask client to explain benefits of breathing exercises.	Client will describe how exercises help prevent pneumonia.

tives. If the evaluation process indicates a knowledge or skill deficit, the nurse repeats or modifies the teaching plan. Evaluation may reveal new learning needs or existence of new factors that may interfere with the client's ability to learn. Alternative teaching methods often help clarify information or skills that the client was unable to comprehend or perform originally. When a client has difficulty in an acute care setting the nurse may make a referral to resources such as home health care for further education and evaluation. Like the nursing process, the teaching-learning process is continuous and changing.

Documentation of Client Teaching

Because client teaching often occurs informally between nurse and client (for example, during medication administration or physical examination), it is difficult to document it consistently. Nurses often fail to take the time to write down material taught. However, because a nurse is legally responsible for providing accurate and timely information to clients, it is essential to document the outcomes of teaching. Barron (1987) suggests the following for documenting client education:

1. Specific content. Specifically describe the material taught so that other nurses can follow up and reinforce teaching (for example, "Insulin injection demonstrated" or "Explained side effects of Inderal"). Avoid generalizations, such as "medications taught," that leave staff confused.

2. Evaluation of learning. Document evidence of the outcomes of the client's learning (for example, a return demonstration or the ability to describe a medication). This informs the health care team about the client's progress and determines information that still needs to be taught.

3. Method of teaching. Describe teaching methods. Knowing the methods used in instruction (for example, demonstrations or discussion) helps nurses follow up more efficiently or offer alternative teaching methods if learning does not occur. When resources such as pamphlets or audiovisual materials are used the nurse documents it in the client's record. Many institutions have special forms that allow easy documentation.

SUMMARY

More than ever, a goal in health care is to engage clients and families in maintaining health and managing health problems. During interactions with clients the nurse has an opportunity to teach. The nurse teaches clients the knowledge and skills needed to maintain health or gain an improved level of function. Client education focuses on the client's unique needs and capacity for learning. The nurse and client work together to define information and skills that the client needs to learn.

Use of the nursing process allows the nurse to first define a client's learning needs. Then the application of the teaching process ensures an individualized teaching plan. The nurse assesses a client's learning needs, readiness, and ability to learn; the teaching environment; and resources for learning. Nursing diagnoses focus on specific types of learning needs. The teaching plan involves the nurse and client in a collaborative effort, setting realistic learning objectives. The nurse selects the teaching approaches and methods based on the client's learning needs and priorities.

A good teacher uses basic teaching principles to promote participation in learning. Teaching begins when the learner is most receptive. The teacher organizes teaching material in a format that progresses from simple to more complex ideas. The teacher's actions and use of instructional resources help stimulate interest in learning. To determine whether a client has gained the necessary knowledge or skills, the nurse evaluates the success of the teaching plan on the basis of expected learning outcomes or objectives.

CHAPTER 16 REVIEW

Key Concepts

- In the health care system today, there is greater emphasis in providing quality health education.

- The nurse must ensure that clients and families receive information needed to maintain optimal health.

- Client education is aimed at the promotion, restoration, and maintenance of health.

- Teaching is a form of interpersonal communication; teacher and student are actively involved in a process that increases the student's knowledge and skills.

- Teaching a client a specific behavior can involve incorporation of behaviors from all three learning domains.

- The ability to learn depends on a person's physical and cognitive attributes.

- The ability to attend to the learning process depends on physical comfort, low anxiety, and the lack of environmental distractions.

- Health beliefs influence the willingness to gain knowledge and skills necessary to maintain health.

- If a nurse can modify a client's perception of the severity of an illness and the client's susceptibility to disease, the client may become receptive to learning.

- Teaching must be timed to coincide with the client's readiness to learn.

- Clients of different ages require different teaching strategies as a result of developmental capabilities.

- When education becomes a part of the nurse's plan of care the teaching process begins.

- The client should be an active participant in a teaching plan, agreeing to the plan, helping choose instructional methods, and recommending times for instruction.

- Learning objectives describe measurable, singular behaviors performed under set conditions and time frames.

- Presentation of teaching content should begin with essential information and progress to more complex ideas.

- A combination of teaching methods improves the learner's attentiveness and involvement.

- A teacher is more effective when presenting information that builds on a learner's existing knowledge.

- A teacher who uses reinforcers such as praise or encouragement for a behavior is trying to increase the probability of the behavior recurring.

- The older adult learns most effectively when information is slow paced and presented in small amounts.

- A nurse evaluates a client's learning by observing performance of expected learning behaviors under desired conditions.

Key Terms

Affective learning, p. 354

Analogies, p. 373

Cognitive learning, p. 353

Compliance, p. 356

Learning, p. 351

Learning objectives, p. 365

Motivation, p. 355

Psychomotor learning, p. 354

Reinforcement, p. 371

Return demonstrations, p. 372

Teaching, p. 351

Critical Thinking Exercises

1. Mrs. Smith is a 40-year-old woman who is married and has three children. She is employed as an insurance agent for one of the top companies in the city. After a routine annual checkup, Mrs. Smith learns that she has diabetes. No one in her family has had the disease. The physician has prescribed daily insulin injections and a special diet. Apply the health-belief model in describing how to prepare a teaching plan for Mrs. Smith.

2. Cy Thomas underwent an amputation of his left lower leg as a result of a traumatic injury. It has been about 3 weeks since the injury. Cy comes to the clinic and usually becomes angry with the nurses and physician. He openly complains about the clinic facilities. How would you as the nurse approach teaching Mr. Thomas?

3. Mr. Taylor, 42 years old, has a right leg cast after repair of a fractured ankle. He is to begin crutch walking tomorrow and must learn about cast care. He is to be discharged in 2 days. What should the nurse assess regarding Mr. Taylor's ability to learn? Develop two learning objectives for Mr. Taylor.

4. The day shift at Mercy hospital begins at 7 AM. Your assignment for the day is the following four clients:
   Ms. Carter—Scheduled for an arteriogram at 7:30 AM, expected to return around noon with postprocedure orders. It is likely she will go home tomorrow with newly prescribed medications.
   Mrs. Simon—Has been evaluated in the hospital for dizziness and headaches. She has yet another diagnostic test scheduled early in the afternoon. She has asked for an explanation of the procedure. The night shift reported that she slept poorly.
   Mr. Lee—Underwent major bladder surgery for cancer 6 days ago. He has been instructed on care of his ileostomy (artificial opening created in the skin for urine drainage). Discharge is scheduled for this morning.
   Mrs. Tally—Underwent surgical removal of a breast mass yesterday. The staff report that her husband spent the night and has been very supportive. She asked about activity restrictions after she goes home.
   Identify in order of priority 1-4, when and how you would instruct each client.

REFERENCES

American Nurses Association: *Nursing's agenda for health care reform,* Kansas City, Mo, 1991, The Association.

Barron S: Documentation of patient education, *Patient Educ Couns* 9:81, 1987.

Bloom BS, editor: *Taxonomy of educational objectives,* vol 1, *Cognitive domain,* New York, 1956, Longman.

Byrne TJ, Edeani D: Knowledge of medical terminology among hospitalized patients, *Nurs Res* 33:178, 1984.

Cronbach LJ: *Educational psychology,* ed 3, New York, 1977, Harcourt Brace Jovanovich.

Cupples SA: *Effects of timing and reinforcement of preoperative education on knowledge and recovery of coronary artery bypass graft patients,* doctoral dissertation, Washington, DC, 1989, Catholic University of America.

Elsberry NL, Sorensen ME: Using analogies in patient teaching, *Am J Nurs* 86:1171, 1986.

Henderson V: *The nature of nursing: a definition and its implication for practice, research, and education,* New York, 1966, McMillan.

Hesse H: How elders view learning, *Geriatr Nurs* 5(1):37, 1984.

Joint Commission on Accreditation of Healthcare Organizations: *Accreditation manual of hospitals,* Chicago, 1992, The Commission.

Kim MJ, McFarland GK, McLane AM: *Pocket guide to nursing diagnoses,* ed 4, St Louis, 1991, Mosby–Year Book.

Klausmeier HJ: *Educational psychology,* ed 5, Philadelphia, 1985, Harper & Row.

Knowles M: *The modern practice of adult education,* Cleveland, 1970, Follett.

Krathwohl DR et al: *Taxonomy of educational objectives: the classification of educational goals, handbook II: Affective domain,* New York, 1964, David McKay.

Kruger S: The patient educator role in nursing, *Appl Nurs Res* 4(1):19, 1991.

Merritt S: Learning style preferences of coronary artery disease patients, *Cardiovasc Nurs* 27(2): 7, 1991.

Miller A: When is the time ripe for teaching? *Am J Nurs* 85:801, 1985.

Noble C: Are nurses good patient educators? *J Adv Nurs* 16:1185, 1991.

Paulish C: A model for situational patient teaching, *J Contin Educ Nurs* 18:163, 1987.

Redman BK: *The process of patient education,* ed 6, St Louis, 1988, Mosby–Year Book.

Rendon DC et al: The right to know, the right to be taught, *J Gerontol Nurs* (12):33, 1986.

Roter D: An exploration of health education's responsibility for a partnership model of client-provider relations, *Patient Educ Couns* 9:25, 1987.

Simpson EJ: The classification of educational objectives in the psychomotor domain. In *Contributions of behavioral science to instructional technology: the psychomotor domain,* Mt Rainer, Md, 1972, Gryphon Press.

Spicer J: Teaching the patient, *Nurs Mirror* 55:51, 1982.

Streiff LD: Can clients understand our instructions? *Image J Nurs Sch* 18(2):48, 1986.

Tanner G: A need to know, *Nurs Times* 85(31):54, 1989.

Whaley LF, Wong DL: *Nursing care of infants and children,* ed 4, St Louis, 1991, Mosby–Year Book.

Whitman NI: Age-related factors influencing selection of teaching strategies. In Whitman NI et al, editors: *Teaching in nursing practice: a professional approach,* Norwalk, Conn, 1986, Appleton-Century-Croft.

ADDITIONAL READINGS

Bartlett EE: Assessing benefits of patient education under prospective pricing, *Patient Education Newsletter,* University of Alabama, 1984.

Bartlett EE: Advocacy skills and strategies for patient education managers, *Patient Educ Couns* 8:397, 1986.

Bennett HL: Why patients don't follow instructions, *RN* 49:45, 1986.

Berg BK, Leisner B: Developing a geriatric patient education program, *Patient Educ Couns* 8:201, 1986.

Boyd CW: Patient education promotes transition from hospital to home, *Patient Educ Couns* 8:295, 1986.

Cunningham MA, Baker D: How to teach patients better and faster, *RN* 49:52, 1986.

Cushing M: Legal lessons on patient teaching, *Am J Nurs* 84:721, 1984.

Fielo SB, Rizzolok MA: Handle with caring: meeting elderly clients' special learning needs, *Nurs Health Care* 9(4):193, 1988.

Foster SD: An innovative documentation tool, *MCN* 11:419, 1986.

Fox V: Patient teaching: understanding the needs of the adult learner, *AORN J* 44:234, 1986.

Hindelang M: Aging: a positive experience of growth, *Patient Educ Couns* 9:209, 1987.

Huss K et al : Computer-assisted reinforcement of instruction: effects on adherence in adult atopic asthmatics, *Res Nurs Health* 14(4):259, 1991.

Kozol J: *Illiterate America,* Garden City, NY, 1985, Doubleday.

Leff EW: Ethics and patient teaching, *MCN* 11:375, 1986.

McHatton M: A theory for timely teaching, *Am J Nurs* 85:798, 1985.

McHugh NG, Christman NJ, Johnson JE: Preparatory information: what helps and why, *Am J Nurs* 82:780, 1982.

Morrison JL: The special needs of the special patient, *RN* 49(7):49, 1986.

Moss RC: Overcoming fear: a review of research on patient, family instruction, *AORN J* 43:1107, 1986.

Nielsen E, Sheppard MA: Television as a patient education tool: a review of its effectiveness, *Patient Educ Couns,* 11(1):3, 1988.

Peterson SK et al: Evaluation of a learning resource center for cancer patients, *Health Educ Res* 4(4):495, 1989.

Rosenstock IM: What research in motivation suggests for public health, *Am J Public Health* 50:295, 1960.

Rosenstock IM: The health belief model and preventive health behavior, *Health Educ Monogr* 2:354, 1974.

Smith C: Patient teaching, it's the law, *Nurs 87* 17:67, 1987.

Theis SL: Using previous knowledge to teach elderly clients, *J Gerontol Nurs* 17(8):34, 1991.

Ward DB: Why patient teaching fails, *RN* 49:45, 1986.

Weston C, Cranton PA: Selecting instructional strategies, *J Higher Educ* 57(3):259, 1986.

Woodard S: *Preoperative patient education seminar presentation,* Denver, 1983, Resource Applications.

CHAPTER 17

Leadership and Management

OBJECTIVES

Mastery of content in this chapter will enable the student to:

- Define the key terms listed.
- Differentiate between leadership and management.
- Compare and contrast management theories in respect to their perspectives for improving productivity.
- Describe and give examples of the four classic leadership styles: authoritarian, democratic, laissez-faire, and situational.
- List and give examples of the four primary types of leadership skills that student nurses can begin to develop.
- Describe three phases of a change process.

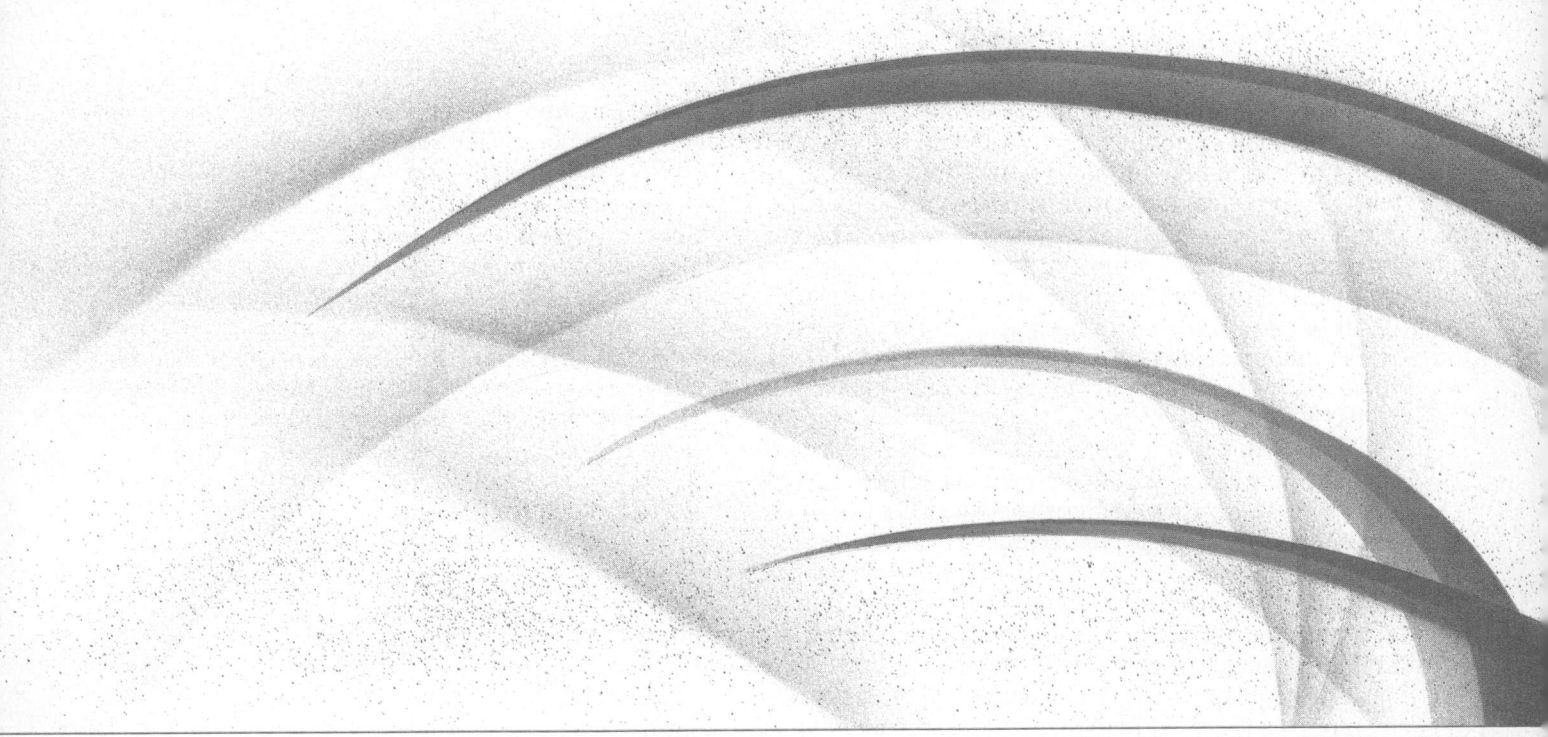

CHAPTER OUTLINE

Definitions of Leadership and Management

Management and Leadership Theories
    Trait development theory
    Scientific management theory
    Human relations movement
    Management process
    Theory X and theory Y
    Theory Z

Leadership and Management Style
    Authoritarian style
    Democratic style
    Laissez-faire style
    Situational leadership

Understanding the Process for Change

Leadership Skills for Student Nurses

uccessful organizations have effective and dynamic leadership. In hospitals and other health care facilities, certain nursing units have reputations for delivering superior nursing care. These units generally have nurse managers who are recognized leaders within their institutions and who motivate the nursing staff to maintain higher standards of care. Effective nursing leaders such as these nurse managers are generally successful because of their early commitment to developing leadership skills.

Peter Drucker (1974), a well-known authority on management, has identified a need for effective leaders in many areas of modern society. Effective leaders are the most basic and scarcest resource in any business, as well as in government and religious, educational, and health care institutions. According to other authorities, there is not only a shortage of leaders who can get the job done effectively but also a scarcity of people willing to assume significant leadership roles (Hersey, Blanchard, 1988). Leadership is also needed in nursing.

Leadership skills are usually developed by individuals early in their careers. To develop into effective leaders, nursing students must understand leadership concepts, so that they can begin to develop leadership skills early in their careers and commit themselves to exercising leadership skills in everyday nursing activities.

DEFINITIONS OF LEADERSHIP AND MANAGEMENT

Leadership is the art of getting others to want to do something you are convinced should be done. (Kranzes, Posner, 1990). The origin of the word *lead* is a word meaning "to go." Leaders typically are the ones who "go first." They have a vision and influence others to follow their lead. Leaders influence others by their actions and their comments. This ability is the essence of leadership.

On the other hand, the origin of the word *manage* comes from a word meaning "hand." Managing then means "handling things." In essence, **managers** get other people to do, but **leaders** get other people to want to do. Leaders are most often associated with times of turbulence, innovation, social transformation, and change. Managers are more often associated with improving productivity, establishing order and stability, and making things run smoothly.

Leaders and managers are needed to make health care institutions function. All managers are to some extent leaders in that their actions influence others.

Ideally, this influence is positive. In this sense, managers have no choice but to be leaders. The only choice is whether they manage and lead consciously or unconsciously and effectively or ineffectively (Manthey, 1990).

A beginning student observes a variety of situations in which managers apply leadership skills. From these observations, the student should learn practical methods for developing a cohesive group, implementing planned change, and enacting innovative ideas. Leadership and managerial skills are acquired in much the same way as clinical skills: theory, application, and practice. The value of carefully selected role models cannot be underestimated.

MANAGEMENT AND LEADERSHIP THEORIES

Leadership has been studied since the turn of the century, when psychological testing became popular and provided tools for objective research. A number of theories about the qualities of leadership have been developed.

Trait Development Theory

Early leadership studies concentrated on the traits and qualities of leaders. **Trait development** theorists generally believed that leaders were born with certain qualities that determine leadership ability and success. These qualities include intelligence, aggressiveness, a high energy level, and friendliness. The trait theorists believed that these leadership traits could be applied to all situations. Effective leaders were studied to identify what traits they had in common. Many attempts were made to put this theory into practice. From a group of job applicants, for example, only those possessing the identified traits were considered potential leaders and were selected for positions requiring leadership. Leadership training was provided only for those who possessed the desired leadership traits. This method of selecting and developing leaders, however, was not particularly effective.

As more research was conducted in the area of leadership, the theory that a leader possesses certain traits has been disproved. Research into necessary leadership traits reveals few consistent findings. The list grew to over 100 traits that were considered essential to successful leadership. Gradually, it became clear that very few successful leaders could possess all of these traits. In a review of this research, Jennings (1961) concluded, "Fifty years of study have failed to produce one personality trait or set of qualities that can be used to discriminate leaders and non-leaders."

Scientific Management Theory

Another approach to the study of leadership was developed by Taylor in the late 1800s. Taylor's theory of **scientific management** emphasized technology as the basis for increasing the productivity of employees. Taylor used the principles of observation, measurement, and scientific comparison to develop work standards. He introduced time-and-motion studies to analyze tasks, based on the belief that improving the performance of tasks would improve the efficiency of the organization. Taylor recommended careful selection and training of workers who could meet the established work standards. Attempts were made to satisfy the needs of employees through various incentives, including increasing wages. If this approach were applied to nursing, a staff could secure cash bonuses for providing efficient client care.

Some critics of this theory believe that the incentives approach is ineffective and simplistic because it emphasizes the performance of the workers and ignores complex human needs. It also encourages shortcuts and short-term goals at the expense of long-term goals. In addition, the leader creates and enforces performance criteria through close supervision, which causes a focus on the needs of the organization rather than the needs of the employees.

Human Relations Movement

Mayo and his associates in the 1920s and 1930s argued that managers attempting to improve productivity must be concerned with human affairs and technological methods. **Human relations management** theorists believe that the real power centers within an organization are the interpersonal relationships established within the work environment. They suggest that organizations be developed around human relationships, including those between leaders and employees. The human relations movement focuses on human feelings and attitudes of the employees.

The leader ensures that employees cooperate to attain their goals and also encourage employees' personal growth and development. The leader focuses more on the workers' needs than the needs of the organization. In this respect the human relations movement directly opposes the scientific management movement.

Management Process

In the mid-1950s, Henri Fayol defined the functions of a manager in a theory that has come to be known as the **management process** theory (Sheridan et al, 1984). Typically the manager's functions include planning, organizing, directing, and controlling. These functions are the same, regardless of the setting. College deans, foremen, bishops, and nurse managers accomplish tasks with and through other people; each must carry out these functions of a manager.

The functions of the management process are similar in many ways to the "nursing process." Both use the same functions. Managers assess the type and amount of work needed and the capabilities of the employees to perform it. Managers also plan and organize work duties, direct staff and customers, and finally control the quality of the work by evaluating and revising plans. Nurses assess their clients' needs, plan and organize client care, direct staff and clients, and control the quality of client care by evaluating and revising care plans.

By placing management functions into a system, Fayol defines the essential activities needed to maintain a functioning organization. These management functions constitute a set of behaviors expected of a manager. When applied to a nursing unit, this would involve the following actions (Clark, Shea, 1979):

1. Planning, including decisions about what to do, in advance, and how to do it: care plans, vacation schedules, department budgets, and long-term goals for the unit (that is, revising all client teaching materials)
2. Organizing, including development of formal structures for work allocation and coordination: designation of "charge nurse" responsibilities or the development of a staff action committee to resolve operational problems at the unit level
3. Directing, including the initiation of action (putting the plan into operation): giving instructions, supervising, facilitating, motivating, and communicating
4. Controlling, including the regulation of activities so that the plans are accomplished: establishing standards, measuring performance, and correcting deviations from the standard

Theory X and Theory Y

McGregor, in the early 1960s, described two kinds of management theories, which he called *theory X and theory Y* (Hersey, Blanchard, 1988). Managers who believe in **theory X** assume that people inherently dislike work and will avoid it when possible. The manager therefore must force employees to work by controlling and directing them continually and threatening them with punishment. Theory X assumes that human beings prefer to be controlled and directed, have little ambition, reject responsibility, and are most concerned about job security. McGregor believed that managers who used the theory X approach would never be able to reach high levels of production because only employees' low-level needs were satisfied.

Theory Y, in contrast, assumes that employees can enjoy physical and mental work just as they enjoy play and rest. Employees are capable of self-motivation and job satisfaction if they are happy in the organization and committed to its goals. Most human beings want responsibility. If employees have responsibility and are not controlled authoritatively, many organizational problems can be solved through group interaction. Theory Y managers believe that the organization is more successful when employees are self-directed and exercise self-control in their work. For this to occur, employees must share the organization's goals and feel commitment to the organization. McGregor suggests that theory Y organizations will satisfy higher human needs, resulting in greater employee responsibility and, in turn, higher productivity (Table 17-1).

In reviewing the assumptions underlying McGregor's theories, it is easy to incorrectly assume that theory X is "bad" and Theory Y is "good." This assumption overlooks the difference between attitude and behavior. Theory X and theory Y are attitudes or predispositions toward people. McGregor believed that most people had the *potential* to be mature and self-motivated. When dealing with employees who function in an immature and unmotivated manner, the manager may need to *behave* in a directive, task-oriented manner until the employee improves. The manager's behavior (theory X in nature) fits the circumstance even though the attitude about human nature may be more oriented toward theory Y (Hershey, Blanchard, 1988).

Theory Z

In recent years, there has been considerable discussion of the ways in which the Japanese have adapted the principles of the human relations theory; this adaptation is commonly known as *theory Z.* The thrust of **theory Z** is participation in management, or involvement of the employees in decisions that affect them. The theory emphasizes group deci-

TABLE 17-1 List of Assumptions of Theory X and Theory Y	
Theory X	**Theory Y**
Work is inherently distasteful to most people.	Work is as natural as play if the conditions are favorable.
Most people are not ambitious, have little desire for responsibility, and prefer to be directed.	Self-control is often indispensable in achieving organizational goals.
Most people have little capacity for creativity in solving organizational problems.	The capacity for creativity in solving organizational problems is widely distributed in the population.
Motivation occurs only at the physiological and security levels.	Motivation occurs at the social, esteem, and self-actualization levels, as well as at the physiological and security levels.
Most people must be controlled and often corrected to achieve organizational objectives.	People can be self-directed and creative at work if properly motivated.

From Hershey P, Blanchard K: *Management of organizational behavior: utilizing human resources,* ed 5, Englewood Cliffs, Prentice-Hall, 1988; adapted from Bennis WG: *Organizational development: nature, origins, prospects,* Reading, Mass, 1969, Addison-Wesley.

sion making, lifetime job security, and a strong commitment to the goals of the organization. The desired results are a greater sense of job commitment, higher productivity, and lower turnover (Ouchi, 1981).

In many ways, this approach to management is a blend of the theories that preceded its development. The importance of employee morale on productivity (as stressed in human relations theory) is reflected in the value placed on group decision making. The functions of management as defined in the management process theory are delegated in an organized way to the employees to manage. McGregor's theory Y is the underlying assumption on which the entire theory revolves. The Japanese brought together key aspects of management theory and used them in a way that others had failed to do. The impact of this approach is now being felt in hospitals through quality improvement and shared governance programs. All of these programs are aimed at increasing employee involvement in decision making.

LEADERSHIP AND MANAGEMENT STYLE

Leadership style is an important factor influencing the extent to which a leader is effective. Style in general involves the ways in which something is said or done, including particular behaviors associated with an individual. Leadership style specifically is the way that the leader influences the group to accomplish goals. Leadership styles, like other behaviors, can be learned, regulated, and developed. Research indicates that no one leadership style is effective in all situations but that each has unique strengths for different situations. The three classic styles of leadership are the authoritarian, democratic, and laissez-faire.

There is no one best leadership style. The effectiveness of each leadership style depends on the situation. As the situation changes, the effective manager adapts by changing leadership behaviors. Hersey (1967) makes the following conclusion about differences in leadership styles:

"The more managers adapt their style of leader behaviors to meet the particular situations and the needs of their followers, the more effective they will tend to be in reaching personal and organizational goals."

Authoritarian Style

The **authoritarian leader** retains all authority and responsibility and is concerned primarily with tasks and goal accomplishment. This type of leader assigns people to clearly defined tasks and establishes one-way communication patterns with the group. The authoritarian leader is firm, insistent, self-assured, and dominating. Such a leader stresses prompt, orderly, and predictable performance from employees or followers. The leader displays little trust or confidence in employees, who generally fear their manager. The authoritarian leader tends to stifle individual initiative and creativity.

The authoritarian leader may also be benevolent and value employees both as people and for their capabilities. This kind of authoritarian leader issues orders but allows employees to comment on them. Employees are permitted some flexibility to carry out their tasks within specific limits and procedures. A benevolent authoritarian leader may give orders, praise employees, demand their loyalty, and make followers feel as though they are participating in the decision-making process, even though they continue to do as the leader directs. The benevolent authoritarian leader generally has a condescending attitude toward employees, who therefore tend to be cautious when dealing with this leader.

Authoritarian leaders have always been present in nursing. The authoritarian nurse leader manages by giving orders and expecting staff members to accept them. The authoritarian manager stresses adherence to hospital policies and procedures. Staff members are expected to conform in nursing practice to the example and direction of the manager (Douglass, 1992).

The authoritarian style of leadership is appropriate in some situations. Some nursing staff members function more productively under the direction of authoritarian leaders because this leadership style meets their needs for security and job satisfaction. In situations in which immediate action is required and there is no time for a group decision-making process, the authoritarian leader is able to take action quickly. Authoritarian leaders excel in times of crisis and in situations of disorder; they often can remain calm while others falter. Authoritarian leaders have the reputation for being able to get difficult assignments completed.

Democratic Style

The **democratic style** is a people-centered approach and allows greater individual participation in the decision-making process. The democratic leader delegates authority but retains ultimate responsibility. The democratic leader maintains active communication that is open, friendly, and trusting with employees.

This management style enhances employees' personal commitment to the organization through group participation. The manager encourages goal setting by the group and has a sense of responsibility for the good of the group and for individual achievements. The democratic manager uses performance standards to assist the group in knowing job responsibilities rather than to control employees.

In nursing practice, democratic nurse managers have introduced a variety of mechanisms to promote staff involvement in the management of the nursing unit. Some examples are staff involvement in the development of the time schedule, group problem solving through quality control circles, and mutual goal setting during performance appraisals.

Laissez-Faire Style

The last classical leadership style is the **laissez-faire style** and is also referred to as the *free-run style* or *permissive leadership*. This type of leader denies responsibility and abdicates authority to the group. The laissez-faire manager may simply tell group members to work things out themselves and do the best they can. Communication between the manager and employees is open and lacks control and direction.

Laissez-faire managers want everyone to feel good, including themselves. This management style allows the group to drift aimlessly because the leader provides no direction. The principal management functions, such as decision making, planning, structuring, and controlling organization goals, are carried out by the group.

This style is not generally useful in the health care system because organization and control are necessary for efficient day-to-day operation. Laissez-faire leadership may be beneficial for employees involved in research projects, however, because self-direction assists in the creative process (Douglass, 1992). This style is probably most beneficial to a staff of highly motivated professionals who have shown the capacity for independent work.

Situational Leadership

Situational leadership combines the style of the leader, the skills needed in the situation, and the maturity of the employees. Situational leadership uses the following leadership styles (Blanchard, Zigarmi, Zigarmi, 1985):

1. Directing. The leader provides specific instructions and supervises task accomplishment.
2. Coaching. The leader directs and closely supervises task accomplishment. The leader also explains decisions, seeks suggestions, and supports progress.
3. Supporting. The leader facilitates and supports the efforts of the subordinates toward task accomplishment. The leader shares responsibility for decision making with employees.
4. Delegating. The leader gives the responsibility for decision making and problem solving to subordinates.

Employees who have limited technical skills or who are unwilling or unable to take responsibility require a directive leadership style. Employees with appropriate skills and who are willing to take responsibility are effectively managed with a democratic or participatory style. This style encourages participation in decision making. With the delegating style, the leader allows employees to make decisions and manage the daily operations. The leader diagnoses

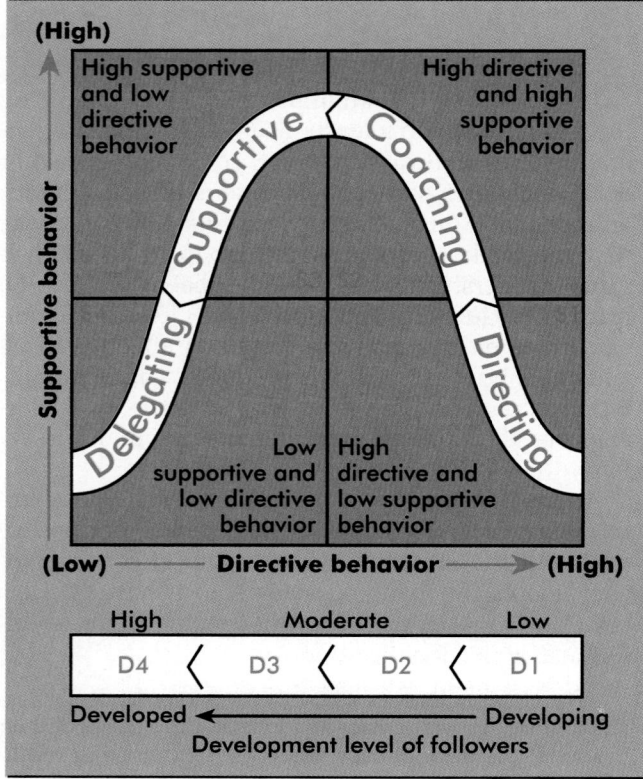

Fig. 17-1 The four leadership styles in the situational leadership model.
From Hersey P, Blanchard K: *Management of organizational behaviors utilizing human resources*, ed 3, Englewood Cliffs, NJ, 1977, Prentice Hall.

the particular situation to determine the correct leadership style (Fig. 17-1).

The following example applies situational leadership to a specific situation. A nursing service institutes a new client-classification system. The nurse manager uses the directing style to introduce the staff to the form. As the nursing staff becomes familiar with the new task, the manager solicits staff participation in working through the details of implementation. Using the coaching and supporting styles, the nurse manager encourages group decision making to resolve problems. Finally, when all staff members have demonstrated that they have the knowledge and ability to continue using the system without direction, the nurse manager uses the delegating style, which allows staff nurses to continue using the new system on their own. If problems occur, the head nurse returns to a directing or coaching style as needed to resolve the problem. Although the nurse uses a delegating style with this situation, another situation may require a directive style.

The key point in situational leadership theory is that leaders must adapt personal style to the needs and developmental level of the group. In that sense, situational leadership theory uses "different strokes for different folks." In typical nursing units, managers may behave in directive manners with the new graduates on the 11-7 shift. They will need to be task-oriented until they are certain that the graduates are functioning in a safe manner. On the other hand, they are likely to use supportive or delegating styles with the 7-3 nurses, who for the most part are very experienced. Because the developmental level of these nurses is much higher, the managers can delegate responsibilities (that is schedules, client teaching materials, and orientation) and in this way meet the needs of these nurses for greater self-direction.

The manager must be aware of the developmental level of the staff and adjust their behaviors accordingly. This ability to be flexible is the mark of effective managers. When managers use the same style with all staff (that is, directive), the more experienced staff members may feel devalued and choose employment elsewhere. On the other hand, managers who delegate responsibility to inexperienced staff may overwhelm them and again result in staff turnover. Managers who know the capabilities of their staff and adjust their styles accordingly will improve the likelihood of retaining capable, competent, satisfied nurses on staff. In this sense, the understanding of situational leadership theory is key to success as a manager.

 ## UNDERSTANDING THE PROCESS FOR CHANGE

No discussion of leadership and management would be complete without reviewing the process for planned change. Implementing and managing a **change process** is an integral part of leadership and management. A number of authors have developed models to describe the process of planned change.

Kurt Lewin, a well-known management theorist, has identified three phases of the change process: unfreezing, change, and refreezing (Hershey, Blanchard, 1988). This model provides a framework in which to view the system or unit as change occurs.

The first step, unfreezing, is described as "disturbing the equilibrium." This step sets the stage for change. For example, the nurse manager may be aware of a number of complaints from clients and families that their needs are not being met during "change of shift" time. The manager investigates further and finds that the average time used for shift reports on the 24-bed unit is 45 minutes. This problem is discussed in a staff meeting, and everyone agrees that time is not being effectively used, there is miscommunication, the overtime budget is adversely affected, and the problem needs attention. The manager has facilitated the beginning phase—creating an awareness of needed change and preparing the way for the acceptance of new alternatives.

The second step involves selecting and implementing the new alternatives, thus actually changing behavior. In this scenario the manager may choose to delegate this issue to the staff action committee and ask them for a plan of action. (This would involve carefully assessing the problem, analyzing its underlying causes, brainstorming possible solutions, and finally agreeing on a plan of action.) The committee decides to revamp their process for shift report and try "walking rounds." The staff agrees to participate in this new approach, giving report outside each client's room, for a 3-month period and evaluating the process at that time.

During this trial period the new behaviors gradually become integrated and are soon seen as normal procedure. This is the refreezing step of change. The committee reports the results of the 3-month trial. There are no client complaints, the time for reports is reduced to 20 minutes, and the staff feel that communication is improved when the nurses caring for the client actually see the client during the report. The change is adopted by the group with a final evaluation to be done 3 months later. This final evaluation ensures that the behavior changes are appropriately reinforced and that the change is sustained over time.

For planned change to be successful, several key concepts about managing change should be addressed. These concepts, if adhered to, will greatly reduce staff resistance. First, change should only be implemented for a good reason. Change for change's sake is rarely successful. A new manager who arbitrarily changes procedures just to "get the staff out of their rut" is overlooking this key aspect of effective change. Second, change should be introduced gradually. This means that it should be orderly and planned in manageable increments so that it is not overwhelming. In the earlier scenario, changing the way in which reports were handled would have been inappropriate if major changes in the charting system were underway at the same time.

A third concept of introducing change is to carefully plan the process. It may involve more time to

Primary Leadership Skills for Nurses

SKILLS OF PERSONAL BEHAVIOR

The effective leader:
- Is sensitive to feelings of the group
- Identifies self with the needs of the group
- Does not ridicule or criticize another's suggestions
- Helps others feel important and needed
- Does not argue

SKILLS OF COMMUNICATION

The effective leader:
- Listens attentively
- Makes sure everyone understands what is needed and the reason why
- Establishes positive communication with the group as a routine part of the job
- Recognizes that everyone's contributions are important

SKILLS OF ORGANIZATION

The effective leader helps the group to:
- Develop long- and short-range objectives
- Break big problems into small ones
- Share responsibilities and opportunities
- Plan, act, follow-up, and evaluate
- Be attentive to details

SKILLS OF SELF-EXAMINATION

The effective leader:
- Is aware of personal motivations
- Is aware of group members' level of hostility so that appropriate countermeasures are taken
- Helps the group be aware of their attitudes and values

enlist the informal leaders in the process or to establish a system for evaluation of the change, but the time spent will be worth it. Sudden changes are rarely sustained over time.

In terms of gaining staff support, it is also important to establish a need for the change. In the earlier scenario the staff was motivated to change the way they gave reports not only because of client complaints but because they recognized that they were not using their time effectively, miscommunicating with each other, and negatively affecting the overtime budget. Staff members are more likely to cooperate with a new approach if they feel some dissonance or discomfort with the current practice. Tying in this discomfort or felt need for change with the alternative approach augments the process and reduces resistance to the change. Giving thought to these basic principles and understanding the process for change in a broad sense greatly enhance the likelihood that the manager will successfully lead the staff (Sullivan, Decker, 1985).

LEADERSHIP SKILLS FOR STUDENT NURSES

Nursing continues to need new, effective leaders in all practice areas. Leadership is most important when changes are occurring in health care, such as the current changes being implemented in financing of the health care system. Changes are coming about in Medicare and private health insurance programs (see Chapter 3). For this and other reasons, it is imperative that student nurses begin early to prepare for future leadership and management roles. The box lists skills that are important for effective leadership and that the student nurse can begin to develop. These skills can be applied by leaders using any leadership style in any situation.

SUMMARY

As the nursing profession and health care agencies become increasingly specialized and complex, the need for effective leadership in nursing is even more important than in the past. Many nursing roles and responsibilities involve group activities, and for a group to function optimally, the leader must be able to motivate and influence the behavior of others. Successful leadership, whether in nursing, business, or another area, depends on an effective leadership style. For this reason, many theorists have analyzed the components of leadership that result in success. Although these theories do not agree entirely about the components of successful leadership, it is clear that the leader must remain flexible and adapt the leadership style to the particular group situation and goals.

In any situation the nurse in a leadership role needs certain skills, including skills related to personal behavior, communication skills, organization skills, and the skills of self-examination. These are all skills that the nursing student can begin to develop while learning other nursing skills. By developing these skills early in their careers, nurses will be better prepared to meet the needs for leadership in professional groups, health care agencies, and practice settings.

CHAPTER 17 REVIEW

Key Concepts

- Leadership involves influencing others toward the accomplishment of a goal.
- The leader moves a group forward with a sense of vision or direction, whereas the a manager improves productivity and makes things run smoothly.
- All managers are leaders to some extent in that their actions influence others, hopefully in a positive way.
- The human relations approach suggests that morale and attention to growth and development of employees are key to improving productivity of staff.
- A manager plans, organizes, directs, and controls activities so that the plan is actually accomplished.
- Theory X and theory Y deal with the manager's attitudes about employees, which are often reflected in management style.
- Theory Z, developed by the Japanese, stresses the importance of employee participation in decision making.
- Rather than focusing on one "best" leadership style, situational leadership stresses that the leadership style is determined by the needs and maturity of the group being led.
- Three phases of the change process according to Lewin are unfreezing, change, and refreezing.
- Leadership skills that the nurse can begin to develop while still a student include those of personal behaviors, communication, organization, and self-examination.

Key Terms

Authoritarian leader, p. 387

Change process, p. 389

Democratic style, p. 387

Human relations management, p. 385

Laissez-faire, p. 387

Leaders, p. 384

Managers, p. 384

Management process, p. 385

Scientific management, p. 385

Situational leadership, p. 388

Theory X, p. 385

Theory Y, p. 385

Theory Z, p. 386

Trait development, p. 384

Critical Thinking Exercises

1. The nursing staff have voiced displeasure regarding their monthly schedule. They feel that they are working too many weekends and that days off are inconsistent. As a head nurse, it is important to be sure all shifts are covered with an adequate complement of staff. To resolve the problem of having a suitable schedule, how might a manager act? How might a leader act?

2. The staff of a general surgical unit has formed a quality-improvement committee. This month they are monitoring their clients' knowledge of discharge restrictions. The head nurse encourages staff involvement and attempts to schedule time for regular meetings. What leadership theory supports this type of employee activity?

3. Consider the following two situations. What style of situational leadership should the head nurse apply in each?
   Joan is a new staff nurse who is in her third month of employment. She is about to perform a tracheostomy dressing change for the first time.
   Eileen is a staff nurse of 10 years. She is an expert clinician and an excellent teacher. Her colleagues consistently work well with her. She has asked to precept a new employee

4. During the last 3 months, eight patients have fallen on 7500. The Head nurse called a staff meeting to share information about each fall. Staff recognize that all falls are occurring between the day and evening shift. Staff immediately began to discuss possible solutions. What phase of change has the head nurse introduced in this situation?

REFERENCES

Blanchard K, Zigarmi P, Zigarmi D: *Leadership and the one-minute manager,* New York, 1985, Morrow.

Clark CC, Shea C: *Management in nursing,* New York, 1979, McGraw-Hill.

Douglass LM: *The effective nurse: leader and manager,* ed 4, St Louis, 1992, Mosby–Year Book.

Drucker PF: *Management: tasks responsibilities, and practices,* New York, 1974, Harper & Row.

Hersey P: *Management concepts and behavior: programmed instruction for managers,* Little Rock, Ark, 1967, Mancin.

Hersey P, Blanchard K: *Management of organizational behavior: utilizing human resources,* ed 5, Englewood Cliffs, NJ, 1988, Prentice Hall.

Jennings EE: The anatomy of leadership, *Manage Personnel Q* 1(1):1, 1961.

Kauzes JM, Posner BZ: *The leadership challenge,* San Franciso, 1990, Jossey-Base.

Manthey M: The nurse manager as leader, *Nurs Manage* 21(6):18, 1990.

Ouchi, W.: *Theory Z: how American businesses can meet the Japanese challenge,* Reading, Mass, 1981, Addison-Wesley.

Sheridan D et al: *The new nurse manager,* Rockville, Md, 1984, Aspen.

Sullivan EJ, Decker PJ: *Effective management in nursing,* Reading, Mass, 1985, Addison-Wesley.

ADDITIONAL READINGS

Adams CE: Leadership behavior of chief nurse executives, *Nurs Manage* 21(8):36, 1990.

Cox S: Retention of staff: the head nurse connection, *Curr Concepts Nurs* 2:5, 1990.

Golmors T: Effective leadership during organization transitions, *Nurs Econ* 8(3):135, 1990.

Orth C: The managers role as coach and mentor, *J Nurs Adm* 20(9):11, 1990.

Rauer R: Practicing participative manager, *Nurs Manage* 21(6):(suppl) 48a, 1990.

Townsend MB: Creating a better work environment, *J Nurs Adm* 21(1):11, 1991.

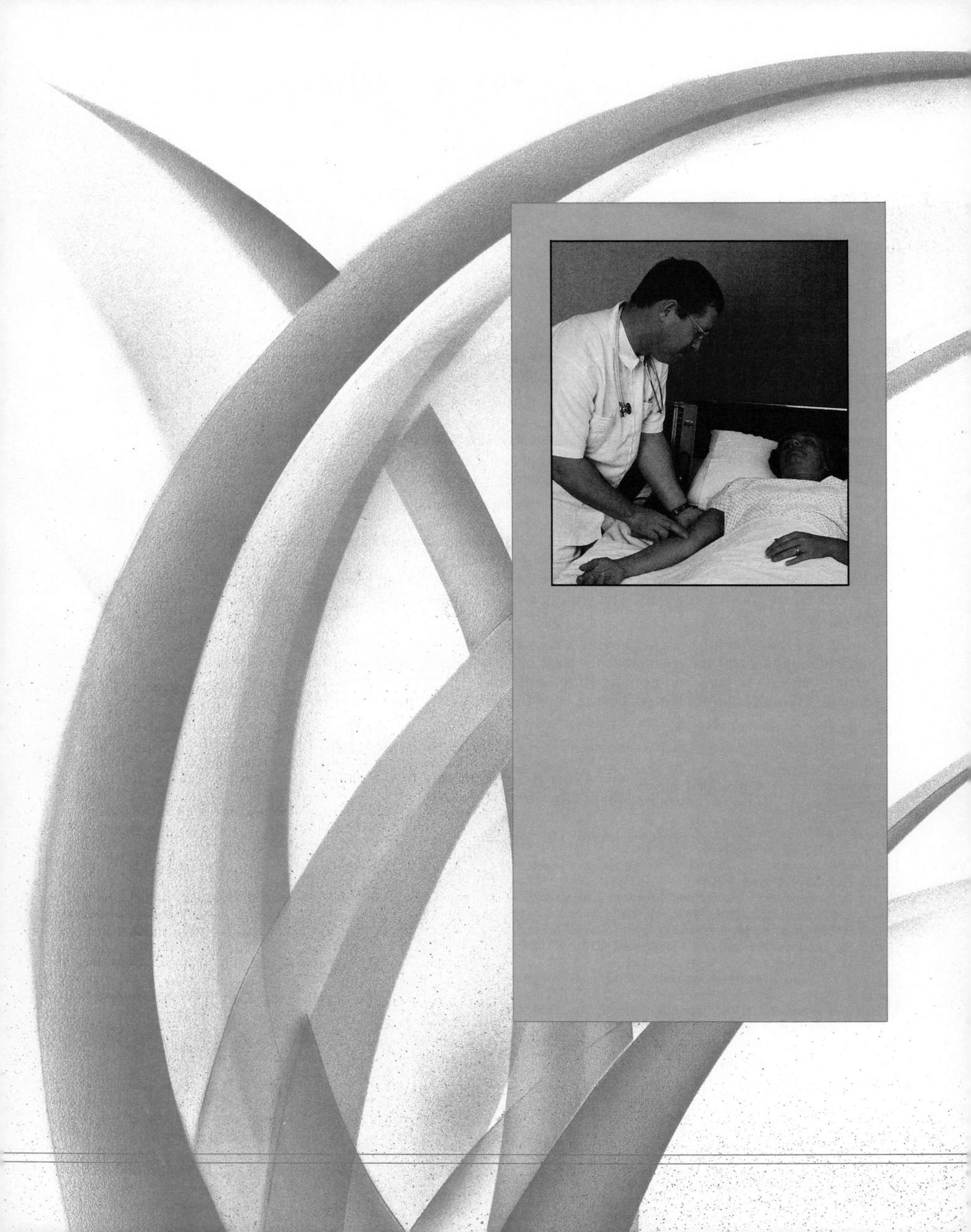

UNIT 4

Professional Nursing Skills

Infection Control

OBJECTIVES

Mastery of content in this chapter will enable the student to:

- Define the key terms listed.
- Explain how each element of the infection-control chain contributes to infection.
- Identify the body's normal defenses against infection.
- Discuss the events in the inflammatory response.
- Explain the difference between cell-mediated and humoral immunity.
- Describe the nature of signs of a localized and systemic infection.
- Identify clients most at risk for acquiring infection.
- Explain conditions that promote the onset of nosocomial infections.
- Explain the difference between medical and surgical asepsis.
- Give an example for preventing infection for each element of the infection chain.
- Compare body substance isolation with universal blood and body fluid precautions.
- Identify principles of surgical asepsis.
- Correctly perform protective isolation techniques.
- Perform proper procedures for handwashing.
- Explain how infection-control measures may differ in the home versus the hospital.
- Properly apply a surgical mask, sterile gown, and sterile gloves.

CHAPTER OUTLINE

ood health depends in part on a safe environment. Infection control practices control or eliminate sources of infection and help protect clients and health care providers from disease. A client entering a health care setting is at risk for acquiring infections because of lowered resistance to infectious **microorganisms,** increased exposure to numbers and types of disease-causing organisms, and invasive procedures. The nurse comes in contact with a variety of microorganisms and thus must practice infection-control techniques to avoid spreading them to clients.

In the home a client must recognize sources of infection and be able to institute protective measures. The nurse is responsible for teaching clients about infection, mode of transmission, reasons for susceptibility, and infection control.

The nurse's knowledge of infection, application of infection control principles, and use of common sense help protect clients from infection. Control of infection is an important part of every action the nurse performs.

NATURE OF INFECTION

An infection is an invasion of the body by **pathogens,** or microorganisms capable of producing disease. If the microorganisms fail to cause serious injury to cells or tissues, the infection is **asymptomatic.** Disease results if the pathogens multiply and cause an alteration in normal tissue function. If the infectious disease can be transmitted directly from one person to another, it is a **communicable** or contagious disease.

Chain of Infection

The presence of a pathogen does not mean that an infection will begin. Development of an infection occurs in a cyclical process that depends on the following elements:

1. An infectious agent or pathogen
2. A reservoir or source for pathogen growth
3. A portal of exit from the reservoir
4. A mode of transmission
5. A portal of entry to host
6. A susceptible host

An infection will develop if this chain remains intact (Fig. 18-1). Nurses use aseptic practices to break an element of the chain so that infection will not develop.

Infectious Agent

Pathogenic organisms include bacteria, viruses, fungi, and protozoa (Table 18-1). Pathogens on the skin are resident or transient. Resident pathogens are normally present and stable in number. They survive and multiply on the skin. Most are found in superficial skin layers, but about 10% to 20% inhabit deep epidermal layers (Garner, Favero, 1985). Resident pathogens are not easily removed by handwashing with plain soaps and detergents unless considerable friction is used. Resident microorganisms in deep skin layers are usually killed only by handwashing with products containing antimicrobial ingredients.

Transient pathogens attach to the skin when a person has contact with another object during normal activities of living. For example, when a nurse touches a bedpan or a contaminated dressing, transient bacteria adhere to the skin. The organisms attach loosely to the skin in dirt and grease or under fingernails. Frequent, thorough handwashing removes transient pathogens easily.

The potential for microorganisms or parasites to cause disease depends on the following factors:

1. Number of organisms
2. **Virulence,** or ability to produce disease
3. Ability to enter and survive in the host
4. Susceptibility of host

Many resident skin microorganisms are not highly virulent and cause only minor skin infections. However, they can cause serious infection when surgery or other **invasive** procedures allow them to enter deep tissues or when a client is severely **immunocompromised** (impaired immune system).

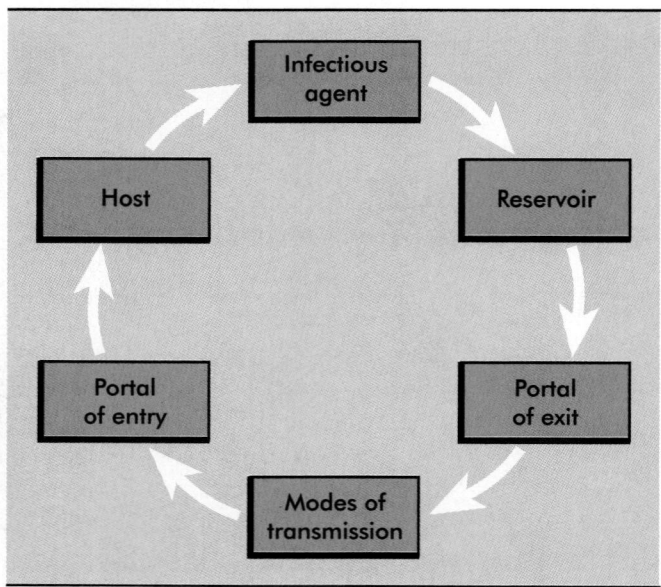

Fig. 18-1 Chain of infection.

TABLE 18-1   Common Pathogens and Some Infections or Diseases They Produce

Organism	Reservoir	Infection or Disease
BACTERIA		
Escherichia coli	Colon	Enteritis
Staphylococcus aureus	Skin, hair, anterior nares	Wound infection, pneumonia, food poisoning, cellulitis
Streptococcus (beta-hemolytic group A) organisms	Oropharynx, skin, perianal area	"Strep throat," rheumatic fever, scarlet fever, impetigo
Streptococcus (beta-hemolytic group B) organisms	Adult genitalia	Urinary tract infection, wound infection, endometritis
Mycobacterium tuberculosis	Lungs	Tuberculosis
Neisseria gonorrhoeae	Genitourinary tract, rectum, mouth, eye	Gonorrhea, pelvic inflammatory disease, infectious arthritis, conjunctivitis
Rickettsia rickettsii	Wood tick	Rocky Mountain spotted fever
Staphylococcus epidermidis	Skin	Wound infection, bacteremia
VIRUSES		
Hepatitis A virus	Feces, blood, urine	Infectious hepatitis
Hepatitis B virus	Feces, blood, all body fluids and excretions	Serum hepatitis
Herpes simplex virus (type 1)	Lesions of mouth, skin, blood, excretions	Cold sores, aseptic meningitis, sexually transmitted disease
Human immunodeficiency virus (HIV)	Blood, semen, vaginal secretions (also isolated in saliva, tears, urine, breast milk but not proven to be sources of transmission)	Acquired immunodeficiency syndrome (AIDS)
FUNGI		
Aspergillus organisms	Mouth, skin, colon, genital tract	Thrush, dermatitis
Candida albicans	Soil, dust	Aspergillosis
PROTOZOA		
Plasmodium falciparum	Mosquito	Malaria

Reservoir

Microorganisms have many sources or reservoirs for growth. One of the most common is the body itself. A variety of organisms lives on the surface of the skin and within body cavities, fluids, and discharges. The presence of microorganisms does not always cause a person to be ill. **Carriers** are persons or animals who show no symptoms of illness but who have pathogens on or in their bodies that can be transferred to others. For example, a person can be a carrier of hepatitis B virus or *Staphylococcus* organisms without having manifestations of infection.

Some areas of the body contain larger populations of resident flora than others. These include the skin, respiratory tract, mouth, vagina, colon, and lower urethra. Areas of the body normally considered sterile, without organism growth, are the bloodstream, spinal fluid, peritoneal cavity, urinary tract, muscles, bones, and chambers of the eye. The entrance of a foreign object into a sterile site increases the risk for infection.

Animals, plants, insects, and inanimate objects are also reservoirs for infectious organisms. Shellfish can become contaminated with *Vibrio cholerae*, the bacterium that causes cholera. The tick is a carrier for the microbe that causes Lyme disease. Suction drainage bottles collect fluids that become a reservoir for microorganisms such as *Pseudomonas* organisms.

Food, water, and milk are additional reservoirs for pathogens. *Clostridium botulinum* toxin survives in improperly stored food such as unrefrigerated milk products to cause botulism. The bacterium, *Legionella pneumophila,* which causes legionnaires' disease, lives in contaminated, pooled water.

To thrive, organisms require food and a proper environment to survive. Characteristics of an environment that supports organism growth include food, oxygen, water, temperature, pH, and light.

FOOD. Microorganisms require nourishment. Some, such as *Clostridium perfringens,* the microbe that causes gas gangrene, thrive on organic matter. Others, such as *E. coli,* consume undigested foodstuffs in the bowel. Carbon dioxide and inorganic material such as soil provide nourishment for other organisms. In a health care setting, bed linens and counter tops soiled with body secretions can become food sources for microorganisms.

OXYGEN. **Aerobic** bacteria require free oxygen for survival and for multiplication sufficient to cause disease. Aerobic organisms tend to cause more infections in humans. Examples of aerobic organisms are *S. aureus* and strains of *Streptococcus* organisms.

Anaerobic bacteria thrive where little or no free oxygen is available. Infections deep within the pleural cavity, in a joint, or in a deep sinus tract are typically caused by anaerobes. Bacteria that cause tetanus, gas gangrene, and botulism are anaerobes.

WATER. Most organisms require water for survival. The spirochete that causes syphilis, *Treponema pallidum,* lives only in a moist environment. Some bacteria assume a form resistant to drying. These spore-forming bacteria, such as those that cause anthrax, botulism, and tetanus, can live without water.

TEMPERATURE. Microorganisms can live only in certain temperature ranges. However, some can survive temperature extremes that would be fatal to humans. Some viruses are resistant to boiling water. Cold temperatures tend to prevent growth and reproduction of bacteria (**bacteriostasis**). A temperature that destroys bacteria is **bacteriocidal.**

pH. The acidity of an environment determines the viability of microorganisms. Most microorganisms prefer an alkaline environment within a pH range of 5 to 8. Bacteria in particular thrive in urine with a high pH. Organisms cannot survive the acid environment of the stomach.

LIGHT. Microorganisms thrive in dark environments such as those under dressings and within body cavities. Ultraviolet light is effective in killing certain forms of bacteria.

Portal of Exit

After microorganisms find a site to grow and multiply, they must find a portal of exit if they are to enter another host and cause disease. When the human is the reservoir, microorganisms can exit through a variety of sites.

SKIN AND MUCOUS MEMBRANES. Normally the skin is considered a portal of entry because any break in the integrity of skin and mucous membranes can lead to an infection. However, as pathogenic organisms grow and multiply within a wound, they create **purulent** drainage. For example, *S. aureus* creates a characteristic yellow drainage, whereas *Pseudomonas aeruginosa* causes a greenish drainage. This drainage is a potential portal of exit.

RESPIRATORY TRACT. Pathogens such as *Mycobacterium tuberculosis* that reside in the respiratory tract can be released from the body when a person sneezes, coughs, talks, or even breathes. Microorganisms exit through the mouth and nose in normal clients. In clients with artificial airways such as tracheostomy or endotracheal tubes (see Chapter 38), organisms easily exit through these devices.

URINARY TRACT. Normally urine is sterile. However, when a client has an infection, microorganisms exit during urination or through urinary diversions such as ileostomies and suprapubic drains (see Chapter 40).

GASTROINTESTINAL TRACT. The mouth is one of the more bacterially contaminated sites of the body, even though most of the organisms are normal flora, bacteria that reside within the body and defend against infection. However, organisms that are normal flora in one person can be pathogens in another. Organisms, for example, exit when a person expectorates saliva. Kissing can also provide a means of exit. Bowel elimination, drainage of bile via surgical wounds or drainage tubes, and escape of gastric contents during vomiting are additional portals of exit.

REPRODUCTIVE TRACT. Organisms such as *N. gonorrhoeae* and human immununodeficiency virus (HIV) may exit through a man's urethral meatus or a woman's vaginal canal. In the man, urine or semen may be the vehicle of pathogens. Discharge from the woman's vaginal canal may carry pathogens.

BLOOD. The blood is normally sterile, but in the case of infectious diseases such as hepatitis B (serum hepatitis) it becomes a reservoir for infectious organisms. A break in the skin by needle puncture or a surgical or traumatic wound allows pathogens to exit the body. Care givers can easily become exposed unless precautions are taken.

Modes of Transmission

There are many vehicles for transmission of microorganisms from the reservoir to the host. Table 18-2 summarizes common modes of transmission. Certain infectious diseases tend to be transmitted more commonly by specific modes. However, the same microorganisms may be transmitted by more than one route. For example, herpes zoster may be spread by the airborne route in droplet nuclei or by direct contact.

Almost any object within the environment (for example, a stethoscope or thermometer) can become a means of transmitting infection. All hospital personnel providing direct care (for example, nurses, physical therapists, and physicians) and performing diagnostic and support services (for example, laboratory technicians, respiratory therapists, and dietary workers) must follow practices to minimize the spread of infection. Each group follows procedures for handling equipment and supplies used by a client. For example, respiratory therapists wash their hands before working with each client and dispose of soiled oxygen equipment in a prescribed manner. Certain medical devices and diagnostic procedures provide avenues for growth and spread of pathogens. Invasive procedures such as cystoscopy (visualization of the bladder) facilitate diagnosis of problems but also increase the risk of transmitting infection. Because so many factors can promote the spread of infection to a client, all health care workers must be conscientious in using infection-control practices.

Portal of Entry

Organisms can enter the body through the same routes they use for exiting. For example, when a con-

---

TABLE 18-2   Modes of Transmission

Route and Means	Examples of Organisms
CONTACT	
Direct contact, or direct physical transfer between infected person and susceptible host (e.g., turning clients, giving baths, having sexual contact with infected person)	*Staphylococcus* organisms, *T. pallidum* (syphilis), herpes simplex virus
Indirect contact, personal contact of susceptible host with contaminated inanimate object (e.g., needles, bedpan, intravenous tubing, instruments and dressings, linen, dishes, silverware)	Measles virus, hepatitis B virus, *Enterococcus* and *Pseudomonas* organisms
Droplet contact or infectious agent coming in contact with conjunctivae, nose, mouth of susceptible host (droplets travel only up to 3 feet and therefore contact is not airborne) (e.g., coughing, sneezing)	Influenza virus, *Mycobacterium tuberculosis* (tuberculosis)
AIR	
Droplet nuclei, or residue of evaporated droplets remaining suspended in air (e.g., coughing, sneezing, talking)	Influenza viruses, pneumococcus (pneumonia, meningitis, other infections), varicella-zoster virus (chickenpox)
Dust (contains infectious agent)	*Aspergillus* organisms (aspergillosis)
VEHICLES	
Contaminated items	*M. tuberculosis* (tuberculosis)
Liquids	
Water	*Bivrio cholerae* (cholera)
Drugs, solutions	*Pseudomonas* organisms
Blood	Hepatitis B virus
Food (improperly handled or stored, fresh fruits and vegetables)	*Salmonella, Staphylococcus, Enterobacter,* and *Klebsiella* organisms
VECTORS	
Insects	
Mosquitoes	*Plasmodium falciparum* (malaria)
Fleas, ticks, lice	*Rickettsia typhi* and *R. prowazekii* (typhus)
Animals (cows, pigs)	*Brucella* organisms (brucellosis)

taminated needle pierces a client's skin, organisms enter the body. Any obstruction to the flow of urine from a urinary catheter allows organisms to travel up the urethra. Mishandling of sterile bandages over an open wound permits pathogens to enter exposed tissues. Factors that reduce the body's defenses enhance the chances of pathogens entering the body.

Susceptible Host

Whether a person acquires an infection depends on susceptibility to an infectious agent. **Susceptibility** is the degree of resistance an individual has to pathogens. Although everyone is constantly in contact with large numbers of microorganisms, an infection will not develop until an individual becomes susceptible to the strength and numbers of those microorganisms. The more virulent an organism, the greater the likelihood of a person's susceptibility. A person's natural defenses against infection, as well as a number of other factors, influence susceptibility (see section on risk factors).

Course of Infection

By understanding the chain of infection, the nurse can intervene to prevent infections from developing. When the client acquires an infection, the nurse is able to observe signs and symptoms of infection and take appropriate actions to prevent its spread. Infections follow a progressive course (see box). The severity of the client's illness depends on the extent of the infection, the **pathogenicity** of the microorganisms, and susceptibility of the host.

If infection is **localized** (limited to a particular area such as a wound infection), proper care will control the spread and minimize the illness. Only localized symptoms such as pain and tenderness at the wound site will develop. An infection that affects the entire body instead of just a single organ or part is **systemic**. A systemic infection can progress and become fatal.

The course of an infection influences the level of nursing care provided. The nurse is responsible for properly administering antibiotics and monitoring the response to drug therapy (see Chapter 21). Supportive therapy includes providing adequate nutrition and rest to bolster defenses against the infectious process. The complexity of care further depends on body systems affected by the infection.

Regardless of whether infection is localized or systemic, the nurse plays a dominant role in minimizing its spread. The organism causing a simple wound infection can spread to involve an intravenous needle insertion site if the nurse uses poor technique during an IV dressing change. Nurses who have breaks in

---

Course of Infection by Stage

INCUBATION PERIOD

- Interval between entrance of pathogen into body and appearance of first symptoms (e.g., chickenpox, 2-3 weeks; common cold, 1-2 days; influenza, 1-3 days; mumps, 18 days)

PRODROMAL STAGE

- Interval from onset of nonspecific signs and symptoms (malaise, low-grade fever, fatigue) to more specific symptoms (During this time, microorganisms grow and multiply, and client is more capable of spreading disease to others.)

ILLNESS STAGE

- Interval when client manifests signs and symptoms specific to type of infection (e.g., common cold manifested by sore throat, sinus congestion, rhinitis; mumps manifested by earache, high fever, parotid and salivary gland swelling)

CONVALESCENCE

- Interval when acute symptoms of infection disappear (Length of recovery depends on severity of infection and client's general state of health; recovery may take several days to months.)

---

their own skin can also acquire infections from clients if their techniques for controlling infection transmission are inadequate.

Defenses Against Infection

The body has normal defenses against infection. Normal body flora that reside inside and outside of the body protect a person from several pathogens. Each organ system has defense mechanisms that minimize exposure to infectious microorganisms. The **inflammatory response** is a protective vascular and cellular reaction that neutralizes pathogens and repairs body cells. Normal flora, body system defenses, and inflammation are all nonspecific defenses that protect against microorganisms regardless of prior exposure. The immune system is composed of separate cells and molecules resistant to disease. Certain responses of the immune system are nonspecific, whereas others are specific defenses against specific pathogens. If any of the body's defenses fail, an infection can quickly progress to a serious health problem.

Normal Flora

The body normally contains microorganisms that reside on the surface and deep layers of skin, in the saliva and oral mucosa, and in the gastrointestinal tract. A person normally excretes trillions of microbes daily through the intestines. The skin also has a large population of resident flora. Normal flora do not cause disease but instead participate in maintaining health.

Flora of the large intestine exist in large numbers without causing injury. These bacterial flora compete with disease-producing microorganisms for food. Flora also secrete antibacterial substances within the intestine's walls. The skin's flora exert a decontaminative action by inhibiting multiplication of organisms landing on the skin. The mouth and pharynx are also protected by flora that impair growth of invading microbes. The mass of normal flora maintains a sensitive balance with other microorganisms to prevent infection. Any factor that disrupts this balance places a person at serious risk for acquiring an infectious disease. For example, the inappropriate use of **broad-spectrum antibiotics** (antibodies effective against gram-positive and gram-negative organisms) for the treatment of infection can lead to suprainfection. Normal bacterial flora are eliminated, allowing disease-producing microorganisms to multiply.

Body System Defenses

A number of the body's organ systems have unique defenses against infection (Table 18-3 on p. 404). The skin, respiratory tract, and gastrointestinal tract are easily accessible to microorganisms. Pathogenic organisms easily adhere to the skin's surface, are inhaled into the lungs, or are ingested with food. Each organ system has defense mechanisms physiologically suited to its structure and function. For example, the lungs cannot completely control the entrance of microorganisms. However, the airways are lined with hairlike projections, or cilia, that rhythmically beat to move a blanket of mucus and adherent organisms up to the pharynx to be swallowed. Conditions that impair an organ's specialized defenses increase susceptibility to infection.

Inflammation

The body's cellular response to injury or infection is inflammation. Inflammation is a protective vascular reaction that delivers fluid, blood products, and nutrients to interstitial tissues in an area of injury. The process neutralizes and eliminates pathogens or dead (**necrotic**) tissues and establishes a means of repairing body cells and tissues. Signs of inflammation include swelling, redness, heat, pain or tenderness, and loss of function in the affected body part.

When inflammation becomes systemic, other signs and symptoms develop, including fever, leukocytosis, malaise, anorexia, nausea, vomiting, and lymph node enlargement.

The inflammatory response may be triggered by physical agents, chemical agents, and microorganisms. Mechanical trauma, exposure to temperature extremes, and radiation are physical agents. Chemical agents include external and internal irritants such as harsh poisons or gastric acid. Microorganisms were previously discussed.

After tissues are injured, a series of well-coordinated events occurs. The inflammatory response includes the following:
1. Vascular and cellular responses
2. Formation of inflammatory exudate
3. Tissue repair

VASCULAR AND CELLULAR RESPONSES. Acute inflammation is an immediate response to cellular injury. Arterioles supplying the infected or injured area dilate, allowing more blood into local circulation. The increase in local blood flow causes the characteristic redness of inflammation. The symptom of localized warmth results from a greater volume of blood at the inflammatory site. If the inflamed area is deep within the body, local warmth does not occur because the maximum body temperature is at the body's core. Local vasodilation delivers blood and white blood cells (WBCs) to injured tissues.

Injury causes tissue necrosis, and as a result the body releases histamine, bradykinin, prostaglandin, and serotonin. These chemical mediators increase the permeability of small blood vessels. Fluid, protein, and cells enter interstitial spaces. Accumulated fluid appears as localized swelling (**edema**).

Another sign of inflammation is pain. The swelling of inflamed tissues increases pressure on nerve endings, causing pain. Chemical substances such as histamine stimulate nerve endings. As a result of physiological changes occurring with inflammation, the involved body part usually undergoes a temporary loss of function. For example, a localized infection of the hand causes the fingers to become swollen, painful, and discolored. Joints may become stiff as a result of swelling, but function of the fingers returns when inflammation subsides.

The cellular response of inflammation involves WBCs arriving at the site. WBCs pass through blood vessels and into the tissues. Through the process of **phagocytosis**, specialized WBCs, neutrophils and monocytes, ingest and destroy microorganisms or other small particles. As inflammation becomes systemic, other signs and symptoms develop. **Leukocytosis,** or an increase in the number of circulating

TABLE 18-3 Normal Defense Mechanisms against Infection		
Defense Mechanisms	Action	Factors That May Alter Defense
SKIN		
Intact multilayered surface (body's first line of defense against infection)	Provides barrier to microorganisms	Cuts, abrasions, puncture wounds, areas of maceration
Shedding of outer layer of skin cells	Removes organisms that adhere to skin's outer layers	Failure to bathe regularly
Sebum	Contains fatty acid that kills some bacteria	Excessive bathing
MOUTH		
Intact multilayered mucosa	Provides mechanical barrier to microorganisms	Lacerations, trauma, extracted teeth
Saliva	Washes away particles containing microorganisms	Poor oral hygiene, dehydration
	Contains microbial inhibitors (e.g., lysozyme)	
RESPIRATORY TRACT		
Cilia lining upper airway, coated by mucus	Trap inhaled microbes and sweep them outward in mucus to be expectorated or swallowed	Smoking, high concentration of oxygen and carbon dioxide, decreased humidity, cold air
Macrophages	Engulf and destroy microorganisms that reach lung's alveoli	Smoking
URINARY TRACT		
Flushing action of urine flow	Washes away microorganisms on lining of bladder and urethra	Obstruction to normal flow by urinary catheter placement, obstruction from growth or tumor, delayed micturition
Intact multilayered epithelium	Provides barrier to microorganisms	Introduction of urinary catheter, continual movement of catheter in urethra
GASTROINTESTINAL TRACT		
Acidity of gastric secretions	Chemically destroys microorganisms incapable of surviving low pH	Administration of antacids
Rapid peristalsis in small intestine	Prevents retention of bacterial contents	Delayed motility resulting from impaction of fecal contents in large bowel or mechanical obstruction by masses
VAGINA		
At puberty, normal flora causing vaginal secretions to achieve low pH	Inhibit growth of many microorganisms	Antibiotics and oral contraceptives disrupting normal flora

WBCs, is the body's response to WBCs leaving blood vessels. A serum WBC count is normally 5000 to 10,000/mm^3 but may rise to 15,000 to 20,000/mm^3 during inflammation. Fever is caused by phagocytic release of pyrogens from bacterial cells that cause a rise in the hypothalamic set point (see Chapter 19). Other systemic signs and symptoms include malaise, anorexia, and lymph node enlargement.

INFLAMMATORY EXUDATE. Accumulation of fluid and dead tissue cells and WBCs forms an **exudate** at the site of inflammation. Exudate may be **serous** (clear like plasma) or **sanguineous** (containing red blood cells). Eventually the exudate is cleared away through lymphatic drainage. Platelets and plasma proteins such as fibrinogen form a meshlike matrix at the inflammation to prevent its spread.

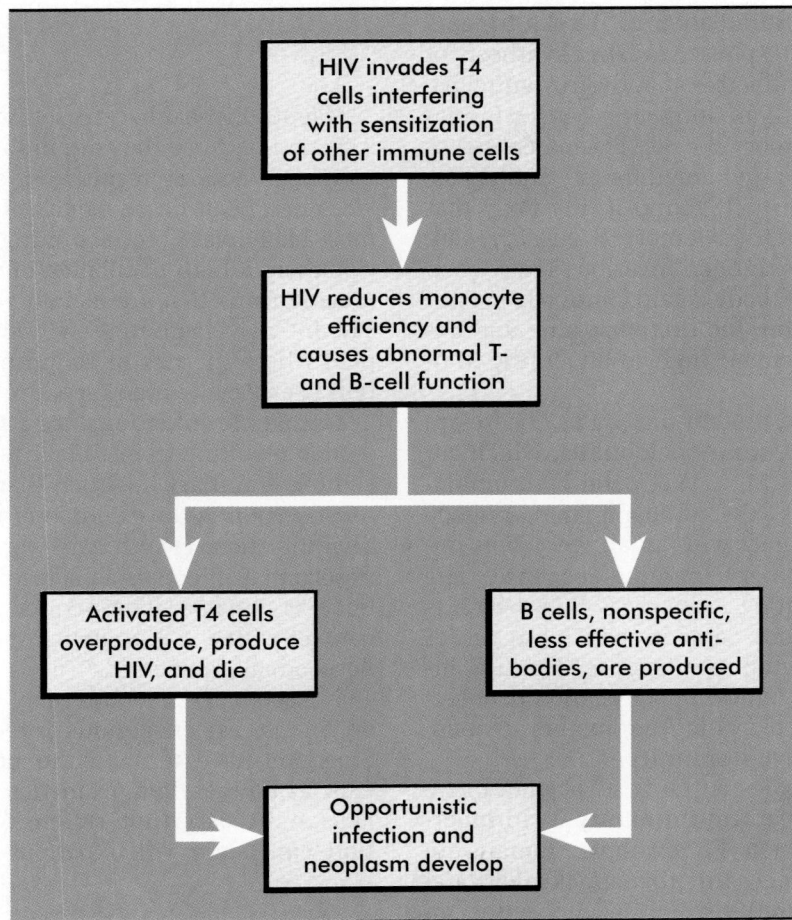

Fig. 18-2   The pathologic responses of HIV.

TISSUE REPAIR. When there is injury to tissue cells, healing involves the defensive, reconstructive, and maturative stages (see Chapter 48). Damaged cells are eventually replaced with healthy new cells. The new cells undergo a gradual maturation until they take on the same structural characteristics and appearance as the previous cells. If inflammation is chronic, tissue defects may fill with fragile **granulation tissue**. Granulation tissue is not as strong as tissue collagen and assumes the form of scar tissue.

Immune Response

When an invading microorganism enters the body, it is first attacked by monocytes. Remnants of the microorganism then trigger the immune response. The remaining foreign material (**antigen**) causes a series of responses that changes the body's biological makeup so that reactions to future exposures are different from the first reaction. These altered responses are known as **immune responses**. In a normal immune response, the antigen is neutralized, destroyed, or eliminated.

Antigens are usually composed of proteins that are not normally found in a person's body. Often, antigens exist as part of the structure of a bacterium or virus. After an antigen enters the body, it travels in the blood or lymph and initiates cell-mediated or humoral immunity.

CELL-MEDIATED IMMUNITY. There are two classes of lymphocytes. These are T lymphocytes (T cells) and B lymphocytes (B cells). T cells play a major role in cell-mediated immunity. There are antigen receptors on the surface membranes of T cells. When an antigen meets a T cell whose surface receptors fit the antigen, a binding occurs. This binding activates the T cell to divide rapidly to form sensitized T cells. Sensitized T cells travel to the area of inflammation or injury, bind with antigens, and release chemical compounds called *lymphokines*. The lymphokines attract macrophages and stimulate them to attack antigens. Eventually the antigens are killed. The cell-mediated response is altered by the HIV, which causes AIDS (Fig. 18-2).

HUMORAL IMMUNITY. Stimulation of B cells triggers the humoral immune response, causing synthesis of immunoglobulins or antibodies that destroy antigens. After a B cell binds with an antigen, it causes formation of plasma and memory B cells. Plasma cells synthesize and secrete large amounts of antibodies, which are proteins normally found in the body that provide general immunity. Memory B cells prepare the body against future antigen invasion. Thus when an antigen enters the body again, antibodies form more rapidly than during the first exposure, and immunoglobulin levels remain high to attack the antigen.

Antibodies are large protein molecules. There are five classes of antibody **immunoglobulins,** which are identified by the letters M, G, A, E, and D. Immunoglobulin M (IgM) is the predominant antibody formed after initial contact with an antigen. This initial contact is the primary immune response. The most abundant circulating antibody is IgG, which is formed after subsequent contacts with antigens or during the secondary immune response. The IgG antibody is important in providing resistance to infection and can cross the placenta from mother to child, giving the infant **passive immunity.**

Formation of antibodies is the basis of immunization against disease. **Natural immunity** is an inherited resistance to infection. For example, humans are resistant to the distemper virus that attacks dogs and cats. Acquired immunity, which occurs after an exposure to a foreign antigen, is the result of antibody production. For example, when children are vaccinated against diseases such as diphtheria or pertussis, the vaccine produces an acquired immunity.

COMPLEMENT. A **complement** is an inactive protein compound found in blood serum. It is activated when an antigen and antibody bind together. After a complement is activated, a rapid sequence of catalytic activity changes the shape of antigenic cells. The foreign bacteria, for example, assume the shape of a doughnut. The complement actually makes a hole through the antigen's cell membrane. Ions and water enter the cell, causing it to burst. This process is called *cytolysis.*

INTERFERON. When certain cells are invaded by viruses, they synthesize the protein interferon. **Interferon** interferes with the ability of viruses to multiply and protects body cells from simultaneous infection with other viruses. Classified as a biological response modifier, interferon also directly inhibits the growth and division of tumor cells (Hood, 1987).

NOSOCOMIAL INFECTIONS

Clients in health care settings can easily acquire infection because they are in high-risk groups. **Nosocomial infections** result from delivery of health services in a health care facility. A hospital is one of the most likely places for acquiring an infection because it harbors a high population of virulent strains of microorganisms that are usually resistant to antibiotics. The intensive care unit (ICU) is one area in the hospital where the risk of acquiring a nosocomial infection is especially high (see box below).

Iatrogenic infections are a type of nosocomial infection resulting from a diagnostic or therapeutic procedure. A urinary infection that develops after catheter insertion is an example of an iatrogenic nosocomial infection. Health care workers may also acquire nosocomial infection as a result of contacting infectious organisms. The acquisition of hepatitis from contact with a contaminated needle is an example of nosocomial infection.

Nosocomial infections may be exogenous or endogenous. An **exogenous infection** arises from microorganisms external to the individual, which do not exist as normal flora; examples are *Salmonella* organisms and *Clostridium tetani*. An **endogenous infection** can occur when part of the client's flora be-

---

Risk of Nosocomial Infection in ICUs

Nurses working in ICUs should be particularly conscious of aseptic practices. Clients are at risk for infection for the following reasons:

- ICU clients are critically ill and often have more underlying disease than other clients.
- More invasive devices such as intravenous or intraarterial lines are used in ICUs.
- More invasive procedures are performed in the ICU than other general-care areas.
- Often, surgical procedures are performed in the ICU instead of the operating room because of a client's critical condition.
- Overuse of broad-spectrum antibiotics causes the formation of resistant microorganisms that later cause infection.
- The busy pace of activities in an ICU can often cause nurses and other health care providers to become less diligent with aseptic technique.

Adapted from Crow S: *Crit Care Nurs Q* 11(4):11, 1989.

comes altered and an overgrowth results. Examples are infections caused by enterococci, yeasts, and streptococci. When sufficient numbers of microorganisms normally found in one body cavity or lining are transferred to another body site, an endogenous infection develops. For example, transmission of enterococci, normally found in fecal material, from the hands to the skin is a common cause of wound infections. The number of microorganisms needed to cause a nosocomial infection depends on the virulence of the organism, the host's susceptibility, and the site affected.

The number of health care employees having direct contact with clients, type and number of invasive procedures, therapy received, and length of hospitalization influence the risk of infection. Major sites for nosocomial infection include the urinary tract, surgical or traumatic wounds, respiratory tract, and bloodstream (see box at right).

Nosocomial infections significantly increase costs of health care. Extended lengths of stay in health care institutions, increased disability, and prolonged recovery times add to the expenses of the client, as well as the health care institution and funding bodies (for example, Medicare). Often, costs for nosocomial infections are not reimbursed; as a result, prevention has a beneficial financial impact.

Concept of Asepsis

The nurse's efforts to minimize the onset and spread of infection are based on the principles of aseptic technique. **Asepsis** is the absence of germs or pathogens. Aseptic technique is the efforts to keep a client as free from hospital microorganisms as possible (Crow, 1989). The two types of aseptic technique the nurse practices are medical and surgical asepsis.

Medical asepsis, or clean technique, includes procedures used to reduce the number of microorganisms and prevent their spread. Changing a client's bed linen daily, handwashing, and using clean medication cups are examples of medical asepsis. Principles of medical asepsis are commonly followed in the home as in the case of washing hands before preparing food.

Surgical asepsis, or sterile technique, includes procedures used to eliminate microorganisms from an area. Sterilization destroys all microorganisms and their spores. Sterile technique is practiced by nurses in the operating room and treatment areas, where sterile instruments and supplies are used.

After an object becomes unsterile or unclean, it is contaminated. In medical asepsis an area or object is considered contaminated if it contains or is suspected

---

Sites and Causes for Nosocomial Infections

URINARY TRACT

- Insertion of urinary catheter
- Closed drainage system becoming open
- Catheter and tube becoming disconnected
- Drainage bag port touching dirty surface
- Poor specimen collection technique
- Obstruction or interference with urinary drainage
- Urine in catheter or drainage tube being allowed to reenter bladder (reflux)
- Poor handwashing technique
- Repeated catheter irrigations with solutions

SURGICAL OR TRAUMATIC WOUNDS

- Improper skin preparation (shaving and bathing) before surgery
- Poor handwashing before and after dressing changes
- Failure to cleanse skin surface properly
- Failure to use aseptic technique during dressing changes
- Use of contaminated antiseptic solutions

RESPIRATORY TRACT

- Contaminated respiratory therapy equipment
- Failure to use aseptic technique while suctioning airway
- Improper disposal of mucous secretions

BLOODSTREAM

- Contamination of intravenous fluids by tubing or needle changes
- Insertion of drug additives to intravenous fluid
- Addition of connecting tube or stopcocks to intravenous system
- Improper care of needle insertion site
- Contaminated needles or catheters
- Failure to change intravenous access site when inflammation first appears
- Poor technique during administration of multiple blood products
- Improper care of peritoneal or hemodialysis shunts

---

of containing pathogens. For example, a used bedpan, the floor, and a wet piece of gauze are contaminated. In surgical asepsis an area or object is considered contaminated if touched by any object that is not sterile. For example, a tear in a surgical glove exposes the outside of the glove to the skin surface, thus contaminating it.

The nurse is responsible for providing the client with a safe environment. Florence Nightingale (1859) wrote that the nurse's first responsibility to the client is to first do no harm. Effectiveness of aseptic practices depends on the nurse's conscientiousness and consistency in using effective aseptic techniques. It is easy to forget key procedural steps or, when hurried, to take shortcuts that break aseptic procedures. However, the nurse's failure to be meticulous will place the client at risk for an infection that can seriously impair recovery.

THE NURSING PROCESS IN INFECTION CONTROL

Assessment

To appropriately prevent or manage an infection, the nurse assesses a client's defenses against infection and susceptibility to infection. A thorough review of the client's clinical condition may detect signs and symptoms of infection. An analysis of laboratory findings provides information about a client's defense against infection. By knowing the factors that increase susceptibility or risk for infection, the nurse is better able to plan preventive therapy that includes aseptic technique. By recognizing early signs and symptoms of infection, the nurse can alert the physician to the potential need for therapy and initiate supportive nursing measures.

Risk Factors for Infection

INADEQUATE PRIMARY DEFENSES

- Broken skin or mucosa
- Traumatized tissue
- Decreased ciliary action
- Obstructed urine outflow
- Altered peristalsis
- Change in pH of secretions

INADEQUATE SECONDARY DEFENSES

- Reduced hemoglobin level
- Suppression of WBCs (drug or disease related)
- Suppressed inflammatory response (drug or disease related)
- Low WBC count (leukopenia)

Status of Defense Mechanisms

A review of physical assessment findings and the client's medical condition reveals the status of normal defense mechanisms against infection. For example, any break in the skin or mucosa is a potential site for infection. Similarly, a chronic smoker is at greater risk for acquiring a respiratory tract infection after general surgery (see Chapter 47) because the cilia of the lung are less likely to be active and able to propel retained mucus from the lung's airways. Any reduction in the body's primary or secondary defenses against infection places a client at risk (see box).

Client Susceptibility

Many factors influence susceptibility to infection. The nurse gathers information about each factor through the nursing history.

AGE. Throughout the life span, susceptibility to infection changes. An infant has reduced defenses against infection. Born with only the antibodies provided by the mother, the infant's immature immune system is incapable of producing the necessary immunoglobulins and WBCs. As the child grows, the immune system matures, but the child is still susceptible to organisms that cause the common cold, intestinal infections, and infectious diseases such as mumps and measles.

The young or middle-age adult has refined defenses against infection. Normal flora, body system defenses, inflammation, and the immune response provide protection against invading microorganisms. Viruses are the most common cause of infectious illness in adults.

Defenses against infection change with aging. The immune response, particularly cell-mediated immunity, declines. Older adults also undergo alterations in the structure and function of the skin, urinary tract, and lungs. For example, the skin loses its turgor and the epithelium thins. As a result, the skin is more easily abraded or torn. This increases exposure to pathogens (Table 18-4).

Alterations in the immune system may even trigger the aging process. Cells of the immune system such as lymphocytes become more diversified with age, and the body undergoes a progressive loss of cellular regulation. When viruses or other antigens and corresponding antibodies lodge in sites such as the kidney and arteries, factors injurious to the tissues are released, and deterioration begins. With aging and autoimmune diseases (alterations of the immune system), cellular changes such as depletion of lymphoid tissues occur. The basic mechanism for the aging process is not understood. However, it is known

TABLE 18-4 Assessing the Risk of Infection in Older Adults

Component	Possible Changes With Age	Outcome
Skin	Thinner dermal and epidermal layers, decreased collagen strength, decreased skin elasticity, decreased sweat	Pressure ulcers
Peripheral nerves	Reduced sensitivity, particularly in clients with history of alcohol abuse, vitamin B$_{12}$ deficiency, and diabetes mellitus	Pressure ulcers, ignored trauma leading to infection
Circulation	Congestive heart failure, calcified mitral and aortic valves	Pneumonia, bacterial endocarditis
Peripheral circulation	More elastic veins, less effective venous valves, blood pooling in lower extremities	Venous stasis ulcers
Mouth	Dehydration, loss of saliva production, functional inability to maintain oral hygiene	Parotid gland infection, peridontal disease, localized abscess, bacteremia
Gastrointestinal tract	Loss of ability to secrete stomach acid in 30% of persons over 70	Salmonellal diarrhea
Pulmonary system	Increased colonization of oropharynx, impaired mucociliary clearance, decreased macrophage function, decreased cough reflex	Viral and bacterial pneumonia
Urinary tract	Prostatic hyperplasia, urethral strictures, age-related hormonal changes in vaginal wall, pelvic floor relaxation, ureterocele or cystocele, degeneration of nerves leading to neurogenic bladder, use of tricyclic antidepressants, dehydration	Asymptomatic bacteriuria, cystitis, pyelonephritis
Nutrition	Malnutrition, vitamin deficiency (vitamin A, pyridoxine, and riboflavin), protein and caloric malnutrition	Impaired immune response to infection
Drug therapy	Corticosteroid and cytotoxic drugs	Impaired immune response to infection
Nursing home residency	Exposure to nosocomial infections, including influenza, *Proteus* and *Providencia* organisms with an indwelling catheter, tuberculosis, and wound infections (Incidence of bacteremia after admission is 50%.)	Frequent serious infection, increased risk of pneumonia

Adapted from Tideiksaar R: *Physician Assist* 11(2):17, 1987.

that immunity to infection decreases with advancing age.

NUTRITIONAL STATUS. When protein intake is inadequate as a result of poor diet or debilitating disease, the rate of protein breakdown exceeds that of tissue synthesis (see Chapter 35). As a result, the body is in a negative nitrogen balance; in other words, the output of nitrogen sources such as protein exceeds nitrogen intake. A reduction in the intake of protein and other nutrients such as carbohydrates and fats reduces the body's defenses against infection and impairs wound healing (see Chapter 48).

Clients with illnesses or problems that increase protein requirements are at further risk. These problems include traumatic injury, extensive burns, and conditions causing fever. Clients who have had surgery also have this problem.

The nurse assesses clients' dietary intakes and abilities to tolerate solid foods. Clients who have difficulty with swallowing, who experience alterations in digestion, or who are too confused or weak to feed themselves are at risk for inadequate dietary intake. A dietitian may be called to assist in calculating the calorie count of foods ingested.

STRESS. The body responds to emotional or physical stress by the general adaptation syndrome (see Chapter 30). During the alarm stage, the basal metabolic rate increases as the body uses energy stores.

Adrenocorticotropic hormone (ACTH) acts to increase serum glucose levels and decrease unnecessary antiinflammatory responses through the release of cortisone. If stress continues or becomes intense, elevated cortisone levels result in decreased resistance to infection. Continued stress leads to exhaustion, wherein energy stores are depleted and the body has no resistance to invading organisms. The same conditions that increase nutritional requirements such as surgery or trauma also increase physiological stress.

HEREDITY. Certain hereditary conditions impair an individual's response to infection. The client's history of preexisting medical problems should reveal known hereditary disorders. For example, agammaglobulinemia is a rare inherited or acquired disorder characterized by the absence of serum antibodies. The client's ability to initiate defenses against infection, such as the formation of antibodies, is virtually absent.

DISEASE PROCESS. Clients with diseases of the immune system are at particular risk for infection. Leukemia, acquired immunodeficiency syndrome (AIDS), lymphoma, and aplastic anemia are examples of conditions that compromise a host by weakening defenses against infectious organisms. Clients with leukemia are unable to produce enough WBCs to ward off infection.

Victims of chronic disease such as diabetes mellitus and multiple sclerosis are also more susceptible to infection because of general debilitation and nutritional impairment. Diseases that impair body system defenses, such as pulmonary emphysema and bronchitis (which impair ciliary action and thicken mucus), cancer (which alters the immune response), and peripheral vascular disease (which reduces blood flow to injured tissues), increase susceptibility to infection. Burn clients have a very high susceptibility to infection because of the damage of skin surfaces. The greater the depth and extent of the burns, the higher the risk for infection.

MEDICAL THERAPY. Some drug and medical therapies compromise immunity to infection. The nurse assesses the client's history to determine whether the client takes medications at home that increase infection susceptibility. A review of therapies received within the health care setting further reveals risks. Adrenal corticosteroids, prescribed for several conditions, are antiinflammatory drugs that cause protein breakdown and impair the inflammatory response against bacteria and other pathogens. Cytotoxic or antineoplastic drugs attack cancer cells but cause side effects of bone marrow depression and normal cell toxicity. With bone marrow depression the body is unable to produce lymphocytes and sufficient WBCs. When normal cells become altered by antineoplastic agents, cellular defenses against infection fail. Cyclosporine and other immunosuppressant drugs, which decrease the body's immune response, are commonly taken by clients who are organ transplant recipients. The immunosuppressants prevent organ and tissue rejection; yet they increase susceptibility to infection.

Cancer clients receiving radiotherapy are also at risk for infection. The massive doses of radiation, which destroy cancerous cells, can also depress the bone marrow and destroy normal cells.

Clinical Appearance

The signs and symptoms of infection are local or systemic. Localized infections are most common in areas of skin or mucous membrane breakdown such as surgical and traumatic wounds, pressure ulcers, and mouth lesions. Infections also develop locally in cavities beneath the skin; an example is an abscess.

To assess an area for localized infection, the nurse first inspects the area for redness and swelling caused by inflammation. There may be drainage from open lesions or wounds. Infected drainage may be yellow, green, or brown, depending on the site of infection. The nurse asks the client about pain or tenderness around the site. The client may complain of tightness caused by edema. If the infected area is large enough, movement of a body part may be restricted. Gentle palpation of an infected area usually results in some degree of tenderness.

Systemic infections cause more generalized symptoms than local infection. They usually result in fever, fatigue, and malaise. Lymph nodes that drain the area of infection often become enlarged, swollen, and tender during palpation. For example, an abscess in the peritoneal cavity may cause enlargement of lymph nodes in the groin. An infection of the upper respiratory tract may cause cervical lymph node enlargement. If an infection is serious and widespread, all major lymph nodes may enlarge. Systemic infections commonly cause a loss of appetite, nausea, and vomiting.

Systemic infections often develop after treatment for localized infection has failed. The nurse should be alert for changes in the client's level of activity and responsiveness. As systemic infections develop, the client may become lethargic and complain of a loss of energy. An elevation in body temperature may lead to episodes of increased heart and respiratory rates. Involvement of major body systems produces specific signs. For example, a pulmonary infection results in a productive cough with purulent sputum. A urinary tract infection may result in cloudy, foul-smelling urine.

An infection in older adults may not present with typical signs and symptoms. Often older adults have advanced infection before it is identified. This is because of their reduced inflammatory and immune responses. Normally older adults have diminished pain sensitivity. A reduced or absent fever response may occur from chronic use of aspirin or nonsteroidal antiinflammatory drugs. Atypical symptoms such as confusion, incontinence, or agitation may be the only symptoms of an infectious illness (Tideiksaar, 1987). An example is pneumonia, the main complication of influenza. As many as 20% of older adults with pneumonia do not have the typical signs and symptoms of fever, shaking, chills, and rusty productive sputum (Finkelstein et al, 1983). The only symptom may be an increased, unexplained heart rate.

Laboratory Data

A review of test results may reveal infection (Table 18-5). Laboratory values, however, are not enough to detect infection. Other clinical signs must be assessed. Factors other than infection may alter test values. For example, trauma and physical stress can cause an elevation in the number of neutrophils.

Clients with Infection

A client with infection may have a variety of health problems. The nurse assesses the influences of the infection on the client's needs, which may be physical, psychological, social, or economic. For example, a client with a sexually transmitted disease such as AIDS may experience serious psychological problems as a result of self-imposed isolation or rejection by family and friends. A client with a chronic infection in need of continuous wound care at home may not be able to afford the cost of medical supplies. The nurse determines the client's ability to adjust to the disease and resources available for managing health problems.

 Nursing Diagnosis

During assessment, the nurse gathers objective findings, such as an open incision or a reduced caloric intake, and subjective data, such as a client's complaint of tenderness over a surgical wound site. Then the nurse interprets the data carefully, looking for clusters of defining characteristics or risk factors that create a pattern suggesting a specific nursing diagnosis (see diagnoses box on p. 412). It may be necessary for the nurse to validate data (for example, by inspecting the integrity of a wound more carefully). Likewise, additional data such as laboratory findings may help. The accuracy of selecting an appropriate nursing diagnosis depends on analyzing and organizing data correctly (see diagnostic process box on p. 412).

TABLE 18-5 Laboratory Tests to Screen for Infection		
Laboratory Value	Normal (Adult) Values	Indication of Infection
WBC count	5000-10,000/mm	Increased in acute infection, decreased in certain viral or overwhelming infections
Erythrocyte sedimentation rate	Up to 15 mm/hr for men and 20 mm/hr for women	Elevated in presence of inflammatory process
Iron level	60-90 g/dl	Decreased in chronic infection
Cultures of urine and blood	Normally sterile, without microorganism growth	Presence of infectious microorganism growth
Cultures of wound, sputum, and throat	Possible normal flora	Presence of infectious microorganism growth
Differential count (percentage of each type of WBC)		
Neutrophils	55%-70%	Increased in acute suppurative infection, decreased in overwhelming bacterial infection (older adult)
Lymphocytes	20%-40%	Increased in chronic bacterial and viral infection, decreased in sepsis
Monocytes	2%-8%	Increased in protozoal, rickettsial, and tuberculosis infections
Eosinophils	1%-4%	Increased in parasitic infection
Basophils	0.5%-1%	Normal during infection

Examples of Nursing Diagnoses Related to Infection

NANDA-APPROVED NURSING DIAGNOSES

High risk for infection related to:
- Altered immunity
- Tissue destruction
- Malnutrition

High risk for injury related to:
- Altered immunity

Impaired tissue integrity related to:
- Altered circulation
- Exposure to irritants

Altered oral mucous membrane related to:
- Traumatic irritation of nasogastric tube
- Ineffective oral hygiene

Altered nutrition: less than body requirements related to:
- Poor diet habits
- Altered gastrointestinal function

Actual or *high risk for impaired skin integrity* related to:
- Shearing force
- Physical immobilization
- Exposure to skin irritants

Social isolation related to:
- Misconceptions about sexually transmitted disease

Body-image disturbance related to:
- Client's aversion to open wound
- Self-perception regarding sexually transmitted disease

 Sample Nursing Diagnostic Process For Infection

Assessment Activities	Defining Characteristics	Nursing Diagnoses
Check results of laboratory tests.	WBC count 5000/mm³	*High risk for infection* related to lowered immunity
Review current medications.	Client receiving azathioprine (Imuran), an immunosuppressant	
Identify potential sites of infection.	Intravenous catheter in right forearm, in place for 3 days / Foley catheter draining amber-colored urine	
Inspect condition of dependent pressure points.	Area 2 cm in diameter, superficial broken skin over sacrum	*Impaired skin integrity* related to pressure and exposure to fecal irritants
Determine client's food intake over 24-72 hr.	Protein and related calorie intake reduced	
Observe for skin contamination.	Client incontinent (semiliquid stool)	

The nurse may diagnose a high risk for infection or make diagnoses that result from the effects of infection on health status. The nurse's success in planning appropriate nursing interventions depends on the accuracy of the diagnosis and the ability to meet the client's needs.

 ## Planning

The nursing diagnoses identified for a client direct the nurse's selection of interventions for a care plan. As always, the nurse involves the client and any family in establishing goals of care and the specific nursing measures required. When there is a high risk for infection or the client has a known infection, common goals of care may include the following:

1. Preventing exposure to infectious organisms
2. Controlling or reducing the extent of infection
3. Maintaining a resistance to infection
4. Understanding infection-control self-care practices

The nurse establishes priorities for the goals of care. For example, a client has developed an open wound, suffers a debilitating disease such as cancer, and has been unable to tolerate solid foods. The priority of administering therapies that promote wound healing exceeds the goal of educating the client to assume self-care therapies at home. When the client's condition improves, the priorities will change, and client education becomes an essential intervention.

The development of a care plan (see care plan) includes measures involving use of aseptic technique. The care plan will also include goals and expected outcomes for reducing or eliminating infection. The nurse may include appropriate referrals such as a dietitian, infection-control nurse, or home health care nurse. When care is being administered in the home, the nurse plans to be sure the environment promotes good infection-control practices. For example, if a cli-

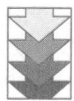

Sample Nursing Care Plan for High Risk for Infection

Nursing diagnosis: *High risk for infection* related to lowered immunity
Definition: High risk for infection is the state in which an individual is at increased risk for being invaded by pathogenic organisms (Kim, McFarland, McLane, 1991).

Goals	Expected Outcomes	Nursing Interventions	Rationale
Client will remain free of nosocomial infection.	Intravenous needle site will not become infected for 72 hr.	Change intravenous peripheral catheters every 48-72 hr; cover site with gauze dressing.	Replacement of peripheral venous catheters every 48-72 hr reduces nosocomial septicemia.
	Client will remain afebrile during hospitalization.		Gauze can be used with low risk of catheter-related infection (Maki, Ringer, 1987).
		When moisture or blood accumulates on dressing, change it and cleanse site with 10% iodine.	Visible moisture or blood beneath dressing is risk factor for catheter-related infection (Maki, Ringer, 1987).
	Client's urine will remain clear, without bacterial growth during hospitalization.	Provide daily perineal hygiene.	Regular periurethral cleansing and reduced urethral manipulation may decrease migration of bacteria up urethra.
		Anchor urinary catheter to avoid up-and-down movement within urethra.	Break in integrity of system can allow introduction of microorganisms and bladder colonization (Classen et al, 1991).
		Keep junction between catheter and drainage bag sealed.	

ent does not have running water, even simple handwashing is difficult to achieve.

Implementation

The nurse's primary goals in controlling infection are preventing the onset and spread of infection and administering measures for treatment of infection. By recognizing and assessing a client's risk factors for infection and implementing appropriate measures, the nurse can reduce the risk of infection.

Through the application of knowledge about the chain of infection, the nurse tries to prevent an infection from developing or spreading by minimizing the numbers and kinds of organisms transmitted to potential infection sites. Eliminating reservoirs of infection, controlling portals of exit and entry, and avoiding actions that transmit microorganisms prevent bacteria from finding a site to grow. Proper use of sterile supplies and protective garments and good handwashing are examples of medically aseptic methods that the nurse uses to control the spread of microorganisms. A final preventive measure is to strengthen a potential host's defenses against infection. Nutritional support, rest, maintenance of physiological protective mechanisms, and immunization protect a client from invasion by pathogens.

When a client develops an infection, the nurse continues preventive care so that health care personnel and other clients are not exposed to the infection. Clients with communicable diseases require isolation techniques that control the environment by forming barriers against bacterial spread.

Treatment of an infectious process includes eliminating the infectious organisms and supporting the client's defenses. The nurse collects specimens of body fluids or drainage from infected body sites for cultures. When the disease process or causative organism has been identified, the physician prescribes the antiinfective or antibiotic drug most effective for the situation. The nurse properly administers antibiotics, watching for allergic reactions and assessing the progress of the infection.

Systemic infections require measures to prevent complications of fever (see Chapter 19). Maintaining intake of fluids prevents dehydration resulting from diaphoresis. The client's increased metabolic rate requires an adequate nutritional intake. Rest preserves energy for the healing process.

Localized infections often require measures to facilitate removal of infectious organisms. The nurse applies principles of wound care (see Chapter 48) to remove infected drainage from wound sites and support the integrity of healing wounds. Special dressings can be applied to facilitate removal of infectious drainage and promote healing of wound margins. Drainage tubes may be inserted to remove infected drainage from body cavities. The nurse uses medical and surgical aseptic techniques to manage wounds and ensures correct handling of infected drainage or body fluids.

During the course of infection the nurse supports the client's body defense mechanisms. For example, if a client has infectious diarrhea, the nurse must maintain skin integrity to prevent breakdown and the entrance of microorganisms. Routine hygiene measures such as cleansing the oral cavity and bathing protect the skin and mucous membranes from organism spread.

A client with an infection has many needs. By monitoring the infection's course carefully, the nurse can choose the most appropriate measures to maintain or restore health.

Medical Asepsis

The nurse follows certain principles and procedures to prevent infection and control its spread. During daily routine care, the nurse uses basic medical aseptic techniques to break the infection chain. Because infections are readily transmissible between clients and care givers, the nurse follows isolation techniques as appropriate. Clients with high susceptibility to infection require special precautions to prevent exposure to pathogens.

CONTROL OR ELIMINATION OF INFECTIOUS AGENTS. Proper cleansing, disinfection, and sterilization of contaminated objects significantly reduce and often eliminate microorganisms. In health care centers a central supply department disinfects and sterilizes reusable supplies. However, the nurse may encounter situations that require use of these techniques. Many principles of cleansing and disinfection also apply to the home.

Cleansing. Cleansing is the removal of all foreign materials such as soil and organic material from objects (Rutala, 1989). Generally, cleansing involves use of water and mechanical action with or without detergents. When an object comes in contact with infectious or potentially infectious material, the object is contaminated. If the object is disposable, it is discarded. Reusable objects must be cleansed thoroughly before disinfection and sterilization.

When cleaning equipment that is soiled by organic material such as blood, fecal matter, mucus, or pus, the nurse applies a mask, protective eyewear, and waterproof gloves. These barriers provide protection from infectious organisms. A stiff-bristled brush and detergent or soap are needed for cleaning. The following steps ensure that an object is clean:

1. Rinse a contaminated object or article with cold running water to remove organic material. Hot water causes the protein in organic material to coagulate and stick to objects, making removal difficult.

Items Requiring Disinfection or Sterilization

CRITICAL ITEMS

Items that enter sterile tissue or the vascular system present a high risk of infection if the items are contaminated with microorganisms, especially bacterial spores. *Critical* items must be *sterile*. Some of these items follow:

- Surgical instruments
- Intravascular catheters
- Urinary catheters
- Needles

SEMICRITICAL ITEMS

Items that come in contact with mucous membranes or skin that is not intact also present risks. These objects must be free of all microorganisms (except bacterial spores). *Semicritical items* must be *disinfected* or *sterilized*. Some of these items follow:

- Respiratory suction tubing and catheters
- Endotracheal tubes
- Gastrointestinal endoscopes
- Thermometers

NONCRITICAL ITEMS

Items that come in contact with intact skin but not mucous membranes must be clean. *Noncritical items* must be *disinfected*. Some of these items follow:

- Bedpans
- Blood pressure cuffs
- Linens
- Stethoscope

2. After rinsing, wash the object with soap and warm water. Soap or detergent reduces the surface tension of water and emulsifies dirt or remaining material. Few household detergents, however, have disinfectant properties. Rinse the object thoroughly to remove the emulsified dirt.
3. Use a brush to remove dirt or material in grooves or seams. Friction dislodges contaminated material for easy removal.
4. Rinse the object in warm water.
5. Dry the object and prepare it for disinfection or sterilization.
6. The brush, gloves, and sink in which the equipment is cleaned should be considered contaminated and should be cleansed.

Disinfection and Sterilization. Disinfection eliminates pathogenic organisms on inanimate objects with the exception of the bacterial spore (Rutala, 1989). Noninfectious microorganisms may or may not be killed. **Sterilization** is the process of eliminating and destroying all microorganisms, including spores and viruses.

The two primary methods for disinfection and sterilization are physical processes, which involve the use of heat or radiation, and chemical processes, which use various solutions or gases. Both disrupt the internal function of microorganisms by destroying cell proteins. Sterilization and disinfection occur when heat reaches a level sufficient to destroy organisms or when a concentration of chemicals has adequate exposure to microorganisms.

A disinfectant is a chemical solution that is used when cleaning only inanimate objects. Examples of disinfectants are alcohol, chlorine, glutaraldehyde, and phenol. The solutions can be caustic and toxic to tissues. A **germicide** (for example, silver sulfadiazine [Silvadene] or isopropyl alcohol) is a chemical preparation that can be applied on skin and tissues, as well as inanimate objects.

The levels of disinfection and sterilization required depends on the type of item contaminated (Spaulding, 1968; Rutala, 1989). There are three categories of instruments and items for client care, and they are based on the degree of risk of infection involved (see box at left). Nurses should be familiar with agency policy and procedures for cleansing, handling, and delivering care items for eventual disinfection and sterilization (Table 18-6). Workers especially trained in disinfection and sterilization perform most of the work. Selection of a method for disinfecting or sterilizing is made after considering the following factors:

TABLE 18-6   Examples of Disinfection and Sterilization Processes

Characteristics	Examples of Use
MOIST HEAT	
Moist heat includes steam (moist heat under pressure) . When exposed to high pressure, water vapor can attain temperature above boiling point to kill all pathogens and spores.	Autoclave is used to sterilize surgical instruments, parenteral solutions, and surgical dressings.
RADIATION	
Ionizing radiation penetrates deeply into objects for effective sterilization and disinfection.	Radiation is used in sterilizing drugs, foods, and other heat-sensitive items.
CHEMICALS	
Chemicals are effective disinfectants because they attack all types of microorganisms, act rapidly, work with water, retain no odor, are stable in light and heat, are inexpensive, are not harmful to body tissues, do not destroy article being disinfected, and are not inactivated by organic material.	Chemicals are used for disinfection of instruments and equipment such as glass thermometers. Chlorine is useful for disinfecting water and for housekeeping purposes.
ETHYLENE OXIDE GAS	
This gas destroys spores and microorganisms by altering cells' metabolic processes. Fumes are released within an autoclave-like chamber. Ethylene oxide gas is toxic to humans.	This gas sterilizes rubber, paper, and plastic items.
BOILING WATER	
Boiling is least expensive for use in home. Bacterial spores and some viruses resist boiling. It is not used in hospitals.	The items (e.g., glass baby bottles) should be boiled for at least 15 minutes.

1. Concentration of solution and duration of contact. A weakened concentration or shortened exposure time may lessen effectiveness.
2. Type and number of pathogens. Certain organisms are killed more easily than others by disruption. The greater the number of pathogens on an object, the longer the required disinfecting time.
3. Surface areas to treat. All dirty surfaces and areas must be fully exposed to disinfecting and sterilizing agents.
4. Temperature of environment. Disinfectants tend to work best at room temperature.
5. Presence of soap. Soap may cause certain disinfectants to be ineffective. Thorough rinsing of an object is necessary before disinfecting.
6. Presence of organic materials. Disinfectants can become inactivated unless blood, saliva, pus, or body excretions are washed off.

Table 18-6 lists processes for disinfection and sterilization and their characteristics.

CONTROL OR ELIMINATION OF RESERVOIRS. To control or eliminate reservoir sites for infection, the nurse eliminates sources of body fluids, drainage, or solutions that might harbor microorganisms. The nurse also carefully discards articles that become contaminated with infectious material (see box). The Occupational Safety and Health Act (OSHA) of 1991 sets standards for minimizing occupational exposure to blood-borne pathogens or other potentially infectious materials (Federal Register, 1991). All health care institutions must have guidelines for the disposal of infectious waste material.

CONTROL OF PORTALS OF EXIT. The nurse follows aseptic practices to minimize or prevent infectious organisms from exiting the body. To control organisms exiting via the respiratory tract, the nurse should avoid talking directly into clients' faces or talking, sneezing, or coughing directly over surgical wounds or sterile dressing fields. The nurse should cover the mouth or nose when sneezing or coughing. The nurse is also responsible for teaching clients to protect others when they sneeze or cough and for providing clients with disposable wipes or tissues to control the spread of microorganisms.

A nurse who has a mild cold and continues to work with clients should wear a mask, especially when changing a dressing or performing a sterile procedure. The same nurse should refrain from working with clients who are highly susceptible to infection.

Another way of controlling the exit of microorganisms is the careful handling of exudate (such as urine, feces, emesis, and blood). Contaminated fluids can easily splash while being discarded in toilets or hoppers. The nurse should wear disposable gloves, gowns, and eye wear if there is a chance of contact with any fluids (see section on body substance isolation). The nurse appropriately bags and disposes of

---

Infection Control to Reduce Reservoirs of Infection

BATHING

Use soap and water to remove drainage, dried secretions, excess perspiration, or sediment from disinfectants.

DRESSING CHANGES

- Change dressings that become wet and soiled (see Chapter 48).

CONTAMINATED ARTICLES

- Place tissues, soiled dressings, or soiled linen in moisture-resistant bags for proper disposal.

CONTAMINATED NEEDLES

- Place syringes and uncapped hypodermic needles and intravenous needles in moisture-resistant, puncture-proof containers, which should be located in client rooms or treatment areas so that exposed, contaminated equipment need not be carried a distance (see Chapter 21).
- Do not recap needles or attempt to break them.

BEDSIDE UNIT

- Keep table surfaces clean and dry.

BOTTLED SOLUTIONS

- Do not leave bottled solutions open for prolonged periods.
- Keep solutions tightly capped.
- Date bottles when opened.

SURGICAL WOUNDS

- Keep drainage tubes and collection bags patent to prevent accumulation of serous fluid under the skin surface.

DRAINAGE BOTTLES AND BAGS

Empty and dispose of drainage suction bottles according to agency policy.

- Empty all drainage systems on each shift unless otherwise ordered by a physician.
- Never raise a drainage system (e.g., urinary drainage bag) above the level of the site being drained unless it is clamped off.

soiled items. Laboratory specimens from all clients are handled as if they were infectious.

CONTROL OF TRANSMISSION. Effective control of infection requires a nurse to remain aware of the modes of transmission and ways to control them. In the hospital, home, or extended care facility a client should have a personal set of care items. Sharing bedpans, urinals, bath basins, and eating utensils can easily lead to transmission of infection. Glass thermometers, even when individually used, warrant special care. Because the client's own mucus can become a source for microorganism growth, after each use the glass thermometer is washed in soap and water and dried.

Because certain microorganisms travel easily through the air, linens or bedclothes should not be shaken. Dusting with a treated or dampened cloth prevents dust particles from entering the air.

To prevent transmission of microorganisms through indirect contact, soiled items and equipment must be kept from touching the nurse's clothing. A common error is to carry dirty linen in the arms against the uniform. Special linen bags should be used, or soiled linen carried with hands held out from the body. Laundry hampers should not be allowed to overflow.

Anything that touches the floor is contaminated. If the nurse accidentally drops a piece of equipment, it should be discarded. When the nurse stoops or bends, the uniform should not touch the floor, and clean or soiled linen should never be put on the floor.

Handwashing. The most important and most basic technique in preventing and controlling transmission of pathogens is handwashing. **Handwashing** is a vigorous, brief rubbing together of all surfaces of hands lathered in soap, followed by rinsing under a stream of water (Garner, Favero, 1985). The purpose is to remove soil and transient organisms from the hands and to reduce total microbial counts over time (Larson, 1989).

Contaminated hands are a prime cause of cross-infection. For example, a nurse caring for a client who has excessive pulmonary excretions assists the client in expectorating mucus and disposes of the tissues in a bedside container. The client's roommate asks the nurse to open containers of food on the meal tray. The nurse then leaves the client's room to pour a dose of medication due in 5 minutes. If the nurse fails to wash hands before each of these actions, organisms from the first client's mucus could easily be transmitted to the roommate's food and to the medication container.

The need for handwashing depends on the type, intensity, duration, and sequence of activity. For example, if a nurse touches an object that is not visibly soiled, handwashing is not required. In contrast, prolonged and intense contact with a client, especially one with wound drainage, requires thorough handwashing. Garner and Favero (1985) recommend that nurses wash hands in the following situations:

1. Before contact with clients who are susceptible to infection (for example, newborn infants or immunosuppressed clients [clients with leukemia, organ transplant recipients, and clients who are HIV-positive])
2. After caring for an infected client
3. After touching organic material
4. Before performing invasive procedures such as administration of injections, catheterization, and suctioning
5. Before and after handling dressings or touching open wounds
6. After handling contaminated equipment
7. Between contact with different clients in high-risk units (for example, nursery and critical care units)

The ideal duration of handwashing is not known. The Centers for Disease Control (CDC) and Public Health Service note that washing times of at least 10 to 15 seconds (Garner, Favero, 1985) will remove most transient microorganisms from the skin. If hands are visibly soiled, more time may be needed. Agency policies often recommend that staff wash hands for 1 to 2 minutes after working in high-risk areas. The frequency of washing also affects the type and number of bacteria on the hands. Larson (1984) has found that nurses who washed their hands 8 times a day were less likely to carry gram-negative bacteria on their hands. Routine handwashing may be performed with liquid or granule soap or soap-impregnated tissue.

Use of antimicrobial soaps is encouraged when nurses work in special care units, emergency departments, and units where many clients are immunosuppressed and when exposure to blood and body fluids is likely (Larson, 1989). There are a number of effective antimicrobial soaps, including alcohols, chlorhexidine glucomate (CHG), and iodophors. Certain soaps can irritate the skin. Procedure 18-1 on pp. 418-419 lists the steps for handwashing.

Health care workers' compliance with handwashing is important. Failure to follow good handwashing techniques may be due to concern over the effects repeated handwashing has on the condition of skin. Larson et al (1986) studied the effects of five different soaps (plain and antimicrobial) on skin damage. The study revealed that although all soaps caused some trauma to the skin, addition of antiseptics to soap caused no greater skin damage. There was no correlation between greater antimicrobial activity and the degree of skin damage.

Handwashing

STEPS

RATIONALE

1. Use easy-to-reach sink with warm running water, soap or disinfectant, paper towels.

   Running water facilitates removal of organisms. Paper towels are easy to discard.

2. Push wristwatch and long uniform sleeves above wrists. Avoid wearing rings. If worn, remove during washing.

   Provides complete access to fingers, hands, wrists. Wearing of rings increases number of microorganisms on hands (Jacobson et al, 1985).

3. Keep fingernails short and filed.

   Most microbes on hands come from subungal region (beneath fingernails) (McGinley et al, 1988).

4. Inspect surface of hands and fingers for breaks or cuts in skin and cuticles. Report such lesions when caring for highly susceptible clients.

   Open cuts or wounds can harbor high concentrations of microorganisms and may serve as portals of exit, increasing client's exposure to infection, or as portals of entry, increasing your risk of acquiring infection.

5. Stand in front of sink, keeping hands and uniform away from sink surface. (If hands touch sink during handwashing, repeat.)

   Inside of sink is contaminated area. Reaching over sink increases risk of touching edge, which is contaminated.

6. Turn on water. Press pedals with foot to regulate flow and temperature (see illustration). Push knee pedals laterally to control flow and temperature. Turn on hand-operated faucets by covering faucet with paper towel.

   When hands contact faucet, they are contaminated. Organisms spread easily from hands to faucet.

7. Avoid splashing water against uniform.

   Microorganisms travel and grow in moisture.

8. Regulate flow of water so that temperature is warm.

   Warm water is more comfortable. Hot water opens skin pores, causing irritation.

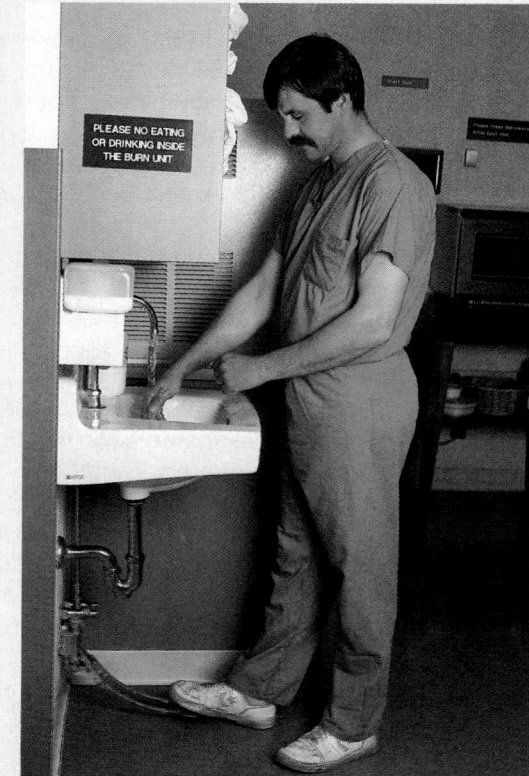

Step 6

STEPS	RATIONALE
9. Wet hands and lower arms thoroughly under running water. Keep hands and forearms lower than elbows during washing.	Hands are most contaminated parts to be washed. Water flows from least to most contaminated area, rinsing microorganisms into sink.
10. Apply 1 ml of regular or 3 ml of antiseptic liquid soap to hands, lathering thoroughly. Soap granules and leaflet preparations may be used.	Bacterial counts drop significantly on hands when using 3 to 5 ml of antimicrobial soap (Larson et al, 1987).
11. Wash hands using plenty of lather and friction for at least 10 to 15 sec. Interlace fingers and rub palms and back of hands with circular motion at least 5 times each (see illustration).	Soap cleanses by emulsifying fat and oil and lowering surface tension. Friction and rubbing mechanically loosen and remove dirt and transient bacteria. Interlacing fingers and thumbs ensures that all surfaces are cleansed. Antimicrobial soap must be in contact with skin at least 10 sec (Garner, 1985).
12. If areas underlying fingernails are soiled, clean them with fingernails of other hand and additional soap or clean orangewood stick. Do not tear or cut skin under or around nail.	
13. Rinse hands and wrists thoroughly, keeping hands down and elbows up (see illustration).	Rinsing mechanically washes away dirt and microorganisms.
14. Optional: repeat steps 10 through 12 but extend period of washing to 1, 2, and 3 min.	Greater the likelihood of hands being contaminated, greater the need for thorough handwashing.
15. Dry hands thoroughly from fingers to wrists and forearms.	Drying from cleanest (fingertips) to least clean (forearms) area avoids contamination. Drying hands prevents chapping and roughened skin.
16. Discard paper towel in proper receptacle.	Prevents transfer of microorganisms.
17. Turn off water with foot and knee pedals. To turn off hand faucet, use clean, dry paper towel.	Wet towel and hands allow transfer of pathogens by capillary action.

CONTINUED

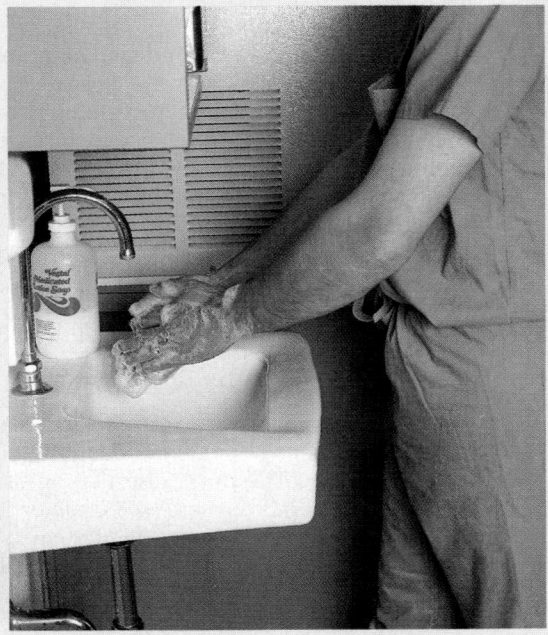

Step 11

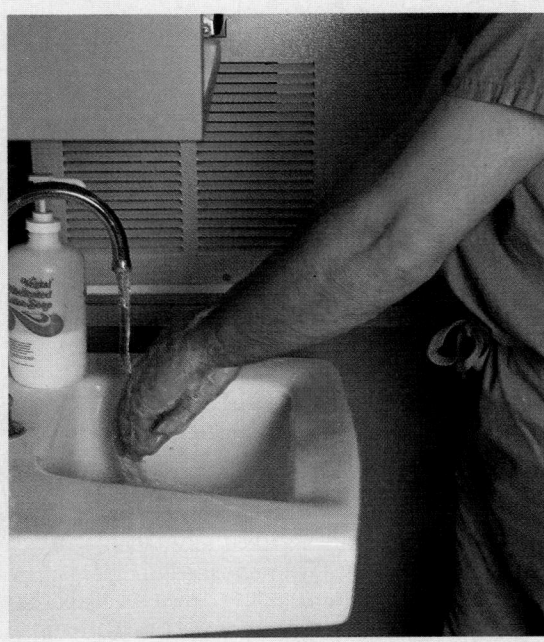

Step 13

The nurse instructs clients and visitors about the proper technique and times for handwashing. Teaching handwashing is particularly important if health care is to continue at home. Clients should wash their hands before eating or handling food; after handling contaminated equipment, linen, or organic material; and before and after elimination. Visitors are encouraged to wash their hands before eating or handling food, after coming in contact with infected clients, and after handling contaminated equipment or organic material.

CONTROL OF PORTALS OF ENTRY. Many measures that control the exit of microorganisms likewise control the entrance of pathogens. Maintaining the integrity of skin and mucous membranes reduces the chances of microorganisms reaching a host. The client's skin should be kept well lubricated by using hand lotion as appropriate (see Chapter 34). Immobilized and debilitated clients are particularly susceptible to skin breakdown. Clients should not be positioned on tubes or objects that might cause breaks in the skin. Dry, wrinkle-free linen also reduces the chances of skin breakdown. Turning and positioning are needed as soon as a client's skin becomes reddened. Frequent oral hygiene prevents drying of mucous membranes. A water-soluble ointment keeps the client's lips well lubricated.

After elimination, a woman should clean the rectum and perineum by wiping from the urinary meatus toward the rectum. Cleansing in a direction from the least to the most contaminated area helps reduce genitourinary infections.

Clients, health care personnel, and even housekeepers are at risk for acquiring infections from accidental needlesticks. After administering an injection or inserting an intravenous catheter, the nurse should carefully dispose of contaminated needles (see Chapter 21). A stray needle lying in bed linen or carelessly thrown into a wastebasket is a prime source for pathogens. Hepatitis B, or serum hepatitis, is the infection most commonly transmitted by contaminated needles. A needlestick should be reported immediately. Health care agencies require the victim

---

Hepatitis B Vaccination and Follow-Up after Exposure

- Health care employers shall make available the hepatitis B vaccine and vaccination series to all employees who have occupational exposure. Evaluation and follow-up care will be available to all employees who have been exposed.
- All medical evaluations and procedures, including the vaccine and vaccination series and evaluation after exposure (prophylaxis), are made available at no cost to employees.
- A confidential written medical evaluation will be available to employees with exposure incidents.
- Hepatitis B vaccinations will be made available to employees within 10 working days of assignment.

From Occupational Safety and Health Act of 1991, Federal Register, 1991.

Infection Control: Protecting the Susceptible Host

PROTECTING NORMAL DEFENSE MECHANISMS

- Regular bathing removes transient microorganisms from the skin's surface. Lubrication helps keep the skin hydrated and intact.
- Regular oral hygiene removes proteins in the saliva that attract microorganisms. Flossing removes tartar and plaque that can cause germ infection.
- Maintenance of an adequate fluid intake promotes normal urine formation and a resultant outflow of urine to flush the bladder and urethral lining of microorganisms.
- For physically dependent or immobilized clients, the nurse encourages routine coughing and deep breathing to keep lower airways clear of mucus.
- The nurse encourages proper immunization of children or adult clients who become exposed to certain infectious microorganisms. Children are vaccinated for smallpox, measles, mumps, rubella, and diphtheria. Adults should have tetanus-diphtheria boosters every 10 years. Influenza vaccines are recommended for health care workers. Older adults should regularly receive influenza and pneumococcal vaccines.

MAINTAINING HEALING PROCESSES

- The nurse promotes intake of a well-balanced diet containing essential proteins, vitamins, carbohydrates, and fats. The nurse also uses measures to increase the client's appetite (see Chapter 35).
- The nurse promotes a client's comfort and sleep so that energy stores are replaced daily (see Chapters 36 and 37).
- The nurse assists the client in learning techniques to reduce stress (see Chapter 30).

of a needlestick to complete an injury report and seek appropriate treatment (see box at far left).

Another cause for entrance of microorganisms into a host is improper handling and management of urinary catheters and drainage sets (See Chapter 40). The point of connection between a catheter and drainage tube should remain closed and intact. As long as such systems are closed, their contents are considered sterile. Outflow of spigots on drainage bags should also remain closed and cleansed to prevent entrance of bacteria. Movement of the catheter at the urethra should be minimized to reduce chances of microorganisms ascending the urethra into the bladder.

The nurse may care for clients with closed drainage systems that collect wound drainage, bile, or other body fluids. In each example, the site from which a drainage tube exits should remain clear of excess moisture or accumulated drainage. All tubing should remain connected throughout use. Drainage receptacles should only be opened when it is necessary to discard or measure volume of drainage.

At times the nurse obtains specimens from drainage tubes or inserts needles into intravenous tubing ports. The nurse disinfects tubes and ports by wiping outward with alcohol or an iodine solution before entering the system. Temporarily placing squares of sterile gauze around the ends of an opened drainage tube adds further protection against bacteria.

A final method for reducing the entrance of microorganisms is the technique for cleansing wounds (see Chapter 48). The wound itself is considered to be sterile. To prevent entrance of microorganisms, into the wound, the nurse should clean outward from a wound site. When applying a disinfectant or cleaning with soap and water, the nurse wipes around the wound edge first and then cleans outward. A clean gauze should be used for each revolution around the wound's circumference.

PROTECTION OF THE SUSCEPTIBLE HOST. A client's resistance to infection improves as the nurse protects normal body defenses against infection. The nurse also intervenes to maintain the body's normal reparative processes (see box at left).

Isolation Practices. The risk of transmitting nosocomial infection or infectious disease among clients is high. When a client has a known source of infection, health care workers become alerted and follow infection-control practices. However, health care workers may not be aware that clients have infections. The majority of organisms causing nosocomial infections are found in the **colonized** body substances of clients regardless of whether a culture has confirmed infection and a diagnosis has been made

(Lynch, Jackson, 1988). Body substances such as feces, urine, mucus, and wound drainage always contain potentially infectious organisms.

Isolation precautions control the transmission of pathogens. Barriers such as protective gowns and gloves, masks, eyewear and private rooms keep pathogens in a confined area. Care givers follow procedures to prevent organisms from leaving the room of clients or to prohibit organisms from entering the rooms of susceptible clients.

There are two systems for isolation precautions used in health care institutions. The first, **body substance isolation (BSI),** is an isolation system that uses generic infection precautions for all clients (Lynch et al, 1990). This system emphasizes the potential infectiousness of all moist body substances. Health care workers use protective apparel based on the kind of client interaction anticipated. The precautions used in BSI are adequate for all clients except for those with diseases spread by the respiratory tract (for example, tuberculosis, rubella, chickenpox, and disseminated herpes zoster). These clients must be cared for in private rooms under a category of isolation called *stop-sign isolation* (Fig. 18-3). The box on p. 422 describes the elements of BSI.

The other system for isolation involves the use of specific guidelines for isolating clients in controlled environments. The CDC (Garner, Simmons, 1984) developed two methods for implementing this isolation system. In the **disease-specific isolation** method, certain practices are followed for each infectious disease. For example, if a client has chickenpox, it is necessary to place the client in a private room and use techniques to prevent respiratory spread. This is a less costly and time-consuming sys-

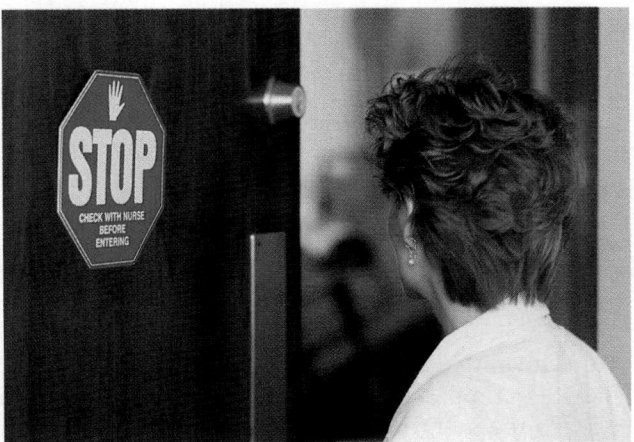

Fig. 18-3   A visible stop sign is placed on the door of a client under special isolation precautions.

Body Substance Isolation

- Personnel wear clean, disposable gloves before contact with mucous membranes, nonintact skin, or moist body substances.
- Personnel change gloves between clients and between activities with the same client when gloves become excessively soiled.
- Personnel wash hands for at least 10 seconds when the hands are soiled, before each new client contact, and after gloves are removed. (Wearing gloves does *not* eliminate the need to wash hands).
- Additional barriers such as gowns or plastic aprons, masks, goggles or glasses, hair covers, and shoe covers are used as needed to keep moist body substances off clothing, skin, and mucous membranes of the wearer. For example, the nurse wears masks and goggles when performing a procedure in which the face can be sprayed with mucus, blood, or any body fluid.
- All sharp instruments and needles are discarded uncapped in a rigid, puncture-proof container located at the point of use such as a client room or treatment area.
- Laboratory specimens from all clients are handled as if they were infectious.
- Handling and reprocessing practices are uniform for all articles and equipment used on all clients. For example, soiled reusable articles are transported in plastic bags or rigid containers.
- Soiled linen is bagged securely before transport.
- Private rooms are used for clients with communicable diseases transmitted via the air or clients who soil their environment uncontrollably with body substances. A large red sign reading *Stop* is placed at the door of this client's room; it also instructs all persons, "Check with the nurse before entering." For certain diseases (e.g., meningococcal meningitis), masks are worn when personnel or family enter the client's room. Roommates who are immune to the client's disease or who are currently infected with the same disease may share rooms (institutional policy may vary on this issue).

---

tem because certain diseases require only minimal precautions. The other method is category-specific isolation. Diseases requiring similar isolation precautions, indicated by the manner in which organisms are transmitted, are grouped in eight categories (Table 18-7 on pp. 424-425). A sign is placed outside the client's room and at the bedside to remind personnel of specific precautions.

The CDC's category-specific isolation categories include the **universal blood and body fluid precau-tions.** Initially developed in 1987 by the CDC and in 1989 by the Bureau of Communicable Disease Epidemiology in Canada, universal precautions were issued to prevent the transmission of blood-borne diseases such as AIDS and hepatitis B in health care settings. Universal precautions are now the minimum standard of practice recommended in the Occuptional Safety and Health Act of 1991 (Federal Register, 1991) for all health care agencies. The HIV virus has become a serious threat that heightens the attention of health care workers and thus warrants special precautions. Universal precautions and BSI are very similar. Both involve the use of the same barrier precautions, but universal precautions are not intended to reduce cross-transmission of organisms among ill clients (Lynch et al, 1990). Specifically the recommendations for glove use differs. BSI requires that clean gloves be worn before contact with body fluids, mucous membranes, nonintact skin, and insertion sites for indwelling devices (moist areas). For universal precautions, gloves are used only for anticipated contact with blood or body secretions containing blood (Lynch et al, 1990). The guidelines for universal precautions for general client care include the following (CDC, 1987a, 1987b, 1988):

1. Universal precautions apply to blood and to other body fluids containing visible blood. Blood is the greatest source of blood-borne pathogens. Precautions also apply to semen, vaginal secretions, tissues, and the following fluids: cerebrospinal, synovial, pleural, peritoneal, pericardial, and amniotic.
2. Universal precautions do not apply to feces, nasal secretions, sputum, sweat, tears, urine, and vomitus unless they contain visible blood.
3. Gloves should be worn when contacting blood and body fluids at risk, mucous membranes, nonintact skin; when handling items or surfaces soiled with blood or body fluids; and for performing venipuncture and other vascular access procedures.
4. Gloves should be changed after contact with each client.
5. Masks and protective eyewear or face shields should be worn during procedures (for example, irrigations) that are likely to generate droplets of blood or other body fluids containing blood to prevent exposure of mucous membranes of the mouth, nose, and eyes.
6. Gowns should be worn during procedures that are likely to generate splashes of blood or other body fluids containing blood.
7. Hands and other skin surfaces should be washed immediately and thoroughly if contaminated with blood or other body fluids containing blood.

8. To prevent needlestick injuries, needles should not be recapped, purposely bent, broken, or removed from disposable syringes. Used needles are placed in puncture-resistant containers near the work area.

9. To reduce the need for mouth-to-mouth resuscitation (see Chapter 38), mouthpieces, resuscitator bags, or other ventilation devices should be used.

10. Health care workers who have exudative lesions should refrain from all direct client care and from handling client care equipment.

11. Universal precautions do not apply to feces, saliva, nasal secretions, sputum, sweat, tears, urine, or vomitus unless it is visibly contaminated with blood.

Regardless of the type of isolation system, the nurse must follow the following basic principles:

1. Hands should be washed thoroughly before entering and leaving the room of a the client receiving isolation.

2. Contaminated supplies and equipment should be disposed of in a manner that prevents spread of microorganisms to other persons.

3. Knowledge of a known disease process and the means of infection transmission should be applied when using protective barriers.

4. All persons who might be exposed during transport of client outside isolation must be protected.

Psychological Implications of Isolation. When a client requires isolation in a private room, normally a sense of loneliness develops because normal social relationships become disrupted. This situation can be psychologically harmful, especially for children.

As a result of the infectious process, clients' body images are altered. They may feel unclean, rejected, lonely, or guilty. Aseptic practices further intensify these beliefs of difference or undesirability. Isolation in a private room limits sensory contact. Unless the nurse acts to minimize feelings of psychological and physical isolation, clients' emotional states can interfere with recovery.

Before isolation measures are instituted, the client and family must understand the nature of the disease or condition, the purposes of isolation, and steps for carrying out specific precautions. If they are able to participate in maintaining asepsis, the chances of reducing the spread of infection are great. The client and family should be taught to wash hands and apply gowns, masks, and gloves. Each procedure should be demonstrated, and the client and family should be given an opportunity for practice. It is also important to explain how infectious organisms can be transmitted so that the client

understands the difference between contaminated and clean objects. Unless family members know that their clothing becomes contaminated by contact with infected secretions, efforts at controlling infection are wasted.

The nurse also takes measures to improve the client's sensory stimulation during isolation. Reading materials, a radio or television set, a clock, and hobby materials should be available. However, if a book or other inanimate object comes in contact with infected material, it must be disinfected or discarded. An object such as a radio can be wrapped in a protective plastic covering. The room environment should be clean and pleasant. Drapes or shades should be opened, and excess supplies and equipment are removed. The nurse must listen to the client's concerns or interests. If the nurse rushes through care or shows a lack of interest, the client will feel rejected and even more isolated. Mealtime is a particularly good opportunity for conversation. Providing comfort measures such as repositioning, a back massage, or a tepid sponge bath increases physical stimulation. If the client's condition permits, the nurse should encourage the client to walk and sit up in a chair.

The nurse must explain to family the client's risk of depression or loneliness. Visiting family members should be encouraged to avoid expressions or actions that convey revulsion or disgust. The nurse discusses ways to provide meaningful stimulation.

Protective Environment. When BSI is in place but a client requires stop-sign isolation because of a respiratory infection or when category- or disease-specific isolation is in place, a private room serves to control microorganisms within the environment. Private rooms used for isolation have negative-pressure air flow to prevent infectious particles from flowing out of the closed environment. There are also special rooms with positive-pressure air flow that are used for highly susceptible clients such as transplant recipients. In this case no organisms are able to enter a room. Health care personnel are especially alerted to use aseptic precautions when clients are placed in isolation rooms. On the door or wall outside the room, the nurse posts a card listing precautions for the client's isolation category. The card is a handy reference for health care personnel and visitors and alerts anyone who might enter the room accidentally that special precautions must be followed.

The isolation room or an adjoining anteroom should contain handwashing, bathing, and toilet facilities. Soap and antiseptic solutions are made available. Personnel and visitors should wash their hands before coming to the client's bedside and again before leaving the room.

TABLE 18-7 Category-Specific Isolation Categories

Category of Isolation	Purpose	Example of Disease or Condition	Room
Strict	Prevents transmission of highly contagious or virulent infections spread by air and contact	Chickenpox, diphtheria	Private room with door closed
Contact	Prevents transmission of highly transmissible infections spread by close or direct contact that do not warrant strict precautions	Acute respiratory infections in infants and young children, impetigo, herpes simplex, infections by multiple resistant bacteria	Private room (Clients infected with same organism may share room.)
Respiratory	Prevents transmission of infectious diseases over short distances through air droplets	Measles, meningitis, mumps, pneumonia, *Haemophilus* influenza (in children)	Private room (Clients infected with same organism may share room.)
Enteric precautions	Prevents infections transmitted by direct or indirect contact with feces	Cholera, diarrhea of an infectious cause, hepatitis A, gastroenteritis caused by highly infectious organism	Private room if client's hygiene is poor (e.g., does not wash hands, shares contaminated items) (Clients with same organism may share room.)
Acid-fast bacillus (AFB) isolation	Prevents spread of pulmonary tuberculosis in clients who have positive results on sputum culture or chest x-ray examination indicating active disease	Laryngeal tuberculosis	Private room with special ventilation (negative pressure) preferred and door closed
Drainage and secretion precautions	Prevents infections transmitted by direct or indirect contact with purulent material or drainage from infected body site	Abscess, burn infection, infected wound, minor infections not included in contact isolation	Private room not indicated
Universal blood and body fluid precautions*	Prevents contact with pathogens transmitted by direct or indirect contact with infective blood or body fluids containing blood	AIDS, hepatitis B, syphillis	Private room if client's hygiene is poor
Care of severely immunocompromised clients†	Protects client with lowered immunity and resistance from acquiring infectious organisms	Leukemia, lymphoma, aplastic anemia	Private room with door closed

*Formerly blood and body fluid precautions (still used by some hospitals).
†Formerly protective or reverse isolation.

Gown	Gloves	Mask	Precautions
Required of all persons entering room	Required of all persons entering room	Required of all persons entering room	Discard or bag and label articles contaminated with infective materials. Send reusable articles for disinfection and sterilization.
Indicated if soiling or contact is likely	Indicated for persons touching infective material	Indicated for persons coming close to client	Discard or bag and label articles contaminated with infective material. Send reusable items for disinfection and sterilization.
Not indicated	Not indicated	Indicated for persons coming close to client	Discard or bag and label articles contaminated with infective material. Send reusable items for disinfection and sterilization. Tell clients that they should not share bathroom.
Indicated if soiling is likely	Indicated when touching infective material	Not indicated	Discard or bag and label articles contaminated with infective material. Send reusable items for disinfection and sterilization. Tell clients that they should not share bathroom.
Indicated only if needed to prevent gross contamination of clothing	Not indicated	Indicated only if client is coughing and does not reliably cover mouth	Send articles to be thoroughly cleansed or disinfected, or discard them even though they are rarely involved in transmission of tuberculosis.
Indicated if soiling or contact with infective material is likely	Indicated when touching infective material	Not indicated unless there is high risk of exposure to splash	Discard or bag and label articles contaminated with infective material. Send for disinfection or sterilization.
Indicated during procedures likely to generate splashes of blood or body fluids	Indicated when touching blood or body fluids containing visible blood, mucous membranes, or nonintact skin of all clients; indicated for touching soiled items	Indicated during procedures likely to generate droplets of blood	Discard or bag and label articles contaminated with blood or body fluids. Disinfect and sterilize articles. Avoid needlesticks. Dispose of used needles in properly labeled, puncture-resistant container. Clean blood spills promptly with 5.25% solution of sodium hypochloride diluted 1:10 with water.
Required of all persons entering room	Required of all persons entering room	Indicated for persons coming in contact with client	For open wound or burns, use sterile gloves.

The nurse makes certain that each isolation room contains a special impervious bag for soiled or contaminated linen, as well as a trash container with plastic liners. Impervious receptacles prevent transmission of microorganisms by preventing seepage to and soiling of the outside surface. A disposable impervious container should be available in the room to discard used needles, syringes, and sharp objects.

The nurse should avoid taking any article or piece of equipment into a client's room that is to be reused outside the isolation area. If such an article becomes contaminated, it must be discarded or disinfected and sterilized. A nurse keeps the chart outside at the nurses' station or on the isolation cart. Equipment such as a sphygmomanometer, stethoscope, or other examination devices should be left in the client's room until isolation precautions are no longer required. Afterward, all reusable equipment is disinfected.

PROTECTION FOR PERSONNEL. Isolation supplies should be readily available for personnel to wear before entering an isolation room. A special anteroom or an isolation cart in the hallway holds supplies of gowns, masks, and gloves.

Gowns. The primary reason for gowning is to prevent soiling clothes during contact with the client. Gowns protect health care personnel and visitors from coming in contact with infected material and also protect clients from organisms on other persons' clothing.

Isolation gowns open at the back and have ties at the neck and waist to keep them closed and secure. Gowns should be long enough to cover all outer garments. Long sleeves with tight-fitting cuffs provide added protection. There is no special technique required for applying clean gowns as long as they are fastened securely. However, the nurse must carefully remove gowns to minimize contamination of the hands and uniform and then discard them after removal (Procedure 18-2).

Masks. A mask protects the nurse from inhaling microorganisms from a client's respiratory tract and prevents transmission of pathogens from the nurse's respiratory tract to the client. The mask protects a wearer from inhaling large-particle aerosols that travel short distances (3 feet) and small-particle droplet nuclei that remain suspended in the air and travel longer distances. At times a client who is susceptible to infection wears a mask to prevent inhalation of pathogens. Clients receiving respiratory precautions who are transported outside of their rooms should wear masks to protect other clients and personnel.

According to the CDC, masks may prevent transmission of infections by direct contact with mucous membranes (Williams, 1983). A mask discourages the wearer from touching the eyes, nose, or mouth.

A properly applied mask fits snugly over the mouth and nose so that pathogens and body fluids cannot enter or escape through the sides (Procedure 18-3 on p. 430). If a person wears glasses, the top edge of the mask fits below the glasses so that they will not cloud over as the person exhales. Talking should be kept to a minimum while wearing a mask to reduce respiratory air flow. A mask that has become moist does not provide a barrier to microorganisms and thus is ineffective. It should be discarded. A mask should never be reused. A safe rule is to change a mask every hour. Clients and family members should be warned that a mask can cause a sensation of smothering. If family members become uncomfortable, they should leave the room and discard the mask.

Before removing a mask, individuals remove gloves (if worn) or wash hands if they have been in contact with infectious material. The mask is disposed of by holding it at the tie, avoiding contact with the soiled surface. It is placed in a waste receptacle.

Gloves. Gloves prevent the transmission of pathogens by direct and indirect contact. The CDC (Williams, 1983) cites the following reasons for wearing gloves:

1. Reduces possibility of personnel coming in contact with infectious organisms that infect clients (for example, handling contaminated dressings or cleaning an incontinent client with hepatitis)
2. Reduces likelihood that personnel will transmit their own endogenous flora to clients
3. Reduces possibility that personnel will become transiently colonized with microorganisms that can be transmitted to other clients (Transient colonization can usually be prevented with handwashing.)

Nurses apply gloves when there is risk of exposure to infected material. Specifically, gloves are recommended when nurses have scratches or breaks in the skin, when performing venipuncture or finger or heel sticks, when they expect to spill blood or other body fluids on the hands, and when they are inexperienced (Dickerson, 1989). The CDC further recommends that gloves be worn only once and then discarded. In most cases, disposable, single-use gloves are worn. When full protective apparel is needed, the nurse first applies a mask, washes and dries hands, applies a gown and then applies gloves. Disposable gloves are easily applied and designed to fit either hand. The glove's thin rubber, however, can be easily torn. The glove cuffs should be pulled up over the wrists or cuffs of a gown.

STEPS	RATIONALE
1. Review the precautions for isolation.	Mode of transmission for infectious microorganism determines type and degree of precautions followed.
2. Explain purpose of isolation and precautions necessary to client, family, visitors.	Improves client's ability to participate in care and minimizes anxiety.

3. Assemble necessary supplies:
  a. Medications
  b. Sphygmomanometer
  c. Thermometer
  d. Hygiene supplies
  e. Linens
  f. Specimen collection equipment with appropriate labels
  g. Water pitcher, cups, water
	Limited number of trips into and out of room reduces risk of breaking isolation procedure.

4. Wash hands.	Reduces transmission of microorganisms.

5. Apply gown, mask, gloves as appropriate:
  a. Apply gown, being sure it covers all outer garments. Pull sleeves down to wrist. Tie securely at neck and waist (see illustration on p. 428).
  b. Apply disposable gloves. If worn with gown, bring cuffs over edge of gown sleeves.
  c. Apply surgical mask around mouth and nose; tie securely.
	Protective garments prevent transmission of organisms from nurse to client and protect nurse from contact with infectious pathogens.

6. Enter client's room. Arrange supplies and equipment. (If equipment will be removed from room for reuse, place on clean paper towel.)	Prevents contamination of items.

7. Assess vital signs:
  a. Place clean paper towel on bedside table. Place additional piece of paper on top.
  b. Place watch on towel positioned for easy visibility.
  c. If equipment remains in room, proceed to assess vital signs by routine procedures. Avoid contact of stethoscope or blood pressure cuff with infective material.
  d. Write vital sign results on or piece of paper without contaminating it.
  e. If stethoscope is to be reused, clean diaphragm or bell with alcohol. Set aside on clean surface.
	Helps avoid contact of clean items with contaminated environment in isolation room.

8. Administer medictions (see Chapter 21):
  a. Give oral medication in wrapper or cup.
  b. Dispose of wrapper or cup in plastic-lined receptacle.
  c. Administer injection, being sure gloves are worn.
  d. Discard syringe and uncapped needle into special container. If reusable syringe (e.g., Carpuject) is used, dispose of inner cartridge and needle in special container.
  e. Place reusable syringe on clean towel for eventual removal and disinfection.
	Supplies are handled and discarded to minimize transfer of microorganisms.
	
	Prevents added contamination of syringe.

9. Administer hygiene (see Chapter 34): a. Avoid allowing your gown to become wet; carry washbasin outward away from gown; avoid leaning against wet table top.	Moisture allows organisms to travel through gown to uniform.

Caring for a Client Under Isolation Precautions

STEPS	RATIONALE
b. Assist client in removing gown; discard in special linen bag.	
c. Remove linen from bed; if excessively soiled, avoid contact with your gown. Dispose in special linen bag.	Linen soiled by client's body fluids is disposed of to prevent contact with clean items.
d. Provide clean bed linen and set of towels.	
e. Change gloves if they become excessively soiled and further care is necessary.	
10. Collect specimens:	
a. Place specimen containers on clean paper towel in client's bathroom.	Specimens of blood and body fluids are placed in well-constructed containers with secure lids to prevent leaks during transport.
b. Follow procedure (see Table 18-8) for collecting specimen of body fluids.	
c. Transfer specimen to container without soiling outside of container. Transfer container to clean plastic bag held outside of room by another care giver (optional).	
d. Check label on specimen for accuracy. Send to laboratory (warning labels may be used, depending on hospital policy).	

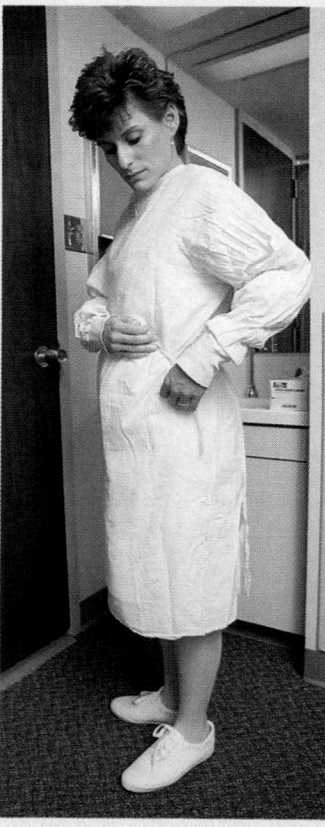

Step 5a

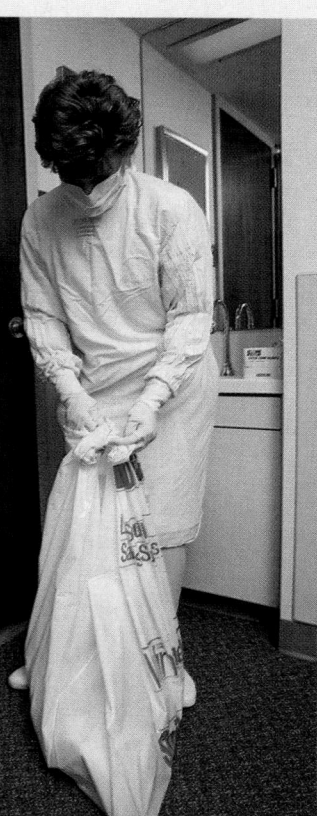

Step 11b

STEPS	RATIONALE

11. Dispose of linen and trash bags as they become full:
  a. Use single bags to contain soiled articles if they are impervious to moisture and are sturdy.
  b. Tie bags securely at top in knot (see illustration).
	Linen or refuse should be totally contained to prevent exposure of personnel to infective material.

12. Resupply room as needed by having another care giver hand over supplies at door.	Limited trips of personnel into and out of room reduces your and client's exposure to microorganisms.

13. Leave isolation room:
  a. Untie gown at waist. Remove one glove by grasping cuff and pulling glove inside out over hand (see illustration). Discard glove. With ungloved hand, tuck finger inside cuff of remaining glove and pull it off, inside out (see illustration).
  b. Untie mask strings; drop mask into trash receptacle.
  c. Untie neck strings of gown. Allow gown to fall from shoulders. Remove hands from sleeves, without touching outside of gown. Hold gown inside at shoulder seams and fold inside out. Discard in laundry bag.
  d. Wash hands minimum of 10 sec.
  e. Retrieve wristwatch and stethoscope and note vital sign values on paper.
  f. Explain to client when you plan to return to room. Ask whether client requires any personal care items.
  g. Leave room and close door.
	Gloves and gown are removed by avoiding contamination of hands.
	
	Clean hands can contact clean items.
	
	Includes client in care plan.

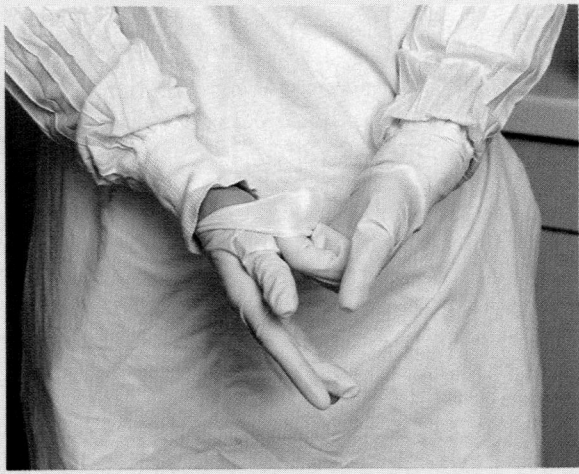

Step 13a

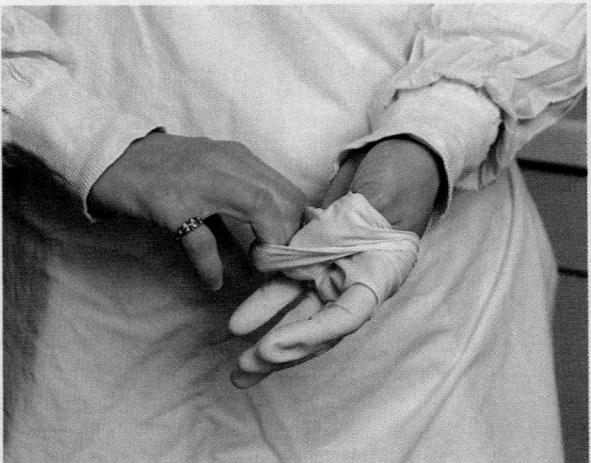

Step 13a

Applying a Surgical Mask

STEPS	RATIONALE
1. Find top edge of mask (usually has thin, metal strip along edge).	Pliable metal fits snugly against bridge of nose.
2. Hold mask by top two strings or loops. Tie two top ties at top of back of head with ties above ears (see illustration) (alternative: slip loops over each ear).	Position of ties at top of head provides tight fit. Ties over ears may cause irritation.
3. Tie two lower ties snugly around neck with mask well under chin (see illustration).	Prevents escape of microorganisms through sides of mask as you talk or breathe.
4. Gently pinch upper metal band around bridge of nose.	Prevents microorganisms from escaping around nose.

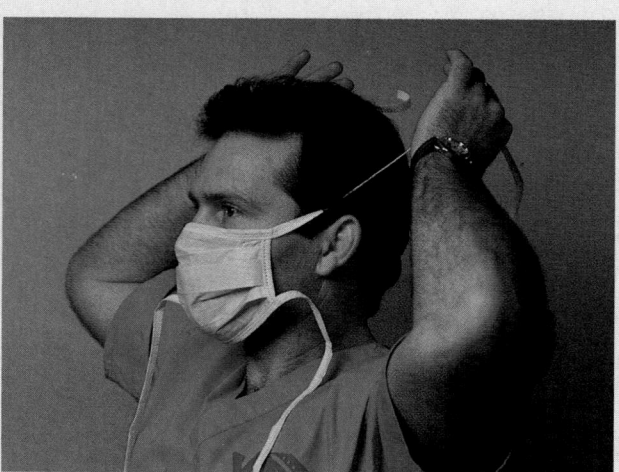

Step 2

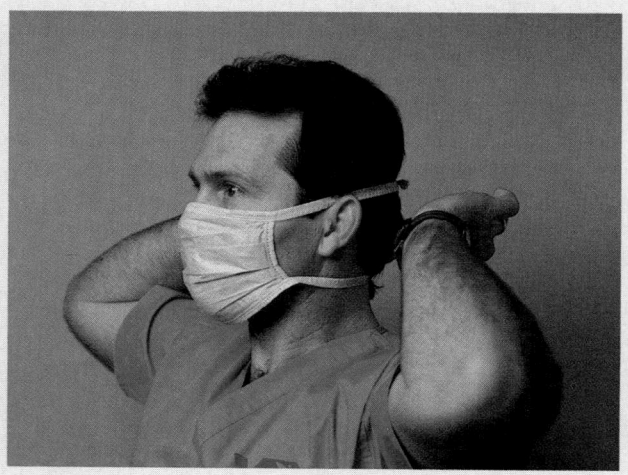

Step 3

After coming in contact with any infected material, the nurse should change gloves if care is not completed. If the nurse does not plan to have more contact with the client, reapplying gloves is unnecessary. Researchers have determined that repeated manipulations of gloved hands can allow bacteria to pass through the rubber. Korniewicz et al (1989) suggest that gloves should perhaps be changed frequently after high-stress use in high-risk situations (see research box).

Family members often believe that they can touch any object after they have applied gloves. The nurse should explain that gloves can also become contaminated after touching infected material or another contaminated object. It is very important to wash hands after removing gloves. Bacteria can cross through rubber gloves, especially if the rubber is thin or if the gloves have been worn a prolonged time under stress (Korniewicz et al, 1989).

Protective Eyewear. When participating in an invasive procedure that creates droplets or splashing of blood or other body fluids, a nurse must wear protective eyewear (CDC, 1987a, 1987b). Examples of invasive procedures include irrigation of a large abdominal wound and insertion of an arterial catheter in which the nurse assists a physician. Eyewear may be available in the form of plastic glasses or goggles. The eyewear should fit snugly around the face so that fluids cannot enter between the face and glasses.

Delivering Care in an Isolation Room. The nurse must remain aware of medical aseptic technique while working with clients in protected environments. The nurse should feel comfortable in performing all procedures and yet remain conscious of infection-control principles. If the nurse brings any article into the room or exposes an article to infected material and then touches or removes the article, the risk of

Research Highlight

In an experimental research study by Korniewicz et al, 28 volunteers were asked to test the integrity of vinyl and latex procedure gloves under in-use conditions. Researchers were interested in determining whether small bacterial molecules could penetrate gloves after three levels of manipulation: no manipulation, partial manipulation (rubbing gloved hands with a washcloth in an established sequence), and full manipulation (attaching a needle to a syringe repeatedly, connecting and disconnecting a syringe to intravenous tubing, and wrapping and unwrapping a blunt object). After the manipulations, subjects immersed their gloved hands into a nutrient broth containing the microorganism *Serratia marcescens*. Cultures of the subject's skin were then used to determine whether the gloves were permeable to bacteria. In 34% of the vinyl gloves and 20% of the latex gloves, bacteria were isolated from the inside of the gloves. Both latex and vinyl gloves provide some barrier protection. The protective effect of both gloves was markedly reduced when the gloves were stressed like they would be in client care activities. Hands should be washed after client care, even if gloves are worn, and after removal of gloves.

Korniewicz DM et al: Integrity of vinyl and latex procedure gloves, *Nurs Res* 38(3):144, 1989.

transmitting infection to other clients or personnel is increased. Procedure 18-2 describes the procedures commonly performed in an isolation room.

Regardless of the form of isolation, the nurse follows certain precautions when handling equipment and supplies. The following guidelines limit transmission of microorganisms:

1. Keep medication carts or trays outside of the client's room.
2. Discard uncapped needles, sharp objects, and syringes in puncture-proof receptacles in the client's room.
3. Keep equipment for assessing vital signs in the client's room for the duration of isolation. Use disposable thermometers. Avoid bringing electronic thermometers into isolation rooms. The units are difficult to clean.
4. Check agency policy for methods for removing regular dishes and eating utensils from isolation rooms.
5. When plastic, rubber, or glass reusable items become soiled, place them in separate bags because methods of sterilization differ.

Specimen Collection. Many laboratory studies may be required when a client is suspected of having an infectious disease. Body fluids and secretions suspected of containing infectious organisms are collected for culture and sensitivity tests. The specimen is placed in a medium that promotes growth of organisms. A laboratory technologist then identifies the microorganisms growing in the culture. Additional test results indicate antibiotics to which the organisms are resistant or sensitive. Sensitivity reports determine the antibiotics used in treatment.

The nurse obtains all culture specimens using disposable gloves and sterile equipment. Collecting fresh material from the site of infection, such as in the case of wound drainage, ensures that the specimen will not be contaminated by neighboring microbes. All specimen containers should be sealed tightly to prevent spillage and contamination of the outside of the container. Table 18-8 on p. 432 describes techniques for collecting specimens from the client with a suspected infection.

Bagging Articles. Nurses use special bagging procedures for removing contaminated items from the client's environment. Bagging articles prevents accidental exposure of personnel to contaminated articles and prevents contamination of the surrounding environment.

The CDC recommends that a single bag is adequate for discarding or wrapping items if the bag is impervious and sturdy and if the article can be placed in the bag without contaminating the outside of the bag (Williams, 1983). The nurse typically discards contaminated reusable equipment such as stethoscopes, forceps, or suction bottles in a single bag. When a linen bag becomes filled, the CDC suggests the following guidelines (Weinstein et al, 1989) for handling isolation linen:

1. Soiled linen should be placed in a laundry bag in the client's room.
2. The bag should be labeled, or it should be a specific color (for example, red) designated for such linen so that it is easily recognized.
3. Linen requires less handling if the bag is soluble in hot water. However, such a bag may need to be double bagged because it punctures or tears easily.

The CDC recommends double bagging, if it is impossible to prevent contamination of the bag's outer surface. Double bagging may still be routine in hospitals. However, studies have shown that this procedure is not necessary to control infection (Maki, Alvarado, Hassemer, 1986; Weinstein et al, 1989). Use of one standard-sized linen bag that is not overfilled and that is tied securely and is intact is adequate to prevent infection transmission. The same rule applies to trash bags.

TABLE 18-8 Specimen Collection Techniques		
Amount Needed*	Collection Device*	Specimen Collection and Transfer
WOUND CULTURE		
As much as possible (after cleaning skin to remove flora)	Cotton-tipped swab or syringe	Place clean test tube or culturette tube on clean paper towel. After swabbing center of wound site, grasp collection tube by holding it with paper towel. Carefully insert swab without touching outside of tube. After washing hands and securing tube's top, transfer labeled tube into bag for transport to laboratory.
BLOOD CULTURE		
10 ml per culture bottle, from two different venipuncture sites (Volume may differ based on collection containers.)	Syringes and culture media bottles	Perform venipuncture at two different sites to decrease likelihood of both specimens being contaminated by skin flora. Inject 10 ml of blood into each bottle. Wash hands. Secure tops of bottles, label specimens, and send to laboratory.
STOOL CULTURE		
Small amount, approximately size of a walnut	Clean cup with seal top (not necessary to be sterile) and tongue blade	Place cup on clean paper towel in client's bathroom. Using tongue blade, collect needed amount of feces from bedpan. Transfer feces to cup without touching cup's outside surface. Wash hands and place seal on cup. Transfer specimen cup into clean bag for transport to laboratory.
URINE CULTURE		
1-5 ml	Syringe and sterile cup	Place cup or tube on clean towel in client's bathroom. Use syringe to collect specimen if client has Foley catheter. Have client follow procedure to obtain clean-voided specimen (see Chapter 40) if not catheterized. Transfer urine into sterile container by injecting urine from syringe or pouring it from used container. Wash hands and secure top of labeled container. Transfer labeled specimen into clean bag for transport to laboratory.

*Agency policies may differ on type of containers, amount of specimen material required, and bagging.

If double bagging is followed, the procedure requires the nurse in the client's room to place all soiled linen into a bag and close it tightly. The nurse then places the first bag into a second bag held by a "clean nurse" or into a self-supporting hamper outside the client's room. The outer bag is specially labeled or colored. The clean nurse secures the outer bag and sends it to the laundry. The nurse should consult agency policy for the proper procedure.

Transporting Clients. Clients infected with virulent organisms should leave their rooms only for essential purposes such as diagnostic procedures or surgery. Before transferring clients to wheelchairs or stretchers, the nurse gives them clean gowns and isolation gowns to serve as robes. Clients infected by organisms transmitted via the respiratory tract must also wear masks. Personnel transporting these clients should also wear masks and gowns as needed.

At times a client being transported may drain body fluids onto a stretcher or wheelchair. When this occurs, the nurse must be sure to have the equipment disinfected after the client returns to the room. An extra layer of sheets may be used to cover the stretcher or seat of the wheelchair.

Personnel in diagnostic areas or the operating room should be notified that the client is on isolation precautions. The nurse explains ways the client can help prevent transmission of infection during transport. A client on respiratory isolation is given tissues and a bag to allow proper disposal of secretions. The nurse records the type of isolation on the client's chart.

ROLE OF THE INFECTION CONTROL NURSE. Many hospitals employ nurses who are specially trained in infection control. These nurses are responsible for advising hospital personnel on safe aseptic practices and for monitoring infection outbreaks within the hospital. Duties of an infection control nurse include the following:

1. Providing staff education on infection control
2. Reviewing infection-control policies and procedures
3. Reviewing client's medical records and laboratory reports to recommend appropriate isolation procedures
4. Screening client records for community-acquired infections
5. Consulting with employee health departments concerning recommendations to prevent and control the spread of infection among personnel such as tuberculosis testing
6. Gathering statistics regarding the **epidemiology** of nosocomial infections
7. Notifying public health department of incidences of communicable diseases
8. Conferring with all hospital departments to investigate unusual events or clusters of infection
9. Educating clients and families
10. Identifying infection-control problems with equipment
11. Checking microorganism sensitivity to antibiotics in use and reminding medical staff of resistance

An infection control nurse can be a valuable resource for controlling nosocomial infections (Rasley, 1989).

INFECTION CONTROL FOR HOSPITAL PERSONNEL. Health care workers are continually at risk for exposure to infectious microorganisms. The Occupational Safety and Health Act (OSHA) of 1991 established rules and regulations to protect employees from in-fectious hazards in the workplace (Federal Register, 1991). The OSHA guidelines are incorporated into the policies and procedures of health care institutions. Elements of the OSHA guidelines include the following:

1. Exposure-control plan. Institutions must have exposure-control plans designed to eliminate or minimize empoloyee exposure. The plan must be accessible to all employees. A list of all tasks and procedures in which an occupational exposure may occur, such as intravenous insertions, tracheal suctioning, or phlebotomy, must be provided. The plan also describes how to avoid exposure to infectious agents, such as when to use protective equipment.
2. Compliance with universal precautions. Employees are to follow universal precautions to prevent contact with blood or other infectious materials during the routine care of clients. Many institutions follow the more stringent BSI precautions. Personal protective equipment must be provided at no cost to employees who are at risk for exposure.
3. Housekeeping. Workplaces are to be maintained in a clean and sanitary condition. Routine cleaning and decontamination procedures are established, depending on surfaces to clean and the procedures performed in the work area. For example, containers of contaminated needles must be replaced regularly and not be allowed to overfill.
4. High-risk exposure. If health care workers have parenteral (needlestick) or mucous membrane exposure to blood or other infectious body fluids, the incident should be reported immediately. Evaluation and preventive treatment for hepatitis B and the HIV is critical. The staff member is screened, and appropriate therapies are provided. If a person is HIV negative, re-screening is recommended at 6 weeks, 3 months, and 6 months after exposure (CDC, 1987a, 1987b). Immunization programs are also to be made available to protect employees from becoming infected. Hepatitis B vaccinations should now be made available after the employee has received initial training. Other vaccinations may be made available by employers. For example, nurses working in obstetrical areas should be immunized against rubella to protect pregnant clients and their unborn children.
5. Training. Employers will ensure that all employees with risk of occupational exposure participate in a training program. The program will present the exposure-control plan for the insti-

tution and specifically explain the measures to be taken by employees for their safety. Written policies and guidelines must be provided for all personnel with respect to infection prevention and infection control activities (JCAHO, 1992). Training is provided at the time that an employee is assigned to an area at risk and at least annually thereafter.

CLIENT EDUCATION. Often clients must learn to use infection-control practices at home (see teaching box). Aseptic technique becomes almost second nature to the nurse who practices it daily. However, the

Client Teaching for Infection Control

OBJECTIVE

- Client will assume self-care using proper infection-control techniques.

TEACHING STRATEGIES

- Instruct client about cleaning equipment using soap and water and disinfecting with chlorine bleach solution.
- Demonstrate proper handwashing, explaining that it should be done before and after all treatments and when infected body fluids are contacted.
- Instruct client about signs and symptoms of wound infection.
- For clients who receive tube feedings at home, explain the importance of preparing enough formula for only 8 hours (commercially prepared) or 4 hours (home prepared). Tell client that contaminated enteral feeding can cause salmonellal or staphylococcal infections. Rinse feeding bag and tubing with mild soap and water daily.
- Instruct client to place contaminated dressings and other disposable items containing infectious body fluids in impervious plastic bags. Place needles in metal containers such as soda cans and tape the openings shut.
- Clean noticeably soiled linen separate from other laundry. Wash in water that is as hot as the fabric will tolerate. Add 1 cup of bleach or Lysol to detergent.

EVALUATION

- Ask client or family member to describe techniques used to reduce transmission of infection.
- Have client demonstrate select techniques.
- Ask client to explain risks for infection based on the condition.

client is less aware of factors that promote the spread of infection or ways to prevent its transmission. The home environment does not always lend itself to the practice of aseptic technique. Often a nurse must help a client improvise with the resources available to maintain hygienic techniques. One factor in a client's favor is the fact that people have a higher resistance to household bacteria than hospital bacteria. Because of this, infection-control practices in the home can be less rigorous. Clean instead of sterile technique can often be used (Roth, Land, 1987).

After clients are at home, nurses determine their compliance with infection-control practices. The nurse educates clients about infection and techniques to prevent or control its spread. Topics the nurse can discuss in a teaching session include the following:

1. Clients' susceptibility to infection
2. The chain of infection with specific reference to means of transmission
3. Hygienic practices that minimize organism growth and spread
4. Preventive health care (for example, diet, immunizations, and exercise)
5. Proper methods for handling and storage of food
6. Family members who are at risk for acquiring infections

Except for the need to administer self-injections, it is more practical for clients to learn clean, medical aseptic techniques than strict sterile techniques. Physicians try not to allow clients to return home with open wounds or conditions that require sterile procedures unless home care is available. Family members who must care for such a client, however, must be involved in the nurse's teaching plan. The nurse teaches clients and family members a commonsense approach to controlling and preventing infection.

Surgical Asepsis

Surgical asepsis or sterile technique requires a nurse to use different precautions from those of medical asepsis. Surgical asepsis requires the absence of all microorganisms, including pathogens and spores, from an object. The nurse working with a sterile field or with sterile equipment must understand that the slightest break in technique results in contamination. The nurse also practices surgical asepsis (for example, filling a syringe or changing a dressing on a wound) to keep microorganisms away from an area.

Although surgical asepsis is commonly practiced in the operating room, labor and delivery area, and major diagnostic areas, the nurse may also use surgical aseptic techniques at the client's bedside. This would include, for example, inserting intravenous or urinary catheters, suctioning the tracheobronchial airway, and reapplying sterile dressings. A nurse in an operating room follows a series of steps to maintain sterile techniques, including applying a mask, protective eyewear, and a cap; performing a surgical handwashing; and applying a sterile gown and gloves. In contrast, a nurse performing a dressing change at a client's bedside may only wash hands and apply sterile gloves. The box lists guidelines for using sterile technique.

CLIENT PREPARATION. Because surgical asepsis requires exact techniques, the nurse must have the client's cooperation. Therefore the nurse must prepare the client before any procedure. Certain clients may fear moving or touching objects during a sterile procedure, whereas others may even try to assist. The nurse explains how a procedure is to be performed and what the client can do to avoid contaminating sterile items, including the following:

1. Avoiding sudden movements of body parts covered by sterile drapes
2. Refraining from touching sterile supplies, drapes, or the nurse's gloves and gown
3. Avoiding coughing, sneezing, or talking over a sterile area

Certain sterile procedures may last a long time. The nurse must assess the client's needs and anticipate factors that may disrupt a procedure. If a client is in pain, the nurse tries to administer analgesics no more than half an hour before a sterile procedure begins. The nurse allows the client to have elimination needs met. Often clients must assume relatively uncomfortable positions during sterile procedures. The nurse helps the client assume the most comfortable position possible. Finally, the client's condition may

---

Indications for Using Sterile Technique

- During procedures that require intentional perforation of a client's skin (e.g., insertion of intravenous catheters, administration of injections)
- When the skin's integrity is broken due to trauma, surgical incision, or burns
- During procedures that involve insertion of catheters or surgical instruments into sterile body cavities

---

result in actions or events that contaminate a sterile field, such as the client with a respiratory infection who transmits organisms by coughing or breathing. The nurse anticipates such a problem and offers the client a mask.

PRINCIPLES OF SURGICAL ASEPSIS. When beginning a surgically aseptic procedure, the nurse follows certain principles to ensure maintenance of asepsis. Failure to follow each principle conscientiously endangers clients, placing them at risk for infection. The following principles are important:

1. A sterile object remains sterile only when touched by another sterile object. This principle guides the nurse in placement of sterile objects and how to handle them.
   a. Sterile touching sterile remains sterile; for example, sterile gloves are worn, or sterile forceps are used to handle objects on a sterile field.
   b. Sterile touching clean becomes contaminated; for example, if the tip of a syringe or other sterile object touches the surface of a clean disposable glove, the object is contaminated.
   c. Sterile touching contaminated becomes contaminated; for example, when the nurse touches a sterile object with an ungloved hand, the object is contaminated.
   d. Sterile touching questionable is contaminated; for example, when a tear or break in the covering of a sterile object is found, it is discarded regardless of whether the object itself appears untouched.

2. Only sterile objects may be placed on a sterile field. All items are properly sterilized before use. Sterile objects are kept in clean, dry storage areas for only a prescribed time; thereafter they are considered unsterile. Before use, all sterile packages are checked for sterilization dates or time periods on labels. The package or container holding a sterile object must be intact and dry. A package that is torn, punctured, wet, or open is unsterile.

3. A sterile object or field out of the range of vision or an object held below a person's waist is contaminated. Nurses never turn their backs on a sterile tray or leave it unattended. Contamination can occur accidentally by a dangling piece of clothing, falling hair, or an unknowing client touching a sterile object. Any object held below waist level is considered contaminated because it cannot be viewed at all times. Sterile objects should be kept in front with hands as close together as possible.

4. A sterile object or field becomes contaminated by prolonged exposure to air. The nurse avoids activities that may create air currents, such as exces-

sive movements or rearranging linen after a sterile object or field becomes exposed. When sterile packages are being opened, it is important to minimize the number of people walking into the area. Microorganisms also travel by droplet through the air. No one should talk, laugh, sneeze, or cough over a sterile field or when gathering and using sterile equipment. A nurse with a cold or other respiratory ailment should never perform sterile procedures unless a double mask is worn. Microorganisms traveling through the air can fall on sterile items or fields if the nurse reaches over the work area. When opening sterile packages, the nurse holds the item or piece of equipment as close as possible to the sterile field without touching the sterile surface. Minimal movement or rearranging of sterile items also reduces contamination by air transmission.

5. When a sterile surface comes in contact with a wet, contaminated surface, the sterile object or field becomes contaminated by capillary action. If moisture seeps through a sterile package's protective covering, microorganisms travel to the sterile object. When stored sterile packages become wet, the nurse discards the objects immediately or sends the equipment for resterilization. When working with a sterile field or tray, the nurse may have to pour sterile solutions. Any spill can be a source of contamination unless the object or field rests on a sterile surface that cannot be penetrated by moisture. Urinary catheterization trays contain sterile supplies that rest in a sterile, plastic container. In this example, sterile solutions spilled within the container will not contaminate the catheter or other objects. In contrast, if a nurse places a piece of sterile gauze in its wrapper on a client's bedside table and the table surface is wet, the gauze is considered contaminated.

6. Fluid flows in the direction of gravity. A sterile object becomes contaminated if gravity causes a contaminated liquid to flow over the object's surface. To avoid contamination during a surgical hand scrub, the nurse holds the hands above the elbows. This allows water to flow downward without contaminating the nurse's hands and fingers. The principle of water flow by gravity is also the reason for drying from fingers to elbows with hands held up, after the scrub.

7. The edges of a sterile field or container are considered to be contaminated. Frequently a nurse places sterile objects on a sterile towel or drape. Because the edge of the drape touches an unsterile surface, such as a table or bed linen, a 2.5-cm

(1-inch) border around the drape is considered contaminated. The edges of sterile containers become exposed to air after they are open and are thus contaminated. After a sterile needle is removed from its protective cap or after forceps are removed from a container, the objects must not touch the container's edge. The lip of an opened bottle of solution also becomes contaminated after it is exposed to air. When pouring a sterile liquid, the nurse first pours a small amount of solution and discards it. The solution washes away microorganisms on the bottle lip. Then the nurse pours a second time on the same side to fill a container with the desired amount of solution.

PERFORMING STERILE PROCEDURES. All the equipment that will be needed should be assembled before a procedure. Thus the nurse avoids having to leave a sterile area unattended because equipment is missing. A few extra supplies should be available in case objects accidentally become contaminated. Before the sterile procedure, each step should be explained so that the client can cooperate fully. If an object becomes contaminated during the procedure, the nurse should not hesitate to discard it immediately.

Donning and Removing Caps, Masks, and Eyewear.
For sterile procedures on a general nursing division, the nurse may wear a surgical mask and eyewear without a cap. Eyewear is worn as a part of BSI or universal precautions if there is a risk of fluid or blood splashing into the nurse's eyes. For sterile surgical procedures in the operating room, the nurse first applies a clean paper or cloth cap that covers all of the hair and then the surgical mask and eyewear.

A mask must fit snugly around the face and nose to prevent contamination by droplet nuclei. After a mask is worn for several hours, the area over the mouth and nose often becomes moist. Moisture promotes the spread of microorganisms. The nurse in the operating room must apply a second mask over the first because removing a mask in a surgical area results in immediate contamination of surrounding objects. Procedure 18-3 describes the steps for applying a mask.

Protective glasses or goggles fit snugly around the forehead and face to fully protect the eyes. Eyewear needs to be worn only for procedures that create the risk of body fluids splashing into the eyes. Before removing a mask, eyewear, and cap, the nurse removes sterile gloves to prevent contamination of the hair, neck, and facial area. After untying the mask, the nurse holds it by the ties and discards it with the cap. Eyewear is removed and cleaned later for reuse. After removing all protective wear, the nurse washes hands thoroughly.

Opening Sterile Packages. Sterile items such as syringes, gauze dressings, or catheters are packaged in paper or plastic containers impervious to microorganisms as long as they are dry and intact. Some institutions wrap reusable supplies in a double thickness of linen or muslin. Paper packages are permeable to steam and thus allow for steam autoclaving. A disadvantage of paper wrappers is that they tear or puncture relatively easily. Sterile items are kept in clean, enclosed storage cabinets and are never in the same room as dirty equipment.

Sterile supplies have dated labels or chemical tapes that indicate the date when the sterilization period expires. The tapes change color during the sterilization process. Failure of the tapes to change color means the item is not sterile. A sterile supply or piece of equipment should never be used after the expiration date. The item is either discarded or returned to the institution's supply area for resterilization.

Before opening a sterile item the nurse washes hands thoroughly. The nurse assembles the supplies in the work area such as the bedside table or treatment room before opening packages. A bedside table or counter top provides a large, clean working area for opening items. The work area should be above waist level. Sterile supplies should not be opened in a confined space where a dirty object might fall on or strike them.

OPENING A STERILE ITEM ON A FLAT SURFACE. Sterile packaged items can be opened without contaminating the contents. Commercially packaged items

are usually designed so that the nurse only has to tear away or separate the paper or plastic cover. The item is held in one hand while the wrapper is pulled away with the other (Fig. 18-4). Care is then taken to keep the inner contents sterile before use. When opening items packed in linen, the nurse uses the following steps:

1. Place the item flat in the center of the work surface.
2. Remove the tape or seal indicating the sterilization date.
3. Grasp the outer surface of the tip of the outermost flap.
4. Open the outer flap away from the body, keeping the arm outstretched and away from the sterile field (Fig. 18-5, *A* on p. 438).
5. Grasp the outside surface of the first side flap.
6. Open the side flap, allowing it to lie flat on the table surface. Keep the arm to the side and not over the sterile surface (Fig. 18-5, *B*). Do not allow flaps to spring back over the sterile contents.
7. Grasp the outside surface of the second side flap and allow it to lie flat on table surface (Fig. 18-5, *C*).
8. Grasp the outside surface of the last and innermost flap.
9. Stand away from the sterile package and pull the flap back, allowing it to fall flat on the surface (Fig. 18-5, *D*).
10. Use the inner surface of the linen package (except for the 1-inch border around the edges) as a sterile field to add additional sterile items. The 1-inch border can be grasped to maneuver the field on the table surface.

If the sterile supplies are not to be used immediately, the nurse can close the sterile package. In this case the nurse should touch only the wrapper's outside surface. To close a package the order of unwrapping is reversed and the nurse does not touch the inside contents or reach over the field.

OPENING A STERILE ITEM WHILE HOLDING IT. To open small, sterile items, the package is held in the nondominant hand while the top flap is opened and pulled away from the nurse. Using the dominant hand the nurse carefully opens the sides and top flaps away from the enclosed sterile item in the same order previously mentioned. The nurse opens items in a hand so that the item can be handed to a person wearing sterile gloves or transferred to a sterile field.

Preparing a Sterile Field. When performing sterile procedures, the nurse needs a sterile work area that provides room for handling and placing of sterile

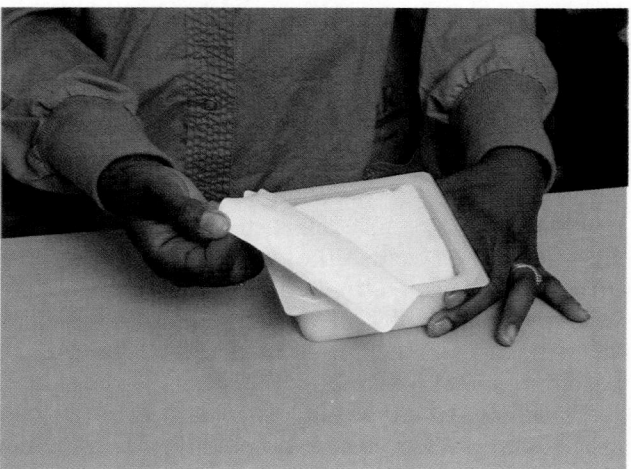

Fig. 18-4 When opening a commercially packaged sterile item, the nurse tears the wrapper away from the body.

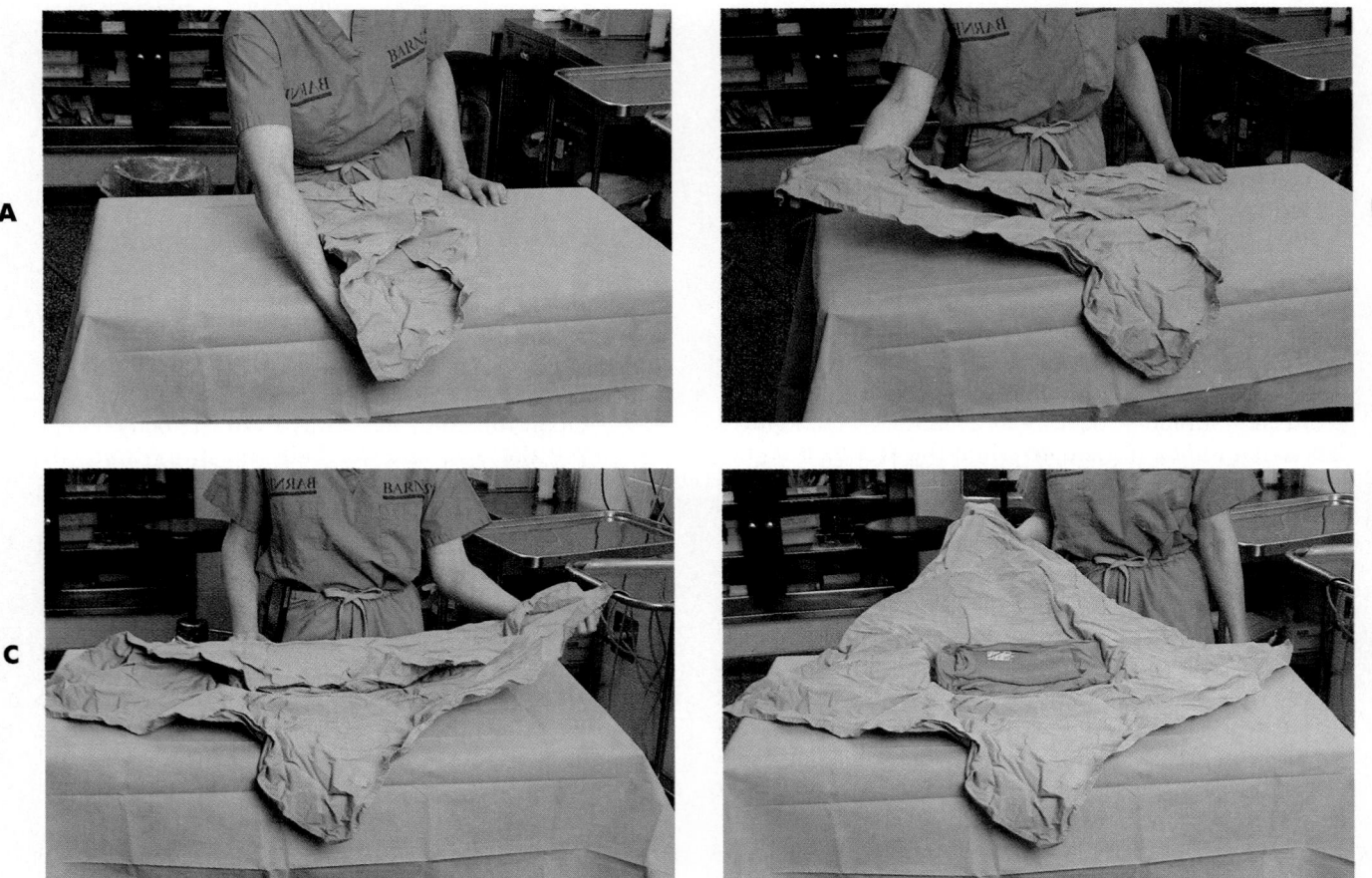

Fig. 18-5   Opening sterile packaged items on a flat surface. **A,** Nurse opens the top flap away from the body. **B,** The nurse's arm is kept out, away from the sterile field while opening a side flap. **C,** The second side flap is opened. **D,** The back flap is opened.

items. A **sterile field** is an area free of microorganisms and prepared to receive sterile items. The field may be prepared by using the inner surface of a sterile wrapper as the work surface or by using a sterile drape. Procedure 18-4 describes preparation of a sterile field. After the surface for the field is created, the nurse adds sterile items by placing them directly on the field or by transferring them with a sterile forceps. When transferring sterile items, the nurse must carefully place objects onto the sterile field. An object that comes in contact within the 1-inch border must be discarded.

The nurse may choose to wear sterile gloves while preparing items on the field. If this is done, the nurse can touch the entire drape, but sterile items must be handed over by an assistant. The nurse's gloves cannot touch the wrappers of sterile items.

Pouring Sterile Solutions. Often the nurse must pour sterile solutions into sterile containers. A bottle containing a sterile solution is sterile on the inside

and contaminated on the outside; the bottle's neck is also contaminated, but the inside of the bottle cap is considered sterile. After a cap or lid is opened, it is held in the hand or placed sterile side (inside) up on a clean surface. This means that the inside of the lid can be seen as it rests on the table surface. A bottle cap or lid should never rest sterile side down on a sterile surface because the outer edge of the cap is unsterile and would contaminate the surface. Likewise, placing a sterile cap down on an unsterile surface increases the chances of the inside of the cap becoming contaminated.

The bottle should be held with its label in the palm of the hand to prevent the possibility of the solution wetting and fading the label. Before pouring the solution into the container, the nurse pours a small amount (1 to 2 ml) into a disposable cap or plastic-lined waste receptacle. The discarded solution cleans the lip of the bottle. The edge of the bottle is kept away from the edge or inside of the receiving con-

STEPS

1. Prepare sterile field just before planned procedure. Supplies are to be used immediately.
2. Select clean work surface above waist level.
3. Assemble necessary equipment:
   a. Sterile drape
   b. Assorted sterile supplies
4. Check dates or labels on supplies for sterility of equipment.
5. Wash hands thoroughly.
6. Place pack containing sterile drape on work surface and open as described on p. 438.
7. With fingertips of one hand, pick up folded top edge of sterile drape (see illustration).
8. Gently lift drape up from its outer cover and let it unfold by itself without touching any object. Discard outer cover with your other hand.
9. With other hand, grasp adjacent corner of drape and hold it straight up and away from your body.
10. Holding drape, first position the bottom half over intended work surface (see illustration).
11. Allow top half of drape to be placed over work surface last (see illustration).

ADDING STERILE ITEMS

12. Open sterile item (following package directions) while holding outside wrapper in nondominant hand.
13. Carefully peel wrapper onto nondominant hand.
14. Being sure wrapper does not fall down on sterile field, place item onto field at angle. Do not hold arm over sterile field (see illustration on p. 440).

RATIONALE

Prevents exposure of sterile field and supplies to air and contamination.

Sterile object held below waist is contaminated.

Preparation of equipment in advance prevents break in technique.

Equipment stored beyond expiration date is considered unsterile.

Prevents transmission of infection.

Ensures sterility of packaged drape.

One-inch border around drape is unsterile and may be touched.

If sterile object touches any other nonsterile object, it becomes contaminated.

Drape can now be properly placed while using two hands. Drape must be held away from unsterile surfaces.

Prevents nurse from reaching over sterile field.

Creates flat, sterile work surface.

Frees dominant hand for unwrapping outer wrapper.

Item remains sterile. Inner surface of wrapper covers hand, making it sterile.

Prevents reaching over field and contaminating its surface.

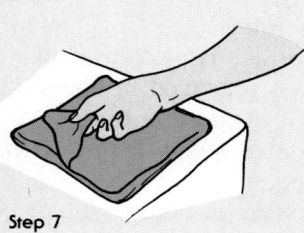

Step 7

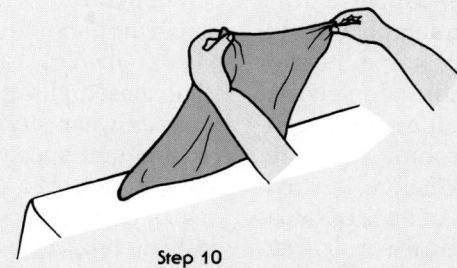

Step 10

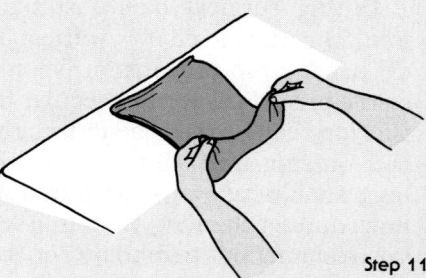

Step 11

Preparing a Sterile Field

STEPS	RATIONALE
15. Dispose of outer wrapper (see illustration).	Prevents accidental contamination of sterile field.
16. Perform procedure using sterile technique.	Prevents transmission of infection to client.

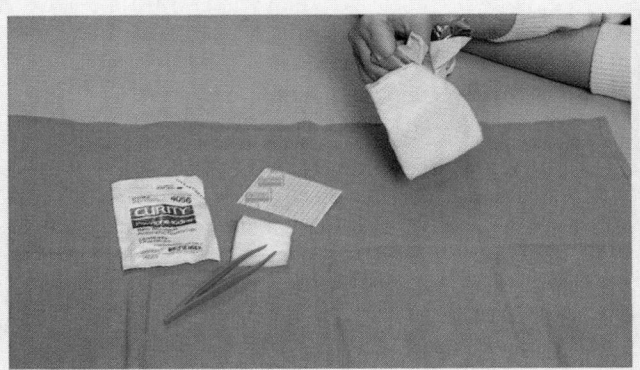

Step 14

tainer. The nurse pours the solution slowly to avoid splashing the underlying drape or field. The bottle should never be held so high above the container that even slow pouring will cause splashing. The bottle should be held outside the edge of the sterile field.

Surgical Handwashing. Clients who undergo operative procedures are at high risk for infection because of open operative wounds. Nurses working in the operating room perform surgical handwashing to decrease microorganisms and suppress their growth to avoid microbial contamination of operative wounds.

During surgical handwashing the nurse scrubs from fingertips to elbows with an antimicrobial surgical hand scrub preparation before each operation or sterile procedure. (NOTE: Regular handwashing is satisfactory before routine sterile procedures on a general nursing unit). Surgical handwashing or scrubbing should take at least 5 minutes before the first procedure of the day (Garner, 1985). The CDC does not recommend a duration for surgical scrubs performed between procedures. However, 2 to 5 minutes is probably acceptable (check agency policies). For maximum elimination of bacteria, the nurse removes all jewelry and keeps fingernails short, clean, and free of polish. Artificial nails should not be worn

because water can easily become trapped between the actual and artificial nail, promoting fungal growth. Staff who have active skin infections should be excluded from the surgical team. Brushes are used during scrubbing. Some experts caution that too much brushing removes outer layers of the epidermis, thereby exposing bacterial flora in the deeper skin layers. Procedure 18-5 describes the steps of the surgical handwashing procedure.

Applying Sterile Gloves. Sterile gloves are an additional barrier to bacterial transfer. There are two gloving methods: open and closed. Nurses who work on general nursing divisions use open gloving before procedures such as dressing changes (see Chapter 48) or urinary catheter insertions (see Chapter 40). The closed gloved method, which is performed when nurses wear sterile gowns, is practiced in operating rooms and special treatment areas. Procedures 18-6 on pp. 443-444 and 18-7 on p. 445-448 review the steps of each gloving technique.

The proper glove size should be selected; the glove should not stretch so tightly that it can easily tear; yet it should be tight enough that objects can be picked up easily.

Donning a Sterile Gown. Nurses must wear sterile gowns in the operating room and delivery

Text continued on p. 448.

STEPS	RATIONALE
1. Remove all jewelry. Ensure that fingernails are short and free of polish and that cuticles are in good condition.	Minimizes number of resident and transient microorganisms.
2. Use deep sink with foot pedals or knee controls for dispensing soap and controlling water temperature and flow.	Minimizes risk of hands and lower arms touching dirty surface.
3. Use appropriate antimicrobial agent such as CHG or iodophor.	Broad-spectrum antimicrobial agents maximally reduce number of microorganisms on hands.
4. Have two disposable hand brushes and disposable nail file available.	Brushes are used to enhance mechanical friction during handwashing.
5. Apply cap, covering hair completely. Contain pierced earrings within cap.	Microorganisms reside on hair. Hair and earrings would act as foreign bodies if allowed to enter operative wound.
6. Apply face mask, making certain to cover nose and mouth snugly.	Mask prevents escape of microorganisms into air, which can contaminate hands.

HANDWASHING

7. Adjust water flow to lukewarm temperature.	Hot water removes protective oils from skin and increases sensitivity to soap.
8. Wet hands and forearms liberally, keeping arms and hands above elbow level during entire procedure. NOTE: Scrub dress or uniform must be kept dry.	Water runs by gravity from fingertips to elbows. Hands become cleanest part of upper extremity. Keeping hands elevated allows water to flow from least to most contaminated area.
9. Dispense liberal amounts of soap (2 to 5 ml) into hands and lather hands and arms to 5 cm (2 in) above elbows.	Washing wide area reduces risk of contaminating overlying gown that is later applied.

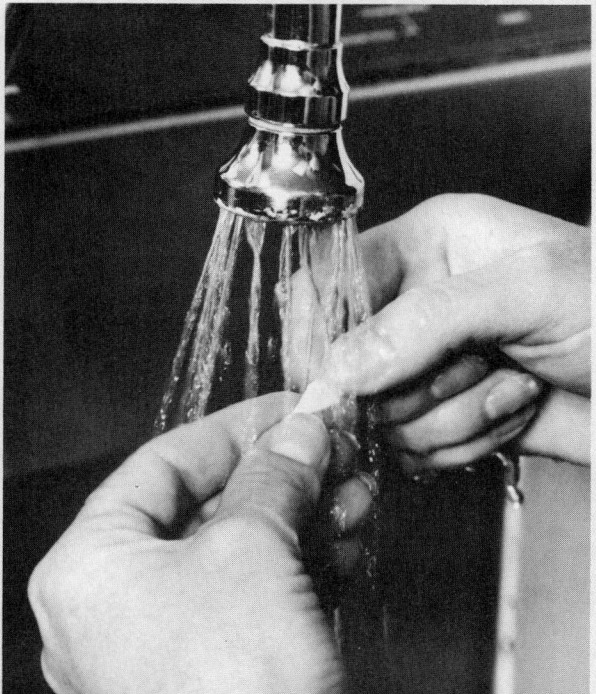

Step 10

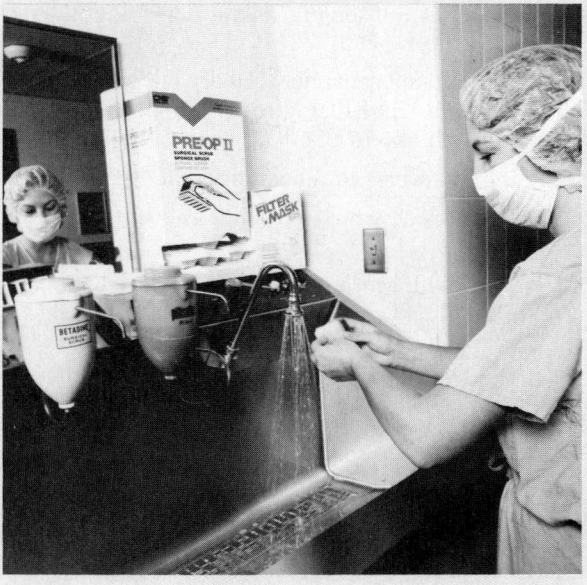

Step 11

Surgical Handwashing:
Preparing for Gowning

STEPS	RATIONALE
10. Clean nails with file under running water (see illustration). Discard file.	Removes dirt and organic material that harbor large numbers of microorganisms.
11. Wet brush and apply antimicrobial soap. Scrub fingernails, hand, arm in following manner (see illustration on p. 441):	Loosens resident bacteria that adhere to skin's surface. Methodical scrub covers all skin surfaces.
a. Scrub nails of hand 15 strokes.	
b. Using circular motion, scrub palm of hand and anterior surface of fingers 10 strokes.	
c. Scrub side of thumb 10 strokes and posterior aspect of thumb 10 strokes.	
d. Scrub sides and back of each finger 10 strokes each area.	
e. Scrub back of hand 10 strokes.	
12. Rinse brush thoroughly. Reapply soap.	Rinsing of brush removes microorganisms and avoids contamination of arms.
13. Mentally divide arms into thirds. Scrub each surface of lower forearm with circular motion for 10 strokes; scrub middle and upper forearm in same manner. Discard brush.	Removes microorganisms over wide area.
14. With arms flexed, rinse thoroughly from fingertips to elbow in one motion, allowing water to run off at elbow (see illustration).	Allows water to flow from least to most contaminated area.
15. Repeat Steps 11 through 14 for second arm.	
16. Keeping arms flexed, discard brush. Turn off water with foot pedal. Proceed to operating room.	After touching skin, brush is contaminated. Rinsing removes resident bacteria.
17. Pick up sterile towel found on top of sterile gown pack. Be sure no one is within arm's reach.	Dry from cleanest to least clean area. Drying prevents chapping, facilitates application of gloves, and prevents contamination of gown.
18. Open towel full length, holding one side away from scrub attire.	Avoids contact with microorganisms on scrub gown.
19. Dry each hand separately. To dry one arm, hold towel in opposite hand; using rotating motion, draw towel from fingers up to elbow.	Drying hands first prevents contaminating hands from areas proximal to elbows.
20. Carefully reverse towel and dry other hand and arm.	
21. Discard towel, which prevents accidental contamination.	
22. Proceed with sterile gowning (see Procedure 18-7).	

Step 14

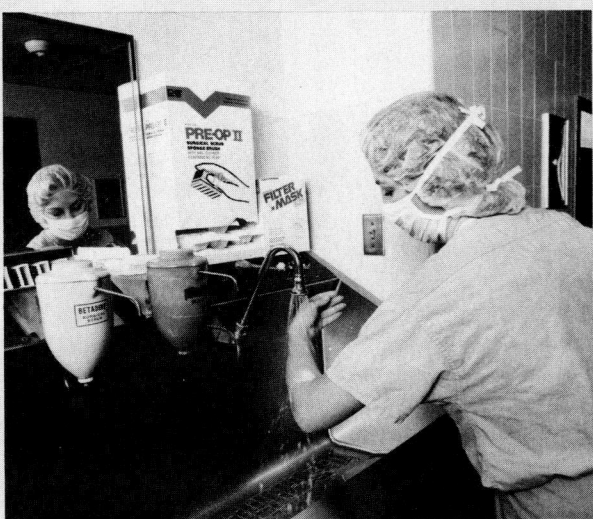

STEPS	RATIONALE
1. Have package of proper-sized sterile gloves at treatment area.	
2. Perform thorough handwashing.	Removes bacteria from skin surfaces and reduces transmission of infection.
3. Remove outer glove package wrapper by carefully separating and peeling apart sides.	Prevents inner glove package from accidentally opening and touching contaminated objects.
4. Grasp inner package and lay it on clean, flat surface just above waist level. Open package, keeping gloves on wrapper's inside surface.	Sterile object held below waist is contaminated. Inner surface of glove package is sterile.
5. If gloves are not prepowdered, take packet of powder and apply lightly to hands over sink or wastebasket.	Powder allows gloves to slip on easily. (Some staff members do not use powder for fear of promoting growth of microorganisms.)
6. Identify right and left glove. Each glove has cuff approximately 5 cm (2 in) wide. Glove dominant hand first.	Proper identification of gloves prevents contamination by improper fit. Gloving of dominant hand first improves dexterity.
7. With thumb and first two fingers of nondominant hand, grasp edge of cuff of glove for dominant hand. Touch only glove's inside surface (see illustration).	Inner edge of cuff will lie against skin and thus is not sterile.
8. Carefully pull glove over dominant hand, leaving cuff and being sure cuff does not roll up wrist. Be sure thumb and fingers are in proper spaces (see illustration).	If glove's outer surface touches hand or wrist, it is contaminated.
9. With gloved dominant hand, slip fingers underneath second glove's cuff (see illustration on p. 444).	Cuff protects gloved fingers. Sterile touching sterile prevents glove contamination.
10. Carefully pull second glove over nondominant hand. Do not allow fingers and thumb of gloved dominant hand to touch any part of exposed nondominant hand. Keep thumb of dominant hand abducted back (see illustration).	Contact of gloved hand with exposed hand results in contamination.

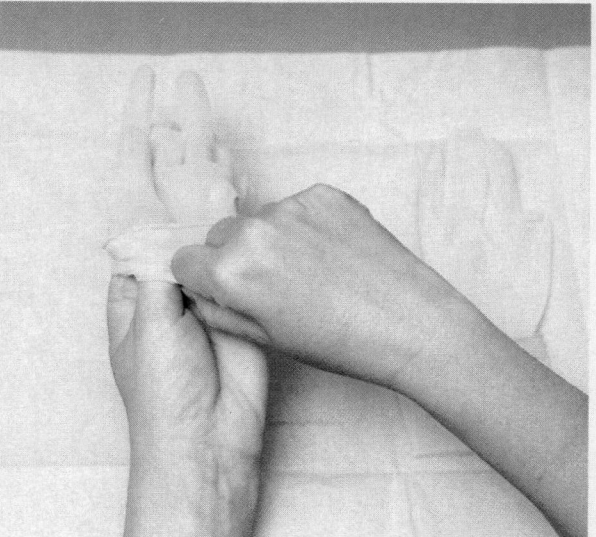

Step 7

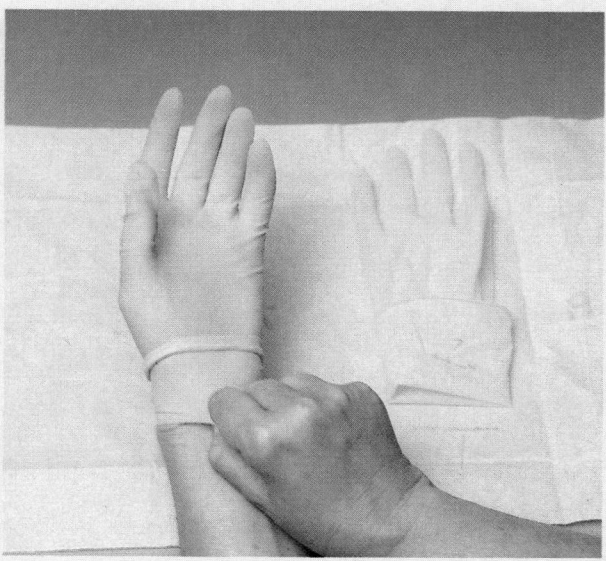

Step 8

Performing Open Gloving

STEPS	RATIONALE
11. After second glove is on, interlock hands together. The cuffs usually fall down after application. Be sure to touch only sterile sides (see illustration on p. 444).	Ensures smooth fit over fingers.

GLOVE DISPOSAL

STEPS	RATIONALE
12. Grasp outside of one cuff with other gloved hand; avoid touching wrist.	Minimizes contamination of underlying skin.
13. Pull glove off, turning it inside out (see Procedure 18-2, Step 13a). Discard in receptacle.	Outside of glove does not touch skin surface.
14. Take fingers of bare hand and tuck inside remaining glove cuff. Peel glove off, inside out (see Procedure 18-2, Step 13a). Discard in receptacle.	

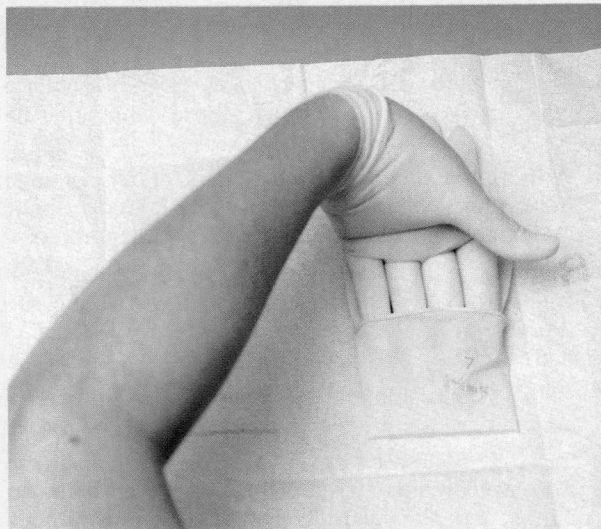

Step 9

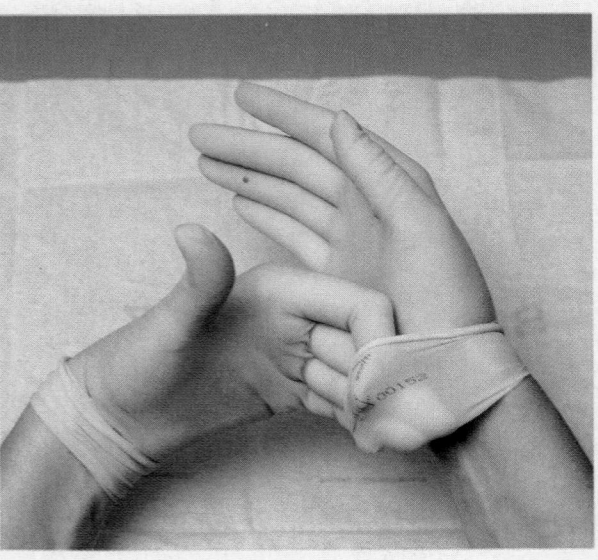

Step 10

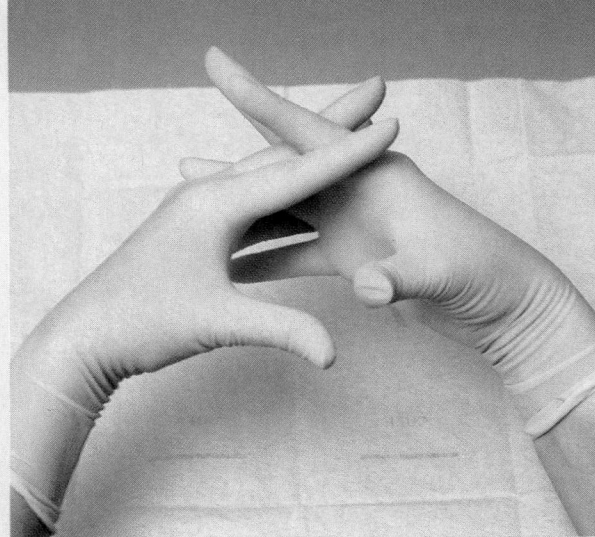

Step 11

STEPS	RATIONALE
GOWNING	
1. Before entering operating room or treatment area, apply cap and face mask. Foot covers are also required in operating room.	Prevents hair and air droplet nuclei from contaminating sterile work areas. Foot covers are paper or cloth and fit over work shoes.
2. Perform thorough surgical handwash (see Procedure 18-5).	Removes transient and resident bacteria from fingers, hands, forearms.
3. Ask circulating nurse to assist by opening sterile pack containing sterile gown (folded inside out).	Gown's outer surface remains sterile.
4. Have circulating nurse prepare glove package by peeling outer wrapper open while keeping inner contents sterile. Inner glove package is then placed on sterile field created by sterile outer wrapper.	Keeps gloves sterile and allows nurse who has scrubbed to handle sterile items.
5. Reach down to sterile gown package; lift folded gown directly upward and step back away from table (see illustrations).	Provides wide margin of safety, avoiding contamination of gown.
6. Holding folded gown, locate neckband. With both hands, grasp inside front of gown just below neckband.	Clean hands may touch inside of gown without contaminating outer surface.

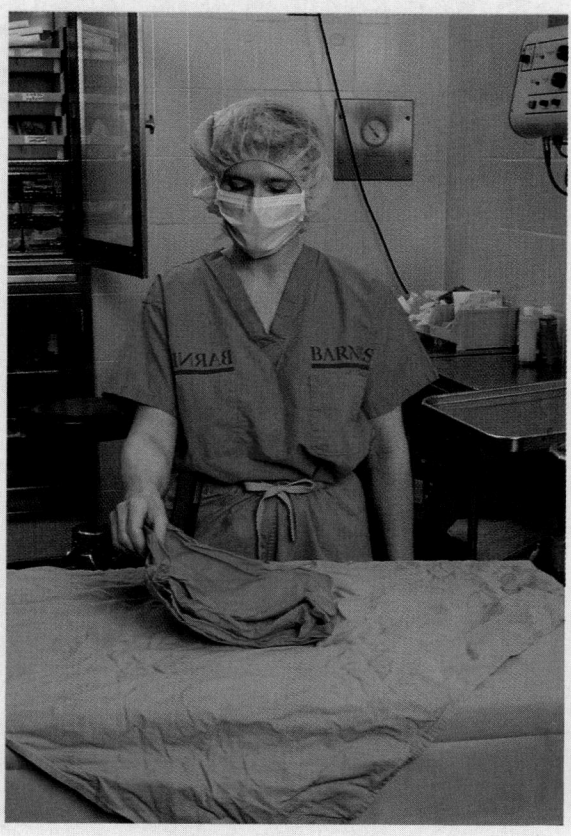

Step 5

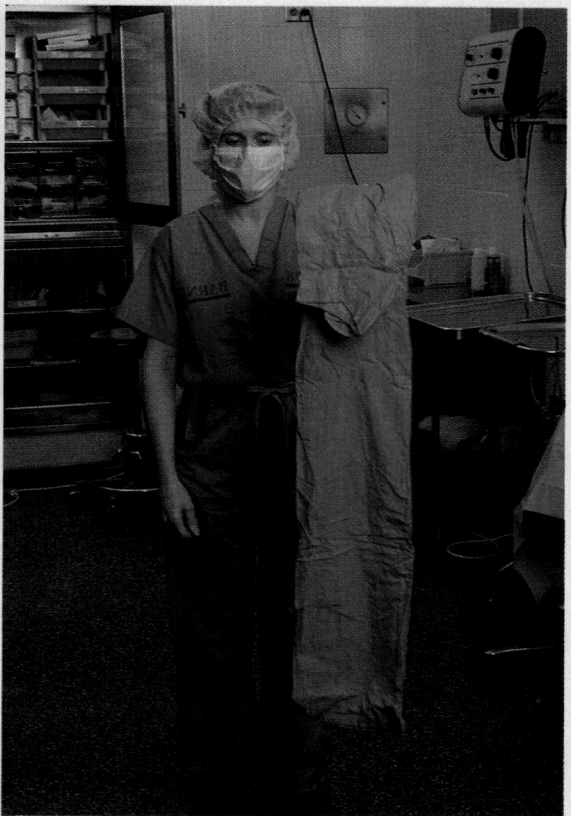

Step 5

Applying a Sterile Gown and Performing Closed Gloving

STEPS	RATIONALE
7. Allow gown to unfold, keeping inside of gown toward body. Do not touch outside of gown with bare hands (see illustration).	Outside of gown will be sterile surface.
8. With hands at shoulder level, slip both arms into armholes simultaneously (see illustration). Ask circulating nurse to bring gown over shoulders by reaching inside to arm seams. Gown is pulled on, leaving sleeves covering hands (see illustrations).	Careful application prevents contamination. Gown covers hands to prepare for closed gloving.
9. Have circulating nurse securely tie back of gown at neck and waist. (If gown is a wraparound style, sterile flap to cover gown is not touched until the nurse has gloved).	Gown must completely enclose underlying garments.

CLOSED GLOVING

10. With hands covered by gown sleeves, open inner sterile glove package.	Hands remain clean. Sterile gown cuff will touch sterile glove surface.
11. With nondominant hand inside gown cuff, pick up glove for the dominant hand by grasping folded cuff.	Sterile gown touches sterile glove.

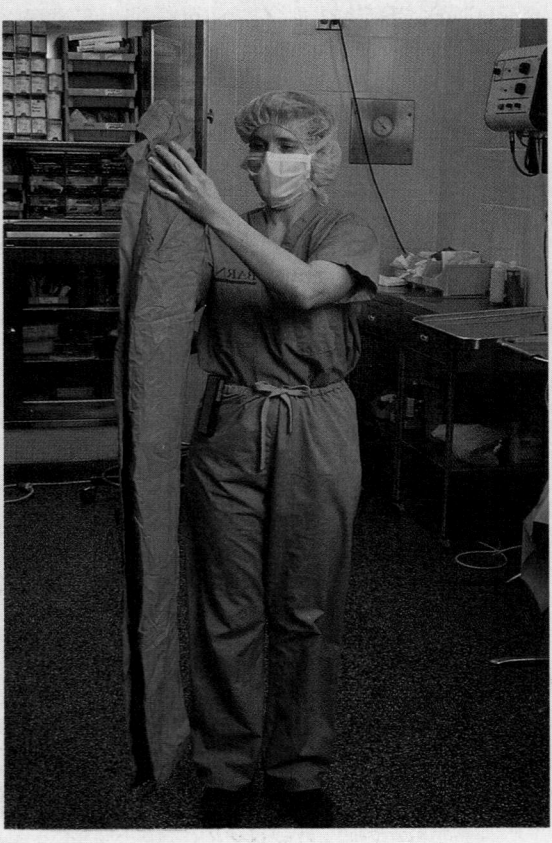

Step 7

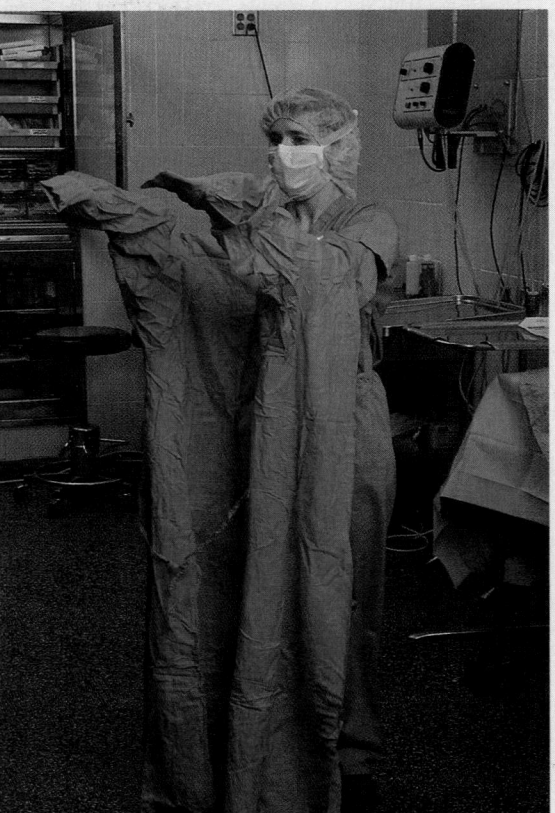

Step 8

STEPS	RATIONALE
12. Extend dominent forearm with palm up and place palm of glove against palm of dominant hand. Glove fingers will point toward elbow.	Positions glove for application over cuffed hand, keeping glove sterile.
13. Grasp back of glove cuff with nondominant hand and turn glove cuff over end of dominant hand and gown cuff (see illustration).	
14. Grasp top of glove and underlying gown sleeve with covered nondominant hand. Carefully extend fingers into glove, being sure glove's cuff covers gown's cuff.	Seal created by glove cuff over gown prevents exit of microorganisms over operative sterile field.
15. Glove nondominant hand in same manner, reversing hands (see illustration). Use gloved right hand to pull on glove. Keep hand inside sleeve (see illustration on p. 448).	Sterile touches sterile.
16. Be sure fingers are fully extended into both gloves.	Ensures that nurse has full dexterity while using gloved hand.

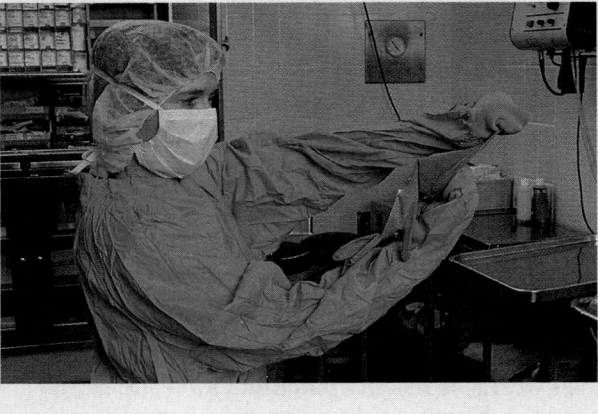

Step 13

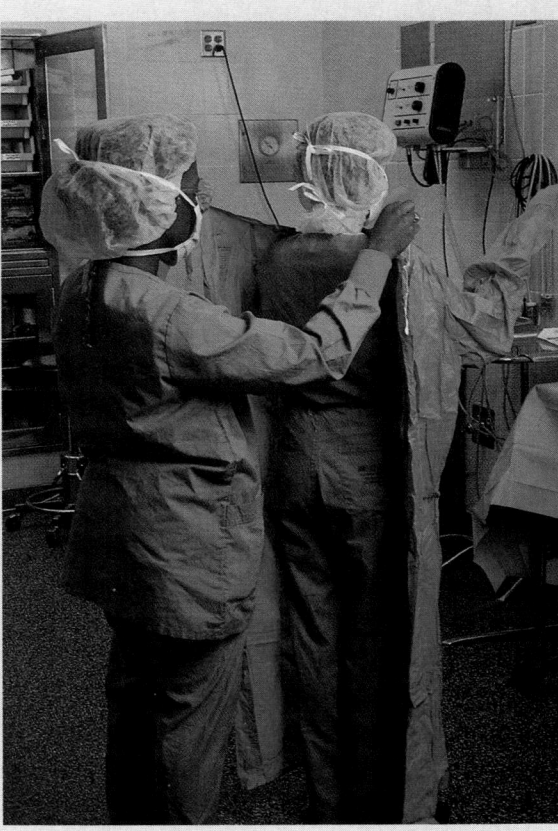

Step 8

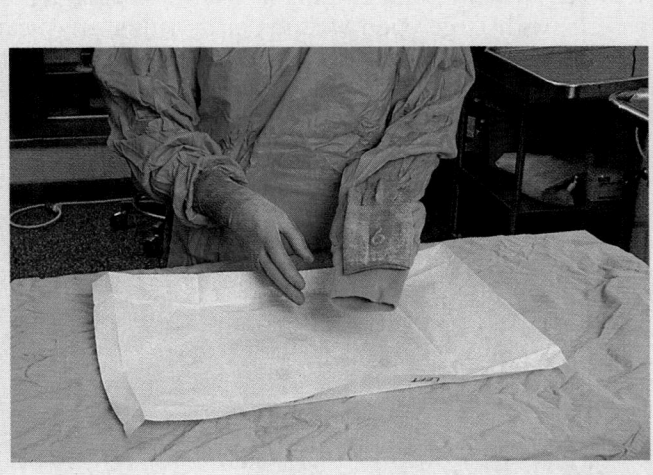

Step 15

CONTINUED

Applying a Sterile Gown and Performing Closed Gloving

STEPS	RATIONALE
17. For wraparound sterile gowns: take gloved hand and release fastener or ties in front of gown.	Front of gown is sterile.
18. Hand tie to sterile team member who stands still. Allowing margin of safety, turn around to the left, covering back with extended gown flap. Take back tie from team member and secure tie to gown.	Contact with team member could contaminate gown and gloves. Gown must be enclosed undergarments.

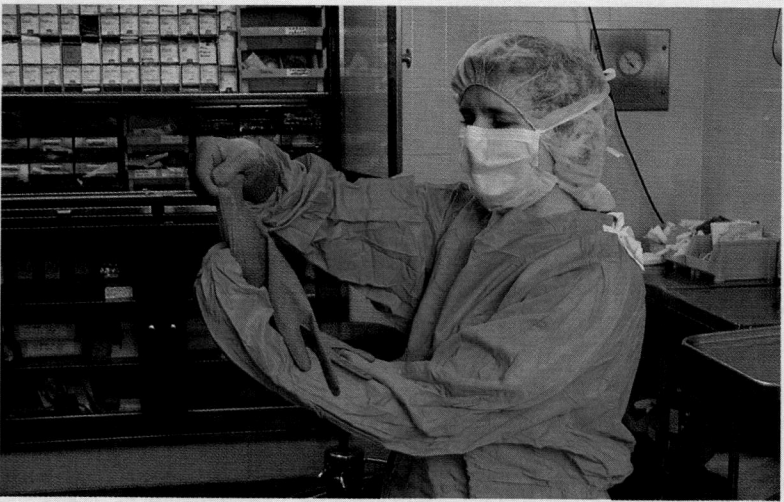

Step 15

room so that sterile objects can be comfortably handled with less risk of contamination. The sterile gown acts as a barrier to decrease shedding of microorganisms from skin surfaces into the air and thus prevents wound contamination. Nurses caring for clients with large open wounds or assisting physicians during major invasive procedures (for example, inserting an arterial catheter) may also wear sterile gowns.

Nurses do not apply sterile gowns until after applying masks and surgical caps and performing surgical handwashing. Nurses pick up the gown from sterile packs or have gowned assistants hand them the gowns. Only a certain portion of the gown—the area from the anterior waist to but not including the collar and the anterior surface of the sleeves—is considered sterile. The back of the gown, the area under the arms, the collar, the area below the waist, and the underside of the sleeves are not sterile because the nurse cannot keep these areas in constant view and ensure their sterility. Procedure 18-7 reviews the steps for applying a gown.

Sample Evaluation for High Risk for Infection

Goals	Evaluative Measures	Expected Outcomes
Client will remain free of nosocomial infection.	Inspect intravenous puncture site for erythema, swelling, purulent drainage. Palpate site for tenderness.	Invasive needle site will not become infected.
	Measure client's body temperature.	Client's condition will remain afebrile.
	Review laboratory test results.	WBC count will remain normal.
Client will practice infection-control techniques at home.	Ask client to describe basic infection control measures used in the home.	Client will identify examples of infection control (e.g., hand-washing before meal preparation) appropriate to home.
	Observe client performing medical aseptic procedures.	Client will correctly perform procedures such as dressing change and self-administration of injections.

 Evaluation

The success of the nurse who practices infection-control techniques is measured by determining whether the goals for reducing or preventing infection are achieved. A comparison of the client's response, such as absence of fever or development of wound drainage, with expected outcomes determines the success of nursing interventions. Similarly, a de-termination is made about whether interventions should be revised or eliminated. The ability to correctly assess wounds for healing (see Chapter 48) and conduct a physical assessment of body systems (see Chapter 20) are important skills in evaluation. The nurse closely monitors clients, especially those at risk, for signs and symptoms of infection. The evaluation box describes criteria used in evaluating the effects of infection-control techniques.

The client at risk for infection must understand the measures needed to reduce or prevent microorganism growth and spread. Providing clients or family members the opportunity to discuss infection-control measures or to demonstrate procedures will reveal their ability to comply with therapy. The nurse may determine that clients require new information or that previously instructed information needs reinforcement.

The nurse documents the client's response to therapies for infection control. A clear description of any signs and symptoms of systemic or local infection is necessary to give all nurses a baseline for comparative evaluation. The efficacy of any intervention in reducing infection must also be reported.

 ## SUMMARY

In every aspect of practice the nurse encounters situations that present a risk of an infection developing or being transmitted. Knowledge of the body's normal defenses against infection helps the nurse recognize clients most at risk for acquiring infections. The nature of the infection chain is a useful concept in identifying nursing interventions for infection control.

Nurses use two types of infection-control practices, medical and surgical asepsis, to prevent infection transmission. Each set of practices calls for a conscientious and knowledgeable application of infection-control principles. The nurse's failure to follow these principles seriously hampers recovery or maintenance of good health.

CHAPTER 18 REVIEW

Key Concepts

- Handwashing is the most important technique in preventing and controlling transmission of infection.

- The potential for microorganisms to cause disease depends on number of organisms, virulence, ability to enter and survive in a host, and susceptibility of the host.

- Normal body flora resist infection by releasing antibacterial substances and inhibiting multiplication of pathogenic microorganisms.

- The signs of local inflammation and infection are identical.

- Immunity to infection is a biological response that changes the body's response to future exposure to antigens.

- An infection can develop as long as the six elements composing the infection chain are uninterrupted.

- Microorganisms are transmitted by direct and indirect contact, by airborne spread, and by vectors and contaminated vehicles.

- Increasing age, poor nutrition, stress, inherited conditions, chronic disease, and treatments or conditions that compromise the immune response increase susceptibility to infection.

- The major sites for nosocomial infections include the urinary and respiratory tracts, bloodstream, and surgical or traumatic wounds.

- Invasive procedures, medical therapies, long hospitalization, and contact with health care personnel increase a hospitalized client's risk for acquiring a nosocomial infection.

- Clients within an intensive care unit have a higher risk for infection than clients who are not in this area.

- Isolation practices prevent personnel and clients from acquiring infections and prevent transmission of microorganisms to other persons.

- Body substance isolation uses generic infection-control precautions for all clients.

- Proper cleansing requires mechanical removal of all foreign material from an object or area.

- Universal blood and body fluid precautions serve to prevent the spread of the HIV virus and other blood-borne pathogens.

- A client in isolation is subject to sensory deprivation because of the restricted environment.

- An infection-control nurse monitors the incidence of infections within an institution and provides educational and consultative services to maintain aseptic practices.

- Surgical asepsis requires more stringent techniques than medical asepsis and is directed at eliminating microorganisms.

- If the skin is broken or if the nurse performs an invasive procedure into a body cavity normally free of microorganisms, surgical aseptic practices are followed.

Key Terms

Aerobic, p. 400

Anaerobic, p. 400

Antibodies, p. 406

Antigen, p. 405

Asepsis, p. 407

Asymptomatic, p. 398

Bacteriocidal, p. 400

Bacteriostasis, p. 400

Body substance isolation (BSI), p. 421

Broad-spectrum antibiotics, p. 403

Carriers, p. 399

Category-specific isolation, p. 422

Colonized, p. 421

Communicable, p. 398

Complement, p. 406

Cytolysis, p. 406

Disease-specific isolation, p. 421

Disinfection, p. 415

Edema, p. 403

Endogenous infection, p. 406

Epidemiology, p. 433

Exogenous infection, p. 406

Exudate, p. 404

Germicide, p. 415

Granulation tissue, p. 405

Handwashing, p. 417

Iatrogenic infections, p. 406

Immune responses, p. 405

Immunocompromised, p. 398

Immunoglobulins, p. 406

Inflammatory response, p. 402

Interferon, p. 406

Invasive, p. 398

Leukocytosis, p. 403

Localized, p. 402

Lymphokines, p. 405

Medical asepsis, p. 407

Microorganisms, p. 398

Natural immunity, p. 406

Necrotic, p. 403

Nosocomial infections, p. 406

Passive immunity, p. 406

Pathogenicity, p. 402

Pathogens, p. 398

Phagocytosis, p. 403

Purulent, p. 400

Sanguineous, p. 404

Serous, p. 404

Sterile field, p. 438

Sterilization, p. 415

Stop-sign isolation, p. 421

Surgical asepsis, p. 407

Susceptibility, p. 402

Systemic, p. 402

Universal blood and body fluid precautions, p. 422

Virulence, p. 398

451

Critical Thinking Exercises

1. It is a busy day on 6300, a general surgery nursing unit. Joe Thomas, RN, enters Mr. Willis' room to administer his 8 AM dose of antibiotic. The physician has ordered a blood test on Mr. Willis, so Joe obtains a blood specimen. While in the room, Joe also prepares the bath water for Mr. Willis to begin morning hygiene. Joe next visits Ms. Marshall, who underwent colon surgery. Her dressing shows drainage, so Joe removes the soiled gauze and applies a new dressing. While in the room, Joe measures Ms. Marshall's temperature. Finally, Joe is called to check Mr. Skiles, who requests a pain medication. Joe prepares an injection and administers it to Mr. Skiles. Which of the activities in the above clinical situation required Joe to use clean, disposable gloves? Which activities required Joe to use sterile gloves?

2. The infection chain consists of six elements. Identify the elements of the infection chain created by the introduction of an intravenous catheter into a client. Explain the risks to the client and nurse.

3. Mrs. Lacson became ill suddenly with fever, chills, and malaise. Her doctor diagnosed viral flu. Describe the phase of the immune response in which the viral cells are attacked by the body.

4. Mrs. Niles is 83 years old and lives alone. She has difficulty walking and relies on a church volunteer group to deliver lunches during the week. Her fixed income limits her ability to buy food. Last week, Mrs. Niles' 79-year-old sister died. The two sisters had been very close. As a home health care nurse, explain the factors that might increase Mrs. Niles' risk for infection.

5. The cleansing of client care equipment breaks which element of the infection chain?

REFERENCES

Centers for Disease Control: Recommendations for prevention of HIV transmission in health care settings, *MMWR* 36:55, 1987a.

Centers for Disease Control: Recommendations for prevention of HIV transmission in health care settings, *MMWR* 36(suppl 25):15, 1987 b.

Centers for Disease Control: Update: universal precautions for prevention of transmission of human immunodeficiency virus, hepatitis B virus, and other bloodborne pathogens in health care settings, *MMWR* 37(24):377, 1988.

Classen DC et al: Prevention of catheter-associated bacteriuria: clinical trial of methods to block three known pathways of infection, *Am J Infect Control* 19(3):136, 1991.

Crow S: Asepsis: an indispensable part of the patient's care plan, *Crit Care Nurs Q* 11(4):11, 1989.

Dickerson M: Protecting yourself from AIDS: infection control measures, *Crit Care Nurse* 9(10)26, 1989.

Federal Register, 58(235):64175-64182, Dec 6, 1991.

Finkelstein MS et al: Pneumococcal bacteremia in adults: age-dependent differences in presentation and outcome, *J Am Geriatr Soc* 31:19, 1983.

Garner JS: *Guidelines for prevention of surgical wound infections*, Bethesda, Md, 1985, Hospital Infections Program, Centers for Disease Control, Public Health Services, and US Department of Health and Human Services.

Garner JS, Favero MS: *Guidelines for handwashing and hospital environmental control*, Bethesda, Md, 1985, Hospital Infections Program, Centers for Disease Control, Public Health Service, and US Department of Health and Human Services.

Garner JS, Simmons BP: CDC guidelines for the prevention and control of nosocomial infections: guidelines for isolation precautions in hospitals, *Am J Infect Control* 12:103, 1984.

Hood LE: Interferon, *Am J Nurs* 87:459, 1987.

Jacobson G et al: Handwashing: ring-wearing and number of microorganisms, *Nurs Res* 34:186, 1985.

Joint Commission on Accreditation of Healthcare Organizations: *Accreditation Manual for Hospitals,* Oakbrook Terrace, Ill, 1992, The Commission.

Kim MJ, McFarland GK, McLane AM: *Pocket guide to nursing diagnoses,* ed 4, St Louis, 1991, Mosby–Year Book.

Korniewicz DM et al: Integrity of vinyl and latex procedure gloves, *Nurs Res* 38(3):144, 1989.

Larson EL: Effects of handwashing agent, handwashing frequency, and clinical area on hand flora, *Am J Infect Control* 12:76, 1984.

Larson EL: Handwashing: it's essential even when you use gloves, *Am J Nurs* 89:934, 1989.

Larson EL et al: Physiological and microbiologic changes in skin related to frequent handwashing, *Infect Control* 7:59, 1986.

Larson EL et al: Quantity of soap as a variable in handwashing, *Infect Control* 8:371, 1987.

Lynch P, Jackson MM: Isolation practices: how much is too much or not enough? *Asepsis* 10(3):12, 1988.

Lynch P et al: Implementing and evaluating a system of generic infection precautions: body substance isolation, *Am J Infect Control* 18(1):1, 1990.

Maki DG, Ringer M: Evaluation of dressing regimens for prevention of infection with peripheral intravenous catheters, *JAMA* 258(17):2396, 1987.

Maki DG, Alvarado C, Hassemer C: Double-bagging of items from isolation rooms is unnecessary as an infection control measure: a comparative study of surface contamination with single and double-bagging, *Infect Control* 7(11):535, 1986.

McGinley KJ et al: Composition and density of micro flora in the subungual space of the hand, *J Clin Microbiol* 26:950, 1988.

Nightingale F: *Notes on nursing: what it is and what it is not,* London, 1859, Harrison.

Rasely DA: Surveillance of nosocomial infections, *Crit Care Nurs Q* 11(4):75, 1989.

Roth MK, Land GK: How to prevent infection in a home care patient, *RN* 50:61, 1987.

Rutala WA: Draft guidelines for selection and use of disinfectants, *Am J Infect Control* 17(1):24A, 1989.

Spaulding EH: Chemical disinfection of medical and surgical materials. In Lawrence CA, Block SS, editors: *Disinfection, sterilization, and preservation,* Philadelphia, 1968, Lea & Febiger.

Tideiksaar R: Infections in the elderly. I. Diagnosis and treatment, *Physician Assist* 11(2):17, 1987.

Weinstein SA et al: Bacterial surface contamination of patient's linen: isolation precautions versus standard care, *Am J Infect Control* 17(5):264, 1989.

Williams WW: CDC guidelines for infection control in hospital personnel, *Infect Control* 4(4):325, 1983.

ADDITIONAL READINGS

Aiken LH: AIDS: the health policy context, *Fam Community Health* 12(2):1, 1989.

Association of Operating Room Nurses: *Standards and recommended practices for perioperative nursing: recommended practices for surgical scrubs,* Denver, 1991, The Association.

Atkinson LJ, Kohn ML: *Berry and Kohn's introduction to operating room technique,* New York, 1986, McGraw-Hill.

Banick B: Light at the end of a decade, *AJN* 90:37, 1990.

Choudhuri M et al: Efficiency of skin sterilization for a venipuncture with the use of commercially available alcohol or iodine pads, *Am J Infect Control* 18(2):82, 1990.

Department of Labor: Joint advisory notice: Department of Labor and Department of Health and Human Services, *HBV/HIV* Oct 30, 1987, p 52.

Ebersole P, Hess P: *Toward healthy aging,* ed 3, St Louis, 1990, Mosby–Year Book.

Forrester DA: AIDS-related risk factors, medical diagnosis, do-not-resuscitate orders and aggressiveness of nursing care, *Nurs Res* 39(6):350, 1990.

Gross PA et al: Nosocomial infection: decade-specific risk, *Infect Control* 4(3):145, 1983.

Hamory B: Nosocomial sepsis related to intravascular access, *Crit Care Nurs Q* 11(4): 58, 1989.

Health Services and Promotion Branch: *Infection control guidelines for isolation precautions,* 1990, Ottawa, Deptartment of National Health and Welfare.

Jackson M et al: *The body substance isolation system, infection prevention and control manual,* San Diego, 1987, University of California, San Diego Medical Center.

Jaffe HW: The acquired immunodeficiency syndrome epidemic: issues for health care professionals, *Am J Infect Control* 14:272, 1986.

McCrary E, Martone WJ: Preventing HIV exposure among patients and staff, *AIDS Patient Care* 1:32, 1987.

MMWR update: Universal precautions for prevention of transmission of HIV, Hepatitis B virus and other bloodborne pathogens in health care settings, *MMWR* 37(24):378, 1988.

Pagana KD, Pagana TJ: *Diagnostic testing and nursing implications,* ed 3, St Louis, 1990, Mosby–Year Book.

Simmons BP: Guidelines for prevention of surgical wound infections, *Am J Infect Control* 11(4):133, 1983.

Thibodeau GA, Patton K: *Anatomy and physiology,* ed 2, St Louis, 1993, Mosby–Year Book.

Vital Signs

OBJECTIVES

Mastery of content in this chapter will enable the student to:

- Define the key terms listed.
- Identify when vital signs should be taken.
- Explain the principles and mechanisms of thermoregulation.
- Discuss the rationale for a care plan for a client with a fever.
- Identify steps used to assess oral, rectal, axillary, and tympanic membrane temperature.
- Explain the physiology for the normal regulation of temperature, blood pressure, pulse, and respirations.
- Describe the types of factors that normally cause variations in body temperature, pulse, respirations, and blood pressure.
- Identify steps used to assess pulse, respirations, and blood pressure.
- Identify normal vital sign values for an adult and an infant.
- Explain variations in technique used to assess an infant's and a child's vital signs.
- Describe the benefits and precautions involving self-measurement of blood pressure.
- Accurately record and report vital sign measurements.

CHAPTER OUTLINE

ital signs—temperature, pulse, respirations, and blood pressure—are indicators of health status. Many factors such as the temperature of the environment, physical activity, and the effects of illness cause vital signs to change, sometimes beyond a normal range. Measurement of vital signs provides data that can be used to determine a client's usual state of health (baseline data), as well as the response to physical and psychological stress and medical and nursing therapy. An alteration from normal may signal the need for medical or nursing intervention.

When a client comes to a health care agency or is seen by a nurse in the home, measurement of vital signs is a routine part of the complete physical assessment (see Chapter 20). Vital signs may also be measured separately as a part of a review of the client's condition. Vital signs are a quick and efficient way of monitoring a condition or identifying the presence of problems. The basic skills required to measure vital signs are simple but should not be taken for granted. Vital signs and other physiological measurements can be the basis for clinical problem solving. Careful technique ensures accurate findings.

GUIDELINES FOR TAKING VITAL SIGNS

Vital signs are a part of the data base that a nurse collects during assessment. The box is a reference for normal values in the adult client. The process of taking vital signs is not routine but is individualized to the client's needs and condition. The nurse must be able to measure vital signs correctly, understand and interpret the values, communicate findings appropriately, and begin interventions as needed. The nurse's judgment helps determine the need for and frequency of vital sign measurement. The following guidelines help the nurse incorporate vital sign measurement into nursing practice:

1. The nurse caring for the client measures vital signs. Throughout a shift, the nurse makes observations of the client's condition. Vital signs give important information about the client's state of health. The nurse who provides care for a client is ideally the one to take vital signs, interpret their significance, and make decisions about care.

2. Equipment is functional and appropriate. Equipment used to measure vital signs (for example, a thermometer or stethoscope) must work properly to ensure accurate findings.

3. The nurse knows the normal range for all vital signs. This knowledge helps the nurse detect abnormalities.

4. The nurse knows the client's normal range of vital signs. A client's normal values may differ from the standard range for that age or physical state. These values serve as a baseline for comparison with findings taken later. Thus a nurse can detect a change in condition over time.

5. The nurse knows the client's medical history and therapies or medications prescribed. Some illnesses or treatments cause predictable vital sign changes.

6. The nurse controls or minimizes environmental factors that may affect vital signs. Measuring a pulse after the client exercises or experiences an emotional upset or checking temperature in a warm, humid room may yield values that are not true indicators of the client's condition.

7. The nurse uses an organized, systematic approach when taking vital signs. For example, many nurses measure temperature first. When using a glass thermometer, the nurse can measure the temperature while checking pulse, respirations, and blood pressure.

8. The nurse and physician decide the frequency of vital sign assessment on the basis of the client's condition. In the hospital the physician orders a

---

Vital Signs: Normal Ranges for Adults

TEMPERATURE

Oral: $C = 37^0$, $F = 98.6^0$ (Range $\pm 1^0$ F)
Rectal: $C = 37.6^0$, $F = 99.6^0$
Axilla: $C = 36.4^0$, $F = 97.6^0$

PULSE

55 - 100 beats/min

RESPRIATIONS

12 - 20 breaths/min

BLOOD PRESSURE

Average: 120/80 mm Hg
Hypertension: Systolic above 140 mm Hg
                        Diastolic above 90 mm Hg
Hypotension: Systolic below 90 mm Hg with
   signs of dizziness and increased pulse
Orthostatic hypotension: Fall in systolic blood pressure of 25 mm Hg systolic and 10 mm Hg diastolic accompanied by signs and symptoms of inadequate cerebral perfusion when arising from lying position to sitting or standing position

minimum frequency of measurement for each client. After a client returns from surgery or a major diagnostic examination such as cardiac catheterization, frequent measurements are taken until the vital signs stabilize to the normal range before the procedure. The nurse may judge whether more frequent assessments are needed. If a client's physical condition begins to worsen, the nurse takes vital signs more often, perhaps as often as every 5 to 10 minutes. For example, the client may experience severe bleeding after cardiac catheterization, and the nurse may monitor vital signs every 5 minutes while applying pressure at the site to prevent hemorrhage. Taking vital signs as a basis for determining changes and trends is useful in making therapeutic decisions.

9. The nurse analyzes the results of vital sign measurement. The nurse is often in the best position to assess all of the clinical findings about a client. Vital signs are not assessed in isolation. The nurse must also know other physical signs or symptoms and be aware of the client's ongoing health status. Vital signs are just a part of the assessment of the client's physical and psychological condition.

10. The nurse verifies and communicates significant changes in vital signs. Baseline measurements allow a nurse to identify changes in vital signs. When vital signs reach an abnormal range, it may help to have another nurse or a physician repeat a measurement to verify it. The nurse reports abnormal vital signs to the physician. The nurse must also record and report any changes to the nurses working the next shift (see Chapter 22).

Vital signs are physiological data that assist the nurse in performing routine care measures and critical interventions. For example, to determine whether a client tolerates exercise, the nurse may assess pulse rate before and during exercise. When a client experiences excessive blood loss after injury or surgery, blood pressure measurement can reveal the seriousness of the hemorrhage. Continued blood pressure checks help determine when the nurse should administer fluids or medications to restore blood pressure to normal. The box provides information about when to assess vital signs.

BODY TEMPERATURE

Physiology

Temperature is the "hotness" or "coldness" of a substance. The body's temperature remains within a relatively narrow range for optimal function. A person's body temperature remains relatively stable despite internal extremes (for example, metabolic changes) or external conditions (for example, climatic temperature). Temperature-control mechanisms keep the body's **core temperature** (temperature of deep tissues) in a relatively constant range, 37° C (98.6° F) ± 1° C. The body's surface temperature rises and falls with the temperature of the environment. Layers of skin, subcutaneous tissues, and fat may fluctuate between 20° and 40° C (68° and 104° F) without damage.

A thermometer registers the body's core temperature. In clinical practice, nurses learn the normal temperature range of individuals. No single temperature is normal for all people. The temperature range for a normal, active adult is higher than might be expected (Fig. 19-1 on p. 458), depending in part on the person's range of activity. When the body's core temperature rises above normal, **hyperthermia** occurs. When the body's core temperature falls below normal, **hypothermia** occurs.

Regulation

The balance of body temperature is precisely regulated by physiological and behavioral mechanisms. For the body temperature to stay constant, heat produced in the body must equal heat lost to the environment. A nurse applies knowledge of temperature-control mechanisms to promote temperature regulation.

When to Take Vital Signs

- On the client's admission to a health care facility
- In a hospital on a routine schedule according to a physician's order or hospital policy
- Before and after a surgical procedure
- Before and after an invasive diagnostic procedure
- Before and after the administration of certain medications that affect cardiovascular, respiratory, and temperature-control functions
- When the client's general physical condition changes (as with loss of consciousness or increased intensity of pain)
- Before and after nursing interventions influencing a vital sign (such as when a client previously on bed rest ambulates or when a client requires tracheal suctioning)
- When the client reports nonspecific symptoms of physical distress (such as feeling "funny" or "different")

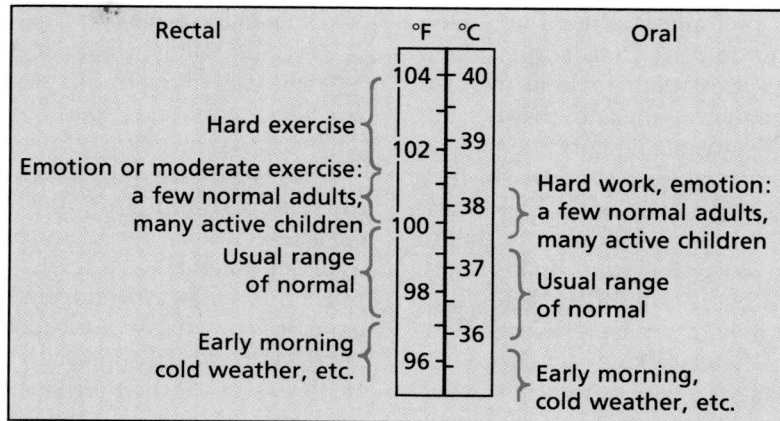

Fig. 19-1   Ranges of rectal and oral temperatures found in normal persons.
Redrawn from Mountcastle VB: *Medical physiology,* vol 2, ed 14, St Louis, 1980, Mosby–Year Book based on Dubois EF: *Fever and the regulation of body temperature,* Springfield, Ill, 1948, Charles C Thomas.

Neural Control

The hypothalamus in the brain controls body temperature the same way that a thermostat works in the home. A comfortable temperature is the "set point" at which a heating system operates. In the home a fall in environmental temperature activates the furnace, whereas a rise in temperature shuts the system down. The hypothalamus senses minor changes in body temperature. When body temperature deviates from the set point, the temperaure center of the hypothalamus activates heat loss (cooling) or heat production so that the core temperature stays in a safe physiological range.

When nerve cells in the hypothalamus become heated, impulses are sent out to reduce body temperature (Fig. 19-2). The body cools itself by sweating, **vasodilation** (widening of blood vessels), and inhibition of heat production. If the hypothalamus senses that the body's temperature is too low, signals are sent out to increase heat production and conservation through **vasoconstriction** (narrowing of blood vessels), muscle shivering, and **piloerection** (erection of hairs). Lesions or trauma to the hypothalamus or spinal cord, which carries hypothalamic messages, can cause serious alterations in temperature control.

HEAT PRODUCTION. Heat is produced in the body by metabolism, which is the chemical reaction in all body cells. Food is the primary fuel source for metabolism. Although heat production increases when a person is active, it is a constant process. Most heat comes from the body's core during quiet times and rest. During work, the main site of heat production is the muscles. Table 19-1 reviews the sources and mechanisms of heat production.

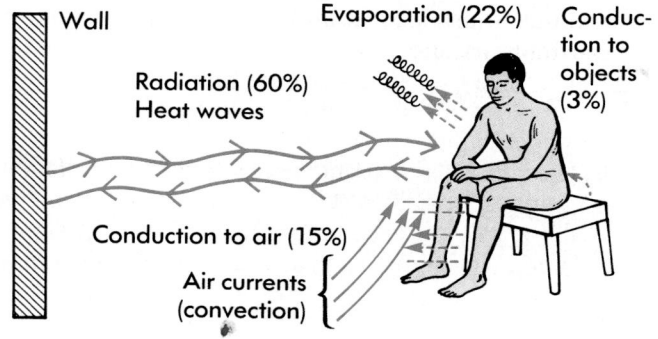

Fig. 19-2   Mechanisms of heat loss from the body.
From Guyton AC: *Textbook of medical physiology,* ed 8, Philadelphia, 1991, Saunders.

Skin in Temperature Regulation

The skin's roles in temperature regulation include insulation of the body, vasoconstriction (which affects the amount of blood flow and heat loss to the skin), and temperature sensation. The skin, subcutaneous tissue, and fat keep heat inside the body. When blood flow between skin layers is reduced, the skin alone is an excellent insulator. Persons with more body fat have more natural insulation than slim and muscular people.

The way that the skin controls body temperature is similar to the way that an automobile radiator controls engine temperature. The engine of an automobile generates a great deal of heat. Water is pumped through the engine's system to collect the heat and carry it to the radiator, where a fan transfers the heat from the water to the outside air. The engine's temperature thus stays within safe limits to prevent dam-

TABLE 19-1 Sources and Mechanisms of Heat Production	
Mechanism	Nursing Implications

METABOLISM

Basal metabolic rate (BMR) is smallest amount of energy expenditure needed to sustain life and maintain normal body temperature in comfortable, warm environment. BMR is measure of kilocalories of energy expended per hour per square meter of surface area. The BMR constitutes 55% to 60% of total metabolic rate, or amount of energy used or expended by the body at any time.

Food intake and exercise influence metabolic rate.
Seriously ill clients benefit from increased calorie intake and reduced activity so that energy is available for healing and vital functions.

MUSCLE ACTIVITY

As exercise levels increase, amount of muscular work increases. Energy of muscular work comes from breakdown of carbohydrates and fats. Even minor muscular activity such as bathing can raise metabolic rate and therefore heat production.

Clients whose energy reserves are minimal and whose body temperatures are already elevated can suffer increased temperature from any physical exertion.

Shivering of skeletal muscles increases heat production.
Maximal shivering can increase heat production 4 to 5 times greater than normal.*

Nurses may give medications that reduce shivering to prevent rise in fever and metabolic rate.

When body temperature becomes too low, tone of all skeletal muscles increases.

Extra clothing or bed coverings are applied to prevent or reduce shivering.

THYROID HORMONES

Thyroxine and triiodothyronine increase basal metabolism by breaking down glucose and fat. Anterior pituitary gland releases thyroid-stimulating hormone (TSH) according to metabolic demands. Both thyroid hormones must be present for maintenance of normal BMR. Deficient thyroid secretion slows metabolism. Excessive thyroid secretion increases metabolism.

Clients with thyroid disorders may have intolerances to heat or cold. Clients with thyroid hormone deficiencies exhibit decreased energy levels.

SYMPATHETIC STIMULATION

Norepinephrine and epinephrine stimulate sympathetic nervous system to increase metabolism when blood glucose levels drop. This results in glycogen metabolism, which makes glucose available to cells for energy.

For ill clients, nutritional maintenance prevents depletion of energy stores and supports normal temperature.

*Data from Guyton AC: *Textbook of medical physiology*, ed 8, Philadelphia, 1991, Saunders.

age from overheating. In the human body the internal organs produce sweat, and during exercise or increased sympathetic stimulation, the amount of heat produced is greater than the normal core temperature. Blood flows from the internal organs, carrying heat to the body surface. The skin is well supplied with blood vessels. In the most exposed areas of the body—the hands, feet, and ears—blood can flow directly from arteries to veins. Blood flow through the more vascular areas of the skin may vary from minimal flow to as much as 30% of the blood ejected from the heart (Guyton, 1991). Heat transfers from the blood, through vessel walls, and to the skin's surface and is lost to the environment through heat-loss mechanisms. The body's core temperature remains within safe limits.

The degree of vasoconstriction determines the amount of blood flow and heat loss to the skin. If the core temperature is too high, the hypothalamus inhibits vasoconstriction. As a result, blood vessels dilate, and more blood reaches the skin's surface. On a hot, humid day the blood vessels in the hands are dilated and easily visible. In contrast, if the core temperature becomes too low, the hypothalamus initiates vasoconstriction and blood flow to the skin lessens. Thus body heat is conserved.

The skin is well supplied with heat and cold receptors. Because cold receptors are more plentiful, however, the skin functions primarily to detect cold surface temperatures. When the skin becomes chilled, its sensors send information to the hypothalamus, which initiates shivering to increase body heat production, inhibition of sweating, and vasoconstriction.

Heat Loss

As the body produces heat, it also loses heat. The skin's structure and exposure to the environment result in constant, normal heat loss through radiation, conduction, convection, and evaporation.

RADIATION. Radiation is the transfer of heat from the surface of one object to the surface of another without actual contact between the two (Thibodeau, Patton, 1993). Heat radiates from the skin to nearby objects that are cooler and radiates to the skin from warmer objects. The amount of heat lost by radiation from the skin varies according to dilation of surface blood vessels when the body is overheated and by vasoconstriction when the body is chilled.

Heat loss through radiation can be reduced by covering the body with clothing, especially dark, closely woven clothes. Radiant heat loss can be enhanced by removing clothing or by wearing light clothing that facilitates heat loss. Body positioning also affects heat loss through radiation. Because of the amount of exposed surface area, a person standing with arms and legs extended radiates more heat than a person lying down in a fetal position.

CONDUCTION. Conduction is the transfer of heat to any object or surface in contact with the body. Conduction accounts for a small amount of heat loss. Heat conducts through solids, gases, and liquids.

When a person sits on a chair, there is heat conduction until the chair's surface temperature begins to rise. When the temperature of the skin and chair temperature are the same, conductive heat loss stops. If the air next to the skin is cooler than the skin's surface, the body's heat warms the air. Wearing several layers of clothing creates layers of warmed air surrounding the body, which keeps a person warm and reduces conductive heat loss. In the client with an elevated temperature, a cooling blanket placed on the bed produces continuous conductive heat loss as the skin tries to equalize temperature with the blanket.

Water conducts heat more than air does. For example, the client exposed to water at 32.2° C (90° F) will lose far more heat than the client exposed to air at 32.2° C (90° F). Thus water used to bathe clients should be above body temperature to prevent conductive heat loss. However, if the client's temperature is abnormally high, the nurse can lower a fever by bathing the person in tepid water that is below body temperature. Conductive heat loss from the body will occur.

CONVECTION. Convection is the transfer of heat away from a surface, such as the skin, by movement of heated air or fluid particles (Thibodeau, Patton, 1993). Normally a warm layer of air exists close to the skin's surface. Heated air rises from the skin and passes to cooler air by convection currents, causing a minimal amount of heat loss from the skin.

As the speed of movement of air surrounding the skin increases, the convection of heat loss from the skin increases. Normally, convective heat loss is minimal, but it can be artificially enhanced by the use of fans to promote heat loss. To help prevent heat-related illnesses, fans may be useful for clients who live in warm climates without air conditioning.

EVAPORATION. Heat energy is needed to change water from a liquid to a gas. For each gram of water that evaporates from the body surface, approximately 0.6 kilocalorie (kcal) of heat is lost (Mountcastle, 1980). The body always loses some heat and water by evaporation. This occurs from the continuous loss of insensible water from the skin and lungs. About 600 ml of moisture that evaporates daily from breathing and skin functions is considered **insensible water loss**. The drying effect from evaporation can cause skin scaling and itching, as well as drying of the nares and pharynx. An average adult may lose 280 to 390 kcal per day from evaporation by insensible loss. However, insensible loss occurs regardless of body temperature and thus plays no major role in temperature regulation.

However, **diaphoresis** (sweating) controls body temperature through evaporative heat loss. Millions of sweat glands lie deep below the dermal layer of the skin. The glands secrete sweat, a watery solution containing sodium and chloride, which passes through tiny ducts on the skin's surface. The glands are controlled by the sympathetic nervous system. When the body's temperature rises, sweat glands release sweat, which evaporates from the skin's surface to promote heat loss. Exercise causes a significant rise in body temperature to stimulate diaphoresis. Emotional or mental stress causes diaphoresis through sympathetic stimulation. When temperatures are cold, sweat gland secretion is inhibited, and body temperature is conserved. Diaphoresis is less efficient when air movement is minimal or when the humidity of the air is high. People who have a congenital absence of sweat glands or who have a serious skin disease that impairs diaphoresis are unable to tolerate warm temperatures because they cannot cool themselves adequately.

Behavioral Control

Behavioral regulation involves the voluntary acts that persons take to maintain comfortable body temperatures. Humans alter their behavior when exposed to temperature extremes. The ability of people to control body temperature depends on the degree of temperature extreme, the ability to sense feeling comfortable or uncomfortable, and thought processes or emotions. When the temperature in the environment falls, people can add clothing, move to warmer places, raise the temperature settings on furnace thermostats, increase muscular activity by running in place, or sit with arms and legs tightly wrapped together. In contrast, when the temperature becomes hot, individuals can remove clothing, stop activity, lower temperature settings on air conditioners, turn on fans, seek cooler places, or take cool showers or baths.

Persons with altered temperature-control mechanisms, such as infants or older adults, have difficulty with maintaining body temperature. These persons may need assistance in changing their environments so that their exposure to temperature extremes is limited. Individuals who are ill or who have injuries that lower consciousness or cause impairment in thought processes may also be unable to recognize the need to change behavior for temperature control. When temperatures become extremely hot or cold, behavioral modifications have a limited effect on controlling temperature loss or gain.

Factors Affecting Body Temperature

To assess temperature variations and evaluate the significance of changes from normal, the nurse must be aware of several factors that affect body temperature.

Age

At birth the newborn leaves a warm, relatively constant environment and enters one in which temperatures fluctuate widely. Temperature-control mechanisms are not fully developed; thus an infant's temperature may change drastically with changes in the environment. Extra care is therefore needed to protect the newborn. Clothing must be adequate, and exposure to temperature extremes must be avoided. A newborn loses up to 30% of body heat through the head and therefore needs to wear a cap at first to prevent heat loss. When protected from environmental extremes, the newborn's body temperature is main-

tained within 35.5° to 37.5° C (96° to 99.5° F). Heat production steadily declines as the infant grows into childhood. Individual differences of 0.25° to 0.55°C (0.5° to 1° F) are normal (Whaley, Wong, 1991).

Temperature regulation is unstable until children reach puberty. The normal temperature range gradually drops as individuals approach older adulthood. Oral temperatures of 35° C (95° F) are not unusual for older adults in cold weather. However, the average body temperature of older adults is approximately 36° C (96.8° F). Older adults are particularly sensitive to temperature extremes because of deterioration in thermoregulation, including poor vasomotor control (control of vasoconstriction and vasodilation), reduced amounts of subcutaneous tissue, reduced sweat gland activity, and reduced metabolism. Some of these clients are especially at risk for hypothermia, in which body temperature falls below 94° F. This drop may occur when environmental temperatures fall if older adults are not physically active or are unable to heat their homes adequately.

Exercise

Muscle activity requires an increased blood supply and an increase in carbohydrate and fat breakdown for more energy. This increased metabolism causes an increase in heat production. Any form of exercise can increase heat production and thus body temperature. After prolonged exercise, such as long-distance running, body temperatures may temporarily reach levels as high as 39° to 41° C (103.2° to 105.8° F) (Petersdorf, 1980).

Hormone Level

Women generally experience greater fluctuations in body temperature than men. Hormonal variations during the menstrual cycle cause body temperature fluctuations. Progesterone levels rise and fall cyclically during the menstrual cycle. Before this cycle, progesterone levels are low, and the body temperature falls a few tenths of a degree below the baseline level. The lower temperature persists until ovulation occurs. During ovulation, greater amounts of progesterone enter the circulatory system and raise the body temperature to previous baseline levels or higher. Plotting temperature variations during the menstrual cycle to determine when ovulation occurs and avoiding sexual intercourse during ovulation is a form of birth control. These temperature variations can be used to predict a woman's most fertile time to achieve pregnancy.

Body temperature changes also occur in women during menopause (cessation of menstruation). Women who have stopped menstruating may experience periods of intense body heat and sweating lasting from 30 seconds to 5 minutes. This is due to the instability of the vasomotor controls for vasodilation and vasoconstriction (Bobak, Jensen, Zalar, 1989).

The amount of thyroxine, triiodothyronine, epinephrine, and norepinephrine circulating in the body also affect heat production and the basal metabolic rate. These are listed in Table 19-1.

Circadian Rhythms

Body temperatures normally change 0.5° to 1° C (0.9° to 1.8° F) during a 24-hour period. However, temperature is one of the most stable rhythms in humans. The temperature is usually lowest between 1 and 4 AM (Fig. 19-3). During the day, body temperature rises steadily, until about 6 PM, and then declines to early morning levels. At one time, daily temperature variations were believed to be a result of greater daytime activity. However, temperature patterns are not automatically reversed in people who work during the night and sleep during the day. It takes 1 to 3 weeks for the cycle to reverse. Each client has a different temperature pattern, which the nurse must assess to identify a change in health.

Stress

Physical and emotional stress increase body temperature through hormonal and neural stimulation. The client may experience an increased heart or respiratory rate or increased diaphoresis. These physiological changes increase metabolism, which increases heat production. The client who is anxious about entering a hospital or a physician's office may register a higher-than-normal temperature. The nurse can obtain a more accurate temperature reading by waiting until the emotional stress subsides.

Environment

Environment influences body temperature. If temperature is assessed in a very warm room, a client may be unable to conduct heat away, and the body temperature will be elevated. If the client has just been outside in the cold without warm clothing, body temperature may be low because of extensive radiant and conductive heat loss. Shivering to raise body temperature would be observed. Infants and older adults are most likely to be affected by environmental temperatures because their temperature-regulating mechanisms are less efficient.

Fever

The simplest definition of a **fever** is a rectal temperature above 38° C (100.4° F) that is measured under resting conditions. However, because each person's temperature range varies, a fever may exist in a person whose temperature is within the normal accepted range. For example, consider an individual whose normal temperature is 97° F. The person would be considered **febrile** if the temperature was 100° F. A true fever results from an alteration in the hypothalamic set point. Bacteria, viruses, fungi, and certain antigens are **pyrogens** (substances that cause a rise in body temperature). After pyrogens enter the body, more white blood cells are produced to help promote the body's defense against infection (Fig. 19-4). They also act on cells in the hypothalamus to raise the set point in the body. After the set point is increased, physiological and behavioral mechanisms work to produce fever. During the chill phase of a fever, the body acts to produce and conserve heat. It may take several hours before the body temperature reaches the new set point. During this time, neural responses cause vasoconstriction. A person experiences chills and shivers and feels cold, even though body temperature is rising. After the body temperature reaches the new set point, the chills subside, and the person then feels warm (Fig. 19-5).

During a fever, the body's metabolism increases 7% for every degree of temperature elevation. Heart and respiratory rates also increase to meet this metabolic demand. If the client has a cardiac or respiratory problem, the stress of fever can be great. A prolonged fever can seriously weaken a client because of exhaustion of energy stores and the increased work of breathing. Older adults are especially at risk for rapid deterioration resulting from fever because they have a diminished response to pyrogens and may already have chronic diseases causing debilitation. Confusion can result from high fevers because of reduced oxygen levels in the brain (although this condition is completely reversible in some cases). The increased metabolism places a client at risk for dehydration from evaporative heat loss and a possible reduced oral intake. Dehydration is a problem,

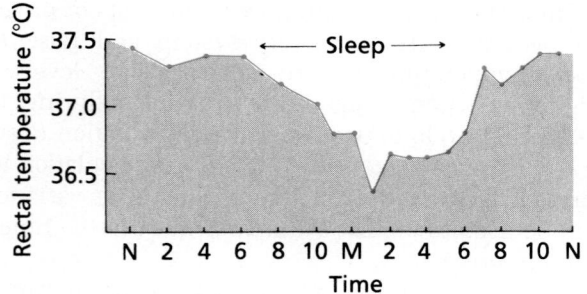

Fig. 19-3   The 24-hour temperature cycle.
From Mountcastle VB: *Medical physiology,* vol 2, ed 14, St Louis, 1980, Mosby–Year Book.

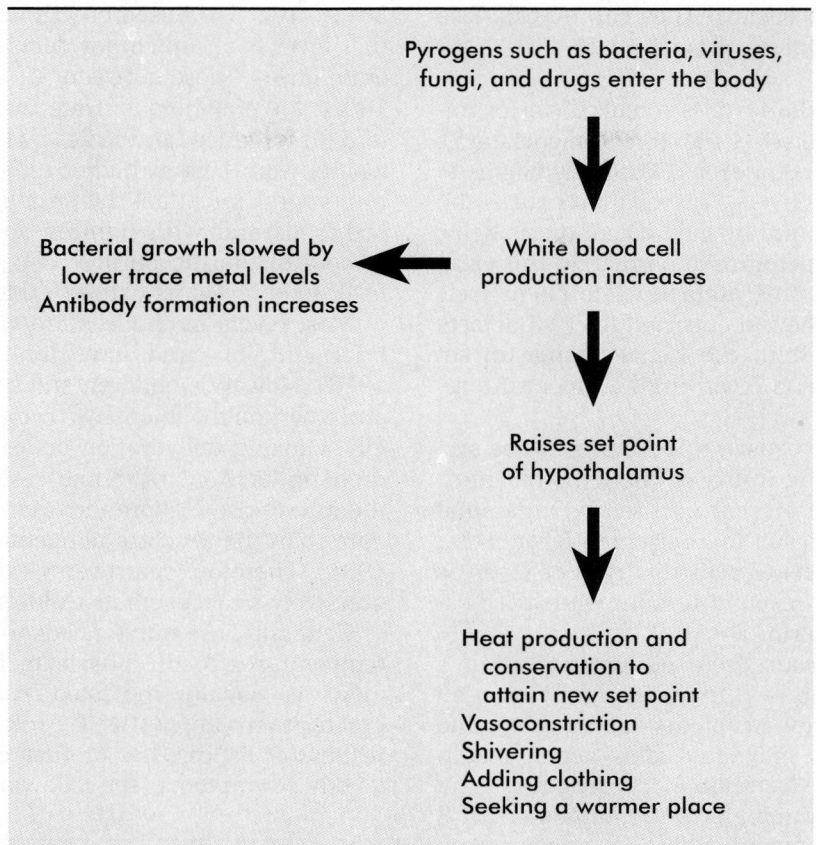

Fig. 19-4   Mechanism of a fever.

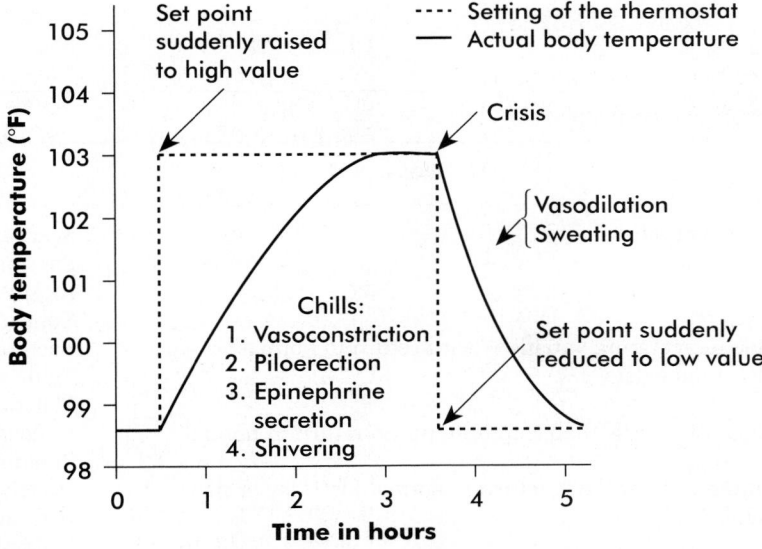

Fig. 19-5   Effects of changing the set point of the hypothalamic temperature control.
From Guyton AC: *Textbook of medical physiology*, ed 8, Philadelphia, 1991, Saunders.

especially for children because they can quickly lose large amounts of fluids in proportion to their body weight.

After the cause of the fever is removed (for example, destruction of bacteria by antibiotic medication), the hypothalamic set point drops. The body begins to initiate heat-loss maneuvers. Vasodilation causes the skin to become warm and flushed. Diaphoresis helps return the body's temperature to normal; in this case, the condition has become **afebrile**. The client feels more alert and has renewed energy. Fig. 19-5 depicts the process of fever from the initial change in set point, through chills and fever, until temperature returns to normal.

Fevers may also be caused by central nervous system problems involving injury to the hypothalamus. Increased intracranial pressure caused by inflammation or bleeding may result in a very high fever, 41° C (106° F) or above. Clients with this type of fever do not sweat and fail to respond to antipyretic medication (for example, aspirin).

Fever may also result from administration of a drug. A drug fever can be a hypersensitivity reaction accompanied by allergy symptoms such as rash and itching. It may be an individual idiosyncrasy resulting from a genetic predisposition, or a drug may have an intrinsic fever-producing activity; amphotericin B (Fungizone) and bleomycin sulfate (Blenoxane) can cause drug fevers. Treatment is usually simple; it is withdrawal of the offending medication (Hanson, 1991).

Treatment Issues

Physicians often disagree about when to treat a fever. A fever is usually not harmful if it stays below 39° C (102° F). Research (Dinarello, 1984) suggests that fever is an important defense mechanism. Moderate fevers, those between 37° and 38° C (98.6° and 100.4° F), may help activate the body's immune system to produce antibodies. These disease-fighting agents work best at higher temperatures. Fever also fights viral infections by stimulating interferon, the body's natural virus-fighting substance. Fevers also serve a diagnostic purpose. The natural pattern of a fever may reveal its cause (Table 19-2).

Most fevers in children are of a viral origin, are of brief duration, and have limited effects (Lovejoy, 1978). However, children still have unstable temperature-control mechanisms. Temperature can rise rapidly, causing dehydration or febrile seizures in children under 5 years. Some researchers believe that the rate of rise is more important in generating a seizure than the absolute temperature (Leung, Robson, 1991). Therefore controversy exists over when to aggressively treat fevers in children.

Generally, the nurse needs to report elevated body temperatures to the physician for all clients. Treatment is usually indicated if the temperature is greater than 38°C (101° F), especially if the client is restless or listless, has profuse diaphoresis, or exhibits other symptoms (see following section).

 ## Assessment

The nurse caring for clients with febrile conditions performs the following assessments through all stages of the febrile episode:
1. Measure vital signs when a fever is suspected and on an ongoing basis as ordered (for example, ev-

TABLE 19-2 Common Fever Patterns		
Type of Fever	Nature of Pattern	Possible Cause
Sustained	Little fluctuation	Scarlet fever Pneumococcal pneumonia Rickettsial fever Central nervous system problems
Intermittent	Wide temperature variations with return to normal at least once daily	Bacterial or viral infection Acute pyelonephritis Malaria
Remittent	Fluctuations less than intermittent; no return to normal	Endocarditis Pneumonia
Recurrent	Duration of few days; return to normal for 1 day or more and then return	Hodgkin's disease Rat-bite fever Yellow fever
Night	Occurrence late in evening or night	Tuberculosis

ery 2 to 4 hours) until body temperature returns to normal. An increase in temperature usually occurs with tachycardia (increased heart rate) and tachypnea (increased respiratory rate). Hypertension (increased blood pressure) may be seen initially with fever, and hypotension (decreased blood pressure) may follow with prolonged, high fevers.

2. Inspect and palpate the client's skin and check for turgor (see Chapter 20). As a fever develops, the skin may feel cool and dry and look pale. At the height of the fever the skin becomes warm. After a fever begins to break, the skin is flushed, warm, and moist from sweating. Reduced skin turgor is a sign of dehydration. Children and older adults are especially prone to dehydration and should be observed closely.

3. Ask how the client feels. Common symptoms of fever include headache, **myalgia** (muscle aches), chills, nausea, **photophobia** (sensitivity of the eyes to light), weakness, fatigue, and loss of appetite. A client often complains of thirst.

4. Note vomiting or diarrhea, which can increase fluid and electrolyte loss (see Chapter 39).

5. Observe the client for behavioral changes such as confusion or disorientation and restlessness or listlessness.

6. Monitor test results for electrolyte levels. An excessive loss of fluids will cause electrolyte imbalance (see Chapter 39). (Sodium, potassium, and chloride levels are most likely to be altered.)

7. Inspect the condition of the oral mucosa (see Chapter 20) for dryness resulting from dehydration. Small herpetic lesions characteristic of a fever may also be found on the mucosa.

Nursing Diagnosis

The nurse reviews assessment findings to identify the nursing diagnoses related to problems caused by fever (see diagnoses box). The diagnosis of *hyperthermia* directs the nurse to a comprehensive approach of care. However, the nurse may choose to separately diagnose problems resulting from fever (see diagnostic process box).

Sample Nursing Diagnostic Process for Fever

Assessment Activities	Defining Characteristics	Nursing Diagnoses
Obtain vital signs, including temperature, pulse, respirations.	High body temperature	*Hyperthermia* related to infectious process
Palpate skin.	Tachycardia	
Observe client's behavior while talking and resting.	Tachypnea Warm skin Restlessness	
Assess temperature, pulse, blood pressure for changes.	Fever Tachycardia Tachypnea Hypotension	*Fluid volume deficit* related to hyperthermia
Observe mucous membranes in mouth, nose, eyes, skin for dryness.	Dry skin and mucous membranes	
Assess skin turgor by gently pinching skin for slow, elastic recoil.	Reduced skin turgor	
Closely monitor intake and output levels for intake less than output.	Reduced fluid intake Vomiting Diarrhea	
Evaluate laboratory values for alterations in sodium, potassium, chloride levels.	Altered electrolyte values	

Examples of Nursing Diagnoses Related to Fever

NANDA-APPROVED NURSING DIAGNOSES

Hyperthermia related to:
- Infectious process
- Central nervous system injury
- Reaction to medication

Pain related to:
- Fever

Activity intolerance related to:
- Reduced energy stores

Impaired gas exchange related to:
- Increased oxygen consumption

Fluid volume deficit related to:
- Increased metabolism

Altered nutrition: less than body requirements related to:
- Increased metabolism

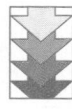

Sample Nursing Care Plan for Hyperthermia

Nursing Diagnosis: *Hyperthermia* related to infectious process
Definition: Hyperthermia is a state in which an individual's body temperature is elevated above the normal range (Kim, McFarland, McLane, 1991).

Goals	Expected Outcomes	Interventions	Rationales
Client will regain normal range of body temperature by 3/21.	Body temperature will decline at least 1° C after therapy (by 3/19).	Keep room temperature at 21°C (70° F) unless shivering develops.	Ambient room temperature can elevate body temperature. However, shivering should be avoided because it increases body temperature (Guyton, 1991).
	Body temperature will remain in normal range for at least 24 hr (by 3/20).	Administer tepid sponge bath (water temperature 32° to 39° C ([89.6° to 102° F]) for 15 min.	Sponge baths enhance conductive heat loss; 15 minutes is enough to cause temperature decline (Enright, Hill, 1989).
		Administer acetaminophen as ordered for temperature higher than 39° C (102° F).	Antipyretics reduce set point (Enright, Hill, 1989).

Nursing Measures for Clients with Fever

CHILL STAGE

- Reduce frequency of activities that increase oxygen demand such as excessive turning and ambulation. Allow rest periods.
- Provide supplemental oxygen therapy as ordered to improve oxygen delivery to body cells.
- Provide measures to stimulate appetite and offer well-balanced meals to meet increased metabolic needs.
- Offer extra blankets and raise room temperature to keep client warm during chills. Remove blankets when client feels warm.
- Provide extra fluids to replace fluids lost through increased metabolism.
- Assess onset and duration of chill. Take temperature immediately after episode.

COURSE OF FEVER

- Provide fluids (at least 3 L per day for client with normal cardiac and renal function) to replace fluids lost through insensible water loss and diaphoresis.
- Bathe client with tepid water to reduce body's surface temperature.
- Encourage oral hygiene because oral mucous membranes dry easily because of dehydration.
- Reduce external covering on client's body to promote heat loss through radiation and conduction. Do not induce chills.
- Keep clothing and bed linen dry to increase heat loss through conduction and convection.
- Control environmental temperature without causing chills. Provide cool, circulating air.
- Limit physical activity to minimize heat production.
- Administer antipyretic medications as ordered to reduce manifestations of fever.

Planning

The nurse will need to plan strategies to assist clients in managing fever (see care plan). Often, other medical problems complicate the care plan. For instance, clients with diabetes may have difficulty in controlling their blood sugar levels. Children with cystic fibrosis may be too exhausted from fever to tolerate chest physiotherapy. The nurse needs to consider all assessment findings when setting goals for clients with fever. Involving clients and families in the care plans and goal setting helps to ensure a successful team approach. Fever involves complex physiological responses from many organ systems. Goals of care for clients with fever include the following:

1. Attaining a sense of comfort and rest
2. Returning to normal body temperature
3. Maintaining adequate nutrition
4. Maintaining fluid and electrolye balance

 ## Implementation

After a client becomes febrile, the physician may try to determine the cause of the fever. The nurse obtains necessary culture specimens (such as urine, blood, and sputum) for diagnostic testing (see Chapter 18). When an infection is suspected, the physician will order antibiotic medications for the nurse to administer. The physician will also order the temperature value for giving antipyretic medications. For example, "Give 10 grains of aspirin for temperature of 39° C or over." Antipyretic medications (aspirin and acetaminophen) act to prevent the hypothalamus from synthesizing prostaglandin E, thus preventing the set point from rising further. The nurse can also provide a number of independent measures (see box) for clients with fever.

 ## Evaluation

After any intervention, the nurse measures the client's temperature to evaluate for change. If therapies are effective, body temperature will decrease.

The nurse also evaluates success at meeting the goals of care. Examples of evaluative criteria used by the nurse are included in the evaluation box.

Thermal Disorders

Thermal disorders are heat-related disorders and are not symptoms of another disease. In other words,

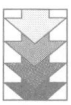 ## Sample Evaluation of Interventions for Hyperthermia

Goals	Evaluative Measures	Expected Outcomes
Client will regain normal body temperature range by 3/21.	Monitor body temperature after intervention (e.g., tepid sponge bath, antipyretic medications). Monitor body temperature every 4 hr.	Body temperature will decline at least 1° C (18° F) after therapy. Body temperature will remain in normal range for at least 24 hr by 3/20.
Fluid electrolyte balance will be maintained by 3/21.	Assess skin turgor and texture. Monitor serum electrolyte values. Measure intake and output levels.	Skin will remain supple with normal texture. Electrolyte level will remain in normal range. Output will not exceed intake.
Client will attain sense of comfort and rest by 3/21.	Question how client feels. Observe for restlessness.	Client will describe sense of relaxation with renewed energy. Client will be able to rest or sleep quietly.

fever and excess heat production are the primary problems rather than indications of infection at another site, such as the blood, lung, or kidney. Thermal disorders include heat exhaustion, heat stroke, and hypothermia, in which the body is unable to maintain adequate heat.

Heat Exhaustion

Heat exhaustion occurs when a person loses excessive amounts of water and sodium from profuse diaphoresis. The reduction in fluid volume and electrolytes causes extreme thirst, nausea, vomiting, weakness, headache, mild disorientation, normal or slightly elevated body temperature, tachycardia, and **postural hypotension** (drop in blood pressure when a person stands or sits). Exposure to high environmental temperature causes this common heat-related illness. Placing a person immediately in a cool environment to rest and stopping diaphoresis is the first treatment. Fluid and electrolyte replacement (see Chapter 39) will restore imbalances.

Heat Stroke

Heat stroke is a dangerous condition because it has a high fatality rate. Persons most at risk include infants and older adults; obese people; clients with cardiovascular disease, hyperthyroidism, diabetes, and alcoholism; clients taking medications that decrease the body's ability to lose heat for example, (phenothiazines, anticholinergics, diuretics, amphetamines, and beta-adrenergic receptor antagonists); and persons who exercise or work strenuously in the heat (for example, athletes, construction workers, and farmers).

Heat stroke with temperatures greater than 105° F produces tissue damage to the cells of all body organs. The brain may be the first organ affected because of its sensitivity to electrolyte imbalances. Permanent central nervous system damage can occur if cooling measures are not initiated rapidly.

A person with heat stroke suddenly becomes giddy, confused, or delirious. Extreme thirst, nausea, muscle cramps, and visual disturbances are common. The most important sign is hot, dry skin. The victim does not sweat because of severe electrolyte loss and impaired hypothalamic function. Vital signs measurement reveal an elevated temperature (sometimes as high as 45° C [120° F]), tachycardia, and hypotension. Clients are often unconscious by the time they reach the emergency room and have incontinence, blotchy redness of the skin, and fixed, unreactive pupils.

Moving the person to a cool environment is not enough to affect heat stroke. Immersion in tubs of ice water is no longer recommended because it causes severe peripheral vasoconstriction and shivering, which raises the body's core temperature. Because most victims are discovered outdoors, Marine Corps physicians recommend placing the client in a mesh hammock and directing an electric fan at the body while spraying the skin with mists of warm water (Barner et al, 1984). If a hammock is unavailable, the number of coverings in contact with the client must be reduced. Undressing the heat stroke victim allows air to circulate around the skin. Placement of wet towels over the skin and ice packs at vascular areas such as the neck, axilla, or groin can promote heat loss (Posey, Caruso, 1986).

The best approach for dealing with heat stroke is prevention. The nurse can teach people to avoid strenuous exercise in hot, humid weather; drink fluids such as clear fruit juices before, during, and after exercise; wear light, loose-fitting, light-colored clothing; avoid exercising in areas with poor ventilation; wear protective covering over the head when outdoors; and expose themselves to hot climates gradually.

Hypothermia

When a person is found ill or injured in cold weather or immersed in cold water, hypothermia should be suspected. This condition usually develops gradually and may not be noticed for several hours. Skin temperature drops to around 35° C (95° F), and uncontrolled shivering begins. A loss of memory, depression, and signs of poor judgment may be early indications. If body temperature falls to below 34.4° C (94° F), heart and respiratory rates and blood pressure begin to fall, and the skin becomes cyanotic. If hypothermia progresses, the client may experience cardiac dysrhythmias, lose consciousness, and become unresponsive to painful stimuli. In cases of severe hypothermia a person may demonstrate clinical signs similar to death (for example, lack of response to stimuli and extremely slow respirations and pulse).

Surface areas of the skin can actually freeze when a client is exposed to extremely cold temperatures without protection. This is called *frostbite*. Areas especially susceptible to frostbite include the earlobes, fingers, and toes. Permanent circulatory and tissue damage may result if ice crystals form inside of the cells (Guyton, 1991).

The priority treatment for hypothermia in the conscious client is prevention of further decrease in body temperature. The nurse should remove wet clothes, replace them with dry ones, and wrap the client in blankets. In emergencies away from a hospital or health care setting, it helps to have the client lie under blankets next to a warm person. A conscious client will benefit from drinking hot liquids such as soup. Placing the client near a fire or in a warm room or placing heating pads next to areas of the body (head and neck) that lose heat the quickest also helps.

While in transit to an emergency department, the client may receive warmed intravenous fluids (see Chapter 39). Once in the emergency department, forms of treatment depend on the severity of the condition. Application of heating blankets and instillation of warm fluids into the stomach may be used. Clients with hypothermia must be watched closely for cardiac irregularities and electrolyte imbalances.

Prevention is the key for clients at risk for hypothermia. Prevention involves education of clients or family and friends. Clients most at risk include infants, older adults, and persons debilitated by trauma, stroke, diabetes, drug or alcohol intoxication, sepsis, and Raynaud's disease (LaVoy, 1985). Mentally ill or handicapped clients may suffer hypothermia because they are unaware of the potential dangers of cold conditions. Persons who have inadequate home heating, poor diet, and lack of warm clothing are also at risk.

TABLE 19-3 Selection of Sites for Temperature Measurement	
Advantages	Disadvantages
MOUTH	
Most accessible site; more comfortable for client	Should not be used for clients who could be injured by thermometer, who are unable to hold thermometer properly, or who might bite thermometer, including infants or small children, confused or unconscious clients, clients who have had oral surgery, clients with trauma to face or mouth, clients experiencing oral pain, clients who breathe only with mouth open, clients with history of convulsions, clients experiencing shaking chills
RECTUM	
Thought to provide most reliable measurement	Should not be used for clients who have had rectal surgery, clients who have a rectal disorder such as tumor or severe hemorrhoids, clients who cannot be positioned for proper thermometer placement such as those in traction, newborns
AXILLA	
Safest method because noninvasive	Requires nurse to hold thermometer in position; is less accurate
TYMPANIC MEMBRANE	
Easy access to vascular tympanic membrane, which reflects core temperature	Is costly and device is less accessible

Assessment of Body Temperature

Sites

The mouth, rectum, and axilla are common sites for measuring body temperature. Special chemically prepared thermometer strips or patches can also be applied to the forehead. Tympanic membrane probes for temperature measurement are currently being studied for measurement at the ear. Each site has advantages and disadvantages (Table 19-3). Oral temperatures can be affected by a number of variables. The nurse waits 20 to 30 minutes to measure oral temperature after a client ingests hot or cold liquids or food, has been smoking, or has been involved in strenuous exercise. An oral thermometer can be reliably used as long as the client is able to close the mouth and breath through the nose. This includes clients using oxygen via nasal cannula or face mask, nasogastric tubes, and nasal endotracheal tubes (Heinz, 1985; Lukasiewicz, 1986). Oral temperature is approximately 0.55° C (1° F) less than core temperature.

The rectal site is believed to provide the most reliable measurement because few factors can alter the results. A rectal thermometer is used for infants and young children; it is not used for newborns, who may experience rectal trauma. Rectal temperature is usually a few tenths of a degree higher than the oral temperature. Even within the rectum, variations of 0.1° to 0.9° C (0.2° to 1.6° F) exist, depending on the position of the thermometer (Mountcastle, 1980).

The axilla is the safest site for temperature measurement, especially with newborns. However, the time required for measurement with a thermometer and the difficulty with thermometer placement makes the axillary area less convenient and accurate. When chemical thermometer strips are used, an axillary temperature can be obtained within a minute. Axillary temperature is approximately 1.1° C (2° F) cooler than core temperature.

The tympanic membrane is an excellent site for temperature measurement because of its highly vascular nature and easy accessibility. The problem lies in the availability of reliable, accurate, cost-efficient equipment. Several tympanic membrane thermometers are available and appear to be accurate, instantaneous, and easy to use. Tympanic membrane temperatures directly reflect core temperature.

Thermometers

The four types of thermometers available for determining body temperature include mercury in glass, electronic, disposable, and tympanic membrane.

The mercury-in-glass thermometer is the most familiar. It consists of a glass tube sealed at one end and a mercury-filled bulb at the other. Exposure of

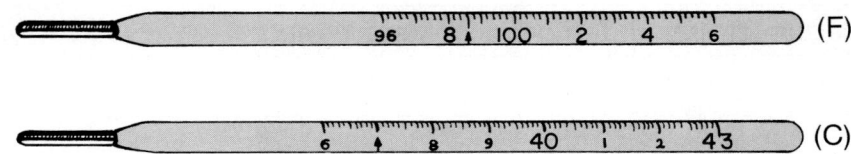

Fig. 19-6   Comparison of Fahrenheit and centigrade calibrations.

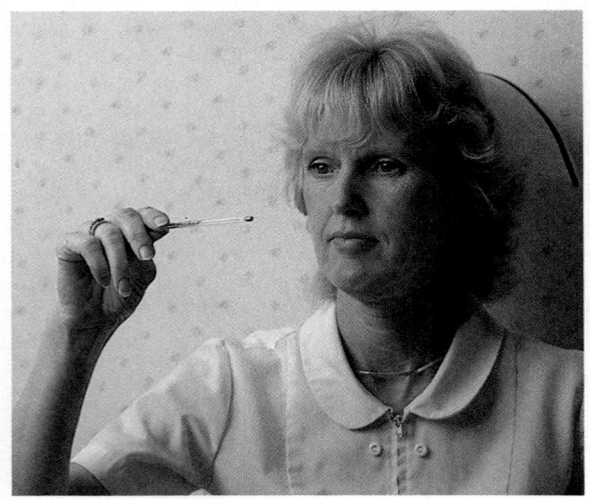

Fig. 19-7   Reading a glass thermometer.

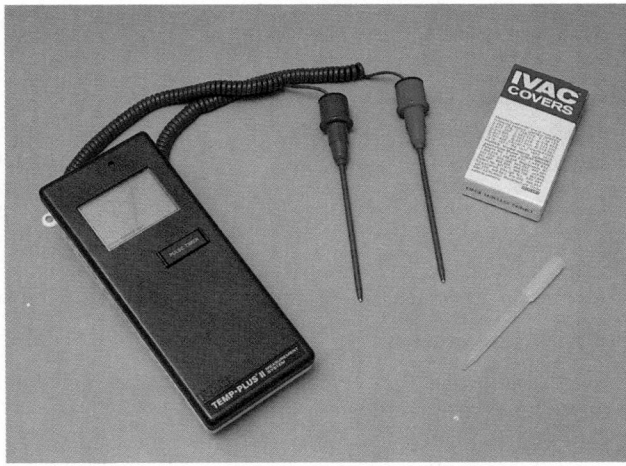

Fig. 19-8   Electronic thermometer.

the bulb to heat causes the mercury to expand and rise in the enclosed tube. The length of the thermometer is marked with Fahrenheit or centigrade calibrations (Fig. 19-6). The mercury will not fluctuate or fall unless the thermometer is shaken vigorously.

A glass thermometer is read by holding it with the fingertips horizontally at eye level, with the bulb pointed to the left (Fig. 19-7). The bulb should not be touched. Touching it might bring the fingers into contact with the client's body secretions and may also cause a change in the thermometer reading. The thermometer is rotated slowly until the column of silver mercury appears. The calibrated line at the end of the mercury column is the temperature reading.

Glass thermometers, the oral or slim tipped, the stubby, and the pear-shaped rectal, are all available with centigrade or Fahrenheit measurements. The oral thermometer is slender, allowing greater exposure of the bulb against the blood vessels in the mouth. It usually has a blue tip. The stubby thermometer is shorter and thicker than the oral type. It

can be used to measure temperature at any site. The pear-shaped rectal thermometer has a blunt end designed to prevent trauma during rectal insertion. It usually has a red tip. Time delay for recordings and easy breakability are disadvantages of mercury-in-glass thermometers. Advantages are low price, wide availability, and reliable accuracy.

The electronic thermometer consists of a battery-powered display unit, a thin wire cord, and a temperature-sensitive probe covered by a disposable plastic sheath to prevent the transmission of infection (Fig. 19-8). Separate probes are available for oral and rectal use. Within only a few seconds of insertion a reading appears on the display unit. Temperature readings appear in Fahrenheit, centigrade, or both. An electronic thermometer is not necessarily more accurate than a glass thermometer (Baker et al, 1984). For example, variables that alter oral temperature measurements affect all types of thermometers. An electronic thermometer may be less accurate because the sensor probe is inserted for a shorter time. However, a study by Baker et al (1984) showed that, although length of insertion may result in different

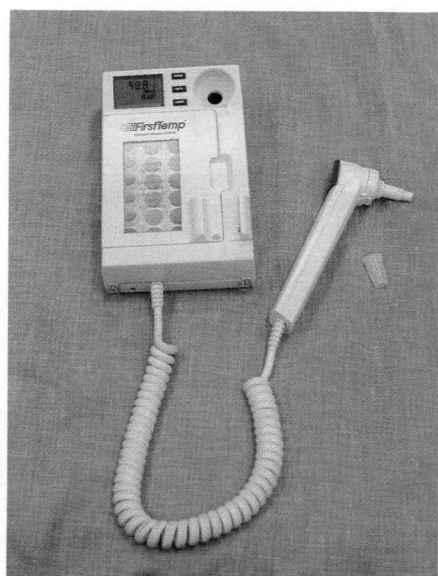

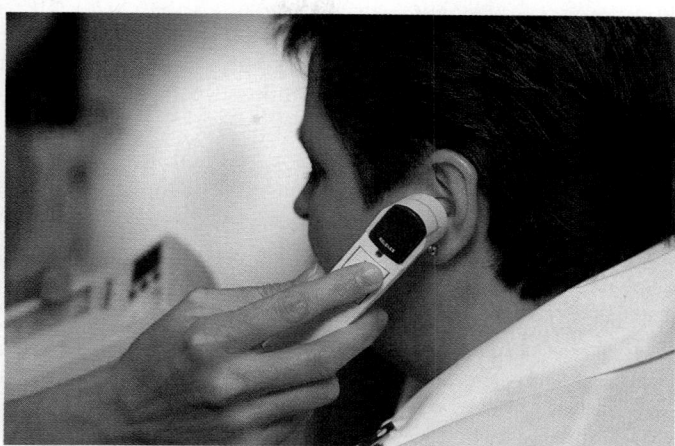

Fig. 19-9 Tympanic membrane thermometer.

temperature values, the difference is not likely to be clinically significant. The study found mercury-in-glass thermometers with insertion times of 2 minutes to be essentially no different than readings on the quicker electronic thermometers.

Electronic thermometers have many advantages. They can be inserted immediately. Their readings appear within seconds, and they are easy to read. The duration of the client's discomfort is also minimized. Lubricant should be avoided with rectal electronic thermometers because it can cause a falsely elevated reading.

Disposable, single-use thermometers are thin strips of plastic with chemically impregnated paper. They are used for oral or axillary temperatures, particularly with children. They can be inserted in the same way as an oral thermometer or can be applied to the skin. The chemical dots on the thermometer change color to reflect the temperature reading. Only 45 seconds are needed to record a temperature. Chemically treated paper thermometers are generally less accurate, but they are useful in providing a general temperature range.

Tympanic membrane thermometers are small hand-held devices similar to otoscopes, with disposable speculums, infrared sensing electronics, and liquid crystal displays. Most are battery operated and rechargeable. Results are displayed 1 to 2 seconds after placing the speculum in the outer third of the ear canal (Fig 19-9). Accuracy appears to be good (Shi-

nozaki, Deane, Perkins, 1988), but studies have been conflicting.

Guidelines for Taking Temperature

When measuring body temperature at any site, the following basic principles should be carefully followed to maintain the client's safety and ensure accuracy in measurement (Procedure 19-1):

1. The most appropriate site for measuring temperature is assessed.
2. All necessary equipment is assembled to ensure an uninterrupted procedure.
3. The hands are washed using medically aseptic technique (see Chapter 18) to prevent spread of infection. Gloves are worn to prevent exposure to microorganisms in saliva.
4. The client is positioned properly, with privacy ensured if necessary, and the purpose and method for the procedure are explained.

When it is necessary to convert temperature readings, formulas can be used. To convert Fahrenheit to centigrade, the nurse subtracts 32° from the Fahrenheit reading and multiplies the result by $\frac{5}{9}$:

$$C = (F - 32°) \times \frac{5}{9}$$

To convert centigrade to Fahrenheit, the nurse multiplies the centigrade reading by $\frac{9}{5}$ and adds 32° to the product.

$$F = (\frac{9}{5} \times C) + 32°$$

Text continued on p. 477.

Measuring Body Temperature

STEPS	RATIONALE
1. Assess for signs and symptoms of temperature alterations and for factors that normally influence body temperature.	Physical signs and symptoms may indicate abnormal body temperature. Nurse can accurately assess nature of temperature variations.
2. Explain way that temperature is to be taken and importance of maintaining proper position until reading is complete.	Clients are often curious as to what their temperatures are and should be cautioned against prematurely removing thermometer to read results.
3. When taking oral temperature, wait 20 to 30 min before measuring temperature if client has smoked or ingested hot or cold liquids or foods.	Smoking and hot or cold substances can cause false temperature readings in oral cavity (Erickson, 1980).
4. Prepare needed equipment and supplies: a. Appropriate thermometer b. Soft tissues c. Lubricant (for rectal glass thermometer only) d. Pen, pencil, flowsheet or record form e. Disposable gloves	Chosen on basis of preferred site for temperature measurement.
5. Wash hands.	Reduces transmission of microorganisms.
6. **Oral temperature—electronic thermometer** a. Assist client in assuming position of comfort that provides easy access to mouth.	Ensures comfort and accuracy of temperature reading.
b. Apply disposable gloves.	Gloves should be worn for handling items soiled with body fluids (e.g., saliva) (CDC, 1987).
c. Attach oral probe (blue tip) to thermometer unit. Grasp top of stem, being careful not to apply pressure to ejection button.	Ejection button releases plastic cover from probe.
d. Slide disposable plastic probe cover over thermometer probe until it locks in place.	Soft plastic cover will not break in mouth and prevents transmission of microorganisms between clients.
e. Ask client to open mouth and gently place probe under tongue in posterior sublingual pocket lateral to center of lower jaw.	Heat from superficial blood vessels in sublingual pocket produces temperature reading. With electronic thermometer, temperatures in right and left posterior sublingual pocket are significantly higher than in area under front of tongue (Erickson, 1980).
f. Ask client to hold thermometer with lips closed.	Maintains proper position of thermometer during recording.
g. Leave probe in place until audible signal occurs. Temperature appears on digital display.	Probe must stay in place until signal occurs to ensure accurate reading.
h. Remove probe from under tongue and inform client of temperature reading.	Promotes participation in care and understanding of health status.
i. Push ejection button on thermometer probe to discard plastic probe cover into proper receptacle.	Reduces transmission of microorganisms.
j. Return probe to storage well.	Protects probe from damage. Automatically causes digital reading to disappear.
k. Remove and dispose of gloves. Wash hands.	Reduces transmission of microorganisms.
l. Return thermometer to charger after temperature reading.	Maintains battery charge.
7. **Oral temperature—glass thermometer** a. Assist client in assuming comfortable position that provides easy access to mouth.	Ensures comfort and accuracy of temperature reading.
b. Apply disposable gloves.	Gloves should be worn for handling items soiled with body fluids (e.g., saliva) (CDC, 1987).
c. Hold color-coded end of glass thermometer with fingertips.	Reduces contamination of thermometer blub.
d. If thermometer is stored in disinfectant solution, rinse in cold water before using.	Removes solution irritating to oral mucosa. Hot water can cause mercury to expand and break bulb.

STEPS	RATIONALE
e. Take soft tissue and wipe thermometer bulb end toward fingers in rotating fashion. Dispose of tissue.	Reduces contamination of bulb end.
f. Read mercury level while holding thermometer at eye level and gently rotating it.	Mercury should be below 35.5° C (96° F). Thermometer reading must be below body temperature before use.
g. If mercury is above desired level, securely grasp tip and stand away from solid objects. Sharply flick wrist downward as through cracking a whip. Continue shaking until reading is below 35.5° C (96° F).	Brisk shaking lowers mercury level in glass tube. Standing in open spot avoids breakage of thermometer.
h. Ask client to open mouth and gently place thermometer under tongue in posterior sublingual pocket lateral to center of lower jaw (see illustration).	Heat from superficial blood vessels in sublingual pocket produces temperature reading.
i. Ask client to hold thermometer with lips closed. Caution against biting down.	Maintains proper position of thermometer during recording. Breakage of thermometer may injure mucosa and cause mercury poisoning.
j. Leave thermometer in place for 2 min or according to agency policy.	Studies about proper length of time for recording vary. Graves and Markarian (1980) found that glass thermometers kept in place for 8 min recorded values averaging only 0.4° C (0.7° F) higher than those kept in place for 3 min. Baker et al (1984) found that 2-min insertions did not cause clinically significant variations.
k. Carefully remove thermometer and read at eye level.	Ensures accurate reading.
l. Inform client of temperature reading.	Promotes participation in care and understanding of health status.
m. Wipe secretions from thermometer with soft tissue. Wipe in rotating fashion from fingers toward bulb. Dispose of tissue.	Wipe from area of least contamination to area of most contamination.
n. Wash thermometer in lukewarm soapy water, rinse in cool water, dry, and replace in storage container.	Mechanically removes organic material that can harbor microorganisms and hinder action of disinfectant. Storage container prevents breakage.
o. Remove and dispose of gloves. Wash hands.	Reduces transmission of microorganisms.
8. Rectal temperature—electronic thermometer	
a. Draw curtain around bed and/or close room door. Keep client's upper body and lower extremities covered with sheet or blanket.	Maintains privacy, minimizes embarrassment, and promotes comfort.

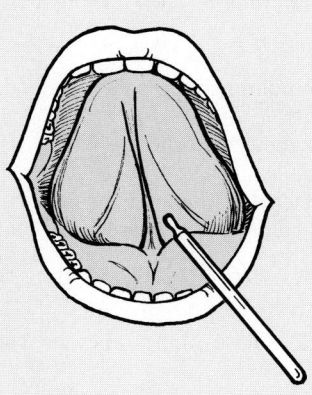

Step 7h

Measuring Body Temperature

STEPS	RATIONALE
b. Assist client in assuming Sims' position with upper leg flexed. Move aside bed linen to expose only anal area.	Exposes anal area for correct thermometer placement.
c. Attach rectal probe (red tip) to thermometer unit. Grasp top of stem, being careful not to apply pressure to ejection button.	Ejection button releases plastic cover from probe.
d. Slide disposable plastic cover over thermometer probe until it locks in place.	Probe cover prevents transmission of microorganisms between clients.
e. Apply disposable gloves.	Gloves should be worn for handling items soiled with body fluids (e.g., feces) (CDC, 1987).
f. With nondominant hand, separate buttocks to expose anus.	Fully exposes anus for thermometer insertion.
g. Ask client to breathe slowly and relax.	Relaxes anal sphincter for easier thermometer insertion.
h. Gently insert probe into anus in direction of umbilicus. Insert 1.2 cm (½ in) for infant and 3.5 cm (1½ in) for adult. Do not force thermometer.	Ensures adequate exposure against blood vessels in rectal wall.
(1) If resistance is felt during insertion, withdraw thermometer immediately. Never force it.	Prevents trauma to mucosa.
i. Hold probe until audible signal occurs. Read temperature on digital display.	Reading occurs within seconds after insertion.
j. Carefully remove probe from rectum and inform client of temperature reading.	Promotes participation in care and understanding of health status.
k. Push ejection button to discard plastic probe cover into receptacle.	Reduces transmission of microorganisms.
l. Return probe to storage well.	Protects probe from damage. Automatically causes digital reading to disappear.
m. Wipe anal area to remove feces. Remove and dispose of gloves.	Provides comfort. Reduces transmission of microorganisms.
n. Help client return to comfortable position.	Restores comfort.
o. Wash hands.	Reduces transmission of microorganisms.

9. **Rectal temperature—glass thermometer**

STEPS	RATIONALE
a. Draw curtain around bed and/or close room door. Keep client's upper body and lower extremities covered with sheet or blanket.	Maintains privacy, mimimizes embarrassment, and promotes comfort.
b. Assist client in assuming Sims' position with upper leg flexed. Move aside bed linen to expose only anal area.	Exposes anal area for correct thermometer placement.
c. Prepare thermometer following Steps 7c to 7g.	Mercury must be below temperature level before insertion.
d. Squeeze liberal portion of lubricant onto tissue. Dip thermometer's blunt end into lubricant, covering 2.5 to 3.5 cm (1 to 1½ in) for adult or 1.2 to 2.5 cm (½ to 1 in) for infant.	Lubrication minimizes trauma to rectal mucosa during insertion. Tissue avoids contamination of all lubricant in container.
a. Apply disposable gloves.	Gloves should be worn for handling items soiled by body fluids (e.g., feces) (CDC, 1987).
f. With nondominant hand, separate buttocks to expose anus.	Fully exposes anus for thermometer insertion.
g. Ask client to breathe slowly and relax.	Relaxes anal sphincter for easier thermometer insertion.
h. Gently insert thermometer into anus in direction of umbilicus. Insert 1.2 (½ in) for infant and 3.5 cm 1½ in) for adult. Do not force thermometer (see illustration).	Ensures adequate exposure against blood vessels in rectal wall.
(1) If resistance is felt during insertion, withdraw thermometer immediately. Never force it.	Prevents trauma to mucosa. Glass thermometers can break.

STEPS	RATIONALE
i. Hold thermometer in place for 2 min or according to agency policy.	Prevents injury to client. Recommended times vary among institutions. Nichols and Kucha (1972) identified optimal placement time as 2 min.
j. Carefully remove thermometer and wipe off secretions with tissue. Wipe in rotating fashion from fingers toward bulb. Dispose of tissue.	Avoids contact with microorganisms. Wipe from area of least contamination to area of most contamination.
k. Read thermometer at eye level.	Ensures accurate reading.
l. Inform client of temperature reading.	Promotes participation in care and understanding of status.
m. Wipe anal area to remove lubricant or feces.	Provides comfort.
n. Help client return to comfortable position.	Restores comfort.
o. Wash thermometer in lukewarm soapy water, rinse in cool water, dry, and replace in storage container.	Mechanically removes organic material that can harbor microorganisms and hinder action of disinfectant. Storage container prevents breakage.
p. Dispose of gloves. Wash hands.	Reduces transmission of microorganisms.

10. Axillary temperature—electronic thermometer

STEPS	RATIONALE
a. Draw curtain around bed and/or close room door.	Provides privacy and minimizes embarrassment.
b. Position client in supine or sitting position.	Provides easy access to axilla.
c. Move clothing or gown away from shoulder and arm.	Provides optimal exposure of axilla.
d. Attach rectal probe (red) to thermometer unit. Prepare electronic thermometer following Steps 8c and 8d.	Probe cover prevents transmission of microorganisms between clients.
e. Insert probe into center of axilla, lower arm over thermometer, and place arm across client's chest.	Maintains proper position of thermometer against blood vessels in axilla.
f. Hold probe in place until audible signal occurs. Read temperature on digital display.	Reading occurs within seconds after insertion.
g. Remove probe from axilla and inform client of temperature reading.	Promotes participation in care and understanding of health status.
h. Push ejection button to discard plastic probe into proper receptacle.	Reduces transmission of microorganisms.
i. Return electronic probe to storage well.	Protects probe from damage. Automatically causes digital reading to disappear.
j. Assist client in replacing clothing or gown.	Restores comfort.
k. Wash hands.	Reduces transmission of infection.

11. Axillary temperature—glass thermometer

STEPS	RATIONALE
a. Draw curtain around bed or close door.	Provides privacy and minimizes embarrassment.
b. Position client lying supine or sitting.	Provides easy access to axilla.

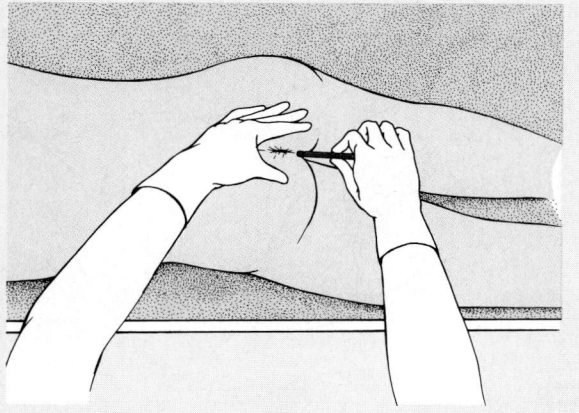

Step 9h

Measuring Body Temperature

STEPS	RATIONALE
c. Move clothing or gown away from shoulder and arm.	Provides optimal exposure of axilla.
d. Prepare glass thermometer following Steps 7c- 7g.	Mercury must be below temperature level before insertion.
e. Insert thermometer into center of axilla, lower arm over thermometer, and place arm across client's chest (see illustrations).	Maintains proper position of thermometer against blood vessels in axilla.
f. Hold thermometer in place for 5-10 min or according to agency policy.	Recommended time varies among institutions. Eoff and Joyce (1981) recommend 5 min for children.
g. Remove thermometer and wipe off any moisture with tissue. Wipe in rotating fashion from fingers toward bulb. Dispose of tissue.	Avoids contact with microorganisms. Wipe from area of least contamination to area of most contamination.
h. Read thermometer at eye level.	Ensures accurate reading.
i. Inform client of temperature reading.	Promotes participation in care and understanding of health status.
j. Wash thermometer in lukewarm soapy water, rinse in cool water, dry, and replace in storage container.	Mechanically removes organic material that can harbor microorganisms and hinder action of disinfectant. Storage container prevents breakage.
k. Assist client in replacing clothing or gown.	Restores sense of well-being.
l. Wash hands.	Reduces transmission of microorganisms.

12. Tympanic membrane thermometer

a. Attach tympanic probe cover to thermometer unit.	Probe cover prevents transmission of microorganisms between clients.
b. Insert probe into ear canal, applying a gentle but firm pressure.	Gentle pressure seals ear canal from ambient air and improves accuracy.
c. Remove thermometer after reading is displayed on digital unit, approximately 2 sec.	Tympanic core temperatures are rapid (less than 2 sec) and extremely accurate (Shinozaki, Deane, Perkins, 1988; Erickson, Yount, 1991).
d. Remove probe cover and place in proper receptacle.	Prevents transmission of microorganisms.
e. Return thermometer to storage unit.	Most units are battery operated and recharge in storage.
f. Wash hands.	Reduces transmission of infection.

13. Compare temperature reading with client's baseline and normal temperature range for age group.

Normal body temperature fluctuates within narrow range. Comparison reveals presence of abnormality.

14. If temperature is abnormal, measure it again.

Improper placement or movement of thermometer can cause inaccuracies. Second reading confirms initial finding of abnormal body temperature.

15. Record temperature on vital sign flowsheet or nurses' notes and report abnormal findings to nurse in charge or physician.

Vital sign measurements should be recorded promptly on flowsheet to avoid omissions from client's record. Abnormalities may require immediate therapy.

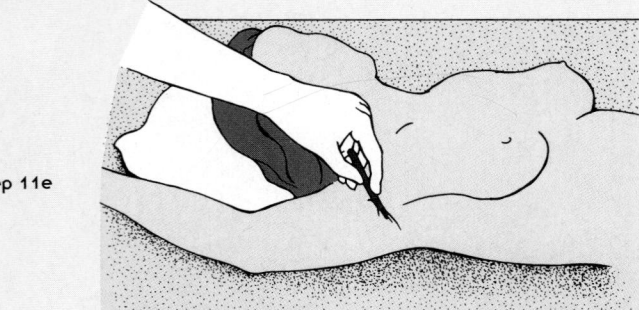

Step 11e

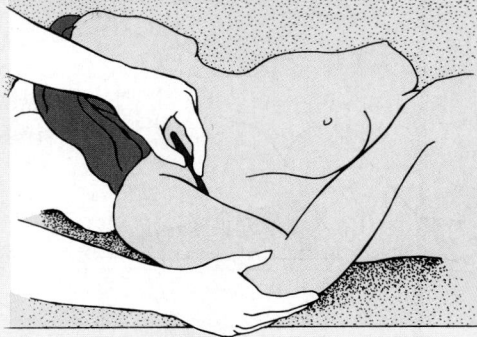

PULSE

The **pulse** is the palpable bounding of blood flow noted at various points on the body. It is an indicator of circulatory status. Circulation is the means by which cells receive nutrients and remove waste products of metabolism. For cells to function normally, there must be a continuous blood flow and an appropriate volume and distribution of blood to cells that need nutrients.

Physiology and Regulation

Blood flows through the body in a continuous circuit. The heart is a pulsatile pump, ejecting blood intermittently into the arterial system. Cardiac centers located in the medulla of the brainstem receive impulses from sensory receptors. These sensory impulses then cause the cardiac centers in the medulla to speed up or slow down the heart rate through sympathetic or parasympathetic innervation. For example, if there is excessive stretch of the aortic arch by an increase in blood volume, sensory impulses travel to the cardiac center. This then triggers a reflex slowing of the heart rate through the action of the vagus nerve. This decrease in heart rate compensates for the increased blood volume. When volume returns to normal, the heart rate returns to baseline .

A person's heart rate varies throughout the day. Nevertheless, the heart functions to maintain a relatively constant circulatory blood flow. Approximately 60 to 70 ml of blood enters the aorta with each ventricular contraction **(stroke volume)**. With each stroke volume ejection, the walls of the aorta distend, creating a pulse wave that travels rapidly toward the distal ends of the arteries. The pulse wave moves 15 times faster through the aorta and 100 times faster through the small arteries than the ejected volume of blood (Guyton, 1991). When a pulse wave reaches a peripheral artery, it can be palpated by palpating the artery lightly against underlying bone or muscle. The pulse rate is an indirect measurement of cardiac output. The volume of blood pumped by the heart during 1 minute is the **cardiac output**, the product of heart rate and the ventricle's stroke volume (HR × SV = CO). In an adult the heart normally pumps 5000 to 6000 ml of blood per minute throughout the circulation.

An abnormally slow, rapid, or irregular pulse may indicate a problem in circulatory regulation. The pathological process causing a change from the normal heart beat may ultimately alter cardiac output. The nurse assesses the heart's function by palpating a peripheral pulse or by using a stethoscope to listen to heart sounds **(apical pulse)**.

Assessment of Pulse

The radial and carotid arteries are the most accessible peripheral pulse sites for assessment. When a client's condition suddenly deteriorates, the carotid artery in the neck is the best site for finding a pulse quickly. The heart will continue delivering blood through the carotid artery to the brain as long as possible, whereas peripheral pulses weaken. The radial and apical pulses are the most common sites for assessment of vital signs. The radial and carotid sites are used by persons learning to monitor their own heart rates (for example, athletes).

Assessment of other peripheral pulse sites (Table 19-4 on p. 478), such as the brachial or femoral artery (see Chapter 20), is unnecessary when routinely taking vital signs. Other peripheral pulses are taken when a complete physical assessment is conducted, when surgery or treatment has impaired blood flow to a body part, or when there are clinical indications of impaired peripheral blood flow. Locations for these pulses are found in Fig 19-10. If the **radial pulse** at the wrist is abnormal or intermittent resulting from dysrhythmias or if it is inaccessible because of a dressing, cast, or other encumbrance, the apical pulse is assessed. When a client takes medication that affects the heart rate, the apical pulse may provide a more accurate assessment of heart function. The apical pulse is the best site for assessing an infant's or young child's pulse because the peripheral pulses are deep and difficult to palpate accurately.

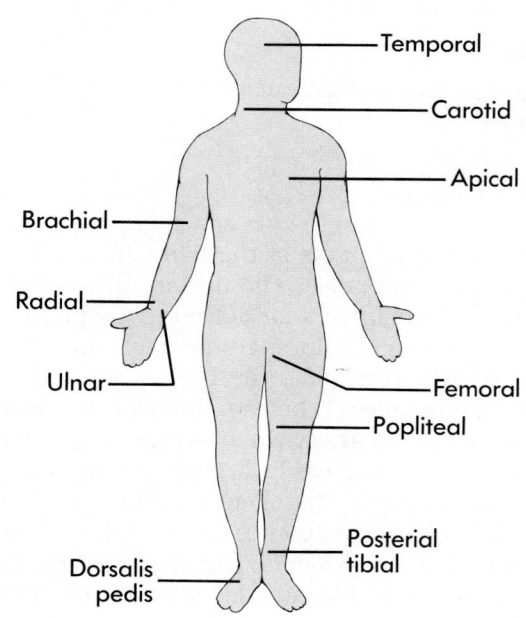

Fig. 19-10   Location of pulse points in the body.

TABLE 19-4 Pulse Sites	
Location	Assessment Criteria
TEMPORAL Over temporal bone of head, above and lateral to eye	Easily accessible site is used to assess pulse in children.
CAROTID Along medial edge of sternocleidomastoid muscle in neck	Easily accessible site is used to assess character of pulse peripherally and is used during shock or cardiac arrest when other sites are not palpable.
APICAL Fourth to fifth intercostal space at midclavicular line	Site is used for auscultation of heart sounds.
BRACHIAL Groove between biceps and triceps muscles at antecubital fossa	Site is used to assess status of circulation to lower arm and auscultate blood pressure.
RADIAL Radial or thumb side of forearm at wrist	Common site is used to assess character of pulse peripherally and status of circulation to hand.
ULNAR Ulnar side of forearm at wrist	Site is used to assess status of circulation to ulnar side of hand and assess Allen's test.
FEMORAL Below inguinal ligament, midway between symphysis pubis and antero superior iliac spine	Site is used to assess character of pulse during physiological shock or cardiac arrest when other pulses are not palpable and to assess status of circulation to leg.
POPLITEAL Behind knee in popliteal fossa	Site is used to assess status of circulation to lower leg.
POSTERIOR TIBIAL Inner side of each ankle, below medial malleolus	Site is used to assess status of circulation to foot.
DORSALIS PEDIS Along top of foot between extension tendons of great and first toe	Site is used to assess status of circulation to foot.

The first two fingers of the hand are used to palpate a peripheral pulse. The tips are the most sensitive parts of the fingers for detecting the pulsation of the arterial wall. Beginning students sometimes apply excessive pressure over the artery and totally obliterate the pulse. It helps to imagine the anatomical position of the artery when attempting to locate it. If the pulse is not easily located on one side, the other can be tried. The client's extremity should be kept in a relaxed position to permit full exposure of an artery. For assessment of the radial artery, the client's wrist should be extended and relaxed. This position ensures that the artery lies superficially above the radius. Procedure 19-2 outlines pulse assessment.

If the nurse is unable to palpate a pulse, a Doppler electronic stethoscope can be used (see Chapter 20). This instrument magnifies sounds produced by the heart and blood vessels for easier evaluation.

Stethoscope

When assessing the apical pulse the nurse uses an acoustical stethoscope. Sound waves originating from an internal organ usually reach the body's surface and are dissipated into the air. Unless the sounds are of a high amplitude, the unassisted ear cannot hear them clearly. The **stethoscope** is a closed cylinder that prevents the dissipation of sound waves as they reach the body's surface and amplifies them for the

STEPS	RATIONALE
1. Before measuring pulse, consider factors that normally influence pulse character (e.g., age, exercise, postural changes).	Allows nurse to accurately assess presence and significance of pulse alterations.
2. Explain to client that pulse or heart rate is to be assessed. Encourage client to relax and not speak. (If client has been active, wait 5 to 10 min.)	Activity and anxiety can cause elevated heart rate. Voice interferes with ability to hear sound when apical pulse is measured.
3. Prepare needed equipment and supplies:	
a. Stethoscope	Used for apical pulse assessment.
b. Pen, pencil, vital sign flowsheet or record form	
c. Wristwatch with second hand or digital display	
d. Alcohol swab	
4. Wash hands.	Reduces transmission of microorganisms.
5. Radial pulse	
a. If client is supine, place forearm across region of lower abdomen or chest with wrist extended and palm down. If client is sitting, bend elbow 90 degrees and support lower arm on chair or on your arm. Slightly extend wrist with palm down (see illustration).	Relaxed position of lower arm and extension of wrist permits full exposure of artery to palpation.
b. Place tips of first two fingers of your hand over groove along radial or thumb side of client's inner wrist (see illustration).	Fingertips are most sensitive parts of hand to palpate arterial pulsation. Thumb has pulsation that may interfere with accuracy.
c. Lightly compress against radius, obliterate pulse initially, and then relax pressure so that pulse becomes easily palpable.	Pulse is more accurately assessed with moderate pressure. Too much pressure occludes pulse and impairs blood flow.
d. After pulse can be felt regularly, look at watch's second hand and begin to count rate: when sweep hand hits number on dial, start counting with *zero,* then *one,* and so on (see illustration on p. 450).	Rate is determined accurately only after assessor is assured that pulse can be palpated. Timing begins with *zero.* Count of *one* is first beat palpated after timing begins.

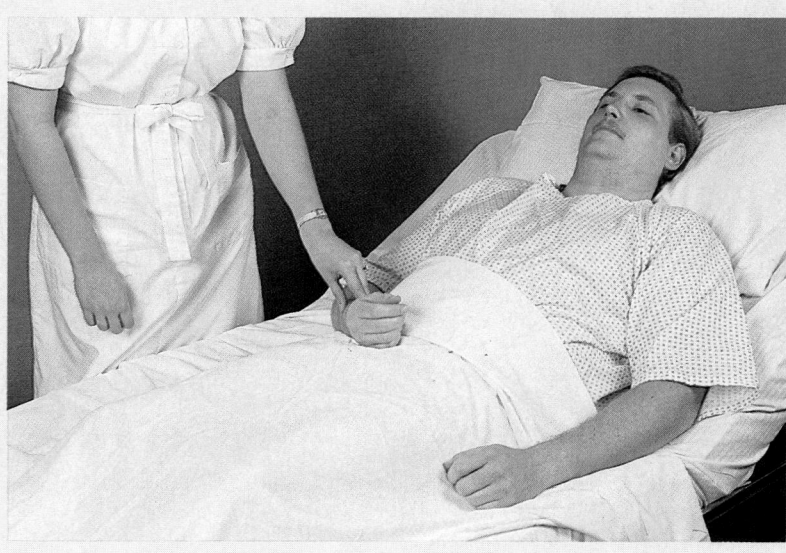

Step 5a

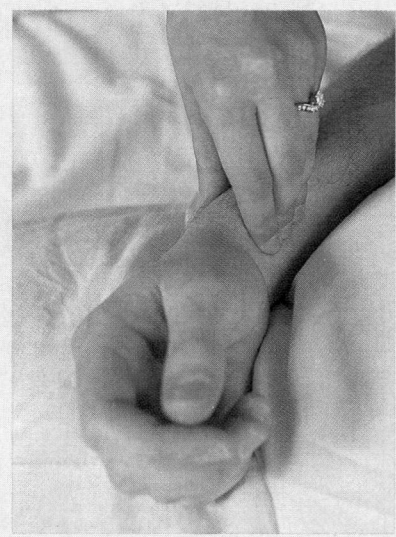

Step 5b

Assessing Pulse Rate

STEPS

RATIONALE

   e. If pulse is regular, count rate for 30 sec and multiply total by 2.

Research indicates that 30-sec check is most accurate for rapid pulse rates and that 15-sec check is often inaccurate for resting and rapid heart rates (Hollerbach, Sneed, 1990).

   f. If pulse is irregular, count for full minute.

Longer time period ensures accurate count.

   g. Assess regularity and frequency of any existing dysrhythmia.

Inefficient contraction of heart fails to transmit pulse wave and can interfere with cardiac output. Determines need to assess for pulse deficit.

   h. Determine strength of pulse. Note thrust of vessel against fingertips.

Strength reflects volume of blood ejected against arterial wall with each contraction.

   i. Palpate with two fingers along course of artery toward wrist to determine elasticity of arterial wall.

Degree of elasticity reflects quality of arterial wall and reveals general condition of peripheral vascular system.

   j. Assist client in returning to comfortable position.

Promotes sense of well-being.

6. **Apical pulse**

   a. Clean earpieces and diaphragm of stethoscope with alcohol swab as needed (optional).

Controls transmission of microorganisms when nurses share stethoscope.

   b. With client in supine or sitting position, turn down bed linen and raise gown to expose sternum and left side of chest.

Exposes portion of chest wall for selection of auscultatory site.

   c. Palpate angle of Louis, located just below suprasternal notch at point where horizontal ridge is felt along body of sternum. Place index finger just to left of sternum and palpate second intercostal space. Place next finger in intercostal space below and proceed downward until fifth intercostal space is located. Move index finger horizontally along fifth intercostal space to left midclavicular line (see illustration). Palpate point of maximal impulse (PMI), also called the *apex*.

Use of anatomical landmarks allows nurse to place stethoscope over apex of heart, which lies just under fifth intercostal space along left midclavicular line. This position enhances ability to hear heart sounds clearly. PMI is over apex of heart.

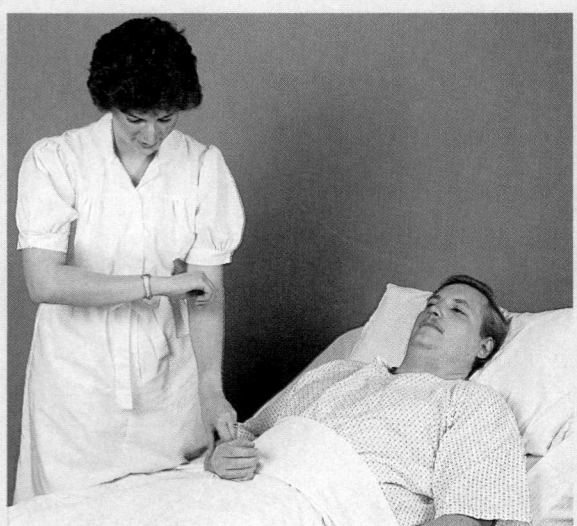

Step 5d

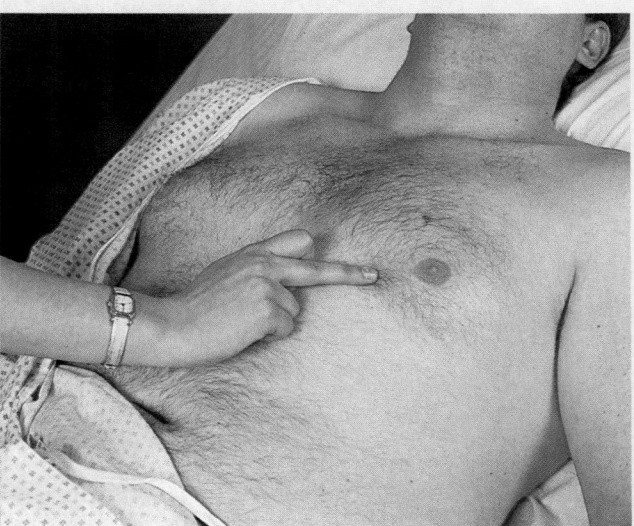

Step 6c

STEPS	RATIONALE
d. Place diaphragm of stethoscope in palm of your hand for 5 to 10 sec.	Warming of metal or plastic diaphragm prevents client from being startled and promotes comfort.
e. Place diaphragm over PMI and auscultate for normal S_1 and S_2 (heard as *lub-dub*) (see illustration).	Heart sounds are caused by movement of blood through heart values.
f. After hearing S_1 and S_2 with regularity, use watch's second hand and begin to count rate: when sweep hand hits number on dial, start with *zero,* then *one,* and so on. Each lub-dub equals one heart beat.	Rate is determined accurately only after nurse is able to auscultate sounds clearly.
g. If heart rate is regular, count for 30 sec and multiply by 2.	Regular apical rate can be assessed within 30 sec.
h. If heart is irregular, count for 1 min.	Rate determined is more accurate when measured over longer interval.
i. Note regularity of any existing dysrhythmia (S_1 and S_2 occur early or later after previous sequence of sounds; S_1 or S_2 is absent for a beat).	Regular occurrence of dysrhythmia within 1 min may indicate need for further cardiac evaluation (see p. 483).
j. Replace gown and bed linen. Assist client in returning to comfortable position.	Maintains comfort.
7. Discuss findings with client.	Promotes participation in care and understanding of health status.
8. Wash hands.	Reduces transmission of microorganisms.
9. Compare pulse rate and character with previous baseline and/or normal pulse range for age group.	Allows assessment for change in condition and for cardiac alteration.
10. Record pulse characteristics on vital signs flowsheet or nurses' notes and report abnormal findings.	Immediate documentation ensures accuracy in medical record. Abnormalities may require therapy.

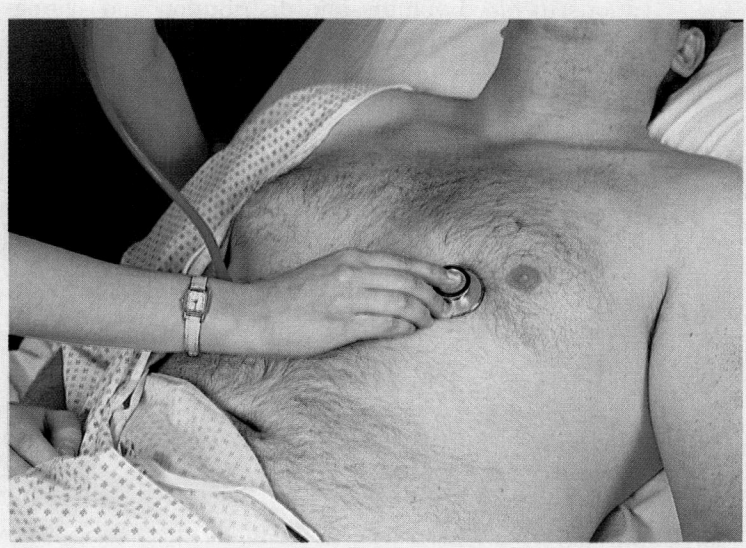

Step 6e

examiner. The four major parts of the stethoscope are the earpieces, binaurals, plastic or rubber tubing, and chestpiece (Fig. 19-11).

The earpieces should fit snugly and comfortably in the nurse's ears. The binaurals should be angled and strong enough so that the earpieces stay firmly in the ears without causing discomfort. To ensure the best reception of sound, the earpieces follow the contour of the ear canal. For most persons therefore the earpieces should point toward the face as the stethoscope is put on.

The rubber or plastic tubing should be flexible and 30 to 40 cm (12 to 18 in) in length. Longer tubing decreases the transmission of sound waves. The tubing should have a thick wall to help eliminate transmission of noises when the tubing rubs against other surfaces.

The chestpiece consists of a bell and a diaphragm. The diaphragm is the circular, flat-surfaced portion of the chestpiece and has a thin plastic disk on the end. It transmits high-pitched sounds, such as bowel and lung sounds, best. The examiner holds the diaphragm firmly against the skin for full sound amplification. The bell transmits low-pitched sounds such as heart and vascular sounds. It is held lightly against the skin. Compressing the bell against the skin reduces sound amplification. The bell and diaphragm are rotated into position on the chestpiece, depending on the part that the nurse chooses to use. The diaphragm or bell must be in proper position during use for the nurse to hear sounds through the stethoscope.

Character of the Pulse

Assessment of the radial pulse includes measurement of the pulse rate, rhythm, strength, and equality. When auscultating an apical pulse, the nurse assesses the heart rate and rhythm only.

Rate

Before measuring a pulse, the nurse should know the baseline heart rate for comparison (Table 19-5). Pulse rates vary, depending on age, level of activity, and a variety of other factors (see box). The sinoatrial (SA) node in the heart is the primary pacemaker of the heart, setting the heart rate faster or slower, depending on the metabolic demands of the body. To obtain a baseline pulse, the client should be at rest during measurement of the pulse because physical activity increases the heart rate. It may be necessary to wait 5 to 10 minutes after activity before measuring the pulse.

Some practitioners prefer to make baseline measurements of the pulse rate as the client assumes sitting, standing, and lying positions. Postural changes cause changes in pulse rate resulting from alterations in blood volume and distribution and sympathetic activity. The heart rate typically increases when a person moves from a lying to a sitting or standing position. To assess peripheral pulse rate, the nurse counts the number of arterial pulsations for a

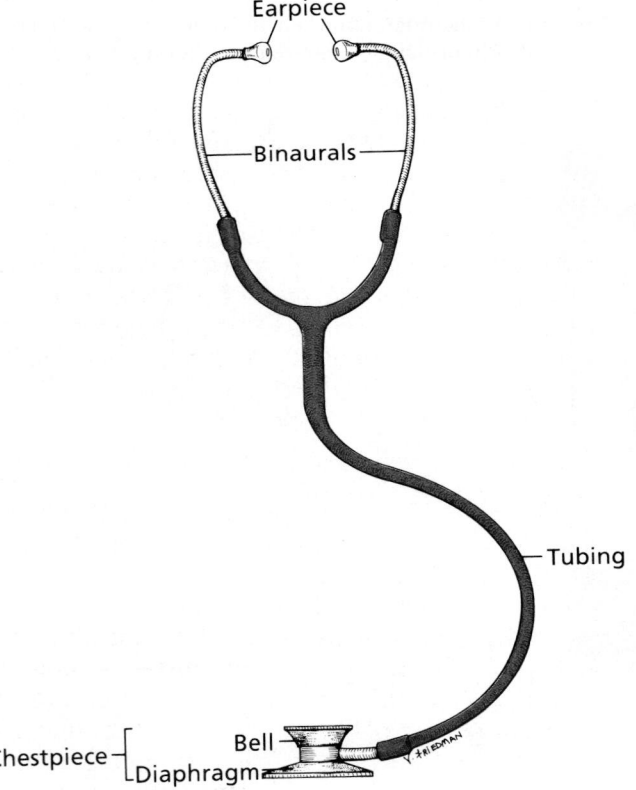

Fig. 19-11 Acoustical stethoscope.

| | Heart Rate* | | |
Age	Resting (Awake)	Resting (Sleeping)	Exercise or Fever
Newborn	100-180	80-160	Up to 220
1 wk to 3 mo	100-220	80-200	Up to 220
3 mo to 2 yr	80-150	70-120	Up to 200
2 yr to 10 yr	70-110	60-90	Up to 200
10 yr to adult	55-90	50-90	Up to 200

TABLE 19-5 Normal Heart Rates

*In beats/min.
From Gillette PC: Dysrhythmias. In Adams FH, Emmanouilides GC, editors: *Moss' heart disease in infants, children, and adolescents*, ed 3, Baltimore, 1983, Williams & Wilkins.

select number of seconds. Then the nurse calculates the number of pulsations that would occur in 60 seconds. If a pulse is irregular, an accurate measurement is made by counting for a full minute.

The nurse assesses an apical pulse by listening for heart sounds (see Chapter 20). The nurse tries to identify the first and second heart sounds (S_1 and S_2). At normal slow rates, S_1 is low pitched and dull in quality, sounding like a "lub." S_2 is a higher pitched and shorter sound and creates the sound "dub." Using the diaphragm or bell of the stethoscope the nurse counts the number of *lub-dubs* occurring in a minute. One *lub-dub* equals one heart beat. For the beginning student a bell may be more difficult to use. However, it is best for detecting vascular sounds.

The nurse may assess common variations in heart rate. **Tachycardia** is an abnormally elevated heart rate, above 100 beats per minute. **Bradycardia** is a rate below 60 beats per minute. The nurse assesses an apical pulse when tachycardia or bradycardia are detected at peripheral pulse sites.

Rhythm

Successive heart beats normally occur at regular intervals. If an interval is interrupted by an early beat or if a beat is late or missed, the individual has an abnormal rhythm (**dysrhythmia**) (see Chapter 20). A dysrhythmia alters the heart's ability to pump properly, particularly if it occurs repetitively. The nurse assesses dysrhythmia by palpating an interruption in the successive pulse waves or auscultating an interruption between sounds. If dysrhythmia is present, the regularity of its occurrence is assessed. It may be intermittent (occasional missed beats) or irregularly irregular (variation in frequency). Children often have a sinus dysrythmia, which is an irregular heart beat that speeds up with inspiration and slows down with expiration. This is a normal finding and can be verified by having the child hold the breath; the heart rate should then become regular.

When palpating for an irregular peripheral pulse, the nurse should also assess for a **pulse deficit,** which occurs when the heart ejects a volume of blood so small that it goes to the brain and peripheral pulse waves cannot be felt. The pulse deficit is evaluated by measuring the **apical-radial pulse.** This is usually done by two people; however, one nurse can do it with some difficulty. One nurse counts the apical impulses heard with a stethoscope while another counts the palpated radial pulse at exactly the same time. Any variation is considered the pulse deficit and should be reported to the client's physician. For example, an apical rate of 92 with a radial rate of 78 leaves a pulse deficit of 14 beats. Chapter 20 also describes the technique used to assess for pulse deficit.

To confirm the presence of a dysrhythmia, the physician may order an **electrocardiogram** to map the electrical activity of the heart for a 12-second interval, or an order for a Holter monitor or cardiac telemetry may be made. **Holter monitoring** records the electrical activity of the heart for 24 hours in a small tape recorder that the client wears. Access to the information recorded is not available until after the 24 hours has passed and the data are printed and reviewed (see Chapter 38).

Cardiac telemetry provides continuous monitoring of the heart's electrical activity transmitted to a stationary monitor, often at the nurses' station. Telemetry permits observation of heart rhythm during all of the client's daily activities and thus allows for immediate treatment if the rhythm becomes erratic or unstable. The client recovering from a myocardial infarction or cardiac surgery is monitored for several

---

Factors Influencing Pulse Rates

- **Exercise.** Short-term exercise increases pulse rate. Long-term exercise strengthens heart muscle, resulting in a lower-than-normal rate at rest and a quicker return to the resting rate after exercise.
- **Fever and heat.** Fever and heat increase the pulse rate because of increased metabolic rate.
- **Acute pain and anxiety.** Pain and anxiety increase the pulse rate because of sympathetic stimulation.
- **Unrelieved severe and chronic pain.** Severe and chronic pain decrease the pulse rate because of parasympathetic stimulation.
- **Medications.** Some medications alter pulse rate. For example, digitalis and beta blockers decreases the pulse rate, whereas atropine increases it.
- **Age.** The pulse rate decreases as the aging process progresses from infancy, through puberty, to adulthood. A newborn infant averages 100 to 180 beats per minute, whereas an adult averages 60 to 80 beats/ min. Pulse rate in elder may be greater than 80 beats/min to compensate for a weakened heart muscle, and it can be higher because of medications.
- **Metabolism.** Certain diseases such as hyperthyroidism or cardiomyopathy can cause a chronic elevated pulse rate. Hypothyroidism can cause a slowing of the pulse.
- **Hemorrhage.** Loss of blood increases the pulse rate because of sympathetic stimulation.
- **Postural changes.** Lying down decreases the pulse rate. Standing or sitting increases it.

days with cardiac telemetry because there is a higher risk for developing complications in this time period.

Strength

The strength or amplitude of a pulse reflects the volume of blood ejected against the arterial wall with each heart contraction. Assessing the pulse strength is a subjective process and requires considerable practice. Normally the pulse strength remains the same with each heart beat. A weak pulse is difficult to palpate and easy for the assessor to lose during palpation. The weak pulse is thready and often rapid. A normal pulse is full, easily palpable, and not easily obliterated by the assessor's fingers. A bounding pulse is easily palpated and difficult to obliterate. Some institutions use a classification system for pulse strength (see Chapter 20).

Equality

Pulses on both sides of the peripheral vascular system should be assessed. The nurse assesses both radial pulses to compare the characteristics of each. A pulse in one extremity may be unequal in strength or absent in many disease states (for example, thrombus [clot] formation, aberrant blood vessels, cervical rib syndrome, or aortic dissection).

 ## RESPIRATIONS

Human survival depends on the ability of oxygen (O_2) to reach body cells and for carbon dioxide (CO_2) to be removed from the cells. **Respiration** involves two distinctly different processes: external respiration, or the movement of air between the environment and lungs, and internal respiration, or the movement of O_2 between hemoglobin and single cells. External respiration further involves the following complex but interrelated processes: ventilation, the mechanical movement of air to and from the lungs and the exchange of respiratory gases; conduction, the movement of air through the airways of the lungs; diffusion, movement of O_2 and CO_2 between alveoli and red blood cells; and perfusion, distribution of blood through the pulmonary capillaries.

The nurse can directly assess only the process of external respiration, specifically by assessing ventilation. The rate, depth, and rhythm of ventilatory movements indicate the quality and efficiency of the respiratory process. Diagnostic tests that measure respiratory function and O_2 and CO_2 levels in arterial blood also provide useful data so that ventilation can be assessed.

Physiological Control

Breathing is generally a passive process. Normally a person thinks little about it. The respiratory center in the brainstem regulates the involuntary control of respirations. Adults normally breathe smoothly and uninterrupted, 19 to 20 times a minute.

Ventilation is regulated by levels of CO_2, O_2, and hydrogen ion concentration (**pH**) in the arterial blood. The most important factor in the control of ventilation is the carbon dioxide pressure (PCO_2) of arterial blood. An elevation in the PCO_2 causes the respiratory center to increase the rate and depth of breathing. The increased ventilatory effort removes excess PCO_2 during exhalation. **Hypercarbia,** a chronic excess of CO_2 in arterial blood, can eventually depress ventilation.

Chemoreceptors located in the aorta and carotid arteries are receptors sensitive to CO_2, pH, and **hypoxia** (low levels of arterial O_2). If arterial O_2 levels fall, the chemoreceptors signal the respiratory center to increase the rate and depth of ventilation. Normally, rising PCO_2 levels stimulate the initiation of inspiration, and falling PO_2 levels have a limited impact on the control of ventilation. However, in clients with chronic lung disease such as emphysema or bronchitis, the hypoxic drive to increase ventilation can become very important. These persons may have chronic hypercarbia, which can suppress the normal stimulus for ventilation. A low level of arterial O_2 then becomes the primary stimulus to breathing for some clients who have chronic lung diseases (see Chapter 38).

Mechanics of Breathing

Although breathing is normally passive, muscular work moves the lung and chest wall. Inspiration is more active than expiration. During inspiration the respiratory center sends impulses along the phrenic nerve, causing the diaphragm, a thin, dome-shaped muscle connected to the lower ribs, to contract. As the diaphragm contracts, the abdominal organs move downward and forward, increasing the length of the chest cavity. At the same time the ribs lift upward and outward, causing transverse expansion of the lungs. Fig. 19-12 shows the way that diaphragmatic movement affects the size of the chest cavity. During expiration, the diaphragm relaxes in the elevated position, and the abdominal organs return to their original positions. The elastic lung and chest wall also return to a relaxed state. Little energy is required to move air out of the lungs. Expiration becomes an active process only during exercise, voluntary **hyper-**

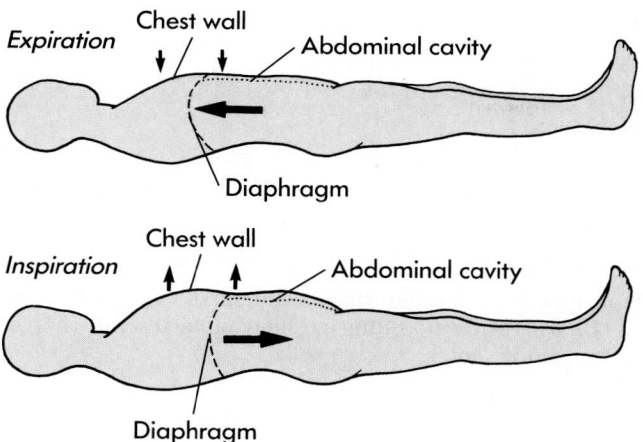

Expiration

Chest wall

Abdominal cavity

Diaphragm

Inspiration

Chest wall

Abdominal cavity

Diaphragm

Fig. 19-12 Illustration of diaphragmatic movement during inspiration and expiration.

Conditions Affecting Ventilatory Movement

- **Chest wall pain.** Pain causes a client to splint or inhibit chest expansion on the painful side. Breaths are shallow.
- **Anemia.** Decreased hemoglobin levels lowers the amount of O_2 carried in the blood. A person breathes faster to increase O_2 delivery.
- **Pneumothorax.** The collapse of all or a portion of a lung lobe reduces chest wall movement on the affected side, causing asymmetry.
- **Emphysema.** This chronic lung condition eventually causes a barrel-shaped appearance of the chest wall. A person actively uses neck and chest wall muscles to forcibly exhale because of air trapped in the lungs.
- **Neuromuscular diseases.** There may be diminished muscle movement due to weakening of chest wall muscles.

---

ventilation (increased ventilation), and certain disease states (see Chapter 38).

The nurse assesses respirations by observing for normal thoracic and abdominal movements and symmetry in chest wall movement. During quiet breathing the chest wall gently rises and falls. Contraction of the intercostal muscles between the ribs or of the accessory muscles in the neck and shoulders is not visible. Passive breathing is more diaphragmatic as the abdominal cavity slowly rises and falls. Breathing during sleep is a good example of passive breathing

using the diaphragm. Infants also use abdominal breathing.

When breathing requires more effort, rib (costal) movement increases. The intercostal and accessory muscles work actively to move air in and out. The shoulders may rise and fall, and the accessory muscles in the neck visibly contract. Diaphragmatic movement is less noticeable when rib movement increases. Certain clinical conditions (see box) affect ventilatory movement. With practice the nurse learns to recognize these conditions.

Assessment of Respirations

Respirations are the easiest of all vital signs to assess but are often the most haphazardly measured. Sometimes a nurse merely estimates the respiratory rate. However, recognition of a subtle change in the character of respirations is important. The following clinical example illustrates this point:

After surgery, Mr. Troy's respirations are 16 per minute, regular, and shallow. Thirty minutes later, he complains of pain across his abdominal incision. The nurse assesses respirations at 28 per minute, regular, and labored. Mr. Troy's physical status has obviously changed, requiring assessment of all vital signs.

A nurse assesses respirations when a client is at rest. If a client is anxious, in pain, or fearful, the respirations will probably be increased in rate and depth. A skillful nurse does not let a client know that respirations are being assessed. A client who is aware of the nurse's intentions may consciously alter the rate and depth of breathing. Assessment is best done immediately after measuring pulse rate, with the nurse's hand still on the client's wrist. The nurse should always assess respirations carefully to avoid overlooking signs that may be relevant to a client's physiological needs. When assessing respirations, the nurse should keep the following factors in mind:

1. The client's normal ventilatory pattern
2. The influences of any disease or illness on respiratory function
3. The relationship between respiratory and cardiovascular function
4. The influence of medical therapies on respirations

Objective measurements composing an assessment of respiratory status include the rate and depth of breathing and the rhythm of ventilatory movements (Procedure 19-3).

Assessing Respirations

STEPS	RATIONALE
1. Assess for factors that normally influence character of respirations.	Allows nurse to accurately assess for presence and significance of respiratory alterations.
2. If client has been active, wait 5 to 10 min.	Exercise increases respiratory rate and depth.
3. Be sure client is in comfortable position, preferably sitting or lying with head of bed elevated 45 to 60 degrees.	Uncomfortable position may cause client to breathe more rapidly. An erect, sitting position promotes full ventilatory movement.
4. Prepare needed equipment and supplies: a. Watch with second hand or digital display b. Pen, pencil, flowsheet or record form	
5. Draw curtain around bed and/or close room door. Wash hands.	Maintains privacy. Prevents transmission of microorganisms.
6. Be sure client's chest is visible. If necessary, move bed linen or gown.	Ensures clear view of chest wall and abdominal movements.
7. Place client's arm in relaxed position across abdomen or lower chest, or place your hand directly over client's upper abdomen (see illustration).	Position is used during assessment of pulse and allows nurse to be inconspicuous. Hand rises and falls during respiratory cycle.
8. Observe complete respiratory cycle (one inspiration and one expiration).	Rate is accurately determined only after you have viewed respiratory cycle.
9. Once cycle has been observed, look at watch's second hand and begin to count rate: when sweep hand hits number on dial, begin time frame, counting *one* with first full respiratory cycle.	Timing begins with count of *one*. Respirations occur more slowly than pulse; thus timing does not begin with *zero*.
10. If rhythm is regular in adult, count number of respirations in 30 sec and multiply by 2. In infant or young child, count respirations for full minute.	Respiratory rate is equivalent to number of respirations per minute. Young infants and children normally breathe irregularly.
11. If adult's respirations have irregular rhythm or are abnormally slow or fast, count for full minute.	Accurate interpretation with irregularities requires assessment for at least 1 min.
12. Note depth of respirations. This can be assessed subjectively by observing degree of chest wall movement while counting rate. Nurse can also objectively assess depth by palpating chest wall excursion (see Chapter 20) after rate has been counted. Depth is shallow, normal, or deep.	Depth of respirations helps reveal volume of air moving to and from lungs. Character of ventilatory movements may reveal specific alterations or disease status.

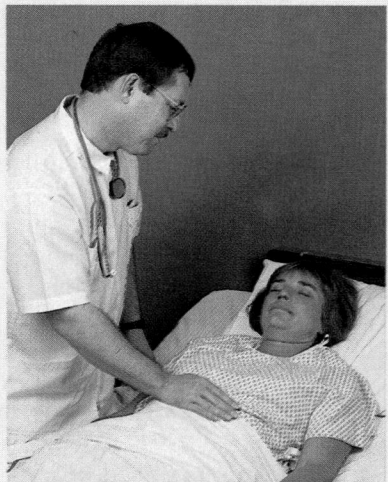

Step 7

CONTINUED

STEPS	RATIONALE
13. Note rhythm of ventilatory cycle. (Normal breathing is regular and uninterrupted.)	Various irregular patterns of ventilations can reveal specific types of alterations.
14. Replace client's gown and cover with bed linen.	Restores comfort.
15. Wash hands.	Reduces transmission of microorganisms.
16. Discuss findings with client as needed.	Promotes participation and understanding of health status.
17. Compare respirations with previous baseline and/or normal respiratory rate for age group.	Allows nurse to assess for change in condition and for respiratory alterations.
18. Record respiratory rate and character on vital sign flowsheet or nurses' notes and report any abnormal findings.	Immediate recording ensures accuracy and inclusion in medical record. Abnormalities may require therapy.

TABLE 19-6 Normal Respiratory Rates by Age

Age Group	Rate	Age Group	Rate
Newborn	35	10 yr	19
1-11 mo	30	12 yr	19
2 yr	25	14 yr	18
4 yr	23	16 yr	17
6 yr	21	18 yr	16-18
8 yrs	20	Adult	12-20

Rate

The nurse observes a full inspiration and expiration when counting a respiration. The respiratory rate varies with age (Table 19-6). An infant normally breathes 30 to 35 times per minute. Throughout childhood, the respiratory rate declines. Among adults, normal rates vary from 19 to 20 respirations per minute. Respiratory rates greater than 20 in adults are called **tachypnea**. Respiratory rates less than 10 are called **bradypnea** and may be seen normally when people sleep. **Apnea** is the absence of breathing, which may be for a few seconds or life threatening if prolonged. The box lists factors affecting character of respirations.

Depth

The depth of respirations is assessed by observing the degree of excursion or movement in the chest wall. The nurse subjectively describes ventilatory movements as *shallow*, *normal*, or *deep*. Chapter 20

Factors Influencing Character of Respirations

- **Exercise.** Exercise increases rate and depth to meet the body's greater O_2 needs.
- **Acute pain.** Pain increases rate and depth as a result of sympathetic stimulation.
- **Anxiety.** Anxiety increases rate and depth as a result of sympathetic stimulation.
- **Smoking.** Long-term smoking changes the lung's airways, resulting in an increased rate.
- **Body position.** Straight, erect posture promotes full chest expansion. Stooped or slumped position impairs ventilatory movement.
- **Medications.** Narcotic analgesics and sedatives depress rate and depth. Amphetamines and cocaine may increase rate and depth.
- **Brainstem injury.** Injury to the brainstem impairs the respiratory center and inhibits respiratory rate and rhythm.

describes a more objective means of measuring chest excursions by palpation of chest wall movement. This technique can be used if the nurse observes that chest excursion is unusually shallow.

During a normal, relaxed breath (**tidal breath**), a person inhales approximately 500 cc of air (tidal volume). The diaphragm moves approximately 1 cm (4/10 inch) down, and the ribs retract upward from the body's midline approximately 1.2 to 2.5 cm (½ to

1 inch). A deep respiration involves a full expansion of the lungs with full exhalation. Respirations are shallow when only a small quantity of air passes through the lungs and ventilatory movement is difficult to see.

The capacity of the lungs to take in air depends on gender and age. Lung capacity is determined by taking as deep a breath as possible and then blowing it all the way out into a **spirometer,** a device that measures air volume. The amount of air exhaled after a minimal full inspiration is the lung's **vital capacity.** Men tend to have a larger vital capacity than women of the same age. Infants and young children have smaller vital capacities than adolescents and adults. With advancing age the lung loses its elasticity, and the capacity for forcible exhalation declines. Nursing care may focus on increasing the client's efforts to breathe deeply. The nurse's knowledge of the client's normal capacity to move air is helpful in planning realistic therapy.

Rhythm

Normal breathing is regular and uninterrupted. A regular interval occurs after each respiratory cycle. An occasional extra deep breath, a sigh, is commonly seen during quiet breathing. Infants tend to breathe less regularly. The young child may breathe slowly for a few seconds and then suddenly breathe more rapidly.

While assessing respirations, the nurse may use some of the advanced technology to make skilled assessments. Noninvasive measurement of CO_2 levels by the transcutaneous method provides a continuous reading of the CO_2 levels in the capillary bed at the level of the skin. This reflects the amount of CO_2 that the lungs are able to effectively clear or ineffectively retain. **End-tidal CO_2 monitoring** measures the amount of CO_2 exhaled by the lungs at the end of a tidal breath. This device is mainly used with clients who have artificial airways.

Noninvasive assessment of oxygenation is simple. An **oximeter** equipped with a probe to clip to the finger or ear can provide continuous or intermittent determinations of **oxygen saturation** (percent of hemoglobin saturated with oxygen). This provides a reliable method of assessing adequacy of oxygenation and indirectly assessing adequacy of ventilation (see Chapter 38).

Another respiratory monitoring device that aids the nurse's assessment is the apnea monitor. This

TABLE 19-7 Alterations in Respiration	
Term	Description
Bradypnea	Rate of breathing is abnormally slow (less than 10 beats/min) but regular.
Tachypnea	Rate of breathing is abnormally rapid (greater than 20 breaths/min) but regular.
Hyperpnea	Respirations are increased in depth and rate. This occurs normally with exercise.
Apnea	Respirations cease for several seconds. Persistent cessation is called *respiratory arrest.*
Hyperventilation	Rate of ventilation exceeds normal metabolic requirements for exchange of respiratory gases. Rate and depth of respirations increase. There is excessive intake of O_2 and blowing off of CO_2.
Hypoventilation	Rate of ventilation entering lungs is insufficient for metabolic needs. Respiratory rate is below normal, and depth of ventilation is depressed. There is decreased O_2 intake and CO_2 exhalation.
Cheyne-Stokes respiration	Respiratory rhythm is irregular, characterized by alternating periods of apnea and hyperventilation. Respiratory cycle begins with slow, shallow breaths that gradually increase to abnormal depth and rapidity. Gradually, breathing slows and becomes shallower, climaxing in 10- to 20-second period of apnea before respiration resumes.
Kussmaul's respiration	Respirations are abnormally deep but regular, similar to hyperventilation. Rate is increased. This is characteristic of clients with diabetic ketoacidosis.
Dyspnea	Breathing is difficult and characterized by increased effort to inhale and exhale. Client actively uses intercostal and accessory muscles to breathe.
Sighing	Not to be confused with abnormal ventilatory rhythm, sigh is protective physiological mechanism for expanding small airways and alveoli not used during a normal tidal breath.
Orthopnea	Orthopnea is respiratory condition in which person must sit or stand to breathe deeply or comfortably.
Biot's respiration	Condition of the central nervous system causes shallow breathing interrupted by irregular periods of apnea.

device has leads that attach to a client's chest wall to sense movement, or more specifically apnea. Apnea monitoring is used frequently with infants in the hospital and at home to observe for prolonged apneic events. Noninvasive monitoring provides information that helps the nurse assess the rate, depth, and rhythm of respiration more knowledgeably.

General Respiratory Characteristics

While assessing the three objective qualities of rate, depth, and rhythm, the nurse also observes factors related to the general character of respirations. Depending on the level of oxygenation, respiratory alterations may cause changes in skin color and level of consciousness. The nail beds, lips, and skin may take on a bluish or cyanotic appearance when arterial O_2 levels are reduced (see Chapter 20). As oxygenation decreases, a person typically becomes more restless and anxious and tries harder to breathe.

Difficulty in breathing is **dyspnea.** As breathing becomes labored a person uses accessory muscles in the chest and neck to breathe. A client with dyspnea usually feels short of breath.

Sounds of breathing may indicate a respiratory disorder. Inflammation or stricture of the trachea or larynx causes obstruction to airflow. As a client inhales, air passing the obstruction creates a harsh, crowing sound, or respiratory stridor, which can easily be heard without a stethoscope. Secretions in the large airways of the trachea and the bronchus can often be heard without a stethoscope. These sounds can occur during inspiration or expiration. They have a gurgling sound and are called *rhonchi* or *gurgles.* Chapter 20 describes in detail the normal and abnormal breath sounds that can be heard by auscultation with a stethoscope.

Respiratory alterations may cause changes in the features or characteristics of breathing. Table 19-7 describes several common respiratory alterations.

BLOOD PRESSURE

To cause blood to flow throughout the circulatory system, the heart pumps blood into the arteries under high pressure. **Blood pressure** is the force exerted by the blood against a vessel wall. The standard unit for measuring blood pressure is millimeters of mercury (mm Hg). The measurement indicates the height to which the blood pressure can raise a column of mercury. During a normal cardiac cycle (see Chapter 20), blood pressure reaches a peak that is followed by a trough. The peak or maximum pressure occurs during **systole** as the left ventricle pumps blood into the aorta. The trough occurs during **diastole** as the ventricles relax. Diastolic pressure is the minimal pressure exerted against the arterial walls at all times. The nurse records blood pressure with the systolic reading before the diastolic (for example, 120/80). The difference between systolic and diastolic pressure is the **pulse pressure.** Thus if the blood pressure is 120/80, the pulse pressure is 40 mm Hg.

Physiology of Arterial Blood Pressure

Blood pressure reflects the balance between various factors, including cardiac output, blood volume, **peripheral vascular resistance** (resistance within the blood vessels in the periphery of the body) and blood viscosity (thickness). Each factor can affect another. For example, an increase in blood volume increases cardiac output. These factors have an impact on blood movement and blood pressure in the body and are known as *hemodynamic factors.* Knowledge of the hemodynamic variables helps the nurse assess blood pressure alterations. The box lists how hemodynamic factors can affect blood pressure.

The complex control of the cardiovascular system normally prevents any single factor from permanently changing blood pressure. For example, if blood volume falls, the body compensates with increased peripheral resistance due to vasoconstriction. This shunts blood to vital organs and maintains the blood pressure at a normal level. When vascular resistance increases, the blood pressure rises. The size of arteries and arterioles changes to adjust blood flow to the needs of local tissues. The smaller the lumen (internal diameter) of a vessel, the greater its peripheral vascular resistance to blood flow. When blood

---

Hemodynamic Effects on Blood Pressure

FACTORS THAT INCREASE BLOOD PRESSURE

- Increased cardiac output
- Increased peripheral vascular resistance
- Increased blood volume
- Increased blood viscosity

FACTORS THAT DECREASE BLOOD PRESSURE

- Decreased cardiac output
- Decreased peripheral vascular resistance
- Decreased blood volume
- Decreased blood viscosity

flow to a major organ falls sharply, peripheral arteries vasoconstrict to shunt blood back to the major vessels supplying the organ. Arterial pressure rises to push blood through narrowed vessels. In contrast, as vessels dilate and vascular resistance falls, blood pressure drops.

The blood pressure (BP) is a product of the cardiac output (CO) and peripheral vascular resistance (R), so BP = CO × R. When volume increases in an enclosed space, the pressure in that space rises. Thus as the cardiac output increases, more blood is pumped against the arterial walls, causing an elevation in blood pressure. Exercise temporarily elevates blood pressure as the demand for cardiac output increases.

The volume of blood circulating within the vascular system affects blood pressure. Most adults have a circulating blood volume of 5000 ml. Normally the blood volume remains constant. However, if volume increases, more pressure is exerted against arterial walls. The rapid, uncontrolled infusion of intravenous fluids is a typical cause of elevated blood pressure. When circulating blood volume falls to a critical level, as in the case of hemorrhage or dehydration, blood pressure falls.

Normally the walls of an artery are elastic and easily distensible. As pressure within the arteries increases, the diameter of vessel walls also increases. Arterial distensibility prevents wide fluctuations in blood pressure. For example, if the volume pumped by the heart suddenly increases, arteries can distend and absorb much of the increase in pressure. However, in certain diseases such as arteriosclerosis the vessel walls lose their elasticity and are replaced by fibrous tissue that cannot stretch well. With reduced elasticity, there is greater resistance to blood flow.

Peripheral vascular resistance increases. As a result, when the left ventricle ejects its stroke volume, the vessels no longer yield to the pressure. Instead, a given volume of blood is forced through the rigid arterial walls, and the pressure rises. Systolic pressure is more significantly elevated than diastolic because of reduced arterial elasticity.

The thickness or viscosity of blood affects the ease with which blood flows through small vessels. The **hematocrit,** or percentage of red blood cells in the blood, determines blood viscosity. When the hematocrit rises and blood flow slows, arterial blood pressure increases.

Factors Influencing Blood Pressure

Blood pressure does not stay constant. Many factors influence it throughout the day. An understanding of these factors ensures a more accurate interpretation of blood pressure readings.

Age

Normal blood pressure levels vary throughout life. They increase during childhood. The level of a child's or adolescent's blood pressure is assessed with respect to body size and age (Task Force on Blood Pressure Control in Children, 1987). An infant's blood pressure ranges from 65-115/42-80. The normal blood pressure for a 7 year old is 87-117/48-64. Larger children (heavier and/or taller) have higher blood pressures than smaller children of the same age.

During adolescence, blood pressure continues to vary according to body size. However, the normal range for 10 to 19 year olds at the 90th percentile is 124-136/77-84 for boys and 124-127/63-74 for girls.

TABLE 19-8 Antihypertensive Medications		
Medication Type	Names	Actions
Diuretics	Furosemide (Lasix), spironolactone (Aldactone), metolazone, polythizide, benzthiazide	Lower blood pressure by reducing reabsorption of sodium and water by the kidneys, thus lowering circulating fluid volume.
Beta-adrenergic blockers	Atenolol (Tenormin), nadolol (Corgard), timolol maleate (Blocadren), propranalol (Inderal)	Combine with beta-adrenergic receptors in the heart, arteries, and arterioles to block response to sympathetic nerve impulses. Reduce heart rate and thus cardiac output.
Vasodilators	Hydralazine hydrochloride (Apresoline), minoxidil (Loniten)	Act on arteriolar smooth muscle to cause relaxation and reduce peripheral vascular resistance.
Calcium channel blockers	Verapamil hydrochloride (Calan), nifedipine (Procardia)	Reduce peripheral vascular resistance by systemic vasodilation.

An adult's blood pressure tends to increase with advancing age. The standard norm for a healthy, middle-age adult is 120/80. A systolic pressure below 140 mm and a diastolic pressure below 90 mm are still considered normal. The older adult's blood pressure range is 140-160/80-90.

Stress

Anxiety, fear, pain, and emotional stress initiate sympathetic stimulation, causing the blood pressure to rise. Sympathetic stimulation increases the heart rate, which increases the cardiac output and vasoconstriction, which results in increased peripheral vascular resistance.

Race

The rate of **hypertension** (high blood pressure) is higher in urban African Americans than in European Americans (National Academy of Science, 1989). Hypertension-related deaths are also higher among African Americans. The tendency for this population to have hypertension is believed to be genetically and environmentally related.

Medications

Some medications can directly or indirectly affect blood pressure. During blood pressure assessment, the nurse asks whether the client is receiving antihypertensive medications, which lower blood pressure (Table 19-8). Another class of medications affecting blood pressure is narcotic analgesics, which can lower blood pressure.

Diurnal Variation

Blood pressure levels vary over the course of a day. The blood pressure is typically lowest in the early morning. It gradually rises during the morning and afternoon, peaking in late afternoon or evening. No two persons have the same pattern or degree of variation. A student may find it interesting to have a friend check blood pressure at intervals during 24 hours.

Hypertension

Hypertension is a major factor underlying death from strokes in the United States, and it also contributes to myocardial infarctions (heart attacks). The Joint National Committee on Detection, Evaluation, and Treatment of High Blood Pressure (1988) has set criteria for determining categories of hypertension (Table 19-9). The diagnosis of hypertension in adults is made when an average of two or more diastolic readings on at least two subsequent visits is 90 mm Hg or higher or when an average of two or more systolic readings on at least two visits is higher than 140 mm Hg. One blood pressure recording does not qualify as a diagnosis of hypertension. However, if the nurse assesses a high reading (for example, 150/90 mm Hg), the client should be encouraged to return for another checkup within 2 months (Table 19-10).

TABLE 19-9   Classification of Blood Pressure

Range*	Category
DIASTOLIC	
<85	Normal blood pressure
85-89	High normal blood pressure
90-104	Mild hypertension
105-114	Moderate hypertension
≥115	Severe hypertension
SYSTOLIC, WHEN DIASTOLIC BP IS <90	
<140	Normal blood pressure
140-159	Borderline isolated systolic hypertension
≥160	Isolated systolic hypertension

*In mm Hg.
From The Joint National Committee on Detection, Evaluation, and Treatment of High Blood Pressure: The 1988 report of the Joint National Committee on Detection, Evaluation, and Treatment of High Blood Pressure, *Arch Intern Med* 148:1023, 1988.

TABLE 19-10   Follow-Up Criteria for First Measurement

Range*	Recommended Follow-Up
DIASTOLIC	
<85	Recheck within 2 yr.
85-89	Recheck within 1 yr.
90-104	Confirm promptly (not to exceed 2 mo).
105-114	Evaluate or refer to source of care (not to exceed 2 wk).
≥115	Evaluate or refer immediately to a source of care.
SYSTOLIC, WHEN DIASTOLIC PRESSURE IS LESS THAN 90	
<140	Recheck within 2 yr.
140-199	Confirm promptly (not to exceed 2 mo).
≥200	Evaluate or refer promptly to source of care (not to exceed 2 wk).

*In mm Hg.
From The Joint National Committee on Detection, Evaluation, and Treatment of High Blood Pressure: 1988 report of the Joint National Committee on Detection, Evaluation and Treatment of High Blood Pressure, *Arch Intern Med* 148:1023, 1988.

When a nurse assesses a client's blood pressure for the first time, an average of two or more measurements should be taken with the client positioned comfortably (Joint National Committee on Detection, Evaluation, and Treatment of High Blood Pressure, 1988).

Hypertension causes thickening and loss of elasticity in the arterial walls. Peripheral vascular resistance increases within the affected vessels. As a result, blood flow to vital organs such as the heart, brain, and kidney decreases. The heart must continually pump against greater resistance.

The nurse can educate clients about their risks for hypertension. Persons with family members who have had hypertension are at significant risk. Other risk factors for hypertension are listed in the box. When clients are diagnosed with hypertension, the nurse helps to educate them about the following factors (Joint National Committee on Detection, Evaluation, and Treatment of High Blood Pressure, 1988):

1. Blood pressure values
2. Long-term follow-up care and therapy
3. The usual lack of symptoms (the fact that it may not be "felt")
4. Therapy's ability to control but not cure hypertension
5. A consistently followed treatment plan that can ensure a relatively normal lifestyle

Hypotension

Hypotension is generally considered present when the systolic blood pressure falls to 90 mm Hg or below. Although some adults have a low blood pressure normally, for the majority of people, low blood pressure is an abnormal finding associated with illness.

Hypotension occurs in disease because of the dilation of the arteries in the vascular bed (that is, shock), the loss of a substantial amount of blood vol-

---

Risk Factors for Hypertension

- Family history of hypertension
- Obesity
- Cigarette smoking
- Heavy alcohol consumption
- Elevated blood cholesterol level
- Continued exposure to stress

---

ume (that is, hemorrhage), or the failure of the heart muscle to pump adequately (that is, myocardial infarction). Hypotension associated with pallor, skin mottling, clamminess, confusion, increased heart rate, or decreased urine output may be life threatening and should be reported to a physician immediately.

Assessment of Blood Pressure

Blood pressure may be measured directly or indirectly. The direct method requires the insertion of a thin intravenous catheter into an artery. Tubing connects the catheter with an electronic sensor. Pressure within the artery transmits pressure along the fluid-filled tubing to the sensor, which then displays a blood pressure reading on an electronic display. Direct monitoring is used only in an operating room or critical care areas.

The indirect method requires use of the sphygmomanometer. The nurse may use auscultation, palpation, or both. Assessing the blood pressure indirectly by auscultation is the most common technique.

Sphygmomanometer

To assess blood pressure the nurse must have equipment that functions properly. The nurse also must be competent and feel comfortable when using a stethoscope and sphygmomanometer.

A **sphygmomanometer** consists of a pressure manometer, an occlusive cloth cuff enclosing an inflatable rubber bladder, and a pressure bulb with a release valve to inflate the cuff (Fig. 19-13). There are two types of manometers, mercury and aneroid. The mercury manometer is the most accurate. It is an upright tube containing mercury. Pressure created by inflation of the compression cuff moves the column of mercury upward against the force of gravity. Millimeter calibrations mark the height of the mercury column. To ensure accurate readings, the mercury column should always be at *zero* when the cuff is deflated, and it should fall freely as pressure is released. Repeated calibrations are not needed as long as this is done. Deviations indicate that the manometer is malfunctioning. Mercury manometers are mounted on the wall or are portable. Accurate readings are made by looking at the mercury meniscus at eye level. This is the point where the crescent-shaped top of the mercury column aligns with the manometer scale. Looking up or down at the mercury results in measurement distortions.

The aneroid manometer has a glass-enclosed circular gauge containing a needle that registers millimeter calibrations. A metal bellows within the gauge expands and collapses in response to pressure varia-

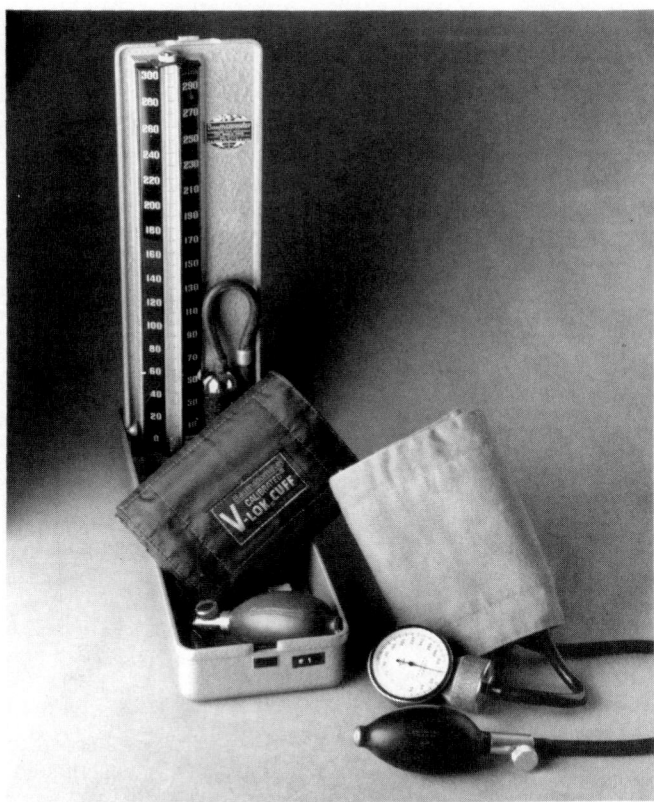

Fig. 19-13 Mercury *(left)* and aneroid sphygmomanometer.

TABLE 19-11 Common Mistakes in Blood Pressure Assessment

Error	Effect
Bladder or cuff too wide	False low reading
Bladder or cuff too narrow	False high reading
Cuff wrapped too loosely	False high reading
Deflating cuff too slowly	False high diastolic reading
Deflating cuff too quickly	False low systolic and false high diastolic reading
Stethoscope that fits poorly or impairment of the examiner's hearing, causing sounds to be muffled	False low systolic and false high diastolic reading
Inaccurate inflation level	False low systolic reading
Multiple examiners using different Korotkoff sounds for diastolic readings	Inaccurate interpretation of systolic and diastolic readings

tions in the inflated cuff. Before using the aneroid model, the nurse must be sure that the needle points to *zero* and that the manometer is correctly calibrated. An aneroid manometer should be recalibrated against a perfectly working mercury manometer at least once a year. Aneroid manometers have the advantages of being lightweight, portable, and compact.

Cloth cuffs used with the sphygmomanometer come in several sizes. Ideally the width of the cuff should be 40% of the circumference (or 20% wider than the diameter) of the midpoint of the limb on which the cuff is to be used (American Heart Association, 1987). The length of the enclosed bladder should be approximately twice the recommended width. A bladder of this length nearly encircles the arm and minimizes the risk of misapplication. In an adult the average bladder width is 12 to 13 cm., and the length is 22 to 23 cm. In children the lower edge of the cuff should be above the antecubital fossa, allowing room for placement of the stethoscope. An improperly fitting cuff causes inaccurate readings (Table 19-11).

Before using a sphygmomanometer the nurse should inspect the parts of the release valve and the pressure bulb. The valve should be clean and freely movable in either direction. If it sticks or becomes too tightly closed, the deflation of the pressure cuff will be hard to regulate. The pressure bulb is made of tough rubber and should be free of leaks.

A third type of sphygmomanometer is used by clients in the community for ambulatory (or home) monitoring. This type of manometer is battery driven and functions by noting oscillations or by auscultating sounds of blood flow. This equipment needs to be carefully calibrated against a mercury manometer for accuracy.

Auscultation

The best environment for blood pressure measurement by auscultation (Procedure 19-4) is a quiet room at a comfortable temperature. The nurse attempts to control the client's pain, anxiety, or exertion and asks the client to refrain from eating or smoking before the assessment because these factors can cause false high readings.

Although the client may lie or stand, sitting is the preferred position. Some clients, especially older adults, may experience postural or **orthostatic hypotension** (a drop of 25 mm Hg in systolic pressure and a drop of 10 mm Hg in diastolic pressure when moving from a lying to sitting or a sitting to standing position). Orthostatic hypotension is a common side effect of antihypertensive medications. To detect orthostatic blood pressure changes, the nurse obtains the

Assessing Blood Pressure by Auscultation

STEPS	RATIONALE
1. Assess for factors that normally influence blood pressure.	Allows nurse to accurately assess blood pressure and significance of pressure changes.
2. Determine best site for assessment. Avoid applying cuff to arm when intravenous catheter is in antecubital fossa and fluids are infusing, when arteriovenous shunt is present, or when breast or axillary surgery has been performed on that side; avoid it also, if arm or hand has been traumatized or diseased or if lower arm is enclosed by cast or bulky bandage.	Inappropriate site selection may result in poor amplification of sounds, causing inaccurate readings. Application of pressure from inflated bladder can temporarily impair blood flow and compromise circulation in extremity that already has impaired circulation.
3. Prepare equipment and supplies and make sure they work:	
a. Mercury sphygmomanometer: control valve should be clear and freely adjustable; when closed, valve should hold mercury constant; when released, valve allows controlled fall in mercury level; air vent at top of mercury manometer should be patent; rubber tubing connecting bladder to manometer should be at least 80 cm (32 in) long with air-tight connections.	Used to measure arterial blood pressure indirectly. Accurate measurements depend on functional equipment.
b. Bladder and cuff: bladder should completely encircle arm without overlapping; tapering cuff should be long enough to encircle arm several times.	Secure-fitting cuff and proper-sized bladder are needed to exert equal pressure around artery being auscultated. Too-narrow bladder causes false high reading.

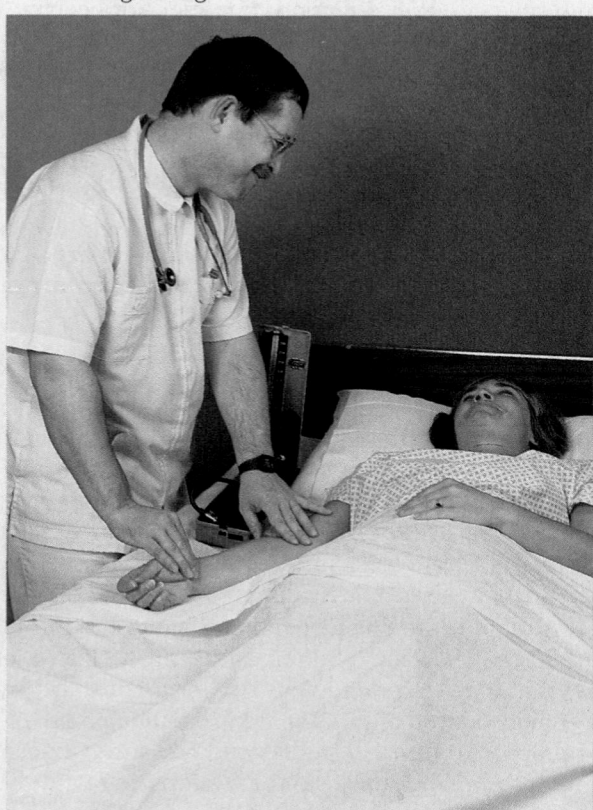

Step 8

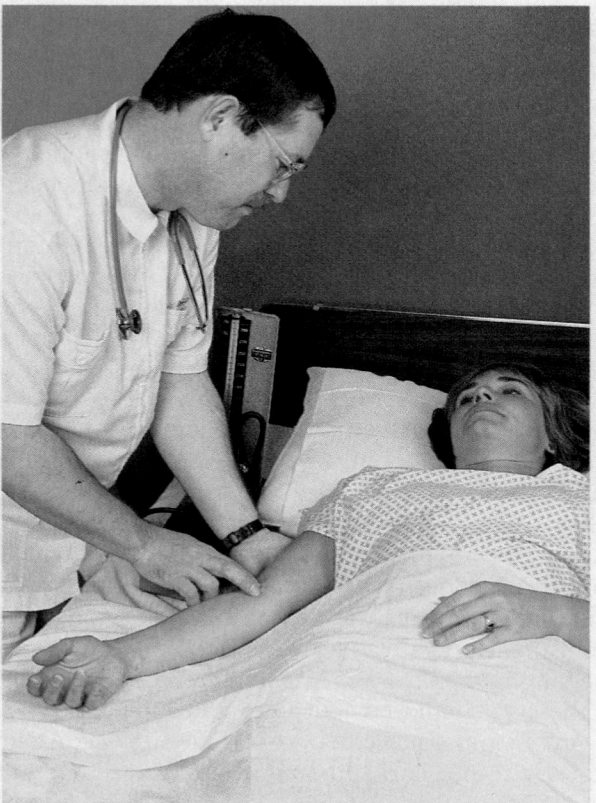

Step 10

STEPS	RATIONALE
c. Stethoscope	Auscultates arterial pressure waves.
d. Pen, pencil, and flowsheet or record form	Provide for timely documentation of findings.
4. Encourage client to avoid exercise and smoking for 30 min before assessment.	These factors can cause false elevations in blood pressure.
5. Have client assume sitting or lying position. Be sure room is warm and quiet.	Maintains comfort during measurement.
6. Explain procedure to client and have client rest at least 5 min before measurement.	Reduces anxiety that can falsely elevate readings. Readings taken at different times can be objectively compared when all are assessed with client at rest.
7. Wash hands.	Reduces transmission of microorganisms.
8. Support client's bare upper arm (while client is sitting or lying) at heart level with palm turned up (see illustration).	If arm is unsupported, client may perform isometric exercise that can increase diastolic pressure 10%. Placement of arm above heart level causes false low reading.
9. Expose upper arm fully by removing constricting clothing.	Ensures proper cuff application.
10. Palpate brachial artery (see illustration). Position cuff 2.5 cm (1 in) above brachial pulsation (antecubital space). Center bladder above artery (see illustration).	Inflating bladder directly over brachial artery ensures that proper pressure is applied during inflation.
11. With cuff fully deflated, wrap cuff evenly and snugly around upper arm (see illustration).	Loose-fitting cuff causes false high readings.

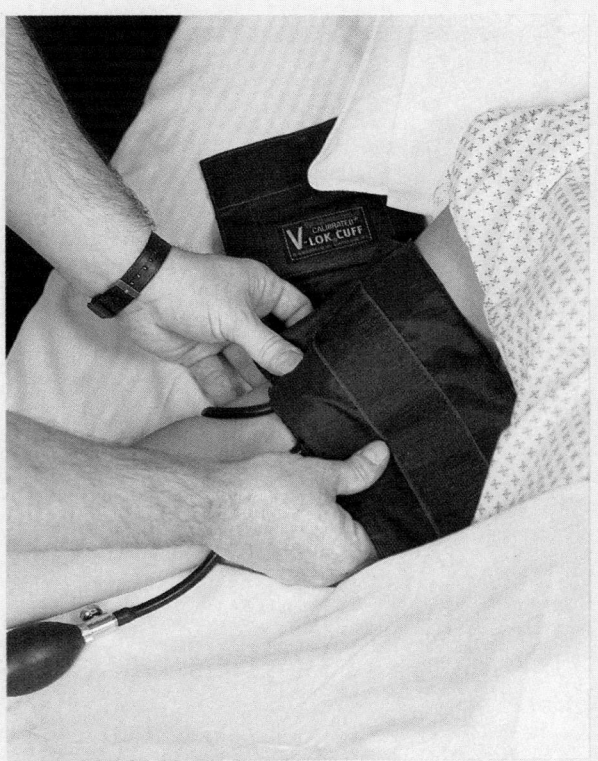

Step 10

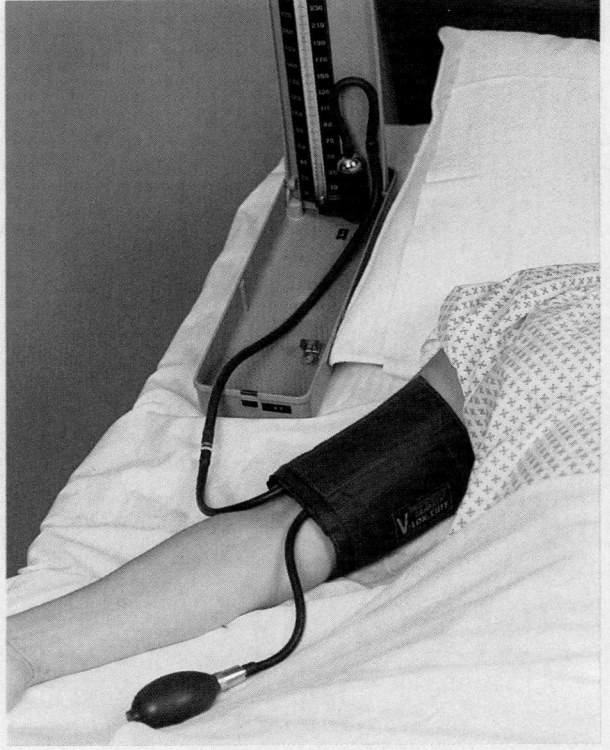

Step 11

Assessing Blood Pressure by Auscultation

STEPS	RATIONALE
12. Be sure manometer is positioned vertically at eye level. Stand no further than 1 m (approximately 1 yd) away.	Eye level placement ensures accurate reading of mercury level.
13. Palpate brachial or radial artery with fingertips of one hand while inflating cuff rapidly to 30 mm Hg pressure above point at which pulse disappears. Slowly deflate cuff and note point when pulse reappears.	Identifies approximate systolic pressure and determines maximum inflation point for accurate reading. Prevents auscultatory gap.
14. Deflate cuff fully and wait 30 sec.	Prevents venous congestion and false high readings.
15. Place stethoscope earpieces in ears and be sure sounds are clear, not muffled.	Each earpiece should follow angle of ear canal to facilitate hearing.
16. Relocate brachial artery and place bell or diaphragm chestpiece over it. Do not allow chestpiece to touch cuff or clothing (see illustration).	Proper stethoscope placement ensures optimal sound reception. Stethoscope improperly positioned causes muffled sounds that often result in false low systolic and false high diastolic readings.
17. Close valve of pressure bulb clockwise until tight.	Tightening of valve prevents air leak during inflation.
18. Inflate cuff to 30 mm Hg above palpated systolic pressure (see illustration).	Ensures accurate measurement of systolic pressure.
19. Slowly release valve and allow mercury to fall at rate of 2-3 mm Hg/sec.	Too rapid or slow a decline in mercury level can cause inaccurate readings.
20. Note point on manometer when first clear sound is heard.	First Korotkoff sound indicates systolic pressure.

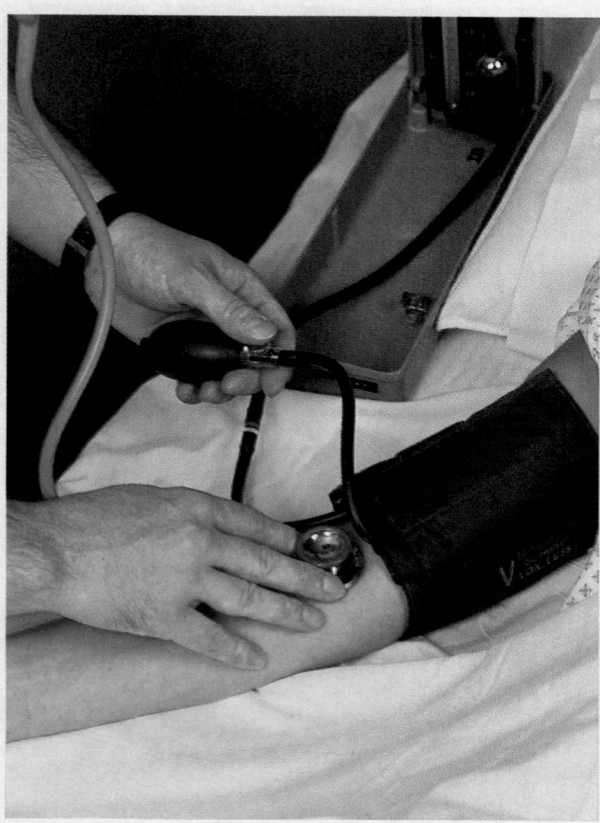

Step 16

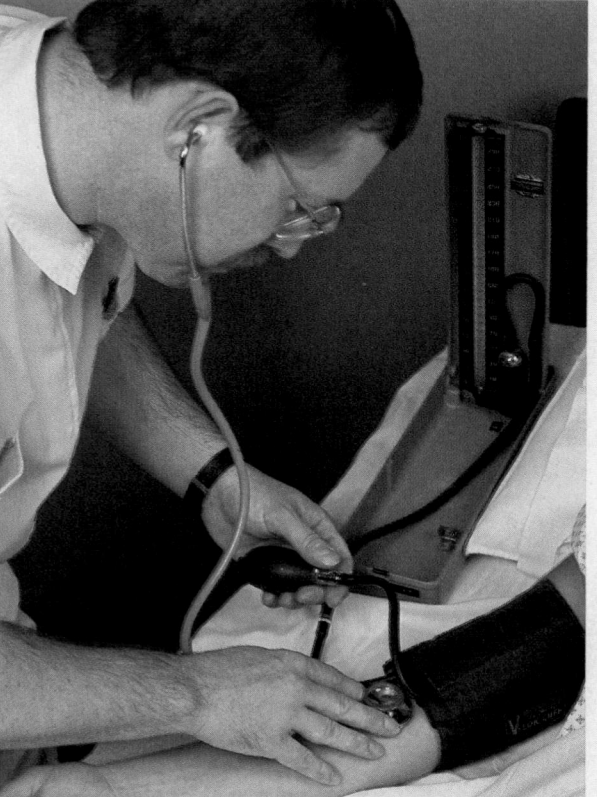

Step 18

STEPS	RATIONALE
21. Continue to deflate cuff gradually, noting point at which muffled or dampened sound appears.	Fourth Korotkoff sound involves distinct muffling of sounds and is recommended by American Heart Association (1987) as indication of diastolic pressure in children.
22. Continue cuff deflation, noting point on manometer at which sound disappears. (Note pressure to nearest 2 mm Hg.)	American Heart Association (1987) recommends recording fifth Korotkoff sound as diastolic pressure in adults.
23. Deflate cuff rapidly and completely. Remove from arm unless you plan to repeat measurement.	Continuous cuff inflation causes arterial occlusion, resulting in numbness and tingling of arm.
24. If this is first assessment of client, repeat procedure on other arm.	Comparison of pressure in both arms serves to detect circulatory problems. (Normal difference of 5 to 10 mm Hg exists between arms.)
25. Assist client in returning to comfortable position and cover upper arm if previously clothed.	Restores comfort.
26. Inform client of reading.	Promotes participation in care and understanding of health status.
27. Wash hands.	Prevents transmission of microorganisms.
28. Compare reading with previous baseline and/or normal average pressure for client's age.	Evaluates for change in condition and presence of blood pressure alterations.
29. Record blood pressure in nurses' notes or flowsheet and report abnormal findings immediately.	Vital signs should be recorded immediately to ensure accuracy.

client's blood pressure in the lying position. The client is then asked to stand if possible. The blood pressure is rechecked in the same arm after 30 to 60 seconds in the upright position. Normally, variations greater than 10 mm Hg systolic pressure, a fall of systolic pressure below 90 mm Hg, or complaints of lightheadedness should be reported to the physician. Normally, blood pressures obtained with a client in different positions are similar.

The nurse should initially measure blood pressure in both arms, especially if the client has heart disease or if the reading in the first arm is abnormal. Normally a difference of 5 to 10 mm Hg exists between the arms. In subsequent assessments the blood pressure should be measured in the arm with the higher pressure. Pressure differences higher than 10 mm Hg indicate conditions such as aortic stenosis or an arterial occlusion in the arm with the lower pressure.

PRESSURE DYNAMICS. Indirect measurement of arterial blood pressure works on a basic principle of pressure. The external application of pressure beyond that which keeps a vessel open causes the vessel to close. For example, in a client with a normal blood pressure of 120/80 mm Hg, blood flows freely through the brachial artery at a systolic pressure of 120 mm Hg. Inflation of the cuff gradually applies pressure to tissues surrounding the brachial artery. When the cuff pressure exceeds 120 mm Hg, the artery collapses, blood flow ceases, and auscultation reveals absence of sounds. When the cuff pressure is released, the point on the manometer at which sounds reappear through auscultation is the systolic pressure.

KOROTKOFF SOUNDS. With the stethoscope placed over the artery the nurse listens for sounds created by blood flowing through it. In 1905, Nikolai S. Korotkoff, a Russian surgeon, first described arterial sounds. The **Korotkoff sounds** are used to assess arterial blood pressure values.

The first Korotkoff sound (phase I) is a clear, rhythmical, tapping sound. *Onset of the sound corresponds to the systolic pressure.* With the second Korotkoff sound (phase II), a murmur or swishing sound appears as the cuff is further deflated. As the artery distends, there is a turbulence of blood flow. With the third Korotkoff sound (phase III), sounds become temporarily crisper and more intense. The fourth Korotkoff sound (phase IV) becomes muffled and low pitched as the cuff is further deflated. Cuff pressure falls below the pressure within the vessel walls. *This sound is the diastolic pressure in infants and children.* The fifth Korotkoff sound (phase V) is a disappearance of all sounds. *In adolescents and adults, this sound corresponds with the diastolic pressure.*

POTENTIAL ERRORS IN AUSCULTATION. Several causes exist for error in blood pressure readings if the auscultation method is not performed correctly. Table 19-11 summarizes common mistakes in measurement.

The nurse records the position of the client and the arm in which the pressure was assessed. Most institutions record only the systolic and diastolic pressures (for example, client sitting in a chair, right arm 120/80). However, if both the fourth and fifth Korotkoff sounds are used for diastolic readings, the pressure may be recorded with three numbers (for example, client sitting in a chair, right arm 110/78/70). When a nurse is unsure of a reading, a colleague should reassess the blood pressure.

Palpation

The indirect palpation technique is useful for clients whose arterial pulsations are too weak to create Korotkoff sounds. Severe blood loss and weakened myocardial contractility are examples of conditions that result in blood pressures that are too low to auscultate accurately.

The blood pressure cuff is applied in the same manner as in the auscultation method. The nurse palpates the radial artery throughout the procedure instead of using a stethoscope. When the cuff is inflated to the desired level, the valve is released and the mercury is allowed to fall 2 mm Hg per second. As soon as the radial pulse is again palpable, the manometer reading is noted. This reading is the systolic blood pressure. The diastolic pressure is difficult to determine by palpation. A subtle change in sensation, usually in the form of a thin, snapping vibration, marks the diastolic level. When the palpation technique is used, the systolic value and the manner in which it was measured are recorded (for example, "90 systolic by palpation").

The palpation technique is used with auscultation in some cases. In clients with hypertension, the sounds usually heard over the brachial artery with high cuff pressure disappear as pressure is reduced and then reappear at a lower level. This temporary disappearance of sound is the **auscultatory gap.** It typically occurs between the first and second Korotkoff sounds. The gap in sound may cover a range of 40 mm Hg and thus may cause an underestimation of systolic pressure or overestimation of diastolic pressure. The examiner must be certain to inflate the cuff high enough to hear the true systolic pressure before the auscultatory gap. Palpation of the radial artery helps determine how high to inflate the cuff. The examiner inflates the cuff 30 mm Hg above the pressure at which the radial pulse was palpated. The range of pressures in which the auscultatory gap occurs is recorded (for example, "BP 190/94, with an auscultatory gap from 190 to 160").

Ultrasonic Stethoscope

If a nurse is unable to auscultate sounds because of a weakened arterial pulse, a Doppler ultrasonic stethoscope can be used (see Chapter 20). This stethoscope allows the nurse to hear low-frequency sounds and is commonly used with adults who have very weak blood pressures and with infants and children.

Assessment of Blood Pressure in Children

The nurse should include blood pressure measurement in the routine assessment of all children. The Task Force on Blood Pressure Control in Children (1987) recommends that all children age 3 through adolescence should have blood pressures checked at least yearly. The nurse can help parents understand the importance of this routine screening to detect children who may be at risk for hypertension. The measurement and interpretation of blood pressure in infants and children is difficult for the following reasons:

1. Various arm sizes require careful and appropriate cuff size selection.
2. Readings are difficult to obtain in restless or anxious infants and children.
3. Placing the stethoscope too firmly on the antecubital fossa can cause errors in auscultation of Korotkoff sounds.
4. Korotkoff sounds are difficult to hear in children because of low frequency and amplitude.
5. Blood pressure in children changes with growth and development.

The nurse can use the same auscultation method used with adults. A Doppler ultrasonic stethoscope may be helpful with small children and infants. Infants or children under 5 years of age should lie supine with the arms supported at heart level. Older children may sit. Children should be relaxed and calm. A delay of at least 15 minutes before taking a reading is recommended to allow children to recover from recent activity or apprehension. Those 15 minutes can be used for other quiet nursing activities. It may help to have parents nearby.

In newborns and small infants whose pressures are difficult or impossible to obtain by other techniques, the flush method is used. This measures the mean blood pressure, which correlates well with the aortic pressure. The flush method involves placing a blood pressure cuff on a wrist or ankle and then wrapping the hand or foot with an elastic wrap toward the cuff to allow for capillary emptying. The blood pressure cuff is inflated, the bandage is removed, and the point where a flush is noted in the blanched extremity while deflating the cuff is the flush pressure.

Assessment of Blood Pressure in Lower Extremities

Occasionally, dressings, casts, intravenous catheters, or other devices make the upper extremities inaccessible, so blood pressure must be measured in the lower extremities. Also, in clients with certain circulatory abnormalities, it helps to compare blood pressure in the upper extremities with that in the legs. The popliteal artery, located behind the knee in the popliteal space, is the site for auscultation. The cuff must be wide and long enough to allow for the larger girth of the thigh and is positioned with the bladder over the posterior aspect of the midthigh. Placing the client in a prone position is best. If such a position is impossible, the client should be asked to flex the knee slightly for easier access to the artery. The procedure is the same as that for brachial artery auscultation. Systolic pressure in the legs is usually higher by 10 to 40 mm Hg than that in the brachial artery, but the diastolic pressure is essentially the same.

Self-Measurement of Blood Pressure

More people measure their own blood pressures because of improved technology in home monitoring devices and a greater interest in health promotion. Two of the more common devices used by the general public include portable home devices and stationary automated machines.

The portable home devices include the mercury and aneroid sphygmomanometers and electronic digital readout devices that do not require use of a stethoscope. The electronic devices inflate and deflate cuffs with the push of a button. The electronic devices may be easier to manipulate but can easily become inaccurate and require recalibration more than once a year. Because of their sensitivity, improper cuff placement or movement of the arm can cause electronic devices to give incorrect readings.

Stationary automated machines can be found in public places such as grocery stores, fitness clubs, banks, airports, or work sites. Users simply rest their arms within the machine's inflatable cuff, which contains a pressure sensor. The cuff fits over the clothing. A visual display tells users their blood pressure within 60 to 90 seconds. The reliability of the stationary machines is limited. Blood pressure values may vary by 5 to 10 mm Hg or more (for both systolic and diastolic values) compared with pressures taken with a manual sphygmomanometer.

The National High Blood Pressure Education Program Coordinating Committee (Hunt et al, 1985) has identified the following benefits of blood pressure self-measurement:

1. Self-administered blood pressure measurement can detect an elevated blood pressure in persons previously unaware of a problem.
2. When persons have borderline hypertension, self-measurement can provide information about the pattern of blood pressure values.
3. Clients with hypertension can benefit from participating actively in their treatment through self-monitoring.
4. For some clients undergoing treatment for hypertension, visual evidence of blood pressure control may help compliance with treatment.

The Coordinating Committee (Hunt et al, 1985) also cites the following concerns about self-measurement of blood pressure:

1. There is the possibility that persons will be inadequately trained in using the devices. Printed instructions accompanying the equipment may be incomplete or written at an inappropriate reading level.
2. One elevated reading is not enough to diagnose hypertension and only indicates that further evaluation is needed by health care personnel. Thus a client may be needlessly alarmed.
3. Clients with hypertension may become overly conscious of their pressures and make inappropriate self-adjustment of medications.

Consumers can learn to use self-measurement devices if they have the information needed to perform the procedure correctly and if they know when to seek medical attention. The nurse can advise clients of possible inaccuracies in the machines, help clients understand the meaning and implications of readings, and teach them proper measurement techniques.

 ## REPORTING AND RECORDING VITAL SIGNS

The nurse is responsible for recording all vital signs accurately and in a timely manner. When a change or abnormality is assessed, the nurse reports the problem to the physician and the nurse on the next shift. The nurse decides when an abnormality has been assessed or reports a problem in response to

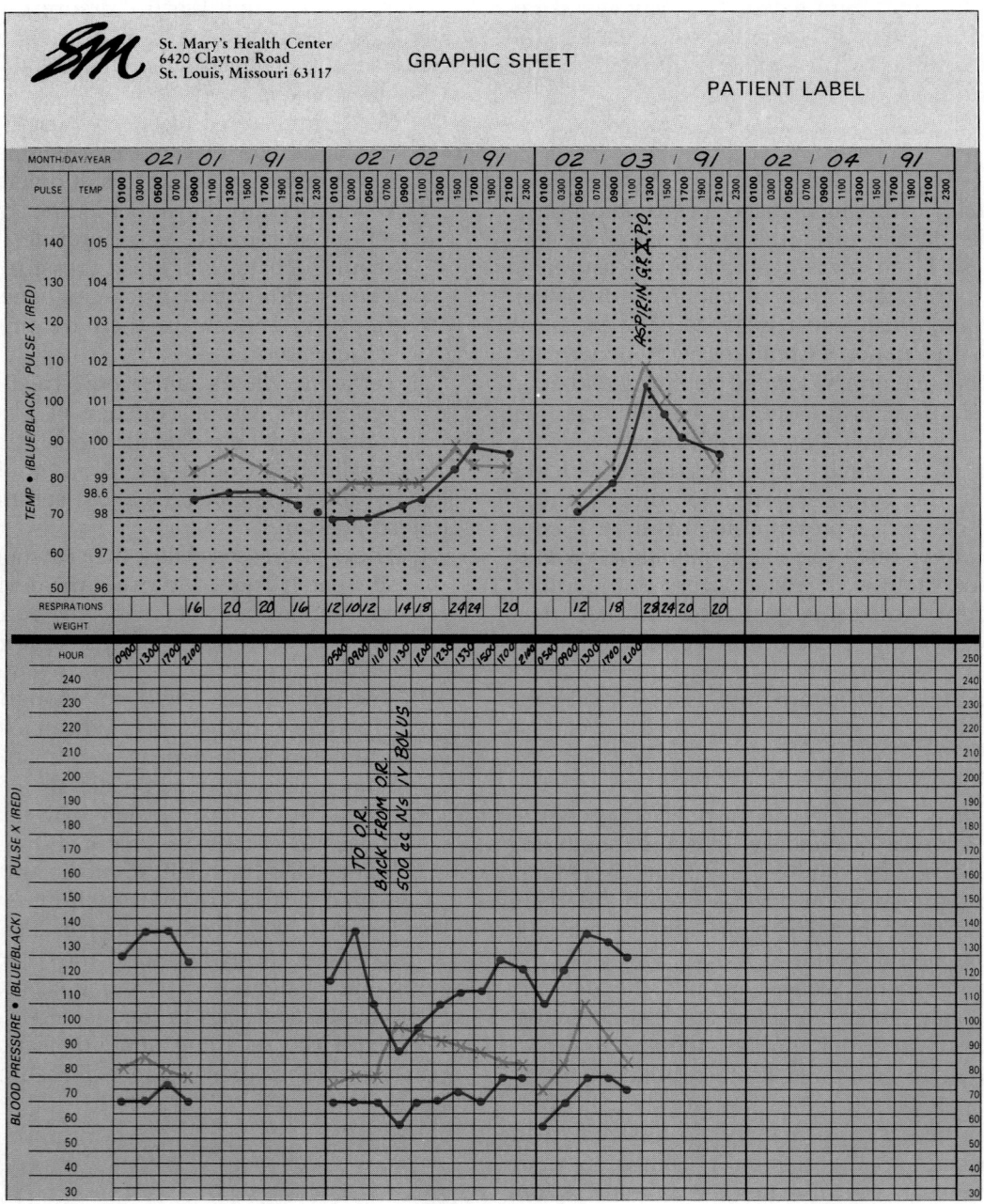

Fig. 19-14   Graphic flow sheet.
Courtesy St Mary's Health Center, St Louis.

a preexisting order such as "Call physician when systolic pressure ≥190 mm Hg or diastolic ≥100 mm Hg or pulse >110 beats per minute."

Special graphic flowsheets exist for recording vital signs (Fig. 19-14). In addition to the actual vital sign values, the nurse records in the nurses' notes any accompanying or precipitating symptoms such as chest pain and dizziness with abnormal blood pressure, shortness of breath with abnormal respirations, or flushing and diaphoresis with elevated temperature. The nurse documents any interventions initiated as a result of vital sign measurement such as administration of tepid sponging or an antihypertensive medication.

 ## SUMMARY

Vital signs measurements are a basic series of physiological assessments reflecting a client's health status. The nurse uses these data to make clinical decisions. Physical and psychological factors can create changes in vital signs. The nurse often decides the need for and frequency of vital sign assessment, which is not simply a routine chore but rather an integral part of a nurse's practice.

Before measuring any vital sign, the nurse should understand the physiological controls governing it. Each physiological control is influenced by certain variables such as age, physical exercise, or hormonal changes. The nurse who understands the effects of these variables is better prepared to anticipate normal variations. A nurse cannot recognize abnormalities without first knowing the norms.

Basic principles apply in the procedures for assessing vital signs accurately. Medical aseptic technique should be used. The client should be placed in the most comfortable position for measurements. Procedures should be explained to the client to reduce anxiety. The nurse should not rush through an assessment and should not estimate values. All characteristics of a vital sign are assessed. Results are recorded promptly and accurately.

CHAPTER 19 REVIEW

Key Concepts

- Vital signs include the physiological measurements of temperature, pulse, respirations, and blood pressure.
- Vital signs may be measured as part of a complete physical examination or more commonly in a review of the client's condition.
- The nurse assesses vital sign changes in conjunction with other physical assessment findings.
- The nurse uses clinical judgment to determine the frequency of vital sign measurement.
- Knowledge of the factors influencing vital signs assists the nurse in interpreting abnormal values.
- Vital sign measurements provide a basis for evaluating response to nursing interventions.
- Assessment of vital signs yields the most accurate values when the client is inactive and the environment is controlled for comfort.
- Normally, heat production balances heat loss to maintain body temperature.
- The nurse assists the client in attaining a normal body temperature by initiating interventions promoting heat loss or production.
- A fever is a normal defense mechanism and often does not require treatment.
- The oral route is the most accessible and acceptable site for temperature measurement.
- Rectal temperature measurements should not be performed on newborn infants or adults with rectal alterations.
- To assess cardiac function, pulse rate and rhythm are most easily and accurately measured using the radial or apical pulse.
- The nurse assesses the presence and character of peripheral pulses to determine the adequacy of local blood flow.
- Assessment of respirations involves observation of ventilatory movements through the whole respiratory cycle.
- Blood pressure levels reflect the relationship among several hemodynamic variables.
- Blood pressure can be measured by auscultation or palpation.
- The diagnosis of hypertension can only be made after averaging pressure readings made on at least two occasions.
- Changes in any vital sign can influence characteristics of the other vital signs.
- Self-measurement of blood pressure can be useful in detecting an elevated blood pressure in persons previously unaware of a problem or in monitoring blood pressure in persons already diagnosed with hypertension.

Key Terms

Critical Thinking Exercises

1. During admission assessment, you need to obtain a temperature measurement on a restless 18-year-old client who had been in a motor vehicle accident. Oral, rectal or tympanic electronic thermometer save available. What criteria do you use to select the most efficient and effect method for obtaining this client's body temperature.

2. You are caring for a client having uncontrolled seizures. What type of thermometer is best for this client?

3. It is raining and your client just ran into the clinic from the parking lot. What effect would you expect this activity to have on vital signs? When would you expect to get vital signs that reflect the clients "true" values for pulse, blood pressure, and respirations?

4. The previous blood pressure for your 280-pound male client was taken with a regular cuff, and the reading was 170/100 mm Hg. What conclusions can you make about the previous reading? What would you do to verify this reading?

5. While obtaining your client's vital signs, you palpate a rapid, irregular heart beat. Your confirm this irregularity with a one-minute apical pulse measurement. The result is a rate of 124 beats per minute with irregular rhythm. What are your anticipated follow-up activities for this client?

REFERENCES

American Heart Association: *Recommendations for human blood pressure determination by sphygomomanometers,* pub no 701005, Dallas, 1987, The Association.

Baker NC et al: The effect of type of thermometer and length of time inserted on oral temperature measurements of afebrile subjects, *Nurs Res* 33:109, 1984.

Barner HB et al: Field evaluation of a new simplified method for cooling of heat casualties in the desert, *Milit Med* 149:95, 1984.

Bobak IM, Jenson MD, Zalar MK: *Maternity and gynecologic care: the nurse and the family,* ed 4, St Louis, 1989, Mosby–Year Book.

Centers for Disease Control: Recommendations for prevention of HIV transmission in health-care settings, *MMWR* 36:(suppl) SS, 1987.

Dinarello C: Interleukin-1, *Rev Infect Dis* 6:51, 1984.

Enright T, Hill MG: Treatment of fever, *Focus Crit Care* 16(2):96, 1989.

Eoff M, Joyce B: Temperature measurements in children, *Am J Nurs* 81:1010, 1981.

Erickson R: Oral temperature differences in relation to thermometer and technique, *Nurs Res* 29:157, 1980.

Erickson R, Yount S: Comparison of tympanic and oral temperatures in surgical patients, *Nurs Res* 40(2):90, 1991.

Graves RP, Markarian MF: Three minute time intervals when using an oral mercury-in-glass thermometer with or without J-temp sheaths, *Nurs Res* 29:323, 1980.

Guyton AC: *Textbook of medical physiology,* ed 8, Philadelphia, 1991, Saunders.

Hanson M: Drug fever: remember to consider it in diagnosis, *Postgrad Med* 89(5)167, 1991.

Heinz J: Validation of sublingual temperatures in patients with nasogastric tubes, *Heart Lung* 14:198, 1985.

Hollerbach AD, Sneed NV: Accuracy of radial pulse assessment by length of counting interval, *Heart Lung* 19(3):258, 1990.

Hunt JC et al: Devices used for self-measurement of blood pressure: revised statement of the National High Blood Pressure Education Program, *Arch Intern Med* 145:2231, 1985.

Joint National Committee on Detection, Evaluation, and Treatment of High Blood Pressure: The 1988 report of the Joint National Committee on Detection, Evaluation, and Treatment of High Blood Pressure, *Arch Intern Med* 148:1023, 1988.

Kim MJ, McFarland GK, McLane AM: *Pocket guide to nursing diagnoses,* ed 4, St Louis, 1991, Mosby–Year Book.

LaVoy K: Dealing with hypothermia and frostbite, *RN* 48:53, 1985.

Leung AKC, Robson WLM: Febrile convulsions: how dangerous are they? *Postgrad Med* 89(5):217, 1991.

Lovejoy FH Jr: Aspirin and acetaminophen: a comparative view of their anti-pyretic and analgesic activity, *Pediatrics* 62(suppl): 904, 1978.

Lukasiewicz P: Rectal temperatures are as accurate as oral temperatures in patients receiving oxygen therapy, *Crit Care Nurse* 6:72, 1986.

Mountcastle VB: *Medical physiology,* vol 2, ed 14, St Louis, 1980, Mosby–Year Book.

National Academy of Sciences, Food and Nutrition Board: *Recommended dietary allowances,* ed 10, Washington, DC, 1989, The Academy. 1989.

Petersdorf RC: Disturbances of heat regulation. In Isselbacher KJ et al, editors: *Harrison's principles of internal medicine,* ed 9, New York, 1980, McGraw-Hill.

Posey, VM, Caruso C: Life-threatening heat-related emergencies, *Dimens Crit Care Nurs* 5(4):216 1986.

Schatz IJ: Orthostatic hypotension, II. Clinical diagnosis, testing, and treatment, *Arch Intern Med* 44:1037, 1984.

Shinozaki T, Deane R, Perkins FM: Infrared tympanic thermometer: evaluation of a new clinical thermometer, *Crit Care Med* 16 (2):148, 1988.

Task Force on Blood Pressure Control in Children: Report of second task force on blood pressure control in children: 1987, *Pediatrics* 79:1, 1987.

Thibodeau GA, Patton K: *Anatomy and physiology,* ed 2, St Louis, 1993, Mosby–Year Book.

Whaley LF, Wong DL: *Nursing care of infants and children,* ed 4, St Louis, 1991, Mosby Year–Book.

ADDITIONAL READINGS

Adelman EM: When patient's blood pressure falls, what does it mean? What should you do? *Nurs 80* 10:26, 1980.

Angerami ELS: Epidemiological study of a body temperature in patients in a teaching hospital, *Int J Nurs Stud* 17:91, 1980.

Atkins E: Fever: a new perspective on an old phenomenon, *New Engl J Med* 308:958, 1983.

Bernheim HA et al: Fever: pathogenesis, pathophysiology, and purpose, *Ann Intern Med* 91:261, 1979.

Birdsall C: How accurate are your blood pressures? *Am J Nurs* 84:1414, 1984.

Birdsall C: How do you handle heat loss? *Am J Nurs* 85:367, 1985.

Birdsall C: How do you interpret pulses? *Am J Nurs* 85:785, 1985.

Davis C, Lentz M: Circadian rhythms: charting oral temperatures to spot abnormalities, *J Gerontol Nurs* 15 (4):34, 1989.

Donaldson JF: Therapy of acute fever: a comparative approach, *Hosp Pract* [off] 9:195, 1981.

Dressler DK et al: A comparison of oral and rectal temperature measurement on patients receiving oxygen by mask, *Nurs Res* 32:393, 1983.

Durham ML: Swanson B, Paulford N:Effect of tachypnea on oral temperature estimation: a replication, *Nurs Res* 35(4):211, 1986.

Electronic thermometers: the better alternative? *Health Devices* 19:19, 1982.

Fraser C, Filler MJ: The assessment factor most nurses forget, *RN* 52:32, 1989.

Giuffre M et al: The relationship between axillary and core body temperatures, *Appl Nurs Res* 3(2):52, 1990.

Griffin JP: Fever: when to leave it alone, *Nurs 86* 16:58, 1986.

Guerevich I: Fever: when to worry about it, *RN* 48:14, 1985.

Hayes KB: Dealing with heat injuries, *RN* 47:41, 1984.

Lim-Levy F: The effect of oxygen inhalation on oral temperature, *Nur Res* 31:150, 1982.

McCarron K: Fever: the cardinal vital sign, *CCQ* 9 (1):15, 1986.

Metzger B, Therrien B: Effect of position on cardiovascular response during the Valsalva maneuver, *Nurs Res* 39(4):198, 1990.

The National High Blood Pressure Education Program Coordination Committee: National high blood pressure education program working group report on ambulatory blood presure monitoring, *Arch Intern Med* 150:2270, 1990.

Nichols GA: Time analysis of afebrile and febrile temperature reading, *Nurs Res* 21:463, 1972.

Nichols GA et al: Oral, axillary, and rectal temperature determinations and relationships, *Nurs Res* 15:307, 1966.

Nichols GA et al: Taking oral temperature of febrile patients, *Nurs Res* 19:448, 1969.

Nichols GA et al: Measuring oral and rectal temperatures of febrile children, *Nurs Res* 21:261, 1972.

Rayburn W et al: Self-monitoring of blood pressure during pregnancy, *Am J Obstet Gynecol* 148(2):159, 1984.

Rebenson-Piano M et al: An evaluation of two indirect methods of blood pressure measurements in ill patients, *Nurs Res* 39:42, 1989.

Reeves-Swift R: Rational management of a child's acute fever, *MCN* 15(2):82, 1990.

Samples, JF et al: Circadian rhythms: basis for screening for fever, *Nurs Res* 34:397, 1985.

Stevens S, Becker KL: How to perform picture-perfect respiratory assessment, *Nurs 88* 19:57, 1988.

Sulzbach LM: Measurement of pulsus paradoxus, *Focus Crit Care* 16:142, 1989.

Thomas DO: Fever in children, *RN* 48:19, 1985.

Thomas SP, Groer MW: Relationship of demographic lifestyle and stress variables to blood pressure in adolescents, *Nurs Res* 35:169, 1986.

Working Group on Hypertension in the Elderly: Statement on hypertension in the elderly, *JAMA* 256(1):70, 1986.

CHAPTER **20**

Physical Examination and Health Assessment

OBJECTIVES

Mastery of content in this chapter will enable the student to:
- Define the key terms listed.
- Discuss the purposes of physical assessment.
- Describe the techniques used with each physical assessment skill.
- Describe the proper position for the client during each phase of the examination.
- List techniques used to promote the client's physical and psychological comfort during an examination.
- Make environmental preparations before an examination.
- Identify information to collect from the nursing history before an examination.
- Discuss normal physical findings in a young and middle-age adult compared with an older adult.
- Discuss ways to incorporate health teaching into the examination.
- Use physical assessment skills during routine nursing care.
- Conduct physical assessments in an organized and proper fashion.
- Describe physical measurements made in the assessment of each body system.
- Identify self-screening examinations commonly performed by clients.
- Document findings on a physical examination form.

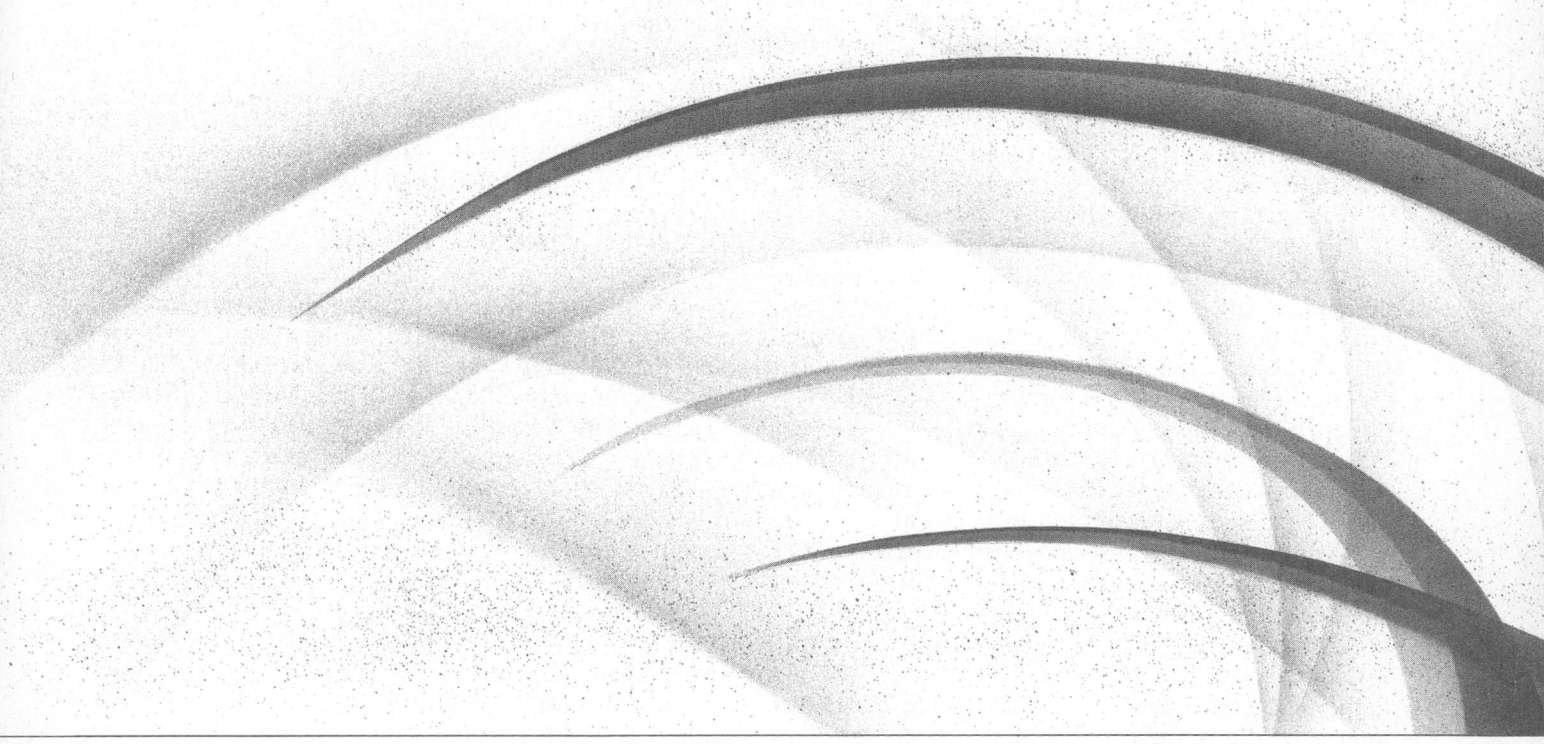

CHAPTER OUTLINE

The nurse works in a variety of settings, seeking information about clients' health status. The nurse conducts health assessments at health fairs, at screening clinics, in physician's offices, or in hospitals to identify clients' physical and psychosocial needs. Health screenings involve measurement of specific physical functions or diagnostic tests to detect persons with high probabilities of having a characteristic (Larson, 1986). For example, blood pressure screenings detect the risk for high blood pressure. Tine tests identify persons who have been exposed to tuberculosis. Information from health screenings determines the need for more comprehensive examinations.

A complete health assessment involves a more detailed review of a client's condition. The nurse collects a nursing history (see Chapter 6) and performs a behavioral and physical examination. The health history involves a lengthy interview with a client to gather subjective data about a condition. During the interview, the nurse can also make important observations about a client's status. A physical examination is a head-to-toe review of each body system that offers objective information about the client. The nurse uses the skills of physical assessment to make clinical judgments. The client's condition and response affect the extent of the examination. The accuracy of a physical assessment influences the choice of therapies a client receives and the determination of the response to those therapies. Continuity in health care improves when the nurse makes ongoing, objective, and comprehensive assessments.

PURPOSES OF PHYSICAL EXAMINATION

An examination should be designed for the client's needs. If a client is acutely ill, the nurse may assess only the involved body systems. A more comprehensive examination is conducted when the client feels more at ease, and the nurse then learns about the client's total health status. A complete physical examination is performed for routine screening to promote wellness behaviors and preventive health care measures; for determination of eligibility for health insurance, military service, or a new job; and for admission to a hospital or long-term care facility. The nurse uses physical assessment for the following reasons:

1. To gather baseline data about the client's health
2. To supplement, confirm, or refute data obtained in the nursing history
3. To confirm and identify nursing diagnoses

4. To make clinical judgments about a client's changing health status and management
5. To evaluate the physiological outcomes of care

Gathering a Data Base

Through the nursing health history, the nurse initially gathers complete and detailed information about the client's health status. However, a client may be unaware of a physical problem, so a thorough assessment of physical status is necessary. Even if a history is complete, a physical assessment reveals information that refutes, confirms, or supplements the existing data base. For example, a client may complain of back pain. The nurse asks several questions to clarify the nature of the pain. However, unless the nurse sees the bruise across the client's back, the symptom of pain could suggest several ailments.

One assessment finding cannot conclusively reveal the nature of an abnormality. A complete assessment is needed to form a definitive diagnosis. The nurse learns to group significant findings into patterns of data that reveal actual or high-risk nursing diagnoses. In addition, each abnormal finding directs the nurse to gather additional information. Information gathered during an initial physical assessment provides a baseline of functional abilities. The baseline is not the normal range of physical findings but rather the pattern of findings identified when the client was first assessed. This baseline serves as a comparison for future assessment findings. During a subsequent assessment, the nurse can determine whether changes in the client's condition have occurred.

Developing Nursing Diagnoses and a Care Plan

The accuracy of the data base allows the nurse to develop individualized nursing diagnoses (Table 20-1). Physical assessment findings help determine the etiology of diagnoses so that the nurse can select the correct type of interventions for the care plan. Physical assessment is ongoing, and thus the care plan changes with the client's condition. The nurse monitors the client's progress and responses to therapies to review existing diagnoses and identify new problems.

Managing Client Problems

When caring for clients, the nurse makes many observations and performs a variety of therapies. Yet the nurse's success in giving care depends on the

TABLE 20-1 Development of Individualized Nursing Diagnoses

Assessment Method	Findings	Patterns	Nursing Diagnosis
Inspection of skin	Skin along sacral area is intact. There is 3-cm area of redness around coccyx. No skin lesions are observed.	There is pressure area around coccyx.	*High risk for impaired skin integrity*
Palpation of skin	Skin is moist from diaphoresis. There is tenderness to palpation around sacral area. There is good skin turgor.	Skin moisture promotes maceration.	
Historical data	Client suffered fractured left leg. Client is immobilized due to left leg traction. Diet history reveals normal caloric and nutrient intake.	Continued pressure is exerted over sacrum.	

ability to recognize change in status and to modify therapies so that clients gain the most desirable outcome. Physical assessment skills allow the nurse to judge the status of the client's health and direct the management of care. For example, the nurse inspects the skin during a routine bath and finds it excessively dry. The nurse does not use soap and applies body lotion to the skin. The nurse revises the written care plan so that other nurses know the type of skin care to provide. Instruction is also given to the client about skin care. Performing the mechanics of physical assessment is relatively simple. The more difficult challenge lies in using findings to make decisions.

Evaluating Nursing Care

Nurses become accountable for their nursing care by evaluating the results of nursing interventions. Physical assessment skills enhance the evaluation of nursing measures through monitoring physiological and behavioral outcomes of care. The same physical assessment skill used to assess a condition (for example, palpation of the client's pulse) can be used as an evaluation measure after care is administered (for example, an evaluation of a client's tolerance to an exercise plan).

Physical assessment skills allow a nurse to make accurate, detailed, objective measurements. The measurements determine whether the expected outcomes of care are met. The nurse does not depend on intuition when physical assessment can be used to evaluate effectiveness of care.

 ## INTEGRATION OF PHYSICAL ASSESSMENT WITH NURSING CARE

Whether a complete or partial physical assessment is performed, an examination should be integrated into routine care. For example, the nurse can assess the condition of the skin and other body parts during a bed bath. When a client undergoes oral hygiene, the nurse can carefully assess oral cavity structures. As a client ambulates down the hall, the nurse assesses range of motion and gait. This practice makes more efficient use of time. The nurse also learns that physical assessment should become an automatic behavior when nurse and client interact. Physical assessment skills enable the nurse to gather more comprehensive and relevant assessment findings.

 ## SKILLS OF PHYSICAL ASSESSMENT

Chapter 6 briefly describes the skills of inspection, palpation, percussion, and auscultation. This chapter provides a more detailed description of those skills and their application in the physical examination.

Inspection

The nurse inspects or looks at body parts to detect normal characteristics or significant physical signs. It helps to know normal physical characteristics before trying to distinguish abnormal findings. It is especially important to know normal characteristics of clients of different ages. Dry, wrinkled, inelastic skin is normal in an older but not in a young adult. Experience is needed to recognize normal variations among clients, as well as ranges of normal in an individual. Inspection is a simple technique, but it is often underused. For example, when hurrying to complete a bath, a nurse may fail to inspect all skin surfaces and overlook a rash under the client's arm. The quality of an inspection depends on the nurse's willingness to spend time doing a thorough job. To inspect body parts accurately the nurse observes the following principles:

1. Make sure good lighting is available.
2. Position and expose body parts so that all surfaces can be viewed.
3. Inspect each area for size, shape, color, symmetry, position, and abnormalities.
4. If possible, compare each area inspected with the same area on the opposite side of the body.
5. Use additional light (for example, a penlight) to inspect body cavities.

After inspection of a body part is completed, findings may indicate further examination. Palpation is often used with or after visual inspection.

Palpation

Further assessment of body parts is made through the sense of touch. The hands can make delicate and sensitive measurements of specific physical signs, so palpation is used to examine all accessible parts of the body (Table 20-2). The nurse uses different parts of the hand to detect characteristics such as texture, temperature, and the perception of movement.

The client should be relaxed and positioned comfortably because muscle tension during palpation impairs the ability to use palpation effectively. For example, tension of the abdominal muscles makes palpation of underlying organs impossible and mimics muscle rigidity. Asking the client to take slow deep breaths enhances muscle relaxation. Tender areas are palpated last. The nurse asks the client to point out the more sensitive areas and notes any nonverbal signs of discomfort.

Clients appreciate warm hands, short fingernails, and a gentle approach. The nurse applies tactile pressure slowly, gently, and deliberately. Light palpation of structures such as the abdomen is performed to determine areas of tenderness. The nurse's hand is placed on the part to be examined and depressed about 1 cm (½ in). Tender areas are examined further. The sensation of touch is best preserved with light, intermittent pressure. Heavy, prolonged pressure causes a loss of sensitivity in the nurse's hand.

After light palpation has been applied, deeper palpation is used to examine the condition of organs,

TABLE 20-2 Examples of Characteristics Measured by Palpation

Area Examined	Criteria Measured
Skin	Temperature
	Moisture
	Texture
	Turgor and elasticity
	Tenderness
	Thickness
Organs (e.g., liver and intestine)	Size
	Shape
	Tenderness
	Absence of masses
Glands (e.g., thyroid and lymph)	Swelling
	Symmetry and mobility
Blood vessels (e.g., carotid or femoral artery)	Pulse amplitude
	Elasticity
	Rate
	Rhythm
Thorax	Excursion
	Tenderness

such as those in the abdomen (Fig. 20-1). The nurse depresses the area being examined approximately 2 cm (1 in). Caution is the rule. A student nurse should not attempt deep palpation without the assistance of a qualified instructor because prolonged pressure could cause internal injury. Deep palpation may be applied with one hand or both hands (bimanually). When the nurse uses bimanual palpation, one hand (called the *sensing hand*) is relaxed and placed lightly over the client's skin. The other hand (called the *active hand*) applies pressure to the sensing hand. The lower hand does not exert pressure directly and thus retains the sensitivity needed to detect organ characteristics.

The most sensitive parts of the hand, the pads of the fingertips, are used to assess texture, shape, size, consistency, and pulsation (Fig. 20-2, *A*). Temperature is best measured using the dorsum or back of the hand (Fig. 20-2, *B*) and fingers, where the skin is thinnest. The palm of the hand (Fig. 20-2, *C*) is more sensitive to vibration. The nurse measures position, consistency, and turgor by lightly grasping the body part with the fingertips (Fig. 20-2, *D*). The nurse must not palpate without considering the client's condition. For example, if the client has a fractured rib, extra care is used to locate the painful area. A vital artery is not palpated with pressure that obstructs blood flow. The nurse also considers the body area being palpated and the reason for using palpation and must be able to discriminate and interpret the significance of what is sensed.

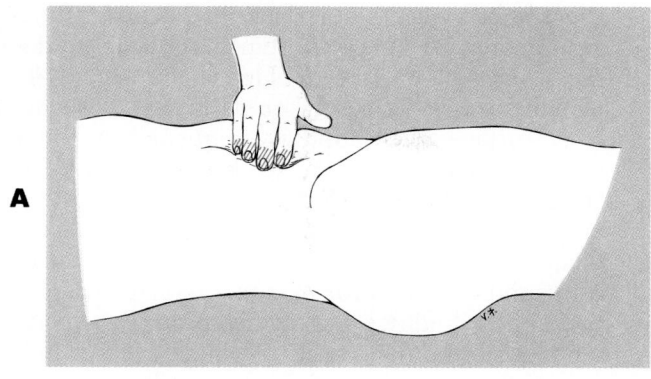

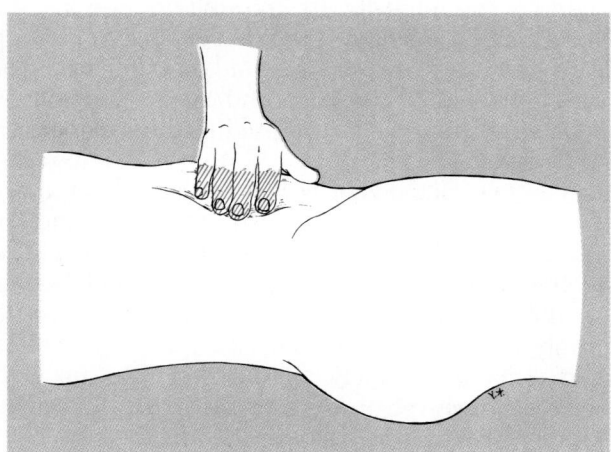

Fig. 20-1 **A,** During light palpation, gentle pressure against underlying skin and tissues can detect areas of irregularity and tenderness. **B,** During deep palpation, the nurse depresses tissue to assess the condition of underlying organs.

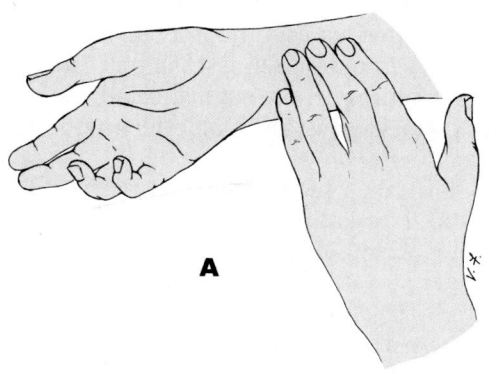

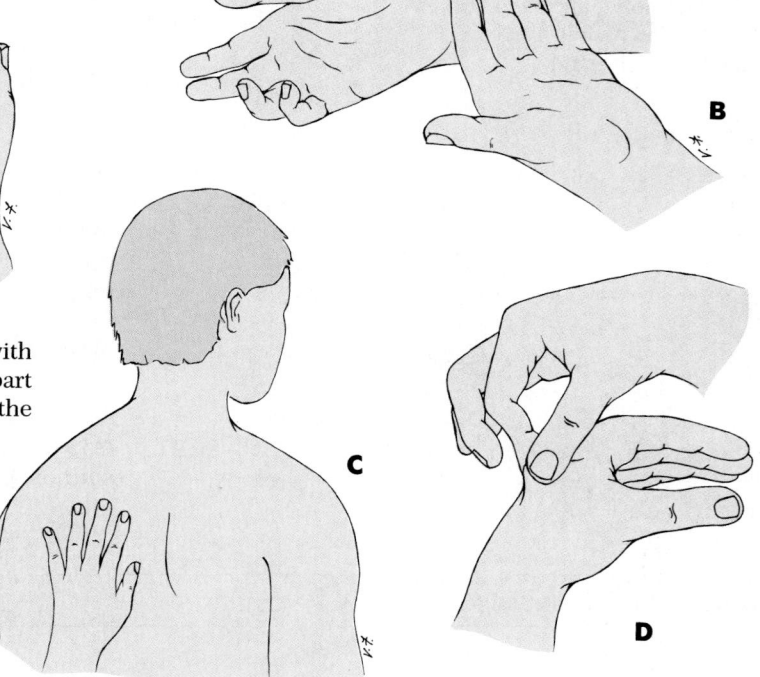

Fig. 20-2 **A,** The radial pulse is detected with the pads of the fingertips, the most sensitive part of the hand. **B,** The dorsum of the hand allows the nurse to detect temperature variations in skin. **C,** The nurse uses the palm of the hand to detect vibration. **D,** The nurse grasps the skin with the fingertips to assess turgor.

Percussion

Percussion requires considerable skill. It is perhaps the least-used assessment skill; however, it can be very helpful in confirming other assessment findings. Through percussion, the location, size, and density of an underlying structure are determined. Percussion helps verify abnormalities reported from x-ray studies or assessed through palpation and auscultation. For example, if the nurse hears abnormal breath sounds when auscultating the lungs, percussion may rule out the presence of consolidated fluids or air in the pleural space.

When the examiner strikes the body's surface with a finger, vibration and sound are produced. This vibration is transmitted through the body tissues, and the character of the sound depends on the density of the underlying tissue. For example, the normal lung transmits sounds with high intensity and low pitch, whereas the more solid liver transmits a high-pitched sound of soft intensity. By knowing the way that densities influence sound, the nurse is able to locate organs or masses, map their boundaries, and determine their size. An abnormal sound suggests a mass or substance such as air or fluid within an organ or body cavity.

The two methods of percussion are direct and indirect. The direct method involves striking the body surface directly with one or two fingers. The indirect technique is performed by placing the middle finger of the nondominant hand (called the *pleximeter*) firmly against the body surface, keeping the palm and remaining fingers off the skin. The tip of the middle finger of the dominant hand (called the *plexor*) strikes the base of the distal joint of the pleximeter (Fig. 20-3). The examiner uses a quick,

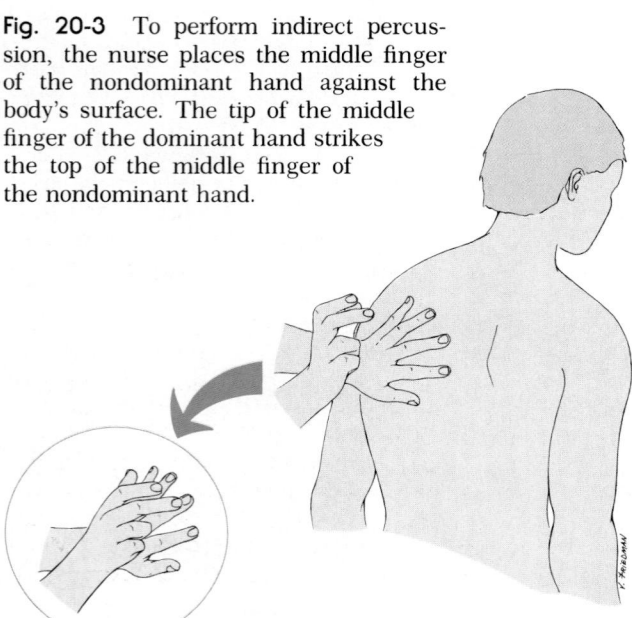

Fig. 20-3 To perform indirect percussion, the nurse places the middle finger of the nondominant hand against the body's surface. The tip of the middle finger of the dominant hand strikes the top of the middle finger of the nondominant hand.

sharp stroke with the plexor finger, keeping the forearm stationary. The wrist remains relaxed to deliver the proper blow. If the blow is not sharp, if the pleximeter is held loosely, or if the palm rests on the body surface, the sound is dampened or softened, preventing transmission of sound to underlying structures. The same force must be applied to each area so that an accurate comparison of sounds can be made. A light, quick blow usually produces the clearest sound. Parrino (1987) cautions that variations in percussion findings commonly occur between two different examiners. Use of direct versus indirect percussion or firm versus light percussion can lead to different interpretation of results.

Percussion produces five types of sounds: tympany, resonance, hyperresonance, dullness, and flatness. Each sound is created by certain types of underlying tissues and is judged by its intensity of pitch, duration, and quality (Table 20-3).

The common use of x-ray studies, computer-assisted tomography (CAT), or magnetic resonance imaging (MRI) provides argument against the need to regularly use percussion for assessment. However, in an emergent setting where sophisticated tests are not available, percussion is a valuable technique to master.

Percussion takes practice. The wrist is flexed by keeping the forearm stationary. For practice, the hand can be placed on the surface of a table and the middle finger struck with the middle finger of the opposite hand. The character of the sound changes when the blow is not light and quick.

Auscultation

Auscultation is listening to sounds created in body organs to detect variations from normal. Some sounds can be heard with the unassisted ear, al-

TABLE 20-3	Sounds Produced by Percussion				
Sound	Intensity	Pitch	Duration	Quality	Percussion
Tympany	Loud	High	Moderate	Drumlike	Enclosed, air-containing space; gastric air bubble, puffed-out cheek
Resonance	Moderate to loud	Low	Long	Hollow	Normal lung
Hyperresonance	Very loud	Very low	Longer than resonance	Booming	Emphysematous lung
Dullness	Soft to moderate	High	Moderate	Thudlike	Liver
Flatness	Soft	High	Short	Flat	Muscle

though most sounds can be heard only through a stethoscope. A student must first become familiar with the normal sounds created by the cardiovascular, respiratory, and gastrointestinal systems, such as the passage of blood through an artery. Abnormal sounds can be recognized only after normal variations are learned. The nurse becomes more successful in auscultation by knowing the types of sounds arising from each body structure and the location in which they can most easily be heard. Likewise, the nurse becomes familiar with the areas that normally do not emit sounds.

To auscultate correctly the nurse needs good hearing acuity, a good stethoscope, and knowledge of how to use the stethoscope properly. Nurses with hearing disorders should purchase stethoscopes with greater sound amplification or ask colleagues to check findings through auscultation.

Chapter 19 describes the parts of the acoustic stethoscope and the general use of the bell and diaphragm. The bell is best for low-pitched sounds, such as vascular and certain heart sounds, and the diaphragm is best for high-pitched sounds, such as bowel and lung sounds.

A nurse must become familiar with the stethoscope before attempting to use it with a client. It helps to practice using it with a friend. A number of extraneous sounds created by movement of the tubing or chestpiece interferes with auscultation of body organ sounds. By deliberately producing these sounds, the nurse learns to recognize and disregard them during the actual examination (see box). Through auscultation, the nurse notes the following characteristics of sounds:

1. Frequency, or the number of sound wave cycles generated per second by a vibrating object. The higher the frequency, the higher the pitch of a sound and vice versa.
2. Loudness, or the amplitude of a sound wave. Auscultated sounds are described as *loud* or *soft*.
3. Quality, or the sounds of similar frequency and loudness from different sources. Terms such as *blowing* or *gurgling* describe the quality of sound.
4. Duration, or the length of time that sound vibrations last. The duration of sound is short, medium, or long. Layers of soft tissue dampen the duration of sounds from deep internal organs.

Auscultation requires concentration, practice, and application of knowledge. The nurse must consider the part of the body auscultated and the causes of the sounds. For example, the first heart sound is caused by closure of the mitral valve. The nurse identifies

---

Exercises to Increase Familiarity with the Stethoscope

- Ensure that the earpiece follows the contour of the ear canal. Learn what fit is best for you by comparing amplification of sounds with the earpieces in both directions.
- Place the earpieces in your ears with the tips of the earpieces turned toward the face. *Lightly* blow into the diaphragm. Again place the earpieces in your ears, this time with the ends turned toward the back of the head. *Lightly* blow into the diaphragm. After you have learned the right fit for the loudest amplification, wear the stethoscope the same way each time.
- Put on the stethoscope and *lightly* blow into the diaphragm. If the sound is barely audible, *lightly* blow into the bell. Sound is carried through only one part of the chestpiece at a time. If the sound is greatly amplified through the diaphragm, the diaphragm is in position for use. If the sound is barely audible through the diaphragm, the bell is in position for use. Rotation of the diaphragm and bell places the chestpiece in the desired position. Leave the diaphragm in position for the next exercise.
- Place the diaphragm over the anterior part of your chest. Ask a friend to speak in a normal conversational tone. Environmental noise seriously detracts from hearing the noise created by body organs. When a stethoscope is used, the client and the examiner should remain quiet.
- Place the stethoscope on and gently tap the tubing. It is often difficult to avoid stretching or movement of the stethoscope's tubing. The examiner should be in a position so that the tubing hangs free. Moving or touching the tubing creates extraneous sounds.

---

where the sound is best heard. The first heart sound is best auscultated at the fifth intercostal space along the midclavicular line. The nurse also considers how the sound is heard normally. The first heart sound has the quality of a loud *lub,* whereas the second sound is a *dub.* After the cause and character of normal auscultated sounds are understood, it becomes easier to recognize abnormal sounds and their origins.

Olfaction

While assessing a client, the nurse should be familiar with the nature and source of body odors (Ta-

TABLE 20-4 Assessment of Characteristic Odors		
Odor	Site or Source	Potential Causes
Alcohol	Oral cavity	Ingestion of alcohol
Ammonia	Urine	Urinary tract infection
Body odor	Skin, particularly in areas where body parts rub together (e.g., under arms, beneath breasts)	Poor hygiene, excess perspiration (hyperhidrosis), foul-smelling perspiration (bromidrosis)
Feces	Wound site	Wound abscess
	Vomitus	Bowel obstruction
	Rectal area	Fecal incontinence
Foul-smelling stools in infant	Stool	Malabsorption syndrome
Halitosis	Oral cavity	Poor dental and oral hygiene, gum disease
Sweet, fruity ketones	Oral cavity	Diabetes acidosis
Stale urine	Skin	Uremic acidosis
Sweet, heavy, thick odor	Draining wound	*Pseudomonas* (bacterial) infection
Musty odor	Casted body part	Infection inside cast
Fetid, sweet odor	Tracheostomy or mucous secretions	Infection of bronchial tree (*Pseudomonas* bacteria)

ble 20-4). Olfaction helps the nurse detect abnormalities that cannot be recognized by any other means. For example, a client with a cast is expected to experience discomfort after an injury. However, the nurse who notes a strong odor will suspect that the discomfort may also be related to wound infection. The discomfort alone does not reveal the presence of infection. Findings from olfaction and other assessment skills allow the nurse to detect serious abnormalities. If a nurse notices an unfamiliar odor, a colleague may be able to identify the problem.

 PREPARATION FOR EXAMINATION

A disorganized approach when preparing for a physical examination can cause errors and incomplete findings. Proper preparation of the environment, equipment, and client ensures a smooth examination with few interruptions.

Environment

A physical examination requires privacy. An examination room that is well equipped for all necessary procedures is preferable. However, often the examination occurs in the client's room, where it may be necessary to use room curtains or dividers around the bed. In the home, the nurse may perform an examination in the client's bedroom.

Any examination room should be well equipped for all necessary procedures. Adequate lighting is needed for proper illumination of body parts. Ideally an examination room is soundproofed so that clients feel comfortable discussing their conditions. The nurse eliminates sources of noise such as televisions or radios and takes steps to prevent interruptions from others. The room should also be warm enough to maintain clients' comfort.

Sometimes, it is difficult to perform a complete examination when clients are in beds or on stretchers. Special examination tables make clients easily accessible and help them assume special positions. The tables are high and narrow, so the nurse must carefully assist clients so that they do not fall while getting on and off them. A confused, combative, or uncooperative client should not be left on an examination table without supervision.

Examination tables are often hard and uncomfortable. When the client lies supine, the head of the table can be raised about 30 degrees. The client may also be given a small pillow. When examining a client in bed, the nurse can raise the bed to reach body parts more easily.

Equipment

Handwashing is done before equipment preparation and the examination. Handwashing reduces the transmission of microorganisms. The equipment needed for an examination should be readily available and arranged in order for easy use (Fig. 20-4). It should be kept warm as appropriate. The diaphragm of the stethoscope may be briskly rubbed between the hands before it is applied to the skin. Warm wa-

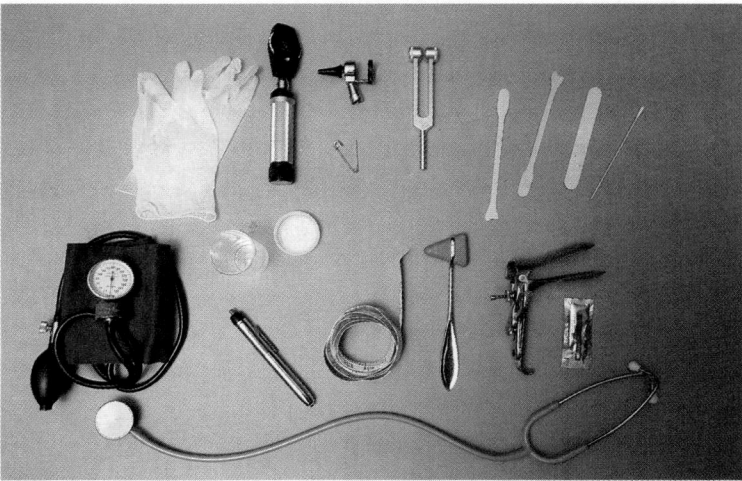

Fig. 20-4   Equipment used during a physical examination *(clockwise from upper left):* Disposable gloves, ophthalmoscope, otoscope attachment, sterile safety pin, tuning fork, cervical spatulas, tongue depressor, cotton-tip swab, lubricant, vaginal speculum, reflex hammer, tape measure, penlight, specimen cup, sphygmomanometer, and stethoscope *(bottom).*

ter should be run over the vaginal speculum. All equipment must be checked to see that it functions properly. The ophthalmoscope and otoscope require good batteries and light bulbs. Equipment typically used is listed in the box.

Client

Physical Preparation

The client's physical comfort is vital to the success of the examination. Before starting, the nurse asks if the client needs to use the toilet. An empty bladder and bowel facilitate examination of the abdomen, genitalia, and rectum and provide the opportunity to collect urine or fecal specimens. The nurse explains the proper method for collecting specimens and ensures that each specimen is properly labeled.

Physical preparation involves being sure the client is dressed and draped properly. A client in the hospital will likely be wearing only a simple gown. An outpatient will have to undress. If the examination is limited to certain body systems, it may be unnecessary for the client to undress completely. The client should have privacy during undressing and plenty of time to finish. Walking into the room as the client undresses causes embarrassment. Drapes and gowns are made of linen or disposable paper. After clients have undressed and donned the gown, they should sit or lie down on the examination table with the drape over the lap or lower trunk. The examiner makes sure that the client stays warm by eliminating drafts, controlling room temperature, and providing warm blankets. A seriously ill client or older adult is

Equipment and Supplies for Physical Assessment

- Cotton applicators
- Cytobrush
- Disposable pad
- Drapes
- Eye chart (e.g., Snellen chart)
- Flashlight and spotlight
- Forms (e.g., physical, laboratory)
- Gloves (sterile or clean)
- Gown for client
- Lubricant
- Ophthalmoscope
- Otoscope
- Papanicolaou smear slides
- Paper towels
- Percussion hammer
- Safety pin
- Scale with height measurement rod
- Spatula
- Specimen containers and microscope slides
- Sphygmomanometer and cuff
- Stethoscope
- Swabs or sponge forceps
- Tape measure
- Thermometer
- Tissues
- Tongue depressor
- Tuning fork
- Vaginal speculum
- Wristwatch with second hand

TABLE 20-5 Positions for Examination

Position		Areas Assessed	Rationale	Limitations
Sitting		Head and neck, back, posterior thorax and lungs, anterior thorax and lungs, breasts, axillae, heart, vital signs, and upper extremities	Sitting upright provides full expansion of lungs and provides better visualization of symmetry of upper body parts.	Physically weakened client may be unable to sit. Examiner should use supine position with head of bed elevated instead.
Supine		Head and neck, anterior thorax and lungs, breasts, axillae, heart, abdomen, extremities, pulses	This is most normally relaxed position. It prevents contracture of abdominal muscles and provides easy access to pulse sites.	If client becomes short of breath easily, examiner may need to raise head of bed.
Dorsal recumbent		Head and neck, anterior thorax and lungs, breasts, axillae, heart	Clients with painful disorders are more comfortable with knees flexed.	Position is not used for abdominal assessment because it promotes contracture of abdominal muscles.
Lithotomy		Female genitalia and genital tract	This position provides maximal exposure of genitalia and facilitates insertion of vaginal speculum.	Lithotomy position is embarrassing and uncomfortable, so examiner minimizes time that client spends in it. Client is kept well draped. Client with severe arthritis or other joint deformity may be unable to assume this position.
Sims'		Rectum and vagina	Flexion of hip and knee improves exposure of rectal area.	Joint deformities may hinder client's ability to bend hip and knee.
Prone		Musculoskeletal system	This position is used only to assess extension of hip joint.	This position is intolerable for client with respiratory difficulties.
Knee-chest		Rectum	This position provides maximal exposure of rectal area.	This position is embarrassing and uncomfortable. Clients with arthritis or other joint deformities may be unable to assume this position.

more susceptible to chills. The nurse should ask if the client is comfortable. The client may become more relaxed if offered a pillow, sip of water, or tissue.

POSITIONING. During the examination, the nurse asks clients to assume proper positions so that body parts are accessible and clients stay comfortable. Table 20-5 lists the preferred positions for each part of the examination and contains figures illustrating these positions. Clients' abilities to assume positions will depend on their physical strength and degree of wellness. Many of the positions, such as the lithotomy and knee-chest, are embarrassing and uncomfortable. Therefore clients should be kept in these positions no longer than necessary. The examiner explains the positions and assists clients in attaining them. The drapes are adjusted to be sure that the area to be examined is accessible and that no body part is unnecessarily exposed. More than one position can be assumed for the same part of an examination (for example, supine and sitting for assessment of the anterior thorax), so the nurse first chooses the position that provides greater accessibility and accuracy in assessing body parts (sitting for anterior thorax). However, if clients are too weak or are physically unable to assume a position, the nurse may choose an alternative position. The nurse uses extra care to position older adults to avoid looking into the source of light, which can cause discomfort from glare.

Psychological Preparation

Clients are easily embarrassed when forced to answer sensitive questions about bodily functions or when body parts are exposed and examined. The possibility that the examiner will find something abnormal also creates anxiety, so reduction of this anxiety may be the nurse's highest priority before the examination. A thorough explanation lets clients know what to expect and what to do so that they can cooperate. The nurse first tells clients about the examination in general terms.

Ms. Bryce, I'm going to do a complete physical examination so that I can have a good idea of whether you have any health problems. As we go along, I'll explain to you exactly what I'll be doing. Feel free to ask any questions. If you become uncomfortable, please tell me.

Then as the nurse examines each body system, a more detailed explanation is given.

As I examine your breasts, I want you to relax lying down. First I want to look at the color, size, and shape of your breasts. Then I'll gently use my hands to feel the breast tissue itself.

The nurse uses simple terms when describing steps of the examination. Complicated terminology confuses clients and adds to their fears. The nurse's manner should be professional. Yet, voice tone and facial expressions should be relaxed to put clients at ease. The nurse encourages clients to ask questions and mention discomfort they feel during the assessment. When the client and examiner are of opposite gender, it helps to have a third person of the client's gender in the room, especially when examination of the sexual organs is required. The presence of a third person assures the client that the examiner will behave ethically, and the third person acts as a witness to the examiner's proper conduct.

During the examination, the nurse watches the client's emotional responses. The nurse observes whether the client's facial expression conveys fear or concern and whether body movements reveal anxiety, such as frequently pulling the drape around the body or tensing up as the examiner touches the body. The nurse must remain calm and clearly explain each step of the assessment. It may be necessary to stop the examination and ask whether the client feels anxious, afraid, or uncomfortable. The client should not be forced to continue. Postponing the examination until a later time may be advantageous because the findings may be more accurate when the client can cooperate and relax. If the fears result from misconceptions, the examiner clarifies the purpose of the examination and how it is to be performed.

Assessment of Age Groups

The nurse uses different interview styles when talking with clients of different ages and with parents of clients. The following tips assist in data collection during physical examination:

1. When obtaining histories on infants and children, gather all or part of the information from parents or guardians.
2. Because parents may think they are being tested by the examiner, offer support during the examination and do not pass judgment.
3. Call children by their first name, and address the parents as "Mr. and Mrs. Brown" rather than by their first names.
4. Use open-ended questions to allow parents to share more information and describe more of the children's problems.

5. Interview older children to allow observation of parent-child interactions.

6. Interview older children, who can often provide details about their health history and severity of symptoms.

7. Treat adolescents as adults and individuals because they tend to respond best when treated as such.

8. Remember that adolescents have the right to confidentiality. After talking with parents about historical information, speak alone with adolescents.

9. Do not stereotype aging clients. Most are able to adapt to change and to learn about their health. Similarly, they are reliable historians.

10. Recognize that sensory or physical limitations can affect how quickly you are able to interview older adults and conduct examinations. Plan for more than one examination session.

 ## ORGANIZATION OF THE EXAMINATION

A physical examination, using the skills of physical assessment, is composed of individual assessments for each body system. The extent of an examination depends on its purpose and a client's condition. A client who comes to a clinic with symptoms of a severe chest cold will not routinely require a neurological assessment. An acutely ill client requires assessment of body systems most at risk for being abnormal. When a client is admitted to the hospital, a complete examination is usually performed. Clients with specific symptoms or needs often require only portions of an examination. The performance of a complete health assessment follows the format of the nursing history (see Chapter 6). The nurse uses information from the history to focus attention on specific parts of the examination. For example, if the history reveals symptoms of abdominal discomfort, the nurse examines the abdomen carefully. Findings from the history generally reveal a pattern of related signs and symptoms. The physical examination supplements information from the history to confirm or refute the data.

The examination should be systematic and well organized so that important assessments are not deleted. A head-to-toe approach includes all body systems and helps the nurse anticipate each step. The examiner begins with an assessment of the head and neck area, progressing methodically down the body to incorporate all body systems. The following tips help the nurse keep an examination well organized:

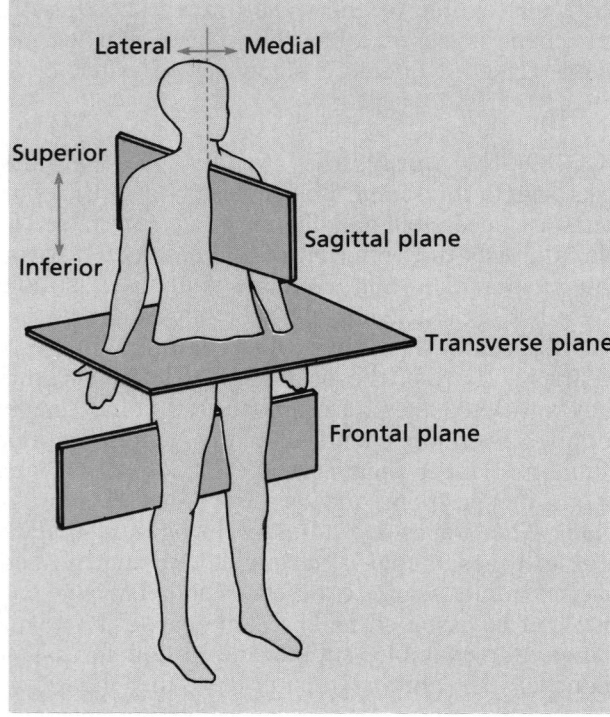

Fig. 20-5 The nurse describes assessment findings in terms of the anatomical position within body planes.

1. Compare both sides of the body for symmetry. A degree of asymmetry is normal (for example, the bicep muscles in the dominant arm may be more developed than the same muscles in the nondominant arm).

2. If a client is seriously ill, first assess the systems of the body more at risk for being abnormal. For example, a client with chest pain should undergo a cardiovascular assessment first.

3. If a client becomes fatigued, offer rest periods between assessments.

4. Perform painful procedures near the end of the examination.

5. Record results of the examination in specific anatomical and scientific terms so that any professional can interpret the findings (Fig. 20-5).

6. Use common and accepted medical abbreviations to keep notes brief and concise.

7. Record quick notes during the examination to avoid keeping the client waiting. Complete any observations at the end of the examination.

8. A physical assessment form allows recording of information in the same sequence it is gathered.

GENERAL SURVEY

As soon as a nurse meets a client, assessment begins. During a client's health history the nurse makes mental notes of the client's behavior and appearance.

The examination begins with a general survey that includes observation of general appearance and behavior and vital sign, height, and weight measurements. If abnormalities are found, the affected body system is closely assessed later during the examination. For example, if a client's appearance is unkempt, the nurse later inspects the skin and nails for adequacy of hygiene.

General Appearance and Behavior

Assessment of appearance and behavior begins while the nurse prepares the client for the examination. Information gained about general features may reveal characteristics of illness (for example, the facial appearance of a depressed client). The nurse's review of general appearance and behavior includes the following:

1. Gender and race. A person's gender affects the type of examination performed and the manner in which assessments are made. Different physical features are related to gender and race.
2. Signs of distress. There may be obvious signs or symptoms indicating a problem such as pain, difficulty in breathing, or anxiety. These findings help to establish priorities regarding what to examine first.
3. Body type. The nurse observes whether a client appears trim and muscular, obese, or excessively thin. Body type can reflect level of health, age, and lifestyle.
4. Posture. Normal standing posture is an upright stance with parallel alignment of hips and shoulders. Normal sitting posture involves some degree of rounding of the shoulders. The nurse observes whether the client has a slumped, erect, or bent posture. Posture may reflect mood or presence of pain. Many older adults assume a stooped, forward-bent posture, with hips and knees somewhat flexed and arms bent at the elbows, raising the level of the arms.
5. Gait. The nurse observes when a client walks into the examination room or at the bedside (if client is ambulatory). Movements are coordinated or uncoordinated. A person normally walks with arms swinging freely at the sides, with the head and face leading the body.

6. Body movements. The nurse observes whether movements are purposeful and notes whether there are any tremors involving the extremities. The nurse also determines whether any body parts are immobile.
7. Age. Age influences the normal features or physical characteristics. The ability to participate in some parts of the examination are also influenced by age.
8. Hygiene and grooming. The client's level of cleanliness is noted by observing the appearance of the hair, skin, and fingernails. The nurse also notes whether the client's clothes are clean. Grooming may depend on the activities being performed just before the examination. The nurse also notices the amount and type of cosmetics used.
9. Dress. Culture, lifestyle, socioeconomic level, and personal preference affect the type of clothes worn. The nurse notes whether the type of clothing worn is appropriate for the temperature and weather conditions. A depressed or mentally ill person may be unable to choose proper clothing. An older adult tends to wear extra clothing because of the sensitivity to cold.
10. Body odor. An unpleasant body odor may be the result of physical exercise. Poor hygiene may result in body odor, and poor oral hygiene may result in bad breath. A breath with alcohol on it does not always mean alcoholism.
11. Affect and mood. Affect is a person's feelings as they appear to others. Mood or emotional state is expressed verbally and nonverbally. The nurse notes whether verbal expressions match nonverbal behavior and observes whether the client's mood is appropriate for the situation. For example, the mood is inappropriate if the client seems unusually happy after recently being diagnosed with cancer. Facial expressions are observed as questions are asked.
12. Speech. Normal speech is understandable and moderately paced and shows an association with the person's thoughts. The nurse notes whether the client talks rapidly or slowly. An abnormal pace may be caused by emotions or neurological impairment. The nurse also observes whether the client speaks in a normal tone with clear inflection of words.
13. Client abuse. The abuse or neglect of a child or older adult is becoming a serious health problem. The nurse may suspect abuse while conducting a general survey. Additional assessment findings that may indicate abuse include the client's fear of the care giver, parent, or child; the care giver's

history of violence, alcoholism, or drug abuse; evidence that the client has suffered obvious physical injury or signs of neglect (for example, evidence of malnutrition); the care giver's unemployment, illness, or frustration in caring for the client (Elder abuse, 1987). Many states now mandate a report to a social service center if abuse or neglect is suspected.

Vital Signs

Most nurses prefer measuring vital signs (see Chapter 19) before the physical examination because positioning or moving the client during the examination can interfere with obtaining accurate values. However, it is also appropriate for the nurse to measure specific vital signs during assessment of individual body systems. For example, the pulse can be assessed during examination of the peripheral pulses or the heart and respirations during examination of the thorax. Body temperature is always measured during the general survey.

Height and Weight

General level of health can be reflected in the ratio of height to weight. Weight is a routine measure for clients visiting physicians' offices or clinics, and many health screenings routinely include height and weight. Both measures are always taken when clients are admitted to hospitals. A nurse measures infants' and children's height and weight to assess growth and development. Before this measurement, the nurse asks clients their height and weight. It may help to know their satisfaction or perceptions of body image. The nurse also determines whether they have had recent weight gains or losses. If a change exists, the nurse determines the amount, the period of time over which weight change occurred, and the cause, including change in diet habits, appetite, or physical symptoms (for example, nausea). A sudden loss in weight may indicate serious disease or a major change in dietary habits. It is normal for a client's weight to vary each day because of fluid loss or retention.

Clients should be weighed at the same time of day, on the same scale, and in the same clothes to allow an objective comparison of subsequent weights. Clients capable of bearing their own weight use a standing scale. The nurse calibrates the scale by setting the weight at *zero* and noting whether the balance beam registers in the middle of the mark. Scales with a digital display should read *zero* before each use. The client stands on the scale platform and remains still (Fig. 20-6). The nurse slowly adjusts the scale weight on the balance beam until the tip of the beam

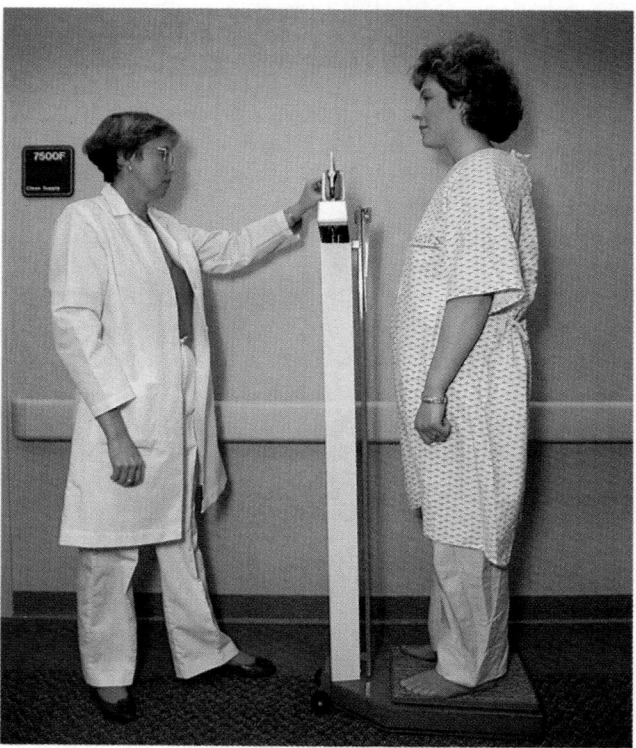

Fig. 20-6 The client stands on the scale as the nurse adjusts the balance.

registers in the middle of the mark. Digital scale readouts display weight in a matter of seconds.

Stretcher and chair scales are available for clients unable to bear weight. After being transferred to the scale, the client is lifted above the bed by a hydraulic device, and the weight is measured on a balance beam or digital display. Caution must be used when transferring clients to and from the scales.

Infants can be weighed in baskets or on platform scales. The nurse removes clothing and diapers to ensure accurate readings. The room should be warm to prevent chills. A light cloth or paper placed on the scale's surface prevents cross-infection from urine or feces. The nurse places infants in baskets or on platforms and holds a hand lightly above them to prevent accidental falls. Weight is measured in grams or pounds.

Different techniques exist for measuring the height of weight-bearing and non-weight-bearing clients. Clients able to stand remove their shoes. Paper towels are placed on the scale platforms or floor so that clients' feet remain clean. A measuring stick or tape is attached vertically to the weight scales or wall. The nurse asks clients to stand erect, exercising good posture. On a standing scale, a metal rod, which is attached to the back of the scale, swings out and over the top of the head (Fig. 20-7). A measuring

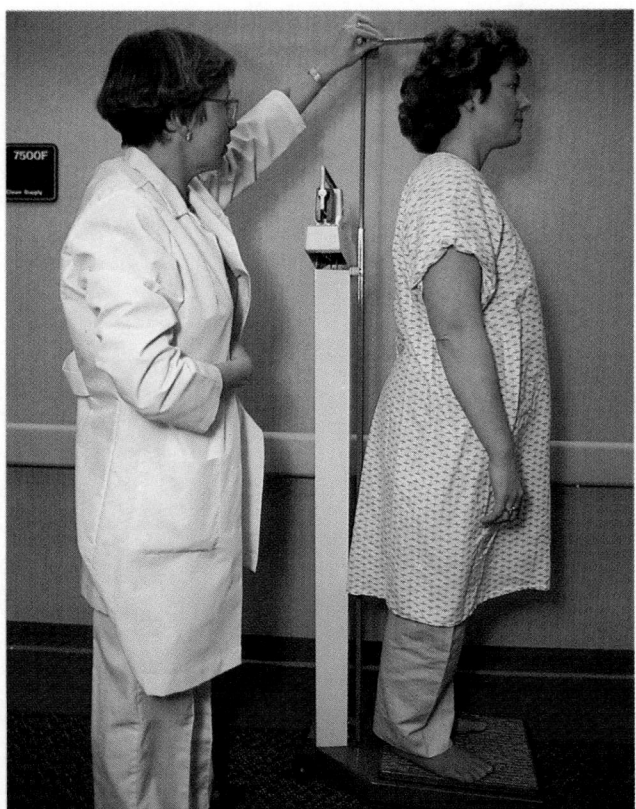

Fig. 20-7 The client stands erect to permit an accurate measurement of height.

stick or flat book can also be placed on the head when a scale is unavailable. With the rod or stick placed level horizontally at a 90-degree angle to the measuring stick, the nurse measures height in inches or centimeters.

A non-weight-bearing client (such as an infant) is positioned supine on a firm surface. The legs are extended straight with the soles of the feet supported upright. The nurse places a tape measure from the soles of the feet to the vertex of the head to measure the recumbent length.

 ## INTEGUMENT

The skin or **integumentary system** provides the body's external protection, regulates body temperature, and acts as a sensory organ for pain, temperature, and touch. Assessment of the integument includes the skin, hair, scalp, and nails. The nurse may initially inspect all skin surfaces or may assess the skin gradually while other body systems are examined.

A greater proportion of hospitalized clients are debilitated or older. As a result there are significant risks for skin lesions resulting from trauma to the skin while administering care, for exposure to pressure during immobilization, or for reaction to the various medications used in treatment. Nurses must routinely assess the skin to look for primary or initial lesions that may develop. Without proper care, primary lesions can quickly deteriorate to become secondary lesions that require more extensive nursing care. The development of a pressure ulcer, for example, can lengthen a hospital stay unless it is prevented or discovered early and treated properly. The nurse uses assessment findings to determine the type of hygiene measures required to maintain integrity of the integument (see Chapter 34). Adequate nutrition and hydration become goals of therapy if the nurse identifies alterations in the integument's status (see Chapter 35). To assess the integument, the nurse uses inspection, palpation, and olfaction.

Skin

Adequate illumination of the skin is required during assessment. If moist or draining skin lesions are present, disposable gloves are needed for palpation. Because the nurse inspects all skin surfaces, the client must assume several positions. The nursing history for skin assessment is outlined in Table 20-6 on p. 522. The examination includes inspection of the skin's color, moisture, temperature, texture and thickness, and turgor. Vascular changes, edema, and any lesions are noted. If abnormalities are seen, the nurse palpates the involved areas. Skin odors are usually noted in the skin folds, such as the axilla or under the female client's breasts. Fig. 20-8 on p. 522 illustrates a normal cross section of the skin.

Color

Skin color varies from body part to body part and from person to person. Despite individual variations, skin color is usually uniform over the body. However, in older adults, **pigmentation** increases unevenly, causing discolored skin. Table 20-7 on p. 523 lists common variations. Normal skin pigmentation ranges in tone from ivory to deep brown, ruddy pink to light pink, or yellow to olive. Race affects skin color. The assessment of color first involves areas of the skin not exposed to the sun, such as the palms of the hands. Exposed areas such as the face and arms will be darker. It is more difficult to note changes such as pallor or cyanosis in clients with dark skin. Usually they have lighter areas of pigmentation in the palms, soles of the feet, lips, and nail beds. Areas of increased color (hyperpigmentation) and decreased color (hypopigmentation) are common.

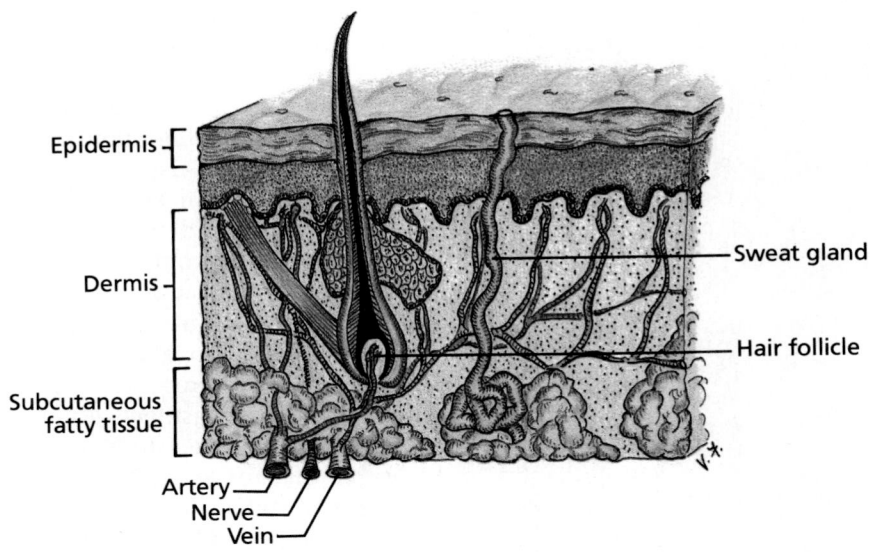

Fig. 20-8 A cross section of the skin reveals three layers: epidermis, dermis, and subcutaneous fatty tissues.

TABLE 20-6 Nursing History for Skin Assessment	
Assessment Category	Rationale
Ask client about history of changes in skin color.	Client is the best source to note change. Skin cancer may first be noticed as localized change in skin color.
Determine whether client works or spends excessive time outside. If so, ask whether a sunscreen is worn and the level of protection.	Exposed areas such as face and arms will be more pigmented than rest of body. Use of sunscreen reduces risk of skin cancer when the sun-protection factor (SPF) is greater than or equal to 15.
Determine whether client has noted lesions or changes in skin.	Most skin changes do not develop suddenly. Change in character of lesion might indicate cancer.
Question client about frequency of bathing and type of soap used.	Excessive bathing and use of harsh soaps can cause dry skin.
Ask if client has had recent trauma to skin.	Injury can cause bruising and changes in skin texture.
Determine whether client has history of allergies.	Skin rashes commonly occur from allergies.
Ask if client uses topical medications or home remedies on skin.	Incorrect use of topical agents may cause inflammation or irritation.
Ask if client goes to tanning parlors, uses sun lamps, or takes tanning pills.	Overexposure of skin to these irritants can cause skin cancer.
Ask if client has family history of serious skin disorders such as skin cancer or psoriasis.	Family history may reveal information about client's condition.

The nurse focuses on sites where abnormalities are more easily identified. For example, pallor is most easily perceived in the buccal (mouth) mucosa, particularly in individuals with dark skin. **Cyanosis** (bluish discoloration) is more readily seen in areas of least pigmentation such as the lips, nail beds, palpebral conjunctivae, and palms. The best site to inspect for **jaundice** (yellow-orange discolorations) is the client's sclera. Localized skin changes, such as pallor or **erythema** (red discoloration), may indicate circulatory changes. For example, an area of erythema may be due to localized vasodilation resulting from a sunburn or fever. An area of an extremity that appears unusually pale may result from arterial occlusion or edema. It is important to ask if the client has noticed any changes in skin coloring (see teaching box). The client usually knows whether a change has occurred.

TABLE 20-7   Skin Color Variations

Color	Condition	Causes	Assessment Locations
Bluish (cyanosis)	Increased amount of deoxy-genated hemoglobin (associated with hypoxia)	Heart or lung disease, cold environment	Nail beds, lips, mouth, skin (severe cases)
Pallor (decrease in color)	Reduced amount of oxyhemoglobin	Anemia	Face, conjunctivae, nail beds, palms of hands
	Reduced visibility of oxyhemoglobin resulting from decreased blood flow	Shock	Skin, nail beds, conjunctivae, lips
	Vitiligo	Congenital or autoimmune condition causing lack of pigment	Patchy areas on skin over face, hands, arms
Yellow-orange (jaundice)	Increased deposit of bilirubin in tissues	Liver disease, destruction of red blood cells	Sclera, mucous membranes, skin
Red (erythema)	Increased visibility of oxyhemoglobin caused by dilation or increased blood flow	Fever, direct trauma, blushing, alcohol intake	Face, area of trauma, sacrum, shoulders, other common sites for pressure ulcers
Tan-brown	Increased amount of melanin	Suntan, pregnancy	Areas exposed to sun: face, arms; areola, nipples

Client Teaching During Skin Assessment

OBJECTIVES

- Client will perform a monthly self-examination of the skin.
- Client will identify factors that increase the risk of skin cancer.
- Client will follow hygiene practices aimed at maintaining skin integrity.

TEACHING STRATEGIES

- Teach client to conduct a monthly self-examination of the skin, noting moles, blemishes, and birth marks. Tell client to inspect all skin surfaces.
- Tell client to report to a physician any changes in the size, shape, or color of lesions or a sore that does not heal. A malignant melanoma (a dangerous disease if not diagnosed early) has warning signs of asymmetry (half of the mole is unlike the other half), border irregularity (edges are scalloped or ragged), color variety (many colors may be present), and diameter measurement (melanoma is usually larger than a pencil eraser).
- Instruct client to prevent skin cancer by avoiding overexposure to the sun: wear wide-brimmed hats and long sleeves, apply sunscreens with SPF greater than or equal to 15 approximately 15 minutes before going into the sun and after swimming or perspiring, avoid tanning under the direct sun at midday (11 AM to 3 PM), and do not use indoor sunlamps, tanning parlors, or tanning pills. Medications such as oral contraceptives and antibiotics can make the skin more sensitive to the sun.
- Instruct client to report any lesion that bleeds or fails to heal to a physician. Especially instruct older adult, who tends to have delayed wound healing.
- To treat "winter itch," tell client to avoid hot water, harsh soaps, and drying agents such as rubbing alcohol.
- Tell client to apply lotion and moisturizers to the skin regularly to reduce itching and drying.

EVALUATION

- Observe client perform skin assessment.
- Have client describe signs of skin cancer and measures to take to prevent skin cancer.
- Ask client to describe methods for keeping the skin lubricated and supple.

Moisture

Moisture in the skin is directly related to the degree of client hydration and the condition of the outer lipid layer of the skin surface (DeWitt, 1990) The hydration of skin and mucous membranes helps reveal body fluid imbalances, changes in the integument's environment, and regulation of body temperature. *Moisture* refers to wetness and oiliness. The skin is normally smooth and dry. Skin folds such as the axillae are normally moist. After excessive exercise or exposure to warm temperatures, the skin may be moist from perspiration. Excessively dry skin is common in older adults and persons who use excessive amounts of soap during bathing. The nurse palpates the skin surface and observes mucous membranes for dullness, dryness, crusting, and flaking. The client is asked about itching. "Winter itch" is a common condition found in climates with low humidity during the winter season (DeWitt, l990). This excessive dryness can worsen existing skin conditions such as **eczema** and **dermatitis**. During palpation the nurse may locate skin lesions. If lesions ooze fluid, the color, odor, amount, and consistency are noted. The nurse must wear gloves to prevent exposure to infectious drainage.

Temperature

The temperature of the skin depends on the amount of blood circulating through the dermis. Increased or decreased skin temperature indicates an increase or decrease in blood flow. Temperature is more accurately assessed by palpating the skin with the dorsum or back of the hand. Skin temperature may be the same throughout the body or may vary in one area, such as the localized warmth at an infected wound site or the coldness of fingers resulting from reduced blood flow. Assessment of skin temperature is a basic assessment when the client is at risk for having impaired circulation (for example, after application of a cast or tight bandage or after vascular surgery). In addition, a nurse can identify a stage I pressure ulcer early when noting warmth and erythema of an area of the skin.

Texture

The character of the skin's surface and the feel of deeper portions are its texture. The nurse determines whether the client's skin is smooth or rough, thin or thick, tight or supple, and **indurated** (hardened) or soft by stroking it and palpating it lightly with the fingertips. The texture of the skin is normally smooth, soft, and flexible in children and adults. However, the texture is usually not uniform throughout. The palms of the hand and soles of the feet tend to be thicker. In older adults, the skin becomes wrinkled and leathery because of a decrease in collagen, subcutaneous fat, and sweat glands.

Localized changes may result from trauma or lesions. When irregularities in texture are found, the nurse asks if the client has experienced any recent injury to the skin. Deep palpation may reveal irregularities such as localized areas of induration commonly caused by repeated intramuscular or subcutaneous injections. If the client has diabetes or receives vitamin B_{12} or iron injections, indurated areas are common.

Turgor

Turgor is the skin's elasticity, which can be diminished by edema or dehydration. Normally the skin loses its elasticity with age. To assess the skin turgor, a fold of skin on the back of the client's hand or over the sternum is pinched between the thumb and forefinger and released (Fig. 20-9). The nurse notes the ease with which the skin moves and the speed at which it returns to place. Normally the skin lifts easily and snaps back immediately to its resting position. Failure of the skin to reassume its normal contour or shape indicates dehydration. The client with poor skin turgor does not have a resilience to the normal wear and tear on the skin. The skin tends to stay pinched or tented when turgor is poor. A decrease in turgor predisposes the client to skin breakdown.

Vascularity

The circulation of the skin affects color in localized areas and the appearance of superficial blood vessels. With aging, capillaries become fragile. Localized pressure area, found after a client has lain or sat

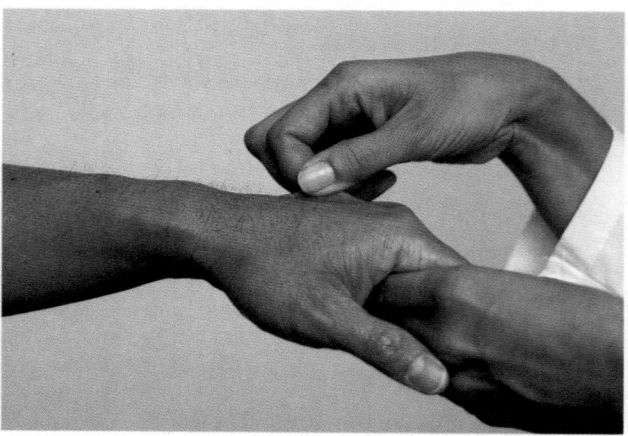

Fig. 20-9 Assessment for skin turgor.
From Canobbio MM: *Cardiovascular disorders*, St Louis, 1990, Mosby–Year Book.

in one position, appear reddened, pink, or pale. **Petechiae** are tiny, pinpoint-sized, red or purple spots on the skin caused by small hemorrhages in the skin layers. Petechiae may indicate serious blood-clotting disorders, drug reactions, or liver disease.

Edema

Areas of the skin become edematous because of a buildup of fluid in the tissues. Direct trauma and impairment of venous return are two common causes of **edema.** Edematous areas should be inspected for location, color, and shape. For the client with dependent edema caused by poor venous return, typical sites of edema are the feet, ankles, and sacrum. The formation of edema separates the skin's surface from the pigmented and vascular layers, masking skin color. The skin often becomes stretched and takes on a shiny appearance. The nurse palpates areas of edema to determine mobility, consistency, and tenderness. When pressure from the examiner's finger leaves an indentation in the edematous area, it is called *pitting edema*. To check the degree of pitting edema the nurse presses the edematous area firmly with the thumb for 5 seconds. The depth of pitting determines the degree of edema. For each centimeter in depth, the nurse records a plus sign (for example, 1 cm equals 1 + edema and 2 cm equal 2 + edema).

Lesions

The skin is normally free of lesions, except common freckles or age-related changes such as skin tags, **senile keratosis,** (thickening of skin), and atrophic warts. When a lesion is detected, it is inspected for color, location, size, type (see box on p. 526), grouping (clustered or linear), and distribution (localized or generalized). Palpation determines the lesion's mobility, contour (flat, raised, or depressed), and consistency (soft or indurated). Certain types of lesions present a characteristic pattern. For example, a tumor is usually an elevated, solid lesion larger than 2 cm. Primary lesions such as macules and nodules arise from some stimulus to the skin. Secondary lesions such as ulcers occur as alterations in primary lesions.

After it is identified, a lesion is closely inspected with good illumination. The lesion is palpated gently, covering its entire area. If the lesion is moist or draining fluid, gloves are worn during palpation because contact with drainage could spread infectious organisms.

It helps to ask clients if they have noticed any lesions, their causes, and any recent changes in their character (see teaching box). Further questioning as to how a lesion bothers a client and what has been done to care for it may reveal how a client feels about the disorder. Many clients react with fear and anxiety to rashes or other lesions. Cancerous lesions frequently undergo changes in color and size. Abnormal lesions are reported to the physician because further examination may be required.

Hair and Scalp

Good lighting allows the nurse to inspect the condition and distribution of hair and integrity of the scalp. Assessment of the hair occurs during all portions of the examination. Clients are sensitive about personal appearance. Thus the nurse explains the need to separate parts of the hair to detect problems. If lesions or lice are probable, the nurse wears disposable gloves to avoid infection. Table 20-8 describes the nursing history for a hair and scalp assessment.

Two types of hair cover the body, terminal hair (long, coarse, thick hair easily visible on the scalp, axillae, and pubic areas) and vellus hair (small, soft, tiny hairs covering the whole body except for palms and soles). The nurse assesses the distribution, thickness, texture, and lubrication of the hair. In addition, the nurse inspects for infection or infestation of the scalp.

Much of the information gathered about characteristics of hair growth comes from the client. In addition, the nurse needs to be aware of the normal distribution of hair growth in a man and a woman. Fine

TABLE 20-8 Nursing History for Hair and Scalp Assessment

Assessment Category	Rationale
Ask client if wig or hairpiece is being worn and request that it be removed.	Wigs or hairpieces interfere with inspection of hair and scalp. (Client may request to omit this part of examination.)
Determine if client has noted change in growth or loss of hair.	Change may occur slowly over time.
Identify type of shampoo, other hair care products, and curling irons used for grooming.	Excessive use of chemical agents and burning of hair causes drying and brittleness.
Determine if client has recently taken chemotherapy (if hair loss noted).	Chemotherapeutic agents kill cells that rapidly multiply, such as tumor cells and normal hair cells.

Types of Skin Lesions

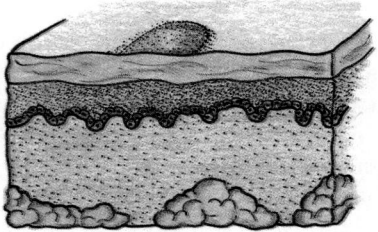

Macule: flat, nonpalpable, change in skin color, smaller than 1 cm (e.g., freckle, petechia)

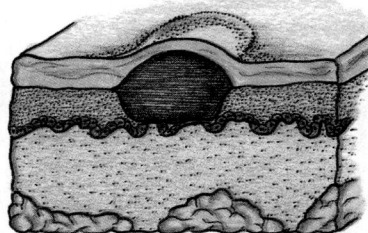

Papule: palpable, circumscribed, solid elevation in skin, smaller than 0.5 cm (e.g., elevated nevus)

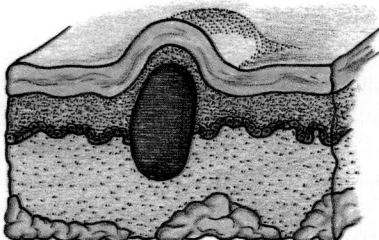

Nodule: elevated solid mass, deeper and firmer than papule, 0.5-0.2 cm (e.g., wart)

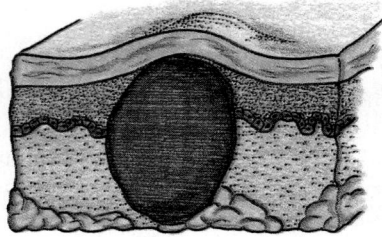

Tumor: solid mass that may extend deep through subcutaneous tissue, larger than 1-2 cm (e.g., epithelioma)

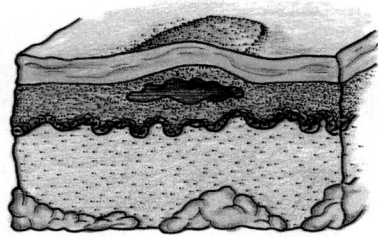

Wheal: irregularly shaped, elevated area or superficial localized edema, varies in size (e.g., hive, mosquito bite)

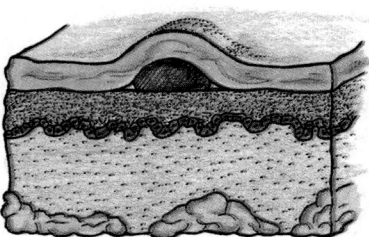

Vesicle: circumscribed elevation of skin filled with serous fluid, smaller than 0.5 cm (e.g., herpes simplex, chickenpox)

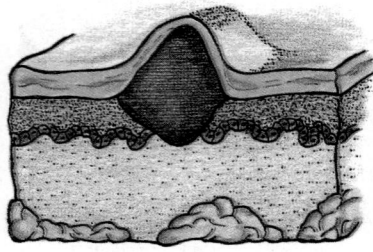

Pustule: circumscribed elevation of skin similar to vesicle but filled with pus, varies in size (e.g., acne, staphylococcal infection)

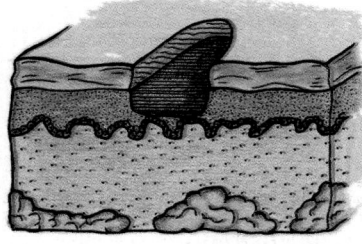

Ulcer: deep loss of skin surface that may extend to dermis and frequently bleeds and scars, varies in size (e.g., venous stasis ulcer)

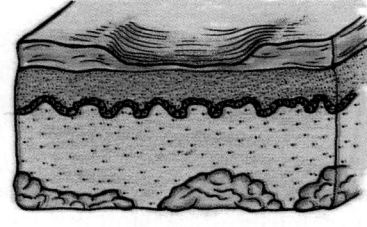

Atrophy: thinning of skin with loss of normal skin furrow with skin appearing shiny and translucent, varies in size (e.g., arterial insufficiency)

vellus hair covers the body and scalp hair, eyebrows, and eyelashes in both sexes. At puberty, a change in the amount and distribution of hair growth occurs. A client with hormone disorders may experience an unusual distribution and growth. A woman with **hirsutism** has hair growth on the upper lip, chin, and cheeks, with vellus hair becoming coarser over the body. A change in hair growth can negatively affect body image and emotional well-being. Asian and African Americans have less hair than European Americans, and Native Americans have little or no hair on their bodies (Rossman, 1979).

Normal, terminal hair is black, brown, red, yellow, or variations of these colors. The hair is coarse or fine. Normal variations exist in the shape of hair fibers. Clients' hair may be straight, curly, spiral, or wavy. The hair of African Americans is usually thicker, curlier, and drier than the hair of European Americans. The hair shaft is usually shiny and pliant.

In older adults, the hair becomes dull gray, white, or yellow. It also thins over the scalp, axillae, and pubic areas. Older men lose facial hair, whereas older women may develop hair on the chin and upper lip.

Changes may occur in the thickness, texture, and lubrication of scalp hair. A number of disturbances in body function, such as a febrile illness, can result in hair loss. Scalp disease can also cause loss of hair. Baldness (**alopecia**), or thinning of the hair, is usually related to genetic tendencies and endocrine disorders such as diabetes, thyroiditis, and even menopause (DeWitt, 1990). The hair is lubricated from the oil of sebaceous glands. Excessively oily hair is associated with androgen hormone stimulation. Dry, brittle hair occurs with aging and with excessive use of shampoo or other chemical agents. Poor nutrition often causes development of dry, coarse, discolored hair.

The amount of hair covering the extremities may be reduced as a result of aging and arterial insufficiency and is most commonly seen over the lower extremities. In women, loss of hair should not be confused with shaven legs.

The nurse inspects hair follicles on the scalp and pubic areas for lice or other parasites. The three types of lice are *Pediculus humanus capitis* (head lice), *Pediculus humanus corporis* (body lice), and *Pediculus pubis* (crab lice). Head and crab lice attach their eggs to hair. The tiny eggs look like oval particles of dandruff. The lice themselves are difficult to see. Head and body lice are very small with grayish white bodies. Crab lice have red legs. The nurse looks for bites or pustular eruptions in the hair follicles and in areas where skin surfaces meet, such as behind the ears and in the groin. The discovery of lice requires immediate treatment (see client teaching box).

When inspecting the scalp, the nurse asks if the client has noticed anything unusual. Lesions can easily go unnoticed in a thick growth of hair. By carefully separating strands of hair the nurse can thoroughly examine the scalp. The nurse assesses any lesion using the guidelines for skin lesions. If lumps or bruises are found, the nurse asks if the client has experienced recent trauma to the head. Moles on the scalp are common. The nurse should warn the client that combing or brushing can cause a mole to bleed. Scaliness or dryness of the scalp is frequently caused by dandruff or psoriasis.

Client Teaching During Hair and Scalp Assessment

OBJECTIVE

- Client will perform proper hygiene practices for care of the hair and scalp.

TEACHING STRATEGIES

- Instruct client about basic hygiene practices for care of the hair and scalp (see Chapter 34).
- Instruct client who has head lice to shampoo thoroughly with pediculicide (shampoo available at drug stores), comb thoroughly with fine-tooth comb (following product directions), and discard comb.
- Instruct client about ways to reduce the transmission of lice:
  - Do not share personal care items with others.
  - Vacuum all rugs, furniture, and flooring thoroughly and discard vacuum bag.
  - Use thorough handwashing.
  - Launder all clothing, linen, and bedding in hot soap and water and dry in hot dryer.

EVALUATION

- Have client describe methods used to care for hair and scalp.
- Have client explain steps taken to reduce lice transmission in the home.

Nails

The nails can reflect an individual's general state of health, state of nutrition, and occupation. Even a person's psychological state may be revealed by evidence of biting at nails. Before assessing the nails the nurse gathers a brief history (Table 20-9 on p. 528). The most visible portion of the nails is the nail plate, the transparent layer of epithelial cells covering the nail bed (Fig. 20-10 on p. 528). The vascularity of the nail bed creates the nail's underlying color. The semilunar, whitish area at the base of the nail bed is called the *lunula*, from which the nail plate develops. The nurse inspects the nail bed color, thickness and shape of the nail plate, texture of the nail, angle between the nail and the nail bed, and condition of the lateral and proximal nail folds around the nail. The nurse also palpates the nail base.

The nails are normally transparent, smooth, and convex, with a nail bed angle of about 160 degrees. The surrounding cuticles are smooth, intact, and without inflammation. In European Americans the

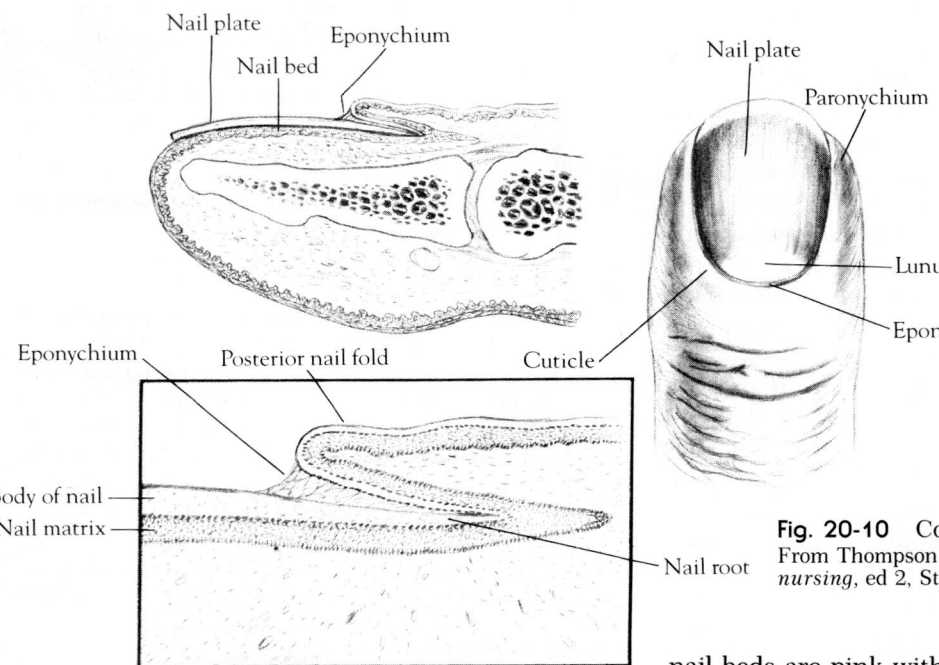

Fig. 20-10   Components of the nail unit.
From Thompson SM et al: *Mosby's manual of clinical nursing*, ed 2, St Louis, 1989, Mosby–Year Book.

TABLE 20-9   Nursing History for Nail Assessment

Assessment Category	Rationale
Ask if client has experienced recent trauma to nails.	Trauma may change shape and growth of nail. All or portion of nail plate can be lost.
Question client's nail care practices.	Chemical agents can cause drying of nails. Improper care may damage nails and cuticles.
Determine if client has noticed changes in nail appearance or growth.	Alterations may occur slowly over time.
Determine if client has risks for nail or foot problems (e.g., diabetes, older adulthood, obesity).	Vascular changes associated with diabetes reduce blood flow to peripheral tissues; foot lesions and thickened nails are common. Older adult may have trouble performing foot and nail care because of poor vision, uncoordination, or inability to bend over. Obese clients have difficulty bending over.

nail beds are pink with translucent white tips. In African Americans a brown or black pigmentation is normally present in longitudinal streaks. The nail bed is normally firm on palpation. Nails normally grow at a constant rate, but direct injury or generalized disease can impair growth. With aging, the nails of the fingers and toes develop longitudinal striations. The rate of nail growth also slows (Jacobs, 1981). Because of insufficient calcium, nails may turn yellow in older adults (Berman, Haxby, Pomerantz, 1988).

The nurse inspects the nail bed for splinter hemorrhages, transverse bands, and abnormal thickness. Splinter hemorrhages can be caused by trauma, cirrhosis, diabetes mellitus, hypertension, and acute bacterial endocarditis (Kpea, 1987). Vitamin, protein, and electrolyte changes can result in various lines or bands forming on the nail beds.

The surrounding nail folds are normally smooth and intact without inflammation. Chronic biting can cause inflammation, drying, and rough surfaces. Abnormalities such as erythema, swelling, and scaling should be reported.

The color of nails is an indicator of blood oxygenation. A bluish or purplish cast to the nail bed occurs with cyanosis. A white cast or pallor is the result of anemia. Thin nails can be a sign of poor circulation and nutritional deficiency. Extremely short nails with rough edges indicate nail biting, which is common in persons who frequently feel anxious. Changes in the shape and curvature of nails are indications of systemic disease (see box). Palpation of the nails also determines the adequacy of circulation or capillary refill. To palpate, the nurse gently grasps the client's

Abnormalities of the Nail Bed

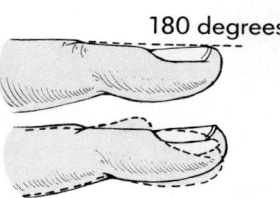

160 degrees

Normal nail: Approximately 160-degree angle between nail plate and nail

180 degrees Clubbing: Change in angle between nail and nail base (eventually larger than 180 degrees); nail bed softening, with nail flattening; often, enlargement of fingertips

180 degrees *Causes:* Chronic lack of oxygen: heart or pulmonary disease

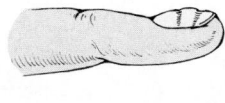

Beau's lines: Transverse depressions in nails indicating temporary disturbance of nail growth (Nail grows out over several months.)
Causes: Systemic illness such as severe infection, nail injury

Koilonychia (spoon nail): Concave curves
Causes: Iron deficiency anemia, syphilis, use of strong detergents

Splinter hemorrhages: Red or brown linear streaks in nail bed
Causes: Minor trauma, subacute bacterial endocarditis, trichinosis

Paronychia: Inflammation of skin at base of nail
Causes: Local infection, trauma

Client Teaching During Nail Assessment

OBJECTIVE

- Client will be able to properly care for fingernails and toe nails.

TEACHING STRATEGIES

- Instruct client to cut nails only after soaking them about 10 minutes in warm water.
- Instruct client to avoid use of over-the-counter preparations to treat corns, calluses, or ingrown toenails.
- Tell client to cut nails straight across and even with the tops of the fingers or toes. If client has diabetes, tell client to file, not cut, nails.
- Instruct client to shape nails with a file or emery board.

EVALUATION

- Inspect client's nails and feet during a follow-up examination.
- Have the client describe nail care measures.

Calluses and corns are commonly found on the toes or fingers. A callus is flat and painless. It results from a thickening of the epidermis. Corns are caused by friction and pressure from shoes and can usually be seen over a bony prominence. During the examination, the nurse instructs clients about proper nail care (see client teaching box).

HEAD AND NECK

An examination of the head and neck reviews the integrity of anatomical structures, including the head, eyes, ears, nose, mouth, pharynx, and neck (lymph nodes, carotid arteries, thyroid gland, and trachea). The carotid arteries can also be assessed during assessment of peripheral arteries. The nurse needs to understand each anatomical area and its normal function. Assessment of the head and neck uses inspection, palpation, and auscultation, with inspection and palpation often used simultaneously.

Head

The nursing history will reveal risk for intracranial injury and local or congenital deformities (Table 20-

finger and observes the color of the nail bed. Next, gentle, firm pressure is quickly applied with the thumb to the nail bed and released. As pressure is applied, the nail bed appears white or blanched. However, the pink color should return immediately after the release of pressure. Failure of the pinkness to promptly return indicates circulatory insufficiency.

TABLE 20-10 Nursing History for Head Assessment	
Assessment Category	**Rationale**
Determine if client experienced recent trauma to head.	Trauma is major cause for lumps, bumps, cuts, bruises, or deformities of scalp or skull.
Ask if client has noticed neurological symptoms such as headaches, dizziness, loss of consciousness, seizures, or blurred vision.	Head trauma may cause damage to brain tissues and change in neurological function.
Determine length of time client has experienced neurological symptoms.	Duration of signs or symptoms may reveal severity of problem.

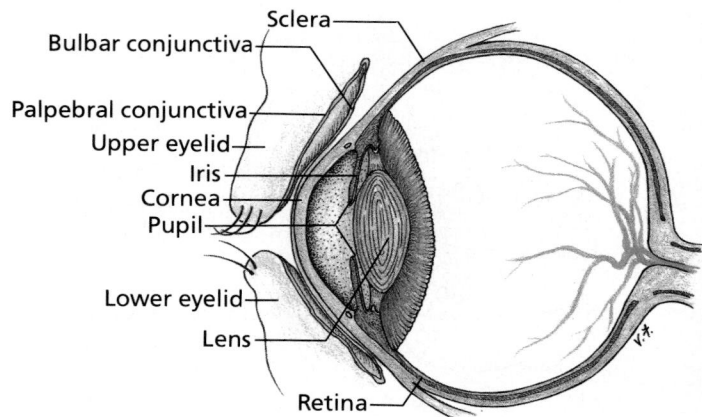

Fig. 20-11 Cross section of the eye.

10). The nurse inspects the client's head, noting the size, shape, and contour. The skull is generally round with prominences in the frontal area anteriorly and the occipital area posteriorly. Local skull deformities are typically caused by trauma. In infants, large heads may result from congenital anomalies or the buildup of cerebrospinal fluid in the ventricles (**hydrocephalus**). Adults may have enlarged jaws and facial bones resulting from **acromegaly,** a disorder caused by excessive secretion of growth hormone. The nurse palpates the skull for nodules or masses. Gentle rotation of the fingertips down the midline of the scalp and then along the sides of the head reveals abnormalities.

Eyes

Examination of the eyes includes assessment of visual acuity, visual fields, extraocular movements, and external and internal eye structures. Fig. 20-11 shows a cross section of the eye.

Assessment is very useful in determining the level of assistance that clients require when ambulating or performing self-care activities. Clients with visual problems may also need special aids for reading teaching materials or instructions (for example, medication labels). Table 20-11 reviews the nursing history for an eye examination. The box describes common types of visual problems.

Visual Acuity

The easiest way to initially assess visual acuity is to ask clients to read printed material under adequate lighting. If clients wear glasses, they should wear

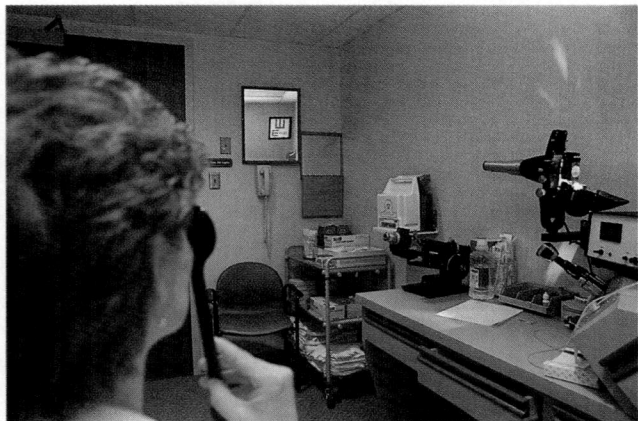

Fig. 20-12 Assessment of visual acuity. The client covers one eye while reading the Snellen chart. Each eye is assessed separately for visual acuity.

them. The nurse should know the language clients speak and whether they are literate and able to read. Asking clients to read aloud can help determine literacy.

For a more accurate assessment of visual acuity, a Snellen chart is used. If clients wear glasses, they wear them during the test but not if the glasses are prescribed for reading. Clients are positioned 20 feet from a chart or screen on which a chart is displayed. The client tries to read the smallest line of print possible three times, once with both eyes, then with each eye separately when the opposite eye is covered (Fig. 20-12). For clients unable to read, the E chart is used. Instead of reading letters, clients tell the examiner which direction each E is pointing. Clients are successful when they read more than half the letters or figures in a line. The visual acuity score is recorded for each eye and both eyes. The Snellen chart

TABLE 20-11 Nursing History for Eye Assessment

Assessment Category	Rationale
Determine if client has history of eye disease, eye trauma, diabetes, or hypertension.	Some diseases or trauma can cause risk for partial or complete visual loss.
Determine problems that prompted client to seek health care. Ask client about eye pain, photophobia (sensitivity to light), burning, itching, excess tearing or crusting, diplopia (double vision), blurred vision, awareness of a "film" over field of vision, floaters (small, black spots that seem to float across the field of vision), flashing lights, or halos around lights.	Common symptoms of eye disease indicate need for physician referral.
Determine whether there is family history of eye disorders.	Certain eye problems such as glaucoma or retinitis pigmentosa are inherited.
Assess client's occupational history.	Performance of close, intricate work can cause eye fatigue. Working with computers may cause eye strain. Certain occupational tasks (e.g., working with chemicals) place persons at risk for eye injury unless precautions are taken.
Ask client if glasses or contacts are normally worn.	Glasses or contacts should be worn during certain portions of examination for accurate assessment.
Determine when client last visited ophthalmologist or optometrist.	Date of last eye examination reveals level of preventive care taken by client.
Assess medications client is taking, including eye medications.	Determines need to assess client's knowledge of medications. Certain medications can cause visual symptoms.

Common Eye and Visual Problems

HYPEROPIA

Hyperopia is farsightedness, a refractive error in which rays of light enter the eye and focus behind the retina. Persons are able to clearly see distant objects but not close objects.

MYOPIA

Myopia is nearsightedness, a refractive error in which rays of light enter the eye and focus in front of the retina. Persons are able to clearly see close objects but not distant objects.

PRESBYOPIA

Presbyopia is impaired near vision in middle-age and older adults, caused by loss of elasticity of the lens and associated with the aging process.

ASTIGMATISM

Astigmatism is a condition in which parallel light rays do not focus on a single point on the retina. An uneven curvature of the cornea or lens causes light to be focused on different points.

STRABISMUS

Strabismus is a congenital problem in which the eyes appear crossed. The muscles controlling movement of the eyes are not coordinated.

CATARACTS

A cataract is the loss of transparency of the lens, which blocks light rays entering the eye. Cataracts may develop slowly and progressively after age 35 or suddenly after trauma. Cataracts are one of the most common eye disorders. By age 70, approximately 90% of the population has some evidence of visual impairment from cataracts.*

GLAUCOMA

Glaucoma is intraocular structural damage resulting from elevated intraocular pressure. It is caused by obstruction of the outflow of aqueous humor. Without treatment the disorder can cause blindness.

MACULAR DEGENERATION

Macular degeneration is blurred central vision often occurring suddenly caused by a progressive degeneration of the center of the retina. It is the most common cause of blindness in older adults. There is no cure.

*Data from Kirton M, Richardson M: *Ophthalmic nursing,* ed 3, Philadelphia, 1987, Bailliere-Tindall.

has standardized numbers at the end of each line of the chart. The numerator is the number 20 or the standard distance the client stands from the chart. The denominator is the distance from which the normal eye can read the chart. Normal vision is 20/20. The larger the denominator, the poorer the visual acuity. For example, a value of 20/40 means the client, standing 20 feet away, can read a line that a person with normal vision can read from 40 feet away. The nurse records visual acuity as s̄c (without correction) or c̄c (with correction), depending on whether clients wear glasses or contact lenses.

If clients cannot read even the largest letters or figures of a Snellen chart, the nurse tests their ability to count upraised fingers or distinguish light. The nurse holds a hand 30 cm (1 ft) from the face and instructs clients to count the upraised fingers. To check light perception, the nurse shines a penlight into the eye and then turns the light off. If clients note when the light is turned on or off, light perception is intact.

Extraocular Movements

Six small muscles guide the movement of each eye. Both eyes move parallel to each other in each direction of gaze. Extraocular movements are measured through the eight cardinal gazes (Fig. 20-13). The nurse stands in front of the client and holds a finger at a comfortable distance (6 to 12 in or 15 to 30 cm) in front of the client's eyes. The client keeps the head in a fixed position facing the nurse and follows the movement of the finger with the eyes only. The client looks to the right, to the left, up, down, and diagonally up and down to the left and right. The examiner's finger stays within the normal field of vision. As the client gazes in each direction, the nurse moves the finger slowly and smoothly.

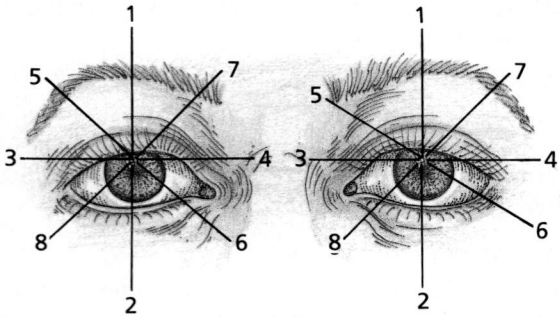

Fig. 20-13 The eight directions of gaze. The nurse directs the client to follow the finger movement through each gaze.

The nurse observes for parallel eye movement, the position of the upper eyelid in relation to the iris, and the presence of abnormal movements. As the eyes move through each direction of gaze, the upper eyelid only covers the iris slightly. By periodically stopping movement of the finger the nurse can assess **nystagmus,** an involuntary, rhythmical oscillation of the eyes. The nurse can also often initiate nystagmus in clients with normal eye movements by having them gaze to the far left or right. Disturbances in eye movement reflect local injury to eye muscles and supporting structures or a disorder of the cranial nerves innervating the muscles.

The nurse can also check the alignment of the eyes by assessing the corneal light reflex. A weakness or imbalance of the extraocular muscles can cause a misalignment. The nurse shines a penlight onto the bridge of the client's nose from 60 to 90 cm (2 to 3 ft) away in a darkened room. The client stares straight ahead. Normally the light reflects on the cornea in the same spot on both eyes. If an abnormality is present, the light shines on a different spot on each eye.

Visual Fields

As a person looks straight ahead, all objects in the periphery can normally be seen. To assess visual fields the nurse has the client stand or sit 60 cm (2 ft) away, facing the nurse at eye level. The client gently closes or covers one eye (such as the left) and looks at the nurse's eye directly opposite. The nurse closes the opposite eye (in this case the right) so that the field of vision is superimposed on that of the client. The nurse moves a finger equidistant from the nurse and client outside the field of vision, then slowly brings it back into the visual field. The client is asked to tell when the nurse's finger is seen. If the nurse sees the finger before the client does, a portion of the client's visual field is reduced. To test temporal field vision, the object should be slightly behind the client. (NOTE: The nurse can see the finger.) The procedure is repeated for each field of vision for the other eye. Clients with visual field problems may be at risk for injury because they cannot see all objects in front of them. Older adults commonly have loss of peripheral vision caused by changes in the lens.

External Eye Structures

To inspect external eye structures, nurses stand directly in front of the client at eye level and asks the client to look at their faces.

POSITION AND ALIGNMENT. The eyes are normally parallel to each other. Bulging (**exophthalmos**) is usually caused by hyperthyroidism when both eyes are involved. Abnormal protrusion of one eye may be caused by a tumor or inflammation of the eye's orbit.

EYEBROWS. The eyebrows are normally symmetrical. The eyebrows are inspected for distribution of hair, alignment, and movement. A loss or absence of hair indicates hormonal disturbance. Aging causes loss of the lateral third of the eyebrows. Flaking of skin around the brows may be a form of dandruff, which can cause chronic eye irritation. The brows should raise and lower symmetrically. Paralysis of the facial nerve exists if a client cannot move the eyebrows.

EYELIDS. The nurse inspects the eyelids for position, color, condition of surface, condition and direction of eyelashes, and the client's ability to close and blink. When the eyes are open in a normal position, the lids do not cover the pupil, and the sclera cannot be seen above the iris. The lids are also close to the eyeball. An abnormal drooping of the lid over the pupil is called *ptosis* (pronounced "toe-sis") and is caused by edema or impairment of the third cranial nerve. Defects in the position of the lid margins may be observed. An older adult frequently has lid margins that turn out (**ectropion**) or in (**entropion**). A disruption of the lid margin may lead to irritation of the conjunctivae. The eyelashes are normally distributed evenly and curved outward away from the eye. If the eyelid becomes inverted the lashes may turn inward and irritate the eye.

To inspect the surface of the upper lids, the nurse asks clients to close their eyes and raises both eyebrows gently with the thumb and index finger to stretch the skin. The lids are normally the same color as the skin. Redness indicates inflammation or infection. Heart and kidney failure and allergies can cause edema of the eyelids, which prevents them from closing. Lesions are inspected for typical characteristics and discomfort or drainage. The lids normally close symmetrically. Failure of the lids to close exposes the cornea to drying.

The nurse asks the client to open the eyes for inspection of the lower lids. The same characteristics noted for the upper lids are assessed. Normally a person blinks involuntarily and bilaterally up to 20 times a minute. The blink reflex helps lubricate the cornea. The nurse reports absent or infrequent, rapid, or monocular (one-eyed) blinking.

LACRIMAL APPARATUS. The anterior surface of the eye, made up of the sensitive cornea and conjunctivae, is moistened or lubricated by tears secreted from the lacrimal gland (Fig. 20-14). The gland is located in the upper outer wall of the anterior part of the orbit. Tears flow from the gland across the eye's sur-

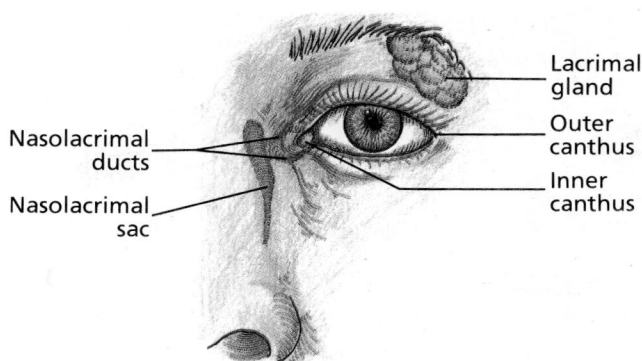

Fig. 20-14 The lacrimal apparatus secretes and drains tears, which moisten and lubricate eye structures.

face to the lacrimal duct, which is located in the nasal corner or inner canthus of the eye. The lacrimal gland can be the site of tumors or infections. The area of the gland is inspected for edema and redness, and it is palpated gently to detect tenderness. Normally the gland cannot be felt.

The nasolacrimal duct may become obstructed, blocking the flow of tears. If the client complains of excess tearing, the nurse looks for evidence of edema in the inner canthus. Mild palpation of the duct at the lower eyelid just inside the lower orbital rim, not on the side of the nose, may cause a regurgitation of tears.

CONJUNCTIVAE AND SCLERAE. The bulbar conjunctiva covers the exposed surface of the eyeball up to the outer edge of the cornea, and the palpebral conjunctiva is the delicate membrane lining the eyelids. Normally the conjunctiva is transparent, enabling the examiner to view the tiny underlying blood vessels that give it a light pink color. The sclera is seen under the bulbar conjunctiva and normally has the color of white porcelain in European Americans and light yellow in African Americans.

Care must be taken when inspecting the conjunctivae. For adequate exposure of the bulbar conjunctivae, the eyelids must be retracted without placing pressure directly on the eyeball. Both lids are gently retracted, with the thumb and index finger pressed against the lower and upper bony orbits. The client is asked to look up, down, and side to side. Many clients begin to blink, making the examination difficult. The nurse inspects for color, texture, and lesions.

To inspect the palpebral conjunctiva the nurse must evert the lower eyelids (Fig. 20-15 on p. 534). The lower lid is gently depressed with the thumb or index finger. Often the client can depress the eyelid to facilitate examination. The conjunctiva's color and

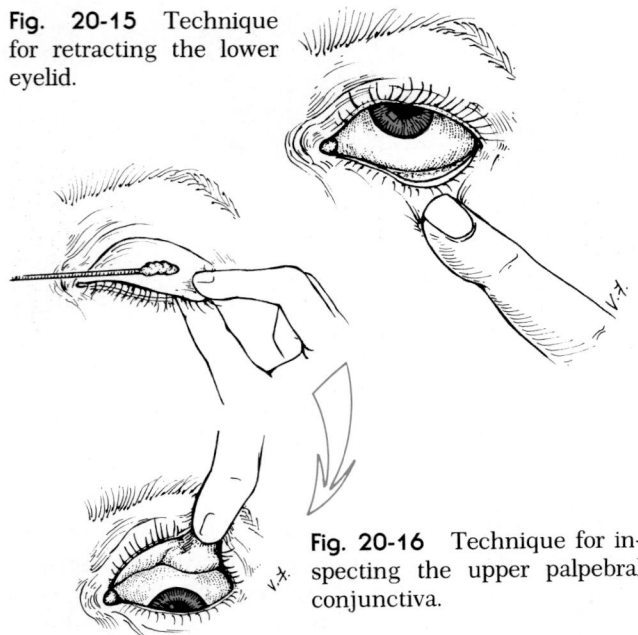

Fig. 20-15 Technique for retracting the lower eyelid.

Fig. 20-16 Technique for inspecting the upper palpebral conjunctiva.

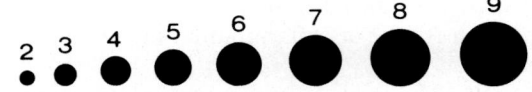

Fig. 20-17 Chart depicting pupillary size in millimeters.

edema or lesions are noted. A pale conjunctiva results from anemia, whereas a fiery red appearance is the result of inflammation (conjunctivitis). **Conjunctivitis** is a highly contagious infection. The crusty drainage that collects on eyelid margins can easily spread from one eye to the other. The nurse should wear gloves during the examination. Thorough handwashing is necessary before and after the examination.

A special technique is used to inspect the upper palpebral conjunctiva (Fig. 20-16) and should not be attempted the first time without qualified assistance. The technique is useful if the nurse suspects a foreign body under the lid. The client is asked to look down, relax the eyes, and avoid any sudden movement. The upper lid is gently grasped with a gloved hand, and the lashes are pulled down and forward. The end of a cotton applicator is placed 1 cm (½ inch) above the lid margin. The nurse pushes down on the upper eyelid, turning it inside out. A light grasp on the upper lashes keeps the lid inverted. After inspection the eyelashes are gently pulled forward, and the client is instructed to look up. The eyelid will return to its normal position. If a foreign body appears to be embedded in the eye, the nurse should *not* attempt to remove it and should notify a physician immediately.

CORNEAS. The cornea is the transparent, colorless portion of the eye covering the pupil and iris. From a side view, the cornea looks like the crystal of a wristwatch. As the client looks straight ahead, the nurse inspects the cornea for clarity and texture while shining a penlight obliquely across the cornea's entire surface. The cornea is normally shiny, transparent, and smooth. However, in an older adult, the cornea loses its luster. Any irregularity in the surface may indicate an abrasion or tear. The color and details of the underlying iris should be easy to see. In an older adult, the iris becomes faded. A thin, white ring along the margin of the iris, called an *arcus senilis,* is common with aging but is abnormal in anyone under age 40.

PUPILS AND IRISES. When a beam of light is shined through the pupil and onto the retina, the third cranial nerve is stimulated and innervates the muscles of the iris to constrict. Any abnormality along the nerve pathways from the retina to the iris alters the ability of the pupils to react to light. Changes in intracranial pressure, lesions along the nerve pathways, locally applied ophthalmic medications, and direct trauma to the eye may alter pupillary reaction.

The nurse observes the pupils for size, shape, equality, accommodation, and reaction to light. The pupils are normally black, round, and equal in size (3 to 7 mm in diameter) (Fig 20-17). Cloudy pupils often indicate cataracts. Dilated pupils can result from glaucoma, trauma, neurological disorders, or eye medications (for example, atropine). Constricted pupils may be caused by inflammation of the iris or drugs (for example, pilocarpine, morphine, or cocaine). The surrounding iris is inspected for defects along its margins.

Pupillary reflexes (to light and accommodation) should be tested in a dimly lit room. As the client looks straight ahead, the nurse brings a penlight from the side of the client's face, directing the light onto the pupil (Fig. 20-18). If the client looks at the light, there will be a false reaction to accommodation. A directly illuminated pupil constricts, and the opposite pupil constricts consensually. The nurse observes the quickness and equality of the reflex.

To test for accommodation, the nurse holds a finger 10 to 15 cm (4 to 6 in) from the client's nose. The client is asked to gaze at the finger and then at a distant object (for example, the wall in the distance). The pupils normally constrict when the client looks at the examiner's finger and dilate when the client looks at the wall; this shows the pupil's ability to accommodate to near and distant vision. Finally the

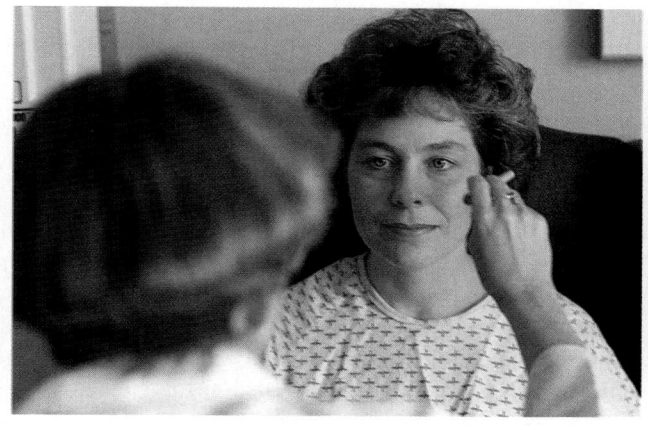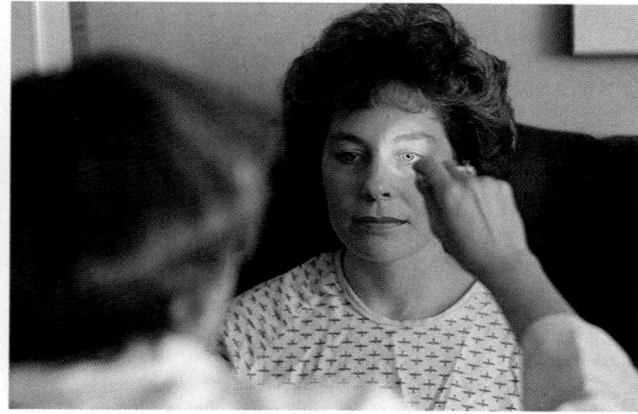

Fig. 20-18   **A,** To check pupil reflexes, the nurse first holds the penlight to the side of the client's face. **B,** Illumination of the pupil causes pupillary constriction.

nurse moves the finger smoothly and symmetrically toward the nasal bridge. The pupils normally converge.

If assessment of pupillary reaction is normal in all tests the nurse records the abbreviation, *PERRLA* (pupils equal, round, reactive to light, and accommodation).

Internal Eye Structures

The internal eye cannot be observed without an instrument to illuminate its structures. The **ophthalmoscope** is used to inspect the fundus, which includes the retina, choroid, optic nerve disc, macula, fovea centralis, and retinal vessels. Clients in greatest need of an examination are those with diabetes, hypertension, and intracranial disorders. The nurse should feel competent in using an ophthalmoscope before attempting this examination.

The ophthalmoscope has a battery tube light source, two dials or disks, and a keyhole viewer (Fig. 20-19). The dial at the top of the battery tube changes the light image. Five lenses are available, but the large white light is used for general examination. The dial at the top of the viewer rotates clockwise for selection of lenses.

The nurse should practice holding the ophthalmoscope in each hand, using the index finger to rotate the lens dial. The nurse turns the white light on, rotates the lens dial to *0*, and looks through the keyhole, focusing on near objects such as the palm of the hand. Reading the newspaper with the ophthalmoscope is useful practice. During an examination the nurse keeps both eyes open when looking through the keyhole.

The examination is performed in a darkened room. The examiner and client sit in comfortable positions

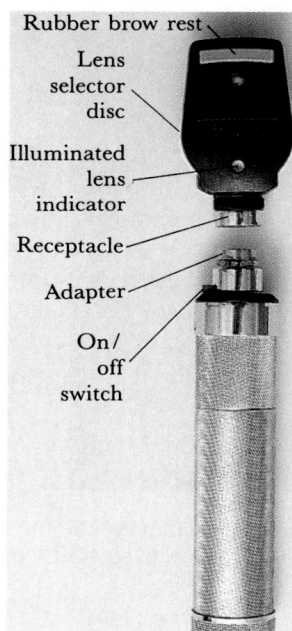

Rubber brow rest

Lens selector disc

Illuminated lens indicator

Receptacle

Adapter

On/off switch

Fig. 20-19   An ophthalmoscope.
From Seidel HM et al: *Mosby's guide to physical examination,* ed 2, St Louis, 1991, Mosby–Year Book.

facing each other with their eyes at the same height. The client removes eyeglasses, but contact lenses may be left in place. The ophthalmoscope's light is switched on and the lens rotated to *0*. The index finger is kept on the lens dial to refocus the ophthalmoscope.

The examiner's right hand and eye are used to examine the client's right eye, and the left hand and eye are used for the client's left eye. The client is asked to gaze straight ahead over the examiner's shoulder, keeping both eyes open through the examination.

The ophthalmoscope is held comfortably against the nurse's face. At a distance of approximately 25 cm (10 in) from the client and 25 degrees lateral to the client's central line of vision, the examiner shines the light on the pupil. A bright, orange glow in the pupil, called the *red reflex*, can then normally be seen. The light from the ophthalmoscope causes the pupil to constrict. The light is slowly moved toward the pupil while the examiner keeps it focused on the red reflex (Fig. 20-20). The nurse must relax and keep both eyes open. As the light approaches the pupil, the nurse begins to see structures of the fundus. Rotating the lens dial brings the internal structures into focus. The examiner inspects the size, color, and clarity of the disc; integrity of vessels; presence of retinal lesions; and appearance of the macula and fovea (Fig. 20-21). Normally the following structures are observed:

1. A clear, yellow optic nerve disc
2. Reddish-pink retina (European Americans) or darkened retina (African Americans)
3. Light red arteries and dark red veins
4. A 3:2 vein to artery ratio in size proportion
5. The avascular macula

If any abnormalities are observed, the client should be examined by an ophthalmologist (see teaching box). The client's fundus should not be illuminated for extended periods. The bright light of the ophthalmoscope is very irritating and can cause discomfort and tearing. During the examination, the nurse assesses the client for discomfort.

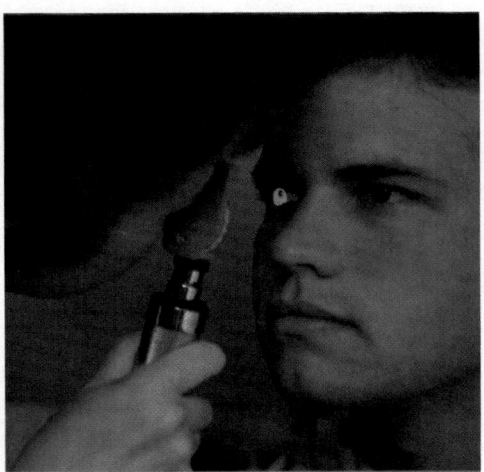

Fig. 20-20   To visualize internal eye structures, the nurse moves in toward the pupil with the light focused on the red reflex.

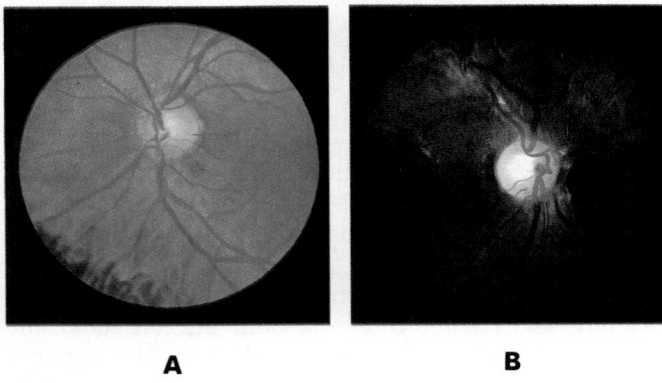

A   B

Fig. 20-21   Normal fundus. **A,** European American adult. **B,** African American adult.
From *Selected topics in ophthalmology,* Medcom clinical lecture guides, Garden Grove, Calif, 1973, Medcom, Inc.

| Client Teaching During Eye Assessment |

OBJECTIVES

- Client will follow recommendations for regular eye examinations.
- Client will be able to recognize warning signs and symptoms of eye disease.
- Client will take appropriate safety precautions for visual deficits.

TEACHING STRATEGIES

- Tell client that persons under age 40 should have complete eye examinations every 3 to 5 years (or more often if family histories reveal risks such as diabetes or hypertension).
- Tell client that persons over age 40 should have eye examinations every 2 years to screen for glaucoma.
- Tell client that persons over age 65 should have yearly eye examinations.
- Describe the typical symptoms of eye disease (see Table 20-11).
- Instruct older adult to take the following precautions because of normal visual changes: avoid or use caution while driving at night, increase lighting in the home to reduce risk of falls, and paint the first and last steps of a staircase and the edge of each step in between a bright color to aid depth perception.

EVALUATION

- Ask client or family member to report on most recent visit to ophthalmologist.
- Have client describe when to have an eye examination.
- Ask client to describe common symptoms of eye disease.
- Observe the home environment of a client with visual deficits.

Ears

The ears are easy to examine because of their accessibility. The three parts of the ear are the external, middle, and inner ear (Fig. 20-22). The nurse inspects and palpates external ear structures, inspects middle ear structures with an otoscope, and tests the inner ear by measuring hearing acuity. External ear structures consist of the auricle, outer ear canal, and tympanic membrane (eardrum). The ear canal is normally curved and approximately 1 inch (2.5 cm) long in an adult. It is lined with skin containing fine hairs, nerve endings, and glands secreting cerumen. The middle ear is an air-filled cavity containing the three bony ossicles (malleus, incus, and stapes). The eustachian tube connects the middle ear to the nasopharynx. Pressure between the outer atmosphere and middle ear is stabilized through the eustachian tube.

The inner ear contains the cochlea, vestibule, and semicircular canals. The nurse assesses the ears to determine the integrity of ear structures and the condition of hearing. Nursing history data (Table 20-12 on p. 538) aid in identifying risks for hearing disorders.

Understanding the mechanisms for sound transmission helps the nurse identify the nature of hearing disorders. Sound travels through the ear by air and bone conduction; the following explains the steps of hearing:

1. Sound waves in the air enter the external ear, passing through the outer ear canal.
2. The sound waves reach the tympanic membrane, causing it to vibrate.
3. Vibrations are transmitted through the middle ear by the bony ossicular chain to the oval window at the opening of the inner ear.
4. The cochlea receives the sound vibration.
5. Nerve impulses from the cochlea travel to the auditory (eighth cranial) nerve and to the cerebral cortex.

Disorders of the ear result from several types of problems, including mechanical dysfunction (blockage by ear wax or foreign body), trauma (foreign bodies or noise exposure), neurological disorders (auditory nerve damage), acute illnesses (viral infection), and toxic effects of medications.

Auricles

With the client sitting comfortably the nurse inspects the auricle's placement, size, symmetry, and color. The auricles are normally level with each other. The upper point of attachment is in a straight line with the lateral canthus, or corner of the eye. Low-set ears are a sign of a congenital abnormality (for example, Down syndrome). The color should be the same as that of the face. Redness is a sign of inflammation or fever. Pallor can indicate frostbite.

The nurse palpates the auricles for texture, tenderness, and skin lesions. The auricle is normally smooth without lesions. If the client complains of pain, the nurse gently pulls the auricle and presses on the tragus and behind the ear over the mastoid process. If palpating the external ear increases the pain, an external ear infection is likely. If palpation of the auricle and tragus do not influence the pain, the client may have a middle ear infection.

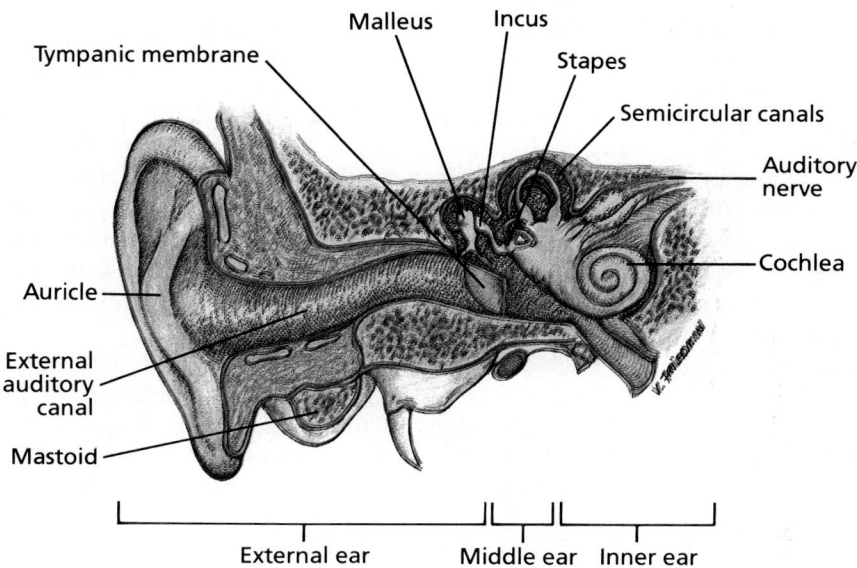

Fig. 20-22 The structures of the external, middle, and inner ear.

TABLE 20-12 Nursing History for Ear Assessment	
Assessment Category	Rationale
Ask if client has experienced ear pain, itching, discharge, tinnitus (ringing in ears), or change in hearing.	These signs and symptoms indicate infection or hearing loss.
Assess risks for hearing problem: hypoxia at birth, meningitis, birth weight less than 1500 g, family history of hearing loss, congenital anomalies of skull or face, nonbacterial intrauterine infections (rubella, herpes), constant exposure to high levels of noise.	Risk factors predispose client to permanent hearing loss. It may be difficult to assess infant's hearing status with examination only.
Determine client's exposure to loud noises at work and availability of protective devices.	Prolonged noise exposure can cause temporary or permanent hearing loss.
Note behaviors indicative of hearing loss such as failure to respond when spoken to, requests to repeat comments, leaning forward to hear, and child's inattentiveness or use of monotonous voice tone.	Persons with hearing loss cope with sensory deficit through variety of behavioral cues.
Assess if client takes large doses of aspirin or antibiotics.	Medications have side effects of hearing disorders.
Determine whether client uses hearing aid.	Determination allows nurse to assess ability to care for device and allows nurse to adjust voice tone to communicate.
If client has had recent hearing problem, note onset, contributing factors, and effect on activities of daily living.	Nature and severity of hearing problem are determined.

The nurse inspects the opening of the ear canal for size and discharge. The meatus should not be swollen or occluded. A yellow, waxy substance called *cerumen* is common. Yellow or green discharge may indicate infection.

Ear Canals and Eardrums

The deeper structures of the external and middle ear can be observed only with an **otoscope,** which is an ophthalmoscope with a special ear speculum attached to the battery tube. Speculums come in different sizes to conform to the size of ear canals. For best visualization the largest speculum that fits comfortably into the ear canal should be used.

Before inserting the speculum, the examiner checks for foreign bodies in the opening of the auditory canal. Clients must not move their heads during the examination to avoid damage to the canal and tympanic membrane. Infants and young children often need to be restrained. Infants should lie supine with their heads turned to one side and their arms held securely at their sides. Young children can sit on their parents' laps with their legs held between the parents' knees.

The nurse turns on the otoscope by rotating the dial at the top of the battery tube. To insert the speculum properly the nurse asks the client to tip the head slightly toward the opposite shoulder. Pulling the auricle gently up, back, and slightly out in the adult or older child straightens the ear canal (Fig. 20-23). In infants the nurse pulls the auricle back and down. The nurse inserts the speculum into the ear canal slightly down and forward. Care is taken not to abrade the sensitive lining of the ear canal. The nurse keeps the otoscope braced against the client's head to avoid sudden movement. Two grips on the otoscope may be used. In one, the examiner holds the battery tube along the neck with the fingers against the neck. In the other grip, the inverted otoscope is lightly braced against the side of the head or cheek. This grip, used commonly with children, prevents accidental movement of the otoscope deeper into the ear canal.

The nurse identifies cerumen and observes for lesions, foreign bodies, or discharge in the canal. Normally cerumen is dry (tan or light yellow) or moist (dark yellow or brown). A reddened canal with discharge is a sign of inflammation or infection. During the examination the examiner asks about methods that the client uses to clean the ear canal (see teaching box).

The light from the otoscope allows visualization of the tympanic membrane. The nurse must be familiar with the common anatomical landmarks and their appearances (Fig. 20-24). This takes practice. The otoscope is slowly moved to see the entire tympanic membrane and its periphery. The nurse methodically visualizes the tympanic membrane as if it were di-

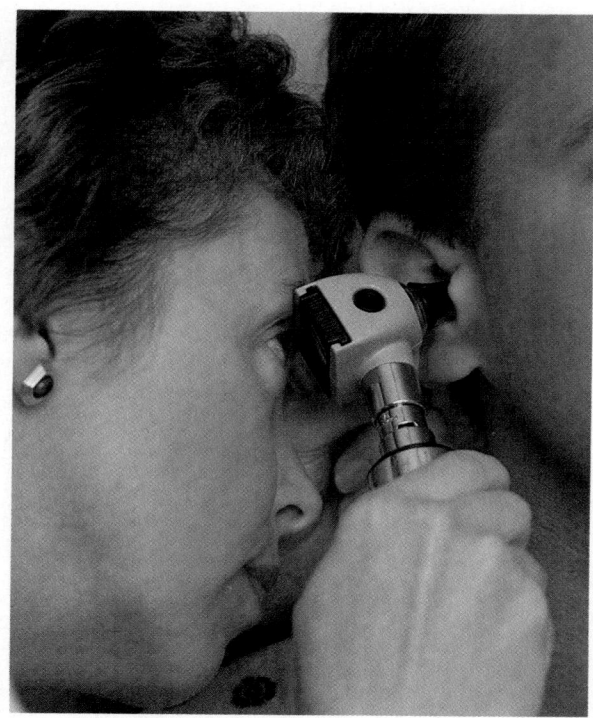

Fig. 20-23 In an adult, pulling the auricle upward and backward straightens the ear canal for easier otoscope placement.

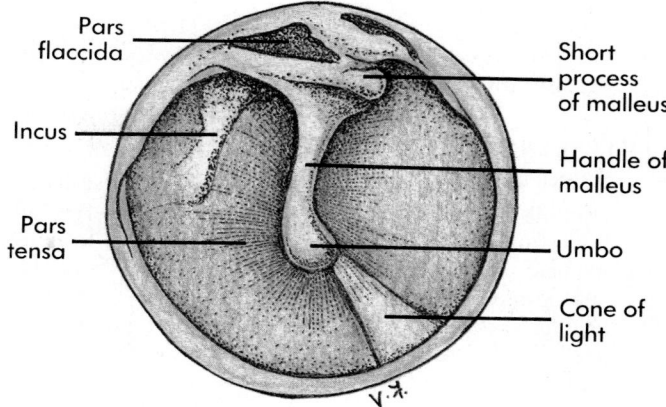

Fig. 20-24 Normal right tympanic membrane.

vided into four quadrants, with a line running through the handle of the malleus. A ring of fibrous cartilage surrounds the oval membrane. The normal tympanic membrane is translucent or pearly gray. A pink or red color indicates inflammation. A white color reveals pus behind it. The membrane is taut, except for the small triangular pars flaccida near the top. Because the tympanic membrane is angled away from the ear canal, the light from the otoscope appears as a cone rather than a circle. The umbo is near the center of the membrane, and the attachment of the malleus is behind it. A knoblike structure at the top of the tympanic membrane is created by the underlying short process of the malleus. The examiner should check carefully to be sure there are no tears or breaks.

Hearing Acuity

Often the nurse can tell whether the client has a hearing loss from a response to conversation. The three types of hearing loss are conduction, sensorineural, and mixed. A conduction loss involves an interruption of sound waves as they travel from the outer ear to the cochlea of the inner ear because the sound waves are not transmitted through the outer

Client Teaching During Ear Assessment

OBJECTIVES

- Client will use proper technique for cleansing the ears.
- Client will follow preventive guidelines for screening of hearing loss.
- Client with hearing loss will communicate effectively.

TEACHING STRATEGIES

- Instruct client about the proper way to clean outer ear (see Chapter 34), avoiding use of cotton-tipped applicators and sharp objects such as hairpins.
- Tell client to avoid inserting pointed objects into the ear canal.
- Encourage clients over 65 to have regular hearing checks. Explain that a reduction in hearing is a normal part of aging (see Chapter 45).
- Instruct family members of clients with hearing losses to avoid shouting, speaking instead in low tones, and to be sure the client can see the speaker's face.

EVALUATION

- Ask client to explain the proper technique for cleansing the ears.
- In a follow-up visit, question client about frequency of hearing checks.
- Observe client with hearing loss interact with family members.

TABLE 20-13 Tuning Fork Tests	
Tests and Steps	**Rationale**

WEBER'S TEST (LATERALIZATION OF SOUND)

Hold fork at its base and tap it lightly against heel of palm.

Place base of vibrating fork on top of client's head or middle of forehead (see figure at right).

Ask client where sound is heard (one or both sides).

Client with normal hearing hears sound equally in both ears or in midline of head. In conduction deafness, sound is heard in impaired ear. In unilateral sensorineural hearing loss, sound is identified only in normal ear.

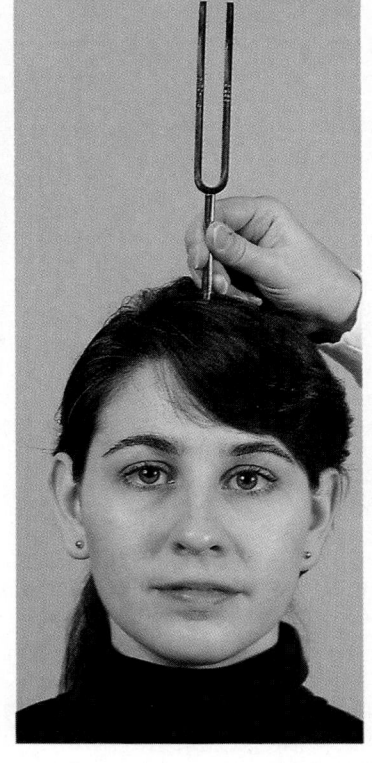

RINNE TEST (COMPARISON OF AIR AND BONE CONDUCTION)

Strike tuning fork against heel of palm.

First hold vibrating fork with tines parallel to auricle and their tips 2 cm from the external meatus* (see figure).

Place stem of vibrating fork on bone of mastoid process (see figure).

Ask client to inform you if sound is louder by air conduction or bone conduction.

If client is believed to have conduction deficit, referral for audiometry is appropriate.

Client first confirms that sound can be heard. Normally, sound can be heard louder through air than through bone (positive test). In conduction deafness, sounds through bone conduction can be heard longer than through air conduction (negative test). In sensorineural deafness, sound is reduced and heard longer through air.

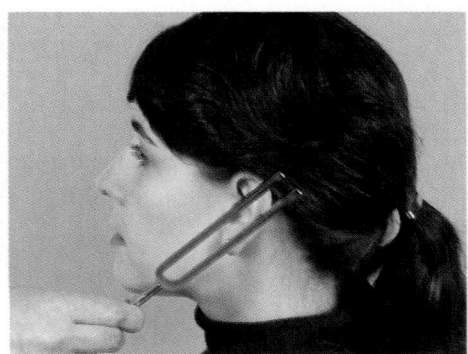
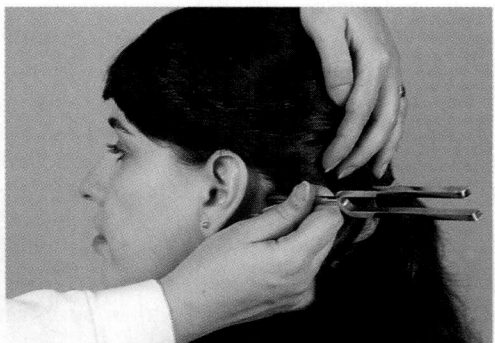

---

*Data from Swan IRC: *Hosp Pract* Sept 30, 1989, p 99.
Illustrations from Seidel HM et al: *Mosby's guide to physical examination,* ed 2, St Louis, 1991, Mosby–Year Book.

and middle ear structures. Examples of causes of a conduction loss are swelling of the auditory canal or tears in the tympanic membrane. A sensorineural loss involves the inner ear, auditory nerve, or hearing center of the brain. Sound is conducted through the outer and middle ear structures, but the continued transmission of sound becomes interrupted at some point beyond the bony ossicles. A mixed loss involves a combination of conduction and sensorineural loss.

Clients working or living around loud noises are at risk for hearing loss. Older adults experience an inability to hear high-frequency sounds and consonants (for example, S, Z, T, and G). Deterioration of the cochlea and a thickening of the tympanic membrane cause older adults to gradually lose hearing acuity. They are especially at risk for hearing loss due to **ototoxicity** (injury to auditory nerve) resulting from high maintenance doses of antibiotics. Aminoglycosides, including amikacin, gentamicin, tobramycin, and vancomycin, are especially toxic (Berman, Haxby, Pomerantz, 1988).

The simplest test for hearing acuity is identification of voice tones, with the client repeating test words spoken by the nurse. One ear is tested at a time, with the nurse occluding the other ear. The ear not being tested is masked by gentle rubbing of the tragus. While standing 6 in (15 cm) and 2 ft (60 cm) away the nurse covers the mouth so that the client is unable to read lips. After exhaling fully, the nurse first whispers softly toward the unoccluded ear, reciting numbers with two equally accented syllables such as *nine-four*. The client is asked to repeat what is heard. The test is repeated in conversational and loud tones if necessary until the client correctly repeats the numbers. A ticking watch may also be used to test hearing acuity, but the spoken word allows for more accuracy and control in testing.

If a hearing loss is present, the nurse can assess for conduction and sensorineural deafness through use of a tuning fork. A tuning fork of 256 to 512 hertz (Hz) is most commonly used because the conductive element of a hearing impairment is greatest in this range of sound frequencies (Swan, 1989). The fork should be lightly vibrated by tapping it on the heel of the palm or on the knee (Table 20-13).

Nose and Sinuses

The nurse uses inspection and palpation to assess the nose and sinuses. A penlight allows the nurse to perform a gross examination of each naris. A more detailed examination requires use of a nasal speculum to inspect the deeper nasal turbinates. A student should not use a speculum unless a qualified practitioner is present. Table 20-14 lists components of the nursing history.

Nose

When inspecting the nose, the nurse observes for asymmetry, inflammation, and deformity. Recent trauma may have caused edema and discoloration. If swelling or deformities exist, the nose is palpated gently for tenderness, swelling, and underlying deviations. Normally the external nose is symmetrical, straight, and nontender without discharge.

Air normally passes freely through the nose as a person breathes. While illuminating the anterior nares, the nurse inspects the mucosa for color, le-

sions, discharge, swelling, and bleeding. Normal mucosa is pink. Discharge resulting from common sinus irritation is clear and watery. A sinus infection results in yellowish or greenish discharge. A pale mucosa with clear discharge is a sign of allergy. For the client with a nasogastric tube, the nurse routinely checks for local skin breakdown (**excoriation**) of the naris, characterized by redness and sloughing of the skin.

The client tips the head back slightly to give the nurse a clearer view of the septum and turbinates. The septum is inspected for deviation, lesions, and superficial blood vessels. Normally the septum is midline. A deviated septum can obstruct breathing and interfere with passage of a nasogastric tube. The turbinates are covered with mucous membranes that warm and moisten inspired air. The nurse notes any **polyps** (tumorlike growth) or purulent drainage.

Sinuses

Examination of the sinuses involves palpation and transillumination. In cases of allergies or infection, the interior of the sinuses becomes inflamed and swollen. The most effective way to assess for tenderness is by externally palpating the frontal and maxillary facial areas (Fig. 20-25 on p. 542). Gentle, upward pressure elicits tenderness easily and reveals the severity of sinus irritation. Pressure should not be applied to the eyes. Fig. 20-26 on p. 542 are cross sections of the nasal sinus cavities.

Another method for examining the sinuses is through transillumination to detect air or fluid in the

---

TABLE 20-14   Nursing History for Nose and Sinus Assessment

Assessment Category	Rationale
Determine if client has experienced trauma to nose.	Trauma can cause deviation of septum and asymmetry of external nose.
Ask if client has history of allergies, nasal discharge, epistaxis (nose bleeds), or postnasal drip.	History is useful in determining source or nature of nasal and sinus drainage.
Ask if client uses nasal spray or drops.	Overuse of over-the-counter nasal preparations can cause physical change in mucosa.
Ask if client snores at night or has difficulty with breathing.	Difficulty with breathing or snoring may indicate septal deviation or obstruction.

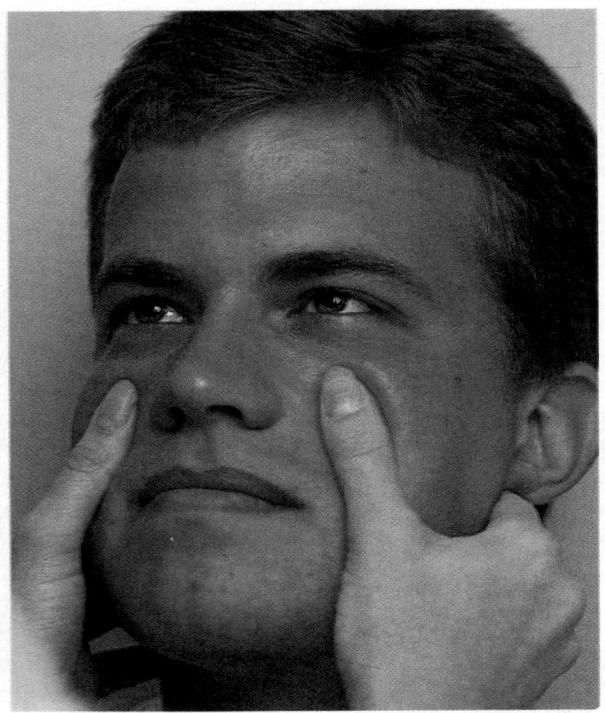

Fig. 20-25 Palpation of maxillary sinuses.

sinuses. To view the frontal sinuses the nurse shines a penlight against the inner aspect of the supraorbital ridge of the frontal bone. The light passes through bone to illuminate the sinus. In a darkened room the light will outline the sinus. Air is normally found within the sinuses; thus a darker color reveals fluid. To illuminate the maxillary sinuses the nurse places the penlight below each orbital ridge while inspect-

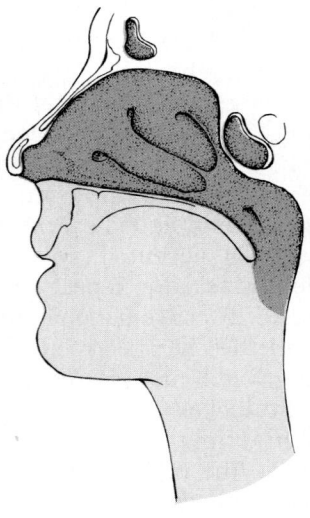

Fig. 20-26 Cross section of nasal sinus cavities.

Client Teaching During Nose and Sinus Assessment

OBJECTIVES
- Client will safely use over-the-counter nasal sprays.
- Parents will take proper measures to stop a child's nosebleed.
- Older adult will take safety precautions for loss of olfaction.

TEACHING STRATEGIES
- Caution client against overuse of over-the-counter nasal sprays, which can lead to "rebound" effect causing excess nasal congestion.
- Instruct parents on care of child with nosebleeds: have child sit up and lean forward to avoid aspiration of blood, apply pressure to anterior nose with thumb and forefinger as child breathes through mouth, and apply ice or cold cloth to bridge of nose if pressure fails to stop bleeding.

EVALUATION
- Have client explain proper use of over-the-counter nasal sprays.
- Have parents demonstrate and describe technique for stopping a nosebleed.

TABLE 20-15 Nursing History for Mouth and Pharynx Assessment

Assessment Category	Rationale
Determine if client wears dentures and if they are comfortable.	Dentures must be removed to visualize and palpate gums. Ill-fitting dentures irritate mucosa and gums and may be risk for mouth cancer.*
Determine if client has had recent change in appetite or weight.	Symptoms may result from painful mouth conditions or poor hygiene.
Assess dental hygiene practices and determine when client last visited dentist.	Assessment reveals client's need for education or financial support.
Determine if client smokes or chews tobacco.	Tobacco users have greater risk for mouth and throat cancers than nonusers.
Review history for alcohol consumption.	Heavy drinkers appear to have greater risk for oral cancer.

*Data from US Department of Health and Human Services: 1985.

ing the hard palate through the client's open mouth. The palate should show a glow of light. The box describes teaching guidelines during nose and sinus assessment.

Mouth and Pharynx

To assess the oral cavity the nurse uses a penlight and tongue depressor or single gauze square. The Centers for Disease Control (CDC) recommends wearing gloves when contacting mucous membranes (see Chapter 18). Assessment of the oral cavity can be made during administration of oral hygiene (see Chapter 34). Table 20-15 describes the nursing history.

Lips

The lips are inspected for color, texture, hydration, contour, and lesions. As the client opens the mouth, the nurse views the lips from end to end. Normally they are pink, moist, symmetrical, and smooth (Fig. 20-27).

Inner and Buccal Mucosas

To view the inner oral mucosa, the nurse has the client open and relax the mouth slightly and then gently pulls the client's lower lip away from the teeth (Fig. 20-28, *A*). This process is repeated for the upper lip. The mucosa is inspected for color, hydration, texture, and lesions such as ulcers, abrasions, or cysts. If lesions are present, the nurse palpates them gently with gloved hand for tenderness, size, and consistency.

To visualize the buccal mucosa, the nurse asks the client to open the mouth and then gently retracts the cheeks with a tongue depressor or gloved finger covered with gauze (Fig. 20-28, *B*). The surface of the mucosa must be viewed from right to left and top to bottom. A penlight illuminates the most posterior portion of the mucosa. Normal mucosa is glistening, pink, soft, moist, and smooth. An increase in color or hyperpigmentation is normal in 10% of European

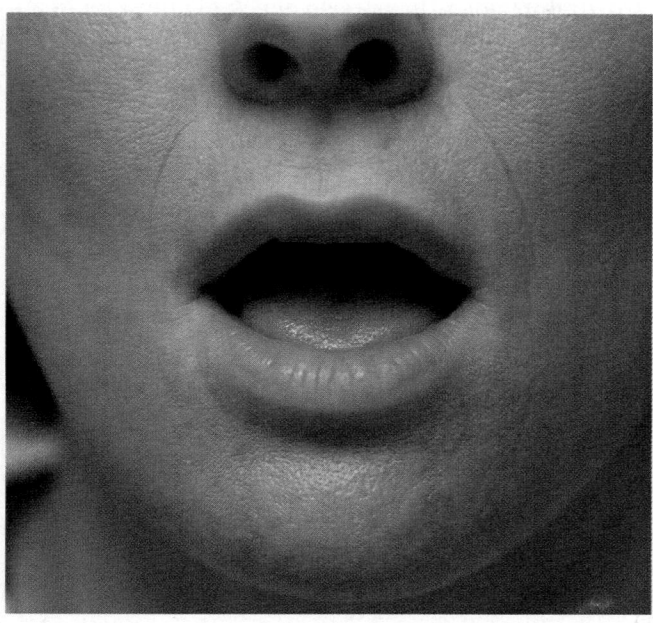

Fig. 20-27 The lips are normally pink, symmetrical, smooth, and moist.

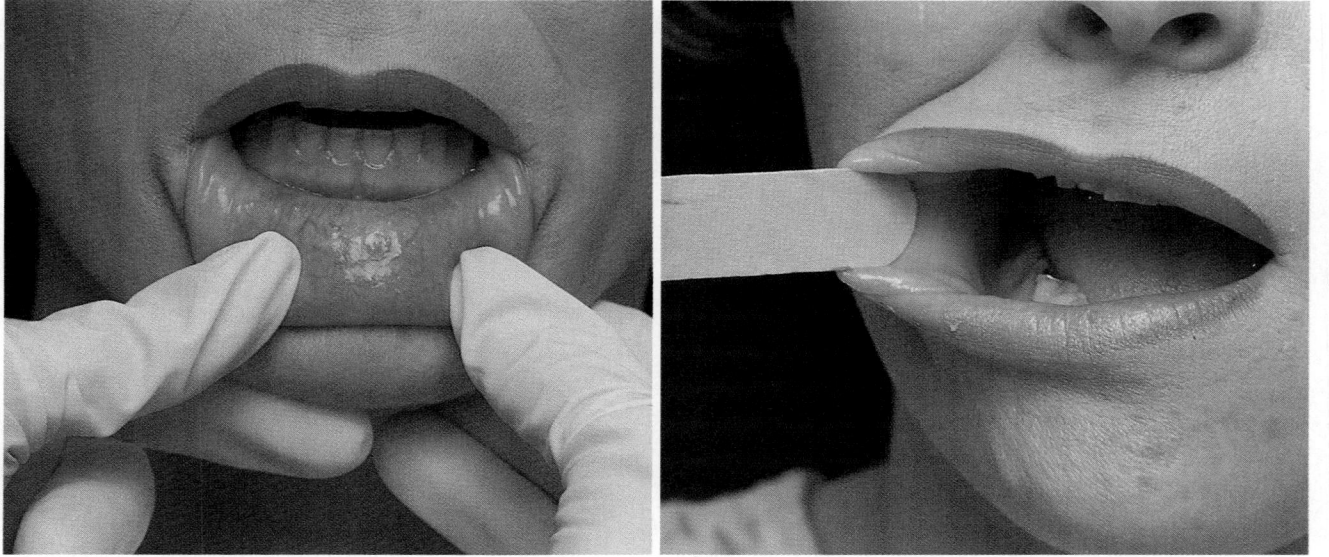

Fig. 20-28   **A,** Inspection of inner oral mucosa of lower lip. **B,** Retraction of the buccal mucosa allows for clear visualization.

Americans after age 50 and up to 90% of African Americans by the same age. For clients with normal pigmentation the buccal mucosa is a good site to inspect for jaundice and pallor. In older adults, the mucosa is normally dry because of reduced salivation. The appearance of thick, white patches (**leukoplakia**) can be seen in heavy smokers and alcoholics. Leukoplakia should be reported because it can also be a precancerous lesion. The nurse palpates the cheek with one finger along the inner mucosa and the thumb along the outside cheek to check for deep-seated lumps or ulcerations.

Gums and Teeth

While the nurse retracts the cheeks, the gums or gingivae are inspected for color, edema, retraction, bleeding, and lesions. The gums around the back molars should be viewed because this is a difficult area to reach when cleaning teeth. Healthy gums are pink, smooth, and moist. African Americans may have patchy pigmentation. In older adults the gums

are usually pale. The nurse palpates the gums with a tongue depressor to determine whether they are firm. Spongy gums that bleed easily indicate periodontal disease and vitamin C deficiency.

If a client wears dentures, irregularity or lesions of the gums can cause discomfort and impair chewing. The nurse asks the client to remove dentures so that a complete assessment can be performed. Roughness on the surface can be smoothed out by a dentist.

The quality of dental hygiene is easily determined by inspecting the teeth. The client should open the lips and clench the teeth (see teaching box). The position and alignment of teeth are noted. To examine the posterior surface of the teeth the nurse has the client open the mouth with lips relaxed. A tongue depressor may be needed to retract the lips and cheeks, especially when viewing the molars. Tartar along the base of the teeth, dental **caries** (cavities), extraction sites, and the teeth's color should be noted. Normal, healthy teeth are smooth, white, and shiny. A chalky white discoloration of the enamel is an early indication of caries formation. Brown or black discolorations indicate formation of caries. In the older adult, loose or missing teeth are common because bone resorption increases. An older adult's teeth often feel rough when tooth enamel calcifies. Yellow or darkened teeth are also common in the older adult because of the general wear and tear that exposes the darker, underlying dentin.

Tongue and Floor of Mouth

The tongue is carefully inspected on all sides, and the floor of the mouth is checked. The client relaxes

---

Client Teaching During Mouth and Pharynx Assessment

OBJECTIVES

- Client will practice proper oral hygiene measures and dental care.
- Client will describe warning signs of oral cancer.
- Older adult will maintain normal solid food intake.

TEACHING STRATEGIES

- Discuss proper techniques for oral hygiene, including brushing (see Chapter 34).
- Explain the early warning signs of oral cancer, including a sore that bleeds easily and does not heal, a lump or thickening, and a red or white patch on the mucosa that persists.*
- Encourage a yearly dental examination for each child and adult. An older adult should visit a dentist every 6 months.
- Identify older client that has difficulty in chewing and changes in the teeth. Teach client to eat soft foods and cut food into small pieces.

EVALUATION

- Ask client to demonstrate brushing.
- Have client identify when to have regular dental checkups.
- Have client identify warning signs of oral cancer.
- Ask older adult to keep diet record for 3 days.

*Data from American Cancer Society: *1991 Cancer facts and figures*, New York, 1991, The Society.

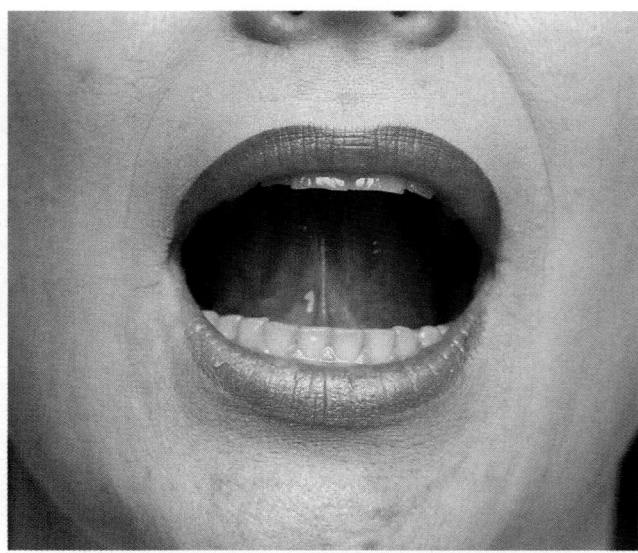

Fig. 20-29 The undersurface of the tongue is highly vascular.

the mouth and sticks the tongue out halfway. If the client is forced to protrude the tongue too far, the gag reflex may be elicited. Using the penlight for illumination, the nurse examines the tongue for color, size, position, texture, and coatings or lesions. The tongue should be medium red or pink in color and moist and smooth along lateral margins with free mobility. When the tongue protrudes, it lies midline. The top surface of the tongue is slightly rough. To test for tongue mobility the nurse asks the client to raise the tongue up and move it side to side. The tongue should move freely.

The tongue is highly vascular, particularly on the undersurface (Fig. 20-29). Extra care is taken to inspect the undersurface, a common site of origin for oral cancer lesions. The client lifts the tongue to permit adequate inspection. The nurse looks for white or red areas, nodules, or cysts. To palpate the tongue, the nurse explains the procedure and then asks the client to protrude the tongue. The nurse grasps the tip with a gauze square and gently pulls it to one side. With a gloved hand the nurse palpates the full length of the tongue and the base for any areas of hardening. The floor of the mouth is also a site for oral cancer. **Varicosities** (swollen, tortuous veins) may be seen. Varicosities rarely cause problems but are common in the older adult. The nurse palpates any lumps or nodules.

Palate

The client should extend the head backward, holding the mouth open so that the nurse can inspect the hard and soft palates (Fig. 20-30). The hard palate or

roof of the mouth is located anteriorly. The soft palate extends posteriorly toward the pharynx. The palates are observed for color, shape, texture, and extra bony prominences or defects. A bonygrowth, or **exostosis**, between the two palates is common. Normal palates are light pink. The soft palate appears smooth, whereas the hard palate is rough.

Pharynx

The pharynx can be a site for infection, inflammation, or lesions. Before examining the pharynx the nurse explains the procedure to the client. The client tips the head back slightly, opens the mouth wide, and says "ah." The nurse places the tip of a tongue depressor on the middle third of the tongue, taking care not to press the lower lip against the teeth. If the tongue depressor is placed too far anteriorly, the posterior part of the tongue mounds up, obstructing the view. The gag reflex is elicited when the tongue depressor touches the posterior tongue.

With a penlight, the nurse inspects the uvula and soft palate (Fig. 20-31). Both structures, which are innervated by the tenth cranial (vagus) nerve, should rise centrally as the client says "ah." The nurse also inspects the arch formed by the anterior and posterior pillars, soft palate, and uvula. The tonsils can be viewed in the cavities between the anterior and posterior pillars and are oval with infoldings of tissue.

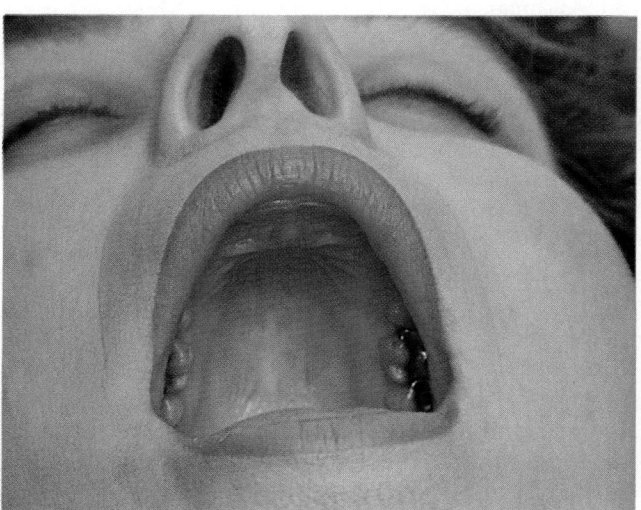

Fig. 20-30 The hard palate is located anteriorly in the roof of the mouth.

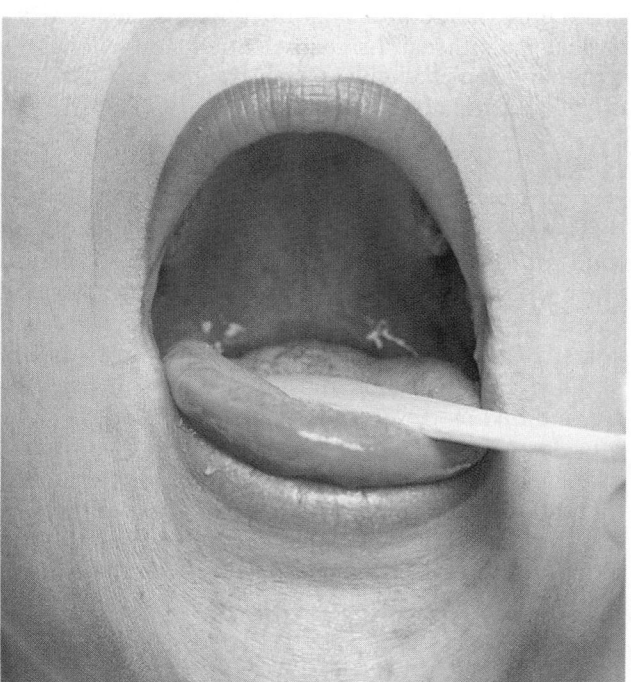

Fig. 20-31 A tongue depressor allows the nurse to visualize the uvula and posterior soft palate.

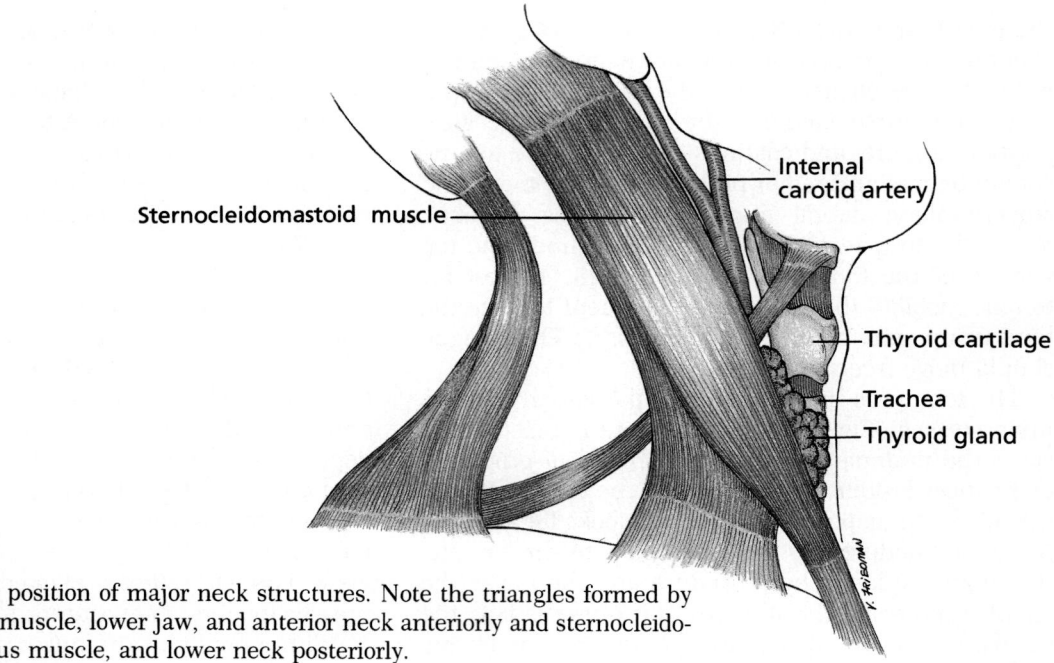

Sternocleidomastoid muscle

Internal carotid artery

Thyroid cartilage

Trachea

Thyroid gland

Fig. 20-32 Anatomical position of major neck structures. Note the triangles formed by the sternocleidomastoid muscle, lower jaw, and anterior neck anteriorly and sternocleidomastoid muscle, trapezius muscle, and lower neck posteriorly.

The posterior pharynx is behind the pillars. The pharyngeal tissues are normally pink and smooth. Edema, ulceration, or inflammation indicates infection or abnormal lesions. Clients with chronic sinus problems frequently exhibit a clear exudate that drains along the wall of the posterior pharynx. Yellow or green exudate indicates infection. A client with a typical sore throat has a reddened and edematous uvula and tonsillar pillars with the possible presence of yellow exudate.

Neck

The neck muscles, lymph nodes of the head, carotid arteries, jugular veins, thyroid gland, and trachea are located within the neck (Fig. 20-32). The nurse inspects and palpates these structures and auscultates the carotid arteries. Examination is best performed with the client sitting. Areas of the neck are outlined by the sternocleidomastoid and trapezius muscles, which divide each side of the neck into two triangles. The anterior triangle contains the trachea, thyroid gland, carotid artery, and anterior cervical lymph nodes. The posterior triangle contains the posterior lymph nodes. Table 20-16 reviews the nursing history for the neck examination.

Neck Muscles

To test the function of the sternocleidomastoid muscle, the nurse asks the client to flex the neck with the chin to the chest. The client hyperextends

TABLE 20-16 Nursing History for Neck Assessment	
Assessment Category	**Rationale**
Assess for history of recent cold or infection.	Colds or infections can cause temporary or permanent lymph node enlargement.
Determine if client has history of thyroid problem or takes thyroid medication.	Disease or medications may influence tissue growth in thyroid gland.
Ask if client has had history of neck pain.	Neck pain may indicate muscle strain, local nerve injury, or enlarged or swollen lymph node.
Review medical history of pneumothorax (collapsed lung) or bronchial tumor.	Conditions place client at risk for tracheal displacement or lateral deviation.

the neck backward so that the nurse can check for trapezius muscle function. Movement of the head sideways so that the ear moves toward the shoulder further tests function of the sternocleidomastoid muscle. Other tests for muscle strength and function can also be performed (see section on musculoskeletal system).

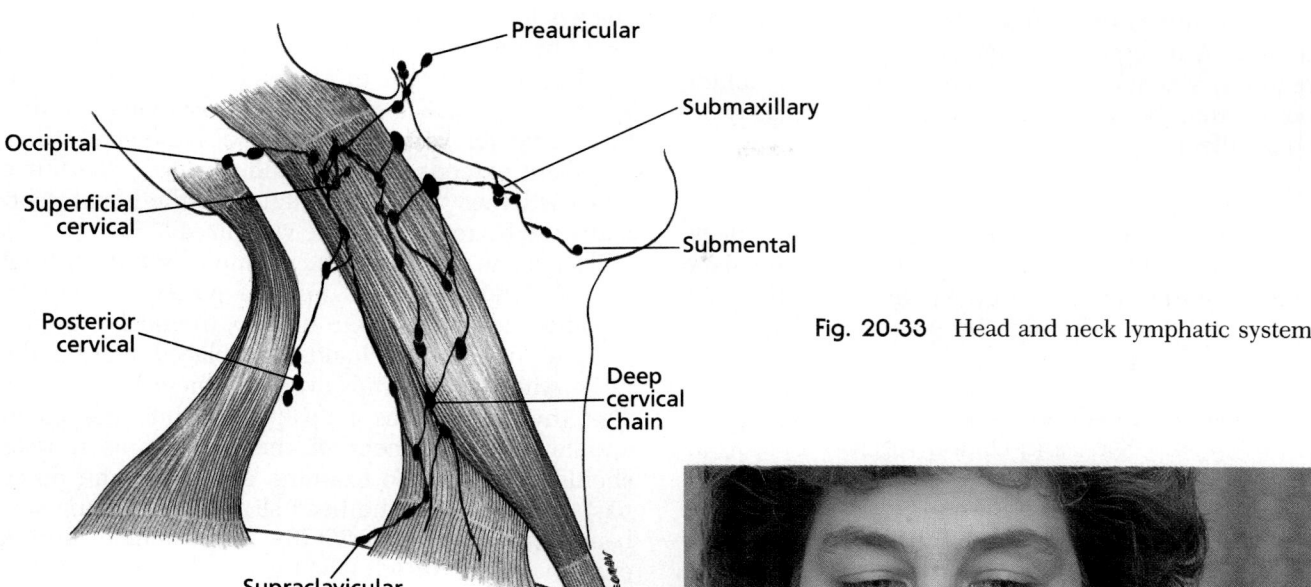

Fig. 20-33   Head and neck lymphatic system.

Lymph Nodes

An extensive system of lymph nodes collects lymph from the head, ears, nose, cheeks, and lips (Fig. 20-33). With the client's chin raised and head tilted backward, the nurse first inspects the neck for symmetry, masses, or scars. If masses are seen, they should be palpated to assess size, shape, tenderness, consistency, and mobility.

Lymph nodes are superficial or deep. The superficial nodes can be palpated; however, deep nodes lying beneath muscular facia are not usually palpable. The nodes may be round, flat, oval, or cylindrical. Normally the number and size of lymph nodes decrease with aging (McConnell, 1988).

A methodical approach is used to examine the lymph nodes to avoid overlooking any single node or chain. The client relaxes with the neck flexed slightly forward and, if needed, toward the side of the examiner. This maneuver relaxes tissues and muscles. Both sides of the neck are inspected and palpated for comparison. During palpation the nurse faces or stands to the side of the client for easy access to all nodes. Using the pads of the middle three fingers of the hand, the nurse palpates gently in a rotary motion over the nodes (Fig. 20-34). It is important to press underlying tissue in each area and not simply move the fingers over the skin. However, if excessive pressure is applied, small nodes are missed and palpable nodes are obliterated. During palpation the nurse notes the location, size, shape, mobility, symmetry, and surface characteristics of the lymph nodes. Lymph nodes that are large, fixed, inflamed,

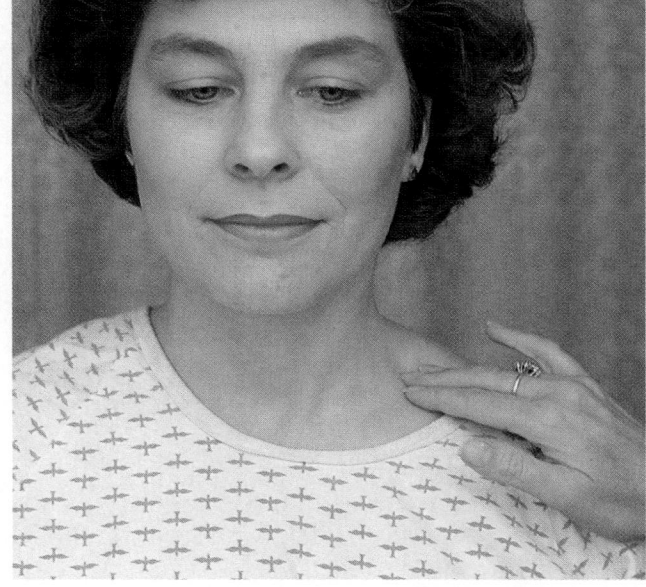

Fig. 20-34   Palpation of cervical lymph nodes.

or tender indicate a problem (McConnell, 1988). Tenderness is usually the result of inflammation. Noting which nodes are enlarged may help locate the site of an infection. For example, ear infections usually drain to the preauricular or deep cervical nodes.

Normally the nodes are not easily palpable. However, small, mobile, nontender nodes are common. After a serious infection, a node may remain permanently enlarged but may not be tender.

To palpate supraclavicular nodes the nurse asks the client to bend the head forward and relax the shoulders. The nurse may have to hook the index and third finger over the clavicle, lateral to the sternocleidomastoid muscle, to palpate nodes. The deep cervical nodes can only be palpated with the nurse's thumb and index finger hooked around the sternocleidomastoid muscle.

The lymph nodes can also be the site of malignant tumors. A malignancy is usually hard, immobile, irregularly shaped, and often nontender (see teaching box). Often the nodes on just one side of the body become affected.

Thyroid Gland

The thyroid gland lies in the anterior lower neck, in front of and to both sides of the trachea. The gland is fixed to the trachea with the isthmus overlying the trachea and connecting the two irregular, cone-

shaped lobes (Fig. 20-35). The nurse assesses the gland by inspection, palpation, and auscultation.

The nurse stands in front of the client and inspects the area of the lower neck overlying the thyroid gland for visible masses and symmetry. While the client extends the neck and swallows, the nurse notes whether there is a bulging of the gland. Normally the thyroid cannot be visualized.

To palpate the gland, the examiner stands in front of or behind the client. For the posterior approach the client lowers the chin to relax the neck muscles. Both of the nurse's hands are placed around the neck, with the fingertips overlying the lower trachea. The thyroid isthmus is palpated while the client swallows. Enlargement of the isthmus as it rises should be noted. To examine each lobe, the nurse has the client turn the head slightly toward the side being examined (Fig. 20-36). For example, during examination of the left lobe the client lowers the chin and turns the head slightly to the left. The examiner's right hand gently displaces the thyroid to the left while the left hand palpates the lobe. This procedure is repeated for the right lobe. Normally the thyroid gland is not enlarged. However, in extremely thin individuals the thyroid is more easily palpable. Enlargement is a manifestation of thyroid dysfunction. Masses or nodules may be signs of malignant disease. However, not all nodules are malignant.

The anterior approach follows the same maneuvers as the posterior approach. The nurse uses the

---

Client Teaching During Neck Assessment

OBJECTIVE

- Client will take proper preventive action if mass is noted in neck.

TEACHING STRATEGIES

- Instruct client about the lymph nodes and how infection can commonly cause node tenderness.
- Instruct client to call the physician when an enlarged lump or mass is noted in the neck.

EVALUATION

- Have client explain when to notify a physician about a neck mass.

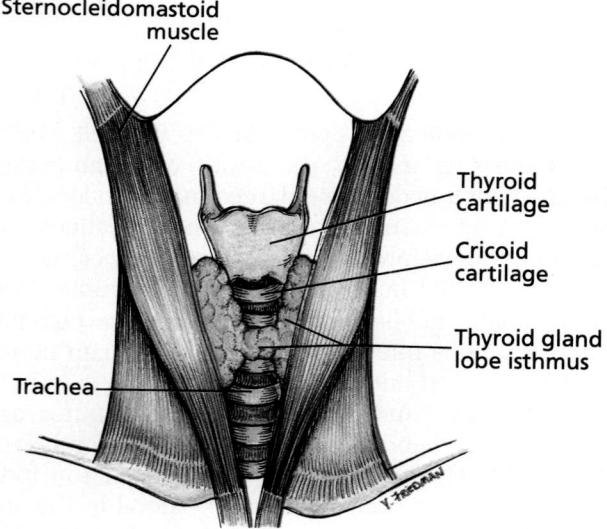

Fig. 20-35 The thyroid gland lies anteriorly in the neck. It is fixed to both sides of the trachea with the isthmus overlying the trachea.

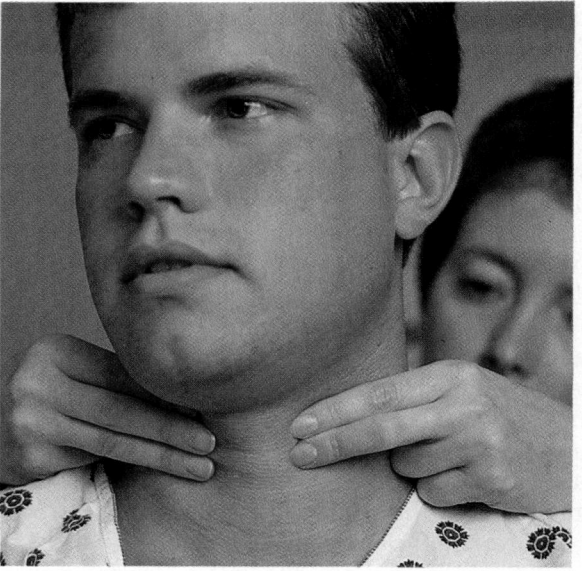

Fig. 20-36 The nurse palpates each thyroid lobe by having the client lower the chin and turn the head toward the side being examined.

index and middle fingers of the dominant hand to palpate the isthmus as the client swallows. Then with the client's head turned alternately to each side, the nurse displaces each lobe and palpates it with the other hand.

When the gland appears enlarged, the nurse places the diaphragm of the stethoscope over the thyroid. If the gland is enlarged, blood flow through the thyroid arteries increases and causes a fine vibration. The nurse can auscultate the vibration, which is heard as a soft, rushing sound, or bruit.

Carotid Artery and Jugular Vein

This portion of the examination is described under examination of the vascular system (see later section).

Trachea

The trachea can be directly palpated and is normally located in the midline of the neck, above the suprasternal notch. Masses in the neck or mediastinum and pulmonary abnormalities can cause displacement laterally. The client may sit or lie down during palpation. The position of the trachea is determined by palpating at the suprasternal notch, slipping the thumb and index fingers to each side. Forceful pressure must not be applied because this action may elicit a cough.

THORAX AND LUNGS

Accurate physical assessment of the thorax and lungs requires consideration of the vital ventilatory and respiratory roles of the lungs. If the lungs are affected by disease, other body systems will reflect alterations. For example, reduced oxygenation can cause changes in mental alertness because of the brain's sensitivity to lowered oxygen levels. The alert nurse uses the data from all body systems to determine the nature of pulmonary alterations.

Before assessing the thorax and lungs, the nurse must be familiar with the landmarks of the chest (Fig. 20-37). These landmarks help the nurse describe the location of findings and use assessment skills correctly. For example, by knowing the position of underlying organs in relation to the landmarks, the nurse can anticipate where to percuss or auscultate the chest wall. The landmarks are a series of imaginary lines and easily identifiable anatomical landmarks such as the ribs and spine. The lungs and thorax are assessed anteriorly, laterally (on both sides), and posteriorly, with the nurse using landmarks to record localized findings.

During the examination, the nurse keeps a mental image of the location of the lobes of the lung (Fig. 20-38 on p. 550). Locating the position of each rib is

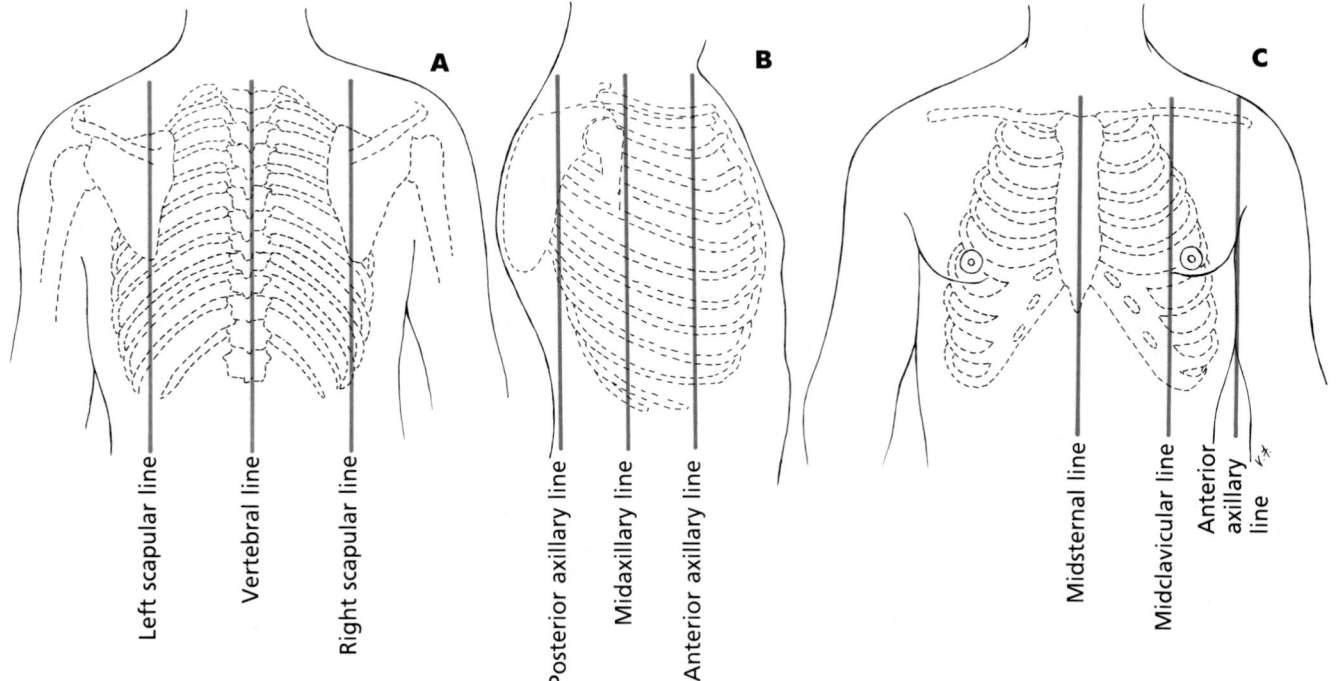

Fig. 20-37 Anatomical chest wall landmarks. **A**, Posterior chest landmarks. **B**, Lateral chest landmarks. **C**, Anterior chest landmarks.

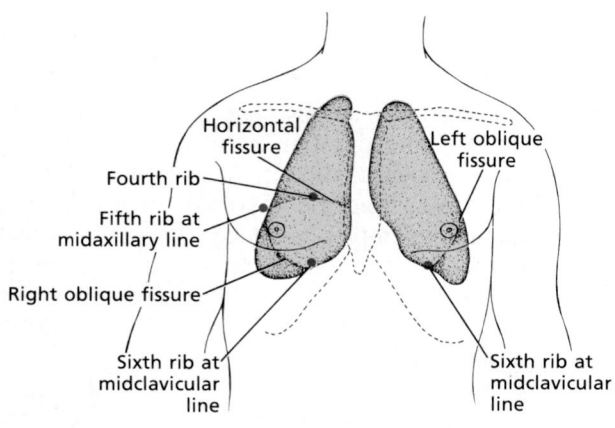

Fig. 20-38 Anterior position of lung lobes in relation to anatomical landmarks.

critical to visualizing the lobe of the lung being assessed. Louis' angle, at the junction between the manubrium and body of the sternum, is the starting point for locating the ribs anteriorly. Knowing that the second rib extends from the angle makes it easy to locate and palpate the intercostal spaces (between the ribs) in succession. The spinous process of the third thoracic vertebra and the fourth, fifth, and sixth ribs help to locate the lung's lobes laterally. The lower lobes project laterally and anteriorly (Fig. 20-39). Posteriorly the tip or inferior margin of the scapula lies approximately at the level of the seventh rib (Fig. 20-40). After identifying the seventh rib the examiner can count upward to locate the third thoracic vertebra and align it with the inner borders of the scapula to locate the posterior lobes.

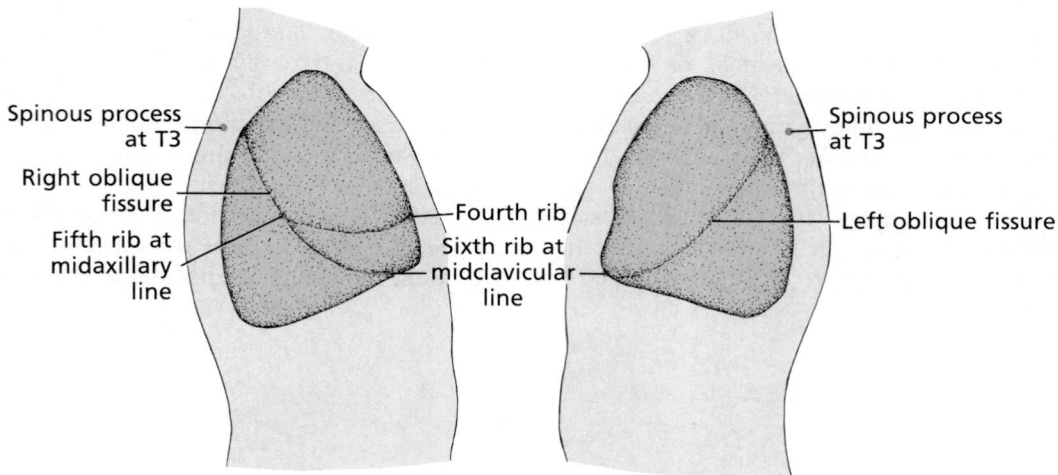

Fig. 20-39 Lateral position of lung lobes in relation to anatomical landmarks.

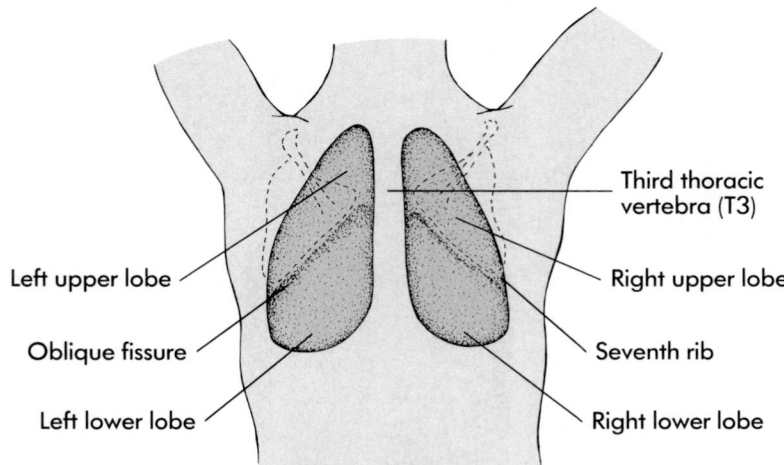

Fig. 20-40 Posterior position of lung lobes in relation to anatomical landmarks.

Examination of the lungs and thorax requires the client to be undressed to the waist. Good lighting is essential. The nurse uses each physical assessment skill in an orderly, systematic fashion. The nurse should assess clients at risk for pulmonary problems, such as the client confined to bed rest or the client with chest pain who cannot fully expand the lungs. The examination begins with the client sitting for assessment of the posterior and lateral chest. For assessment of the anterior chest, the client sits or lies. Table 20-17 reviews the nursing history for lung examination.

Posterior Thorax

The nurse first inspects the shape of the client's chest and posture. Shape or posture can significantly impair ventilatory movement. Normally the chest contour is symmetrical, and the chest is twice as wide as deep (anteroposterior diameter in a 1:2 ratio)

(Fig. 20-41). A small infant has a 1:1 ratio, with the chest having an almost round shape. Abnormal contours are caused by congenital and postural alterations. Aging and chronic lung disease are characterized by a barrel-shaped chest; the anteroposterior to lateral diameter is 1:1. A client may assume a posture such as leaning over a table or splinting the side of the chest as a result of a breathing problem. Splinting or holding the chest wall as a result of localized pain causes a client to bend toward the side affected. Such a posture impairs ventilatory movement.

Standing at a midline position behind the client, the nurse looks for deformities, position of the spine, slope of the ribs, retraction of the intercostal spaces on inspiration, and bulging of the intercostal spaces on expiration. The scapulae are normally symmetrical and closely attached to the thoracic wall. The normal spine is straight without lateral deviation. Posteriorly, the ribs tend to slope across and down. The

TABLE 20-17 Nursing History for Lung Assessment	
Assessment Category	Rationale
Assess history of smoking, including number of years smoked, number of cigarettes per day, cigar or pipe-smoking, and length of time since smoking stopped.	Smoking is risk factor for lung cancer, heart disease, and emphysema or bronchitis. Cigarette smoking accounts for 30% of all cancer deaths.*
Ask if client has had *persistent cough* (productive or nonproductive), *sputum production, chest pain,* shortness of breath, orthopnea, dyspnea during exertion, poor activity tolerance, and *recurrent attacks of pneumonia or bronchitis.*	Symptoms of respiratory alterations may help nurse localize objective physical findings. (Warning signals for lung cancer are in italic type.)
Determine if client works in environment containing pollutants, (e.g., asbestos, coal dust, chemical irritants).	These risk factors increase chance for various lung diseases.
Assess history of allergies to pollens, dust, or other airborne irritants and to foods, drugs, or chemical substances.	Symptoms such as choking feeling, bronchospasm with respiratory stridor, wheezes on auscultation, and dyspnea may be caused by allergic response.
Review family history for cancer, tuberculosis, allergies, or chronic obstructive pulmonary disease.	These conditions may place client at risk for lung disease.

*Data from American Cancer Society: *1991 cancer facts and figures,* New York, 1991, The Society.

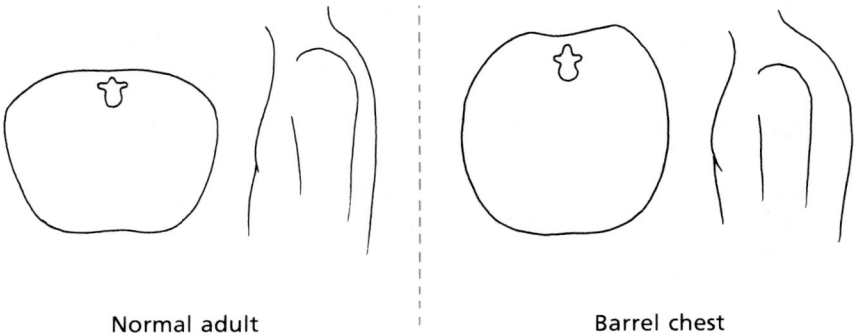

Normal adult   Barrel chest

Fig. 20-41   Anteroposterior diameter of normal adult and barrel chest.

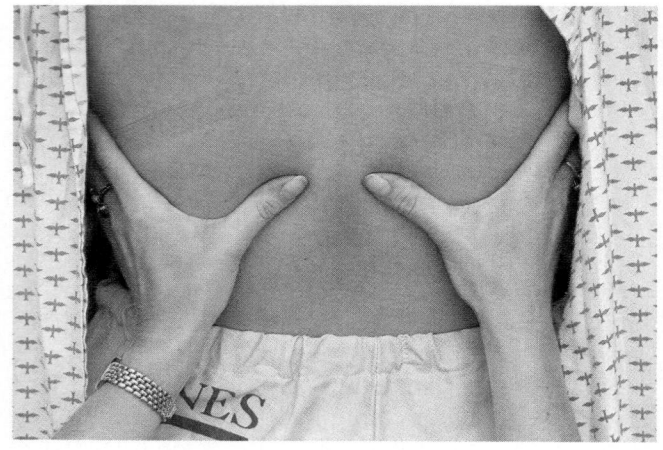 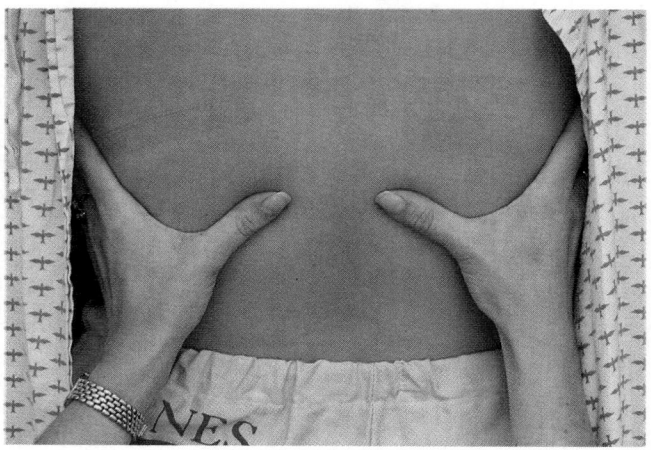

Fig. 20-42 A, Position of nurse's hands for palpation of posterior thorax excursion. B, As the client inhales, the movement of chest excursion separates the nurse's thumbs.

ribs and intercostal spaces are easier to see in a thin person. Normally, no bulging or active movement occurs within the intercostal spaces during breathing. Bulging indicates that the client is using great effort to breathe.

The nurse may also inspect the posterior thorax to determine the rate and rhythm of breathing (see Chapter 19). The thorax as a whole is observed. The entire thorax normally expands and relaxes regularly with equality of movement. In healthy adults the normal respiratory rates vary from 12 to 20 respirations per minute.

Palpation of the posterior thorax assesses further characteristics and confirms or supplements assessment findings. The chest is palpated to detect lumps or masses, identify areas of tenderness, and measure chest excursion and tactile fremitus.

If a suspicious mass or swollen area is detected, it is lightly palpated for size, shape, and the typical qualities of a lesion. When pain or tenderness is elicited, deep palpation is not used because deep palpation of a fractured rib segment could displace the bone fragment against vital organs.

Chest excursion is used to determine the depth of breathing. While standing behind the client, the nurse places the hands on the lower portion of the rib cage. The hands are held parallel with the thumbs at the level of the tenth ribs, 2 in apart and pointing toward the spine (Fig. 20-42, A). The fingers point out laterally. The hands are pressed toward the spine that so a small fold of skin appears between the thumbs. The nurse does not slide the hands over the skin. After exhalation, the client takes a deep breath and the movement of the examiner's thumbs is noted. Normally the thumbs are separated 1½ to 2 in (3 to 5 cm) during excursion. The two sides of the

thorax normally expand equally (Fig. 20-42, B). The nurse normally feels symmetry of respiratory movement during excursion. In the older adult, chest movement declines because of costal cartilage calcification and respiratory muscle atrophy.

During speech the sound created by the vocal cords is transmitted through the lung to the chest wall. The sound waves create vibrations that can be palpated externally. These vibrations are called vocal or *tactile fremitus*. The accumulation of mucus, the collapse of lung tissue, or the presence of lung lesions can block the vibrations from reaching the chest wall.

To palpate for tactile fremitus, the nurse places the ball or lower palm of the hand over an intercostal space, beginning at the lung apex (Fig. 20-43, A). The nurse asks the client to repeat the words, *ninety-nine* or *one-one-one*. Normally there is a faint vibration as the client speaks. Both sides of the thorax are compared, moving from top to bottom. Only one hand is used to ensure accuracy. If fremitus is faint, it may be necessary to ask the client to speak in a louder or lower tone of voice. Symmetry of fremitus is normal. Vibrations are strongest at the top, near the level of the tracheal bifurcation. It is easy to assess for tactile fremitus in a crying infant because strong vibrations can be felt through the chest wall.

Percussion of the chest wall is a difficult assessment technique that determines whether underlying lung tissue is filled with air or fluid or is solid. Percussion reaches only 5 to 7 cm (2 to 3 in) into the chest wall and thus cannot detect deep lesions. The client folds the arms forward across the chest. This position separates the scapulae further to expose more lung to assessment. Using the indirect technique, the nurse percusses in the intercostal spaces

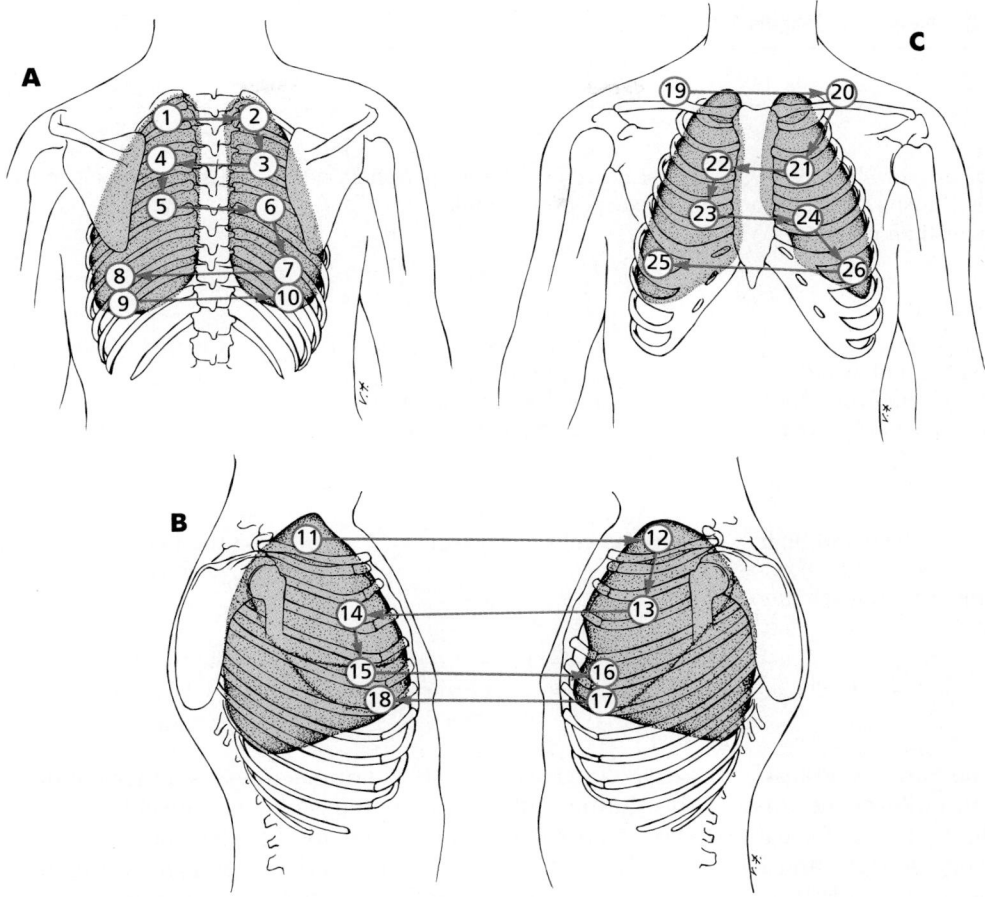

Fig. 20-43 A to C, The nurse follows a systematic pattern (posterior-lateral-anterior) when comparing fremitus, percussion notes, and auscultation.

over symmetrical areas of the lungs. Resonance, the sound created by air-filled lungs, is heard over the posterior thorax. The chest is normally more resonant in the child than in the adult. If the nurse percusses over the scapulae, ribs, spine, or muscle, the percussion note will sound flat. A lung mass also causes a flat sound.

Auscultation assesses the movement of air through the tracheobronchial tree. Normally air flows through the airways in an unobstructed pattern. Recognizing the sounds created by normal airflow allows the nurse to detect sounds caused by obstruction.

In an adult the diaphragm of the stethoscope is placed over the posterior chest wall between the ribs (Fig. 20-44). The bell works best in a child because of the small chest. The client should take slow, deep breaths with the mouth slightly open. The examiner listens to an entire inspiration and expiration at each position of the stethoscope. If sounds are faint, as in the case of the obese client, the client should be

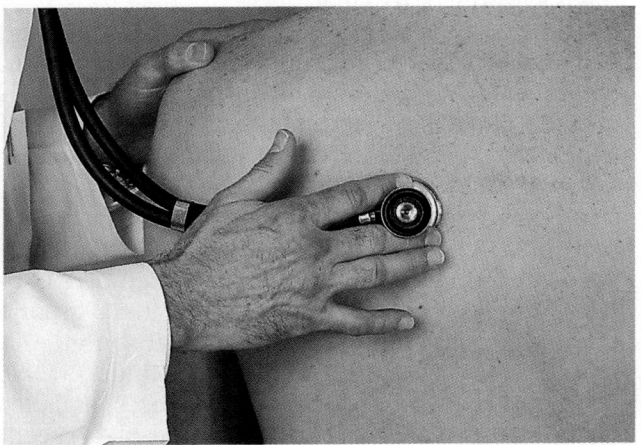

Fig. 20-44 In an adult the nurse uses the diaphragm of the stethoscope to auscultate breath sounds.
From Seidel HM et al: *Mosby's guide to physical examination*, ed 2, St Louis, 1991, Mosby–Year Book.

TABLE 20-18 Normal Breath Sounds

Description	Location	Origin
VESICULAR		
Vesicular sounds are soft, breezy, and low pitched. Inspiratory phase is 3 times longer than expiratory phase.	Best heard over lung's periphery (except over scapula)	Created by air moving through smaller airways
BRONCHOVESICULAR		
Bronchovesicular sounds are medium-pitched and blowing sounds of medium intensity. Inspiratory phase is equal to expiratory phase.	Best heard posteriorly between scapula and anteriorly over bronchioles lateral to sternum at first and second intercostal spaces	Created by air moving through large airways
BRONCHIAL		
Bronchial sounds are loud and high pitched with hollow quality. Expiration lasts longer than inspiration (3:2 ratio).	Best heard over trachea	Created by air moving through trachea close to chest wall

asked to breathe harder and faster. Breath sounds are much louder in children because of the thinness of the chest wall. A systematic pattern should be used when comparing the right and left sides (Fig. 20-43, A). An inexperienced student may attempt to auscultate all of the left side and then return to the right side. This is incorrect. The examiner compares the sounds in one region on one side of the body with sounds in the same region on the opposite side. It is impossible to remember the quality of all sounds noted on one side of the body and then compare them with the other side.

The nurse auscultates for normal breath sounds and abnormal or **adventitious sounds.** Normal breath sounds differ in character, depending on the area of lungs being auscultated. Sounds normally heard over the posterior thorax include bronchovesicular and vesicular sounds (Table 20-18).

Abnormal sounds result from air passing through moisture, mucus, or narrowed airways; from alveoli suddenly reinflating; or from an inflammation between the lung's pleural linings. Adventitious sounds often occur superimposed over normal sounds. The four types of adventitious sounds include crackles (previously called *rales*), rhonchi, wheezes, and pleural friction rub. Each sound is caused by a specific entity and is characterized by typical auditory features (Table 20-19). The location and characteristics of the sounds should be noted, as should the absence of breath sounds (found in clients with collapsed or surgically removed lobes).

If the nurse assesses abnormalities in tactile fremitus, percussion, or auscultation, another test is performed for spoken and whispered voice sounds. With the stethoscope placed over the same locations used to assess breath sounds, the client says, *ninety-nine* or *eee* in a normal voice tone. Normally the sounds are muffled. If fluid is compressing the lung, vibrations from the client's voice are transmitted to the chest wall and the sounds become clear (**bronchophony**). The nurse then asks the client to whisper, *ninety-nine.* The whispered voice is usually faint and indistinct. Certain lung abnormalities may cause the whispered voice to become clear and distinct (**whispered pectoriloquy**).

Lateral Thorax

The client sits during examination of the lateral chest. Usually the nurse extends the assessment of the posterior thorax to the lateral sides of the chest. The client is asked to raise the arms up, which improves access to lateral thoracic structures. The nurse uses all four assessment skills to methodically examine the lateral thorax (Fig. 20-43, B). Excursion cannot be assessed laterally. Normally, percussion notes are resonant, and breath sounds are vesicular.

Anterior Thorax

The anterior thorax is inspected for the same features as the posterior thorax. The client sits or lies

TABLE 20-19	Adventitious Sounds		
Sound	**Site Auscultated**	**Cause**	**Character**
Crackles (previously called *rales*)	Are most commonly heard in dependent lobes: right and left lung bases	Random, sudden reinflation of groups of alveoli*	Are fine, short, interrupted crackling sounds heard during inspiration, expiration, or both; vary in pitch: high or low; may or may not change with coughing*
Rhonchi	Are primarily heard over trachea and bronchi; if loud enough, can be heard over most lung fields	Fluid or mucus in larger airways, causing turbulence	Are low-pitched, continuous musical sounds heard more during expiration; may be cleared by coughing
Wheezes	Can be heard over all lung fields	Severely narrowed bronchus	Are high-pitched, continuous musical sounds heard during inspiration or expiration; do not clear with coughing†
Pleural friction rub	Is heard over anterior lateral lung field (if client is sitting upright)	Inflamed pleura, parietal pleura rubbing against visceral pleura	Has grating quality heard best during inspiration; does not clear with coughing

*Data from Forgacs P: *Chest* 73:399, 1978.
†Data from Wilkins RL, Hodgkin JE, Lopez B: *Lung sounds: a practical guide,* St Louis, 1988, Mosby–Year Book.

down. Anteriorly, the width of the costal angle is noted. It is usually larger than 90 degrees between the two costal margins. The nurse observes the breathing pattern. Normal breathing is quiet and barely audible near the open mouth. Clients with **chronic obstructive pulmonary disease (COPD)** (emphysema and chronic bronchitis) breathe noisily and may produce a grunting sound (see teaching box on p. 556).

The accessory muscles of breathing—sternocleidomastoid and trapezius muscles in the neck and abdominal muscles—are observed. Breathing is usually a passive activity with little effort required to ventilate. When the client is forced to use effort to venti-

late, the accessory muscles are used and can be seen contracting.

Respiratory rate and rhythm are more often assessed anteriorly (see Chapter 19). A man's respirations are usually diaphragmatic, whereas a woman's are more costal. Accurate assessment occurs as a client breathes passively.

The examiner palpates anteriorly for areas of abnormality, tenderness, chest excursion, and tactile fremitus. To measure chest excursion anteriorly, the nurse places the hands over each lateral rib cage, with the thumbs approximately 5 cm (2 in) apart and angled along each costal margin (Fig. 20-45, *A* on p. 556). The thumbs are pushed toward the midline to

Client Teaching During Lung Assessment

OBJECTIVES

- Client will describe warning signs of lung disease.
- Older adult will receive influenza and pneumonia vaccines annually.

TEACHING STRATEGIES

- Explain the risk factors for chronic lung disease and lung cancer, including cigarette smoking, history of cigarette smoking for over 20 years, exposure to certain industrial substances (e.g., arsenic, asbestos), and radiation exposure from occupational, medical, and environmental sources. Residential radon exposure may increase risk for lung cancer, especially in cigarette smokers.*
- Share brochures on lung cancer from American Cancer Society with client and family.

- Discuss the warning signs of lung cancer, such as a persistent cough, sputum streaked with blood, chest pains, and recurrent attacks of pneumonia or bronchitis.
- Counsel older adult on benefits from receiving annual influenza and pneumonia vaccinations because of a greater susceptibility to respiratory infection.

EVALUATION

- Have client describe risk factors for lung disease and cancer.
- Ask client to identify any known risks for cancer.
- Ask client to name warning signs for cancer.
- In a follow-up visit, review client's immunization record.

*Data from American Cancer Society: *1991 cancer facts and figures*, New York, 1991, The Society.

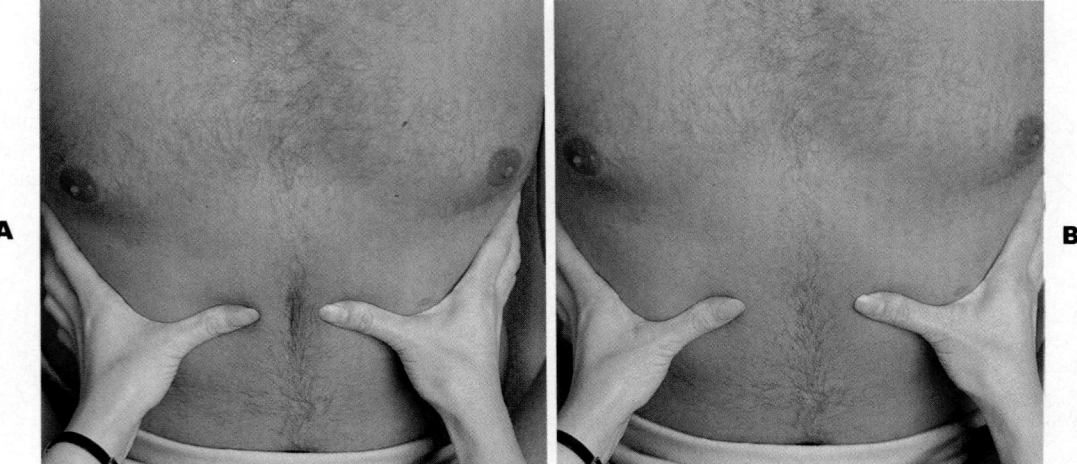

Fig. 20-45   A, Position of nurse's hands before excursion of the anterior chest wall. B, As the client inhales, the nurse's hands normally separate 3 to 5 cm (1½ to 2 in).

create a fold of skin between the thumbs. As the client inhales deeply, the thumbs should normally separate approximately 3 to 5 cm (½ to 2 in), with each side expanding equally (Fig. 20-45, *B*).

Tactile fremitus is assessed over the chest wall. Anterior findings differ from posterior findings because of the heart and female breast tissue. Fremitus is decreased over the precordium (area over the heart and lower thorax). The nurse will not be able to sense vibrations over breast tissue and thus must retract the breasts gently during palpation. If the breasts are large, this portion of the examination may be omitted.

Percussion of the anterior thorax follows a systematic pattern. The nurse must imagine the location of all internal organs anteriorly accessible to examina-

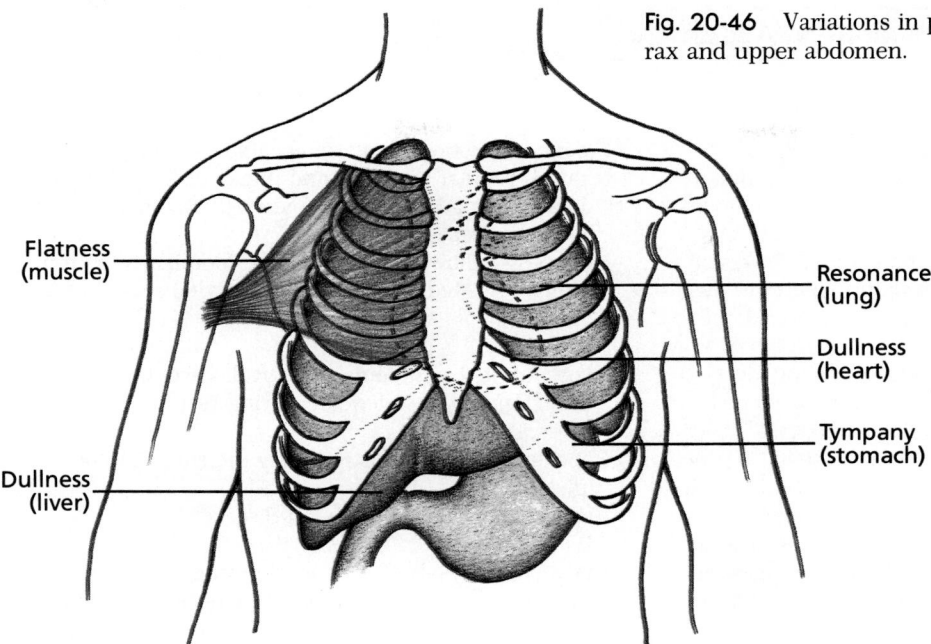

Fig. 20-46   Variations in percussion notes in the normal thorax and upper abdomen.

Flatness (muscle)

Dullness (liver)

Resonance (lung)

Dullness (heart)

Tympany (stomach)

tion. The underlying liver, heart, and stomach create percussion notes characteristically different from those of the lung (Fig. 20-46). Percussion may be conducted with the client in a sitting or lying position. However, the procedure is easier for the examiner if the client lies down. The examiner starts above the clavicles and moves across and then down. The female breasts are displaced as needed. The normal lung is resonant. As the examiner proceeds downward, the areas of heart and liver dullness and the tympanic gastric air bubble will be detectable.

Auscultation of the anterior thorax follows the same pattern as percussion (Fig. 20-43, *C*). The client should sit if possible to maximize chest expansion. In addition to bronchovesicular and vesicular sounds, a normal breath sound can be heard anteriorly. This bronchial sound is loud and high pitched and normally heard only over the trachea.

 ## HEART

The assessment of heart function involves a review of signs and symptoms from the nursing history, pulse assessment (see Chapter 19), and direct examination of the heart. A client who has signs or symptoms of heart (cardiac) problems (for example, chest pain and irregular heart rate) may be suffering a life-threatening condition requiring immediate attention. The nurse must sense which portions of an

examination are absolutely necessary. When a client's condition is stable, assessment can reveal baseline heart function and any risks for heart disease. Abnormal findings require a physician's attention. The nurse performing a cardiac assessment compares findings with those made in the vascular examination (see later section). The nursing history (Table 20-20 on p. 558) provides data that help the nurse interpret physical findings.

Assessment of cardiac function is performed through the anterior thorax. The nurse forms a mental image of the heart's exact location. In the adult, it is in the center of the chest (precordium), behind and to the left of the sternum, with a small section of the right atrium extending to the sternum's right. The base of the heart is the upper portion, and the apex is the bottom tip. The surface of the right ventricle composes most of the heart's anterior surface. A section of the left ventricle shapes the left anterior side of the apex. The apex actually touches the anterior chest wall at approximately the fourth to fifth intercostal space along the midclavicular line, known as the *point of maximal impulse (PMI)*.

An infant's heart is positioned more horizontally and has a larger diameter compared with that of an adult. The apex of the heart in an infant is at the third or fourth intercostal space, just to the left of the midclavicular line. By the age of 7 a child's PMI is in the same location as the adult's.

To understand the significance of assessment findings, the nurse must first understand timing

TABLE 20-20 Nursing History for Heart Assessment	
Assessment Category	Rationale
Determine history of smoking, alcohol intake, use of drugs, exercise habits, and dietary patterns and intake.	Smoking, alcohol ingestion, cocaine use, absent or reduced regular exercise, and intake of foods high in carbohydrates and cholesterol are risk factors for cardiovascular disease.
Determine if client is taking medications for cardiovascular function (e.g., antidysrhythmics, antihypertensives) and if client knows their purpose, dosage, and side effects.	Knowledge allows nurse to assess compliance with drug therapies. Medications may affect vital sign values.
Assess for chest pain, palpitations, excess fatigue, dyspnea, edema of feet, cyanosis, fainting, and orthopnea. Ask if symptoms occur at rest or during exercise.	These are key symptoms of heart disease. Cardiovascular function may be adequate during rest but not during exercise.
Determine whether client has a stressful lifestyle.	Repeated exposure to stress may increase risk for heart disease.
Assess family history for heart disease, high cholesterol levels, hypertension, stroke, or rheumatic heart disease.	Factors increase risk for heart disease.
Ask client about history of heart trouble (e.g., congestive heart failure, congenital heart disease, coronary artery disease, dysrhythmias, murmurs).	Knowledge reveals client's level of understanding of condition. Prexisting condition influences examination techniques used by nurse, as well as findings to expect.
Determine whether client has preexisting diabetes, lung disease, obesity, or hypertension.	These disorders may alter heart function.
Determine whether client drinks excessive amounts of coffee, tea, or caffeine-containing soft drinks.	Caffeine can cause heart dysrhythmias.

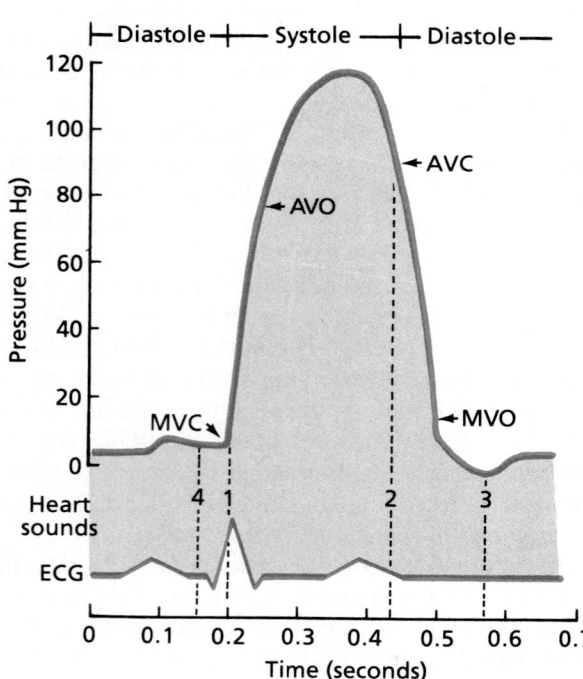

Fig. 20-47 Cardiac cycle. *MVC*, Mitral valve closes; *AVO*, aortic valve opens; *AVC*, aortic valve closes; *MVO*, mitral valve opens.

in relation to the cardiac cycle (Fig. 20-47). The heart normally pumps blood through its four chambers in a methodical, even sequence. As blood flows through each chamber, the valves open and close, the pressures within chambers rise and fall, and the chambers contract. Each event creates a physiological sign that can be detected by an examiner. Both sides of the heart function in a coordinated fashion. Blood flows from the right atrium to the right ventricle and from the left atrium to the left ventricle through the atrioventricular valves. The tricuspid valve separates the right atrium and ventricle, and the mitral valve separates the left atrium and ventricle. Blood passes from the right ventricle through the pulmonic valve to the pulmonary artery. Similarly, blood leaves the left ventricle through the aortic valve into the aorta.

Events occurring on the left side of the heart have the most dramatic effect on assessment findings. Pressure is greatest on the left side, so longer and louder sounds are created. Events on the left side slightly precede those on the right. When the left ventricle is at rest (diastolic phase), the pressure in the left atrium exceeds that in the ventricle, creating a pressure gradient that moves blood through the opened mitral valve. During ventricular filling, pressure rises in the ventricle to exceed the pressure in the left atrium. Just before the ventricle contracts, the mitral valve closes to prevent regurgitation of blood into the atrium, creating the first heart sound (S_1). Ventricular pressure builds, causing the aortic valve to open as the ventricle contracts (systolic phase). Blood flows into the aorta, elevating aortic pressure. When the ventricle empties, pressure within the chamber falls. To prevent regurgitation from the aorta into the left ventricle, the aortic valve closes, creating the second heart sound (S_2). As ventricular pressure continues to fall, it drops below that of the left atrium. The mitral valve reopens to again allow ventricular filling. The rapid filling of the ventricle may create a third heart sound (S_3), heard more often in children and young adults. An S_3 can also be heard as an abnormality in older adults. When the atria contract to enhance ventricular filling, a fourth heart sound (S_4) is produced. The S_4 is not normally heard in adults.

Inspection and Palpation

Before beginning the examination, the nurse ensures that the client is relaxed and comfortable. An anxious or uncomfortable client can have mild tachycardia that may lead the nurse to misinterpret the findings. An alteration in heart function can also result in changes affecting other body systems; for example, cyanosis can indicate poor arterial oxygenation resulting from heart disease. Edema in the feet, ankles, or sacrum can be the result of right-sided heart failure. Crackles or rhonchi can develop from left-sided heart failure.

The nurse uses inspection and palpation simultaneously. The examination begins with the client in the supine position or with the upper body elevated 45 degrees because clients with heart disease frequently suffer shortness of breath while lying flat. The nurse stands on the client's right side. The client must refrain from talking, especially after the nurse begins auscultation of heart sounds. The nurse directs attention to the anatomical sites best suited for assessment of cardiac function. Louis' angle lies between the sternal body and manubrium and can be felt as a prominence on the sternum. The nurse can slip the fingers down each side of the angle, until the second intercostal spaces are felt (Fig. 20-48, *dots 1* and *2*). The second intercostal space on the right is the aortic area (*dot 1*), and the left second intercostal space is the pulmonic area (*dot 2*). Deeper palpation is required to feel the spaces in obese clients or those with well-developed chest muscles.

The aortic and pulmonic areas are inspected for pulsations. Viewing these areas at an angle to the side improves the likelihood of detecting pulsation, which may arise from abnormalities in major vessels of the heart or improper valve closure. Pulsations are more easily felt with the fingertips. A vibration, felt best with the ball of the hand, is caused by loud murmurs. If pulsations or vibrations are palpated, the nurse times their occurrence in relation to systole or diastole by auscultating heart sounds simultaneously.

Inspection and palpation continue over the other anatomical sites. After the pulmonic area is located (*dot 2*), the nurse simply moves the fingers along the client's left sternal border to the third intercostal space, called *Erb's point* (Fig. 20-48, *dot 3*). The tricuspid area (Fig. 20-48, *dot 4*) is located at the fifth intercostal space along the sternum. To find the apical area the nurse locates the fifth intercostal space just to the left of the sternum and moves the fingers laterally to the left midclavicular line (Fig. 20-48, *dot 5*). Some examiners are able to locate the apical area with the palm of the hand, but others use their fingertips. Normally, at the PMI the apical pulse is a light tap felt in an area 1 to 2 cm (½ in) in diameter at the apex (Fig. 20-49 on p. 560). When the apical pulse is more forceful, like a heave, it can be a sign of left ventricular failure. If the PMI cannot be found with the client in the supine position, the nurse asks the client to roll onto the left side, which moves the heart closer to the chest wall. The nurse estimates the heart's size by noting the diameter of the PMI and its position relative to the midclavicular line. In cases of serious heart disease, the cardiac muscle enlarges, with the PMI found to the left of the midclavicular line. The PMI may be difficult to find in the

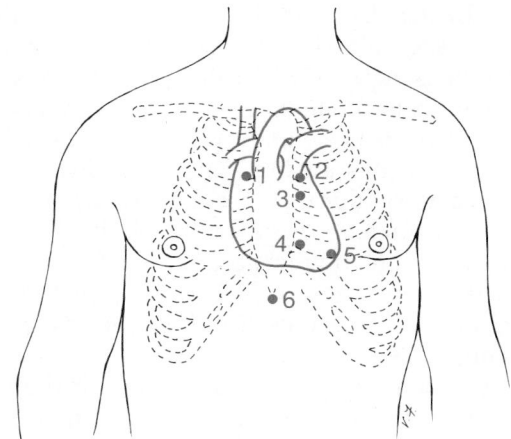

Fig. 20-48   Anatomical sites for assessment of cardiac function.

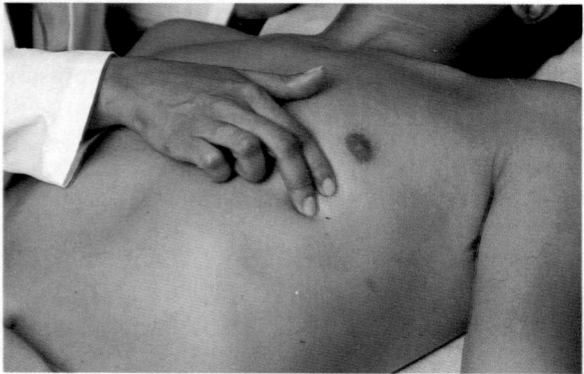

Fig. 20-49 Palpation of PMI at the fourth to fifth intercostal space along the midclavicular line.
From Canobbio MM: *Cardiovascular disorders,* St Louis, 1990, Mosby–Year Book.

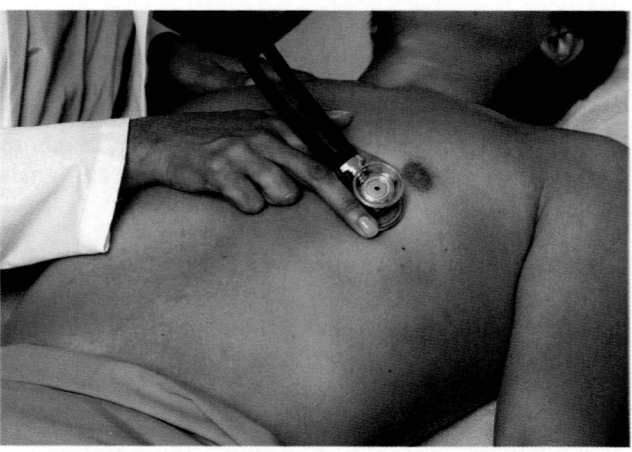

Fig. 20-50 Auscultation of heart sounds at the PMI using the diaphragm of the stethoscope.
From Canobbio MM: *Cardiovascular disorders,* St Louis, 1990, Mosby–Year Book.

older adult because the chest deepens in its anteroposterior diameters. It may also be difficult to locate in a client who is very muscular or overweight. The PMI of an infant can usually be found near the third or fourth intercostal space. It is easy to palpate the child's PMI because of the thin chest wall.

The final area to inspect and palpate is the epigastric area at the tip of the sternum (Fig. 20-48, *dot 6*). In clients with normal aortic structure and function, the pulsation of the abdominal aorta may be seen and felt.

Auscultation

Auscultation of the heart detects normal heart sounds, extra heart sounds, and murmurs. The nursing student should first become skilled in detecting normal heart sounds. These low-intensity sounds, created by the closing of the valves, are often difficult to hear, especially if breath sounds are noisy. Concentration is needed when detecting heart sounds. To begin auscultation the nurse eliminates all sources of room noise and explains the procedure to relieve the client's anxiety. The nurse follows a systematic pattern during auscultation moving across each of the anatomical sites (Fig. 20-48). The nurse usually must lift the female client's left breast to listen better to the chest wall. The nurse first identifies the first (S_1) and second (S_2) heart sounds using the following steps:

1. Auscultate using the diaphragm of the stethoscope because S_1 and S_2 are high-pitched sounds.
2. Begin auscultating at the apex or PMI (Fig. 20-50) and then move systematically to the tricuspid area, Erb's point, and the pulmonic and aortic areas.

A methodical approach ensures that all areas are assessed. At normal slow rates, S_1 is high pitched and dull in quality and sounds like a *lub*. It is heard best and more loudly at the apex and precedes the short systolic phase of heart contraction. If it is difficult to detect S_1, it should be timed in relation to the carotid pulse (see next section). It occurs just before the carotid pulsation at systole.

S_2 follows the short systolic phase, precedes the long diastolic phase, and sounds like *dub*. Examiners learn to hear the sound of S_2 best at the aortic area. The nurse should become familiar with hearing both heart sounds clearly. By slowly inching the stethoscope diagonally toward the apex and keeping the sound in focus, the nurse notes that S_2 begins to diminish in sound and S_1 gets louder. After both sounds are heard clearly as *lub dub,* the nurse assesses heart rate and rhythm using the following steps:

1. Count each combination of S_1 and S_2 as one heart beat. Assess the apical pulse for 1 minute.
2. To assess heart rhythm, note the time between S_1 and S_2 (systole) and then the time between S_2 and the next S_1 (diastole). Listen to the full cycle at each auscultation area. A regular rhythm involves regular intervals of time between each sequence of beats. There should also be a distinct silent pause between S_1 and S_2.
3. Listen for dysrhythmias. Failure of the heart to beat at regular successive intervals is a **dysrhythmia.** Some dysrhythmias can be life threatening (see Chapter 38).
4. When the heart rhythm is irregular, compare apical and radial pulse rates to determine

whether a pulse deficit exists. Auscultate the apical pulse first and then immediately palpate the radial pulse (see Chapter 19). A colleague can assess the apical pulse as the examiner simultaneously measures the radial pulse. Compare the two rates. When a client has a **pulse deficit,** the radial pulse is slower than the apical because ineffective contractions fail to send pulse waves to the periphery.

Next, the nurse auscultates for extra heart sounds using the following steps:

1. Apply the bell of the stethoscope, and listen for low-pitched extra heart sounds such as S_3 and S_4 gallops, clicks, and rubs. Auscultate over all five anatomical areas.
2. S_3 or a **ventricular gallop,** occurs just after S_2 at the end of ventricular diastole. It may be caused by a premature rush of blood into a ventricle that is stiff or dilated due to failure and hypertension. S_4, or an **atrial gallop,** occurs just before S_1 or ventricular systole. Physiologically it may be due to an atrial contraction pushing against a ventricle that is not accepting blood because of heart failure or other alterations. S_3 and S_4 are common in children, young adults, and athletes. They are not considered normal in persons over age 30.
3. The nurse often hears S_3 and S_4 best with the client on the left side with the bell placed over the apex or PMI (Fig. 20-48, *dot 5*).
4. Further auscultate for clicks and rubs. Clicks are short, high-pitched, extra heart sounds created by mitral valve prolapse, aortic stenosis, or prosthetic valves. In contrast, rubs result from a rubbing of inflamed visceral and parietal layers of the pericardium against one another. Myocardial infarction and infection of the pericardium can predispose to inflammation of the tissues surrounding the heart.

The final portion of the examination includes assessment for heart murmurs. **Murmurs** are sustained swishing or blowing sounds heard at the beginning, middle, or end of the systolic or diastolic phase. They are caused by increased blood flow through a normal valve, forward flow through a stenotic valve or into a dilated vessel or heart chamber, or backward flow through a valve that fails to close. A murmur can be asymptomatic or a sign of heart disease (see teaching box). Murmurs are common in children. The nurse keeps the following factors in mind when auscultating to detect murmurs:

1. When a murmur is detected, the nurse auscultates the mitral, tricuspid, aortic, and pulmonic valve areas for its place in the cardiac cycle (timing), place it is heard best (location), radiation, loudness, pitch, and quality.

2. If a murmur occurs between S_1 and S_2, it is a systolic murmur. If it occurs between S_2 and the next S_1, it is a diastolic murmur.
3. The location of a murmur is not necessarily directly over the valves. With experience, a nurse can learn where each type of murmur is best heard. For example, mitral murmurs are heard best at the apex of the heart.

Client Teaching During Heart Assessment

OBJECTIVES

■ Client will know risks of heart disease and take steps to eliminate risks from lifestyle.
■ Client with risk for heart disease will seek support from appropriate care givers.

TEACHING STRATEGIES

■ Explain the risk factors for heart disease, including high dietary intake of cholesterol, lack of regular aerobic exercise, smoking, stressful lifestyle, and family history of heart disease.
■ Refer client (if appropriate) to resources available for controlling or reducing risks (e.g., nutritional counseling, exercise class, stress-reduction programs).
■ Explain that research shows clinical benefit from reducing dietary intake of cholesterol and saturated fats. Tell client that about 70% to 75% of saturated fatty acids come from meats, poultry, fish, and dairy products and that the one-step diet recommended by the National Institutes of Health includes an intake of total fat less than 30% of calories, saturated fatty acids less than 10% of calories, and cholesterol less than 300 mg/100 ml.*
■ Encourage client to have regular measurement of total blood cholesterol levels. Desirable levels are 150-200 mg/100 ml.† More than one cholesterol measurement is needed to assess the blood cholesterol level accurately. Low-density lipoprotein (LDL) cholesterol is the major component of atherosclerotic plaques. Separate measurement of LDL cholesterol is wise in a client with high total blood cholesterol levels. An LDL cholesterol level of 160 mg/dl or higher is high risk.

EVALUATION

■ Ask client to identify risk factors for heart disease.
■ Have client develop a meal plan low in saturated fat and cholesterol.
■ Check client's cholesterol level during follow-up appointments at clinic or physician's office.

*Data from Ernst ND: *Fam Community Health* 12(1):23, 1989.
†Data from Bullock B, Rosenthal pp: *Pathophysiology: adaptation and alteration*, ed 3, 1992, Lippincott.

4. To assess for radiation the nurse listens for a murmur over areas besides where it is heard best. Murmurs can also sometimes be heard over the neck or back.

5. Intensity or loudness is related to the rate of blood flow through the heart or the amount of blood regurgitated. In serious murmurs the nurse may feel a thrust or intermittent palpable sensation at the auscultation site. A **thrill** is a continuous palpable sensation like the purring of a cat. Intensity is recorded in the following grades:

Grade 1   Barely audible
Grade 2   Audible immediately but faint
Grade 3   Loud, without thrust or thrill
Grade 4   Loud, with thrust or thrill
Grade 5   Very loud, with thrust or thrill; audible with stethoscope only partially applied
Grade 6   Louder, may be heard without stethoscope

6. A murmur may be low, medium, or high in pitch, depending on the velocity of blood flow through the valves. A low-pitched murmur is heard best with the bell of the stethoscope. If it is heard best with the diaphragm, a murmur is high pitched.

7. The quality of a murmur refers to its characteristic pattern and sound. A crescendo murmur starts softly and builds in loudness. A decrescendo murmur starts loudly and then becomes less intense. A crescendo-decrescendo murmur starts softly, becomes louder, and then softens again. Finally, a plateau murmur sounds the same throughout its duration (Miracle, 1988).

VASCULAR SYSTEM

Examination of the vascular system includes measurement of the blood pressure (see Chapter 19) and a thorough assessment of the integrity of the peripheral vascular system. Table 20-21 reviews the nursing history data collected before the examination. The nurse may perform portions of the vascular examination during assessment of other body systems. For example, the carotid pulse may be checked after palpation of cervical lymph nodes. As the nurse inspects the skin, signs and symptoms of arterial and venous insufficiency are noted. An experienced nurse integrates vascular assessment with other portions of the examination if it is important to minimize time spent in the total examination.

TABLE 20-21 Nursing History for Vascular Assessment	
Assessment Category	**Rationale**
Determine if client experiences leg cramps, numbness, pain, or burning in extremities or edema around ankles.	These signs and symptoms indicate vascular disease.
If client experiences pain or cramping in lower extremities, ask if it is relieved or aggravated by walking.	Relationship of symptoms to exercise can clarify whether problem is vascular or musculoskeletal. Pain caused by vascular condition tends to increase with activity.
Ask women if they wear tight-fitting garters or knee-length nylons.	Tight clothing around lower extremities can impair venous return.
Assess medical history for heart disease, hypertension, phlebitis, diabetes, or varicose veins.	Circulatory and vascular disorders influence findings gathered during examination.

Blood Pressure

The nurse auscultates the blood pressure at the brachial artery site in both arms. Systolic readings that differ by 15 mm Hg or more suggest atherosclerosis or disease of the aorta. The nurse also compares the blood pressure with the client in the lying position with that in the sitting or standing position. This maneuver assesses for orthostatic (postural) hypotension (see Chapter 19). A fall in systolic blood pressure of at least 25 mm Hg and a fall in diastolic pressure of at least 10 mm Hg accompanied by signs and symptoms of inadequate cerebral perfusion signals the condition (Schatz, 1984).

Arteries and Veins

Examination of the vascular system involves palpation, inspection, and auscultation. The nurse begins with an assessment of the integrity of accessible arteries and veins. In addition, the nurse notes the condition of the extremities perfused by the vascular system. Abnormalities interfering with arterial perfusion or venous return cause changes in the skin and tissues of affected extremities.

Carotid Arteries

When the left ventricle pumps blood into the aorta, pressure waves are transmitted through the ar-

Fig. 20-51 Anatomical position of the carotid artery.

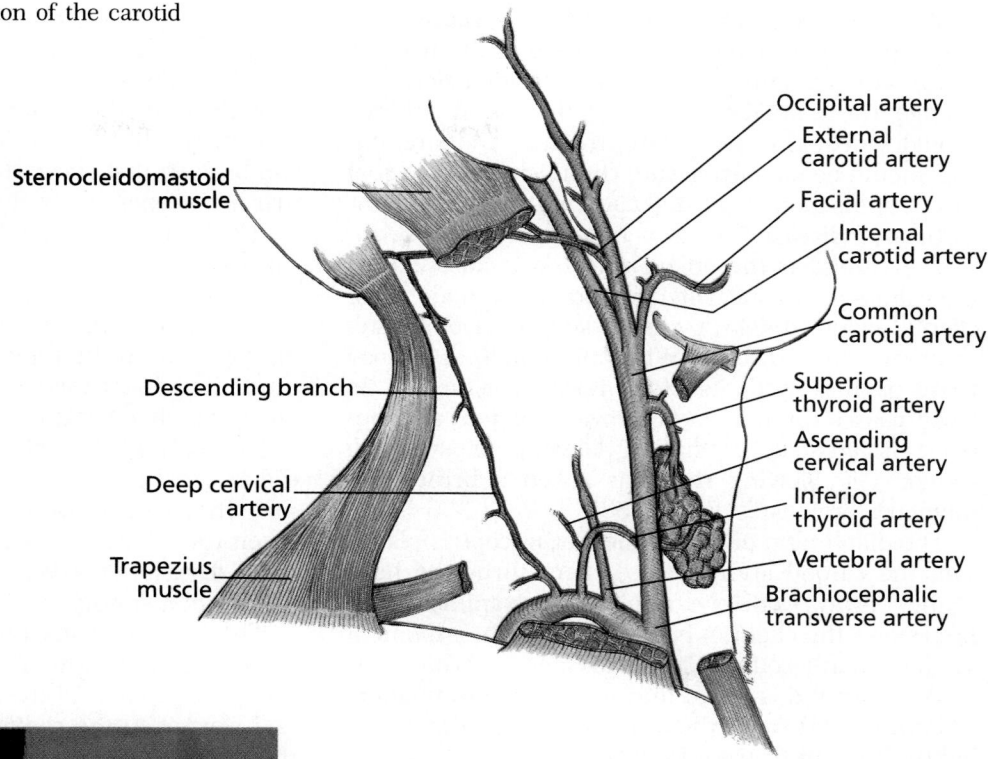

Sternocleidomastoid muscle

Descending branch

Deep cervical artery

Trapezius muscle

Occipital artery

External carotid artery

Facial artery

Internal carotid artery

Common carotid artery

Superior thyroid artery

Ascending cervical artery

Inferior thyroid artery

Vertebral artery

Brachiocephalic transverse artery

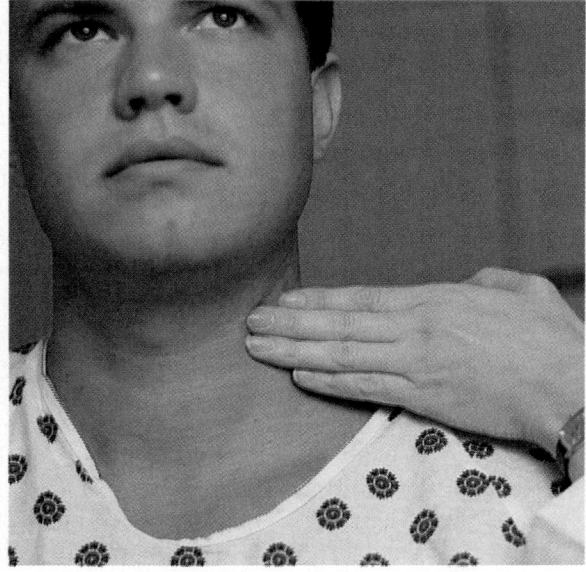

Fig. 20-52 Palpation of internal carotid artery along the margin of the sternocleidomastoid muscle.

terial system. Pressure waves are manifested as pulses that are palpable in arteries close to the skin or overlying bone. The carotid arteries reflect heart function better than peripheral arteries because their pressure correlates with that of the aorta.

The carotid arteries supply oxygenated blood to the head and neck (Fig. 20-51) and are protected by the overlying sternocleidomastoid muscle. To examine the carotid arteries, the nurse has the client sit or lie supine with the head of the bed elevated 30 degrees. One carotid artery is examined at a time. If both arteries were to be occluded during palpation, the client could lose consciousness as a result of inadequate circulation to the brain. The carotids must not be vigorously palpated or massaged. The carotid sinus is located at the bifurcation of the common carotid arteries in the upper third of the neck. The sinus sends impulses along the vagus nerve. Its stimulation can cause a reflex drop in heart rate and blood pressure, which cause **syncope** or circulatory arrest.

The neck is first inspected for obvious pulsation of the artery. The client turns the head slightly away from the artery being examined. Sometimes, the wave of the pulse can be seen. The carotid is the only site for assessing the quality of a pulse wave. Only an experienced assessor can evaluate the quality of the wave in relation to systole and diastole of the cardiac cycle. An absent pulse wave can indicate arterial **occlusion** (blockage) or **stenosis** (narrowing).

For palpation of the pulse, the client turns the head slightly toward the side being examined. This maneuver relaxes the neck muscles for easier palpation. The nurse slides the tips of the index and middle fingers around the medial edge of the sternocleidomastoid muscle. Gentle palpation avoids occlusion of circulation (Fig. 20-52).

The normal carotid pulse is localized rather than diffuse. A strong pulse, the carotid has a thrusting quality. As the client breathes, no change occurs during inspiration or expiration. Rotation of the neck or a shift from a sitting to a supine position does not change the carotid's quality. Both carotid arteries should be equal in pulse rate, rhythm, and strength and should be equally elastic. Diminished or unequal carotid pulsations can indicate **atherosclerosis** or aortic arch disease.

The carotid is the only pulse that is auscultated. Auscultation is especially important for middle-age clients, older adults, or clients suspected of having cerebrovascular disease. When the lumen of a blood vessel is narrowed, its blood flow is disturbed. As blood passes through the narrowed section, a turbulence is created, causing a blowing or swishing sound. The blowing sound is called a **bruit** (pronounced "brew-ee") (Fig. 20-53).

The diaphragm or bell of the stethoscope is placed over the carotid artery as the client turns the head slightly away from the side being examined. The nurse asks the client to hold the breath for a moment so that breath sounds do not obscure a bruit. Normally, no sound is heard during carotid auscultation. If a bruit is heard, the nurse palpates the artery lightly for a thrill (palpable bruit).

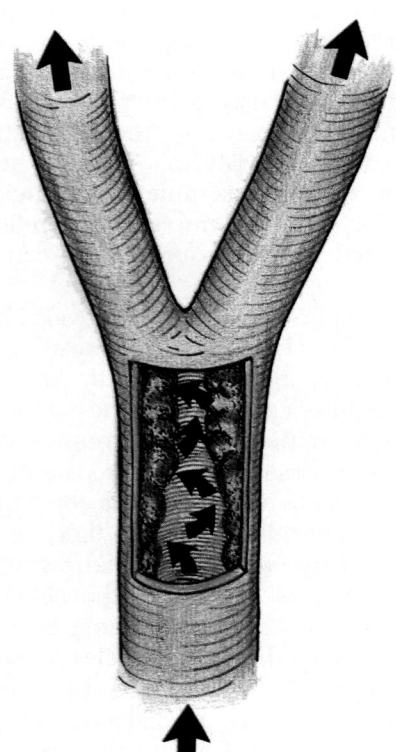

Fig. 20-53 Occlusion or narrowing of the carotid artery disrupts normal blood flow. The resultant turbulence creates a sound (bruit) that the nurse can auscultate.

Jugular Veins

The most accessible veins are the internal and external jugular veins in the neck. Both veins drain bilaterally from the head and neck into the superior vena cava. The external jugular lies superficially and can be seen just above the clavicle. The internal jugular lies deeper, along the carotid artery.

It is best to examine the right internal jugular because it follows a more direct anatomical path to the right atrium of the heart. The column of blood inside the internal jugular serves as a manometer, reflecting pressure in the right atrium. The higher the column, the greater the venous pressure. Raised venous pressure reflects right-sided heart failure.

Normally when a client lies in the supine position, the external jugular distends and becomes easily visible. In contrast the jugular veins normally flatten when the client is in a sitting position. A client with heart disease, however, may have distended jugular veins when sitting.

The jugular veins are inspected to measure venous pressures, which are influenced by blood volume, the capacity of the right atrium to receive blood and send it to the right ventricle, and the ability of the right ventricle to contract and force blood into the pulmonary artery. Any factor resulting in greater blood volume within the venous system results in elevated venous pressure. The nurse assesses venous pressure by using the following steps:

1. Have the client lie supine with head elevated 30 to 45 degrees (semi-Fowler's position).
2. Be sure the neck and upper thorax are exposed. Use a small pillow to align the head. Avoid neck hyperextension or flexion to ensure that the vein is not stretched or kinked (Fig. 20-54).
3. Look for the usual position of the internal jugular vein, just visible 2 to 3 cm (1 in) above the sternal angle or suprasternal notch. Measure venous pressure by finding the highest visible point of the internal jugular vein.
4. Use two rulers. Line up the bottom edge of a regular ruler with the top of the area of pulsation in the jugular vein. Then take a centimeter ruler and align it perpendicular to the first ruler at the level of the sternal angle. Measure in centimeters the distance between the second ruler and the sternal angle (Fig. 20-55).
5. Repeat the same measurement on the other side. Bilateral pressures higher than 3 cm (1 in) are considered elevated and are a sign of right-sided heart failure. One-sided pressure elevation can be caused by obstruction.

Peripheral Arteries and Veins

To examine the peripheral vascular system the nurse first assesses the adequacy of blood flow to the

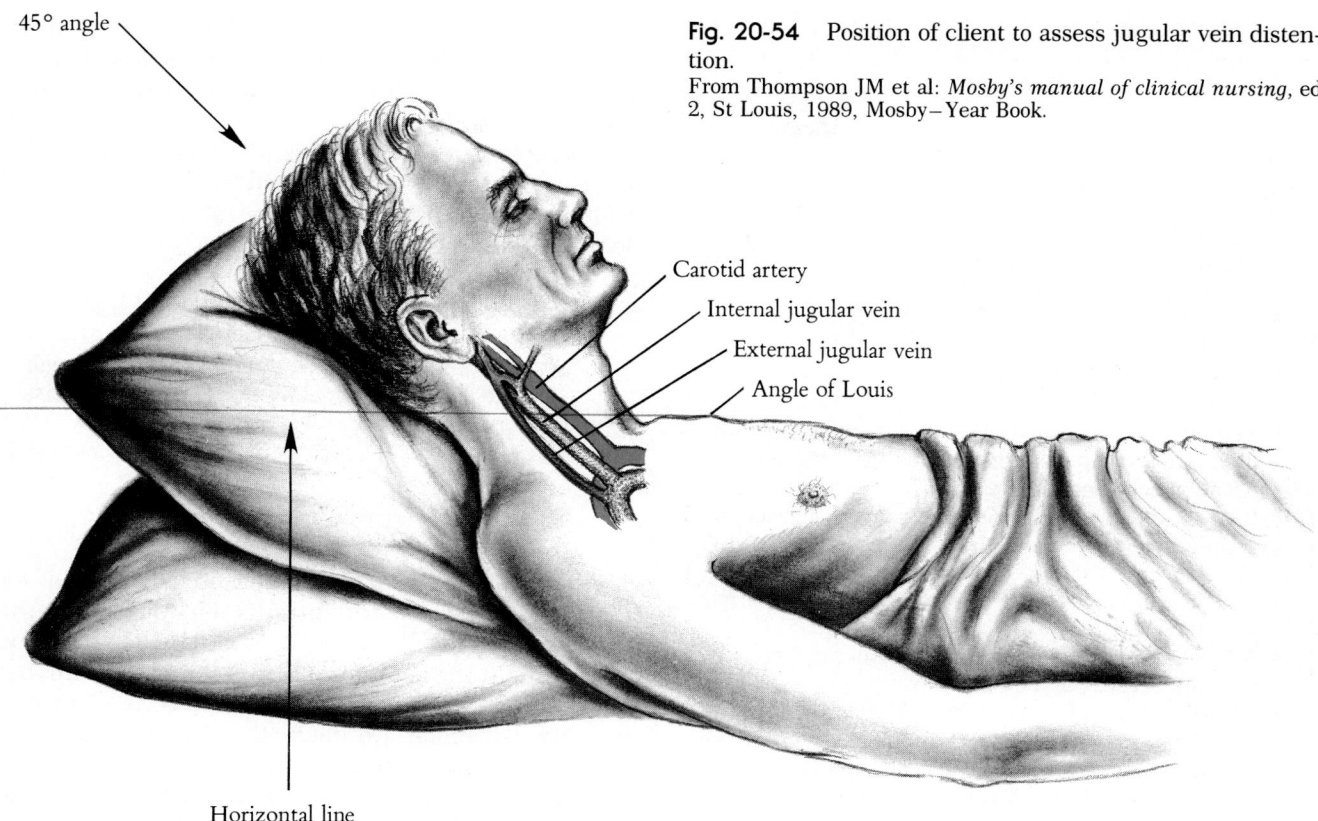

45° angle

Horizontal line

Fig. 20-54   Position of client to assess jugular vein distention.
From Thompson JM et al: *Mosby's manual of clinical nursing,* ed 2, St Louis, 1989, Mosby–Year Book.

Carotid artery
Internal jugular vein
External jugular vein
Angle of Louis

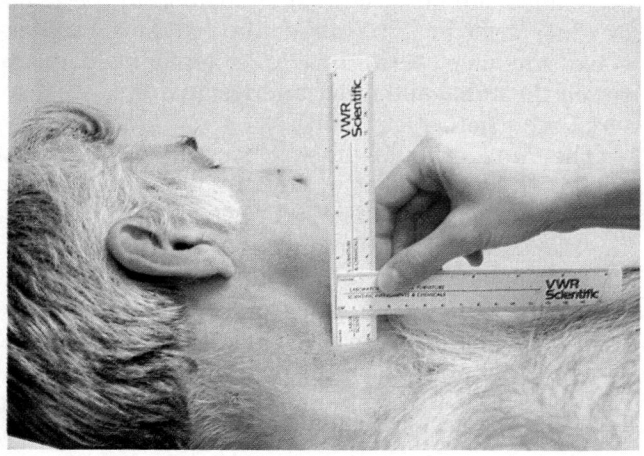

Fig. 20-55   Measurement of jugular vein distention.
From Seidel HM et al: *Mosby's guide to physical examination,* ed 2, St Louis, 1991, Mosby–Year Book.

TABLE 20-22 Indicators for Assessing Local Blood Flow	
Indicator	Rationale
Systemic diseases (e.g., arteriosclerosis, atherosclerosis, diabetes)	Disease results in changes in integrity of walls of arteries and smaller blood vessels.
Coagulation disorders (e.g., thrombosis, embolus)	Blood clot causes mechanical obstruction to blood flow.
Local trauma or surgery (e.g., contusion, fracture, vascular surgery)	Direct manipulation of vessels or localized edema impairs blood flow.
Application of constricting devices (e.g., casts, dressings, elastic bandages, restraints)	Constriction causes tourniquet effect, impairing blood flow to areas below site of constriction.

extremities by measuring arterial pulses and inspecting the condition of the skin and nails. The integrity of the venous system is also assessed, with attention given to determining whether the client has abnormalities. A number of factors can impair circulation to the extremities (Table 20-22). Altered blood vessel integrity, mechanical obstruction to blood flow, and overlying constriction on vessel walls reduce perfusion of tissues. The nurse should anticipate risk of circulatory impairment (see teaching box on p. 566). Some clients, such as older adults and diabetic persons, suffer physical changes in blood vessel walls that increase the risk of perfusion problems.

Client Teaching During Vascular Assessment

OBJECTIVES

- Client will know normal blood pressure range for age and compare it with own blood pressure readings to identify normalcy of blood pressure.
- Client with vascular insufficiency will avoid activities that worsen circulatory status.

TEACHING STRATEGIES

- Tell the client the blood pressure reading. Explain the normal reading for the client's age. Discuss implications of abnormalities.
- Instruct the client with risk or evidence of vascular insufficiency in the lower extremities to avoid tight clothing over the lower body or legs, to avoid sitting or standing for long periods, to walk regularly, and to elevate feet when sitting.
- Advise client to avoid cigarette smoking because nicotine causes vasoconstriction.
- Identify older adult with hypertension who may benefit from regular monitoring of blood pressure (daily, weekly, or monthly). Teach client how to use home monitoring kits (see Chapter 19).

EVALUATION

- Ask client to identify if blood pressure reading is within normal limits for age.
- Have client with vascular insufficiency describe precautions to take to avoid further circulatory deficiency.
- Have older adult demonstrate self-monitoring of blood pressure.

ARTERIAL PULSES. The nurse palpates peripheral arteries for elasticity of the vessel wall, rate and rhythm of pulse, strength of pulse, type of pulse, and equality of pulses. A systematic technique is useful, starting with the temporal arteries in the head and moving down to the arteries in the upper and lower extremities.

The wall of an artery is normally elastic, making it easily palpable. After the artery is depressed, it will spring back to shape when pressure is released. An abnormal artery may be described as *hard, inelastic,* or *calcified.*

The peripheral pulse rate is measured for 1 minute. The radial artery is usually chosen as the site to determine pulse rate when the nurse measures vital signs (see Chapter 19). To check for local circulatory perfusion the nurse may palpate a peripheral pulse long enough to assess its presence. With palpa-

tion the nurse normally feels the pulse wave at regular intervals. When an interval is interrupted by an early, late, or missed beat, the pulse rhythm is irregular.

The strength of a pulse is a measurement of the force at which blood is ejected against the arterial wall. Some examiners use a scale rating from 0 to 4 + for the strength of a pulse:

0   No pulse is palpable.
1+   Pulse is difficult to palpate, weak, and thready in character and is easy to obliterate.
2+   Pulse is difficult to palpate, and light pressure will locate it. A discriminating touch senses that it is stronger than 1+.
3+   This is a normal pulse, easy to palpate and not easily obliterated.
4+   Strong pulse is easily palpated, seems to bound against fingertips, and cannot be obliterated.

All peripheral pulses are measured bilaterally for equality and symmetry. In addition, pulses on the same side of the body can be assessed for equality. For example, the left radial pulse is compared with that of the right, and the left brachial pulse is compared with the left radial. An inequality may indicate localized obstruction or an abnormally positioned artery.

In the upper extremities the primary artery is the brachial, which channels blood to the radial and ulnar arteries of the forearm and hand. If circulation in the brachial artery is blocked, the hands will not receive adequate blood flow. If circulation in the radial or ulnar arteries is impaired, the hand will still receive adequate perfusion. An interconnection between the radial and ulnar arteries guards against arterial occlusion (Fig. 20-56).

The nurse should practice locating pulses on a friend. To locate pulses in the arm, the nurse has the client sit or lie down. The radial pulse is found along the radial side of the forearm, at the wrist. In a thin individual, a groove is formed lateral to the flexor tendon of the wrist. The radial pulse can be felt with light palpation in the groove (Fig. 20-57).

The ulnar pulse is on the opposite side of the wrist and tends to feel less prominent than the radial pulse (Fig. 20-58). An examiner palpates the ulnar pulse only when arterial insufficiency to the hand is expected.

To palpate the brachial pulse, the nurse finds the groove between the biceps and triceps muscles above the elbow at the antecubital fossa (Fig. 20-59). The artery runs along the medial side of the extended arm. The nurse palpates the artery with the fingertips of the first three fingers in the muscle groove.

The femoral artery is the primary artery in the leg, delivering blood to the popliteal, posterior tibial, and dorsalis pedis arteries (Fig. 20-60). It is one of the strongest arteries in an infant or small child. An in-

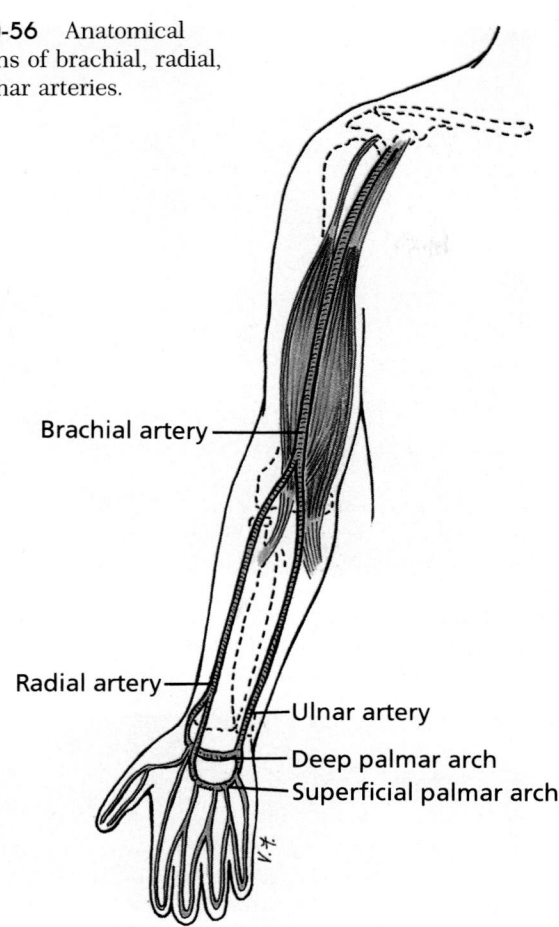

Fig. 20-56 Anatomical positions of brachial, radial, and ulnar arteries.

Brachial artery

Radial artery

Ulnar artery

Deep palmar arch

Superficial palmar arch

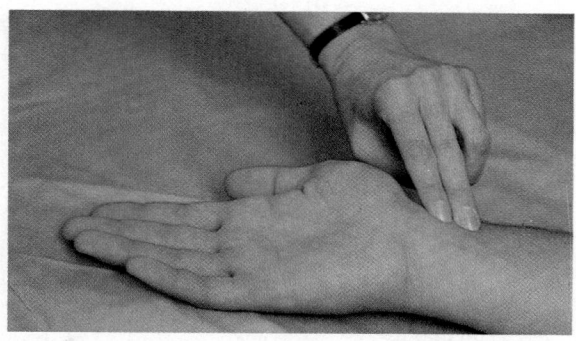

Fig. 20-57 Palpation of the radial pulse along the radial side of the forearm.

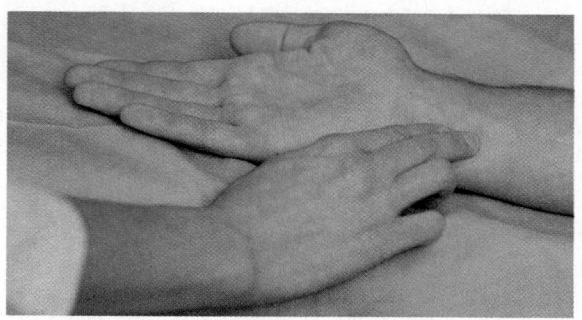

Fig. 20-58 Palpation of the ulnar pulse.

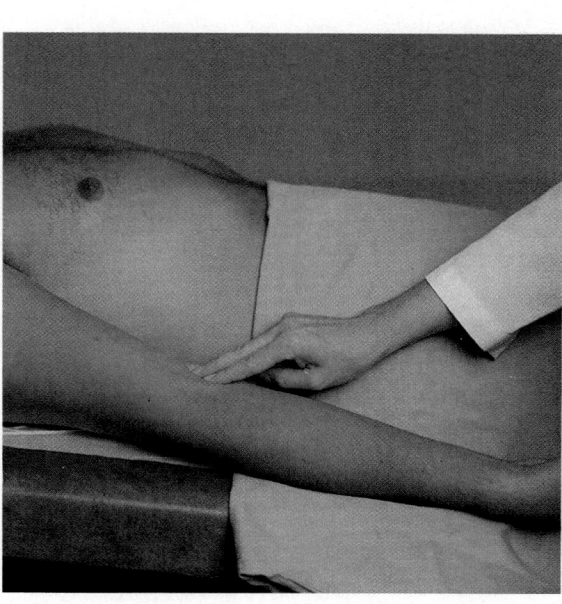

Fig. 20-59 The nurse palpates the brachial pulse by placing the fingertips in the groove between the biceps and triceps muscle.

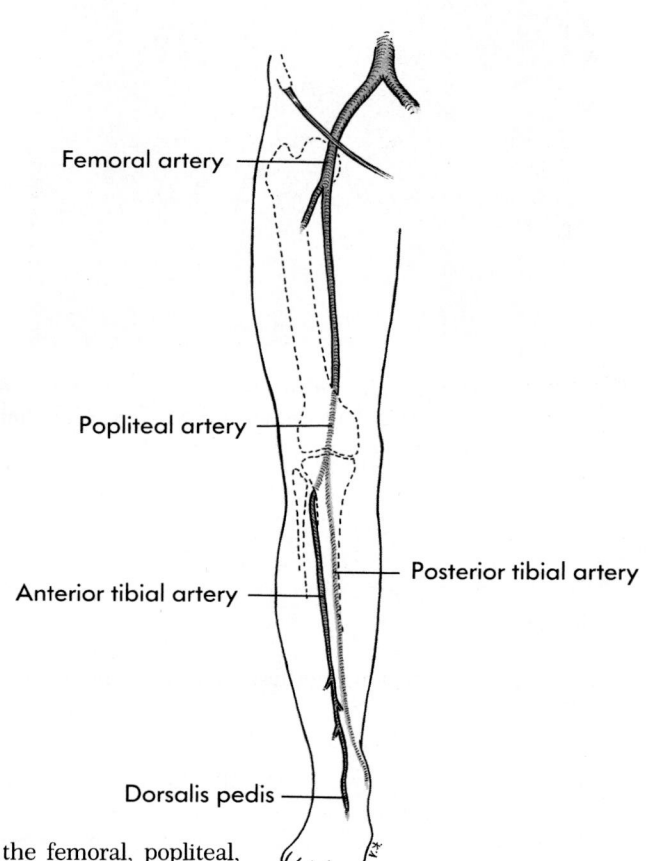

Femoral artery

Popliteal artery

Anterior tibial artery

Posterior tibial artery

Dorsalis pedis

Fig. 20-60 Anatomical position of the femoral, popliteal, dorsalis pedis, and posterior tibial arteries.

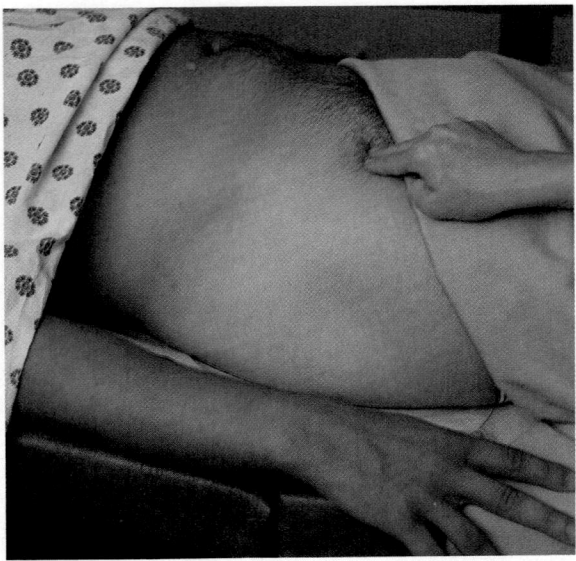

Fig. 20-61 The femoral pulse is usually palpated at the inguinal area midway between the symphysis pubis and anterosuperior iliac spine.

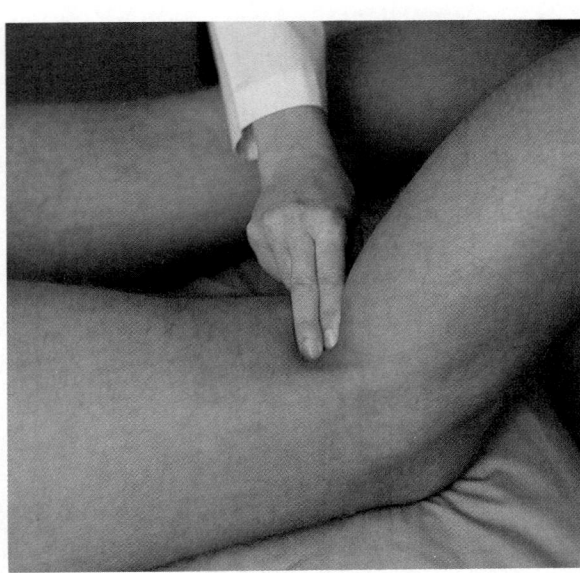

Fig. 20-62 The client lies with knee flexed to give the nurse access to the popliteal pulse.

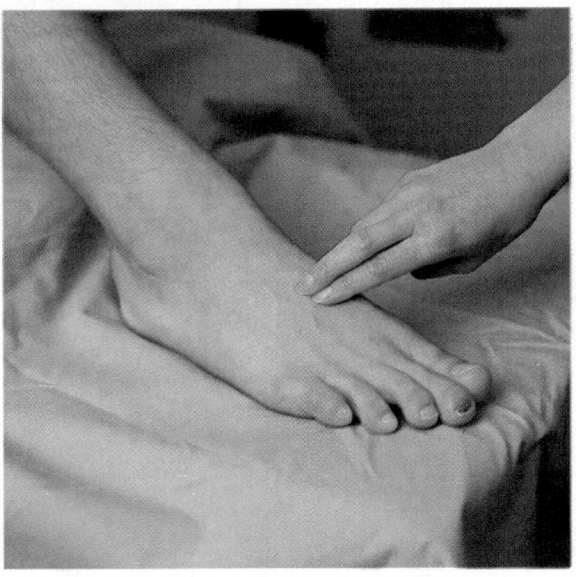

Fig. 20-63 The dorsalis pedis pulse is palpated at a point along a line with the groove between the extensor tendons of the great and first toes.

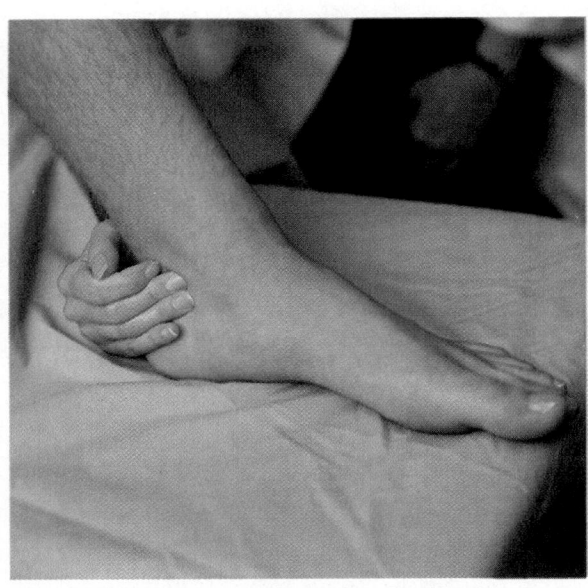

Fig. 20-64 Palpation of posterior tibial pulse below the medial malleolus.

Fig. 20-65 Ultrasound stethoscope in position on brachial artery.

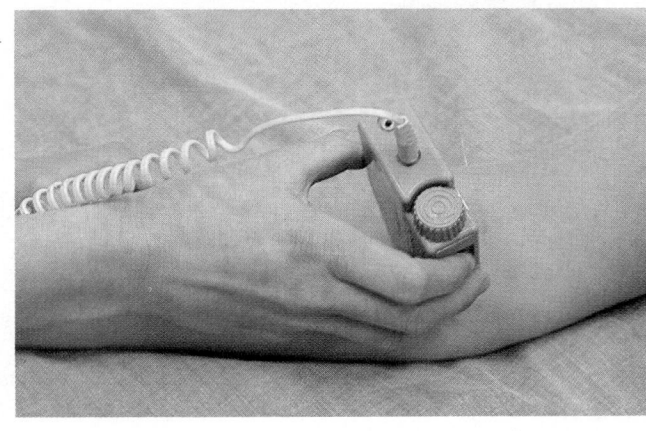

terconnection between the posterior tibial and dorsalis pedis arteries guards against local arterial occlusion.

The femoral pulse is found best with the client lying down with the inguinal area exposed (Fig. 20-61). The femoral artery runs below the inguinal ligament, midway between the symphysis pubis and the anterosuperior iliac spine. Deep palpation may be required to feel the pulse. Bimanual palpation is effective in obese clients. This technique differs from the previous description of bimanual palpation. The nurse places the fingertips of both hands on opposite sides of the pulse site. A pulsatile sensation can be felt as the fingertips are pushed apart by arterial pulsation.

The popliteal pulse is found behind the knee. The client should slightly flex the knee, with the foot resting on the examination table. The client may also assume a prone position with the knee slightly flexed (Fig. 20-62). The client is instructed to keep leg muscles relaxed. The nurse palpates with the fingers of both hands deeply into the popliteal fossa, just lateral to the midline. The popliteal pulse is difficult to locate.

With the client's foot relaxed the nurse locates the dorsalis pedis pulse. The artery runs along the top of the foot in a line with the groove between the extensor tendons of the great toe and first toe (Fig. 20-63). Often an examiner finds the pulse by placing the fingertips between the great and first toe and slowly inching up the foot. This pulse may be congenitally absent.

The posterior tibial pulse is found on the inner side of each ankle (Fig. 20-64). The nurse places the fingers behind and below the medial malleolus (ankle bone). The artery is easily located with the foot relaxed and slightly extended.

Ultrasound Stethoscopes. Occasionally a nurse has difficulty palpating a pulse. A pulse wave may not be manually palpable if the client is obese, if the heart's stroke volume is seriously reduced, if the blood volume is diminished, or if there is an obstruction of the artery. An ultrasound stethoscope will amplify sounds, allowing the nurse to hear low-velocity blood flow. Use of the stethoscope involves the following steps:

1. Connect the stethoscope headset to the ultrasound probe.
2. Apply transmission gel to the client's skin at the pulse site or directly onto the transducer tip of the probe. (The gel creates an airtight seal for transmission of sound waves).
3. Turn the stethoscope's volume control to *on*.
4. Gently apply the probe at a 45- to 90-degree angle on the skin at the pulse site (Fig. 20-65). (Excess pressure might obliterate the pulse.)

5. Move the probe over the pulse site until a pulsating whooshing sound, which indicates arterial blood flow, is heard. Do not be fooled by more intermittent and faint venous sounds.

TISSUE PERFUSION. The condition of the skin, mucosa, and nail beds offers useful data about the status of circulatory blood flow. The nurse first examines the face and upper extremities, looking at the color of the skin, mucosa, and nail beds. The presence of cyanosis requires special attention. Central cyanosis, which indicates poor arterial oxygenation, may be due to heart disease. It can be noted by a bluish discoloration of the lips, mouth, and conjunctivae. Peripheral cyanosis, which indicates peripheral vasoconstriction, is noted by blue lips, earlobes, and nail beds. When cyanosis is present, the nurse refers to available laboratory data on oxygen saturation to determine the severity of the problem. Examination of the nails involves inspection for **clubbing**, a bulging of the tissues at the nail base. Clubbing is due to insufficient oxygenation at the periphery resulting from conditions such as chronic emphysema and congenital heart disease.

The nurse inspects the lower extremities for changes in color, temperature, and condition of the skin indicating either arterial or venous alterations (Table 20-23). If an arterial occlusion is present, the client has signs resulting from an absence in blood flow. Venous congestion causes tissue changes indicating an inadequate circulatory flow back to the heart.

During examination of the lower extremities, the nurse also inspects skin and nail texture; hair distri-

TABLE 20-23	Signs of Venous and Arterial Insufficiency	
Assessment Criterion	Venous	Arterial
Color	Normal or cyanotic	Pale; worsened by elevation of extremity; dusky red when extremity lowered
Temperature	Normal	Cool (blood flow blocked to extremity)
Pulse	Normal	Decreased or absent
Edema	Often marked	Absent or mild
Skin changes	Brown pigmentation around ankles	Thin, shiny skin; decreased hair growth; thickened nails

bution on the lower legs, feet, and toes; venous pattern; and scars, pigmentation, or ulcers. The absence of hair growth over the legs may indicate circulatory insufficiency. The nurse should not be misled by women who shave their lower legs. Chronic recurring ulcers of the feet or lower legs is a serious sign of circulatory insufficiency and requires a physician's intervention.

PERIPHERAL VEINS. The status of the peripheral venous system is examined when the nurse inspects for varicosities, peripheral edema, and phlebitis. Varicosities are superficial veins that become dilated, especially when the legs are in a dependent position. They are common in older adults because the veins normally fibrose, dilate, and stretch. They are also common in people who stand for prolonged periods. Varicosities in the anterior or medial part of the thigh and the posterolateral part of the calf are abnormal.

Dependent edema around the area of the feet and ankles can be a sign of venous insufficiency and right-sided heart failure. Dependent edema is common in older adults and persons who spend a lot of time standing (for example, waitresses, security guards, or nurses). To assess for pitting edema the nurse uses a thumb to press firmly for at least 5 seconds over the medial malleolus or shin. A permanent depression left in the skin indicates edema. The depth of the depression is estimated in millimeters (2 to 8) to determine the severity of the edema. Two millimeters, for example, is rated as 1 + and 8 millimeters is rated as 4 +.

Phlebitis is an inflammation of a vein that occurs commonly after trauma to the vessel wall, infection, prolonged immobilization, and prolonged insertion of intravenous catheters (see Chapter 39). Phlebitis promotes clot formation, a potentially dangerous situation because a clot within a deep vein of the leg can become dislodged and travel through the heart, causing a pulmonary embolus. To assess for phlebitis the nurse inspects the calves for localized redness, tenderness, and swelling over vein sites. Gentle palpation of calf muscles reveals tenderness and firmness of the muscle. The nurse may also check for Homans' sign by supporting the leg while flexing the foot upward. If phlebitis is present in the lower leg, forceful dorsiflexion of the foot often causes pain in the calf.

LYMPHATIC SYSTEM. Assessment of the lymphatic drainage of the lower extremities is performed during examination of the vascular system. The nurse may also perform this examination just before the female or male genital examination. The legs are drained by superficial and deep nodes, but only the two groups of superficial nodes are palpable. The nurse palpates

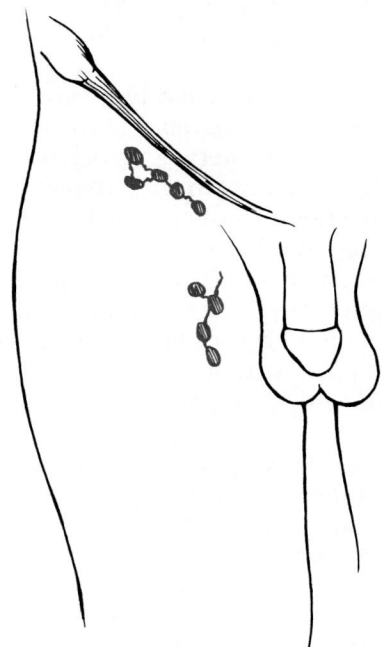

Fig. 20-66 Inguinal lymph nodes.

the area of the superficial inguinal nodes (Fig. 20-66), beginning in the groin area and moving down toward the inner thigh. The vertical group of nodes lies close to the upper portion of the great saphenous vein. The horizontal group lies below the inguinal ligament. The nurse uses a firm but gentle pressure when palpating over each lymphatic chain. Multiple nodes are not normally palpable, although a few soft, nontender nodes are not unusual. Enlarged, hardened, tender nodes can reveal potential sites of infection or metastatic disease. An infection site can be identified by drainage collected by the nodes. For example, the horizontal group drains lymph from the skin of the lower abdominal wall, the external genitalia, anal canal, and lower vagina.

 BREASTS

It is important to examine the breasts of female and male clients. A small amount of glandular tissue, a potential site for the growth of cancer cells, is located in the male breast. In contrast, the majority of the female breast is glandular tissue.

Female Breasts

Breast cancer affects one out of every nine women in the United States (American Cancer Society,

The purpose of Champion's descriptive study was to identify the relationship of knowledge, teaching methods, confidence, and social influence to a woman's intent, frequency, and proficiency of BSE. A sample population ($N = 380$) of women ages 35 years and over was selected. Subjects were interviewed in their homes. The mean age of the group was 50.8 years, with a range of 35 to 81 years. Most of the women participating were European Americans (81%), 18% were African Americans, and 0.3% were Asian Americans.

The frequency of BSE was variable: 30% did not examine, 20% examined every 6 months, 12% examined 4 times a year, 8% examined 1 or 2 times a year, 4% examined 3 times a year, 17% examined monthly, and 10% examined more often than monthly.

Knowledge correlated significantly with a woman's intent to practice BSE and with proficiency in examination. The scores on knowledge were higher for persons taught by a physician or nurse, as well as those who had their technique checked. Individualized teaching with return demonstration resulted in higher scores on intent, frequency, and proficiency. Surprisingly, being taught BSE by a physician resulted in higher scores for intent, frequency, and proficiency than if taught by a nurse. The researcher questioned that perhaps the characteristics of teaching are more important than the person who teaches because earlier studies showed nurses to be more effective than physicians. Social influence was not a significant factor in the practice of BSE.

Champion VS: Effect of knowledge, teaching method, confidence and social influence on breast self-examination behavior, *Image J Nurs Sch* 21(2):76, 1989.

1991). The disease is second to lung cancer as the leading cause of death in women with cancer. Early detection is the key to cure. A major responsibility for nurses is to teach clients health behaviors such as breast self-examination (BSE). Studies suggest that a minority of women actually perform BSE, particularly older women (Leather, Roberts, 1985). Nurses should know factors that increase the likelihood of a woman performing BSE (see research highlight). Incorporating these interventions into teaching strategies may improve the likelihood of a client detecting breast cancer early (Champion, 1989). The American Cancer Society (1991) recommends the following guidelines for the early detection of breast cancer:

1. BSE should be performed monthly by women 20 years of age and older.
2. An examination by a physician should be performed every 3 years from ages 20 to 40, and after 40, the examination should be performed every year.
3. Women with a family history of breast cancer should have a yearly physician's examination.
4. A diagnostic mammogram (x-ray study of the breast) should be performed every year for women who have no symptoms of problems who are age 50 and over, and a baseline mammogram should be performed for women 35 to 39. Women who have no symptoms who are 40 to 49 years old should have a mammogram every 1 to 2 years. For women age 40 or over with a family history of breast cancer and for women age 35 or over with a history of breast cancer, a yearly examination is recommended.

During an examination the nurse explains how to perform a BSE. While assessing the client's breasts, the nurse uses many of the same techniques the client will adapt for home use (see box on p. 572).

If the client already performs BSE, the nurse can ask about the method she uses and times she does the examination in relation to her menstrual cycle. The best time for a BSE is on the last day of the menstrual period, when the breast is no longer swollen or tender from hormone elevations. If the woman has already experienced menopause, she should check her breasts the same time each month. The pregnant woman also must check her breasts on a monthly basis.

Older women may require special attention when reviewing the need for regular BSE. Many older adults are limited by fixed incomes and thus fail to pursue regular clinical breast examination and mammography. Unfortunately, many older women ignore changes in their breasts, assuming that they are a part of aging. The normal physiological changes that affect the breast as a result of aging can often mimic breast cancer (Williams, Edwards, Hane, 1987). In addition, physiological factors can affect the ease at which older women can perform a BSE. Musculoskeletal limitations, diminished peripheral sensation, reduced eyesight, and changes in joint range of motion can limit palpation and inspection abilities. The nurse should find resources for older women, including free screening programs. Often family members can be taught to perform examinations.

The client's history (Table 20-24 on p. 572) should alert the nurse to any signs of breast disease and normal developmental changes. Because of its glandular structure, the breast undergoes changes during a woman's life. Knowledge of these changes (see box) helps the nurse complete an accurate assessment.

Breast Self-Examination

Instruct client on BSE. All women 20 years and older should perform this self-examination monthly using the following steps:

- Stand before a mirror. Look at both breasts for anything unusual, such as discharge from the nipples, puckering, dimpling, or scaling of the skin.
- To note changes in the shape of the breasts, perform the following measures (see figure 2):
  - Watch in the mirror while raising the arms above the head.
  - Press hands firmly on the hips and bow slightly toward the mirror when pulling the shoulders and elbows forward.
- In the shower or in front of the mirror, palpate each breast. Raise the left arm and use three or four fingers of the right hand to explore the breast carefully (see figure 1). Then start at the outer edge, pressing the flat part of the fingers in small circles, moving the circles slowly around the breast, gradually working toward the nipple. Pay close attention to the area between the breast and armpit and feel for unusual lumps or masses. Repeat the process for the right breast (see figure 3).
- Gently squeeze each nipple, looking for discharge (see figure 3).
- Repeat the third and fourth steps lying down. Lie flat on the back with the left arm over the head and a small pillow under the left shoulder. Palpate the left breast. Repeat the process on the right breast.
- Call your physician if you find a lump.

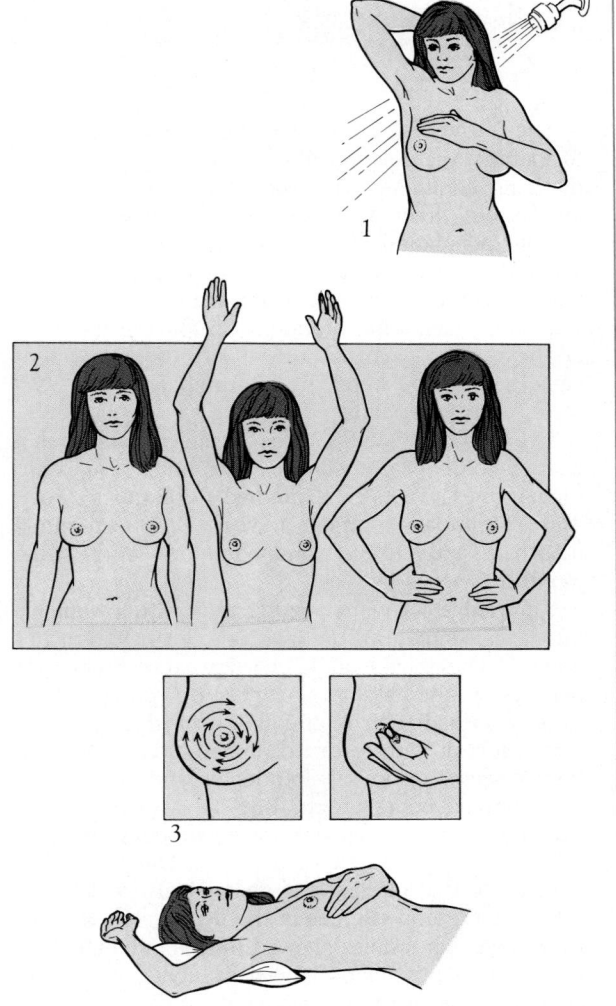

Illustrations from Payne WA, Hahn DB: *Understanding your health*, ed 2, St Louis, 1989, Mosby–Year Book.

TABLE 20-24 Nursing History for Breast Assessment

Assessment Category	Rationale
Determine if woman is over age 50, has family history of breast cancer, had previous breast cancer, never had children, or had first child after age 30.	These are risk factors for breast cancer.
Ask if client (both sexes) has noticed lump, thickening, pain, or tenderness of breast; discharge, distortion, retraction, or scaling of nipple; or change in size of breast.	Potential signs and symptoms of breast cancer allow nurse to focus on specific areas of breast during assessment.
Ask if client performs monthly BSE. If so, determine time of month she performs examination in relation to menstrual cycle. Have client describe method used.	Nurse's role is to educate client about breast cancer and techniques for BSE.
Assess client's age at menarche, menopause, and first pregnancy.	Risk of cancer is greater in women who reach menarche early (before age 13), have menopause late (after age 50), and who had their first children after age 30.
Determine if client is taking oral contraceptives, digitalis, diuretics, steroids, or estrogen hormones.	Medications may cause nipple discharge. Hormones may cause fibrocystic changes in breast.

Inspection

The client removes the top gown or drape to allow simultaneous visualization of both breasts. The client may stand or sit with arms at her side. If possible, the nurse places a mirror in front of the client so that she can see what to look for when performing a BSE. To recognize abnormalities, the client must be familiar with the normal appearance of her breasts.

The nurse describes observations or findings in relation to imaginary lines that divide the breast into four quadrants and a tail. The lines cross at the center of the nipple. Each tail extends outward from the upper outer quadrant (Fig. 20-67).

The breasts are inspected for size and symmetry. One breast is commonly larger than the other. However, a difference in size may be caused by inflammation or a mass. The breasts usually extend in area from the third to the sixth ribs. The nipple is usually at the level of the fourth intercostal space. As the woman becomes older, the ligaments supporting the breast tissue weaken, causing the breasts to sag and the nipples to lower (see box).

The nurse observes the contour or shape of the breasts and notes masses, retraction, or flattening. Retraction or dimpling results from invasion of underlying ligaments by tumors. The ligaments become fibrotic and pull the overlying skin inward toward the tumor. Edema also changes the breasts' contour. To elicit retraction or changes in the shape of breasts, the nurse asks the client to raise her arms above her head or press her hands against her hips. Each maneuver causes a contraction of the pectoral muscles, which will accentuate retraction.

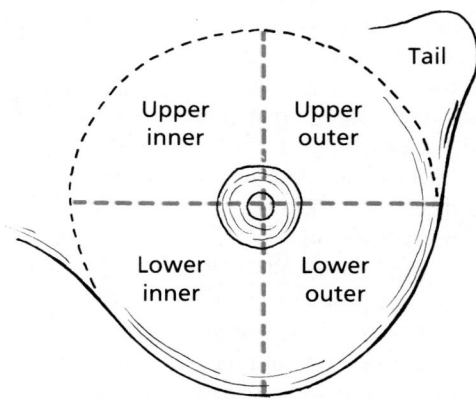

Fig. 20-67   The nurse localizes assessment findings by dividing each breast into four quadrants and an axillary tail.

Normal Changes in the Breast During a Woman's Life Span

PUBERTY (8 TO 20 YEARS)

Breasts mature in five stages. One breast may grow more rapidly than the other.

Stage 1 (Preadolescent)

- This stage involves elevation of the nipple only.

Stage 2

- The breast and nipple elevate as a small mound, and the areolar diameters enlarge.

Stage 3

- There is further enlargement and elevation of the breast and areola, with no separation of contour.

Stage 4

- The areola and nipple project into the secondary mound above the level of the breast.

Stage 5 (Mature Breast)

- Only the nipple projects, and the areola recedes (may vary in some women).

YOUNG ADULTHOOD (20 TO 30 YEARS)

- Breasts reach full (nonpregnant) size. Shape is generally symmetrical. Breasts may be unequal in size.

PREGNANCY

- Breast size gradually enlarges to 2 to 3 times the previous size. Nipples enlarge and may become erect. Areolae darken. Superficial veins become prominent. A yellowish fluid (colostrum) may be expelled from the nipples.

MENOPAUSE

- Breasts shrink. Tissue becomes softer, sometimes flabby.

OLDER ADULTHOOD

- Breasts become elongated, pendulous, and flaccid as a result of glandular tissue atrophy.* The skin of the breasts tends to wrinkle, appearing loose and flabby.

*Data from Rumpler C: Breast problems. In Griffth-Kinney J, editor: *Contemporary women's health: a nursing advocacy approach*, Menlo Park, Calif, 1986, Addison-Wesley.

The overlying skin is carefully inspected for color and venous pattern. Venous patterns are more easily seen in thin clients or pregnant women. Edema or inflammation is noted. For women with large breasts the nurse should be sure to look carefully at the undersurface, a common site for redness and excoriation caused by rubbing of skin surfaces.

The normal areolae and nipples of a European American are pink, becoming brown with pregnancy. In dark-skinned clients, the nipple is darker than other skin surfaces. Pregnancy causes an even darker color to develop. The nipple and areola are inspected for size and shape. A slight asymmetry is common. The nurse also observes the direction in which the nipples point. Normally they point in symmetrical directions. A recently inverted (turned inward) nipple may indicate an underlying growth. Rashes or ulcerations are not normal. Bleeding or discharge from the nipple is noted. The color of a discharge may range from clear yellow to green.

While inspecting the breasts, the nurse explains the characteristics observed. The client must be taught the significance of abnormal signs or symptoms.

Palpation

Palpation allows the nurse to determine the condition of underlying breast tissue and lymph nodes. Breast tissue consists of glandular tissue, fibrous supportive ligaments, and fat (Fig. 20-68). Glandular tissue is organized into lobes that end in ducts that open onto the nipple's surface. The largest portion of glandular tissue is in the upper outer quadrant and

tail of each breast. Suspensory ligaments connect to skin and fascia underlying the breast to support the breast and maintain its upright position. Fatty tissue is located superficially and to the sides of the breast.

A large portion of lymph from the breasts drains into axillary lymph nodes. If cancerous lesions **metastasize** (spread), the nodes are commonly involved. The nurse must know the location of supraclavicular, infraclavicular, and axillary nodes (Fig. 20-69). The axillary nodes drain lymph from the chest wall, breasts, arms, and hands. A tumor of one breast may also involve nodes on the opposite side.

The lymph nodes are best palpated when the client sits, although the examination can be performed with the client supine. Easy access is gained to the axillary nodes with the client's arms at her sides and muscles relaxed. The nurse faces the client and supports her arm, while abducting that arm away from the chest wall. Then the nurse places a hand against the client's chest wall and high in the axilla. The axillary nodes are palpated, with the fingertips of the nurse's hand pressing gently down over the surface of the ribs and muscles (Fig. 20-70).

The following areas of the axilla are palpated:
1. The edge of the pectoralis major muscle along the anterior axillary line
2. The chest wall in the midaxillary area
3. The upper part of the humerus
4. The anterior edge of the latissimus dorsi muscle along the posterior axillary line

Each area must be assessed carefully because these nodes are easily missed. The nurse notes their number, consistency, movability, and size.

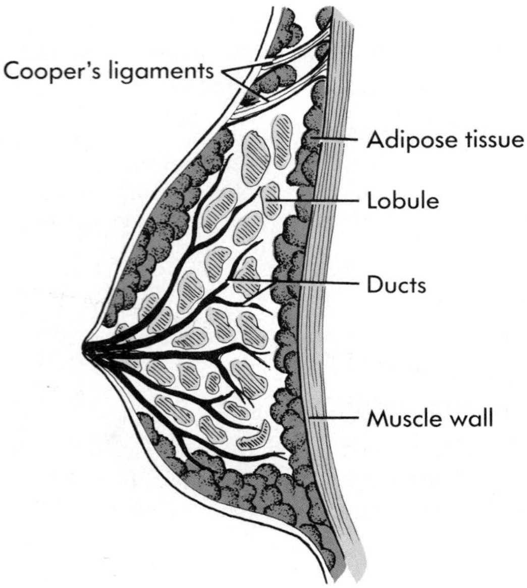

Fig. 20-68 Cross section of breast tissue.

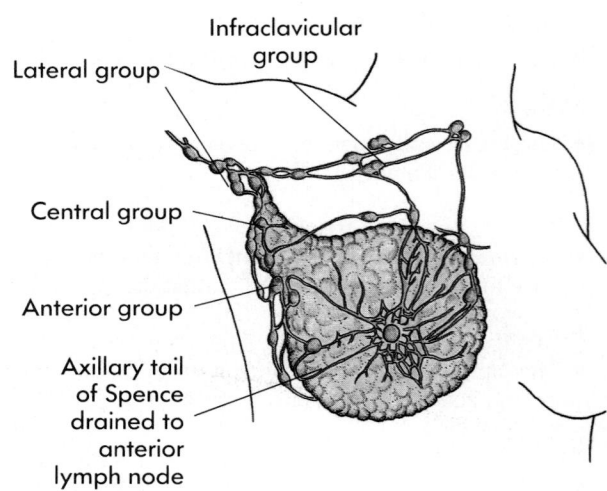

Fig. 20-69 Anatomical position of axillary and clavicular lymph nodes.

Normally lymph nodes are not palpable. However, one or two small, soft, nontender nodes may be normal. A palpable node feels like a small mass that may be hard, tender, and immobile. The supraclavicular and infraclavicular nodes are also palpated as the nurse stands at the client's right side. The procedure is reversed for the left side.

It may be difficult for the client to learn to palpate for lymph nodes. Lying down with the arm abducted makes the area more accessible. The client is instructed to use her left hand for the right axillary and clavicular areas. The nurse can take the client's fingertips and move them in the proper circular fashion. The client then uses her right hand to palpate left-sided nodes.

Palpation of breast tissue is performed with the client in the supine or sitting position. The supine position allows the breast tissue to flatten evenly against the chest wall. The client should raise her hand and place it behind the neck to further stretch and position breast tissue evenly (Fig. 20-71). The examiner often places a small pillow or towel under the shoulder blade to further position breast tissue.

The consistency of normal breast tissue varies widely. The breasts of a young client are firm and elastic. In an older client the tissue may feel stringy and nodular. The client's familiarity with the texture of her own breasts is very important. This familiarity is gained through monthly BSE (see teaching box on p. 576).

If the client complains of a mass, the nurse examines the opposite breast first to ensure an objective comparison of normal and abnormal tissue. The palmar surface of the first two fingers is used to compress breast tissue gently against the chest wall (Fig. 20-72). Palpation is performed using variable pressure in an organized and complete pattern. Some examiners start in the upper outer quadrant, where tumors develop most frequently. After the entire quadrant is palpated, the nurse moves systematically to the lower outer, lower inner, and upper inner quadrants. Another method is to proceed in and out, starting at the nipple. This pattern of palpation appears

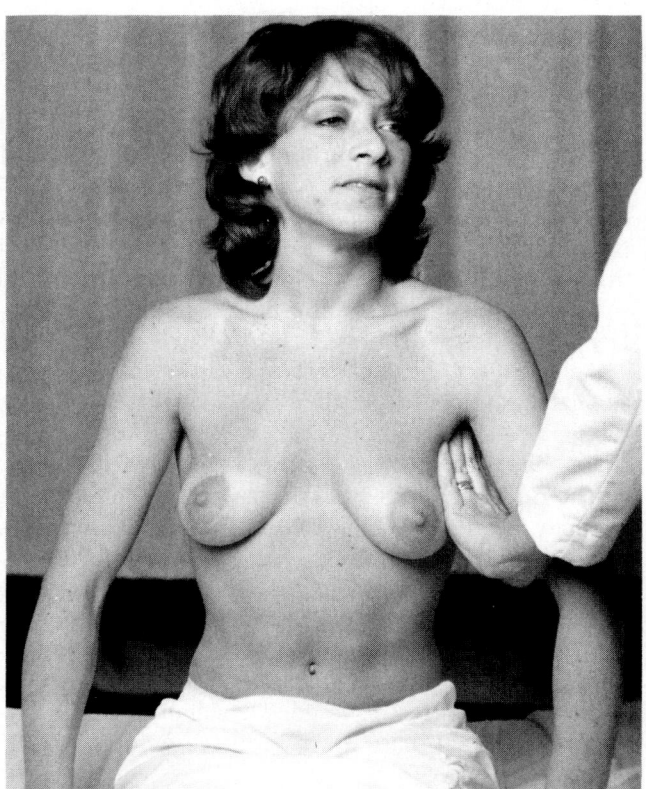

Fig. 20-70   The nurse supports the client's arm and palpates axillary lymph nodes.

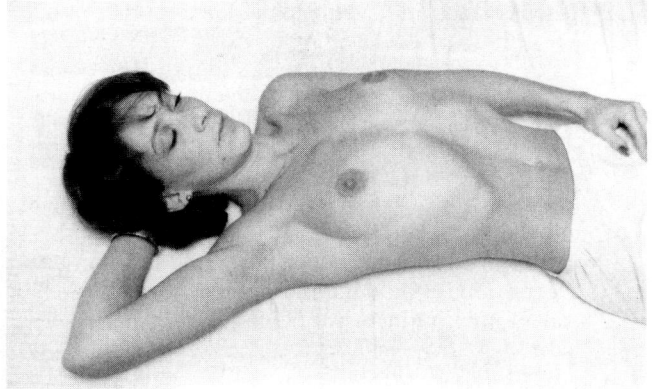

Fig. 20-71   The client lies flat with arm abducted and hand under head to help flatten breast tissue evenly over the chest wall.

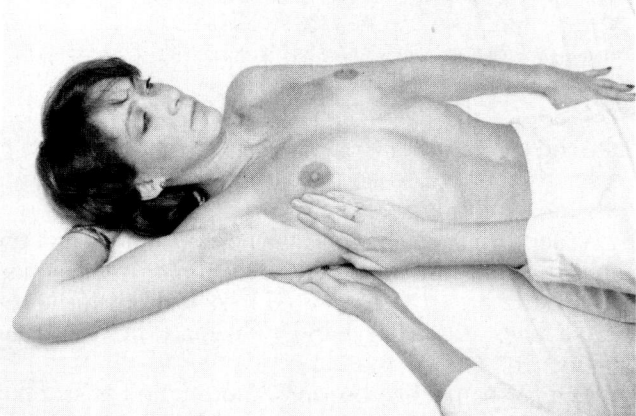

Fig. 20-72   The nurse palpates each breast quadrant using a rotary motion of the fingerpads.

Client Teaching During Female Breast Assessment

OBJECTIVES

- Client will perform BSE (see box on p. 572).
- Client will have mammography performed at recommended intervals.
- Client will identify signs and symptoms of breast cancer.
- Client will identify signs and symptoms of fibrocystic disease.
- Client will follow a low-fat diet.

TEACHING STRATEGIES

- Have client perform return demonstration of BSE and offer the opportunity to ask questions.
- Explain recommended frequency of mammography and BSE by a health care provider.
- Discuss signs and symptoms of breast cancer.
- Discuss signs and symptoms of fibrocystic disease.
- Inform a woman who is obese or who has a family history of breast cancer that she is at higher risk for the disease.* Encourage dietary changes, including limiting meat consumption to well-trimmed, lean beef, pork, or lamb; removing skin from cooked chicken before eating it; selecting tuna and salmon packed in water and not oil; and using low-fat dairy products.
- Encourage client to reduce intake of caffeine and theophyllines. Although this approach is controversial, it may reduce symptoms of fibrocystic disease.†

EVALUATION

- Have client demonstrate BSE.
- During follow-up visit, determine whether client has had mammography performed.
- Ask client to explain frequency of mammography.
- Have client describe signs and symptoms of breast cancer compared with fibrocystic disease.

*Data from Willett W et al: *N Engl J Med* 316:22, 1987.
†Data from Cerrato P: *RN* 50:63, 1987.

like the spokes of a wheel. The nurse must be sure to cover the entire breast and tail, directing attention to any areas of tenderness.

When palpating large, pendulous breasts, the nurse uses a bimanual technique. The inferior portion of the breast is supported in one hand while the nurse uses the other hand to palpate breast tissue against the supporting hand.

During palpation the nurse notes the consistency of breast tissue. The lobular feel of glandular tissue is normal. The lower edge of each breast may feel firm and hard. This is the normal inframammary ridge and not a tumor. It may be helpful to move the cli-

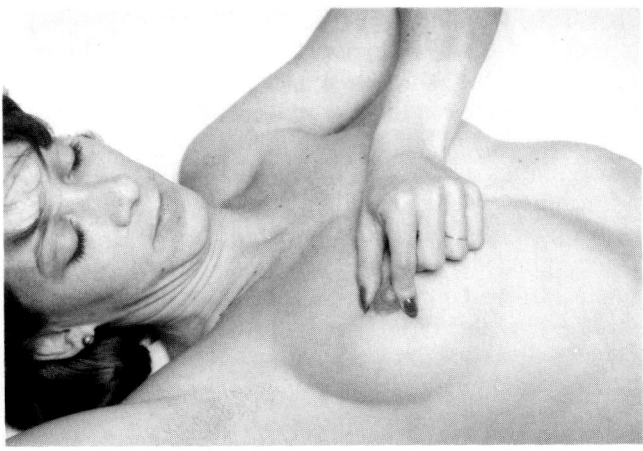

Fig. 20-73 The client palpates the nipple for discharge.

ent's hand so that she can feel normal tissue variations. Abnormal masses are palpated to determine the following:

1. Location in relation to quadrants
2. Size in centimeters
3. Shape (for example, round or discoid)
4. Consistency (soft, firm, or hard)
5. Tenderness
6. Mobility
7. Discreetness (whether boundaries of mass are easily detected)

Cancerous lesions are hard, fixed, nontender, and irregular in shape. A common benign condition of the breast is **fibrocystic disease**. This disease is characterized by lumpy painful breasts and sometimes nipple discharge. Symptoms are more apparent during the menstrual period. When palpated, the cysts (lumps) are soft, well differentiated, and movable. Deep cysts may feel hard.

As the nurse or client continues the examination, special attention is given to gentle palpation of the nipple and areola. The thumb and index finger compress the nipple, and the nurse notes any discharge. As the nurse examines the nipple and areola, the nipple may become erect with wrinkling of the areola. These changes are normal.

After the nurse completes the examination, the client can demonstrate self-palpation (Fig. 20-73). Observing the client's technique helps the nurse emphasize the importance of a systematic approach. The client is urged to see her physician if she discovers an abnormal mass during routine monthly BSE.

Male Breasts

Examination of the male breast is relatively easy. The nipple and areola are inspected for nodules,

theophyllines = bronchodilator

TABLE 20-25 Nursing History for Abdomen Assessment	
Assessment Category	Rationale
If client has abdominal or low back pain, assess character of pain in detail (location, onset, frequency, precipitating factors, aggravating factors, type of pain, severity, course).	Pattern of characteristics of pain help determine its source.
Carefully observe client's movement and position, including lying still with knees drawn up, moving restlessly to find comfortable position, and lying on one side or sitting with knees drawn to chest.	Positions assumed by client may reveal nature and source of pain, including peritonitis, renal stone, and pancreatitis.
Assess normal bowel habits.	Data compared with physical findings can help identify cause and nature of elimination problems.
Determine if client has had abdominal surgery or trauma.	Surgical or traumatic alterations of abdominal organs may cause changes in expected findings (e.g., position of underlying organs).
Assess if client has had recent weight changes or intolerance to diet (e.g., nausea, vomiting, cramping, especially in last 24 hours).	Data may indicate alterations in upper gastrointestinal tract (stomach or gallbladder) or lower colon.
Assess for difficulty in swallowing, belching, flatulence, bloody emesis (hematemesis), black or tarry stools (melena), heartburn, diarrhea, or constipation.	These characteristic signs and symptoms indicate gastrointestinal alterations.
Ask client to locate tender areas.	Nurse assesses painful areas last to minimize discomfort and anxiety.
Inquire about family history of cancer, kidney disease, alcoholism, hypertension, or heart disease.	Data may reveal risk for alterations identifiable during examination.
Determine if female client is pregnant; note last menstrual period.	Pregnancy causes changes in abdominal shape and contour.
Assess client's usual intake of alcohol.	Chronic alcohol ingestion can cause gastrointestinal and liver problems.

edema, and ulceration. An enlarged male breast may result from obesity or glandular enlargement. Fatty tissue feels soft, whereas glandular tissue is firm. Any masses are palpated for the same characteristics as the female breast. Because breast cancer in men is relatively rare, routine self-examinations are unnecessary.

 ABDOMEN

The abdominal examination can be complex because of the organs located within and near the abdominal cavity. A thorough nursing history (Table 20-25) helps the nurse interpret physical signs. A client with abdominal pain may suffer problems involving abdominal organs (for example, liver, stomach, and colon) or tissues and bones outside the abdominal cavity (for example, spine and muscles). Familiarity with common signs and symptoms, as well as the location of organs, helps the nurse make an accurate assessment (Fig. 20-74 on p. 578). Landmarks help the nurse map out the abdominal region. The xiphoid process (tip of the sternum) marks the upper boundary of the abdominal region, and the symphysis pubis delineates the lowermost boundary. By dividing the abdomen into four imaginary quadrants (Fig 20-74, A) the nurse can refer to assessment findings and record them in relation to each quadrant. For example, the nurse may determine that the client is experiencing tenderness over the left lower quadrant (LLQ) with normal bowel sounds present.

Assessment of the abdomen involves examination of organs and tissues anteriorly and posteriorly (Fig. 20-74, B). Posteriorly the kidneys are protected by the lower ribs and heavy back muscles. The costovertebral angle formed by the last rib and vertebral column is a landmark used during kidney palpation.

Clients must be relaxed for abdominal examinations. A tightening of abdominal muscles hinders accuracy with palpation and auscultation. To help clients relax, the nurse asks if they need to void. The room should be warm, and clients' upper chests and legs are draped. Abdomens are exposed from just above the xiphoid process down to the symphysis pu-

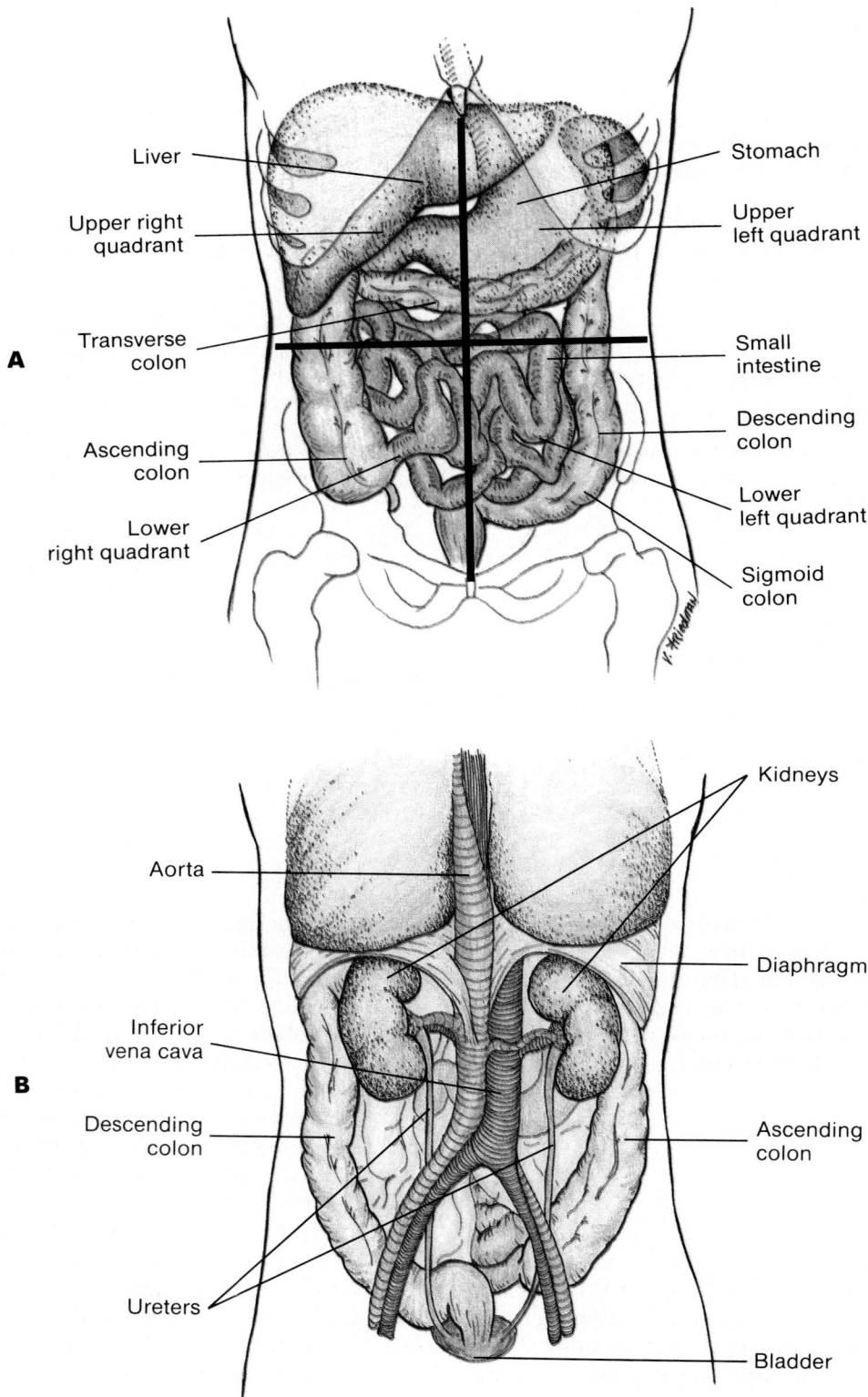

Fig. 20-74   A, Anterior view of abdomen divided by quadrants. **B,** Posterior view of abdominal sections.

bis. A good examination light is essential. Clients lie in the supine position with arms down at the sides and knees slightly bent. Small pillows can be placed beneath the knees (McConnell, 1990). If the nurse allows clients to place their arms under their heads, the abdominal muscles may tighten. Small pillows may also be placed under the heads. Warm hands and stethoscope further promote relaxation. Maintaining conversation except during auscultation helps to distract clients. The nurse performs the examination slowly and calmly. Clients should be asked to report pain and point out tender areas.

The order of an abdominal examination differs slightly from previous assessments. The nurse begins with inspection and then follows with auscultation. It is important to auscultate before palpation and percussion because palpation and percussion may alter frequency and character of bowel sounds. The nurse will also need a tape measure.

Inspection

The nurse stands on the client's right side and inspects the abdomen and then sits to look across the abdomen's surface. Standing helps detect abnormal shadows and movement. The sitting position provides a horizontal view that allows detection of abnormal protuberances. The examination light is directed over the abdomen.

Skin

The location of scars, venous patterns, rashes, lesions, pigmentation changes, and **striae** (stretch marks) are noted. An artificial opening may indicate a drainage site resulting from surgery (see Chapter 47) or an ostomy (see Chapter 41). Scars indicate past trauma or surgery that may have created permanent changes in underlying organ anatomy. Venous patterns are usually faint, except in very thin clients. Striae result from stretching of tissue by obesity or pregnancy.

Umbilicus

The position, shape, color, and signs of inflammation, discharge, or protruding masses are noted. Normally the umbilicus is a flat or concave hemisphere positioned midway between the xiphoid process and symphysis pubis. The color is the same as that of the surrounding skin. Underlying masses can cause displacement of the umbilicus. An everted (pouched out) umbilicus usually indicates distention. **Hernias** (protrusions of abdominal organs through the muscle wall) cause upward protrusion of the umbilicus. Normally, no discharge is emitted from the umbilical area.

Contour and Symmetry

A flat abdomen forms a horizontal plane from the xiphoid process to the symphysis pubis. A round abdomen protrudes in a convex sphere from the horizontal plane. A concave abdomen appears to sink into the muscular wall. Each of these findings is normal if the abdomen's shape is symmetric. The presence of masses on only one side, or asymmetry, may indicate an underlying pathological condition.

Intestinal gas, tumor, or fluid in the abdominal cavity may cause **distention** (swelling). When distention is generalized, the entire abdomen protrudes. The skin often appears taut, as if it were stretched over the abdomen. When gas causes distention, the flanks do not bulge. However, if fluid is the source of the problem, the flanks bulge. The client should be asked to roll onto one side. A protuberance forms on the dependent side if fluid is the cause of the distention. The nurse asks the client if the abdomen feels unusually tight. The nurse must be careful not to confuse distention with obesity. In obesity the abdomen is large, rolls of adipose tissue are often present along the flanks, and the client does not complain of tightness in the abdomen. If abdominal distention is expected, the nurse may choose to measure the abdomen's girth by placing a tape measure around the abdomen at the level of the umbilicus. Consecutive measurements will show any increase or decrease in distention.

Enlarged Organs or Masses

The nurse observes the abdominal contour while asking the client to take a deep breath and hold it. This maneuver forces the diaphragm downward and reduces the size of the abdominal cavity. Any enlarged organs in the upper abdominal cavity (for example, liver or spleen) may descend below the rib cage to cause a bulge. Closer examination can be performed with palpation.

To evaluate the abdominal musculature, the nurse has clients raise their heads. This position causes superficial abdominal wall masses, hernias, and muscle separations to become more apparent. Visual identification is followed with palpation.

Movement or Pulsations

The nurse should remember that a man breathes abdominally and a woman breathes more costally. If the client has severe pain, respiratory movement is diminished, and the client tightens abdominal muscles to guard against the pain. On closer inspection the nurse may see peristaltic movement and aortic pulsation by looking across the abdomen from the side to detect movement. It may take several minutes to see a peristaltic wave. In contrast, aortic pulsations occur with each beat of systole and appear in the midline above the umbilicus (epigastric area).

Auscultation

The nurse asks the client to refrain from talking. If a client has a nasogastric or intestinal tube connected to intermittent suction, it should be momentarily turned off. Sound from the suction will obscure bowel sounds.

Bowel Motility

Peristalsis, or intestinal motility, is a normal function of the small and large intestine. Bowel sounds are the audible passage of air and fluid created by peristalsis. The warmed diaphragm of the stethoscope is placed lightly over each of the four quadrants to detect normally high-pitched bowel sounds. Air and fluid move through the intestines, creating soft gurgling, tinkling, or bubbling sounds that normally occur every 5 to 15 seconds in each quadrant. Sounds may last ½ second to several seconds. It may take as long as a minute to hear bowel sounds. The best time to auscultate is between meals. When the nurse auscultates just after meals or long after the client eats, bowel sounds tend to be increased.

Sounds are generally described as normal, audible, absent, hyperactive, or hypoactive. The nurse must listen 3 to 5 minutes before deciding that bowel sounds are absent in any one quadrant. Absent sounds indicate a cessation of gastrointestinal motility that may result from late-stage bowel obstruction, **paralytic ileus,** or **peritonitis.** Hyperactive sounds are loud, "growling" sounds called **borborygmi,** which indicate increased gastrointestinal motility. Inflammation of the bowel, anxiety, diarrhea, bleeding, excess ingestion of laxatives, and reaction of the intestines to certain foods cause increased motility (see teaching box).

Vascular Sounds

The nurse applies the bell of the stethoscope over the epigastrium for bruits. These whooshing or blowing sounds often originate from a narrowing of the thoracic or abdominal aorta. Renal artery bruits can be heard by placing the stethoscope over each upper quadrant anteriorly or the costovertebral angle posteriorly (which can be done when the client sits). A bruit should be reported immediately to a physician.

Friction Rubs

An inflamed liver or spleen may rub against the peritoneum during inspiration, creating a grating sound with respiratory variations. Friction rubs are heard best with the stethoscope's bell placed above the liver and spleen.

Client Teaching During Abdomen Assessment

OBJECTIVES
- Client will maintain normal bowel elimination.
- Client will achieve pain relief.

TEACHING STRATEGIES
- Explain factors such as diet, regular exercise, and fluid intake that promote normal bowel elimination (see Chapter 41).
- Caution clients about dangers of excessive use of laxatives or enemas.
- If client has chronic pain, explain measures used for pain relief (e.g., relaxation exercises, positioning) (see Chapter 37).
- If client has acute pain, explain activities or positions to avoid.

EVALUATION
- Reassess client's bowel elimination pattern and stool character after therapies are started.
- Observe client use pain-relief measures and reassess character of pain.

Percussion

Percussion of the abdomen maps out underlying organs, bone, and masses and helps reveal the presence of air or fluid-filled structures within the abdomen. The beginning student uses this skill in a limited fashion. Practice is needed to ensure accuracy.

Organs and Masses

The nurse systematically percusses each quadrant to assess areas of tympany and dullness. Potentially painful areas are always percussed last. Tympany usually predominates because of air in the stomach and intestines. A dull percussion note is a medium-to-high-pitched short sound heard over solid masses such as an enlarged liver or spleen, tumors, or a full bladder. When dullness is noted, it may be useful to also use palpation to complete a detailed assessment.

Liver Size

Percussion allows the nurse to identify borders of the liver to detect organ enlargement. The nurse starts at the right iliac crest and proceeds upward on the right midclavicular line. As the nurse slowly percusses upward, the percussion note changes from tympanic to dull at the liver's lower border. Usually the border is at the right costal margin. The nurse

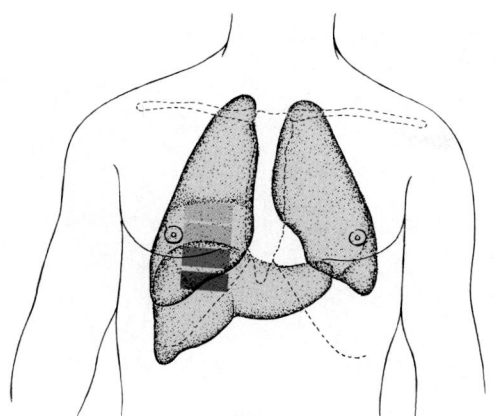

Fig. 20-75   To locate the liver's upper border, the nurse percusses downward, noting the change in sound from resonance (lung) to dullness (liver).

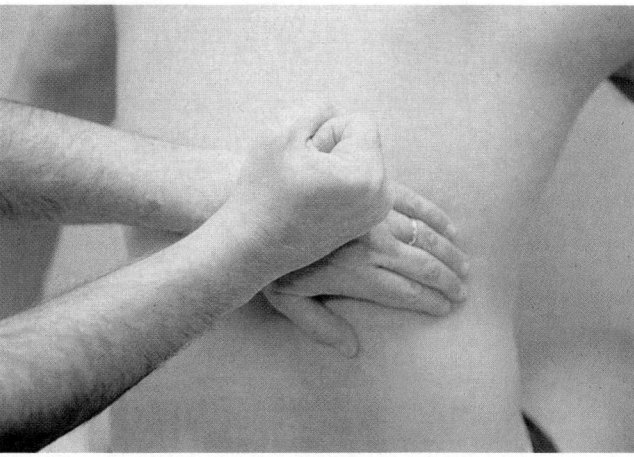

Fig. 20-76   Percussion for kidney tenderness along costovertebral angle.
From Seidel HM et al: *Mosby's guide to physical examination,* ed 2, St Louis, 1991, Mosby–Year Book.

may mark the point of the lower border on the client's abdomen with a water-soluble pencil. The upper border is found by percussing down from the nipple along the midclavicular line. While the nurse percusses in the intercostal spaces, the note changes from resonant to dull (Fig. 20-75). The liver's upper border is usually found in the fifth, sixth, or seventh intercostal space. The distance between the points where dullness is percussed along the midclavicular line should be 6 to 12 cm (½ to 5 in). Diseases such as **cirrhosis,** cancer, and **hepatitis** cause liver enlargement.

Stomach Position

With practice the nurse can locate the tympanic air bubble of the stomach by percussing over the left lower anterior rib cage. The bubble's size varies.

Kidney Tenderness

With the client sitting or standing erect, the nurse uses direct or indirect percussion to assess for kidney inflammation. With the ulnar surface of the partially closed fist, the nurse percusses the costovertebral angle at the scapular line (Fig. 20-76). If the kidneys are inflamed, the client feels tenderness during percussion.

Palpation

With palpation, nursing students are primarily concerned with detecting areas of abdominal tenderness and noting the quality of abnormal distentions or masses. As students become more skilled, they learn to palpate for specific organs such as the liver, spleen, and kidney. Light and deep palpation are used by the nurse.

After rubbing the hands together, the nurse uses light palpation over each quadrant. Again the nurse waits to palpate painful areas last. The palm of the hand and forearm are kept horizontal as the nurse places the hand on the abdomen (Fig. 20-77 on p. 582). The pads of the fingertips depress gently into the abdomen, approximately 1 cm (½ in), moving smoothly through the quadrants. The nurse avoids quick jabs. If the client is ticklish, the nurse places the hand under the client's until the touch is tolerated.

A systematic palpation of each quadrant assesses for muscular resistance, distention, tenderness, and superficial organs or masses. If the nurse palpates a sensitive area, guarding or muscle tenseness may occur. If tightening remains after the client is helped to relax, peritonitis, acute **cholecystitis,** or appendicitis may be the cause. A distended bladder is easy to detect with light palpation. Normally the bladder lies below the umbilicus and above the symphysis pubis. The nurse routinely checks for a distended bladder if a client has been unable to void.

A nurse must have experience to perform deep palpation successfully. Short fingernails are needed. One or two hands may be used (Fig. 20-78 on p. 582). The client must be relaxed as the nurse's hands are depressed approximately 2.5 to 7.5 cm (1 to 3 in) into the abdomen. Deep palpation is never used over a surgical incision or over extremely tender organs. It is also unwise to use palpation on abnormal masses.

Each quadrant is surveyed systematically. Masses palpated are assessed for size, location, shape, consistency, tenderness, mobility (for example, during respiration), and texture. If tenderness is found, the ex-

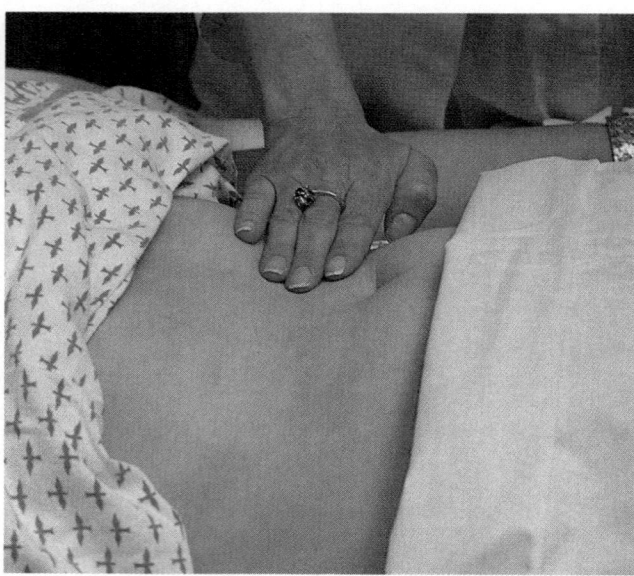

Fig. 20-77   Light palpation of the abdomen.

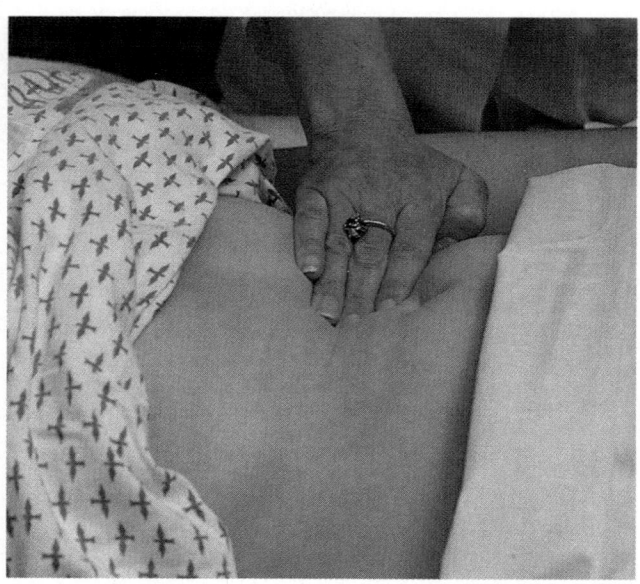

Fig. 20-78   Deep palpation of the abdomen.

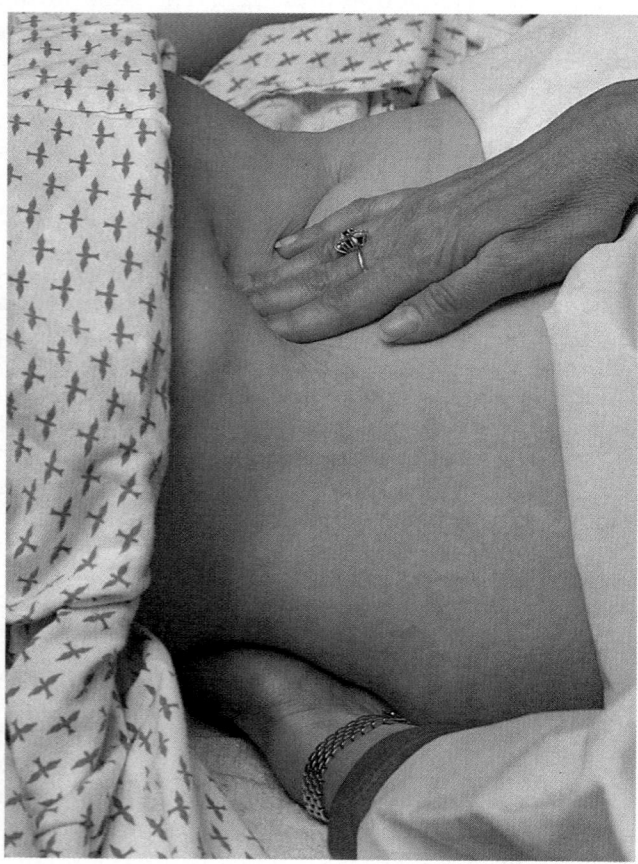

Fig. 20-79   The nurse's left hand is placed under the client's posterior thorax at the eleventh and twelfth ribs. The nurse's right hand palpates in and up to feel the liver's edge as the client inhales.

aminer checks for rebound tenderness. With this test the examiner presses a hand slowly and deeply into the involved area and then lets go quickly. If pain is aggravated with the release of the hand, the test is positive. Rebound tenderness occurs in clients with peritoneal irritation such as in appendicitis, **pancreatitis,** or any peritoneal injury causing bile, blood, or enzymes to enter the peritoneal cavity.

Liver

The liver normally lies in the right upper quadrant under the rib cage. The nurse uses deep palpation to locate the liver's lower edge. This technique detects liver enlargement. To palpate the liver, the nurse places the left hand under the client's right posterior thorax at the eleventh and twelfth ribs and then applies upward pressure. This maneuver makes it easier to feel the liver anteriorly. With the fingers of the right hand pointing toward the right costal margin, the nurse places the hand on the right upper quadrant well below the liver's lower border. As the nurse presses gently in and up (Fig. 20-79), the client takes a deep abdominal breath. As the client inhales, the nurse tries to palpate the liver's edge as it descends. A normal liver may not be palpable. However, it is nontender and has a firm, regular, and sharp edge. If the liver is palpable, the nurse traces its edge medially and laterally by repeating the maneuver.

Aortic Pulsation

To assess aortic pulsation, the nurse palpates with the thumb and forefinger of one hand deeply into the upper abdomen, just left of the midline. Normally a pulsation is transmitted forward. If there is enlargement of the aorta from an **aneurysm** (localized dilation of a vessel wall), the pulsation expands laterally. In obese clients, it may be necessary to palpate with both hands, one on each side of the aorta.

Bladder

It is usually unnecessary to palpate the bladder. However, clients who are still under the effects of anesthesia, who have received large doses of analgesic medications, who have spinal cord injuries, or who suffer incontinence should be examined for bladder retention. The nurse places one hand just above the symphysis pubis and palpates, feeling for the smooth bladder dome. An empty bladder is not palpable.

 ## FEMALE GENITALIA AND REPRODUCTIVE TRACT

An examination of the female genitalia and rectum can be embarrassing for many women. The gynecological examination is one of the most difficult experiences for adolescents. Cultural background may further add to apprehension (see Chapter 4). The lithotomy position assumed during the examination is an additional source of embarrassment, so the nurse uses a calm, reassuring, and attentive approach. Comfort is established through correct positioning and draping. Each portion of the examination is explained in advance so that clients can anticipate the nurse's actions. Adolescents may choose to have parents present in the examination room. Delays that might aggravate embarrassment should be avoided.

The client may require a complete examination of the female reproductive organs, which includes assessment of external genitalia and a vaginal examination. Most nurses do not perform a vaginal examination until they become nurse practitioners with extensive experience. However, it is important for the nurse to understand the procedure because a physician will require the nurse's assistance. Frequently a client will undergo an examination of external genitalia during routine nursing care. For example, while performing routine hygiene measures or preparing to insert a urinary catheter, a nurse uses the opportunity to examine the external genitalia.

Adolescents and young adults should be examined because of the growing incidence of sexually transmitted diseases. The nurse collects a history (Table 20-26) before an examination to assess client anxiety. The examination is relatively simple and should be a part of preventive health care because uterine and vaginal cancer have a high incidence rate. Rectal and anal assessments are easily combined with this examination because the client can assume a lithotomy or dorsal recumbent position.

Preparation of the Client

If a complete examination will be performed, the following special equipment will be needed:
1. Examination table with stirrups
2. Vaginal speculum
3. Adjustable light source
4. Sink
5. Clean, disposable gloves
6. Glass microscopic slides and coverslips
7. Sponge forceps or swabs
8. Plastic spatulas and/or cytobrush
9. Specimen bottles with fixative spray

Equipment must be ready before the examination begins. Often it is necessary to collect a urine specimen. If only the vaginal examination will be performed, the client should empty her bladder before it begins. The client should be placed in a lithotomy position. This position allows full visualization of the genital area. The client lies on her back, the thighs are flexed and abducted, the knees are flexed, and the feet rest in stirrups. The client's arms should be at her sides or folded across the chest to prevent tightening of abdominal muscles.

A square drape or sheet is given to the client. She holds one corner over her sternum, the adjacent corners fall over each knee, and the fourth corner covers the perineum. After the examination begins, the drape over the perineum is lifted.

If only the external genitalia will be examined, the nurse helps the client assume the lithotomy position in bed or on the examination table. The client flexes her knees perpendicular to the bed and is then asked to relax her thighs, allowing each leg to abduct to the side. The client's head may be elevated for comfort. A woman suffering pain or deformity of the joints may be unable to assume a lithotomy position. In this situation it may be necessary to have the client abduct only one leg or to have another nurse assist in separating the client's thighs.

The male examiner should always have another woman in attendance during the examination. A female examiner may prefer to work alone but should have a female attendant if the client is particularly anxious or emotionally unstable. Adolescents being examined for the first time tend to prefer a female examiner (Seymour et al, 1986).

External Genitalia

The perineal area must be well illuminated. The nurse gloves both hands to facilitate the assessment and prevent the spread of infection.

TABLE 20-26 Nursing History for Female Genitalia and Reproductive Tract Assessment	
Assessment Category	**Rationale**
Determine if client has previous illness or surgery involving reproductive organs, including sexually transmitted disease.	Illness or surgery can influence appearance and position of organs being examined.
Review menstrual history, including age at menarche, frequency and duration of menstrual cycle, character of flow (e.g., amount, presence of clots), presence of dysmenorrhea (painful menstuation), pelvic pain, dates of last two menstrual periods.	This information helps to reveal level of reproductive health, including normalcy of menstrual cycle.
Ask if client has had signs of bleeding outside of normal menstrual period or after menopause or has had unusual vaginal discharge.	These are warning signs for cervical cancer.
Ask client to describe obstetrical history, including each pregnancy and history of abortions or miscarriages.	Observed physical findings will vary, depending on woman's history of pregnancy.
Ask client to describe current and past contraceptive practices and problems encountered. Determine whether client uses safe sex practices. Discuss risk of STDs and HIV infection.	Use of certain types of contraceptives may influence reproductive health (e.g., sensitivity reaction to spermicidal jelly).
Determine if client has symptoms or history of genitourinary problems, including burning during urination, frequency, urgency, nocturia, hematuria, incontinence, or stress incontinence (see Chapter 40).	Urinary problems may be associated with gynecological disorders, including sexually transmitted diseases.
Assess client's sexual history.	Sexual history reveals risk for and understanding of sexually transmitted disease.
Assess if client has signs and symptoms of vaginal discharge, painful or swollen perianal tissues, or genital lesions.	These signs and symptoms indicate sexually transmitted disease.

The perineum is extremely sensitive and tender. The area is not touched without warning the client. It is best to touch the neighboring thigh first before advancing to the perineum.

To assess sexual maturity, quantity and distribution of hair growth is noted. A preadolescent has no pubic hair except for fine body hair like that on the abdomen. During adolescence, hair grows along the labia, becoming darker, coarser, and curlier as it spreads over the pubic symphysis. Hair growth eventually forms a triangle over the female perineum and along the medial surfaces of the thighs. Hair growth should not spread up over the abdomen. The nurse also inspects the skin of the pubic hair for lice, inflammation, irritation, or lesions.

The skin of the perineum is slightly darker than the skin of the rest of the body. The mucous membranes appear dark pink and moist. The labia majora are usually plump and well formed in a normal adult. After childbirth the labia majora are separated, causing the labia minora to become more prominent. When a woman reaches menopause, the labia majora become thinned, and with advancing age, they be-

come atrophied. The labia majora are normally without inflammation, edema, lesions, or lacerations.

To inspect the remaining external structures, the nurse gently places the thumb and index finger of the nondominant hand inside the labia minora and retracts the tissues outwardly (Fig. 20-80). The nurse should have a firm hold to avoid repeated retraction against the sensitive tissues. The clitoris, labia minora, urethral orifice, hymen, and vaginal orifice are then examined, paying attention to discharge, inflammation, edema, ulceration, or lesions.

The size of the clitoris is variable. However, it normally is 0.5 cm (⅕ in) in diameter. If inflamed, the clitoris will be a bright cherry red. In young women it is a common site for syphilitic lesions or **chancres,** which appear as small open ulcers that drain serous material. Older women may have malignant changes that result in dry, scaly, nodular lesions.

The labia minora are normally thinner than the labia majora. One side is usually larger than the other. In the female who is a virgin, the labia normally lie together. As a result of vaginal childbirth or intercourse, they tend to gape more and fall to the sides.

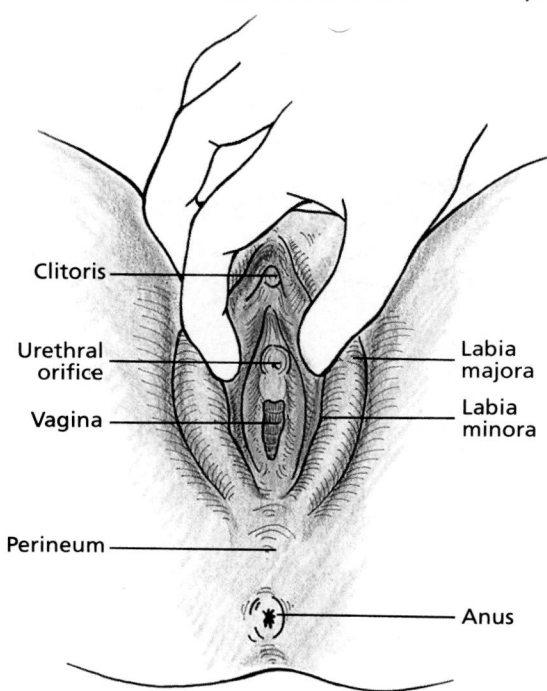

Fig. 20-80   Female external genitalia.

Clitoris

Urethral orifice

Vagina

Labia majora

Labia minora

Perineum

Anus

When inspecting the vaginal orifice (introitus), the examiner notices the condition of the hymen, which is just inside the introitus. In the virgin the hymen may restrict the opening of the vagina. Only remnants of the hymen remain after sexual intercourse.

If inflammation and edema are found near the posterior end of the introitus, Bartholin's glands may be infected. The glands cannot normally be palpated. To attempt palpation the nurse places a thumb and index finger between the labia majora and introitus and palpates one side at a time.

The urethral orifice is carefully observed for inflammation. The urethra is often difficult to locate. It is a small slit or pinhole opening just above the vaginal canal. In women who have had several vaginal childbirths, the opening to the vaginal canal often extends upward, interfering with the view of the urethra.

Minute openings of the Skene's gland are around the urethra. The nurse suspecting inflammation checks for urethral discharge. The nurse gently places an index finger 2.5 cm (1 in) in the vaginal orifice and milks the urethra gently from inside outward. Drainage will be manually expressed if inflammation is present. If drainage is found, the nurse changes gloves for the remainder of the examination to prevent transmission of infection.

With the gloved index and middle fingers in the vaginal orifice, the nurse asks the client to strain downward as if she were voiding. If the client lacks ade-

quate muscular support, the vaginal walls bulge, blocking the introitus. A portion of the vaginal wall and bladder may prolapse or fall into the orifice anteriorly; this is a **cystocele**. Bulging of the posterior wall may be caused by prolapse of the rectum (**rectocele**). Normally when a client is asked to constrict or close the vaginal orifice, the nurse palpates tension in the muscles. A woman who has undergone vaginal childbirth has less muscle tone than one who has not.

The nurse may also inspect the anus at this time, looking for lesions and hemorrhoids (see section on rectal examination). If the nurse performs only the external examination, the examination gloves are disposed of at this time. The client is then offered perineal hygiene if the skin is soiled with secretions.

Speculum Examination of Internal Genitalia

To view the internal walls of the vagina and the cervix a speculum examination is needed. Nurses are *unlikely* to perform a speculum examination because the procedure requires considerable practice. The procedure should *not* be attempted without supervision of an experienced examiner because incorrect use of the speculum can cause trauma to vaginal tissues. A nurse often assists the physician during the procedure. During the examination, specimens are collected for testing for cervical and vaginal cancer (Papanicolaou smears) (see later section).

The speculum consists of two blades: the top, which is movable, and the bottom, which is fixed. The blades are attached by a thumbscrew that can be adjusted to open or close the blades. It helps to practice opening and closing the speculum before using it with a client. The nurse must select the proper size speculum to avoid causing discomfort. The smallest size will fit a virgin. If the woman is sexually active, a medium-sized speculum is best. For women who have had children vaginally, the examiner uses a medium-to-large speculum.

All equipment for a speculum examination should be easily accessible. To begin the examiner applies a new pair of disposable gloves and places the speculum blades under warm running water. Water is the ideal lubricant; commercially prepared lubricants interfere with Papanicolaou studies. The examiner sits on a stool facing the client's perineum. The adjustable light is placed over the examiner's shoulder, directed at the examination site.

The examiner holds the speculum in the dominant hand and explains the procedure to the client. If the woman has never been examined, two fingers are gently inserted into the vagina to explore for abnor-

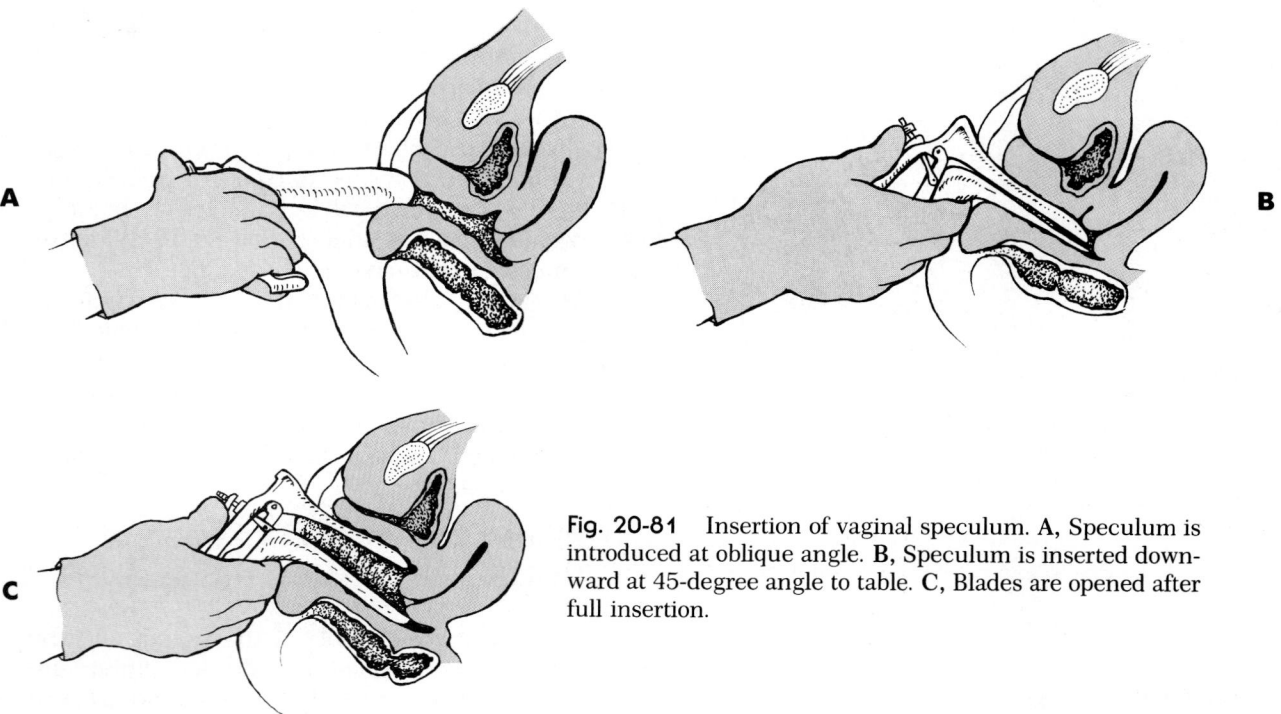

Fig. 20-81 Insertion of vaginal speculum. **A,** Speculum is introduced at oblique angle. **B,** Speculum is inserted downward at 45-degree angle to table. **C,** Blades are opened after full insertion.

malities. Then with two fingers the examiner presses down on the perineal body just inside the introitus. After checking to be sure that the speculum blades are closed, the examiner introduces the closed speculum obliquely (rotated 50 degrees counterclockwise from the vertical position) past the fingers (Fig. 20-81). The speculum is inserted downward at a 45-degree angle toward the examination table to avoid trauma to the urethra (this maneuver corresponds with the normal downward slope of the vaginal canal). Care is taken to avoid pulling the pubic hair or pinching the labia.

After the wide portions of the blades have passed the introitus, the speculum is rotated so that the blades are horizontal. The blades are opened slowly after full insertion and the speculum is moved to visualize the cervix. When the cervix is in full view, the blades are locked in the open position.

Cervix

The examiner inspects the cervix and its opening, or os. The cervix is the thick, funnel-shaped organ that serves as the narrow corridor between the internal and external sex organs (see Chapter 32). The normal cervix is a glistening pink color (Fig. 20-82). The cervical diameter is approximately 2.5 to 3 cm (1 to 1²⁄₁₀ in) in a normal young woman. In an older

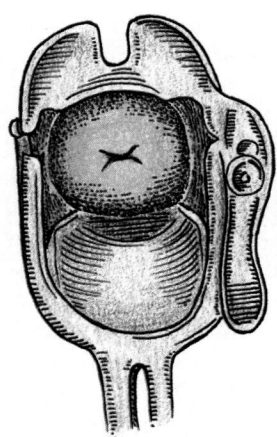

Fig. 20-82 Appearance of cervix through vaginal speculum.

woman the cervix is smaller. In a woman who has not vaginally delivered a fetus, the cervix is round. In women who have delivered one or more newborns, it is slitlike.

Discharge, lacerations, ulcerations, or lesions are abnormal. Cancerous lesions tend to bleed easily, and the margins are difficult to identify. A bluish appearance of the cervix (**Chadwick's sign**) is an early sign of pregnancy. Any discharge is examined carefully for color, odor, quantity, and consistency. Chronic yeast infections yield thick, malodorous discharges.

Client Teaching During Female Genitalia and Reproductive Tract Assessment

OBJECTIVES

- Client will pursue routine gynecological examinations based on her level of risk for cervical cancer.
- Client with a sexually transmitted disease will follow safe sexual practices.
- Client will use measures to prevent acquisition and transmission of sexually transmitted disease.

TEACHING STRATEGIES

- Instruct client about purpose and recommended frequency of Pap smears and gynecological examinations.
- Counsel client with sexually transmitted disease about diagnosis and treatment.
- Teach measures to prevent sexually transmitted disease, including preventive measures (e.g., male partner's use of condoms, restricting number of sexual partners, avoiding sex with persons who have several other partners, perineal hygiene measures).
- Tell client with sexually transmitted diseases that they must inform sexual partner of the need for an examination.
- Reinforce the importance of perineal hygiene (as appropriate).

EVALUATION

- Ask client to explain when she should routinely have a gynecological examination.
- Have client describe ways to prevent transmission of sexually transmitted diseases.
- For client with sexually transmitted diesase, determine during follow-up visit if safe sexual practices have been followed (use nonthreatening inquiry).

Papanicolaou Smear

The surface of the cervix, at the cervical canal opening, is lined with layers of vaginal squamous cells. These cells meet a different group of cells, known as *columnar cells*. The columnar cells secrete mucus and line the passageway that leads up into the central cavity of the uterus. The squamous cells have a protective role for the cervix, and the columnar cells have a reproductive role (assisting the sperm to enter the uterus for fertilization). A **Papanicolaou (PAP) smear** is a painless screening test for cervical cancer. Specimens are taken of squamous and columnar cells. The test is simple and has no side effects. Women who are or have been sexually

TABLE 20-27   Methods for Obtaining Pap Smears

Location	Technique
Endocervical	Use cervical brush (cytobrush). Gently insert brush through os. Rotate brush 180-360 degrees. Apply cells by rolling and twisting brush on glass slide. Apply fixative solution and label slide. WARNING: Do *not* use on pregnant clients.

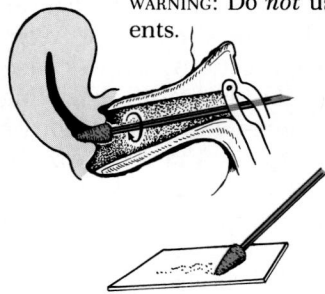

| Outer cervix | Use plastic spatula. Place tip of longer arm in os. Rotate spatula, scraping outer surface of cervix. Apply cells to glass slide. Apply fixative solution and label slide. |

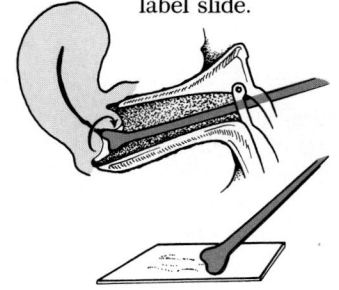

active and women who have reached the age of 18 who do not have symptoms of disease are advised to have annual tests until three smears are negative. Thereafter, tests are done at the discretion of the physician. Women at high risk for cervical cancer should have annual checkups (see teaching box). The National Institutes of Health recommend that women who have reached age 60 and have had two consecutive negative Pap smears need to undergo no further screening (Henderson, 1989).

The examiner collects smear samples from the endocervical area (columnar cells at the cervical opening) and the outer cervix (squamous cells) (Table 20-27). After specimens are obtained, the nurse prepares slides with the fixative solution. Each specimen is labeled with the client's name and source of the specimen. The results of a Pap smear are reported as stages and takes a few days for accurate interpretation.

Vagina

The vaginal walls are viewed more easily as the speculum is withdrawn. As the speculum leaves the cervix, the thumbscrew is loosened, but the blades are kept open with the thumb. During the withdrawal, the nurse inspects the vaginal wall's texture, color, and support. Discharge or lesions are noted. The color is normally pink throughout. Women commonly acquire yeast infections, which cause a thick, white, patchy, curdlike discharge that clings to the vaginal walls. The nurse closes the blades gradually as the speculum is removed to avoid excess stretching and pinching of the mucosa. The blades should be closed completely as the speculum emerges from the introitus. The nurse removes the disposable gloves and discards them in a proper receptacle. Perineal hygiene is provided for the client.

MALE GENITALIA

An examination of the male genitalia includes assessment of the external genitalia and the inguinal ring and canal. The examination begins with the client lying supine with the chest, abdomen, and lower legs draped. Inspection and palpation are used. The nurse applies disposable gloves to prevent the chance of cross-infection from urethral discharge.

The nurse must learn to relax during because anxiety would make the procedure highly embarrassing for the nurse and client. If the examiner feels uncomfortable, it helps to ask another nurse to witness the examination. The nurse should not discuss the client's sexual activity during the examination because the client might perceive this as evaluative or judgmental (see teaching box). The client's modesty must be preserved. In this case, teaching is done after the examination. The genitalia are gently manipulated to avoid causing erection or discomfort.

Client Teaching During Male Genitalia Assessment

OBJECTIVES

- Client will perform testicular self-examination correctly (see box on p. 590).
- Client will describe methods to prevent transmission of sexually transmitted diseases.
- Client with sexually transmitted disease will follow safe sexual practices.

TEACHING STRATEGIES

- Instruct client about testicular self-examination (see box, p. 590).
- Counsel client with sexually transmitted diseases about diagnosis and treatment.
- Teach measures to prevent sexually transmitted diseases, including using condoms, restricting the number of sexual partners, avoiding sex with persons who have several other partners, and using perineal hygiene.
- Tell client with sexually transmitted disease that sexual partners must be informed of the need for examination.

EVALUATION

- Have client perform return demonstration of testicular self-examination.
- Ask client to describe methods for preventing transmission of sexually transmitted disease.
- During a follow-up visit, determine whether client with sexually transmitted disease has used safe sexual practices (use nonthreatening inquiry).

TABLE 20-28   Nursing History for Male Genitalia Assessment

Assessment Category	Rationale
Review normal urinary elimination pattern, including frequency of voiding; history of nocturia; character and volume of urine; daily fluid intake; symptoms of burning, urgency, frequency; difficulty starting stream; hematuria (see Chapter 40).	Urinary problems can be directly associated with genitourinary problems because of anatomical structure of men's reproductive and urinary systems.
Assess client's sexual history and use of safe sex habits.	Sexual history reveals risk for and understanding of sexually transmitted disease.
Determine if client has had previous surgery or illness involving urinary or reproductive organs, including sexually transmitted disease.	Alterations resulting from disease or surgery may be responsible for symptoms or changes in organ structure or function.
Ask if client has noted penile pain or swelling, genital lesions, or urethral discharge.	These signs and symptoms indicate sexually transmitted disease.
Determine if client has noticed heaviness or painless enlargement of testis.	These signs and symptoms are early warning sign for testicular cancer.

Because the incidence of sexually transmitted disease in adolescents and young adults is high, an assessment of the genitalia should be a routine part of any health maintenance examination for this age group (see teaching box). If this is the only assessment to be performed on a client, the nurse must be sure to collect a thorough nursing history (Table 20-28).

Sexual Maturity

The nurse begins by assessing the sexual maturity of the client, noting the size and shape of the penis and testes, the color and texture of the scrotal skin, and the character and distribution of pubic hair. The first sign of puberty, involving an increase in the size of the testes, begins between 9.5 and 13.5 years of age. During the preadolescent stage, there is no pubic hair except for the fine body hair found on the abdomen. By puberty the pubic hair extends from the base of the penis over the symphysis pubis and becomes coarse and curly. The testes and penis have enlarged to adult size and shape. The scrotal skin darkens and becomes wrinkled in texture. The nurse inspects the skin covering the genitalia for lice, rashes, excoriations, or lesions.

Penis

The nurse inspects the structures of the penis, including the shaft, corona, prepuce (foreskin), glans, and urethral meatus (Fig. 20-83). The penile structures should not be excessively manipulated because an erection may be caused.

In uncircumcised males the foreskin is retracted to reveal the glans and urethral meatus. The foreskin should retract easily. A small amount of thick, white secretion between the glans and foreskin is normal. If there is evidence of abnormal discharge, a culture is usually obtained. The urethral meatus should be positioned at the tip of the glans. In some congenital conditions the meatus is displaced along the penile shaft. Gentle compression of the glans between the nurse's thumb and index finger opens the urethral meatus to allow inspection for discharge. The meatus is also inspected for lesions, edema, and inflammation.

The glans is carefully checked around its entire circumference for lesions. The area between the foreskin and glans is a common site for venereal lesions. Any lesion is palpated gently to note tenderness, size, consistency, and shape. When inspection of the glans is completed, the foreskin is pulled down to its original position.

The nurse continues to inspect the entire shaft of the penis, including the undersurface, looking for lesions, scars, and edema. The shaft is palpated between the thumb and first two fingers to detect any localized areas of hardness.

Scrotum

The nurse must be particularly cautious when inspecting and palpating the scrotum because the structures lying within the scrotal sac are very sensitive. The scrotum is a saclike structure divided internally into two halves. Each half contains a testicle, epididymis, and the vas deferens, which travels upward into the inguinal ring. Normally the left testicle is lower than the right. The nurse inspects the scrotum's size, shape, and symmetry while observing for lesions or edema. The scrotum is gently lifted to view

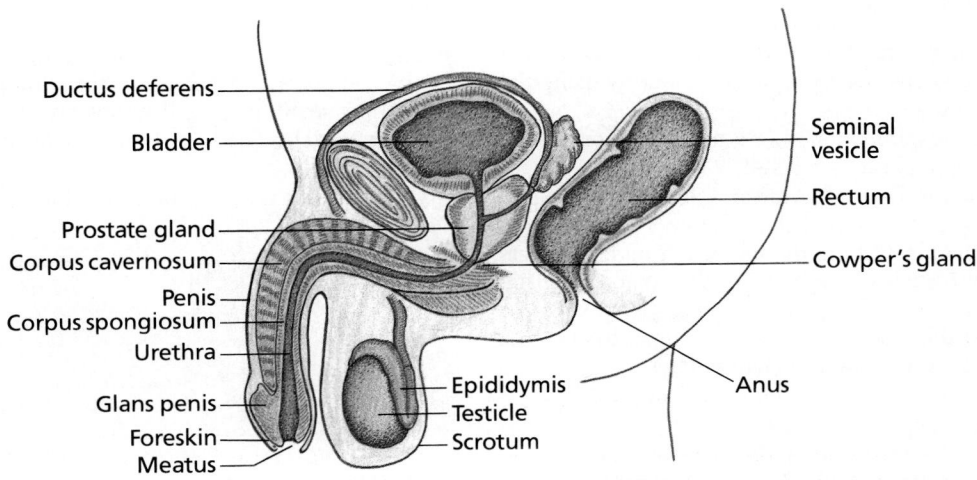

Fig. 20-83   External and internal male sex organs.

the posterior surface. The scrotal skin is usually loose. A tightening of the skin may reveal edema. The scrotum's size normally changes with temperature variations as its dartos muscle contracts in cold and relaxes in warm temperatures. Testicular cancer has become a common solid tumor among young men aged 18 to 34 years. Early detection is critical, and thus clients must learn to perform testicular self-examinations (TSE) (see box). The nurse can explain the technique while examining the client. The underlying testicles are normally ovoid and approximately 2×4 cm (⅘ × 1⅗ in) in size. The testicles and epididymis are gently palpated between the nurse's thumb and first two fingers. The most common symptoms of testicular cancer are a painless enlargement of one testis and appearance of a palpable small, hard lump, about the size of a pea, on the front or side of the testicle. The size, shape, and consistency of the organs are noted. The testicles normally feel smooth and firm. The epididymis is resilient. In the older adult the testicles decrease in size and are less firm during palpation. The client should be asked about any unusual tenderness. The nurse continues palpating the vas deferens separately as it forms the spermatic cord toward the inguinal ring, noting the presence of nodules or swelling.

Inguinal Ring and Canal

The external inguinal ring provides the opening for the spermatic cord to pass into the inguinal canal. The canal forms a passage through the abdominal wall, a potential site for hernia formation. An intestinal loop may even enter the scrotum. The client stands during this portion of the examination.

Both inguinal areas are inspected for signs of obvious bulging. During inspection the client is asked to strain or bear down. The maneuver helps make a hernia more visible.

The nurse completes an examination by palpating for inguinal lymph nodes. Small, nontender, mobile horizontal nodes may be normally found. Normally the nodes are not palpable. Any abnormality may indicate local or systemic infection or metastatic disease.

 ## RECTUM AND ANUS

An examination of the rectum and anus can be conducted separately or as a continuation of the examination of the genitalia and reproductive organs. Usually the examination is not performed in young children or adolescents. The examination can detect colorectal cancer in its early stages. In men the rectal examination can also detect prostatic tumors. The nurse collects a thorough history (Table 20-29) to detect risk for bowel or rectal disease or prostatic disease.

The rectal examination can be uncomfortable and embarrassing, so the nurse uses a calm, gentle approach. Explanation of steps of the procedure helps clients to relax and lessens discomfort during the digital examination. Women can be examined immediately after examination of genitalia while still in

---

Testicular Self-Examination

Instruct client on TSE. All men 15 years and older should perform this self-examination monthly using the following steps:
- Perform the examination after a warm bath or shower when the scrotal sac is relaxed.
- Stand naked in front of a mirror and look for swelling of or lumps in the skin of the scrotum.
- Use both hands, placing the index and middle fingers under the testicles and the thumbs on top (see figure).
- Gently roll the testicle, feeling for lumps, thickening, or a change in consistency (hardening).

- Find the epididymis (a cordlike structure on the top and back of the testicle; it is *not* a lump).
- Feel for small, pea-sized lumps on the front and side of the testicle. The lumps are usually painless and are abnormal.
- Call your physician if you find a lump.

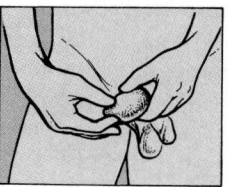

Illustration from Payne WA, Hahn DB: *Understanding your health,* ed 2, St Louis, 1989, Mosby–Year Book.

dorsal recumbent positions. Otherwise the left lateral sidelying (Sims') position is preferred. Men are best examined by having the client bend over forward with his hips flexed and upper body resting across the examination table. A nonambulatory client can be examined in the Sims' position. Clients are draped with only the anal area exposed. The nurse applies disposable gloves for the examination.

Inspection

Using the nondominant hand the nurse gently retracts the buttocks as needed to visualize the perianal and sacrococcygeal areas. Anal tissues are normally moist and hairless compared with perianal skin. The anus is held closed by the voluntary external muscle sphincter. The nurse inspects perianal tissue for lesions, **hemorrhoids** (dilated veins that appear as reddened protrusions), ulcers, inflammation, rashes, or discoloration. The perianal skin is normally intact, more pigmented, and coarser than skin overlying the buttocks. Next, the nurse asks the client to bear down as though having a bowel movement. Any internal hemorrhoids or fissures will appear at this time. Normally the anal lining is intact.

Digital Palpation

Some institutions do not permit nurses to perform digital examinations. When policy permits, the nurs-

ing student should have a qualified examiner present during the first examination.

The nurse lubricates the index finger of the gloved dominant hand. The procedure is explained, and then the client is asked to bear down gently as if having a bowel movement. As the anal sphincter relaxes, the nurse's fingertip is gently inserted into the anal canal in a direction toward the umbilicus. Normally the client feels as though stool is being passed. The nurse never forces digital insertion, so mucosal tissues are not injured.

The anal canal is the distal portion of the gastrointestinal tract. The canal extends in a line toward the umbilicus before turning into the mucus-lined rectum. The anus contains a rich supply of sensory nerve fibers. Thus digital manipulation can be painful. At the junction of the anal canal and rectum, the rectum balloons out and turns posteriorly into the hollow of the coccyx and sacrum. The nurse notes the tone of the anal sphincter as the muscle closes snugly around the finger. Beyond the anal canal the nurse palpates each side of the rectal wall for tenderness, irregularities, or nodules. After the finger is advanced fully, the client is asked to bear down again. High lesions within the rectum will descend against the fingertip (see teaching box on p. 592).

In men the nurse turns the hand so that the finger palpates the anterior rectal wall. The prostate gland is palpable anteriorly as a rounded, heart-shaped structure about 2.5 to 4 cm (1 to 1½ in) in length

TABLE 20-29 Nursing History for Rectum and Anus Assessment	
Assessment Category	Rationale
Determine whether client has experienced bleeding from rectum, black or tarry stools (melena), rectal pain, or change in bowel habits (constipation or diarrhea).	These are warning signs of colorectal cancer or other gastrointestinal alterations.
Determine whether client has personal or family history of colorectal cancer, polyps, or inflammatory bowel disease. Ask if client is over age 40.	These are risk factors for colorectal cancer.*
Assess dietary habits for high-fat intake or deficient fiber content.	Bowel cancer may be linked to dietary intake of fat or insufficient fiber intake.*
Determine whether client has undergone screening for colorectal cancer (digital examination, stool blood slide test, proctosigmoidoscopy).	Undergoing this screening reflects understanding and compliance with preventive health care measures.
Assess medication history for use of laxatives or cathartic medications.	Repeated use can cause diarrhea and eventual loss of intestinal muscle tone.
Assess for use of codeine or iron preparations.	Codeine causes constipation. Iron turns the color of feces black and tarry.
Ask male client if weak or interrupted urine flow, inability to urinate, difficulty in starting or stopping urine flow, polyuria, nocturia, hematuria, or dysuria has been experienced.	These are warning signs of prostatic cancer.*

*Data from American Cancer Society: *1991 cancer facts and figures*, New York, 1991, The Society.

Client Teaching During Rectal and Anal Assessment

OBJECTIVES

- Client will have a regular digital examination performed appropriate to age.
- Client will be able to identify symptoms of colorectal and prostatic cancer.
- Client will follow a diet of increased fiber and reduced fat.

TEACHING STRATEGIES

- Discuss the American Cancer Society's guidelines for early detection of colorectal cancer:
  - Digital rectal examination yearly after age 40
  - Stool blood test (guaiac test) yearly after age 50
  - Proctosigmoidoscopy (visual inspection of the rectum and lower colon with a hollow, lighted tube) performed by a physician, every 3 to 5 years after age 50 on the advice of a physician
  - Warning signs of colorectal cancer (see Table 20-29)
- Discuss dietary planning to reduce fat and increase fiber content.

- Warn client against problems caused by overuse of laxatives, cathartic medications, codeine, or enemas.
- Discuss with male client the American Cancer Society's guidelines for early detection of prostatic cancer:
  - Digital rectal examination performed annually after age 40
  - Possible prostate ultrasound testing for men at high risk of smaller tumors
  - Warning signs of prostatic cancer
- Inform client about a new blood test that may detect prostate-specific antigen (PSA), which can be an early indicator of prostate disease (see Table 20-29).

EVALUATION

- During follow-up visits, determine whether client has had a rectal examination performed.
- Have client explain warning signs of colorectal and prostatic cancer.
- Ask client to describe foods high in fiber and low in fat.

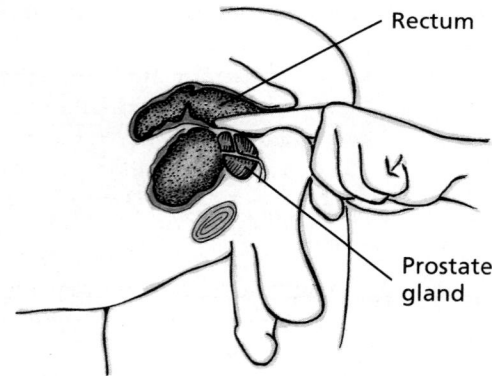

Fig. 20-84 Palpation of prostate gland during rectal examination.

(Fig. 20-84). A small medial groove separates the gland into two lateral lobes. The nurse palpates the size, shape, and consistency of the prostate. The gland normally is firm, without bogginess, tenderness, or nodules. Hardness or nodules may indicate presence of a cancerous lesion.

In women, it may be possible to palpate the cervix through the anterior rectal wall. It is common to mis-take the cervix or an inserted tampon for a rectal tumor.

After palpation is completed the nurse gently withdraws the finger and observes it for feces. Feces are normally brown. The presence of mucus, blood, or black, tarry stool should be reported. A sample of the feces is tested for occult blood (see Chapter 41). For women suspected of having sexually transmitted disease, a rectal culture may be taken to rule out cross-infection from vaginal discharge. The nurse cleans the perianal area before continuing to the next part of the examination.

MUSCULOSKELETAL SYSTEM

The nurse can learn to integrate portions of the musculoskeletal assessment when the client walks, moves in bed, or performs any type of physical activity. The assessment of musculoskeletal function focuses on determining range of joint motion, muscle strength and tone, and joint and muscle condition. Assessment of musculoskeletal integrity is especially important when the client reports pain or loss of function in a joint or muscle. Frequently, muscular

TABLE 20-30 Nursing History for Musculoskeletal System Assessment

Assessment Category	Rationale
Ask client to describe history of alteration in bone, muscle, or joint function (e.g., recent fall, trauma, lifting of heavy objects, history of bone or joint disease with sudden or gradual onset, location of alteration).	History assists in assessing nature of musculoskeletal problem.
Assess nature and extent of pain, including location, duration, severity, predisposing and aggravating factors, relieving factors, and type.	Alterations in bone, joints, or muscle are frequently accompanied by pain, which has implications for not only comfort but also ability to perform activities of daily living.
Determine how alteration influences ability to perform activities of daily living (e.g., bathing, feeding, dressing, toileting, and ambulating) and social functions (e.g., household chores, work, recreation, sexual activities).	Level of nursing care will be determined by extent to which client is able to perform self-care. Type and degree of restriction in continuing social activities influence topics for client education and ability of nurse to identify alternative ways to maintain function.
Assess height loss of woman over age 50 by subtracting current height from recall of maximum adult height.*	Measurement may be useful screening tool to predict osteoporosis. In study by Reed and Birge,* 75% of clients who had lost 2 in or more in height were later found to have osteoporosis on x-ray films.

*Data from Reed AT, Birge SJ: *J Gerontol Nurs* 14(7):18, 1988.

disorders are manifestations of neurological disease. For this reason a neurological assessment is often conducted simultaneously.

It is important to review the anatomy of bone and muscle placement and joint structure (see Chapter 43). Joints vary in their degree of mobility. Some, as in the knee, are freely movable. The spinal vertebrae are examples of slightly movable joints.

The examination uses inspection and palpation. The muscles and joints should be exposed and free to move. Depending on the muscle groups assessed, the client assumes a sitting, supine, prone, or standing position. Table 20-30 lists the information gathered in the nursing history.

General Inspection

The nurse observes gait and posture as the client walks into the examination room. When the client is unaware of the nature of the observations, gait is more natural. Later a more formal test involves having the client walk in a straight line away from the nurse and then return. The nurse looks for foot dragging, limping, shuffling, and the position of the trunk in relation to the legs. Normally the client walks with arms swinging freely at the sides and the head and face leading the body. An older adult often walks with smaller steps and a wider base of support.

The normal standing posture is an upright stance with parallel alignment of the hips and shoulders (Fig. 20-85 on p. 594). Looking sideways at the client, the nurse notes the normal cervical, thoracic, and lumbar curves. The head is held erect. As the client sits, some degree of rounding of the shoulders is normal. Common postural abnormalities include lordosis, kyphosis, and scoliosis (Fig. 20-86 on p. 594). **Kyphosis,** or hunchback, is an exaggeration of the posterior curvature of the thoracic spine. This postural abnormality is common in the older adult. **Lordosis,** or swayback, is an increased lumbar curvature. A lateral spinal curvature is called *scoliosis* (see teaching box on p. 594). Loss of height is frequently the first clinical sign of **osteoporosis,** in which height loss occurs in the trunk as a result of vertebral fracture and collapse (Reed, Birge, 1988). Although a small amount of height loss is to be expected with aging, if the amount of loss is greater than that expected through aging, osteoporosis is likely (see Chapter 43).

During general inspection the nurse looks for symmetry of joints, muscles, and extremity length and obvious musculoskeletal deformities. A general review pinpoints areas requiring specialized assessment.

Range of Joint Motion

The nurse asks the client to put each joint through its full range of motion. If the client is weakened by illness, the nurse assesses range of motion passively by gently supporting and moving the extremities through their range of movement. The nurse must learn the correct terminology for the

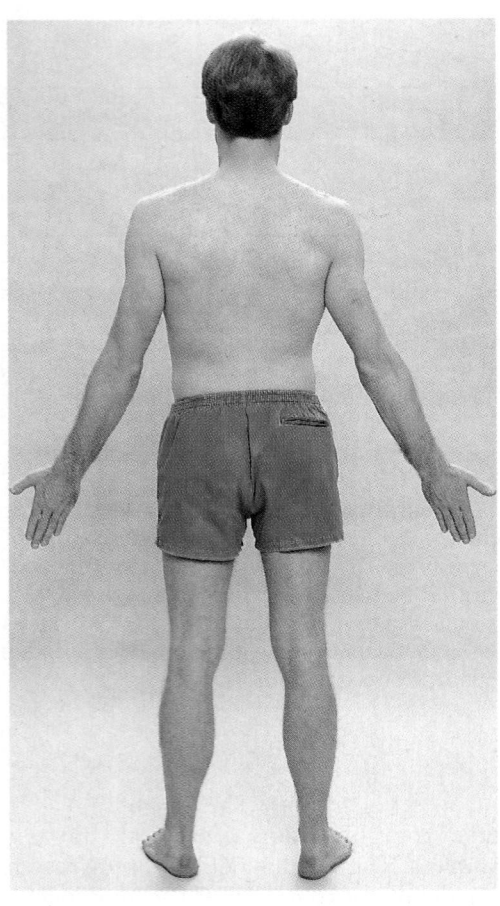

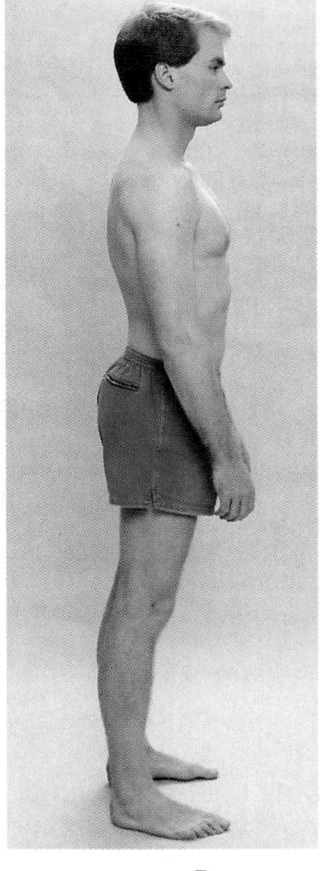

A   **B**

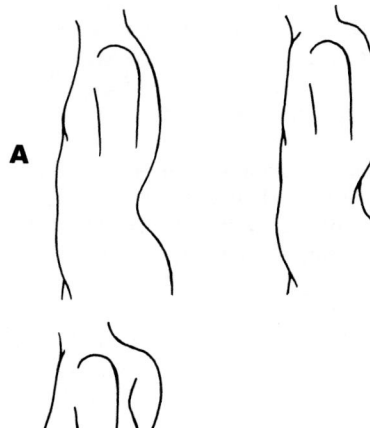

Fig. 20-85 **A,** Normal standing position. Client's hips and shoulders are aligned in parallel. **B,** Viewing the client sideways allows the nurse to observe the cervical, thoracic, and lumbar curves.
From Seidel HM et al: *Mosby's guide to physical examination,* ed 2, St Louis, 1991, Mosby–Year Book.

Fig. 20-86 Common postural abnormalities. **A,** Lordosis, **B,** Kyphosis. **C,** Scoliosis.

Client Teaching During Musculoskeletal Assessment

OBJECTIVES
- Female client will follow measures to prevent or minimize osteoporosis.
- Client will assume proper body posture.
- Client will be able to perform self-care measures.

TEACHING STRATEGIES
- Instruct client about correct postural alignment. Consult with physical therapist to provide client with exercises for improving posture.
- To reduce bone demineralization, instruct older client about a proper exercise program (e.g., walking) to be followed 3 or more times a week. Also encourage intake of calcium to meet the recommended daily allowance. Increased vitamin D will aid calcium absorption. Recommendations for calcium supplements are 1000 mg before and 1500 mg after menopause.

- For client with osteoporosis, instruct on proper body mechanics (see Chapter 43) and range of motion and moderate-weight-bearing exercises (swimming and walking) to minimize trauma and subsequent fracture of bones.
- When client is unable to perform self-care, instruct on use of assistive devices (e.g., zippers on clothing instead of buttons, elevation of chairs to minimize bending of knees and hips).
- Instruct older client to pace activities to compensate for loss in muscle strength.

EVALUATION
- Observe client's posture.
- Ask client to describe therapies for preventing osteoporosis.
- Observe client perform range of motion exercises.
- Have client keep log of regular weight-training exercises.
- Ask client or family members to describe client's use of self-care aids.

TABLE 20-31   Terminology for Normal Range of Motion Positions

Term	Range of Motion	Examples of Joints
Flexion	Movement decreasing angle between two adjoining bones; bending of limb	Elbow, fingers, knee
Extension	Movement increasing angle between two adjoining bones	Elbow, knee, fingers
Hyperextension	Movement of body part beyond its normal resting extended position	Head
Pronation	Movement of body part so that front or ventral surface faces downward	Hand, forearm
Supination	Movement of body part so that front or ventral surface faces upward	Hand, forearm
Abduction	Movement of extremity away from midline of body	Leg, arm, fingers
Adduction	Movement of extremity toward midline of body	Leg, arm, fingers
Internal rotation	Rotation of joint inward	Knee, hip
External rotation	Rotation of joint outward	Knee, hip
Eversion	Turning of body part away from midline	Foot
Inversion	Turning of body part toward midline	Foot
Dorsiflexion	Flexion of toes and foot upward	Foot
Plantar flexion	Bending of toes and foot downward	Foot

movements that the joints are capable of making (Table 20-31). It also helps to practice range of motion of one's own joints to learn the limits of mobility. The same body parts are compared for equality in movement.

When assessing range of motion, the nurse does not force a joint into a painful position. The nurse must know the joint's normal range and the extent to which it can be moved (see Chapter 43). Ideally, the normal range is assessed to determine a baseline for assessing later change.

A **goniometer** measures the precise degree of motion in a particular joint and is used mainly in clients who have a suspected reduction in joint movement. The instrument has two flexible arms with a 180-degree protractor in the center. The center of the protractor is positioned at the center of the joint being measured (Fig. 20-87). The arms extend along the body parts on each side of the protractor. A measurement is taken of the joint angle before moving the joint. After taking the joint through a full range of motion, the nurse measures the angle again to determine the degree of movement (Fig. 20-87). The reading is compared with the normal degree of joint movement.

When putting each joint through its range of motion, the nurse makes a number of basic observations, noting swelling, stiffness, instability, deformity, or tenderness. Normal joints are nontender, without swelling, and move freely. In older adults, joints often become swollen and stiff, with reduced range of motion resulting from cartilage erosion and fibrosis of synovial membranes (see Chapter 43).

The nurse also palpates for unusual joint movement and for nodules. **Crepitus** (a crackling sensation and noise caused by rubbing of bone fragments)

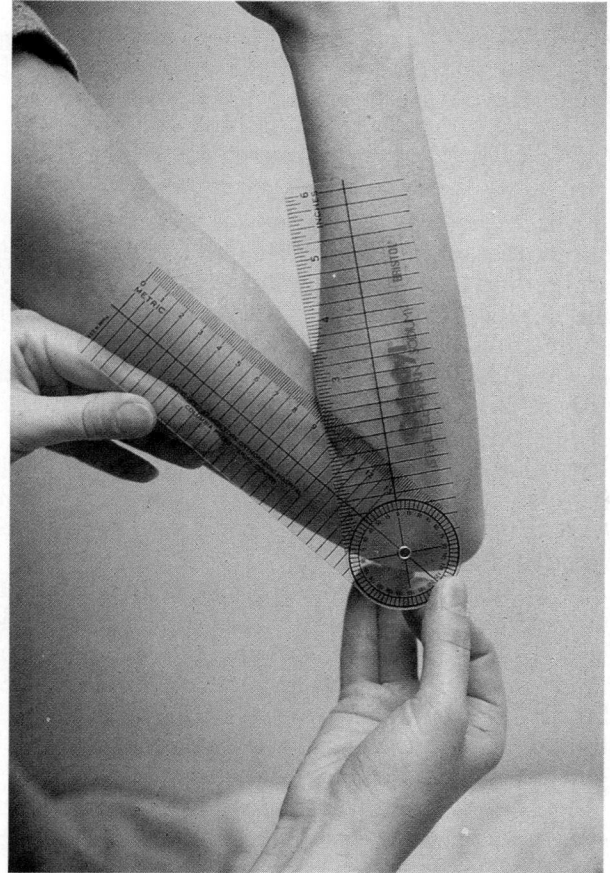

Fig. 20-87 After the client flexes the arm the goniometer measures the degree of joint flexion.
From Seidel HM et al: *Mosby's guide to physical examination*, ed 2, St Louis, 1991, Mosby–Year Book.

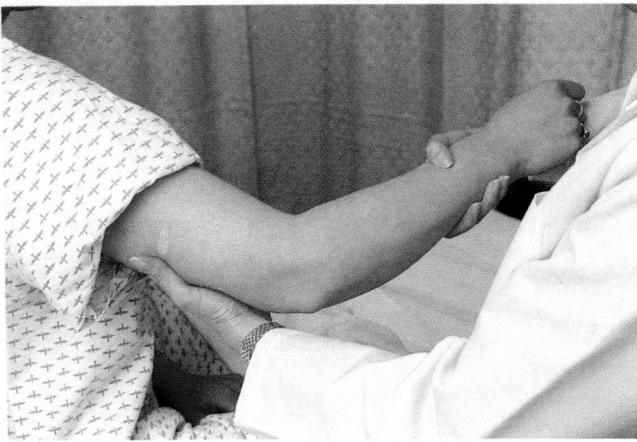

Fig. 20-88 The nurse palpates muscle tone when moving the extremity passively.

may be noted. A normal joint has no nodules or crepitus. If a joint appears swollen and inflamed, the nurse may be able to detect warmth in the tissues.

Muscle Tone and Strength

The nurse may assess muscle strength and tone during measurement of range of motion. Tone is the slight muscular resistance felt by the examiner as the relaxed extremity is passively moved through its range of motion.

The client is asked to allow an extremity to relax or hang limp. This is often difficult, particularly if the client feels pain in the extremity. The extremity is supported, and each limb grasped, moving it through the normal range of motion (Fig. 20-88). Normal tone causes a mild, even resistance to movement through the entire range.

If a muscle has increased tone, or **hypertonicity,** any sudden passive movement of a joint is met with considerable resistance. Continued movement eventually causes the muscle to relax. A muscle that has little tone (**hypotonicity**) feels flabby. The involved extremity hangs loosely in a position determined by gravity.

For assessment of muscle strength, the client assumes a stable position. The client performs maneuvers demonstrating strength of major muscle groups (Table 20-32). Symmetrical muscle pairs are compared. The arm on the dominant side is normally stronger than the arm on the nondominant side. In the older adult a loss of muscle mass causes bilateral weakness.

Each muscle group is examined. The examiner applies a gradual increase in pressure to a muscle group (for example, elbow extension). The client re-

TABLE 20-32 Maneuvers to Assess Muscle Strength	
Muscle Group	Maneuver
Neck (sternocleido-mastoid)	Place hand firmly against client's upper jaw. Ask client to turn head laterally against resistance.
Shoulder (trapezius)	Place hand over midline of client's shoulder, exerting firm pressure. Have client raise shoulders against resistance.
Elbow	
Biceps	Pull down on forearm as client attempts to flex arm.
Triceps	As client's arm is flexed, apply pressure against forearm. Ask client to straighten arm.
Hip	
Quadriceps	When client is sitting, apply downward pressure to thigh. Ask client to raise leg up from table.
Gastrocnemius	Client sits, holding shin of flexed leg. Ask client to straighten leg against resistance.

sists the pressure applied by the examiner by attempting to move against resistance (for example, elbow flexion). The client resists until instructed to stop. As the examiner varies the amount of pressure applied, the joint moves.

If a weakness is identified, the muscle's size is compared to its opposite counterpart by measuring the muscle body's circumference with a tape measure. A muscle that has **atrophied** (reduced in size) may feel soft and boggy when palpated.

 NEUROLOGICAL SYSTEM

The neurological system is responsible for many functions, including initiation and coordination of movement, reception and perception of sensory stimuli, organization of thought processes, control of speech, and storage of memory. A close integration exists between the neurological system and all other body systems. For example, urine production relies in part on the adequacy of blood flow to the kidneys, and the size of arterioles supplying the kidneys is under neural control.

An assessment of neurological function can be time consuming. An efficient nurse integrates neuro-

TABLE 20-33 Nursing History for Neurological System Assessment	
Assessment Category	Rationale
Determine if client is taking analgesics, sedatives, hypnotics, antipsychotics, antidepressants, or nervous system stimulants.	These medications can alter level of consciousness or cause behavioral changes.
Screen client for headache, seizures, tremors, dizziness, vertigo, numbness or tingling of body part, visual changes, weakness, pain, or changes in speech.	These symptoms frequently originate from alterations in central nervous system or peripheral nervous system function. Identification of specific patterns may aid in diagnosis of pathological condition.
Discuss with spouse, family members, or friends any recent changes in client's behavior (e.g., increased irritability, mood swings, memory loss).	Behavioral changes may result from intracranial pathological states.
Assess client for history of change in vision, hearing, smell, taste, or touch.	Major sensory nerves originate from brainstem. These symptoms may help to localize nature of problem.

logical measurements with other parts of the physical examination. For example, cranial nerve function can be tested during the survey of the head and neck. Mental and emotional status is observed as the nursing history is collected.

Many variables must be considered when deciding the extent of the examination. A client's level of consciousness influences the ability to follow directions. A person's general physical status influences tolerance to assessment. For example, an inability to walk makes a detailed assessment of coordination difficult. The client's chief complaint also helps determine the need for a thorough neurological assessment. If the client complains of headache or a recent loss of function in an extremity, a complete neurological review is needed. Table 20-33 reviews the data collected in the nursing history. If a complete examination will be given, the following special equipment will be needed:

1. Reading material
2. Vials containing aromatic substances (for example, vanilla and coffee)
3. Safety pins (sterile)
4. Snellen chart
5. Penlight
6. Vials containing sugar or salt
7. Tongue blade
8. Two test tubes, one filled with hot water and the other with cold water
9. Cotton balls or cotton-tipped applicators
10. Tuning fork
11. Reflex hammer

Mental and Emotional Status

A great deal can be learned about mental capacities and emotional state by simply interacting with a client. A nurse can ask questions throughout an examination to gather data and observe the appropriateness of emotions and ideas.

To ensure an objective assessment the nurse considers the client's cultural and educational background, values, beliefs, and previous experiences. Such factors will influence the client's response to questions. An alteration in mental or emotional status may reflect a disturbance in cerebral functioning. The cerebral cortex controls and integrates intellectual and emotional functioning. Primary brain disorders, medication, and metabolic changes are examples of factors that may change cerebral function.

Level of Consciousness

The level of consciousness exists along a continuum, from full awakening, alertness, and cooperation to unresponsiveness to any form of external stimuli. A fully conscious client responds to questions spontaneously. As consciousness lowers, a client may show irritability, a shortened attention span, or an unwillingness to cooperate. To avoid ambiguity in the assessment of the level of consciousness, the Glasgow coma scale (GCS) measures consciousness by an objective numerical scale (Table 20-34 on p. 597). Caution is needed in using the scale with clients who have sensory losses. For example, a client may not respond to a nurse's presence if both sight and hearing are impaired.

As consciousness deteriorates, a client becomes disoriented to name, time, and place. The nurse asks questions regarding information that the client knows and that are short and to the point (for example, "Tell me your name," "What's the name of this place?" and "What day is this?") The client's ability to understand and answer questions has a direct effect on the nurse's ability to perform a complete examina-

TABLE 20-34 Glasgow Coma Scale		
Action	**Response**	**Score**
Eyes open	Spontaneously	④
	To speech	3
	To pain	2
	None	1
Best verbal response	Oriented	⑤
	Confused	4
	Inappropriate words	3
	Incomprehensible sounds	2
	None	1
Best motor response	Obeys commands	⑥
	Localized pain	5
	Flexion withdrawal	4
	Abnormal flexion	3
	Abnormal extension	2
	Flaccid	1
	Total Score	⑮

Client Teaching During Neurological Assessment

OBJECTIVES

- Client's family will understand relationship of client's behavioral and mental changes to physical status.
- Client with sensory or motor impairment will select safety measures for self-care.
- Older adult will routinely inspect skin for injuries.

TEACHING STRATEGIES

- Explain to family or friends the neurological implications of any behavioral or mental impairment shown by the client.
- If the client has sensory or motor impairments, explain measures to ensure safety (e.g., use of ambulation aids or safety bars in bathrooms or stairways).
- Teach the older adult to plan enough time to complete tasks because reaction time is slowed.
- Teach older adult to observe skin surfaces for areas of trauma because perception of pain is reduced.

EVALUATION

- Ask family to discuss client behaviors that result from neurological impairments.
- Have client explain safety measures used to avoid injury from sensory and motor limitations.
- Have older client explain reason for inspecting skin surface routinely.

tion. The client must be aroused to full alertness before the assessment can be conducted.

Eventually a client may be unable to follow simple commands such as "Squeeze my finger" or "Move your toes." At this lowered level of consciousness the client often is responsive only to painful stimuli. The nurse tests the client by applying firm pressure with the thumb over the root of the fingernail. The client should withdraw the hand from the painful stimulus. In cases of serious neurological impairment a client exhibits abnormal posturing in response to pain. A flaccid response indicates an absence of muscle tone in the extremities and severe injury to brain tissue.

The GCS allows the nurse to evaluate a client's neurological status over time. The higher the score, the more improved or normal the level of functioning.

Behavior and Appearance

Behaviors, moods, hygiene, grooming, and choice of dress reveal pertinent information about a client's mental status. The nurse must be perceptive of mannerisms and actions during the entire physical assessment. The nurse notes whether the client responds appropriately to directions and observes the mood throughout the examination. The nurse notices the manner of speech and level of participation in the examination procedures (see teaching box).

Appearance reflects how a client feels about the self. Personal hygiene, such as unkempt hair, a dirty body, or broken, dirty fingernails, should be noted. The nurse observes the cleanliness, fit, and state of

repair of clothes. Also the nurse observes whether the client's choice of clothing is appropriate to the setting or type of weather. An unkempt appearance can result from a poor self-image, an unexpected emergency, an inability to keep clothing clean, or an inability to perform grooming, rather than a mental problem.

Older adults frequently wear clothing that fits improperly. Many ready-to-wear garments are not designed to fit physical changes resulting from aging. Often older adults ignore their appearances because of a lack of energy, finances, incentive, or reduced vision. The nurse considers these factors before assuming that older adults have altered mental function.

Language

The ability of an individual to understand spoken or written words and to express the self through writing, words, or gestures is a function of the cerebral cortex. An injury to the cortex may result in a disorder known as *aphasia.* There are three types of aphasia: sensory (or receptive), motor (or expressive), and global (mixed sensory and motor). With receptive aphasia a person cannot understand written or verbal speech. With expressive aphasia a person understands written and verbal speech but cannot write or speak appropriately when attempting to communicate. A client with global aphasia is unable to understand speech or express the self.

The nurse assesses language capabilities when it is clear that communication with the client is ineffective. Some simple assessment techniques include the following:

1. Asking the client to name a familiar object to which the nurse points
2. Asking the client to respond to simple verbal and written commands such as "Stand up" or "Sit down"
3. Asking the client to read simple sentences out loud

Intellectual Function

Intellectual function includes memory (recent, immediate, and past), knowledge, abstract thinking, association, and judgment. Each aspect of intellectual function is tested through a specific assessment technique. However, because cultural and educational background has a significant bearing on the ability to respond to the test questions, the nurse should not ask questions related to concepts or ideas with which the client is unfamiliar.

Memory

The nurse assesses immediate recall and recent and remote memory. Often a problem with memory becomes apparent when the nurse takes the nursing history. To assess immediate recall, the nurse has the client repeat a series of numbers (for example, 7, 4, 1) or repeat a series of numbers backward.

The nurse gradually increases the number of digits (for example, 7, 4, 1, 8, 6) until the client fails to repeat the digits correctly. Normally an individual is able to repeat a series of 5 to 8 digits forward and 4 to 6 digits backward.

To assess recent memory, the nurse asks clients to recall events occurring during the same day (for example, what they had for breakfast or lunch and how they came to the hospital or health care facility). Accuracy of this information should be validated with a family member or witness. The nurse also has clients recall information shared earlier during the interview (for example, name of nurse). To assess past memory, the nurse asks clients to recall their previous medical histories or family histories. The nurse also

asks the client when their birthdays or anniversaries are.

It is common for older adults to show symptoms of confusion and forgetfulness because of normal neurological changes. Sudden confusion, however, is usually not related to age. Older adults are simply at greater risk to become confused by acute conditions such as dehydration, infection, drug toxicity, or hypoglycemia. In addition, hearing loss often falsely leads to a decision that older adults are confused. When an older adult experiences gradual, progressive deterioration in mental function, Alzheimer's disease should be suspected (see Chapter 27).

Knowledge

The nurse can assess knowledge by asking clients what they know about their illnesses or the reason for seeking health care. By assessing knowledge, the nurse determines clients' abilities to learn or understand. If an opportunity to teach exists, the nurse can test mental status by asking for feedback during a follow-up visit.

Abstract Thinking

Interpreting abstract ideas or concepts reflects the capacity for abstract thinking. A higher level of intellectual functioning is required for an individual to explain such phrases as "A stitch in time saves nine" or "Don't count your chickens before they're hatched." The nurse notes whether the explanations are relevant and concrete. The client with altered mentation will likely interpret the phrase literally or merely rephrase the words.

Association

Another higher level of intellectual function involves finding similarities or associations between concepts: a dog is to a beagle as a cat is to a Siamese. The nurse names related concepts and asks the client to identify their associations. It is sufficient to use simple concepts.

Judgment

Judgment requires a comparison and evaluation of facts and ideas to understand their relationships and to form appropriate conclusions. The nurse attempts to measure the ability to make logical decisions. By assessing judgment the nurse also measures the ability to organize thought processes. The nurse may choose to ask clients why they decided to seek health care or how they plan to adjust to limitations after returning home. A simpler test would involve asking what the clients would do if placed in a situation such as being locked out of their homes or suddenly becoming ill when alone at home.

Cranial Nerve Function

The nurse may assess all 12 cranial nerves or test a single nerve or related group of nerves. A test of the oculomotor nerve measures pupillary response. Assessment of the glossopharyngeal and vagus nerves reveal integrity of the gag reflex. Measurements used to assess the integrity of organs within the head and neck also assess cranial nerve function. For example, the cochlear branch of the eighth cranial nerve is tested during a hearing assessment. The function of the ninth and tenth nerves can be assessed during examination of the pharynx. A dysfunction in any nerve reflects an alteration at some point along the cranial nerve's distribution. Cranial nerve assessment is easy after the nurse is familiar with the nerve's normal functions. To remember the order of the 12 nerves, the nurse can use this simple phrase, "On old Olympus' towering tops, a Finn and German viewed some hops." The first letter of each word in the phrase is the same as the first letter of the names of the cranial nerves (Table 20-35).

TABLE 20-35 Cranial Nerve Function and Assessment

Number	Name	Type	Function	Method
I	Olfactory	Sensory	Sense of smell	Ask client to identify different non-irritating aromas such as coffee and vanilla.
II	Optic	Sensory	Visual acuity	Use Snellen chart or ask client to read printed material while wearing glasses.
III	Oculomotor	Motor	Extraocular eye movement	Assess directions of gaze.
			Pupil constriction and dilation	Measure pupil reaction to light reflex and accommodation.
IV	Trochlear	Motor	Upward and downward movement of eyeball	Assess directions of gaze.
V	Trigeminal	Sensory and motor	Sensory nerve to skin of face	Lightly touch cornea with wisp of cotton. Assess corneal reflex. Measure sensation of light pain and touch across skin of face.
			Motor nerve to muscles of jaw	Palpate temples as client clenches teeth.
VI	Abducens	Motor	Lateral movement of eyeballs	Assess directions of gaze.
VII	Facial	Sensory and motor	Facial expression	As client smiles, frowns, puffs out cheeks, and raises and lowers eyebrows look for asymetry.
			Taste	Have client identify salty or sweet taste on front of tongue.
VIII	Auditory	Sensory	Hearing	Assess ability to hear spoken word.
IX	Glossopharyngeal	Sensory and motor	Taste	Ask client to identify sour or sweet taste on back of tongue.
			Ability to swallow	Use tongue blade to elicit gag reflex.
X	Vagus	Sensory and motor	Sensation of pharynx	Ask client to say "ah." Observe palate and pharynx movement.
			Ability to swallow	Use tongue blade to elicit gag reflex.
			Movement of vocal cords	Assess speech for hoarseness.
XI	Spinal accessory	Motor	Movement of head and shoulders	Ask client to shrug shoulders and turn head against passive resistance.
XII	Hypoglossal	Motor	Position of tongue	Ask client to stick out tongue to midline and move it from side to side.

Sensory Function

The sensory pathways of the central nervous system conduct sensations of pain, temperature, position, vibration, and crude and finely localized touch. Different nerve pathways relay the sensations. For most clients a quick screening of sensory function is sufficient. However, clients who have symptoms of altered or decreased sensation, who have motor impairment, or who have paralysis require more extensive examinations.

Normally a client has sensory responses to all stimuli that are tested. Sensations along the body's surface are felt equally on both sides of the face, trunk, and extremities. A nurse can assess the major sensory nerves by knowing the sensory dermatone zones (Fig. 20-89). Some areas of the skin are innervated by specific dorsal root cutaneous nerves. For example, if the nurse notes reduced sensation when checking for light touch along an area of the skin (for example, the lower neck), the nurse can determine, in general, where a neurological lesion may exist (for example, fourth cervical spinal cord segment).

All sensory testing is performed with the client's eyes closed so that the client is unable to see when or where a stimulus strikes the skin (Table 20-36 on p. 602). Stimuli are applied in a random, unpredictable order to maintain the client's attention and prevent detection of a predictable pattern. The client is asked to say when the particular stimulus is felt. The nurse compares symmetrical areas of the body while applying stimuli to the client's arms, trunk, and legs.

Motor Function

An assessment of motor function includes the same measurements made during the musculoskeletal examination. In addition, cerebellar function is assessed. The cerebellum coordinates muscular activity by producing smooth, steady, and efficient movements of muscle groups. The maintenance of balance and equilibrium is also a function of the cerebellum. Sensory impulses from the vestibular portion of the inner ear travel to the cerebellum, where impulses are relayed to proper motor nerves to maintain body equilibrium. The cerebellum also controls posture.

CUTANEOUS INNERVATION FOR SENSORY ASSESSMENT

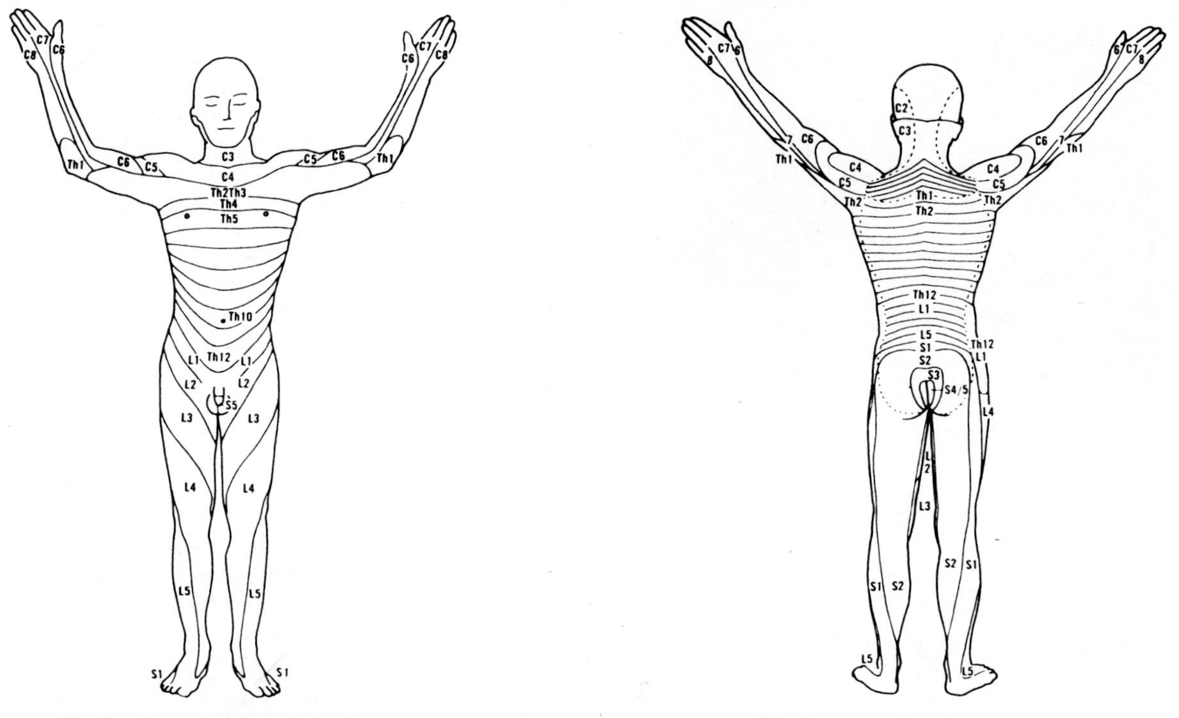

The dermatomes from the anterior view.

The dermatomes from the posterior view.

Fig. 20-89   Sensory dermatone areas overlying the human body.
From Thelan LA, Dane JK, Urden LD: *Textbook of critical care nursing: diagnosis and management*, St Louis, 1990, Mosby–Year Book.

TABLE 20-36	Assessment of Sensory Nerve Function		
Function	**Equipment**	**Method**	**Precautions**
Pain	Safety pin	Ask client to voice when dull or sharp sensation is felt. Alternately apply pointed and blunt ends of pin to skin's surface. Note areas of numbness or increased sensitivity.	Remember that areas where skin is thickened, such as heel or sole of foot, may be less sensitive to pain.
Temperature	Two test tubes, one filled with hot water and other with cold	Touch skin with tube. Ask client to identify hot or cold sensation.	Omit test if pain sensation is normal.
Light touch	Cotton ball or cotton-tip applicator	Apply light wisp of cotton to different points along skin's surface. Ask client to voice when sensation is felt.	Apply at areas where skin is thin or more sensitive (e.g., face, neck, inner aspect of arms, top of feet and hands).

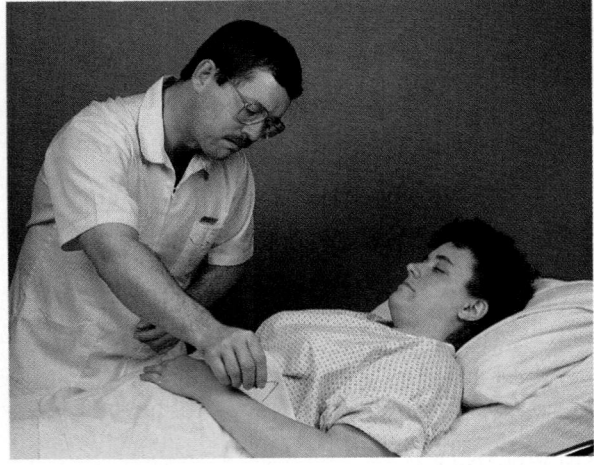

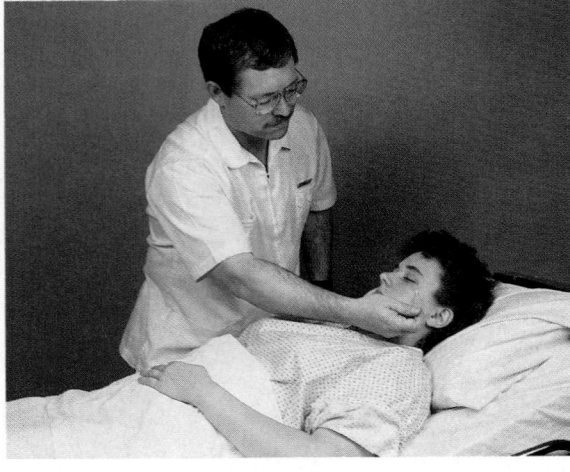

Coordination

It is difficult for the nurse to explain the tests used to measure coordination. To avoid confusion the nurse demonstrates each maneuver and then has clients repeat it after determining that their mobility is normal and they are physically able to make the necessary movements. The nurse observes the smoothness and balance of movements (see teaching box on p. 598). In older adults a slow reaction time may cause movements to be less rhythmical.

Performing rapid, rhythmical, alternating movements demonstrates coordination in the upper extremities. First, the client pats a hand against the thigh as fast as possible while sitting. The client should be able to strike the thigh rapidly and evenly without hesitation. Next the client alternately strikes the thigh with the hand supinated and then pronated. The speed and symmetry of movement are noted. An additional maneuver for upper extremity coordination involves touching each finger with the

TABLE 20-36	Assessment of Sensory Nerve Function—cont'd		
Function	Equipment	Method	Precautions
Vibration	Tuning fork	Apply vibrating fork to distal interphalangeal joint of fingers and interphalangeal joint of great toe. Have client voice when the vibration stops.	Be sure client feels vibration and not merely pressure.
Position		Grasp finger, holding it by its sides with thumb and index finger. Alternate moving finger up and down. Ask client to state when finger is up or down. Repeat with toes.	Avoid rubbing adjacent appendages as finger or toe is moved.
Two-point discrimination	Two safety pins	Lightly apply points of two safety pins simultaneously to skin's surface. Ask client if one or two pinpricks are felt.	Apply pins to same anatomical site (e.g., fingertips, palm of hand, or upper arms). Minimum distance at which client can discriminate two points varies (2-3 mm on fingertips).

thumb of the same hand in rapid sequence. The client's dominant hand is slightly less awkward when performing this movement.

A final measurement of upper extremity coordination involves the point-to-point test. The nurse stands in front of clients holding an index finger 2 feet in front of their faces. Clients are instructed to touch the nurse's finger with their index fingers and then to touch their noses. Clients move their fingers back and forth repeatedly. The nurse looks for any tremor of the hands or awkwardness in movement. The test may be repeated with clients' eyes closed.

Lower extremity coordination is tested with the client lying supine. The nurse places a hand at the ball of the client's foot. The client taps the nurse's hand with the foot as quickly as possible. Each foot is tested for speed and smoothness. The feet do not move as rapidly or evenly as the hands.

A final test involves having the client sit with eyes closed and placing the heel of the foot on the opposite knee. The client then slides the heel down the opposite leg to the foot. This maneuver normally is performed evenly without the heel sliding off the leg.

Balance

The nurse may use one or two of the following tests to assess balance and gross motor function:
1. Have the client perform a Romberg test by standing with feet together and eyes closed.

While protecting the client's safety by standing at the side, observe swaying. Slight swaying is normal in an older adult. The client normally does not have to break the stance.
2. Have the client close the eyes and stand on one foot and then the other.
3. Ask the client to walk a straight line by placing the heel of one foot directly in front of the toes of the other foot.

Reflexes

Eliciting reflex reactions allows the nurse to assess the integrity of sensory and motor pathways of the reflex arc and specific spinal cord segments. Assessment of reflexes does not determine higher neural center functioning. Fig. 20-90 on p. 604 traces the pathway of the reflex arc. Each muscle contains a small sensory unit called a *muscle spindle,* which controls muscle tone and detects changes in the length of muscle fibers. By tapping a tendon with a reflex hammer, the nurse stretches the muscle and tendon, lengthening the spindle. The spindle sends nerve impulses along afferent nerve pathways to the dorsal horn of the spinal cord segment. Within milliseconds the impulses reach the spinal cord and synapse to travel to the efferent motor neuron in the spinal cord. A motor nerve sends the impulses back to the muscle, causing the reflex response.

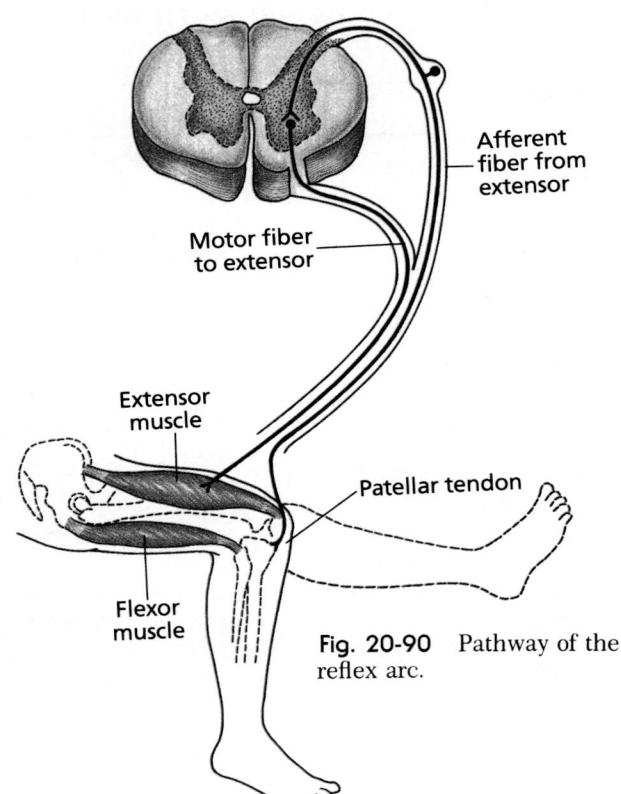

Fig. 20-90 Pathway of the reflex arc.

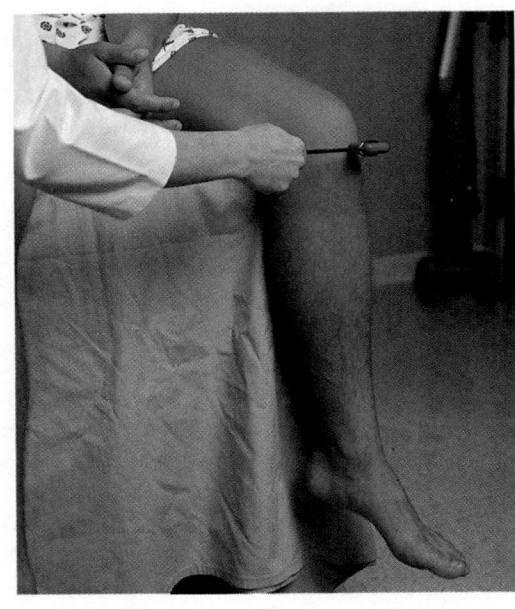

Fig. 20-91 Position for eliciting the patellar tendon reflex. The lower leg normally extends.

TABLE 20-37 Assessment of Common Reflexes

Type	Procedure	Normal Reflex
DEEP TENDON REFLEXES		
Biceps	Flex client's arm at elbow with palms down. Place your thumb in antecubital fossa at base of biceps tendon. Strike thumb with reflex hammer.	Flexion of arm at elbow
Triceps	Flex client's elbow, holding arm across chest, or hold upper arm horizontally and allow lower arm to go limp. Strike triceps tendon just above elbow.	Extension at elbow
Patellar	Have client sit with legs hanging freely over side of bed or chair or have client lie supine and support knee in flexed position. Briskly tap patellar tendon just below patella.	Extension of lower leg at knee
Achilles	Have client assume same position as for patellar reflex. Slightly dorsiflex client's ankle by grasping toes in palm of your hand. Strike Achilles tendon just above heel.	Plantar flexion of foot
Plantar (Babinski's)	Have client lie supine with legs straight and feet relaxed. Take handle end of reflex hammer and stroke lateral aspect of sole from heel to ball of foot, curving across ball of foot toward big toe.	Bending of toes downward
CUTANEOUS REFLEXES		
Gluteal	Have client assume side-lying position. Spread buttocks apart and lightly stimulate perineal area with cotton applicator.	Contraction of anal sphincter
Abdominal	Have client stand or lie supine. Stroke abdominal skin with base of cotton applicator over lateral borders of rectus abdominis muscle toward midline. Repeat test in each abdominal quadrant.	Contraction of rectus abdominis muscle with pulling of umbilicus toward stimulated side

The two categories of normal reflexes are deep tendon reflexes, elicited by mildly stretching a muscle and tapping a tendon, and cutaneous reflexes, elicited by stimulating the skin superficially. Reflexes are graded as follows:

0   No response
1+   Low normal with slight muscle contraction
2+   Normal with visible muscle twitch and movement of the arm or leg
3+   Brisker than normal; may not indicate disease
4+   Hyperactive and very brisk; often associated with spinal cord disorders

When reflexes are being assessed, the client should relax as much as possible to avoid voluntary movement or tensing of muscles. The nurse positions the limbs to slightly stretch the muscle being tested. The reflex hammer is held loosely between the nurse's thumb and fingers so that it can swing freely and tap the tendon briskly (Fig. 20-91). The nurse compares the symmetry of the reflex from one side of the body to the other. In the older adult, reflexes are normally slowed. Practitioners often use stick figures to record reflexes. Table 20-37 summarizes common deep tendon and cutaneous reflexes.

 ## AFTER THE EXAMINATION

The nurse may choose to record findings from the physical assessment during the examination or at the end. Most institutions have special forms that make it easy to record examination data. The nurse reviews all findings before assisting the client with dressing, in case there is a need to recheck any information or gather additional data. Findings from physical assessment are integrated into the care plan.

After completing the assessment, the nurse assists the client in dressing if necessary. The hospitalized client may need help in returning to bed and assuming a comfortable position. When the client is comfortable, it helps to share a summary of the assessment findings. If the findings have revealed serious abnormalities such as a mass or highly irregular heart rate, the client's physician should be consulted before any findings are revealed. It is the physician's responsibility to make definitive medical diagnoses. The nurse can explain the type of abnormality found and the need for the physician to conduct an additional examination.

The nurse also cleans the examination area, storing all reusable equipment and disposing of materials that cannot be reused. Infection-control practices are used in removing materials or instruments soiled with potentially infectious wastes (see Chapter 18). Afterward, the nurse washes hands. If the client's

bedside was the examination site, the nurse clears away soiled items from the table and makes sure the bed linen is dry and clean. The client may appreciate a clean gown and the opportunity to wash the face and hands.

The nurse checks to be sure the recording of the assessment is complete. If entry of items into the assessment form was delayed, the nurse records them at this time to avoid forgetting any important information. If entries were made periodically during the examination, they are reviewed for accuracy and thoroughness. Significant findings are communicated to appropriate medical and nursing personnel, either verbally or in the written care plan.

The client often needs a number of ancillary examinations such as x-ray examinations, laboratory tests, or ultrasonography after a physical examination. These tests provide additional screening information to rule out the presence of abnormalities and help in the diagnosis of specific abnormalities found during the examination.

 ## SUMMARY

Through physical assessment, the nurse makes insightful clinical decisions that contribute to the client's health management. Each body system is reviewed following a methodical sequence of observations and measurements. Information gathered during physical assessment supplements data obtained in the nursing history and from ongoing nurse-client interactions. As a result of more thorough data gathering, the nurse is able to make nursing diagnoses with greater precision. Therefore the care plan becomes more individualized and comprehensive. Physical assessment findings also reveal whether specific nursing measures were successful in managing client problems.

Before an examination begins, the nurse takes the necessary steps to prepare the client and setting. Measures are taken to ensure privacy and psychological and physical comfort and reduce the transmission of microorganisms. Clients become active participants as the nurse carefully explains each step of the examination. It is important to organize the examination. Each system review entails many observations. Basic principles for a thorough examination include comparing both sides of the body for symmetry, completing each system before moving to the next, using each skill as appropriate, and recognizing the observations that have priority for clients. The nurse can use time during an assessment to provide important information about how clients can maintain or improve their health.

CHAPTER 20 REVIEW

Key Concepts

- Baseline assessment findings reflect functional abilities when the nurse first assesses the client and serve as the basis for comparison with subsequent assessment findings.

- Assessment data can be used to evaluate the physiological outcomes of nursing care.

- Physical assessment of a child or infant requires the nurse to apply principles of physical growth and development.

- The nurse recognizes that the normal process of aging affects physical findings collected from an older adult.

- Client teaching should be integrated throughout the examination to help clients understand the implications of all findings.

- The nurse can use time more efficiently by integrating physical assessment with routine nursing care.

- Inspection requires good lighting, full exposure of the body part, and a careful comparison of the part with its counterpart on the opposite side of the body.

- A good stethoscope should have earpieces that fit snugly, a flexible thick-walled tubing of the proper length, and a chestpiece with a bell and diaphragm.

- A physical examination should be performed only after proper preparation of the environment and equipment and after preparing the client physically and psychologically.

- Throughout the examination the nurse should keep the client warm, comfortable, and informed of each step of the process.

- The client assumes various positions during the physical examination to provide greater accessibility of body parts and to increase accuracy in assessment.

- The nurse uses a systematic approach when conducting a physical assessment.

- When assessing a seriously ill client, the nurse concentrates on the body systems most likely to be affected.

- Information from the nursing history helps the nurse focus on specific parts of the examination.

- Accuracy in assessing the thorax, heart, and abdomen is enhanced by creating a mental image of internal organs in relation to external anatomical landmarks.

- When assessing heart sounds, the nurse imagines events occurring during the cardiac cycle.

- The carotid arteries should never be palpated simultaneously.

- When examining a woman's breasts, the nurse explains the techniques for breast self-examinations.

- The abdominal assessment differs from other portions of the examination in that auscultation follows inspection.

- If the client and nurse are of opposite sexes, a nurse of the same sex as the client should be present during examination of the genitalia.

- During assessment of the male genitalia, the nurse explains the techniques for testicular self-examination.
- Assessment of musculoskeletal function can easily be conducted when observing the client ambulate or participate in other active movements.
- The nurse assesses mental and emotional status by interacting with the client throughout the examination.

Key Terms

Critical Thinking Exercises

1. You inspect Mr. Smiley's skin overlying the right forearm and find it to be reddened. Identify two possible causes for the skin color change. Describe any additional assessment you would measure to further understand the cause.

2. When assisting a client in setting up a meal tray and preparing for a meal, identify four different body systems you might choose to assess during this time.

3. The nurse finds Mr. Wilson experiencing acute abdominal pain during admission to the emergency room. His family is present and reports that he fell from a tree while pruning and was briefly kocked unconscious. What three major body systems would you assess as a priority for Mr. Wilson?

4. Two body systems are assessed when determining the nature of edema; identify each.

5. What physical examination measures would you use to evaluate chest pain, application of a warm moist pack to the lower back, range of motion exercises, and tingling of the fingers?

6. An elderly woman with reduced visual acuity would have difficulty performing what aspect of a breast self-examination?

7. Explain the difference you would expect in examining the skin and vision of a 40-year-old man and 78-year-old man.

REFERENCES

American Cancer Society: *1991 Cancer facts and figures,* New York, 1991, The Society.

Berman R, Haxby JV, Pomerantz RS: Physiology of aging. I. Normal changes, *Patient Care* 22:20, 1988.

Cerrato P: Can a low-fat diet prevent breast cancer? *RN* 50:63, 1987.

Champion VL: Effect of knowledge, teaching method, confidence and social influence on breast self-examination behavior, *Image J Nurs Sch* 21(2):76 1989.

DeWitt S: Nursing assessment of the skin and dermatologic lesions, *Nurs Clin North Am,* 25(1): 235, 1990.

Elder abuse common: clues help identify high-risk patients, *Geriatrics* 42:26, 1987.

Geriatrics: 1987.

Henderson M: Less frequent screening? perhaps, for some, *Consultant* 28(2):209, 1989.

Jacobs R: Physical changes in the aged. In Devereaux M et al, editors: *Elder care: a guide to clinical geriatrics,* New York, 1981, Grune & Stratton.

Kpea NT: Easily observed signs of systemic disease, *Consultant* 27(8):47, 1987.

Larson E: Evaluating validity of screening tests, *Nurs Res* 35:186, 1986.

Leather DS, Roberts MM: Older women's attitudes toward breast disease, self-examination, and screening facilities: implications for communication, *BMJ* 290:668, 1985.

McConnell E: Getting the feel of lymph node assessment, *Nurs 88* 18:55, 1988.

McConnell E: Auscultating bowel sounds, *Nurs 90* 20:106, 1990.

Miracle VA: Get in touch and tune with cardiac assessment. I. *Nurs 88* 18:41, 1988.

Parrino TA: The art and science of percussion, *Hosp Pract,* 15:25, 1987.

Reed AT, Birge SJ: Screening for osteoporosis, *J Gerontol Nurs* 14(7):18, 1988.

Rossman I: Anatomy of aging. In Rossman I, editor: *Clinical geriatrics,* ed 2, Philadelphia, 1979, Lippincott.

Schatz IJ: Orthostatic hypotension. II. Clinical diagnosis, testing, and treatment, *Arch Intern Med* 144:1037, 1984.

Seymour C et al: Influence of position during examination and sex of examiner on patient anxiety during pelvic examination, *J Pediatr* 108:312, 1986.

Swan IRC: The Rinne tuning fork test, *Hosp Pract* 17:99, 1989.

Williams ED, Edwards D, Hane N: Barriers to breast cancer screening in older women, *Fam Community Health* 10(3):51, 1987.

ADDITIONAL READINGS

Baas L, Kretten C: Valvular heart disease: its causes, symptoms and consequences, *RN* 50:30, 1987.

Becker KL, Stevens SA: Performing in-depth abdominal assessment, *Nurs 88* 18(6):59 1988.

Berliner H: Aging skin. I. *Am J Nurs* 86:1208, 1986.

Berliner H: Aging skin. II. *Am J Nurs* 86:1259, 1986.

Berman R, Haxby JV, Pomerantz RS: Physiology of aging. II. Clinical implications, *Patient Care* 23:39, 1989.

Blair JD: A quick, high-yield mouth exam, *Patient Care* 20:33, 1985.

Burggraf V, Donlon B: Assessing the elderly, system by system, *Am J Nurs* 85:974, 1985.

Calvani D: Assessing the elderly. II. *Am J Nurs* 85:1103, 1985.

Casey MP: Testicular cancer: the worst disease at the worst time, *RN* 50:36, 1987.

Cerrato PL: Can a low-fat diet prevent breast cancer? *RN* 50:63, 1987.

Cerrato PL: Spotting the patient who looks healthy but isn't, *RN* 52:81 1989.

Dennison R: Cardiopulmonary assessment, *Nurs 86* 16:34, 1986.

Durham CF: The no-fault way to assess carotid arteries, *Nurs 88,* 18:65, 1988.

Ebersole P, Hess P: *Toward healthy aging: human needs and nursing response,* ed 3, St Louis, 1990, Mosby–Year Book.

Erickson BA: Detecting abnormal heart sounds, *Nurs 86* 16:58, 1986.

Ernst ND: The national cholesterol education program's recommendations for treatment of high blood cholesterol, *Fam Community Health* 12(1):23, 1989.

Forgacs P: The functional basis of pulmonary sounds, *Chest* 73:399, 1978.

Fraser MC, McGuire DB: Skin cancer's early warning system, *Am J Nurs* 84:1232, 1984.

Handerhan B: How to measure jugular venous distension, *Nurs 87* Sept 1987, p 48.

Hays AM, Borger F: Assessing the elderly: a test in-time, *Am J Nurs* 85:1107, 1985.

Henderson M: Less frequent screening? Perhaps, for some, *Consultant* 28(2):209, 1989

Henderson ML: Assessing the elderly: altered perception, *Am J Nurs* 85:1104, 1985.

Hurst JW et al: Noises in the neck, *N Engl J Med* 302:862, 1980.

Kirton M, Richardson M: *Ophthalmic nursing,* ed 3, Philadelphia, 1987, Baillière-Tindall.

Lewis R: Pap smears: a closer look, *Health* 19(4):69, 1987.

Lindsey M: Abdominal assessment, *Orthop Nurs* 8(4):34, 1989.

Mahboub E, Sayed GM: oral cavity and pharynx. In Schottenfeld D, Fraumeni JF Jr, editors: *Cancer epidemiology and prevention,* Philadelphia, 1982, Saunders.

McHugh J, McHugh W: How to assess deep tendon reflexes, *Nurs 90* 20:62, 1990.

Memmer MK: Acute orthostatic hypertension, *Heart Lung,* 17(2):4, 1988.

Miracle VA: Anatomy of a murmur, *Nurs 86* 16:26, 1986.

National Institutes of Health: Osteoporosis: cause, treatment, prevention, *Orthop Nurs,* Nov/Dec 1985, p 29.

Phipps W et al: *Medical-surgical nursing: concepts and clinical practice,* ed 4, St Louis, 1991, Mosby–Year Book.

Prigel CLB: How to spot melanoma, *Nurs 87* June 1987, p 60.

Rubin D: Gynecologic cancer: cervical, vulvar, and vaginal malignancies, *RN* 50:56, 1987.

Rubin D: Gynecologic cancer: uterine and ovarian malignancies, *RN* 50(6):52, 1987.

Rudolph A, McDermott RJ: The breast physical examination: its value in early cancer detection, *Cancer Nurs* 10(2):100, 1987.

Rumpler C: Breast problems. In Griffith-Kennney J, editor: *Contemporary women's health: a nursing advocacy approach,* Menlo Park, Calif, 1986, Addison-Wesley.

Rutledge DN: Factors related to women's practice of breast self-examination, *Nurs Res* 36:117, 1987.

Santo-Novak DA: Seven keys to assessing the elderly, *Nurs 88,* 18(8):60, 1988.

Seidel HM et al: *Mosby's guide to physical examination,* ed 2, St Louis, 1991, Mosby–Year Book.

Smith C: Assessing bowel sounds: more than just listening, *Nurs 88* 18:42, 1988.

Stanford J: Testicular self-examination: teaching, learning and practice by nurses, *J Adv Nurs* 12:13, 1987.

Swanson DA: Why you should conscientiously promote self-examination, *Consultant* April 1987, p 142.

Wech E: Taking a look at eye exams, *FDA Consumer* May 1987, p 14.

Weinrich SP et al: Timely detection of colorectal cancer in the elderly: implications of the aging process, *Cancer Nurs* 12(3):170, 1989.

Whaley LF, Wong DL: *Nursing care of infants and children,* ed 4, St Louis, 1991, Mosby–Year Book.

Wilkins, RL: *Lung sounds: a practical guide,* St Louis, 1988, Mosby–Year Book.

Willett W et al: Dietary fat and the risk of breast cancer, *N Engl J Med* 316:22, 1987.

Yacone LA: Cardiac assessment: what to do, how to do it, *RN* 50:42, 1987.

CHAPTER 21

Administration of Medications

OBJECTIVES

Mastery of content in this chapter will enable the student to:

- Define the key terms listed.
- Discuss the nurse's legal responsibilities in drug prescription and administration.
- Describe the physiological mechanisms of drug action, including absorption, distribution, metabolism, and excretion.
- Differentiate among toxic, idiosyncratic, allergic, and side effects of drugs.
- Discuss developmental factors that influence drug pharmacokinetics.
- Discuss factors that influence drug actions.
- Discuss methods of educating a client about medications.
- Describe the roles of the pharmacist, physician, and nurse in drug administration.
- Describe factors to consider in choosing routes of administration.
- Correctly calculate a prescribed drug dosage.
- Assess the client's need for and response to drug therapy.
- List the "five rights" of drug administration.
- Correctly prepare and administer subcutaneous, intramuscular, and intradermal injections and intravenous medication; insulin injections; oral medications; topical skin preparations; eye, ear, and nose drops; vaginal instillations; rectal suppositories; and inhalants.

CHAPTER OUTLINE

The safe and accurate administration of medications is one of the nurse's most important responsibilities. Drugs are a primary means of therapy for clients with health problems, but any drug has the potential for causing harmful effects when administered improperly. The nurse is responsible for understanding a drug's action and its side effects, administering it correctly, monitoring the client's response, and helping the client self-administer drugs correctly and knowledgeably.

In addition to knowing about a specific drug's action, the nurse must also understand the client's previous and current health problems to determine whether a particular medication is safe to give. The nurse's judgment is critical for proper and safe drug administration.

DRUG NOMENCLATURE AND FORMS

A drug or **medication** is a substance used in the diagnosis, treatment, cure, relief, or prevention of disease. Health care personnel use the term *drugs* and *medications* interchangeably. Lay persons commonly refer to medications as *medicines*.

Physicians and dentists prescribe the majority of medications in the United States and Canada. However, in a few states, nurse practitioners and physician assistants may prescribe selected medications with the supervision of a physician.

Names

A single medication may have as many as four different names. The *chemical name* provides an exact description of the drug's composition. An example of a chemical name is acetylsalicylic acid, known commonly as *aspirin*. The generic name is given by the manufacturer who first develops the drug before it receives official approval. Protected by law, the generic name is given before a drug receives official approval. Aspirin and verapamil hydrochloride are examples of generic names. Federal legislation in 1962 mandated that there be one official name for each drug. The official name of a drug is the name under which the drug is listed in official publications such as the *United States Pharmacopeia (USP)*. A drug's generic name often becomes its official name, as with aspirin.

The trade name, brand name, or proprietary name is the name under which a manufacturer markets a drug. A generic drug may have many different trade names. For example, aspirin is known by the trade name Bufferin, and verapamil hydrochloride is known by the trade names Calan and Isoptin. The

trade name has the symbol ® at the upper right of the name, indicating that the drug has been registered. Manufacturers try to choose trade names that are easier to pronounce and spell to help the lay person recognize and remember the medications more readily. Because many companies may produce the same drug, similarities in trade names can be confusing. The nurse encounters medications under a variety of different nomenclatures or names and must be careful to obtain the exact name and spelling for a particular drug.

Classification

Nurses categorize medications with similar characteristics by their class. Drug classification indicates the effect on a body system, the symptoms relieved, or the desired effect. Each class contains drugs prescribed for similar types of health problems. The physical and chemical composition of drugs within a class is not necessarily the same. A drug may also belong to more than one class. For example, aspirin is an analgesic, an antipyretic, and an antiinflammatory drug.

Nurses should know the general characteristics of medications in each class. Each class has nursing implications for proper administration and monitoring. For example, nursing implications related to diuretic administration include monitoring intake and output, weighing the client daily, assessing the development of edema in body tissues, and monitoring serum electrolyte levels. Nursing implications for all drugs within a class provide guidelines for safe and effective care.

Drug Forms

Drugs are available in a variety of forms or preparations. The form of the drug determines its route of administration. For example, a capsule is taken orally, and a solution may be given intravenously. The composition of a drug is designed to enhance its absorption and metabolism within the body. Many drugs are available in several forms such as tablets, capsules, elixirs, and suppositories. When administering a medication, the nurse must be certain to give the medication in the proper form (Table 21-1).

DRUG LEGISLATION AND STANDARDS

Drug Standards

In 1906, the U.S. government set standards for drug quality and purity as a result of the Pure Food

TABLE 21-1 Forms of Medication	
Form	Description
Caplet	Solid dosage form for oral use; shaped like capsule and coated for ease of swallowing
Capsule	Solid dosage form for oral use; medication in powder, liquid, or oil form and encased by gelatin shell; capsule colored to aid in product identification
Elixir	Clear fluid containing water and/or alcohol; designed for oral use; usually has sweetener added
Enteric-coated tablet	Tablet for oral use coated with materials that do not dissolve in stomach; coatings dissolve in intestine, where medication is absorbed
Extract	Concentrated drug form made by removing active portion of drug from its other components (e.g., fluid extract is drug made into solution from vegetable source)
Glycerite	Solution of drug combined with glycerin for external use; contains at least 50% glycerin
Liniment	Preparation usually containing alcohol, oil, or soapy emollient that is applied to skin
Lotion	Drug in liquid suspension applied externally to protect skin
Ointment (salve)	Semisolid, externally applied preparation, usually containing one or more drugs
Paste	Semisolid preparation, thicker and stiffer than ointment; absorbed through skin more slowly than ointment
Pill	Solid dosage form containing one or more drugs, shaped into globules, ovoids, or oblong shapes; true pills rarely used because they have been replaced by tablets
Solution	Liquid preparation that may be used orally, parenterally, or externally; can also be instilled into body organ or cavity (e.g., bladder irrigations); contains water with one or more dissolved compounds; must be sterile for parenteral use
Suppository	Solid dosage form mixed with gelatin and shaped in form of pellet for insertion into body cavity (rectum or vagina); melts when it reaches body temperature, releasing drug for absorption
Suspension	Finely divided drug particles dispersed in liquid medium; when suspension is left standing, particles settle to bottom of container; commonly oral medication and not given intravenously
Syrup	Medication dissolved in concentrated sugar solution; may contain flavoring to make drug more palatable
Tablet	Powdered dosage form compressed into hard disks or cylinders; in addition to primary drug, contains binders (adhesive to allow powder to stick together), disintegrators (to promote tablet dissolution), lubricants (for ease of manufacturing), and fillers (for convenient tablet size)
Transdermal disk or patch	Medication contained within semipermeable membrane disk or patch, which allows medications to be absorbed through skin slowly over long period
Tincture	Alcohol or water-alcohol drug solution
Troche (lozenge)	Flat, round dosage form containing drug, flavoring, sugar, and mucilage; dissolves in mouth to release drug

and Drug Act. Official publications—the *USP* and the *National Formulary*—set standards for drug strength, quality, purity, packaging, safety, labeling, and dosage form. In Canada the *British Pharmacopoeia (BP)* sets similar standards. Physicians, nurses, and pharmacists depend on these standards to ensure that clients receive pure drugs in safe and effective dosages. Accepted standards must be met in the following areas:

1. Purity. Manufacturers must meet purity standards for the type and concentration of other substances allowed in drug products.
2. Potency. The concentration of active drug in the preparation affects strength or potency.
3. Bioavailability. The ability of a drug to be released from its dosage form and dissolved, absorbed, and transported by the body to its site of action is its **bioavailability.**

4. Efficacy. Detailed laboratory studies can help determine a drug's effectiveness.
5. Safety. All drugs should be continually evaluated to determine their side effects.

Legislation and Control

In the United States, drug legislation began with the Pure Food and Drug Act of 1906. The act focused attention on the purity of food but also set official standards for drugs. Manufacturers were required to label drugs accurately and ensure that the strength and purity of drugs conformed to their claims. Since that time, federal law has extended and refined government controls on drug sales and distribution; drug testing, naming, and labeling; and the regulation of controlled substances (Tables 21-2 and 21-3 on p. 614).

TABLE 21-2 Federal Drug Laws in the United States

Date	Title of Law	Provisions
1906	Pure Food and Drug Act	Designated official standards for drugs (*USP* and the *National Formulary*); specified standards for drug labeling
1912	Sherley Amendment	Prohibited manufacturers from making fraudulent claims about drug efficacy and therapeutic effects
1914	Harrison Narcotic Act	Legally classified drugs believed to be habit forming as *narcotics;* regulated importation, manufacture, sale, and use of narcotic substances
1938	Federal Food, Drug, and Cosmetic Act	Added the *Homeopathic Pharmacopeia of the United States* as a third drug standard; required that drug preparation be approved as safe by the Food and Drug Administration (FDA) before marketing; further outlined criteria for drug labeling
1945	Amendment to the Food and Drug Act	Provided for certification of biological products used as drugs (e.g., insulin, antibiotics) on batch basis; allowed for direct supervision and inspection of drug production
1952	Durham-Humphrey Amendment	Distinguished between prescription ("legend") and nonprescription drugs
1962	Kefauver-Harris Amendment	Authorized FDA to supervise drug production to ensure safety and efficacy and to establish official drug names; specified greater controls on investigational drugs
1970	Comprehensive Drug Abuse Prevention and Control Act (Controlled Substances Act)	Set strict controls on manufacture and distribution of controlled drugs (possession of controlled substances unlawful without prescription); established government programs to promote prevention and treatment of drug dependence

TABLE 21-3 Canadian Drug Legislation

Date	Title of Law	Provisions
1908	Proprietary or Patent Medicine Act	Set standards to protect consumers from unsafe and ineffective nonprescription drugs
1953	Canadian Food and Drug Act	Prohibited sale of contaminated, unsafe drugs and of improperly labeled drugs; designated official standards (*Pharmacopoeia Internationalis, BP,* and *Canadian Formulary*); defined certain controlled drugs; prohibited advertising of prescription and controlled drugs to general public; set standards for labeling
1961	Canadian Narcotic Control Act	Restricted sale, possession, and use of narcotics; set guidelines for reporting loss of theft of narcotics; set standards for labeling and record keeping

State drug laws must conform with federal legislation. States can also impose additional controls, including control of substances not regulated by the federal government. For example, local governments can regulate the sale and use of alcohol and tobacco.

Health care institutions establish policies that conform to federal, state, and local regulations. The size of an institution, the types of services it provides, and the types of professional personnel it employs influence policies for drug control, distribution, and administration. Institutional policies are often more restrictive than government controls. An institution is primarily concerned with preventing health problems resulting from drug use. For example, a common institutional policy is the automatic discontinuation of antibiotic therapy after a set number of days. Although a physician may reorder an antibiotic, this policy helps to control unnecessarily prolonged drug therapy, which may lead to sensitivity or toxic reactions.

Federal, state, and local legislation governs nursing practice, including the administration of medications. State nurse practice acts define and set limits on the scope of a nurse's professional functions and responsibilities. These acts are joint policy statements made by nursing, medical, and hospital associations in a state. Institutions and agencies may interpret specific actions allowed under the acts but cannot modify, expand, or restrict the act's intent. The nurse practice acts protect the public from unskilled, undereducated, and unlicensed nurses.

Nurses must know the regulations affecting drug administration in their practice areas. When moving from one state to another, nurses may discover significant differences in the laws governing drug administration. For example, laws vary concerning the prescription and administration of intravenous (IV) drugs. In the past, only physicians prescribed medications. Today, several states have recognized the expanding role of the nurse and have revised nurse practice acts to include prescription of medications. In most cases, this privilege is limited to licensed nurse practitioners under the supervision of a physician.

Before assuming the responsibility of administering IV medications, the nurse should be aware of the nurse practice act of the state and administrative policies of the employing institution. Because IV injection of medications may cause serious adverse effects, nurses who perform this function must be qualified through proper training, education, and experience.

The nurse is responsible for following legal provisions when administering **controlled substances** (drugs that affect the mind or behavior), which can be dispensed only with a prescription. Violations of the Controlled Substances Act are punishable by fines, imprisonment, and loss of nurse licensure. Hospitals and other health care institutions have policies for the proper storage and distribution of controlled substances, including **narcotics** (see box).

Nontherapeutic Drug Use

Despite legislative controls, some people use drugs for purposes other than their proper purpose. Nontherapeutic drug use poses serious health problems for the user, family, and community. In the past, the misuse or abuse of medications was related to use for therapeutic qualities, such as the relief of pain or reduction in anxiety. Today, factors such as peer pressure, curiosity, and the pursuit of pleasure are motivators for drug use. Problems with drug use are not

---

Guidelines for Safe Narcotic Administration and Control

- Store all narcotics in a locked, secure cabinet or container. (Computerized, locked cabinets are now available.)
- Nurses in charge carry a set of keys (or a special computer entry code) for the narcotics cabinet.
- During an institution's change-of-shift, the nurse going off duty counts all narcotics with the nurse coming on duty. Both nurses sign the narcotic record to indicate that the count is correct.
- Discrepancies in narcotic counts are reported immediately.
- A special inventory record is used each time a narcotic is dispensed.
- The record is used to document the client's name, date, time of drug administration, name of drug, dosage, and signature of nurse dispensing the drug.
- The form provides an accurate ongoing count of narcotics used and remaining.
- If only one part of a premeasured dosage of a controlled substance is given, a second nurse witnesses disposal of the unused portion and documents such on the record form.

---

limited to heroin, cocaine, and other "hard" drugs. Millions of people in the United States and Canada consume alcohol daily. Our society is drug conscious, as shown by the frequent advertisements for pain relievers, decongestants, and antacids on television.

Nurses have ethical and legal responsibilities to understand the problems of persons using drugs improperly. When caring for clients with suspected **drug abuse** or **drug dependence,** nurses must be aware of their own values and attitudes about the willful use of potentially harmful substances. Nurses cannot develop therapeutic relationships with clients if personal values interfere with acceptance or understanding of their needs. Knowing the physical, psychological, and social changes resulting from drug abuse allows nurses to identify clients with drug problems.

A problem involving the misuse of drugs by health professionals also exists. Stress in the work place, personal problems, and the strong desire to perform well are some of the factors that may cause nurses to rely on drugs. Nurses must recognize and understand the problems of colleagues who suffer from drug abuse (see box on p. 616). Today, many pro-

---

Terms Associated with the Nontherapeutic Use of Drugs

ABUSE

- A maladaptive pattern of substance use indicated by at least one of the following: continued substance use despite knowledge of having a persistent or recurrent social, occupational, psychological, or physical problem caused or exacerbated by use of the substance
- Some symptoms of the disturbance persisting for at least 1 month or occurring repeatedly over a longer period

DEPENDENCE

- Dependence is indicated by at least three of the following:
  - Substance often taken in larger amounts or over a longer period than the person intended
  - Persistent desire or one or more unsuccessful efforts to cut down or control substance use
  - A great deal of time spent in activities necessary to get the substance, taking the substance, or recovering from its effects

DEPENDENCE—CONT'D

- Frequent intoxication or withdrawal symptoms when expected to fulfill major role obligations at work, school, or home
- Important social, occupational, or recreational activities given up or reduced because of substance use
- Continued substance use despite knowledge of having a persistent or recurrent social, psychological, or physical problem caused or exacerbated by the use of the substance
- Marked tolerance, need for markedly increased amounts of the substance to achieve intoxication or desired effect, or markedly diminished effect with continued use of the same amount
- Characteristic withdrawal symptoms
- Substance often taken to relieve or avoid withdrawal symptoms
- Some symptoms of the disturbance persisting for at least 1 month or occurring repeatedly over a longer period

---

Modified from American Psychiatric Association: *Diagnostic and statistical manual of mental disorders (DSM-IIIR)*, rev 3, Washington, DC, 1987, The Association.

grams are available to assist these nurses toward recovery. These programs may be offered through the Employee's Assistance Program, the state board of nursing, or other community agencies.

 ## NATURE OF DRUG ACTIONS

Medications act to produce therapeutically useful effects. A drug does not create a function in a tissue or organ but rather alters physiological functions. Drugs may protect cells from the influence of other chemical agents, promote cell function, or accelerate or slow cell processes. A medication may replace a substance that is missing (for example, insulin, thyroid hormone, or estrogen).

Mechanisms of Action

Drugs produce actions by altering body fluids or cell membranes or interacting with receptor sites. The drug aluminum hydroxide gel exerts its effect by altering the chemical properties of a body fluid (specifically, neutralizing the stomach's acid contents.) Drugs such as general anesthetic gases interact with cell membranes. After properties of the cells become altered, the drug exerts its effects. The most common mechanism of drug action is binding to a cell's receptor sites. Receptors localize drug effects. Sites on the receptors interact with drugs because of similar chemical shapes. The drug and receptor bind together like a lock-and-key fit. When receptors and drugs lock together, the therapeutic effects are realized. Each tissue or cell in the body possesses a unique group of receptors. For example, receptors in the myocardial cells respond to digitalis preparations.

Pharmacokinetics

Pharmacokinetics is the study of how drugs enter the body, reach their site of action, are metabolized, and exit the body. The physician and nurse use the knowledge of pharmacokinetics when timing drug administration, selecting the route of administration, judging the risk for alterations in drug action, and observing client response.

Absorption

Absorption is the passage of drug molecules into the blood. Most drugs, except those applied topically for local effects, must enter the systemic circulation to exert therapeutic effect. Factors influencing absorption include route of administration, ability of the drug to dissolve, and conditions at the site of absorption.

Each route has a different influence on drug absorption, depending on the physical structure of the tissues. The skin is relatively impermeable to chemicals, making absorption slow. The mucous membranes and respiratory airways allow quick drug absorption because of the high vascularity of mucosal and alveolar-capillary surfaces. Because orally administered drugs must pass through the gastrointestinal tract to be absorbed, the overall rate of absorption may be slowed. IV injection produces the most rapid absorption because this route provides immediate access to the systemic circulation.

The ability of an oral medication to dissolve after ingestion depends largely on its form or preparation. Solutions and suspensions already in a liquid state are absorbed more readily than tablets or capsules. Solid dosage forms must first disintegrate to expose the chemical to gastric and intestinal secretions. Acidic drugs pass through the gastric mucosa rapidly. Drugs that are basic are not absorbed before reaching the small intestine.

Conditions at the site of absorption influence the ease with which medications enter the systemic circulation. When skin is abraded, topical drugs are absorbed easily. Topical substances normally prescribed for local effect can cause serious reactions when absorbed through the skin's layers. The formation of edema in mucous membranes slows drug absorption because medications take longer to diffuse to blood vessels. The absorption of parenterally administered medications depends on the blood supply of the tissues. Before administering a drug by injection, the nurse should assess for local factors, such as edema, bruising, or scarring, which might impair the absorption of the medication. Because muscles have a richer blood supply than subcutaneous (SQ) tissues, a drug given intramuscularly is absorbed more quickly than one injected subcutaneously. In some instances a delayed SQ absorption is preferable to produce long-lasting drug effects. If a client's tissue perfusion is poor, as in the case of circulatory shock, the IV route is best. IV administration provides the most rapid and dependable absorption.

Oral medications are absorbed more easily when administered between meals. When the stomach is filled with food, the contents are emptied slowly into the duodenum, thus slowing drug absorption. Certain foods and antacids cause drugs to bind into complexes that cannot pass through the gastrointestinal tract lining. For example, milk interferes with the absorption of iron and tetracycline. Some drugs are destroyed by the increased acidity of gastric contents and protein digestion during a meal. Enteric coatings on certain tablets resist dissolution in gastric juices and prevent certain medications from being digested in the upper gastrointestinal tract. The coating also protects the stomach lining from irritation by the medication.

The route of drug administration is prescribed by the physician. Nurses may need to request medication be given by an alternate route or in a different form, based on physical assessments of the client. For example, a client may not be able to swallow tablets; therefore the nurse would request the medication as an elixir or syrup. Knowledge of factors that alter or impair drug absorption helps the nurse administer drugs correctly. There are no rules about giving medications before, during, or after meals. The nurse should be aware of the nursing implications for each medication given. For example, drugs such as aspirin, iron, and phenytoin sodium (Dilantin) irritate the gastrointestinal tract and should be administered with or immediately after a meal. However, food may interfere with the absorption of drugs such as cloxacillin sodium and penicillin; therefore they should be given 1 to 2 hours before meals or 2 to 3 hours afterward.

Distribution

After a drug is absorbed, it is distributed within the body to tissues and organs and ultimately to its specific site of action. The rate and extent of distribution depend on the physical and chemical properties of the drug and the physiological makeup of the person taking the drug.

BODY SIZE. A direct relationship exists between the amount of drug administration and the amount of body tissue in which it is distributed. Most medications are distributed to body fat or water (Simonson, 1984). An increase in the percentage of body fat may cause a longer duration of drug action because of slower distribution throughout the body. In an obese client a lower concentration accumulates in the body tissues that are the targets for drug action. The less a client weighs, the greater the concentration of a drug in tissues and the more powerful the drug's effects. The older adult experiences a reduction in both tissue mass and height and often requires a lower drug dosage than a younger client.

CIRCULATORY DYNAMICS. Drugs pass more easily from interstitial to intravascular spaces than between body compartments. Blood vessels are permeable to most dissolved substances unless drug particles are large or bound to serum proteins. The concentration of a drug at a specific site depends on the number of blood vessels in tissues, the degree of local vasodilation or vasoconstriction, and the rate of blood flow to a tissue site. Exercise, warming, and chilling alter local circulation. For example, if a client applies a warm compress to an intramuscular (IM) injection site, the resultant vasodilation increases drug distribution.

PROTEIN BINDING. The degree to which drugs bind to the protein albumin in the bloodstream affects drug distribution. Most medications bind to this protein to some extent. When drug molecules are bound to albumin, they cannot exert any pharmacological activity. Unbound or "free" drug is the active form of the drug. Older adults have a decreased albumin level in the bloodsteam, probably caused by a change in liver function. The same is true for clients with liver disease or malnutrition. Because of this, older adults may be at risk for an increase in drug activity, toxicity, or both.

Metabolism

After a drug reaches its site of action, it is metabolized into an inactive form that is more easily excreted. This **biotransformation** occurs under the influence of enzymes that detoxify, degrade (break down), and remove biologically active chemicals. Most biotransformation occurs within the liver, although the lungs, kidneys, blood, and intestines also metabolize drugs.

The liver is especially important because its specialized structure oxidizes and transforms many toxic substances. The liver degrades many harmful chemicals before they are distributed to the tissues. The decrease in liver function that occurs with aging or with liver disease influences the rate at which a drug is eliminated from the body. The resultant slowing of metabolism causes the drug to accumulate in the body. Thus a client would be at greater risk for drug toxicity. If any of the organs that participate in drug metabolism are altered, a client is at risk for drug toxicity.

Excretion

After drugs are metabolized, they exit the body through the kidneys, liver, bowel, lungs, and exocrine glands. The chemical makeup of a drug determines the organ of excretion. Gaseous and volatile compounds such as ether, nitrous oxide, and alcohol exit through the lungs. Deep breathing and coughing help the postoperative client eliminate anesthetic gases more rapidly.

The exocrine glands excrete lipid-soluble drugs. When medications exit through sweat glands, the skin may become irritated. The nurse assists the client in good hygiene practices to promote cleanliness and skin integrity. If a drug exits through the mammary glands, a nursing infant may absorb the chemicals. Nursing mothers should check on the safety of each drug. The risk to the infant receiving the drug and the risk of the mother not taking the drug must be given careful consideration.

The gastrointestinal tract is another route for drug excretion. Many drugs enter the hepatic circulation to be broken down by the liver and excreted into the bile. After chemicals enter the intestines through the biliary tract, they may be reabsorbed by the intestines. Factors increasing peristalsis, such as laxatives and enemas, accelerate drug excretion through the feces, whereas factors slowing peristalsis, such as inactivity and improper diet, may prolong a drug's effects.

The kidneys are the main organs for drug excretion. Some drugs escape extensive metabolism and exit relatively unchanged in the urine. Others undergo biotransformation in the liver before they are excreted by the kidney. If renal function declines, a common change in aging, the risk for drug toxicity increases. If the kidneys cannot adequately excrete a drug, it may be necessary to reduce the dosage. Maintenance of a normal fluid intake promotes proper elimination of drugs.

Types of Drug Actions

Because of its chemical makeup and physiological action, a drug may produce more than one effect.

Therapeutic Effects

The **therapeutic effect** is the intended or predicted physiological response that a drug causes. Each drug has a desired or therapeutic effect for which it is prescribed. For example, the nurse administers codeine phosphate to create analgesia and gives theophylline to dilate narrowed respiratory bronchioles. A single medication may have many therapeutic effects. For example, aspirin is an analgesic, antipyretic, and antiinflammatory, and it reduces platelet aggregation (clumping).

Side Effects

Predictably a drug will cause unintended, secondary effects. These **side effects** may be harmless or injurious. For example, with codeine phosphate, a client may also experience constipation, and theophylline may cause headache and dizziness; these side effects may be considered harmless. However, digoxin may cause cardiac dysrhythmias that could be lethal. If the side effects are serious enough to negate the beneficial effects of a drug's therapeutic action, the physician may discontinue it. Clients often stop taking medications without consulting their physicians because of side effects.

Toxic Effects

Generally, **toxic effects** develop after prolonged intake of high doses of medication, after prolonged use of a drug intended for external application, or after a drug accumulates in the blood because of impaired metabolism or excretion. *One* dose of medication can have toxic effects for some clients. Excess amounts of a drug within the body may have lethal effects, depending on the drug's action. For example, morphine, a narcotic analgesic, relieves pain by depressing the central nervous system. However, toxic levels of morphine cause severe respiratory depression and death.

Idiosyncratic Reactions

Medications may cause an **idiosyncratic effect;** this occurs when a client overreacts or underreacts to a drug or has a reaction different from normal. It is impossible to predict which client will have an idiosyncratic response.

Allergic Reactions

An **allergic reaction** is another unpredictable response to a drug; allergic reactions compose 5% to 10% of all drug reactions. Exposure to an initial dose of a medication may cause an immunological response. With repeated administration the client may also develop an allergic response to the drug, its chemical preservatives, or a metabolite. In this case the drug or chemical acts as an antigen, triggering the release of antibodies.

A drug allergy may be mild or severe. Allergic symptoms vary, depending on the individual and the drug; for example, antibiotics cause many allergic reactions. Common allergy symptoms are summarized in Table 21-4. Severe or anaphylactic reactions are characterized by sudden constriction of bronchiolar muscles, edema of the pharynx and larynx, and severe wheezing and shortness of breath. The client may also become severely hypotensive, necessitating emergency resuscitation. A client with a known history of an allergy to a medication should wear an identification bracelet or medal that alerts nurses and physicians to the allergy if the client is unconscious.

Drug Tolerance

Some persons have unusually low metabolisms in response to a drug. An increase in dosage may be needed to cause a therapeutic effect. Clients that are taking various pain medications may develop a tolerance over time. Frequently, clients require increasing dosages of morphine over time to relieve pain.

TABLE 21-4 Allergic Reactions	
Symptom	Description
Urticaria (hives)	Raised, irregularly shaped skin eruptions with varying sizes and shapes; have reddened margins and pale centers
Eczema (rash)	Small, raised vesicles that are usually reddened; often distributed over entire body
Pruritus	Itching of skin; accompanies most rashes
Rhinitis	Inflammation of mucous membranes lining nose; causes swelling and clear, watery discharge

Drug Interactions

When one drug modifies the action of another, a **drug interaction** occurs. Drug interactions are common in individuals taking many medications. A drug may potentiate or diminish the action of other drugs and may alter the way in which another drug is absorbed, metabolized, or eliminated from the body.

When two drugs are given simultaneously, they can have a synergistic or addictive effect. With a **synergistic effect** the physiological action of the two drugs in combination is greater than the effect of the drugs when given separately. Alcohol is a central nervous system depressant that has a synergistic effect on antihistamines, antidepressants, and narcotic analgesics.

Often a physician orders combination drug therapy to create a drug interaction for therapeutic benefit. A drug interaction may create a therapeutic effect. For example, a client with moderate hypertension may receive combination drug therapy, such as diuretics and vasodilators, that act together to keep the blood pressure at a desirable level.

Drug Dose Responses

After the nurse administers a drug, it undergoes absorption, distribution, metabolism, and excretion. Except when administered intravenously, drugs take time to enter the bloodstream. The quantity and distribution of a drug in different body compartments change constantly.

When a medication is prescribed, the goal is to achieve a constant blood level within a safe therapeutic range. Repeated doses are required to achieve a constant therapeutic concentration of a medication because a portion of a drug is always being excreted.

When absorption ceases, only metabolism, excretion, and distribution continue. The highest **serum concentration** (peak concentration) of the drug usually occurs just before the last of the drug is absorbed. After peaking, the serum concentration falls progressively. With IV drug infusions, the peak concentration occurs quickly, but the serum level also begins to fall immediately.

All drugs have a **serum half-life,** or the time it takes for excretion processes to lower the serum concentration by half. To maintain a therapeutic plateau, the client must receive regular, fixed doses. After an initial medication dose the client receives each successive dose when the previous dose reaches its half-life (Fig. 21-1). In this way an almost constant therapeutic drug concentration is maintained.

The client and nurse must follow regular dosage schedules and adhere to prescribed doses and dosage intervals. Knowledge of the following time intervals of drug action also helps to anticipate a drug's effect:

1. Onset of drug action, or period of time it takes after a drug is administered for it to produce a response
2. Peak action, time it takes for a drug to reach its highest effective concentration
3. Duration of action, or length of time during which the drug is present in a concentration great enough to produce a response

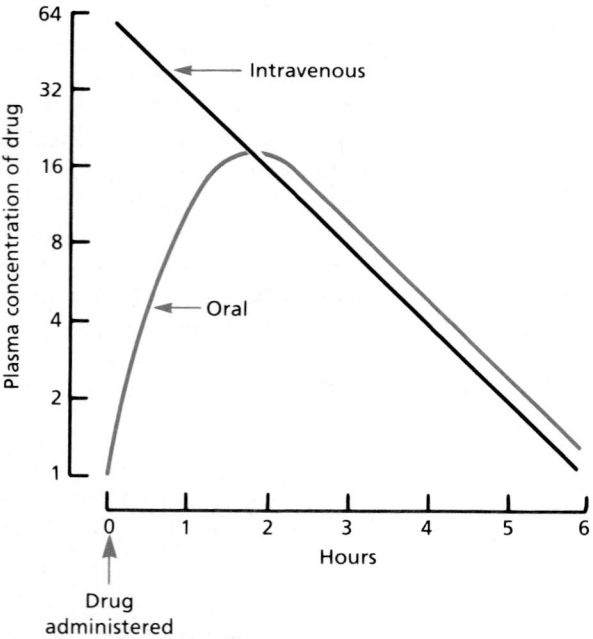

Fig. 21-1 Curve showing therapeutic blood levels. From Clark J, Queener S, Karb V: *Pharmacologic basis of nursing practice,* ed 4, St Louis, 1993, Mosby–Year Book.

4. Plateau, blood serum concentration reached and maintained after repeated, fixed doses of the medication

The ideal way to achieve a constant therapeutic drug level is continuous IV infusions, which eliminate the fluctuating effects of intermittent dosages.

 FACTORS INFLUENCING DRUG ACTIONS

Because of differences in the manner in which drugs act and their types of action, responses to medications vary considerably. Factors other than characteristics of the medication also influence drug actions. A client may not respond in the same way to each successive dose of a medication. Likewise, the same drug dosage may cause very different responses in different clients.

Genetic Differences

Genetic makeup affects the manner in which biotransformation of drugs occurs. Metabolic patterns are often similar within families. Genetic factors determine whether naturally occurring enzymes are present to assist in drug degradation. As a result, members of a family may share a sensitivity to a medication.

Physiological Variables

Hormonal differences between men and women alter the metabolism of certain drugs. Hormones and drugs compete with each other in biotransformation because they are degraded by the same metabolic processes. Diurnal variations in estrogen secretion may be responsible for cyclic fluctuations in drug reactions experienced by women.

Age has a direct effect on drug action. Infants lack many of the enzymes necessary for normal drug metabolism. A number of physiological changes accompanying the aging process influence the response to drug therapy (Table 21-5). Body systems undergo functional and structural changes that alter the influence of drugs. The nurse initiates actions that minimize a drug's harmful effects and promote the client's remaining functional capacities.

If a client's nutritional status is poor, proper cell function for biotransformation cannot occur. Like all body functions, drug metabolism relies on adequate nutrition for enzyme and protein formation. Most drugs bind with proteins before being distributed to their sites of action.

TABLE 21-5   Influence of Drug Actions in Older Adults

Physiological Change	Drug Action/Client Response	Nursing Interventions
GASTROINTESTINAL TRACT **Oral cavity**		
Loss of elasticity in oral mucosa, which becomes dry and easily abraded	Difficulty in swallowing tablets or capsules; sensitivity to drugs that cause dryness of mouth; suscepti-bility to gum disease and dental caries	Rinse client's oral cavity frequently with tepid clear water. Floss daily. Brush teeth and gums gently. Use substitute saliva.
Esophagus		
Delayed esophageal clearance be-cause of weakened contractions and failure of lower esophageal sphincter to relax	Difficulty in swallowing large tablets or capsules; tissue erosion caused by drugs such as aspirin and un-coated potassium chloride	Position client upright. Administer full glass of liquid with drug. Crush tablets and mix with food (if gastric pH does not affect ab-sorption).
Stomach		
Decrease in gastric acidity and peri-stalsis	Potentiation of irritating effects of highly acidic drugs (e.g., aspirin); alteration of solubility of certain drugs	Have client drink full glass of water and take medication with nonfat snack to reduce gastric distress.
Large intestine		
Reduced colon muscle tone; loss of defecation reflex; decreased intes-tinal blood flow	Slowing of drug excretion; overuse and abuse of laxatives by client; delayed drug absorption	Provide normal fluid intake. Instruct client to eat bulk-forming foods and avoid use of constipating drugs.
SKIN AND VASCULAR SYSTEM		
Reduced SQ skin fold thickness in extremities (less body fat); re-duced elasticity in skin and vascu-lar system	Fragile blood vessels; client prone to bleeding after injection	Avoid using veins in hand for IV injections. Apply pressure to in-jection sites after administration. Observe injection sites for bleed-ing.
LIVER		
Reduced liver size; decline in he-patic blood flow	Longer biotransformation time; longer-than-normal duration of drug action; greater risk for drug sensitivity and toxicity	Monitor for signs of liver impair-ment (jaundice, pruritus, dark urine). Question dosages for cli-ents with known liver disease.
KIDNEYS		
Reduced glomerular filtration; de-creased tubular function and re-nal blood flow	Risk of drug accumulation and tox-icity	Prevent urinary retention (keep catheters free flowing and observe frequency of urination). Monitor for signs of renal impairment (re-duced output and difficulty in uri-nating). Question dosages for clients with renal disease.

Any disease state that impairs the function of organs responsible for normal pharmacokinetics also impairs drug action. Altered skin integrity, reduced gastrointestinal absorption or motility, and impaired renal or hepatic function are just some of the disease-related conditions that can reduce a drug's efficacy or place a client at risk for drug toxicity.

Environmental Conditions

A client's exposure to severe physical and emotional stress triggers a hormonal response that eventually may interfere with drug metabolism. Ionizing radiation creates a similar effect by altering the rate of enzyme activity.

Exposure to heat and cold can affect responses to drugs. Hypertensive clients receive vasodilators to control blood pressure. In hot weather, it may be necessary to reduce vasodilator dosages because the temperature adds to the medication's effects. Cold weather tends to promote vasoconstriction, necessitating an increase in vasodilator dosage.

A reaction to a medication may vary, depending on the setting in which it is taken. Clients in protective isolation often receive less pain relief from an analgesic than clients in rooms where their families can visit them. Similarly, when drinking alcohol alone, persons may only become sleepy. However, drinking with a group of friends can cause people to become playful and outgoing.

Psychological Factors

A number of psychological factors influence the use of drugs and response to a medication. A person's attitude about drugs may stem from early experiences or familial influences. Seeing a parent use medications frequently may cause a child to accept drugs as a normal part of life.

The meaning or significance that a drug or taking a drug has for clients influences the response to therapy. A drug may serve as a means for overcoming feelings of insecurity. In this situation, clients depend on drugs as a means of coping with life. In contrast, if clients resent their physical conditions, anger and hostility may result in adverse reactions to medications. Medications often provide a sense of security. The regular use of nonprescription medications, or **over-the-counter drugs,** such as vitamins, laxatives, and aspirin, gives many people a sense of control over their health.

The nurse's behavior when administering a drug can have a significant impact on the client's response to a medication. If the nurse conveys a sense that the medication can be helpful, it is more likely that the drug will have a positive effect. If the nurse seems uncaring when the client experiences discomfort, the medication administered may prove relatively ineffective.

Diet

Drug and nutrient interactions can alter a drug's action or the effect of a nutrient. For example, vitamin K (found in green leafy vegetables) is a nutrient that antagonizes the effect of warfarin sodium (Coumadin), decreasing its effect on clotting mechanisms. Mineral oil decreases the absorption of fat-soluble vitamins. Clients may be required to take nutritional supplements when taking drugs that reduce a nutrient's effect. Similarly, withholding certain nutrients may ensure a drug's therapeutic effect.

 ## ROUTES OF ADMINISTRATION

The route chosen for administering a drug depends on its properties and desired effect and the client's physical and mental condition (Table 21-6). The nurse frequently is involved in judging the best route for a medication, as in the following hypothetical situation:

The client, Mr. Bush, has progressively worsened physically. His temperature is 39.2° C. He complains of nausea and is unable to tolerate oral fluids. The nurse checks Mr. Bush's order, which reads, "Aspirin 600 mg orally for temperature above 38.5° C." On the basis of the assessment, the nurse believes that Mr. Bush will be unable to tolerate an oral dose of aspirin. By consulting the physician, the nurse acquires an order for a rectal suppository instead.

Oral Routes

Oral Administration

The oral route is the easiest and the most commonly used. Medications are given by mouth and swallowed. Orally administered medications are less expensive than many other preparations. They have a slower onset of action and a more prolonged effect. Clients generally prefer the oral route.

Sublingual Administration

Sublingual drugs are designed to be readily absorbed after being placed under the tongue to dissolve. A drug given sublingually should not be swallowed. Otherwise the desired effect will not be achieved. Nitroglycerin is commonly given sublin-

TABLE 21-6   Factors Influencing Choice of Administration Routes

Advantages	Disadvantages or Contraindications
ORAL, BUCCAL, SUBLINGUAL ROUTES	
Routes are convenient and comfortable for client.	These routes are avoided when client has alterations in gastrointestinal function (e.g., nausea, vomiting), reduced motility (after general anesthesia or bowel inflammation, and surgical resection of portion of gastrointestinal tract.
Routes are economical.	
Medications may produce local or systemic effects.	
Routes rarely cause anxiety for client.	Some drugs are destroyed by gastric secretions. Oral administration is contraindicated in clients unable to swallow (e.g., clients with neuromuscular disorders, esophageal strictures, mouth lesions).
	Oral medications cannot be given when client has gastric suction and are contraindicated in clients before some tests or surgery.
	Unconscious or confused client is unable or unwilling to swallow or hold medication under tongue.
	Oral medications may irritate lining of gastrointestinal tract, discolor teeth, or have unpleasant taste.
SQ, IM, IV, INTRADERMAL ROUTES	
Routes provide means of administration when oral drugs are contraindicated.	There is risk of introducing infection, drugs are expensive, and these routes are avoided in clients with bleeding tendencies.
More rapid absorption occurs than with topical or oral routes.	There is risk of tissue damage with SQ injections.
IV infusion provides drug delivery when client is critically ill. If preipheral perfusion is poor, IV route is preferred over injections.	IM and IV routes are dangerous because of rapid absorption.
	These routes cause considerable anxiety in many clients, especially children.
SKIN	
Topical	
Topical skin applications primarily provide local effect.	Extensive applications may be bulky and cause difficulty in maneuvering.
Route is painless.	Clients with skin abrasions are at risk for rapid drug absorption and systemic effects.
Limited side effects occur.	
Transdermal	
Transdermal applications provide prolonged systemic effects, with limited side effects.	Application leaves oily or pasty substance on skin and may soil clothing.
MUCOUS MEMBRANES*	
Therapeutic effects are provided by local application to involved sites.	Mucous membranes are highly sensitive to some drug concentrations.
Aqueous solutions are readily absorbed and capable of causing systemic effects.	Insertion of rectal and vaginal medication often causes embarrassment.
Mucous membranes provide route of administration when oral drugs are contraindicated.	Client with ruptured eardrum cannot receive irrigations.
	Rectal suppositories are contraindicated if client has had rectal surgery or if active rectal bleeding is present.
INHALATION	
Inhalation provides rapid relief for local respiratory problems.	Some local agents can cause serious systemic effects.
Route provides easy access for introduction of general anesthetic gases.	

*Includes eyes, ears, nose, vagina, rectum, buccal, sublingual routes.

gually. A drink should not be taken by the client until the drug is completely dissolved.

Buccal Administration

Administration of a drug by the **buccal** route involves placing the solid medication against the mucous membranes of the cheek until the drug dissolves. Clients should be taught to alternate cheeks with each subsequent dose to avoid mucosal irritation. Clients are also warned not to chew or swallow the drug or to take liquids with it. A buccal medication acts locally on the mucosa or systemically as it is swallowed in saliva.

Parenteral Routes

Parenteral administration involves giving a drug by a route through injection into body tissues. Parenteral administration of medication involves four major types of injections:
1. **Subcutaneous (SQ),** or injection into tissues just below the dermis of the skin
2. **Intradermal (ID),** or injection into the dermis just under the epidermis
3. **Intramuscular (IM),** or injection into a muscle body
4. **Intravenous (IV),** or injection into a vein

A physician often uses additional routes for parenteral injections, including intrathecal or intraspinal, intracardiac, intrapleural, intraarterial, and intraarticular.

The nurse uses strict sterile technique when preparing medications for parenteral injection. Contamination of the medication solution, syringe needle, or the syringe itself can lead to infection.

Topical Administration

Drugs applied to the skin and mucous membranes principally have local effects. The **topical** medication is applied to the skin by painting or spreading it over an area, applying moist dressings, soaking body parts in a solution, or giving medicated baths. Systemic effects can occur if a client's skin is thin, if the drug concentration is high, or if skin contact is prolonged.

Some medications (for example, nitroglycerin, scopolamine, and estrogens) are applied topically by a transdermal disk or patch. The disk secures the medicated ointment to the skin. These topical applications may be applied for as little as 24 hours or up to 7 days. Medications delivered by this route have systemic effects.

Drugs can also be applied to mucous membranes. They are quickly absorbed. If the drug concentration is high enough or applied in great quantities, systemic effects may occur.

Mucous membranes differ in their sensitivity to medications. The cornea of the eye and nasal mucous membranes are particularly sensitive. The client may complain of a burning sensation when the nurse administers eye drops or nose drops. Medications are generally less irritating to vaginal or rectal mucosa. The nurse uses the following methods for applying medications to mucous membranes:
1. Direct application of liquid (for example, applying eyedrops, having the client gargle, swabbing the throat)
2. Insertion of the drug into a body cavity (for example, placing a suppository in the rectum or vagina or inserting medicated packing into the vagina)
3. **Instillation** (slow introduction) of fluid into a body cavity (for example, instilling eardrops, nose drops, and bladder and rectal fluids)
4. **Irrigation** (washing out) of body cavity (for example, flushing the eye, ear, vagina, bladder, or rectum with medicated fluid)
5. Spraying (for example, instilling medication into nose and throat)

Inhalation

The deeper passages of the respiratory tract provide a large surface area for drug absorption. The vascular alveolar-capillary network readily absorbs gases and mists introduced through the airways. Medications introduced into the lung's airways must not interfere with normal gas exchange such as constricting bronchioles. Inhaled medications may have local effects. Drugs such as oxygen and general anesthetics create general systemic effects. Some medications given by inhalation are designed to produce local effects but have potentially dangerous systemic side effects. Oxygen must be administrated with the appropriate oxygen delivery equipment (see Chapter 38). Administration of local-acting medications with hand-operated inhalers must be carefully taught to the client by the nurse.

 ## SYSTEMS OF DRUG MEASUREMENT

The proper administration of medication depends on the nurse's ability to compute drug dosages accurately and measure medications correctly. A careless mistake in placing a decimal point or adding a zero to a dosage can lead to a fatal error. The nurse is responsible for checking the dose before giving a drug and teaching clients about prescribed doses.

The metric, apothecary, and household systems of measurement are used in drug therapy. Most nations of the world, including Canada, use the metric system as their standard of measurement. Although the U.S. Congress has not officially adopted the metric system, most health professionals in the United States use it and the apothecary system. Prescriptions to be self-administered are often written in household measures for clients.

Metric System

Because it is a decimal system, the **metric system** is the most logically organized of the measurement systems. Metric units can easily be converted and computed through simple multiplication and division. Each basic unit of measurement is organized into units of 10. Multiplying or dividing by 10 forms secondary units. In multiplication, the decimal point moves to the right; in division, the decimal moves to the left. For example,

$$10.0 \text{ mg} \times 10 = 100.\text{mg}$$
$$10.0 \text{ mg} \div 10 = 1.00 \text{ mg}$$

The basic units of measurement in the metric system are the meter (length), liter (volume), and gram (weight). For drug calculations the nurse uses primarily volume and weight units. In the metric system, small and large letters are used to designate the basic units (for example, gram = g or Gm and liter = l or L). Small letters are abbreviations for subdivisions of major units (for example, milligram = mg and milliliter = ml).

A system of Latin prefixes designates subdivision of the basic units: *deci-* (1/10 or 0.1), *centi-* (1/100 or 0.01), and *milli-* (1/1000 or 0.001). Greek prefixes designate multiples of the basic units: *deka-* (10), *hecto-* (100), and *kilo-* (1000). When writing drug dosages in metric units, physicians and nurses use fractions or multiples of a unit. Fractions are always in decimal form (for example, 500 mg or 0.5 g, *not* ½ g and 10 ml or 0.01 L, *not* 1/100 L). When fractions are used, a zero is always placed in front of the decimal to prevent error.

Apothecary System

The **apothecary system** of measurement is familiar to most people in the United States and Canada. The standards for measurement are commonly used in the home; for example, milk is bottled in pints and quarts, a yardstick has inches and feet, and a bathroom scale weighs in pounds.

The basic unit of weight is a grain. In colonial days the grain represented the weight of one grain of wheat. Units of weight derived from the grain are the dram, ounce, and pound. The apothecary unit for volume of fluid measurement is the minim. The minim is the approximate quantity of water that weighs a grain. The fluidram, fluid ounce, pint, quart, and gallon are measures derived from the minim.

In the apothecary system, small letters or symbols are used for measurement units: grain = gr, ounce = oz or ℥, fluid ounce = f℥, minim = ♏, and dram = ℨ. Lowercase Roman numerals designate the quantities of the apothecary units. The Roman numeral follows the unit of measure (for example, 3 grains = gr iii). Physicians often use fractions and symbols with apothecary units (for example, 2½ fluid ounces = f℥ iiss and ½ fluid ounce = f℥ ½ or f℥ ss).

Household Measurements

Household units of measurement are also familiar to most people. Household measures include drops, teaspoons, tablespoons, and cups for volume and ounces and pounds for weight. Although pints and quarts are considered household measures, they are also used in the apothecary system. The disadvantage with household measures is their inaccuracy. Household utensils such as teaspoons and cups often vary in size. Scales to measure pints or quarts are often not well calibrated.

The advantage of household measurements is their convenience and familiarity. When accuracy is not critical, it is safe to use household measures. For example, many over-the-counter drugs, such as laxatives, antacids, and cough syrups, can safely be measured by this method. Table 21-7 gives common equivalents from each measurement unit.

TABLE 21-7   Equivalents of Measurement

Metric	Apothecary	Household
1 ml	15-16 minims (m)	15 drops (gtt)
4-5 ml	fluidram (fℨ)	1 teaspoon (tsp)
15 ml	4 fluidrams (fℨ)	1 tablespoon (tbsp)
30 ml	1 fluid ounce (f℥)	2 tablespoons (tbsp)
240 ml	8 fluid ounces (f℥)	1 cup (c)
480 ml (approximately 500 ml)	1 pint (pt)	1 pint (pt)
960 ml (approximately 1 L)	1 quart (qt)	1 quart (qt)
3840 ml (approximately 5 L)	1 gallon (gal)	1 gallon (gal)

Solutions

In clinical practice the nurse uses solutions of various concentrations for injections, irrigations, and infusions. The nurse should understand terms that describe concentrations of solutions. A **solution** is a given mass of solid substance dissolved in a known volume of fluid or a given volume of liquid dissolved in a known volume of another fluid. When a solid is dissolved in fluid, the **concentration** is in units of mass per units of volume (for example, g/ml, g/L, mg/ml). A concentration may also be expressed as a percentage. A 10% solution, for example, is 10 g of solid dissolved in 100 ml of solution. A proportion also expresses concentrations. A 1:1000 solution is a solution containing 1 g of solid in 1000 ml of liquid or 1 ml of liquid with 1000 ml of another liquid.

 ## CONVERTING MEASUREMENT UNITS

A pharmacist does not always dispense a medication in the unit of measure in which it is ordered. Drug companies package and bottle certain standard equivalents. For example, the physician may order 250 mg of a medication that is available only in grams. The nurse is responsible for converting available units of volume and weight to the desired dosages. The nurse must know the standardized equivalents in all of the major measurement systems.

Drug administration is not the only function in which nurses use conversions (see box). They are used in many nursing activities.

Conversions Within One System

Converting measurements within one system is relatively easy. In the metric system the nurse simply divides or multiplies. To change milligrams to grams the nurse divides by 1000, moving the decimal 3 points to the left (for example, 1000 mg = 1 g and 350 mg = 0.35 g). To convert liters to milliliters the nurse multiplies by 1000 or moves the decimal 3 points to the right (for example, 1 L = 1000 ml and 0.25 L = 250 ml).

To convert units of measurement within the apothecary or household system, the nurse must consult a conversion table. For example, when converting fluid ounces to quarts, the nurse must first know that 32 ounces is the equivalent of 1 quart. To convert 8 ounces to a quart measurement, for example, the nurse divides 8 by 32 to get the equivalent, ¼ or 0.25 quart.

Conversion Between Systems

Frequently the nurse must determine the proper dosage of a medication by converting weights or volumes from one system of measurement to another. Commonly, apothecary and metric units must be converted to equivalent household measures for use at home. When the time comes to make actual drug calculations, it is necessary to work with units in the same measurement system.

Tables of equivalent measurements are available in all health care institutions. The pharmacist is also a good resource.

Before making a conversion, the nurse compares the measurement system available with that ordered. For example, a physician orders, "Morphine gr ⅙ IM." The medication is available only in milligrams. To convert grains to milligrams the nurse must know the equivalents, 1 mg = 1/60 gr or 60 mg = 1 gr. Therefore by converting gr ⅙ to milligrams, the nurse has the measurements needed to make the eventual dosage calculation. The nurse divides by 6:

$$60 \text{ mg} \div 6 = 1/6 \text{ gr}$$
$$10 \text{ mg} = 1/6 \text{ gr}$$

After calculating that the physician's order for "morphine gr ⅙" is the same as 10 mg of morphine, the nurse can accurately prepare the medication based on the available dosage.

Dosage Calculations

The nurse can use a simple formula in many types of dosage calculations. The following formula can be applied when preparing solid or liquid forms of medications:

$$\frac{\text{Dose ordered}}{\text{Dose on hand}} \times \text{Amount on hand} = \text{Amount to administer}$$

Common Reasons for Drug Conversions

- Converting fluid ounces to milliliters for measurement of intake and output
- Converting body weight from pounds to kilograms and vice versa
- Converting volume equivalents to calculate IV flow rates and prepare wound irrigation solutions, enemas, or bladder irrigations

The dose ordered is the amount of pure drug that the physician prescribes for a client. The dose on hand is the weight or volume of drug available in units supplied by the pharmacy; it may be expressed on the drug label as the contents of a tablet or capsule or the amount of drug dissolved per unit volume of liquid. The amount on hand is the basic unit or quantity of the drug containing the dose on hand. For solid drugs the amount on hand may be 1 tablet or capsule; the amount of liquid on hand may be a milliliter or liter. The amount to administer is always expressed in the same unit as the amount on hand.

The following example illustrates how to apply the formula. The physician orders the client to receive Demerol 50 mg IM. Thus the *dose ordered* is 50 mg. The medication is available only in ampules containing 100 mg per 2 ml. Thus the *dose on hand* is 100 mg in an *amount on hand* of 2 ml. The formula is applied as follows:

$$\frac{50 \text{ mg}}{100 \text{ mg}} \times 2 \text{ ml} = \text{Volume to administer in milliliters}$$

The numerator and denominator cancel out and can be ignored. To simplify the fraction, divide numerator and denominator by 50:

$$\frac{1}{2} \times 2 \text{ ml} = 1 \text{ ml to administer}$$

Another example demonstrates how the formula applies with solid dosage forms. The physician orders 0.125 mg PO* of digoxin. The drug is available in tablets containing 0.25 mg.

$$\frac{0.125 \text{ mg}}{0.250 \text{ mg}} \times 1 \text{ tablet} = \text{Number of tablets to administer}$$

The fraction $^{0.125}\!/_{0.250}$ equals ½ or 0.5. Therefore

$$0.5 \times 1 \text{ tablet} = 0.5 \text{ or } \frac{1}{2} \text{ tablet to be administered}$$

Many tablets come with scores or indentations across the center of the tablet. A scored tablet is easy to break for divided dosages. The nurse should never attempt to estimate the amount of medication in a broken, unscored tablet. The potential for giving a dangerously low or high dosage of medication is likely if the nurse attempts to estimate dosage by breaking unscored tablets.

Liquid medications often come prepared in volumes greater than 1 ml. In this situation the formula still applies. For example, the medication order is, "Erythromycin suspension 250 mg PO." The pharmacy delivers 100-ml bottles with the labels stating, "5 ml contains 125 mg of erythromycin."

---

*PO is the abbreviation for the Latin phase, *per orum,* "by mouth."

$$\frac{250 \text{ mg}}{125 \text{ mg}} \times 5 \text{ ml} = \text{Volume to administer}$$

The fraction $^{250}\!/_{125}$ equals 2. Therefore

$$2 \times 5 \text{ ml} = 10 \text{ ml to administer}$$

In this situation the nurse ignores the total volume of medication available and instead uses the dosage values noted on the label. If the nurse calculated the dosage on the basis of 100 ml available, the following error would occur:

$$\frac{250 \text{ mg}}{125 \text{ mg}} \times 100 \text{ ml} = 200 \text{ ml to administer}$$

On the basis of this calculation the client would receive 20 times the desired dosage. The nurse should always double check calculations or check with another professional if the answer seems unreasonable.

Pediatric Dosages

Calculating a child's drug dosages requires caution. A child is unable to metabolize many drugs as readily as an adult. The child's body size also necessitates smaller dosages. In most cases physicians calculate the safe dosage for a child before ordering the medication. However, nurses should be aware of the formula used to calculate pediatric dosages and recheck all dosage before administration. Most drug references list the normal ranges for pediatric dosages.

The most accurate method of calculating pediatric dosages is based on body surface area. Body surface area is estimated on the basis of weight. Standard nomograms, or charts, list body surface area by weight and approximate age (Fig. 21-2 on p. 628). The formula is a ratio of the child's body surface area compared with the body surface area of an average adult (1.7 square meters, or 1.7 m^2).

$$\text{Child's dose} = \frac{\text{Surface area of child}}{1.7 \text{ m}^2 \times \text{Normal adult dose}}$$

For example, a physician orders ampicillin for a child weighing 12 kg, but the normal single adult dose is 250 mg. The nomogram chart shows that a child weighing 12 kg has a surface area of 0.54 m^2.

$$\text{Child's dose} = \frac{0.54 \text{ m}^2}{1.7} \text{ m}^2 \times 250 \text{ mg}$$

The m^2 units cancel out and can be ignored.

$$\text{Child's dose} = \frac{0.54}{1.7} \times 250 \text{ mg}$$

$$\frac{0.54}{1.7} = 0.3$$

$$\text{Child's dose} = 0.3 \times 250 \text{ mg} = 75 \text{ mg}$$

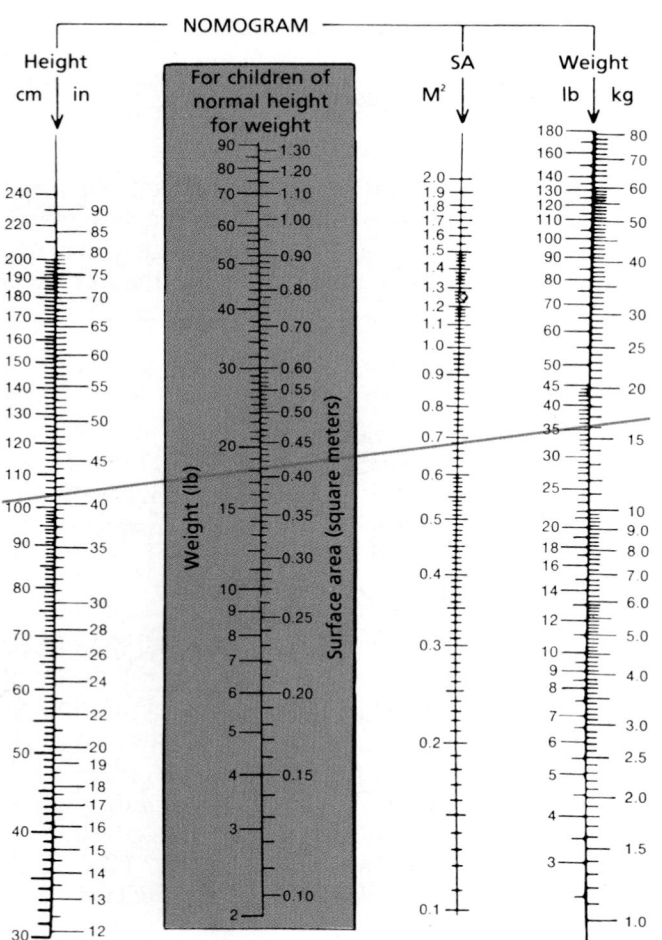

NOMOGRAM

Fig. 21-2 West nomogram for estimation of surface areas in children. A straight line is drawn between height and weight. The point where the line crosses the surface area column is the estimated body surface area.

From Behrman RE, Vaughan VC, editors: *Nelson textbook of pediatrics*, ed 13, Philadelphia, 1987, Saunders; modified from data of Boyd E, by West CD.

ADMINISTERING MEDICATIONS

The nurse does not bear sole responsibility for drug administration. The physician and pharmacist play key roles in ensuring that the right medication gets to the right client. However, the nurse giving the medications bears responsibility and accountability of accuracy of the five rights.

Physician's Role

The physician prescribes medications (unless a state's nurse practice act allows nurse practitioners to

Components of Drug Orders

A medication order is incomplete unless it has the following parts:

- Client's full name. The client's full name distinguishes the client from other persons with the same last name.
- Date that the order is written. The day, month, year, and time must be included. Designating the time that an order is written helps clarify when certain orders are to stop automatically. If an incident occurs involving a medication error, it is easier to document what happened when this information is available.
- Drug name. The physician will order a generic or trade-name drug. Correct spelling is essential in preventing confusion with drugs with similar spelling.
- Dosage. The amount or strength of the medication is included.
- Route of administration. The physician uses common abbreviations for drug routes. Accuracy is important because some drugs are administered by more than one route.
- Time and frequency of administration. The nurse needs to know when to initiate drug therapy. Orders for multiple doses establish a routine schedule for drug administration.
- Signature of physician or nurse practitioner. The signature makes the order a legal request.

prescribe in specific situations). The physician writes an order on a designated form in the client's medical record, in a physician's order book, or on a legal prescription pad. In some situations a physician may also order a medication by telephone or by giving the nurse a verbal order. The nurse enters and signs all telephone and verbal orders writes the time, date, and name of the physician ordering the drug; and later has the physician countersign the order. Most institutions require a physician's signature within 24 hours after the order is given. Institutional policies vary as to which personnel can take verbal or telephone orders. In many institutions, nursing students cannot take medication orders. *No* medication is given without an order.

Common abbreviations (see end paper) are used when writing orders. The abbreviations indicate dosage frequencies or times, routes of administration, and special information for the nurse to follow in giving the drug.

Types of Orders

The four common types of medication orders are based on the frequency of drug administration.

STANDING ORDERS. A standing order is carried out until the physician cancels it by another order or until a prescribed number of days elapse. A standing order may have a final date. Many institutions have policies for automatically discontinuing standing orders. The following are examples of standing orders: "tetracycline 500 mg PO q6h"* and "Decadron 10 mg qd† × 5 days."

PRN ORDERS. The physician may order a drug on a prn basis (when a client requires it). The nurse uses discretion in determining the client's need. Often the physician sets minimal intervals for the time of administration. The nurse may decide to lengthen the interval if the client does not need the drug. Examples of prn orders are "morphine sulfate gr ¼ IM q3-4h prn for incisional pain" and "Maalox 30 ml prn for gastric discomfort."

SINGLE (ONE-TIME) ORDERS. A physician may order a drug to be given only once at a specified time. This is common for preoperative drugs or drugs given before diagnostic examinations. Examples include the following: "Valium 10 mg PO at 0900" and "Stadol 4 mg IM on call to OR."

STAT ORDERS. A stat order signifies that a single dose of a medication is to be given immediately and only once. Often stat orders are written for emergencies when a client's condition changes suddenly. An example follows: "Give Apresoline 10 mg IM stat."

Some conditions change the status of a client's medication orders. Surgery automatically cancels all preoperative medications (see Chapter 47). Because the client's condition is generally changed after surgery, the physician must write new orders. When a client is transferred to another health care agency or a different medical service within a hospital or is discharged, the physician should review the medications and rewrite them to reflect the medication regimen desired. Various institutions have policies regarding the frequency and circumstances under which medications must be reviewed and reordered.

Prescriptions

The physician writes prescriptions for clients to take medications outside the hospital. The prescription includes more detailed information than a regular order because the client must understand how to take the medication and when to refill the prescription if necessary (Fig. 21-3). Parts of a prescription include the following:

1. Superscription. The client's name, address, and age and the date are given for identification purposes. The symbol ℞ ("take thou") is at the top of the form.
2. Inscription. This is the drug name, strength, and dose.
3. Subscription. Directions about the number of tablets or amount to be dispensed are given to the pharmacist.
4. Signature. Information to be written on the label, such as directions to the client (for example, take with full glass of water or take between meals), directions for refilling the prescription, and whether the drug name should be on the label, is included.
5. Personal data. The physician signs the prescription. If the drug is a controlled substance, the physician includes registration number and address.

Pharmacist's Role

The pharmacist prepares and distributes prescribed drugs. The pharmacist is responsible for fill-

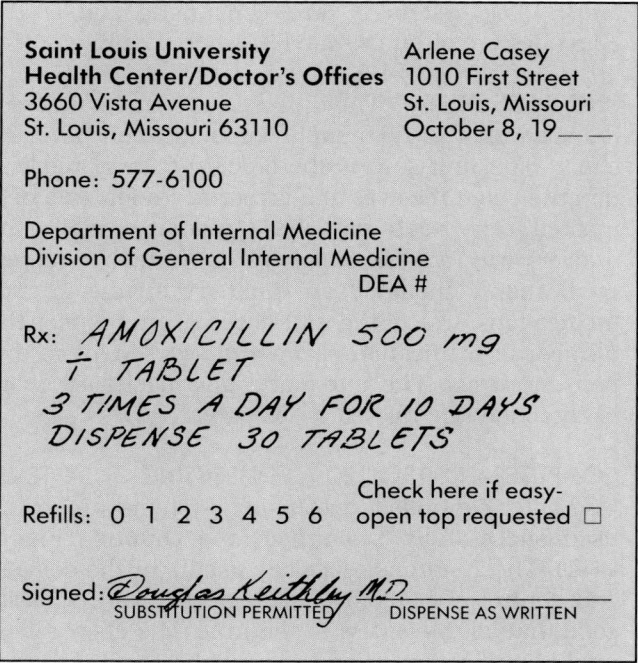

Saint Louis University
Health Center/Doctor's Offices
3660 Vista Avenue
St. Louis, Missouri 63110

Arlene Casey
1010 First Street
St. Louis, Missouri
October 8, 19___ ___

Phone: 577-6100

Department of Internal Medicine
Division of General Internal Medicine
DEA #

Rx: *AMOXICILLIN 500 mg*
ī TABLET
3 TIMES A DAY FOR 10 DAYS
DISPENSE 30 TABLETS

Refills: 0 1 2 3 4 5 6   Check here if easy-open top requested ☐

Signed: *Douglas Keithly M.D.*
SUBSTITUTION PERMITTED   DISPENSE AS WRITTEN

Fig. 21-3 Example of a medication prescription.
Courtesy Saint Louis University Medical Center, St Louis.

*q (every) 6h (hours)
†qd, every day.

ing prescriptions accurately and for being sure that prescriptions are valid. If there is any question that a prescription is forged or that the prescribing physician is unlicensed, the pharmacist should not fill the prescription. The pharmacist calls the physician if an ordered dose seems outside the safe therapeutic range.

The pharmacist in a health care agency today rarely has to mix compounds or solutions except in the case of IV additive solutions. Most drug companies deliver drugs in a form ready for administration. Dispensing the correct drug, in the proper dosage and amount, with an accurate label is the pharmacist's chief responsibility. The pharmacist can also provide information about drug side effects, toxicity, interactions, and incompatibilities.

Distribution Systems

Systems for the storage and distribution of medications vary among health care agencies. Institutions providing nursing care have a designated area for stocking and dispensing drugs. Special medication rooms, portable locked carts, and individual storage units adjacent to clients' rooms are some of the facilities used. Nurses should keep close watch on the supply of medications, making sure that storage areas are locked when unattended.

STOCK SUPPLY. With a stock system, medications are available in quantity in stock containers. A nurse prepares individual doses from a large stock supply container. The system is time consuming and costly. Narcotics are often provided in stock supply.

UNIT-DOSE SYSTEM. The unit-dose system consist of a drawer with a 24-hour supply of medications for each client. The unit-dose is the ordered dose of medication the client receives at a prescribed hour. At a designated time each day the pharmacist refills the drawers with a fresh supply of individually wrapped medications. Included are limited amounts of prn medications. Use of the unit-dose system reduces the number of medication errors and saves steps in dispensing drugs. The nurse and pharmacist are more likely to identify missed doses earlier.

COMPUTER-CONTROLLED DISPENSING SYSTEMS. Computer-controlled dispensing systems are being used successfully throughout the country (Figure 21-4). The system is especially useful for the delivery and control of narcotics. Each nurse has a security code that allows access to the unit. The client's hospital identification number is then entered. In some systems the nurse is then allowed to select the desired drug, dose, and route. The system delivers the

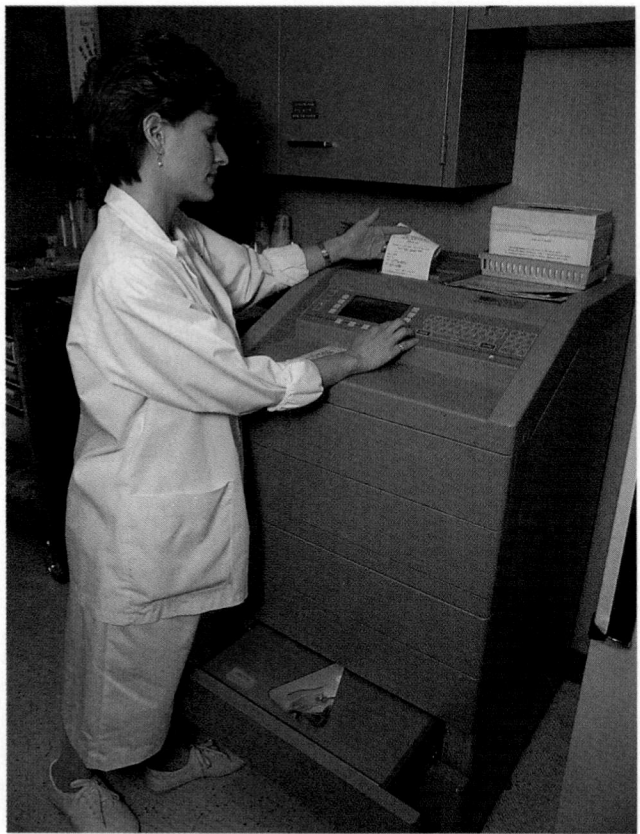

Fig. 21-4 Computer-controlled dispensing system.

medication to the nurse, records it, and charges it to the client. For example, the following narcotics are entered into the computer for Mr. Svoda:

1. Morphine 2 mg IM q3h
2. Morphine 5 mg IM q3h
3. Percodan II PO q̄ 4°*
4. Halcion 0.125 mg PO HS†

The nurse first enters the security code number and the client's identification number and then reviews the orders. The nurse may then enter 1, and a single unit dose of Morphine 2 mg for IM injection would be delivered with opening.

Nurse's Role

The nurse's role extends beyond simply giving drugs to a client. The nurse must determine whether a client should receive a drug at a given time, assess the client's ability to self-administer drugs, provide

---

*q̄, Before.

†HS, Hour of sleep.

medications at the proper time, and monitor the effects of prescribed medications. Client and family education about proper drug administration and monitoring is also the nurse's role. The nurse uses the nursing process to integrate drug therapy into care.

 ## Assessment

To determine the need for and potential response to drug therapy, the nurse assesses many factors.

MEDICAL HISTORY. A medical history provides indications or contraindications for drug therapy. Disease or illness may place clients at risk for adverse drug effects. For example, if a client has a gastric ulcer or bleeding tendency, compounds containing aspirin or anticoagulants will increase the likelihood of bleeding. Long-term health problems such as diabetes or arthritis, which require medications, suggest to the nurse the type of drugs a client is taking. A client's surgical history may indicate use of medications. For example, after a thyroidectomy a client may require hormone replacement. From this history, nurses may need to request orders for drugs the client takes routinely (for example, Synthroid and antihypertensives) if they are not ordered on admission.

HISTORY OF ALLERGIES. If the client has a history of allergies to medication, the nurse informs other members of the health care team. Food allergies should also be carefully documented because many drugs have ingredients found in food sources. One example is shellfish. If clients are allergic to shellfish, the client may be sensitive to any product containing iodine. In a hospital, clients wear identification bands listing medications to which they are allergic. All allergies should be noted on the nurse's admission notes, medication records, and physician's history.

DRUG DATA. The nurse assesses information about each drug, including action, purpose, normal dosages, routes, side effects, and nursing implications for administration and monitoring. Common questions to ask include the following: "Is this the smallest possible dose ordered (a question pertinent to older adults)?" "Can a certain drug interact with other drugs being used?" and "Are there special instructions for administering the drug?"

Often, several resources must be consulted to gather needed information. Pharmacology textbooks, nursing journals, the *Physicians' Desk Reference (PDR)*, drug package inserts, and the pharmacist are valuable resources. The nurse is responsible for knowing as much as possible about each drug given. Many nursing students prepare or purchase cards and or books containing drug data to use as a quick resource.

DIET HISTORY. A diet history reveals the client's usual eating patterns. The nurse can then plan the dosage schedule more effectively.

CLIENT'S CURRENT CONDITION. The ongoing physical or mental status of a client may affect whether a drug is given or how it is administered. The nurse should assess a client carefully before giving any drug. For example, the nurse checks blood pressure before giving an antihypertensive. If the client is nauseated, it is unlikely a tablet can be swallowed. Assessment findings can also serve as a baseline in evaluating the effects of drug therapy.

CLIENT'S PERCEPTUAL OR COORDINATION PROBLEMS. For a client with perceptual or coordination limitations, self-administration may be difficult. The nurse must assess the client's ability to prepare dosages and take medications correctly. If the client is unable to self-administer drugs, the nurse learns whether family members or friends are available to assist.

CLIENT'S ATTITUDE ABOUT THE USE OF DRUGS. The client's attitude about drugs may reveal the level of drug dependence. Clients are often reluctant to express feelings about drugs, particularly if drug dependence is a problem. To assess attitudes, the nurse may have to observe the client's behavior for evidence of dependence.

CLIENT'S KNOWLEDGE AND UNDERSTANDING OF DRUG THERAPY. The client's knowledge and understanding of drug therapy influence the willingness or ability to follow a drug regimen. Unless a client understands a drug's purpose, the importance of regular dosage schedules and proper administration methods, and the possible side effects, compliance is unlikely. When assessing knowledge of a drug, the nurse asks the client the following questions:
1. What is it for?
2. How and when is it taken?
3. What side effects have there been?
4. Have you ever stopped taking doses?
5. Is there anything else you do not understand and would like to know about the drug?

CLIENT'S LEARNING NEEDS. By assessing the client's level of knowledge about a medication, the nurse determines the need for instruction. It may be necessary for the nurse to explain the action and purpose of the drug, expected side effects, correct administration techniques, and ways to remember the drug regimen. If a client has been placed on a newly prescribed drug, instruction may need to be more involved.

Nursing Diagnosis

Assessment provides data on the client's condition, ability to self-administer drugs, and drug use patterns, which can be used to determine actual or potential problems with drug therapy (see diagnoses box). If the nurse diagnoses *knowledge deficit* or factors interfering with drug therapy compliance, client education becomes a part of the nursing care plan. If the client has physical limitations that interfere with drug administration, the nurse plans strategies to ensure safety. The identification of appropriate defining characteristics ensures that an accurate diagnosis is made (see diagnostic process).

Planning

The nurse organizes care activities to ensure that safe administrative techniques are used. Hurrying to give clients medications can lead to errors. The nurse can also plan to use time during drug administration to teach clients about their medications.

In situations in which clients learn to self-administer medications, the nurse plans to use all available teaching resources. Inclusion of family members or friends in instruction is very important. Clients may be unable to consistently self-administer medications. There may be other non-health-related reasons. When there is little time for instruction, brochures or pamphlets describing drug therapy are available. If clients have been newly diagnosed and require a medicine such as insulin, a home health referral is an important option of the care plan. Home health nurses can assist clients in establishing medication schedules to fit home routines.

Whether a client attempts self-administration or the nurse assumes responsibility for administering

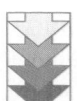

Examples of Nursing Diagnoses Related to Drug Therapy

NANDA-APPROVED NURSING DIAGNOSES

Knowledge deficit regarding drug therapy related to:
- Lack of exposure and inexperience
- Cognitive limitations
- Unfamiliarity with information resources

Noncompliance regarding drug therapy related to:
- Limited economic resources
- Health beliefs
- Cultural influences

Impaired physical mobility related to:
- Musculoskeletal impairment
- Decreased strength
- Pain and discomfort

Sensory/perceptual alterations: visual related to:
- Blurred vision

Anxiety related to:
- Threat to or change in health status
- Threat to or change in socioeconomic status
- Threat to or change in interaction patterns

Impaired swallowing related to:
- Neuromuscular impairment
- Irritated oral cavity
- Limited awareness

Sample Nursing Diagnostic Process for Drug Therapy

Assessment Activities	Defining Characteristics	Nursing Diagnoses
Ask client about previous use of prescribed medication.	Client denies use. Inquires about purpose of medication	*Knowledge deficit regarding drug therapy* related to newly prescribed medication
Check client's medical record for new orders.	New drug ordered in morning. No previous history of taking prescribed medication	
Observe client swallow medication.	Coughs when attempting to swallow capsule	*Impaired swallowing* related to right facial paralysis
Ask if client is able to perceive food in the mouth.	Food retained in mouth after eating	
Perform neurological assessment of ninth and tenth cranial nerves (see Chapter 20)	Reduced gag reflex	

medications (see care plan), the following goals should be met:

1. Absence of complications related to the route of administration
2. Achievement of the therapeutic effect of the prescribed medications safely while maintaining the client's comfort
3. Understanding on the part of the client and family members regarding drug therapy
4. Safe self-administration of medications

 Implementation

CORRECT TRANSCRIPTION AND COMMUNICATION OF ORDERS. The nurse or a designated unit secretary writes the physician's complete order on the appropriate medication forms or tickets (Figs. 21-5 at right and 21-6 on p. 634). The transcribed order includes client's name, room, and bed number; drug name, dosage, and time; and route of administration. Each time a drug dosage is prepared, the nurse refers to the medication form or ticket. With the unit-dose system, only one transcription is necessary, limiting the opportunity for errors. When transcribing orders, the nurse should be sure that names, dosages, and symbols are legible. The nurse rewrites any smudged or illegible transcriptions.

In some institutions a computer printout lists all currently ordered medications with dosage information. Orders are entered directly into the computer, preventing the need for transcription of orders. The same printout may be used to record medications given.

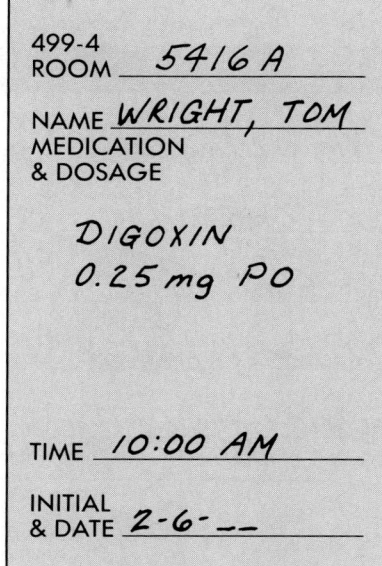

499-4
ROOM _5416 A_

NAME _WRIGHT, TOM_
MEDICATION
& DOSAGE

DIGOXIN
_0.25 mg PO_

TIME _10:00 AM_

INITIAL
& DATE _2-6-__

Fig. 21-5 Sample medication ticket.

 Sample Nursing Care Plan for Knowledge Deficit

Nursing Diagnosis: *Knowledge deficit regarding drug therapy* related to newly prescribed medication
Definition: Knowledge deficit is the state in which specific information is lacking (Kim, McFarland, McLane, 1991).

Goal	Expected Outcomes	Interventions	Rationale
Client will correctly self-administer insulin by day of planned discharge (2/18).	Client will correctly prepare proper insulin dose (2/16). Client will correctly state rationale and implications for insulin dose (2/16).	Provide syringe and allow client to manipulate parts. Explain and demonstrate aseptic technique for preparing dosage from vial.	Client becomes familiar with working parts of syringe. Explanation provides learner with clear mental image of how skill is performed; demonstration is method most suited for teaching psychomoter skill (Redman, 1988).
	Client will state rationale for rotating injection sites (2/17). Client will correctly self-administer subcutaneous insulin 3 times before discharge 2/18.	Discuss importance of proper dosage. Explain and demonstrate method for administering subcutaneous injection (have client stand behind nurse).	Insulin can create serious side effects if improper dosage is administered. Demonstration provides image of injection technique; over-the-shoulder view provides clear image of how to do action (Redman, 1988).

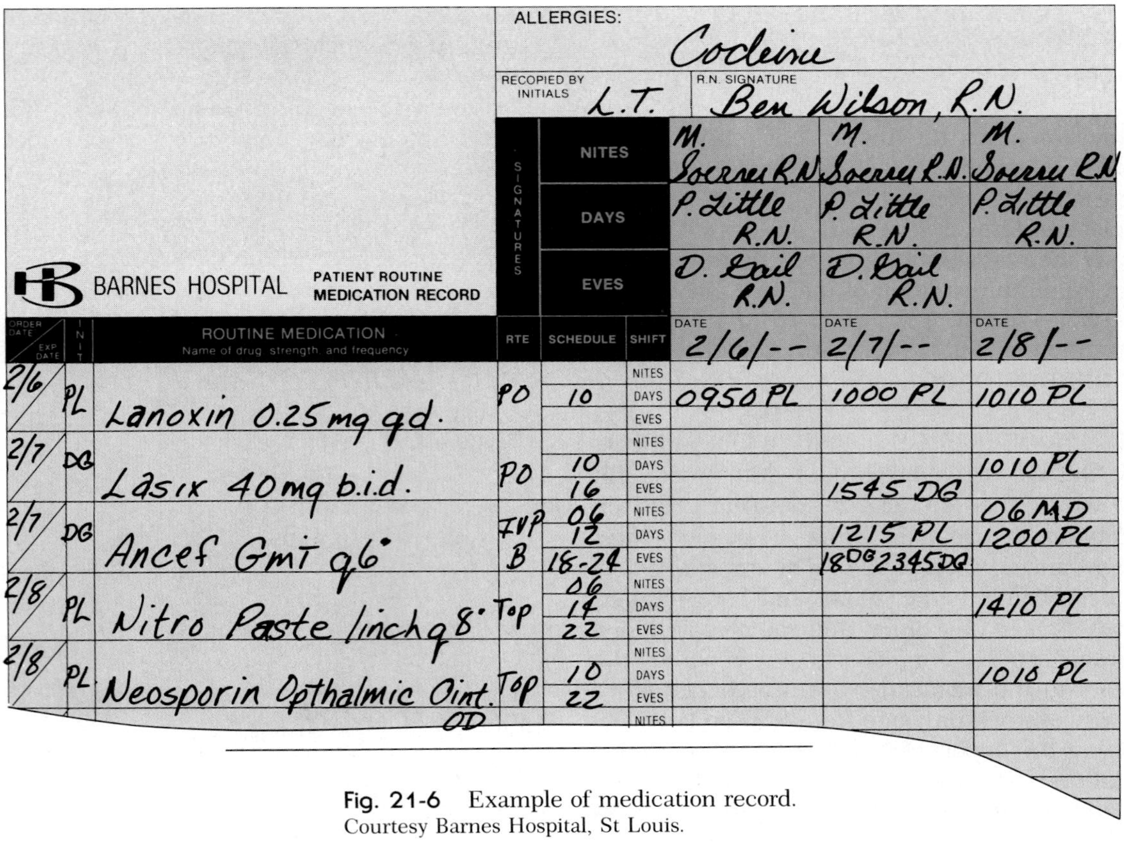

ALLERGIES: Codeine

RECOPIED BY INITIALS: L.T. R.N. SIGNATURE: Ben Wilson, R.N.

BARNES HOSPITAL PATIENT ROUTINE MEDICATION RECORD

SIGNATURES			
NITES	M. Socrrei R.N.	M. Socrrei R.N.	M. Socrrei R.N.
DAYS	P. Little R.N.	P. Little R.N.	P. Little R.N.
EVES	D. Gail R.N.	D. Gail R.N.	

ORDER DATE / EXP DATE	INIT	ROUTINE MEDICATION Name of drug, strength, and frequency	RTE	SCHEDULE	SHIFT	DATE 2/6/--	DATE 2/7/--	DATE 2/8/--
2/6	PL	Lanoxin 0.25mg qd.	PO		NITES			
				10	DAYS	0950 PL	1000 PL	1010 PL
					EVES			
2/7	DG	Lasix 40mg b.i.d.	PO		NITES			
				10	DAYS			1010 PL
				16	EVES		1545 DG	
2/7	DG	Ancef Gm q6°	IVPB	06	NITES			06 MD
				12	DAYS		1215 PL	1200 PL
				18-24	EVES		18 DG 2345 DG	
2/8	PL	Nitro Paste 1 inch q8°	Top	06	NITES			
				14	DAYS			1410 PL
				22	EVES			
2/8	PL	Neosporin Opthalmic Oint. OD	Top		NITES			
				10	DAYS			1010 PL
				22	EVES			

Fig. 21-6 Example of medication record.
Courtesy Barnes Hospital, St Louis.

A registered nurse checks all transcribed orders against the original order for accuracy and thoroughness. If an order seems incorrect or inappropriate, the nurse consults the physician. The nurse who gives the wrong medication or an incorrect dosage is legally responsible for the error.

ACCURATE DOSAGE CALCULATION AND MEASUREMENT. When measuring liquid drugs, the nurse uses standard measuring receptacles. The procedure for drug measurement is systematic to lessen the chance of error. The nurse calculates each dose when preparing the drug, pays close attention to calculation, and avoids interference from other nursing activities.

CORRECT ADMINISTRATION. The nurse uses aseptic technique and proper procedures when handling and giving medications. Certain drugs require the nurse to perform assessments at the time of administration, such as assessing heart rate before giving antidysrhythmic medications.

RECORDING DRUG ADMINISTRATION. To avoid having another nurse give a medication without knowing that the client had already received a dose, the nurse documents medications at the time of administration. When a nurse forgets to record medications, double doses can easily be given. Agency policy determines whether a nurse should document while preparing the medication for a client or immediately after administering the medications (Fig. 21-6). If the nurse records a drug but the medication is not given due to client refusal or physical assessment findings contraindicating drug use, the medication record must be revised.

The recording of a drug includes the name of the drug, dosage, route, and exact time of administration. Often the drug forms are prepared and the nurse needs to record only the time. Agency policies may also require that the nurse record the location of an injection.

If a client refuses a drug or is undergoing tests or procedures that result in a missed dose, the nurse explains in the nurses' notes the reason that the drug was not given. Some agencies require the nurse to circle and initial the prescribed administration time on the drug record when a dose is missed.

CLIENT AND FAMILY TEACHING. Unless clients are properly informed about drugs, they may take the drugs incorrectly or not at all. The nurse provides information about the purpose of medications and their actions and effects. Many health care institutions offer easy-to-read leaflets on specific types of drugs. Clients must know the way to take drugs properly and the effects if they fail to do so. For example, a client receiving a prescription for an antibiotic must understand the importance of taking the full prescription. Failure to do this can lead to a worsening of the condition, as well as the development of bacterial resistance to the drug.

Nurses teach proper self-administration of drugs to clients who depend on daily injections. The client learns to prepare and administer injections correctly using aseptic technique. Family members should be taught to give injections in case clients become ill or physically unable to handle syringes. For clients with visual alterations, nurses can provide specially designed equipment such as syringes with enlarged calibrated scales for easier reading or braille-labeled medication vials. Many older clients are responsible for self-medication, so instructions should include detailed information about medications and dosage schedules that help them remember to take medications regularly.

Clients must be aware of the symptoms of drug side effects or toxicity. For example, clients taking anticoagulants learn to notify the physician immediately when signs of bleeding or frequent bruising develop. Family members should be informed of drug side effects, such as changes in behavior, because they are often the first persons to recognize such effects. Clients are better able to cope with problems caused by drugs if they understand how and when to act. All clients should learn the following basic guidelines for drug safety in the home:

1. Keep each drug in its original, labeled container.
2. Be sure labels are legible.
3. Discard any outdated medications.
4. Always finish a prescribed drug unless otherwise instructed. Never save a drug for future illnesses.
5. Dispose of drugs in a sink or toilet. Do not place drugs in the trash within reach of children.
6. Do not give a family member or friend a drug prescribed for another.
7. Refrigerate medications that require it.
8. Read labels carefully and follow all instructions.

MAINTAINING CLIENTS' RIGHTS. In 1973 the American Hospital Association issued a Patient's Bill of Rights (see Chapter 14), a comprehensive statement defining the rights and responsibilities for a broad area of medical and nursing practice. The Patient's Bill of Rights helps to clarify the rights of clients in an area

of practice such as medication administration. Because of the potential risks related to drug administration, a client has the right to the following:

1. Be informed of drug name, purpose, action, and potential undesired effects
2. Refuse a medication regardless of the consequences
3. Have qualified nurses or physicians assess a drug history, including allergies
4. Be properly advised of the experimental nature of any drug therapy and give written consent for its use
5. Receive labeled medications safely without discomfort in accordance with the "five rights" of drug administration (see section on medication delivery)
6. Receive appropriate supportive therapy in relation to drug therapy
7. Not receive unnecessary medications

The nurse must be aware of these rights and handle all inquiries by clients and families courteously and professionally. A nurse should not become defensive if a client refuses drug therapy. The nurse must have the knowledge and skill to satisfy the responsibilities of safe and effective drug administration.

 ## Evaluation

The nurse monitors a client's response to medications on an ongoing basis. To do this the nurse knows the therapeutic action and common side effects of each medication. A change in a client's condition can be physiologically related to health status, may result from medications, or both. The nurse must be alert for reactions when a client takes several medications.

The goal of safe and effective drug administration involves a careful evaluation of technique and the client's response to therapy and ability to assume responsibility for self-care. To evaluate the effectiveness of nursing interventions when meeting established goals of care, the nurse uses evaluative measures to identify actual outcomes. Examples of evaluative measures for determining absence of complications related to the route of administration include the following and those listed in the evaluation box on p. 636:

1. Observing injection sites for bruises, inflammation, localized pain, or bleeding
2. Questioning the client about localized numbness or tingling at injection sites
3. Assessing the client for gastrointestinal disturbances, including nausea, vomiting, and diarrhea

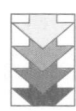 Sample Evaluation of Interventions for Knowledge Deficit

Goals	Evaluative Measures	Expected Outcomes
Client will correctly self-administer insulin by day of planned discharge. (2/18).	Observe client perform return demonstration of preparing dose in syringe. Ask client to describe ordered insulin dosage and implications of receiving incorrect dose. Observe client perform return demonstration of self-administration of injections.	Client will correctly prepare proper insulin dose. Client will correctly state rationale and implications for insulin dose. Client will correctly self-administer insulin.
Client will not experience complication related to route of administration.	Inspect injection sites for localized tenderness, inflammation, hardness, or bruising. Inspect IV sites for redness, swelling, tenderness, or cool or warm skin. Ask client if gastric distress follows oral intake of medication.	Injection sites will have no inflammation and minimal bruising. IV sites will have no signs of phlebitis or infiltration. Client will deny symptoms of gastric distress.
Client will achieve therapeutic effect of prescribed medications.	Monitor or have client monitor desired effect of medication (e.g., relief of discomfort after analgesic, lowering of body temperature after antipyretic, lowering or maintenance of blood pressure after antihypertensive).	Medication will exert measurable therapeutic effect.
Client will be safe and comfortable.	Note positioning of client before administration (e.g., sitting up for oral medication ingestion, lying on side before ventrogluteal injection). Monitor IV infusion rate regularly. Observe for potential side or toxic effects.	When sitting, client will be able to swallow oral medications without difficulty, or when lying on side, injection will be given correctly in proper tissue. IV medication will infuse over prescribed time. Client will deny side effects, and no adverse effects will be observed.
Client will understand drug therapy.	Ask client or family member to explain purpose of medication and all pertinent information related to drug administration.	Client or family member will explain information needed to demonstrate understanding of drug regimen.

4. Inspecting IV sites for phlebitis, including fever, swelling, and localized tenderness

Examples of evaluative measures for determining whether the therapuetic effect of prescribed medication has been achieved safely include the following:
1. Questioning the client for expected response to the drug (for example, pain relief, or reduction in symptoms)
2. Monitoring client's physical response to medication (for example, antidysrhythmic medication, regular heart rhythm; hypertension medication, lowered blood pressure; diuretics, increased urine output).

Examples of evaluative measures for maintaining the client's safety and comfort include the following:
1. Monitoring the client for potential side or toxic effects, allergic reactions, or interactions

2. Assessing the client up to 30 minutes after administration of medications for symptoms of discomfort

Examples of evaluative measures for understanding drug therapy include the following:
1. Asking the client to explain the drug's purpose, action, dosage, schedule of administration, and possible side effects
2. Asking the client to describe when each medication is taken during the day

Examples of evaluative measures for determining the client's ability to self-administer medications safely include the following:
1. Observing the client preparing an ordered dose of medication
2. Observing the client administering the ordered dose of medication

MEDICATION DELIVERY

Preparing and administering medications requires accuracy by the nurse. The nurse must pay full attention to preparing medications and must not attempt to do other tasks simultaneously. The nurse uses the following guidelines, the "five rights" of drug administration, to ensure safe drug administration:

1. The *right* drug
2. The *right* dose
3. The *right* client
4. The *right* route
5. The *right* time

Right Drug

When drugs are first ordered, the nurse compares the medicine ticket or unit-dose recording form with the physician's written orders. When administering drugs, the nurse compares the label of the drug container with the form or medicine ticket. The nurse does this three times: (1) before removing the container from the drawer or shelf, (2) as the amount of drug ordered is removed from the container, and (3) before returning the container to storage. With single-dose prepackaged drugs the nurse checks the label with the medicine ticket or form three times even though the medication is not being taken from a bulk container (Fig. 21-7). Nurses administer *only* the drugs they prepare. If an error occurs, the nurse administering the drug is responsible for its effects.

If a client questions the medication, the nurse does not ignore these concerns. An alert client will know whether a drug is different from those received before. In most cases the drug order has been changed. However, the client's questions might reveal an error. The nurse should withhold the drug until the preparation can be rechecked against physician's orders. Clients who self-administer drugs should keep them in their original labeled containers, separate from other drugs, to avoid confusion.

The nurse never prepares medications from unmarked containers or containers with illegible labels. If a client refuses a drug, the nurse should never return the medication to the original container or transfer the drug to another container. Single-dose prepackaged drugs can be returned to storage areas if they are unopened.

Right Dose

The unit-dose system of drug distribution minimizes errors because most medications come pre-

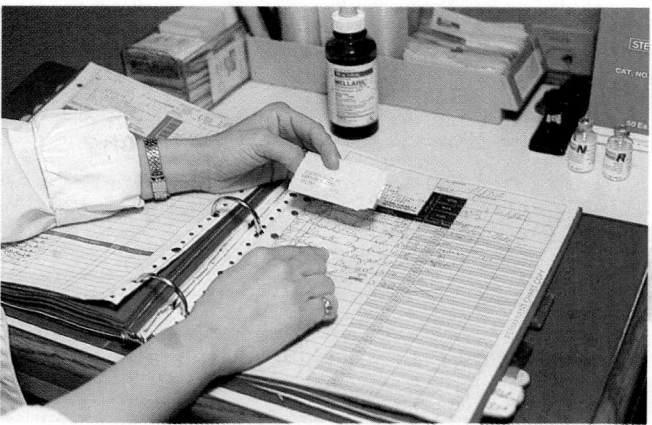

Fig. 21-7 The nurse checks the label of the medication with the transcribed medication order.

pared in proper doses. When a medication must be prepared from a larger or smaller volume or strength than needed or when a physician orders a system of measurement different from what the pharmacist supplies, the chance of error increases. In these situations, a nurse should check another nurse's dosage calculations. For example, some institutions require two nurses to check all insulin and anticoagulant dosages.

After calculating dosages the nurse prepares the medication by using standard measurement devices. For example, many liquid pediatric medications come with a scaled dropper. Graduated cups, syringes, and specially designed spoons can be used to measure medications accurately. In the home, clients should use standard kitchen measuring spoons rather than flatware teaspoons and tablespoons, which vary in volume.

To break a scored tablet, the nurse makes sure that the break is even. A tablet may be cut in half by using a knife edge or by folding a tissue over the tablet and breaking it with the fingers. Any tablets that do not break evenly are discarded. After a tablet is split, the nurse may give the two halves in successive doses, but only if the second half has been repackaged and labeled.

Often a nurse prepares a tablet by crushing it in a mortar with a pestle or in a special tablet crusher so that it can be mixed in food, especially when a client has difficulty with swallowing and an injection is unnecessary or undesirable. The mortar should always be cleaned out completely before the tablet is crushed. Remnants of previously crushed drugs may increase a drug's concentration or result in the client receiving a portion of an unprescribed drug. Crushed medications should be mixed with very small amounts of food or liquid. Foods and liquids that clients are taking well or especially liked foods should not be used because a medication may decrease a clients desire for a food after it has been altered with "bitter" and "bad-tasting" medications. Some suggestions are jelly, syrup, and chocolate syrup or other ice cream toppings, which must be sugar free for diabetic persons.

Right Client

An important step in administering drugs safely is being sure that the medication is given to the right client. The nurse working in a hospital or extended care setting is frequently responsible for administering drugs to several clients. Clients often have similar last names, and it is difficult to remember every name and face, especially if a nurse has been off duty for several days. To identify clients correctly, the nurse checks the medicine tickets, forms, or printouts against clients' identification bracelets (Fig. 21-8) and asks clients to state their names.

If an identification bracelet becomes smudged or illegible, the nurse should replace it with a new one. When asking for a name, the nurse should not speak the name and then assume that the response indicates that the client is the right person. Instead, the nurse asks the client to state a full name. This is vital even if the nurse has been caring for a client for several days. To avoid making the client feel uneasy, the

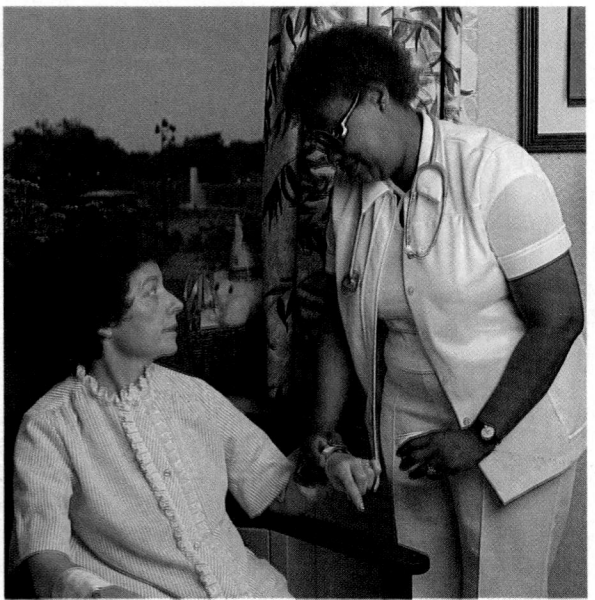

Fig. 21-8 Before administering any medication, the nurse checks the client's identification and allergy bracelet.

nurse simply says that the routine for giving a medication requires identification by name.

Clients who self-administer medications at home should be cautioned to never give a family member or friend one of their medications. A physician should be consulted before one person uses a prescription meant for another because a drug that is safe for one person can be dangerous for another.

Right Route

If a medication order does not designate a route of administration, the nurse consults the physician. Likewise, if the specified route is not the recommended route, the nurse should alert the physician immediately.

When administering injections (see the section on parenteral routes), the nurse ensures that medications are given correctly. It is also important to prepare injections only from preparations designed for parenteral use. The injection of a liquid designed for oral use can produce local complications such as a sterile abscess or fatal systemic effects. Drug companies label parenteral drugs for "injectable use only."

Right Time

The nurse must know why a drug is ordered for certain times of the day and whether the time schedule can be altered. For example, two drugs are ordered, one q8h (every 8 hours) and the other tid (3 times a day). Both medications are given 3 times within 24 hours. The physician intends the q8h medication to be given around the clock to maintain therapeutic blood levels of the drug. In contrast, the tid medication is given during the waking hours. Each institution has a recommended time schedule for medications ordered at frequent intervals. For example, qid (4 times a day) medications may be given at 0800, 1200, 1600, and 2000; tid medications may be given at 0800, 1400, and 2000.

The physician often gives specific instructions about when to administer a medication. A preoperative medication to be given on call means that the nurse is to administer the drug when the operating room notifies the nursing division. A drug ordered pc (after meals) is to be given within half an hour after a meal, when the client has a full stomach. A stat medication is to be given immediately.

When a nurse is responsible for administering several medications, drugs that must act at certain times are given priority. For example, insulin should be administered at a precise interval before a meal. All routinely ordered medications should be given within 30 minutes of the times ordered.

Some medications require the nurse's clinical judgment in determining the proper time for administration. A prn sleeping medication should be administered when the client is prepared for bed. Many hospitalized clients prefer to go to sleep earlier than they might normally at home. However, if the nurse is aware that a procedure might interrupt the client's sleep, it is appropriate to withhold the drug until a time when the client can gain full benefit from the medication. A nurse also uses judgment in administering prn analgesics. When a client's order reads q3-4h, the nurse may give the medication as often as every 3 hours. The nurse assesses the client's level of pain to determine the degree of discomfort. If a client is made to wait until the pain becomes severe, the analgesic effect may not be sufficient. The nurse may then need to obtain an order from the physician to supplement the prn analgesic. (For more about analgesia, see Chapter 37)

In the home a client may have to take several medications throughout the day. The nurse can help plan medication schedules based on the preferred drug intervals and the client's daily schedule. For example, the schedule for drugs to be given around mealtime can be easily adjusted to client preferences. For clients who have difficulty remembering when to take medications, the nurse can make a chart that lists the times when each drug is to be taken.

Avoiding Errors

Most medication errors occur when a nurse fails to follow routine procedures (Table 21-8). Unfortunately, many medication errors are never identified.

An error should be acknowledged immediately. The nurse has the ethical and professional responsibility for reporting the error to the physician and the risk manager of the employing institution (see Chap-

---

TABLE 21-8 Ways to Prevent Drug Administration Errors

Precaution	Rationale	Precaution	Rationale
Read drug labels carefully.	Many products come in similar containers, colors, and shapes.	When new or unfamiliar drug is ordered, consult resource.	If physician is also unfamiliar with drug, there is greater risk of inaccurate dosages being ordered.
Question administration of multiple tablets or vials for single dose.	Most doses are one or two tablets or capsules or one single-dose vial. Incorrect interpretation of order may result in excessively high dose.	Do not administer drug ordered by nickname or unofficial abbreviation.	Many physicians refer to commonly ordered medications by nicknames or unofficial abbreviations. If nurse or pharmacist is unfamiliar with name, wrong drug may be dispensed and administered.
Be aware of drugs with similar names.	Many drug names sound alike (e.g., digoxin and digitoxin, Keflex and Keflin, Orinase and Ornade).		
Check decimal point.	Some drugs come in quantities that are multiples of one another (e.g., Coumadin in 2.5 and 25 mg tablets, Thorazine in 30 and 300 mg spansules).	Do not attempt to decipher illegible writing.	When in doubt, ask physician. Unless nurse questions order that is difficult to read, chance of misinterpretation is great.
Question abrupt and excessive increases in dosages.	Most dosages are made gradually so that physician can monitor therapeutic effect and response.	Know clients with same last names. Also have clients state their full names. Check name bands carefully.	It is common to have two or more clients with same or similar last names. Special labels on Kardex or medication book can warn of potential problem.
		Do not confuse equivalents.	When in hurry, it may be easy to misread equivalents (e.g., milligram instead of milliliter).

ter 14). Measures to counteract the effects of the error, such as administering an antidote when the wrong drug is given, withholding a dose when a previous medication has been given too soon, or monitoring the effects when an unusually high dosage is given, may be necessary.

The nurse is also responsible for completing an incident report describing the nature of the incident. The report is not an admission of guilt or the basis for punishment and is not a part of the client's legal medical record. The report provides an objective analysis of what went wrong and is a means for the institution's risk management team to monitor such occurrences. Incident reports assist nursing supervisory personnel in identifying errors and solving recurrent problems affecting care.

Special Considerations for Age Groups

A client's developmental level is a factor in the way in which nurses administer medications. Knowledge of a client's developmental needs helps the nurse anticipate responses to drug therapy.

Infants and Children

Children vary in age, weight, body surface area, and the ability to absorb, metabolize, and excrete medications. Children's dosages are lower than those of adults, so special caution is needed in preparing medications for them. Drugs are usually not prepared and packaged in standardized dosage ranges for children. Preparing an ordered dosage from an available amount requires careful calculation.

A child's parents are valuable resources for learning the best way to give a child medications. Sometimes it is less traumatic for the child if a parent gives the drug and the nurse supervises.

All children require special psychological preparation before receiving medications. Supportive care is needed if a child is expected to cooperate. The nurse explains the procedure to a child, using short words and simple language appropriate to the child's level of comprehension. Long explanations may increase anxiety, especially for painful procedures such as an injection. The nurse must approach a child with confidence and act as though the child is expected to cooperate (Whaley, Wong, 1991). If it is possible to involve the child, the nurse may have greater success giving a medication. For example, saying "It's time to take your pill now. Do you want it with water or juice?" allows a child to make a choice. The nurse *never* gives the child the option of not taking a medication. After a drug is given, the nurse praises the child and may even offer a simple reward such as a star or token. Depending on the route of administra-

tion, the nurse can use several tips when administering drugs to children (see box).

Older Adults

Older adults also require special consideration during drug administration. Age has an effect on the absorption, distribution, metabolism, and excretion of drugs (see earlier section). In addition to physiological changes of aging, behavioral and economic factors influence older persons' use of drugs.

Noncompliance with drug therapy is the failure of clients to follow instructions regarding the use of medication, which is a problem more complicated than simply forgetting to take a medication. Noncompliance may involve failure to take a medication by choice, intentional reduction in drug dosage, failure

---

Tips for Administering Drugs to Children

ORAL MEDICATIONS

- Liquid forms are safer to swallow to avoid aspiration.
- Juice, a soft drink, or a frozen juice bar is offered after a drug is swallowed.
- Carbonated beverages poured over finely crushed ice reduce nausea.
- When mixing drugs with palatable flavorings such as syrup or honey, the nurse uses only a small amount. The child may refuse to take all of a larger mixture. The nurse avoids mixing a drug with foods or liquids that the child is taking well because the child may in turn refuse them.
- A plastic, disposable syringe is the most accurate device for preparing liquid dosages, especially those less than 10 ml. (Cups, teaspoons, and droppers are inaccurate.)
- When administering liquid drugs, a spoon, plastic cup, or oral syringe (without needle) are useful.

INJECTIONS

- The nurse is very careful when selecting IM injection sites. Infants and small children have underdeveloped muscles.
- Children can be unpredictable and uncooperative. Someone should be available to restrain a child if needed.
- The nurse always awakens a sleeping child before giving an injection.
- Distracting the child with conversation or a toy may reduce pain perception.
- The nurse gives the injection quickly and does not fight with the child.

to take a drug at the right time, increasing the frequency or dosage of medication, or discontinuing use of a drug prematurely. Older clients may also deny the presence of an illness and therefore choose not to take a medication.

Although noncompliance may occur in any age group, it is a special problem for older adults. Older persons are more prone to suffer serious physical effects from particular diseases when medications are not taken. Simonson (1984) summarizes the following client-related factors that may cause noncompliance with drug therapy in older adults:

1. Lack of understanding of drug therapy. Older adults can easily become confused when prescribed several medications.
2. Poor self-medication practices. Clients may consume more nonprescription drugs than needed. These drugs can interfere with the action of prescription drugs.
3. Lack of social supervision. Persons living alone are less likely to comply with prescribed medication therapy than those living with another person.
4. Feeling too ill or tired to take medication. These feelings may be complicated by older persons' difficulty with ambulating and adverse effects of certain drugs.
5. Sensory losses. Visual alterations make it difficult to read prescriptions. Hearing problems may alter the ability to understand oral instructions.
6. Keeping old prescriptions and self-dosing. Old medications may be inappropriate or have little therapeutic effect.
7. Economic status. The high costs of certain medications are not affordable for many clients on a fixed income.

Compliance can be improved by offering clients simple, realistic plans for drug therapy. The least possible number of medications should be prescribed and complement daily habits (for example, meal and bedtime). Eliopoulos (1987) makes the following recommendations for instructing and assisting older adults with drug regimens:

1. Provide detailed written and oral descriptions to clients and care givers. Outline the drug's name, dosage schedule, route of administration, action, special precautions, incompatible foods or drugs, and adverse reactions.
2. Offer a color-coded dosage schedule for persons who have visual deficits or are illiterate.
3. Be sure that all medication labels are typed in large print.
4. Provide medicine containers with easy-to-remove caps for weak or arthritic hands.

5. Offer memory aids to remind clients of medication schedules (for example, partitioned plastic box containing prescribed doses for 1 week, labeled plastic baggies holding each timed dose, or a color-coded chart describing each drug and time to be taken).

 ORAL DRUG ADMINISTRATION

The most desirable way to administer medications is by mouth (Procedure 21-1 on pp. 642-644). Unless the client has impaired gastrointestinal functioning or is unable to swallow, an oral medication is the safest and easiest to give.

Most tablets and capsules should be swallowed and administered with an adequate amount of fluid, providing an opportunity for the nurse to increase a client's fluid intake. For clients with nasogastric feeding tubes, liquid medications are preferred, but some tablets can be crushed and capsules opened to mix in a solution for administration (see box).

When administering medications orally, the nurse must protect the client against possible aspiration. Positioning the client in a sitting or side-lying position will prevent accumulation of a liquid or a solid

---

Guidelines for Giving Drugs Through a Nasogastric Tube, J-Tube, G-Tube, or Small-Bore Feeding Tube

- Administer medications in a liquid form (suspension, elixer, or solution) when possible to prevent tube obstruction.
- Read medication labels carefully before crushing a tablet or opening a capsule.
- Do *not* crush buccal or sublingual tablets.
- Do not crush enteric-coated or sustained-action medications.
- Dissolve crushed tablets and powders in warm water.
- Dissolve soft, gelatin capsules in warm water.
- Irrigate the tube before and after all medication is given with 50-150 ml of water.
- Avoid giving syrups or medications with a pH of less than 4.
- Do not attempt to give whole or undissolved medications.

Adapted from Petrosin BM et al: *Crit Care Nurs Q* 12:1, 1989.

Administering Oral Medications

STEPS

RATIONALE

1. Assess for contraindications to client receiving oral medication, including difficulty in swallowing, nausea or vomiting, bowel inflammation or reduced peristalsis, recent gastrointestinal surgery, reduced or absent bowel sounds, gastric suction.

   Alterations in gastrointestinal function interfere with drug distribution, absorption, and excretion. When gastric suction is in place, medication can be suctioned out before it can be absorbed.

2. Determine client's preferences and tolerances for fluids.

   Offering fluids can increase fluid intake unless it is contradicted by heart, lung, or renal diseases.

3. Prepare needed supplies and equipment:
   a. Medication cards, record forms, or printout
   b. Medication cart or tray
   c. Disposable medication cups
   d. Glass of water, juice, or preferred liquid
   e. Drinking straw
   f. Mortar and pestle (optional)

   Used to crush tablets for clients who have difficulty in swallowing.

   g. Paper towels

4. Check accuracy and completeness of each medication card, form, or printout with physician's written medication order. Check client's name and drug name, dosage, route of administration, and time for administration. Report discrepancy in order to charge nurse or physician.

   Physician's order is most reliable source and only legal record of drugs client is to receive.

5. Prepare drug:
   a. Wash hands.

   Reduces transfer of microorganisms from your hands to medications and equipment.

   b. Arrange medication tray and cups in medicine room or move medication cart to position outside client's room.

   Saves time and reduces error.

   c. Unlock medicine drawer or cart (see illustration). (Narcotics are generally stored in double-locked box separate from medicine drawers or carts.)

   Medications are safeguarded when locked in cabinet or cart.

   d. Prepare medications for one client at a time. Keep medication tickets or forms for each client together.

   Prevents preparation errors.

   e. Select correct drug from stock supply or unit-dose drawer. Compare label of medication with medication form, card, or printout.

   Reduces error.

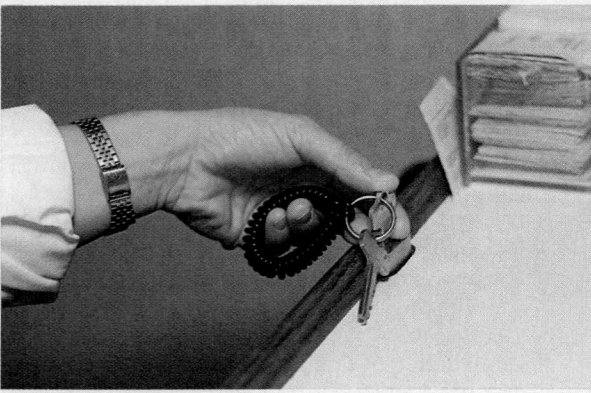

Step 5c

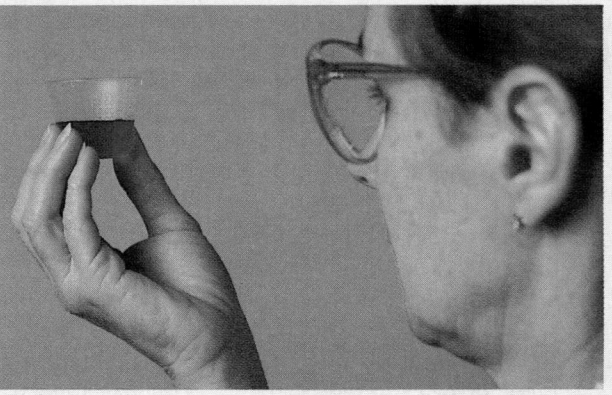

Step 5k

STEPS	RATIONALE
f. Calculate correct drug dose. Take time. Double check calculation.	Calculation is more accurate when information from drug label is at hand.
g. To prepare tablet or capsules from bottle, pour required number into bottle cap and transfer to medication cup. Do not touch with fingers. Extra tablets or capsules may be returned to bottle.	Maintains cleanliness of drugs.
h. To prepare unit-dose tablets or capsules, place packaged tablet or capsule directly into medicine cup. (Do not remove wrapper.) (See illustration.)	Wrappers maintain cleanliness and identification of medications. Unopened medications may be returned to pharmacy if they are refused.
i. Place all tablets or capsules given at same time in one cup except for those requiring preadministration assessments (e.g., pulse rate or blood pressure).	Keeping medications that require preadministration assessments separate from others makes it easier for you to withhold drugs as necessary.
j. If client has difficulty in swallowing, grind tablets in mortar with pestle. Place tablet in bottom of mortar and grind. Continue to crush fragments until smooth powder remains. Alternative method is to place tablet between two medication cups and grind with blunt instrument. Again, continue to crush fragments until fine powder is achieved. Mix crushed tablet in small amount of soft food, such as custard or applesauce. Caution: Do not crush enteric-coated or sustained-action medications.	Large tablets can be difficult to swallow. Ground tablet mixed with palatable soft food is usually easy to swallow. Verify that medication can be crushed before doing so; enteric-coated medications are not designed to be absorbed in stomach.

Step 5h

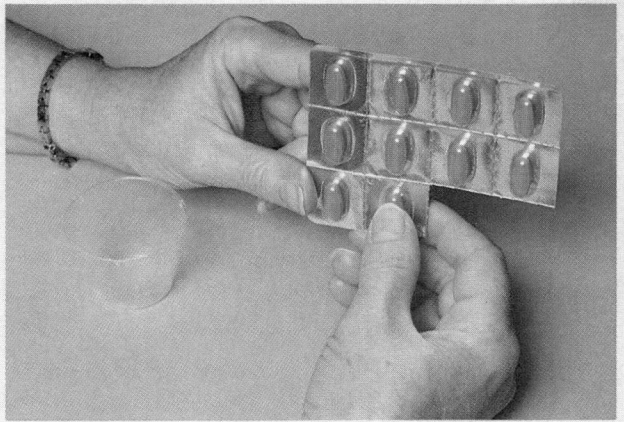

STEPS	RATIONALE
k. Prepare liquids:	
(1) Remove bottle cap from container and place cap upside down.	Prevents contamination of inside of cap.
(2) Hold bottle with label against palm of hand while pouring.	Spilled liquid will not soil or fade label.
(3) Hold medication cup at eye level and fill to desired level on scale. (see illustration) (Scale should be even with fluid level at its surface or base of meniscus, not edges.)	Ensures accuracy of measurement.
(4) Discard excess liquid in cup into sink. Wipe lip of bottle with paper towel.	Prevents contamination of bottle's contents and prevents bottle cap from sticking.
(5) Draw volumes of less than 10 ml in syringe (without needle). To prevent accidental ingestion, during administration, never use needle to draw up oral medication.	
l. When preparing narcotic, check narcotic record for previous drug count, compare with supply available, remove drug, and complete necessary information on narcotic form and sign.	Controlled substance laws require careful monitoring of dispensed narcotics.
m. Compare medication form, card, or printout with prepared drug and container.	Reading label second time reduces error.

Administering Oral Medications

STEPS	RATIONALE
n. Return stock containers or unused uni.-dose medications to shelf or drawer and read label again.	Third check of label reduces errors.
o. Place medications and cards, forms, or printouts together on tray or cart.	Drugs are labeled at all times for identification.
p. Do not leave drugs unattended.	Nurse is responsible for safekeeping of drugs.
6. Administer medications:	
a. Take medications to client at correct time.	Medications are given within 30 min before or after prescribed time to ensure intended effect. Stat or single-order medications should be given at time ordered.
b. Identify client by comparing name on card, form, or printout with name on client's identification bracelet. Ask client to state full name.	Identification bracelets are made at time of client's admission and are most reliable source of identification. Missing or faded bracelets are replaced to avoid errors.
c. Perform necessary preadministration assessment for specific medications (e.g., blood pressure or pulse).	Assessment data determine whether specific medications should be given at that time.
d. Explain purpose of each medication and its action to client. Allow client to ask questions about drugs.	Client has right to be informed, and understanding of medication improves compliance with therapy.
e. Assist client to sitting or side-lying position.	Prevents aspiration during swallowing.
f. Administer drugs properly:	
(1) Ask if client wishes to hold solid medications in hand or cup before placing in mouth.	Client can become familiar with medications by seeing each drug.
(2) Offer full glass of water or juice with drugs to be swallowed.	Choice of fluid promotes comfort and can improve fluid intake.
(3) For sublingual administered drugs, have client place medication under tongue and allow it to dissolve completely. Caution client against swallowing.	Drug is absorbed through blood vessels of undersurface of tongue. If swallowed, drug is destroyed by gastric juices or is so rapidly detoxified by liver that therapeutic blood levels are not attained.
(4) Mix powdered medications with liquids at bedside and give to client to drink.	When prepared in advance, powdered drug forms may thicken and even harden, making swallowing difficult.
(5) Caution client against chewing or swallowing lozenges.	Drug acts through slow absorption through oral mucosa, not gastric mucosa.
(6) Give effervescent powders and tablets immediately after dissolving.	Effervescence helps improve unpleasant taste of drug and often has therapeutic value for gastrointestinal problems.
g. If client is unable to hold medications, place medication cup to lips and gently introduce each drug into mouth, one at a time. Do not rush.	Prevents contamination of medications. Administering single tablet or capsule eases swallowing and prevents aspiration.
h. If tablet or capsule falls to floor, discard it and repeat preparation.	Drug is contaminated when it touches floor.
i. Stay with client until each medication has been swallowed. If uncertain whether medication has been swallowed, ask client to open the mouth.	Nurse assumes responsibility for ensuring that client receives ordered dosage. If left unattended, client may not take dose or may save drugs, causing risk to health.
j. For highly acidic medications (e.g., aspirin), offer nonfat snack (e.g., crackers).	Reduces gastric irritation.
k. Assist client in returning to comfortable position.	Maintains comfort.
l. Dispose of soiled supplies and wash hands.	Reduces transmission of microorganisms.
m. Return medication cards, forms, or printouts to appropriate file for next administration time.	Cards, forms, and printouts are used as reference for when next dose is due. Loss can lead to administration error.
n. Replenish stock such as cups and straws, return cart to medicine room, and clean work area.	Clean working space assists other staff in completing duties efficiently.
7. Record actual time that each drug was administered on medication record or computer. Include initials or signature (see Fig. 21-6).	Prompt documentation prevents errors such as repeated doses. Signature establishes accountability for administration.
8. Return within 30 min to evaluate response to medications.	Used to assess drug's therapeutic benefit and detect onset of side effects or allergic reactions.

medication in the back of the throat. A client who swallows slowly should not be forced to take a large amount of liquid with each swallow. Likewise, a client should swallow only one pill or capsule at a time. If a client begins to cough while taking a medication, the nurse withholds the remaining portion of the drug until the client can breathe more easily. If the client has difficulty with swallowing tablets, other forms of the medication should be considered.

 ## ADMINISTRATION OF INJECTIONS

Administering an injection is an invasive procedure that must be performed using aseptic techniques (see box). After a needle pierces the skin, the risk of infection exists. The nurse administers drugs parenterally by the SQ, IM, ID, and IV routes. Each type of injection requires certain skills to ensure that the drug reaches the proper location. The effects of a parenterally administered drug can develop rapidly, depending on the rate of drug absorption. The nurse closely observes the client's response.

Equipment

A variety of syringes and needles are available; each is designed to deliver a certain volume of a drug to a specific type of tissue. The nurse uses judgment when determining which syringe or needle will be the most effective.

Preventing Infection During an Injection

- To prevent contamination of solution, draw medication from ampule quickly. Do not allow it to stand open.
- To prevent needle contamination, avoid letting needle touch contaminated surface (e.g., outer edges of ampule or vial, outer surface of needle cap, nurse's hands, counter top, table surface).
- To prevent syringe contamination, avoid touching length of plunger or inner part of barrel. Keep tip of syringe covered with cap or needle.
- To prepare skin, wash skin soiled with dirt, drainage, or feces with soap and water and dry. Use friction and a circular motion while cleaning with an antiseptic swab. Swab from center of site, and move outward in a 2-inch radius.

Syringes

Syringes consist of a cylindrical barrel with a tip designed to fit the hub of a hypodermic needle and a close-fitting plunger (Fig. 21-9). Most health care institutions use disposable, single-use plastic syringes that are inexpensive and easy to manipulate. The syringes are packaged separately, with or without a sterile needle in a paper wrapper or rigid, plastic container. Glass syringes are also available, although they are not commonly used.

The nurse fills a syringe by aspiration, pulling the plunger outward while the needle tip remains immersed in the prepared solution. The nurse may handle the outside of the syringe barrel and the handle of the plunger. To maintain sterility the nurse avoids letting any unsterile object touch the tip or inside of the barrel, the shaft of the plunger, or the needle.

Syringes come in a number of sizes, from 0.5 to 60 ml (Fig. 21-10). It is unusual to use a syringe larger than 5 ml for an SQ or IM injection. A 2- to 3-ml syringe is adequate. A larger volume creates discom-

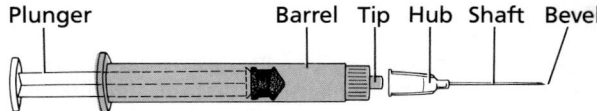

Fig. 21-9 Parts of a syringe and hypodermic needle.

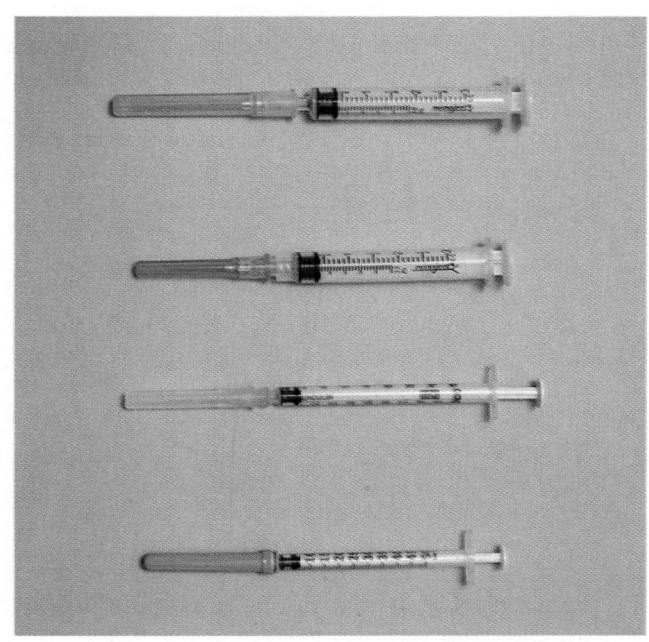

Fig. 21-10 Types of syringes. *From top to bottom:* disposable 3-ml hypodermic syringe (intramuscular), 3-ml hypodermic syringe (subcutaneous), insulin syringe, and tuberculin syringe.

fort. Larger syringes are used to prepare IV drugs. The 2.5- or 3-ml hypodermic syringe often comes packaged with a needle attached. However, the nurse may change needle sizes. The hypodermic has two scales on the barrel. One scale is divided into minims and the other into tenths of a milliliter.

Insulin syringes (Fig. 21-10) hold 0.5 to 1 ml and are calibrated in units. Insulin syringes that hold 0.5 ml are known as *low-dose syringes* (50 μ per 0.5 ml) and are easier to read. Insulin syringes in the United States and Canada are U-100s, designed for use with U-100 strength insulin. Each milliliter of solution contains 100 units of insulin.

The tuberculin syringe (Fig. 21-10) has a long, thin barrel with a preattached thin needle. The syringe is calibrated in sixteenths of a minim and hundredths of a milliliter and has a capacity of 1 ml. The nurse uses a tuberculin syringe to prepare small amounts of potent drugs. A tuberculin syringe is useful in preparing small, precise doses for infants or young children. The nurse uses large hypodermic syringes to administer certain IV drugs and add medications to IV solutions.

Needles

Needles come packaged in individual sheaths to allow flexibility in choosing the right needle. Some needles are preattached to standard-size syringes. Most are made of stainless steel and are disposable.

The needle has three parts: the hub, which fits onto the tip of a syringe; the shaft, which connects to the hub; and the bevel or slanted tip (see Fig. 21-9). The nurse may handle the needle hub to ensure a tight fit on the syringe. However, the shaft and bevel must remain sterile.

Each needle has three characteristic features: the slant of the bevel, the length of the shaft, and the needle gauge or diameter. Long bevels are sharper, which minimizes discomfort caused by SQ and IM injections. Needles vary in length from ¼ to 5 inches, although 1½ inches is most commonly used to give IM injections to adults. The nurse chooses needle length according to client size and weight and the type of tissue into which the drug is to be injected. A child or a slender adult generally requires a shorter needle. The nurse uses a longer needle (usually 1 to 1½ inches) for IM injections and a shorter needle (usually ⅜ to ⅝ inch) for SQ injections.

The smaller the gauge, the larger the needle diameter (Fig. 21-11). The selection of a gauge depends on the viscosity of the fluid to be injected or infused. An IM injection usually requires a 19- to 23-gauge needle, depending on the viscosity of the medication. SQ injections require smaller-diameter needles, such as a 25-gauge needle. For an ID injection a 26-gauge needle is used.

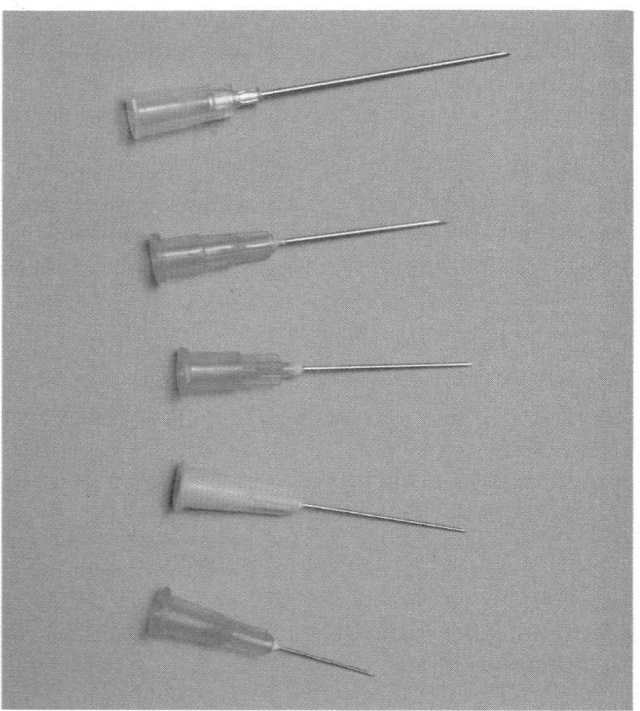

Fig. 21-11 Hypodermic needles arranged in order of gauge. *Top to bottom:* 19-, 20-, 21-, 23-, and 25-gauge.

Disposable Injection Units

Disposable, single-dose, prefilled syringes are available for many medications. The nurse must be careful to check the medication and concentration because all prefilled syringes appear very similiar.

The Tubex and Carpuject injection systems include reusable plastic mechanisms that hold prefilled, disposable, sterile cartridge-needle units (Fig. 21-12). The nurse slips the cartridge into the mechanism, secures it (following package directions), and checks for air bubbles in the syringe. The nurse advances the plunger to expel the medication as in a regular syringe. These systems are designed to decrease the chance of accidental needlesticks if used according to the manufacters' recommendations.

Preparing an Injection from an Ampule

Ampules contain single doses of medication in a liquid and are available in several sizes, from 1 ml to 10 ml or more (Fig. 21-13, *A*). An ampule is made of glass with a constricted neck that must be snapped off to allow access to the medication. A colored ring around the neck indicates where the ampule is prescored to break easily. Aspiration of the drug into a syringe should be done with a filter needle. This is a relatively easy procedure (Procedure 21-2).

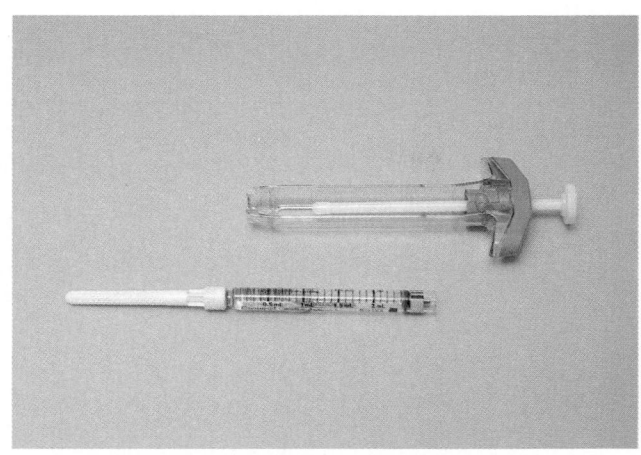

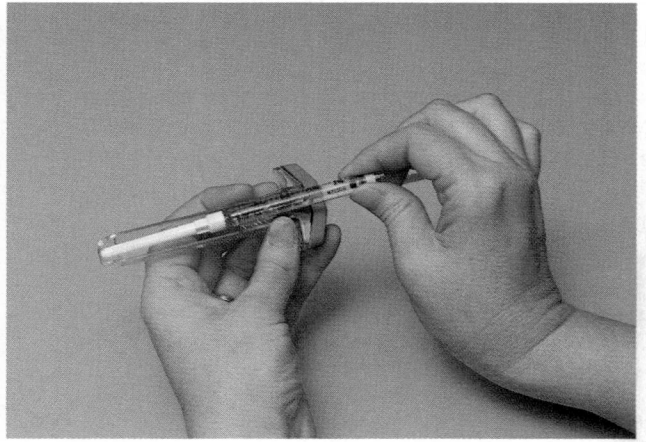

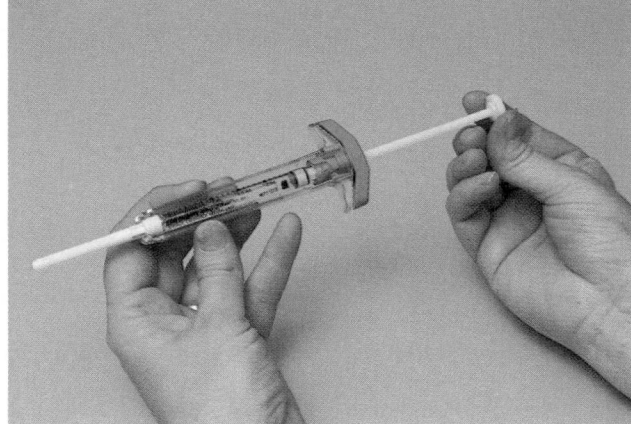

Fig. 21-12 A, Carpuject syringe and prefilled sterile cartridge with needle. B, Assembling the carpuject. C, The cartridge slides into the syringe barrel, turns, and locks at the needle end. The plunger then screws into the cartridge end.

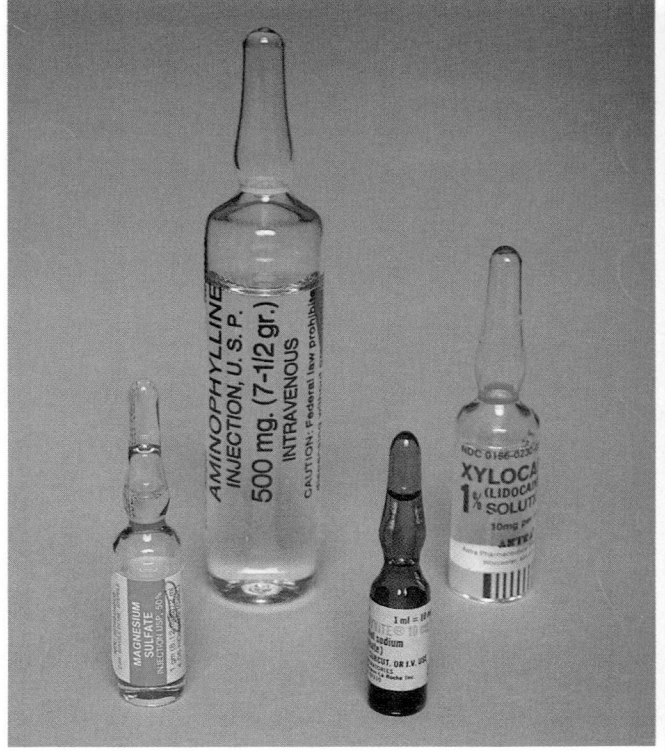

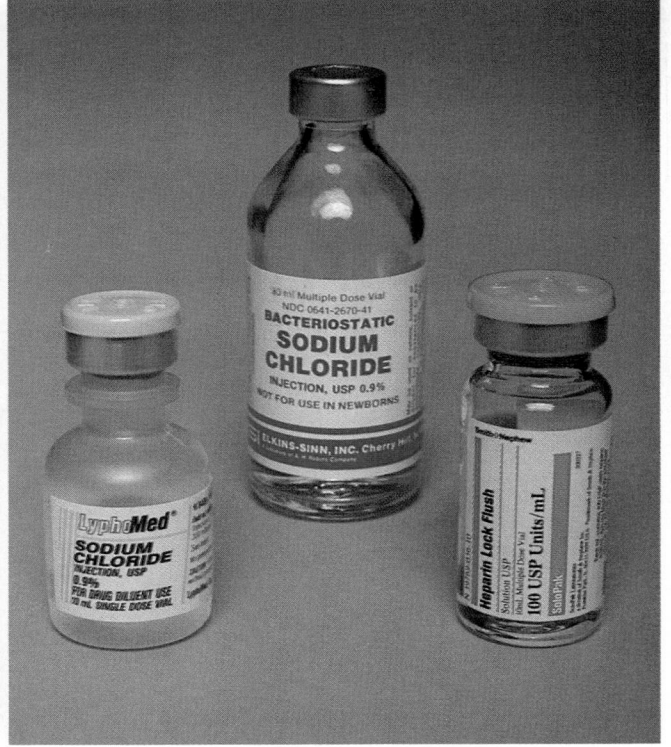

Fig. 21-13   A, Ampules.   B, Vials.

Preparing Injections from Ampules and Vials

STEPS	RATIONALE
1. Wash hands.	Reduces transmission of infection.

2. Prepare needed equipment and supplies:
  a. Ampules:
    (1) Ampule containing medication
    (2) Syringe and needle
    (3) Small gauze pad or alcohol swab
    (4) Container for disposing of glass
  b. Vials:
    (1) Vial with medication
    (2) Syringe and needle
    (3) Alcohol swab
    (4) Solvent (e.g., normal saline or sterile water)
  c. Medication cards, forms, or printouts
	Used to dissolve drugs in dry form.
	Verifies order.

3. Assemble supplies at work area in medicine room.	Makes procedure orderly.
4. Check each medication card, form, or computer print-out against label on each ampule or vial.	Ensures that right drug and dosage are prepared.
5. Prepare injection from ampule: a. Tap top of ampule lightly and quickly with finger until fluid leaves neck (see illustration).	Dislodges fluid that collects above neck. All solution moves into lower chamber.
b. Place small gauze pad or dry alcohol swab around neck of ampule.	Protects your fingers from trauma as glass tip is broken off.
c. Snap neck quickly and firmly away from hands (see illustration).	Prevents shattering glass toward or in your fingers or face.
d. Draw up medication quickly. Hold ampule upside down or set it on flat surface. Insert syringe needle into center of ampule opening (see illustration). Do not allow needle tip or shaft to touch rim of ampule.	Broken rim of ampule is considered contaminated. As long as needle tip or shaft does not touch rim, solution does not dribble out.
e. Aspirate medication into syringe by gently pulling back on plunger (see illustration).	Withdrawal of plunger creates negative pressure within syringe barrel, which pulls fluid into syringe.
f. Keep needle tip below surface of liquid. Tip ampule to bring all fluid within reach of needle.	Prevents aspiration of air bubbles.

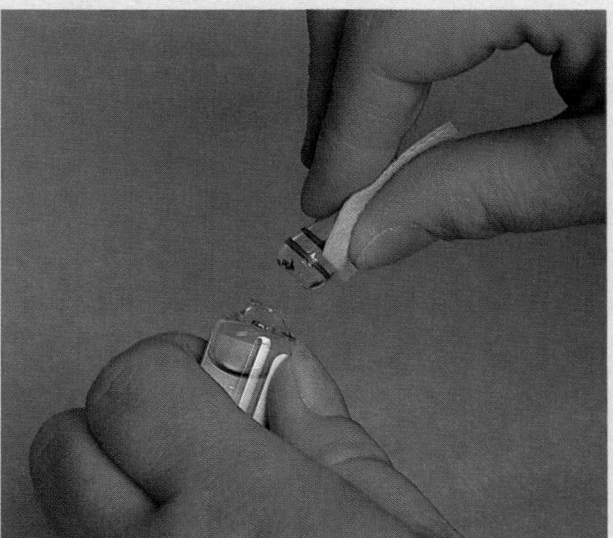

Step 5a   Step 5c

STEPS	RATIONALE
g. If air bubbles are aspirated, do not expel air into ampule.	Air pressure may force fluid out of ampule, and medication will be lost.
h. To expel excess air bubbles, remove needle. Hold syringe with needle pointing up. Tap side of syringe to cause bubbles to rise toward needle. Draw back slightly on plunger, and push plunger upward to eject air. *Do not eject fluid.*	Withdrawing plunger too far will pull it from barrel. Holding syringe vertically allows fluid to settle in bottom of barrel. Pulling back on plunger allows fluid within needle to enter barrel so that fluid is not expelled. Air at top of barrel and within needle is then expelled.
i. If syringe contains excess fluid, use sink for disposal. Hold syringe vertically with needle tip up and slanted slightly toward sink. Slowly eject excess fluid into sink. Recheck fluid level in syringe by holding it vertically.	Medication is safely dispersed into sink. Position of needle allows medication to be expelled without flowing down needle shaft. Rechecking fluid level ensures proper dose.
j. Cover needle with sheath or cap. Change needle on syringe.	Prevents contamination of needle and protects you from needlestick. Changing needle is required if you suspect that medication is on needle shaft. New needle prevents tracking medication through skin and SQ tissues.
k. Dispose of soiled supplies. Place broken ampule in special container for glass.	Controls transmission of infection. Proper disposal of glass prevents accidental injury to personnel.
6. Prepare injection from vial:	
a. Remove metal cap covering top of unused vial. Expose rubber seal.	Vial comes packaged with cap to prevent contamination of rubber seal.
b. Wipe off surface of rubber seal with alcohol swab, if vial had been previously opened.	Removes dust or grease but does not sterilize surface.
c. Take syringe and remove needle cap. Pull back on plunger to draw amount of air into syringe equivalent to volume of medication to be aspirated from vial (see illustration on p. 650).	To prevent buildup of negative pressure in vial when aspirating medication, air must first be injected into vial.
d. Insert tip of needle, with bevel pointing up, through center of rubber seal (see illustration on p. 650). Apply pressure to tip of needle during insertion.	Center of seal is thinner and easier to penetrate. Keeping bevel up and using firm pressure prevents cutting rubber core from seal.
e. Inject air into vial, holding on to plunger.	Air must be injected before aspirating fluid. Plunger may be forced backward by air pressure within vial.
f. Invert vial while keeping firm hold on syringe and plunger (see illustration on p. 651). Hold vial between thumb and middle fingers of nondominant hand. Grasp end of syringe barrel and plunger with thumb and forefinger of dominant hand.	Inverting vial allows fluid to settle in lower half of container. Position of hands prevents movement of plunger and permits easy manipulation of syringe.

CONTINUED

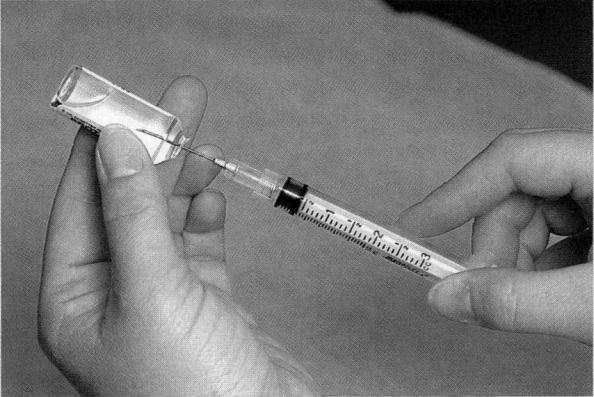

Step 5d

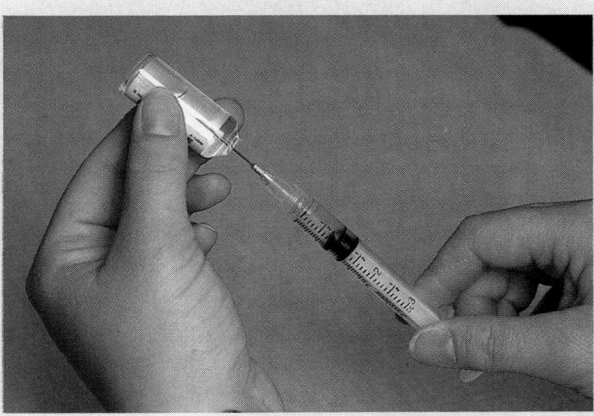

Step 5e

Preparing Injections from Ampules and Vials

STEPS	RATIONALE
g. Keep tip of needle below fluid level.	Prevents aspiration of air.
h. Allow air pressure to fill syringe gradually with medication. Pull back slightly on plunger if necessary.	Positive pressure within vial forces fluid into syringe.
i. Tap side of syringe barrel carefully to dislodge air bubbles. Eject air remaining at top of syringe into vial.	Forefully striking barrel while needle is inserted in vial may bend needle. Accumulation of air displaces medication and causes errors.
j. After correct volume is obtained, remove needle from vial by pulling back on barrel of syringe.	Pulling plunger rather than barrel causes separation from barrel and loss of medication.
k. Remove remaining air from syringe by holding it and needle upright. Tap barrel to dislodge air bubbles (see illustration). Draw back slightly on plunger, and then push plunger upward to eject air. Do not eject fluid.	Holding syringe vertically allows fluid to settle in bottom of barrel. Pulling back on plunger allows fluid within needle to enter barrel so that fluid is not expelled. Air at top of barrel and within needle is then expelled.
l. Change needle and cover.	Inserting needle through rubber stopper may blunt bevel. New needle is sharper, and because no fluid is along shaft, it will not track medication through tissues.
m. For multidose vial, make label that includes date of mixing, concentration of drug per milliliter, and your initials.	Ensures that future doses will be prepared correctly. Certain drugs should be discarded after set number of days after mixing of vial.
n. Dispose of soiled supplies in proper containers.	Reduces transmission of microorganisms.

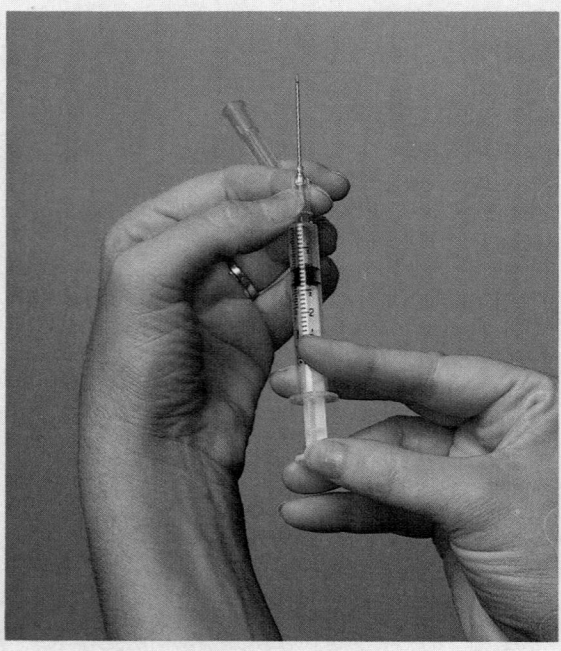

Step 6c

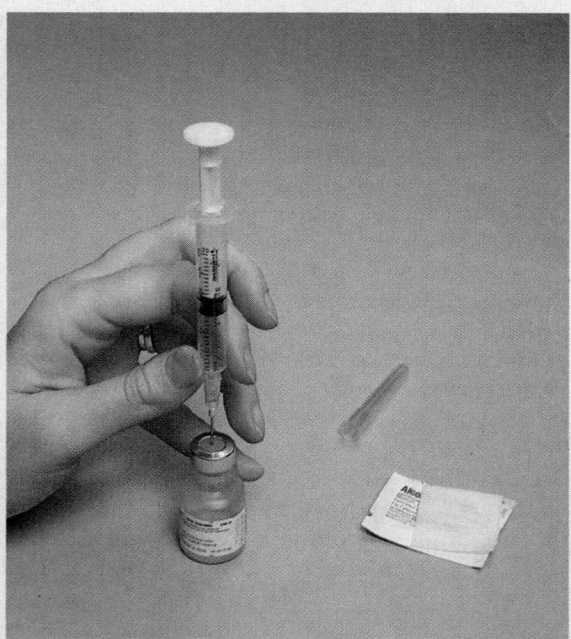

Step 6d

STEPS	RATIONALE
7. Clean work area. Wash hands.	Reduces transmission of microorganisms.
8. Check fluid level in syringe and compare with desired dose.	Ensures that accurate dose has been prepared.

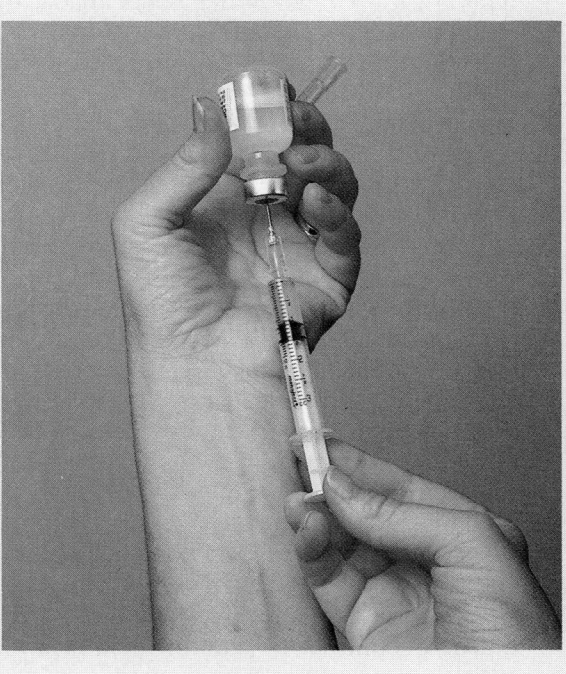

Step 6f

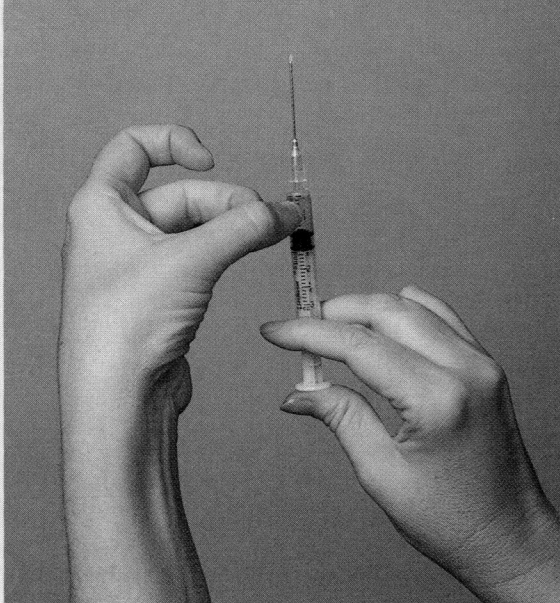

Step 6k

Preparing an Injection from a Vial

A vial is a single-dose or multidose glass container with a rubber seal at the top (Fig. 21-13, *B*). A metal cap protects the seal until it is ready for use. Vials contain liquid and/or dry forms of medications. Drugs that are unstable in solution are packaged dry. The vial label specifies the solution (solvent) used to dissolve the drug and the amount needed to prepare a desired drug concentration. Normal saline and sterile distilled water are solutions commonly used to dissolve drugs.

Unlike the ampule, the vial is a closed system, and air must be injected into it to permit easy withdrawal of the solution. Failure to inject air before withdrawing the solution leaves a vacuum within the vial that makes withdrawal difficult (Procedure 21-2).

To prepare a powdered drug, the nurse draws up the amount of solvent recommended on the vial's label. The nurse injects the solvent into the vial in the same manner as injecting air into the vial. Most powdered drugs dissolve easily, but it may be necessary to withdraw the needle to mix the contents thoroughly. Gently shaking or rolling the vial between the hands will dissolve the powdered drug. The needle is reinserted to draw up the dissolved medication.

After mixing multidose vials the nurse makes a label that includes the date of mixing and concentration of drug per milliliter. Multidose vials may require refrigeration after contents are reconstituted.

Mixing Medications

If two drugs are compatible, it is possible to mix them together into one injection if the total dosage is within accepted limits. A client will appreciate not having to receive more than one injection at a time. Most nursing units have charts that list common compatible drugs. If there is any uncertainty about drug compatibilities, a pharmacist should be consulted.

Mixing Medications from Two Vials

The nurse follows the following principles when mixing medications from two vials:
1. Do not contaminate one medication with another.
2. Ensure that the final dosage is accurate.
3. Maintain aseptic technique.

Only one syringe is needed to mix medications from two vials (Fig 21-14). The nurse takes a syringe and aspirates the volume of air equivalent to the first drug's dosage (vial A). The nurse injects air into vial A, making sure that the needle does not touch the solution. The nurse withdraws the needle, aspirates air equivalent to the second drug's dose (vial B), and then injects the volume of air into vial B. The nurse immediately withdraws the required medication from vial B into the syringe. At this point the drug from vial A has not contaminated vial B.

The nurse applies a new, sterile needle to the syringe and inserts it into vial A, being careful not to push the plunger and expel the drug within the syringe into the vial. The nurse then withdraws the desired amount of drug from vial A into the syringe. If a vial has excess positive pressure, the plunger may begin to move before the nurse is ready. This can cause an accidental withdrawal of too much of the drug. After withdrawing the necessary amount of solution, the nurse withdraws the needle, applies a new needle, and sheaths the syringe.

Mixing Medications from One Vial and One Ampule

Mixing medications from a vial and an ampule is simple because it is unnecessary to add air to withdraw medication from an ampule. The nurse prepares medication from the vial first and then, using the same syringe and needle, withdraws medication from the ampule. This technique prevents contamination of solutions from the needle.

Preparing Insulin

Insulin is the hormone used to treat diabetes. The drug must be administered by injection because it is a protein and therefore would be digested and destroyed in the gastrointestinal tract. Most clients with diabetes requiring insulin learn to self-administer injections. In the United States and Canada, the drug is in 100 units per milliliter of solution. When preparing insulin, a 100-unit scaled syringe is used to prepare 100-unit insulin.

Insulin is classified by its rate of action, as *rapid, intermediate,* and *long acting.* Each type has a different onset, peak, and duration of action. A client with diabetes may require more than one type of insulin. For example, by receiving a rapid-acting (regular) insulin and an intermediate-acting insulin (isophane [NPH Insulin]), a client receives more sustained control of blood glucose levels over a 24-hour period.

Regular, unmodified insulin is a clear solution that can be given subcutaneously or intravenously. The other types of insulin are cloudy solutions because of the addition of a protein, which slows absorption. These slower-acting, modified types of insulin can only be given subcutaneously.

Insulin can be stored safely for about 1 month at room temperature, but it requires refrigeration for longer time periods (Clark, Queener, Karb, 1993). The drug should not be administered cold but is allowed to warm to room temperature.

Before mixing different types of insulin, each vial should be rotated for at least 1 minute between both hands. This resuspends the modified insulin preparations and helps warm the medication. The nurse should not shake insulin vials. Shaking causes foaming and bubbles to form, which may trap particles of insulin and alter the dosage. Insulin is ordered by specific dosages at select times or by a sliding scale. (Only regular insulin is used for sliding scales.) With a sliding scale order, the physician orders different insulin doses based on a client's blood glucose reading. Several doses may thus be given throughout the day. The following are some simple guidelines for mixing two kinds of insulin in the same syringe:
1. Regular insulin can be mixed with any other type of insulin.
2. Insulin zinc suspensions (Lente Insulins) can be mixed with each other and regular insulin. They should not be mixed with other types of insulin.

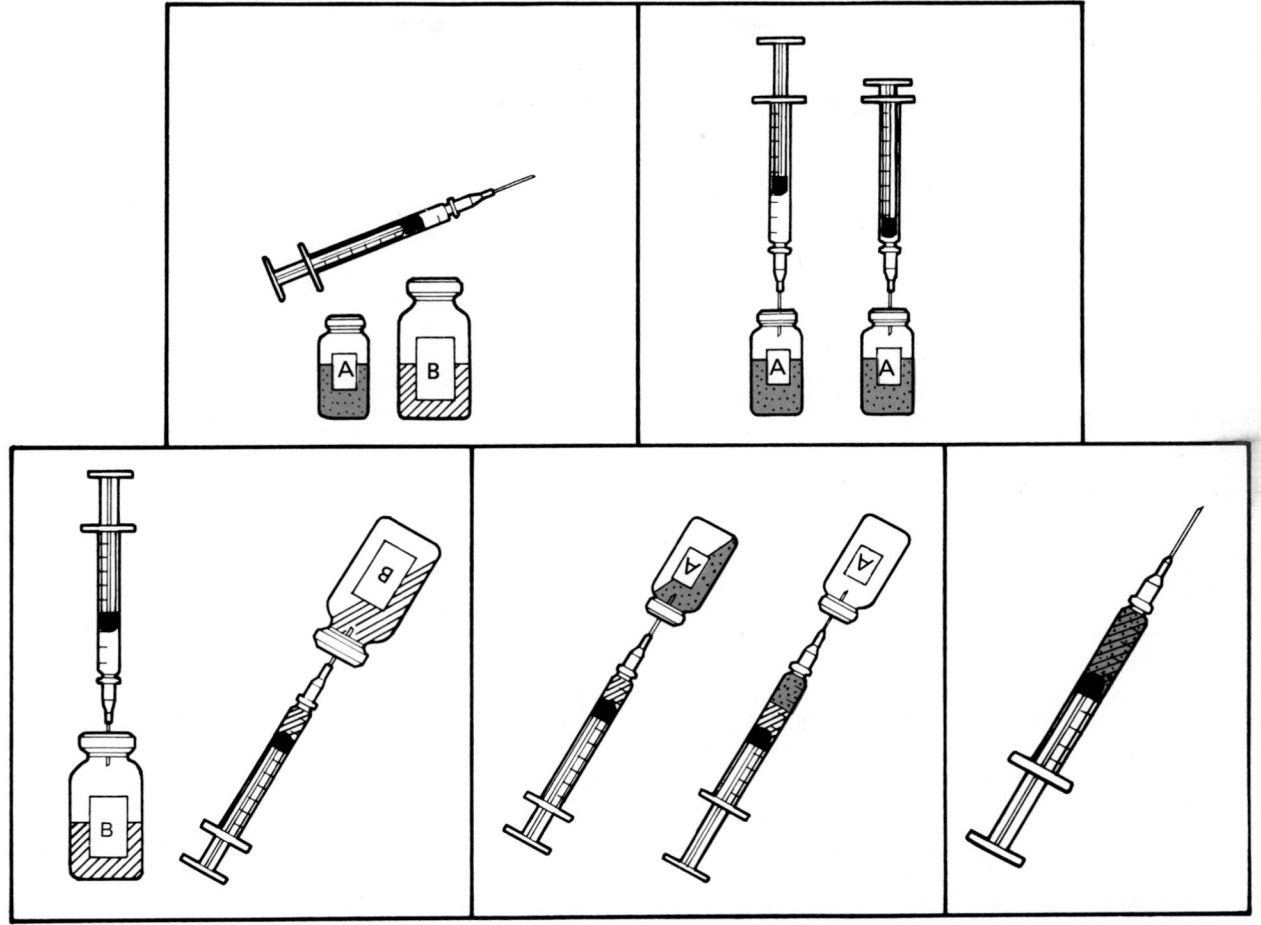

Fig. 21-14   Steps in mixing medications from two vials.

To prepare insulin from two vials the nurse or client follows the following steps:

1. With a syringe and needle, inject air equal to the dose of insulin to be withdrawn into the vial of modified (NPH) insulin (cloudy vial). Do not touch tip of needle to the solution.
2. Remove the syringe from the vial of modified insulin.
3. With the same syringe, inject air equal to the dose of insulin to be withdrawn into the vial of unmodified (regular) insulin (clear vial). Then withdraw the correct dose.
4. Remove the syringe from the unmodified (regular) insulin. Carefully remove air bubbles in the syringe.
5. Return to the vial of modified (NPH) insulin, and withdraw the correct dose.
6. Administer mixture of insulins within 5 minutes of preparing it. Regular insulin binds with

the modified (NPH) insulin, and the action of the regular insulin is reduced.

Always prepare the unmodified (regular) insulin first. This prevents adding modified insulin to the unmodified (regular) vial. If two modified forms are mixed, it makes no difference which vial is prepared first.

Administering Injections

Each injection route is unique in regard to the type of tissues into which the medication is injected. The characteristics of the tissues influence the rate of drug absorption and thus the onset of drug action. Before injecting a drug, the nurse should know the volume of the drug to administer, the drug's characteristics and viscosity, and the location of anatomical structures underlying injection sites (Procedure 21-3).

Text continued on p. 658.

Administering Injections

STEPS	RATIONALE
1. Assess indications for proper route for medication.	Ensures proper drug absorption and distribution through tissues to enhance drug action. Ensures proper route appropriate for client per physician orders.
2. Assess medical history and history of allergies.	May influence certain drugs. Parenteral medications often create sensitivities in form of allergies.
3. Observe verbal and nonverbal responses toward receiving injection.	Injections can be painful. Clients may experience considerable anxiety, which can increase pain.
4. Wash hands.	Reduces transmission of microorganisms.

5. Prepare needed equipment and supplies:
  a. Proper-size syringe:
    (1) SQ: 1 to 2 ml
    (2) IM: 2 to 3 ml for adult, 1 to 2 ml for child
    (3) ID: 1-ml tuberculin
  b. Proper-size needle:
    (1) SQ: 25- to 27-gauge and ⅜ to ⅝ in in length
    (2) IM: 18- to 23-gauge and 1 to 1½ in in length for adults, 25- to 27-gauge and ½ to 1 in in length for child and ⅝ for newborn (Whaley, Wong, 1991)
    (3) ID: preattached 26- to 27-gauge
  c. Antiseptic swab (Betadine or alcohol)
  d. Disposable gloves
  e. Medication ampule or vial
  f. Medication card, forms, or printouts
	Volume injected should be compatible with tissue type.
	
	Prevents injury to client and ensures distribution of drug.
	
	Used to cleanse skin.
	
	Identifies medication dose ordered and client's name.

6. Check medication order.	Ensures accuracy of order.
7. Prepare correct medication dose from ampule or vial. (Procedure 21-2). Check carefully. Be sure all air is expelled. (For IM medications that are particularly irritating to tissues, draw 0.2 cc of air into syringe, being careful not to expel drug dose. See Z-track method.)	Ensures that medication is sterile. Preparation techniques differ for ampule and vial.
8. For IM injection, change needle if medication is irritating to SQ tissue.	Prevents tracking of irritating substance through tissues as needle passes into muscle.
9. Apply disposable gloves.	Injections could cause mild seepage of blood at injection site. Gloves reduce risk of exposure.
10. Identify client by checking identification armband and asking name.	Ensures that correct client is receiving prescribed medication.
11. Explain procedure to client and proceed in calm, confident manner.	Helps client anticipate actions. Calm approach minimizes anxiety.
12. Close room curtains or door.	Provides for privacy.
13. Keep sheet or gown draped over body parts not requiring exposure.	Proper selection of injection site may require exposure of body parts.

14. Select appropriate injection site. Inspect skin surface over sites for bruises, inflammation, or edema:
  a. SQ: palpate sites for masses of tenderness.
  b. IM: note integrity and size of muscle and palpate for tenderness.
  c. ID: note lesions or discolorations of forearm.
	Injection sites should be free of abnormalities that may interfere with drug absorption. ID site should be clear so that results of skin test can be seen and interpreted correctly.

15. If injections are given frequently, rotate sites.	Site used repeatedly can become hardened from lipohypertrophy (increased growth in fatty tissue).

CONTINUED

STEPS	RATIONALE
16. Assist client to comfortable position:	
a. SQ: have client relax arm, leg, or abdomen, depending on site chosen.	Relaxation of site minimizes discomfort.
b. IM: have client lie flat, on side, or prone or have client sit, depending on site chosen.	Reduces strain on muscle and minimizes discomfort of injections.
c. ID: have client extend elbow and support it and forearm on flat surface.	Stabilizes site for easiest accessibility.
17. Relocate site using anatomical landmarks.	Accurate injection requires insertion in correct site to avoid injury to underlying tissues, blood vessels, nerves, or bone.
18. Cleanse site with antiseptic swab. Apply swab at center of site and rotate outward in circular direction for about 5 cm (2 in) (see illustration).	Mechanical action of swab removes secretions containing microorganisms.
19. Hold swab between third and fourth fingers of nondominant hand.	Swab remains readily accessible when needle is with drawn.
20. Remove cap from needle by pulling it straight off.	Prevents contamination.
21. Hold syringe correctly between thumb and forefinger of dominant hand:	Quick, smooth injection requires proper manipulation of syringe parts.
a. SQ: hold as dart (see illustration) at 45- or 90-degree angle.	
b. IM: hold as dart.	
c. ID: hold bevel of needle pointing up.	With bevel up, medication will less likely be deposited into tissues below dermis.
22. Administer injection:	
a. SQ:	
(1) For average-size client, spread skin tightly across injection site or pinch skin with nondominant hand.	Needle penetrates tight skin easier than loose skin. Pinching skin elevates SQ tissue.

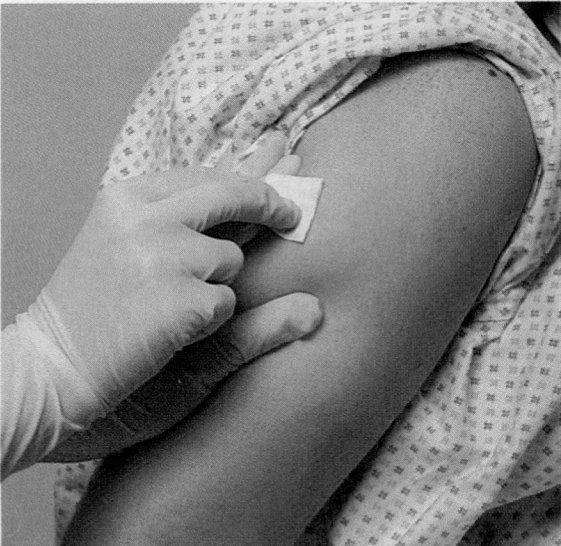

Step 18

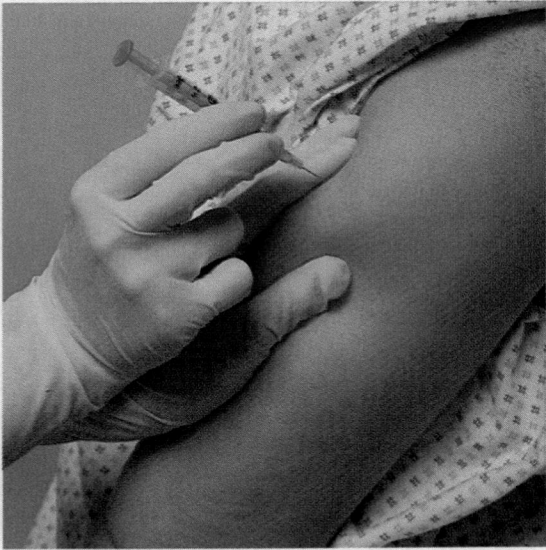

Step 21a

Administering Injections

STEPS	RATIONALE

    (2) Inject needle quickly and firmly at 45- to 90-degree angle (see illustration). (Then release skin, if pinched.)

Quick, firm insertion minimizes discomfort. (Injecting medication into compressed tissue irritates nerve fibers.)

    (3) For obese client, pinch skin at site and inject needle below tissue fold.

Obese clients have fatty layer of tissue above SQ layer.

  b. IM:

    (1) Position nondominant hand at proper anatomical landmarks and spread skin tightly. Inject needle quickly at 90-degree angle into muscle.

Speeds insertion and reduces discomfort.

    (2) If client's muscle mass is small, grasp body of muscle between thumb and other fingers.

Ensures that medication reaches muscle mass.

    (3) If medication is irritating, use Z-track method (see section on Z-track methods).

Used to prevent tracking of drug through SQ tissue.

  c. ID:

    (1) With nondominant hand, stretch skin over site with forefinger or thumb.

Needle pierces tight skin more easily.

    (2) With needle almost against client's skin, insert it slowly at 5- to 15-degree angle until resistance is felt. Then advance needle through epidermis to approximately 3 mm (⅛ in) below surface. Needle tip can be seen through skin.

Ensures that needle tip is in dermis.

23. After needle enters site of SQ or IM injections *only,* grasp lower end of syringe barrel with nondominant hand. Move dominant hand to end of plunger. Avoid moving syringe while slowly pulling back on plunger to aspirate drug (see illustration). If blood appears in syringe, remove needle, discard medication and syringe and repeat procedure. (It is unnecessary to aspirate ID injection.)

Properly performed injection requires smooth manipulation of syringe parts. Movement of syringe may displace needle and cause discomfort. Aspiration of blood into syringe indicates IV placement of needle. SQ and IM injections are not for IV use. Do not aspirate when giving heparin by SQ route. (Dermis is relatively avascular.)

24. Inject medication slowly. (For ID injections, it is normal to feel resistance; if not, needle is too deep.)

Minimizes discomfort and trauma at site. (Dermal layer is tight and does not expand easily.)

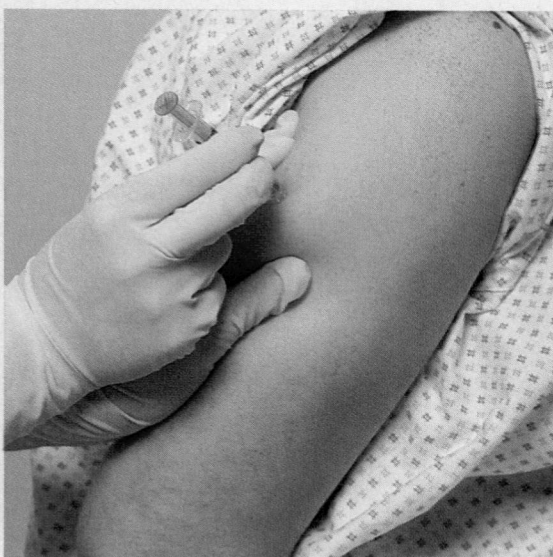

Step 22a(2)

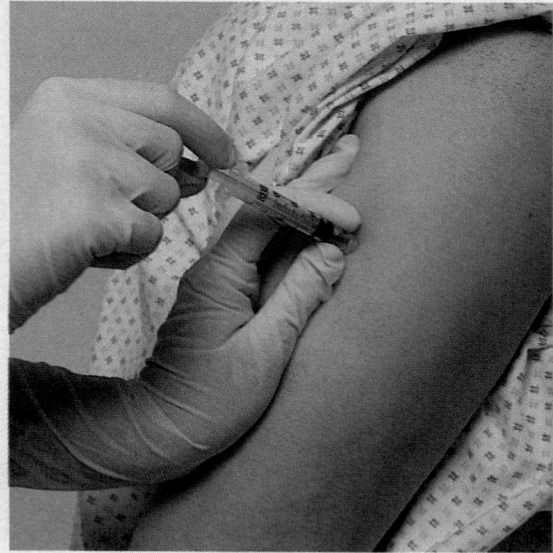

Step 23

STEPS	RATIONALE
25. During ID injection, note formation of small bleb on skin's surface (see illustration).	Indicates that medication is deposited into dermis.
26. Withdraw needle while applying alcohol swab gently above or over injection site.	Supports tissues around injection site to minimize discomfort during needle withdrawal.
27. For SQ or IM injections, massage skin lightly. OPTIONAL: apply bandage For ID injections, *do not massage site*.	Stimulates circulation and improves drug distribution. (NOTE: Do not massage after SQ injection of heparin.) Massage of ID site may disperse medication into underlying tissue layers and alter test results. (e.g., tuberculin test).
28. Assist client to comfortable position.	Gives client sense of well-being.
29. Discard unsheathed needle and attached syringe into appropriately labeled receptacles.	Prevents injury to clients and health care personnel. Centers for Disease Control no longer recommends capping needles before disposal.
30. Remove disposable gloves. Wash hands.	Reduces transmission of microorganisms.
31. Return to room and ask if client feels acute pain, burning, numbness, or tingling at injection site. Observe for allergic reaction after ID injection.	Continued discomfort may indicate injury to underlying bones or nerves. Anaphylactic reaction may occur suddenly after ID injection due to drug's toxicity.
32. Return to evaluate response to medication in 10 to 30 min.	IM medications absorb quickly; undesired effects may also develop rapidly. Observations determine efficacy of drug action.
33. For ID injection, draw circle around perimeter of injection site with skin pencil.	Site must be read at various intervals to determine test results. Pencil mark makes site easier to find.
34. For SQ and IM injections, chart medication dose, route, and site and time and date given in medication record. Correctly sign according to institutional policy.	Timely documentation prevents administration errors.
35. For ID injections, record area of injection, amount and type of testing substance, and date and time on medication record.	Timely documentation prevents administration errors.

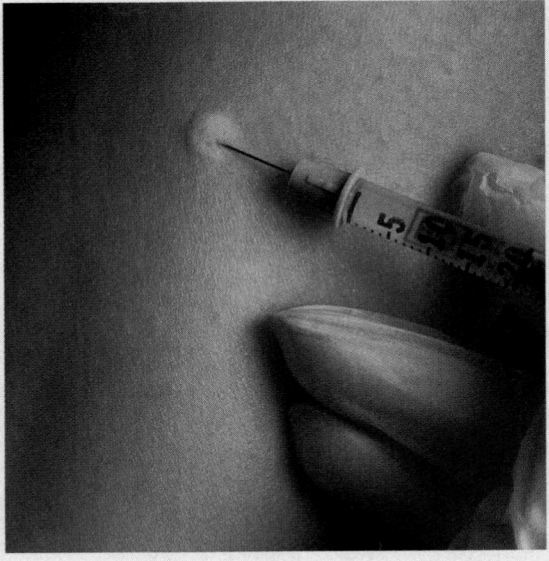

Step 25

Serious consequences may occur if an injection is administered incorrectly (see research highlight). Failure to select an injection site in relation to anatomical landmarks can result in nerve or bone damage during needle insertion. If the nurse fails to aspirate the syringe before injecting a drug, the drug may accidentally be injected directly into an artery or vein. Injecting too large a volume of medication for the site selected can cause extreme pain and may result in local tissue damage.

Many clients, particularly children, fear injections. Clients with serious or chronic illness often are given multiple injections daily. The nurse can attempt to minimize discomfort in the following ways:

1. Use a sharp, beveled needle in the smallest suitable length and gauge.
2. Position the client as comfortably as possible to reduce muscular tension.
3. Select the proper injection site, using anatomical landmarks.
4. Apply ice to the injection site to create local anesthesia before needle insertion.
5. Divert the client's attention from the injection through conversation.
6. Insert the needle smoothly and quickly to minimize tissue pulling.
7. Hold the syringe steady while the needle remains in tissues.
8. Massage the injected area gently for several seconds unless contraindicated.

SQ Injections

SQ injections involve placing medication into the loose connective tissue under the dermis (Procedure 21-3). Because SQ tissue is not as richly supplied with blood as the muscles, drug absorption is some- what slower than with IM injections. However, drugs are absorbed completely if circulatory status is normal. Because SQ tissue contains pain receptors, the client may experience some discomfort.

The best sites for SQ injections include vascular areas around the outer aspect of the upper arms, the abdomen from below the costal margins to the iliac crests, and the anterior aspect of the thighs. These areas are easily accessible, especially for clients with diabetes who self-administer insulin. The site most frequently recommended for heparin injections is the abdomen. Other sites include the scapular areas of the upper back and the upper ventral or dorsal gluteal areas. The injection site chosen should be free of infection, skin lesions, scars, bony prominences, and large underlying muscles or nerves (see research highlight). Clients with diabetes regularly rotate daily injection sites to prevent hypertrophy (thickening) of the skin and **lipodystrophy** (atrophy of tissue). No injection site should be used more than every 6 to 7 weeks. An injection diagram allows nurses and clients to record daily injections to be sure that sites are rotated (Fig. 21-15).

Only small doses (0.5 to 1 ml) of water-soluble medication should be given by the SQ route. SQ tissue is sensitive to irritating solutions and large vol-

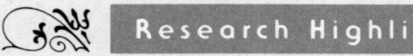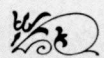

Research Highlight

Woodridge and Jackson, in 1988, conducted a study using 50 medical-surgical clients. Two injection methods were used; each client received one injection using both tested techniques. Smaller areas of bruising and induration resulted from a technique using a 3-ml syringe with a 25-gauge, ⅝-inch needle; a change of needle after drawing up the medication into the syringe; use of a 0.2-ml air bubble; and use of a drug sponge afterward.

Woodridge JB, Jackson JG: Evaluation of brusies and areas of induration after two techniques of subcutaneous heparin injection, *Heart Lung* 17:476, 1988.

Research Highlight

Vanbree et al studied the effect of techniques for administering SQ, low-dose heparin on the formation of bruises at the injection site. The following variables were held constant for all injections: (1) site (lower abdomen at least 2 inches from umbilicus), (2) preinjection skin preparation (gentle alcohol wipe), (3) grasping a roll of tissue, (4) drug dose and syringe, (5) angle of needle insertion (90 degrees), (6) withdrawal of needle (same angle as inserted), and (7) postinjection skin preparation (pressing site lightly with alcohol swab for 1 minute). The following methods were used to study needle manipulation and tracking of medication through tissues: (1) standard SQ injection technique using aspiration, (2) nonaspiration techniques, and (3) air-lock technique.

Forty-three clients received 129 injections each; each technique was used 43 times on each client. The study revealed that none of the three techniques was clearly superior in ensuring smaller or fewer bruises.

Vanbree NS et al: Clinical evaluation of three techniques for administering low-dose heparin, *Nurs Res* 33:15, 1984.

umes of medication. Collecting of medication within the tissues can cause sterile abscesses, which appear as hardened, painful lumps under the skin.

Body weight indicates the depth of the SQ layer. Therefore the nurse must choose the needle length and angle of insertion based on the client's weight. Generally a 25-gauge ⅝-inch needle inserted at a 45-degree angle (Fig. 21-16) deposits medication into the SQ tissue of a normal-size client. A child may require a ½-inch needle. If the client is obese, the nurse pinches the tissue and uses a needle long enough to insert through fatty tissue at the base of the skinfold. The preferred needle length is half the

width of the skinfold. With this method the angle of insertion may be between 45 and 90 degrees.

Thin, cachectic clients may have insufficient tissue for SQ injections. The upper abdomen is the best site for injection with this client. Insulin syringes usually come with 26-gauge needles. To ensure that the insulin reaches SQ tissue, the nurse follows this simple rule: if 2 inches of tissue can be grasped, the needle should be inserted at a 90-degree angle, and if 1 inch of tissue can be grasped, the needle should be inserted at a 45-degree angle.

IM Injections

The IM route provides faster drug absorption than the SQ route because of a muscle's greater vascularity. The danger of causing tissue damage is less when drugs enter deep muscle, but there is the risk of inadvertently injecting drugs directly into blood vessels. The nurse uses a longer and heavier-gauge needle to pass through SQ tissue and penetrate deep muscle tissue (Procedure 21-3). However, weight influences selection of needle size. For example, a client weighing 100 pounds may only require a needle 1¼ to 1½ inches long, whereas a child weighing 50 pounds usually requires a 1-inch needle. The angle of insertion for an IM injection is 90 degrees (Fig. 21-16). Muscle is less sensitive to irritating and viscous drugs. A normal, well-developed client can safely tolerate as much as 3 ml of medication in larger-developed muscles such as the dorsogluteal or vastus lateralis. Smaller muscles can tolerate only smaller amounts of medication without severe muscle discomfort. Children, older adults, and thin clients tolerate less than 2 ml of medication. Whaley and Wong (1991) recommend giving no more than 1 ml to small children and older infants.

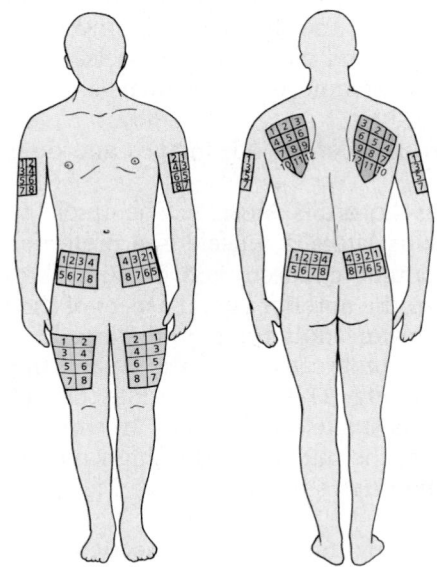

Fig. 21-15   Common sites for SQ injections. Note how sites might be rotated.

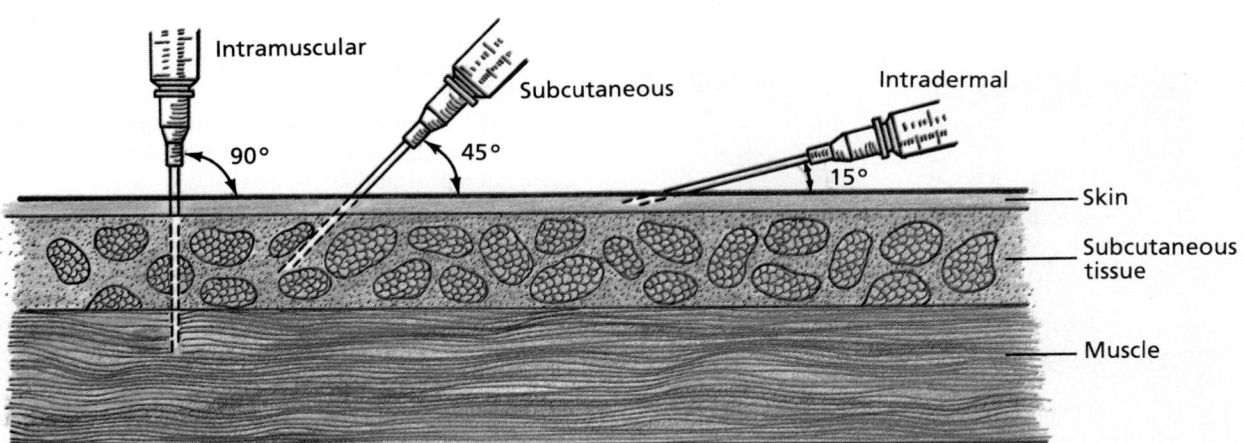

Fig. 21-16   Comparison of the angles of insertion for IM (90 degrees), SQ (45 degrees), and ID (15 degrees) injections.

Characteristics of IM Sites

VASTUS LATERALIS MUSCLE

- This large, developed muscle lacks major nerves and blood vessels.
- Rapid drug absorption occurs.

VENTROGLUTEAL MUSCLE

- A deep site, the ventrogluteal muscle is situated away from major nerves and blood vessels.
- There is less chance of contamination in incontinent clients or infants because it is away from the rectum.
- It is easily identified by a prominent bony landmark.

DORSOGLUTEAL MUSCLE

- The nurse runs the risk of striking the underlying sciatic nerve, greater trochanter, or major blood vessels.
- This site is not used with infants or children under 3 years of age due to underdeveloped muscle.
- This site must be clean to avoid contamination.

DELTOID MUSCLE

- This site is easily accessible, but the muscle is not well developed in most clients.
- Nurses use this site for small amounts of medications.
- The nurse avoids using the deltoid muscle in infants or children with underdeveloped muscles.
- There is potential for injury to radial and ulnar nerves or brachial artery.
- Less discomfort is felt in the deltoid, and this site is less likely to impair circulation.

The nurse assesses the integrity of a muscle before giving an injection. The muscle should be free of tenderness. Repeated injections in the same muscle cause considerable discomfort. By asking the client to relax, the nurse can palpate the muscle to rule out the presence of hardened lesions. Normally a muscle feels soft when relaxed and firm when tense. The nurse can minimize discomfort during an injection by helping the client assume a position that will help reduce the strain on the muscle.

SITES. When selecting an IM site, the nurse asks the following questions:

1. Is the area free of infection or necrosis?
2. Are there local areas of bruising or abrasions?
3. What is the location of underlying bones, nerves, and major blood vessels?
4. What volume of medication is to be administered?

Each site has certain advantages and disadvantages (see box).

Vastus Lateralis Muscle. The thick, well developed vastus lateralis muscle is a preferred injection site for adults, children, and infants. The muscle is located on the anterior lateral aspect of the thigh and extends in an adult from a handbreadth above the knee to a handbreath below the greater trochanter of the femur (Fig. 21-17). The middle third of the muscle is the best site for injection. In width the site extends from the midline of the thigh's top to the midline of the thigh's outer side. See Fig. 21-18 for children.

With young children or cachectic clients, it helps to grasp the body of the muscle during injection to be sure the drug is deposited in muscle tissue. To help relax the muscle, the nurse asks the client to lie flat with the knee slightly flexed or in a sitting position.

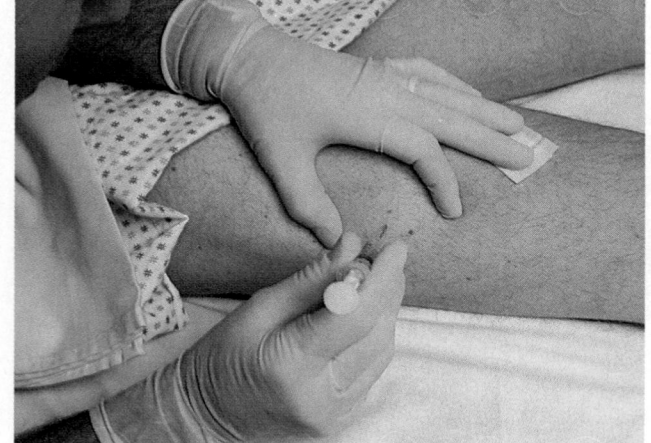

A

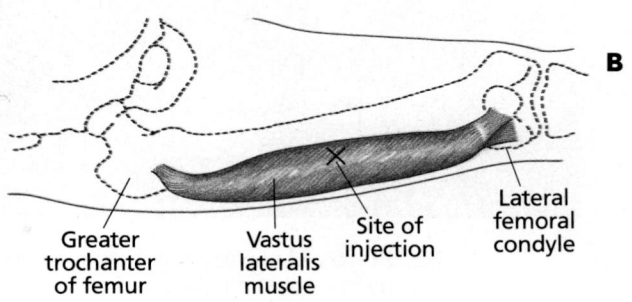

B

Fig. 21-17 **A,** Injection site into the vastus lateralis muscle. **B,** Anatomical view of the site for IM injection into the vastus lateralis muscle.

Ventrogluteal Muscle. The ventrogluteal muscle involves the gluteus medius and minimus. The nurse locates the muscle by placing the heel of the hand over the greater trochanter of the client's hip. The right hand is used for the left hip, and the left hand is used for the right hip.

The nurse points the thumb toward the client's groin and fingers toward the head, places the index finger over the anterior superior iliac spine, and extends the middle finger back along the iliac crest toward the buttock. The index finger, the middle finger, and the iliac crest form a V-shaped triangle, and the injection site is the center of it (Fig. 21-19). The client may lie on the side or back. Flexing of the knee and hip helps the client relax this muscle.

Dorsogluteal Muscle. The dorsogluteal muscle has been a traditional site for IM injections. However, accidental insertion of a needle into the sciatic nerve can cause permanent or partial paralysis of the involved leg. Major blood vessels and bone are also near the site. In clients with flabby, sagging tissues, the site is difficult to locate.

The dorsogluteal site is located in the upper outer aspect of the upper outer quadrant of the buttock, approximately 5 to 8 cm (2 to 3 in) below the iliac crest. Clients may lie in the prone position with toes turned medially or in a side-lying position with the upper leg flexed at the hip and knee. To locate the dorsogluteal site, the nurse palpates the posterosuperior iliac spine and the greater trochanter of the femur. An imaginary line is drawn between the two anatomical landmarks. The sciatic nerve runs parallel and below the line. The injection site is above and lateral to the line (Fig. 21-20 on p. 662). Nurses may use the dorsogluteal injection site in adults and children (at least 3 years of age) with well-developed gluteal muscles.

Deltoid Muscle. In infants and children the deltoid muscle is not well developed. The radial and ulnar nerves and brachial artery lie within the upper arm along the humerus. The nurse rarely uses the deltoid site unless other injection sites are inaccessible because of dressings, casts, or other obstructions.

To locate the deltoid muscle the nurse has the client fully expose the upper arm and shoulder. A tight-fitting sleeve should not be rolled up. The nurse has

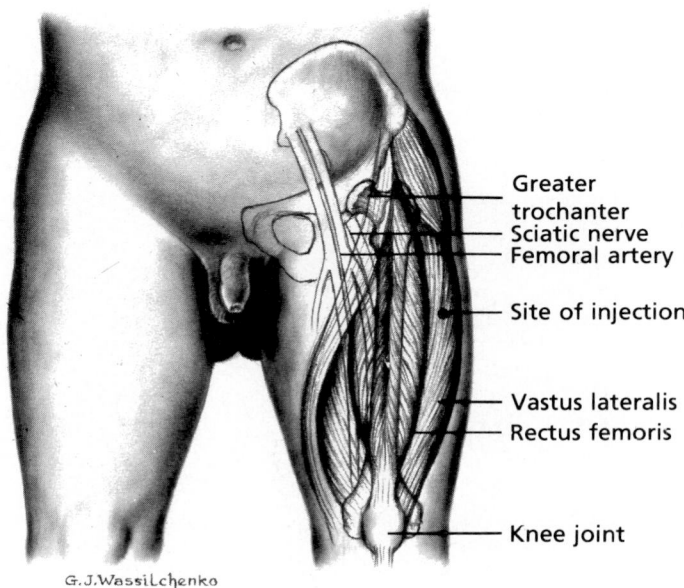

G.J.Wassilchenko

Fig. 21-18 Acceptable IM site for children, the vastus lateralis muscle.
From Whaley LF, Wong DL: *Nursing care of infants and children,* ed 4, St Louis, 1991, Mosby–Year Book.

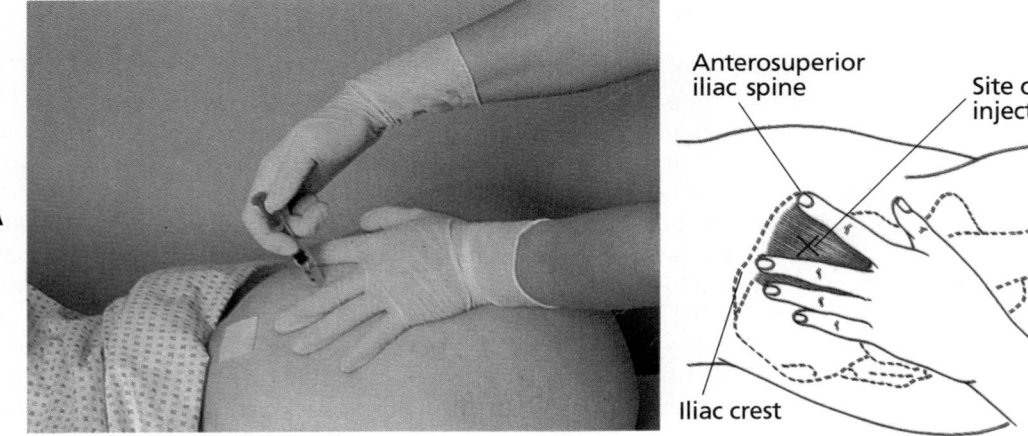

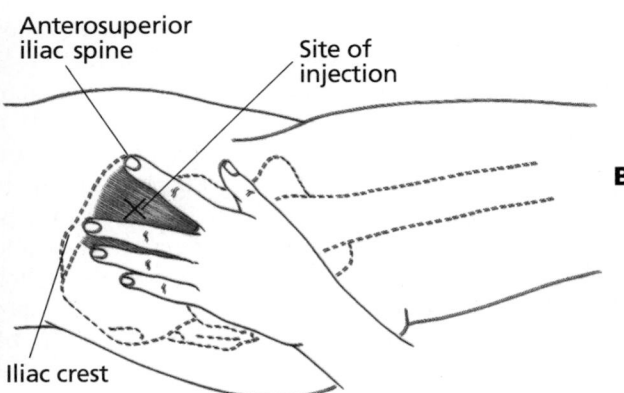

Fig. 21-19 **A,** Injection site into ventrogluteal muscle avoids major nerves and blood vessels. **B,** Anatomical view of ventrogluteal muscle injection site.

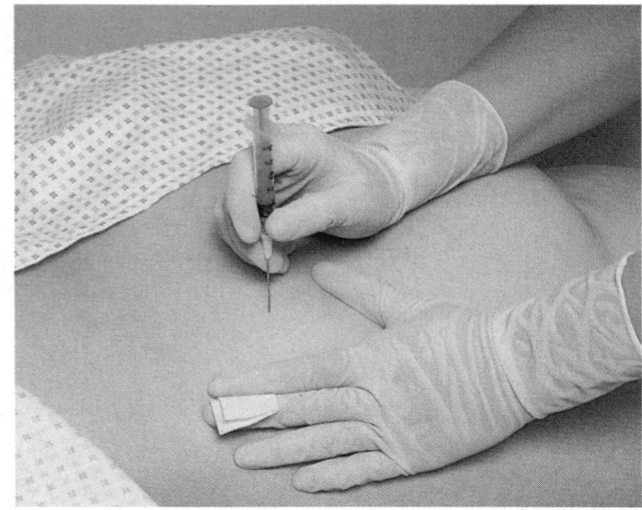

A

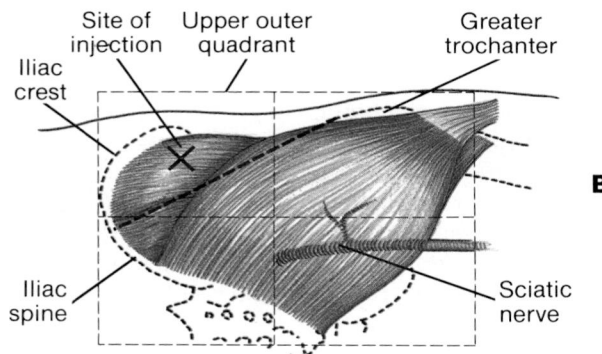

B

Fig. 21-20   **A,** Site of injection into the left dorsogluteal muscle. **B,** Imaginary diagonal line extending from the posterior superior iliac spine to the greater trochanter is the landmark for selecting the dorsogluteal injection site.

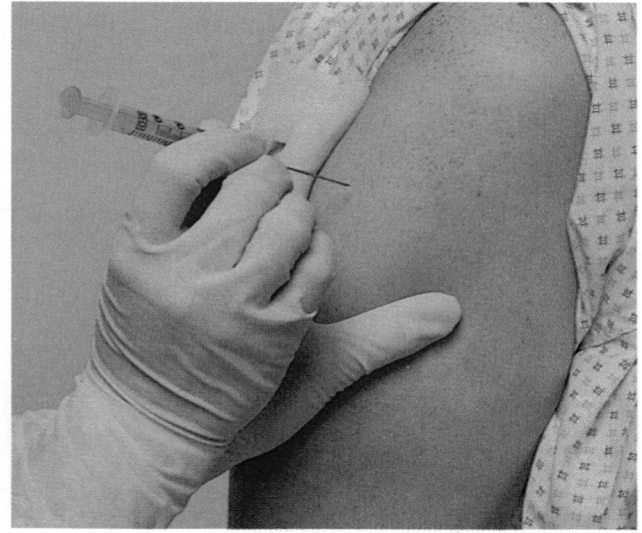

A

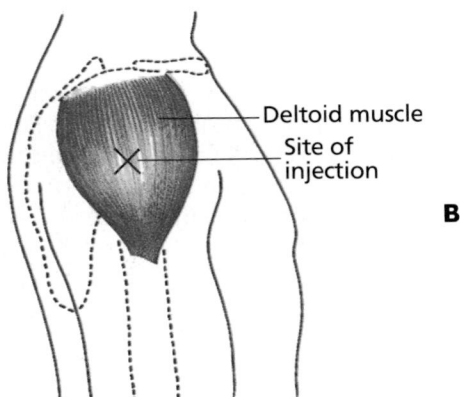

B

Fig. 21-21   **A,** Site of IM injection into the deltoid muscle. **B,** Site of deltoid muscle injection below acromion process.

the client relax the arm at the side and flex the elbow (Fig. 21-21, *A*). The client may sit, stand, or lie down. The nurse palpates the lower edge of the acromion process, which forms the base of a triangle in line with the midpoint of the lateral aspect of the upper arm (Fig. 21-21, *B*). The injection site is in the center of the triangle, about 2.5 to 5 cm (1 to 2 in) below the acromion process. The nurse may also locate the site by placing four fingers across the deltoid muscle, with the top finger along the acromion process. The injection site is then 3 fingerbreadths below the acromion process.

Z-TRACK METHOD. When irritating preparations (for example, iron) are given intramuscularly, the **Z-track**

method of injection minimizes tissue irritation by sealing the drug within the muscle tissues. The nurse selects an IM site, preferably in larger, deeper muscles such as the ventrogluteal muscle. A new needle must be applied to the syringe after preparing the drug so that no solution remains on the outside needle shaft. The nurse draws up 0.2 ml of air to create an air lock. After preparing the site with an antiseptic swab, the nurse pulls the overlying skin and SQ tissues approximately 2.5 to 3.5 cm (1 to 1½ in) laterally to the side. Holding the skin taut with the nondominant hand, the nurse injects the needle deep into the muscle. With practice the nurse learns to hold the syringe and aspirate with one hand. The nurse injects the drug and air slowly if there is no

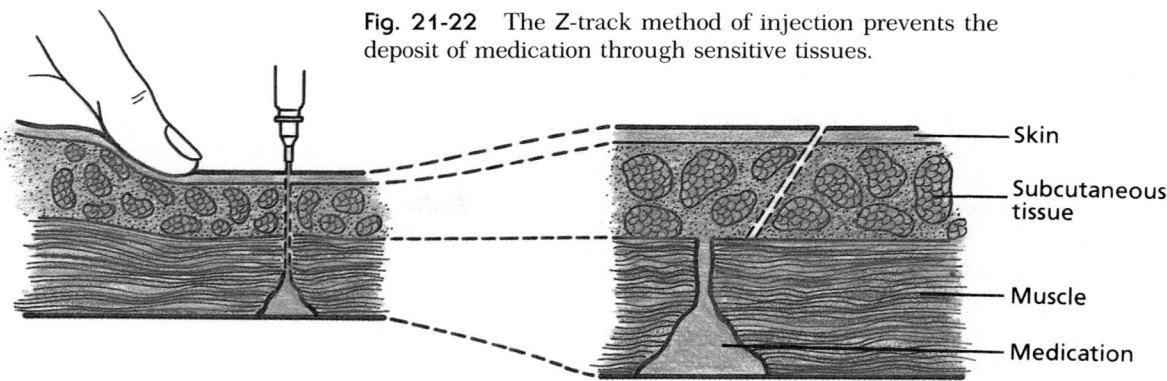

Fig. 21-22   The Z-track method of injection prevents the deposit of medication through sensitive tissues.

Skin

Subcutaneous tissue

Muscle

Medication

blood return on aspiration. The needle remains inserted for 10 seconds to allow the medication to disperse evenly. The nurse releases the skin after withdrawing the needle, which leaves a zigzag path that seals the needle track wherever tissue planes slide across each other (Fig. 21-22). The drug cannot escape from the muscle tissue.

AIR-LOCK TECHNIQUE. IM injections using the **air-lock technique** are less irritating to SQ tissues. When a small volume of air is injected behind a bolus of medication, the air clears the needle of medication, preventing tracking of the drug through SQ tissues. This technique is specifically recommended in the drug information insert of only a few medications. Examples include Inferon, Wyeth's vaccines prepared with aluminum adjuvant, diphtheria and tetanus toxoid vaccines, and the pertussis (whooping cough) vaccine.

After preparing the proper dose, the nurse draws up 0.2 ml of air. The needle then must be injected downward at a 90-degree angle so that the air rises to the top of the drug toward the plunger (Fig. 21-23). As the nurse injects the drug into the muscle, the air follows the medication, creating an air lock (Fig. 21-23). If the nurse administers the drug with the needle at an angle less than 90 degrees, the air collects along the barrel of the syringe and enters the muscle too soon. Medication can then easily leak back into SQ tissues.

ID Injections

The nurse typically gives ID injections for skin testing (for example, tuberculin screening and allergy tests). Because these medications are potent, they are injected into the dermis, where the blood supply is reduced and drug absorption occurs slowly. A client may have a severe anaphylactic reaction if the medications enter the circulation too rapidly. For clients with a history of numerous allergies, the physician often performs skin testing.

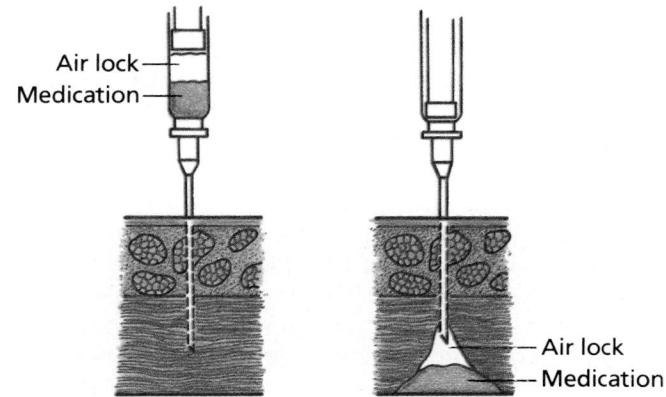

Air lock

Medication

Air lock

Medication

Fig. 21-23   Administering IM injection by the air-lock technique prevents tracking of medication through SQ tissues.

Skin testing requires the nurse to be able to clearly see the injection sites for changes in color and tissue integrity. ID sites should be lightly pigmented, free of lesions, and relatively hairless. The inner forearm and upper back are ideal locations.

The nurse uses a tuberculin or small hypodermic syringe for skin testing. The angle of insertion is 5 to 15 degrees (Fig. 21-16). As the nurse injects the drug, a small bleb resembling a mosquito bite should appear on the skin's surface (Procedure 21-3). If a bleb does not appear or if the site bleeds after needle withdrawal, there is a good chance the medication entered SQ tissues. In this case, skin test results will not be valid.

Data from an ID injection include a description of the precise location and time of administration. The injected site must be "read" within a prescribed time.

IV Administration

The nurse administers drugs intravenously by the following methods:

1. As mixtures within large volumes of IV fluids

2. By injection of a bolus, or small volume, of medication through an existing IV infusion line or heparin lock

3. By "piggyback" **infusion** of a solution containing the prescribed drug and a small volume of IV fluid through an existing IV line

In all three methods the client has an existing IV infusion line or an IV access site such as a heparin lock. In most institutions, policies and procedures list persons who may give IV medication and the situations in which they may be given. These policies are based on the drug, capability and availability of staff, and the type of monitoring equipment available.

Chapter 39 describes the technique for performing venipuncture and establishing continuous IV fluid infusions. Medication administration is only one reason for supplying IV fluids. IV fluid therapy is used primarily for fluid and electrolyte replacement in clients unable to take oral fluids.

The nurse must observe clients closely for symptoms of adverse reactions when using any method of IV drug administration. After a drug enters the bloodstream, it begins to act immediately, and there is no way to stop its action. Thus the nurse takes special care to avoid errors in dosage calculation and preparation. The nurse should double-check the "five rights" of safe drug administration and know the desired action and potential side effects. If the drug has an antidote, the nurse must have it available during administration. When administering potent drugs, the nurse assesses vital signs before, during, and after infusion.

Administering drugs by the IV route has advantages. In emergencies when a fast-acting drug must be delivered quickly, the IV route is most desirable. The IV route is also best when constant therapeutic blood levels must be established. Some medications are highly alkaline and irritating to muscle and SQ tissue. Therefore giving these drugs intravenously causes less discomfort.

LARGE-VOLUME INFUSIONS. Of the three methods of administering IV medications, mixing drugs in large volumes of fluids is the safest and easiest. Drugs are diluted in large volumes (500 ml or 1000 ml) of compatible IV fluids such as normal saline or Ringer's lactate solution. In most institutions the pharmacist adds drugs to the primary container of IV solution to ensure asepsis. Because the drug is not in a concentrated form, the risk of side effects or fatal reactions is minimal. Vitamins and potassium chloride are two types of drugs commonly added to IV fluids. The danger with continuous infusion is that the client may suffer circulatory fluid overload if the IV fluid is infused too rapidly (see Chapter 39 and Procedure 21-4).

INTRAVENOUS BOLUS. An **IV bolus** involves introducing a concentrated dose of a drug directly into systemic circulation (see box). The IV bolus is used during emergencies, with critically unstable clients, and as a route of administration when rapid and predictable responses are required (Burman, Berkowitz, 1986). An IV bolus may be given directly into a vein, into an existing IV line through an injection port, or through a heparin lock.

Because only a small amount of fluid is required to deliver a drug, use of a bolus is an advantage when the amount of fluid the client can take is restricted.

Guidelines for Giving Medications by IV Bolus

- Check physician's order for type of medication to be administered, dose, and route.
- Wash hands. Apply gloves.
- Prepare ordered medication. Carefully read package directions for proper dilution.
- Prepare syringe with small-gauge needles (21- to 25-gauge) to insert through ports.
- Carefully check client's identification by looking at armband and asking name.
- Assess IV insertion site for signs of infiltration or phlebitis. If present, do not give medication; restart IV line in another site.
- Start IV push through IV lock:
  - Clean off injection port with antiseptic swab.
  - Clear lock with 1 ml of saline.
  - Administer medication.
  - Clear lock with 1 ml of saline.
  - Inject 10 μ/ml of heparin (may be omitted).
- Start IV push through existing line:
  - Select injection port closest to client.
  - Clean off injection port with antiseptic swab.
  - Occlude IV line by pinching tubing just above injection port.
- Gently aspirate for blood return and inject medication.
- Administer medication over specified time recommended. (Check manufacturer's directions.) Use a watch to time administration.
- Dispose of gloves and wash hands.
- Observe client closely for adverse reactions as the drug is administered and for several minutes thereafter.
- Dispose of uncapped needles and syringes in proper container.
- Record drug, dose, route, time administered, and length of time medication given on medication form. Note adverse reactions.

STEPS	RATIONALE
1. Check physician's order for type of IV solution, medication, and dose.	Overall physical condition determines type of solution to use. Ensures safe and accurate drug administration.
2. When more than one medication is to be added to solution, assess for drug compatibility.	Certain drugs are incompatible when mixed. May result in clouding or crystallization of fluids or cause drug interaction that is not visible.
3. Prepare equipment and supplies: a. Vial or ampule of prescribed medication b. Syringe of appropriate size (5 to 20 ml) c. Sterile needle (1 to 1½ in, 19- to 21-gauge) with special filters (optional) d. Correct solvent (e.g., sterile water or normal saline) e. Sterile IV fluid container (bag or bottle, 500 to 1000 ml in volume) f. Alcohol or antiseptic swab g. Label to attach to IV bag or bottle	Larger needle gauge ensures easy aspiration of drugs from vial or ampule. Filter prevents solid material from entering syringe and thus avoids transfer to fluid container. Certain IV medications are prepared in dry powder form. Solvent must be added for mixing. Solution bags are kept sterile by being stored in separate intact plastic bag. Bottles have plastic or metal seal over bottle cap. Continuously infusing medication must be labeled properly for all nurses to observe.
4. Wash hands thoroughly.	Reduces transfer of microorganisms when handling sterile equipment.
5. Assemble supplies in medication room.	Ensures that procedure will be orderly with less likelihood of contaminating supplies.
6. Prepare prescribed medication from vial or ampule (Procedure 21-2). (If filter needle is used, replace it with regular needle before injecting medication into IV fluid container.)	Different techniques are used for each type of container.
7. Identify client by reading identification band and asking name.	Ensures that correct client receives ordered medication.
8. Prepare client by explaining that medication is to be given through existing IV line or one to be started. Explain that no discomfort should be felt during infusion. Encourage client to report symptoms of discomfort.	Allows client to understand procedure and minimizes anxiety. Most IV medications will not cause discomfort when diluted. However, potassium chloride can be irritating. Pain at insertion site may be early indication of infiltration.

9. Add medication to new container:
a. Locate medication injection port on IV solution bag:
  (1) Remove plastic cover over port. Port has small rubber stopper at end. Do not select port for IV tubing insertion or air vent.
b. Locate injection site on IV solution bottle:
  (1) Remove metal or plastic cap and rubber disk. Place cap upside down on counter top.
  (2) Locate medication injection site on bottle's rubber stopper. Site is usually marked by X, circle, or triangle.
c. Wipe off port or injection site with alcohol or antiseptic swab (see illustration on p. 666).
d. Remove needle cap from syringe and insert needle of syringe through center of injection port or site, and inject medication (see illustration on p. 666).
	Medication injection port is self-sealing to prevent introduction of microorganisms after repeated use.
	
	Cap seals bottle to maintain sterility. Inside of cap may remain sterile for reuse.
	Accidental injection of medication through main tubing port or air vent can alter pressure within bottle and cause fluid leaks through air vent.
	Reduces risk of introducing microorganisms into bag during needle insertion.
	Injection of needle into sides of port may produce leak and lead to fluid contamination.

Adding Medications to IV Fluid Containers

STEPS	RATIONALE
e. Withdraw syringe from bag or bottle. Cover glass bottle top with antiseptic swab and sterile bottle cap.	Open tubing port in bottle provides direct route for microorganisms to enter solution. Bags have self-sealing port.
f. Mix medication and IV solution by holding bag or bottle and turning it gently end to end.	Allows medication to be distributed evenly.
g. Complete medication label with name and dose of medication, date, time, and your initials. Stick it upside down on bottle or bag (see illustration).	Label can be easily read during infusion of solution. Informs nurses and physicians of contents of bag or bottle.
h. Spike bag or bottle with IV tubing and hang (see Chapter 39). Regulate infusion at ordered rate.	Prevents rapid infusion of fluid.

10. Add medication to existing container:

    a. Prepare vented IV bottle or plastic bag:

(1) Check volume of solution remaining in bottle.	Proper volume is needed to dilute medication adequately.
(2) Verify dilution of medication desired (amount of medication per milliliter).	
(3) Close off IV infusion clamp.	Prevents medication from directly entering circulation as it is injected into bag or bottle.

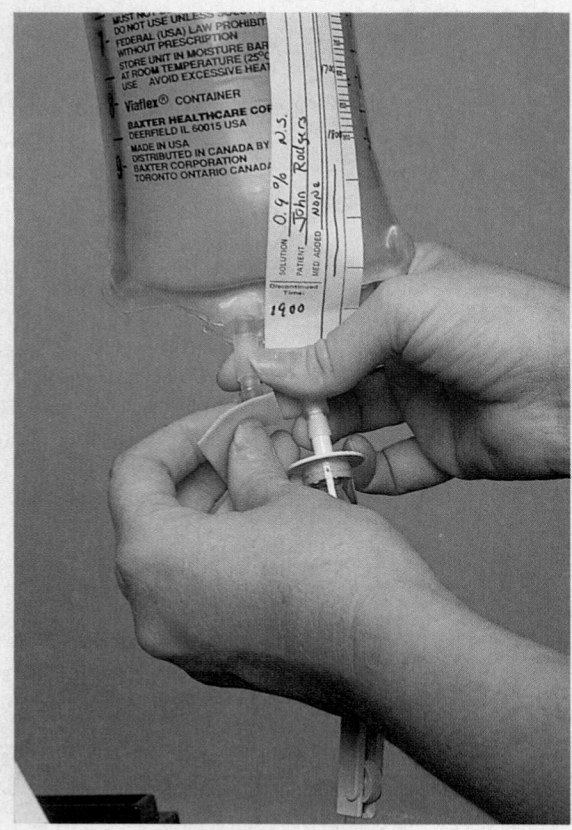

Step 9c

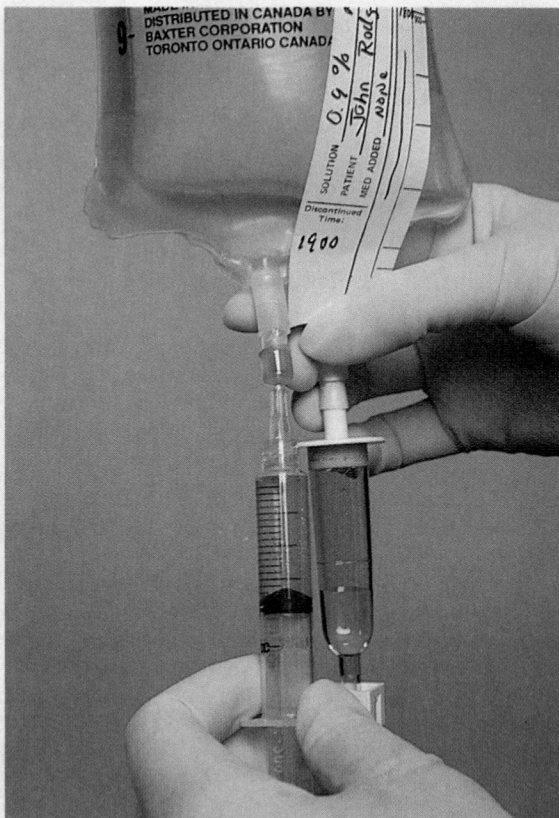

Step 9d

STEPS	RATIONALE

(4) Wipe medication port with alcohol or antiseptic swab.

Mechanically removes microorganisms that could enter container during needle insertion.

(5) Lower bag or bottle from IV pole. Insert syringe needle through injection port and inject medication.

Injection port is self-sealing and prevents fluid leaks.

(6) Gently mix bottle or bag.

Ensures that medication is evenly distributed.

(7) Rehang bag and regulate infusion to desired rate.

Prevents rapid infusion of fluid.

b. Complete medication label and stick it to bag or bottle.

Informs nurses and physicians of contents of bag or bottle.

11. Properly dispose of equipment and supplies.

Reduces transmission of microorganisms.

12. Record solution and medication added to parenteral fluid on appropriate form (see illustration).

Information used to monitor type of solutions client receives and fluid intake over 24 hours.

13. Report side effects (e.g., change in pulse rate, noisy respirations, or change in blood pressure) to nurse in charge or physician.

Reaction may require therapeutic intervention.

CONTINUED

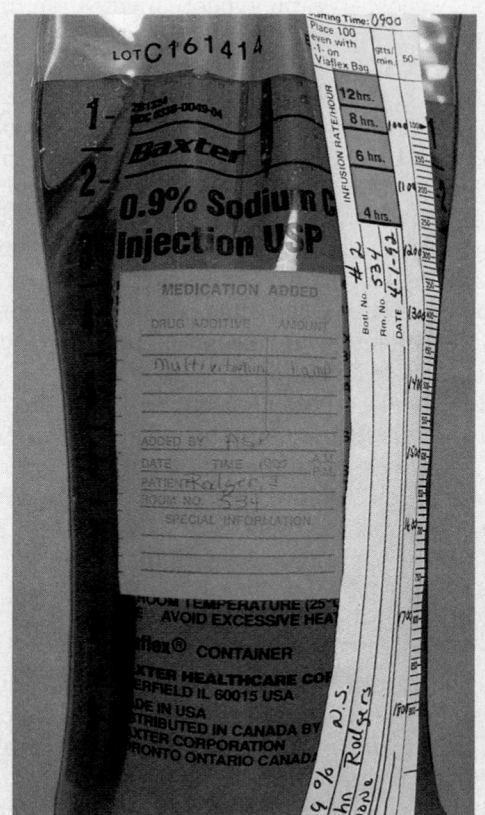

Step 9g

PARENTERAL FLUID

AMT.	TYPE OF FLUID	MEDICATION ADDED	DATE/ HR START	RN INIT	DATE/ HR COMP	RN INIT	AMT. REC'D	SITE	IV SITE CARE DATE/HR	TUBING CHANGE DATE/HR	RN INIT
1L	D5W	20 meq. KCl	1/8 0900	PL	1/8 1800	T.M.	1000 ml	✓	1/8 1000		
1L	LR	20 meq. KCl	1/8 1800	T.M.							

Step 12

The IV bolus is the most dangerous method for administering drugs because there is no time to correct errors. In addition, a bolus may cause direct irritation to the lining of blood vessels. Before administering a bolus, the nurse confirms placement of the IV line. This involves obtaining a blood return through the IV catheter or needle. The inability to obtain a blood return may suggest that the needle or catheter is in tissues or resting against the vein wall. A drug should never be given intravenously if the insertion site appears puffy or edematous or the IV fluid cannot flow at the proper rate. Accidental injection of a medication into the tissues surrounding a vein can cause pain, sloughing of tissues, and abscesses, depending on the drug's composition.

The rate of administration of an IV bolus medication is usually determined by the amount of drug that can be given each minute. The nurse should look up each medication to be given to determine the maximum concentration and rate of administration recommended. The standard rate is 1 ml/min if no specific rate of administration is recommended (Burman, Berkowitz, 1986). The purpose for which a drug is prescribed and any potential adverse effects related to the rate or route of administration must be considered when a nurse gives a drug IV push.

VOLUME-CONTROLLED INFUSIONS. Another way of administering IV medications is through small amounts (50 to 100 ml) of compatible IV fluids. The fluid is within a secondary fluid container separate from the primary IV fluid bag. The container connects directly to the primary IV line or to a separate tubing that inserts into the primary IV line. Two types of containers are volume-control administration sets (for example, Volutrol or Pediatrol) and piggyback sets (see Chapter 39). There are several advantages to using volume-controlled infusions, including the following:

1. Reduces risk of rapid-dose infusion by IV push; IV medications are diluted and infused over longer time intervals (for example, 30 to 60 minutes)
2. Allows administration of drugs that are incompatible with drugs in the primary IV solution
3. Allows administration of drugs (for example, antibiotics) that are stable for a limited time in solution
4. Allows control of IV fluid intake

Volume-control administration sets are small (100 to 150 ml) containers that attach just below the primary infusion bag or bottle (Procedure 21-5). The set is attached and filled in a manner similar to a regular IV infusion (see Chapter 39). However, the priming or filling of the set is different, depending on the type of filter (floating valve or membane) within the set. Package directions should be followed during priming, or the set will not function properly.

PIGGYBACK IV ADMINISTRATION. **Piggyback sets** are small (50 or 100 ml) IV bags or bottles connected to short tubing lines that connect to the upper Y-port of a primary infusion line or an intermittent venous access. The piggyback tubing is a microdrip or macrodrip system.

INTERMITTENT VENOUS ACCESS. A **heparin lock**, or saline lock, is an IV infusion device with a male adapter covered by a rubber diaphragm. Special rubber-seal injection caps serve as adapters and can be inserted into most IV catheters (see Chapter 39). Advantages to intermittent venous access include the following:

1. Cost savings resulting from the omission of continuous IV therapy
2. Convenience to the nurse by eliminating constant monitoring of flow rates
3. Increased mobility, safety, and comfort for the client

After an IV bolus or piggyback medication has been administered through a heparin lock, the lock must be flushed with a solution to keep it **patent** (free of clots). Disagreement exists as to the type of solution to use to keep heparin locks free of clots. Cyganski et al (1987) demonstrated that a heparin flush solution (1 ml = 100 units), given after an IV drug, was effective in minimizing phlebitis of IV sites and clotting of IV catheters. However, Dunn and Lenihan (1987), Harrigan (1985), and Taylor et al (1989) showed that regular flushes of normal saline were just as effective in keeping heparin locks patent. Agency policies differ.

Normally, checking for a blood return in an IV lock before bolus administration is unnecessary. However, if the needle site becomes puffy or the client complains of discomfort, the "well" must be aspirated for a blood return. Procedure 21-6 on pp. 672-674 describes the technique for administering an IV medication bolus.

Disposal of Equipment

After administering injections, the nurse must properly dispose of used equipment. A stray needle can injure the client, nurse, housekeeper, or other health care personnel. A needlestick can be the source of hepatitis or acquired immunodeficiency syndrome (AIDS).

The Centers for Disease Control (CDC) recommends that needles should not be capped before disposal. Covering a needle may predispose the nurse to a needlestick. The nurse discards the needle and sy-

Text continued on p. 675.

STEPS	RATIONALE
1. Check physician's order to determine type of medication and dosage.	Client's overall physical condition determines type of solution used. Ensures safe and accurate drug administration.
2. Assess patency of existing IV infusion line (see Chapter 39) by noting infusion rate of main IV line.	IV line must be patent and fluids must infuse easily for medication to reach venous circulation effectively.
3. Assess insertion site for signs of infiltration or phlebitis (see Chapter 39).	Confirmation of placement of needle or catheter and integrity of surrounding tissues ensure that medication is administered safely.
4. Prepare following equipment and supplies:	
a. Piggyback set:	
(1) Medication prepared in a 50- to 100-ml, labeled infusion bag with IV line, microdrip or macrodrip infusion tubing set	Used for piggyback administration. Most piggybacks are prepared by pharmacies.
(2) Needle (21- or 23-gauge)	Medication is "piggybacked" or connected to main infusion line by needle inserted through injection port. Larger needle would cause leakage at Y-port connector.
(3) Adhesive tape (optional)	
(4) Antiseptic swab	
(5) Metal hook (optional)	Used to lower primary infusion bag below smaller infusion bag (only if tubing is shorter than primary tubing).
(6) Disposable gloves	
b. Volume-control administration set:	
(1) Volutrol, Pediatrol, or Burette	Graduated container connects to main IV solution.
(2) Infusion tubing	Connected to administration set used to inject medication into set.
(3) Syringe (5 to 20 ml)	
(4) Needle (1 to 1½ in, 21- or 23-gauge)	
(5) Vial or ampule of ordered medication	
(6) Medication label	
5. Wash hands and apply gloves.	Reduces transmission of microorganisms. During handling of IV equipment, there is some risk of blood exposure.
6. Administer medications by piggyback set:	
a. Assemble supplies at bedside.	Drug preparation is usually not required. May assemble infusion tubing and bag of medication in medication or client's room.
b. Connect infusion tubing to medication bag (see Chapter 39). Allow solution to fill tubing by opening regulator flow clamp.	Infusion tube should be filled with solution and free of air bubbles to prevent air embolus.
c. Hang medication bag at or above level of main fluid bag. Hook may be used to lower main bag (see illustration on p. 670).	Height of fluid bag affects rate of flow to client.
d. Connect covered sterile needle to end of infusion tubing.	Cover keeps needle sterile before connecting it to main line.
e. Check client's identification by looking at armband and asking name.	Ensures that drug is administered to correct client.
f. Clean injection Y-port of main line with antiseptic swab.	Prevents introduction of microorganisms during needle insertion.
g. Remove cover and insert needle of secondary piggyback line through injection port of main line. Secure with strip of adhesive tape if necessary. If available, use needle-lock devices to secure needle of secondary piggyback line through injection port of main line (see illustrations on pp. 670-671).	Establishes route for medication to enter main IV line. Needle-lock devices or tape prevents needle from slipping out of port which could result in improper dose of medication and increased risk of needlestick injury to health care workers.

Administering IV Medications by Piggyback or Volume Administration Sets

STEPS

h. Regulate flow rate appropriate or as ordered by physician, pharmacist, or manufacturer.

i. After medication has infused, check flow regulator on primary infusion. Piggyback set hung at level of primary bag has backcheck valve that automatically stops flow of primary infusion until medication infuses. Primary infusion should automatically begin to flow after piggyback is empty.

j. Regulate main infusion line to desired rate, if necessary.

k. Leave secondary bag, tubing, and inserted needle in place for future drug administration or discard in appropriate containers.

7. Administer medication by volume-control administration set (e.g., Volutrol:)

   a. Assemble supplies in medication room.

   b. Prepare medication from vial or ampule (Procedure 21-2).

   c. Check client's identification by looking at armband and asking name.

   d. Fill Volutrol with desired amount of fluid (50 to 100 ml) by opening clamp between Volutrol and main IV bag (see illustrations).

RATIONALE

Intermittent infusion of medication maintains therapeutic blood levels. For optimal effect, drug should infuse in prescribed time interval.

Valve prevents backup of medication into main infusion line. Checking flow rate ensures proper administration of fluids.

Infusion of piggyback may interfere with main line infusion rate.

Establishment of secondary line produces route for microorganisms to enter main line. Repeated changes in tubing or needles increase risk of infection transmission.

Controls risk of contaminating IV solution.

Ensures drug administered to correct client.

Small volume of fluid dilutes medication and reduces risk of too-rapid infusion.

Step 6g

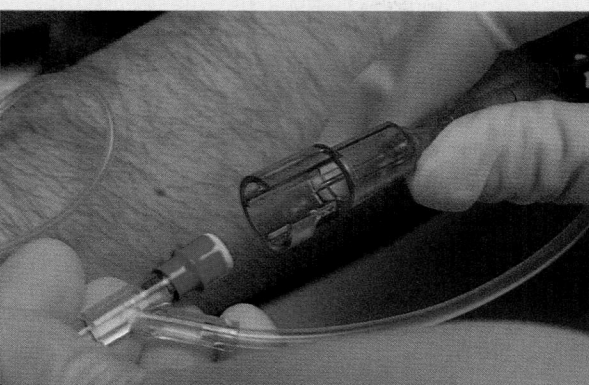

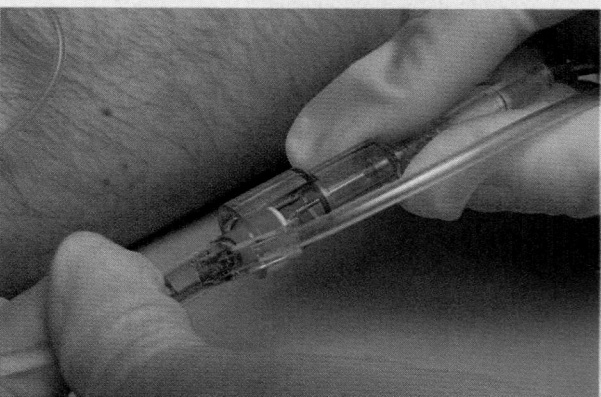

Step 6g

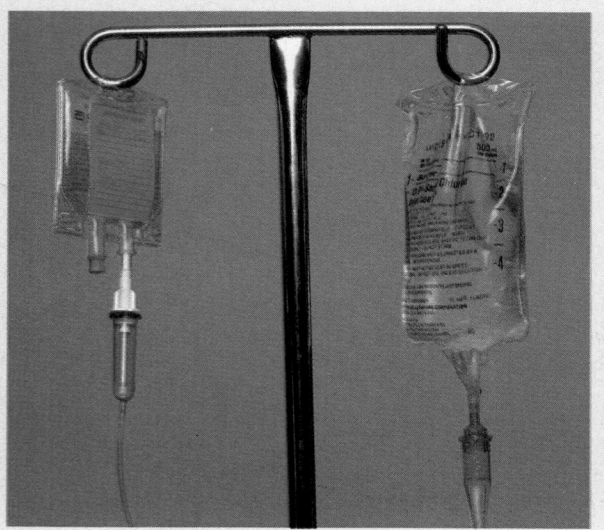

Step 6c

CONTINUED

STEPS	RATIONALE
e. Close clamp and check to be sure clamp in air vent of Volutrol chamber is open.	Prevents additional leakage of fluid into Volutrol. Air vent allows fluid in Volutrol to exit at regulated rate.
f. Clean injection port on top of Volutrol with antiseptic swab.	Prevents introduction of microorganisms during needle insertion.
g. Remove needle cap and insert syringe needle through port, and then inject medication (see illustration). Gently rotate Volutrol between hands.	Rotating mixes medication with solution in Volutrol to ensure equal distribution.
h. Regulate IV infusion rate appropriate for medication. Follow physician, pharmacist, or manufacturer recommendations for infusion rates.	For optimal therapeutic effect, drug should infuse in prescribed time interval.
i. Label Volutrol with name of drug, dose, total volume including diluent, and time of administration.	Alerts nurses to drug being infused. Prevents other medications from being added to Volutrol.
j. Dispose of uncapped needle and syringe in proper container.	Prevents accidental needlesticks.
8. Remove and dispose of gloves. Wash hands.	Prevents transmission of microorganisms.
9. Observe client for signs of adverse reactions.	IV medications act rapidly.
10. During infusion, periodically check infusion rate and condition of IV site.	IV line must remain patent for proper drug administration. Development of infiltration necessitates discontinuing infusion.
11. Record drug, dose, route, and time administered on medication form (Fig. 21-6). Record volume of fluid in medication bag or Volutrol on intake and output form (see Chapter 39).	Timely documentation prevents medication errors (e.g., repeated doses). Fluid balance is regulated and monitored on basis of total fluid intake.

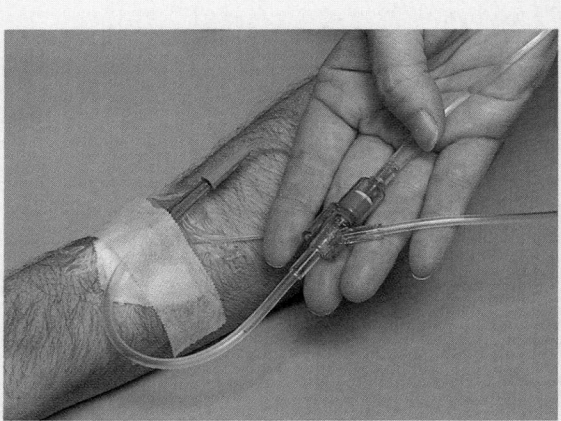

Step 6g

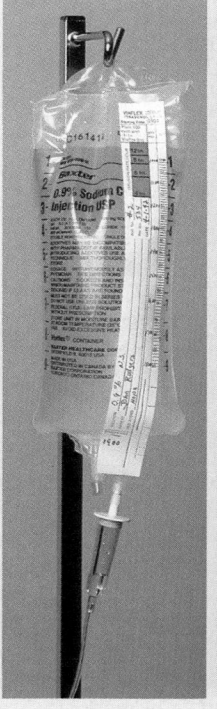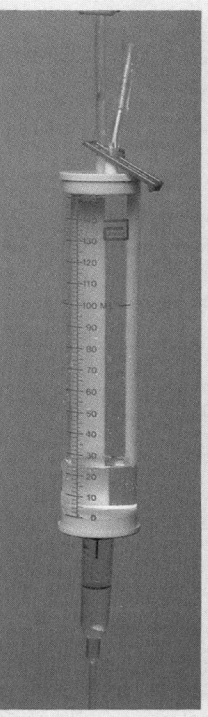

Step 7d

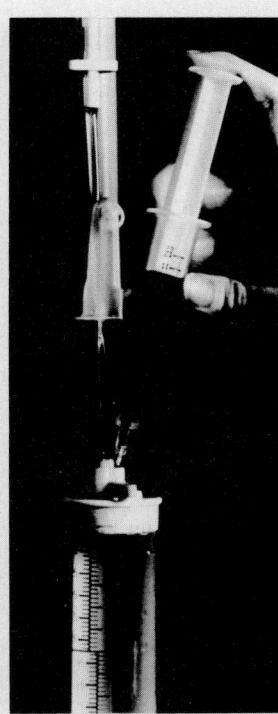

Step 7g

Administering Medications by IV Bolus (Push)

STEPS	RATIONALE
1. Check physician's order for type of medication to be administered, dosage, and route.	Ensures safe and accurate drug administration.
2. Assess IV or heparin (saline) lock insertion site for signs of infiltration or phlebitis (see Chapter 39).	Confirmation of placement of IV needle or catheter and integrity of surrounding tissues ensure that medication is administered safely.
3. If medication is to be pushed into IV line, assess patency of line by noting infusion rate.	IV line must be patent and fluids must infuse easily for medication to reach venous circulation effectively.

4. Prepare equipment and supplies:
a. IV push (existing line)
  (1) Medication in vial or ampule
  (2) Syringe (3 to 5 ml)
  (3) Sterile needles (21- and 25-gauge)
	Large-gauge needles are used to draw up medication. Small-gauge needles are used to insert through Y-port of tubing.

(4) Antiseptic swab
  (5) Watch with second hand or digital readout
b. IV push (IV lock):
  (1) Medication in vial or ampule
  (2) Syringe (3 to 5 ml)
  (3) Syringe (3 ml)
  (4) Vial of heparin flush solution (1 ml = 100 units or 1 ml = 10 units) or vial of normal saline (depending on agency policy)
  (5) Sterile needles (21- and 25-gauge)
	Used for medication preparation.
	Used for heparin flush or saline solution.
	Keeps heparin lock patent and free of clots. Studies have not shown clear advantage of using heparin instead of saline (Dunn, Lenihan, 1987; Harrigan, 1985).
	Large-gauge needles are used to draw up medication. Small-gauge needle are used to insert through heparin (saline) lock.

(6) Antiseptic swab
  (7) Watch with second hand or digital readout
  (8) Disposable gloves	

5. Wash hands. Apply gloves.	Reduces transmission of infection. During IV bolus administration, risk of blood exposure is low. However, nurse may have to manipulate IV dressing or expose site while completing other activities. Gloves reduce exposure.
6. Prepare ordered medication from vial or ampule (Procedure 21-2). Read package directions carefully for proper IV dilution of medication.	
7. After preparing medication, apply small-gauge needle to syringe.	Used to insert through IV line or heparin (saline) lock.
8. Administer medication by IV push (existing line): a. Check client's identification by looking at armband and asking name.	Ensures that drug is administered to correct client.
b. Select injection port of IV tubing closest to client. (Circle on port may indicate site for needle insertion.)	Allows for easier fluid aspiration to obtain blood return. Injection ports are self-sealing and will not leak.
c. Clean off injection port with antiseptic swab.	Prevents introduction of microorganisms during needle insertion.
d. Insert small-gauge needle of syringe containing prepared drug through center of port.	Prevents damage to port's diaphragm and subsequent leakage.
e. Occlude IV line by pinching tubing just above injection port. Pull back gently on syringe's plunger to aspirate for blood return (see illustration).	Final check ensures that medication is being delivered into bloodstream.

STEPS	RATIONALE
f. After noting blood return, inject medication slowly over several minutes. (Read directions on drug package.) Use watch to time administrations (see illustration).	Ensues safe drug infusion. Rapid injection of IV drug can prove fatal.
g. After injecting medication, release tubing, withdraw syringe, and recheck fluid infusion rate.	Injection of bolus may alter rate of fluid infusion. Rapid fluid infusion can cause circulatory fluid overload.

9. Administer medications by IV push (IV lock):

   a. Check client's identification by looking at armband and asking full name.

      Ensures that drug is administered to correct client.

   b. Heparin flush:

     (1) Prepare syringe with 1 ml of heparin flush solution.

      Flush solution keeps heparin lock patent after drug is administered.

     (2) Prepare syringe with 3 ml of normal saline. Attach 25-gauge needle to syringe.

      Used to assess for blood return in heparin lock.

   c. Saline only:

     (1) Prepare 2 syringes with 2 ml of normal saline each. Attach 25-gauge needle to each syringe.

      Normal saline is effective in keeping IV locks patent.

   d. Heparin and saline:

     (1) Clean lock's rubber diaphragm with antiseptic swab.

      Prevents introduction of microorganisms during needle insertion.

     (2) Insert needle of syringe containing normal saline through center of diaphragm. Pull back gently on syringe plunger and look for blood return.

      Determines whether IV needle or catheter is positioned in vein. (At times heparin lock will not yield blood return even though it is patent.)

     (3) Flush reservoir with 1 ml saline by pushing slowly on plunger.

      Cleans needle and reservoir of blood.

     (4) Remove needle and saline-filled syringe.

     (5) Clean lock's diaphragm with antiseptic swab.

      Prevents transmission of infection.

     (6) Insert needle of syringe containing prepared drug through center of diaphragm.

      Using center of diaphragm prevents leakage.

     (7) Inject medication bolus slowly over several minutes. (Each medication has recommended rate for bolus administration. Check package directions.) Use watch to time administration (see illustration on p. 674).

      Rapid injection of IV drug can result in death.

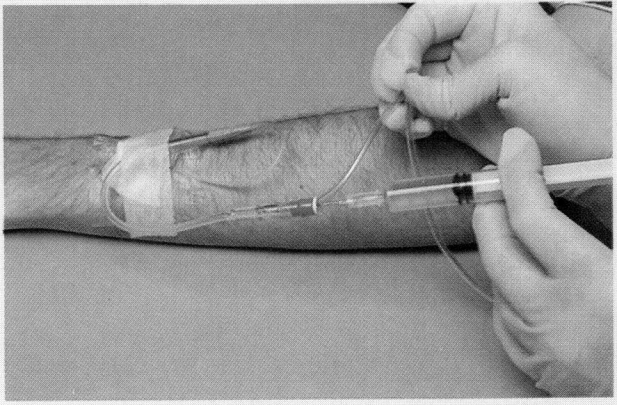

Step 8e

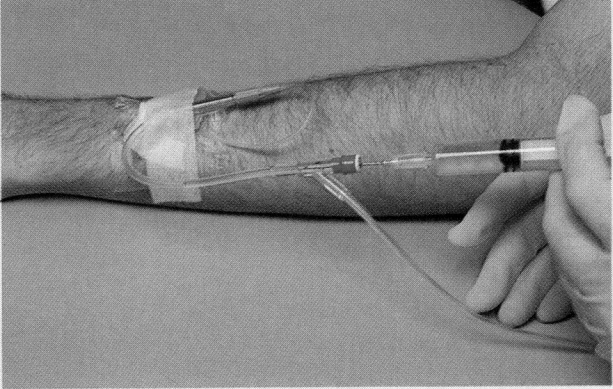

Step 8f

Administering Medications by IV Bolus (Push)

STEPS	RATIONALE
(8) After administering bolus, withdraw syringe.	Prevents transmission of infection.
(9) Clean lock's diaphragm with antiseptic swab.	Flushes reservoir and needle of medication.
(10) Repeat injection of 1 ml of normal saline.	Maintains patency of needle by inhibiting clot formation.
(11) *Heparin flush:* Insert needle of syringe containing heparin through diaphragm. Inject heparin slowly, and remove syringe. *Saline flush:* If using only saline to flush reservoir, use 2 ml of saline before and after each use of IV lock.	Diluted heparin avoids anticoagulation.

10. Remove and dispose of gloves. Wash hands.

Reduces transmission of microorganisms.

11. Observe client closely for adverse reaction as drug is administered and for several minutes thereafter.

IV medications act rapidly.

12. Dispose of uncapped needles and syringes in proper receptacle.

Prevents accidental needlesticks.

13. Record drug, dose, route, and time administered on medication form (Fig. 21-6). Also note adverse reactions.

Timely documentation prevents medication errors.

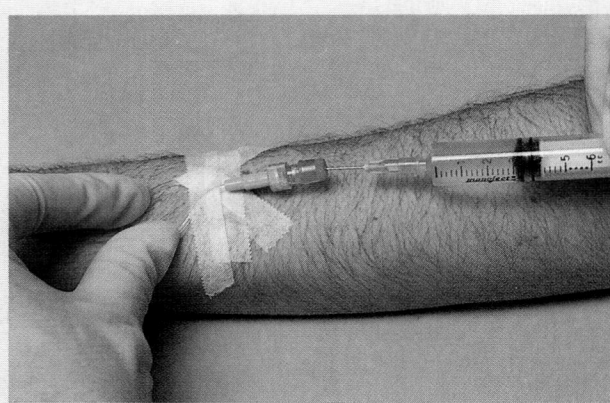

Step 9d(7)

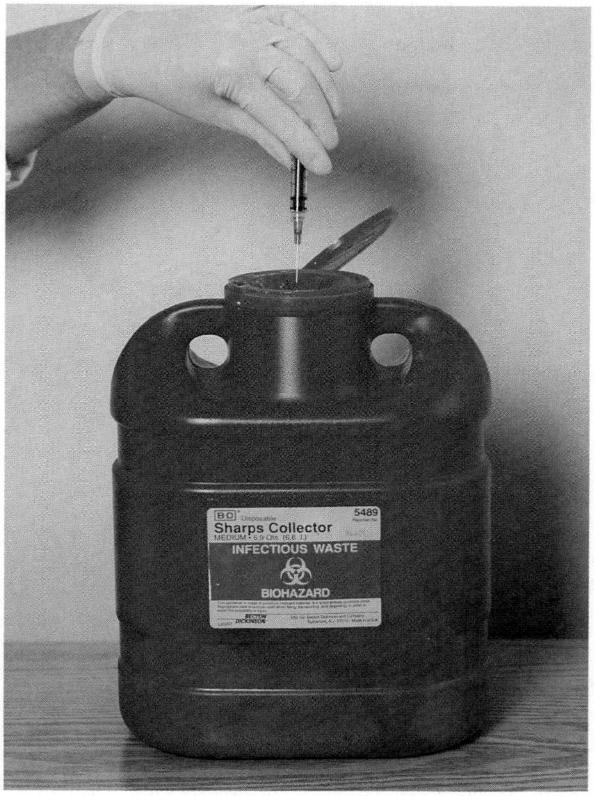

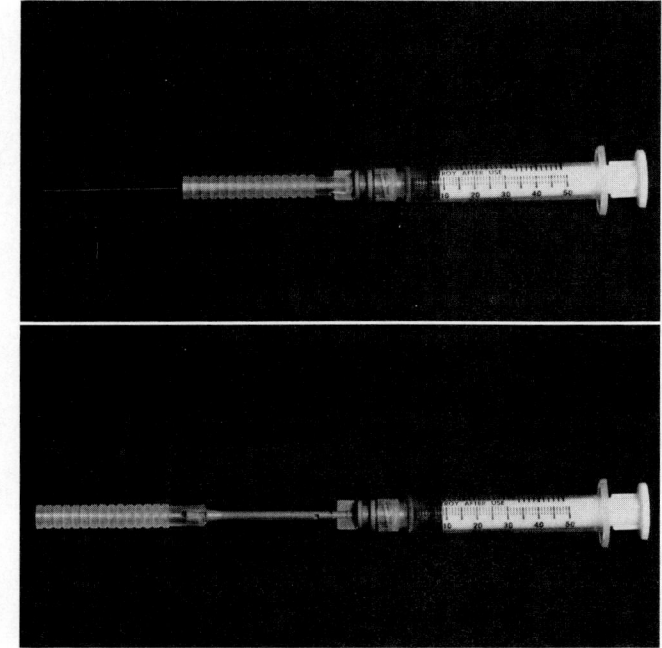

Fig. 21-24 Special containers are available in nursing units for the disposal of contaminated syringes.

Fig. 21-25 Needle with plastic guard to prevent needlesticks. **A,** Position of guard before injection. **B,** After injection, the guard locks in place, covering the needle.

ringe intact into clearly marked, a ers (Fig. 21-24). Containers shoula leak-proof. Needles and plungers s ken. A needle should never be forcea full needle disposal receptacle. Used ringes should not be placed in any was nurse's pocket, or at the client's bedsid

A new needle especially designed to sucks is now available. It is equipped with a plastic guard shield that slips over the needle as it is withdrawn from the skin. The guard locks in place, preventing accidental needlesticks and eliminating the need to recap the needle. The guard and needle are disposed of as a single unit (Fig. 21-25).

TOPICAL DRUG APPLICATIONS

Skin Applications

Because many locally applied drugs such as lotions, pastes, and ointments can create systemic and local effects, the nurse should apply these drugs using gloves and applicators. Sterile technique is important, especially if the client has an open wound.

Skin encrustations and dead tissues harbor microorganisms and block contact of medications with the tissues to be treated. Simply applying new medications over previously applied drugs does little to prevent infection or offer therapeutic benefit. Before applying medications, the nurse cleans the skin thoroughly by washing the area gently with soap and water, soaking an involved site, or locally debriding tissue.

When applying ointments or pastes, the nurse spreads the medication evenly over the involved surface and covers the area well without applying an overly thick layer. Opaque ointments prevent visualization of underlying skin. Physicians often order a gauze dressing to be applied over the medication to prevent soiling of clothes and wiping away of the drug.

Each type of medication—ointment, lotion, powder, or other type—should be applied a specific way to ensure proper penetration and absorption. The nurse applies lotions and creams by smearing them lightly onto the skin's surface. Rubbing may cause irritation. A liniment is applied by rubbing it gently but firmly into the skin. A powder is dusted lightly to cover the affected area with a thin layer. During any skin application the nurse should assess the skin thoroughly. To record administration the nurse notes the area applied, name of medication, and condition of skin.

STEPS	RATIONALE
1. Review physician's medication order, including client's name, drug name, concentration, number of drops (if a liquid), time, and eye (right or left) to receive medication.	Ensures correct administration of medication.
2. Wash hands.	Reduces transmission of microorganisms.

3. Prepare equipment and supplies:
  a. Medication bottle with sterile eye dropper or ointment tube
  b. Medication card, form, or printout
  c. Cotton ball or tissue
  d. Wash basin filled with warm water and wash cloth
  e. Eye patch and tape (optional)
  f. Disposable gloves
	Ophthalmic drops come in plastic or glass bottles. Ointments are prepared in small tubes.

4. Check client's identification by looking at identification bracelet and asking name.	Ensures that correct client receives medication.
5. If eye patch is present, remove it.	
6. Assess condition of external eye structures (see Chapter 20).	Provides baseline to later determine whether local response to medications occurs. Also indicates need to clean eye before drug application.
7. Explain procedure to client.	Client often becomes anxious about medication being instilled into eye because of potential for discomfort.
8. Arrange supplies at bedside and apply gloves.	Ensures smooth, orderly procedure. Gloves reduce exposure to infectious drainage.
9. Ask client to lie supine or sit back in chair with head slightly hyperextended.	Provides easy access to eye for medication instillation and minimizes drainage of medication through tear duct.
10. If crusts or drainage are present along eyelid margins or inner canthus, gently wash away. Soak crusts that are dried and difficult to remove by applying damp washcloth or cotton ball over eye for few minutes. Always wipe clean from inner to outer canthus.	Crusts and drainage harbor microorganisms. Soaking allows easy removal, thus preventing pressure from being applied directly over eye. Cleansing from inner to outer canthus avoids entrance of microorganisms into lacrimal duct.
11. Hold cotton ball or clean tissue in nondominant hand on client's checkbone just below lower eyelid.	Cotton or tissue absorbs medication that escapes eye.
12. With tissue or cotton resting below lower lid, gently press downward with thumb or forefinger against bony orbit.	Technique exposes lower conjunctival sac. Retraction against bony orbit prevents pressure and trauma to eyeball and prevents fingers from touching eye.
13. Ask client to look at ceiling.	Action retracts sensitive cornea up and away from conjunctival sac and reduces stimulation of blink reflex.
14. Instill eyedrops: a. With dominant hand resting on client's forehead, hold filled medication eye dropper approximately 1 to 2 cm (½ to ¾ in) above conjunctival sac (see illustration).	Helps prevent accidental contact of eyedropper with eye structures, thus reducing risk of injury to eye and transfer of infection to dropper. Ophthalmic medications are sterilized.
b. Drop prescribed number of drops into conjunctival sac.	Conjunctival sac normally holds 1 to 2 drops. Applying drops to sac provides even distribution across eye.
c. If client blinks or closes eye or if drops land on outer lid margins, repeat procedure.	Therapeutic effect is obtained only when drops enter conjunctival sac.

CONTINUED

STEPS	RATIONALE
d. When administering drugs that cause systemic effects, protect your finger with clean tissue and apply gentle pressure to client's nasolacrimal duct for 30 to 60 sec.	Prevents overflow of medication into nasal and pharyngeal passages. Prevents absorption into systemic circulation.
e. After instilling drops, ask client to close eye gently.	Helps distribute medication. Squinting or squeezing of eyelids forces medication from conjunctival sac.
15. Instill eye ointment:	
a. Holding ointment applicator above lid margin, apply thin stream of ointment evenly along inside edge of lower eyelid on conjunctiva.	Distributes medication evenly across eye and lid margin.
b. Ask client to look down.	Reduces blinking reflex during ointment application.
c. Apply thin stream of ointment along upper lid margin on inner conjunctiva.	Distributes medication evenly across eye and lid margin.
d. Have client close eye and rub lid lightly in circular motion with cotton ball.	Further distributes medication without traumatizing eye.
16. If excess medication is on eyelid, gently wipe it from inner to outer canthus.	Promotes comfort and prevents trauma to eye.
17. If client has eye patch, apply clean one by placing it over affected eye so that entire eye is covered. Tape securely without applying pressure to eye.	Reduces chance of infection.
18. Dispose of soiled supplies in proper receptacle. Remove and dispose of gloves. Wash hands.	Maintains neat environment at bedside and reduces transmission of microorganisms.
19. Observe response to medication, noting signs and symptoms of potential systemic effects and condition of eye.	Evaluates reaction to medication.
20. Record drug, concentration, number of drops, time of administration, and eye (left, right, or both) that received medication.	Timely documentation prevents drug errors (e.g., repeated or missed doses).

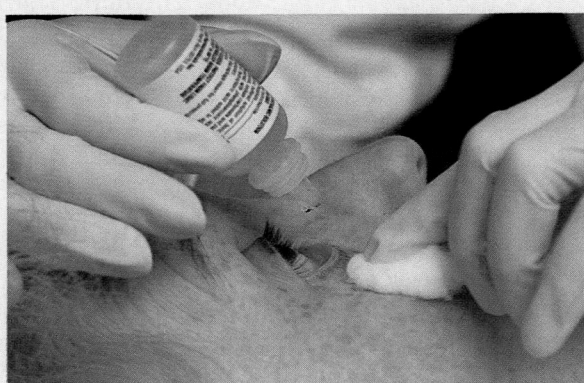

Step 14a

Eye Applications

A common medication used by clients is eye drops and ointments, including over-the-counter preparations such as artificial tears and vasoconstrictors (for example, Visine and Murine). However, many clients receive prescribed ophthalmic drugs for eye conditions such as glaucoma and for treatment after procedures such as cataract extraction. A large percentage of clients receiving eye medications are older adults. Age-related problems, including poor vision, hand tremors, and difficulty in grasping or manipulating containers, affect the ease with which older adults can self-administer eye medications. The nurse instructs clients and family members about the proper techniques for administering eye medications. Donnelly (1987) suggests showing clients each step of the procedure for instilling eye drops to improve compliance. The following principles can be followed when administering eye medications:

1. The cornea of the eye is richly supplied with pain fibers and thus is very sensitive to anything applied to it. As a result the nurse avoids instilling any form of eye medication directly onto the cornea.
2. The risk of transmitting infection from one eye to the other is high. The nurse avoids touching the eyelids or other eye structures with eye droppers or ointment tubes.
3. The nurse uses eye medication only for the affected eye.
4. The nurse never allows a person to use another's eye medications.

Procedure 21-7 reviews the steps for administering eye medications.

Ear Instillations

Internal ear structures are very sensitive to temperature extremes. Failure to instill ear drops or irrigating fluid at room temperature may cause vertigo (severe dizziness) or nausea. Although the structures of the outer ear are not sterile, it is wise to use sterile drops and solutions in case the eardrum is ruptured. Entrance of nonsterile solutions into middle ear structures could result in infection. With ear drainage, the nurse can also check with the physician to be sure that the client does not have a ruptured eardrum. A nurse should never occlude the ear canal with the dropper or irrigating syringe. Forcing medication into an occluded ear canal creates pressure that may injure the eardrum.

The external ear structures of children are different from those of adults. When instilling drops or irrigating the canal (Procedure 21-8), the nurse must straighten the ear canal. In infants and young children the nurse straightens the cartilaginous canal by grasping the auricle of the ear and pulling it gently *down* and backward. In adults the ear canal is longer and composed of underlying bone and is straightened by pulling the auricle *upward* and backward. Failure to straighten the canal properly may prevent medicinal solutions from reaching the deeper external ear structures.

Nasal Instillations

Clients with nasal sinus alterations may receive drugs by spray, drops, or tampons (Procedure 21-9 on pp. 681-682). The most commonly administered form of nasal instillation is decongestant spray or drops, which are used to relieve symptoms of sinus congestion and colds. Clients must be cautioned to avoid overuse because it can lead to a rebound effect in which the nasal congestion worsens. When excess decongestant solution is swallowed, serious systemic effects may also develop, especially in children. Saline drops are safer as a decongestant for children than nasal preparations that contain sympathomimetics (for example, Afrin or Neo-Synephrine).

It is easier to have the client self-administer sprays. In the supine position with the head tilted back, the client holds the tip of the container just inside the nares. The client inhales as the spray enters the nasal passages. For clients who use nasal sprays repeatedly, the nurse checks the nares for irritation. In children, nasal sprays should be given with the head in an upright position so that excess spray will drip anteriorly from the nostrils and not be swallowed.

Nasal drops are effective in treating sinus infections. The nurse learns the proper way of positioning clients to permit the medication to reach the affected sinus. Severe nose bleeds are usually treated with packing or tampons. Tampons are treated with epinephrine, which causes peripheral vasoconstriction, to reduce blood flow. Usually a physician places nasal tampons.

Vaginal Instillations

Vaginal medications are available as suppositories, foam, jellies, or creams. Suppositories come individually packaged in foil wrappers. Storage in a refrigerator prevents the solid, oval-shaped suppositories from melting. After a suppository is inserted into the vaginal cavity, body temperature causes it to melt and be distributed and absorbed. Foam, jellies, and creams are administered with an inserter or applicator (Pro-

STEPS	RATIONALE
1. Review physician's medication order for client's name, drug name, concentration, time of administration, number of drops to instill, and ear (right or left) to receive medication.	Ensures safe and correct administration of medication.
2. Wash hands.	Reduces transmission of microorganisms.
3. Prepare equipment and supplies: a. Medication bottle and dropper b. Medication card, form, or printout c. Cotton-tipped applicator d. Tissue e. Cotton ball (optional) f. Disposable gloves (optional)	Used to remove cerumen or drainage.
4. Identify client by reading identification bracelet and asking name.	Ensures that correct client receives medication.
5. Apply gloves if client has ear drainage.	Reduces exposure to microorganisms
6. Assess condition of external ear structures and canal (see Chapter 20).	Provides baseline to determine whether local response to medication occurs, client's condition improves, or cleansing will be necessary before instillation.
7. Explain procedure to client.	Reduces anxiety.
8. Arrange supplies at bedside.	Ensures smooth procedure.
9. Have client assume side-lying position with ear to be treated facing up.	Provides easy access to ear for instillation of medication. Ear canal is in position to receive medication.
10. If cerumen or drainage occludes outermost portion of ear canal, wipe out gently with cotton-tipped applicator. Do *not* force wax inward to block or occlude canal.	Cerumen and drainage habor microorganisms and can block distribution of medication into canal. Occlusion of canal interferes with normal sound conduction.
11. Straighten ear canal by pulling auricle down and back (children) or upward and outward (adult).	Straightening of ear canal provides direct access to deeper external ear structures.
12. Instill prescribed drops holding dropper 1 cm (½ in) above ear canal (see illustration on p. 680).	Forcing drops into occluded canal can cause injury to eardrum.
13. Ask client to remain in side-lying position 2 to 3 min. Apply gentle massage or pressure to tragus of ear with finger (see illustration on p. 680).	Allows complete distribution of medication. Pressure and massage move medication inward.
14. At times, physician orders placement of cotton ball into outermost part of canal. Do not press cotton into innermost part of canal.	Inserting cotton into outer canal prevents escape of medication when client sits or stands. Cotton should not block canal to impair hearing.
15. Remove cotton in 15 min.	Promotes drug distribution and absorption.
16. Dispose of soiled supplies and gloves and wash hands.	Keeps bedside neat. Reduces transmission of infection.
17. Assist client to comfortable position after drops are absorbed.	Restores comfort.
18. Evaluate condition of external ear between drug instillations.	Determines response to medication.
19. Record drug, concentration, number of drops, time administered, and ear into which drops were instilled on medication form.	Timely documentation prevents drug errors (e.g., repeated doses).

Administering Eardrops

STEPS	RATIONALE
20. Record condition of ear canal in nurses' notes.	Documents client's status and response to therapy.

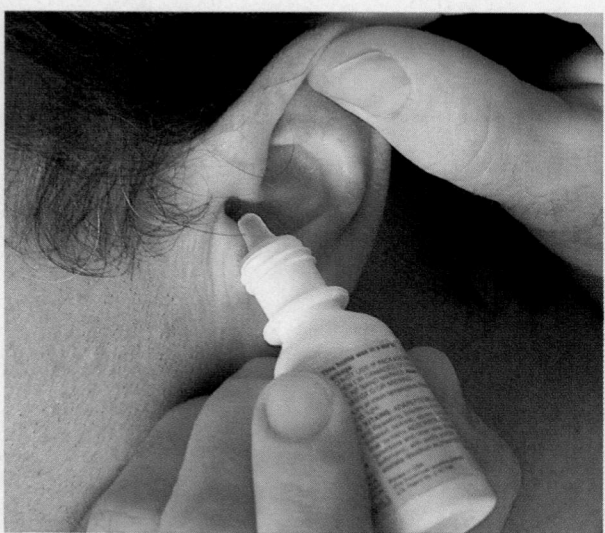

Step 12

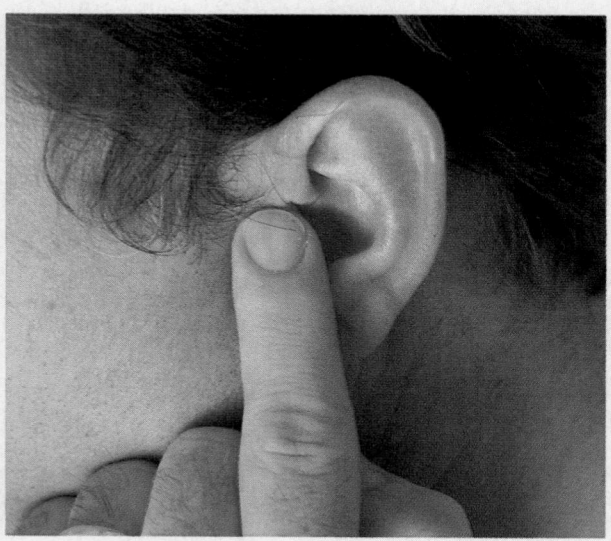

Step 13

cedure 21- 10 on pp. 683-684). A suppository is given with a gloved hand. Clients often prefer administering their own vaginal medications and should be given privacy. After instillation, client may wish to wear perineal pads to collect excess drainage. Because vaginal medications are frequently given to treat infection, any discharge may be foul smelling. Good aseptic technique should be followed, and clients should be offered frequent opportunities to maintain perineal hygiene (see Chapter 34).

Rectal Instillations

Rectal suppositories differ in shape from vaginal suppositories; they are thinner and bullet shaped. The rounded end prevents anal trauma during insertion. Rectal suppositories contain medications that exert local effects, such as promoting defecation, or systemic effects, such as reducing nausea. Rectal suppositories are stored in the refrigerator until they are administered.

During administration the nurse must place the suppository past the internal anal sphincter and against the rectal mucosa (Procedure 21-11 on p. 685). Otherwise the suppository may be expelled before it can dissolve and be absorbed into the mucosa. With practice a nurse learns to recognize the sensation of the sphincter relaxing around the finger. The suppository should not be forced into a mass of fecal material. It may be necessary to clear the rectum with a small cleansing enema before a suppository can be inserted.

 ## ADMINISTERING DRUGS BY INHALATION

Drugs administered with hand-held inhalers are dispersed through an aerosol spray, mist, or powder that penetrates lung airways. The alveolar-capillary network absorbs medications rapidly. Metered-dose inhalers (MDIs) are usually designed to deliver medications that produce local effects such as bronchodilation. The advantage of MDIs is that drugs can be delivered into the airways in high concentrations and systemic side effects are usually avoided. The major

STEPS	RATIONALE
1. Review physician's medication order for client's name, drug name, concentration of solution, number of drops, and time of administration.	Ensures safe and correct administration of medication.
2. Refer to medical record to determine which sinus is affected.	Will affect positioning that client assumes during drug instillation.
3. Wash hands.	Reduces transmission of microorganisms.
4. Prepare equipment and supplies: a. Prepared medication with clean dropper b. Medication card, form, or printout c. Facial tissue d. Small pillow (optional) e. Washcloth (optional)	Dropper or applicator need not be sterile but should be clean. Used in positioning client. Used to clean nares.
5. Check client's identification by reading identification bracelet and asking name.	Ensures that correct client receives medication.
6. Inspect condition of nose and sinuses (see Chapter 20). Palpate sinuses for tenderness.	Findings provide baseline to monitor effect of medication. Discharge will interfere with drug absorption.
7. Explain procedure regarding positioning and sensations to expect, such as burning or stinging of mucosa or choking sensation as medication trickles into throat.	Helps reduce anxiety.
8. Arrange supplies and medications at bedside.	Ensures smooth, orderly procedure.
9. Instruct client to blow nose unless contraindicated (e.g., risk of increased intracranial pressure or nose bleeds).	Removes mucus and secretions that can block distribution of medication.

10. Administer nasal drops:
a. Assist client to supine position.
b. Position head properly:
  (1) Posterior pharynx—tilt client's head backward.
  (2) Ethmoid or sphenoid sinus—tilt head back over edge of bed or place pillow under shoulder and tilt head back (see illustration on p. 682).
  (3) Frontal and maxillary sinus—tilt head back over edge of bed or pillow with head turned toward side treated (see illustration on p. 682).
Support client's head with nondominant hand.
c. Instruct client to breathe through mouth.
 	
d. Hold dropper 1 cm (½ in) above nares and instill prescribed number of drops toward midline of ethmoid bone.
e. Have client remain in supine position 5 min.
f. Offer facial tissue to blot runny nose, but caution against blowing nose for several minutes.
	Position provides access to nasal passages.
	Position allows medication to drain into affected sinus.
	
	Prevents straining of neck muscles.
	Reduces chance of aspirating nasal drops into trachea and lungs.
	Avoids contamination of dropper. Instilling toward ethmoid bone facilitates distribution of medication over nasal mucosa.
	Prevents premature loss of medication through nares.
	Allows maximum amount of medication to be absorbed.

11. Assist client to a comfortable position after drug has been absorbed.	Restores comfort.
12. Dispose of soiled supplies in proper container and wash hands.	Maintains neat, orderly environment. Reduces spread of microorganisms.

Administering Nasal Drops

STEPS	RATIONALE
13. Record medication administration, including drug name, concentration, number of drops, nostril into which drug was instilled, and time of administration.	Timely documentation prevents drug errors (e.g., repeated doses).
14. Observe client for side effects 15 to 30 min after administration.	Drugs absorbed through mucosa can cause systemic reaction.

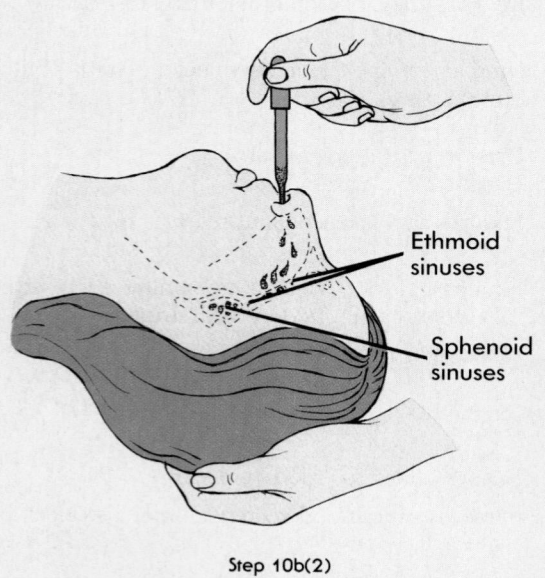

Ethmoid sinuses

Sphenoid sinuses

Step 10b(2)

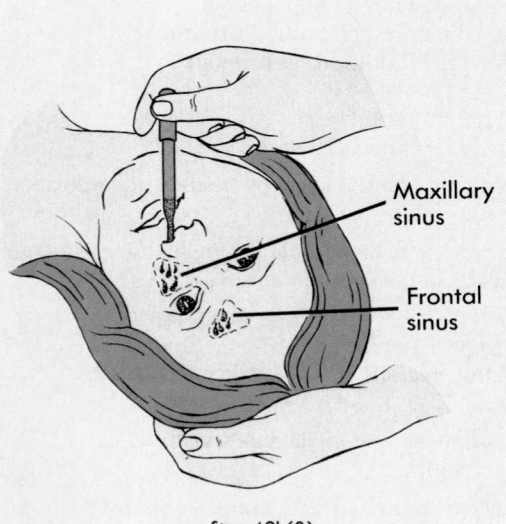

Maxillary sinus

Frontal sinus

Step 10b(3)

disadvantage of MDI therapy is that training and skill are required to coordinate activation of the metered-dose inhaler with inhalation of the drug (Mellins, 1989).

Clients who receive drugs by inhalation frequently suffer chronic respiratory disease such as chronic asthma, emphysema, or bronchitis. Drugs given by inhalation provide these clients with control of airway obstruction, and because these clients depend on medications for disease control, they must learn about them and their safe administration.

An MDI (Procedure 21-12 on pp. 686-687) delivers a measured dose of drug with each push of a canister. Approximately 5 to 10 pounds of pressure must be used to activate the aerosol. However, hand strength diminishes with age and from chronic respiratory disease. Statz (1984) found that MDI works best when clients use a three-point or lateral hand position to activate canisters. Manufacturers indicate that the two-point hand position is least effective.

IRRIGATIONS

Medications may be used to irrigate or wash out a body cavity and are delivered through a stream of solution. Irrigations are most commonly performed with sterile water, saline, or antiseptic solutions on the eye, ear, throat, vagina, and urinary tract. When there is a break in the skin or mucosa, the nurse uses aseptic technique to perform an irrigation. When the cavity to be irrigated is not sterile, as in the case with the ear canal (Procedure 21-13 on p. 688), vagina, or eye, clean technique is acceptable. In health care settings, however, sterile solutions are used. An irrigation can be used to cleanse an area or apply a medication or heat or cold to injured tissue. When performing irrigations, the nurse follows the following principles:

1. Avoid further injury to tissue.
2. Prevent the transmission of infection.
3. Maintain the client's comfort.

Text continued on p. 689.

STEPS	RATIONALE
1. Review physician's order including client's name, drug name, form (cream or suppository), route, dosage, and time of administration.	Ensures safe and correct administration of medication.
2. Wash hands.	Reduces transfer of microorganisms.
3. Prepare supplies: a. Suppository insertion: (1) Vaginal suppository (2) Clean, disposable gloves (3) Lubricating jelly (4) Clean facial tissues (5) Perineal pad (optional) (6) Medication ticket, form, or printout b. Cream or foam instillation: (1) Vaginal cream or foam (2) Plastic applicator (3) Clean, disposable gloves (4) Paper towel (5) Perineal pad (optional) (6) Medication ticket, form, or printout	Stored in refrigerator to maintain solid shape. Eases insertion of suppository. Prepared in plastic tube or can.
4. Check client's identification by reading identification bracelet and asking name.	Ensures that correct client receives medication.
5. Inspect condition of external genitalia and vaginal canal (see Chapter 20).	Findings provide baseline to monitor effect of medication.
6. Assess client's ability to manipulate applicator or suppository and to position self to insert medication.	Mobility restriction indicates level of assistance required from nurse.
7. Explain procedure to client. Be specific if client plans to self-administer medication.	Promotes understanding. Will enable client to self-administer drug if physically able.
8. Arrange supplies at bedside.	Ensures smooth procedure.
9. Close room curtain or door.	Provides privacy.
10. Assist client to lie in dorsal recumbent position.	Provides easy access to and good exposure of vaginal canal. Also allows suppository to dissolve without escaping through orifice.
11. Keep abdomen and lower extremities draped.	Minimizes embarrassment.
12. Apply disposable gloves.	Prevents transmission of infection between you and client.
13. Be sure vaginal orifice is well-illuminated by room light or gooseneck lamp.	Proper insertion requires visualization of external genitalia.
14. Insert suppository with gloved hand: a. Remove suppository from foil wrapper and apply liberal amount of petroleum jelly to smooth or rounded end. Lubricate gloved index finger of dominant hand. b. With nondominant gloved hand, gently retract labial folds. c. Insert rounded end of suppository along posterior wall of vaginal canal entire length of finger (7.5-10 cm or 3-4 in) (see illustration on p. 684). d. Withdraw finger and wipe away remaining lubricant from around orifice and labia.	Lubrication reduces friction against mucosal surfaces during insertion. Exposes vaginal orifice. Proper placement ensures equal distribution of medication along walls of vaginal cavity. Maintains comfort.

Administering Vaginal Instillations

STEPS	RATIONALE
15. Apply cream or foam:	
a. Fill cream or foam applicator following package directions.	Dosage is prescribed by volume in applicator.
b. With nondominant gloved hand, gently retract labial folds.	Exposes vaginal orifice.
c. With dominant gloved hand, insert applicator approximately 5-7.5 cm (2-3 in). Push applicator plunger to deposit medication into vagina (see illustration).	Allows equal distribution of medication along vaginal walls.
d. Withdraw applicator and place on paper towel. Wipe off residual cream from labia or vaginal orifice.	Residual cream on applicator may contain microorganisms.
16. Remove gloves by pulling them inside out and discard in appropriate receptacle. Wash hands.	Reduces transfer of microorganisms.
17. Instruct client to remain on back for at least 10 min.	Medication will be distributed and absorbed evenly throughout vaginal cavity and not be lost through orifice.
18. If applicator is used, wash with soap and warm water, rinse, and store for future use.	Vaginal cavity is not sterile. Soap and water assist in removal of bacteria and residual cream.
19. Offer client perineal pad when she resumes ambulation.	Provides comfort.
20. Inspect condition of vaginal canal and external genitalia between applications.	Evaluates whether vaginal medication effectively reduced irritation or inflammation of tissues.
21. Record drug name, dosage, route, and time of administration on medication record.	Timely recording prevents drug errors.

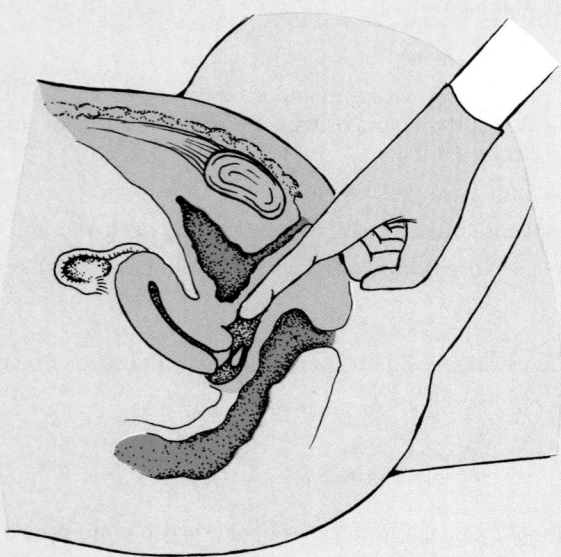

Step 14c

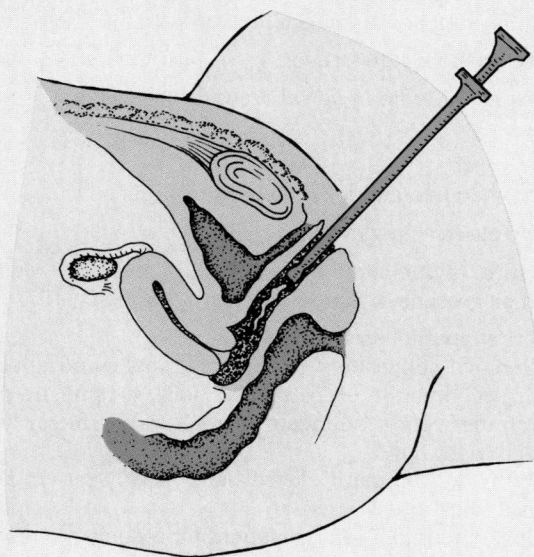

Step 15c

STEPS	RATIONALE
1. Review physician's order, including client's name, drug name, form, route, and time of administration.	Ensures safe and correct administration of medication.
2. Review medical record for rectal surgery or bleeding.	Conditions contraindicate use of suppository.
3. Wash hands.	Reduces transfer of microorganisms.
4. Prepare equipment and supplies: a. Rectal suppository b. Lubricating jelly c. Clean, disposable gloves d. Tissue e. Medication ticket, form, or printout	
5. Apply disposable gloves.	Prevents contact with infected fecal material.
6. Check client's identification by reading identification bracelet and asking name.	Ensures that correct client receives medication.
7. Explain procedure. Be specific if client wishes to self-administer drug.	Promotes understanding and cooperation. Will enable client to self-administer drug if physically able.
8. Arrange supplies at bedside.	Ensures smooth procedure.
9. Close room curtain or door.	Maintains privacy and minimizes embarrassment.
10. Assist client in assuming Sims' position. Keep client draped with only anal area exposed	Exposes anus and helps client relax external anal sphincter. Maintains privacy and facilitates relaxation.
11. Examine condition of anus externally and palpate rectal walls as needed (see Chapter 20). If gloves become soiled, dispose of them by turning them inside out and placing them in proper receptacle.	Determines presence of active rectal bleeding. Palpation determines whether rectum is filled with feces, which may interfere with suppository placement. Reduces transmission of infection.
12. Apply disposable gloves (if previous gloves were discarded).	Minimizes contact with fecal material and reduces transmission of microorganisms.
13. Remove suppository from wrapper and lubricate rounded end. Lubricate index finger of dominant hand.	Lubrication reduces friction as suppository enters rectal canal.
14. Ask client to take slow deep breaths through mouth and relax anal sphincter.	Forcing suppository through constricted sphincter causes pain.
15. Retract buttocks with nondominant hand. Insert suppository gently through anus, past internal sphincter and against rectal wall, 10 cm (4 in) in adults, 5 cm (2 in) in children and infants.	Suppository must be placed against rectal mucosa for eventual absorption and therapeutic action.
16. Withdraw finger and wipe anal area with tissue.	Provides comfort.
17. Discard gloves by turning them inside out, and dispose of them in appropriate receptacle.	Reduces transfer of microorganisms.
18. Ask client to remain flat or on side for 5 min.	Prevents expulsion of suppository.
19. If suppository contains laxative or fecal softener, place call light within reach.	Provides client with sense of control over elimination. Allows client to obtain assistance to bedpan or toilet.
20. Wash hands.	Reduces risk of transfer of infection.
21. Return within 5 min to determine whether suppository was expelled.	Reinsertion may be necessary.
22. Record drug name, dosage, route, and time of administration on medication record.	Timely recording prevents errors.
23. Observe for effects of suppository (e.g., bowel movement, relief of nausea) 30 min after administration.	Evaluates effectiveness of medication and relief of client's symptoms.

Using Metered Dose Inhalers

STEPS	RATIONALE
1. Review physician's medication order, including client's name, drug name, dosage, number of inhalations, and time of administration.	Ensures safe and correct administration of medication.
2. Assess client's ability to hold and manipulate inhaler.	Impairment of grasp, muscle strength, or tremors of hands interfere with ability to depress inhaler canister.
3. Assess drug schedule and number of inhalations prescribed for each dose.	Influences explanations nurse provides for use of inhaler.

4. Have client prepare equipment and supplies:
  a. MDI with medication canister
  b. Facial tissues (optional)
  c. Wash basin or sink with warm water
  d. Paper towel
	
	Used to clean inhaler.

5. Instruct client in comfortable environment by sitting in chair in hospital room or at kitchen table in home.	Client will be more likely to remain perceptive of explanation.
6. Allow client to manipulate inhaler and canister. Explain and demonstrate how canister fits into inhaler.	Client must be familiar with how to use equipment.
7. Explain *metered dose* and warn client about overuse of inhaler, including drug side effects.	Client must not arbitrarily decide to administer excessive inhalations because of risk of serious side effects. If given in recommended doses, side effects are uncommon.

8. Explain steps used to administer inhaled dose of medication. (Demonstrate steps when possible.)
  a. Remove cap and hold inhaler upright, grasping it with thumb and first two fingers..
  b. Shake inhaler.
 	
  c. Tilt head back slightly and breathe out.
  d. Position inhaler in one of following ways:
    (1) Open mouth with inhaler 0.5-1 cm (1-2 in) away from mouth (see illustration).
    (2) OPTION: attach spacer to mouthpiece of inhaler (see illustration).
	Use of simple, step-by-step explanations allows client to ask questions at any point during procedure. Nurse demonstrates depression of canister without self-administering drug dose.
	Mixes medication evenly within solution so that aerosol drug concentration is even.
	Maximizes airway exposure to medication from inhaler.
	
	Avoids rapid influx of inhaled medication and subsequent airway irritation.
	Eliminates rapid influx of particles from inhaled drugs, which reduces irritant properties and tendency to cough. Spacer is recommended for young children (National Heart, Lung, and Blood Institute, 1991).

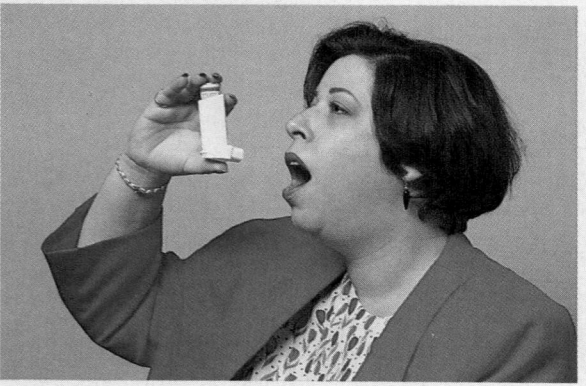

Step 8d(1)

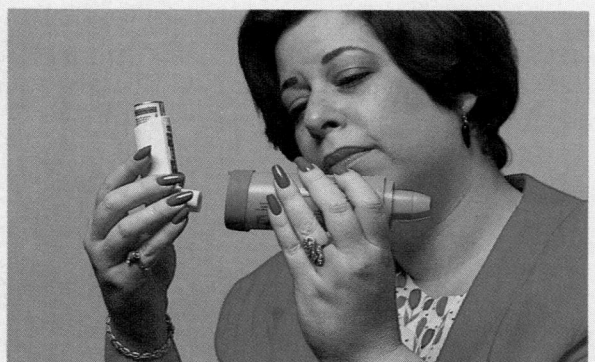

Step 8d(2)

CONTINUED

STEPS	RATIONALE
(3) Place mouthpiece of inhaler or spacer in mouth.	
e. Press down on inhaler to release medication (one puff) while inhaling slowly (see illustration).	Medication is distributed to airways during inhalation. Inhalation through mouth rather than nose draws medication more effectively into airways.
f. Breathe in slowly for 2 to 3 sec.	As client inhales, particles of medication are delivered to airway (National Heart, Lung, and Blood Institute, 1991).
g. Hold breath for approximately 10 sec.	Allows tiny drops of aerosol spray to reach deeper branches of airways.
h. Repeat puffs as ordered, waiting 1 min between puffs.	Allows maximal airway effect from first puff of medication. Therefore airways are more open for second delivery. Thus more particles are delivered directly to airways.
9. If two inhaled medications are prescribed, wait 5 to 10 min between inhalations or as ordered by physician.	Drugs must be inhaled sequentially. Usually bronchodilator are given first to maximize airway opening, followed by other inhaled medications such as steroids.
10. Explain that client may feel gagging sensation in throat caused by droplets of medication on pharynx or tongue.	Results when inhalant is sprayed and inhaled incorrectly.
11. Instruct client in removing medication canister and cleaning inhaler in warm water.	Accumulation of spray around mouthpiece can interfere with proper distribution during use. Accumulation at mouthpiece increases risk of microorganism accumulation and oral infections.
12. Ask if client has questions.	Allows clarification of misconceptions or misunderstanding.
13. Have client demonstrate use of inhaler and explain drug schedule.	Provides feedback for measuring learning. Improves likelihood of compliance with therapy (Redman, 1988).
14. Instruct client against repeating inhalations before next scheduled dose.	Drugs are prescribed at intervals during day to provide constant bronchodilation and minimize side effects.
15. Describe in nurses' notes content of skill taught and client's ability to perform skill.	Provides continuity to teach plan so that other members of nursing staff will not teach same material.

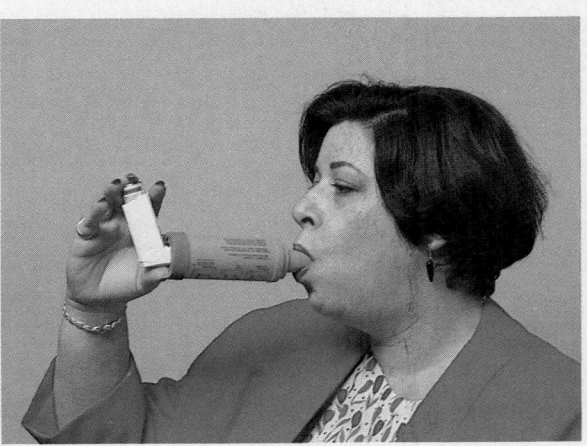

Step 8d(3)

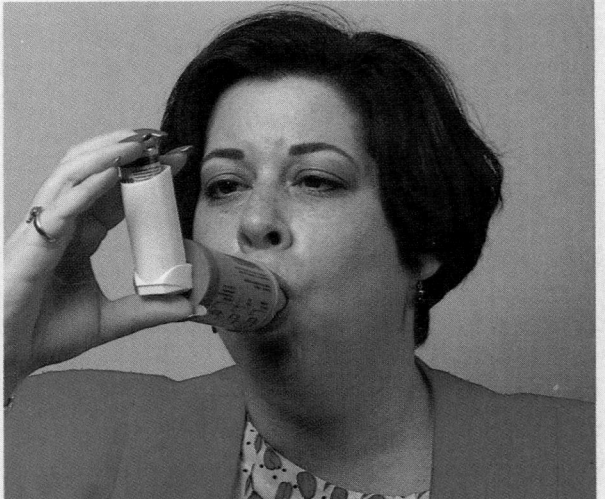

Step 8e

Ear Irrigations

STEPS	RATIONALE
1. Review physician's order for client name, purpose of irrigation, type of irrigant ordered, and time of administration.	Ensures safe and correct administration of irrigation.
2. Check client's identification by reading identification bracelet and asking name.	Ensures that correct client receives irrigation.
3. Wash hands.	Reduces transfer of microorganisms.
4. Assess condition of external ear structures and canal for redness, swelling, and discharge (see Chapter 20).	Evidence of signs of infection serves as baseline data in determining effectiveness of irrigation.
5. Determine whether client is experiencing localized tenderness or discomfort.	Indicates inflammation of outer ear structures.
6. Prepare equipment and supplies:	
a. Container of sterile irrigating solution warmed to room temperature	Warmed solution minimizes chance of causing client to feel dizzy when solution comes in contact with tympanic membrane.
b. Irrigating syringe (rubber bulb or Asepto)	Used to introduce solution under low pressure.
c. Kidney-shaped basin	Used to collect irrigating solution.
d. Towel	
e. Applicator swab and cotton balls	Used to clean and dry ear canal.
7. Explain procedure. Warn that irrigation may cause sensation of dizziness, fullness, and warmth.	Prepares client to anticipate effects of irrigation and promotes cooperation.
8. Arrange supplies at bedside.	Ensures smooth procedure.
9. Close curtain or room door.	Maintains privacy.
10. Assist client to assume sitting or lying position with head tilted or turned toward affected ear. Place towel under client's head and shoulder and have client hold basin under affected ear.	Position minimizes leakage of fluids around neck and facial area for comfort. Solution will flow from ear canal to basin.
11. Gently clean auricle and ear canal with cotton applicator. Do *not* force drainage or cerumen into ear canal.	Prevents infected material from reentering ear canal.
12. Fill irrigating syringe with solution (approximately 50 ml).	Enough fluid is needed to provide steady irrigating stream.
13. Gently grasp auricle and straighten ear canal by pulling it down and back (children) or upward and outward (adult).	Allows fluid to flow length of canal.
14. Slowly instill irrigating solution by holding tip of syringe 1 cm (½ inch) above opening of ear canal. Allow fluid to drain out during instillation. Continue until canal is cleansed or all solution is used.	Slow instillation prevents buildup of pressure in ear canal and ensures contact of medication with all of canal surfaces.
15. Do *not* occlude canal with tip of syringe.	Buildup of fluid in canal under forced pressure could cause rupture of tympanic membrane.
16. Dry off outer ear canal with cotton ball. Leave cotton loosely in place for 5 to 10 min.	Maintains comfort. Absorbs excess moisture in ear canal.
17. Assist client to sitting position.	Maintains comfort.
18. Wash hands and dispose of supplies.	Reduces transmission of infection.
19. Record and report irrigation solution used, character of ear structures, appearance of fluid return or discharge, and client's response.	Documents response to therapy.

SUMMARY

The nurse is responsible for safely and effectively administering medications, which requires understanding of legal guidelines affecting drug prescription and administration. The nurse's care of clients also involves making decisions about the need for drug therapy.

The nurse must have detailed knowledge about a drug and the client receiving it. A thorough assessment of the client's physical condition, medical history, allergies, diet, and medication history ensures that accurate judgments are made about drug therapy.

Preparation of medication requires accurate calculation and a methodical approach. Application of physiological, anatomical, and aseptic principles ensures safe administration of drugs. When monitoring a response to medications, the nurse uses physical assessment skills and knowledge of expected drug effects. The nurse also teaches clients and families to administer drugs safely and to follow schedules for drug therapy. A client's well-being depends on the nurse's application of all the principles of drug administration.

CHAPTER 21 REVIEW

Key Concepts

- Learning drug classifications improves the understanding of nursing implications for administering drugs with similar characteristics.
- Nurse practice acts define and set limits on the scope of a nurse's professional functions and responsibilities in giving medications.
- All controlled substances are handled according to strict procedures that account for each drug.
- The nurse applies understanding of the physiological action of drug action when timing administration, selecting routes, initiating actions to promote drug efficacy, and observing responses to drugs.
- Clients with alterations in organs that metabolize or excrete drugs are at risk for drug toxicity.
- The older adult's body undergoes structural and functional changes that alter drug actions and influence the manner in which nurses provide drug therapy.
- Children's drug dosages are computed on the basis of body surface area.
- Repeated doses of a drug are required to achieve constant therapeutic blood levels.
- Drugs given parenterally are absorbed more quickly than drugs administered by other routes.
- Each drug order should include the client's name, order date, drug name, dosage, route and frequency of administration, and physician's signature.
- A teaching plan for drug therapy should include guidelines for drug safety.
- The "five rights" of drug administration ensure accurate preparation and administration of drug dosages.
- Nurses administer only medications they prepare.
- The nurse never administers a drug without accurately identifying a client.
- Drugs should be charted immediately after administration.
- A nurse uses clinical judgment in determining the best time to administer prn medications.
- The nurse reports a drug error immediately.
- When preparing medications, the nurse checks the drug container label against the medication card, form, or printout three times.
- The nurse never leaves a prepared medication unattended.
- The nurse rotates injection sites when giving repeated parenteral administrations.
- Failure to select injection sites by anatomical landmarks may lead to tissue, bone, or nerve damage.

Key Terms

Critical Thinking Exercises

1. During assessment, you note that your client is taking two types of antihypertensive medications prescribed by two different physicians. What actions do you need to take?

2. You are preparing to give a parenteral injection of preoperative atropine. You check the order and calculate the dose. You note that your calculations result in a 3-ml dose. You recognize that this is an excessive dose, and you recalculate the dose and obtain the same answer. You check the dosing information against the physician's order and realize that the order is excessive. You verify this information with the charge nurse, who says "The order is okay." What action do you take at this point?

3. When preparing to give a narcotic injection to your client you observe that the narcotic count for that particular drug is wrong. What do you do?

4. You need to give an injectable pain medication to a client with metastatic cancer. The client's pain increases with change of position, the client is cachexic, and is receiving multiple injections. What information do you need to prepare the medication, the syringe, and the needle and to determine the site of injection?

5. You are caring for a septic client, and the physician writes two new intravenous antibiotic orders in addition to the two intravenous antibiotics the client is already receiving. In planning care, you and the physician agree that there could be potential drug interactions with these antibiotics. What do you do to reduce the risk of drug interactions for this client?

REFERENCES

Burman R, Berkowitz H: IV bolus: effective but potentially hazardous, *Crit Care Nurs* 6(1):22, 1986.

Clark JB, Queener SF, Karb GB: *Pharmacologic basis of nursing practice,* ed 4, St Louis, 1993, Mosby–Year Book.

Cyganski JM et al: The case for the heparin flush, *Am J Nurs* 87:796, 1987.

Donnelly D: Instilling eye drops: difficulties experienced by patients following cataract surgery, *J Adv Nurs* 12:235, 1987.

Dunn DL, Lenihan SF: The case for the saline flush, *Am J Nurs* 87:798, 1987.

Eliopoulos C: Geriatric pharmacology. In Eliopoulos C: *Gerontological nursing,* ed 2, Philadelphia, 1987, Lippincott.

Harrigan CA: Intermittent IV therapy without heparin: a study, *NITA* 8:519, 1985.

Kim MJ, McFarland GK, McLane AM: *Pocket guide to nursing diagnosis,* ed 4, St Louis, 1991, Mosby–Year Book.

Mellins RB: Patient education is key to successful management of asthma, *J Respir Dis* 10:8 S47 (suppl), 1989.

National Heart, Lung, and Blood Institute: *Guidelines for the diagnosis and management of asthma,* National Asthma Education Program, Expert Panel Report, Pub No 91-3042, Bethesda, Md, 1991, The Institute.

Redman BK: *The process of patient education,* ed 6, St Louis, 1988, Mosby–Year Book.

Simonson W: *Medications and the elderly: a guide for promoting proper use,* Rockville, Md, 1984, Aspen.

Statz E: Hand strength and metered dose inhalers, *Am J Nurs* 84:800, 1984.

Taylor N et al: Comparison of normal versus heparinized saline for flushing infusion devices, *J Nurs Qual Assur* 3: 49, 1989.

Whaley LF, Wong DL: *Nursing care of infants and children,* ed 4, St Louis, 1991, Mosby–Year Book.

ADDITIONAL READINGS

Albanese JA, Nutz PA: *Mosby's nursing drug cards,* ed 2, St Louis, 1991, Mosby–Year Book.

American Psychiatric Association: *Diagnostic and statistical manual of mental disorders (DSM-IIIR),* rev 3, Washington, DC, 1987, The Association.

Beecroft PC, Redick S: Possible complications of intramuscular injections on the pediatric unit, *Pediatr Nurs* 15:333, 1989.

Birdsall C, Uretsky S: How do I administer medication by NG? *Am J Nurs* 84:1259, 1984.

Clayton M: The right way to prevent medication errors, *RN* 50(6):30, 1987.

Cushing M: Drug errors can be bitter pills, *Am J Nurs* 86:895, 1986.

Gahart BL: *Intravenous medications*, ed 8, St Louis, 1992, Mosby–Year Book.

Hasselbalch H et al: Alternative to optimal administration of tablets, *Acta Med Scand* 217:527, 1985.

Hayes JE: Normal changes in aging and nursing implications of drug therapy, *Nurs Clin North Am* 17:253, 1982.

Hergert MJ: New aids for low-vision diabetics, *Am J Nurs* 89:1319, 1989.

Jones NH: Creative analgesic dosing in the elderly, *Am J Nurs* 89:1285, 1989.

Keen MF: Comparison of intramuscular injection techniques to

Keithley JK, O'Donnell J: Look out for these drug-nutrient interactions, *Nurs 86* 16(2):42, 1986.

Kolcaba K, Miller CA: Geropharmacology treatment, *J Gerontol Nurs* 15:29, 1989.

Labar C: Filling in the blanks of prescription writing, *Am J Nurs* 86:30, 1986.

Lent-Wunderlich E, Ott MJ: Helping your patient through eye surgery, *RN* 49:43, 1986.

MacIsaac AM, Rivers R, Adamson CB: Multiple medications: is your elderly patient caught in the storm? *Nurs 89* 19:61, 1989.

McCaffery M: Narcotic analgesia for the elderly, *Am J Nurs* 85:296, 1985.

McGovern K: Ten steps for preventing medication errors, *Nurs 86* 16(12):36, 1986.

McPherson ML: Medicating the elderly in home health care, *Home Health Care Pract* 2:16, 1989.

Megal ME et al: Nursing student's performance: administrating injections in laboratory and clinical area, *J Nurs Educ* 26:288, 1987.

Mellema SJ, Poniatowski BC: Geriatric IV therapy, *J Intravenous Nurs* 11:56, 1988.

Miyares MV: Medication aids your elderly patient will love, *RN* 48:44, 1985.

Moree NA: Nurses speak out on patients and drug regimens, *Am J Nurs* 85:51, 1985.

Nurses Drug Alert: Hazards of nasal decongestants in young children, *Am J Nurs* 84:1265, 1984.

Perez S: Reducing injection pain, *Am J Nurs* 84:7, 1984.

Petrosin BM et al: Implications of selected problems with nasoenteral tube feedings, *Crit Care Nurs Q* 12:1, 1989.

Rettig FM, Southby JR: Using different body positions to reduce discomfort from dorsogluteal injection, *Nurs Res* 31:219, 1982.

Woodridge JB, Jackson JG: Evaluation of bruises and areas of induration after two techniques of subcutaneous heparin injection, *Heart Lung* 17:476, 1988.

Saxton AF, O'Neill NE: *Basic mathematics and calculation of drugs and solutions: a programmed approach*, St Louis, 1986, Mosby–Year Book.

Scharf L: Safe needle disposal: a timely reminder, *RN* 49:42, 1986.

Schwertz DW, Buschmann MT: Pharmacogeriatrics, *Crit Care Nurs Q* 12:26, 1989.

Shepherd MJ, Swearingen P: Z-track injections, *Am J Nurs* 84:746, 1984.

Skidmore-Roth L: *Mosby's 1992 nursing drug reference*, ed 5, St Louis, 1992, Mosby–Year Book.

Smith JB: The patient who can't remember to take her meds, *RN* 49(9):38, 1986.

Thatcher G: Insulin injections: the case against random rotation, *Am J Nurs* 85:690, 1985.

Todd B: Drugs and the elderly: using eye drops and ointments safely, *Geriatr Nurs* 4(1):55, 1983.

Todd B: Intravenous drug hazards: interactions, absorption, and inadequate mixing, *Geriatr Nurs* 9:20, 1988.

Vanbree NS et al: Clinical evaluation of three techniques for administering low-dose heparin, *Nurs Res* 33:15, 1984.

Wayland MA: "Safe learning": helping students learn to give team medications, *AD Nurse* 3:34, 1988.

Westfall LK, Pavlis RW: Why the elderly are so vulnerable to drug reactions, *RN* 50:39, 1987.

Williams PJ: How do you keep medicine from clogging feeding tubes? *Am J Nurs* 89:181, 1989.

Wong DL: Significance of dead space in syringes, *Am J Nurs* 82:1237, 1982.reduce site discomfort and lesions, *Nurs Res* 35:207, 1986.

Woodridge JB, Jackson JG: Evaluation of bruises and areas of induration after two techniques of heparin injection, *Heart Lung* 17:476, 1988.

CHAPTER **22**

Documentation and Reporting

OBJECTIVES

Mastery of content in this chapter will enable the student to:

- Define the key terms listed.
- Describe guidelines for effective documentation and reporting.
- Discuss the relationship between documentation and health care financial reimbursement.
- Identify ways to maintain confidentiality of records and reports.
- Describe the purpose of a change-of-shift report.
- Present a change-of-shift report on a client.
- Explain how to verify telephone orders.
- Identify seven purposes of a health care record.
- Discuss legal guidelines for recording.
- Describe the different methods used in record keeping.
- Discuss the advantages and disadvantages of standardized documentation forms.
- Identify elements to include when documenting a client's discharge plan.
- Identify computerized applications for documentation.

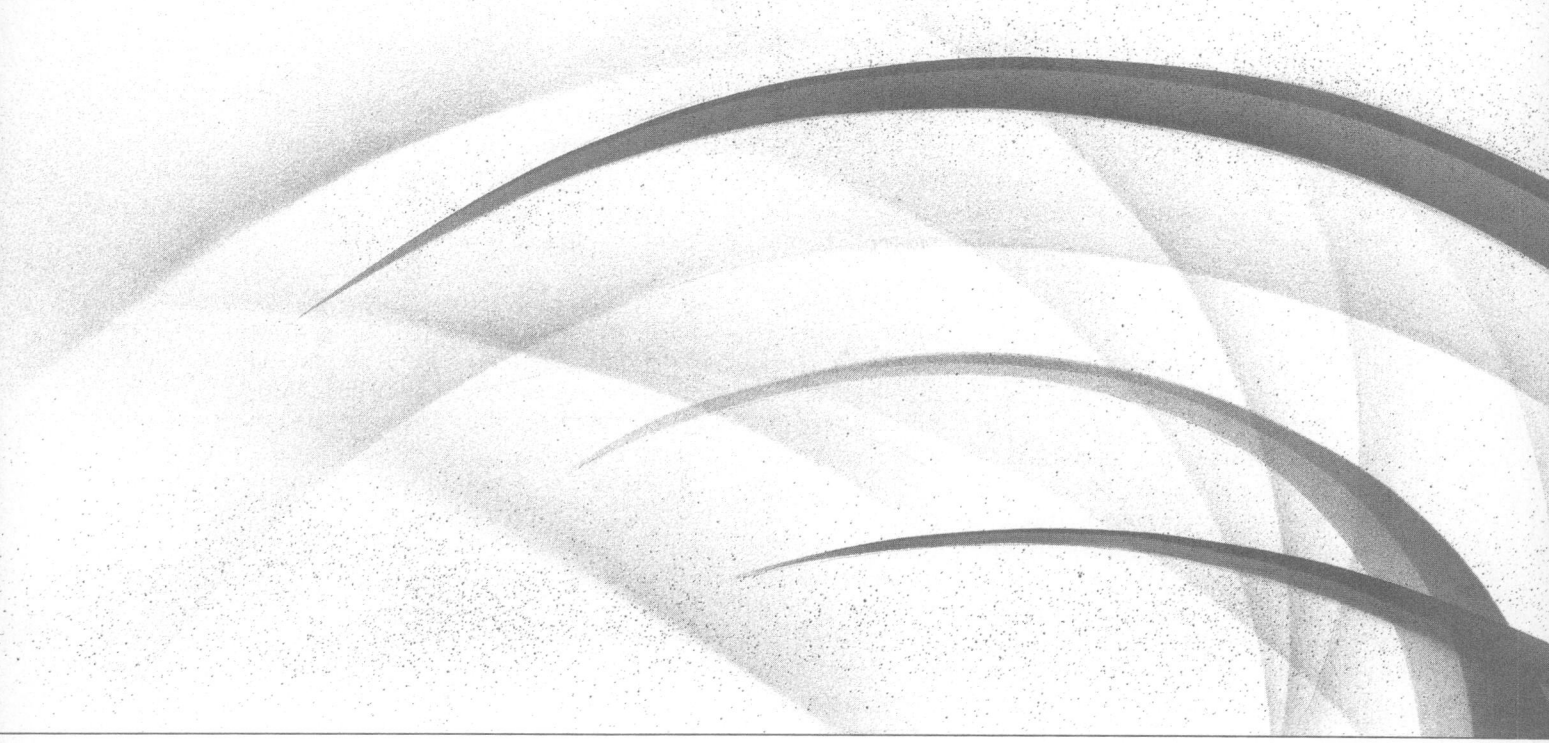

CHAPTER OUTLINE

Nurses as members of the health care team must communicate information about clients accurately and completely and in the most timely and effective way possible. A client depends on care givers to communicate to one another to ensure the best quality of care. All health care providers require the same information about clients so that they can plan an organized, comprehensive care plan. For example, when a client experiences pain, all care givers should be informed about the nature of the pain and the most effective therapies that benefit the client. Unless the client's care plan is communicated to all members of the health care team, care becomes fragmented, repetition of tasks occurs, and therapies are often delayed or even deleted. The result of poor communication is often poor client outcomes such as delayed recovery and complications that could have been avoided.

The health care environment creates many challenges for accurately documenting and reporting the care delivered to clients. Regulations require health care institutions to monitor and evaluate the quality and appropriateness of client care. Such monitoring requires a thorough review of the documentation in a client's medical record. **Accreditation** agencies such as the Joint Commission on Accreditation of Healthcare Organizations (JCAHO) specify guidelines for information to be documented. Under the prospective payment system, hospitals are reimbursed a set dollar amount by Medicare for each **diagnosis-related group (DRG)**. Everything that is done for a client should be documented in the medical record. If the documentation is incomplete, a health care institution will not recover its costs. Finally, the medical record is a legal document. Nurses are accountable for their actions, and as a result, information in the record must be clear and logical, describing exactly all care delivered.

The quality of care deserved by clients, the standards of regulatory agencies, the reimbursement structure in the health care system, and the legal guidelines for nursing practice make documentation and reporting two of the most important functions of a nurse. Any information about a client's care should be communicated with careful thought. All members of the health care team depend on recorded and reported information. Accurate information ensures continuity and quality of care.

COMMUNICATION WITHIN THE HEALTH CARE TEAM

It is difficult for staff members caring for a specific client to communicate with one another. The more that care givers know about a client, the better prepared they are to provide high-quality care. Care givers use a variety of ways to communicate information about clients. **Reports** are oral or written exchanges of information shared between care givers in a number of ways. After completing a work shift, nurses give a verbal report to nurses on the next shift. A physician may call a nursing unit to receive a verbal report on a client's progress for the day. The laboratory submits a written report describing the results of diagnostic tests for inclusion in the permanent medical record.

A **record** is a permanent written communication that documents information relevant to a client's health care management. An example is a clinic record or chart. After each clinic visit, information about the client's health care is recorded. With each successive visit the record is available to the physician and other members of the health team. It is a continuing account of the client's health care status and needs.

Another way that information is communicated is through discussions among team members. Discussions may be informal or formal. They allow a review of information so that problems are identified and solutions are recommended. An example is a discharge planning conference, in which members of all disciplines (for example, nursing, social work, medicine, and physical therapy) meet to discuss the client's progress toward established discharge goals. **Consultations** are a form of discussion whereby one professional care giver gives formal advice about the care of a client to another. For example, a clinical nurse specialist confers with a staff nurse about the best choice of therapies for controlling the side effects of chemotherapy, or a physician consults with a dietitian to select the best diet therapy for a client. Both consultations and conferences should be documented in a client's permanent record so that all care givers can benefit from the information and plan care accordingly.

GUIDELINES FOR GOOD DOCUMENTATION AND REPORTING

When nurses fail to take documentation and reporting seriously, many problems can arise, such as those in the following situations:

Mrs. Blake has recently been diagnosed with diabetes. She must learn to give herself insulin injections before going home. A nurse on the day shift fails to document the teaching session about syringe parts and the method for preparing insulin doses. During the evening shift, another nurse spends time assessing Mrs. Blake's learning needs because the teaching plan was not communicated. Valuable time is wasted, and Mrs. Blake becomes frustrated with the nurses' failure to know her needs.

Mr. Ryan returned from major abdominal surgery just before change of shift. The day nurse, Mr. Wells, measures the client's vital signs and gives a medication for pain. The evening nurse, Miss Tally, learns during the report that Mr. Ryan received an analgesic medication but is not told his response to the drug. When Miss Tally enters Mr. Ryan's room, she measures his blood pressure at 90/60. She leaves the room to check the chart because she is concerned that the pain medication has lowered Mr. Ryan's blood pressure. If Mr. Wells had given a thorough report, Miss Tally would have known the client's blood pressure was normally low.

Both case examples demonstrate that quality documentation and reporting are necessary to enhance efficient, individualized client care. Six important guidelines must be followed for quality documentation and reporting. Documentation and reports must be factual, accurate, complete, current, organized, and confidential.

Fact

Information about clients and their care must be factual. A record should contain descriptive, objective information about what a nurse sees, hears, feels, and smells (Bergerson, 1988). An objective description (for example, "Respirations 14 per minute, regular, with normal breath sounds bilaterally") is the result of direct observation and measurement. Factual information is less likely to be misleading or cause misinterpretation. The use of words such as *appears, seems,* or *apparently* are not acceptable because they lead to conclusions that cannot be supported by objective information. If a nurse documents inferences or conclusions without factual information, errors in care can occur.

The nurse should also document subjective information but only when it is supported by facts. For example, the description, "the client seems depressed" does not communicate helpful information. The description does not tell another care giver whether the client is withdrawing from conversation or is threatening to injure the self. The phrase, *seems depressed,* is a conclusion without supported facts. Documentation should clearly explain the nurse's observations of the client's behaviors and not interpret those observations. If a client reports information to the nurse, it should be charted as a subjective entry, in the client's own words. For example, "Client states, 'I feel so helpless being unable to do anything for myself. Sometimes I wish I could stop all of this.' " The nurse can then add any objective findings that more clearly describe the client's depression, such as crying or difficulty with sleeping.

Accuracy

A client's record must be reliable. In other words, information must be accurate so that health team members have confidence in it. The use of precise measurements ensures that a record is accurate. The nurse makes descriptions such as "Intake, 360 ml of water" rather than "Client drank an adequate amount of fluid." Measurements are later used as a means to determine whether a client's condition has improved or worsened. Charting that an abdominal wound is "5 cm in length" is more accurate than "large and gaping." Use of an institution's accepted abbreviations, symbols, and system of measures (for example, metric) ensures that all staff members will use the same language in their reports and records (see end sheet).

It is also important to use abbreviations that will not be misinterpreted. For example, o.d. (once daily) can be interpreted to mean OD (right eye). To avoid any chance of error, abbreviations should be spelled out when terminology is confusing.

Correct spelling is also important for accurate documentation and reporting. Terms can easily be confused or misinterpreted (for example, *dysphagia* or *dysphasia* and *dram* or *gram*). Simple spelling mistakes can also cause serious treatment errors. Medications such as digitoxin or digoxin and morphine or Numorphan must be spelled carefully. If a mistake is made on a medication record, a client may receive the wrong medication.

An accurate entry in a record must reflect what nurses do during the time frame of the entry. Nurses never chart for anyone else or let anyone chart for them (exception is when nurses call their units to report on medication or therapy that had not been charted). In a court of law, it would be easy for a lawyer to create doubt about care when a recorded note did not truly reflect what was done by the nurses. It is acceptable for nurses to later call and ask colleagues to chart information after they leave work. However, the entry must clearly show what was done and by whom (for example, "At 11 AM Sam Turner, RN, called and reported that at 8 AM Demerol 100 mg IM was administered to client for abdominal pain" (Bergerson, 1988).

Another way to ensure accuracy of records is to correctly countersign entries. Agency policies explain how and when to countersign. An example might include registered nurses being required to countersign a note entered into the record by a nursing student. When a nurse countersigns another nurse's entry, it means that the entry was reviewed and the care given was approved. When a nurse countersigns an entry, it is important that the person administering care is clearly identified. If the record is inaccurate, both nurses can share liability for any client injury that might result (Bergerson, 1988).

Any descriptive entry in a client's record ends with the care giver's full name and status, such as "Sharon Day, RN." Nicknames are not used. A nursing student enters the full name and current program status, such as "Tom Neely, Junior nursing student." The signature holds a nurse accountable for information recorded.

Completeness

The information within a recorded entry or a report should be complete, containing concise and thorough information about a client's care. Concise data are easy to understand. Lengthy notes are difficult to read. Sketchy or abbreviated notes may leave

TABLE 22-1 Examples of Criteria for Reporting and Recording	
Topic	Items to Report or Record
Symptom (e.g., pain, nausea, headache, dizziness)	Description of episode Location of symptom Severity Onset Precipitating factors Frequency and duration Aggravating and relieving factors Associated symptoms
Sign (e.g., rash, tenderness on palpation of body part, decreased breath sounds)	Location of sign Description or quality of findings Aggravating or relieving factors Onset
Nursing care measures (e.g., enema, bath, dressing change)	Time administered Equipment used if appropriate Client's response (positive* or negative†) Nurse's observations
Client behavior (e.g., anxiety, confusion, hostility)	Onset Behaviors exhibited Precipitating factors Nursing response or action Client's response
Medication administration	Time administered Any required preliminary observations (e.g., pulse and blood pressure measurements) Client's response or effect of medication (positive‡ or negative§) Nursing measures taken for negative response
Client teaching	Information or topic presented Method of instruction (e.g., discussion, role playing, demonstration) Resources used (e.g., videotape, booklet) Evidence that client understands instruction (e.g., return demonstration, change in behavior)
Discharge planning	Client goals or expected outcomes Progress toward goals Need for referrals or resources Client's involvement in care plan

*For example, client denied pain during dressing change.
†For example, client experienced severe abdominal cramping during enema.
‡For example, client reports that pain is reduced after analgesic.
§For example, rash is noted over lower abdomen.

an impression that nursing care was hurried or incomplete. A long report wastes time and is often boring. Clear, succinct recording and reporting gives only essential information and avoids the use of unnecessary words or irrelevant detail. A comparison of a concise and lengthy record entry follows:

Concise Entry	Lengthy Entry
Left toes are warm, color pink; nail beds show capillary return within 2 sec; dorsalis pedis pulse strong 4+ bilaterally; no inflammation; client denies pain.	The client's left toes appear to be warm with color pink. There is no inflammation. There is good capillary return present. Dorsalis pedis pulse in left foot is strong. The client denies pain.

A good report or record is thorough, with complete information about a client. Criteria for thorough communication exist for certain health problems or nursing activities (Table 22-1). The nurse makes written entries in the client's medical record, describing nursing care administered and the client's response. An example of a thorough nurses' note follows:

7:15 PM: Client verbalizes sharp, throbbing pain localized along radial side of right wrist, beginning approximately 15 minutes ago. Pain increased with movement of wrist, slightly relieved with elevation of hand on pillow. Radial pulses equal bilaterally. Right wrist circumference 1 cm larger than left wrist. Dr. Kent notified at 7:10. Percocet 2 tabs given for pain. Lee Turno, RN.

Currentness

Delays in recording or reporting can result in serious omissions and untimely delays for needed care. For example, failure to report a drop in blood pressure can delay the administration of a critically needed medication. Legally, a late entry in a chart may be interpreted as negligence (see Chapter 14). Ongoing decisions about care must be based on currently reported information. Activities or findings to communicate at the time of occurrence include the following:

1. Vital signs
2. Administration of medications and treatments
3. Preparation for diagnostic tests or surgery
4. Change in status
5. Admission, transfer, discharge, or death of a client
6. Treatment for a sudden change in status

Routine activities such as bathing or giving oral hygiene do not need to be charted immediately. This information is often included in flowsheets (p. 718).

When describing an aspect of care, a nurse should refer to the client's problem, nursing intervention, and client's response. A revision or update of a care plan should occur when the client's condition changes. It is impossible and unnecessary for a nurse to document every aspect of care in the record when it happens. Therefore it may help to keep a worksheet or notepad close at hand when caring for several clients. Writing notes while they are fresh in the mind ensures that an entry recorded later in the record will be accurate.

Each institution uses a system to report the time of day. Military time, a 24-hour system, avoids misinterpretation of AM and PM times that occur with the 12-hour system. A 4-digit number indicates the hours and minutes (Table 22-2).

Organization

The nurse communicates information in a logical format or order. Health team members understand information better when it is given in the order in which it occurred. The following example compares a well-organized note with a disorganized note:

Organized Note	Disorganized Note
7/17 6:30 AM Client reports sharp pain in left lower quadrant of abdomen, worsened by turning onto right side. Positioning on left side offers minimal relief. Abdomen is tender to touch, rigid, dull to percussion. Bowel sounds are absent. Dr. Phillips notified; Demerol 75 mg IM given as ordered for pain, client taken to x-ray department for CT scan of abdomen — Tim Reis, RN.	7/17 6:30 AM Client experiences sharp pain in lower quadrant of abdomen. MD notified. Abdomen tender to touch, rigid with bowel sounds absent. Pecussion note is dull. Demerol 75 mg IM ordered for pain. Positioning on left side offers minimal relief of pain. CT scan ordered of the abdomen — Jill Ames, RN.

TABLE 22-2 Comparison of Military and Civilian Times			
Military	Civilian	Military	Civilian
0100	1:00 AM	1420	2:20 PM
0200	2:00 AM	1800	6:00 PM
0215	2:15 AM	2400	midnight
1200	Noon	0001	12:01 AM

The organized note describes the client's pain, nurse's assessment and interventions, and the physician's order in a logical order of occurrence. The disorganized note is fragmented and does not clearly explain what happened first. Poorly organized notes can lead to confusion about whether proper care was given.

Confidentiality

A confidential communication is information given by one person to another with trust and confidence that such information will not be disclosed. The law protects information about clients that is gathered by examination, observation, conversation, or treatment. Nurses should not discuss clients' status with other clients or staff uninvolved in their care. Nurses are legally and ethically obligated to keep information about clients' illnesses and treatments confidential. A legal suit can be brought against nurses who disclose information about clients without their consent (see Chapter 14). Only staff members directly involved in care have legitimate access to the records. Nurses and other health care professionals may have reason to use records for data gathering, research, or continuing education. These are not breaks in confidentiality as long as the records are used as specified and permission is granted from hospital internal review boards.

A client's record is accessible to many personnel. Nurses are responsible for protecting records from unauthorized readers such as visitors. The nurse should know the location of the record at all times. If it is misplaced, every effort should be made to find it. The record is stored by the health care agency after treatment ends.

 ## REPORTING

Information about clients is exchanged between health care team members, clients, and family members. Nurses communicate information about clients so that all team members can make the best decisions about them and their care. Reports offer a summary of activities or observations seen, performed, or heard. Four types of reports made by nurses include the change-of-shift report, telephone reports, transfer reports, and incident reports.

Change-of-Shift Reports

The **change-of-shift report** occurs 2 or 3 times a day on every type of nursing unit in all types of health care settings. At the end of each shift, nurses report information about their assigned clients to the nurses working on the next shift. The report is a system of communication aimed at transferring essential information necessary for safe and holistic client care (Riegel, 1985). The purpose of the report is to provide better continuity of care among nurses car-

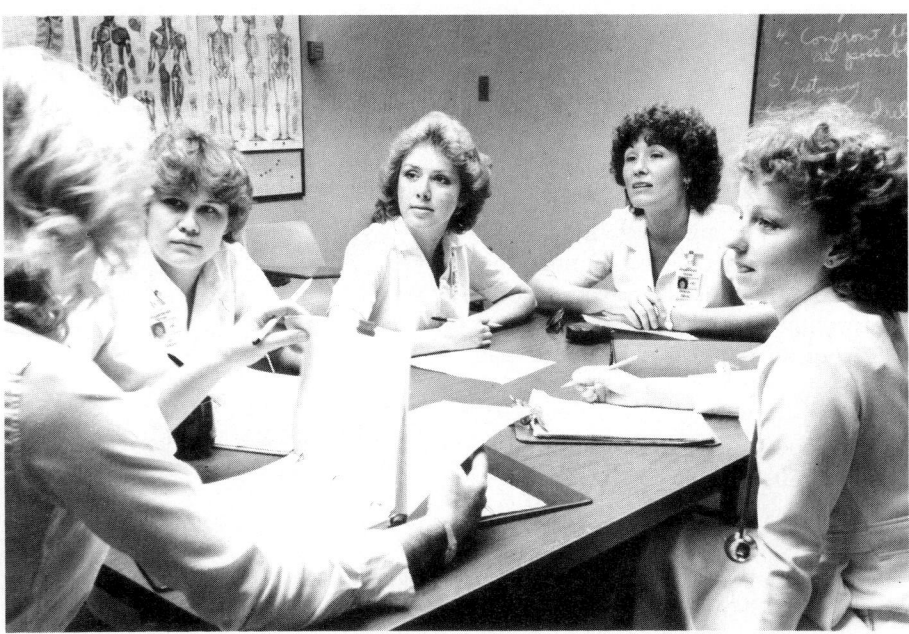

Fig. 22-1 Members of the nursing team meet at change of shift for a report on each client's progress and specific health care needs.

ing for a client. If a dressing is changed a certain way during the day shift, it should be changed the same way on the evening shift unless the client's condition changes or a physician's order changes the procedure. If one nurse finds a certain pain-relief measure more effective for a client, it is important that the information be relayed to the next nurse caring for the client so that pain control can be maintained. This information is also incorporated into the written care plan to further enhance communication across shifts. A complete report establishes the nurses' accountability in being sure that client care is uninterrupted. A client who sees different nurses performing care in the same manner will likely trust the care givers more.

A change-of-shift report may be given orally in person, by audiotape recording, or during rounds at the client's bedside. Oral reports are given in conference rooms (Fig. 22-1), with staff members from both shifts participating. An audiotape report is given by the nurse who has completed care for the client and left for the nurse on the next shift to review. Taped reports can improve efficiency by allowing staff to report when time is available. A disadvantage of a taped report is that it does not allow staff members to ask questions or clarify explanations. Reports given in person or during rounds permit nurses to obtain immediate feedback when questions are raised about a client's care. Rounds may involve two or more nurses going to a client's bedside to discuss the care plan. When nurses make rounds, the client and family members have the opportunity to participate in any decisions. Likewise the nurses can see the client together to perform needed assessments, evaluate progress, and determine the interventions best suited to the client's needs. During rounds, any information that might alarm the client is reported out of hearing. The nurse giving the report ensures privacy by speaking in a low voice to prevent others from overhearing. A disadvantage to rounds is the lengthy time it takes to complete a report on all clients.

Because of the many responsibilities nurses have to assume, it is important that a change-of-shift report be conducted quickly and efficiently (Table 22-3). Time taken during the report keeps the nurse away from clients. A good report describes clients' health status and lets staff on the next shift know exactly what kind of care the clients will require. Significant facts about clients are reviewed (for example, the condition of wounds or episodes of chest pain) to provide a baseline for comparison during the next shift. Any data about clients should be objective and concise. Interpretation, the result of selecting, comparing, and summarizing, is important because the nurse can report the clinical significance of the shift's events.

TABLE 22-3   Do's and Don'ts of Intershift Report

Do's	Don'ts
Provide only essential background information about client (i.e., name, sex, age, physician's diagnosis, and medical history).	Don't review all routine care procedures or tasks (e.g., bathing, scheduled medications).
Identify client's nursing diagnosis or health care problems and their related causes.	Don't review all biographical information already available on Kardex.
Describe objective measurements or observations about client's condition and response to health problem. Stress recent changes.	Don't use critical comments about client's behavior, such as "Mrs. Wills is so demanding."
Share significant information about family members as it relates to client's problems.	Don't make assumptions about relationships between family members.
Continuously review ongoing discharge plan (e.g., need for resources, client's level of preparation to go home).	Don't engage in idle gossip.
Relay to staff significant changes in the way therapies are given (e.g., different position for pain relief, new medication).	Don't describe basic steps of a procedure.
Describe instructions given in teaching plan and client's response.	Don't explain detailed content unless staff members ask for clarification.
Evaluate results of nursing or medical care measures (e.g., effect of backrub or analgesic administration).	Don't simply describe results as "good" or "poor." Be specific.
Be clear on priorities to which oncoming staff must attend.	Don't force oncoming staff to guess what to do first.

An organized report follows a logical sequence. To prepare for the report the nurse gathers information from worksheets, the client's Kardex, and the client's care plan. The nurse giving the report should avoid reading forms that the next nurse can easily do independently. Instead the reporting nurse provides a brief overview of the client's reason for hospitalization in case the nurse reporting for duty has never cared for the client. Then the nurse provides a detailed description of the client's progress during the shift. A systematic approach such as using the nursing process can provide staff with critical information needed to continue care. The basis for the report is the client's health problems. The following is an example of a change-of-shift report:

1. *Background information:* Cy Tolan, a 32-year-old client of Dr. Lang in bed 4, is scheduled for a colon resection this morning. He has had ulcerative colitis for 2 years. This is his first experience with surgery. He knows he may require a colostomy.
2. *Assessment:* Mr. Tolan expressed difficulty falling asleep last night. He had several questions about surgery. Early in the night he called for assistance several times.
3. *Nursing diagnosis:* His chief nursing care problems are *knowledge deficit* related to inexperience with surgery and *anxiety* related to potential body change.
4. *Teaching plan:* He asks appropriate questions about surgery. Dr. Lang has explained to him that a colostomy may be needed. Staff on evenings explained postoperative routines. I reinforced information with him early in the night. He stated that he felt less anxious.
5. *Treatments:* A cleansing enema was administered till clear at 9 PM; no blood was noted in the return. He complained of some abdominal cramping immediately afterward, but that disappeared. He received a Dalmane 15 mg PO at 11:30 PM, and I gave him a backrub. He fell asleep after midnight.
6. *Family information:* His wife remained with him last evening until the end of visiting hours. She has returned and is in the room this morning.
7. *Discharge plan:* Mr. Tolan is a very active person at home. He plays tennis & basketball and swims. Mrs. Tolan is concerned about how he might react to a colostomy. I suggest making a referral to the enterostomal therapist early if the colostomy is performed.
8. *Priority needs:* Right now, Mr. Tolan is relaxing in his room. The operative permit has been signed. All preoperative procedures have been completed except for his pre-op medications, due on call to the operating room.

In the previous example, the nurse gave a clear picture of Mr. Tolan's anxiety about surgery and need for information. The nurse assuming Mr. Tolan's care has a clear picture of the client's immediate needs. If Mr. Tolan presents new information during the next shift the nurse will know that a change in Mr. Tolan's condition has occurred or new problems have developed. An organized and comprehensive approach to reporting helps nurses anticipate the client's needs early and lessens the chance of important information being forgotten or overlooked.

When giving a report, the nurse discusses clients or family members in a professional manner. It is often necessary to describe the interactions between clients, nurse, and family members in behavioral terms. The nurse avoids using labels such as *uncooperative, difficult,* or *bad* when describing such behaviors. Any derogatory statements overheard by clients could lead to lawsuits against the nurse (see Chapter 14). A good report is objective and nonjudgmental. Value-laden terms do not establish working relationships between staff members and clients. Staff members may unintentionally form a prejudicial opinion about clients before even meeting them. The content of reports should be pertinent to clients' health care.

Telephone Reports

Health care team members frequently talk to one another by telephone. For example, a nurse informs a physician of changes in a client's condition, a nurse from one unit communicates information to a nurse on another unit about a client transfer, or the laboratory staff or a radiologist reports results of diagnostic tests. Information in a telephone report should be permanently documented in written form if significant events or changes in a client's condition have occurred. Thus the persons involved with a telephone report should be sure that the information is clear, accurate, and concise. If any doubt exists about the information conveyed over the telephone, the receiver repeats the message back to the sender.

Nurse: This is Ms. Towns from 7 south. Do you have the potassium results for Mr. Tom Rush in room 702A?
Laboratory technician: Yes. Mr. Tom Rush's potassium level is 3.2.
Nurse: Let me repeat that, 3.2?
Laboratory technician: Yes, that's correct.
Nurse: And may I have your name?
Laboratory technician: Yes, Ms. Sue Thomas.

To document a phone call, the nurse includes when the call was made, who made it (if other than the writer of the information), who was called, to whom information was given, what information was given, and what information was received (Feutz-Harter, 1989). An example would be, "At 10:22 AM, called laboratory; S. Thomas, technician, reported Mr. Rush's potassium at 3.2—C. Towns, RN."

Telephone Orders

Telephone orders (TOs) involve a physician stating a prescribed therapy over the phone to a registered nurse. Clarifying messages is important when a nurse accepts physician's orders over the telephone. The order must be verified by repeating it clearly and precisely. Then the nurse writes the order on the physician's order sheet in the client's permanent record and signs it. An example follows: "1/16/93: 7:20 PM: Darvocet-N PO 1 tab now and q4h prn— T.O. Dr. Reiss/Carol Towns, RN." The physician later verifies the telephone order legally by signing it within a set time period (for example, 24 hours). Telephone orders are frequently given at night or during an emergency. Telephone orders should only be used when absolutely necessary and not for the sake of convenience. The box provides guidelines that the nurse can use to prevent errors in receiving telephone orders.

It is important to be as courteous as possible when making or receiving phone calls (see box). Anyone calling a nursing unit should be treated as a consumer needing a service. Courtesy conveys a sense of caring and professionalism and promotes cooperation of all health team members.

Transfer Reports

Clients frequently transfer from one unit to another to receive different levels of care. For example, clients transfer from intensive care units to general nursing units after the level of care no longer requires intense monitoring. A **transfer report** involves communication of information about clients from the nurse on the sending unit to the nurse on the receiving unit. The receiving unit must know the most current information about clients and their progress. For example, if a client has undergone a surgical procedure, the receiving unit will want to know the type of procedure, information about any complications, and the client's current health status. A complete and accurate transfer report is essential for continuity of care from one unit to the next.

Transfer reports may be given by phone or in person. A transfer form is completed for nurses to document the client's status at the time of transfer. It is

---

Telephone Order Guidelines

- If the physician sounds hurried over the phone, use clarification questions to avoid misunderstanding.
- Clearly determine the client's name, room number, and diagnosis.
- Repeat any prescribed orders back to the physician.
- Write a telephone order to include date and time given; name of client, nurse, and physician; and the complete order.
- Follow agency policies; some institutions require telephone (and verbal) orders to be reviewed and signed by two nurses.
- Have the physician cosign the order within the time frame required by the institution (usually 24 hours).

Telephone Techniques

INCOMING CALLS

- Cue yourself to smile before picking up the phone.
- Identify the nursing division and yourself.
- Be natural. Use your real voice, tone, and volume.
- Treat each call as important.
- Give the caller your full attention.
- Listen carefully.
- Use words of courtesy and politeness.
- Take notes as pertinent information is communicated.
- If there are any questions, ask them after the caller has finished speaking.
- End the call graciously.
- Let the caller hang up first.

OUTGOING CALLS

- Place your call.
- When the other person answers, identify yourself by name and title.
- Use the person's name. State the reason that you are calling.
- If the report is lengthy, have notes in front of you.
- Ask if the other person has any other questions.
- End the call graciously.

also important for the medical record to be up-to-date. When giving a transfer report, nurses include the following information:

1. Client's name, age, primary physician, and medical diagnosis
2. Summary of medical progress up to the time of transfer
3. Current health status (physical and psychosocial)
4. Current nursing diagnoses or problems and care plan
5. Any critical assessments or interventions to be completed shortly after transfer (helps receiving nurse to establish priorities of care)
6. Need for any special equipment

After the sending nurse completes the transfer report, the receiving nurse should have time to ask any questions about the client's status.

Incident Reports

An incident is any event not consistent with the routine operation of a health care unit or routine care of a client (Blake, 1984). The client, visitor, or employee may be at risk when anything unusual occurs in a health care area. Examples of incidents include client falls, accidental needlestick injuries, a visitor experiencing symptoms of illness, medication administration errors, accidental deletion of ordered therapies, or carelessness in performance of a procedure that led to actual or a high risk for client injury. Reporting of incidents helps the identification of high-risk trends in nursing care or daily unit operations that warrant correction. Changes in policies and procedures, in-service seminars about nursing care practice, & changes in the operation of a nursing unit are ways in which repeated incidents can be corrected. Incident reports are an important part of a unit's quality-assurance program (see Chapter 10).

When an incident occurs, the nurse involved in the incident or the nurse who witnesses an injury completes an **incident report.** The report is completed even though an injury does not occur or is not apparent (Feutz-Harter, 1989). Most institutions have specific incident report forms (Fig. 22-2). The report typically goes to the institution's risk-management office for review. Further review may occur, depending on the nature of the incident. For example, the employee health department might review all incidents involving employee needlesticks. The hospital's legal department may review incidents when possible lawsuits against the hospital are expected.

When a client or visitor is involved in an incident, the nurse observing the incident takes steps to remove the individual from risk and then begins a report describing details of the incident. A physician examines the individual to determine whether any injury has been suffered. If a client is affected, the physician documents the examination and findings in the client's medical record. The nurse documents only an objective description of what happened and any follow-up care that occurred. The nurse reports what was actually observed. The following example compares an accurate and an inaccurate note.

Accurate Note	Inaccurate Note
Client found on floor, complained of pain in left hip. Noted external rotation and shortening of left leg. Lifted back into bed with assistance from orderlies. VS: BP, 142/88; P, 90°; R, 22. Side rails up, call light within reach, instructed to remain in bed. Dr. Smith notified, portable x-ray ordered stat.	Client fell out of bed, complained of pain in left hip. Noted external rotation and shortening of left leg. Dr. Smith notified.

An incident report should be concise and accurate, reporting exactly what the nurse observes and administers in the way of care.

The nurse does not specify in the medical record that an incident, report was prepared. When the victim of an incident, the nurse reports details of the incident and then seeks medical attention according to institutional policy.

Nurses usually become involved in client-related incidents at some point in their careers. They must understand the purpose of incident reports and the correct way to report information. The following list provides some guidelines for correctly completing an incident report:

1. The nurse who witnessed the incident or who found the client at the time of the incident should file the report.
2. The nurse describes specifically what happened in concise, objective terms.
3. The nurse does not interpret or attempt to explain the cause of the incident.
4. The nurse describes objectively the client's condition when the incident was discovered.
5. Any measures taken by the nurse, other nurses, or physicians at the time of the incident are reported.
6. No nurse is blamed in an incident report.
7. The report is submitted as soon as possible to the appropriate administrator.
8. The nurse should never make a photocopy of the incident report for a personal file because the copy could be subpoenaed in court.

INCIDENT REPORT / Patient-Visitor

Barnes Hospital — St. Louis, Missouri

THIS DATA IS PROVIDED FOR THE LEGAL COUNSEL OF THE DIRECTORS OF BARNES HOSPITAL IN THE EVENT OF POSSIBLE LITIGATION AND IS TO BE CONSIDERED CONFIDENTIAL AND PRIVILEGED INFORMATION.

USE ADDRESSOGRAPH IF PATIENT

REPORT NO.

PERSON INVOLVED

PETERS   RON   L
(Last Name)   (First Name)   (M.I.)

Age **68**
Sex **M**

Date of Incident **1/8/--**
Date Reported **1/8/--**

Time (Military) **0915**
Exact location of incident **Room 6201A**

Tele. No.

PATIENT ☒

Rm. No. **6201A**
Reason for hospitalization (Diagnosis) **ALZHEIMERS WORK UP**
Attending Physician **ROGERS**

Mental condition of patient before incident:

Normal ☐ Senile ☐
Disoriented ☒ Sedated ☐ Other_____

Bedrails: Up ☒ Down ☐ Restraints: Yes ☐ No ☒
Activity Orders: Restraints ☐ Bed Rest ☐
Up privileges with assistance ☒ Without assistance ☐

Brief description of incident: PATIENT FOUND ON FLOOR AT SIDE OF BED. SMALL, 2CM ABRASION NOTED OVER Ⓛ FOREHEAD. CONSCIOUS AND RESPONDS TO VOICE.

VISTOR ☐
OTHER ☐

By whom employed_____
Home Address_____
Nature of Incident

Occupation_____
Home Phone_____
Reason in Hospital

ACCIDENT
FACTS

Name, Address, Tele. No. of Witnesses, if any:

Was patient seen by physician: Yes ☒ No ☐ Not indicated ☐
Time called **1000** a.m. p.m. Time arrived **1030** a.m. p.m.

Physician's Name.

Was treatment initiated by physician: Yes ☒ No ☐ X-Rays: Yes ☒ No ☐

I DO NOT WISH TO BE EXAMINED BY A PHYSICIAN: Signed:_____

DESCRIPTION
OF
INCIDENT

State what you saw and/or what you were told. Give names and addresses of all individuals who provided information concerning this incident.

ENTERED ROOM. FOUND PT. ON FLOOR AT SIDE OF BED. STATED "WHERE IS MARIE?" NOTED SMALL, 2CM ABRASION OVER Ⓛ FOREHEAD. AREA TENDER TO PALPATION. PT. ABLE TO MOVE ALL EXTREMITIES FULL ROM. ABLE TO RAISE FROM FLOOR INDEPENDENTLY. CALLED DR. ROGERS. SKULL-FILM ORDERED.

Date of Report **1/8/--**
Signature of person preparing report *Rita Woods RN*

PROPERTY
DAMAGE ☐

Owner of Property
Home Address

If theft, what day   and hour   last seen.
Tele. No.

MISSING
ARTICLE ☐

Nature and Extent of Damage or Loss

Estimated replacement or repair cost: $

Fig 22-2 Incident report form.
Courtesy Barnes Hospital, St Louis.

DOCUMENTATION

Documentation is very important in health care today. Edelstein (1990) defines **documentation** as anything written or printed that is relied on as a record of proof for authorized persons. A medical record should be a comprehensive description of the client's health status and needs, as well as the services provided for the client's care. Good documentation reflects not only quality of care but also evidence of each health care member's accountability in giving care.

Several types of records are used to communicate information about clients. Although each agency uses a different record format, all records contain basically the following information:

1. Client identification and demographic data
2. Informed consent for treatment and procedures
3. Admission nursing history
4. Nursing diagnoses or problems
5. Nursing care plan
6. Record of nursing care treatment and evaluation
7. Medical history
8. Medical diagnosis
9. Therapeutic orders
10. Medical and health discipline's progress notes
11. Reports of physical examinations
12. Reports of diagnostic studies
13. Summary of operative procedures
14. Discharge plan and summary

Purpose of Records

A record is a valuable source of data used by all members of the health care team. Its purposes include communication, financial billing, education, assessment, research, auditing, and legal documentation.

Communication

The record is a means by which health team members communicate contributions to the client's care, including individual therapies, client education, and use of referrals for discharge planning. A care plan should be clear to anyone reading the chart. When a staff member is caring for a client, the record should explain the measures needed to maintain continuity and consistency of care.

Financial Billing

The medical record is a document that shows the extent to which hospitals should be reimbursed for services; it is a client's bill. To obtain reimbursement the medical record must reflect that all physicians' orders were carried out adequately and correctly, and it must reflect results of those orders (Feutz-Harter, 1989). DRGs have become the basis for establishing reimbursement to hospitals (see box). If a hospital treats a client for less than the price attached to the DRG, a profit is made (see Chapter 3). If it costs the hospital more to treat a client than the DRG-reimbursed amount, the hospital absorbs a loss (Hines, 1988).

Nursing documentation can make a difference to ensure high standards of quality care and maximum reimbursement to health care agencies. Detailed recording helps in establishing codable diagnoses used to determine a DRG (Fig. 22-3). Although this is largely determined by a physician's documentation, the nurse's contribution to documentation can help interpret the type of treatment a client received. To be coded as an active problem, a client must receive treatment for a condition such as respiratory distress or phlebitis or the condition must have an impact on the client's current illness (Hines, 1988). Good documentation has become the foundation for DRG assignments.

Education

A client's record contains a variety of information, including medical and nursing diagnoses, signs and symptoms of disease, successful and unsuccessful therapies, diagnostic findings, and client behaviors. Students of nursing, medicine, and other health-related disciplines use these records as educational resources. An effective way to learn the nature of an illness and the response to it is to read the medical record. Although no two clients have identical

---

Diagnosis-Related Groups

- A DRG is a series of decision trees designed to cluster groups of clients together by diagnosis, surgical procedures, complications, comorbidities (preexisting illness), and age.
- The statistical weight of a DRG is multiplied by a hospital's specific rate of reimbursement.
- The hospital is reimbursed a fixed amount for every client grouped into the DRG regardless of length of stay or cost of treatment.
- An assigned DRG may change on the basis of documentation.

records, patterns of information can be identified in records of clients who have similar medical problems. With this information, students learn the patterns to look for in various health problems or diseases and become better able to anticipate the type of care required for a client.

Assessment

The record provides data that nurses use to identify and support nursing diagnoses and plan proper interventions for care. Information from the record adds to the nurse's own observations and assessment. The medical history, for example, is in the

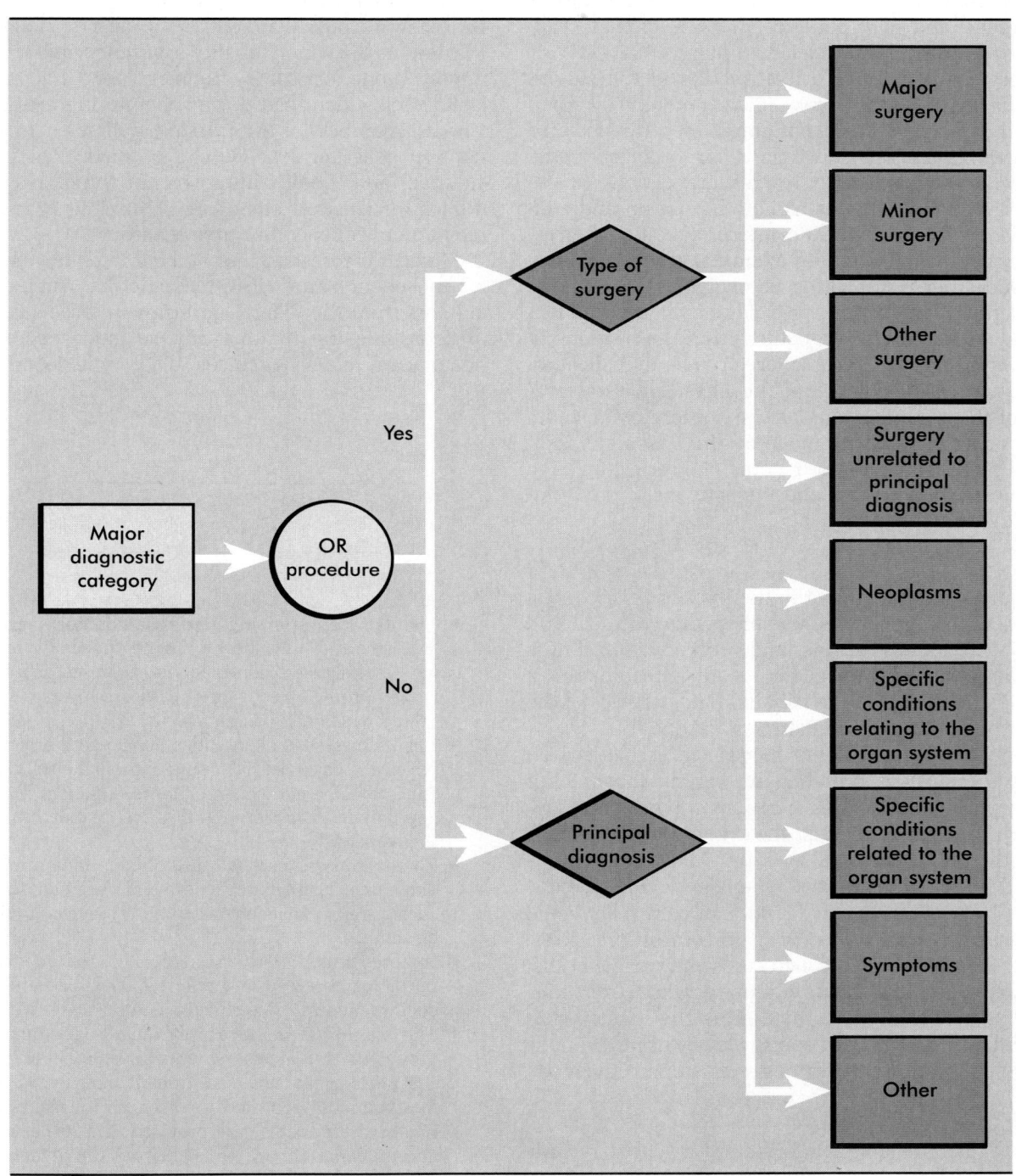

Fig. 22-3   Example of DRG structure for a major diagnostic category. Multiple DRGs are identified for each major diagnostic category.

record. Thus it is unnecessary for the nurse to collect information that is already available unless there is reason to believe that the information is inaccurate. The medical progress notes detail the physician's findings at the time of assessment. Before caring for any client, the nurse refers to the medical record for new and relevant assessment findings. The nurse is able to enter a client's room, anticipate the status of the client, and then conduct an assessment to validate or confirm the physician's findings.

The record provides a total picture of the client's health status. Assessment data entered by each health care member do not simply describe isolated happenings. Each observation is part of a larger puzzle, which when solved reveals the client's health status. The record contains data to explain and confirm observations or refute interpretations. After inspection of a wound, for example, the nurse may conclude that it is healing poorly; the nurse checks the record, which may give additional information, including the client's appetite, other descriptions of the wound's appearance, laboratory results indicating the onset of infection, and the physician's observation of the wound in the last 24 hours. Any observations or interpretations made by the nurse are compared with data from the record. The record helps to explain the reasons for and implications of any findings the nurse gathers.

Research

Statistical data relating to the frequency of clinical disorders, complications, use of specific medical and nursing therapies, deaths, and recovery from illness can be gathered from client records. Records are a valuable resource for describing characteristics of the client populations in a health care agency.

A nurse may use clients' records during a research study to collect information on certain factors. For example, if a nurse uses a new method of pain control on a group of clients, the records could provide data on the success of therapy. Recording entries that describe the number of analgesic medications used or clients' subjective reports of pain relief could be used to evaluate new pain-control measures. Nurses may also research records of previously discharged clients to identify nursing care problems. For example, a study to determine the incidence of infection in clients with specific types of intravenous catheters might be performed with a chart review.

Auditing and Monitoring

A regular review of information in client records gives a basis for evaluation of the quality and appropriateness of care provided in an institution. The JCAHO requires hospitals to establish quality-assur-

ance and quality-improvement programs to conduct objective, ongoing reviews of client care. The JCAHO has standards for types of information to be found in the client's record, such as indications that a care plan is developed with the client as a participant and that discharge planning and client education have occurred. The JCAHO asks institutions to establish standards for quality care (see box). Nurses monitor or review records throughout the year to determine the degree to which quality-assurance and quality-improvement standards are met (see Chapter 10). Deficiencies identified during monitoring are shared with all members of the nursing staff so that corrections in policy or practice can be made. Quality-assurance and quality-improvement programs keep nurses informed of standards of nursing practice to maintain excellence in nursing care.

Medical records are also audited to review charges for the client's care. Private insurance carriers and auditors from the federal government review records to determine the reimbursement that a client or a health care agency receives. Thorough documenta-

---

Examples of JCAHO Nursing Service Standards

- Clients receive nursing care based on documented assessment of their needs. Clients' needs for nursing care related to admission are assessed by a registered nurse. Needs are reassessed when warranted by clients' conditions.
- Clients' assessment includes consideration of biophysical, psychosocial, environmental, self-care, educational, and discharge-planning factors. When appropriate, data from families are included in the assessment.
- Clients' nursing care is based on identified nursing diagnoses, client care needs, and care standards; such care is consistent with the therapies of other disciplines.
- In preparation for discharge, continuing care needs are assessed and referrals for such care are documented in the medical records.
- The clients' medical records include documentation of the initial assessments and reassessments, the nursing diagnoses and client care needs, the interventions identified to meet the nursing care needs, the nursing care provided, the response to and outcome of care provided, and the abilities of the clients and families to manage continuing care needs after discharge.

tion of supplies and equipment used ensures that costs are recovered and that clients receive the care they require.

Legal Documentation

A medical record must be accurate because it is a legal document (see Chapter 14). In the case of a lawsuit, the medical record, not the nursing care, is on trial. The record serves as a description of exactly what happened to a client. Nursing care may have been excellent; however, care not documented is care not done in a court of law. Clients frequently request copies of their medical records, and they have the right to read those records. Each institution has

policies for controlling the manner in which records are shared.

Recording should not become merely routine or superficial. Nor should nurses wait until the end of a tiring day to record the client's care. Good documentation should be done in a timely manner with careful thought. Table 22-4 provides guidelines to ensure that a client's record is legally sound.

Methods of Recording

The quality of documentation is constantly under review by nursing managers as they attempt to find ways to help nurses improve their documentation. Documentation must follow standards dictated by the

TABLE 22-4 Legal Guidelines for Recording		
Guidelines	Rationale	Correct Action
Do not erase, apply correction fluid, or scratch out errors made while recording.	Charting becomes illegible. It may appear as though you were attempting to hide information or deface record.	Draw single line through error, write word *error* above it. and sign your name or initials. Then record note correctly.
Do not write retaliatory or critical comments about client or care by other health care professionals.	Statements can be used as evidence for nonprofessional behavior or poor quality of care.	Enter only objective descriptions of client's behavior. Client comments should be quoted.
Correct all errors promptly.	Errors in recording can lead to errors in treatment.	Avoid rushing to complete charting. Be sure information is accurate.
Record only facts.	Record must be accurate and reliable.	Be certain entry is factual. Do not speculate or guess.
Do not leave blank spaces in nurse's notes.	Another person can add incorrect information in space.	Chart consecutively, line by line. If space is left, draw line horizontally through it and sign your name at end.
Record all entries legibly and in ink.	Illegible entries can be misinterpreted, causing errors and lawsuits. Ink can not be erased. Records are photocopied and stored on microfilm.	Never erase entries or use correction fluid, and never use pencil.
If order is questioned, record that clarification was sought.	If you perform order known to be incorrect, you are just as liable for prosecution as physician.	Do not record "physician made error." Instead chart that "Dr. Smith was called to clarify order for—"
Chart only for yourself.	You are accountable for information you enter into chart.	Never chart for someone else (exception: if care giver has left unit for day and calls with information).
Avoid using generalized, empty phrases such as "status unchanged" or "had good day."	Specific information about client's condition or case can be accidentally deleted if information is too generalized.	Use complete, concise descriptions of care.
Begin each entry with time and end with your signature and title.	This ensures that correct sequence of events is recorded. Signature documents who is accountable for care delivered.	Do not wait until end of shift to record important changes that occurred several hours earlier. Be sure to sign each entry.

JCAHO to maintain institutional accreditation, to lessen liability, and to justify the need for nursing services (Edelstein, 1990). For example, the JCAHO (1992) requires that all clients admitted to a health care institution have an assessment of physical, psychosocial, environmental, self-care, client education, and discharge-planning needs. In addition, the JCAHO stresses the importance of evaluating client outcomes, including the client's response to treatments, teaching, or preventive care. Such standards can make documentation time consuming.

Nurses involved in the direct care of clients often have difficulty in fully documenting their client's care. Lack of time, the feeling that no one reads notes, excess duplication, and a concern about the meaningfulness of information in charts are just some of the attitudes nurses have about documentation (Edelstein, 1990; Montemuro, 1988). These problems have led to more bedside charting and the creation of flowsheets (see later section). Bedside graphics offer nurses the convenience of entering information immediately after it is collected from a client. There is no need to leave the bedside, jot information down on a reminder sheet, and then enter the data in the record at the nurse's station.

The nursing service department of each health care agency selects the method used for documentation of client care. The method should reflect the philosophy of the nursing service and incorporate the standards of care and practice for the department. For example, if a nursing department's standards of practice use nursing diagnosis or a framework such as Gordon's functional health patterns (Gordon, 1991), the documentation system uses nursing diagnoses and health patterns in care plans and other forms.

Professional care is reflected by professional charting, which proves what the nurse has done and effectively communicates the client's status and progress (Edelstein, 1990). Because the nursing process shapes a nurse's approach and direction of care, good documentation reflects the nursing process. Assessment data are recorded to offer to all health care members a data base from which to draw conclusions about the client's problems. Information describing the client's problems or diagnoses then directs care givers to choose an appropriate care plan with nursing therapies. Evaluation of care communicates the client's status, degree of progress, and success in meeting expected outcomes of care.

A challenge exists to find a record-keeping method that ensures optimal communication and yet simplifies the charting process. The JCAHO requires documentation of nursing diagnoses or problems within the context of the nursing process, as well as evidence of client and family teaching and discharge planning. If more than one discipline regularly cares for a client, the JCAHO also expects a multidisciplinary care plan.

Many record-keeping methods are found within health care institutions. The difference between them is the manner in which information is organized.

Problem-Oriented Medical Records

The **problem-oriented medical record (POMR)** is a method of documentation that places emphasis on the client's problems. The method corresponds to the nursing process and facilitates communication of client needs (Gawlinski, Rasmussen, 1984). Data are organized by problem or diagnosis. Narrative notes incorporate assessment, planning, intervention, and evaluative information specific to the client's health status. Each member of the health care team contributes to a single list of identified client problems. With the POMR, the client's problems are easy to recognize and locate, data are well coordinated, and each discipline records progress notes on the same form. The client benefits from this charting method because all health care team members contribute to a common, coordinated plan of care. If there is an argument against POMR documentation, it is the lengthiness of narrative notes for each problem. Many nurses find it takes considerable time to write complete POMR progress notes. The POMR has the following major sections: data base, problem list, care plan, and progress notes. The box describes advantages of the POMR method.

Advantages of POMR Charting Method

- Places emphasis on clients and their problems
- Increases efficiency in gathering data about clients from all care givers
- Gives emphasis to clients' perceptions of their problems
- Requires continuous evaluation and revision of the care plan
- Provides greater continuity of care among health care team members
- Enhances effective communication among health care team members
- Provides easy to read information in chronological order
- Reinforces for nurses the use of the nursing process

DATA BASE. This section contains all available assessment information pertaining to the client (for example, the physician's physical examination and medical history, the nurse's admission history and ongoing assessment, the dietitian's assessment, laboratory reports, and radiological test results). The data base is the foundation for identifying client problems and planning care. The data base should remain active and current with revisions made as new data become available. The data base accompanies clients through successive hospitalizations or clinic visits. An active data base ensures continuity of care.

PROBLEM LIST. After data are analyzed, problems are identified, and a single list is made (Fig. 22-4). The problems are listed in chronological order according to the date each was identified (not in order of priority). The list is an organizing guide by which all health care disciplines plan the client's care.

A problem may be well defined, such as a specific medical or nursing diagnosis. Signs, symptoms, or syndromes such as pain or diarrhea may be stated as problems when insufficient data have been recorded to diagnose a problem or when complications of a medical diagnosis arise. Problems include the client's physiological, psychological, social, cultural, spiritual, developmental, and environmental needs.

It is important to avoid listing problems that are vague or not supported by data. The nurse lists a diagnosis, if one can be established, rather than a less specific term. For example, the nursing diagnosis of *ineffective airway clearance* is characterized by a cough, dyspnea, and abnormal breath sounds. *Impaired breathing* or *coughing* would be an unacceptable nursing diagnosis. Clinical manifestations or defining characteristics for diagnoses or problems should not be listed separately. This can cause a fragmentation of care. Integration of data to form specific, well-defined diagnoses or problems results in goal-directed care.

The list of problems is filed in the front of the client's record to serve as an organizer or table of contents. New problems are added as they are identified. After a problem has been resolved, the date is recorded and a line is drawn through the problem and its number. The number for a resolved problem is not used again. This system keeps the problem list simple and meaningful. After a problem list is developed, succeeding record entries such as progress notes are coded by the problem number.

Problem number	Date onset	Problem	Inactive or resolved	Date resolved
~~1~~	~~7/8/--~~	~~R breast mass~~	~~Resolved~~	~~7/9/--~~
2	7/8/--	Anxiety related to inexperience with surgery		
3	7/9/--	R Sub-total mastectomy		
4	7/9/--	Pain related to incisional swelling	Controlled	7/12/--
5	7/10/--	Self-esteem disturbance		
6	7/11/--	Inadequate family support systems		

Fig. 22-4 · POMR problem list.

CARE PLAN. A care plan is developed for each problem. The plan may be diagnostic, therapeutic, or educational, or it may contain all three interventions.

1. Diagnostic plan. The physician indicates diagnostic studies to be performed. Setting priorities prevents duplication of efforts and delay in dealing with the client's needs. During a time of cost containment in health care, a coordination of diagnostic testing is very important.
2. Therapeutic plan. The physician orders specific medical therapies by problem. The orders may include medications, activity restrictions, diet, & special treatments. If the original problem is a nursing diagnosis, the nurse outlines proposed interventions (independent, interdependent, or dependent) such as pain-relief measures, wound care techniques, or the timing of prn (as needed) medications. The format of a POMR allows each health care worker to understand the rationale for all orders.
3. Educational plan. Health team members identify the types of information or skills required by a client to assume self-care or adapt to any health-related problems.

PROGRESS NOTES. Health team members monitor and record the progress of a client's problems. Narrative notes, flowsheets, and discharge summaries are forms used to document the client's progress. Narrative notes often follow a special format (for example, SOAP, SOAPE, or PIE) so that information about each client problem is communicated clearly (Fig. 22-5). **SOAP** is an acronym for subjective data, objective data, assessment, and plan. SOAPE is used by various institutions; *E* represents evaluation. The logic for SOAP notes is similar to that of the nursing process. Data are collected about each of the client's problems, a conclusion is made, and a care plan is developed. Each SOAP note is numbered and titled according to the problem on the list it addresses. The numbering system makes it easy to find notes about the same problem. The notes communicate an ongoing plan of care.

S—This section includes subjective data or information gathered from the client. For example, the client will describe a symptom such as pain or discuss an interest in learning about a medication. Whether the progress note includes subjective data depends on the acuteness of the client's illness or the nature of the problem.

O—Objective data consist of information that can be observed or measured. Physical findings, laboratory results, observations, & results of x-ray examinations are examples of objective data.

A—The individual who writes a SOAP note takes the subjective and objective data and forms conclusions. The assessment is an interpretation of the client's condition or level of progress. It is a statement of the status of the diagnosis or problem. The assessment describes whether the problem has been resolved or further care is required.

P—Depending on the assessment of the situation, the health care member then develops a care plan. Plans may include specific orders designed to manage the client's problem, collection of additional data about the problem, individual or family education, and goals of care. The plan in each SOAP note is compared with the plan in previous notes. A decision is made to revise, modify, or continue previously proposed interventions.

E—If the SOAPE format is used, the nurse evaluates the client's response to therapies, present status, and progress toward goals of care.

PIE is an acronym for problem-intervention-evaluation. This format simplifies documentation by unifying the care plan and progress notes into a complete record (Siegrist et al, 1985). The PIE format differs from SOAP because the narrative note does not include assessment information. Daily assessment data appear instead on special flowsheets, thus preventing

---

1/19/___ ___   Knowledge deficit related to inexperi-
4:30 PM   ence regarding surgery

S—"I'm worried about what it will be like after surgery."

O—Client asking frequent questions about surgery. Has had no previous experience with surgery. Wife present, acts as a support person.

A—Knowledge deficit regarding surgery related to inexperience. Client also expressing anxiety.

P—Explain routine preoperative preparation. Demonstrate and explain rationale for TCDB exercises. Provide explanation and teaching booklet on postoperative nursing care.—S. Lazarus, RN

P—Knowledge deficit regarding surgery related to inexperience.

I—Explained to client normal preoperative preparations for surgery. Demonstrated TCDB exercises. Provided booklet to client on postoperative nursing care.

E—Client able to demonstrate TCDB exercises correctly. Needs review of postoperative nursing care.—S. Lazarus, RN

Fig. 22-5 Examples of progress notes written in the SOAP and PIE formats.

duplication of information. The PIE notes can be numbered or labeled according to the client's problems. Resolved problems are dropped from daily documentation after the nurse's review. Continuing problems are documented daily.

P—Problem or nursing diagnosis applicable to client

I—Interventions or actions taken

E—Evaluation of the outcomes of nursing interventions and the client's response to nursing therapies

Modified POMRs

In some institutions the POMR method of charting may only be used in the nursing notes record section. POMR takes the place of narrative notes seen in the traditional source record (see next section).

At admission, an initial nursing assessment identifies the client's nursing diagnoses or problems. The diagnoses are dated and then numbered in order of occurrence or priority on the basis of the initial assessment. The nurse then lists the problem number or writes out the problem name each time the problem is recorded in the SOAP or PIE notes. It is also acceptable to underline the number, diagnosis, or problem in the notes so that it can easily be spotted. After a diagnosis is resolved the nurse enters the date, notes that the problem is resolved, and initials it.

Nurses record SOAP or PIE notes on each pertinent problem when the client's condition changes or at least daily or every shift, depending on agency policy. This continues until problems are resolved. The SOAP or PIE format helps nurses to be aware of the care plan and the client response to interventions. New problems may be added as they are identified.

A disadvantage to SOAP or PIE notes is that the nurse's note focuses exclusively on a single client problem. Throughout the day a client may undergo changes or experience care activities that are not directly related to an indentified problem. For example, a client may accidentally fall. In this case a SOAP or PIE note may not be an ideal format. Many hospitals use standard narrative notes for such occurrences. Narrative notes are descriptive summaries that describe the circumstances of the client's care.

Source Records

In a **source record** the client's chart is organized so that each discipline (for example, nursing, medicine, social work, or respiratory therapy) has a separate section in which to record data. Unlike POMR the information is not organized by client problems. However, an advantage of a source record is that care givers can easily locate the proper section of the record in which to make entries. Table 22-5 lists the components of a source record.

TABLE 22-5   Organization of Traditional Source Record

Sections	Contents
Admission sheet	Specific demographic data about client: legal name, identification number, sex, age, birthdate, marital status, occupation and employer, health insurance, nearest relative to notify in an emergency, religious preference, name of attending physician, date and time of admission
Physician's order sheet	Record of physician's orders for treatment and medications, with date, time, and physician's signature
Nurse's admission assessment	Summary of nursing history and physical examination
Graphic sheet and flowsheet	Record of repeated observations and measurements such as vital signs, daily weights, and intake and output
Medical history and examination	Results of initial examination performed by physician, including findings, family history, confirmed diagnoses, and medical plan of care
Nurses notes'	Narrative record of nursing process: assessment, nursing diagnosis, planning, implementation, and evaluation of care
Medication records	Accurate documentation of all medications administered to client: date, time, dose, route, and nurse's signature
Physician's progress notes	Ongoing record of client's progress and response to medical therapy and review of disease process
Health care discipline's records	Entries made into record by all health-related disciplines: physical therapy, dietary, radiology, social work, and laboratories
Discharge summary	Summary of client's condition, progress, prognosis, rehabilitation, and teaching needs at time of dismissal from hospital or health care agency

A disadvantage of the source record is that information is fragmented. Because information is not organized by client problems, any details about a specific problem may be distributed throughout the record. It may become necessary to locate data from several different sections before identifying the client's problems and the care plan. For example, the nurse describes the character of abdominal pain and use of relaxation therapy and analgesic medication in the nurses' notes. The physician's notes describe the progress of the client's bowel obstruction and the plan for surgery in a separate section of the record. The results of x-ray examinations showing the location of the bowel obstruction is in the test results section of the record. The method by which source records are organized does not show how information from the disciplines is related or how care is coordinated to meet all of the client's needs.

The nurses' notes section is where nurses enter a narrative description of nursing care and the client's response (see box). It is also a section for documenting care provided by the physician in the nurse's presence. The nurse may record key diagnostic test results from other sections of the record in the nurses' notes if they are of major importance in the care of the client.

Charting by Exception

Recently, an innovative approach has been created to streamline documentation by reducing repetition and time spent charting. **Charting by exception** is a shorthand method for documenting normal findings

and routine care based on clearly defined standards of practice and predetermined criteria for nursing assessments and interventions (Murphy, Burke, 1990). Clearly defined standards of practice that define nurses' responsibilities to clients provide the framework for routine care of all clients. With standards integrated into documentation forms such as predefined normal assessment findings or predetermined interventions, a nurse needs only to document significant findings or exceptions to the predefined norms. In other words, the nurse writes a longhand note only when the standardized statement on the form is not met. Assessments are standardized on forms so that all care givers evaluate and document findings consistently (Murphy, Burke, 1990).

Because the standard assessments are located in the chart, client data are already present on the permanent record, so nurses do not have to keep temporary notes for later transcription and care givers have easy access to current data (Murphy, Burke, 1990). The assumption with charting by exception is that all standards are met with a normal or expected response unless otherwise documented. When nurses see entries in the chart, they know that something out of the ordinary has been observed or occurred. For that reason, it is easy to track when changes in a client's condition have developed.

Focus Charting

One additional approach to charting is **focus charting** (Lampe, 1988). This charting format reduces the lengthy notes often seen with SOAP charting and provides a format to document any client situation, even one unrelated to a specific client problem. Focus charting structures progress notes according to the focus of the note: a sign or symptom, a condition, a nursing diagnosis, a behavior, a significant event, or an acute change in a client's condition. Each note includes data, actions, and client response (**DAR**) (see box) for the particular client situation. The system is easily understood by all care givers and adaptable to most health care settings.

Common Record-Keeping Forms

A client's medical record may use a variety of forms to make documentation easy, quick, and comprehensive. Many forms eliminate the need to duplicate repeated data in the nursing notes. The forms present special types of information in a format more accessible than long, detailed progress notes.

Nursing History Forms

A nursing history form is a special form completed at the time a client is admitted to a nursing care unit (Fig. 22-6 on pp. 716–717). The form usually con-

---

Sample Nurses' Note

8/6   1100   Client states, "I'm having a hard time catching my breath." Respirations, labored at 28/min; P, 96; BP, 112/70. Client using intercostal muscles during inhalation, breathing primarily costal. Breath sounds auscultated, crackles over both lower lobes. Chest excursion equal bilaterally. Elevated head of bed to Fowler's position. Obtained arterial blood gas analysis at 1045 per order. Results are pH, 7.34; Pco_2, 44mm Hg; Po_2, 80mm Hg. Dr. Stein called. Applied O_2 at 4 L/min per mask as ordered. Remained at bedside to calm client—P. Haske, RN.

Examples of Focus Charting

Date	Time	Focus	
6/20	8:20 AM	Hypotension	D—BP in left arm 90/60, right arm 94/60, client's skin diaphoretic, client responds to name.
			A—Placed client in Trendelenburg position, increased IV fluid rate to 100 ml/hr per protocol, called Dr. Akin.
			R—Client remains responsive, BP in left arm 94/68 3 min after increasing fluids—S. Wilson, RN.
6/30	4:20 PM	Pain	D—Twisting in bed, grimacing with movement, states has sharp lower back pain.
			A—Administered morphine sulfate 10 mg IM.
			R—Verbalized relief within 15 minutes, lying quietly—T. Newson, RN.

---

tains basic biographical data (for example, age, method of admission, and physician), the admitting medical diagnosis or chief complaint, a brief medical-surgical history (for example, previous surgeries or illnesses, allergies, and medication history), the client's perceptions about illness or hospitalization, and a physical assessment of all body systems. The form allows the admitting nurse to make a thorough assessment to identify relevant nursing diagnoses or problems for the client's care plan. Data on history forms provide baseline data that can be compared with changes in the client's condition. Each institution designs a nursing history form differently, depending on the standards of practice and philosophy of nursing care.

Graphic Sheets and Flowsheets

Flowsheets are forms that allow nurses to record specific measurements or routine observations on a repeated basis. It is unnecessary to chart a narrative progress note each time that vital signs are checked, a bath is given, or a drug is administered. The flowsheet is a quicker and more efficient way to record information. Fig. 22-7 on pp. 718-719 is a nursing assessment and activity flowsheet.

The only time that the nurse may wish to duplicate information from a flowsheet into a narrative or progress note is when a significant change that results in specific therapies occurs. For example, if a client's blood pressure becomes dangerously high, the nurse may record the pressure and the medication administered in the narrative progress note.

A flowsheet provides a quick and easy reference to nurses and physicians to assess a client's status. It becomes unnecessary to locate data from several different sources. Critical care units commonly use flowsheets for all types of physiological data.

Nursing Kardex

Nursing information needed for the daily care of clients is readily accessible in the nursing **Kardex** (see Chapter 8). The Kardex is a flip-over card usually kept in a portable index file or notebook at the nurses' station. Most Kardex forms have two parts, an activity and treatment section and a nursing care plan section. Nurses refer to the Kardex throughout the day. It organizes information in a useful manner as nurses give change-of-shift reports or make walking rounds. The Kardex contains pertinent information about clients and their ongoing care plans. An updated Kardex eliminates the need for continual referral to the chart for routine information. Information commonly found in the Kardex includes the following:

1. Basic demographic data (for example, age and religion)
2. Primary medical diagnosis
3. Current physician's orders to be carried out by the nurse
4. A written nursing care plan (based on the nursing process and used when a formal plan is not found in the client's record)
5. Nursing orders
6. Scheduled tests and procedures
7. Safety precautions to be used in the client's care
8. Factors related to activities of daily living

In many institutions, nurses make Kardex entries in pencil because it is usually necessary to make frequent revisions as the client's needs change. However, entries should be made in ink if the Kardex is a permanent part of the client's record. The Kardex provides the nurse an opportunity to communicate useful information to the nursing team about the client's unique needs. Within the care plan or the order-

Barnes Hospital

NURSES ADMISSION NOTE   C-2

Date 10/13/-- Time 1400 Informant _PATIENT_ Age 71

T 36⁸ P 92 R 22 B/P ¹⁶⁰/90 Ht. 5'4" Wt. 165 LB

Chief Complaint and History of Present Illness:

"_I'VE HAD THIS SORE ON MY FOOT FOR_
2 MONTHS AND IT WON'T HEAL."
ADMITTED FOR EVALUATION OF
VASCULAR DISEASE.

ADDRESSOGRAPH

Type of previous illness/surgery	Date	Type of previous illness/surgery	Date
DIABETES	1968		
HYSTERECTOMY	1958		

Has received blood products in the past: ☐ Yes ☒ No If yes, List dates _____ Reactions: ☐ Yes ☐ No

Allergies: _PENICILLIN_

Medication Name	Dose/Frequency	Time of Last Dose	Name	Dose/Frequency	Time of Last Dose
INSULIN (NPH)	30 UNITS q AM	0800			
INSULIN (REG)	8 UNITS q AM	0800			
METAMUCIL	ī Tbsp q AM	0900			

Patient Provided: ☒ Admission Kit   ☒ I.D. Band   ☒ Sensitivity/Allergy Band

Patient Instructed: ☒ Valuables Policy   ☒ Waiver signed   ☒ Smoking/Visitor policy   ☒ Nurses Call/Emergency/TV/Phone
☒ Chaplain availability   ☐ Patient rights (Psych. only)   SIGNATURE: _L. Reed RN_

DIRECTIONS: Circle those that apply. Comment on those circled if needed.

Sensory

Sensory Alteration

- EYES: (Decreased acuity) (Blurred vision) Photophobia Discharge Prosthesis
  EARS: Tinnitus Discharge Hard of hearing (R or L)
  NOSE: Congestion Obstruction Discharge Epistaxis
  THROAT: Sore throat Hoarseness   TOUCH: (Reduced) absent tactile perception
  ASSIST DEVICES/MEASURES: (Glasses) Contacts Hearing aid Tracheostomy
  Comments: _ABLE TO READ ONLY LARGE PRINT WITH GLASSES._
  HAS REDUCED SENSATION IN BOTH FEET UP TO ANKLE LEVEL.

Skin/Mucous Membrane

Impaired Skin Integrity
Alt. in mucous membranes

- Poor hygiene Poor turgor Diaphoretic Bruises Scars Erythema Petechiae Rash
  Itching Jaundice (Wound (describe)) Pale/dry membranes Coated tongue Stomatitis
  Carious teeth Halitosis
  Comments: _3 CM OPEN AREA OVER Ⓛ METATARSAL OF Ⓛ FOOT,_
  DRAINING MODERATE AMOUNT OF YELLOW DISCHARGE.

Respiratory

Ineffective airway clearance
Ineffective breathing patterns
Impaired gas exchange

- Cough Hemoptysis Dyspnea Orthopnea Cyanosis Restlessness Home 02 ___ L/min
  Use of accessory muscles Pursed lip breathing Pain with breathing
  Smoker (packs/day ___ years ___) (Lung sounds (describe))
  Comments: _LUNGS CLEAR TO AUSCULTATION BILATERALLY_

Circulatory

Decreased cardiac output
Alt. periph. tissue perfusion
Alt. fluid volume

- Fatigue Chest pain Palpitations Syncope (Numbness) (Tingling) Edema
  (Weak) absent peripheral pulse Capillary refill (describe) (Extremities (describe color/temperature))
  Comments: _BOTH LOWER FEET COOL TO PALPATION, MOTTLING NOTED_
  AROUND Ⓛ FOOT ULCER, DORSALIS PEDIS PULSES WEAK BILATERALLY.

Nutrition

Alt. in nutrition

- Diet: _1800 CAL ADA DIET AT HOME._
  Dysphagia Heartburn Nausea Vomiting Appetite increase/decrease Decreased taste
  Weight gain/loss ___ lbs. (Difficulty chewing) (Dentures - lower/upper)
  Comments: _DENTURES LOOSE FITTING._

Fig. 22-6 Nursing history form.
Courtesy Barnes Hospital, St Louis.

Elimination
Alt. in bowel elimination
Alt. in urinary elimination

- BOWEL: Constipation Diarrhea Incontinence Melena Tarry stools Ostomy
Abd. pain/cramps/gas Hemorrhoids (Last BM) *10/12* Usual pattern *(describe)* *EVERY OTHER DAY*
Medications/Enemas *METAMUCIL* (Bowel Sounds) *(describe)*
Comments: *NORMAL IN ALL 4 QUADRANTS*

URINARY: (Frequency) Urgency Incontinence Polyuria Dysuria Hematuria
(Nocturia) Anuria Retention Urinary appliance
Comments: *URINE PALE YELLOW, CLEAR. PATIENT REPORTS THAT SHE VOIDS HOURLY. VOIDS AT LEAST TWICE NIGHTLY.*

Activity/Exercise Alteration
Impaired physical mobility
Self care deficit
Activity intolerance

- Self Care *(describe limitations to eat/bathe/dress/toilet/ambulate)* Fatigue Purposeful movement limited/absent
Decreased strength (Altered weight bearing) Limited ROM Abnormal gait Impaired coordination
Exercise routine *MILE A DAY, PRIOR TO ILLNESS* Assist devices used
Comments: *DISCOMFORT WHILE BEARING WEIGHT ON L FOOT. HAS BEEN UNABLE TO WALK REGULARLY IN LAST 3 WEEKS.*

Comfort
Alteration in comfort
Alteration in sleep pattern

- Pain *(describe character and patient behaviors)* Restlessness Sleep pattern *(Describe)* *7-8 HRS NIGHTLY*
Pain control/sleeping aids used *ENJOYS HOT CHOCOLATE @ BEDTIME*
Comments:

Immune Function
Potential for infection

- Fever in last 48° Lymphadenopathy Transplant history Chemotherapy *(date)*
Radiation therapy *(date)* Venous access device
Comments: *NO ABNORMAL FINDINGS*

Sexuality/Reproductive
Alt. in sexual function/ response

- Vaginal/urethral discharge Pap smear *UNSURE* LMP *AGE 48* Mammogram *1985*
(Knowledge of self breast exam) testicular exam Change in relationship with partner
Limitation imposed by disease/therapy
Comments: *DOES PERFORM A SELF-BREAST EXAM, BUT NOT REGULARLY*

Neuro/Cerebral Function
Alt. in thought process
Alt. in communication
Potential for violence

- (Alert) Oriented x *3* Memory impairment Impaired attention span H/A Dizziness
Inappropriate behavior Inaccurate interpretation of environment Difficulty expressing self verbally
Numbness Impaired judgement/perception
Comments:

Cognitive Response
Lack of knowledge

- Foreign language Poor understanding Inexperience with therapy (Requests information)
Comments: *DESIRES TO HAVE MORE INFORMATION REGARDING SKIN CARE TO ULCER SITE AND ASSISTANCE WITH MENU PLANNING.*

Emotional Response
Alt. in coping mechanism
Alt. in self concept

- VERBALIZES: (Fear) of therapy or surgery Loss of control Inability to cope Poor self-esteem
Identifies stressors *(describe)* (Anxious) Angry Crying Irritable Inappropriate affect Low mood
Comments: *EXPRESSES CONCERN REGARDING IMPLICATIONS IF FOOT ULCER DOES NOT HEAL.*

Social System
Alt. in support system

- Employed/unemployed Lives: *FOUR-ROOM APARTMENT*
In nursing home/other Support person *HUSBAND, JOHN OWENS*
Ability to assist after discharge *HUSBAND IS ABLE TO ASSIST WITH ADL*
Home environment affecting self-care
Comments: *HUSBAND'S HOME PHONE 427-1060*

Values/Beliefs
Value/belief conflict

- Expresses attitudes/beliefs re: Hospitalization (Implications of care)
Inappropriate perceptions of illness *(patient/family)*
Patient preference for spiritual assistance *CATHOLIC, REQUESTS VISIT BY PRIEST*
Comments: *DOES NOT WANT TO BECOME DEPENDENT PHYSICALLY.*

Health Management Pattern
Alt. in health maintenance
Potential for injury

- Last physical *1/88* Alcohol use *DENIES* Drug Use *DENIES*
Noncompliance with therapies Lack of knowledge *(describe)* Needs equipment/finances/resources
Comments:

Referrals

- (Dietitian) Social service (Nurse specialist) AT/OT/PT (Pastoral care) Speech therapy
Nurse Signature *L. Read RN*

Fig. 22-6, cont'd   Nursing history form.

BARNES HOSPITAL

Nursing Assessment Flowsheet

Date 10/14/88   C-10b

Instructions: Circle if Present.
Write in Assessment.
Indicate N/A if not applicable or not assessed.

Code: S - Self, A - Assist, T - Total
I - Instructed, C - Collected

Addressograph

		NIGHT	DAY
NEURO/ CEREBRAL	NEURO/ CEREBRAL	(Alert) Confused Memory Loss Agitated Oriented x 3 _____ ASKS QUESTIONS ABOUT ULCER CARE	(Alert) Confused Memory Loss Agitated Oriented x 3 NOTES BURNING @ ULCER SITE DURING DRESSING CHANGE
COMFORT/ SLEEP	Discomfort Intervention	N/A	
	Sleep Status	Awake (Slept at intervals) Slept	(Awake) Slept at intervals Slept
ACTIVITY/ EXERCISE	MOBILITY Limitations/ Devices	(Independent) Assist Dependent	(Independent) Assist Dependent
	ACTIVITY	UP TO BATHROOM x2	UP TO CHAIR IN ROOM x3
SKIN/ MUCOSA	Appearance	Warm (Dry) Turgor _____ SKIN INTACT AROUND BONY PROMINENCES	Warm Dry Turgor REDUCED SKIN DRY, INTACT EXCEPT FOR ULCER LOTION APPLIED TO BONY PROMINENCES
	Mattress/ Equipment	Foam Air (Heel Protectors) Aqua K pad Teds	Foam Air (Heel Protectors) Aqua K pad Teds
WOUND	LOCATION Appearance	(L) FOOT ULCER 3CM DIAMETER, DRAINING YELLOW DISCHARGE	(L) FOOT ULCER CONTINUES TO DRAIN YELLOW DISCHARGE, 3CM ULCER INFLAMED ALONG MARGINS
	Dressing Change	X1 WET-TO-DRY SALINE, FINE MESH GAUZE	X2 WET-TO-DRY, SALINE AND FINE MESH GAUZE
NUTRI-TION	MEALS Tube Feeding Infusion Device	Continuous Bolus Flush X _____	% Eaten B: 90% (S) A T L: 80% (S) A T Continuous Bolus Flush X _____
ELIMINATION	URINE	(Continent) x2 Incontinent Foley CLEAR, YELLOW URINE	(Continent) x4 Incontinent Foley CLEAR, YELLOW URINE
	BOWEL Bowel Sounds	Continent Incontinent Guaiac _____ Freq X: N/A Absent Present _____ Abdomen _____	(Continent) Incontinent Guaiac _____ Freq X: 1 SOFT FORMED STOOL Absent (Present) ALL QUADRANTS Abdomen SOFT, NON-TENDER
RESPIRATORY	Auscultation	N/A	CLEAR TO AUSCULTATION IN ALL LOBES
		O₂ _____ Cough/Secretion _____	O₂ _____ Cough/Secretion _____
CIRC	CIRCULATION	FEET COOL, DORSALIS PEDIS PULSES WEAK BILATERALLY	PEDAL PULSES WEAK BILATERALLY
OTHER	Specimen	I C Test _____ GLUCOMETER READING AT 10:00 PM - 110	I C Test _____ GLUCOMETER READING AT 8:30 AM - 165 GLUCOMETER READING AT 12:30 PM - 180

Signature/Status S. Tucker, RN   Signature/Status

HYGIENE: (S) A T	SAFETY	HYGIENE: (S) A T	SAFETY
Bath Tub Shower Shave Hair Nails (Oral) x1	ID Band on ✓ Siderails in Use ✓	(Bath) Tub Shower Shave (Hair) Nails (Oral) x2	ID Band on ✓ Siderails in Use ✓

Fig. 22-7 Nursing assessment flowsheet.
Courtesy Barnes Hospital, St Louis.

Nursing Assessment Flowsheet

Date _10/14/88_   C-10b

Instructions: Circle if Present.
              Write in Assessment.
              Indicate N/A if not applicable or not assessed.

Code: S - Self, A - Assist, T - Total
      I - Instructed, C - Collected

EVENING
(Alert)   Confused   Memory Loss   Agitated
Oriented x _3_ _____
BURNING AT ULCER SITE MORE
INTENSE; PRN ANALGESIC AT 7:00 PM
RELIEVED DISCOMFORT
Awake   (Slept at intervals)   Slept
(Independent)   Assist   Dependent
UP TO CHAIR x2
(Warm)   (Dry)   Turgor _____
TURNS SELF WELL
Foam   Air   (Heel Protectors)   Aqua K pad   Teds
MINIMAL DRAINAGE NOTED AT ULCER
SITE. WOUND APPEARS CLEAN. SLIGHT
INFLAMMATION ALONG MARGINS
X _1 WET-TO-DRY SALINE, FINE MESH GAUZE_
% Eaten D: _90%_   (S) A T
Continuous   Bolus   Flush X _____
(Continent) _x2_ Incontinent   Foley
CLEAR, YELLOW URINE
Continent   Incontinent   Guaiac _____
Freq X: _N/A_
Absent (Present) _ALL QUADRANTS_
Abdomen _SOFT, NON-TENDER_
_N/A_
O₂ _____
Cough/Secretion _____
PEDAL PULSES WEAK BILATERALLY
I   C   Test _____
GLUCOMETER READING AT 5PM
_155_
Signature/Status

HYGIENE: (S) A T	SAFETY
Bath Tub Shower	ID Band on ✓
Shave (Hair) Nails	Siderails in Use ✓
(Oral)	

entries sections, the nurse can communicate information such as preferences and diet, specific methods to perform a treatment, methods to incorporate client participation in care, or preferred times to perform a nursing order. Information within the Kardex should not simply be a reflection of routine nursing responsibilities or standardized care.

For example, a client with the nursing diagnosis of *altered patterns of urinary elimination* has a urinary tract infection and is required to drink large amounts of fluids. A Kardex entry of "increase fluid intake" is relevant but not particularly individualized. If, however, the nurse's assessment has revealed that the client prefers iced tea and cranberry juice, a Kardex entry of "offer cranberry juice and iced tea, 1000 ml per shift" addresses the client's preferences and tailors the care plan to the client's needs. The box provides a summary of guidelines for Kardex care plans.

The Kardex care plan has some disadvantages. Access is usually limited to nurses. Also, the Kardex does not offer space for writing an extensive plan for the client with multiple problems.

Standardized Care Plans

Although every professional nurse is responsible for developing an individualized care plan for a cli-

---

Tips on Writing Kardex Care Plans

WHEN TO WRITE A CARE PLAN

- During a report as nurses discuss client problems and needs
- On rounds after client problems are identified and reviewed
- After discussions with other health team members responsible for client care
- After interactions with the client and family members

WHAT TO INCLUDE

- Pertinent nursing assessment data
- Nursing diagnoses
- Nursing orders and collaborative interventions
  - Observations to make and frequency required
  - Nursing measures aimed at restoring, maintaining, or promoting health
  - Specific methods used to implement nursing measures
  - Appropriate inclusion of family participation
  - Discharge planning
- Expected outcomes of nursing care

ent, the process of writing the plan is time consuming. Nurses caring for several clients may need to write extensive care plans. Many institutions have attempted to make documentation easier for nurses with **standardized care plans.** The plans, based on the institution's standards of nursing practice, are preprinted, established guidelines that are used to care for clients who have similar health problems. After a nursing assessment is completed, the staff nurse identifies the standard care plans appropriate to the client. The care plans are placed in the client's medical record. Modifications can be made in ink to the standardized plans to individualize the therapies. Most standardized plans also allow the nurse to write in specific goals or desired outcomes of care, as well as the dates when these outcomes should be achieved.

There are several advantages and disadvantages of standardized care plans. One advantage is the establishment of clinically sound standards of care for similar groups of clients. These standards can be useful when quality-assurance audits are conducted. Standardized plans are easy to locate in a client's record, and thus all staff can quickly refer to them. Another advantage is the education. Nurses learn to recognize the accepted requirements of care for clients. The standardized plans can also improve continuity of care among professional nurses. Finally, even though the plans must be modified for each client, documentation takes less time.

Controversy exists over the use of standardized care plans. The major disadvantage is the risk that the standardized plans inhibit nurses' identification of unique, individualized therapies for clients. A second disadvantage is the need to formally update the plans on a routine basis to ensure that content is current and appropriate. Staff members often develop many standardized plans for clients seen in their institutions. Large numbers of plans take up space for storage and are more costly to print than one common care plan form. There is the trend among many hospitals to computerize care plans. With such a system, daily computer-generated care plans are printed and incorporate several nursing diagnoses or problems in a single care plan. Such a streamlined system improves the daily revision and updating of plans.

When standardized care plans are used in a health care facility, the nurse remains responsible for an individualized approach to care. Therefore if a standardized plan has an intervention that is not specifically tailored to the client's need, there should be a method for the nurse to revise or alter the intervention to make it individualized. Standardized care plans are not meant to replace the nurse's professional judgment and decision making.

Critical Pathways

With the arrival of managed care as a delivery of care model (see Chapter 3), documentation tools that integrate the standards of care of multiple disciplines have been developed. These tools or **critical pathways** allow staff from all disciplines to develop integrated care plans for a projected length of stay for clients of a specific case type. For example, the critical pathway for a client who has had a total hip repair will recommend on a day-by-day basis the level of activity, advancement in diet, and topics for education required for a normal recovery. The critical pathway lists client problems, key interventions, and expected outcomes. The nurse and other team members such as physical or respiratory therapists use the critical pathway to monitor the client's progress during each shift. All care givers use one critical pathway as a monitoring and documentation tool (see Chapter 3). Critical pathways incorporated into documentation tools can be developed to eliminate other nursing forms and thus reduce duplication and the amount of charting.

Discharge Summary Forms

Much emphasis is placed on preparing a client for an efficient and timely discharge from a health care institution. A prospective payment system based on DRGs encourages health care institutions to be more efficient and discharge the client as soon as possible. However, it is important to ensure that a client's discharge results in desirable outcomes. The earlier a client is discharged, the more likely a hospital will be fully reimbursed. The Healthcare Financing Administration (HCFA) requires multidisciplinary involvement in discharge planning to ensure that a client leaves the hospital in a timely manner with the necessary resources.

Ideally, discharge planning begins at admission. Nurses revise the plan as the client's condition changes. There should be evidence of the client's and family members' involvement in the discharge-planning process. There should be no surprises by the time the client is discharged. The client should have the necessary information and resources to return home. The box includes tips on completing discharge summary forms.

At discharge the nurse and other health team members summarize the client's condition and review the care plan for the home. The client's status should be described in relation to planned outcomes of discharge. Discharge summary forms (Fig. 22-8 on p. 722) make the summary concise and instructive. Many forms include a copy that is given to a client, family member, or home health care nurse. This transfer of information ensures better continuity of self-care in the home. A summary form emphasizes

---

Tips on Writing Discharge Summary Forms

INFORMATION FOR HOME HEALTH CARE NURSES

- Describe nursing interventions (e.g., dressing changes, step-by-step wound care).
- Describe information presented to client.
- Describe client's ability to perform health care skills (e.g., administering medications, use of crutches).
- Explain family members' involvement in care.
- Describe resources needed in home (e.g., Meals on Wheels, self-help devices).

INFORMATION FOR CLIENTS

- Use clear, concise descriptions in client's own language.
- Provide step-by-step description of how to perform a procedure (e.g., home drug administration). Reinforce explanation with printed instructions.
- Identify precautions to follow when performing self-care or administering medications.
- Review signs and symptoms of complications that should be reported to physician.
- List names and phone numbers of health care providers that client can contact.

Charting for Home Care Reimbursement

- Document the reason a client is homebound. Record objective, measurable criteria such as, "Client experiences pain after walking 10 ft" instead of "tolerates ambulation poorly."
- Clearly document complications (actual or potential) that relate to a client's diagnosis. For example, record how a diabetic client is having difficulty following a diet therapy or how a client who has suffered a heart attack is poorly complying with medication therapy.
- Specifically describe any skilled care that a client receives such as observation and assessment, teaching, case management, parenteral medications, tube feedings, venipuncture, and wound, catheter, or ostomy care. Explain how the skill relates to the primary diagnosis and why it is reasonable and necessary.
- If clients have been taught skills, explain the degree of assistance required to be sure that they are performed correctly, such as, "Client has difficulty inserting catheter tip into stoma, repeat instruction given with wife present." Avoid words such as *reinforce* or *monitor*.

---

previous learning by the client and family. The form may be attached to pamphlets or teaching brochures. In many institutions the social worker also contributes to the discharge summary.

Home Care Documentation

The home health care business (see Chapter 5) continues to grow as clients are discharged home earlier with significant health care problems. Medicare has specific guidelines for establishing eligibility for home care reimbursement. To fulfill Medicare guidelines, documentation by home health care nurses must clearly describe the clients' health status and levels of nursing care required.

Clients need home health care if they have limited mobility or are blind, senile, or otherwise unable to go out unassisted (Magliozzi, 1990). Activity restrictions after discharge also qualify clients for homebound status. The nurse documents the extent to which clients remain homebound throughout the period that visits are made. The potential for complications after discharge can also make clients eligible for home care reimbursement for 3 weeks after discharge. The nurse documents how potential problems are linked to the primary condition (see box).

(Magliozzi, 1990). When clients require skilled care, such as tasks performed or supervised by a registered nurse, Medicare will pay for home health care services. Specific descriptions of the skills required by clients are entered into their medical records.

Computerized Documentation

Computers have been widely used in hospitals and other health care facilities for over a decade. Automated technology improves the integration of informational resources and the accessibility of the information to all health care personnel. The results of laboratory and diagnostic tests can be stored within the computer and displayed on the computer terminal screen with a mere push of a key.

In the past, most hospital information systems have included ordering programs and communication systems. Nurses have been the primary users of these systems. Supplies, equipment, stock medications, and diagnostic testing are examples of services nurses may order through a computer. Computerized communication systems relay information about clients quickly and accurately. For example, client classification data, quality-assurance monitoring scores, and test results can be organized within the com-

Barnes Hospital

PATIENT DISCHARGE SUMMARY

C-16

Date _10/17/--_ Time _1030_

MEANS: ☐ Ambulatory ☒ Wheelchair ☐ Stretcher

METHODS: ☒ M.D. order ☐ AMA with release ☐ AMA without release   Addressograph Plate

Afebrile 24 hours? ☒ Yes ☐ No TPR 36^8–72–16 _____   B/P _124/72_

☐ Physician notified of irregularities

DISCHARGED TO: ☐ Home ☐ Nursing Home ☒ Home with Home Health Care ☐ Other

If discharged to Nursing Home or other facility/service:

Name _____   Address/Phone _____

☐ Release of Information form signed   ☐ Chart copied   ☐ Transfer form completed   ☐ Transportation Arranged

DISCHARGE CONSIDERATIONS:

☐ Valuables from cashier   ☐ PTA meds returned   ☐ Scripts given
☒ NA   ☒ NA   ☒ NA

DISCHARGE INSTRUCTIONS

FOR PROBLEMS OR FOLLOW-UP:

Physician _Dr. Stan Jones_   Phone _362-5000_ Appt. _10/24/91_

Other: _____

_____

Activity: _To remain in bed with (L) foot elevated on two pillows. May be up only_
to go to the bathroom.

Diet: _To follow 1800 calorie ADA diet as instructed by the dietitian. For questions_
about diet, call the dietitian (Sue Marlin) 362-3184.

Medications: _To take usual dosage of 30 units NPH insulin and 8 units of regular_
insulin every morning before breakfast.

Wound Care: _Change dressings to (L) foot daily using moistened fine mesh gauze_
with dry 4x4 gauze and wrap dressings with 4 kling gauze.

Teaching Materials Given: _Copy of "Controlling Your Diabetes" and "Diabetic Menu_
Planning."

Special Instructions: _Call doctor for increased pain, redness, swelling or drainage from_
(L) foot wound. Barnes Home Health nurses will be visiting daily to change
dressing to (L) foot.

My discharge instructions have been explained and a copy has been given to me.

Patient/Significant Other _John Owens_   Relation _HUSBAND_

Nurse _B. Rand, RN_

Fig. 22-8 Discharge summary form.
Courtesy Barnes Hospital, St Louis.

puter for all clients and made accessible when the nurse enters a name or identification number.

Today, computers are changing the way nurses practice. The new information systems that are now available can relieve nurses of repetitive clerical and monitoring tasks and increase the time available for direct client care. Some programs allow nurses to quickly enter specific assessment data one time, with the information automatically transferred to different reports. For example, after a nurse enters intake and output measurements for a specific time, the data are automatically transferred to shift total and daily summary records. Computers also help reduce errors, standardize nursing practice (for example, care plans and test preparation protocols), and document client care (Ford, 1990; Schroeder, 1987). Instead of writing lengthy nurses' notes, nurses can select choices on a screen that automatically builds a comprehensive record of an event.

The American Nurses Association's design criteria for computerized information systems identify the need for systems to support the nursing process (ANA, 1988). Additional criteria identify the need for systems that integrate elements of the client's automated record, permit electronic transport of data to other computer systems, and allow easy data retrieval (McLaughlin et al, 1990). These criteria aim to establish an efficient information system designed to support professional nursing practice. Most computer systems have been developed using medical, management, or systems models. McLaughlin et al (1990) describe one nursing information system that incorporates nursing theory and is data driven. The model supports the process by which nurses make clinical decisions and manage care. As nurses enter data about a client's health status, data drive the selection of screens so that ultimately a nursing diagnosis is made and a plan of care is created.

Nurses must know the benefits and risks of computerized documentation. All members of the health care team can access and enter data and thus generate a comprehensive data base. McNeil (1979) describes the computer as a source of information superior to face-to-face reporting because the input of all individuals caring for a client is available in an integrated and more complete manner than what previous shift members choose to report. Computers can reduce many tasks that burden nurses. It is likely that the logic integrated into computers will hasten decision-making activities and track the outcomes resulting from select nursing care protocols.

There are legal risks associated with computerized documentation. Computers open the way for access to information by almost everyone. The password used to enter and sign off computer files should not be shared with another care giver. A good system requires frequent changes in personal passwords to prevent unauthorized persons from tampering with records. Nurses must know how to correct charting errors on a computer. Any data that has been permanently saved as part of the record should not be deleted. However, any incorrect entries or misspelled words that have not been stored can be deleted or corrected (Collins, 1990). If information is accidentally deleted, a brief explanation can be entered into the computer. Some institutions may request an incident report. Finally, printouts of computerized records should be protected. Shredding of printouts or the logging of the number of copies generated by each care giver are ways to minimize duplicate records and protect the confidentiality of clients.

Nurses should be familiar with basic computer skills because most hospitals now have automated systems. Hospitals have large mainframe computer systems or individualized personal computers. A mainframe system consists of one centrally located computer with a huge memory capacity to power a variety of programs throughout the hospital. Each nursing division or hospital department has a computer screen or cathode-ray tube (CRT) with a keyboard attached to the main computer. Information may be entered or retrieved by using the keyboard by pressing a light-sensitive pen directly onto the CRT screen, or by using a mouse to guide a cursor on a screen. Most computer programs give the user information that helps make the proper keyboard or light-pen selections on the screen. More progressive hospitals have small CRTs or individual computers at each client's bedside. Nurses can enter assessment findings or document interventions that are quickly transmitted for storage. Documentation is timely, and fewer errors occur because the nurse does not have to leave the bedside to record information.

 ## SUMMARY

Documentation and reporting are methods of communicating information related to health care management. In any setting the success of a care plan depends on accurate and complete reporting and precise record documentation. Good reporting and documentation create a high level of communication that helps health team members have a common view of the client's problems. Nurses are the primary care providers because they have the most contact with clients. The use of basic principles for accurate and comprehensive documentation and reporting will ensure the delivery of safe and effective nursing care.

CHAPTER 22 REVIEW

Key Concepts

- A client's health care record is written documentation of the care received.
- Accurate record keeping requires an objective interpretation of data with precise measurements, correct spelling, and proper use of abbreviations.
- The medical record is a legal document and requires information describing exactly the care delivered to a client.
- A nurse's signature on an entry in a record designates accountability for the contents of that entry.
- Any change in a client's condition warrants immediate documentation to keep a record accurate.
- An organized record presents information logically, in order of the occurrence of events.
- All information pertaining to a client's health care management that is gathered by examination, observation, conversation, or treatment is confidential.
- The major purpose of the change-of-shift report is to maintain continuity of care.
- Rounds allow nurses to perform needed assessments, evaluate clients' progress, and determine the best interventions for a client's needs.
- Any oral report is delivered in a professional manner emphasizing objectivity and a nonjudgmental viewpoint.
- When information pertinent to care is communicated by telephone, the information must be verified.
- Incident reports objectively describe any event not consistent with the routine care of a client.
- The client's record serves as a resource to explain and confirm observations or refute interpretations of data.
- Errors made while recording should never be erased or made illegible.
- The medical record is a client's bill or financial record that serves as the basis for reimbursement to hospitals.
- Problem-oriented medical records are organized by the client's health care problems.
- Flowsheets eliminate the need to write narrative notes for repeated observations or measurements.
- The logic of SOAP, SOAPE, or PIE narrative notes is to organize entries in the progress notes by the nursing process.
- Medicare guidelines for establishing a client's home care reimbursement is the basis for documentation by home health nurses.
- Computerized information systems provide information about clients in an organized and easily accessible fashion.

Key Terms

Accreditation, p. 696

Change-of-shift report, p. 700

Charting by exception, p. 714

Consultations, p. 696

Critical pathways, p. 720

DAR, p. 714

Diagnosis-related group (DRG), p. 696

Documentation, p. 706

Flowsheets, p. 715

Focus charting, p. 714

Incident report, p. 704

Kardex, p. 715

PIE, p. 712

Problem-oriented medical record (POMR), p. 710

Record, p. 696

Reports, p. 696

SOAP, p. 712

Source record, p. 713

Standardized care plans, p. 720

Transfer report, p. 703

Critical Thinking Exercises

1. Mrs. Brown has the nursing diagnosis of *knowledge deficit regarding impending surgery related to inexperience*. The nurse instructed her on turning, coughing, and deep breathing (TCDB). In addition the nurse explained routine postoperative monitoring procedures. The client asked questions and was especially concerned about whether she would have anything offered for pain. Mrs. Brown was able to demonstrate TCDB to the nurse. Summarize the above description in PIE, SOAP, and FOCUS charting formats.

2. Ms. Voss is scheduled to receive an antibiotic at 10 AM. What criteria should the nurse use to completely document medication administration?

3. Review the following incident report and identify what is missing: "Mr. James was administered Lasix 400 mg at 9:30 AM. The prescribed dose was 40 mg. Dr. Millis was notified—B. Sims, RN."

4. If you discover an order written by a physician that you believe is incorrect, how would you document it in the medical record?

REFERENCES

American Nurses Association: *Design for computerized information systems,* Kansas City, Mo, 1988, The Association.

Bergerson SR: Charting with a jury in mind, *Nurs 88* 18:51, 1988.

Blake P: Incident investigation: a complete guide, *Nurs Manage* 15:37, 1984.

Collins HL: Legal risks of computer charting, *RN* 53:81, 1990.

Edelstein J: A study of nursing documentation, *Nurs Manage* 21:40, 1990.

Feutz-Harter S: Documentation principles and pitfalls, *JONA* 19(12):7, 1989.

Ford J: Computers and nursing, possibilities for transforming nursing, *Comput Nurs* 8(4):160, 1990.

Gawlinski A, Rasmussen S: Improving documentation through the use of change theory, *Focus Crit Care* 11:12, 1984.

Gordon M: *Manual of nursing diagnosis: 1991-1992,* St Louis, 1991, Mosby–Year Book.

Hines GL: DRGs: nursing documentation contributes to the bottom line, *Nurs Clin North Am* 23:579, 1988.

Joint Commission on Accreditation of Healthcare Organizations: *Accreditation manual for hospitals,* Chicago, 1992, The Commission.

Lampe S: *Focus charting: a patient-centered approach,* ed 4, Minneapolis, 1988, Creative Nursing Management.

Magliozzi HM: Charting that makes it through the Medicare maze, *RN* 53:75, 1990.

McLaughlin K et al: Shaping the future, the marriage of theory and informatics, *Comput Nurs* 8(4):174, 1990.

McNeil DG: Developing the complete computer-based information system, *JONA* 9:34, 1979.

Montemuro M: CORE documentation: a complete system for charting nursing care, *Nurs Manage* 19(8):28, 1988.

Murphy J, Burke LJ: Charting by exception, a more efficient way to document, *Nurs 90* 21:65, 1990.

Riegel B: A method of giving intershift report based on a conceptual model, *Focus Crit Care* 12:12, 1985.

Schroeder MA: Computers in nursing: applications for ambulatory care, *Nurs Econ* 5(1):27, 1987.

Siegrist LM et al: The PIE system: complete planning and documentation of nursing care, *QRB* 11:186, 1985.

ADDITIONAL READINGS

Albrecht CA, Lieske AM: Automating patient care planning, *Nurs Manage* 16:21, 1985.

Atwood J et al: The POR: a system for communication, *Nurs Clin North Am* 9:229, 1974.

Budziszewski W: Reports: vital links to communication, *Hosp Prog* 41:60, 1960.

Costello S, Summers BY: Documenting patient care: getting it all together, *Nurs Manage* 16:31, 1985.

Dobberstein K: Attacking fuzzy documentation, *Am J Nurs* 6:559, 1986.

Gamberg D et al: Outcome charting, *Nurs Manage* 12:36, 1981.

Harkins B: Keep your eye on the patient's problems, *RN* 49(12):30, 1986.

Hoke JL: Charting for dollars, *Am J Nurs* 85:658, 1985.

Kitto J, Dale B: Designing a brief discharge planning screen, *Nurs Manage* 16:28, 1985.

Kleiber C, Chase L: Solving documentation problems with a pediatric flow sheet, *Pediatr Nurs* 15(3):253, 1989.

Miller P, Pastorino C: Daily nursing documentation can be quick and thorough, *Nurs Manage* 20(11):47, 1990.

Nadzam DM: Documentation evaluation system: streamlining quality of care and personnel evaluations, *Nurs Manage* 18(11):38, 1987.

Napiewocki JK: Documentation: a nurse's best defense, *Prof Nurs* 1:321, 1985.

Reiley PJ, Stengrevics SS: Change-of-shift report: put it in writing! *Nurs Manage* 20(9):54, 1989.

Sanborn CW, Blount M: Standard plans for care and discharge, *Am J Nurs* 84:1294, 1984.

Thielman DE: Report: how to say it all in a few words, *RN* 50:15, 1987.

Vaughan-Wrobel BD, Henderson BS: *The problem-oriented system in nursing*, ed 3, St Louis, 1986, Mosby–Year Book.

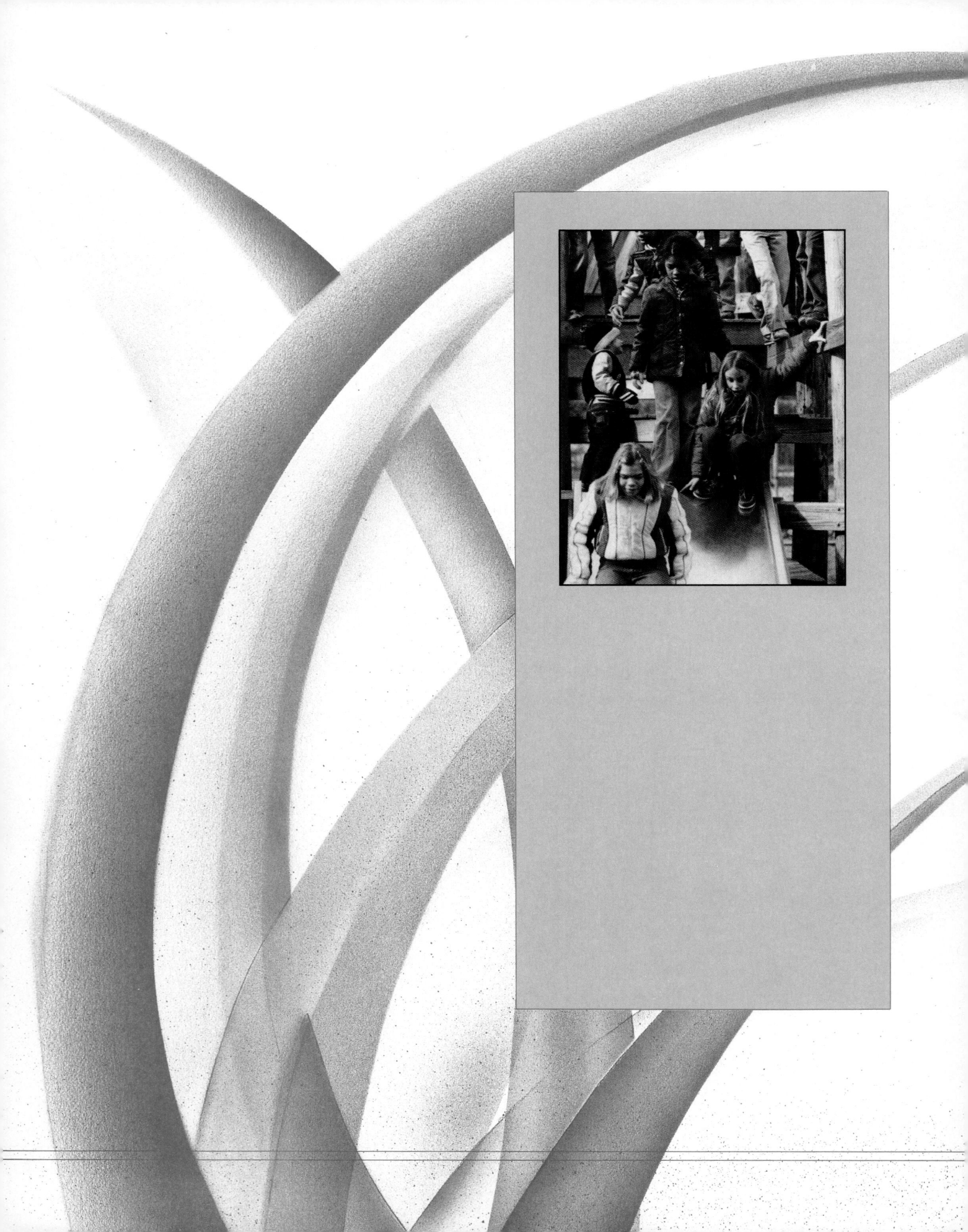

UNIT 5

Growth and Development for the Individual and Family

CHAPTER 23

The Family

OBJECTIVES

Mastery of content in this chapter will enable the student to:
- Define the key terms listed.
- Discuss the way family members influence one another's health.
- Describe current trends in the American family.
- Define the family in terms applicable to all family forms.
- Describe four common family forms and discuss the relevant health concerns of each.
- Explain the way that family structure and pattern of functioning affect the health of family members and the family as a whole.
- Compare family as context to family as client, and explain the way that these perspectives influence nursing practice.
- Describe the family nursing process in terms of assessment, nursing diagnosis, planning, intervention, and evaluation.
- Describe the attributes of effective and ineffective families.
- Describe how the health of the family is influenced by its relative position in society.

CHAPTER OUTLINE

Despite many challenges, the family remains the central institution in society. Within this social unit, individuals grow and develop and seek health. Twenty years ago, many people felt that the family was an endangered species. Some social scientists predicted that family influence on individual members would decline. They anticipated that rapid social change and a mobile population would cause psychological and physical distancing of family members. However, although family members today may be geographically farther from each other than in the past and may be living in nontraditional families, family ties remain strong between and within generations. For example, although America's older adults are often portrayed as isolated and alone, this is not the reality for most of them. More than two thirds of older persons see their children or communicate with them by telephone or letter at least once a week. In addition, approximately 58% of those with two or more children live within a 30-minute drive from them (Chiriboga, 1987).

The influence of the family is important in American society, and this must always be considered during interactions with clients. The family shapes early health beliefs and values, and family members have an impact on each other's health practices and status. The nurse views clients as individuals and as people who are integral parts of families. All family members need to be incorporated into the nursing process whenever possible because the family environment significantly influences health outcomes.

 ## CURRENT TRENDS

Although the institution of the family remains strong, the family itself is changing, and the emerging patterns are having a major effect on society. As Berardo (1990) notes, the new family forms and expanding range of alternative types of marriages are bringing a combination of new freedoms, responsibilities, and problems. Although some family scientists argue that the future will bring even more types of lifestyles, others believe that we are approaching a conservative era that will emphasize traditional family patterns. It is clear, however, that current statistics reveal fundamental changes from the traditional family form. People are marrying later, women are delaying childbirth, and couples are choosing to have fewer children. Divorce rates have tripled since the 1950s, and if current rates continue, half of all marriages will end in divorce. Some research suggests that the divorce level may have peaked and is starting to decline, and it is speculated that the threat of acquired immunodeficiency syndrome (AIDS) may

cause more early and permanent marriages (Norton, Moorman, 1987). Although divorce occurs often, marriage continues to be a desired state; most people who end a marriage enter another one. About 90% of young Americans are likely to marry, and between 66% and 75% of those who divorce remarry (Glick, 1989). The median interval between divorce and remarriage is about 3 years (Coleman, Ganong, 1990). Men are more likely to remarry than women, younger persons are more likely to remarry than older persons, and divorcees are more likely to remarry than widows (Eshleman, 1991). Remarriage often results in a blended family, with a complex set of relationships between step-parents and step-children and half brothers and sisters. There may also be new extended family members. Researchers are beginning to investigate the extended families.

The majority of women work outside the home, and about 57% of this work force have at least one child under 6 years of age (Eshleman, 1991). Although there appears to be few direct effects on the mother-child relationship, there is a growing need for consistent substitute child care. The division of labor within the home has become a major issue in many families today. Research demonstrates that, although equal division receives verbal approval, the majority of household tasks remains "women's work."

The number of one-person households is growing rapidly. Although some people choose a single lifestyle, it is not always a matter of choice. Demography and culture have created a "marriage squeeze," a shortage of men compared in the prime marrying ages (Zinn, Eitzen, 1990).

The fastest growing age group is 65 and over. Only a few decades ago, long-term generational ties were the exception rather than the rule. Currently, however, there are more people who live through their 60s, and the number of people who have reached 80 has increased significantly (US Bureau of the Census, 1987). This "graying" of America has an impact on the family life cycle and society as a whole. For example, the emergence of an older society has increased the likelihood of grandparents (and great-grandparents) being regular members of the family. Although it is often assumed that a large number of older adults live in nursing homes, this is not the case. Most retirees live with spouses or alone. Only about 6% reside in a health care institution.

An increase in the number of people 85 and over is having consequences for middle-age adults. This generation is finding that they must balance the needs of their offspring and the needs of their aging parents, sometimes at the expense of their own well-being and resources. Caring for a frail or chronically ill relative is a major concern in a growing number of families. Family care givers often develop significant

Research Highlight

The psychological well-being of 87 family care givers of impaired older adults were examined. Ballie, Norbeck, and Barnes conclude that care givers are at a high risk for psychological distress or depression when they have been providing care for an extended period of time and have little social support. The authors suggest that nursing interventions should also focus on the needs of the care giver, perhaps through the care giver's own network. This type of intervention strategy can decrease care giver illness and elder abuse.

Ballie V, Norbeck JS, Barnes LE: Stress, social support, and psychological distress of the family caregivers of the elderly, *Nurs Res* 37(4):217, 1988.

problems related to the stresses of this role (see research highlight). In addition, young adults often return to their parents' home because of economic necessity or convenience. Called *yo-yos* or *boomerangs* in the literature, these adult children need to renegotiate household rules and responsibilities and can cause a strain on the parent-child relationship.

 CONCEPT OF FAMILY

A popular conception exists about what the family is or at least what it should be. This "ideal" model dictates that the family is a nuclear unit; consists of a father, mother, and their children; and exhibits a sexual division of labor (that is, the mother cooks, cleans, and is responsible for child-rearing, and the father works outside the home). Family evokes a visual impression, a mental image of adults and children living together in a satisfying, harmonious fashion (Zinn, Eitzen, 1990). Families are, however, as diverse as the individuals that compose them. Nurses, like all people, have feelings and values rooted deeply in their family, which influence their definition of family. Unless nurses recognize these values, they may inhibit their understanding and acceptance of the client's perspective and definition.

The definition of family has received much attention from a variety of scholars and organizations. The **family** can be viewed as a biological entity, a legal unit, or a social network with personally constructed ties and ideologies. According to the U.S. Bureau of Census, it is two or more individuals related by blood, marriage, or adoption, who reside in the same household (Ross et al, 1990). Although this is an efficient definition and one that works for census data, it clearly does not include the varying concepts of family that individual clients may hold and is not flexible enough for nursing practice. In fact, a definition that is sufficiently broad to encompass all possible client situations offers little in terms of helping the nurse incorporate the concept of family into practice. Thus the nurse must think of family as defined by each individual. In other words, the nurse can think of the family as a set of relationships that the *client* identifies as family or as a network of individuals who influences each other's lives.

To effectively provide care, nurses must understand that individual attitudes about family are deeply ingrained and deserve respect. To some clients, family may include only persons related by marriage, birth, or adoption, whereas to others, aunts, uncles, close friends, and cohabitating persons are family. The nurse's personal beliefs do not have to coincide with those of the client. To provide individualized care the nurse recognizes and accepts the client's view. The attitudes of many clients are based on common family forms. The nurse should know about these forms and their health implications.

 FAMILY FORMS

Family forms are patterns of people considered by family members to be included in the family. Although all families have some things in common, each family form has unique problems and strengths. The nurse needs to have an open mind about family forms so that potential resources and concerns are not overlooked.

Nuclear Family

Although the nuclear family is not the dominant family form in North America, health care professionals often consider it to be the usual and ideal form. The **nuclear family** consists of the husband, wife, and perhaps one or more children. For the children, this family is often referred to as the **family of origin**. For the parents, it is the **family of procreation**. Many couples in American society choose to not have children. Others are unable to have children because of infertility.

Extended Family

The **extended family** includes members of the nuclear family and other relatives. Aunts, uncles, grandparents, and cousins are all part of the extended family. The extended family can be psychologically and geographically close or separated. The closer the extended family, the greater the influence on the client and the greater the importance of incorporating extended family members into the health care plan. Extended families often provide a larger range of experience and talents and therefore a more diverse support base than the nuclear family. After the birth of a child with a physical deformity, for example, the grandparents may provide comfort to the parents when they feel extremely vulnerable and unable to give each other emotional support. Other relatives can be recruited to cook meals to give the parents more time together or to be with the child.

Single-Parent Family

Single-parent families are formed when one parent leaves the nuclear family because of divorce, desertion, or death. The circumstances of the separation influence its impact on the family. In the past, most single-parent families existed because of the death of one parent. Today, these families are most commonly the result of a divorce, unwed parents living alone, or the decision of a single person to adopt a child. Children of divorce are most often placed in the custody of the mother, which contributes to the fact that female-headed households are the fastest growing type of family today (Zinn, Eitzen, 1990). Although all single-parent families are not poor, the vast majority are at a disadvantage compared with other family groups. Single-parent families are characterized by a high rate of poverty, relatively low education, a high rate of mobility, and a high percentage of minority representation (Eshleman, 1991). All of these factors suggest that the pursuit of health in these families is a challenge. Single parents tend to be more depressed, have lower self-esteem, and are overwhelmed by meeting all the physical and emotional needs within the family. Even a routine illness may cause a crisis because income may be inadequate for health care and few alternatives exist for carrying out all tasks within the family. Thus extended family and a social network are particularly important because family members may be able to provide the necessary emotional and financial support.

Blended Family

Blended families are formed when parents bring unrelated children from prior marriages into a new, joint-living situation because of remarriage or cohabitation. With the rate of divorce and remarriage, one out of every five children belongs to a blended family (Romanczuk, 1987). Although studies have in general failed to demonstrate that divorce and remarriage have long-term negative effects on children, subtle changes appear to occur in children's relationships with fathers, mothers, siblings, and other family members (see research highlight). The nature of the prior living situations and rapidity with which the family members must adapt to changes can influence health. Multiple, rapid changes severely tax coping resources. Stress experienced during the earlier family dissolution, the length of time in which each family functioned with one parent, and the extent of the members' familiarity with one another influence the blended family's coping capabilities.

The key to healthy stepfamily functioning is establishment of a strong couple bond, which provides the foundation of the new family unit (Engebretson, 1982). The mental health of family members during adjustment to the new family pattern is of primary interest. This adjustment period can last up to 2 years. The long-term impact of stress on the health of the individual members and of the family as a whole during this extended period requires assessment. The nurse can assure families that this period is a normal phase and can help the family identify its resources to prevent or lessen stressful situations.

Other Family Forms

The "typical" family has become a rarity. In 1983, only 6% of American families consisted of a bread-

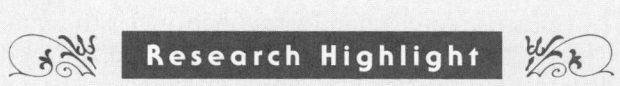

Research Highlight

Amato investigated the effects of divorce and remarriage on the adjustment and development of children in three types of families: mother-custody one-parent, mother-custody step-parent, and intact families. Interviews were conducted with 402 children (195 primary and 207 secondary) at school and with the children's parents in the home. The interviews dealt with family relationships and activities and contained open- and close-ended questions. The author concluded that children in one-parent homes have more demands placed on them but also have corresponding privileges. Children in step-parent families also had many household responsibilities but no more autonomy than in intact families. In one-parent and step-parent families, the author perceived low cohesion in family life.

Amato P: Family processes in one-parent, stepparent, and intact families: the child's point of view, *J Marriage Fam* 49(2):327, 1987.

winning husband, a full-time housewife, and two children (Skolnick, 1987). The diversity in lifestyles and new living arrangements is an outgrowth of economic and family trends. This rise in alternatives is associated with new patterns of divorce and remarriage and new expectations about individual fulfillment and personal life (Zinn, Eitzen, 1990). Many individuals structure their lives differently than their parents did.

In the early 1980s an estimated 1.8 million couples cohabitated, and since then the number has risen substantially (Berardo, 1990). Some couples choose to live together as an alternative to marriage. However, the majority see it as a temporary arrangement and as a pretrial for marriage.

Approximately half of all gay male couples live together, compared to three fourths of lesbian couples. Although sometimes unable to marry by law, many homosexual couples define their relationship in family terms. They have become more open about their sexual preferences and more vocal about their legal rights. Some homosexual families include children, either through adoption, through artificial insemination, or from prior relationships. Less controversial but more significant departures from the past include dual-earner families, commuter marriages, and couples who are voluntarily childless. It has been suggested that these departures from the more traditional form of family can result in added stress. However, evidence exists that this is not the case and that certain lifestyles do not threaten family health (see research highlight).

 Research Highlight

Sund and Ostwald investigated personal and lifestyle-related variables and stress levels in dual-earner families in the preschool stage of development. In a sample consisting of 92 families, family stress levels were measured by The Family Inventory of Life Events and Changes. The conclusion that dual-earner families in this study had only a moderate amount of family stress compared to national stress level norms contraindicated the notion that the mother's employment outside the home increases stress. The authors suggest that the advantages resulting from a dual-earner lifestyle help maintain equilibrium within the family.

Sund K, Ostwald SK: Dual-earner families' stress levels and personal lifestyle–related variables, *Nurs Res* 34(6):357, 1985.

 STRUCTURE AND FUNCTION

Families have a structure and a way of functioning. Structure and function are closely related and continually interact with one another. Structure is based on organization (that is, the ongoing membership of the family and the pattern of relationships). Relationships can be numerous and complex. For example, a woman's relationships may include wife-husband, mother-son, and mother-daughter, each with different demands, roles, and expectations. Although the definitions of structure vary, the nurse asks the following questions when assessing the structure of a client's family:

1. Who is included in the family?
2. Who performs which tasks?
3. Who makes which decisions?

Structure may enhance or detract from the family's ability to respond to stressors. Very rigid or very flexible structures can be detrimental to functioning. A rigid structure specifically dictates who is permitted to accomplish a task and may also limit the number of persons outside the immediate family allowed to assume these tasks. For example, the mother might be considered the only acceptable person to provide emotional support for the children or the husband the only one to provide financial support. A change in the health status of the person responsible for a task places a burden on the family because no other person is available or considered acceptable to assume that task. An extremely open structure can also present problems for the family. An underlying stability that otherwise leads to automatic action during a crisis or rapid change is often absent.

Friedman (1986) describes functioning as what the family does. Family functioning involves the processes used by the family to achieve its goals. These processes include communication among family members, goal setting, conflict resolution, nurturing, and use of internal and external resources. The reproductive, sexual, economic, and educational goals that were once considered central family goals no longer apply to all families. Although many families pursue these goals at various times during their development, they provide psychological support to their members throughout the life span. When the psychological needs of family members are not met, symptoms of family dysfunction are the usual consequence. These symptoms include emotional responses such as anger, delinquent behavior, somatic complaints, and depression (Friedman, 1986).

Goals are more easily achieved when communication is clear and direct. Clear communication enhances problem solving and conflict resolution. Another family process facilitating goal achievement is the ability to nurture and promote growth. Families need to have available and must be able to use internal and external resources. A social network is useful as an external support system. Social relationships act as buffers, particularly during times of stress, and reduce a family's vulnerability.

 DEVELOPMENTAL STAGES

Families, like individuals, change and grow over time. Although families are far from identical to one another, they all go through predictable stages. Each developmental stage has its own challenges, needs, and resources and includes tasks that need to be completed before the family can successfully move on to the next stage. McGoldrick and Carter (1985) have developed a model of family life stages based on expansion, contraction, and realignment of family relationships that support the entry, exit, and development of the members. This model provides the nurse with the emotional aspects of transition and the changes and tasks necessary for the family to proceed developmentally (Table 23-1). Consequently, the nurse can promote behaviors to achieve essential tasks and help families prepare for later transitions. This model does not take into account diverse family forms. However, other researchers suggest alternative models. For example, Aldous, as reported in McCubbin and Dahl (1985), has devised a six-stage system for single-mother families resulting from divorce.

TABLE 23-1 Stages of the Family Life Cycle

Family Life Cycle Stage	Emotional Process of Transition: Key Principles	Changes in Family Status Required to Proceed Developmentally
Between families: unattached young adult	Accepting parent-offspring separation	Differentiating self in relation to family of origin Developing intimate peer relationships Establishing self in work
Joining of families through marriage: newly married couple	Commitment to new system	Forming marital system Realigning relationships with extended families and friends to include spouse
Family with young children	Accepting new generation of members into system	Adjusting marital system to make space for children) Taking on parenting roles Realigning relationships with extended family to include parenting and grandparenting roles
Family with adolescents	Increasing flexibility of family boundaries to include children's independence	Shifting parent-child relationships to permit adolescents to move in and out of system Refocusing midlife marital and career issues Beginning shift toward concerns for older generation
Launching children and moving on	Accepting multitude of exits from and entries into family system	Renegotiating marital system as dyad Developing adult-to-adult relationships between grown children and parents Realigning relationships to include in-laws and grandchildren Dealing with disabilities and death of parents (grandparents)
Family in later life	Accepting shifting of generational roles	Maintaining own and/or couple functioning and interests in face of physiological decline; exploration of new familial and social role options Supporting a more central role for middle generation Making room in system for wisdom and experience of older adults; supporting older generation without overfunctioning for them Dealing with loss of spouse, siblings, and other peers and preparation for own death; dealing with view and integration

From McGoldrick M, Carter E: The stages of the family life cycle. In Henslin J, editor: *Marriage and family in a changing society*, New York, 1985, Free Press; and Walsh F: *Normal family processes*, New York, 1982, Guilford Press.

The initial stage is the establishment of the single-parent family, and the final stage is retirement of women from their work life or from the responsibilities of parenthood.

 FAMILY AND HEALTH

The health status of family members influences family functioning, and family functioning, in turn, influences its own and society's perceptions of its health. When the family satisfactorily meets its goals through adequate functioning, its members tend to feel positive about themselves and their family. Conversely, when they do not meet goals, families view themselves as ineffective. Constant stress resulting from inadequate functioning can also adversely affect a family member's health. Constant stress may alter cardiovascular function, blood pressure, and circulating neuroendocrine substances. Stressors are suspected precursors of poor health (see Chapter 30). In addition, even stress that occurs over a relatively short time period (such as a high-risk pregnancy) can adversely affect long-term family functioning and health (see research highlight). Maladaptive behaviors within the family have a negative impact on the health of its members and the overall ability of the family to meet its goals. A lack of communication or poor communication inhibits the family's ability to make decisions and solve problems. Good health may not be highly valued, and in fact, detrimental practices may be accepted. In some cases a family member may provide mixed messages about health. For example, a parent may continue to smoke while telling children that smoking is bad for them. Family environment is crucial because health behavior reinforced in early life has a strong influence on later health practices.

Ruebin Hill noted nearly 30 years ago that it is possible to explain the reactions of crisis-proof and crisis-prone families (Adams, 1986). The crisis-proof or effective family is able to integrate the need for stability with the need for growth and change. This family has a flexible structure that allows adaptable performance of tasks and acceptance of help from outside the family system. The structure is flexible enough to allow adaptability but not so flexible that the family lacks cohesiveness and a sense of stability. The effective family has control over the environment and exerts influence on the immediate environs of home, neighborhood, and school. The ineffective family may lack or believe it lacks control over these environs. Effective families demonstrate a combination of strengths that help them withstand crisis and manage change. McCubbin and McCubbin (1988) have identified eleven strengths of the resilient family (see box).

The health of the family is influenced by its relative position in society. Although American families share the same culture, they live in very different ways. The structure, function, and health of any family is a reflection and result of its social class, economic resources, and racial and ethnic background. For some minority groups and the poor, patterned differences in family living are consequences of

 Research Highlight

A causal model was tested to examine the effects of stress on family functioning for four groups of parents at 8 months after the birth of a child. Women who had high-risk pregnancies and their partners were compared with women who had low-risk pregnancies and their partners. Mercer and Ferketich conclude that a high-risk pregnancy had direct effects on family functioning at 8 months. This long-term effect of poorer family functioning concurs with the hypothesized relationship between health status and family functioning.

Mercer RM, Ferketich SL: Predictors of family functioning eight months following birth, *Nurs Res* 39(2):76, 1990.

 Family Strengths

- Accord, or relationships that foster problem solving and management of conflict
- Celebrations, or special events (e.g., birthdays, religious holidays)
- Communication, or ability to convey personal beliefs and emotions
- Good financial management
- Hardiness, or commitment to family and belief that members have control over their lives
- Health (physical and mental)
- Shared leisure activities
- Acceptance of each member's personality and behavior
- Social support network of relatives and friends
- Shared routines such as meals and chores
- Traditions that carry over from one generation to another

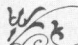 **Research Highlight**

Using data from a 1985 epidemiological survey of 2115 adults, Ulbrich, Warheit, and Zimmerman examined the influence of race and socioeconomic status (SES) on mental health and the effect of economic problems and undesirable life events on psychological distress. Using multiple indicators of mental health, the authors concluded that SES interacts with race to increase psychological symptoms of distress. For example, lower-class SES blacks were more vulnerable than middle-class SES blacks to the impact of undesirable events.

Ulbrich PM, Warheit GJ, Zimmerman RS: Race, socioeconomic status, and psychological distress: an examination of differential vulnerability, *J Health Soc Behav* 30(1):131, 1989.

 **Research Highlight**

Gillis explored stress in the family during and after coronary artery bypass surgery. The purpose was to compare clients' stress with spouses' report the major sources of stress, and examine the couples' social processes of recovery. The scores of 71 clients were compared with their spouses' scores. The spouses reported higher stress levels than the clients. The author concluded that it is essential to include the family in nursing intervention.

Gilliss CL: Reducing family stress during and after coronary artery bypass surgery, *Nurs Clin North Am* 19(1):103, 1984.

inequalities deeply rooted in society. Class and ethnicity can produce differences in the access of families to society's resources and rewards, and this access creates differences in family life and most significantly in different life chances for its members (Zinn, Eitzen, 1990) (see research highlight). Distribution of wealth greatly affects the capacity to maintain health. "Low education, poverty, and low support feed on each other, magnify each other's impact *on* sickness in the family, and magnify the impact of sickness *in* the family," according to Ross et al (1990). Economic stability creates more opportunity for nutrition, rest, education, lack of stress, and better access to health care (Estes et al, 1984). Higher infant mortality rates and shortened life span of the poor and some minority groups show how inequality has an impact on health (see Chapter 2).

FAMILY NURSING: FAMILY AS CONTEXT AND AS CLIENT

The family can be approached as the environment or context within which the individual strives for health or as the client itself. The approach depends on the situation. If only one family member is receptive to nursing care, it is realistic and practical to view the family as context. When all family members are involved in the day-to-day care of one another, nursing intervention with one individual necessitates some change in the activities of the others. Both approaches—family as context and family as client—can be useful in providing effective nursing care.

Friedman (1986) suggests that care must be directed to the family as a whole, as well as to its members.

When nurses view the **family as context,** their primary focus is the health and development of an individual member existing within a specific environment (that is, the client's family). Although assessment, nursing diagnosis, planning, implementation, and evaluation concentrate on the individual's health status, the nurse also assesses the extent to which the family provides the individual's basic needs (see Chapter 29). These needs vary, depending on the individual's developmental level and situation. Families provide more than just material essentials, so their ability to help the client meet psychological needs must also be considered. Family members often need direct interventions themselves. For example, the hospitalized child's parents feel a great deal of stress, as does a spouse whose partner is undergoing surgery (see research highlight). Chronic illness is often particularly debilitating for family members because of feelings of powerlessness and changes in family relationships (Miller, 1983).

Although nurses have cared for families for years, it is only recently that nurse researchers have begun to study the **family as client** (Murphy, 1986). The family is viewed as more than the sum of its individual members. The family unit is the primary focus of nursing care because any nursing intervention with one member ultimately influences all members. Family patterns versus individual characteristics are studied. For example, a single, 25-year-old man lives at home with his parents and two younger siblings. He requests the assistance of the nurse in altering his diet and developing stress-management techniques to help him cope with his borderline hypertension, which is thought to be related to high-sodium intake, a stressful job, and continuing expectations by his family for participation in their activities. If the family is viewed as environment, the nurse focuses on the client as an individual. The nurse might assess the client's knowledge of high-sodium foods, strategies for reducing the number of high-sodium foods in the diet, realistic opportunities to reduce the number and extent of perceived stressors in work and family environments, and knowledge and skill in stress management such as relaxation or biofeedback techniques. If the family is viewed as client, the nurse would assess the family's current dietary patterns and its desire and resources for changing the patterns. The nurse also determines the demands placed on the hypertensive family member and explores the potential for redistributing the demands among other family members. The family's capabilities to support the hypertensive member's development and use of stress management are also assessed. The structure of the American health care system can make it difficult to provide effective nursing care to the family as a whole because the system focuses on individual health. However, the nurse must always be aware that clients are affected by their families and that clients affect their families.

 ## NURSING PROCESS FOR THE FAMILY

Family nursing process is the same, whether the focus is family as client or as environment. The nursing process is used in the same way as with individuals (that is, assessment, nursing diagnosis, planning, intervention, and evaluation). Friedman (1986) notes that the only difference is that the individual and family receive care. Assumptions underlying the family approach to the nursing process are that all individuals must be viewed within their family context, and families have an impact on individuals and individuals have an impact on families.

The goal of the family nurse is to help the family reach and maintain its maximum health in any given situation. Gillis et al (1989) point out that it is necessary to understand the distinction between family nursing and family therapy. They suggest that when a family is demonstrating overtly dysfunctional behavior patterns that require a dramatic change in the system, they must be referred to a family therapist. The nurse, however, can intervene with families whose behavioral patterns need some adjustment to cope with transitions or crises.

Bomar (1989) correctly notes that there are a number of highly sophisticated family assessment instruments available from a variety of disciplines; however, the ones developed by nurses lack adequate clinical testing. She has designed a tool for assessing

and measuring family health, and the reader is referred to her book, *Nurses and Family Health Promotion: Concepts, Assessment, and Interventions,* for an example of an in-depth measure that may be used in advanced nursing practice and a list of other family assessment tools.

 ## Assessment

Family assessment is an essential component of the nursing process (see box on p. 740). Although the family as a whole differs from individual members, the measure of family health must be more than a summation of the health of all members. Areas included in family assessment are the form, structure, and function of the family; its developmental stage; and its progress toward or accomplishment of developmental tasks. Cultural background is an important variable when assessing the family because race and ethnicity have an impact on structure and function and influence health beliefs and values.

The nurse begins assessment by determining the client's definition of and attitude toward family and the extent to which the family can be incorporated into the nursing process. To determine family form and membership, the nurse can ask whom the client considers family or with whom the client shares strong emotional feelings. If the client is unable to express a concept of family, the nurse can ask with whom the client lives, spends time, and shares confidences and then ask whether the client considers them to be family or like family. To further assess the family structure, the nurse asks questions that determine the power structure and patterning of roles and tasks. Examples include the following:

1. How are the tasks divided in your family?
2. Who does the laundry?
3. Who mows the lawn?
4. Who decides on where to go on vacation?

Because a moderately flexible structure is generally most beneficial to the family, nursing interventions may involve modulating the family patterns away from extremely rigid or flexible structures if either extreme causes problems in the health of an individual or the family. However, the nurse attempts to work within the family structure when providing care and does not attempt to change the structure.

The nurse assesses family functions such as the ability to provide emotional support for members, the ability to cope with its current health problem or situation, and the appropriateness of its goal setting (that is, whether the goals are realistic and obtainable considering the family's status and developmental stage). Although families' goals vary, measures of family health care must be flexible. The nurse also

Assessment Tool

The family assessment tool is used when the beginning student interviews family members and observes family interaction. It is only a *guideline* and is not meant to be all inclusive. The student must also assume that individual health histories accompany this assessment.

FAMILY FORM AND STRUCTURE

Names of adults _____ Ages_____
Relationship _____
Names of children   Ages

_____
_____
_____

Others living in home (include age, sex, relationship)
_____

Cultural background (include any pertinent health beliefs, child-rearing practices, related health concerns)
_____

Developmental stage _____
Progress toward accomplishment of developmental tasks _____
Concerns related to developmental stage _____

RESOURCES

Significant relatives and friends not occupying immediate residence _____
Strengths and coping skills _____
Ways the family obtains health services _____
Membership in community groups (e.g., church affiliation) _____
Education (formal and informal) _____
Finances (ability to meet current and future needs) _____

FAMILY PATTERNS

Persons working outside the home _____
Type of work _____ Number of hours _____
Satisfaction with work _____
Ways the housekeeping tasks are accomplished _____
Family members' satisfaction with the way tasks are divided _____
Ways that child-rearing responsibilities are divided _____
Person who makes the major decisions in the family _____
Person who makes day-to-day decisions _____
Family members' satisfaction with the way decisions are made _____

FAMILY FUNCTION
Goals

Long term _____
Short term _____
Individual family members' goals _____
Are individual and family goals appropriate, considering their current health problem and status? _____
How are individual family members and the family as a whole coping with their current health problem and status?
_____ _____ _____

Communication

Do husband and wife communicate regularly and effectively with each other? _____
Are family members able to communicate openly and honestly with each other? _____
Is conflict openly expressed and discussed? _____
Do family members respect each other's point of view? _____
Do family members offer emotional support to each other? _____

assesses whether the family is able to provide and allocate sufficient economic resources and whether its social network is extensive enough to provide support. Attainment of family developmental tasks is also a useful criterion of family health.

Nursing Diagnosis

Nursing assessment results in clustering pertinent data that support the nursing diagnosis and identifies inadequate or deficient functioning and interventions needed. The diagnostic label may include the family's health needs, current and potential health problems, level of wellness, or a combination of the above. In addition, the diagnostic statement should indicate possible causes and etiologies. Friedman (1986) notes the difficulty in defining discrete nursing diagnoses because information about the family is interrelated (see diagnoses and diagnostic process boxes).

The nursing diagnoses often focus on the family's ability to cope with its current situation, whether it is an acute illness or an anticipated developmental transition. Coping strategies can be adaptive or maladaptive. Appropriate use of external and internal resources allows the family to cope with day-to-day stressors and with unexpected occurrences that threaten its equilibrium and health. To cope effectively, the family needs to coordinate its member's

positive adaptive responses. A health crisis can be a growth experience and can result in greater family cohesiveness. Barbarin et al (1985) identify the following coping techniques used by parents of children with cancer: information seeking, problem solving, help seeking, maintenance of emotional balance, reliance on religion, optimism, denial, and acceptance. They suggest that parents' coping styles determine whether the experience of childhood cancer is destructive or produces growth.

Planning

When nursing diagnoses have been formulated, the next step is to plan a course of action with the family. Planning includes setting goals, identifying potential internal and external resources, choosing effective approaches, and setting priorities. The plan of care must be clearly understood by the family, and they must agree to it. Goal setting must be a mutual endeavor. The goals must be concrete and realistic, compatible with the developmental stage, and acceptable to family members. The nurse's care plan should include the following goals:

1. The client will use appropriate resources within the family.
2. The family will accomplish appropriate developmental tasks.

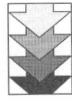

Examples of Nursing Diagnoses for a Family with a Hospitalized Adult Member

NANDA-APPROVED NURSING DIAGNOSES

Altered family processes related to:
- Sudden, unexpected illness
- Financial concerns
- Inability to problem solve
- Inadequate communication

Fear (individual family members) related to:
- Hospitalization
- Knowledge deficit

Powerlessness (individual family members) related to:
- Hospitalization
- Knowledge deficit

Ineffective family coping: compromised or *disabled* related to:
- Chronic illness
- Family disorganization

Impaired home maintenance management related to:
- Dysfunctional grieving
- Alteration in communication skills

Sample Nursing Diagnostic Process for a Family with a Hospitalized Adult Member

Assessment activities	Defining characteristics	Nursing diagnosis
Observe wife and husband interact during care activity.	Basic human needs of wife are neglected. Husband displays facial tension, poor eye contact, and quivering voice while interacting with wife.	*Ineffective family coping: compromised* related to husband's inadequate understanding of wife's physical limitations
Have husband describe personal reaction to wife's illness.	Husband expresses guilt over wife's illness. Husband describes inadequate understanding of wife's illness.	

3. Family members will understand the client's health problems.

4. The client will return to a functional state within the family environment.

At times, family members may need to take on the roles of care givers. Many of these care givers are older adults taking care of spouses (Chappell, 1991). In such cases, every health care decision has profound impact on both of their lives (Phillips, 1989). Illness often disrupts well-established family patterns and necessitates short- and long-term planning. The following scenario and care plan illustrate this point:

Mr. and Mrs. Smith, in their 70s, have recently celebrated their 50th wedding anniversary and have been living in Florida since Mr. Smith retired 10 years before. They have two married sons living in Iowa. Mr. and Mrs. Smith's marriage has been very traditional, with Mrs. Smith performing all the household tasks. They have many friends and are active in various church groups. Both have been comparatively healthy until 3 weeks before, when Mrs. Smith suffered a stroke that left her with left-sided weakness. Mrs. Smith participates in rehabilitation therapy daily, demonstrates a great deal of determination, and is making good progress. She is to be discharged in about a month to the care of her husband. Although Mr. Smith is anxious to take her home, his behavior suggests that he has unrealistic expectations of her current and future abilities. For example, he becomes impatient with her slowness at performing activities such as feeding herself and has stated that he expects her to "be her old self" as

soon as she goes home. Mrs. Smith has stated that their relationship is "strained" and that her husband often tells her that she is "just not trying hard enough to get well."

The nurse decides to include Mr. Smith in the care plan and develops short- and long-term goals for the couple. Short-term planning includes actions that will help Mr. Smith better understand the effects of the stroke and to recognize his wife's limitations. Long-term planning focuses on new adaptive patterns so that the couple can reach their maximal individual health and family functioning. For example, Mr. Smith will have to assume the majority of household tasks and essentially change roles with Mrs. Smith. The nurse realizes that this may difficult for both of them and refers them to a family therapist and family social worker. The nurse keeps in mind the couple's long marital history, their developmental stage, and the limitations and strengths inherent in both.

Implementation

After goals and actions have been defined, implementation begins. Interventions are strategies that help families adjust goals or are the processes by which the family attains them. Family interventions include nursing actions that increase members' abilities in a certain area, remove barriers to health care, and do things that the family cannot do for itself (Friedman, 1986). The nurse guides family members

---

 Sample Nursing Care Plan for Ineffective Family Coping: Compromised

Nursing diagnosis: *Ineffective family coping: compromised* related to husband's inadequate understanding of wife's physical limitations

Definition: Ineffective family coping: compromised is insufficient, ineffective, or compromised support, comfort, or assistance—usually by a supportive primary person (family member or close friend); client may need it to manage or master adaptive tasks related to his/her health challenge (Kim, McFarland, McLane, 1991).

Goals	Expected Outcomes	Interventions	Rationale
Husband will gain improved understanding of wife's physical limitations (3/25).	Husband will be able to identify activities appropriate for his wife to perform and activities with which he will have to assist her (3/21).	Discuss with husband effects of stroke and reasons it occurs, and provide reading material designed for family members of clients with strokes.	Accurate information will assist husband in interpreting wife's limitations (Phillips, 1989).
Husband will accept wife's physical limitations (3/30).	Husband will not demonstrate impatient behavior (such as telling his wife to "hurry up") while she performs activities (3/27).	Provide list of care giver support groups.	Group support allows care giver to share experiences, stresses, and coping methods.

in problem solving and provides practical service and concrete aid. In the previous example, one of the roles the nurse will need to adopt is that of educator. Providing accurate health information about diagnosis and prognosis helps the care giver to not "blame" the client and to interpret behavior correctly (Phillips, 1989). As a general framework, effective interventions for Mr. and Mrs. Smith focus on the needs of the care giver as an older adult. As Phillips (1989) states, "Caregivers are not born with the knowledge of how to be caregivers and elders are not born with the knowledge of how to accept dependency."

One approach for meeting goals is the use of family strengths. The nurse can help the family become aware of its own unique strengths, thereby increasing its potential and capabilities. Family strengths include clear communication, adaptability, healthy child-rearing practices, support and nurturing among family members, and the use of crisis for growth. The nurse can help the family focus on these strengths instead of its problems and weaknesses. For example, the nurse can point out that the Smiths' 50-year marriage must have endured many crises and transitions. Therefore they are likely to be able to adapt to this latest challenge.

 ## Evaluation

When the client's family functions as an environment, evaluation is client centered, although nursing measures may have involved assisting the client to adapt to the family environment. The response of the client is compared with predetermined outcomes.

When the family receives care as the client, the measure of family health must be more than a summation of the health of all family members. For example, the family's attainment of family developmental tasks may be a useful criterion. The nurse evaluates the family's change in functioning and its satisfaction with the new level of functioning.

Evaluation is an ongoing process. Goals and interventions are modified as needed. In addition to the evaluation box, examples of evaluative measures to determine whether a client uses appropriate family resources include the following:

1. Observing family members performing care-centered activities
2. Asking the client to identify ways to include family members in care

Examples of measures to determine accomplishment of developmental tasks include the following:

1. Observing the manner in which the family adjusts to the hospitalized client's return home

 ## Sample Evaluation of Interventions for Ineffective Family Coping: Compromised

Goal	Evaluative Measures	Expected Outcomes
Husband will gain improved understanding of wife's physical limitations by end of home visits (3/25).	Observe husband and wife interact.	Husband will be able to identify activities with which he will need to assist her by first home visit.
	Ask husband about activities wife will be able to perform and activities that will require assistance.	Husband will be able to identify activities that his wife will be able to perform on her own by second home visit.

2. Asking the client to discuss ways to incorporate care measures within the family's lifestyle
3. Observing family members' abilities to maintain current roles and relationships

Examples of evaluative measures to determine the family members' understanding of the client's health problem include the following:

1. Observing the family members regarding the nature and implications of the client's illness
2. Asking family members about the nature and implications of the client's illness

Examples of evaluative measures to determine whether a client has returned to a functional state within the family environment include the following:

1. Observing the client perform self-care at home
2. Observing the client discuss ways that care measures have been adapted to the home

 ## SUMMARY

Although the structure and form of the American family are changing, the family's impact on health is as significant now as ever. Different family forms often involve many health concerns and resources for resolving those concerns. When the family faces health problems, the nurse assesses its structure and function and applies the nursing process, whether the family is viewed as a significant environment within which the client maintains health or viewed as the client itself. The nurse maximizes therapeutic effectiveness by recognizing the family's influence and using its resources to promote individual and family health.

CHAPTER 23 REVIEW

Key Concepts

- The family has a significant impact on the lives of its members.
- Family members influence one another's health beliefs, practices, and status.
- Because the concept of family is highly individual, the nurse should base care on the client's attitude toward family rather than on an inflexible definition of the family.
- Specific family forms tend to have typical family health problems with which the nurse should be familiar.
- The family's structure and functioning and relative position in society significantly influence its health and ability to respond to health problems.
- The nurse can view the family as an important context for the individual family member or can view the family unit as the client. The approach for any family depends in part on the situation.
- Measures of family health involve more than a summation of individual members' health.

Key Terms

Blended families, p. 734
Extended family, p. 733
Family, p. 733
Family as client, p. 738
Family as context, p. 738

Family of origin, p. 733
Family of procreation, p. 733
Nuclear family, p. 733
Single-parent families, p. 734

Critical Thinking Exercises

1. After your assessment, you note that Mr. Jones has recently become unemployed, his wife has chronic health problems, and there are two school-age children at home. What are the potential threats to the family from these stressors? What anticipatory interventions can be designed to minimize these threats?

2. Mrs. Weber is 31 years old and newly widowed with three children under the age of 10. What resources can nurses use to assist this mother in adapting to the abrupt transition to being a single parent?

3. Mr. and Mrs. Kline are in their mid-40s with two teenage children. Both sets of the Klines' parents are in their 80s and have chronic health problems. How can you assist Mr. and Mrs. Kline in developing extended resources to aid in caring for their parents and at the same time maintain the responsibilities of their own family unit?

REFERENCES

Adams BN: *The family: a sociological interpretation*, New York, 1986, Harcourt Brace Jovanovich.

Barbarin O et al: Stress, coping, and marital functioning among parents of children with cancer, *J Marriage Fam* 47:473, 1985.

Berardo FM: Trends and directions in family research, *J Marriage Fam* 52(4):809, 1990.

Bomar PJ: *Nurses and family health promotion: concepts, assessment, and interventions*, Baltimore, 1989, Williams & Wilkins.

Chappell NL: Living arrangements and sources of caregiving, *J Gerontol* 46(1):S1, 1991.

Chiriboga DA: Social supports. In Maddox G, editor: *The encyclopedia of aging*, New York, 1987, Springer.

Coleman M, Ganong LH: Remarriage and stepfamilies, *J Marriage Fam* 52(4):925, 1990.

Engebretson JC: Stepmothers as first-time parents: their needs and problems, *Pediatr Nurs* 8:387, 1982.

Eshleman JR: *The family*, ed 6, Boston, 1991, Allyn & Bacon.

Estes C et al: *Political economy, health, and aging*, Boston, 1984, Little, Brown.

Friedman M: *Family nursing: theory and assessment*, ed 2, New York, 1986, Appleton-Century-Crofts.

Gillis CL et al: *Toward a science of family nursing*, New York, 1989, Addison-Wesley.

Glick P: The family life cycle and social change, *Fam Relations* 34:123, 1989.

Kim MJ, McFarland GK, McLane AM: *Pocket guide to nursing diagnoses*, ed 4, St Louis, 1991, Mosby–Year Book.

McCubbin H, Dahl B: *Marriage and family: individuals and life cycles*, New York, 1985, Free Press.

McCubbin HR, McCubbin M: Typologies of resilient families: emerging roles of social class and ethnicity, *Fam Relations* 37:247, 1988.

McGoldrick M, Carter E: The stage of the family life cycle. In Henslin J, editor: *Marriage and family in a changing society*, New York, 1985, Free Press.

Miller JF: *Coping with chronic illness*, Philadelphia, 1983, Davis.

Murphy S: Family study and nursing research, *Image J Nurs Sch* 18(4):170, 1986.

Norton AJ, Moorman JE: Current trends in marriage and divorce among American women, *J Marriage Fam* 49:3, 1987.

Phillips LR: Elder-family caregiver relationships, *Nurs Clin North Am* 24(24):795, 1989.

Romanczuk A: Helping the stepparent parent, *MCN* 12:106, 1987.

Ross CE et al: Impact of family on health, *J Marriage Fam* 52(4):1059, 1990.

Skolnick A: *The intimate environment: explaining marriage and the family*, 1987, Little, Brown.

US Bureau of the Census: *Statistical abstract of the United States: 1987*, ed 108, Washington, DC, 1987, US Government Printing Office.

Zinn MB, Eitzen DS: *Diversity in American families*, ed 2, New York, 1990, Harper & Row.

ADDITIONAL READINGS

Amato P: Family processes in one-parent, stepparent, and intact families: the child's point of view, *J Marriage Fam* 49(2):327, 1987.

Ballie V, Norbeck JS, Barnes LE: Stress, social support, and psychological distress of the family caregivers of the elderly, *Nurs Res* 37(4):217, 1988.

Gillis CL: Reducing family stress during and after coronary artery bypass surgery, *Nurs Clin North Am* 19(1):103, 1984.

Gillis CL: Family nursing research: theory and practice, *Image J Nurs Sch* 23(1):19, 1991.

Glenn ND, Coleman MT: *Family relations: a reader*, Belmont, Calif, 1988, Dorsey Press.

Lauer RH, Lauer JC: *Marriage and family: the quest for intimacy*, Dubuque, Ia, 1991, Wm C Brown.

Mercer RT, Ferketich SL: Predictors of family functioning eight months following birth, *Nurs Res* 39(2):76, 1990.

Sprey J: *Fashioning family theory: new approaches*, London, 1990, Sage.

Sund K, Ostwald SK: Dual-earner families' stress levels and personal and life-style–related variables, *Nurs Res* 34(6):357, 1985.

Sussman MB, Steinmetz SK: *Handbook of marriage and the family*, New York, 1987, Plenum.

Ulbrich PM, Warheit GJ, Zimmerman RS: Race, socioeconomic status, and psychological distress: a vulnerability, *J Health Soc Behav* 30(1):131, 1989.

CHAPTER 24

Conception Through Preschool

OBJECTIVES

Mastery of content in this chapter will enable the student to:

- Define the key terms listed.
- Describe seven principles of growth and development.
- Discuss the factors influencing growth and development.
- Compare and discuss theories of growth and development.
- Discuss physiological and psychosocial health concerns during the transition of the child from intrauterine to extrauterine life.
- Explain the concept of critical periods of development and identify factors that can disturb or promote optimal development of the child.
- Describe characteristics of the physical growth of the unborn child, infant, toddler, and preschooler.
- Describe cognitive and psychosocial development from birth to 6 years.
- Describe the bonding that occurs between parent and child.
- Describe variables influencing how children learn about and perceive their health status.
- Identify areas in which the parents of well and hospitalized children can benefit from the nurse's anticipatory guidance.
- Describe the use of the nursing process to individualize the nursing care plan for the hospitalized child.

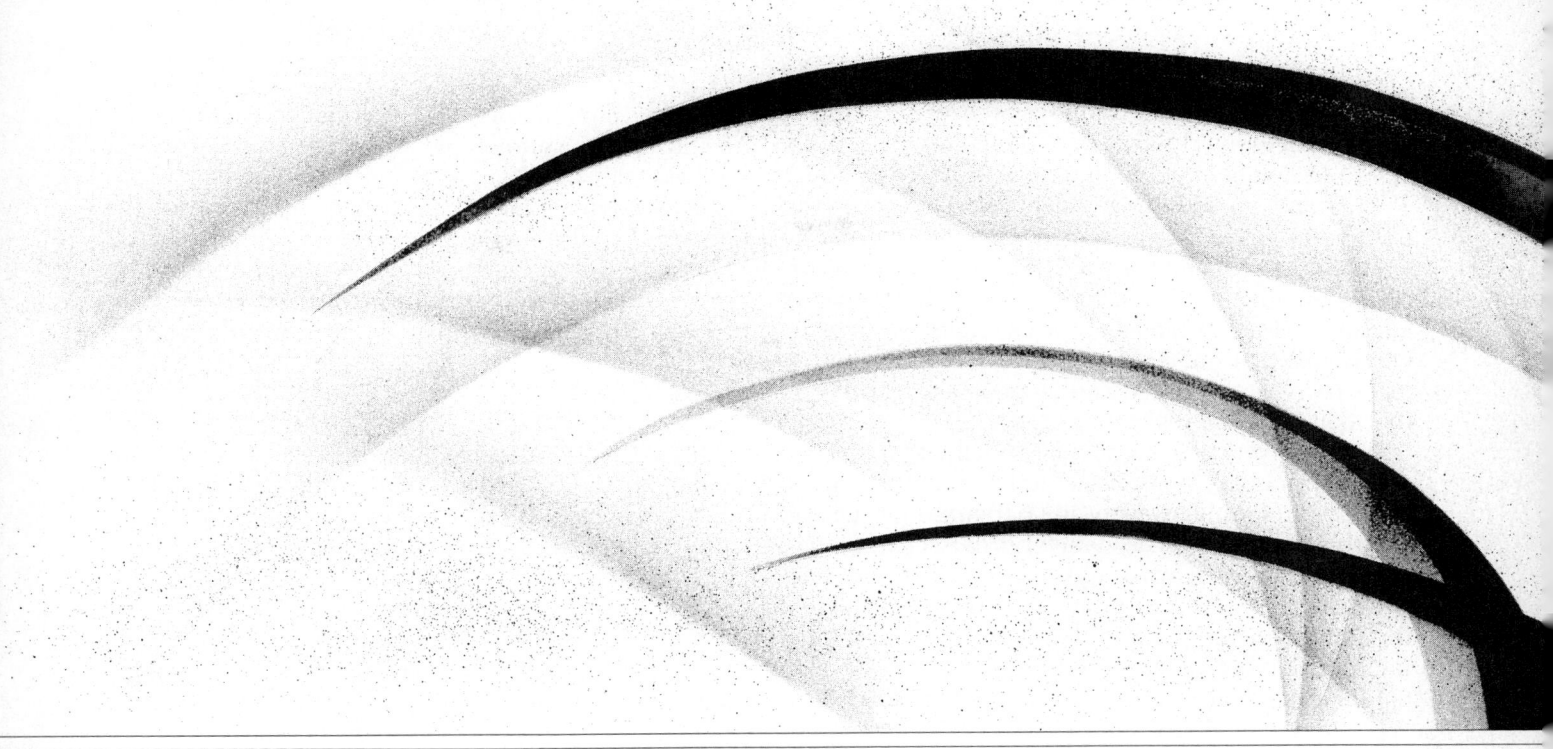

CHAPTER OUTLINE

Growth and Development Theory
    Definitions
Principles of Growth and Development
Stages of Growth and Development
    Major factors influencing growth and development
Theories of Human Development
Selecting a Developmental Framework for Nursing
Conception
    Intrauterine life
    Physical development
    Cognitive development
    Psychosocial development
Transition from Intrauterine to Extrauterine Life
    Physical health concerns
    Psychosocial concerns
Neonate
    Physical development
    Cognitive development
    Psychosocial development

Infant
    Physical development
    Cognitive development
    Psychosocial development
    Perception of health
Toddler
    Physical development
    Cognitive development
    Psychosocial development
    Perception of health
Preschooler
    Physical development
    Cognitive development
    Psychosocial development
    Perception of health
Hospitalization and Illness
Nursing Process and the Child
    Assessment
    Nursing diagnosis
    Planning
    Implementation
    Evaluation

Children are the future of the world. Understanding children and their growth and development is essential to promoting health and establishing healthful patterns. The nurse must have a clear understanding of normal or expected growth and behavior in early developmental stages to guide and promote normalcy and to detect and prevent abnormalities. For example, without the knowledge that the average 2½- to 3-year old child is toilet trained, the nurse cannot promote learning of this skill at an appropriate age.

Nursing practice based on principles of growth and development is organized and directed at helping children and families adapt to changing internal and external conditions. This chapter discusses principles and concepts of growth and development and their application to health promotion from conception through preschool. It also demonstrates that a good understanding of growth and development is essential for individualizing the care of ill children.

 ## GROWTH AND DEVELOPMENT THEORY

Human growth and development are orderly, predictable processes beginning with conception and continuing until death. All persons progress through definite phases of growth and development, but the pace and behavior of this progression are highly individual. Children must learn to walk before they can run, but one child may walk at 10 months, and another may not walk until 15 months.

The ability to progress through each developmental phase influences a person's health. The success or failure experienced within a phase affects the ability to complete subsequent phases. If an individual repeatedly fails to develop, inadequacies result and thus health may be threatened. However, if the individual experiences repeated successes, competencies that help maintain and promote health result. A child not learning to walk by 18 or 20 months, for example, demonstrates delayed gross motor ability that slows exploration and manipulation of the environment. A child walking by 10 months is able to explore and find stimulation in the environment, thereby enhancing learning.

Because nursing promotes the health of individuals of all ages, the nurse must understand the growth and development process, understand its theories and principles, identify its stages, identify factors influencing it, and assess the individual's ability to respond in a healthy manner. Knowledge and understanding of these concepts provide a foundation for delivering health care. A developmental approach allows the nurse to organize knowledge about human behavior into common patterns that can be applied to individuals.

A developmental perspective helps the nurse understand *why* commonalities and variations exist and how they influence health. With this knowledge the nurse can provide care in a manner that addresses the client's unique needs and developmental level.

Definitions

Growth and development are synchronous processes that are interdependent in the healthy individual. A person experiences quantitative and qualitative changes in growth and development.

Physical Growth

Physical **growth** is the quantitative, or measurable, aspect of an individual's increase in physical measurements. Measurable growth indicators include height, weight, and dental, skeletal, and sexual age. Increases in these indicators demonstrate growth. For example, children generally double birth weight by 6 months of age and double height by 36 months. Also children usually have all their primary teeth before 3 years of age and begin to lose them at the end of the preschool period.

Development

The qualitative, or behavioral, aspects of progressive adaptation to the environment are called ***development***. An example of these qualitative changes is increased functioning capacity resulting from mastery of several smaller skills. For instance, a significant qualitative and observable change for preschoolers is participating in telephone conversations with their parents. Before developing this capacity, they must develop a small vocabulary, learn to put words together in phrases and sentences, and develop a cognitive understanding of **object permanence** (that a person or object out of sight still exists).

Maturation

Maturation is the process of becoming fully developed and grown. It involves an individual's biological ability, physiological condition, and desire to learn more mature behaviors. To mature, the individual may have to relinquish previous behaviors and learning, integrate new patterns into existing behaviors, or both. Maturation influences the sequence and timing of the changes associated with growth and development. For example, the infant relinquishes crawling for walking because it permits more extensive investigation of the environment and more learning. However, the infant cannot walk until the biological ability and structures to perform the action (that is, increased muscle cells and tone) have developed.

Critical Periods of Development

Stages of growth and development involve the concept of "critical periods of development." A **critical period** is a specific span of time during which the environment has its greatest impact on the individual (Papalia, Olds, 1989). During these critical periods, some form of sensory stimulation is necessary for developmental progression. Without stimulation, task completion is difficult or unattainable. For example, the toddler who has not been encouraged to learn to walk during a set time period may have difficulty learning to walk at another time. Therefore develop-mental progression depends on the timing and degree of stimulation, as well as on the readiness to be stimulated by the environment. A stimulus provided too early may not be useful. For example, an 18-month-old child cannot learn to write, regardless of the intensity of the stimuli, whereas a 6-year-old has the maturational readiness and ability to learn to write if stimulated to do so.

PRINCIPLES OF GROWTH AND DEVELOPMENT

Some principles of growth and development are true for all people. These commonalities are expressed by the following concepts:

Developmental Age Periods

PRENATAL PERIOD: CONCEPTION TO BIRTH

GERMINAL: conception to approximately 2 wk

EMBRYONIC: 2-8 wk

FETAL: 8-40 wk (birth)

A rapid growth rate and total dependency make this one of the most crucial periods in the developmental process. The relationship between maternal health and certain manifestations in the newborn emphasizes the importance of adequate prenatal care to the health and well-being of the infant.

INFANCY PERIOD: BIRTH TO 12 OR 18 MO

NEONATAL: Birth to 28 days

INFANCY: 1 to approximately 12 mo

The infancy period is one of rapid motor, cognitive, and social development. Through mutuality with the care giver (parent), the infant establishes a basic trust in the world and the foundation for future interpersonal relationships. The critical first month of life, although part of the infancy period, is often differentiated from the remainder because of the major physical adjustments to extrauterine existence and the psychological adjustment of the parent.

EARLY CHILDHOOD: 1-6 YR

TODDLER: 1 to 3 yr

PRESCHOOL: 3 to 6 yr

This period, which extends from the time children attain upright locomotion until they enter school, is characterized by intense activity and discovery. It is a time of marked physical and personality development. Motor development advances steadily. Children at this age acquire language and wider social relationships, learn role standards, gain self-control and mastery, develop increasing awareness of dependence and independence, and begin to develop self-concepts.

MIDDLE CHILDHOOD: 6-11 OR 12 YR

Frequently referred to as the "school age," this period of development is one in which the child is directed away from the family group and is centered around the wider world of peer relationships. There is steady advancement in physical, mental, and social development, with emphasis on developing skill competencies. Social cooperation and early moral development take on more importance with relevance for later life stages. This is a critical period in the development of self-concept.

LATE CHILDHOOD: 11-21 YR

PREADOLESCENCE: 10-13 yr

LATE ADOLESCENCE: 18-21 yr

The tumultuous period of rapid maturation and change known as *adolescence* is considered a transitional period that begins at the onset of puberty and extends to the point of entry into the adult world, which may occur after high school graduation, college graduation, or later. Biological and personality maturation are accompanied by physical and emotional turmoil, and there is a redefining of the self-concept. In late adolescence the child begins to internalize all previously learned values and focus on an individual, rather than a group, identity.

Modified from Whaley LF, Wong DL: *Nursing care of infants and children,* ed 4, St Louis, 1991, Mosby–Year Book.

1. Individuals have adaptive potential for qualitative and quantitative changes by receiving stimuli from and giving stimuli to the environment.
2. Individuals derive uniqueness from the interaction of heredity and environment.
3. The primary goal of development is achievement of potential (self-realization or self-actualization).

The basic principles of growth and development follow:

1. Development is orderly and follows a set sequence.
2. Development is directional and proceeds along the following body axes:
   a. Cephalocaudal, in which growth proceeds from the head to the lower parts of the body
   b. Proximodistal, in which development proceeds from the central (proximal) areas of the body to the outer (peripheral)
   c. Differentiation, in which development proceeds from simple to complex
3. Development is complex, yet predictable, occurring with a consistent pattern and chronology.
4. Development is unique to individuals and their genetic potential, and each individual tends to seek a maximal potential for development.
5. Development occurs through conflict and adaptation, and different aspects develop at different rates, creating periods of equilibrium and disequilibrium.
6. Development involves challenges for individuals in the form of certain tasks specific to age and ability.
7. Developmental tasks require practice and energy, the focus of which varies with each developmental stage and task accomplished.

STAGES OF GROWTH AND DEVELOPMENT

Human growth and development are intricate, complex processes. Although these processes are continuous, they are often divided into stages organized by age groups. Although this chronological division is arbitrary, it is based on the timing and sequence of developmental tasks that the individual must accomplish to progress to another stage. Developmental periods are listed in the box on p. 749.

Major Factors Influencing Growth and Development

The human being is a complex, open system influenced by natural forces from within and from the en-

vironment. Interaction between these forces affects development. In general, natural factors set the limits for development, whereas external factors present opportunities for achieving that potential. The most influential forces of nature are heredity and temperament, whereas family and peers are the primary external forces (Table 24-1).

THEORIES OF HUMAN DEVELOPMENT

Since the beginning of this century, research into human growth and development has led to a number of developmental theories. These theories vary in the way humans are viewed and in the aspect of development emphasized. Some theories view development as a continuous process, moving from the simple to the more complex. Others consider it as discontinuous, with alternating periods of relative equilibrium and disequilibrium. When providing care, health care professionals often use different theoretical frameworks, which may complicate communication between them. Therefore to communicate effectively with other health professionals when providing coordinated health care, the nurse must be familiar with the common theories (Table 24-2 on pp. 752-755). No one framework addresses all developmental areas.

According to Freud, pleasure shifts from one bodily erogenous zone to another. A child's maturation level determines when shift occurs. If gratified too much or too little, the child may become emotionally stuck (fixated) at that stage. Freud did not specifically define "too much or too little."

According to Erikson (1963), each stage has a personality crisis involving a major conflict that is critical at that time. The developing ego is greatly affected by societal and cultural influences, and the successful outcome of each crisis includes development of a particular virtue. The successful mastery of each conflict is built on satisfactory completion of the previous core conflict. This theory recognizes the importance of heredity and environment and has epigenetic basis. Development is predetermined by genetic principles and proceeds along an age-stage pathway influenced by persons and events in the environment.

In Maslow's theory of human needs (1971), the hierarchical order of needs flows upward from basic human needs.

Piaget views the development of the mind as occurring through adaptation to the environment via assimilation (fitting new information into existing cognitive structure [schema]) and accommodation

TABLE 24-1   Major Factors Influencing Growth and Development

Factors	Relevant Influences
FORCES OF NATURE	
Heredity	Genetic endowment includes sex, race, hair and eye color, physical growth, and stature.
Temperament	Temperament is characteristic psychological mood with which child is born and includes behavioral styles of easy, slow-to-warm, and difficult.
EXTERNAL FORCES	
Family	Family purpose is to protect its members.
	Family functions include means for survival, security, assistance with emotional and social development, assistance with maintenance of relationships, instruction about society and world, and assistance in learning roles and behaviors.
	Family influences through its values, beliefs, customs, and specific patterns of interaction and communication.
	Ordinal position and sex influence individual's interaction and communication in family.
Peer group	Peer group provides new and different learning environment.
	Peer group provides different patterns and structures of interaction and communication necessitating different style of behavior.
	Functions of peer group include allowing individual to learn about success and failure; to validate and challenge thoughts, feelings, and concepts; to receive acceptance, support, and rejection as unique person apart from family; and to achieve group purposes by meeting demands, pressures, and expectations.
Life experiences	Life experiences and learning processes allow individual to develop by applying what has been learned to what needs to be learned.
	Learning process involves series of steps: recognition of need to know task; mastery of skills to perform task; mastery of task; expertise in performing task, which expands capabilities; integration into whole functioning; and use of accumulated skills and experiences to develop repertoire of effective behavior.
Health environment	Level of health affects individual's responsiveness to environment.
Prenatal health	Preconception (e.g., genetic and chromosomal factors, maternal age, health) and postconception (e.g., nutrition, weight gain, use of tobacco and alcohol, medical problems, use of prenatal services) factors affect fetal growth and development.
Nutrition	Growth is regulated by dietary factors. Adequacy of nutrients influences whether and how physiological needs, as well as subsequent growth and development needs, are met.
Rest, sleep, and exercise	Balance between rest or sleep and exercise is essential to rejuvenating body. Imbalances diminish growth, whereas equilibrium reinforces physiological and psychological health.
State of health	Illness or injury potentially hampers growth and development. Nature and duration of health problem influence its impact. Prolonged injury or illness leaves individual less able to cope and respond to demands and tasks of developmental stage.
Living environment	Factors affecting growth and development include season, climate, housing, and socioeconomic status.

(changing schema to deal with new information). Striving for balance between the organism and the outside environment occurs through these two processes. Cognitive development within and between stages is a function of maturation, experience, social interaction, and equilibration. Piaget emphasizes genetics in his theory based on epigenesis. Piaget also emphasizes interaction by stressing that the environment provides "food for thought." This theory places humans in an active learning role.

Kohlberg (1969) contends that cognitive development underlies the progression of a person's morality from level to level. These stages occur in the same order, regardless of culture. Individuals differ in how quickly and how far they progress through these stages.

TABLE 24-2 Summary of Development According to Stage Theorists

Stages and Ages	Characteristics of Stages	Theory Addendum
FREUD'S PSYCHOSEXUAL THEORY		
Oral-sensory (birth to 12-18 mo) (infancy)	Activities involving mouth such as sucking, biting, and chewing are chief source of pleasure.	Child deprived of sufficient sucking might attempt to satisfy this need later in life through activities such as gum chewing, smoking, and overeating.
Anal-muscular (12-18 mo to 3 yr) (toddlerhood)	Sensual gratification is derived from retention and expulsion of feces. Smearing is common activity.	External conflicts may be encountered when toilet training is attempted and later result in behaviors such as constipation, tardiness, or stinginess.
Phallic-locomotion (3-6 yr) (preschool)	Manipulation of genitalia results in pleasurable sensations. Masturbation begins and sexual curiosity becomes evident.	Emergence of Oedipus and Electra complexes for males and females respectively, occurs. Brashness, bashfulness, and timidity may be expressions of fixation at this stage.
Latency (6 yr to puberty) (school-age)	This is tranquil period when Freud believed sexual drives were dormant; however, child may engage in erogenous activities with same-sex peers.	Child's use of coping and defense mechanisms emerge at this time; any sexual interest may be sublimated through vigorous play and skill acquisition.
Genital (puberty through adulthood) (adolescence and adulthood)	Genitalia become center of sexual tension and pleasure. Sexual hormone production stimulates development of heterosexual relationships.	This is time of biological upheaval, when immature emotional interactions often occur in early phase. In time, ability to give and receive mature love develops.
ERIKSON'S PSYCHOSOCIAL THEORY		
Trust versus mistrust (birth to 1 yr) (infancy) Mode: taking in and getting Virtue: hope	Care giver's satisfaction of infant's basic needs for food and sucking, warmth and comfort, and love and security in consistent and sensitive manner results in trust.	When basic needs of infant are not met or are met inadequately, infant becomes suspicious, fearful, and mistrusting. This is evidenced by poor eating, sleeping, and elimination behaviors.
Autonomy versus doubt and shame (1-3 yr) (toddlerhood) Mode: holding on and letting go Virtue: will	Child develops beginning independence while gaining control over bodily functions of undressing and dressing, walking, talking, feeding self, and toileting. Self-control begins.	If toddler's developing independence is discouraged by parents, child may doubt personal abilities; if child is made to feel bad when attempts to be autonomous fail, child develops shame.
Initiative versus guilt (3-6 yr) (preschool) Mode: intrusive attack and conquest Virtue: purpose	Child develops initiative when planning and trying out new things. Behavior of child is characterized as vigorous, imaginative, and intrusive. Conscience and identification with same-sex parent develop.	Parental restrictiveness may prevent child from developing initiative. Guilt may arise when child undertakes activities in conflict with those of parents. Child must learn to initiate activities without infringing on rights of others.
Industry versus inferiority (6-12 yr to puberty) (school-age) Mode: doing and producing Virtue: competence	Child wins recognition by demonstration of skill and production of things and develops self-esteem through achievements. Child is greatly influenced by teachers and school.	Feelings of inferiority may occur when adults perceive child's attempt to learn how things work through manipulation to be silly or troublesome. Lack of success in school, development of physical skills, and making of friends also contribute to inferiority.

TABLE 24-2 Summary of Development According to Stage Theorists—cont'd		
Stages and Ages	Characteristics of Stages	Theory Addendum
Identify versus role confusion or diffusion (puberty to 18-21 yr) (adolescence) Virtue: fidelity	Individual develops integrated sense of "self." Peers have major influence over behavior. Major decision is to determine vocational goal.	Failure to develop sense of personal identity may lead to role confusion, which often results in feelings of inadequacy, isolation, and indecisiveness. Psychosocial moratorium provides extra time for making vocational decision.
Intimacy versus isolation (18-21 to 40 yr) (young adulthood) Mode: loving Virtue: love	Task is to develop close and sharing relationships with others, which may include sexual partner.	Individual unsure of self-identity will have difficulty developing intimacy. Person unwilling or unable to share self will be lonely.
Generativity versus self-absorption or stagnation (40-65 yr) (middle adulthood) Mode: nurturing Virtue: care	Mature adult is concerned with establishing and guiding next generation. Adult looks beyond self and expresses concern for future of world in general.	Self-absorbed adult will be preoccupied with personal well-being and material gains. Preoccupation with self leads to stagnation of life.
Ego integrity versus despair (65 yr to death) (older adulthood) Mode: acceptance Virtue: wisdom	Older adult can look back with sense of satisfaction and acceptance of life and death.	Unsuccessful resolution of this crisis may result in sense of despair in which individual views life as series of misfortunes, disappointments, and failures.
MASLOW'S THEORY OF HUMAN NEED		
Physiological needs Safety needs Belongingness and love needs Esteem needs Self-actualization	Physiological needs include food, beverages, and sleep. Satisfying safety needs allows individual to feel safe and secure. Belongingness allows individual to affiliate with and be accepted by others. Esteem allows individual to gain approval of others. Self-fulfillment potential is recognized.	Theory of motivation depicts individual driven to fulfill potential, capacities, and talents to become unique being. Person moves up and down hierarchy as life situations change.
PIAGET'S THEORY OF COGNITIVE DEVELOPMENT		
Sensorimotor (birth to 2 yr)	Child learns about world through sensory and motor activities.	Child slowly develops concept that people and objects have permanence, even though they are no longer visible.
Reflex activities (birth to 1 mo)	Child exercises inborn reflexes and gains some control over them.	Modified reflexes become more efficient. Sucking is more effective and selective.
Primary circular reactions (1-4 mo)	Infant repeats pleasurable actions that first occur by chance. Activities focus on body of infant; coordination begins.	Eye, eye-ear, and hand-mouth coordination develop, and activities such as thumb sucking and bottle sucking become more intentional and proficient.
Secondary circular reactions (4-8 mo)	Child attempts to reproduce interesting, pleasant events in environment. Interest goes beyond body.	Infant searches for object dropped and recognizes partially hidden object. Child begins to associate two behaviors such as cradle position and feeding.

Continued.

TABLE 24-2 Summary of Development According to Stage Theorists—cont'd

Stages and Ages	Characteristics of Stages	Theory Addendum
Coordination of secondary schemes (8-12 mo)	Child puts together skills used earlier to reach goal in new situation.	Child will crawl across room to get desired toy and search for hidden objects where they were previously hidden.
Tertiary circular reactions (12-18 mo) ("trial and error")	Child actively explores world and varies actions to see novelty of object, event, or situation. Trial and error are used to problem solve.	Child might try to get toy out of small opening of container with hand first and then turn it upside down and hit it so that toy falls out. Child comprehends series of object displacements if visible.
Invention of new means through mental combinations (18-24 mo) ("representation")	Toddler begins creating mental images and thus can devise new ways to deal with environment. Child begins to think about events without resorting to action.	Child attains true object permanence and will search for objects they have not seen hidden; for example, toddler will look many places for bottle. Insight is demonstrated by looking for bottle in refrigerator.
Preoperational (2-7 yr)	Child develops representational system and uses symbols such as words to represent people, places, and objects.	Preoperational concepts are limited by ability to focus on only one aspect at time (centration), and thought often seems illogical because child reasons from one specific to another (e.g., car hit dog because boy was mad at it).
Preconceptual (2-4 yr)	Child is primarily egocentric. Perceptual-bound and transductive thinking begin; child is animistic.	Deferred imitation (imitation of observed action after time has passed) demonstrates use of symbolism.
Intuitive (4-7 yr)	Child begins to figure things out but cannot explain them rationally. Child is unable to consider parts as composing whole.	Intuitive concepts allow classification of items by one attribute, usually color or shape (e.g., inability to focus on more than one characteristic at time).
Concrete operations (7-11 yr)	Ability to understand law of conservation results in logical thought patterns and mental operations such as reversibility, decentering, seriation, transformation, classification of two or more attributes, and inductive and deductive reasoning.	Limitations are inability of child to understand abstractions. Child's thinking is restricted to immediate and physical. School-ager can reason about what is but cannot hypothesize about what may be and thus cannot think about future problems (e.g., ability to play game of checkers).
Formal operations (develops 11-15 yr, used throughout life)	Ability to think in abstract manner develops, and scientific reasoning emerges. Initially, thought is rigid, but it becomes adaptable and flexible.	Adolescent may confuse ideal with practical but, when confronted with problem (real or hypothetical), can suggest number of solutions. Ability to consider moral and political issues from variety of perspectives is present.

KOHLBERG'S THEORY OF MORAL REASONING

Premoral level (birth to 9 yr)	There is little awareness, which is socially acceptable moral behavior. Control is external.	Infant defers to power and authority. Life is valued for number and power of possessions.
Punishment and obedience orientation (birth to 6 yr)	Rules of others are followed to avoid punishment.	Child integrates labels of *good* and *bad* and *right* and *wrong* into

TABLE 24-2 Summary of Development According to Stage Theorists—cont'd

Stages and Ages	Characteristics of Stages	Theory Addendum
Naively egoistic orientation (6-9 yr)	Child conforms to rules out of self-interest; child reasons that reward or favor will be earned.	behavior in terms of the consequences of actions. Elements of bargaining, equal sharing, and fairness are evident. Life is valued for how child can satisfy needs of others.
Conventional morality (9-13 yr)	Efforts are made to please other persons. Control is becoming internal.	Child is loyal and concerned with maintaining family expectations regardless of consequences.
"Good boy, nice girl" (9-10 yr)	Desire to please and help others is foremost. Child conforms to avoid rejection.	Life is valued for how good interpersonal relationships are (identify with emotionally important persons).
Authority maintaining morality	Child does duty to avoid criticism by authorities.	Identification shifts to religious or social institutions such as school.
Postconventional level of morality (13 yr to death)	Individual attains true morality. Conduct control is internal.	Attainment of true morality occurs after formal operations have been reached. Not everyone reaches this level.
Contractual and legalistic orientation	Individual selects moral principles by which to live and obeys laws.	Individual is careful not to violate rights and wills of others. Moral and legal views conflict. Person will work to change laws.
Universal ethical-principle orientation	Individual behaves in way that respects dignity of all.	This stage is rarely attained. If internal set of ideas are violated, guilt results.

SELECTING A DEVELOPMENTAL FRAMEWORK FOR NURSING

Providing nursing care to clients of all developmental stages is easier when planning is based on a theoretical framework. An organized, systematic approach ensures that client needs are assessed and met by the care plan. If nursing care is delivered only as a series of isolated actions, some of the client's developmental needs may be overlooked. A developmental approach encourages organized care directed at the client's current level of functioning to motivate self-direction and health promotion. For example, understanding an adolescent's need to be independent should prompt the nurse to establish a contract about the care plan and its implementation.

The developmental approach also has advantages for clients. Their capabilities are used, and they are actively involved in their own care. Total health is also promoted because the nurse is aware of clients' developmental stages and the directions in which they are headed. Therefore the nurse can focus on

activities that foster developmental task completion. For example, nurses might encourage toddlers to feed themselves to advance their developing independence and thus promote their sense of autonomy.

CONCEPTION

From the moment of conception, human development proceeds at a rapid rate. Most intrauterine health problems are caused by genetic and environmental factors. During the prenatal period, the embryo grows from a single cell to a complex, physiological being. All major organ systems develop in utero, with some functioning before birth. The psychosocial being also begins to emerge during gestation.

Intrauterine Life

Intrauterine life generally lasts 9 calendar or 10 lunar months. The organism's life begins after sexual

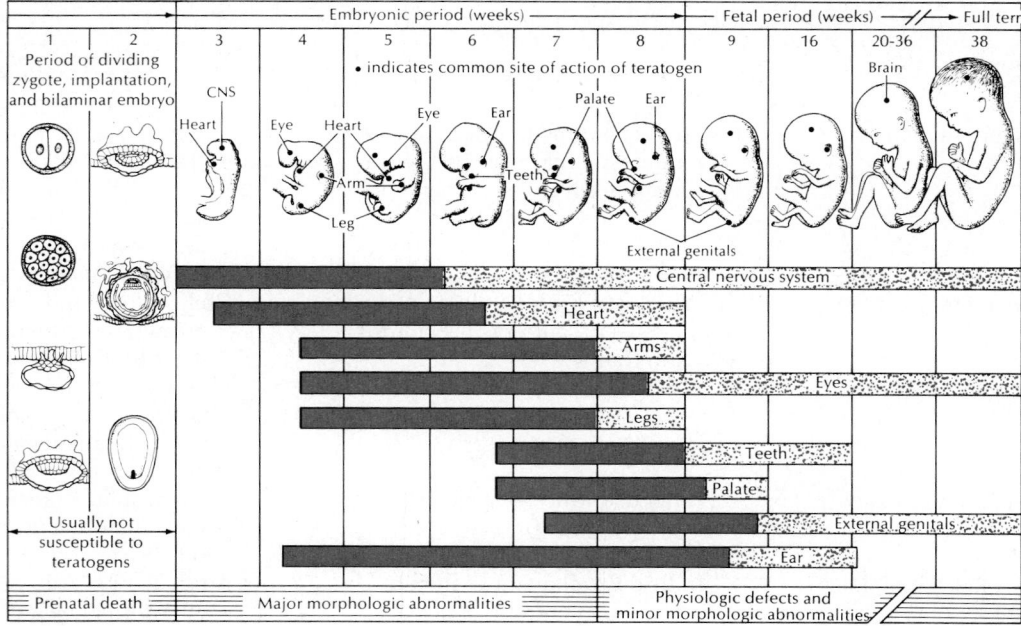

Fig. 24-1   Periods of organ differentiation.
From Whaley LF, Wong DL: *Nursing care of infants and children*, ed 4, St Louis, 1991, Mosby–Year Book.

intercourse has occurred, when the ovum is penetrated by one sperm. Fertilization often takes place in the fallopian tube, usually within 12 to 24 hours after the ovum is released from the ovary. The ovum and sperm fuse, and the material from both cell nuclei unites. The organism then has its full genetic complement in one pair of sex chromosomes and 22 pairs of autosomal chromosomes. The ovum and the sperm each contribute one chromosome to each pair. It is through this mechanism that genetically programmed diseases (such as Down syndrome) and genetically determined characteristics (such as eye color) are transmitted from parent to child.

The fertilized ovum, or **zygote**, passes through the fallopian tube to the uterus within 4 days. During this time the zygote continues to divide. By the third day a solid ball of cells, the **morula**, has formed. This solid ball soon develops a central cavity, or **blastocyst**. Even at this early stage, cells begin to differentiate in structure and function. Cells at one end of the blastocyst develop into the **embryo,** and those at the opposite end form the **placenta.** By day 4 the embryo has traveled through the fallopian tube into the uterus and is implanted in the uterine wall.

Before implantation the embryo is relatively protected from the external environment, but with im-

plantation, it becomes more vulnerable to the larger maternal environment via exchange of materials through the placenta. The placenta produces essential hormones that help maintain the pregnancy and that permit transfer of material between the embryo and mother, including oxygen, carbon dioxide, nutrients, and waste products. Because the placenta is extremely porous, noxious materials such as viruses and drugs can also pass from mother to child. The effect of noxious agents on the unborn child depends on the developmental stage in which exposure takes place.

The period of gestation is frequently divided into three time periods called *trimesters*. Because the developing baby, or **fetus,** is in a different stage of development in each trimester, interference with the development process has different outcomes in each.

Physical Development

First Trimester

The first trimester is the first 3 calendar months. After implantation, fetal cells continue to differenti-

Research Highlight

Coste et al evaluated the potential etiological role of cigarette smoking in the occurrence of ectopic pregnancy. The findings revealed that maternal cigarette smoking at conception was associated with an increased risk of ectopic pregnancy, whereas paternal smoking did not show this same association.

Coste J et al: Increased risk of ectopic pregnancy with maternal cigarette smoking, *Am J Public Health* 81(2):199, 1991.

ate and develop into essential organ systems. These processes of cellular change (differentiation) and staged organ change (development) occur at different rates and times, and each organ is extremely vulnerable to environmental insult. Interference with growth can cause the congenital absence of an organ system or extensive structural or functional alterations. Because several organ systems develop at the same time, disruption of one system often occurs with disruption of others. The nurse should consider this simultaneous development when conducting the initial newborn nursing assessment. Fig. 24-1 shows the approximate times of critical differentiation for some of the major organ systems and their overlapping of development.

HEALTH CONCERNS. Agents capable of producing adverse effects in the fetus are called *teratogens*. Some teratogens produce defects only if the fetus is exposed to the agent when the vulnerable organ is developing. One such teratogen is the rubella or measles virus, which can cause abortion, stillbirth, or defects of the eyes, ears, and heart, primarily when exposure is in the first trimester.

Many drugs are teratogenic during rapid organ growth (**organogenesis**) in the first trimester. Barbiturates, alcohol, hydantoins, anticonvulsants, and anticoagulants are only a few of the chemical agents associated with fetal abnormalities, and many other agents are under investigation. Benefits of any drug needed to maintain the mother's health must be weighed against potential harm to the fetus. Abuse of drugs, such as cocaine, results in infants with low birth weight and congenital abnormalities. Studies show that mothers who smoke deliver infants with lower birth weights than infants delivered by non-

Research Highlight

Free et al investigated 20 infants and toddlers from 15 families and their care givers. These children had measurable levels of alcohol or drugs in their urine or blood at birth or were identified by confirmed history of prenatal substance abuse. Only 11 of the care givers were the biological mothers; the other 9 were maternal grandmothers (5) and aunts (4) because the mothers had neglected or abandoned their children or because they were in prison. The findings confirmed literature reports that many children exposed prenatally to alcohol or drugs fail to grow normally. Three children (born to alcoholic mothers) had microcephaly, and eight children were below the 5th percentile for height and weight. Of the nine children born prematurely, five were below the 5th percentile for height, and five were below the 5th percentile for weight. The incidence of developmental delay was 34%, much higher than in general population, where incidence is thought to be 3% to 5%. Greatest lags were in language and other cognitive skills, a pattern usually associated with mental retardation. Few differences were found between mothers' and other care givers' interactions with the children, suggesting that family members who take care of infants relinquished by substance-abusing mothers are as much in need of support as the mothers.

Free T et al: A descriptive study of infants and toddlers exposed prenatally to substance abuse, *MCN* 15(4):245, 1990.

smoking mothers (Warshaw, 1986; Williams, 1986); more recent studies suggest that maternal smoking is associated with ectopic pregnancy (see research highlights). With this knowledge, the nurse should explore lifestyle changes that can help the woman maintain abstinence from tobacco, alcohol, and medications.

Second Trimester

During the second trimester, months 3 through 6, some organ systems continue basic development, and the functional capabilities of others are refined. By the end of this trimester, most organ systems are complete and can function. The fetus is therefore considered viable, or capable of life outside the uterus, if given intensive environmental support. The fetus weighs about 0.7 kg (1½ lb) and is approximately 30 cm (12 in) long. Fingers and toes are differentiated, a rudimentary kidney functions, and the sex of the fetus can be determined.

The fetus is covered with **vernix caseosa,** a cheese-like substance coating the skin. **Lanugo,** or fine hair, covers most of the body. These substances protect the thin, fragile skin and decrease in amount as gestation lengthens; thus prematurely born infants have more of these protective coverings than full-term infants.

HEALTH CONCERNS. In the second trimester the fetal heart beat becomes audible to stethoscope auscultation, and the mother becomes aware of fetal movement. Both events are highly significant to the parents because they provide tangible evidence of the pregnancy and reassure them that the fetus is alive. Therefore the nurse should focus on these events during prenatal care.

Changes in maternal behavior during this period include planning for the birth, concern for personal safety, and preoccupation with health and appearance. The nurse can help the woman adapt to these changes and plan for the impending birth. This is often a good time for education about gestational events and appropriate maternal rest and nutrition. Discussing birth alternatives and providing support and reassurance about the pregnancy's progression are appropriate nursing actions at this stage.

Third Trimester

During the last 3 months of intrauterine life the fetus grows to approximately 50 cm (19 to 20 in) in length. Subcutaneous fat is stored, and weight increases to between 3.2 and 3.4 kg (7 and 7½ lb). The skin thickens, lanugo begins to disappear, and the fetal body becomes rounder and fuller.

A tremendous spurt in brain growth begins during this trimester and lasts well into the first few years of life. The central nervous system has established its total number of neurons and connections between neurons, and myelination of nerve fibers progresses at a rapid rate. Exposure to noxious agents and the absence of essential nutrients are the most common causes of damage to the central nervous system during this trimester. The nurse can teach the woman about these factors, particularly through nutritional counseling.

At the end of the third trimester the normal fetus is physically able to make the transition from intrauterine to extrauterine life. The cardiac system can change its circulation to end bypassing of the lungs. The lungs are capable of maintaining the inflated state for gas exchange. The primitive temperature maintenance systems, reflexes, and sensory organs are ready for use.

HEALTH CONCERNS. Exposure to noxious agents and the absense of essential nutrients can cause damage to the central nervous system and result in alteration of high-level cognitive functions. The nurse can increase the mother's awareness of these dangers through counseling and help her evaluate the quality of her nutritional intake. Thoughts of delivering a healthy infant are foremost in the mother's mind as she focuses on preparing her mind and body for the delivery. Parents often seek information.

Cognitive Development

Relationships between prenatal events and cognitive development are difficult to establish. However, periods of diminished oxygen (anoxia) during fetal life can cause deficits in later cognitive functioning (Westwood et al, 1983). Some research shows an association between severely inadequate prenatal nutrition and subsequent lower brain weight, head circumference, and specific cognitive abilities. However, other studies show that, unless the malnutrition is severe and long term, the deficiencies can be averted by later supplemental nutrition. Until more is known, the nurse intervenes to support adequate prenatal nutrition and prevent fetal anoxia.

Psychosocial Development

Little information is available about the relationship between prenatal experiences and the child's psychosocial development. Some authorities believe that the biochemical environment of the uterus can significantly influence later psychosocial development. Because the biochemical environment is influenced by the mother, her emotional and physical states may have significant psychosocial consequences for the unborn child. Furthermore, the mother's emotional state may influence her behavior after childbirth, which in turn influences the child's psychosocial development.

 ## TRANSITION FROM INTRAUTERINE TO EXTRAUTERINE LIFE

The transition from intrauterine to extrauterine life requires rapid changes in the neonate. The nurse assesses the neonate's ability to make these changes and intervenes if necessary to ensure success. Gestational age, exposure to depressant drugs before or during labor, and the neonate's own behavioral style influence adjustment to the external environment. Therefore initial assessment encompasses a variety of physical and psychosocial elements. The nurse also provides opportunities for the parents and child to develop close emotional ties.

Physical Health Concerns

An immediate assessment of the neonate's condition is performed because the first concern is the physiological functioning of the major organ systems. Nursing care is then directed at maintaining an open airway, stabilizing body temperature, and protecting the neonate from infection.

Airway patency is best ensured by removing nasoóoropharyngeal secretions with suction or a bulb syringe. After the airway is open, the nurse stabilizes body temperature. Wrapping the neonate in small, soft blankets usually provides adequate heat preservation. For neonates unable to sustain body temperatures, Isolettes and incubators, which supply radiant heat, can be used.

Prevention of infection is a major concern in the care of the neonate, whose immune system is immature. Gloves are worn to handle the neonate in the delivery room and later when handling other body fluids. Good handwashing technique is the most important factor in protecting the neonate and nurse from infection. Although it is not recommended by the Centers for Disease Control, some nurses also wear gloves during diaper changes.

The most commonly used prophylactic treatment against opthalmia conjunctivitis is erythromycin (0.5%) because it prevents *Neisseria gonorrhoeae* and other infections, which can be transmitted during passage through the infected vaginal canal. The traditional use of 1% silver nitrate solution is uncommon today because of chemical irritation to the eyes and its more narrow action against bacteria.

The stump of the umbilical cord is an excellent medium for bacterial growth and should be swabbed with an antibacterial agent such as triple dye (a solution of brilliant green, proflavine hemisulfate, and crystal violet) shortly after birth. Stump drying is encouraged by application of alcohol at each diaper change and folding the diaper away from it.

The nurse is frequently responsible for assessing the newborn's physiological functioning. The most widely used assessment tool is the **Apgar score,** which rates heart rate, respiratory effort, muscle tone, reflex irritability, and color to determine overall status. The Apgar assessment is generally conducted at 1 and 5 minutes after birth and may be repeated until the newborn's condition stabilizes. Table 24-3 outlines the scoring criteria of physiological functioning. A total score of 0 to 3 signifies severe distress, a score of 4 to 6 represents moderate difficulty, and a score of 7 to 10 indicates little difficulty in adjusting to extrauterine life. The nurse can use the Apgar score to determine areas requiring further assessment and careful observation. In addition, the nurse monitors the neonate's body temperature and continues to closely monitor vital signs until they stabilize.

Psychosocial Concerns

After immediate physical evaluation and application of identification bracelets, the nurse assesses the parents' and newborn's needs for close physical contact. Early parent-child interaction encourages parent-child attachment. Physical factors (for example, fatigue, hunger, and health) and emotional factors (for example, happiness and needs for affection and touch) are assessed.

Merely placing the family together does not promote closeness. The parents and neonate must be capable and desirous of exploring and responding to each other. Most healthy neonates are awake and alert for the first half hour after birth, and if the parents are receptive, this is an opportune time for parent-child interaction to begin. Close body contact, often including breast-feeding, is a satisfying way for most families to start. If immediate contact is not possible, the nurse incorporates it into the care plan

TABLE 24-3	Apgar Scoring			
Sign	Score 0	Score 1	Score 2	
Heart rate	Absent	Slow (below 100)	Over 100	
Respiratory effort	Absent	Slow, irregular, hypoventilation	Good, crying lustily	
Muscle tone	Flaccid	Some flexion of extremities	Active motion, well flexed	
Reflex irritability	No response	Crying, some motion	Vigorous cry	
Color	Blue, pale	Pink body, blue hands and feet	Completely pink	

From Krones S: *High-risk newborn infants: the basis for intensive nursing care,* St Louis, ed 4, 1986, Mosby–Year Book.

as early as possible, which may mean bringing the newborn to an ill parent or bringing the parents to an ill or premature child.

Bonding occurs when parents and newborn elicit reciprocal and complementary behaviors. Parental bonding behaviors include attentiveness and physical contact. Neonate bonding behavior involves maintenance of contact with the parent. Preterm and ill neonates and their parents have more difficulty forming this bond if separation is prolonged. The bonding process is further complicated if parents are unable to care for the usual infant needs. The nurse should give the parents support throughout the early attachment process, particularly if the newborn is ill or separated from the parents.

 ## NEONATE

The **neonatal period** is the first month of life. During this stage the newborn's physical functioning is mostly reflexive, and stabilization of major organ systems is the body's primary task. Behavior greatly influences interaction between the newborn and the environment and care givers. For example, the average 2-week-old smiles spontaneously and is able to regard mother's face. The impact of these reflexive behaviors is generally a surge of maternal feelings of love that prompt the mother to cuddle the baby.

Nurses can apply their knowledge of this stage of growth and development to promote newborn and parental health. If the nurse understands, for example, that the newborn's cry is generally a reflexive response to an unmet need (such as hunger), parents can be assisted in identifying ways to meet those needs, such as counseling the parents to feed their baby on demand rather than on a rigid schedule.

Physical Development

A comprehensive nursing assessment is performed as soon as the neonate's physiological functioning is stable, generally within a few hours after birth. At this time the nurse measures height, weight, head circumference, temperature, pulse, and respirations and observes general appearance, body functions, sensory capabilities, and responsiveness. In addition, the nurse coordinates screening tests and other laboratory tests as indicated by the neonate's state of health. Blood tests such as those for hypothyroidism and phenylketonuria (PKU) allow early detection and treatment, thereby preventing permanent central nervous system damage. These and other screening tests are required by law in many states.

The average newborn weighs 3200 g (7 lb, 1 oz), is 50 cm (20 in) in length, and has a head circumference of 35 cm (14 in). Up to 10% of birth weight is lost in the first few days of life, primarily through fluid losses by respiration, urination, defecation, and decreased intake. Birth weight is usually regained by the second week of life, and a gradual pattern of increase in weight, height, and head circumference is evident. During the first month, these increases average 4 to 8 oz in weight per week, 0.6 to 2.5 cm (¼ to 1 in) in length, and 2 cm in head circumference.

The neonate's heart rate gradually decreases from the fetal rate of 130 to 160 beats per minute to 120 to 140 beats per minute. Systole and diastole are of shorter duration, greater intensity, and higher pitch. The average blood pressure is 70/55 mm Hg. The newborn's respiratory movements are primarily abdominal and vary in rate and rhythm, but the average rate is 30 to 50 breaths per minute. Because a neonate breathes through the nose, it is important to keep the nasal passages clear. Their axillary temperature ranges from 36.5° to 37.5° C (97.7° to 99.5° F) and generally stabilizes within 24 hours after birth.

Normal physical characteristics include the continued presence of lanugo on the skin of the back; cyanosis of the hands and feet, especially during activity; and a soft, protuberant abdomen. Skin color varies according to racial and genetic heritage and gradually changes during infancy. **Molding,** or overlapping of the soft skull bones, is common during birth. The bones readjust in a few weeks, producing a more rounded appearance. The linear breaks, sutures, and fontanels, are usually palpable at birth. The diamond shape of the anterior fontanel and the triangular shape of the posterior fontanel between the unfused bones of the skull are shown in Figure 24-2.

Normal behavioral characteristics of the newborn include periods of sucking, crying, sleeping, and activity. Movements are generally sporadic, but they are symmetrical and involve all four extremities. The relatively flexed position of intrauterine life continues as the neonate attempts to maintain an enclosed, secure feeling. Newborns normally watch the care giver's face, reflexively smile, and respond to sensory stimuli, particularly the primary care giver's face, voice, and touch.

Neurological function is assessed by observing the neonate's level of activity, alertness, irritability, and responsiveness to stimuli and the presence and strength of reflexes. Normal reflexes include blinking in response to bright lights and startling in response to sudden, loud noises. Table 24-4 describes other commonly evaluated reflexes. Their absence indicates possible trauma or central nervous system

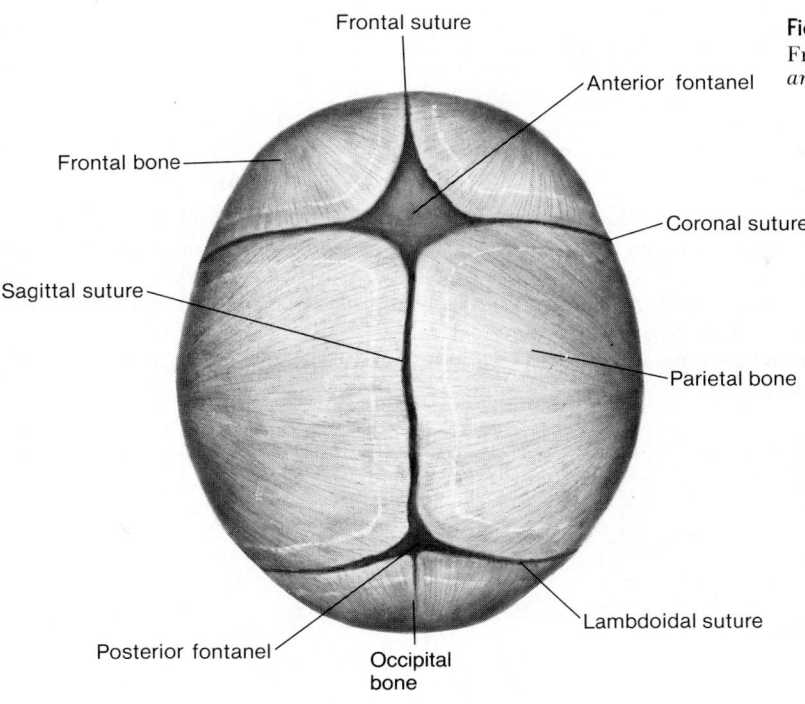

Frontal suture

Anterior fontanel

Frontal bone

Coronal suture

Sagittal suture

Parietal bone

Lambdoidal suture

Posterior fontanel

Occipital bone

Fig. 24-2   Fontanels and suture lines.
From Whaley LF, Wong DL: *Nursing care of infants and children*, ed 4, St Louis, 1991, Mosby–Year Book.

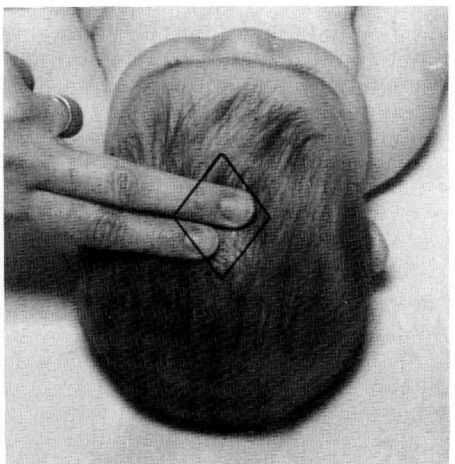

TABLE 24-4   Assessment of Reflexes in the Newborn

Reflexes	Expected Behavioral Responses
LOCALIZED	
Eyes	
Blinking or corneal reflex	Infant blinks at sudden appearance of bright light or at approach of object toward cornea. Reflex persists throughout life.
Pupillary	Pupil constricts when bright light shines toward it. Reflex persists throughout life.
Doll's eye	As head is moved slowly to right or left, eyes lag behind and do not immediately adjust to new position of head. Reflex disappears as fixation develops. Persistent occurrence indicates neurological damage.
Nose	
Sneeze	Nasal passages respond spontaneously to irritation or obstruction. Reflex persists throughout life.
Glabellar	Tapping briskly on glabella (bridge of nose) causes eyes to close tightly.
Mouth and throat	
Sucking	Infant begins strong sucking movements of circumoral area in response to stimulation. Reflex persists throughout infancy, even without stimulation, such as during sleep.
Gag	Stimulation of posterior pharynx by food, suction, or passage of tube causes infant to gag. Reflex persists throughout life.
Rooting	Touching or stroking cheek along side of mouth causes infant to turn head toward that side and begin to suck. Reflex should disappear at about age 3-4 mo but may persist up to 12 mo.
Extrusion	When tongue is touched or depressed, infant responds by forcing it outward. Reflex disappears by 4 mo.
Yawn	Spontaneous response to decreased oxygen increases amount of inspired air. Reflex persists throughout life.
Cough	Irritation of mucous membranes of larynx or tracheobronchial tree causes coughing. Reflex persists throughout life and is usually present first day after birth.

From Whaley L, Wong D: *Nursing care of infants and children*, ed, 4, St Louis, 1991, Mosby–Year Book.
Illustrations from Moore KL: *The developing human: clinically oriented embryology*, ed 2, Philedelphia, 1977, Saunders.

Continued.

TABLE 24-4   Assessment of Reflexes in the Newborn—cont'd

Reflexes	Expected Behavioral Responses

Extremities

Grasp — Touching palms of hands or soles of feet near base of digits causes flexion of hands and toes. Palmar grasp lessens after 3 mo and is replaced by voluntary movement. Plantar grasp lessons by 8 mo. (see Figure A).

Babinski — Stroking outer sole of foot upward from heel and across ball of foot causes toes to hyperextend and hallux to dorsiflex. Reflex disappears after age 1 yr (see Figure B).

Ankle clonus — Briskly dorsiflexing foot while supporting knee in partially flexed position results in one or two oscillating movements ("beats"). Eventually, no beats should be felt.

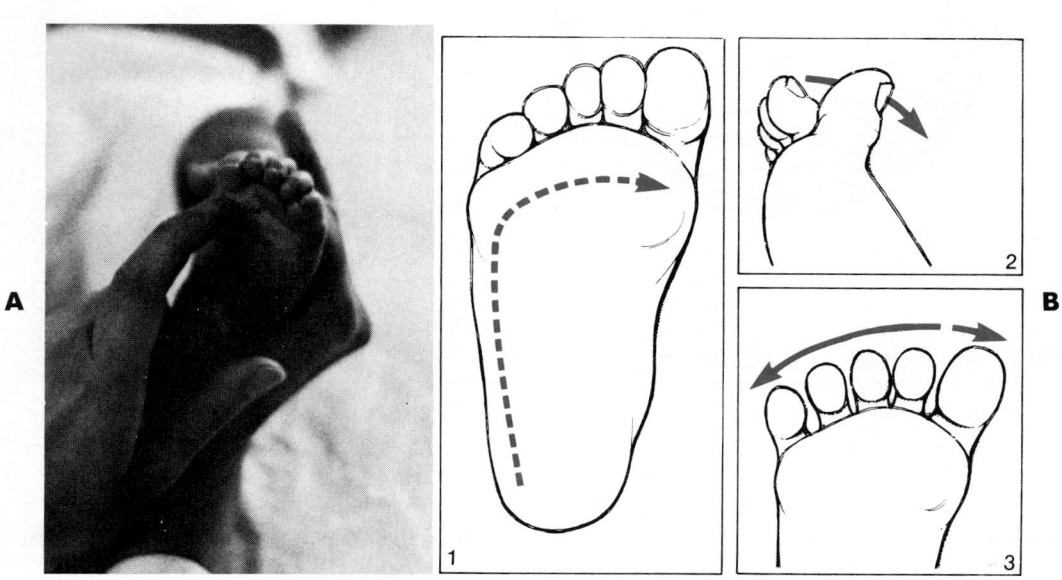

Mass

Moro — Sudden jarring or change in equilibrium causes sudden extension and abduction of extremities and fanning of fingers, with index finger and thumb forming C shape, followed by flexion and adduction of extremities. Legs may weakly flex. Infant may cry. Reflex disappears after 3-4 mo and is usually strongest during first 2 mo.

Startle — Sudden, loud noise causes abduction of arms with flexion of elbows. Hands remain clenched. Reflex disappears by 4 mo.

Perez — While infant is prone on firm surface, thumb is pressed along spine from sacrum to neck; infant responds by crying, flexing extremities, and elevating pelvis and head. Lordosis of spine, as well as defecation and urination, may occur. Reflex disappears by 4-6 mo.

Asymmetrical tonic neck — When infant's head is quickly turned to one side, arm and leg extend on that side, and opposite arm and leg flex. Reflex disappears by age 3-4 mo and is replaced by symmetrical positioning of both sides of body.

Trunk incurvation (Galant) reflex — Stroking infant's back alongside spine causes hips to move toward stimulated side. Reflex disappears by 4 wk.

Dance or step — If infant is held so that sole of foot touches hard surface, there is reciprocal flexion and extension of leg, simulating walking. Reflex disappears after 3-4 wk and is replaced by deliberate movement.

Crawl — When placed on abdomen, infant makes crawling movements with arms and leg. Reflex disappears at about 6 wk.

Placing — When infant is held upright under arms and dorsal side of foot is briskly placed against hard object, such as table, leg lifts as if foot is stepping on table. Age of disappearance varies.

complications. Because the newborn depends largely on reflexes for response to environment, assessment of these response characteristics is vital.

Cognitive Development

Early cognitive development begins with innate behaviors, reflexes, and sensory functions. During this time, newborns initiate reflex activities, assimilate new objects into behavior, and accommodate these behaviors to achieve their desires. For example, neonates learn to turn to the nipple. Although the infants behave of their own volition, activities learned are limited to reflex and sensory function (Nelms, Mullins, 1982).

Sensory functions contribute to cognitive development in the newborn. At birth, children can focus on objects about 8 to 10 in from their faces and can perceive forms. A preference for the human face is apparent. Auditory and vestibular systems function from birth. These sensory capabilities allow neonates to elicit stimuli rather than simply receive it. Parents should be taught the importance of providing sensory stimulation, such as talking to their babies and holding them to see their faces. This allows infants to seek or take in stimuli, thereby enhancing learning and promoting cognitive development.

It is debatable whether infant crying is the precursor of refined language. However, crying elicits a response, and care givers discriminate cry patterns. Crying therefore has significance to newborns and parents. For neonates, crying is a means of communication. They cry for a reason, although at times this reason is difficult to determine. Some babies cry because their diapers are wet or they are hungry or want to be held. Others cry just to make noise. Crying may frustrate the parents if they cannot see an apparent cause. With the nurse's help, parents can learn to define infants' cry patterns to take appropriate action when necessary.

Psychosocial Development

During the first month of life, parents and newborns normally develop a strong bond that grows into a deep **attachment.** Interactions during routine care enhance or detract from the attachment process. Feeding, hygiene, and comfort measures consume much of infants' waking time. These interactive experiences provide a foundation from which deep attachments form. Neonates are active participants in this process.

If parents or children experience health complications after birth, bonding may be compromised. In-

fants' behavioral cues may be weak or absent. Care and care giving are less mutually satisfying. Tired, ill parents have difficulty interpreting and responding to their infants. Children who have congenital anomalies, are too weak to be responsive to parental cues, or require special care need supportive nursing care. For example, infants born with heart defects may tire easily during feedings. They may rest frequently after several bursts of sucking and fall asleep after taking 1 to 1½ oz. Infants may awaken after 1½ hours, crying because they are hungry again. Mothers, not understanding that the crying is a physiologically dictated sequence of events, may think that the infants are being fussy or that they are inadequate. Both infants and mothers derive decreasing pleasure from feeding experiences. In this case, however, bonding is not enhanced and may even be reduced unless nursing intervention breaks the sequence of events.

INFANT

Infancy is the period from 1 month to 1 year of age. Rapid physical growth and change characterize this stage. Psychosocial development advances, aided by the progression from reflexive to more purposeful behavior. Interaction between infants and the environment is greater and more meaningful. Infants who purposefully giggle and roll over in response to tickling are interacting more with their social environments and are receiving a greater response than when they merely smile in response to a hug. During this phase of growth and development the nurse can observe the children's adaptive potential because qualitative and quantitative changes occur rapidly.

Physical Development

Steady and proportional growth of the infant is more important than absolute growth values. Charts of normal age- and sex-related growth measurements enable the nurse to compare growth with norms for a child's age. Using growth charts, the nurse can also evaluate growth patterns by recording measurements of weight, length, and head circumference at intervals. Measurements recorded over time are the best way to monitor growth and identify problems. For example, an infant with a growth problem may be generally below the expected norms at all intervals or may experience an acute, brief interference with growth.

Size increases rapidly during the first year of life; birth weight doubles before 6 months and triples by 12 months. Height increases an average of 1 in during each of the first 6 months and ½ in the next 6 months. This 50% increase in birth height occurs primarily in the trunk, with the chest diameter approximating that of the head by the first birthday (Whaley, Wong, 1991). The fontanels become smaller; the posterior fontanel closes at about 2 months.

Physiological functioning stabilizes, and by the end of the first year, the heart rate is 80 to 130 beats per minute, the blood pressure is 72-110/38-72 mm Hg, and respiratory rate is 30 to 35 breaths per minute. Patterns of body function also stabilize, as evidenced by predictable sleep, elimination, and feeding routines. Motor development proceeds steadily in a head-to-foot direction. Table 24-5 identifies milestones in gross motor and fine motor development.

Nutrition

The quality and quantity of nutrition influence the infant's growth and development. The nurse helps parents select and provide a nutritionally adequate diet for their infant. The nurse must understand that nutrition is influenced by many variables (such as family culture, food preferences, slow eating, or food allergies) and that no diet is effective for all children or for one age group.

FEEDING ALTERNATIVES. Supplying essential nutrients to the infant is the nurse's and parents' goal. Breast-feeding is recommended for infants because it contains the essential nutrients of protein, fats, car- bohydrates, and immunoreactive proteins that bolster the ability to resist infection. However, milk other than human milk may be successfully used. Commercially prepared formulas are popular because they are convenient, contain standard ingredients, and are fortified with vitamins and minerals. The nurse supports the parents' choice of feeding methods and helps them feed the infant successfully.

The 1-month-old infant takes *approximately* 28 ounces of milk per day. This amount increases slightly during the first 6 months and drops to about 24 ounces per day by the end of the first year. Cereals, fruits, vegetables, and meats are important sources of nutrients during the second 6 months of life. However, the amount and frequency of feedings vary among infants, so the nurse should discuss differences in feeding patterns with parents.

SUPPLEMENTATION. The need for dietary vitamin and mineral supplements depends on the infant's diet. Full-term infants are born with some iron stores. The breast-fed infant absorbs adequate iron from breast milk during the first 4 to 6 months of life. After 6 months, iron-fortified cereal is generally considered an adequate supplemental source. Because iron in formula is less readily absorbed than that in breast milk, formula-fed infants should receive iron-fortified formula throughout the first year. Adequate concentrations of fluoride to protect against dental caries are not available in human milk, and therefore fluoridated water or supplemental fluoride is generally recommended. The presence of fluoride in formula depends on the type of formula and the source of water used in preparing the concentrated forms, and sup-

---

TABLE 24-5 Milestones in Infant Motor Development

Month 3	Month 6	Month 9	Month 12	Month 15
GROSS MOTOR				
Lifts head and chest while prone	Rolls over	Attains sitting position independently	Walks holding onto walls and furniture (cruising)	Walks alone
Sits with support	Sits without support	Creeps on all four extremities	Stands alone	
	Crawls on abdomen with arms	Pulls self to standing position	Takes 1-2 steps	
FINE MOTOR				
Grasps and briefly holds objects and takes them to mouth	Uses palm grasp with fingers encircling object	Picks up small objects with thumb-and-finger pincer motion	Places tiny object, such as raisin, into container	Scribbles with crayon
	Transfers object from hand to hand		Makes marks with crayon	Builds tower of two cubes

plementation may be necessary. In general, cow's milk is not recommended in the first year because of inadequate amounts of essential nutrients, particularly fats and carbohydrates.

The association between overfeeding, infant obesity, and later adult obesity is still controversial. However, early feeding experiences can influence later eating habits. The nurse should therefore emphasize balanced nutrition and good dietary habits through feeding experiences mutually satisfying for the parents and infant.

Cognitive Development

The infant learns much by experiencing and manipulating the environment. Developing motor skills and increasing mobility expand an infant's environment and, with developing visual and auditory skills, enhance cognitive development. For these reasons, Piaget (1952) has named his first stage of cognitive development, which extends until around the second birthday, the *sensorimotor period*. The characteristics of each of the four substages are described in Table 24-3. Before the acquisition of language the extraordinary development of the mind occurs through the child's developing senses and motor abilities. For example, a 1-month-old can follow the path of a moving object. Improved visual acuity and eye-hand coordination allow grasping and exploration of objects. In addition, rudimentary color vision begins by 2 months and improves throughout the first year, making the environment more interesting to see and explore. The infant's hearing also progresses, allowing localization and discrimination of sounds.

Speech is an important aspect of cognition that develops during the first year. Infants proceed from crying, cooing, and laughing to imitating sounds, comprehending the meaning of simple commands, and repeating words with knowledge of their meaning. By 1 year, infants not only recognize their own names but also have two- or three-word vocabularies including *Da-Da*, *Ma-Ma*, and *no*. The nurse can promote language development by encouraging mothers to name objects on which their infants' attention is focused.

Infants need opportunities to develop and use their senses. Nurses must evaluate the appropriateness and adequacy of these opportunities. For example, ill or hospitalized infants may lack the energy to interact with their environments, thereby slowing their cognitive development. On the other hand, continuous stimulation can overwhelm and confuse infants. Infants need to be stimulated according to their temperament, energy, and age. Visual, sensory, and tactile stimulation are as necessary for healthy develop-

ment as food. The nurse uses stimulation so that maximize the development of infants while conserving their energy and orientation (that is, talking to and encouraging them to suck on pacifiers while administering tube feedings).

Psychosocial Development

During their first year, infants begin to differentiate themselves from others as separate beings capable of acting on their own. Initially, infants are unaware of the boundaries of self, but through repeated experiences with the environment, they learn where the self ends and the external world begins. This process is slow, and infants occasionally experience brief frustrations with more frequent and consistent satisfactions. As infants determine their physical boundaries, they begin to respond to others. Two- and three-month-old infants begin to smile responsively rather than reflexively. Similarly, they can recognize differences in people when their sensory and cognitive capabilities improve. By 8 months, most infants can differentiate a stranger from a familiar person and respond differently to the two. Close attachment to the primary care givers, most often parents, is usually established by this age. Infants seek out these persons for support and comfort during times of stress. The ability to distinguish self from others allow infants to interact and socialize more within their environments. By 9 months, for example, infants play simple social games such as pat-a-cake and peek-a-boo. More complex interactive games such as hide-and-seek involving objects are possible by age 1.

Erikson (1963) describes the psychosocial developmental crisis for the infant as *trust versus mistrust*. He explains that the quality of parent-infant interactions determines development of trust or mistrust. Parents who meet needs for warmth and comfort, love and security, and food when infants express these needs promote a sense of trust, whereas those that meet the needs of infants at their own convenience or not at all allow a sense of mistrust to develop (Erikson, 1963).

The nurse assesses the availability and appropriateness of experiences contributing to psychosocial development. Hospitalized infants may have difficulty establishing physical boundaries because of repeated bodily intrusions and painful sensations. Limiting these negative experiences and providing pleasurable sensations are interventions that support early psychosocial development. Extended separations from parents complicate the attachment process and increase the number of care givers with whom the infant must interact. Ideally, the parents should provide the majority of care during hospitalization. When parents are not present, an attempt should be made to limit the number of care givers who have contact with the infant and to follow the parents' directions for care. These interventions will foster the infant's continuing development of trust.

Perception of Health

The foundation for children's perceptions of their health status is laid early in life. Internal body sensations and experiences with the outside world affect self-perceptions. The nature of this influence and the value of nursing interventions to alter later perceptions are unknown. It is known, however, that parents tend to label children who are ill in early life as more vulnerable than their siblings and that this labeling may affect the children's perceptions of their own health. In addition, because infants and children depend on others for their health care, their experiences with care givers influence their health attitudes and behaviors. The nurse has a responsibility to educate parents and other care givers about health-promotion behaviors that will positively affect perception of health and self.

 TODDLER

Toddlerhood ranges from the time when children begin to walk independently until they walk and run with ease, which is approximately from 12 to 36 months. Toddlerhood is characterized by increasing independence bolstered by greater physical mobility and cognitive abilities. Toddlers are increasingly aware of their abilities to control and are pleased with successful efforts with this new skill. This success leads them to repeated attempts to control their environments. Unsuccessful attempts at control may result in negative behaviors and temper tantrums. These behaviors are most common when parents thwart the initial independent action. Parents cite these as the most problematic behaviors during the toddler years and at times express frustration with trying to set consistent and firm limits while simultaneously encouraging independence.

Physical Development

The rapid development of motor skills allows the child to participate in self-care activities such as feeding, dressing, and toileting. In the beginning the toddler walks in an upright position with a broad-stanced gait, protuberant abdomen, and arms out to the sides for balance. Soon the child begins to navigate stairs, using a rail or the wall to maintain balance while progressing upward, placing both feet on the same step before continuing. Success provides courage to attempt the upright mode for descending the stairs in the same manner. Locomotion skills soon include running, jumping, standing on one foot for several seconds, and kicking a ball. Most toddlers can ride tricycles, climb ladders, and run well by their third birthday. Fine motor capabilities move from scribbling spontaneously to drawing circles and crosses accurately. By 3 years the child draws simple stick people and can usually stack a tower of small blocks. Improved mobility, the ability to undress, and development of sphincter control allow toilet training if the toddler has developed the necessary cognitive abilities. Parents often consult nurses for an assessment of readiness for toilet training. The nurse needs to remind parents that patience, consistency, and a nonjudgmental attitude, in addition to the child's readiness, are essential to successful toilet training.

The cardiopulmonary system becomes stable in the toddler years. The heart and respiratory rates slow to 110 beats and 24 to 26 breaths per minute, and the blood pressure rises slightly to an average of 92/56 mm Hg.

The anterior fontanel closes between 12 and 18 months of age, ending the period of most rapid growth of the skull and brain. Routine measurement of head circumference is usually not continued past this age.

The rate of increase in weight and length slows. By 2 years the child weighs 4 times the birth weight. Height during toddlerhood increases 3 to 5 inches a year, mainly as a result of increases in leg length. Slowed growth rates are accompanied by decreased caloric need and smaller food intake (**physiological anorexia**), which leads some parents to worry about the adequacy of dietary intake. The nurse can reassure parents by confirming the child's pattern with growth charts.

TABLE 24-6 Daily Dietary Requirements of the Healthy Toddler		
Food	Servings	Size of Serving
Milk	3-4	6-8 oz
Meat	2-3	1-3 tbsp
Vegetables and fruits	4	1-3 tbsp
Cereals and breads	4 or more	½ slice of bread ½ c of rice or cereal

Most toddlers change from breast milk or formula to milk, consuming 3 to 4 glasses per day. Nutritional requirements are increasingly met by solid foods in the remaining three basic food groups. Because the consumption of more than a quart of milk per day decreases the child's appetite for these essential solid foods, the nurse should advise parents to limit milk intake to 28 ounces per day. The healthy toddler requires the daily intake of the foods in Table 24-6. Because parents frequently overestimate the size of a normal serving for their child, the nurse can reduce their anxiety about inadequate intake by pointing out the normal serving size.

Children who are ill, are undergoing surgery, or have diseases involving ingestion, absorption, or use of nutrients require special dietary considerations. Alterations in the type of foods and caloric requirements may be necessary. Children on strict vegetarian diets also require careful planning to ensure adequate, balanced protein intake.

Regardless of children's health status, several basic principles of nutrition apply. Mealtime has psychosocial and physical significance. If the parents struggle to control toddlers' dietary intake, problem behaviors and conflicts may result. Toddlers often develop "food jags" or the desire to eat one food repeatedly. Rather than becoming disturbed by this behavior, parents should be encouraged by the nurse to offer a variety of nutritious foods at meals and to provide only nutritious snacks between meals. Serving finger foods to toddlers allows them to eat by themselves and to satisfy their need for independence and control. Small, *reasonable* servings allow toddlers to eat all of their meals.

Cognitive Development

Toddlers' completion of the development of object permanence, their ability to remember events, and their beginning ability to put thoughts into words at about 2 years of age signals their transition from Piaget's sensorimotor stage of cognitive development to the **preoperational thought** stage (Piaget, 1952). Table 24-3 outlines the basic characteristics of the three substages of cognitive development through which toddlers move between 12 and 36 months. Toddlers recognize that they are separate beings from their mothers, but they are unable to assume the view of another. They use symbols to represent objects, places, and persons. This function is demonstrated when children imitate the behavior of another that they viewed earlier (for example, pretend to shave like daddy), pretend one object is another (use a finger as a gun), and use language to stand for absent objects (for example, requests bottle).

The 18-month-old child uses approximately 10 words. The 24-month-old child has a vocabulary of up to 300 words and is generally able to speak in short sentences. "Who's that?" and "What's that?" typify questions asked during this period. Verbal expressions such as "me do it" and "that's mine" demonstrate the 2-year-old child's use of pronouns and desire for independence and control. Despite the expanded vocabulary of an older toddler, most parents comment that their child's favorite word is *no* until well into the third year.

Because children's moral development is closely associated with their cognitive abilities, the moral development of toddlers is only beginning and is also egocentric. Toddlers do not understand concepts of right and wrong. However, they do grasp the fact that some behaviors bring pleasant results (positive reinforcement) and others elicit unpleasant results (negative reinforcement). Therefore until toddlers achieve a higher level of cognitive function, they behave simply to avoid the unpleasant and seek out the pleasant.

Psychosocial Development

According to Erikson (1963), a sense of autonomy emerges during toddlerhood. Children strive for independence by using their developing muscles to do everything for themselves and become the master of their bodily functions. Their strong wills are frequently exhibited in negative behavior when care givers attempt to direct their actions. Temper tantrums may result when toddlers are frustrated by parental restrictions. Parents need to provide toddlers with graded independence, allowing them to do things that do not result in harm to themselves or others. This prevents them from doubting their ability to do things that they are capable of learning or feeling a sense of shame for those things they have done. Firm limits, patience, and support allow toddlers to develop socially acceptable behavior, which is the goal of parental guidance. Young toddlers who wants to learn to hold their own cups may benefit from two-handled cups with spouts and plastic bibs with pockets to collect the milk that spills during the learning process.

Socially, toddlers remain strongly attached to their parents and fear separation from them. In their presence, they feel safe, and their curiosity is evident in their exploration of the environment. However, they do not want their mothers to close the bathroom door, and if the mothers do so, the children may cry incessantly until the door is opened.

The child continues to engage in solitary play during toddlerhood but also begins to participate in parallel play, which is playing beside rather than with another child. An example would be two toddlers sitting beside each other, each playing with his or her own doll in his or her own independent fashion. Toddlers who are just learning what belongs to them are often possessive of their toys. They learn the joy of sharing when they offer parents toys to hold and the parents express pleasure.

The newly developed locomotion abilities and insatiable curiosity of toddlers make them a danger to their own well-being. Toddlers need close supervision at all times and particularly when in environments that have not been "child-proofed." Poisonings occur frequently because children near 2 years of age are interested in placing any object or substance in their mouths to learn about it. Fortunately, these ingestions do not always result in death, but they do have many negative consequences such as chemical pneumonia from tasting charcoal lighter fluid. The wise parent removes or locks up all possible poisons, including plants, cleaning materials, and medications (see Chapter 42). These parental actions create a safer environment for exploratory behavior. Toddlers' lack of awareness regarding the danger of water and their newly developed walking skills combine to make drowning a major cause of accidental deaths in this age group. Limit setting is extremely important for toddlers' safety. Automobile safety requires toddlers to remain in car seats, even though they say (often loudly) that they would prefer to move freely about the car. Children often learn to release the car restraints, and parents must be firm in their resolve not to drive unless the children are securely restrained. Toddlers completely depend on their parents for physical safety.

Perception of Health

Toddlers' perceptions of their own health are limited by their cognitive capabilities. Children increasingly recognize internal body sensations but have difficulty pinpointing their location. Therefore children often associate generalized responses with illness. Children who deviate radically from their usual patterns of eating, sleeping, or playing require assessment to determine whether these alterations result from illness.

During this stage, children begin to internalize the labels that parents or health care professionals give to the somatic states. That is, if the parents label particular sensations, such as abdominal discomfort, an "illness," children begin to label related sensations similarly. At the same time, children observe and mimic parents' health care practices. Health beliefs and practices are therefore being significantly shaped, even in these early years.

PRESCHOOLER

The **preschool years** are a transition between toddlerhood and the school-age years. The period spans the ages between 3 and 6. Many people consider these the most intriguing years of parenting because children are less negative, can more accurately share their thoughts, and can more effectively interact and communicate. Physical development continues to slow, whereas cognitive and psychosocial development are rapid.

Physical Development

Several aspects of physical development continue to stabilize in the preschool years. Heart and respiratory rates decrease only slightly to approximately 90 beats and 22 to 24 breaths per minute. Blood pressure rises slightly to an average of 95/58 mm Hg. Children gain about 5 lb per year; the average weight at 5 years is about 42 lb, approximately 6 times the birth weight. Preschoolers grow 2 to 3 in per year, double their birth length around 4 years, and stand an average of 43 in tall by their fifth birthday. The elongation of the legs results in more slender appearing children. The head has attained 90% of its adult size by the sixth birthday. Little difference exists between the sexes, although boys are slightly larger with more muscle and less fatty tissue. The most common nutritional deficiencies in children under 6 are vitamins A and C and iron. Ingestion of large amounts of carbohydrates and fats from junk foods may result in overweight and undernourished preschoolers. Parents and health care providers need to make a conscious effort to help preschoolers develop healthy eating habits that prevent deficiencies and excesses.

Large and fine muscle coordination improves. Preschoolers run well, walk up and down steps with ease, and learn to hop. By 6 years, they can usually skip and throw and catch balls. Improving fine motor skills allow intricate manipulations. Children can copy circles, crosses, squares, and triangles. These skills make printing of letters and numbers possible.

Children need opportunities to learn and practice these physical skills. Nursing care of healthy and ill children includes an assessment of the availability of these opportunities. Although children with acute illnesses benefit from rest and exclusion from usual daily activities, children who have chronic conditions or who have been hospitalized for long periods need ongoing exposure to developmental opportunities. The parents and nurse weave these opportunities into the children's daily experiences, depending on their abilities, needs, and energy level.

Cognitive Development

Preschoolers continue to master the preoperational stage of cognition. The first phase of this period, known as *preconceptual thought* (2 to 4 years), is characterized by perceptual-bound thinking, in which children judge persons, objects, and events by their outward appearance or what seems to be (Piaget, 1952). For example children may determine that an 8-ounce glass full of fluid contains more than a 10-ounce glass that also contains 8 ounce of fluid because they center their thoughts on the fullness of the glass. Even if they watch the 8 ounces of fluid from the full glass being poured into the 10-ounce glass and the 8-ounce glass refilled, they will still assert that the full 8-oz glass contains more because they cannot attend to the transfer. Thinking is hindered by their limited attention and attending skills. **Artificialism,** the misconception that everything in the world has been created by humanity, may result in children asking who built the mountains. Another misconception, **animism,** the attribution of life to inanimate objects, often results in statements such as "Trees cry when their branches are broken." A third misconception is a type of reasoning called *immanent justice,* the notion that the world is equipped with a built-in code of law and order. It may result in children's beliefs that they were burned by matches because they were not supposed to handle them.

Around the age of 4 years, the intuitive phase of preoperational thought develops and children's ability to think more complexly is demonstrated by their ability to classify objects according to size or color and questions such as "Why do they call it the 31st day of the month instead of the thirty last?" Egocentricity persists, but during these 3 years, it begins to be replaced with social interaction as is illustrated by the 5-year-old child who offers a bandage to a child with a cut finger. Children become aware of cause-and-effect relationships as illustrated by the statement "The sun sets because people want to go to bed." Early causal thinking is also evident in preschoolers' transductive thoughts (reasoning occurs from one particular to another). If two events are related in time or space, children link them in a causal fashion. The hospitalized child, for example, may reason, "I cried last night, and that's why the nurse gave me the shot." As children near age 5, they begin to use or can be taught to use rules to understand causation. They then begin to reason from the general to the particular. This forms the basis for more formal logical thought. The child can now reason, "I get a shot twice a day, and that's why I got one last night."

Preschoolers' knowledge of the world remains closely linked to concrete experiences. Even their rich fantasy life is grounded in the perception of reality. The mixing of the two aspects can lead to many childhood fears and may be misinterpreted by adults as lying when children are actually presenting reality from their perspective.

The greatest fear of this age group appears to be that of bodily harm, and it can be seen in children's fear of the dark, animals, thunderstorms, and medical personnel. This fear often interferes with their willingness to allow nursing interventions such as measurement of vital signs. They may cooperate if they are allowed to help the nurse measure the blood pressure of a parent.

The preschooler's moral development expands to include a beginning understanding of behaviors considered socially right or wrong. The child continues to be motivated, however, by the wish to avoid punishment or the desire to obtain a reward. The primary difference between this stage of moral development and that of a toddler is that a preschooler is better able to identify behaviors that elicit rewards or punishment and begins to label these behaviors as *right* or *wrong.*

Preschoolers' vocabularies continue to increase rapidly, and by the age of 5, children have more than 2000 words that they can use to define familiar objects, identify colors, and express their desires and frustrations. Language is more social, and questions expand to "Why?" and "How come?" in the quest for information. Phonetically similar words such as *die* and *dye* may confuse preschool children. The nurse avoids such words when preparing children for procedures and assesses comprehension of explanations.

Psychosocial Development

The world of preschoolers expands beyond the family into the neighborhood where children meet other children and adults. Their unquenchable curiosity and developing initiative lead to the active exploration of the environment, the development of new skills, and the making of new friends. Preschoolers have a surplus of energy that permits them to plan and attempt many activities that may be beyond their capabilities, such as pouring milk from a gallon container into their cereal bowls. Guilt arises within children when they overstep the limits of their abilities and feel they have not behaved correctly. Children who in anger have wished their sibling were dead experience guilt if that sibling becomes ill. Children need to be taught that "wishing" for something to happen does not make it occur. Erickson (1963) recommends that parents help their children strike a healthy balance between initiative and guilt by allowing them to do things on their own while setting firm limits and providing guidance.

During times of stress or illness, preschoolers may revert to bedwetting or thumbsucking and want the parents to feed, dress, and hold them continuously. These dependent behaviors are often confusing and embarrassing to parents, who can benefit from the nurse's reassurance that they are normal coping behaviors. The nurse should accept regressive behavior and yet help children understand and gain control of the new situation. The nurse should provide experiences that these children can master. Such successes give children the motivation and strength to return to their prior level of independent functioning.

The play of preschool children becomes more socially interactive after the third birthday as it shifts from parallel to associative play, which involves a borrowing and lending of play material. All participants engage in similar if not identical activity; however, there is no division of labor, and all children do as they wish. Most 3-year-old children are able to play with one other child in a cooperative manner in which they make something or play designated roles such as mother and baby. By age 4, children play in groups of two or three, and by 5 years the group has a temporary leader for each activity.

In many play activities, preschoolers display awareness of social context. Sex-role identification is strengthening, and children most often assume roles of persons of their own sex. Children frequently mimic or repeat social experiences. This tendency is especially significant for the nurse working with hospitalized children. Through play, children may express questions, fears, anger, and misunderstanding about their illnesses and care. The nurse should be alert to such clues and ensure that children can play within energy limits. Play can provide a healthy outlet for frustration when children have been subjected to painful or restrictive experiences against their will.

Pretend play involving imaginary situations depends on children's ability to retain images of things they have seen or heard. This sociodramatic play involving other children occupies about a third of 5-year-old childrens' playtime. Pretending allows children to learn to understand other's points of view, develop skills in solving social problems, and become more creative. Children who watch a great deal of television engage less frequently in imaginative play, possibly because they develop the habit of passively absorbing images rather than generating their own.

Perception of Health

Little research has explored preschoolers perceptions of their own health. Parental beliefs about health, childrens' bodily sensations, and their ability to perform usual daily activities help children's develop attitudes about their health. Preschoolers are usually quite independent in washing, dressing, and feeding. Alterations in this independence can influence their feelings about their own health.

HOSPITALIZATION AND ILLNESS

For children, hospitalization and illness are stressful experiences, primarily because of separation from the normal environment and significant others, a limited selection of coping behaviors, and altered states of health. In this case the nurse should try to make the experience a positive one.

NURSING PROCESS AND THE CHILD

Assessment

A child's reaction to illness and hospitalization is based on developmental age, previous experiences with hospitalization, available support persons, coping skills, and the seriousness of the diagnosis (Whaley, Wong, 1991). Table 24-7 identifies areas to assess and information to obtain. Thorough assessment of factors in each of these areas assists nurses in providing care that will promote resolution of illness and the general well-being of children and their families.

TABLE 24-7 Assessment of Hospitalized Child	
Assessment Area	Assessment Aims
Development	Identify current developmental level and skills achieved.
Observation of response to hospitalization	Identify current coping behaviors and their intensity.
History of previous illness, hospitalization, and separation	Identify previous patterns of coping and their effects.
Medical history	Identify seriousness of problem and its effect on developmental abilities.
Available support systems	Identify availability and willingness of family to participate in care and provide support.

Developmental Assessment

Developmental assessment aims to identify specific attributes of the child so that the nurse can individualize the care plan and enhance the child's coping abilities. Examination of the child's motor skills reveals the amount of assistance the child needs with eating, brushing teeth, bathing, dressing, elimination, and ambulation. If the toddler is accustomed to climbing out of the crib at home, special measures should be taken to prevent a fall during hospitalization. Special equipment brought to the hospital with the child, such as a splint or brace, can be identified and labeled with the child's name. When doing the sensory assessment, the nurse can identify and label any aids that the child uses such as hearing aids or eyeglasses.

It is also appropriate to determine the child's eating, sleeping, and elimination habits. It is also important to address appetite, favorite foods and drinks, use of bottle and favored utensils, and frequency of feedings because distinct preferences become more important to the child at times of stress. Toileting habits and special words for urine and stool need to be clarified. Sleep assessment should include frequency of naps, bedtime, sleeping positions, security items, and occurrence of any night terrors or nightmares.

The Denver Developmental Screening Test (DDST) is a widely used screening tool for children from birth through 6 years. It assesses personal-social, fine motor adaptive, language, and gross motor skills. This tool has been designed for use with well children, and the nurse may find that interventions such as intravenous fluids and casts, as well as children's illnesses, interfere with performance level. Although assessment at this time may not be a true picture of children's abilities, it can indicate how illness and hospitalization interfere with their achievement or display of expected development. Findings from the assessment provide the nurse with a basis on which to plan care that maintains and promotes development.

Observation of Response to Hospitalization

Separation anxiety, loss of control, and fear of bodily injury and pain are the primary causes of behavioral reactions of hospitalized children. Age dictates the specific manifestation, as evidenced by infants who loudly cry and protest separation from parents and toddlers who kick, bite, or hit to protest loss of autonomy. Loss of control behaviors is more apparent in toddlers and preschoolers, who may have frequent temper tantrums or exhibit regressive behaviors. Fear of bodily injury and pain occur in all children, including newborns. Infants react to pain with body rigidity, thrashing, and facial grimacing,

whereas preschoolers loudly protest and can become physically and verbally aggressive (Whaley, Wong, 1991).

Temperament, or how a child behaves or responds to a situation, is a key element in the child's coping style. The nurse assesses temperament by asking the parents questions about the child's usual activity level, general mood, persistence, and general response to new situations. When there is congruence between temperament and environment, the best possible development occurs (Ruddy-Wallace, 1987). The difficult child who seeks activity during stress will have more of a problem adjusting to immobility than the child who is an avid reader and seeks to be alone during stress.

Behaviors such as crying for parents, being uncooperative, and regressing in toileting habits are reactions to an interruption in the preschool child's achieved developmental tasks. The observation of various behavioral reactions to hospitalization allow the nurse to identify coping behaviors and plan care accordingly.

History of Previous Illness, Hospitalization, and Separation

The nurse gathers data about the way a child coped with a previous hospitalization (specific behavior reactions such as protests, withdrawal, aggression, and regression). The nurse also determines the effect that the hospitalization had on subsequent behavior (negative behaviors after discharge such as nightmares, aloofness, clinging, and temper tantrums).

Medical History

From the medical history the nurse should determine the seriousness of the health problem and its effect on development and nursing care. The nurse should also determine the effects of therapies on developmental achievements. For example, toddlers whose activities are severely restricted because of their illnesses or therapies (for example, spica casts) will have difficulty maintaining their independence. Restricting or limiting movement interferes with exploration needed to develop a sense of autonomy.

Available Support Persons

The availability and willingness of families to participate in the care of their children are determined at admission. Parents are encouraged to remain with young children as much as possible so that separation behaviors are minimized. Parents' willingness to stay depends on their involvement with children at home, their work situations, their degree of comfort with the hospital, and the amount of support that they receive from extended family members and friends in meeting the needs of other family members. Based on the information that the parents give, the nurse helps families plan their support of the child during hospitalization.

Assessment Tool

An effective tool for collection of data in the five areas just discussed would include systematic checklists ensuring that essential data are collected. The tool provides a guideline for the student until these assessment skills become automatic. It can also be used as a checklist so that significant data are not omitted. One such tool has been described by Kennedy, Gyr, and Garst (1991). The tool can assist the nurse to elicit, observe, and record essential subjective and objective data regarding the child's physiological, psychosocial, and developmental needs; daily routines; and family situation, concerns, and expectations.

 ### Nursing Diagnosis

Assessment reveals how the child copes with hospitalization and whether this experience will result in other health problems (see diagnoses box). The following case study provides an example:

Assessment data for a 3-year-old on the second day of hospitalization reveal that she continues to cry for her parents in their absence, is not eating, has relinquished her

---

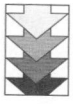 ## Examples of Nursing Diagnoses for Hospitalized Children

NANDA-APPROVED NURSING DIAGNOSES

Altered nutrition: less than body requirements related to:
- Response to hospitalization
- Separation from family
- Effect of illness
- Prescribed dietary restrictions
- Cultural food practices
- Pain

High risk for infection related to:
- Procedures and therapies
- Illness
- Decreased body defenses
- Insufficient knowledge to avoid pathogens

High risk for injury related to:
- Change in environment
- Broken skin
- Nosocomial agents
- Altered mobility

Social isolation related to:
- Separation from significant others
- Effects of illness
- Interruption of developmental task progress
- Hospitalization and routines

Altered family processes related to:
- Hospitalization
- Chronic illness

Activity intolerance related to:
- Conditions of illness
- Hospitalization

Sleep pattern disturbance related to:
- Unfamiliar environment
- Separation from family

- Procedure and therapies
- Pain
- Illness

Diversional activity deficit related to:
- Hospitalization
- Effects of illness
- Pain

Altered growth and development related to:
- Hospitalization and response
- Illness
- Pain
- Separation from family
- Multiple care givers

Powerlessness related to:
- Unfamiliar environment
- Illness

Knowledge deficit related to:
- Cognitive limitations of age
- Lack of information
- Limited experiences

Fear related to:
- Separation from significant care givers
- Potentially threatening situation of hospital

Pain related to:
- Illness
- Procedures and therapies

Anxiety related to:
- Unfamiliar environment
- Strange care givers

Ineffective individual coping related to:
- Inadequate support system
- Strange environment of hospital
- Vulnerability of age

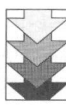

Sample Nursing Diagnostic Process for the Hospitalized Child

Assessment Activities	Defining Characteristics	Nursing Diagnoses
Observe child's behavior in response to hospital room and bed. Observe behavior as mother leaves child's side to use bathroom. Observe child in playroom with toys. Observe child's sleep behavior. Note child's ability to control bowel and bladder. Note child's eating behavior.	Insists on being held Protests strongly with cries and struggle No exploratory activity Uncooperative with blood pressure measurement, even with mother's help Regressive behaviors Child awoke sobbing at 2 AM Wet bed during night Refused to eat breakfast until father arrived and then allowed him to feed her	*Fear* related to threatening hospital environment, separation from parents, stage of cognitive development, fear of bodily harm, and strange care givers *Ineffective individual coping* related to strange environment and care givers, inadequate support system, and vulnerability of age

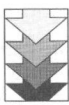

Sample Nursing Care Plan for Fear

Nursing diagnosis: *Fear* related to separation from family, threatening hospital environment, strange care givers, cognitive stage of development, and fear of bodily harm

Definition: Fear is a feeling of dread related to an identifiable source that the person validates (Kim, McFarland, McLane, 1991).

Goals	Expected Outcomes	Interventions	Rationale
Parents will actively participate in care of child each day.	One parent will remain with child (4/2). Parents will participate in child's feeding, hygiene, and play activities each day.	Encourage parent to room-in or have other family member with child. Ask parents how they wish to participate in child's care. Anticipate parents' need for assistance and guidance. Orient parents to nursing division and supplies. Provide appropriate items for these activities.	Parent provides security and prevents development of mistrust. Object permanence is not complete until 2 yr of age. Parental anxiety will decrease (Alexander et al, 1988). Strange environment undermines confidence of parents and results in fatigue. Parents who know events to expect experience less anxiety (Schepp, 1991). Provision of articles gives parents incentive to proceed.
Child will cope effectively with fear associated with hospitalization before discharge.	Child will use coping and defense mechanisms daily to combat fear (4/4). Child's use of regressive behavior will decrease (4/2).	Accept regressive behavior. Ask parent to bring to hospital items comforting to child (e.g., pacifier, blanket). Explain normalcy of this behavior to parents. Encourage information-seeking activities. Provide child with opportunities to "play out" fears, feelings, and concerns.	Comfortable earlier behaviors provide sense of security. Child should have access to familiar items that bring comfort and security. People of all ages combat fear and anxiety with regression after crisis behavior disappears. Explanation allows parents to know that this is coping behavior (Ritchie et al, 1988). Play is medium through which child can express inner feelings.

normal toilet habits, and does not respond favorably to attention from the nurse. The parents found it impossible to spend the night because of the needs of their 3-month-old twins. The maternal grandmother lives nearby and made it possible for the mother to visit during the evening. The father visited in the morning on his way home from work.

The diagnostic process for the hospitalized child (see box on p. 773) demonstrates how analysis of data from the assessment activities identifies the defining characteristics of two nursing diagnoses. The diagnostic statements identify the problems and their probable causes. This identification allows the nurse to plan specific interventions for resolution.

 ## Planning

After identifying nursing diagnoses, the nurse develops a care plan (see box on p. 773). The determination of goals of care for each nursing diagnosis is the first step. Because the child often cannot articulate feelings and needs, it is essential to also involve the parents and sometimes other family members in the establishment of these goals. Goals of care for a hospitalized child should reflect consideration of the following concerns:
1. Minimizing separation anxiety
2. Establishing trust
3. Reducing fear
4. Minimizing physical discomfort
5. Fostering normal growth and development
6. Incorporating play and diversional activity into daily care

Determining Priorities of Care

Children's and parents' responses to illness and hospitalization help the nurse determine priorities among goals. In situations in which family members do not remain with their children who refuse to eat or play and sleep poorly, priority must be given to the goal that deals with minimizing separation anxiety. Often the nurse can assist the parents in considering alternatives and mobilizing their resources.

 ## Implementation

Implementation of interventions are performed by nurses, the child, or the family. The nurse wishes to make the hospitalization a positive experience. This can be accomplished by remembering that each child is unique and by being sensitive to individual responses to nursing measures.

The nurse's organization and management of the child's care can acknowledge the individuality of the child and family by allowing them to have some control over bathtime, menus, bedtime, and certain procedures. For instance the child who is accustomed to taking a bath at bedtime or having a nighttime snack of cereal should be allowed to maintain this ritual in the hospital unless contraindicated by a necessary medical regimen. Each day the nurse should ascertain whether the parents would prefer to do the child's bath, like the nurse to do it, or enjoy all of them doing it together. Bathtime is a good time to continue assessment of the child and family. It is also often an appropriate time for teaching about some aspect of the child's care or to do anticipatory guidance (see teaching box)

Minimizing Separation Anxiety

Parents are more likely to remain with their young hospitalized infant when the nurse makes them feel comfortable and describes the accommodations the hospital has provided for them. When parents cannot continuously be with their child at the hospital, the nurse and parents need to plan together to make this situation more tolerable for the child. Appropriate guidelines include the following:
1. Parents should tell the child when they are leaving and when they will return in terms that the child can comprehend, such as "when daddy comes home from work." Then they should leave quickly.
2. The primary nurse should be with the child when the parents leave to provide some support and distraction.
3. The nurse should explain to the parents that protest is normal behavior and demonstrates a strong relationship with the parents.
4. Parents should leave some item that the child knows belongs to them because it will assure the child that they will return and provide comfort.
5. A child should have favorite toys from home or familiar objects such as a "special blanket" that provides comfort.
6. Parents should be encouraged to tape pictures of family members where the child can easily see them. Health care providers can discuss the photographs with the child.
7. Telephone calls from family members provide a link between home and hospital.
8. The child might be comforted by cassette tape recordings of family members reading stories, singing, or talking.

Establishing Trust

The nurse's establishment of a trusting relationship with the child and family requires careful planning. The nurse who is friendly and informative,

Client Teaching for Car-Seat Safety

OBJECTIVE

- Child will ride correctly restrained in the car and be protected from injury and death.

TEACHING STRATEGIES

- Discuss these measures with parents.
- Tell parents that motor vehicle accidents are the most common cause of death in children.
- Inform parents that the younger the child, the greater the risk of death from automobile accidents. This is because the child is often held by the mother in the front seat and the child's proportionally large head and higher center of gravity causes him or her to be propelled head-first into the dashboard or windshield.
- Demonstrate how an infant rides facing the rear in a semireclining position.
- Demonstrate the use of a convertible car seat model, which allows infant to ride in a rear-facing position and a toddler in a forward-facing position (see figure A). Tell the parents that the child is switched to forward position when weight nears 20 lb.

TEACHING STRATEGIES—cont'd

- Tell parents that a preschool child who outgrows the convertible restraint should ride in a booster seat until the midpoint of the head is higher than the back of the vehicle seat (see figure B).
- Encourage parents to purchase a crash-tested, government-approved car seat and follow manufacturer's directions carefully to achieve maximal protection. Some communities have resources that loan car seats to families who cannot afford to purchase them.
- Inform parents that the child should ride in car seats until they are outgrown. The child can use the regular car restraint system when weight reaches 40 lb or height reaches 40 in.
- Explain that the car should not be started until everyone is properly restrained.
- Tell parents to ensure that child remains in car seat and that cooperative behavior should be rewarded.

EVALUATION

- Observe how parents place child in car seat when leaving hospital.

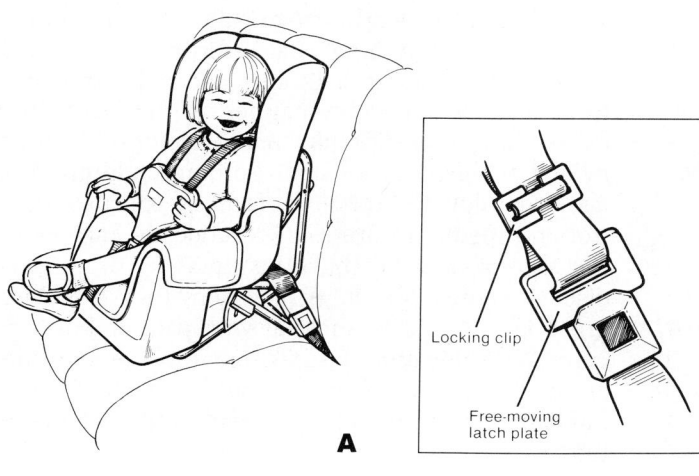

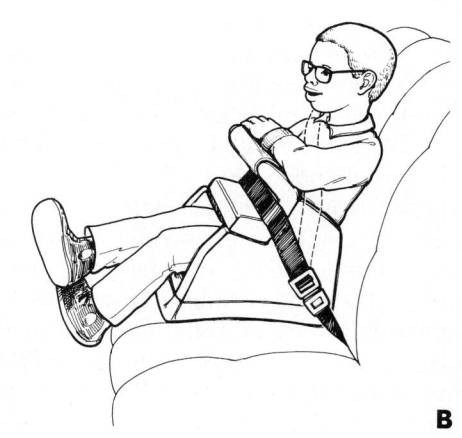

Locking clip

Free-moving latch plate

A

B

Data from US Preventive Services Task Force: Counseling to prevent household and environmental injuries, *Ann Fam Pract* 42(1): 136, 1990.
Illustrations from Whaley LF, Wong DL: *Nursing care of infants and children*, ed 4, St Louis, 1991, Mosby–Year Book.

listens well to the concerns of the family, and is not threatening to the child has laid the foundation for a positive relationship. A few suggestions for non-threatening communication techniques for the young child include the following:

1. Allow the child to observe friendly interaction between the parents and nurse before directly approaching the child.
2. Approach the child at eye level.
3. Communicate through a stuffed animal or doll before directly addressing the child.
4. Allow the child to become accustomed to the nurse through some type of play activity, such as balloon play, before touching the child.
5. Avoid gestures such as broad smiles and extended eye contact.

6. Speak in a clear manner that is unhurried and confident.

7. Incorporate parents into initial assessment activities such as vital sign measurement.

The parent's trust of the nurse will be enhanced by the efforts made to make their child comfortable. Parents often appreciate the opportunity to complete an assessment form that describes their child's eating, sleeping, toileting, and play routines. Providing parents with frequent opportunities to ask questions assures them of the nurse's interest in keeping them well informed and allows the trusting relationship to develop.

Reducing Fear

The nurse who is serious about reducing the fears of pediatric clients must be familiar with the fears' origins. These fears, which are based on cognitive and perceptual development, vary considerably at different ages. According to Servonsky and Opas (1987) the common fears according to age groups follow:

1. Infants from birth to 3 months: sudden movements, loud noises, and loss of physical support

2. Infants from 4 to 12 months: strangers, strange objects, heights, and anticipation of previous uncomfortable situations

3. Toddlers from 1 to 3 years: the dark, being alone, separation from parent, some animals such as barking dogs, and loud machines

4. Preschoolers from 3 to 6 years: body mutilation, supernatural beings, monsters, ghosts, separation from trusted adults and familiar routines, and abandonment

Some fears are associated with health care; these include being stuck with needles; having to take bad-tasting medications; experiencing invasive procedures (those that violate body surfaces) such as ear, nose, and throat examinations; being forced to lie down; and being subjected to the unknown such as x-ray procedures, electrocardiograms, and electroencephalograms.

Many of the plans appropriate for reduction of fear have already been discussed. However, the nurse should plan to use the following additional measures to reduce fear in the hospitalized child:

1. Allow the child to sit up for assessments and procedures whenever possible.

2. Demonstrate the exact steps of a procedure on a doll, another nurse, or parent before beginning the procedure on the child.

3. Allow the child to see and handle equipment or use it on a doll (for example, a sphygmomanometer).

4. Describe sensations that the child will experience such as "The x-ray table will be hard and cold when you lie on it."

5. Encourage parents' presence during procedures and treatments.

6. Provide the child with the opportunity to "play through" experiences and release pent-up feelings of anger and frustration in an acceptable fashion (for example, syringe play, pounding toys, substances to be molded, and percussion instruments).

7. Allow the child to assist with the procedure (for example, cleansing the skin with an alcohol wipe before an injection).

8. Plan for therapeutic play sessions.

Minimizing Physical Discomfort

Children of all ages, including newborns, experience pain. The nurse is often unable to prevent pain but can do much to reduce the physical discomfort. The expression of pain is influenced by the children's culture and parents' child-rearing practices. Children's perception of pain varies according to their pain threshold and degree of anxiety regarding it.

Pain in infants can be differentiated from hunger and general discomfort by crying that does not decrease with comfort measures, increased restlessness, and increased random movements. Toddlers who still perceive sensations in generalized ways cannot indicate clearly where pain is felt. In addition, toddlers find anything that is intrusive or causes pressure to be painful. Infants and toddlers respond to restraint in the same manner as physical pain because they have difficulty using motor activity as a means of releasing tension. Forcing children of any age to lie down is threatening to their sense of control and results in protest. Preschoolers can point to the area of pain but have insufficient vocabulary to discuss or describe it. In addition, they associate a great deal of anxiety and fear with pain and may perceive that the pain is a punishment for some misdeed or "bad" thought. Nurses should use the following guidelines to minimize children's physical discomfort:

1. Keep periods of restraint or immobility to a minimum. This can be facilitated by having at the bedside a care giver whose watchfulness prevents the accidental removal of catheters and tubes.

2. Comfort infants and toddlers by talking in a soft voice or singing and with physical contact such as holding and rocking, hugging, cuddling, and caressing.

3. Provide young children with items that provide security and comfort (for example, special blanket, favorite toy, or mother's scarf).

4. Reassure children that it is OK to cry, and emphasize the helpful things they do, such as keeping their arms very still during shots.

5. Allow choices that are acceptable such as which finger to stick for a blood glucose test or which bandage to put on afterward.
6. Encourage participation in a procedure that may result in discomfort, which is exaggerated by anxiety (for example, removing the tape when intravenous fluids are being discontinued).
7. Provide incentives that encourage cooperation with uncomfortable nursing actions (for example, allowing children to choose surprises from a special box each time they cooperate with fingersticks for blood sugar measurement).
8. Use a pain assessment tool that allows children to use colors to describe the degree of pain.
9. Use a variety of techniques such as positioning, distraction, relaxation, and rhythmic breathing with imagery to alleviate pain.
10. Provide adequate analgesic control of pain to provide comfort and promote cooperation with painful procedures such as coughing, turning, and deep breathing.

Fostering Normal Growth and Development

Illness and hospitalization of children have a disrupting effect on their development. When the illness is mild and hospitalization is short, the effect may be mimimal, but a serious illness can have a more significant impact. The illness is often accompanied by physical restrictions, enforced dependency, and interruption of daily routines for eating, sleeping, elimination, and play. Regression to earlier behaviors that provide security is the most common defense mechanism used by young children to cope with these stresses. Use of the following guidelines will help the nurse plan for fostering of normal growth and development:

1. Provide an environment of acceptance for regressive behavior.
2. Provide favorite toys from home.
3. Encourage participation in self-care activities such as bathing, dressing, and feeding self.
4. Provide intermittent auditory and visual stimulation. (For example, take children for rides in wheelchairs or wagons, play sing-along records, read to children, and look at picture books with children.)
5. Provide opportunities for children to socially interact with other children. (For example, take children to playroom in wagons or wheelchairs, encourage sibling visits, and have other clients visit children.)
6. Provide toys and play equipment that promote development of fine and gross motor activities.

7. Encourage development of new vocabulary by learning names for hospital items and personnel.
8. Encourage participation in assessment and procedures.
9. Discuss the effects of hospitalization on growth and development with parents and explain how they can help children regain and attain optimal levels of growth and development.

Incorporation of Play and Diversional Activity into Care

For children, play is work. It can be one of the most effective tools for managing hospitalized children. Play in the hospital brings a normalacy to the strange and sometimes hostile-appearing environment and provides an avenue for the release of tension. Diversional play allows children to focus their attention on pleasurable experiences and to downplay situations that result when a child combines reality with imagination.

Play helps children deal with strains and stresses, develop their capacities, and strengthen their defenses (Servonsky, Opas, 1987). The nurse may find the following guidelines helpful when planning play for the hospitalized child:

1. Incorporate play into the daily activities of bathing, dressing, feeding, and measurement of vital signs.
2. Provide opportunities for all children, especially those who are immobilized, to go to the playroom or engage in play with other children.
3. Keep the playroom as a "safe" area by prohibiting the administration of medications or performance of any procedures.
4. Provide materials that encourage creativeness (for example, paper, paint, paste, playdough, crayons, and other art materials).
5. Provide sense-pleasure play that allows infants and young children to enjoy sound, movement, smells, tastes, touch, and color through activities and objects such as water play, mobiles, and stuffed toys.
6. Promote motor development through skill play such as putting objects in a container and dumping them out.
7. Promote cognitive development through activities such as reading, hiding and seeking of objects, and counting games.
8. Plan special activities for children whose activities are limited by their health problems or medical regimen. (For example, have children with eye patches identify familiar objects by feel or provide a sense of mobility to children in traction by playing a game of ring toss.)

9. When children are confined to their rooms by isolation, have parents select toys and games from the playroom to take to their child.

10. Request visits by volunteers or the child life worker when children are confined.

11. Prepare children for procedures through play with hospital equipment.

12. Use children's cognitive levels as bases for choosing appropriate play activities for teaching purposes.

13. Provide for judicious television watching.

Collaboration with other health team members is often an important step in providing optimal care for the child. If the preschooler is having difficulty cooperating with the respiratory therapist for a breathing treatment, the nurse might request that the therapist leave the mask with the child for examination and play between treatments. If the toddler refuses to keep the nasal prongs in place and continuously fights a mask, the nurse and respiratory therapist might discuss the situation with the physician and decide that a Croupette would be a more satisfactory delivery system for oxygen. Each hospital has its own guidelines for recording and exchanging information about clients, but regardless of the methods used, it's important to always include the following:

1. Assessments and nursing actions related to nursing diagnoses

2. The child's and parents' response to teaching

3. Questions asked by the child or parents and the nurse's response

4. Social behavior of the child

 ## Evaluation

Each child reacts differently to hospitalization; as a result, it is necessary to evaluate the response of the child and family to nursing interventions to determine whether the goals of care have been met. The statement of expected outcomes and evaluative measures (see evaluation box) provides a method by which to measure the response to interventions. For instance, a goal may have been the active participation of the parents in the care of the child, but the outcome may have been that the mother demonstrated no interest or initiative in bathing the child. The nurse must review the goals and interventions to determine whether and how they should be revised. Modification of the care plan should reflect input from the child and parents. For example, infusion of intravenous fluids might have caused the mother to feel inadequate or afraid to disturb the child, and as a result she needed further support from the nurse.

SUMMARY

Providing nursing care is a highly complex and individualized process. The nurse must first understand the individual's growth and development. The nurse must assess the factors in the individual's life that influence growth and development. Only then can the nurse and client or family make decisions about developmental needs and plan and implement nursing interventions that promote health.

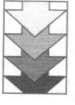 ### Sample Evaluation of Interventions for Fear

Goals	Evaluative Measures	Expected Outcomes
Parents will actively participate in care of child each day.	Observe presence of and activity of family in child's room.	Parent or significant other will remain with child. Parent will participate in feeding, hygiene, and play each day.
Child will cope effectively with anxiety associated with hospitalization before discharge.	Observe child's use of self-comforting measures. Observe child for evidence of regressive behavior. Observe child's play.	Child will use coping and defense mechanisms to combat anxiety daily. Child's use of regressive behavior diminishes. Child's play activities demonstrate feelings toward hospitalization.

The complexities of growth and development are interrelated and influenced by many factors. Developmental theories can be applied by the nurse to assess strengths and weaknesses and plan care accordingly.

A developmental approach is used to individually examine the different stages of growth and development. The physical, psychosocial, and cognitive dimensions of development, as well as the way that developmental factors function, are relevant in assessment, nursing diagnosis, planning, implementation, and evaluation.

REFERENCES

Alexander D et al: Anxiety levels of rooming-in and non-rooming-in parents of young hospitalized children, *Matern Child Nurs J* 12(2):79, 1988.

Erikson EH: *Childhood and society,* ed 2, New York, 1963, Norton.

Freud S: *A general introduction into psychoanalysis,* New York, 1969, Pocket Books.

Kennedy CM, Gyr PM, Garst KF: A nursing tool to assess children upon hospital admission, *MCN* 16(2):78, 1991.

Kim MJ, McFarlane GK, McLane AM: *Pocket guide to nursing diagnoses,* ed 4, St Louis, 1991, Mosby–Year Book.

Kohlberg L: Stages and sequence: the cognitive-developmental approach to socialization. In Goslin DA, editor: *Handbook of socialization theory and research,* Chicago, 1969, Rand McNally.

Maslow AH: *Motivation and personality,* ed 2, New York, 1970, Harper & Row.

Nelms BC, Mullins R: *Growth and development: a primary health care approach,* Englewood Cliffs, NJ, 1982, Prentice Hall.

Papalia DC, Olds SW: *Human development,* ed 4, St Louis, 1989, McGraw-Hill.

Piaget J: *The origins of intelligence in children,* New York, 1952, International Universities Press.

Ritchie JA et al: Coping behaviors of hospitalized preschool children, *Matern Child Nurs J* 17(3):153, 1988.

Ruddy-Wallace M: Temperament: assessing individual differences in hospitalized children, *J Pediatr Nurs* 2:30, 1987.

Schepp KG: Factors influencing the coping effort of mothers of hospitalized children, *Nurs Res* 40(1):42, 1991.

Servonsky J, Opas SR: Nursing management of children, Monterey, Calif, 1987, Jones & Bartlett.

Warshaw JB: Intrauterine growth retardation, *Pediatr Rev* 8:107, 1986.

Westwood M et al: Growth and development of full term nonasphyxiated small-for-gestational-age newborns: follow-up through adolescence, *Pediatrics* 71:376, 1983.

Whaley LF, Wong DL: *Nursing care of infants and children,* ed 4, St Louis, 1991, Mosby–Year Book.

Williams JK: Counseling adolescents about environmental teratogens, *Pediatr Nurs* 12:292, 1986.

ADDITIONAL READINGS

Bergmann T, Freud A: *Children in the hospital,* New York, 1965, International Universities Press.

Birchfield MD: Nursing care for hospitalized children based on different stages of illness, *Matern Child Nurs J* 6(1):46, 1981.

Brown M, Murphy M: *Ambulatory pediatrics for nurses,* ed 2, New York, 1981, McGraw-Hill.

Chess S, Thomas A: Temperamental differences: a critical concept in child health care, *Pediatr Nurs* 11(3):167, 1985.

Chow MP et al: *Handbook of pediatric primary care,* ed 2, New York, 1984, Wiley.

Clatworthy S: Therapeutic play: effects on hospitalized children, *Child Health Care* 9(4):108, 1981.

Coste J et al: Increased risk of ectopic pregnancy with maternal cigarette smoking, *Am J Public Health* 81(2):199, 1991.

Craft MJ, Wyatt N: Effect of visitation of siblings on hospitalized children, *Matern Child Nurs J* 15(1):47, 1986.

Foster RLR et al: *Family-centered nursing care of children,* Philadelphia, 1989, Saunders.

Frankenburg WK et al: The newly abbreviated and revised Denver Developmental Screening Test, *J Pediatr* 106(2):343, 1985.

Free T et al: A descriptive study of infants and toddlers exposed prenatally to substance abuse, *MCN* 15(4):245, 1990.

Furstenberg F: *Unplanned pregnancy: the social consequences of teenage pregnancy,* New York, 1981, Free Press.

Kelley SJ, Walsh JH, Thompson IC: Birth outcomes, health problems, and neglect with prenatal exposure to cocaine, *Pediatr Nurs* 17(2):130, 1991.

Korones S: *High-risk newborn infants: the basis for intensive nursing care,* ed 4, St Louis, 1986, Mosby–Year Book.

Kramer NA: Comparison of therapeutic touch and casual touch in stress reduction of hospitalized children, *Pediatr Nurs* 16(5):483, 1990.

Petitti DB, Coleman C: Cocaine and the risk of low birth weight, *Am J Public Health* 80(1):25, 1990.

Robertson J: *Young children in hospital,* ed 2, London, 1970, Tavistock Publications.

Turner JS, Helms DB: *Lifespan development,* ed 3, New York, 1987, Holt, Rinehart & Winston.

US Preventive Services Task Force: Counseling to prevent household and environmental injuries, *Ann Fam Pract* 42(1):136, 1990.

CHAPTER 24 REVIEW

Key Concepts

- Growth and development are orderly, directional, predictable, interdependent, and complex processes that continue throughout life.

- People progress through similar chronological stages of growth and development but at an individual pace and with individual behaviors.

- A developmental perspective helps the nurse understand commonalities and variations in each stage and the impact that they have on the client's health.

- During critical periods of development, a variety of experiences can foster or hinder optimal physical, cognitive, and psychosocial development.

- Growth and development are influenced by the inner forces of heredity and temperament and the outer forces of family, peers, life experiences, and environmental elements.

- Because the embryo and fetus grow and develop throughout the intrauterine period, impairments in any body system may occur in utero.

- Health risks for the unborn child include genetic impairments and environmental factors (teratogens).

- Physiological health concerns during childbirth include adequate functioning of all systems and prevention of infection.

- A psychosocial health concern that begins at childbirth is the establishment of parent-child attachment.

- Physiological, cognitive, and psychosocial development continues throughout the neonate, infant, toddler, and preschool periods, and the nurse must be familiar with normal parameters to determine potential problems and promote normal development.

- The nurse recognizes that the child's perception of health and health behaviors begins early and assists the parent and child in establishing healthful patterns that will continue for the entire life span.

- The nurse educates the parents about risk factors and the child's health needs, provides emotional support to the parents in the prenatal period, and helps them understand the changes and needs of the developing child.

- The developmental theories of Freud, Erikson, Maslow, Piaget, and Kohlberg help explain the individual aspects of development for each client.

- The nursing care plan for the hospitalized child is based on assessment of development, response to illness and hospitalization, previous experiences with separation, medical history, and available support system.

- In addition to implementing physician's orders to assist the child in becoming well, the nurse should focus on minimizing separation anxiety, reducing fears, minimizing physical discomfort, providing diversional activities, and promoting growth and development.

- Nursing strategies for the ill and hospitalized child include incorporating the parents into the child's care and fostering the child's continued development.

Key Terms

Animism, p. 769

Apgar score, p. 759

Artificialism, p. 769

Attachment, p. 763

Blastocyst, p. 756

Bonding, p. 760

Critical period, p. 749

Development, p. 748

Embryo, p. 756

Fetus, p. 756

Growth, p. 748

Immanent justice, p.769

Infancy, p. 763

Lanugo, p. 758

Maturation, p. 748

Molding, p. 760

Morula, p. 756

Neonatal period, p. 760

Object permanence, p. 748

Organogenesis, p. 757

Physiological anorexia, p. 766

Placenta, p. 756

Preconceptual thought, p. 769

Preoperational thought, p. 767

Preschool years, p. 768

Temperament, p. 771

Teratogens, p. 757

Toddlerhood, p. 766

Vernix caseosa, p. 758

Zygote, p. 756

Critical Thinking Exercises

1. Two-day old Sally has been admitted to the hospital because she has had a seizure. Newborns have very poor resistance to infection. What measures should the nurses take to be sure that Sally does not develop an infection during hospitalization?

2. Six-month-old Jimmy has been admitted to the hospital because of bronchiolitis. His parents wish to participate in his care when they are present but will not be able to be with him continuously. The mother plans to spend the late evening and night at the hospital but will continue to work during the day. The father will visit on his way home from work in the evening. Identify nursing measures that will assist Jimmy to continue developing his sense of trust.

3. Describe the procedure you would follow to measure six month old Jimmy's vital signs.

4. Two-year-old Johnny has been admitted to the hospital for periorbital cellulitis of his right eye and is receiving intravenous antibiotic therapy. What strategies can the nurse use in his daily care to promote his developing autonomy?

5. Johnny's mother will not be able to spend the night at the hospital with him. What measures could the nurse and mother take to comfort him and help him cope with this separation?

6. The nurse needs to measure 4-year-old Jenny's blood pressure, but Jenny is resistant to having the blood pressure cuff placed on her arm. What strategies might the nurse use to gain Jenny's cooperation?

CHAPTER 25

School Age Through Adolescence

OBJECTIVES

Mastery of content in this chapter will enable the student to:

- Define the key terms listed.
- Describe the normal physical changes that occur during the school-age years and adolescence.
- Discuss behaviors reflecting psychosocial and cognitive development of the school-age child and adolescent.
- Contrast the cognitive abilities of the school-ager and adolescent.
- Identify factors that contribute to self-esteem in youth.
- Describe the influence of the school environment on the development of the school-age child and adolescent.
- Discuss ways in which the nurse can help parents meet their children's developmental needs.
- Compare and contrast the ways by which a school-age child and adolescent develop moral values.
- Discuss the development of identity in the adolescent.
- Explain the significance of Erikson's psychosocial moratoriums to the adolescent.
- Identify health concerns of the school-age and adolescent.
- Describe nursing interventions to promote optimal health in the school-ager and adolescent.
- Describe the use of the nursing process to individualize the nursing care of youth.

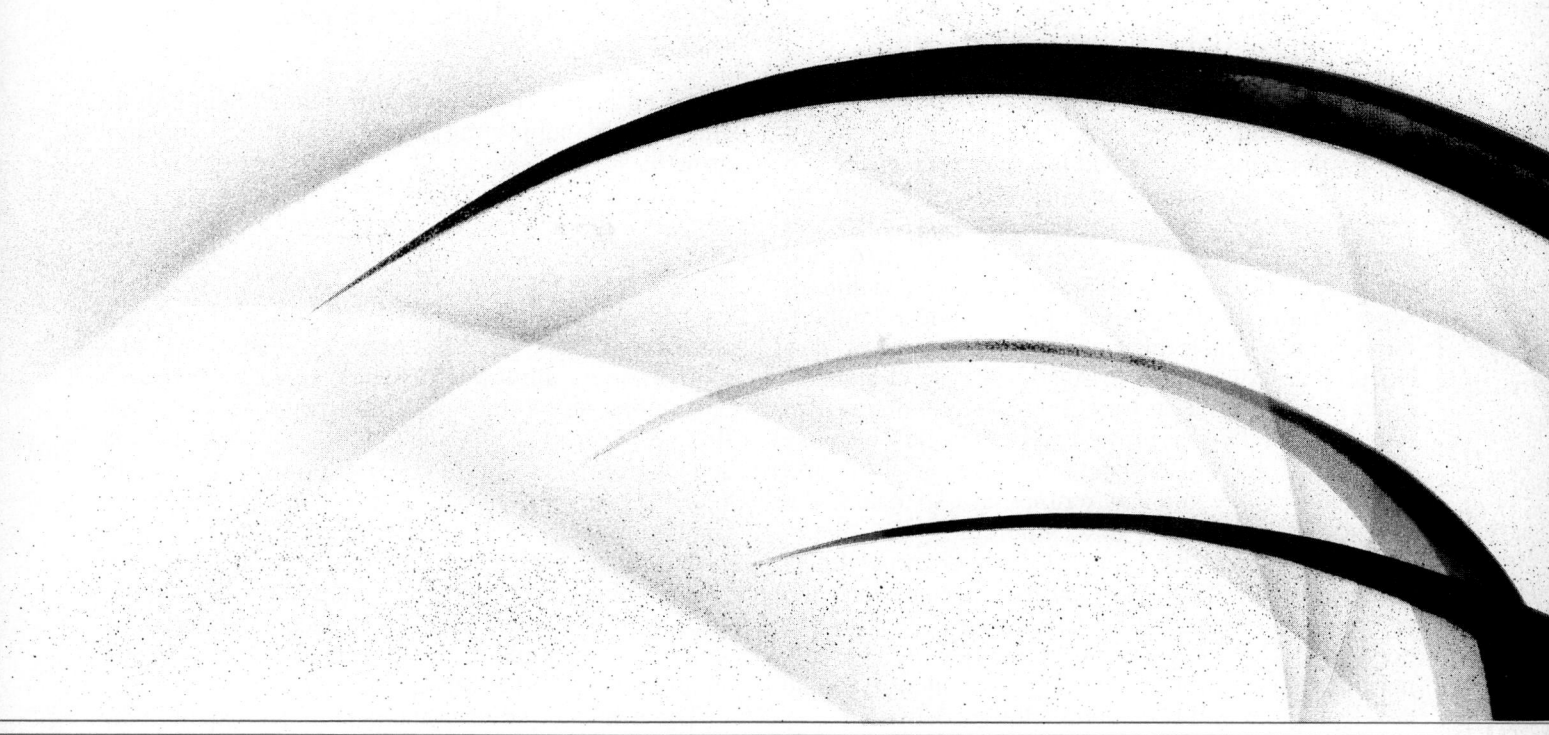

CHAPTER OUTLINE

chool-age children and adolescents lead demanding, challenging lives. The developmental changes of individuals between age 6 and 18 are diverse and span all areas of growth and development. Physical, psychosocial, cognitive, and moral skills are developed, expanded, refined, and synchronized so that the individual may become an accepted and productive member of society. The environment in which the individual develops skills also expands and diversifies. Instead of the principal limits of family and close friends, the environment may include the school, community, and church. Because of expectations for development, increasing skill and knowledge base, and environmental expansion, the individual experiences new difficulties and dilemmas. For proper assessment the nurse must know the appropriate developmental expectations for each age group. For example, before assessing risk-taking behaviors, the nurse must know that adolescents normally strive to achieve a sense of identity while developing a moral code compatible with society.

The nurse needs to direct school-age children and adolescents toward normal developmental behaviors, assisting them in maximizing their abilities and using them to cope. By helping children and adolescents achieve a necessary developmental balance, the nurse promotes health. Table 25-1 provides an overview of developmental behaviors typical of school-age children and adolescents. The nurse must also increasingly involve the child or adolescent in charting a developmental course. Because school-age children have increased cognitive and social skills, they are better able to plan developmental activities. Not only can they describe their feelings about the changes, but they can also think through these changes. Problem solving becomes more purposeful and sophisticated and results in the achievement of the outcomes that they desire. This paced, active participation may initiate a style of involvement in lifelong self-care.

School-age children and adolescents must cope with changes involving all areas of development and frequently occurring at the same time. For example, 6-year-old children are confronted with new authority figures, teachers; new cultures with varying mores; new rules and restrictions; the need to cooperatively work and play with a large group of children; and the challenge of developing cognitive skills that enhance their reasoning and allow them to learn to read, write, and manipulate numbers.

Because of the stress of these changes, a child may develop physical and psychosocial health problems (for example, increasing susceptibility to upper respiratory infections, school maladjustment, inadequate peer relationships, or learning disorders). The nurse helps the child avoid or minimize health problems while supporting the child's developmental growth.

 ## SCHOOL-AGE CHILD

During these "middle years" of childhood, the foundation for adult roles in work, recreation, and social interaction is laid. In industrialized countries, this period begins when the child starts elementary school around the age of 6 years; puberty, around 12 years of age, signals the end of middle childhood. Great developmental strides are made during these early school years when children develop competencies in physical, cognitive, and psychosocial skills. During these years, children become "better" at things; for example, they can run faster and farther as proficiency and endurance develop.

The school or educational experience expands the child's world and is a transition from a life of relatively free play to a life of structured play, learning, and work. The school and home influence growth and development, requiring adjustment by the parents and child. The child must learn to cope with rules and expectations presented by the school and peers. Parents must learn to allow their child to make decisions, accept responsibility, and learn from life's experiences.

While the child goes through this adjustment, the nurse promotes health. The nurse helps the parents and child identify stresses before they occur and plans to minimize stress and the child's reaction to it. This intervention must include parent, child, and teacher for maximal success. Table 25-2 on p. 787 provides an overview of stressors commonly encountered by school-age children and the appropriate nursing interventions.

Physical Development

Height and Weight

The rate of growth during these early school years is slower than any time since birth but continues in a steady manner; however, a particular child may not follow it precisely. Growth accelerates at different times for different children. The average increase in height is 2 inches per year, and the weight, which is more variable, increases by 4 to 7 pounds per year. Many children double their weight during these middle years. Children lose their babylike contours and appear slimmer because fat decreases in thickness and changes in its overall distribution (Turner, Helms, 1987).

TABLE 25-1 Developmental Behaviors of School-Age Children and Adolescents	
School-Age Children	**Adolescents**

RELATIONSHIPS WITH PARENTS

Children gradually learn that parents are less than perfect; they can be disillusioned with them and wish that friends' parents were their own. Sometimes they believe that they must be adopted. They rely on parents for unconditional love, security, guidance, and nurturing.

Adolescents' desire for increasing independence and autonomy and continuing need for some dependence and limit setting by parents place strain on their relationship. Effective communication and democratic parenting are best tools for meeting this challenge.

RELATIONSHIPS WITH SIBLINGS

School-agers seem to be at odds with one another at home; yet they are each others' best defenders away from home. Younger children often idolize older siblings, and this frequently leads to competition. Older children may envy attention that younger siblings require and be quite bossy and somewhat abusive.

Younger siblings rarely understand their adolescent siblings' need for privacy to think, dream, and talk with peers. Adolescents often enjoy interacting with and guiding younger brothers and sisters when timing is convenient for them and they can remain in control.

RELATIONSHIPS WITH PEERS

During primary grades (6-7 years), children of both sexes play together, depending on who is available and interested. Around age 8, social groupings of same-sex peers form. These "gangs" allow children to declare their independence from parental rules and establish their own secret codes or languages and rules of membership and behavior. This period is often referred to as *secret society* of childhood. Preadolescent (10-12 years) friendships are characterized by having best friend of same sex. These relationships may be transient, but they are intense and allow discussion of all areas of life. Some interest in heterosexual relationships develop, but they usually are not reciprocal.

Peer group is factor of critical influence to adolescents who have increasing need for recognition and acceptance. Companionship offered by peer groups provides secure environment for individuals to try out new ideas and share similar feelings and attitudes. Adolescents often form cliques with peers from same socioeconomic group with similar interests. Cliques, which are highly exclusive, help their members, who have strong emotional bonds, develop their identities. The crowd, which is more impersonal than clique, offers opportunities for heterosexual interaction and social activities. The crowd also maintains rigid membership requirements; clique membership is usually prerequisite for crowd membership.

SELF-CONCEPT

Children's feelings of competence regarding mastery of tasks are key element in forming self-esteem. Children need to receive positive feedback from teachers and parents regarding their efforts. It is important for children to develop skills in at least one area such as reading, music, or swimming. Pets that require children's care and attention reward them with unconditional love and promote feelings of self-worth.

Formal and informal peer groups are primary force in shaping self-concept of group members. Popularity and recognition within peer group enhance self-esteem and reinforce self-concept. Total immersion in peer group may make it appear that adolescents have no original thoughts and are incapable of making decisions. Adolescents who withdraw from peers into isolation struggle with developing identity.

FEARS

There is decline in fears related to body safety such as storms, dogs, darkness, noises, scrapes, and scratches. Fears of supernatural such as ghosts and witches persist and decline slowly. New fears related to school and family occur. They fear ridicule from teachers and friends and disapproval and rejection of parents. They also become frightened about death and items that they hear on news such as war and destruction of environment.

Fears in this age group center around peer group acceptance, body changes, loss of self-control, and emerging sexual urges. Adolescents constantly examine their bodies for changes and signs of imperfection. Any defect, real or imagined, is cause of endless worry. Adolescents' developing awareness of economic and political problems may result in fear of going to war with its resulting death and destruction.

Continued.

TABLE 25-1   Developmental Behaviors of School-Age Children and Adolescents—cont'd

School-Age Children	Adolescents
COPING PATTERNS	
To deal with stress, school-agers use problem solving and defense mechanisms, including regression, denial, aggression, and supression. Several categories of coping behaviors of hospitalized school-agers include inactivity (total silence, lack of activity, and apathy), orientation or precoping (looking and listening, walking around and exploring, and asking questions), cooperation (compliance with care), resistance (attempt to get away from the situation by turning away or making physical or verbal attacks), and controlling (assuming responsibility for self-care and suggesting how things could be done).	Repertoire of coping behaviors has expanded with experiences adolescents have gained from life and from developing cognitive maturity. By age 15, most use full range of defense mechanisms, including rationalization and intellectualization. Adolescents' problem-solving abilities have matured, and they can reason through philosophical discussions and complex situations that require abstract thinking and proposition of hypotheses. Some adolescents use avoidance coping strategies in which the problem is denied or repressed and an attempt to reduce tension is made by engaging in chemical abuse or avoiding people.
MORALS	
Children learn rules from parents, but their understanding of rules or reasons for them is limited until about 10 years. Before that, they are concerned with own needs first and may cheat to win. After 10, justice is based on "eye for an eye," and punishment should correct situation (e.g., if children break something, they should pay to have it fixed).	According to Kohlberg (1964), as youths approach adolescence, they reach conventional level where internalization of expectations of their family and society begins. Initially, there is considerable comformity to rules to win praise or approval from others and to avoid social disapproval or rejection; later, they seek to avoid criticism from persons of authority in institutions.
DIVERSIONAL ACTIVITY	
School-agers play cooperatively in group activities such as jumping rope, hopscotch, soccer, and baseball. Play becomes competitive, and children often have difficulty learning to lose. Teasing, insults, dares, superstitions, and increased sensitivity are characteristics of this age.	Many teenagers develop special interests in certain sports and concentrate on developing maximal skills therein. Recreational activities are often determined by what is popular with peers and what can provide independence from parents (e.g., computers, cars).
NUTRITION	
Children have definite likes and dislikes. Few nutritional deficiencies occur in this age group. Children have voracious appetites after school and need quality snacks such as fruit and sandwiches to avoid the empty calorie foods such as chips and candy.	Total nutritional needs become greater during adolescence. Girls' caloric needs decrease, and their need for protein increases slightly. Iron needed by adolescents is almost twice that of adult men, and growth spurt increases calcium demand.

School provides children with the opportunity to compare themselves with large numbers of children of the same age. The physical examination for first grade is an excellent opportunity for the nurse to discuss with the child and parents the influences of genetic endowment, nutrition, and exercise on height and weight. Regular measurement of height and weight may reveal alterations in growth that are symptoms of the onset of a variety of childhood diseases.

Boys are slightly taller and heavier than girls during these early school years. Approximately 2 years before puberty, these school-agers experience a rapid acceleration in skeletal growth, and girls, who reach puberty first, begin to surpass boys in height and weight, which causes embarrassment to both sexes. These changes may begin as early as 9 years in girls but do not usually occur in boys before 12 years.

Cardiovascular Functioning

Cardiovascular functioning is refined and stabilized during the school-age years. The heart rate averages 70 to 90 beats per minute, the blood pressure normalizes to approximately 110/70 mm Hg, and the respiratory rate stabilizes to 19 to 21 breaths per minute. Lung growth is minimal. However, by the end of this period the heart is 6 times the size it was at birth and has generally reached its adult size.

TABLE 25-2   Potential School-Related Stressors

Stressor	Nursing Intervention
AGE 6-8	
Adjusting to teacher's disciplinary approach	Promote parent-teacher-nurse communication through conferences aimed at identifying expectations, encouraging parental involvement in school or classroom activities, and mediating in conflicts or difficult situations.
Meeting teacher's behavioral expectations	Encourage communication between child and parent about school expectations, events, and adjustments.
Competing with peers for teacher's attention	Promote fair and equal treatment of children in classroom. Discourage favoritism and performance comparisons and encourage appropriate individual attention and praise.
Maintaining self-concept	Evaluate parent-child relationship for interaction problems that may transfer to classroom; communicate these to teacher.
Coping with hurtful honesty of peers	Promote close supervision of peer activities and behaviors. Discuss peer relationships, their nature, and characteristics with parents and teacher.
Testing out new ideas and behaviors at home	Set limits on destructive or antisocial behaviors. Allow exploration of new behaviors and ideas with guidance.
Coping with being away from home for extended period of time and adjusting to school rules and routines	Assist child in identifying physical setup of school and daily routines in first few days.
AGE 8-10	
Concentrating on cognitive pursuits, meeting cognitive expectations of school, and meeting own and family's cognitive expectations to best of ability	Encourage communication about child's performance among parent, child, and teacher. Assist in identifying skills mastered and those in need of mastery. Assist in identifying early problems. Assess level of health, particularly sensory function, as it may relate to school difficulties. Accept child, performance, and behaviors as individual when considered within norm.
Integrating peer values into behavior without interference with family values	Observe peer activities and interactions. Reinforce positive behaviors and performance. Provide education for parents and teachers regarding normal behaviors.
AGE 10-12	
Assuming responsibility for own learning	Encourage allocation of learning responsibilities and allow child to carry them out. Encourage child's participation in identifying learning needs.
Deriving satisfaction from own cognitive performance	Positively reinforce good performance and guide child when performance is optimal; do not punish.
Participating in organized school or peer activities	Assist in identifying school or peer group activity that child enjoys and in which child can be successful. Assist parents in realizing need for extracurricular activities and encouraging child's appropriate participation (avoid excessive demands to win and promote honest, fair play). Encourage teachers to recognize importance of after-school activities and avoid overloading child with homework.
Beginning to develop set of behavioral standards that reflect being in control and requiring little or no adult supervision	Promote good conduct through praise and example. Encourage parents to trust child, recognizing that not all behaviors will be "perfect."

Modified from Laige J: The school age child and his family. In Hymovich D, Barnard M, editors: *Family health care: developmental and situational crises,* New York, 1973, McGraw-Hill; and McElroy E, Tackett JJ: Growth and development needs of the family with school age children: maintaining wellness. In Tackett JJ, Hunsberger M, editors: *Family centered care of children and adolescents,* Philadelphia, 1981, Saunders.

Gross Motor Coordination

School-age children become more graceful during the school years because their large muscle coordination improves and strength doubles. Most children practice the basic gross motor skills of running, jumping, balancing, throwing, and catching during play, resulting in refinement of neuromuscular function and skills. Individual differences in the rate of mastering skills and ultimate skill achievement become apparent. Individual differences in motor skills are established by participation in activities and games requiring coordinated muscle movements and innate ability.

Fine Motor Coordination

Fine motor skills lag behind gross motor skills but progress at approximately the same rate. As control is gained over fingers and wrists, children become proficient in a wide range of activities.

Most 6-year-old children can hold a pencil adeptly and print letters and words, but by age 12 the child can make detailed drawings and write sentences in script. Painting, drawing, playing computer games, and modeling allow children to practice and improve newly refined skills. Nurses should encourage children and have parents encourage them to pursue these activities. Table 25-3 describes specific gross

---

TABLE 25-3 Motor Development in the School-Ager		
6-7 Years	8-10 Years	11-12 Years
FINE MOTOR SKILLS		
Uses knife to butter bread and learns to cut tender meat. Cuts, folds, and pastes paper. Prints with pencil. Draws man with 12-16 details. Copies triangle at 6 years and diamond by 7 years. Colors within lines of picture. Needs assistance to clean teeth thoroughly.	Uses knife and fork simultaneously. Learns to thread needle and tie knot. Uses hammer, saw, and screwdriver. Becomes proficient at writing cursive. Uses symbols in drawing (e.g., bird, star). Builds simple models of cars and planes and does simple handcrafts. Learns to play jacks and marbles. Can learn to floss teeth effectively and be independent in tooth care.	Learns to peel apples and potatoes. Sews simple garments on machine. Builds simple objects like birdhouse. Enjoys using decorative script. Begins to use creative and artistic talents. Builds complex models of cars and planes and does complex handcrafts. Learns to play musical instrument. Becomes proficient in caring for teeth with braces and other appliances.
GROSS MOTOR SKILLS		
Remains in constant motion. Moves more cautiously at 7 years than at 6 years. Hops and jumps into small squares. Learns to roller skate, skip rope, ride bicycle, and swim.	Can catch, throw (70 feet), and hit baseball. Engages in alternate rhythmic hopping in 2-2, 2-3, or 3-3 pattern. Engages in complex styles of skipping rope accompanied by verbal jingles.	Can do standing broad jump of 5 feet. Can do standing high jump of 3 feet. Plays games involving simultaneous use of two or more complex motor skills such as roller skating, ice hockey, or dance skating.
SELF-CARE		
Takes bath without supervision. Often returns to finger feeding. Learns to brush and comb hair in acceptable fashion without help. Puts on most clothes but may need assistance with shirttails, sashes, and final adjustments.	Learns to clean bathroom after bath. Enjoys fixing own snacks and sack lunch. Learns to part hair and insert hair ribbons and barrettes. Dresses self completely and can help younger siblings with clothes. Can make own bed.	Dusts, vacuums, and straightens own room. Learns to cook simply prepared foods. Washes, dries, and fixes own hair in braids, curls, and ponytails. Learns to sort, wash, dry, and press own clothing. Learns to care for fingernails and toenails.

motor and fine motor skills and their use in self-care activities.

The improved fine motor capabilities of youngsters in middle childhood allow them to become very independent in bathing, dressing, and taking care of other personal needs, and they develop strong personal preferences in the way these needs are met. Illness and hospitalization threaten children's control in these areas. Therefore it is important to allow them to participate in care and maintain as much independence as possible. Children whose care demands restriction of fluids cannot be allowed to decide the amount of fluids they will drink in 24 hours, but they can help decide the type of fluids and keep an accurate record of intake.

Assessment of neurological development is often based on fine motor coordination. This assessment may include penmanship, stacking ability, and performance of sequential, rapid, alternating movements such as touching the finger to the nose and then to the examiner's finger (smooth movement without tremors is the normal response). Fine motor coordination is critical to success in the typical American school, where children must be able to hold pencils and crayons and use scissors and rulers. Teachers frequently ask school nurses to conduct fine motor assessment of children with questionable ability. To perform this neurological screening, nurses need to know about normal fine motor functioning. Nurses should refer children with deviations from normal for more comprehensive assessments.

Nutrition

The school-age period is one with relatively few nutritional problems. When deficiencies exist, they are usually in iron, vitamin A, or calcium. Obesity may become a problem because children often rush into the home after school or play and eat the most easily obtainable and appealing foods. Unfortunately, these foods are often nutritionally poor and calorie laden. Providing nutritious snacks is often the best way for a parent to ensure good nutritional intake. When parents do not have chips, snack cakes, ice creams, and candies and instead provide ready access to fresh fruit, raw vegetables, cheese, popcorn, and high-protein snacks such as skim-milk pudding and hot chocolate, children readily choose them. Children can learn a great deal about the basic four food groups and a balanced diet by helping to prepare their own lunches and snacks (see teaching box). Nurses should encourage parents to provide children with a variety of foods in adequate amounts to support growth and energy for play. Activity levels vary from day to day, and children's appetites and consumption of food vary accordingly. When children are overweight, they

should be encouraged to increase their expenditure of calories through exercise and vigorous play. Children who become overweight have lower self-esteem, have difficulty in keeping up with other children in physical activities, and are often rejected by their peers. Nurses should help families and children prevent obesity.

Today's families often eat in fast-food restaurants where the food is high in fat, calories, and salt. Nurses need to encourage these restaurants to offer meats that are not breaded and are broiled, shakes that are made with low-fat yogurt or skim milk, and fruits and vegetables that are fresh or prepared in a low-calorie manner. Children need the opportunity to learn about selecting foods that are "heart healthy," that are "cancer preventive" (see research highlight on p. 790), and that promote the body's general well-being (Strecher et al, 1988).

Other Changes

Other physical changes take place during the school-age years. A steady skeletal growth in the trunk and extremities occurs, and small- and long-bone ossification is present but not complete by age 12. Facial bones grow and remodel, as indicated by the presence of frontal sinuses by age 8 or 9. Dental growth is prominent during the school-age years. By 12 years, all primary teeth have been shed, and the

---

| Client Teaching for Nutrition | |

OBJECTIVE

- Child will select nutritious foods that are "heart healthy" and "cancer preventive" for snacks and sack lunches.

TEACHING STRATEGIES

- Discuss with child why and how foods are divided into the basic four groups.
- Discuss foods that are heart healthy and cancer preventive.
- Have the child select desired snacks and foods from pictures or baskets of plastic models of food.
- Help the child discuss selected snacks and foods that are the most beneficial to the body and the reasons.

EVALUATION

- Observe menu selections made by child for the next day.
- Have child ask for particular foods for after-school snacks and school sack lunches.

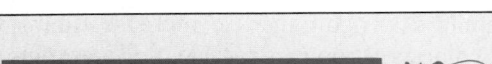

Research Highlight

A survey design was used to identify the relationships among the health locus of control (HLOC), health beliefs about colon cancer, and dietary practices of parents and their sixth-, seventh-, and eighth-grade children. A multiple regression model showed significant relationships between HLOC and fat and fiber intake and between health beliefs and fiber intake. Parents and children with a higher fat intake had a more external HLOC, and those with an internal HLOC had higher fiber intake. The results suggest that knowledge alone does not change behavior; thus nurses need to develop a cancer-prevention curriculum focusing on enhancement of self-esteem and decision making that may lead to reinforcement of internal HLOC, promoting healthy self-care.

Strecher VJ et al: Assessing cancer prevention learning needs of parents and their 6th, 7th, and 8th grade children, *Oncol Nurs Forum* 15(1):59, 1988.

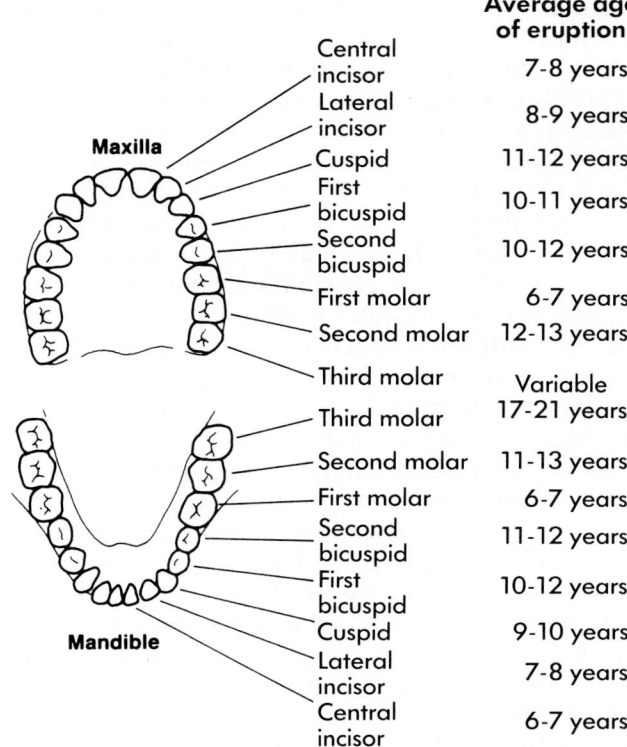

Fig. 25-1   Sequence of eruption of secondary teeth. From Whaley LF, Wong DL: *Nursing care of infants and children,* ed 4, St Louis, 1991, Mosby–Year Book.

majority of permanent teeth have erupted. Fig. 25-1 illustrates the pattern and timing of dental shedding and eruption. Infrequent or inadequate dental care remains a persistent need of many American children.

As skeletal growth progresses, body appearance and posture change. Earlier posture, which was characterized by a stoop-shouldered, slightly lordotic stance and prominent abdomen, changes to a more erect posture (see Chapter 43).

Eye shape alters because of skeletal growth. This improves visual acuity, and normal adult 20/20 vision is achievable. Screening for vision and hearing problems is easier, and results are more reliable because school-age children can more fully understand and cooperate with the test directions. The school nurse typically assesses the dental, visual, and auditory status of school-age children biannually and refers those with possible deviations to a pediatrician.

Cognitive Development

Cognitive changes provide the school-age child with the ability to think in a logical manner about the here and now but not about abstraction. The thoughts of school-agers are no longer dominated by their perceptions, and thus their ability to understand the world greatly expands. Around 7 years of age, children enter Piaget's third stage of cognitive development, known as *concrete operations,* in which they are able to use symbols to carry out operations (mental activities) in thought rather than in action (see Chapter 24). They begin to use logical thought processes with concrete materials (objects, people, and events they can touch and see). A summary of each stage of cognitive development according to Piaget is in Table 24-2.

Children in the concrete operational stage are considerably less egocentric than younger children and develop the ability to **decenter,** which enables them to concentrate on more than one aspect of a situation. Decentering has developed when children can look at two lines of dots unequal in length and recognize that they have the same number of dots even though the spaces in between dots differ (. . . . and . . . .). They also develop **reversibility,** the ability to trace their line of thinking back to where it originated. An example would be the recognition that not only does 3 + 2 = 5 but that 5 − 3 = 2 and 5 − 2 = 3.

Decentering and reversibility allow the child to use **conservation** (that is, the ability to recognize that the amount or quantity of a substance remains the same even when its shape or appearance changes). For instance, two balls of clay of equal size remain the same amount of clay even when one is flattened and the other remains in ball shape.

Seriation, the ability to place objects in order according to their increasing or decreasing size, develops by 7 or 8. This is easily measured by asking the child to arrange a group of pencils according to their length. The younger child usually aligns the tops of the pencils, whereas the child of 7 or 8 uses a methodical approach to line them up from the longest to the shortest.

The mental process of classification becomes more complex during the school years. The young child can separate objects into groups according to shape or color, but the school-age child understands that the same element can exist in two classes at the same time. For example: The school-ager could be shown a group of 16 wooden green beads and 4 wooden red beads and asked if there were more green beads or more wooden beads. The school-ager would recognize there were three classes of beads (red, green, and wooden) and would answer there were more wooden beads, whereas the preschool child would recognize only two classes of beads and answer green.

Middle childhood youngsters can use their newly developed cognitive skills to solve problems. Some individuals are better than others at problem solving because of native intelligence, education, and experience, but all children can improve these skills. Middle school-agers who are good problem solvers demonstrate the following characteristics: a positive attitude that the problem can be solved with persistence, a concern for accuracy, the ability to divide the problem into parts for study, and the ability to avoid guessing while searching for facts. Techniques that adults can use to help children improve their problem-solving strategies include helping them define the problem and its nature, plan their solution carefully, and evaluate their plan and the solution (Dacey, Travers, 1991). Nurses can use these strategies to help school-agers understand their illness and assume responsibility for their general health.

Language Development

Language growth is so rapid during middle childhood that it is no longer possible to match age with language achievements. The average 6-year-old child has a vocabulary of about 3000 words that quickly expands with exposure to peers and adults and reading ability. Children improve their use of language and expand their structural knowledge. They become more aware of the rules of **syntax,** the rules for linking words into phrases and sentences. They can also identify generalizations and exceptions to rules. They accept language as a means for representing the world in a subjective manner and realize that words have arbitrary, rather than absolute, meanings. They

can use different words for the same object or concept, and they understand that a single word may have many meanings. Many school-agers use "bad language" to gain peer status and to shock adults. It often begins with bathroom language and progresses to sexual or genital words. By the end of this period, their use of language is similar to adults.

Psychosocial Development

Moral Development

The need for a moral code and social rules becomes more evident as school-age children's cognitive abilities and social experiences increase. For example, 12-year-old children are able to consider what society would be like without rules because of their ability to reason logically and their experiences with group play. They view rules as necessary principles of life, not just dictates from authorities. In the early school years, children strictly interpret and adhere to rules. As they develop, they make more flexible judgments and evaluate rules for applicability to a given situation. School-age children consider motivations and the actual behavior when making judgments about the way that their behaviors affect themselves and others. The ability to be flexible when applying rules and to take the perspective of others is essential in developing moral judgments. These abilities are present at times in earlier years but are more consistently displayed in later school years.

Peer Relationships

Group and personal achievements become important to the school-age child. Success is important in physical and cognitive activities. Play involves peers and the pursuit of group goals. Although solitary activities are not eliminated, they are overshadowed by group play. Learning to contribute, collaborate, and work cooperatively toward a common goal becomes a measure of success.

The school-age child prefers same-sex peers to opposite-sex peers. This strong gender identity is evidenced by the close network of same-sex companions that a child maintains, often referred to as the *gang*. In general, girls and boys view the opposite sex negatively. Peer influence becomes quite diverse during this stage of development. Conformity is evidenced in mannerisms, clothing styles, and speech patterns that are reinforced and influenced by contact with peers. Group identity increases as the school-age child approaches adolescence.

Sexual Identity

Freud described middle childhood as the *latency period* because he felt that children of this period had

Date _____

Child's first name _____

Child's age _____ Grade _____

Lifestyle Questionnaire for School-Age Children*

Activities that promote health	Yes	No	Sometimes
1. I sleep at least 8 hours every night.			
2. I brush my teeth twice a day.			
3. I visit the dentist every year.			
4. I watch less than 2 hours of TV every day.			
5. I exercise (running, biking, swimming, active sports) one hour every day.			
6. I eat fruits.			
7. I eat vegetables.			
8. I limit my intake of salty snacks and high-sugar snacks.			
9. I have a physical examination every 2 or 3 years.			
10. I stay away from cigarettes.			
11. I stay away from alcohol.			

Injury prevention	Yes	No	Sometimes
12. I wear a seat beat in an automobile.			
13. I look both ways when crossing streets.			
14. I follow bike safety rules.			
15. I stay away from lighters or matches.			
16. I never ride ATVs (all-terrain vehicles).*			
17. I wear a helmet when I go on bike trips.			
18. I swim with a buddy.			
19. I wear a life jacket when I ride in a boat.			
20. I take medicine only with my parent's permission.			
21. I stay away from real guns.			
22. I tell my parents where I am going.			
23. I say "no" to drugs.			
24. Our home has a smoke detector that works.			
25. Our home has a fire extinguisher.			
26. If there is a fire, I know a safe way out of my house.			

Feelings	Yes	No	Sometimes
27. I think it is okay to cry.			
28. I enjoy my family.			
29. It is easy for me to fall asleep at night.			
30. My appetite is good.			
31. I like myself just the way I am.			

*The American Academy of Pediatrics recommends that children do not ride on these vehicles.

Fig. 25-2 Lifestyle questionnaire for school-age children.
From Antwerp CV, Spaiolo AM: *MCN* 16(3):144, 1991.

little interest in their sexuality (see Chapter 24). Today, many contemporary researchers believe that school-agers have a great deal of interest in their sexuality and engage in sex play and masturbation; they hide it, however, because of adult disapproval. Children's confiscation of their parents' magazines, such as *Playboy,* and their interest in looking up certain words, such as *fornicate,* in the dictionary are evidence of their sexual interest.

Self-Concept and Health

During the school-age years, identity and self-concept become stronger and more individualized. Perception of wellness is based on readily observable facts such as presence or absence of illness and adequacy of eating or sleeping. Functional ability is the standard by which personal health and the health of others are judged.

Promotion of good health practices is a nursing responsibility. Programs directed at health education are frequently organized and conducted in the school. During these programs, the nurse focuses on the development of behaviors that positively affect children's health status. Examples of topics that encourage positive behaviors by children are dental health, good nutrition and eating habits, and treatment for a cold.

Antwerp and Spaniolo (1991) have developed a questionnaire that can be used as a tool to assess and promote healthy lifestyles among school-agers (Fig. 25-2). This tool increases children's and parents' awareness of activities that promote health and prevent injury. It also provides data that allow the nurse or health educator to assess the health education needs of children.

Specific Health Concerns

Accidents and injuries are a major health problem affecting school-age children. Motor vehicle accidents and accidents related to recreational activities or equipment are the leading causes of death or injury.

Although falls account for a major portion of pediatric hospital admissions, they account for less than 5% of pediatric deaths resulting from injury. More children die from automobile accidents than from all major preventable childhood diseases. According to the US Preventive Services Task Force, safety belt use by children over age 5 could reduce fatalities by 50% and injuries by 65%. Nurses can contribute to the general health of children by providing education about safety measures to prevent accidents (see Chapter 42).

School-age children are also significantly affected by cancer, birth defects, homicide, and heart disease (Department of Health and Human Services, 1989). In this age group, these problems have a relatively low mortality rate but a high morbidity rate compared to accidents. Infections account for nearly 80% of all childhood illnesses; respiratory infections are the most prevalent. The common cold remains the chief illness of childhood. Certain groups of children are more prone to disease, often as a result of barriers to health care. These include homeless children, children of poverty, children with chronic illness, children who were low-birth-weight infants, foreign-born adopted children, and children in day-care centers (Bell et al, 1989). Involvement with social reform, environmental change, and the method of delivery of health care are necessary if the nurse wants to positively influence the health of children. Children's developing cognitive and psychomotor skills make it possible for them to become more involved in the promotion of their own health and the management of chronic illness.

 ## PREADOLESCENT

Today, children experience more emotional and social pressures than youngsters 30 years ago. As a result, children 10 to 12 years old are now having experiences that were once unique to 13- and 14-year-old youths. This transitional period between childhood and adolescence is often referred to as *preadolescence* by professionals in behavioral science. Others have referred to this period as *late childhood, early adolescence, pubescence,* and *transescence.* Physically it refers to the beginning of the second skeletal growth spurt, when the physical changes such as the development of pubic hair and female breasts begin. These physical changes that announce the approach of puberty begin about 2 years earlier in girls than boys. In addition, children become much more social, and their predictable behavioral patterns become much less predictable. This preparatory period often includes experimentation with makeup by girls and an interest in music and performers that are popular among older adolescents. Both sexes usually develop "best friends" with whom they share intimate feelings. New interest in the opposite sex develops, but little activity other than talk usually occurs. Youths of both sexes often develop a friendship with adults other than their parents (ego ideal), which allows them to acquire information about grown-ups.

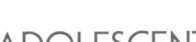

ADOLESCENT

Adolescence is the period of development during which the individual makes the transition from childhood to adulthood, usually between 13 and 21 years. The term *adolescent* usually refers to psychological maturation of the individual, whereas *puberty* refers to the point at which reproduction becomes possible. The hormonal changes of puberty result in changes in the appearance of the young person, and mental development results in the ability to hypothesize and deal with abstractions. Adjustments and adaptations are needed to cope with these simultaneous changes and the attempt to establish an adult sense of identity. In the past, many have referred to adolescence as a stormy and stressful period filled with inner turmoil, but today it is recognized that most teenagers successfully meet the challenges of this period. Adaptations required by this period push the adolescent to develop coping mechanisms and styles of behaviors that will be used or adapted throughout life. These challenges may cause the adolescent to be moody and difficult.

The nurse's understanding of development provides a unique perspective for helping teenagers and parents anticipate and cope with the stresses of adolescence. Nursing activities, particularly education, can promote healthy development. These activities occur in a variety of settings and can be directed at the adolescent, parents, or both. For example, the nurse can conduct seminars in a high school to provide practical suggestions for solving problems of concern to a large group of students, such as treating acne or making responsible decisions about drugs or alcohol use. Similarly, a group education program for parents about how to cope with teenagers would promote parental understanding of adolescent development. These programs can be held in the school, clinic, private office, or community center. To learn more about specific topics or problems, the nurse must identify teenagers' needs and desires. Involvement produces more active, interested learners.

Physical Changes and Sexual Maturation

Physical changes occur rapidly in adolescence. Sexual maturation occurs with the development of primary and secondary sexual characteristics. Primary characteristics are physical and hormonal changes necessary for reproduction, and secondary characteristics externally differentiate males from females. Four main focuses of the physical changes are summarized by Tanner (1974):

1. Increased growth rate of skeleton, muscle, and viscera
2. Sex-specific changes, such as changes in shoulder and hip width
3. Alteration in distribution of muscle and fat
4. Development of the reproductive system and secondary sex characteristics

A wide variation exists in the timing of physical changes associated with puberty, and girls tend to begin their physical changes earlier than boys.

Weight and Skeletal Changes

Height and weight increases usually occur during the prepubertal growth spurt. The growth spurt for girls generally begins between 8 and 14. Height increases 2 to 8 inches, and weight increases by 15 to 55 pounds. The male growth spurt usually takes place between 10 and 16. Height increases approximately 4 to 12 inches, and weight increases by 15 to 65 pounds.

Girls attain 90% to 95% of their adult height by **menarche** (the onset of menstruation) and reach their full height by 16 to 17 years of age, whereas boys continue to grow taller until 18 to 20 years of age. Fat is redistributed into adult proportions as height and weight increase, and gradually the adolescent torso takes on an adult appearance.

Although there are individual and sex differences, growth follows a similar pattern for both sexes. Growth in the length of the extremities occurs earliest, making the hands and feet appear very large and the legs very long; the individual often appears awkward and clumsy. At the same time the lower jaw and nose become longer and the forehead higher and wider as the baby face of childhood disappears. Next the thighs widen; then the shoulders broaden, and growth of the trunk proceeds. Widening of the female hips and broadening of the male shoulders continue throughout adolescence.

Personal growth curves help the nurse assess physical development. The individual's sustained progression along the curve, however, is more important than a comparison to the norm. The nurse charts growth measurements during routine health assessments to evaluate changes.

Effects of Physical Changes on Peer Interaction

Adolescents are sensitive about physical changes that make them different from peers. For this reason, they are generally interested in the normal pattern of growth and their personal growth curves. Consequently, the nurse should share this information to reassure adolescents that their own patterns are normal.

The number of eating disorders is on the rise in adolescent girls, and knowledge of growth progression may be a way to discourage radical weight-reduction activities. If an adolescent deviates radically from the usual pattern, further assessment is necessary to identify the cause. Weight extremes resulting from excessive or inadequate caloric intake are common during the adolescent years. Allowing the adolescent to see when and how the weight curve changed can be a first step in identifying the problem and implementing dietary changes.

Puberty

TIMING. A wide variation exists between the sexes and within the same sex as to when the physical changes of **puberty** begin. This variation is more pronounced in boys (Tanner, Whitehouse, 1982).

Boys who mature early have been shown by some research to be more poised, relaxed, good-natured, skilled in athletic activities, and more likely to be school leaders than boys who mature late. In contrast, girls who mature early have been found to be less sociable and more shy and introverted, perhaps from feeling so conspicuous (Papalia, Olds, 1989).

SEQUENCE. The sequence of pubertal growth changes is the same in most individuals (Table 25-4). The ranges of *normal* are stressed. As with increases in height and weight, the pattern of sexual changes is more significant than their time of onset. Large deviations from normal frames require investigation. For example, a 17-year-old girl who has not menstruated requires assessment and referral.

Being like peers is extremely important for adolescents. Any deviation in the timing of the physical changes can be extremely difficult for them to accept. The nurse should therefore provide emotional support for adolescents undergoing assessment of early or delayed puberty. Even adolescents whose physical changes are occurring at the normal times may seek confirmation of and reassurance about their normalcy.

HORMONAL CHANGES. Visible and invisible changes take place during puberty. All of these changes are created by hormonal changes within the body when the hypothalamus begins to produce gonadotropin-releasing hormones, which signal the pituitary to secrete gonadotropic hormones. Gonadotropic hormones stimulate ovarian cells to produce **estrogen** and testicular cells to produce **testosterone**. These hormones contribute to the development of secondary sex characteristics such as hair growth and voice changes and play an essential role in reproduction. The changing concentrations of these hormones are also linked to acne and body odor. Understanding these hormonal changes enables the nurse to reassure adolescents and educate them about body care needs.

Cognitive Development

Changes that occur within the mind and the widening social environment of the adolescent result in

TABLE 25-4	Average Sequence of Physiological Changes in Adolescence	
Girls*	Characteristics	Boys*
8-14½ (peak: 12)	Beginning of skeletal growth spurt	10½-16 (peak: 14)
8-13	Beginning of breast development	
	Enlargement of testes and scrotal sac	10-13½
8-14	Appearance of straight, pigmented pubic hair, which gradually becomes curly	10-15
	Early voice changes (cracks)	11-14½
	Enlargement of penis and prostate gland	11-14½
10-18 (average: 12¼)	Menarche	
	Spermatogenesis (ejaculation of sperm)	11-17 (average: 13½)
14-18 (average: 15½)	Ovulation and completion of breast development	
	Appearance of downy facial hair	12-17
10-16	Appearance of axillary (underarm) hair and increased output of oil and sweat-producing glands, which may lead to acne	12-17
10-18	Widening and deepening of female pelvis, with deposition of subcutaneous fat that gives rounded appearance to body	
	Increase in shoulder width	11-21
	Deepening of voice, appearance of coarse and pigmented facial hair, and appearance of chest hair	16-21

*Age range is in years.

formal operations, the highest level of intellectual development, according to Piaget (see Chapter 24). Young persons who possess sufficient neurological development to reach this stage may not attain it if they do not receive sufficient support from their cultural and educational environment, and those who are guided toward rational thinking may reach this stage early.

During this period of cognitive development, the teenager develops the ability to solve problems through logical operations. The teenager can think abstractly and deal effectively with hypothetical problems. When confronted with a problem, the teenager can consider an infinite variety of causes and solutions. For the first time the young person can move beyond the physical or concrete properties of a situation and use reasoning powers to understand the abstract. School-agers think about what is, whereas adolescents can imagine what might be. These newly developed abilities allow the individual to have more insight and skill in playing games such as checkers and *Clue* and to learn new games such as chess and bridge that require abstract thinking and deductive reasoning about many possible strategies. A teenager can even solve problems requiring simultaneous manipulation of several abstract concepts. Development of this ability is important in the pursuit of an identity. For example, newly acquired cognitive skills allow the teenager to define appropriate, effective, and comfortable sex-role behaviors and to consider their impact on peers, family, and society. The ability to think logically about these behaviors and their outcomes encourages the adolescent to develop personal thoughts and means of expressing sexual identity. In addition, a higher level of cognitive functioning makes the adolescent receptive to more detailed and diverse information about sexuality and sexual behaviors. For example, sex education can include an explanation of physiological sexual changes and birth control measures.

The complex development of thought during this period leads adolescents to question society and its values. Although teenagers have the capability to think as well as an adult, they do not have experiences on which to build. It is common for teenagers to consider their parents too narrow minded or too materialistic. Cognitive abilities and performance vary greatly among adolescents. In fact, an adolescent may perform at different levels in different situations based on their past experiences, formal education, and motivation in the use of logic and effective deductive reasoning.

Language Skills

Language development is fairly complete by adolescence, although vocabulary continues to expand. The primary focus becomes communication skills that can be used effectively in various situations. Adolescents need to communicate thoughts, feelings, and facts to peers, parents, teachers, and other persons of authority. The skills used in these diverse communication situations are varied. Adolescents must select the person with whom to communicate, decide on the exact message, and choose the way to transmit the message. For example, the way teenagers tell parents about failing grades is not the same as the way that they tell friends. Adolescents develop different skills and styles of communication and learn how and when to use them most effectively. These diverse communication skills are used and refined throughout life. Good communication skills are critical so that adolescents can overcome peer pressures to participate in nonhealthy behaviors.

Psychosocial Development

The search for personal identity is the major task of adolescent psychosocial development. Teenagers must establish close peer relationships or remain socially isolated. Erikson sees identity (or role) confusion as the prime danger of this stage and suggests that the cliquishness and intolerance of differences seen in adolescent behavior are defenses against identity confusion (Erikson, 1968). Teenagers must become emotionally independent from their parents and yet retain family ties. In addition, they need to develop their own ethical systems based on personal values. Choices about vocation, future education, and lifestyle are other decisions that must be made. The various components of total identity evolve from these tasks and comprise an adult personal identity that is unique to the individual.

Sexual Identity

Achievement of sexual identity is enhanced by the physical changes of puberty. In Freud's view, these physiological changes of puberty reactivate the libido, the energy source that fuels the sex drive (see Chapter 24). This is evidenced by the teenager's interest in heterosexual relationships with partners outside of the family and the practice of masturbation. The physical evidence of maturity encourages the development of masculine and feminine behaviors. If these physical changes involve deviations, the person has more difficulty developing a comfortable sexual identity. Adolescents depend on these physical clues because they want assurance of maleness or femaleness and because they do not wish to be different from peers. Without these physical characteristics, achieving sexual identity is difficult. Other influences are cultural attitudes and expectations of sex-role behavior and available role models. The masculine and feminine behaviors that teenagers see affect the way that they express sexuality. Adolescents master age-appropriate sexuality after feeling comfortable with sexual behaviors, choices, and relationships.

Group Identity

Adolescents seek a group identity because they need esteem and acceptance. Similarity in dress or speech is common in teenage groups. Popularity is a major concern. Trends in the desire for popularity have not changed much in recent years. Girls of middle-class status, more than any other group, regard popularity as particularly important. Conforming to group activities, being friendly, being oneself, and having a good personality are considered by teenagers to be the most important factors in gaining popularity (Padin, Lerner, Spiro, 1981). Popularity with opposite-sex and same-sex peers is important. The strong need for group identity seems to conflict at times with the search for personal identity. It is as though adolescents require close bonds with peers so that they can later redefine themselves against this group identity.

Family Identity

The movement toward stronger peer relationships is contrasted with adolescents' movements away from parents. Although financial independence for adolescents is not the norm in American society, many adolescents work part-time, using their income to bolster independence. When adolescents cannot have a part-time job because of studies, school-related activities, and other factors, parents can provide allowances for clothing and incidentals, which encourage adolescents to develop decision-making and budgeting skills.

Some adolescents and families have more difficulty during these years than others. The differences can result from the number, extent, and nature of the movements from independence to relative dependence. Adolescents need to make choices, act independently, and experience the consequences of actions. This testing, however, is best done against a firm, supportive, family foundation. The family needs to allow independence while providing a haven in which adolescents can contemplate actions. Families unable to provide this support complicate movement toward identity formation. Support to the family and adolescent may be essential to their success.

Nurses can provide this support by assisting families to consider ways that are appropriate for them to foster the independence of their adolescent while maintaining family structure. Many of these discussions often involve curfews, use of family car or purchase of personal car, and participation in family chores. Emancipation from the immediate family is most successful when accomplished gradually, resulting in separation from the family and family ties that last a lifetime.

Vocational Identity

The selection of an occupation or a vocational direction in life provides a goal for adolescents. Because of society's changing needs, adolescents must be future oriented when making these choices. However, adolescents do not know which jobs will be available or which jobs will be rewarding 10 or 20 years in the future, so selecting a career is a complicated task. The nurse should provide emotional support during this process and should help adolescent clients select courses of action that promote self-satisfaction, identity, and continued opportunity for growth.

Health Identity

Another component of personal identity is perception of health. This component is of specific interest to health care providers. Healthy adolescents evaluate their own health according to feelings of well-being, ability to function normally, and absence of symptoms. Interventions to improve health perception might therefore concentrate on these areas. Health problems causing severe or long-term alteration of these factors may permanently alter self-identity.

Moral Identity

The development of moral judgment depends heavily on cognitive and communication skills and peer interaction. Although moral development begins in early childhood, it is consolidated in adolescence because of the presence of certain skills. Adolescents learn to understand that rules are cooperative agreements that can be modified to fit the situation, rather than absolutes. Regarding rules, adolescents learn to use their own judgments rather than use the rules to avoid punishment as in the earlier years.

Kohlberg (1964) explains moral developments in terms of stages (see Chapter 24). Adolescents can achieve the highest level of moral judgment. At this level, morality is derived from individual principles of conscience. Adolescents judge themselves by internalized ideals, which often leads to conflict between personal and group values. Group values become less significant in later adolescence.

Not all adolescents attain the same level of moral development. There is, however, a general forward movement through the stages of moral development, and the sequence of the stages is similar for all individuals, even when their time of achievement varies.

Psychosocial Moratorium

According to Erikson (1968), the period of adolescence provides a "time-out period" when society allows the physically mature teenager to delay the assumption of adult responsibilities. This is a time for youth to try a variety of ideological and vocational roles before making a commitment. This **psychosocial moratorium** culminates in the selection of values and a consolidation of identity.

Specific Health Concerns

Accidents remain the leading cause of death in adolescence (about 70%). Motor vehicle accidents, which are the most common cause of death, result in almost half the fatalities of 16 to 19 year olds (Rivara, 1988). Such accidents are often associated with alcohol intoxication or drug abuse. Other frequent causes of accidental death in teenagers are drowning, firearms, and poisoning. Feelings of being indestructible lead to risk-taking behaviors. Nurses can play an important role in preventing accidental deaths by supporting organizations that promote responsible behavior, including Mothers Against Drunk Driving (MADD) and Drug Abuse Resistance Education (DARE), and encouraging students to participate in Students Against Drunk Driving (SADD). Stimulating adolescents to discuss alternatives to driving when under the influence of drugs or alcohol prepares them to consider alternatives when such an occasion arises.

Substance abuse is in fact a major concern to those who work with teenagers. Teenagers may believe that mood-altering substances create a sense of well-being or improve level of performance. All adolescents are at risk for experimental or recreational substance use, but those who have unconventional values or come from unstable homes are more at risk for chronic use and physical dependency. Some adolescents believe that substance use makes them more mature. The nurse must identify those at risk, provide education to prevent accidents related to substance abuse, and provide counseling to those in rehabilitation.

Suicide is the third leading cause of death in adolescents between 15 and 24 years of age (Valente, Saunders, 1987); accidents and homicides are the leading causes. Depression and social isolation commonly precede a suicide attempt, but suicide probably results from a combination of several factors. Nurses should be alert to the following warning signs, which often occur for at least a month before suicide is attempted (Mattsson, 1992):

1. Decrease in school performance
2. Withdrawal
3. Loss of initiative
4. Loneliness, sadness, and crying
5. Appetite and sleep disturbances
6. Verbalization of suicidal thoughts

Immediate referrals to mental health professionals need to be made when assessment suggests that adolescents may be considering suicide. Guidance can help them focus on the positive aspects of life and strengthen coping abilities.

Another area of concern is the formation of healthy habits of daily living. Emphasis on exercise, sleep, nutrition, and stress-reduction habits is increasing. The nurse must recognize the importance of these habits and identify ways to adapt them to each adolescent. To do this the nurse must assess the individual's positive and negative habits and attitudes about health. Accidents and the formation of healthy habits have psychological and physical components and effects. Extensive and long-term follow-up is required if individualized interventions are to succeed. The nurse needs to be aware of the prevalence of these problems and make assessments accordingly.

Sexual experimentation is common among adolescents. Peer pressure, physiological and emotional changes, and societal expectations contribute to early heterosexual and homosexual relations. According to Hofferth, Kahn, and Ballwin (1987), 25% of girls are sexually active by 16 years, and the majority of girls and boys are sexually active by 19 years. The nurse must provide sex education and counseling. The degree of sexual activity among teenagers may not change significantly, but the degree of informed, consenting participation can. Two prominent consequences of adolescent sexual activity are sexually transmitted disease and pregnancy.

Sexually transmitted disease (STD) annually afflicts around 10 million persons under the age of 25 years. Nearly 25% of the million cases of gonorrhea reported each year involve adolescents. This high degree of incidence makes it imperative that sexually active adolescents be screened for STDs, even when they have no symptoms (see Chapter 32). The annual physical examination of a sexually active adolescent should include careful examination of the genitalia so that condylomata acuminata (genital warts), herpes, *Phthirus pubis* (crab lice), primary syphilitic chancres, and other STDs are not missed. Recommended tests for women include Papanicolaou (Pap) smears, cervical cultures for gonorrhea and *Chlamydia* species, and syphilis tests; for men, urethral cultures for gonorrhea and *Chlamydia* species and syphilis tests are recommended. If men have participated in homosexual activities, rectal and pharyngeal cultures also need to be taken to check for gonorrhea. Adolescents who have placed themselves at risk for acquired immunodeficiency syndrome (AIDS) should also be tested for the human immunodeficiency virus (HIV). Extensive educational efforts to prevent the spread of AIDS and other STDs in this age group are a responsibility.

Adolescent pregnancy is a common occurrence in the United States; 1 of every 10 women under the age of 20 years get pregnant, and many choose to keep their babies. Pregnancy does not pose a physical risk to teenage mothers unless they are under 16 years of age or do not receive thorough prenatal care; however, there are many social, educational, and economical ramifications for the mothers (and to a lesser degree, the fathers). Nurses play a key role in counseling teenagers on ways to avoid pregnancies. After pregnancy has occurred, the nurse can assist them in obtaining thorough medical care and developing skills that will enhance their infants' development.

 NURSING PROCESS

The nursing process can be readily applied to the care of children, regardless of age. To illustrate the use of the nursing process in organizing and documenting the care of children and adolescents, an example will be provided from the case of a 10-year-old boy with an acute attack of asthma requiring treatment in the emergency room.

 Assessment

Nursing assessment of the school-age child and adolescent includes developmental level, response to care, history of prior health care, medical history, and available support persons. Assessment provides information about the ability of the child to understand, cooperate with, and assume limited responsibility for immediate and long-term care. It focuses on cognitive, motor, and psychosocial abilities and limitations. In an emergency (such as the child with an asthma attack), cognitive and psychosocial information might initially be assessed indirectly from parental report. Information can be confirmed with the child when dyspnea (difficulty breathing) lessens and the child becomes more verbal. Motor abilities can be assessed by observing the child unbuttoning a coat or removing pieces of clothing in preparation for the physical examination. Cognitive assessment might be based on the report of school grades, favorite activities, ability to describe the onset of illness, and the responses to questions from parents and health care providers. A history of prior health care will enlighten

the nurse's understanding of the child's response to current care.

In the sample care plan, the 10-year-old child had been diagnosed with asthma 6 years before and has had multiple exacerbations in the last 6 months. The boy has been on daily cromolyn sodium for 1 year but has taken no other medications. For the past 3 days the entire family had been "fighting off a cold." At 8 PM the child's cough increased, he felt tired, and he decided to go to bed. At 1:30 AM, he woke with audible wheezing and complaints of a "tight chest, like a brick laid on top of me." Shortness of breath continued to increase rapidly, so the parents took the child to the nearest emergency room. During the ride to the hospital the boy began to cry.

Knowing that the child had three exacerbations of asthma in the past 6 months, two of which required hospitalization, assists the nurse in interpreting the child's insistence that he is feeling better, despite objective physiological signs and symptoms of a worsening condition. Knowing that the child told his parents he "hated the hospital" and begged them not to "leave me at the hospital this time" emphasizes the importance of not minimizing deteriorating physiological parameters. It also stresses the importance of reassuring the child that hospitalization is not planned and that he will be informed of any change in this decision.

Assessment data may also guide long-term planning that will assist the child in learning to replace his wish for improvement with a realistic assessment of his status so that he might take self-care actions at an earlier time. Earlier action might then minimize the exacerbation and avert the need for hospital treatment.

Data about the availability of supportive significant others and the child's ability to use this support are critical. For example, the nurse may observe the child reaching for the father's hand for providing physical comfort but responding best to the mother's firm directions for cooperating with nebulizer treatment. This information will guide the selection of strategies that can maximize the support that each parent can offer. Sharing these observations with the parents can lessen their feelings of helplessness, which are related to the child's ability to cooperate with therapies. It is also useful to identify the internal supports that the child believes are effective. For example, the child might find reading, listening to soft music, or using guided relaxation therapies helpful. School-age children and adolescents can often be helped to identify their internal support systems and taught to use them at appropriate times.

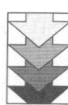 Examples of Nursing Diagnoses for a School-Age Child Having an Acute Episode of Asthma

---

NANDA-APPROVED NURSING DIAGNOSES

Altered oral mucous membranes related to:
- Mouth breathing
- Dehydration

Anxiety related to:
- Unknown progressive nature of the exacerbation
- Unknown personal response to treatment

Diversional activity deficit related to:
- Fatigue
- Dyspnea

Fear related to
- Potential treatments (e.g., injections, hospitalization)
- Recurrence of exacerbation

Fluid volume deficit related to:
- Vomiting
- Lack of desire or ability to drink secondary to dyspnea
- Increased insensible loss of fluid secondary to rapid, labored breathing

Impaired gas exchange related to:
- Airway hyperreactivity
- Increased airway secretions
- Swelling of airway tissues

Impaired verbal communication related to:
- Shortness of breath
- Treatment regimen (e.g., oxygen, nebulizer mask)

Ineffective airway clearance related to:
- Airway constriction
- Thickened secretions
- Reduced force of cough

Ineffective breathing pattern related to:
- Alteration in exchange of oxygen and carbon dioxide
- Weakened breathing muscles

Knowledge deficit related to:
- Inexperience with management of asthma at home

Powerlessness related to:
- Inability to terminate exacerbation without assistance of health care team
- Inability to prevent past and future exacerbations

Sleep pattern disturbance related to:
- Dyspnea
- Fear
- Nursing and medical interventions

 Sample Nursing Diagnostic Process for a School-Age Child Having an Acute Episode of Asthma

---

Assessment Activities	Defining Characteristics	Nursing Diagnosis
During admission, observe child's respiratory behavior regarding rate, rhythm, and depth of respirations.	Increasingly rapid and shallow respirations Dyspnea Use of assessory muscles Nasal flaring	*Ineffective airway clearance* related to thick secretions due to hypersecretion of mucus, airway constriction due to bronchospasm and mucosal edema, and weak cough due to fatigue

Monitor breath sounds.	May become diminished
	  Crackles (rales)
	  Rhonchi (inspiratory or expiratory wheezing)	

Assess coughing.	Effective or ineffective With or without sputum Sputum producing	
Observe client's color.	Pallor progressing to cyanosis	
Evaluate oxygen saturation tests.	Hypoxemia, restlessness, decreased capillary refill Tachycardia	
Observe position that client assumes.	Orthopneic (upright)	

Nursing Diagnosis

The diagnoses box lists examples of potentially relevant nursing diagnoses for the school-age child having an acute episode of asthma. Any or all of the nursing diagnoses may be applicable to a youth. The diagnostic process box selects one of these diagnoses, states related factors, and gives examples of pertinent assessment activities and defining characteristics. *Ineffective airway clearance* represents the primary physiological diagnosis for the school-age child having an acute episode of asthma. No one exhibits all of the possible defining characteristics for any particular nursing diagnosis but instead displays a combination of the defining characteristics. A typical scenario would be a youth with a weak, ineffective cough but a large amount of thick secretions. Assessment of respirations might reveal abnormal breath sounds (crackles and wheezing on expiration), bilateral and loud throughout an initial nebulizer treatment. Dyspnea was identified by observing that the youth sat leaning forward with hands on the thighs, used accessory breathing muscles, had flared nostrils, and commented with effort that it felt "like someone laid a brick on top of me."

Planning

The nursing care plan on p. 802 demonstrates further application of the nursing process for *ineffective airway clearance* and provides goals with related nursing interventions and expected outcomes. Their focus and content clearly relate them to the nursing diagnostic statement.

This plan is based on the nurse's prior knowledge of nursing care, physiology, pathophysiology, human development, and the assessment of the child and family. Airway clearance is essential to improvement of the child's health. Thus the nurse plans interventions to reduce this problem after an initial, medically prescribed, 15-minute nebulizer treatment. The nurse waits until after the treatment so that the medication given by the nebulizer can relax the smooth muscles of the respiratory system and so that the child can rest before the clearing efforts, which require active cooperation.

The plan to improve the airway also incorporates actions to maintain adequate hydration because this is the key to liquefying secretions. Dehydration often occurs in the child experiencing an acute attack because of vomiting, lack of desire or ability to drink fluids, and increased insensible water loss that accompanies rapid, labored breathing (Mansmann et al, 1988). Nursing strategies that structure coughing sessions that actively involve the child, teach the most effective techniques, and provide supplemental passive drainage are also planned.

Planning must also show consideration for social and psychological nursing problems that accompany physical nursing problems. An example of a social nursing problem accompanying an asthmatic attack is impaired verbal communication that arises from dyspnea and the medical therapeutic regimen that usually includes a nebulizer and mask. When planning care, the nurse structures verbal communication to require only brief responses from the youth or devises an alternative communication system. Writing responses is an alternative for the adolescent, whereas drawing may provide a means of communication for the younger school-age child.

Fear of hospitalization, a psychological nursing problem, may exist in the youth experiencing an acute asthma attack. The youth may dread the repetitive injection of epinephrine and the venipunctures for blood gas analysis and intravenous fluids. Planning often needs to go beyond the immediate situation; for example, for the child with asthma, the major emphasis should be prevention of future attacks. After the allergies are identified the nurse needs to assist the family in modifying their environment to reduce the youngster's exposure to them. The most common allergies are specific foods (such as milk), food additives (such as monosodium glutamate), dust, animal dander (for example, feathers or fur), pollen, molds, mildew, and smoke. In addition, the youngster needs to be protected from infections that trigger and aggravate the asthma. The child and family need to be taught breathing exercises and controlled breathing to improve proper diaphragmatic breathing and mobility of the chest wall. The child and family also need to learn stop-and-start activities that encourage regular exercise and that do not overtax the respiratory mechanism (such as swimming), improve ventilatory capacity, and promote normal peer relationships. Self-care is the aim of effective asthma management, and nurses can assist children in learning about methods of preventing attacks and of coping during attacks.

Implementation

Implementation of the care plan must be highly individualized. In the sample care plan for the school-ager having an acute asthmatic episode, the oral fluids offered depend on the child's preference and will probably change during therapy. Having the child add up his own oral intake contributes to his active involvement and a potential sense of mastery over at least one aspect of his illness. Thus this intervention and its outcome could also contribute to the

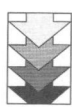

Sample Nursing Care Plan for Ineffective Airway Clearance

Diagnosis: *Ineffective airway clearance* related to thick secretions due to hypersecretion of mucus, airway constriction due to bronchospasm and mucosal edema, and weak cough due to fatigue

Definition: Ineffective airway clearance is the state in which an individual is unable to clear secretions or obstructions from the respiratory tract to maintain airway patency (Kim, McFarland, McLane, 1991).

Goals	Expected outcomes	Nursing interventions	Rationale
Child will cough effectively (6/20).	Lung auscultation will reveal increased air exchange and decrease in wheezing and crackles (6/18). Retractions will diminish. Pulse and respirations will return to normal rate and depth for age (6/18). Child will expectorate mucus (6/18). Child will have normal color, capillary refill, and oxygen saturation values (6/18). Child will breathe comfortably in supine position (6/18). Child's difficulty in breathing will not interfere with ability to communicate verbally (6/18). Child will cooperate and participate with breathing treatments (6/14).	Note during frequent auscultation of lungs whether wheezing clears with change of position or coughing. Demonstrate and monitor performance of desirable coughing attempts (sitting and taking 1 or 2 deep breaths and tightening stomach muscles before coughing and then expectorating sputum).	Wheezing that clears with change of position or coughing is due to increased mucus production that narrows large airways. Effective coughing is necessary to clear airway of thick mucus. Elevation of head of bed or sitting promotes increased lung expansion. Deep breaths and tightening of abdominal muscles increase force of cough and ability to expectorate (Whaley, Wong, 1991).
		Collaborate with physician regarding intravenous administration of aminophylline while monitoring for its side effects and toxicity (tachycardia, nausea, and irritability) and serum level.	Therapeutic level of theophylline, which relieves bronchospasm, is between 10 and 20 μg/ml. Toxicity develops rapidly; thus pulse and blood pressure must be monitored every 5 min during bolus administration (Alexander et al, 1991).
		Administer oxygen (per order) via nasal mask or prongs according to blood gas value and respiratory symptoms.	Hypoxemia is common consequence of airway obstruction. Prongs are effective only if child is breathing nasally. Oxygen saturation value should remain above 93% (Brown, Murphy, 1981).
		Teach child to inhale deeply with nebulization and exhale through pursed lips.	This action increases penetration and effect of medication on bronchial tree.
		Perform chest percussion and postural drainage.	After bronchospasms have subsided, chest physiotherapy will help clear airway of thick secretions (Alexander et al, 1991).
		Administer expectorants and corticosteroids.	Expectorants enhance coughing, and corticosteroids relieve edema.
Child will remain well dehydrated (6/20).	Child will have good skin turgor, moist mucus membranes, and adequate urine output (6/19). Bronchial secretions will become thinner and less tenacious (6/20).	Measure specific gravity.	Keeping urine specific gravity between 1.010 and 1.020 indicates good hydration.
		Offer child 3 to 4 oz of favorite liquid every 30 min.	Small amounts of preferred liquids are more acceptable to child who may be nauseated and dyspneic. Good hydration results in thinned secretions.
		Encourage child to help record fluid intake.	School-agers respond positively when given responsibility and may drink more.

improvement of another nursing diagnosis, powerlessness, which is listed in the diagnoses box. The nurse in the acute-care setting is directly involved not only in the symptomatic relief of the acute attack but also in the support and education of the family to promote adaptive coping and effective home management.

 ## Evaluation

The nursing process is incomplete unless a continuing evaluation is performed as a basis for revision of the care plan. The evaluation box suggests evaluative measures and expected outcomes that the nurse can use to determine the success of the interventions. In this case the effectiveness of the nursing interventions are indicated by good skin turgor, moist mucous membranes, adequate urine output with specific gravity values between 1.010 and 1.020, optimal fluid intake, and thinned bronchial secretions. If these expected outcomes are not attained, the nurse modifies the care plan. It may be appropriate to consult with the physician regarding the flow rate for intravenous fluids or to discuss with the child other fluids preferred. Further teaching regarding the importance of fluid intake might be necessary to gain the child's cooperation. New interventions are often developed as a response to the evaluative process.

 ## SUMMARY

Significant progress occurs in growth and development throughout the school-age and adolescent periods. At the beginning of the school-age years, children are slightly egocentric, inquisitive, and reality oriented, and their physical and cognitive abilities do not always measure up to their psychosocial needs and desires. By age 12, they have become intellectually and physically adept, have established social spheres, have begun to develop moral codes, and have started to mature sexually.

Adolescence is a transitional period when individuals move from childhood into adulthood. It is preceded by preadolescence, when skeletal growth spurts and hormones trigger the beginning of secondary sexual changes. Puberty is often recognized as the onset of adolescence. The end of adolescence is not well defined in Western culture. Although many 18 year olds demonstrate formal cognitive abilities and mature moral development, begin education for their vocational choices, and show ability to sustain interpersonal relationships, few have firm identities and are ready to assume the responsibilities of adulthood.

The school-age and adolescent stages are challenging because of the diversity and simultaneous development of changes in all spheres. The ability to examine and assess all components of these and other developmental stages is an essential skill of nursing.

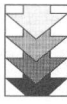 ### Sample Evaluation of Interventions for Ineffective Airway Clearance

Goals	Evaluative Measures	Expected Outcomes
Child will cough effectively (6/20).	Observe effectiveness or ineffectiveness of cough with or without sputum.	Lung ascultation will reveal increased air exchange and decrease or absense of crackles and wheezing after coughing (6/18).
		Coughing will produce sputum (6/18).
	Observe respiratory behavior.	Respirations will return to normal rate and depth for age (6/18).
		Retractions will diminish and gradually cease.
		Child will have normal skin color, quick capillary refill, and oxygen saturation value above 93% (6/18).
	Observe child's ability to verbally communicate.	Child's respirations will not interfere with ability to verbally communicate or with ability to assume desired position (6/19).
	Observe positions child assumes for breathing comfort when awake and sleeping.	
	Observe child's cooperation with and participation in breathing treatments.	Child will hold nebulizer and breathe in appropriate manner. Child will readily assume various positions for chest physiotherapy (6/19).

CHAPTER 25 REVIEW

Key Concepts

- The major psychosocial developmental task of the school-age child is the development of a sense of industry, which is gained through personal achievements and results in positive self-esteem.

- School provides a new cultural environment for the child, with a new authority figure, new rules and restrictions, and a greater need to cooperate with numerous peers.

- Cognitively, the young school-age child develops conservation, the mental operation which allows thought processes to become more logical.

- Language development is very rapid during middle childhood; reading greatly increases vocabulary and the understanding of syntax.

- Physical growth during the school years is slow and steady until the skeletal growth spurt just before puberty.

- The prepubertal growth spurt usually occurs 2 years earlier in girls than in boys; during this time, development of secondary sexual changes begins.

- Development of muscle strength and coordination allows the school-ager to participate in complex gross and fine motor activities.

- Changes in growth pattern may indicate the onset of disease.

- The extent to which school-agers develop physically and cognitively will influence their psychosocial development.

- The school-age child continues to develop the idea of what is morally right and wrong and respects the role of authority.

- Preadolescents move forward to the last stage of cognitive development, formal operations, in which they begin to think in an abstract manner, reflect on thought processes, and plan for the future.

- The adolescent is able to solve complex mental problems, use deductive reasoning, and hypothesize about the future.

- Adolescence begins with puberty, when primary sexual characteristics begin to develop and secondary sexual characteristics complete development.

- The physical changes of puberty do not occur at the same time among members of the same sex.

- The adolescent's rapid change in physical appearance heightens self-consciousness and concerns regarding body image.

- Motor vehicle accidents are the major cause of accidental death in adolescence.

- Sexually transmitted diseases are the most common communicable diseases among adolescents.

- Adolescents spend a great deal of time in thought as they develop their personal philosophy of life and sense of identity.

- The adolescent's sense of right and wrong evolves from the application of moral rules to daily decision making.

- Peer relationships are very important to the adolescent's psychosocial development and to the development of self-esteem.

- Adolescents begin the long process of emancipation from their parents and need parental support to accomplish this in a timely manner.

Key Terms

Adolescence, p. 794

Concrete operations, p. 790

Conservation, p. 790

Decenter, p. 790

Estrogen, p. 795

Menarche, p. 794

Preadolescence, p. 793

Puberty, p. 795

Psychosocial moratorium, p. 798

Reversibility, p. 790

Seriation, p. 791

Sexually transmitted disease (STD), p. 798

Syntax, p. 791

Testosterone, p. 795

Critical Thinking Exercises

1. Seven-year-old Carlos has been admitted to the hospital with an asthma attack and is receiving aminophylline intravenously and oxygen through nasal prongs. Therefore he is confined to his room and spends most of the time in bed. Considering his illness and his development (physical, psychosocial, and cognitive dimensions), choose at least six play activities and explain why they are appropriate for this 7-year-old.

2. According to Erikson, the development crisis for the school-ager is industry versus inferiority. What experiences could the nurse plan to promote the school-ager's development of industry during hospitalization?

3. During the years between 7 and 11, children develop concrete operations, according to Piaget. How could the nurse assess the progress that a particular client is making toward this development?

4. Explain why many professionals assert that adolescence is the most difficult period of life to be hospitalized.

5. What nursing strategies can be used to help the adolescent cope with hospitalization in a positive manner?

6. Sixteen-year-old Jane is in skeletal traction with a fractured femur. During her hospitalization, she begins her monthly menstrual period. Discuss what Jane's concerns might be and how the nurse might help her to cope with the situation.

REFERENCES

Alexander JD et al: Effectiveness of a nurse-managed program for children with chronic asthma, *J Pediatr Nurs* 3(5):312, 1988.

Antwerp CV, Spaniolo AM: Checking out children's lifestyles, *MCN* 16(3):144, 1991.

Bell D et al: Illness associated with child day care: as study of incidence and cost, *Am J Public Health* 79(4):479, 1989.

Brown MS, Murphy MA: *Ambulatory pediatrics for nurses*, ed 2, New York, 1981, McGraw-Hill.

Dacey J, Travers J: *Human development across the lifespan*, Dubuque, Iowa, 1991, Wm C Brown.

Department of Health and Human Services: *Health, United States, 1989 and prevention profile*, DHHS Pub No (PHS) 89-1232, Hyattsville, Md, 1989, US Department of Human Services, National Center for Health Statistics, 1989.

Erikson EH: *Identity: youth and crises*, New York, 1968, Norton.

Hofferth SL, Kahn JR, Ballwin W: Premarital sexual activity among US teenage women over the past three decades, *Fam Plann Perspect* 19:46, 1987.

Kim MJ, McFarland GK, McLane AM: *Pocket guide to nursing diagnoses*, ed 4, St Louis, 1991, Mosby–Year Book.

Kohlberg L: Development of moral character and moral ideology. In Hoffman ML, Hoffman LNW, editors: *Review of child development research*, vol 1, New York, 1964, Russell Sage Foundation.

Mansmann HC et al: Treatment of acute asthma in children. In Bierman C, Pearlman D, editors: *Allergic diseases of infancy, childhood, and adolescence*, ed 2, Philadelphia, 1988, Saunders.

Mattsson A: Adolescent depression and suicide. In Hoekelman R et al, editors: *Primary pediatric care*, ed 2, St Louis, 1992, Mosby–Year Book.

Padin M, Lerner R, Spiro A: Stability of body attitudes and self-esteem in late adolescence, *Adolescence* 61:371, 1981.

Papalia DE, Olds SW: *Human development*, ed 4, St Louis, 1989, McGraw-Hill.

Rivara FP: Motor vehicle injuries during adolescence, *Pediatr Annu* 17:107, 1988.

Strecher VJ et al: Assessing cancer prevention learning needs of parents and their 6th, 7th, and 8th grade children, *Oncol Nurs Forum* 15(1):59, 1988.

Tanner JM: Sequence and temps in the somatic changes of puberty. In Grunbach MM et al, editors: *Control of the onset of puberty*, New York, 1974, Wiley.

Tanner JM, Whitehouse RH: *Atlas of children's growth: normal variation and growth diseases*, New York, 1982, Academic.

Turner JS, Helms DB: *Lifespan development*, ed 3, New York, 1987, Holt, Rinehart & Winston.

US Preventive Services Task Force: Counseling to prevent household and environmental injuries, *Ann Fam Pract* 42(1):136, 1990.

Valente S, Saunders JM: High school suicide prevention programs, *Pediatr Nurs* 13(2):108, 1987.

Whaley LF, Wong DL: *Nursing care of infants and children*, ed 4, St Louis, 1991, Mosby–Year Book.

ADDITIONAL READINGS

Biro FM et al: Hormonal studies and physical maturation in adolescent gynecomastia, *J Pediatr* 116:450, 1990.

Chow M et al: *Handbook of pediatric primary care,* ed 2, New York, 1984, Wiley.

Dickey S: *A guide to the nursing of children: clinical nursing diagnosis series,* Baltimore, 1987, Williams & Wilkins.

Falkner E, Tanner M, editors: *Human growth: a comprehensive treatise,* ed 2, New York, 1986, Plenum.

Foster RLR et al: *Family-centered nursing care of children,* Philadelphia, 1989, Saunders.

Guilleminault C, editor: *Sleep and its disorders in children,* New York, 1987, Raven.

Hayes CD, editor: *Risking the future: adolescent sexuality, pregnancy, and childbearing,* vol 1, Washington, DC, 1987, National Academy Press.

Jenista J, Chapman D: Medical problems of foreign-born adopted children, *Am J Dis Child* 141(3):298, 1987.

Kelly B et al: Safety education in a pediatric primary care setting, *Pediatrics* 79(5):818-829, 1987.

Laige J: The school aged child and his family. In Hymovich D, Barnard M, editors: *Family health care: developmental and situational crises,* New York, 1973, McGraw-Hill.

Lee E et al: Stressful life events and accidents at school, *Pediatr Nurs* 15(2):140, 1989.

Lundholm K, Littrett J: Desire for thinness among high school cheerleaders: relationship to disordered eating and weight control behaviors, *Adolescence* 21:573, 1986.

Marshall W, Tanner J: Variations in the patterns of pubertal changes in girls, *Arch Dis Child* 44:291, 1969.

Marshall W, Tanner J: Variations in the patterns of pubertal changes in boys, *Arch Dis Child* 45:13, 1970.

Masten AS et al: Many variables determine the effects of stress, *J Child Psychol Psychiatry* 29:745, 1988.

McElroy E, Tackett JJ: Growth and development needs of the family with school age children: maintaining wellness. In Tackett JJ, Hunsberger M, editors: *Family centered care of children and adolescents,* Philadelphia, 1981, Saunders.

Meller J, Shermata D: Falls in urban children, *Am J Dis Child* 14(2):1271, 1987.

Miller C et al: Monitoring children's health: key indicators, Washington, DC, 1986, American Public Health Association.

Muscari ME: *Identification and management of children,* Monterey, Calif, 1987, Jones & Bartlett.

National Center for Health Statistics: *Advance report of final mortality statistics (1987),* Monthly vital statistics report 138 (suppl 5) DHHS Pub No (PHS) 89-1120, 1989.

Rew L: The relationship between self-care behaviors and selected psychosocial variables in children with asthma, *J Pediatr Nurs* 2(5):333, 1987.

Scherer P: Childhood asthma: twice the risk if mom smokes, *Am J Nurs* 90:112, 1990.

Servonsky J, Opas SR: *Nursing management of children,* Monterey, Calif, 1987, Jones & Bartlett.

Shen J, editor: *The clinical practice of adolescent medicine,* New York, 1980, Appleton-Century-Crofts.

Vance CJ et al: *Preventing adolescent injury: roles for the health professionals,* Newton, Mass, 1989, Education Development Center.

CHAPTER 26

Young and Middle Adult

OBJECTIVES

Mastery of content in this chapter will enable the student to:
- Define key terms listed.
- Discuss developmental theories of young and middle adults.
- List and discuss major life events of young and middle adults and the childbearing family.
- Describe developmental tasks of the young adult, the childbearing family, and the middle adult.
- Discuss the significance of family in the life of the adult.
- Describe normal physiological changes in young and middle adulthood and in pregnancy.
- Discuss cognitive and psychosocial changes occurring during the adult years.
- Describe health concerns of the young adult, the childbearing family, and the middle adult.
- List nursing diagnoses appropriate for young and middle adults.
- Use the nursing process to administer care to young and middle adults.

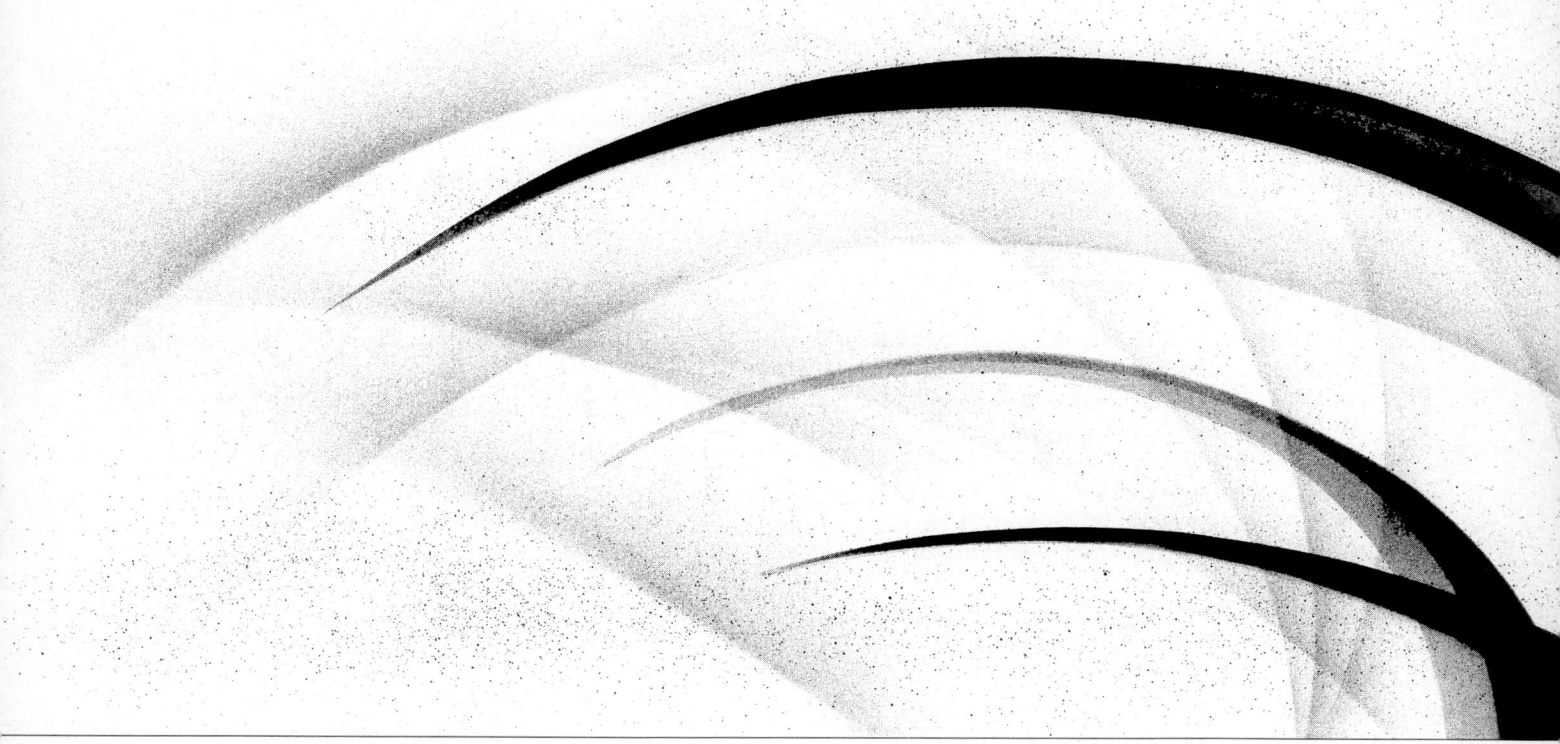

CHAPTER OUTLINE

oung and middle adulthood is a period of challenges, rewards, and crises. Adults have the challenge of entering the work force, the reward of a job well done, and the crises associated with caring for parents and rearing a family or remaining single.

Adult development involves orderly changes in characteristics and attitudes. Developmental changes are based on earlier characteristics that help shape subsequent behavior and characteristics (Beck, Rawlins, Williams, 1988). The changes experienced by young adults include the natural processes of maturation and socialization. Young adults pass through alternating periods of stability and change. During periods of stability, they make certain choices and build structures around them. In periods of change, they reevaluate these choices and consider new alternatives (Erikson, 1968, 1982).

Young adulthood is the period between the late teens and the mid-to late-thirties (Edelman, Mandle, 1990). Young adults comprise approximately 35% of the population. During young adulthood, individuals increasingly separate from their families of origin, establish career goals, and decide whether to marry and begin families or remain single. Young adults are active and must adapt to new experiences. The transition into middle age occurs when young persons become aware that changes in reproductive and physical abilities signify the beginning of another stage in life. During this transition period, individuals may reassess their goals in life and add new goals.

MATURITY AND ADULTHOOD

People are said to have reached **maturity** when they have attained a balance of growth in physiological, psychosocial, and cognitive areas. Mature individuals feel comfortable with the abilities, knowledge, and responses that they have developed over the years. They look at the world with a broad perspective, based on a blend of insight, emotion, and imagination. They take on problems that can be solved but recognize and learn to live with unsolvable problems.

Mature people are open to suggestions and can accept constructive criticism without a major loss of self-esteem. They weigh other persons' input and recommendations when making decisions but are not overly influenced or intimidated by others. Above all, mature people develop by learning from their own and other's experiences.

Other characteristics of maturity are related to interpersonal communication and behavior. Mature persons acknowledge accomplishments and shortcomings. Mature adults confront tasks openly, use decision-making techniques to solve problems, and are accountable and responsible for their actions (Schuster, Ashburn, 1986).

 YOUNG ADULT

Theories of Young Adulthood

Many theorists have attempted to describe the phases of young adulthood and related developmental tasks. Three theorists are presented in this section. Classic research by Levinson has identified the following phases of young and middle adult development (Levinson et al, 1978):

1. Early adult transition (ages 18 to 20), when the person separates from the family and desires independence
2. Entrance into the adult world (ages 21 to 27), when the person tries out careers and lifestyles
3. Transition (ages 28 to 32), when the person may modify life activities greatly
4. Settling down (ages 33 to 39), when the person experiences greater stability
5. The pay-off years (ages 45 to 65), a time for maximal influence, self-direction, and self-appraisal

Theorists propose that intellectual and moral development differs between men and women. According to Gilligan (1982), women struggle with the issues of care and responsibility, and in turn their relationships progress toward a maturity of interdependence. As women progress toward adulthood the moral dilemma changes from how to exercise their rights without interfering in the rights of others to "how to lead a moral life" that includes obligations to themselves and their families and people in general (Gilligan, 1982).

As women entered the professional arenas, they hoped to develop the caring and nurturing roles in their male colleagues (Gordon, 1991). Women have long recognized that, without caring, the perceived quality of life is changed. As a result women maintained caring in the home and educational and work environments. However, women became frustrated in their development because the responsibility of caring was not shared, and frequently nurturing became a gender-specific responsibility (Benner, Wrubel, 1989).

Another theory for young adult development has been developed by Diekelmann (1976). Diekelmann proposes that young adults experience the following developmental tasks:

1. They achieve independence from parental controls.
2. They begin to develop strong friendships and intimate relationships outside the family.
3. They establish a personal set of values.
4. They develop a sense of personal identity.
5. They prepare for life work and develop the capacity for intimacy.

These theories, along with the works of Erikson (1963, 1982), provide nurses with a basis for understanding the life events and developmental tasks of the young adult. Each young adult, however, brings unique characteristics and needs to this developmental stage. A client in this developmental stage presents challenges to nurses who themselves may be young adults coping with the demands of this period. Young adult nurses must be careful to recognize the needs of a young adult client even if they are not experiencing the same challenges and events.

 MIDDLE ADULT

In middle adulthood, the adult makes lasting contributions through involvement with others. Generally the middle adult years begin around 35 and last through the late 60s (Edelman, Mandle, 1990). Personal and career achievements have often already been experienced, and middle adults have socioeconomic stability. Many find particular joy in assisting their children and other young people to become productive and responsible adults. During this period, they may also begin to help aging parents. Using leisure time in satisfying and creative ways is a challenge that, if met satisfactorily, will enable middle adults to prepare for retirement.

Men and women must adjust to inevitable biological changes. As in adolescence, middle adults use considerable energy to adapt self-concept and body image to physiological realities and changes in physical appearance. High self-esteem, a favorable body image, and a positive attitude toward physiological changes are fostered when adults engage in physical exercise, balanced diets, adequate sleep, and good hygiene practices that promote vigorous, healthy bodies.

Theories of Middle Adulthood

Erikson's Theory

According to Erikson's developmental theory, the primary developmental task of the middle years is to achieve generativity (Erikson, 1968, 1982). Generativity is the willingness to care for and guide others.

Middle adults can achieve generativity with their own children or the children of close friends or through guidance in social interactions with the next generation. If middle adults fail to achieve generativity, stagnation occurs. This is manifested by excessive concern with themselves or destructive behavior toward their children and the community.

Havighurst's Theory

Havighurst's developmental theory has been summarized in terms of the following seven developmental tasks for the middle adult (Havighurst, 1972; Beck, Rawlins, Williams, 1988):
1. Achieving adult civic social responsibility
2. Establishing and maintaining a standard of living
3. Helping teenage children become responsible and happy adults
4. Developing leisure activities
5. Relating to one's spouse as a person
6. Accepting and adjusting to the physiological changes of middle age
7. Adjusting to aging parents

 THE NURSING PROCESS AND YOUNG AND MIDDLE ADULTHOOD

 Assessment

The nurse must assess young and middle adults in different ways because they are in different stages of the development process.

Young Adult

PHYSIOLOGICAL DEVELOPMENT. The young adult has achieved physical growth by the age of 20. An exception to this is the pregnant or lactating woman. The physical, cognitive, and psychosocial changes and the health concerns of the pregnant woman and the childbearing family are extensive and are detailed in a later section.

Young adults are usually quite active, experience severe illnesses less commonly than older age groups, tend to ignore physical symptoms, and often postpone seeking health care. Physical characteristics of young adults begins to change as middle age approaches. Unless clients have illnesses, assessment findings are generally within normal limits.

Nonetheless, clients in this developmental stage may benefit from a personal lifestyle assessment (see Chapter 2). A personal lifestyle assessment can help nurses and clients identify habits that increase the risk for cardiac, malignant, pulmonary, renal, or other chronic diseases.

COGNITIVE DEVELOPMENT. Rational thinking habits increase steadily through the young and middle adult years. Formal and informal educational experiences, general life experiences, and occupational opportunities dramatically increase the individual's conceptual, problem-solving, and motor skills.

Identifying preferred occupational areas is a major task of young adults. When people know their educational preparation, skills, talents, and personality characteristics, occupational choices are easier, and they are generally more satisfied with their choices.

An understanding of how adults learn assists the nurse in developing teaching plans for them. Adults enter the teaching-learning situation with a background of unique life experiences. Therefore the nurse always views adults as individuals. Their compliance with regimens, such as medications, treatments, or lifestyle changes, involves decision-making processes. The nurse should present as much information as they need to make decisions about the prescribed course of therapy.

Because young adults are continually evolving and adjusting to changes in the home, workplace, and personal lives, their decision-making processes should be flexible. The more secure that young adults are in their roles, the more flexible and open that they are to change. Insecure persons tend to be more rigid in making decisions.

PSYCHOSOCIAL DEVELOPMENT. The emotional health of the young adult is related to the individual's ability to address and resolve personal and social tasks. Certain patterns or trends are relatively predictable. Between the ages of 23 to 28, the person refines self-perception and ability for intimacy. From 29 to 34 the person directs enormous energy toward achievement and mastery of the surrounding world. The years from 35 to 43 are a time of vigorous examination of life goals and relationships. Alterations are made in personal, social, and occupational lives. Often the stresses of this reexamination result in a "midlife crisis" in which marital partner, lifestyle, and occupation may change.

During the young adult years, people generally give more attention to occupational and social pursuits. During this period, individuals attempt to improve their socioeconomic status. Upward mobility is possible through career choices. Career and personal counseling can help individuals identify career choices and set realistic goals.

Ethnic and gender factors have a sociological and psychological influence in an adult's life. An understanding of ethnicity, race, and gender differences enables the nurse to provide individualized care (see Chapter 4).

Support from the nurse, access to information, anticipatory guidance, and appropriate referrals provide opportunities for achievement of a client's potential. Because health is not merely the absence of disease but involves wellness in all human dimensions, the holistic, humanistic nurse acknowledges the importance of the young adult's psychosocial needs and needs in other dimensions.

The young adult must make decisions concerning career, marriage, and parenthood. Although each person makes these decisions based on individual factors, the nurse should understand the general principles involved in these aspects of psychosocial development to assess the young adult's psychosocial status.

Career. Many adults devote a major portion of their energy and interest to their chosen career. Therefore a successful vocational adjustment is important in the lives of most men and women. Successful employment not only ensures economic security but also leads to friendships, social activities, support, and respect from co-workers.

Two-career marriages are increasing. The two-career marriage has benefits and liabilities. In addition to increasing the family's financial base, the person who works outside the home is able to expand friendships, activities, and interests. However, stresses may occur in a two-career family. These stressors result from a transfer to a new city; increased expenditures of physical, mental, or emotional energy; child care demands; or household needs.

Male and female stereotypes of the past are decreasing. Men are becoming more involved in child-rearing and homemaking duties. Women are becoming active in house and automobile maintenance. To avoid stress in a two-career family, neither partner can assume all responsibilities. For some families a solution may be to limit recreational expenses and instead hire someone to do routine housework. Others may set up an equal division of household, shopping, and cooking duties.

Sexuality. The development of secondary sexual characteristics occurs during the adolescent years (see Chapter 25). Physical development is accompanied by the ability to perform sexual acts. The young adult usually has emotional maturity to complement the physical ability and is therefore able to develop mature sexual relationships.

Masters and Johnson (1970) have contributed important information about the physiological characteristics of the adult sexual response. Detailed discussion of the sexual response occurs in Chapter 32.

The psychodynamic aspect of sexual activity is as important as the type or frequency of sexual intercourse to young adults. Psychological beliefs and expectations give feelings of pleasure and satisfaction to adults. To maintain total wellness, adults should be encouraged to explore various aspects of their sexuality and be aware that their sexual needs and concerns evolve. Today young adults are at risk for sexually transmitted diseases; as a result, they need education regarding the mode of transmission, prevention, and symptom recognition and management.

Childbearing Cycle. Conception, pregnancy, birth, and **lactation** (breastfeeding) are the major phases of the childbearing cycle. The changes during these phases are complex. Fawcett et al (1986) and Whall and Fawcett (1991) have demonstrated that women perceive significant changes in physiological condition, emotion, and perception of body image during the second trimester of pregnancy and immediately after birth, but men do not perceive these changes to be as significant.

Education such as Lamaze classes can prepare the couple to participate in the birthing process. Brown (1986) reported that social support and stressors have an impact on the health of the expectant mother and father. In this study the expectant father appeared to need partner support, but the expectant woman seemed to need both partner and social support. Another study identified a decrease in delivery-room anxiety when the labor room nurse offered support to the woman (Mackey, Lock, 1989). Last, chronic illness and stress had a greater impact on the health of the expectant mother than on the father.

The personal and social changes occurring in the lives of a couple after the birth of a baby cannot be underestimated. The nursing assessment of the couple's response to the birthing experience and parent-child bonding are detailed in a later section of this chapter.

Family. Young adults go through a period of singlehood before getting married. While they are married, a couple experiences several stages and shares responsibilities. The couple may decide to become parents, as well.

Singlehood. Social pressure to get married is not as great as it once was. Today it is socially acceptable for a young adult to leave home and live in an apartment or to own a home without first marrying.

Another cause for the increased single population is the expanding career opportunities for women. Women enter the job market with greater career potential and have greater opportunities for financial independence. It is also becoming more socially acceptable for single individuals to live together outside of marriage. Similarly, it has become more socially ac-

ceptable for married couples to separate or divorce if they find their marital situation unsatisfactory.

Marriage. Every couple's relationship is unique. Although no rules guarantee a successful marriage, some guidelines are useful for building a happy marriage. Before marriage the couple ideally should complete five tasks. First, they should make certain that their emotions are based on love rather than physical or sexual attraction. Second, both partners should explore their motivation for wanting to marry. Third, they should focus on developing clear communication. Fourth, they should understand that any annoying behavior patterns and habits are unlikely to change after marriage. Last, they should determine their compatibility in important beliefs and values.

When establishing a household and family, the married couple must begin to work as a team. They have the following tasks:

1. Establishing an intimate relationship
2. Deciding on and working toward mutual goals
3. Establishing guidelines for power and decision-making issues
4. Setting standards for extrafamily interactions
5. Finding companionship with other people for a social life
6. Choosing morals, values, and ideologies acceptable to both

These major tasks of adults require considerable maturity and self-esteem. When accomplished, however, they provide the foundation for a stable relationship. Growth in marriage extends over many years. Success in solving the formidable problems that occur in any marriage offers marital partners insight into each other.

A marital relationship generally passes through three developmental stages. The establishment stage begins at the wedding and continues as the couple attempts to function as a dyad (pair). They learn patterns of sexual expression and ways to live intimately with each other. They must learn styles of conflict resolution, decision making, and role patterns. In addition, each partner may experience a sense of loss of individuality and self in the transition from *me* to *we*.

The family orientation stage is directed at childbearing and child-rearing activities. Parenting roles must be defined and practiced. Nurturing and socialization needs of the children can put pressure on the couple's intimate relationship. In addition, parents' images of the "perfect parent" conflicts with reality.

In the middle adult years, as children depart from the household, the family enters the postparental family stage. Time and financial demands on the parents decrease, and the couple faces the task of redefining their own relationship. As grandchildren arrive, grandparenting styles must be chosen.

Parenthood. The availability of contraception makes it easier for today's couples to decide when and if to start a family. One factor influencing this decision is the reason for wanting a child. Social pressures may encourage a couple to have a child or may influence them to limit the number of children they have. Economic considerations frequently enter into the decision-making process because having and bringing up children is expensive. General health status and age are also considerations in decisions about parenthood because couples are getting married later and are postponing pregnancies.

Hallmarks of Emotional Health. Most young adults have the physical and emotional resources and support systems to meet the many challenges, tasks, and responsibilities that they face. During psychosocial assessment of young adults, the nurse can assess for 10 hallmarks of emotional health (see box) that indicate successful maturation in this developmental stage.

HEALTH CONCERNS
Physiological Concerns. Young adults are generally active and have no major health problems. However, their lifestyles may put them at risk for illnesses or disabilities during their middle or older adult years. In addition, infertility is a problem for many young adults.

Risk Factors. Risk factors for the young adult's health originate in the community, lifestyle, and family history. These risk factors fall into the following categories

1. Violent death and injury
2. Substance abuse
3. Unwanted pregnancies
4. Sexually transmitted diseases
5. Environmental or occupational factors.

Lifestyle habits such as smoking, stress, lack of exercise, and poor personal hygiene increase the risk of future illness; family history of cardiovascular, renal, endocrine, or neoplastic disease increase the risk of illness, as well. Research has demonstrated that changing unhealthy lifestyle behaviors reduces selected risk factors (see research highlight).

Violence is the greatest cause of mortality and morbidity in the young adult population. Death and injury can occur from physical assaults, motor vehicle or other accidents, and suicide attempts. In the 20- to 48-year-old group, homicides account for approximately 10% of deaths, motor vehicle accidents account for 48.7% of deaths, and suicides account for 32.5% of deaths.

Substance abuse directly or indirectly contributes to mortality and morbidity in young adults. Intoxicated young adults may be severely injured in motor-vehicle accidents that may result in death or permanent disability to other young adults, as well.

Dependence on stimulant or depressant drugs can result in death. Overdose of a stimulant drug ("upper") can stress the cardiovascular and nervous systems to the extent that death occurs. The use of depressants ("downers") can lead to an accidental or intentional overdose and death.

It is a misconception that drug abuse occurs only among adolescents. Cocaine is increasingly used by young adults who have families and responsible jobs. Chapter 46 discusses the many physiological and psychosocial problems resulting from substance abuse.

Ten Hallmarks of Emotional Health

- A sense of meaning and direction in life
- Successful negotiation through transitions
- Absence of feelings of being cheated or disappointed by life
- Attainment of several long-term goals
- Satisfaction with personal growth and development
- When married, feelings of mutual love for partner; when single, satisfaction with social interactions
- Satisfaction with friendships
- Generally cheerful attitude
- No sensitivity to criticism
- No unrealistic fears

Modified from Stanhope M, Lancaster J: *Community health nursing: process and practice for promoting health*, ed 3, St Louis, 1992, Mosby–Year Book.

 **Research Highlight**

Bonheur and Young asked whether there was a difference between people who exercised and those who did not. The researchers studied 105 college students' self-esteem, perceived benefits and barriers to exercise, exercise behavior, and demographic data. The results demonstrated that the exercisers had greater self-esteem and perceived more benefits and less barriers to exercise. In addition, they had more exercise behaviors and perceived exercise as a health-promotion activity.

Bonheur B, Young S: Exercise as a health-promoting life-style choice, *Appl Nurs Res* 4(1):2, 1991.

Unplanned pregnancies, although more common among adolescents, can also have long-term physical and emotional effects if they occur in the young adult years. Unplanned pregnancies are a continual source of stress. Often young adults have educational and career goals that take precedence to family development. Interference with these goals can affect future relationships and affects later parent-child relationships.

Sexually transmitted diseases include syphilis, gonorrhea, genital herpes, and acquired immunodeficiency syndrome (AIDS). These diseases may occur in sexually active persons. Recently, sexual activity with multiple partners has decreased. Many young adults are seeking to establish meaningful relationships before engaging in sexual activity (see Chapter 32). In addition, partners are encouraged to know one another's previous sexual history and sexual practices (Hayes, Sharp, Miner, 1989; Khabbaz et al, 1990).

Sexually transmitted diseases have immediate effects such as discharge, discomfort, and infection. They may also lead to chronic disorders, which can result from genital herpes; infertility, which can result from gonorrhea; or even death, which results from AIDS.

A common environmental or occupational risk factor is exposure to airborne particles, which may cause lung diseases and cancer. Such lung diseases include silicosis from inhalation of talcum and silicon dust, pneumoconiosis from inhalation of coal dust, and emphysema from inhalation of smoke. Cancers resulting from occupational exposures may involve the lung, liver, brain, blood, or skin (Table 26-1).

Lifestyle. Lifestyle habits, particularly those that activate the stress response (see Chapter 30), increase the risk of illness. Smoking is a well-documented risk factor for pulmonary, cardiac, and vascular diseases in smokers and the individuals who receive second-hand smoke. Inhaled cigarette pollutants increase the risk of lung cancer, emphysema, and chronic bronchitis. The nicotine in tobacco is a vasoconstrictor that acts on the coronary arteries, increasing the risk of angina, myocardial infarction, and coronary artery disease. Nicotine also causes peripheral vasoconstriction and may lead to vascular problems such as Raynaud's or Buerger's disease.

Prolonged stress increases wear and tear on the body's adaptive capacities. Stress-related diseases such as ulcers, emotional disorders, and infections can occur (see Chapter 30).

Exercise patterns can affect health status (see research highlight). Exercise that produces a sustained increase in the pulse rate for 15 to 20 minutes 3 times a week improves cardiopulmonary function by

TABLE 26-1 Occupational Hazards Associated with Cancers

Occupational Chemical	Cancer
Asbestos	Mesothelioma (pleural and peritoneal)
	Lung cancer
Vinyl chloride (plastics)	Liver cancer (hemangiosarcoma)
	Brain cancer
	Lung cancer
Benzene	Leukemia, predominantly acute myelogenous
Bischloromethane ether	Oat cell carcinoma
Chromium	Cancer of nasal or paranasal sinus, lung, larynx
Arsenic	Lung cancer
Coal tar pitch, coke oven emissions	Cancer of lung, larynx, skin
Iron oxide	Cancer of lung, larynx
Nickel	Lung cancer
Petroleum distillates	Cancer of lung, larynx

From Stanhope M, Lancaster J: *Community health nursing: process and practice for promoting health*, ed 3, St Louis, 1992, Mosby–Year Book.

decreasing blood pressure and heart rate. In addition, exercise decreases fatigability, insomnia, tension, and irritability.

Personal hygiene habits can be risk factors. Sharing eating utensils with a person who has a contagious illness increases the risk of illness. Poor dental hygiene increases the risk of periodontal disease. These diseases—gingivitis (inflammation of the gums) and periodontitis (loss of tooth support)—can be avoided through oral hygiene (see Chapter 34).

A familial history of a disease may put a young adult at risk for developing it in the middle or older adult years. For example, a young man whose father and paternal grandfather had myocardial infarctions (heart attacks) in their 50s has a risk for a future myocardial infarction. As noted in Chapter 6, the presence of certain chronic illnesses in the family increases the family members' risk of developing a disease. This family risk is distinct from hereditary disease.

Poor adherence to routine screening examinations can put the client at risk for severe illnesses because of failed early detection. Clients should be encouraged to perform monthly breast self-examination (BSE) or testicular self-examination (TSE) (see Chapter 20). Women should be informed of the benefits and suggested schedule for routine mammography. A recent study by the National Cancer Institute

(NCI) reinforces the nurse's role in educating clients about BSE and the current breast screening recommendations (NCI, 1990).

Infertility. **Infertility** is the man's, woman's, or couple's involuntary inability to conceive. To most health professionals, it is the inability to conceive after a year or more of regular sexual intercourse. An estimated 10% to 15% of all couples are infertile (Bobak, Jensen, 1991). However, about half of the couples evaluated and treated in infertility clinics become pregnant. In about 10% to 20% of couples the cause of infertility is unknown, and they remain infertile. In the remaining 30% the cause of the infertility is diagnosed, but they remain infertile because of endometriosis, blocked fallopian tubes, or decreased sperm motility.

For some infertile couples, the nurse may be the first resource identified. Couples often turn to the nurse to express fears and concerns. When fertility problems exist, couples frequently experience a variety of "stages," including disbelief, denial, and anger, in trying to deal with the stress (Blenner, 1990). To effectively intervene with a couple who has a fertility problem, the nurse should be familiar with the fertility problem and the couple's stage of coping.

PSYCHOSOCIAL CONCERNS. The psychosocial health concerns of the young adult are often related to stress, such as job or family stress. As noted in Chapter 30, stress can be valuable because it motivates a client to change. However, if the stress is prolonged and the client is unable to adapt to the stressor, health problems can develop.

Job Stress. Job stress can occur every day or from time to time. Most young adults are able to handle day-to-day crises. Situational job stress may occur when a new boss enters the workplace, a deadline is approaching, or the worker is given new responsibilities. Job stress also occurs when a person becomes dissatisfied with a job or responsibilities. Because individuals perceive jobs differently, the types of job stressors vary from client to client.

Family Stress. Family stressors can occur at any time in family life (see Chapter 23). Family life has peaks, when everyone in the family works together, and valleys, when everyone appears to pull apart. Situational stressors occur during events such as births, deaths, illnesses, marriages, and job losses.

Each family has certain predictable roles or jobs for members. These roles enable the family to function and be an effective part of society. One necessary role is the family leader. In most families, one parent is the leader, or both parents act as co-leaders. In single-parent families the parent or occasionally a member of the extended family is the family leader.

PREGNANT WOMAN AND CHILDBEARING FAMILY. A developmental task for most young adult couples is the decision to begin a family. Although the physiological changes of pregnancy and childbirth occur only in the woman, cognitive and psychosocial changes and health concerns affect the entire childbearing family, including the husband, siblings, and grandparents.

Physiological Changes. Women who are anticipating pregnancy benefit from good health practices before conception; these include a balanced diet, exercise, dental checkups, avoidance of alcohol, and cessation of smoking. Women trying to become pregnant should not try weight-reduction diets. The physiological changes and needs of the pregnant woman vary with each trimester (Table 26-2).

Prenatal Care. **Prenatal care** is the routine examination of the pregnant woman by an obstetrician, nurse practitioner, or certified nurse-midwife. During the prenatal visit the pregnant woman's weight and blood pressure are taken; her urine is checked for glucose, acetone, and protein; and the fundus is measured. In addition, the pregnant woman may be counseled about exercise patterns, diet, and child care. Regular health care can address health concerns such as preeclampsia, eclampsia, excessive weight gain, and the high-risk infant.

First Trimester. All woman experience some physiological changes in the first trimester, but some changes affect only certain women. These changes include morning sickness, increased urination, lack of energy, and changes in nutritional intake. The nurse must be familiar with these physiological changes, their causes, and helpful interventions.

During this period, signs of pregnancy are usually not observable by others. If a woman frequently has **morning sickness,** however, her family, friends, and co-workers may suspect that she is pregnant.

The newly pregnant woman needs routine prenatal care. The first visit includes a pelvic examination. After the thirteenth week of pregnancy, pelvic examinations are not done. Instead the physician or certified nurse-midwife measures fetal growth by palpating the abdomen to determine the size of the uterine fundus.

Second Trimester. During the second trimester, growth of the uterus and fetus results in some of the physical signs of pregnancy. Morning sickness has usually disappeared, and the woman's energy level is restored if her nutritional intake has caught up with her metabolic demands. The urinary frequency ceases, and she is able to sleep through the night.

If this is the woman's first pregnancy, she may be able to see and feel the enlarged uterus. However, it is common for her abdomen to stay relatively flat. In

TABLE 26-2	Major Physiological Changes During Pregnancy	
Signs and Symptoms	Causes	Appropriate Nursing Interventions

FIRST TRIMESTER

Amenorrhea (missed periods)	Fertilization of egg by sperm	Instruct woman to have pregnancy test.
Positive pregnancy test done at home or in laboratory	Presence of human chorionic gonadotropin (HCG) in first voided urine specimen of day	Instruct woman to obtain prenatal care, avoid all medications, avoid alcohol intake, and maintain good nutritional habits.
Morning sickness (nausea or vomiting from sixth week to end of fourth month, which occurs in morning, evening, or all day)	Increased serum hormone levels	Instruct client to eat dry crackers and cold fluids such as ice and popsicles and have small, frequent meals to reduce nausea. Have client inform physician if prolonged vomiting results in weight loss of over 5 lb, abdominal pain, or tenderness.*
Breast enlargement and tenderness, darkened and enlarged nipples	Increased estrogen levels	Instruct woman to wear supportive bra at all times, even while asleep. Tell client that application of ice packs decreases tenderness.
Urinary frequency	Pressure of uterus on bladder	Reassure client that frequency decreases as enlarging uterus moves from pelvis up to abdominal region. Prepare client for return of frequency as head of fetus moves into pelvis in middle to late third trimester.
Fatigue	Increases in hormone levels Increased nutritional demands Decreased nutritional intake resulting from morning sickness	Ensure that client has proper nutrition, sleep patterns, and rest periods to help decrease fatigue. Instruct client to take prenatal vitamins as prescribed.

SECOND TRIMESTER

Pigmented nipple and breast, hyperpigmentation of abdominal line (linea nigra), mottling of cheeks or forehead (chloasma or "mask of pregnancy"), local or generalized pruritus	Increased levels of melanocyte-stimulating hormone	Reassure client that skin changes are normal and temporary. Instruct client to avoid hot baths and use of soap or lotions, which can dry skin and increase itching.
Hypertrophy of gums (pregnancy epulis), causing gingival swelling and bleeding	Proliferation of interdental papillary blood vessels, resulting in local inflammation and hyperplasia	Teach client good flossing technique. Instruct client to get routine dental checkups.
Increasing size of uterine fundus: at level of symphysis pubis at 9 weeks, at intraabdominal organs at 12 weeks, between symphysis pubis and umbilicus at 16 weeks, at umbilicus at 20-22 weeks	Growth of fetus	Reinforce nutrition teaching.
Sensation of movement of gaslike movements (quickening)	Fetal motion	Instruct client to notify physician if they are absent or decline.

*Data from Fogel CI, Woods NF: *Health care of women: a nursing perspective,* St Louis, 1981, Mosby–Year Book.
Data from Bobak IM, Jensen MD: *Essentials of maternity nursing,* ed 3, St Louis, 1991, Mosby–Year Book.

Continued.

TABLE 26-2 Major Physiological Changes During Pregnancy—cont'd		
Signs and Symptoms	Causes	Appropriate Nursing Interventions
SECOND TRIMESTER—cont'd		
Braxton Hicks contractions	Expanding uterus and preparation of uterus for labor	Explain that they are irregular, short contractions, not early labor, and that they will continue throughout pregnancy. Instruct client to notify physician if contractions become regular and increase in frequency and duration.
THIRD TRIMESTER		
Increased colostrum (precursor of true milk)	Preparation of breasts for lactation by hormones	Instruct client to express colostrum to prevent clogged milk ducts.
Increasing size of fundus: at xiphoid process at 36 weeks; downward position of baby's head by month 9 as determined by palpation (Mother may feel that baby has "dropped" and that pressure on xiphoid process, diaphragm, and stomach is relieved)	Descent of baby's head into pelvis (engagement), which may occur at any point from week 36 to onset of labor	Reassure client of baby's growth. Reassure client that baby can be safely repositioned in utero if needed. Reassure client that pregnancy is ending.
Increased urinary frequency, constipation	Pressure on bladder from enlarged fetus; pressure and displacement of colon and decreased gastric motility	Instruct client to reduce fluid intake after 8 PM and increase roughage in diet.

subsequent pregnancies she may "show" as early as the beginning of the second trimester.

Third Trimester. During the third trimester an increase in **Braxton Hicks contractions** (irregular, short contractions), fatigue, and urinary frequency occur. Close to the onset of labor, the woman may experience a burst of energy during which she cleans house and prepares for the baby by shopping for baby supplies. This period is called *nesting*. Many experts in obstetrics and seasoned veterans of pregnancy believe that nesting indicates a rapidly approaching time of delivery.

Puerperium. The **puerperium** is a period of approximately 6 weeks after delivery. During this time the uterus involutes, returning to approximate prepregnancy size.

Cognitive Changes. Cognitive changes during pregnancy, primarily involving sensory perception and needs for education, affect both parents and may occur gradually or quickly.

Sensory Perception. The pregnant woman generally experiences changes in sensory perception. Temporary changes occur in visual and hearing acuity, taste, and smell. Many pregnant women frequently stroke the abdomen, possibly because of a change in

the sensation of touch or other sensory need. The woman may be using the sensation of touch to initiate bonding with her child (Bobak, Jensen, 1991).

Needs for Education. The entire childbearing family needs education about pregnancy, labor, delivery, breastfeeding, and integration of the newborn into the family structure. Childbirth classes help parents plan for the birth of the child. Such classes focus on the normal physiological changes of pregnancy and the processes of labor and delivery. The classes prepare the expectant parents for natural childbirth or childbirth with anesthesia. Other types of classes may emphasize newer advances in obstetrics, such as birthing rooms.

Many health care centers also have sibling and grandparent preparation classes. Sibling classes explain the processes of pregnancy, birth, and integration of the baby into the family structure to the baby's siblings at their level of comprehension. Grandparenting classes help potential grandparents in acquiring grandparenting skills, such as how to childproof their homes and how to support new parents.

Psychosocial Changes. Like the physiological changes of pregnancy, psychosocial changes may occur at various times during the 9 months of pregnancy and in the puerperium. The major categories of psychosocial changes involve body image, role, sexuality, coping mechanisms, and stresses during the puerperium.

Body Image. Although the physical changes of pregnancy are not obvious to others until the second trimester, the woman generally perceives changes in her body during the first 3 months. One change that some women consider positive is an increase in breast size, which may make the woman feel more feminine and sexually appealing. Also, because she is pregnant, the woman may take extra time with her hygiene and grooming, trying new hairstyles and makeup.

The woman having difficulty with morning sickness and fatigue may have a poor body image. She may be too tired or ill to care about her appearance. Her major goal is often just getting through morning sickness and fatigue.

Most women, particularly those who are pregnant for the first time, enjoy the second trimester. They are beginning to "show" and start planning their maternity wardrobe. Their energy level has returned to normal, and they have a general feeling of well-being. Because they can feel the baby move and hear the heart beat, the baby becomes real to them, and they fantasize about the infant's features.

During the third trimester the fetus grows more rapidly. Toward the end of the pregnancy the woman may feel big, awkward, and unattractive. Family and friends should help her feel more attractive.

Role Changes. As the pregnancy advances, both partners think about their role changes. It is normal for expectant parents to feel ambivalent about the upcoming event and to wonder whether it is the right time to begin or to enlarge a family. Both partners may also be concerned about their ability to be parents. They may observe the interactions between parents and children in their friends' families and wonder whether they can cope. The nurse can help them overcome their insecurities by emphasizing that the infant and parent grow together, learning about each other's habits, moods, and behaviors.

Another role change can involve the choice to remain employed or to stay home after the baby's birth. This is no longer solely a woman's decision. An increasing number of men are becoming "househusbands." This may occur when the wife earns more money than the husband and therefore needs to remain in the workforce for the family to remain financially secure. In addition, a husband may choose to remain home or may be laid off or become unemployed near the time of the child's birth.

Sexuality. Pregnancy does not alter a woman's basic sexual response, and sexual activity is not harmful to a normally developing fetus. Often the pregnant woman and her partner need to be reassured about these facts.

However, the woman's perception of her body image influences her desire for sexual activity. Some women may feel more attractive and sexually desirable. Others perceive the changes in their bodies as unattractive. A woman may desire cuddling and holding rather than sexual intercourse.

Coping Mechanisms. Pregnancy requires many adjustments. The pregnant woman and her partner need to remember that, although childbirth and child-rearing are natural positive experiences, they are also stressful. Often parents are unable to cope with a particular stressor such as finding new housing, preparing the nursery, or participating in childbirth classes.

Stresses During the Puerperium. It is common for the new mother to bring the baby home from the hospital, place him or her in the crib, sit down, and wonder, "Now what do I do?" The current trend is for discharge within 24 to 48 hours after birth. A visiting nurse can help the new parents during the transition from hospital to home.

A second stressor during the puerperium may be the mother's return to work. She may feel guilt, anxiety, relief, or a sense of freedom. Even when a return to work is necessary, the mother has mixed emotions about leaving her child. Parents selecting child care need assistance in obtaining references of reliable care givers and agencies. Community organizations and churches can be a good beginning for parents needing child care.

Health Concerns. The pregnant woman and her partner have many health questions. For example, they may wonder whether the pregnancy and baby will be normal. The majority of the health needs related to pregnancy can be met with proper prenatal care.

Middle Adult

PHYSIOLOGICAL DEVELOPMENT. Major physiological changes occur between 40 and 65 years of age. Table 26-3 on p. 820 summarizes these normal developmental changes.

The most visible changes are graying of the hair, wrinkling of the skin, and thickening of the waist. Balding commonly begins during the middle years, but it may also occur in young adults. Often these physiological changes have an impact on self-concept and body image. The most significant physiological changes during middle age are menopause in women and the climacteric in men.

Menopause. Menstruation and ovulation occur in a cyclical rhythm in the woman from adolescence into middle adulthood. **Menopause** is the disruption

TABLE 26-3   Physiological Changes in the Middle Adult as Found During Physical Assessment

Body System	Findings
Integument	Intact condition
	Appropriate distribution of pigmentation
	Slow, progressive decrease in skin turgor
	Graying and loss of hair (Baldness patterns in males are established by age 55; hair loss after this time might have other causes.)
Head and neck	Symmetry of scalp, skull, and face
	Normal accessory organs of vision
Eyes	Visual acuity by Snellen chart that is less than 20/50
	Pupillary reaction to light and accommodation
	Normal visual fields and extraocular movements
	Normal retinal structures
Ears	Normal auditory structures and acuity
Nose, sinuses, and throat	Patent nares and intact sinuses, mouth, and pharynx
	Location of trachea at midline
	Nonpalpable lateral thyroid lobes
Thorax and lungs	Increased anteoposterior diameter
	Respiratory rate 16-21 breaths per minute and regular
	Ratio of respiratory rate to heart rate: 1:4
	Normal tactile fremitus, resonance, and breath sounds
Heart and vascular system	Normal heart sounds
	Systole: S_1 less than S_2 at base
	Diastole: S_1 greater than S_2 at apex
	Point of maximal impulse: at fifth intercostal space in midclavicular line and 2 cm or less in diameter
	Vital signs
	Temperature: 36.7°-37.6° C (97°-99.6° F)
	Pulse: 60-100 (conditioned athlete ≈ 50)
	Blood pressure: 95-140/60-90 mm Hg
	All pulses palpable
Breasts	Decreased size resulting from decreased muscle mass
	Normal nipples
Abdomen	No tenderness or organomegaly
	Decreased strength of abdominal muscles
Female reproductive system	Change in menstrual cycle and in duration and quality of menstrual flow
	"Hot flashes"
	Change in cervical mucosa
Male reproductive system	Normal penis and scrotum
	Prostatic enlargement in some individuals
Musculoskeletal system	Decreased muscle mass
	Decreased range of joint motion
Neurological system	Appropriate effect, appearance, and behavior
	Lucidity and appropriate level of cognitive ability
	Intact cranial nerves
	Adequate motor responses
	Responsive sensory system

of this cycle, primarily because of the inability of the neurohumoral system to maintain its periodic stimulation of the endocrine system. The ovaries no longer produce estrogen and progesterone, and the blood levels of these hormones drop markedly. Menopause typically occurs between 45 and 60 years of age (see Chapter 32).

Climacteric. The **climacteric,** or andropause, occurs in men in their late 40s or early 50s (see Chapter 32). It is caused by decreased levels of androgens. Throughout this period and thereafter, a man is still capable of producing fertile sperm and fathering a child. However, penile erection is less firm, ejaculation is less frequent, and the refractory period is longer.

COGNITIVE DEVELOPMENT. Changes in the cognitive function of middle adults are rare except with illness or trauma. The middle adult can learn new skills and information. Some middle adults enter educational or vocational programs to prepare themselves for entering the job market or changing jobs.

PSYCHOSOCIAL DEVELOPMENT. The psychosocial changes in the middle adult may involve expected events, such as children moving away from home, or unexpected events, such as a marital separation or the death of a spouse. These changes may result in stress that can affect the middle adult's overall level of health.

Career Transition. Career changes may occur by choice or as a result of changes in the workplace or society. In recent decades, middle adults more often change occupations because they are bored with their present employment. In some cases, technological advances or other changes force middle adults to seek new jobs. Such changes, particularly when unanticipated, may result in stress that can affect health, family relationships, self-concept, and other dimensions.

Sexuality. The onset of menopause and the climacteric can affect the sexual health of the middle adult. Menopause results in cessation of ovulation and the ability to conceive. A woman may desire more sexual activity because pregnancy is no longer possible. A man may notice changes in the strength of his erection and a decrease in his ability to experience repeated orgasm. Both may experience stresses related to sexual changes or a conflict between their sexual needs and self-perceptions and social attitudes or expectations (see Chapter 32).

Family. Psychosocial factors involving the family may include marital changes, transition of the family as children leave home, and the care of aging parents.

Marital Changes. Marital changes that may occur during middle age include death of a spouse, separation, divorce, and the choice of remarrying or remaining single. A widowed, separated, or divorced client goes through a period of grief and loss in which it is necessary to adapt to the change in marital status.

If a single middle adult decides to marry, the stressors of marriage are similar to those for the young adult. In addition, the couple may have to cope with the social expectations and pressures related to marriage.

Family Transitions. The departure of the last child from the home may be a stressor. Many parents welcome freedom from child-rearing responsibilities, whereas others feel lonely or without direction because of this change. Eventually parents must reassess their marriage and are able to resolve conflicts and plan for the future. Occasionally this readjustment phase may lead to marital conflicts, separation, and divorce (Beck, Rawlins, Williams, 1988).

Care of Aging Parents. Increasing life spans in the United States and Canada have led to increased numbers of older adults in the population. Therefore greater numbers of middle adults must address the personal and social issues confronting their aging parents. The needs of the care givers is an area that will continue to grow (Scharlach, 1990).

Housing, employment, health, and economic realities have altered the traditional social expectations between generations in families. The middle adult and the older adult parent may have conflicting priorities related to their relationship. Negotiations and compromises are useful in defining and resolving such problems. Nurses deal with middle and older adults in the community, long-term care facilities, and hospitals. The nurse can help identify the health needs of both groups and can assist the multigenerational family in determining the health and community resources available to them as they make decisions and plans.

HEALTH CONCERNS

Physiological Concerns. Physiological concerns include stress, level of wellness, and the formation of positive health habits.

Stress. Because middle adults are experiencing physiological changes and face certain health realities, their perceptions of health and health behaviors are often important factors in maintaining health. Today's complex world makes individuals more prone to stress-related illnesses such as heart attacks, hypertension, migraine headaches, ulcers, colitis, autoimmune disease, backache, arthritis, and cancer.

When adults seek health care, the nurse's focus on the goal of wellness can guide clients to evaluate health behaviors, lifestyle, and environment. Attention to risk factors that can be altered to improve the client's health can increase the quality of life and add years to it.

Levels of Wellness. The nurse must be able to assess the health status of the middle adult client. Such assessment offers direction for planning nursing care and is useful in evaluating the effectiveness of nursing interventions. Table 26-3, which shows the physiological changes of the middle adult, can be used with other standard assessment techniques as a guide for physical assessment (see Chapter 20).

Forming Positive Health Habits. A habit is a person's usual practice or manner of behavior. This behavior pattern is reinforced by frequent repetition until it becomes the individual's customary way of behaving. Some habits support health, such as exercise and brushing and flossing the teeth each day. Other habits involve risk factors to health, such as smoking or eating foods with little or no nutritional value.

During the assessment phase of the nursing process, the nurse frequently obtains data indicating positive and negative health behaviors by the client. In the planning, implementation, and evaluation phases, the nurse helps the client maintain habits that protect health and offers healthier alternatives to poor habits.

Psychosocial Concerns. Two common psychosocial health concerns of the middle adult are anxiety and depression.

Anxiety. Adults often experience anxiety in response to the physiological and psychosocial changes of middle age. Such anxiety can motivate the adult to rethink life goals and can stimulate productivity. For some adults, however, this anxiety precipitates psychosomatic illness and preoccupation with death. In this case the middle adult views life as being half or more over and thinks in terms of the time left to live (Beck, Rawlins, Williams, 1988).

Clearly a life-threatening illness, marital transition, or job stressor increases the anxiety of the client and family. The nurse may need to use crisis-intervention or stress-management techniques to help the client adapt to the changes of the middle adult years (see Chapter 30).

Depression. Depression is common among adults in the middle years and may have many causes. The risk factors for depression are listed in Table 26-4. Menopause is no longer believed to be the only cause

of depression. Depression that occurs during the middle years, often referred to as *agitated depression,* is characterized by moderate-to-high anxiety, bizarre physical complaints, and paranoid ideation (formation of a mental concept or image). Depression may be worsened by the abuse of alcohol or other substances. The nurse may need to refer a severely depressed client for specialized psychological therapy.

Nursing Diagnosis

The nursing assessment of the young or middle adult reveals clusters of data that indicate potential or actual nursing diagnoses (see diagnoses box). The nursing diagnostic statement should include expected or anticipated causes or etiologies for the statement. For example, the assessment of two clients and their families resulted in the identification of *ineffective individual coping.* However, in one family the stressor was the death of a spouse, but in the second family the stressor was a new baby within the home. The inclusion of the etiology statement enables the nurse to quickly target specific goals and interventions of causative factors for each diagnostic statement.

The diagnostic statements require appropriate defining characteristics that provide the rationale for

Examples of Nursing Diagnoses for Young and Middle Adults

TABLE 26-4 Risk Factors for Depression in the Middle Years	
Risk Factor	Characteristics
Sex	Female
Age	Women: declines after early 50s
	Men: increases after late 50s
Social isolation	Absence of intimate, confiding relationships after change in nature of relationship with parents, children, and spouse
Losses	Parental deprivation or loss of mother before age 14
	Other losses during midlife such as job loss, career difficulties, marital problems, and physical changes
	Departure of last child from home
Family history	History of depression in family of origin

From Beck CM, Rawlins RP, Williams SR: *Mental health—psychiatric nursing: a holistic life-cycle approach,* ed 2, St Louis, 1988, Mosby—Year Book.

NANDA-APPROVED NURSING DIAGNOSES

Impaired adjustment related to:
■ Changes in physical appearance
■ Changes in body image

Ineffective family or individual coping related to:
■ Infertility
■ Death of spouse
■ Adjustment to baby
■ Loss of job

Altered family processes related to:
■ Chronic or acute illness
■ Death of spouse
■ Marital problems
■ Financial problems

Altered sexuality patterns related to:
■ Infertility
■ Pregnancy
■ Menopause or climacteric

Altered health maintenance related to:
■ Risk factors (e.g., smoking, substance abuse)
■ Lack of knowledge of positive health behaviors

the diagnosis (see diagnostic process box). The defining characteristics are identified from assessment data obtained by the nurse.

 ## Planning

The identification and formulation of nursing diagnoses are followed by the development of a nursing care plan (see care plan). When providing nursing care for young and middle adults, the nurse must recognize that the needs of clients, families, and communities are interconnected. Nursing interventions are individualized for the client and are modified accordingly for home- or hospital-based nursing care.

General nursing goals for young or middle adults reflect their reactions to day-to-day life events as opposed to nursing goals that result from their responses to specific illnesses or physiological, psychosocial, emotional, or spiritual needs. The goals of nursing for the young or middle adult can include the following:

1. Improved knowledge about the impact of risk factors on level of health
2. Improved health-promotion activities
3. Improved communication within their family structures
4. Fewer experiences of illnesses and inability to problem solve

 ### Sample Nursing Diagnostic Process for Young and Middle Adults

Assessment Activities	Defining Characteristics	Nursing Diagnoses
Ask client about diet, exercise, and self-examination patterns.	Lack of knowledge regarding basic health practices Poor diet	*Altered health maintenance* related to excessive alcohol use
Ask client about use of alcohol, non-prescription drugs, and tobacco.	Verbalizes need for alcohol	
Review previous medical record.	Motor vehicle accident with minor trauma (High blood alcohol level) Hospitalizations for alcohol abuse	
Observe family's interaction with ill family member.	Family system unable to meet physical, emotional, social, or spiritual needs of members	*Altered family process* related to chronic illness of spouse
Listen to family discussion.	Family unable to adapt	
Observe nonverbal interactions.	Poor communication	

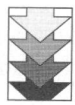 ### Sample Nursing Care Plan for Altered Health Maintenance

Nursing diagnosis: *Altered health maintenance* related to excessive use of alcohol
Definition: Altered health maintenance is the inability to identify, manage, and/or seek out help to maintain health (Kim, McFarland, McLane, 1991).

Goals	Expected Outcomes	Interventions	Rationale
Client will verbalize impact of alcohol excess on level of health by next home visit.	Client will reduce alcohol intake. Client will state three physiological, emotional, and psychosocial effects of alcohol excess.	Provide client with information about 12-step support groups for alcohol abuse within community.	Twelve-step support groups provide education, counseling, and support for clients who want to abstain from alcohol.
Client will modify behavior and remain free of alcohol by 6 mo.	Client will remain free of alcohol intake. Family and significant others verify abstinence from alcohol abuse.	Client enrolls in 12-step program. Teach family about their role in supporting client through program.	Client must enroll self into program. Family evolvement increases support and behavior change.

Client Teaching for Positive Health Habits

OBJECTIVE

- Client will increase exercise patterns to include three 1-mile walks per week to assist weight loss and improve cardiopulmonary function.

INTERVENTIONS

- Review with client the daily work schedule and identify potential times for exercise.
- Inform client about the effect of exercise on weight control and improved cardiac function.
- Demonstrate how to calculate target heart rate and assess pulse correctly.
- Provide warm-up and cool-down exercises and demonstrate how to do them.
- Instruct client about supportive shoes for walking exercises.

EVALUATION

- Have client keep log of exercise periods.
- Have client demonstrate pulse measurement.
- Have client demonstrate warm-up and cool-down exercises.
- Inspect clients feet for blisters or sores.

Barriers to Change

EXTERNAL BARRIERS

- Lack of facilities
- Lack of materials
- Lack of social supports

INTERNAL BARRIERS

- Lack of knowledge
- Lack of motivation
- Insufficient skills to affect change in health habits
- Undefined short- and long-term goals

Implementation

Nursing interventions for the young or middle adult are generalized into changing health habits and teaching health promotion and stress management.

Changing Health Habits

Health teaching and health counseling are often directed at improving health habits (see teaching box). The more fully the nurse understands the dynamics of behavior and habits, the more likely interventions will help the client to achieve or reinforce health-promoting behaviors (see box).

To help clients form positive health habits the nurse becomes a teacher and facilitator. By providing information about how the body functions and how habits are formed and changed, the nurse raises clients' levels of knowledge regarding the potential impact of behavior on health. A nurse cannot change clients' habits. Clients have control of and are responsible for their own behaviors. The nurse can explain psychological principles of changing habits and offer information about health risks. The nurse can also offer positive reinforcement (such as praise and rewards) for health-directed behaviors and decisions. Such reinforcement increases the likelihood that the behavior will be repeated. Ultimately, however, the client decides which behaviors will become habits of daily living.

Barriers to change do exist (see box). Unless these barriers are minimized or eliminated, it is futile to encourage the client to take actions that are going to be blocked.

Health Promotion

Community health programs for young and middle adults are designed to prevent illness, promote health, and detect disease in the early stages. Nurses can make valuable contributions to the community's health by taking an active part in the planning of screening and teaching programs (see Chapter 2).

Family planning, birthing, and parenting skills are program topics in which adults might be interested. Health screening for diabetes, hypertension, eye disease, and cancer is a good opportunity for the nurse to perform assessment and provide health teaching and health counseling.

Health education programs can promote changes in behavior and lifestyle. The nurse as health teacher offers information that will enable the client to make decisions about health practices. During health counseling the nurse and client design a plan of action that addresses the client's health and well-being. Through objective problem solving, the nurse helps the client grow and change.

Regardless of the age of its members and its structure, the family faces certain health tasks. The nurse

Dynamics of Behavior and Habits

- Habits are frequently repeated behaviors.
- The more often that a behavior is repeated, the more likely that it will be repeated thereafter.
- Habits can be a stress-reduction mechanism for the individual (e.g., nail biting) but may be simultaneously detrimental to health (e.g., alcohol consumption).
- Habits often meet some basic need for the person.
- Changing a habit requires a significant motivation by the client. Changing the habit must provide greater pleasure or satisfaction than the habit itself.
- Any change in habits or behavior patterns creates stress.

Sample Evaluation of Interventions for Altered Health Maintenance

Goals	Evaluative Measures	Expected Outcomes
Client will verbalize impact of alcohol excess on level of health.	Ask client about frequency of attendance at alcohol-abstinence support groups.	Client will report 24-hour intake of all food and beverages. Client will name physiological, emotional, and social effects of alcohol.
Client will modify behavior.	Client will supply proof of attendance at alcohol-abstinence support groups.	Client will reduce alcohol intake.

as health teacher and counselor understands the autonomy of the family and supports it while promoting family health.

Nursing roles include community-centered care, hospital-based acute care, and care of the chronically ill. Participation in community health programs for the adult or family often requires many nursing roles and skills.

Stress Reduction

Throughout life, people are exposed to many stressors (see Chapter 30). After these stressors are identified, the client and nurse can work together to intervene and modify the stress response. Specific interventions for stress reduction can fall into three categories (Pender, 1987). First, the frequency of stress-producing situations is minimized. Together the nurse and client identify approaches to prevent stressful situations, such as habituation, change avoidance, time blocking, time management, and environmental modification (Pender, 1987). The second category is psychophysiological preparation to increase stress resistance, such as increasing self-esteem, improving assertiveness, redirecting goal alternatives, and reorienting cognitive appraisal (Pender, 1987). Last, the physiological response to stress is avoided. The nurse uses relaxation techniques, imagery, and biofeedback to recondition the client's response to stress. Chapter 30 explains these general interventions in greater detail.

Evaluation

Each young or middle adult has different health goals. The success of the nurse and client in achieving these goals is determined in the evaluation component. Although it is not practical to describe all evaluation techniques for the care of the client, the evaluation box includes some of these measures.

SUMMARY

Transitional periods and developmental tasks of the young and middle adult can be a source of stress and conflict that can threaten health.

The nurse must understand the interrelationship of physiological, cognitive, and psychosocial needs and their influence on overall health. Anticipatory guidance can provide the client with insight into normal life events within a family. The nurse can inform the client about the normal growth and development patterns of young and middle adulthood.

With an understanding of the norms and common problems faced by others in the same developmental period, young and middle adult clients are better able to put health-related events into perspective. When the client experiences more complex difficulties, the nurse can make a referral for counseling.

CHAPTER 26 REVIEW

Key Concepts

- Adult development involves orderly and sequential changes in characteristics and attitudes that adults experience over time.
- Many changes experienced by the young adult are related to the natural process of maturation and socialization.
- Maturity is reached when the young adult attains a balance of growth in the physiological, psychosocial, and cognitive areas.
- Young adults are in a stable period of physical development, except for changes related to pregnancy.
- Cognitive development continues throughout the young and middle adult years.
- Emotional health of young adults is correlated with the ability to address and resolve personal and social problems.
- Young adults must choose a career and decide whether to remain single or marry and begin a family.
- Pregnant women need to understand physiological changes occurring in each trimester.
- Cognitive and psychosocial changes and health concerns during pregnancy and the puerperium affect the parents, the siblings, and often the extended family.
- Prenatal care reduces maternal and fetal mortality and morbidity.
- Midlife transition begins when a person becomes aware that physiological and psychosocial changes signify passage to another stage in life.
- Erikson and Havighurst have described the primary developmental tasks of the middle adult.
- Two significant physiological changes of the middle years are menopause in women and the climacteric in men.
- Cognitive changes are rare in middle age except in cases of illness or physical trauma.
- Psychosocial changes for middle adults may be related to career transition, sexuality, marital changes, family transition, and care of the aging parent.
- Health concerns of middle adults commonly involve stress-related illnesses, health assessment, and adoption of positive health habits.

Key Terms

Braxton Hicks contractions, p. 818

Climacteric, p. 820

Infertility, p. 816

Lactation, p. 813

Maturity, p. 810

Menopause, p. 819

Morning sickness, p. 816

Nesting, p. 818

Prenatal care, p. 816

Puerperium, p. 818

Critical Thinking Exercises

1. You are providing health education to a couple in their mid-30s. What information do you need to obtain during your initial assessments to determine the general health risks and the risks that are specific to their developmental stage?

2. Your client confides that she wants to get pregnant. However, before getting pregnant, she wants to modify her lifestyle to include more positive health habits. What do you need to know before you can intervene and assist this client in changing her lifestyle habits?

3. You suspect that your middle-age client is having difficulty adjusting to the fact that the children are out on their own and that both he and his wife are retiring. What do you need to know before designing a care plan to ease these role transitions?

REFERENCES

Beck CM, Rawlins RP, Williams SR: *Mental health— psychiatric nursing: a holistic life-cycle approach*, ed 2, St Louis, 1988, Mosby—Year Book.

Benner P, Wrubel J: *The primacy of caring: stress and coping in health and illness*, Menlo Park, Calif, 1989, Addison-Wesley.

Blenner J: Passage through infertility treatment: stage theory, *Image* 22(3):153, 1990.

Bobak IM, Jensen MD: *Essentials of maternity nursing*, ed 3, St Louis, 1991, Mosby—Year Book.

Brown MA: Social support, stress, and health: a comparison of expectant mothers and fathers, *Nurs Res* 35:72, 1986.

Diekelmann JL: The young adult: the choice is health or illness, *Am J Nurs* 76:1276, 1976.

Edelman CL, Mandle CL: *Health promotion throughout the lifespan*, ed 2, St Louis, 1990, Mosby—Year Book.

Erikson EH: *Childhood and society*, ed 2, New York, 1963, Norton.

Erikson EH: *Identity: youth and crisis*, New York, 1968 Norton.

Erikson EH: *The life cycle completed: a review*, New York, 1982, Norton.

Fawcett J et al: Spouses' body image changes during and after pregnancy: a replication and extension, *Nurs Res* 35:220, 1986.

Gilligan C: *In a different voice*, Cambridge, Mass, 1982, Harvard University Press.

Gordon S: *Prisoners of men's dreams: striking out for a new feminine future*, Boston, 1991, Little, Brown.

Havighurst RJ: Successful aging. In Williams RH, Tibbits C, and Donahue W, editors: *Process of aging*, vol 1, New York, 1972, Atherton.

Hayes C, Sharp E, Miner K: Knowledge, attitudes and beliefs of HIV seronegative women about AIDS, *J Nurse Midwife* 34(5):318, 1989.

Khabbaz R et al: Seroprevalence and risk factors for HTLV-I/II infection among female prostitutes in the United States, *JAMA* 263(1):60, 1990.

Kim MJ, McFarland GK, McLane AM: *Pocket guide to nursing diagnoses*, ed 4, St Louis, 1991, Mosby—Year Book.

Levinson D et al: *The seasons of a man's life*, New York, 1978, Knopf.

Mackey M, Lock S: Woman's expectations of the labor and delivery nurse, *JOGNN* 18(6):505, 1989.

Masters WH, Johnson VE: *Human sexual response*, Boston, 1970, Little, Brown.

National Cancer Institute, Breast Cancer Screening Consortium: Screening mammography: a missed clinical opportunity? Results of the NCI breast cancer screening consortium and National Health interview survey studies, *JAMA* 264(1):54, 1990.

Pender NJ: *Health promotion in nursing practice*, ed 2, Norwalk Conn, 1987, Appleton-Lange.

Scharlach A: A comparison of employed caregivers of cognitively and physically impaired elderly persons, *Res Aging* 11(2):225, 1989.

Schuster CS, Ashburn SS: *The process of human development: a holistic approach*, ed 2, Boston, 1986, Little, Brown.

Whall AL, Fawcett J: *Family theory development in nursing: state of the science and art*, Philadelphia, 1991, Davis.

ADDITIONAL READINGS

Bonheur B, Young S: Exercise as a health-promoting lifestyle choice, *Appl Nurs Res* 4(1):2, 1991.

Fife B: A model for predicting the adaptation of families to medical crises: an analysis of role integration, *Image J Nurs Sch* 17(4):108, 1985.

Laffrey SC: Normal and overweight adults: perceived weight and health behavior characteristics, *Nurs Res* 35:173, 1986.

Sandelowski M, Pottock C: Women's experiences of infertility, *Image J Nurs Sch* 18(40):140, 1986.

Stanhope M, Lancaster J: *Community health nursing: process and practice for promoting health*, ed 3, St Louis, 1992, Mosby.

Sund K, Ostwald SK: Dual-earner families' stress levels and personal and life-style related variables, *Nurs Res* 34:357, 1985.

Walker LO, Crain H, Thompson E: Maternal role attainment and identity in the postpartum period: stability and change, *Nurs Res* 35:68, 1986.

CHAPTER 27

Older Adulthood

OBJECTIVES

Mastery of content in this chapter will enable the student to:

- Define the key terms listed.
- Describe common myths and stereotypes about older adults.
- Discuss nurses' attitudes toward older adults.
- Discuss biological and psychosocial theories of aging.
- State and discuss developmental tasks of the older adult.
- Describe physiological changes of aging.
- Describe cognitive changes of dementia and delirium found in some older adults.
- Describe common causes of dementia and delirium.
- Discuss psychosocial changes of retirement, social isolation, sexuality, housing, and death to which older adults must adjust.
- Discuss physical and psychosocial health concerns of older adults and related nursing interventions.
- Describe community and institutional health care services available to older adults.
- Formulate a plan of care and interventions for an older adult with selected nursing diagnoses.
- Evaluate the plan of care and interventions for an older adult with selected nursing diagnoses.

CHAPTER OUTLINE

Myths and Stereotypes

Nurses' Attitudes Toward Older Adults

Theories of Aging
 Biological theories
 Psychosocial theories

Growth and Development

**Community and Institutional Health Care
 Services**
 Home care
 Hospice care

Day care
Respite care
Long-term care

The Nursing Process and Older Adults
 Assessment
 Nursing diagnosis
 Planning
 Implementation
 Evaluation

Older adulthood traditionally begins after retirement, usually between 65 and 75 years of age. The number of people in this age group is increasing at a dramatic rate, and demographers project a continuing increase in the older adult population well into the next century (Table 27-1). Health professionals are spending increasingly more time with older persons in all health care settings; therefore they must focus on identifying and meeting their special needs. Older adults are seeking greater participation in identification, definition, and resolution of issues affecting them. A greater incidence of chronic health problems, technological advances, and contemporary economic, social, ethical, and health issues have prompted health care professionals to focus on improving the duration and quality of life (Stanhope, Lancaster, 1992).

Increased life expectancy and decreased birth rate have contributed to the increase of this "graying" population. Demographic projections estimate continued growth. In addition, the number of persons 85 and over is expected to steadily increase, totaling more than 5% of the U.S. population by 2050 (U.S. Bureau of the Census, 1984). The life expectancy at birth for men born in the urban United States is 71 years; for women it is 79 years (Ebersole, Hess, 1990). The older adult population is expanding in all cultural and ethnic groups in the United States and Canada. In the United States, African Americans compose approximately 8% of persons 65 years and older. This is expected to increase to 11% by 2000 (Stanhope, Lancaster, 1992). Growth of the other races' population (primarily consisting of Asian, Pacific Islander, and Native Americans) is rapid. This group has tripled in number since 1970 and is expected to be 50% of the population or larger by 2000 (US Bureau of the Census, 1990). Older adults are distributed among the states in the same pattern as the total population. However, concentrations are found in some larger states, as well as the northeast and northcentral regions (Yurick et al, 1989).

Nursing care of older adults poses special challenges because of the diversity in physiological, cognitive, and psychosocial health. Older adults vary in their levels of function and productivity as members of society. Many are physically active, intelligent, socially engaging, and productive members of their communities. On the other hand, some older adults have lost the ability to care for themselves, are confused or withdrawn, and are unable to make decisions concerning their needs.

Before assessing an older adult the nurse should be aware of the expected physical and psychosocial findings. Normal changes of aging should also be considered. A comparison of expected and actual findings prevents the nurse from focusing on abnormal assessment data. In other words, the nurse should not assume that all older adults have signs, symptoms, or behaviors representing the lower end of the health continuum. By remembering that each older adult is an individual, the nurse avoids stereotyping this age group.

 MYTHS AND STEREOTYPES

In recent years a health specialty has been developed for older adults. **Geriatrics** is the branch of medicine dealing with the physiological and psychological aspects of aging and with diagnosis and treatment of diseases affecting older adults. **Gerontology** is the study of all aspects of the aging process and its consequence in humans and animals. Gerontological nursing applies the nursing process to older adults to achieve a level of wellness consistent with the changes of aging (Yurick et al, 1989). The term *gerontological nursing* is used because geriatrics is concerned with diseases of old age. Also, gerontological nurses have a broader focus, assisting older adults in maximizing their functional capabilities.

Although researchers are performing more health-related studies and scientific knowledge has expanded, many false stereotypes persist. Some persons believe that older persons lack understanding and are forgetful, rigid, bored, and unpleasant. Furthermore, older adults are often stereotyped as ill, crippled, hard of hearing, and bald. Many people believe that most older adults are institutionalized. In fact, only about 5% of the older adult population resides in institutional settings (Ebersole, Hess 1990).

TABLE 27-1 Population Growth and Projections for Older Adults		
Year	Number*	Total Population†
1960	16.6	5.8
1970	20.1	7.1
1980	25.7	8.3
1990	31.5	10.3
2000	34.8	13.3
2010	38.3	15.5
2020	52.0	12.5
2030	85.6	17.4
2040	85.1	18.0

*In millions.
†Percentage.
From US Bureau of the Census: *Statistical abstract of the United States,* Washington, DC, 1990, The Bureau.

Although financial constraints on older adults are significant, 85% of people 65 years and older have incomes above poverty level (Ebersole, Hess 1990). However, the incomes of most older persons are fixed or do not rise as quickly as inflationary increases in the cost of basic necessities.

Many people incorrectly believe that older adults have decreased learning ability. As a result, health care professionals often fail to provide health education opportunities for them because they wrongly assume that older clients cannot learn to care for themselves (Stanhope, Lancaster, 1992).

There are many misconceptions concerning older adults and sex. Older adults are thought to have no sexual desire (see box). In reality, older adults experience sexual drive and activity, although they are altered because of physiological changes and sociocultural expectations. Health problems, medications, availability of mates, privacy, and living arrangements may alter sexual activity.

Society values attractiveness, energy, and youth. As people age, their contributions become less appreciated. Some people believe that older adults no longer possess worth after they leave the workforce.

These notions have led to the concept of **ageism,** which is discrimination against people because of increasing age, just as people who are racists and sexists discriminate because of skin color and gender. However, sexists or racists never become concerned about changing their attitudes because neither their own gender nor skin color will change. In contrast, an ageist will eventually become old. This realization produces anxiety and a reluctance to accept aging as a normal process.

Unfortunately, when a youth image dominates society, the most diversified segment of our population is ignored. Older adults have a unique perspective on social, economic, and technological developments. In 100 years, society has progressed from riding horse-drawn carriages to space shuttle flights. Older adults may have experienced two world wars, the Spanish Civil, the Korean, the Vietnam, and the Gulf Wars.

In regard to health care, older adults have lived from the era of the family doctor into the age of specialization. They have seen the establishment of our first national health insurance, the Medicare and Medicaid systems.

Older adults are valuable to society, even though society fails to take advantage of their potential. The dramatic increases in the older adult population, however, may mean a change in the impact that they have on society.

A nurse may enter the profession with preconceptions about older adults. To provide appropriate nursing care for these clients, the nurse may first need to clarify personal values about them (see Chapter 12). The nurse must learn to distinguish between myth and reality and be able to identify clients' strengths and limitations.

 ## NURSES' ATTITUDES TOWARD OLDER ADULTS

It is important for nurses to assess their attitudes toward aging because these attitudes influence nursing care. To provide effective care, nurses must foster positive attitudes toward the aged.

Negative attitudes may result in a reduction in clients' sense of security, adequacy, and well-being. Furthermore, such attitudes may lead to a decline in the quality of care. Clients in long-term care facilities present a special challenge for the nurse. They are often considered losers by themselves, by society, or both. The nurse can promote independence and self-esteem of clients who feel that life is not worth living.

The nurse must clarify personal attitudes and values about older adults to provide the most effective care (see Chapter 12). A nurse's age, education, employment experience, and employing institution influence stereotypes. Personal experiences with older adults such as family members can also affect attitudes. Because older adults are becoming more prevalent in health care settings, it becomes imperative for the nurse to perform a self-examination so that ageist attitudes can be eliminated.

Nurses who work with older adults must collect complete assessment data, including clients'

Common Myths and Misconceptions about Sex and Aging

- Sex does not matter. The later years are supposed to be (and usually are) sexless.
- Interest in sex is abnormal for older people.
- Remarriage after the loss of a spouse should be discouraged.
- It is all right for older men to seek younger women as sex partners, but it is ridiculous for older women to be sexually involved with younger men.
- In institutions, older people should be separated according to sex to avoid problems for the staff and criticism by families and the community.
- Emission of semen during sexual activity weakens men and therefore should be avoided in old age.
- Masturbation is a childish activity that should not continue after adolescence.

strengths, resources, and limitations. For example, the nurse should consider clients' hobbies, work histories, and methods of dealing with stress. Information about such resources helps the nurse engage in meaningful interactions with clients. Clients sense the nurse's interest in them as unique individuals.

The nurse's interventions should attempt to incorporate the client's routines or rituals. The older adult often feels more secure when familiar rituals are continued in a hospital or institution. For example, if the nurse learns that the client follows certain practices at bedtime, including these in the care plan will alleviate anxiety and provide an opportunity to remain independent.

Gerontological nursing has expanded to provide nurses with creative approaches for maximizing the potential of older clients. With knowledge that is available regarding the older adult's needs and problems, nurses working in this specialty can better maintain their clients' physical abilities and create an environment for psychosocial health.

 # THEORIES OF AGING

Theorists have tried to describe the complex biopsychosocial process of aging. No theory fully explains the aging process; all of these theories are in various stages of development and have limitations. However, nurses can use them to understand phenomena affecting the health and well-being of aged clients.

Aging is not a simple progression, so there is no universally accepted theory that can predict and explain the complexities of older adults. The nurse must be aware of uncertainties about aging, the scientific attempts to explain these phenomena, and the many environmental factors involved.

Biological Theories

Free Radical Theory

The free radical theory emphasizes the mechanism of oxygen use at the cellular level. Free radicals are molecules with an extracellular charge. This charge creates a reaction that alters the structure or function of the cell membrane. Oxidation of fat, protein, and carbohydrates within the body produces free radicals. Environmental pollutants are external sources of free radicals (Ebersole, Hess, 1990). Research is being conducted on the role that free radical scavengers and antioxidants play in aging.

Cross-Link Theory

The cross-link and connective tissue theory asserts that the molecules of collagen and elastin, connective tissue components, form bonds that increase cell rigidity. Cross-linkage is thought to result from chemical reactions that create bonds between normally separate molecules (Ebersole, Hess, 1990). Research efforts are directed at the factors that cause, reduce, and impede cross-linkage.

Immunological Theory

Some theorists suggest that the immune system is responsible for aging. Erratic cellular mechanisms are thought to cause attacks on body tissues through autoaggression or immunodeficiencies (Ebersole, Hess, 1990). Investigation in immunoengineering attempts to control, moderate, or eliminate the effects of autoimmunity and immunodeficiency.

Psychosocial Theories

In the past, psychosocial theories of development have focused primarily on the child and adolescent. There is no adequate evidence to support theories about aspects of psychosocial aging. Researchers have demonstrated that genetics is not the primary determinant of longevity. Lifestyle, personality, and environmental factors are also influences (Murray, Huelskoetter, O'Driscoll, 1980).

Disengagement Theory

The disengagement theory formulated by Cummings and Henry (1961) states that aging people withdraw from customary roles and engage in more introspective, self-focused activities. This theory includes four basic concepts (Maddox, 1974):
1. Aging persons and society mutually withdraw from each other.
2. Disengagement is biologically and psychologically intrinsic and inevitable.
3. Disengagement is considered necessary for successful aging.
4. Disengagement is beneficial for older adults and society.

The disengagement theory remains controversial because it does not indicate whether society or the aging person initiates disengagement or whether personality, health, culture, and other factors influence disengagement.

Activity Theory

The activity theory disagrees with the disengagement theory and asserts that the continuation of middle-adult activities is necessary for successful aging. Most members of the aging population maintain a high level of activity. This activity level is influenced by past lifestyle and by present social and economic forces. According to this perspective, the maintenance of optimal physical, mental, and social activity is necessary for successful aging (Havighurst, 1963). This theory also assumes that older adults have the same needs as middle-age persons. The activity theory does not address the impact of biopsychosocial changes or the presence of multiple losses on the ability of older people to continue or replace activities.

Continuity Theory

The continuity or developmental theory (Neugarten, 1964) states that personality remains the same and behavior becomes more predictable as people age. Personality and behavior patterns developed during a lifetime determine the degree of engagement and activity in older adulthood. This is a promising psychosocial theory because it addresses the complexities of the aging process and people's adaptive ability.

 GROWTH AND DEVELOPMENT

As in other stages of life, older adults have specific developmental tasks. These are described by Burnside (1979), Duvall (1977), and Havighurst (1953) and include seven major categories (see box).

The older adult must adjust to physical changes. As each body system ages, changes in appearance and functioning occur. These are not associated with a disease but are normal. Structural and functional changes associated with aging are described in the section on physiological development.

Older adults are commonly retired from full-time employment and therefore may need to adjust to boredom, decreased socialization, and reduced or fixed income. However, because retirement is usually anticipated, persons may plan ahead to participate in consultation or volunteer activities. Although most older adults are above the poverty level, they are on fixed incomes and find it difficult to meet basic needs.

The majority of older adults are faced with the deaths of spouses, friends, and sometimes children. These losses are often difficult to resolve. By assisting older adults through grief the nurse can help them adjust to the loss (see Chapter 28). When the grieving process has ended, clients may need help in identifying resources to fill the void.

It is often difficult for older adults to perceive themselves as aging. Some older adults may demonstrate their inability to cope by denying upcoming retirement, requesting that their grandchildren not call them "Grandma" or "Grandpa," or choosing to live like a young or middle adult. This is different from merely remaining active and can pose a threat to health if physical limitations are exceeded.

An older adult may have to change living arrangements. For example, physical impairments may necessitate relocation to a smaller, single-level home. Severe health problems may require the older adult to live with relatives or friends. A change in living arrangements for the older adult may require an extended period of adjustment during which assistance and support from health care professionals and family are needed.

Older adults often need to redefine relationships with adult children. The issues of role reversal, dependence, conflict, guilt, and loss require recognition and resolution. Frequently, adult children must cope with guilt if they feel that they should have "come sooner" or made older parents move into their homes. Often, adult children must realize that some of these behaviors are symptoms rather than meanness or stubbornness.

Older adults must learn to acquire new activities and interests to maintain their quality of life. People who were socially active throughout life may find it relatively easy to meet new people and acquire new interests. However, people who were somewhat introverted, with limited socialization, may have difficulty meeting new people during retirement.

These developmental tasks are common to older adults. The way that older adults adjust to the changes of aging, however, depends on the individual. For some, adaptation and adjustment are relatively easy. For others, each developmental task requires nursing intervention. Many of these tasks are associated with loss, which occurs with greater frequency in older adulthood. The most common losses are health, income, usefulness, socialization, loved ones, and independent living. The nurse must be sensitive to the effect of such losses on the older adult and be prepared to offer support.

Developmental Tasks of the Older Adult

- Adjusting to decreasing health and physical strength
- Adjusting to retirement and reduced or fixed income
- Adjusting to death of a spouse
- Accepting self as aging person
- Maintaining satisfactory living arrangements
- Realigning relationships with adult children
- Finding meaning in life

COMMUNITY AND INSTITUTIONAL HEALTH CARE SERVICES

General health care services were described in Chapter 3. However, five services are frequently used by the older population.

Home Care

Home health care and homemaker services prevent or delay institutionalization for older adults who need assistance with daily living. These agencies may be governmental, private, or voluntary. Home health care is covered by Medicare and health insurance. Care is provided by professional nurses or nonprofessional staff, such as homemaker aides.

Hospice Care

A hospice is a resource for the terminally ill. A hospice can be an independent unit within the community that provides support to the client and family in the home, or it may be contained within an institution. The program focuses on meeting the needs of the dying client and family. It provides pain control and maintains quality of life. The hospice does not attempt to prolong life.

Day Care

Day care provides an alternative to institutionalization, offering health and rehabilitative services. Day-care center clients are usually not seriously ill, although they may have chronic conditions or disabilities that limit independence. A typical participant lives with a family member who must be away during the day. Day care thus enables the family to maintain employment and other activities (Stanhope, Lancaster, 1992).

Respite Care

Respite care is temporary relief for the primary care giver of a dependent older adult. Service is provided in the home or institution. Respite care enables the care giver to be away from home for a few hours.

The continual demand for care of a seriously ill or dependent family member can create emotional and physical stress. Studies indicate that respite services reduce care giver stress.

Long-Term Care

Declining health, decreased physical and human resources, and increased dependence may require an older adult to stay in a long-term care facility. Such a facility provides extended nursing care, medical care, and personal or psychosocial services.

The decision for such care is not easily made, and the family requires much support. In addition, a nurse's help may be needed in locating a proper facility. When possible, the facility should be close to the client's and family's home to make visiting easier.

 ## THE NURSING PROCESS AND OLDER ADULTS

 ### Assessment

The nurse assesses for changes in physiological development, cognition, and psychosocial behavior.

Physiological Changes

Perception of well-being can define quality of life. Understanding the older adult's perceptions about health status is essential for accurate assessment and development of clinically relevant interventions.

Older adults' concepts of health generally depend on personal perceptions of functional ability. Therefore older adults engaged in activities of daily living usually consider themselves healthy, whereas those whose activities are limited by physical, emotional, or social impairments may perceive themselves as ill.

Physiological changes vary with each client. Table 27-2 describes general physiological changes anticipated in older adults. These physiological changes are not pathological processes. They occur in all persons but at different rates and depend on circumstances in life. The nurse should know about these changes to provide appropriate care for older adults and to assist them in adapting to the changes.

The nurse should also consider potential sensory changes that may influence data gathering. For example, the nurse must consider visual problems from cataracts or hearing impairments from nerve deafness when choosing communication techniques. If clients are unable to understand the nurse's visual or auditory cues, assessment data may be inaccurate. For example, if clients have difficulty hearing the nurse's questions, inappropriate responses may lead the nurse to believe that they are confused.

The physiological changes of aging can be anticipated. Some older clients may experience all of these changes, and others experience only a few. The body changes continuously with age, but the effects on clients depend on health, lifestyle, stressors, and environmental conditions.

GENERAL SURVEY. The general survey begins during the initial nurse-client encounter and includes a concise written description of a quick but careful head-

TABLE 27-2 Normal Physical Changes of Aging	
System	Normal Findings
Integument	
Skin color	Spotty pigmentation in areas exposed to the sun; pallor even in absence of anemia
Moisture	Dry, scaly condition
Temperature	Cooler extremities; decreased perspiration
Texture	Decreased elasticity; wrinkles; folding, sagging condition
Fat distribution	Decreased amount on extremities; increased amount on abdomen
Hair	Thinning and graying on scalp; often, decreased amount of axillary and pubic hair and hair on extremities; decreased facial hair in men; possible chin and upper lip hair in women
Nails	Decreased growth rate
Head and neck	
Head	Sharp and angular nasal and facial bones; loss of eyebrow hair in women; bushier eyebrows in men
Eyes	Decreased visual acuity; decreased accommodation; reduced adaptation to darkness; sensitivity to glare
Ears	Decreased pitch discrimination; diminished light reflex; diminished hearing acuity
Nose and sinuses	Increased nasal hair; decreased sense of smell
Mouth and pharynx	Use of bridges or dentures; decreased sense of taste; atrophy of papillae of lateral edges of tongue
Neck	Nodular thyroid gland; slight tracheal deviation resulting from muscle atrophy
Thorax and lungs	Increased anteroposterior diameter; increased chest rigidity; increased respiratory rate with decreased lung expansion; increased airway resistance
Heart and vascular system	Significant increase in systolic pressure with slight increase in diastolic pressure; usually insignificant changes in heart rate at rest; common diastolic murmurs; easily palpated peripheral pulses; weaker pedal pulses and colder lower extremities, especially at night
Breasts	Diminished breast tissue; pendulous, flabby condition
Gastrointestinal system	Decreased salivary secretions, which may make swallowing more difficult; decreased peristalsis; decreased production of digestive enzymes, including hydrochloric acid, pepsin, and pancreatic enzymes; constipation; reduced motility
Reproductive system	
Female	Decreased estrogen; decreased uterine size; decreased secretions; atrophy of epithelial lining of vagina
Male	Decreased levels of testosterone; decreased sperm count; decreased testicular size
Urinary system	Decreased renal filtration and renal efficiency; subsequent loss of protein from kidney; nocturia; decreased bladder capacity; increased incontinence
Female	Urgency and stress incontinence resulting from decrease in perineal muscle tone
Male	Urinary frequency and retention resulting from prostatic enlargement
Musculoskeletal system	Decreased muscle mass and strength; bone demineralization (more pronounced in women); shortening of trunk as result of intervertebral space narrowing; decreased joint mobility; decreased range of joint motion; enhanced bony prominences
Neurological system	Decreased rate of voluntary or automatic reflexes; decreased ability to respond to multiple stimuli; insomnia; shorter sleeping periods

Modified from Ebersole P, Hess P: *Toward healthy aging: human needs and nursing response*, ed 3, St Louis, 1990, Mosby–Year Book.

to-toe scan of the client. An initial inspection of an older adult might reveal eye contact and facial expression appropriate to the situation, facial wrinkles, gray hair, loss of tissue on the extremities, and an increase in tissue and fat on the trunk.

INTEGUMENTARY SYSTEM. The skin loses resilience and moisture in older adulthood. The epithelial layer thins, and elastic collagen fibers shrink and become rigid. Wrinkles of the face and neck reflect lifetime patterns of muscle activity and facial expressions, the pull of gravity on tissue, and diminished elasticity.

Spots and lesions may also be present on skin. Smooth, brown, irregularly shaped spots (age spots, or **senile lentigo**) initially appear on the backs of the hands and on forearms. Small, round, red or brown cherry angiomas may be found on the trunk. Seborrheic lesions or keratosis may appear as irregular, round or oval, brown, watery lesions.

Pressure ulcers are common in this population and are primarily due to chronic unrelieved pressure. Multiple factors play a role in pressure ulcer formation, including mobility and activity, sensory perception, moisture, friction and shearing, nutritional status, and arteriolar pressure (see Chapter 44).

HEAD AND NECK. The facial features of the older adult become more pronounced from loss of fat and skin elasticity. Facial features may appear asymmetrical because of missing teeth or improperly fitting dentures. In addition, changes in voice pitch (usually a rise) occur from decline in power and range.

The older adult's visual acuity declines. This may be the result of retinal damage, reduction in pupillary diameter, reduction in opacity of the lens, or loss of lens elasticity. **Presbyopia,** a decline in the ability of the eyes to accommodate for close, detailed work, is common. Presbyopia begins early in the fourth decade and continues throughout life. The older adult also has a reduced ability to see in darkness, and glare can cause pain and limit the ability to see.

Auditory changes are subtle and may be noted as difficulty in hearing. Age-related changes in auditory acuity are called *presbycusis.* It affects ability to hear high-pitched sounds and sibilant consonants such as *s, sh,* and *ch.* The assessment of an older client's hearing is best accomplished using a tuning fork with frequencies of 500 to 1000 cycles per second (cps) to screen for high-frequency losses.

Taste buds atrophy and lose efficiency. The older adult is able to discern salty, sweet, sour, and bitter tastes less acutely. Sense of smell is also decreased, further reducing taste. Salivary secretion is reduced.

THORAX AND LUNGS. Because of changes in the musculoskeletal system, the configuration of the thorax sometimes changes. There is an increase in the anteroposterior diameter. Kyphosis is a subtle, progressive change in the vertebral structure that is permanent when accompanied by osteoporosis. Calcification of the costal cartilage can cause decreased mobility of the ribs.

Decreased muscle mass and tone lead to decreased lung expansion. Decreased elasticity of lung alveoli results in emphysematous changes in the lungs, and hyperresonance may be present on percussion. If kyphosis or chronic obstructive lung disease is present, breath sounds are distant.

HEART AND VASCULAR SYSTEM. Decreased contractile strength of the myocardium results in a decreased cardiac output. The decrease is significant when the older adult is stressed by anxiety, excitement, illness, or strenuous activity. The body tries to compensate for decreased cardiac output by increasing the heart rate during exercise. However, after exercise, it takes longer for the client's rate to return to baseline.

Frequently the older adult's baseline blood pressure rises. This is the result of vascular changes and the accumulation of sclerotic plaques along the walls of the vessels. Peripheral pulses are palpable but frequently weaker in the lower extremities. The lower extremities are cold, particularly at night.

BREASTS. Decreased muscle mass, tone, and elasticity result in smaller breasts in older women. In addition, the breasts sag. Atrophy of glandular tissue, coupled with more fat deposits, results in a slightly smaller, less dense, and less nodular breast.

GASTROINTESTINAL SYSTEM AND ABDOMEN. Aging leads to an increase in the amount of fatty tissue in the trunk and abdomen. As a result, the abdomen increases in size. Because muscle tone and elasticity decrease, it also becomes more protuberant.

The older adult also experiences changes in gastrointestinal function. Some changes may be slight, such as the sudden development of intolerance to certain foods. Because of decreased peristalsis an older adult experiences delayed gastric emptying and may be unable to consume large meals. Decreased peristalsis also affects emptying of the colon, resulting in constipation.

REPRODUCTIVE SYSTEM. Changes in the structure and function of the reproductive system occur as the result of hormonal alterations. Female menopause is related to a reduced responsiveness of the ovaries to pituitary hormones and a resultant decrease in estrogen and progesterone levels. In men, there is no definite cessation of fertility associated with aging. Spermatogenesis begins to decline during the fourth decade but continues into the ninth.

The changes in reproductive structure and function do not affect libido. Less frequency of sexual activity can result from illness, death of a sexual partner, decreased socialization, or loss of sexual interest.

URINARY SYSTEM. Hypertrophy of the prostate gland may develop in older men. This hypertrophy enlarges the gland, and pressure is displaced to the neck of the bladder. As a result, urinary tract infections, frequency, incontinence, and retention of urine occur. In addition, prostatic hypertrophy can result in difficulty initiating and maintaining a stream.

Older women, particularly those who have had children, can experience stress incontinence, in which an involuntary release of urine occurs when they cough, sneeze, or lift an object. This is a result of a weakening of the perineal and bladder muscles. In addition, older women notice urgency in voiding.

MUSCULOSKELETAL SYSTEM. Older adults who exercise regularly do not lose as much bone and muscle mass or tone as those who are inactive. Muscle fibers are reduced in size, and muscle strength diminishes in proportion to the decline in muscle mass.

Postmenopausal women have a greater rate of bone demineralization than older men. Women who maintain calcium intake throughout life and into menopause have less bone demineralization than those who do not.

NEUROLOGICAL SYSTEM. The number of neurons in the nervous system begins to decrease in the middle of the second decade (Ebersole, Hess, 1990). These neurons do not regenerate, and decrease or damage can lead to functional changes. The changes can affect the special senses described earlier. In addition, the client may experience a decreased sense of balance or uncoordinated motor responses.

The sleep-wake cycle is also influenced by the brain (see Chapter 36). Characteristically, older adults do not sleep through the night. This disruption has the following causes:

1. The sleep cycle is shortened.
2. Sleep disruption can be the result of frequent bladder emptying, pain, or psychological upsets.
3. Medication may affect the sleep-wake cycle.

Cognitive Changes

Much of the psychological and emotional trauma of older adulthood arises from the misconception that older adults have cognitive impairments—that all older people are senile. However, the structural and physiological changes occurring in the brain during aging do not necessarily affect adaptive and functional abilities (Ebersole, Hess, 1990).

Neurophysiological cellular changes vary among individuals, and even with obvious cellular loss some older adults do not demonstrate mental deterioration. Furthermore, some clients with significant cerebral cell loss respond well to therapy.

Occasionally when cerebral dysfunction is present, preexisting behavioral tendencies are magnified. Therefore persons who were compulsive as young and middle adults become more compulsive when older. Cognitive changes occur in older adults when cerebral dysfunction or trauma is present. The nurse must understand these changes so that clients can be helped to maintain optimal functioning.

A nurse who cares for an older adult with cognitive impairments is challenged to meet physical needs and to improve or maintain cognitive functioning. To achieve this, the nurse may use reality orientation, resocialization, and remotivation.

DEMENTIA. Dementia is a syndrome involving progressive impairment of memory, other cognitive abilities (that is, thinking and judgment), and personality change, which can have a variety of causes (Zarit, Orr, Zarit, 1985). Senile dementia of the Alzheimer type (SDAT), or Alzheimer's disease, is the most frequent cause of irreversible dementia. Causes of reversible dementia include infection, drug reactions, a variety of metabolic disorders, and even depression. These conditions are often mistaken for irreversible dementia in the older adult. Consequently, older clients with such disorders may not be appropriately assessed and treated, and a reversible dementia may become irreversible.

DELIRIUM. Delirium, or acute confusional state, is a syndrome resembling irreversible and reversible dementia but is distinguished by clouding of consciousness (American Psychiatric Association, 1987). Other features include attentional deficits, illusions, hallucinations, occasional incoherent speech, disturbed sleep-wake cycle, and disorientation. The onset of delirium is typically sudden, and there are rapid fluctuations in symptoms and severity. Delirium and reversible dementia resemble irreversible dementia. However, their causes can usually be treated, and recovery is possible. The box on p. 838 summarizes frequent causes of delirium and reversible dementia.

Cognitive changes are not normal, expected outcomes of aging. Mental changes frequently considered irreversible often respond to treatment. Distinguishing among irreversible dementia and delirium and reversible dementia is necessary when planning care for promotion of functional ability.

CHRONIC DISORDERS. Chronic brain disorders are irreversible and usually progressive. However, with careful and supportive nursing management, clients with chronic brain disorders can be helped to maintain function.

Alzheimer's Disease. Alzheimer's disease is a disorder of brain cells characterized by senile plaques, neurofibrillary tangles (abnormal, tangled protein fibers), and an overall loss of neurons (Zarit, Orr, Zarit, 1985). These tissue changes occur mainly in the cortex and hippocampus. The cause is not known, and although several theories are being investigated, none are definitive.

Alzheimer's disease involves a gradual, progressive deterioration in functioning. Symptoms have been grouped according to the stage of dementia (see box on p. 839) (Wolanin, Phillips, 1981).

Reversible Causes of Dementia Symptoms and Delirium

CAUSES OF DEMENTIA

- Depression
- Cushing's syndrome
- Normal-pressure hydrocephalus
- Lifelong alcoholism
- Deficiencies of nutrients (vitamin B_{12}, folic acid, niacin)

CAUSES OF DELIRIUM

- Hypernatremia (dehydration, intravenous saline)
- Acid-base disturbance
- Hyperglycemia (diabetic ketoacidosis, hyperosmolar coma)
- Pneumonia
- Pyelonephritis
- Cholecystitis
- Diverticulitis
- Acute myocardial infarction
- Pulmonary embolus
- Transient vascular ischemia of brain
- Concussion or contusion
- Intracerebral hemorrhage
- Epidural hematoma
- Acute meningitis (pyogenic, viral)
- Pain secondary to urinary retention
- Pain secondary to fracture
- Pain secondary to abdominal incision
- Acute hallucinosis
- Delirium tremens
- Accidental hypothermia

CAUSES OF DEMENTIA, DELIRIUM, OR BOTH

- Therapeutic drug intoxication
- Azotemia or renal failure (dehydration, diuretics, obstruction, hypokalemia)
- Hyponatremia (diuretics, excess antidiuretic hormone, salt wasting, intravenous fluids)
- Volume depletion (diuretics, bleeding, inadequate fluids)

- Hypoglycemia (insulin, oral hypoglycemics, starvation)
- Hepatic failure
- Hypothyroidism
- Hyperthyroidism (especially apathetic)
- Hypercalcemia
- Hypopituitarism
- Viral infection or fever
- Tuberculosis
- Endocarditis
- Congestive heart failure
- Dysrhythmia
- Vascular occlusion
- Stroke
- Subdural hematoma
- Chronic meningitis (tuberculous, fungal)
- Neurosyphilis
- Subdural empyema
- Brain abscess
- Tumors
  - Metastatic to brain
  - Primary in brain
- Pain secondary to fecal impaction
- Sensory deprivation states (blindness, deafness)
- Anesthesia or surgery
- Environmental change and isolation
- Alcoholism new in older adulthood
- Decreased alcohol tolerance with age, producing increasing intoxication
- Anemia
- Tumor (systemic effects of nonmetastatic malignant neoplasm)
- Chronic lung disease with hypoxia or hypercapnia
- Chemical intoxications
  - Heavy metals (arsenic, lead, mercury)
  - Consciousness-altering agents
  - Carbon monoxide

Adapted from Zarit SH, Orr NK, Zarit JM: *The hidden victims of Alzheimer's disease: families under stress*, New York, 1985, New York University Press.

Nursing management of clients with Alzheimer's disease is complex. Limited mobility increases the client's risk of hazards of immobility. Therefore the nurse must continually meet the client's physical needs (see Chapter 43). Confusion usually increases at night, and wandering through the home or hospital may increase. As the client progresses through the three stages, communication becomes more difficult. The client may easily misperceive the environment and feel threatened. Typical behavioral re-

sponses of the client who feels threatened include aggressive gestures or acts, increased voice volume, restlessness, agitation, and hostility (Bartol, 1979). Nursing care objectives are individualized to help this client use remaining functional abilities (see box at far right).

Multiinfarct Dementia. Multiinfarct dementia is the second most common cause of dementia, accounting for 10% to 20% of cases (Terry, 1978; Heyman, 1978). Although clients with this form of de-

Stages of Irreversible Dementia

EARLY STAGE

- Attention difficulties occur.
- Client experiences decreasing interest in life.
- Client is indifferent to ceremony and courtesy.
- Client forgets nouns in speech.
- Client is vague, uncertain, and hesitant.

ADVANCED STAGE

- Deficits in memory, retention, and recall occur.
- Client hesitates when responding to questions.
- Time disorientation and day and night confusion occur.
- Client misplaces belongings and forgets regular responsibilities.
- Client forgets dates and appointments.
- Cient has difficulty remembering simple directions.
- Client neglects personal health and hygiene.

LATER STAGE

- Disorientation to place and wandering occur.
- Client loses possessions.
- Client forgets and misidentifies people.
- Client is immodest.
- Client has no sense of time and loses short-term memory.
- Client experiences communication difficulties.

FINAL OR TERMINAL STAGE

- Urinary and fecal incontinence occur.
- Severe motor impairments and extreme psychomotor retardation occur; client loses ability to walk.
- Client is unable to communicate and has little or no response to stimuli.
- Overall marked physical deterioration occurs.

Modified from Wolanin MO, Phillips LR: *Confusion: prevention and care,* St Louis, 1981, Mosby–Year Book.

Comprehensive Nursing Care Objectives for the Client with Alzheimer's Disease

- Keep client ambulating as long as possible.
- Protect client from physical injuries.
- Maintain daily exercise program.
- Maintain optimal nutritional status.
- Maintain integrity of gums and mucous membranes to preserve dental function.
- Assess and evaluate the need for psychotropic medications.
- Provide cognitive stimuli.
- Provide regular social interaction.
- Maintain client's self-esteem through involvement with activities of daily living.
- Maintain reality orientation.
- Maintain a structured milieu.
- Avoid translocation syndrome (physiological and psychological disturbances due to transfer from one setting to another).
- Maintain nonverbal and verbal communication patterns.
- Reduce negative behavior through behavior modification.
- Provide ongoing support for family members.
- Protect client from infection.
- Prevent the hazards of immobility.

Modified from Bartol M: *J Gerontol Nurs* 5:21, 1979.

mentia may display symptoms of SDAT, multiinfarct dementia is distinguished by periods of remission, preservation of personality, insight, lability of emotion, and epileptoid attacks. Multiinfarct dementia may be related to vascular disorders within the brain and may result from the following conditions:

1. Arteriosclerotic plaques blocking cerebral circulation
2. Cerebrovascular accident (stroke)
3. Systemic emboli lodging in cerebrovascular pathways
4. Transient ischemic attacks
5. Decreased cerebral circulation resulting from decreased cardiac output or rupture of cerebral aneurysm
6. Severe hypertension

The causes of multiinfarct dementia are not known, but may have the same risk factors as heart disease and stroke. These include high blood pressure, high-cholesterol diet, obesity, smoking, and lack of exercise. The client with cognitive impairment resulting from multiinfarct dementia usually has a history of hypertension, diabetes mellitus, blackouts, falls, or seizures. In addition, a physical impairment such as hemiplegia or hemiparesis may be present. Nursing management of clients is similar to that described in the box above.

Substance Abuse and Cognitive Impairment.
The abuse of alcohol and other drugs occurs in the older adult population, but the exact incidence is difficult to determine. Studies of substance abuse in older adults indicate that it can be a long-standing or recent problem, making it difficult to determine prevalence. However, most studies indicate that it is a serious problem in older adults because of the stress

and loss associated with aging, such as retirement, loss of spouse, boredom, and loneliness.

Long-term abuse of alcohol and drugs can affect cognitive functioning. After 15 to 20 years of alcohol abuse, tolerance for drinking declines. Prolonged use of large amounts of alcohol creates cerebral, cerebellar, sensory, and peripheral nervous system damage. Many chronic alcoholics also have vitamin B_1 deficiency. A prolonged deficiency can cause neuropathy, myopathy, and encephalopathy, exhibited as Wernicke's syndrome or Korsakoff's syndrome. **Wernicke's syndrome** is present in advanced stages of vitamin B_1 depletion and is characterized by nystagmus, pupillary abnormalities, ataxia, tremor, and stupor. **Korsakoff's syndrome** is a psychosis characterized by disorientation of time, place, and person; amnesia for recent events; and confabulation. **Confabulation** is a defense mechanism in which the person fabricates experiences or situations and recounts them in a detailed and plausible way to fill in memory gaps.

The effects of prolonged drug abuse on the older adult have not been clearly described, but cognitive impairments like those associated with alcohol abuse may occur. In addition, a drug overdose may cause cerebral impairment, so cognitive impairment may result from a decrease of oxygen to the brain.

Psychosocial Changes

The older adult must adapt to psychosocial changes that occur with aging. Although these vary, some are common to the majority of older adults.

RETIREMENT. Retirement often has associations of passivity and seclusion and often leads to psychosocial stresses. These include role changes with the spouse or family and problems of social isolation (see next section).

Mandatory retirement age varies. For example, in a state civil service job, it may be 65, whereas a federal employee may not be required to retire until 70. In private industry the mandatory retirement age is usually between 62 and 70. It is common for people to retire at age 55. More companies are developing early retirement plans to provide advancement for younger employees. One popular program is the "30 and out" plan, which allows workers to retire with full pension, and in some cases large bonuses, after 30 years.

Preretirement planning is advisable during middle age and essential in late middle age (see Chapter 26). People who plan retirement activities generally adjust better. For example, an individual may plan volunteer work, home remodeling, travel, or other activities. Meaningful retirement planning is critical because retirement can last for up to 30 years.

Retirement also has an impact on the spouse. Tension can occur because of role changes in the relationship and because the homemaker may feel that the workload is increased.

The most powerful factors that influence the retired person's satisfaction with life are health status, the option to continue working, and sufficient income. (Ebersole, Hess, 1990). The nurse can help the client and family prepare for retirement by asking questions that may help them make decisions (see box). The nurse should particularly ask the following questions (Diekelman, 1978):

1. What provisions have they made for retirement income? Will these financial resources be enough to meet necessities? How long will these resources meet the needs—5 years, 10 years, or indefinitely?
2. What retirement activities are available after retirement? On what abilities, skills, and interests can the client draw (Fig. 27-1)? Will any of these be a source of income?
3. What living arrangements may be needed? Is the present house too large, difficult, or expensive? Should relocation be considered? Ideally the client should spend several months in a new location before making a commitment.

Questions to Consider When Planning for Retirement

- Will retirement income be adequate to provide a lifestyle that includes things that are currently satisfying?
- Are peer or health pressures significant factors in the decision?
- Is the job depleting to health and energy?
- What are the chief work-related satisfactions, and what might compensate for their loss?
- Are friendship networks tied to the job?
- How do spouse and family enter into the decision-making process?
- Is there an opportunity to test partial work status or nonworking status before retirement?
- Has sufficient information been available regarding retirement planning?
- Is the work situation more stressful than satisfying?
- How much of the self is defined by job status?
- Is competitive activity an important source of satisfaction?

From Ebersole P, Hess P: *Toward healthy aging: human needs and nursing response*, ed 3, St Louis, 1990, Mosby–Year Book.

4. What preparations have been made for role changes? Have the marriage partners discussed how they will spend time together? Will they divide household tasks, spend more time with grandchildren, or become involved in volunteer activities?

5. What provisions have been made to meet health care needs? How will the retired couple meet exercise, nutrition, and other health needs?

6. How will the retired person attend to legal affairs? Estate planning, education in legal affairs, and ability to cope with bureaucratic procedures are essential. Community colleges, offices on aging, and legal aid services may provide guidance.

SOCIAL ISOLATION. Many older adults experience social isolation, which increases as they age. The types of social isolation are attitudinal, presentational, behavioral, and geographical. Some older adults may be affected by all four, and others are affected by only one (Ebersole, Hess, 1990).

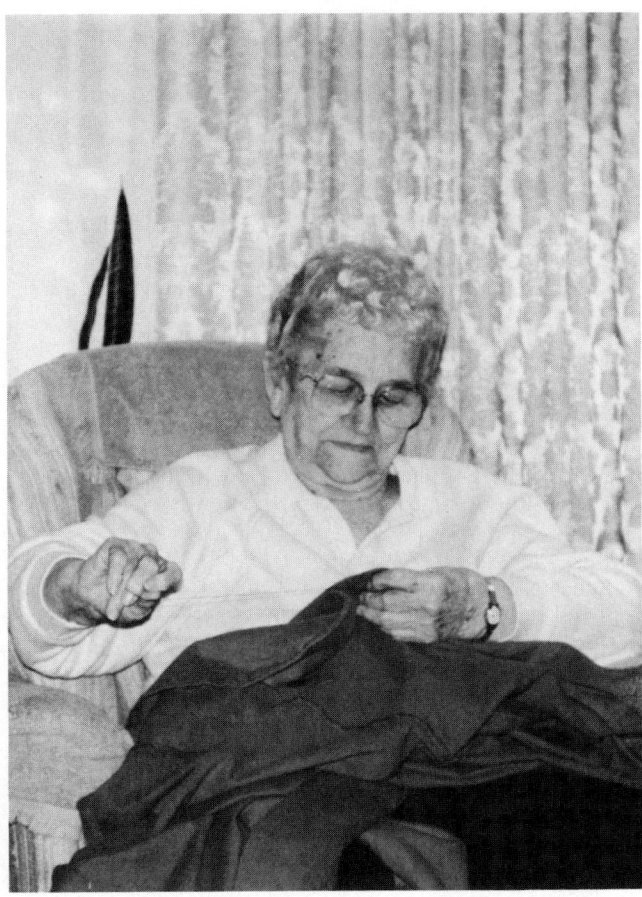

Fig. 27-1   Sewing is this older adult's favorite activity.

Attitudinal isolation occurs because of personal or cultural values. Ageism is a prevailing attitude that stigmatizes the older adult. It is a bias against and rejection of older people. Therefore attitudinal social isolation occurs when the older adult is not easily accepted into social interactions because of society's bias. A vicious circle may result. As the older adult is increasingly rejected, self-esteem may diminish, leading to fewer attempts to socialize.

Presentational isolation results from unacceptable appearance or other factors involved in presenting the self to others. Contributing factors are body image, hygiene, and visible signs of illness or functional loss (Ebersole, Hess, 1990). The person becomes isolated because of rejection by others or because little interaction is sought as a result of self-consciousness.

Behavioral isolation results from unacceptable behaviors. In all age groups and particularly with older adults, socially unacceptable behaviors cause others to withdraw. Behaviors commonly associated with isolation of older adults include confusion, dementia, alcoholism, eccentricity, egocentricity, incontinence, and deviant behavior. The nurse can use behavior-modification techniques to help decrease the frequency of these behaviors in older adults (Ebersole, Hess, 1990).

Geographical isolation occurs because of distance from family, urban crime, and institutional barriers. In today's mobile society, it is common for children to live great distances from parents. Thus the opportunity to visit children decreases. This leads to even further isolation when parents have physical limitations or experience the death of a spouse.

In urban areas a high crime rate can deter older adults from socializing. Living in a high-crime area may result in unwillingness to leave home because it might be vandalized or robbed while unoccupied.

One institutional barrier is lack of easy access for persons who use wheelchairs, walkers, canes, or crutches. Also, when older adults require institutional care, segregation from friends occurs. Social interaction depends on those who come to visit.

Nurses need to determine whether clients who are alone are lonely or merely prefer to be alone. The effects of loneliness and social isolation depend on how the person is able to meet basic human needs. Fig. 27-2 on p. 842 shows the relationship of basic human needs to loneliness and isolation. Loneliness is often associated with poor health, dissatisfaction with housing and other environmental factors, and the loss of a spouse.

The nurse can assist lonely older adults in rebuilding social networks. One resource is outreach programs designed to make contact with isolated older adults. The program may meet nutritional needs, such

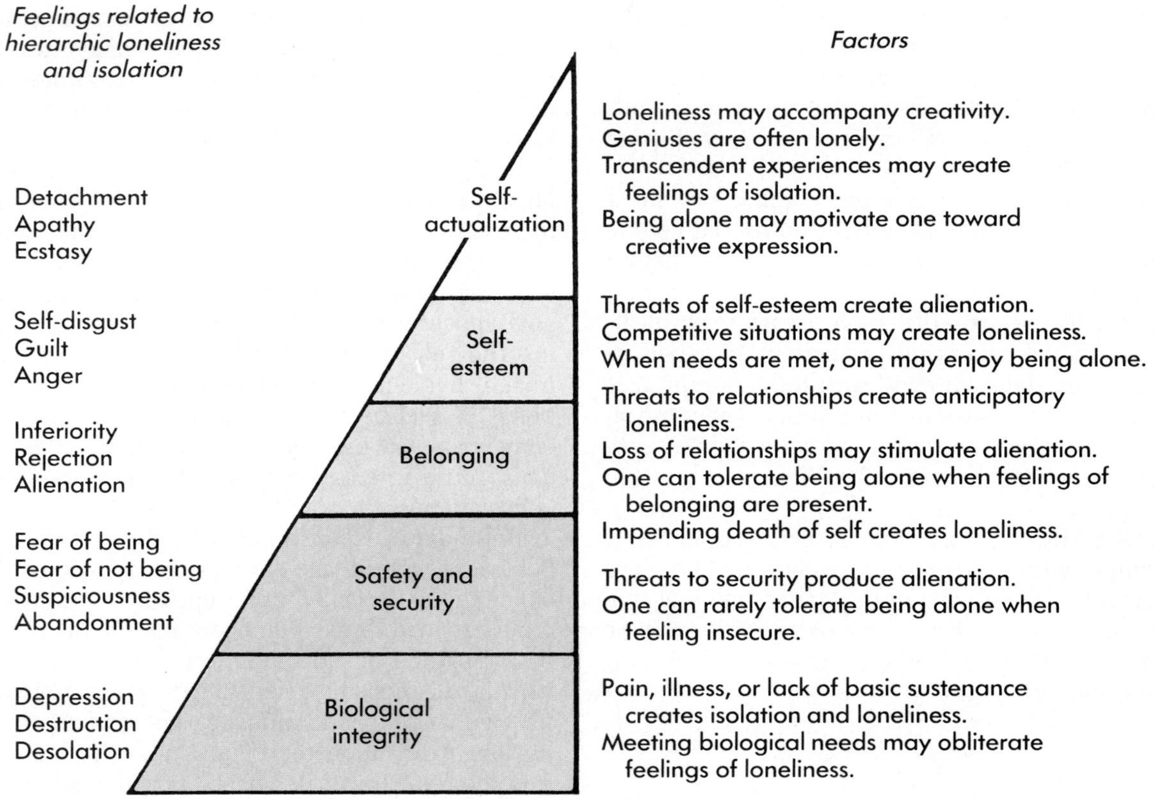
Feelings related to hierarchic loneliness and isolation
Factors
Detachment
Apathy
Ecstasy
Self-actualization
Loneliness may accompany creativity.
Geniuses are often lonely.
Transcendent experiences may create feelings of isolation.
Being alone may motivate one toward creative expression.
Self-disgust
Guilt
Anger
Self-esteem
Threats of self-esteem create alienation.
Competitive situations may create loneliness.
When needs are met, one may enjoy being alone.
Inferiority
Rejection
Alienation
Belonging
Threats to relationships create anticipatory loneliness.
Loss of relationships may stimulate alienation.
One can tolerate being alone when feelings of belonging are present.
Impending death of self creates loneliness.
Fear of being
Fear of not being
Suspiciousness
Abandonment
Safety and security
Threats to security produce alienation.
One can rarely tolerate being alone when feeling insecure.
Depression
Destruction
Desolation
Biological integrity
Pain, illness, or lack of basic sustenance creates isolation and loneliness.
Meeting biological needs may obliterate feelings of loneliness.

Fig. 27-2 Loneliness and isolation in relation to Maslow's hierarchy.
From Ebersole P, Hess P: *Toward healthy aging: human needs and nursing response,* ed 3, St Louis, 1990, Mosby–Year Book.

Contacts Increasing Social Networks of the Older Adult

FORMAL

- Church
- Grandparenting
- Foster Grandparents
- Vista
- Peace Corps
- Retired Senior Volunteer Program
- National Retired Teachers Association
- Unions
- Friends of the Library
- Volunteers
- Public school
- Senior centers
- Title VII nutrition sites
- Involvement in social issues for seniors

INFORMAL

- Neighbors
- Maids, waitresses
- Beauty salons, restaurants, bars, service personnel, shops, laundromats
- Sports
- Buses for older adults
- Special tours
- Education, arts, and crafts courses
- Trailer courts
- Retirement communities
- Pets
- Dancing
- Physicians' offices, clinics
- Nursing home—social corridor
- General social touching
- Radio shows

Modified from Ebersole P, Hess P: *Toward healthy aging: human needs and nursing response,* ed 3, St Louis, 1990, Mosby–Year Book.

as Meals on Wheels; socialization needs, such as daily telephone calls by volunteers; or need for activities, such as outings. In addition, the nurse can investigate networks within older adults' communities (see box). These increase the opportunity to meet people with similar activities, interests, and needs.

SEXUALITY. Sexuality is increasingly recognized as important in the care of older adults. All older adults, whether healthy or frail, need to express sexual feelings. Sexuality involves love, warmth, sharing, and touching, not just the act of intercouse. Sexuality is linked with identity and validates the belief that people can give to others and have the gift appreciated.

The nurse ensures that care is directed at helping the client maintain sexual health. It requires integration of somatic, emotional, intellectual, and social aspects of the sexual being. Success will enhance personality, communication, and love (Woods, 1983).

To help the older adult achieve or maintain sexual health, the nurse needs to understand the physical changes in sexual response. Knowledge of the changes described in Table 27-3, as well as the physical changes in male and female genitalia, enables the nurse to educate the older adult about changes in sexual functioning.

As discussed earlier, the libido does not decrease, although frequency of sexual activity may decline. An older woman who does not understand physical changes affecting sexual activity may be concerned that her sex life is nearly over with the onset of menopause. The older man may feel the same when he discovers a change in the firmness of his erection, has a decreased need for ejaculation with each orgasm, or has a longer recovery period between episodes of intercourse.

In addition to physical changes affecting sexual functioning, many older adults take drugs that de-

---

TABLE 27-3 Physical Changes in Sexual Response in the Older Adult

Female	Male
EXCITATION	
Diminished vaginal lubrication (1-3 min may be required for adequate amounts to appear.)	Less intense and slower erection (which can be maintained longer without ejaculation)
Diminished flattening and separation of labia majora	Less vasocongestion of scrotal sac
Disappearance of elevation of labia majora	Less pronounced elevation and congestion of testicles
Decreased vasocongestion of labia minora	Decreased muscle tension
Decreased elastic expansion of vagina (depth and breadth)	
Slower and less prominent uterine elevation or tenting	
Decreased muscle tension	
PLATEAU	
Decreased capacity for vasocongestion	Less frequent nipple erection and sexual flush
Decreased areolar engorgement	Lack of color change at coronal edge of penis
Less evident labial color change	Decrease or absence of secretory activity (lubrication) by Cowper gland before ejaculation
Less intense swelling or orgasmic platform	
Decreased secretions of Bartholin's glands	
ORGASM	
Fewer contractions of orgasmic platform	Fewer penile contractions
Rectal sphincter contractions with severe tension only	Fewer rectal sphincter contractions
	Decreased force of ejaculation with decreased amount of semen (seepage of semen with long ejaculation)
RESOLUTION	
Observably slower subsidence of nipple erection	Slow subsidence of vasocongestion of nipples and scrotum
Quicker subsidence of vasocongestion of clitoris and orgasmic platform	Loss of erection and descent of testicles shortly after ejaculation
	Extended refractory time (time before another erection: several to 24 hr, occasionally longer)

Modified from Ebersole P, Hess P: *Toward healthy aging: human needs and nursing response*, ed 3, St Louis, 1990, Mosby–Year Book.

press sexual activity, such as antihypertensives, antidepressants, sedatives, or hypnotics. In addition, some drugs increase libido in older adults. Phenothiazines increase sexual desire in women, and levodopa has a similar effect in men (Woods, 1983).

The nurse assists older adults in achieving sexual health. However, a counselor for one or both partners may be needed to describe methods for sexual satisfaction. In addition, the nurse may help other health care professionals understand the sexual behavior of older adults.

Not all nurses feel comfortable counseling clients about sexual health. The nurse need not feel obligated to do so. However, the nurse should recognize the need for assistance. If the nurse is uncomfortable in discussing sexuality, another health care professional should be consulted.

The nursing student needs to recognize that knowledge of clients' sexual needs will increase with professional growth. As information is gained, the nurse will be able to incorporate this information into the nursing care plan.

HOUSING AND ENVIRONMENT. Changes in social roles, family responsibilities, and health status influence older clients' living arrangements. Some choose to live with family members. Others prefer their own homes or apartments near their families. Leisure or retirement communities provide older people with living and social opportunities in a one-generation setting. Federally subsidized housing, where available, offers apartments with communal, social, and, in some cases, eating arrangements. Housing most appropriate for older adults depends on their level of independence (Fig. 27-3).

When assisting older adults with housing needs, the nurse should assess their activity level, financial status, accessibility of public transportation and community activities, environmental hazards, and support systems. In addition, the nurse should help clients determine the length of the arrangement. For example, an older adult with recently diagnosed angina may not be able to live in a second-floor apartment and should be advised to find one on the first floor.

Housing and environment are important because they can have a major impact on the health of older adults. The environment can support or hinder physical and social functioning, enhance or drain energy, and complement or tax existing physical changes such as vision and hearing. For example, red, orange, and yellow are easiest for older adults to see. Pastels, green, blue, violet, white, and dark colors are the most difficult. Some older adults in health care settings have difficulty finding their rooms, but painting the door frames a bright color to contrast with the wall helps them see it at a distance. Painting a stripe along the bottom of a wall makes the boundaries of a hall or room visible. The glare of highly polished floors should be eliminated.

Furniture should be comfortable and address musculoskeletal changes of older adults. It should be easy to get into or out of and provide back support. A dining room chair should be tested for comfort during meals and height in relation to the table. Older clients should examine furniture carefully for size, comfort, and function before purchasing it.

The nurse assesses environmental needs of older adults in the home and institution. The environment should be modified to increase independence and functional ability and thus the quality of life.

DEATH. Birth and death are universal but unique events in life. The death of a young or middle-age person is viewed as tragic because life goals are un-

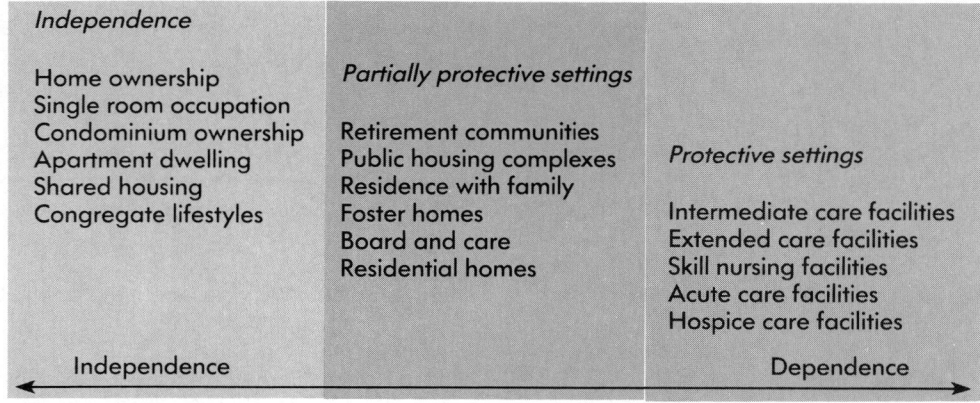

Fig. 27-3 Continuum of housing security.
From Ebersole P, Hess P: *Toward healthy aging: human needs and nursing response*, ed 3, St Louis, 1990, Mosby–Year Book.

completed. A common misconception is that the death of an older adult is a blessing and the culmination of a full life. Many dying older adults still have goals, and they are not emotionally prepared to die. Families and friends are often unable to cope with dying and loss of a loved one.

With knowledge and skills the nurse can help make the dying process a time of fulfillment and growth while enlisting the support, understanding, and assistance of family and friends of the dying client. Chapter 28 describes the work of Kübler-Ross and the five stages of dying. It also describes nursing interventions for a dying client and the family.

Health Concerns

Older adults particularly value good health. A state of wellness provides energy, vitality, and a zest of life. The nurse is in a unique position to establish health maintenance programs that promote older adults' wellness. Senior citizens' centers, churches, schools, shopping malls, libraries, and hospital lobbies can be used to conduct screening tests and present information on health topics. Using creative approaches, the nurse can include health-promotion activities in assessments of older adults.

PHYSIOLOGICAL HEALTH CONCERNS. Approximately 80% of adults over 65 have at least one chronic health problem. The effect of the problem on mobility and independence depends on the individual. The nurse should be familiar with chronic health problems common in the older adult population.

Most older adults are interested in their health and are capable of taking charge of their lives. They like to remain independent and prevent disability. Initial screenings establish baseline data that can be used to determine wellness, identify health needs, and design health-maintenance programs.

Nursing students will find it challenging to test their knowledge and skills in screening sessions. Under the direction of an instructor, students make presentations on nutrition, arthritis, hypertension, foot and skin care, Heimlich maneuver, medications, and exercise. Other topics, such as consumer affairs, safety precautions, and Medicare reimbursement policies, are also of interest. Nurses can significantly improve the quality of life and health of older adults by health promotion, teaching, advising, and counseling. The use of self-help strategies is appropriate because of older adults' limited financial and social resources. Many older adults monitor their own or their spouses' blood pressures, attend health fairs, plan special diets, and care for spouses with chronic disease. The self-help network of older adults is extensive. For example, while shopping, older adults may exchange information about the best physician for cataract surgery, a hospital that provides the best care, and nursing homes to avoid.

As part of health screening, the nurse encourages older adults to complete a stress inventory scale. Individuals at risk for illness resulting from stress should receive teaching. The nurse needs to know about relaxation and stress-reduction techniques to assist the client in selecting the best one.

Cardiovascular Problems. Cardiovascular problems frequently associated with aging are hypertension, angina pectoris, myocardial infarction, and cerebrovascular accident. Hypertension is diagnosed when repeated blood pressure measurements of 95 mm Hg diastolic and 160 mm Hg systolic are present. Risk factors include smoking, obesity, lack of exercise, and stress. African Americans are at a greater risk than European Americans, and men are at greater risk than women. Treatment of hypertension includes weight reduction, decreased salt intake, exercise, stress management, and drugs (Stanhope, Lancaster, 1992). The nurse can teach the client about medications prescribed for hypertension, including drug action and adverse effects, and can evaluate the response to the prescribed therapy.

Angina pectoris is a coronary artery disease in which chest pain is induced by exercise or stress. Risk factors include family history of heart disease, obesity, hyperlipidemia, smoking, and stress. Treatment usually includes vasodilator therapy, exercise, smoking cessation, weight reduction, and stress management. The nurse counsels and teaches the older adult about recommended lifestyle changes.

Myocardial infarction (heart attack) is a condition in which the coronary artery becomes occluded, thus depriving the myocardium of oxygen and blood supply. Myocardial ischemia then occurs. Risk factors include family history of cardiac disease, angina pectoris, diabetes mellitus, smoking, obesity, hypertension, hyperlipidemia, lack of exercise, and stress. Treatment involves hospitalization, followed by a rehabilitation in which habits are modified. These include weight reduction, exercise, smoking cessation, dietary changes, and stress management.

Cerebrovascular accident (stroke) occurs when vessels supplying blood to a portion of the brain become occluded, resulting in decreased circulation. Risk factors include hypertension, hyperlipidemia, diabetes mellitus, history of transient ischemic attacks, and family history of cardiovascular disease. Treatment usually includes hospitalization for days or months, depending on the degree of brain damage.

Cancer. Malignant neoplasms are the second most common cause of death among older adults. The nurse can develop programs to educate clients about early detection and treatment and risk factors. Examples include encouraging smoking cessation, teaching female clients to perform breast self-examination and have routine Papanicolaou (Pap) smears, and teaching male clients to perform testicular self-examination (see Chapter 20). It is also important to educate clients about the signs of cancer. Detection is not easy because symptoms may be mistakenly identified as part of the normal aging process. Careful assessment is necessary before concluding that clients' problems are a normal result of aging.

Arthritis. Approximately 44% of older adults have arthritis. It is more common in women than in men (Stanhope, Lancaster, 1992). The degree to which the mobility of older adults is impaired depends on the extent of the disease and joints affected. Arthritis has no cure, but recently developed pharmacological agents can decrease pain and swelling and therefore increase joint motion. Treatment depends on the nature of the degeneration and deformity. Nursing interventions are aimed at promoting comfort, functional ability, and safety. Education about self-care, exercise, and socialization is also important.

Sensory Impairments. The older adult usually has changes in vision, hearing, taste, and smell. These are often the result of normal aging. The nurse can help the older client identify resources to help correct visual and auditory problems (see Chapter 45). Seasonings can help make food more palatable. Depending on the degree of impairment, the consequences of age-related sensory alterations can be serious. The goal of nursing care is to help the client achieve an optimal level of sensory stimulation.

Dental Problems. Dental problems are common in the older adult. When present, there can also be changes in taste and a decrease in nutritional intake. Because of missing teeth or poorly fitting dentures, the older adult may eat only soft foods.

The nurse can help prevent dental and gum disease through education about routine dental care (see Chapter 34). The nurse can also help the client find dental services that offer reduced rates.

MORTALITY. Common causes of death in older adults are heart disease, malignant neoplasms, cerebrovascular disease, and chronic obstructive pulmonary disease (Table 27-4). Health screenings and fairs can identify older adults at risk so that prevention can be initiated. In addition, older adults, especially those with chronic disease, should be encouraged to obtain a yearly influenza shot. Older adults with histories of pneumonia should be encouraged to get Pneumovax vaccinations, which provide lifelong immunity against pneumococcal pneumonia.

DRUG EFFECTS. As a group, adults over 65 are the greatest users of prescription medications. The most frequently prescribed medications are for heart and

TABLE 27-4 Common Causes of Death Among Persons 75 Years and Older		
Cause of Death	Men*	Women*
Heart disease	3498	2245
Malignancies	1840	948
Cerebrovascular accident	661	572
Chronic obstructive pulmonary disease	505	164
Pneumonia and flu	338	184
Accidents	149	83
Diabetes	129	128
Suicide	53	7
Liver disease	43	25

*Per 100,000.
From Ebersole P, Hess P: *Toward healthy aging: human needs and nursing response,* ed 3, St Louis, 1990, Mosby–Year Book.

vascular disease, hypertension, arthritis, mental health disorders, urinary tract infections, diabetes mellitus, respiratory diseases, chronic skin disorders, and gastrointestinal disorders (Ebersole, Hess, 1990).

Medications may interact with one another, potentiating or negating the effect of another drug. In addition, prescription medications may cause confusion; affect balance; cause dizziness, nausea, and vomiting; or promote constipation or urinary frequency. Some older adults are unwilling to take prescribed drugs because of side effects.

Sedatives and tranquilizers may cause an acute confusional state. Ironically, these drugs are frequently administered to confused older clients. Confusion that varies with time is referred to as *sundown syndrome* and occurs most frequently in an institutional setting. Older clients with clear mental status by day suddenly become disoriented at night. Drugs used to manage this behavior should be carefully administered, taking into account age-related changes in body systems that can affect the drugs' pharmacokinetic activity. In addition, the nurse can use creative measures, such as making the environment more meaningful, providing adequate light, encouraging use of prostheses, or even making telephone calls to friends or family members to let clients hear reassuring voices (Wolanin, Phillips, 1981).

Other frequently occurring drug-induced pathological conditions include incontinence, immobility, and falls. The nurse's role with an older client undergoing drug therapy is to ensure the greatest therapeutic benefit with the least amount of harm.

NUTRITION. Minimum nutritional needs for the older adult are the same as those of younger adults, except that greater amounts of calcium, vitamin C, and vitamin A are required. Total caloric intake usually declines in response to illness, changes in metabolic rate, and physical activity. Nutritional needs of older adults are described in Chapter 35.

EXERCISE. The older adult should be encouraged to maintain physical exercise and activity. Before beginning a formal exercise program, the client should have a physical examination, which may include a stress cardiogram or stress test. This provides information about cardiovascular function during sustained exercise. The nurse should plan an exercise program that meets physical needs while allowing for physical impairments.

Regular exercise to promote functional ability can be incorporated into the older adult's activities of daily living. For example, arm circles and leg circles can be performed while watching television.

PSYCHOSOCIAL HEALTH CONCERNS. Psychosocial health concerns vary among older adults. Many role transitions occur between middle age and older adulthood. Because of this and the cognitive, social, and physical effects of aging, many older adults require assistance to maintain psychosocial health.

Interventions for psychosocial health of older adults resemble those of other age groups. However, some interventions are more crucial for older adults experiencing social isolation, cognitive impairment, or other psychosocial problems. These interventions include therapeutic communication, touch, reality orientation, resocialization, validation therapy, reminiscence, and interventions to improve body image.

Therapeutic Communication. With therapeutic communication the nurse perceives and respects the client's uniqueness. The nurse who communicates effectively will be accepted as one who shares a genuine concern for the client's welfare.

The nurse cannot simply enter a client's environment and immediately establish a therapeutic relationship. The nurse must first be knowledgeable and skilled in communication techniques. The nursing student can practice these techniques with other students (see Chapter 15).

Touch. Touch is the first sense to become functional. It provides knowledge about others throughout life. In all cultures, gentle touch conveys affection and friendliness. Often, older adults who are victims of social isolation are deprived of the touching that was an important part of earlier life.

Touch is a therapeutic tool that nurses can use to help comfort the older adult. It can provide sensory stimulation, reduce anxiety, orient the person to reality, relieve physiological and emotional pain, and give comfort during the dying process (Barnett, 1972).

An older adult who is isolated, dependent, or ill; who fears death; or who lacks self-esteem has a greater need for touch. The client may invite touch by reaching for a nurse's hand. Often, older men are wrongly accused of sexual advances when they demonstrate this need. The nurse should recognize that the client may be suffering from touch deprivation. Nurses should not use touch in a condescending way, however, such as a pat on the head or a gentle pinch. Touch should convey respect and sensitivity. The nurse should not be surprised if the client reciprocates because of an unmet need for intimacy.

Reality Orientation. Reality orientation, first described by Taulbee and Folsom in 1966, is a communication technique used to make a client aware of time, place, and person. The purposes of reality orientation include restoring sense of reality, improving level of awareness, promoting socialization, elevating independent functioning, and minimizing confusion, disorientation, and physical regression.

The nurse can use reality-orientation techniques anywhere. The older adult experiencing a change in environment, surgery, illness, or emotional stress is at risk for becoming disoriented. Environmental changes, such as the bright lights and lack of windows in specialized units of a hospital, often lead to disorientation and confusion. The environment and nursing personnel often change in a hospital, so the client's environment is unstable. This makes adaptation difficult. For this reason, many older clients lose track of time and become confused while in the hospital. The problem is compounded by sedatives, tranquilizers, anesthesia, and restraints that take away dignity.

The nurse should anticipate and monitor for disorientation and confusion as possible consequences of hospitalization, relocation, surgery, loss, or illness and incorporate reality orientation into the care plan. These interventions are based on seven principles (see box on p. 848). Though not a remedy, reality orientation can diminish moderate confusional states when used with other therapies (Burnside, 1986).

Resocialization. Resocialization helps older adults expand their social networks. It is especially beneficial to older adults whose social interaction depended primarily on employment. Similarly, resocialization is important for older adults whose spouses or close friends have died.

The key to resocialization is knowing resources easily available to clients. Many older adults eagerly participate in senior citizens' groups, foster grandparent programs, or hospital volunteer work. However, they may not know how to make the initial contact. The nurse can provide older adults with names or can personally contact the agency. The nurse and clients must work together for effective resocialization.

Guidelines for Reality Orientation

REALISM

- Use reality information such as time, date, place, and name in conversation.
- Refer clients to clocks and other reality-orientation props when necessary.
- Do not reinforce delusions or hallucinations.
- Direct clients back to reality-oriented endeavors if they ramble in conversation or talk unrealistically.
- If erratic behavior is shown, such as picking at clothes, give clients purposeful things to do.

INDEPENDENCE

- Express confidence in clients' ability to be self-directing.
- Encourage clients to perform tasks and make decisions, assisting only when necessary.
- Make sure clients have needed aids, such as glasses, dentures, and hearing aids, and that they work.
- Provide bowel and bladder training when necessary.
- Provide speech or physical therapy when necessary.
- Reduce medication to a minimum.

INDIVIDUALIZATION

- Keep reality-orientation classes small to permit individual attention.
- Allow clients to keep familiar treasures and objects.
- Encourage meaningful object relationships.

REINFORCEMENT

- Watch for small changes in behavior that indicate progress, and reward them.
- Reward correct behavior with verbal praise, touch, or smiles.
- Reinforce achievement with increased responsibility.
- Encourage special talents or interests.

REPETITION

- Repeat information, directions, statements, and questions as necessary.
- Be patient and allow time for responses or replies.
- Give clues to the answer when asking a question; if clients are unable to answer, provide the correct response and allow them to repeat it.

CLARITY

- Enunciate clearly and speak slowly.
- Reword statements and questions if necessary.
- Give directions in clear, simple, short statements.

CONSISTENCY

- Maintain continuity of care.
- Adhere to scheduling.
- Use the same personnel when possible.

From Beck CM, Rawlins RP, Williams SR: *Mental health—psychiatric nursing: a holistic life-cycle approach*, ed 2, St Louis, 1988, Mosby–Year Book.

Developing Secondary Relationships. Just as socialization is important for older adults who are at risk for isolation, secondary relationships are important for those who maintain primary relationships. Family and friends provide long-term support for many older adults. However, reliable secondary relationships with peers must be developed to provide a social group not bound by emotions frequently experienced in families. For example, older persons in a day-care center enjoy socializing with peers and younger staff. They share their experiences and concerns but are related only by common feelings or ideas.

The nurse can help form secondary relationships by promoting discussion on topics of mutual interest at day-care centers, nutrition program sites, or long-term care centers. For example, clients with arthritis may benefit from discussing ways to maintain activity. The following are guidelines for conducting discussion sessions:

1. Select a small, quiet room that is well lit and has comfortable furniture. Consider visual, hearing, or musculoskeletal impairments.
2. Keep meetings short enough to promote learning and reduce exhaustion (20 minutes).
3. Choose participants who are able to participate.
4. Consider older adults' sensory deficits when using visual aids (such as brightly colored posters with large print).
5. Present one topic for discussion at each meeting.
6. Make it clear that participation is voluntary.

Peer group meetings allow participants to develop secondary relationships. Older adults learn to share ideas and solve problems without dwelling on physical ailments or feelings of hopelessness.

TABLE 27-5 Reminiscence Group Strategies

Cognitively Impaired	Psychologically Disturbed	Depressed
CLIENT SELECTION		
Choose no more than five members of same age but both sexes.	Choose 10 members of varied ages and both sexes.	Choose 8 to 10 members of both sexes. Choose persons with similar problems (e.g., grieving, retirement).
STRUCTURE		
Choose consistent place and time. Conduct frequent, 30-min meetings. Use coleaders.	Choose consistent place and time. Conduct biweekly, 1-hr meetings. Use one leader consistently.	Choose varied meeting places. Meet weekly, for 1 hr. Vary leaders.
PROCESS		
Connect specific events, things, and places common to group.	Connect members through shared feelings and survival strategies.	Focus on successful coping during life span; encourage mutuality.
GOALS		
Stimulate memory, enhance identity, raise self-esteem, and increase socialization skills.	Recognize feelings and meaning of suppressed conflicts, enlarge coping strategies, integrate self-view, and promote universality.	Reduce feelings of hopelessness, restore personal control, increase affectual responsiveness, develop sense of integrity and acceptance of life as lived, and promote caring between members.
NURSE'S FUNCTION		
Provide comfortable, mildly stimulating environment. Select props that will stimulate memories. Assist members by giving specific information, reminders, and clues. Give praise and recognition for participation.	Establish private meeting and closed group. Focus on specific developmental stages or critical life events. Accept and validate all expressions of feeling. Clarify multiple meanings of events. Reduce anxiety.	Provide comfortable, stimulating environment. Appeal to sensory memories. Focus on evidence of caring and sharing. Demonstrate caring attitude. Allow time to complain.

From Ebersole P, Hess P: *Toward healthy aging: human needs and nursing response*, ed 3, St Louis, 1990, Mosby–Year Book.

Validation Therapy. **Validation therapy** is a technique used with severely confused and disoriented older adults. The goal is to provide a sense of dignity and self-worth and validate clients' feelings. Clients are not confronted with their inappropriate behaviors. Rather, the nurse attempts to meet older adults in their reality and find the meaning behind the behaviors. Confused older adults gain a positive sense of self because the nurse validates feelings.

Reminiscence. **Reminiscence** is recalling the past to assign new meanings to experiences (Beck, Rawlins, Williams, 1988). It is an adaptive function of older adults. As a therapy, reminiscence is an elaboration of the natural way that older adults revive their pasts to give meaning or reconcile conflicts and

disappointments as they prepare for death (Butler, 1963). Reminiscing contributes to successful adaptation by maintaining self-esteem, reaffirming identity, and working through loss.

Reminiscence can be used for impaired, disturbed, or depressed older adults. The nurse organizes the group and selects strategies. The group's size, structure, process, goals, and activities are adapted to meet its members' needs. Table 27-5 details the techniques of reminiscence.

Body-Image Interventions. The way that older adults present themselves has a significant impact on body image and feelings of isolation. Some physical characteristics of older adulthood are socially desirable, such as distinguished-looking gray hair. Other

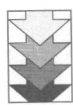

Examples of Nursing Diagnoses for the Older Adult

NANDA-APPROVED NURSING DIAGNOSES

Altered nutrition: less than body requirements related to:
- Altered sense of taste
- Social isolation

Altered thought processes related to:
- Loss (e.g., of control, routine, familiar surroundings)
- Progressive cognitive impairment

Anxiety related to:
- Impending retirement
- Hospitalization

Constipation related to:
- Medication side effect
- Immobility

Sexual dysfunction related to:
- Decreased vaginal lubrication
- Joint pain

features are also impressive, such as a lined face that displays character or wrinkled hands that convey a lifetime of hard work. Too often, however, society sees older people as incapacitated, deaf, obese, or shrunken in stature. When older adults have acute or chronic illnesses, the related physical dependence makes it difficult for them to maintain body image. A nurse with stereotypes about the appearance of older adults may give little attention to grooming or hygiene. Consequences of illness and aging that threaten the older adult's body image include invasive diagnostic procedures, pain, surgery, prosthesis, loss of sensation in a body part, skin changes, dependence on life-sustaining medication, denture odor, loss of scalp hair, and incontinence.

The nurse has a direct influence on the client's appearance. The importance to the older adult of presenting a socially acceptable image must be considered. It takes little effort to assist the client with combing hair, cleaning dentures, shaving, or changing clothing. The older adult does not choose to have an objectionable appearance. The nurse should also be sensitive to odors in the environment. Odors cre-

Sample Nursing Diagnostic Process for the Older Adult

Assessment Activities	Defining Characteristics	Nursing Diagnoses
Determine client's level of consciousness.	Alert and able to interact verbally.	*Altered thought processes* related to progressive cognitive impairment
Observe client's ability to interact with others.	Client responds to conversational dialogue in argumentative fashion; confabulates.	
Observe client's ability to follow 1-step and 2-step commands.	Unable to follow commands: unable to close eyes and unable to pick up piece of paper and fold in half.	
Conduct formal mental status examination; examples include Mini-Mental State Examination (MMSE) and Short Portable Mental Status Questionnaire (SPMSQ).	Score reflects moderate cognitive impairment: impaired judgment, easily distracted, unable to perform calculations, cannot name place.	
Obtain history of typical meal pattern, appetite changes, taste acuity, and diseases affecting nutritional intake (e.g., depression, cancer, arthritis).	Reports "I eat when I feel like it," 2-3 times/day, eats alone at home. Client reports, "Not hungry anymore." Client reports "Food doesn't taste that good." Client reports that joint pain affects ability to prepare meals at home or join friends for meals out.	*Altered nutrition: less than body requirements* related to social isolation
Take height and weight measurements, determine weight change over past 6 mos.	15-lb weight loss in past 3 mos.	

ated by urine and some illnesses are often present. By controlling odors, the nurse may prevent visitors from shortening their stay or not coming at all.

Nursing Diagnosis

Data are systematically collected during assessment. Assessment is essential in gerontological nursing, in which client status changes often. Data regarding the physiological, cognitive, and psychosocial status of the older adult yield actual or potential problems (see diagnoses box). Any nursing diagnosis can have a variety of related factors. Identification of the related factor or probable cause for each diagnosis gives direction in developing nursing interventions. For example, interventions for constipation are different if the probable cause is a medication rather than immobility.

Analysis of data requires consideration of individual strengths and limitations, as well as the older client's perception of health status. Validations of data with family, friends, nursing colleagues, other health professionals, and client records may be necessary.

Assessment data contain subjective and objective characteristics necessary for validation of a nursing diagnosis. Accurate assessment is essential because care is built on this foundation. The diagnostic process box includes examples with defining characteristics and related factors.

Planning

The older adult client often has multiple physical and psychosocial problems. Accurate identification of these in a nursing diagnosis is followed by development of a nursing care plan (see care plan on p. 852).

A care plan for the older adult focuses on activities to prevent, improve, reduce, or eliminate problems. Priorities of care are established, client goals are determined, and interventions are selected. This is done with the client's participation so that the interventions are understood and conflicts in approaches or priorities can be avoided. Consideration by the nurse of the experiences of a lifetime, as well as values and sociocultural patterns developed, should serve as the basis for planning individual care.

Goals of care established with the older adult should reflect consideration of factors that influence normal aging, maintain independence as much as possible, and facilitate an optimal level of comfort and coping. Although it is sometimes more time consuming and difficult, including the older client in the

care planning process and allowing maximal independence in self-care activities can promote physical and psychosocial health.

In the sample care plan for clients with the nursing diagnosis of *altered thought processes,* the emphasis is on promoting remaining functional ability and preventing injury. Because the clients' cognitive status prevents participation in establishing goals and planning interventions, families must be included. Families and friends are rich sources of data when developing individualized care plans because they knew the clients before the impairment. Frequently, they can provide explanations for clients' behaviors and suggest methods of management.

Implementation

Nursing interventions for older adults can encompass health maintenance, recovery, restoration, adaptation, adjustment, and preservation. Interventions generally are aimed at facilitating independence and supporting abilities. Care activities require more time because of slower responses, the number of problems, and the close relationship between physical and psychosocial aspects of aging.

In the sample care plan for a client with altered thought processes the nurse's role is to compensate for reduced abilities by promoting an environment that supports and compensates for the altered functioning. The degree of assistance required by the client varies, depending on the stage of the disease, but the nurse should be careful not to do more for the client than the condition warrants. Preservation of ability despite the cognitive impairment is crucial to client self-esteem.

The nurse also cares for families of cognitively impaired older adults. Families experience much distress and need support, assistance with problem solving, and education about the progressive nature of the disease and the clients' care needs. This can be accomplished through many support groups (see research highlight on p. 853), in family meetings, or in a nurse-client interaction (see teaching box on p. 853).

Evaluation

Evaluation measures the degree to which the plan and interventions were effective in meeting the expected outcomes. The nurse determines whether goals have been met and what changes have occurred in the client's status as a result of the inter-

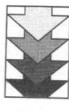

Sample Nursing Care Plan for Altered Thought Processes and Altered Nutrition

Nursing diagnoses: *Altered thought processes* related to progressive cognitive impairment and *altered nutrition: less than body requirements* related to social isolation

Definitions: Altered thought processes is the state in which an individual experiences a disruption in cognitive operations and activities, and altered nutrition: less than body requirements is the state in which an individual experiences an intake of nutrients insufficient to meet metabolic needs (Kim, McFarland, McLane, 1991).

Goals	Expected Outcomes	Interventions	Rationale
Client will effectively communicate needs to staff throughout hospital stay.	Client's communication during hospital stay will be characterized by decreased restlessness and agitation and reduced hostility and striking out.	Approach client in calm, gentle manner; be friendly and relaxed.	Clients with Alzheimer's disease may respond in kind to manner in which they perceive those around them.
		Establish eye contact and introduce self; use touch as necessary to augment spoken word.	Client may lack ability to comprehend, so getting attention will promote meaning. Words combined with touch and stroking reduce frustration.
		Use short, simple, 1-step commands and sentences; use yes and no questions and active tense. Allow time for response and repeat as necessary.	This approach reduces overstimulation, which could lead to catastrophic reaction. Techniques reduce overstimulation, misinterpretations, and agitation. Demented client may require lengthy period to respond.
Client will eat diet consisting of essential nutrients and calories sufficient to meet metabolic demands within 1 mo.	Client will participate in social activities that include meals at least twice a week by 6/10.	Assist client in identifying resources and barriers to social contact.	Food and meal experience have social meaning. Eating alone can promote disinterest in food; eating with someone promotes sense of belonging and can foster development of relationships. Involving client in problem solving promotes active participation and commitment.
	Client will demonstrate adequate oral nutritional intake by 6/17 as demonstrated by 7-day diet log.	Contract with client to keep record for 1 wk of foods eaten, times and places, others present during meals, and feelings associated with meals.	Contracting promotes self-respect, problem-solving skills, autonomy, and motivation.
			By writing down foods, persons present, and feelings, client's awareness will be heightened, which can promote positive changes in health behaviors.

ventions. Goals may be revised or eliminated, or new goals may be developed. Implementation may be affected as goals change. Just as the family was included in developing the care plan, their input in evaluating outcomes of care should be sought.

The frequency of evaluation with an older adult is highly individual. Change is often slow and subtle. Thus infrequent or frequent evaluations may be performed (Yurick et al, 1989). The type of problems, goals established, and interventions used determine frequency of evaluations. For example, if the goal is for the client to be free from skin complications of immobility, evaluation should be frequent and regular. If the intervention is a weight-reduction diet,

Research Highlight

The purpose of this study by Oklay and Volland was to evaluate the effectiveness of a support program for frail older adults and their care givers. Two groups of hospital-discharged clients were compared. The first, or comparison group, did not participate in the program. The second, or treatment group, was provided coordinated health and social services by the program a year after discharge. Both groups were interviewed 5 times during this year to assess care giver stress and use of health services. The treatment group showed an annual estimated cost savings of $4585 per client, primarily because of fewer hospital stays. Care giver stress was only slightly reduced for this same group. Because family care givers provide the largest percentage of home care to older adults, their needs are an important aspect of discharge planning.

Oklay J, Volland P: Post-hospital support program for the frail elderly and their caregivers: a quasi-experimental evaluation, *Am J Public Health* 60(1):39, 1989.

Client Teaching for Catastrophic Reaction

OBJECTIVE

- Client (spouse) will identify factors that place the cognitively impaired client at risk for experiencing a catastrophic reaction.

TEACHING STRATEGIES

- Define *catastrophic reaction.*
- Describe factors that typically precipitate a catastrophic reaction.
- Discuss interventions to avoid or minimize a catastrophic reaction.

EVALUATION

- Client will be able to identify the signs of an impending catastrophic reaction for the cognitively impaired family member.

evaluation of the client should be weekly. The nurse plays a major role in encouraging the older adult to participate in evaluating the plan, interventions, and progress. The evaluation box includes such measures.

Sample Evaluation of Interventions for Altered Thought Processes and Altered Nutrition

Goals	Evaluative Measures	Expected Outcomes
Client will effectively communicate needs to staff throughout hospital stay.	Observe client for emotional lability, excessive crying, anger, increasing restlessness, pacing and stubbornness. Review progress notes of client communication daily. Assess client for ability to perform self-care tasks when coached with 1-step commands.	Client's communication will have no evidence of hostility, restlessness, or agitation.
Client will eat foods with essential nutrients and calories to meet metabolic demands within 1 mo.	Review client's 7-day diet log to include appropriate intake. Ask client to report number of meals eaten at friends' homes during 7 days.	Client demonstrates adequate nutritional intake. Client participates in social activities that include meals.

SUMMARY

Nursing care for the older adult is challenging and rewarding. The older adult must learn to adapt to physical, cognitive, and social changes. The degree of these changes varies from one person to another. Likewise, adaptive capacities are different for each client.

Nurses must develop care plans to meet the individual needs of the older adult while trying to maintain an optimal level of physical and cognitive function. The nurse also incorporates family and community resources to assist in the care of the older adult.

The older adult's independence depends on physical health, cognitive abilities, and social support network. When any are absent or dysfunctional, the older adult's ability to maintain independence decreases, and more extensive health care services are needed.

CHAPTER 27 REVIEW

Key Concepts

- Myths and stereotypes portray older adults as ill, rigid in thinking, institutionalized, poor, unable to learn, and without sexual needs.
- A nurse's attitudes toward older adult affects the quality and level of care.
- Physiological and biological theories of aging rely on physiological explanations for the aging process; these include the free radical, cross-link, and immunological theories.
- The psychosocial theories of aging, which include the disengagement, activity, and continuity theories, attempt to describe the effects of lifestyle, personality, and environmental factors on longevity.
- The older adult must adjust to physical changes in body systems.
- The older adult must adjust to retirement.
- The death of a spouse, a friend, or children affects adaptation to aging.
- Many older adults have difficulty perceiving themselves as old.
- Some older adults require changes in living arrangements.
- Realignment of relationships between older adults and their children is necessary.
- The older adult may need to acquire new activities and interests to maintain quality of life.
- Physiological changes are a normal part of aging and are not the result of illness.
- Structural and physiological changes that occur in the brain during aging do not necessarily impair the older adult's adaptation and functional ability.
- Cerebral dysfunction can magnify preexisting behavioral tendencies.
- Characteristics of dementia include decreased intellectual function, personality change, impaired judgment, and change in affect.
- Cognitive impairment includes acute, potentially reversible disorders and chronic, irreversible, progressive disorders.
- Classic symptoms of dementia and delirium include decreases in attention span, learning, and memory. Some clients have hallucinations, illusions, aphasias, emotional lability, and depression.
- Chronic brain disorders include Alzheimer's disease and multiinfarct dementia.
- Cognitive impairment can result from chemical substance abuse.
- Psychosocial changes affecting the older adult include retirement, social isolation, change in housing, death, and sexual changes.1

- Sexuality is linked with identity and validates the belief that a person can give to others and have the gift appreciated.

- In addition to physical changes, drugs prescribed for the older adult may affect sexual functioning.

- Changes in social roles, family responsibility, and health status influence the choice of living arrangements appropriate for the older adult.

- The older adult and family require nursing interventions to help them cope with the dying process.

- The major health problems of the older adult include hypertension, angina pectoris, myocardial infarction, cerebrovascular accident, cancer, arthritis, sensory impairments, and dental problems.

- The four leading causes of death in the older population are heart disease, malignant neoplasms, cerebrovascular disease, and chronic obstructive pulmonary disease.

- Nursing interventions for psychosocial problems should be individualized; they include therapeutic communication, touch, reality orientation, resocialization, validation therapy, reminiscence, and interventions to improve body image.

- Health care services for older adults are available in the community and institutional settings.

Key Terms

Ageism, p. 831

Alzheimer's disease, p. 837

Attitudinal isolation, p. 841

Behavioral isolation, p. 841

Confabulation, p. 840

Delirium, p. 837

Dementia, p. 837

Geographical isolation, p. 841

Geriatrics, p. 830

Gerontology, p. 830

Korsakoff's syndrome, p. 840

Presbycusis, p. 836

Presbyopia, p. 836

Presentational isolation, p. 841

Reality orientation, p. 847

Reminiscence, p. 849

Resocialization, p. 847

Senile lentigo, p. 835

Sundown syndrome, p. 846

Validation therapy, p. 849

Wernicke's syndrome, p. 840

Critical Thinking Exercises

1. The "graying" of the population has resulted in an increased number of older persons on medical-surgical units in most hospitals. Describe how a nurse's ageist attitudes could influence the care provided to these older clients.

2. Mr. X., a 78-year-old client who was admitted through the emergency room after a fall at home, had surgery yesterday to repair a hip fracture. While giving his morning care, the nurse observes that Mr. X. is acutely confused. Identify three possible causes of his delirium. List six possible interventions aimed at promoting his safety and feelings of security.

3. An older female client comes to the clinic with 11 medications prescribed by her primary physician and two specialists. She complains of not feeling well, despite taking the medications as prescribed. What actions should the nurse take in counseling this client about her medications?

4. You are planning a health screening fair for an area Senior Center. Identify three possible screenings you could offer, including appropriate health-teaching strategies.

5. You are conducting a physical examination on a 73-year-old woman who has noted a gradual decrease in mobility in recent years. What musculoskeletal system changes will you expect to find?

REFERENCES

American Psychiatric Association: *Diagnostic and statistical manual of mental disorders (DSM-III-R)*, Washington, DC, 1987, The Association.

Barnett K: A survey of the current utilization of touch by health team personnel with hospitalized patients, *Int J Nurs Stud* 9:195, 1972.

Bartol M: Dialogue with dementia: non-verbal communication in patients with Alzheimer's disease, *J Gerontol Nurs* 5:21, 1979.

Beck CM, Rawlins RP, Williams SR: *Mental health–psychiatric nursing: a holistic life-cycle approach*, ed 2, St Louis, 1988, Mosby–Year Book.

Burnside IM: Transition to later life: developmental theories and research. In Burnside IM, Ebersole P, Monea HE, editors: *Psychosocial caring through the life span*, New York, 1979, McGraw-Hill.

Burnside IM: *Working with the elderly: group process and techniques*, ed 2, Boston, 1986, Jones & Barlett.

Butler R: Life review: an interpretation of reminiscence in the aged, *Psychiatry* 26:65, 1963.

Cummings E, Henry WE: *Growing old: the process of disengagement*, New York, 1961, Basic Books.

Diekelman N: Pre-retirement counseling, *Am J Nurs* 78:1337, 1978.

Duvall EM: *Family development*, ed 5, Philadelphia, 1977, Lippincott.

Ebersole P, Hess P: *Toward healthy aging: human needs and nursing response*, ed 3, St Louis, 1990, Mosby–Year Book.

Havighurst RJ: *Human development and education*, New York, 1953, David McKay.

Havighurst RJ: Successful aging. In Williams RH, Tibbits C, Donahue W, editors: *Process of aging*, vol 1, New York, 1963, Atherton.

Heyman A: Differentiation of Alzheimer's disease from multi-infarct dementia. In Katzman R, Terry RD, Bick KL, editors: *Alzheimer's disease: senile dementia and related disorders*, New York, 1978, Raven.

Kim MJ, McFarland GK, McLane AM: *Pocket guide to nursing diagnoses*, ed 4, St Louis, 1991, Mosby–Year Book.

Maddox GL: Disengagement theory: a critical evaluation, *Gerontologist* 4:80, 1974.

Murray RB, Huelskoetter MMW, O'Driscoll DL: *The nursing process in later maturity*, Englewood Cliffs, NJ, 1980, Prentice-Hall.

Neugarten BL: *Personality in middle and late life*, New York, 1964, Atherton.

Stanhope M, Lancaster J: *Community health nursing: process and practice for promoting health*, ed 3, St Louis, 1992, Mosby–Year Book.

Taulbee LA, Folsom JC: Reality orientation for geriatric patients, *Hosp Community Psychiatry* 17(5):1966.

Terry RD: Aging, senile dementia, and Alzheimer's disease. In Katzman R, Terry RD, Bick KL, editors: *Alzheimer's disease: senile dementia and related disorders*, New York, 1978, Raven.

United States Bureau of the Census: *Statistical Abstract of the United States*, Washington, DC, 1984, 1988, The Bureau.

Wolanin MO, Phillips LR: *Confusion: prevention and care*, St Louis, 1981, Mosby–Year Book.

Woods NF: *Human sexuality in health and illness*, ed 3, St Louis, 1983, Mosby–Year Book.

Yurick AG et al: *The aged person and the nursing process*, ed 3, Norwalk, Conn, 1989, Appleton & Lange.

Zarit SH, Orr NK, Zarit JM: *The hidden victims of Alzheimer's disease: families under stress*, New York, 1985, New York University Press.

ADDITIONAL READINGS

Boynton PR: Health maintenance alterations: a nursing diagnosis of the elderly, *Clin Nurse Spec* 3(1):5, 1989.

Evans LK, Strumpf NE: Myths about elder restraint, *Image* 22(2):124, 1990.

Gropper-Katz EI: Reality orientation research, *J Gerontol Nurs* 13:13, 1987.

Hamilton J: Comfort and the hospitalized chronically ill, *J Gerontol Nurs* 15(4):28, 1989.

Johnston L, Gueldner SH: Remember when . . .? Using mnemonics to boost memory in the elderly, *J Gerontol Nurs* 15(8):22, 1989.

Kee CC: Sensory impairment: factor X in providing nursing care to the older adult, *J Community Health Nurs* 7(1): 45, 1990.

Lappe JM: Reminiscing: the life review therapy, *J Gerontol Nurs* 13:12, 1987.

McPherson ML: Medicating the elderly in home health care, *J Home Health Care Practice* 2(1):16, 1989.

Nagley SJ: Predicting and preventing confusion in your patients, *J Gerontol Nurs* 12:27, 1986.

Office of Human Development Services: *Need for long-term care: information and issues*, Washington, DC, 1981, Department of Health and Human Services.

O'Leary P et al: Gerontological research: is it useful for nursing practice? *J Gerontol Nurs* 16(5):28, 1990.

Public Health Service: *Health United States: 1976-1977*, Washington, DC, 1977, Health Resources Administration, National Center for Health Statistics, and Department of Health, Education and Welfare.

Rebenson-Piano M: The physiologic changes that occur with aging, *Crit Care Nurs Q* 12(1):1, 1989.

Rodgers BL: Loneliness: easing the pain of the hospitalized elderly, *J Gerontol Nurs* 15(8):16, 1989.

Schank M, Lough M: Maintaining health and independence of elderly women, *J Gerontol Nurs* 15(6):8, 1989.

CHAPTER **28**

Loss, Death, and Grieving

OBJECTIVES

Mastery of content in this chapter will enable the student to:
- Define the key terms listed.
- Identify the nurse's role in assisting clients with problems related to loss, death, and grief.
- Describe and compare the phases of grieving from Engel, Kübler-Ross, and Martocchio.
- Discuss five basic categories of loss and six dimensions of hope.
- Assess a client's reaction to loss and ability to cope.
- Describe the characteristics of a person experiencing grief.
- Compare and contrast grief after loss, anticipatory grief, and resolved grief.
- Develop a care plan for a client or family experiencing grief.
- Implement interventions for grieving clients to provide therapeutic communication, maintain self-esteem, and promote a return to normal activities.
- Describe how a nurse meets a dying client's need for comfort.
- Explain ways for the nurse to assist a family in caring for a dying client.
- Discuss the purposes of a hospice.
- Discuss important factors in caring for the body after death.
- Discuss the role of the nurse's own loss experience as it influences care of the grieving.
- Identify two ways nurses can meet their needs related to loss.

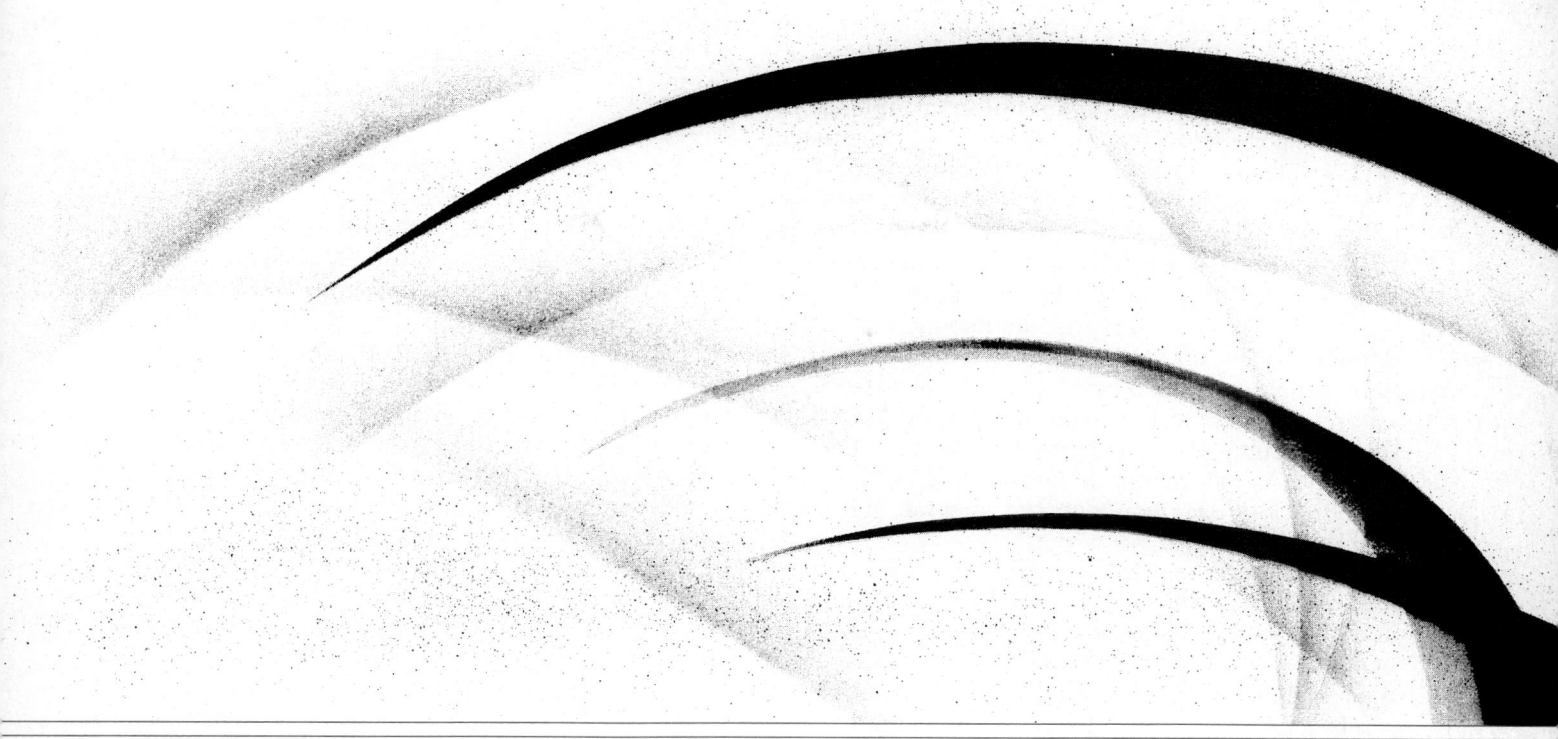

CHAPTER OUTLINE

Birth, loss, and death are universal and individually unique events of the human experience. Life is a series of losses and gains. A child beginning to walk gains independence with mobility. An older person with visual and hearing changes may lose self-reliance. Illness and hospitalization frequently cause losses.

A nurse works with many clients who experience different types of loss. Coping mechanisms determine people's ability to face and accept loss. Grief is a natural response to loss. The nurse assists clients in understanding and accepting loss so that life can continue. When clients do not do grief work after a profound loss, serious emotional, mental, and social problems can occur.

Humans can anticipate death. This causes anxiety, planning, denial, love, loneliness, achievement, and lack of achievement. Death can be an overwhelming experience that affects dying persons and their families, friends, and care givers. When a person becomes terminally ill, others can be reminded of their mortality. The style of dying reflects a person's style of living, and attitudes about death depend on a person's beliefs and emotional strengths.

LOSS, DEATH, GRIEF, AND NURSING

Nurses need to understand loss and grief. Because death is a frequent reality in many nursing care settings, most nurses interact daily with clients and families experiencing loss and grief. While caring for clients and their families, nurses also experience personal loss as client-family-nurse relationships end through transfer, discharge, recovery, or death. Nurses may find that it is easy to relieve physical symptoms associated with illness and death; however, it is difficult to become involved in meaningful interpersonal relationships to support a person who is suffering or dying. Personal feelings, values, and experiences influence the extent to which nurses can support clients and families during loss or death. Self-assessment—exploring personal attitudes, feelings, and values—is necessary before nurses can use a sensitive, therapeutic approach with others. Developing the art of being with the grieving and dying requires an inner strength that arises from knowledge of and a positive belief in self. Formulation of a philosophy of life helps nurses function during difficult times. Knowledge of the concepts of loss and the grieving process enables nurses to use creative interventions to promote health, prevent illness, and support dying clients.

Loss

A person experiences loss in the absence of an object, person, body part or function, or emotion that was formerly present. Losses may be actual or perceived. Actual losses are easily identified, as with the child whose playmate moves away or the adult who loses a marriage partner through divorce. Perceived losses are less tangible and are easily misunderstood, such as the loss of confidence or prestige. The more invested in what is lost, the greater the feeling of loss. The client may experience **maturational loss** (loss resulting from normal life transitions such as a child going off to school for the first time), **situational loss** (loss occurring suddenly in response to a specific external event such as the sudden death of a loved one), or both. The child learning to walk loses the infantlike body image, the woman experiencing menopause loses the ability to bear children, and the unemployed man may lose self-esteem.

Personal loss is any significant loss that requires adaptation through the grieving process. Loss occurs when something or someone can no longer be seen, felt, heard, known, or experienced. The type of loss influences the degree of stress. For example, the loss of an object might not generate the same stress as the loss of a significant other. However, individuals respond to loss differently. The death of a family member would be expected to cause more stress than the loss of a pet, but for an older woman living alone, the death of a pet that has been a constant companion would possibly cause more emotional stress than that of a cousin she had not seen for years. The type of loss is significant to the grieving process; yet the nurse must recognize that each person's interpretation of a loss is highly individualized.

Five categories of loss are loss of external objects, loss of a known environment, loss of a significant other, loss of an aspect of self, and loss of life. Nurses may encounter a client who has experienced more than one type. For the hospitalized chronically ill adult, Lewis (1983) describes many potential permanent losses (see box). Loss threatens self-concept, self-esteem, and security and sense of worth. The nurse must recognize the meaning of each loss to a client and its impact on physical and psychological functioning.

Loss of External Objects

Loss of an external object involves any possession that is worn out, misplaced, stolen, or ruined by disaster. For a child the object may be a toy or a blanket; for an adult it may be jewelry or an article of clothing. The extent of grieving a person feels for a

Potential Losses in Chronic Illness

- Health
- Independence
- Sense of control over life
- Privacy
- Modesty
- Body image
- Relationships
- Established roles inside and outside of the home
- Social status
- Self-confidence
- Possessions
- Financial security
- Means of productivity and self-fulfillment
- Lifestyle
- Plans or fantasies for the future
- Fantasy of immortality
- Money
- Daily routine
- Sleep
- Sexual functioning
- Leisure activities

Modified from Lewis K: *J Rehabil* 49:8, 1983.

lost object depends on its value, the sentiment the person attaches to it, and the object's usefulness.

Loss of a Known Environment

The loss associated with separation from a known environment includes leaving a familiar setting for a period or relocating permanently. Examples include moving to a new neighborhood or city, taking a new job, or hospitalization. Loss through separation from a known environment may occur through maturational or situational circumstances and through injury or illness.

Confinement within an institution results in isolation from routine events. The rules of a hospital create an environment that is often impersonal and demoralizing. The loneliness of an unfamiliar setting may threaten self-esteem and makes grieving more difficult.

Loss of a Significant Other

Significant others include parents, spouses, children, siblings, teachers, clergy, friends, neighbors, and work associates. Entertainment figures and well-known athletes may be significant others for young

people. Research shows that many people regard pets as significant others. Loss occurs as a result of separation, moving, running away, promotion at work, and death.

Loss of an Aspect of Self

The loss of an aspect of self may include a body part, physiological function, or psychological function. Loss of a body part may include a limb, eye, hair, teeth, or breast. Loss of physiological function includes loss of urinary or bowel control, mobility, strength, or sensory function. Loss of psychological function includes loss of memory, humor, self-esteem, self-confidence, power, respect, or love. The loss of these aspects of self may result from illness, injury, or developmental and situational changes. Such a loss lessens the individual's well-being. A person not only experiences grief over the loss but may experience permanent changes in body image and self-concept (see Chapter 31).

Loss of Life

Persons who face death live, feel, think, and respond to events and people around them until the moment of death. Concern is often not about death itself but about pain and loss of control. Although most people are afraid of and anxious about death, the same issues will not be equally important to each person. Each person responds differently to death. For people who have lived alone and suffered long terminal illnesses, death may be a relief. Some perceive death as an entry into an afterlife to be reunited with loved ones in paradise. Others fear separation, abandonment, loneliness, or mutilation. The threat of death often causes individuals to become dependent. The helplessness and shame of dependence experienced by some clients create a challenge for the nurse.

Grief, Mourning, and Bereavement

Bereavement is the state of thought, feeling, and activity that follows loss. It includes grief and mourning. **Grief** is a form of sorrow that follows the perception or anticipation of a loss of one or more valued or significant objects. These responses often include helplessness, loneliness, hopelessness, sadness, guilt, and anger. **Mourning** is the process that follows a loss and includes working through grief. The processes of grief and mourning are intense, internal, painful, and lengthy. The terms *grief, mourning,* and *bereavement* are often used interchangeably.

Grief involves thoughts, feelings, and behaviors. Its purpose is to achieve more effective functioning, which takes time. The grieving person tries a variety of strategies to cope. Worden (1982) describes the following tasks of grief that facilitate healthy adjustment to loss:

1. Accepting the reality of the loss
2. Experiencing the pain of grief
3. Adjusting to an environment that no longer includes the lost person, object, or aspect of self
4. Reinvesting emotional energy into new relationships

These tasks are not sequential. In fact, grieving people may work on all four tasks simultaneously, or only one or two may be priorities. Nurses can assist clients and families in working through these tasks.

In the past, society discouraged openness during grief. Unhappy children were told not to cry when playmates moved away; awkward adolescents were told not to be embarrassed about sudden growth spurts, and dying persons were told to remain calm and dignified. Changes in attitudes, beliefs, and values have promoted more open expressions of grief. For example, nurses learn to seek support from peers in expressing their concerns about dealing with terminally ill clients. Similarly, family members seek support from care givers to express anger and fear over loss. Grieving can lead to new understandings that promote growth. A person can grow from experiences of loss through openness, encouragement of others, and adequate support.

Concepts and Theories of the Grieving Process

Grief is a normal response to any loss. Behaviors and feelings associated with the **grieving process** occur in individuals suffering losses such as physical deformities or deaths of close friends. They also occur when individuals face their own deaths. The person undergoing loss and the family experience grief.

There is no right way to grieve. The concept and theories of grief are only tools that can be used to anticipate the emotional needs of clients and families and plan interventions to help them understand their grief and deal with it.

A nurse should not classify the client's grief; that is, the nurse should not identify a client as experiencing a certain phase of grief or working on a certain grief-related task. The nurse's role is to assess grieving behaviors, recognize the influence of grief on behavior, and provide empathetic support.

Engel's Theory

Engel (1964) proposes that the grieving process has three phases (Table 28-1) that can be applied to grieving and dying persons.

TABLE 28-1 Comparison of Three Theories of the Grieving Process

Engel (1964)	Kübler-Ross (1969)	Martocchio (1985)
Shock and disbelief	Denial	Shock and disbelief
	Anger	Yearning and protest
Developing awareness	Bargaining	Anguish, disorganization, and despair
	Depression	Identification in bereavement
Reorganization and restitution	Acceptance	Reorganization and restitution

In the first phase the individual denies reality of the loss and may withdraw, sit motionless, or wander aimlessly. To observers, it may seem that the person has not realized the implications of the loss. Physical reactions may include fainting, diaphoresis, nausea, diarrhea, rapid heart rate, restlessness, insomnia, and fatigue.

In the second phase the individual begins to feel the loss acutely and may experience desperation. Suddenly, anger, guilt, frustration, depression, and emptiness occur. Crying is typical as the individual becomes preoccupied with the loss. Crying seems to involve "both an acknowledgement of the loss and the regression to a more helpless and childlike status" (Engel, 1964).

In the third phase, inevitability of the loss is acknowledged. Anger or depression is no longer needed. The loss is clear to the individual, who begins to reorganize life. By experiencing these phases a person moves from a lower to a higher level of emotional and intellectual integration. New self-awareness is also developed.

Kübler-Ross' Stages of Dying

The framework provided by Kübler-Ross (1969) is behavior oriented and includes five stages. In the denial stage the individual acts as though nothing has happened and may refuse to believe that a loss has occurred. Statements such as "No, that can't be so," and "It can't be happening to me!" are common.

In the anger stage the individual resists the loss and may "act out" to everyone and everything in the environment. In the bargaining stage, there is postponement of the reality of the loss. The individual may attempt to make a deal in a subtle or overt way to prevent the loss. The client frequently seeks opin-

TABLE 28-2 Nursing Implications of Martocchio's Phases of Grief and Kübler-Ross' Stages of Dying

Behaviors	Nursing Implications
SHOCK AND DISBELIEF **Denial**	
Denial is immediate response to news of loss or impending loss. Physiological responses may include muscular weakness, tremors, deep sighs, flushed or cold and clammy skin, diaphoresis, anorexia, and discomfort. Individuals avoid accepting reality of situation by not making decisions; they may attempt activities that they are no longer able to do, fail to comply with treatment, search for evidence that loss has not or will not occur, and appear artificially happy. Mood swings are common. Individuals isolate themselves from sources of accurate information or reject offers of comfort and support.	Support emotional needs without reinforcing denial. Offer to remain with clients, without discussing reasons for behavior or need to cope, unless they bring it up. Offer regressive care, such as food, drink, and safety.
YEARNING AND PROTEST **Anger**	
Individuals may express anger and retaliate against family, staff, physicians, or supreme being. Bereaved may express anger toward deceased. Individuals become demanding and accusing. Anger may precipitate guilt and lead to anxiety and lowered self-esteem. Individuals may feel resentful and jealous of others who still have lost object or loved one. Individuals may be reluctant to share feelings and thoughts.	Provide anticipatory guidance about feelings and their intensity experienced as part of grief; focus especially on anger. Do not take anger personally. Meet needs that cause angry response.
Bargaining	
Individuals are willing to do anything to avoid loss or change prognosis or fate. Individuals make bargains with supreme being. Individuals accept new forms of therapy.	Provide information needed for decision making.
ANGUISH, DISORGANIZATION, AND DESPAIR **Depression**	
Reality and permanence of loss become recognized. Confusion, lack of motivation, disinterest, indecision, and crying are common. Withdrawal from relationships and activities occurs. Individuals may become quiet and noncommunicative. Feelings of loneliness surface. Reminiscence about past and lost object begins. Individuals may lose interest in appearance. Individuals may bcome suicidal or cope by beginning unhealthy behaviors such as excess drug use.	Provide support and empathy. Support crying by offering touch that communicates caring. Listen attentively. Assess risk of harm to self and refer to mental health professional if needed.
ACCEPTANCE **Reorganization and Restitution**	
Individuals accept terms of loss and death and begin plans for it. Individuals can share feelings about loss. Reminiscence about past occurs. Periods of depression and well-being occur. Good times begin to outweigh bad. Life begins to stabilize.	Offer opportunities to share feelings verbally, in writing or art, or by tape recordings. Allow and encourage review as often as clients want to talk. Show acceptance of lability of feelings. Assist in discussing future plans.

ions of others during this stage. A hospitalized client may show model behavior because of a belief that the staff will find a cure if he or she is a "good patient."

The depression stage occurs when the loss is realized and the full impact of its significance is apparent. This stage may be accompanied by overwhelming loneliness and withdrawal. The depression stage provides an opportunity to work through the loss and begin problem solving.

In the fifth stage, acceptance is reached. Physiological reactions cease, and social interactions resume. Kübler-Ross defines *acceptance* as coming to terms with the situation rather than submitting to resignation or hopelessness.

Martocchio's Phases of Grieving

Although the grieving process has a predictable course and distinctive symptoms, no two persons progress through it in the same way or over the same time. A person progresses and then regresses until the loss is finally resolved. Martocchio (1985) describes five phases of grief that have overlapping boundaries and no expected order. The duration of grief is variable and depends on the factors influencing the grief response. Intense reactions of grief usually subside within 6 to 12 months, and active mourning may continue 3 to 5 years. The saying "Once bereaved, always bereaved" remains true. To expect clients to progress in some specified manner over a specified time would be incorrect, inappropriate, and possibly harmful. Table 28-2 on p. 863 shows nursing implications based on Kübler-Ross' stages of dying and Martocchio's phases of grief.

NURSING PROCESS AND GRIEF

Assessment

During assessment, caution should be taken to avoid forcing a preconceived expectation of grief on the client or family. The nurse should not assume that a particular behavior indicates grief; the nurse should not base such an assumption on inadequate information or a subjective evaluation of the situation.

Assessment of the client and family begins by exploring the meaning of the loss to them. This is done by collecting objective and subjective data. The nurse interviews the client and family, observes their responses and behaviors, and uses open communication, emphasizing listening skills. The nurse should be alert for nonverbal cues. Initial impresssions are validated with the client and family so that nursing diagnoses and effective interventions can be developed.

The nurse must assess not how the client *should be* reacting but how the client *is* reacting. Sequences of behavior or phases may occur in order, they may be skipped, or they may recur. Many variables affect grief. Assessment of these variables gives the nurse a broad data base from which to individualize care.

Personal Characteristics

Personal characteristics influence the response to loss. These include age, sex, socioeconomic status, and education. The nature of the relationship to the lost object, the characteristics of the loss, cultural and spiritual beliefs, support systems, and the potential for goal achievement affect the response to loss.

AGE. Age plays a role in the recognition and reaction to loss. An infant is not generally able to understand loss and death. Loss, separation, and death have little meaning to infants until they are able to recognize familiar persons, form an attachment to a consistent care giver (usually the mother), and demonstrate anxiety concerning strangers. After a trust bond forms between parent and child, even a temporary loss can cause profound anxiety and resistance.

A toddler's cognition is still not sufficiently developed to understand death. The child's self-centeredness and difficulty in separating fact from fantasy prevent comprehension of an absence of life. The toddler experiences anxiety over loss of objects, such as a favorite toy, and separation from parents or the familiar setting of the home.

Between the ages of 3 and 5 years, the preschool years, the child's psychosocial development involves finding a personal purpose and direction; preschool children are also concerned about how parents may perceive them. Loss of parental approval is paramount at this time. One of the fears that may surface during this stage is bodily mutilation. Preschoolers are gaining control over their bodies, which are very important to their self-image (DeSpelder, Strickland, 1987). The processes and responses of grieving of children at this age differ little from their elders, although they lack the capacity to put their thoughts, feelings, and memories into words. Their grief responses are quite variable (Raphael, 1983). The preschooler may not fully comprehend the finality of death. They may ask seemingly inappropriate questions and for weeks repeatedly inquire about the whereabouts of the dead person (Rando, 1984).

School-age children are aware of their bodies and suffer grief over loss of a body part or function. At this age, children are conscious of differences in themselves and others and are strongly affected by such a loss. The school-age child associates misdeeds or bad thoughts with causing death and may feel intense guilt over loss of a significant other. Unlike younger children, however, the school-age child can understand logical explanations about death. The child's concept of death is one of destruction. At the age of 6 or 7 the child associates death with "ghosts" or "evil spirits." By 9 or 10 the child recognizes the universality of death. The child may acquire an unusual fear of the unknown when a death in the family occurs or when faced with a terminal illness.

Physical attributes and strengths are important to most adolescents. Acute grief may be felt when loss of a body part or function occurs. The adolescent fears rejection by peers and views such a loss as interfering with plans. Adolescents have an adult comprehension of the concept of death. Yet they are the least likely of any age group to accept the loss of life, particularly their own. The rejection of death is related to the adolescent's developmental task of establishing identity and purpose in life.

The young adult relates loss to its significance for status, role, and lifestyle. A loss of job or economic well-being, divorce, or a physical impairment causes considerable grief and threatens success. A young adult's concept of death is largely a product of religious and cultural beliefs. The death of a young adult is perceived as especially tragic by society because it is the loss of a life at the brink of realized potential.

During middle age a person begins to realize that youthfulness and physical fitness cannot be taken for granted. The adult begins to reexamine life to consider the options available to gain fulfillment. The person becomes sensitive to the physical changes of aging. Any loss in physical function can create grief. A middle-age adult usually associates actively with friends because children are at an age to move away. Loss of significant others creates a significant threat to lifestyle. The career-oriented adult has usually reached a professional peak. Any loss of job or ability to perform a job causes considerable grief. The middle-age adult knows that time is at a premium and life is finite. Adults often take time to consider life and death.

An older adult experiences anticipatory grief as a result of physical changes accompanying aging and fear of losing capabilities for self-care. The reaction of an older person to death is a reflection of the sense of fulfillment and the contributions made to others. Acceptance of death depends on personality traits, feelings of self-worth, and the amount of functional ability retained. Older adults often fear events surrounding death more than death itself. They may perceive loneliness, isolation, loss of social role, prolonged illness, and loss of self-determination and dignity as worse than death (Gonda, 1971; McGrory, 1978).

SEX ROLES. Reaction to loss is influenced by social expectations of male and female roles. In many cultures in the United States and Canada, it is generally more difficult for men than women to express grief openly. The nurse must be alert to this and verify with the client feelings, reactions, and the personal meaning attached to a loss. Men and women attach different significance to body parts, functions, interpersonal relationships, and objects.

The nurse's own personal thoughts and feelings in regard to sex roles should also be assessed. Such a self-assessment helps a nurse be more supportive. The nurse's expectations should never influence a nurse's attitude toward the client and family.

SOCIOECONOMIC STATUS. Loss is universal, experienced by everyone regardless of socioeconomic status. Assessment of socioeconomic status is essential because it influences the ability to build options and use support mechanisms when coping with loss. Generally, a lack of financial education or occupational skills magnifies the stresses on the griever. The nurse should assess the socioeconomic status of the client to determine realistic options and provide appropriate resource information.

Nature of Relationships

The characteristics of the relationship severed and the functions that the deceased person performed in the griever's life are critical variables in the grief experience. It has been said that to lose your parents is to lose your past, to lose your spouse is to lose your present, and to lose your child is to lose your future. Empirical evidence in literature supports the theory that the loss of a child creates the most intense grief response (Rando, 1984). A child's death is often traumatic because it is premature. Parents often feel guilt and blame themselves.

The reaction to the loss of a parent depends on the quality of the relationship. The death of a parent who was the most nurturing will likely cause the greatest grief for a child. The loss of a parent in adulthood is influenced by the psychological relationship and degree of attachment.

The meaning of the relationship to the griever will influence the grief response, whether the loss is due to death, separation, or divorce. Those who strongly depend on the lost person often have more problems than others as they try to part with the lost relationship and establish new ones. A relationship characterized by extreme ambivalence is more difficult to resolve than one that is not.

One of the most stressful events in life is loss of a spouse. If marital partners usually shared household responsibilities, the loss of one leaves the other with incomplete skills and total responsibility. If children still live at home, the remaining parent may become emotionally overloaded with the extra responsibilities. The loss of a sexual partner may affect the remaining spouse's perception of sexuality and desire for sex. The loss of a spouse also makes it difficult for the survivor to establish new friendships.

Hampe (1975) studied needs of spouses when attempting to cope with their mate's impending death. The needs identified include the need:

1. To be with the dying person
2. To be helpful to the dying person
3. For assurance of the spouse's comfort
4. To be informed of the spouse's condition
5. To be informed of the impending death
6. To ventilate emotions
7. For comfort and support of the family
8. For acceptance, support, and comfort from health care professionals

The nurse who is able to anticipate a family's needs during loss and grief and assess the manner of adjustment to the loss is better equipped to provide emotional support. The nurse can assist by obtaining from physicians the information sought by families about their loved one's condition.

Social Support System

The support that clients receive is based on their value to the members of the social system and the manner and circumstances of their loss. The visibility of a loss, such as the loss of a home resulting from disaster, often brings support from unexpected sources. The visibility of a loss, such as a facial deformity, may cause the loss of support from family or friends, thus augmenting its severity. Persons experiencing less visible or invisible losses, such as early miscarriage, or losses that are often considered socially unacceptable, such as the imprisonment of a family member or the death of a gay partner, often experience the lack of or loss of support from family or friends. When clients do not receive nonjudgmental compassion and support, they lose the vital aid that allows them to handle grief. Lack of support usually leads to difficulty in successful grief resolution (Rando, 1984).

The timing of social support is crucial. Support must be available and used as the griever advances through the mourning process. This requires active sharing by the bereaved individual and the supporters. However, it is common for grievers to not use the support offered (Rando, 1984).

Nature of the Loss

The ability to resolve grief depends on the meaning of the loss and the situation surrounding the loss. The ability to accept help influences whether the bereaved will be able to cope with the loss. The visibility of the loss influences the support received. The duration of a change (that is, whether it is temporary or permanent) affects the amount of time spent in reestablishing physical, psychological, and social equilibrium.

Rando (1984) coined the term *death surround* to describe factors that influence the survivor's ability to do grief work. This includes the location, type, and reason for the death and degree of the preparation for it. Ideally, the survivor feels that the circumstances are appropriate; for example, the deceased had a fulfilled life and died in familiar surroundings, and the mourner had the opportunity and time to prepare for the loss and complete unfinished business. However, sudden and unexpected loss can lead to slower recovery from grief. Deaths by violence through suicide, homicide, or self-neglect are even more difficult to accept. A prolonged, painful illness may leave the survivor emotionally exhausted. Studies show that survivors of clients who died from short-term chronic illnesses (less than 6 months in duration) coped better than those whose loved ones died of a prolonged chronic illness (longer than 6 months in duration) (Rando, 1984).

Cultural and Spiritual Beliefs

Values, attitudes, beliefs, and customs are cultural aspects that influence reaction to loss, grief, and death. The expression of grief generally arises from cultural background and family dynamics. Culture influences each person differently (see Chapter 4). A nurse avoids stereotyping clients by culture and uses self-assessment so that judgmental or prejudicial reactions can be avoided.

Spiritual or religious beliefs include practices, rites, and rituals. An individual may find solace and meaning in losses through spiritual beliefs. Frequently a grieving person turns to religion for strength and support. The nurse should be alert to the significance of religious practices, not only for the client but also for the family (see research highlight). Using words and actions, the nurse can indicate sensitivity to these needs. Through openness in responses, the nurse can determine coping mechanisms used and plan appropriate interventions. For example, members of the Jewish faith remain in a dying person's presence to witness death and be assured that everything possible is done. If Catholic clients are seriously ill, a priest should be notified to provide the sacrament of Anointing of the Sick, which is offered to strengthen them so that they can be restored to health or make their act of death a final sharing in the union with Christ.

For some clients, loss triggers questions about the meaning of life, personal values, and beliefs. Typically this is shown by the "why me?" response. Inter-

Research Highlight

One of the most notable characteristics of the last years of life is the spiritual or religious dimension of human experience. Reed examined the religious perspectives of terminally ill adults who were ambulatory and not in need of hospitalization. The researcher hypothesized that these clients report a greater religiousness than healthy adults. Reed also studied the sense of well-being perceived by the terminally ill.

Reed studied 57 terminally ill adults and 57 healthy adults, matched by age, gender, education, and religious affiliation. Each completed a Religious Perspective Scale and an Index of Well-Being. Terminally ill subjects rated themselves considerably poorer on health status than the healthy group. The terminally ill also indicated awareness of having a shorter life span. The study also found that the terminally ill indicated significantly greater religiousness than the healthy group. Terminally ill women indicated the greatest degree of religiousness.

Reed PG: Religiousness among terminally ill and healthy adults, *Res Nurs Health* 9:35, 1986.

nal conflicts concerning religious beliefs may also occur.

Goals

Loss is any change in a person's situation that reduces the probability of achieving goals. It is critical to understand the client's goals in relation to the loss experienced. Important goal characteristics include the number of goals, centrality of particular goals, number of pathways to goal achievement, compatibility of goals, and change in goal characteristics (temporary or permanent). The more goals a person has, the more likely the person is able to adapt to the loss of only one. The more central the goal, the greater the grief; for example, the amputation of the leg of a woman who has worked her whole life to become a ballerina can be more devastating than death. If a client has many pathways or options to achieving goals, then the client has more than one coping strategy. If one is not available, the client can use another. Goals shift with loss and change; for clients to make this shift, they must have hope (see research highlights).

Hope

Hope is a multidimensional, changing life force. It is characterized by a confident, yet uncertain expec-

 Research Highlight

This descriptive study by O'Connor et al investigated the personal search for meaning conducted by clients recently diagnosed with breast, lung, or colorectal cancer. Six common themes were identified from interviews of 30 clients: seeking an understanding of the personal signficance of the diagnosis; looking at the consequences of the cancer diagnosis; reviewing life; change in outlook toward self, life, and others; living with the cancer; and hope. These 30 randomly selected subjects were interviewed in their homes within the first 6 months of the diagnosis. The data were analyzed using content analysis. The two most significant factors influencing the clients search for meaning were faith and social support.

O'Connor AP et al: Understanding the cancer patient's search for meaning, *Cancer Nurs* 13(3):167, 1990.

 Research Highlight

The purpose of Hearth's descriptive study was to investigate the relationship between hope using the Hearth Hope Scale and coping using the Jalowiec Coping Scale in 120 adults undergoing chemotherapy. The study found a significant relationship ($p < 0.05$) between level of hope and level of coping. They also found that strength of religious convictions and performance of family role responsibilities were significantly related to the variables of hope and coping.

Hearth KA: The relationship between level of hope and level of coping responses and other variables in patients with cancer, *Oncol Nurs Forum* 16(1):67, 1989.

tation of achieving a goal (Dufault, Martocchio, 1985). Hope is not a single act but a complex series of thoughts, feelings, and actions that change often. Clients facing terminal illness or serious loss, as well as their families, experience different dimensions of hope. According to Dufault and Martocchio, hope has six dimensions: affective, cognitive, behavioral, affiliative, temporal, and contextual (Fig. 28-1 on p. 868).

The process of hope involves moving through these dimensions. Dufault and Martocchio also describe two spheres of hope, generalized and particu-

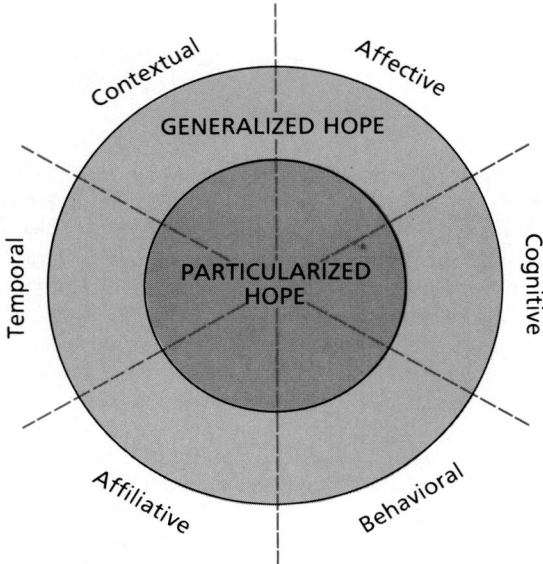

Fig. 28-1 Spheres and dimensions of hope.
From Dufault K, Martocchio BC: *Nurs Clin North Am* 20:379, 1985.

larized. Generalized hope is broad and directed at a future beneficial development. For example, a person with generalized hope may often say "I always hope for the better." Particularized hope is concerned with a specific outcome or state of being (for example, living until a couple's anniversary or a loved one's birthday). A person with particularized hope specifies something as important and is motivated to cope with obstacles that interfere with it.

Awareness of the dimensions of hope (see box) helps the nurse support a client's hope. This can help facilitate grieving associated with terminal illness.

Phase of Grief

Observation of grieving clients allows the nurse to make inferences about effects of the loss. People do not grieve in exactly the same way. However, there are distinct patterns. People in shock and disbelief act differently from those who achieve reorganization and restitution. Clients may move back and forth through phases of grief until final resolution.

The ability to recognize behaviors characteristic of grieving helps the nurse formulate nursing diagnoses and identify means of communicating with and supporting clients and families. The box lists characteristics of dysfunctional grief for an actual or perceived loss, as identified in NANDA-approved defining characteristics, that are also seen in normal grieving. The distinguishing factors are intensity, duration, and the degree to which they interfere with functioning.

Grief of Dying Clients and Their Families

The meaning of death varies widely for individuals because of many variables, including the setting in which death occurs. Most nurses care for dying clients in hospitals. However, as hospice organizations develop, nurses also work with the terminally ill in their homes. Nurses observe client behaviors toward staff and families. Clients' responses to death influence the choice of therapies.

The intensity of coping and the rate at which clients pass through the experience of grief are influenced by the time between their first awareness that they are going to die and the moment of death. In an intensive care unit, clients generally recover or die quickly. Death is sudden and unexpected, and clients and families have little time for expressing grief. In contrast, the process of dying is usually gradual in units for terminally ill clients. Clients have more time to work through grief.

A client experiences many emotions, depending on the phase of dying or grief. Each emotion serves a purpose. The nurse must not identify the client's grief phase on the basis of a single behavior or emotion. However, the client's responses determine techniques used by the nurse to relate to the client. For example, as the client and family begin to come to terms with the inevitability of death, the nurse can encourage the client to discuss feelings about leaving

---

NANDA-Approved Characteristics of Dysfunctional Grief

- Verbal expression of distress at loss
- Denial of loss
- Expression of guilt
- Expression of unresolved issues
- Anger
- Sadness
- Crying
- Difficulty in expressing loss
- Alterations in eating habits
- Alterations in sleep patterns
- Alterations in dream patterns
- Alterations in activity level
- Alterations in libido
- Idealization of lost object
- Reliving of past experiences
- Interference with life functioning
- Developmental regression
- Labile affect
- Alterations in concentration or pursuit of tasks

From Kim MJ, McFarland GK, McLane AM: *Pocket guide to nursing diagnoses*, ed 3, 1991, Mosby–Year Book.

---

family members behind. This would not work if the client is expressing feelings of anguish and despair.

The nurse observes for behaviors that may indicate grief. Physical symptoms should also be noted. Gastrointestinal disturbances such as indigestion, nausea and vomiting, anorexia, or a recent change in weight may indicate grieving. Persons experiencing bereavement also may complain of sleep difficulty. Fatigue and a reduced activity level may also be present. A single physical symptom does not lead to a nursing diagnosis related to grief.

The client's death takes place in a social context. Even during the dying phase the family begins to reorganize itself; the client is no longer available to fulfill the same number and types of roles. The nurse assesses the family's grief process, recognizing that they may be dealing with different aspects of grief than the client.

Risk Factors in Survivors

Numerous risk factors influence whether a person in grief will suffer psychological or physical illness during bereavement. Early identification of risk factors and appropriate nursing interventions can improve a survivor's ability to grieve effectively. Martoc-

chio (1985) lists the following risk factors for survivors:

1. Low socioeconomic status
2. Poor health
3. Sudden death or short illness
4. Perceived lack of available social support
5. Lack of support from religious beliefs
6. Lack of a supportive family or one that discourages grief expressions
7. Strong tendency to cling to the person before death or preoccupation with the deceased's image
8. Strong reactions of distress, anger, and self-reproach
9. History of psychiatric illness or suicidal intention

Nurse's Grief

Nurses may also experience grief when working with clients, especially with dying clients; as a result, their roles in supporting grieving clients and family can become complicated. However, they should never allow their grief to influence clients and families. Nurses who are not aware of their own grief issues have more difficulty in relating to clients as unique individuals; for example, a dying client may remind the nurse of a beloved grandparent, and the nurse may become overly emotionally involved. Other requisites for working with dying clients include coming to grips with mortality, understanding the grief process and appreciating the experience of the dying client, using effective listening skills, acknowledging personal limits, and knowing when there is a need to get away and take care of the self.

 ## Nursing Diagnosis

The nurse gathers data to make a nursing diagnosis regarding grief or a client's reaction to it. Clustering of client or family behaviors, characteristics, and data involving the loss leads to an individualized nursing diagnosis (see diagnoses box on p. 870). Identification of defining characteristics provides the stimulus for development of interventions in the care plan (see diagnostic process box on p. 870).

The diagnosis of **anticipatory grief** refers to accomplishing part of the grief work before the actual loss. For example, a hospitalized woman scheduled for a mastectomy may have begun the grieving process when the breast mass was discovered. Before admission, she may have worked through the phases of disbelief and anger. When the nurse meets her, she may be developing awareness of the significance of the loss. In the same way, a family member com-

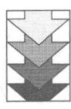

Examples of Nursing Diagnoses Related to Grieving

NANDA-APPROVED NURSING DIAGNOSES

Anticipatory grieving related to:
- Perceived potential loss of significant other
- Perceived potential loss of physiopsychosocial well-being
- Perceived potential loss of personal possessions

Dysfunctional grieving related to:
- Actual or potential object loss
- Thwarted grieving response
- Absence of anticipatory grieving
- Chronic fatal illness
- Lack of resolution of previous grieving response
- Loss of significant other
- Loss of physiopsychosocial well-being
- Loss of personal possessions

Impaired adjustment related to:
- Incomplete grieving

Altered nutrition: less than body requirements related to:
- Depressed grief response

Ineffective family coping: compromised related to:
- Temporary preoccupation by a significant person who is trying to manage emotional conflicts and personal suffering (anticipatory grieving) and is unable to perceive or act effectively in regard to client's needs

Altered family processes related to:
- Situational transition or crisis

Hopelessness related to:
- Failing or deteriorating physiological condition
- Long-term stress
- Abandonment
- Loss of belief in transcendent values or supreme being

Social isolation related to:
- Inadequate personal resources

Spiritual distress (distress of the human spirit) related to:
- Separation from religious and cultural ties

Sleep pattern disturbance related to:
- Stress of grief response

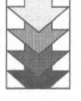

Sample Nursing Diagnostic Process for Grieving

Assessment Activities	Defining Characteristics	Nursing Diagnoses
Observe client's nonverbal behavior when discussing loss.	Client becomes silent and looks away when topic of loss is raised.	*Dysfunctional grieving* related to loss of health and terminal illness
Ask client and family to discuss their understanding of loss situation.	Client and family believe that illness is minor and client will fully recover.	
Observe client's behavior related to treatment.	Client attempts activities prohibited by physical condition and refuses to follow prescribed treatment.	
Assess daily activity level.	Client reports difficulty in sleeping, decreased appetite, and difficulty in concentrating.	
Assess ability to perform roles	Client withdraws from usual decision-making role in family.	
Ask client to discuss future goals and plans.	Client sighs and says, "I have no future."	*Hopelessness* related to failing physical condition
Observe client's nonverbal behavior.	Client becomes passive with little affect and turns away from speaker.	
Offer client choices and observe responses.	Client shrugs and says, "What does it matter?"	
Assess activity level.	Client refuses to eat. Client sleeps all the time, keeping blinds pulled and lights out. Client refuses to participate in care.	

monly experiences anticipatory grief before the loss of a loved one. Nurses also feel anticipatory grief while caring for clients who are dying. Anticipatory grief can be beneficial if it helps progression to a healthier emotional state after the loss.

Some behavioral manifestations of unresolved or **dysfunctional grief** include the following:

1. Overactivity without a sense of loss
2. Alteration in relationships with friends and family
3. Hostilities against specific persons
4. Agitated depression with tension, agitation, insomnia, feelings of worthlessness, extreme guilt, and even suicidal tendencies
5. Diminished participation in religious and ritual activities related to the client's culture
6. Inability to discuss the loss without crying (particularly over a year after the loss)

7. False euphoria

Exaggerated or prolonged grief responses should be identified (see care plan) (Kim, McFarland, McLane, 1991).

The nurse may also diagnose health problems common to a grieving client (for example, sleep pattern disturbance). These may be significant enough to require close attention.

Dying clients require special consideration when nursing diagnoses are formulated. The need to grieve is one of these clients' many problems. Clients with terminal illnesses that cause deformities or physical disabilities are likely to undergo alterations in body image or self-concept. Examples are clients with leukemia who receive drugs that cause loss of hair and clients with bone cancer who become disabled because of chronic pain. As the clients' conditions worsen, the nurse makes diagnoses relevant to basic

 Sample Nursing Care Plan for Dysfunctional Grieving

Nursing diagnosis: *Dysfunctional grieving* related to loss of health and terminal illness
Definition: Dysfunctional grieving is the state in which actual or perceived object loss (a term used in the broadest sense) exists. Objects include people, possessions, a job, status, home, ideals, and parts and processes of the body (Kim, McFarland, McLane, 1991).

Goal	Expected Outcomes	Interventions	Rationale
Client will experience resolution of dysfunctional grieving within 1 mo.	Client will acknowledge awareness of loss.	Acknowledge client's grief through empathetic presence.	Accepting client's feelings as valid allows gradual acceptance of reality and all feelings of grief (Rando, 1986).
	Client will express thoughts and feelings related to loss within 1 week.	Listen to client and encourage sharing of emotions, such as anger, guilt, or depression, in ways most comfortable for client (e.g., verbal or nonverbal, in writing or through art).	Expression of feelings is unique to individual. Listening to client without judgment promotes development of therapeutic relationship that will support further trust and sharing (Rando, 1984).
		Arrange meetings with others who share same experience as client.	Sharing with those experiencing similar situations decreases feelings of isolation (Lewis et al, 1989).
	Client will participate in decision making and cooperate with recommended treatments within 2 weeks.	Offer family time to be with client as possible and assist with care as they wish.	Encouraging time for family to be with and participate in care promotes opportunities for sharing of feelings and completion of unfinished business (Rando, 1984).
		Offer as many choices and opportunities for decision making as possible.	It is important to client's self-esteem to continue making decisions as long as possible (Leavitt et al, 1989).

needs such as alterations in comfort, alterations in elimination, ineffective breathing, or sensory alterations. Because of the nature and severity of terminal illness, physical assessment data are collected frequently and can be used to validate diagnoses.

Planning

Grieving is the natural response to loss. Grieving has a therapeutic value, enabling people to think through their losses, recollect their thoughts, and resume life with new insights and direction. In addition, the physiological, emotional, developmental, and spiritual needs of the client must be met.

Goals for a client dealing with loss are to resolve grief, accept the reality of the loss, regain a sense of self-esteem, and renew normal activities or relationships. Physiological needs must also be met. During planning, the nurse has several resources, including family members, significant others, other team members, and community support groups. The box outlines a sample care plan.

When caring for dying clients, the nurse's responsibilities extend to physical needs and unique psychological and social problems. The nurse must be tolerant and willing to spend more time with dying clients, to listen to expressions of grief, and to maintain their quality of life. Additional goals for dying clients include the following:

1. Gaining and maintaining comfort
2. Maintaining independence in daily activities
3. Maintaining hope
4. Achieving spiritual comfort
5. Gaining relief from loneliness and isolation

The three most crucial needs of the dying client are control of pain, preservation of dignity and self-worth, and love and affection (Rando, 1984). Nurses are in a unique position to address these needs. Their presence can bring comfort and reduce anxiety. They can structure schedules and surroundings so that the client has a sense of security and control over life and the environment. Nurses can support the client's self-esteem by asking for opinions regarding care. Although nurses do not allow families to make decisions for the client, they encourage mutual decision making. This may help prepare the family for when the client may not be able to make choices. As circumstances and the illness change, the client changes, as well. Each client and family should be treated as unique, with recognition that their needs, fears, hopes, expectations, and concerns will change throughout the illness. Continuing re-evaluation and planning is mandatory.

The dying client may be concerned with the circumstances and grief of those left behind. In addition to needing help with problems related to the illness and its emotional stresses, clients often need assistance with financial problems, changes in social and sexual relationships, and difficulties in dealing with the hospital. The formation of an interdisciplinary team is critical. The team usually involves the client, family, physicians, nurses, psychologists, social workers, clergy, pharmacists, physical and occupational therapists, dietitians, and volunteers. Using an interdisciplinary perspective, the nurse can address many potential practical problems before they become overwhelming.

Implementation

Therapeutic Communication

Nursing care of the grieving client begins with establishing the significance of the loss. This is difficult if the client is unwilling to express feelings or is experiencing shock or denial. The nurse observes the response to loss and then attempts to identify the client's strengths in dealing with it. To identify strengths the nurse uses open-ended questions and reflective statements such as "You appear concerned about your brother's condition" or "When the doctor informed you about the test results, you appeared frightened. What were you thinking?" These responses are respectful and give importance to the person's feelings. The nurse must schedule adequate private time with the client and family to promote open communication. The nurse should convey acceptance of all grief reactions. For example, if a client begins to cry, the nurse quietly remains ready to offer comfort, rather than abandoning the client at the time of greatest need. Acknowledging grief through touch and concern promotes trust.

If clients choose not to share feelings or do not wish to be touched, the nurse conveys a willingness to be available when needed. When the nurse acknowledges clients' beliefs and values, a therapeutic relationship may evolve. Sometimes, clients need to begin resolving grief before they can discuss the loss. It is also important to recognize clients' normal styles of dealing with difficult situations. If they do not normally talk about their feelings, they are unlikely to discuss feelings regarding loss.

When considering a client's potential reactions to loss, the nurse is alert to expressions of denial, anger, depression, or guilt. Initial denial is normal. If the nurse encourages the client to face the loss too soon, the nurse may precipitate a reaction that can cause depression, emotional disorganization, or further withdrawal from reality. The nurse often becomes the target of client or family anger. Because it is difficult not to take anger personally, the nurse may avoid expressions of anger or guilt. In an effective relationship the nurse must deal with personal feelings before encouraging the client's expression of anger. The nurse must let the client and family know that such expressions are normal. For example, the nurse might say, "You are obviously upset. So are most people in this situation. I just want to let you know I'm available to talk if you'd like."

The nurse should not erect barriers to communication (see Chapter 15). Communication is blocked by denying the client's grief, providing false reassurance, or avoiding discussion of the problem. For example, when a client expresses anger about a terminal illness, the nurse avoids making statements such as "Don't worry, you'll probably outlive us all" or "Since you're upset, why don't we discuss something else?" Instead the nurse should support the client's expressions of anger by staying close and making statements such as, "It doesn't seem fair" or "Go ahead and let your feelings out, I'll stay with you." The nurse should maintain eye contact and silently stay near. At times, it is most appropriate to do nothing and just be present.

The nurse also does not give advice or analyze causes for loss or behavior. Statements such as "It was God's will" or "You'd feel better if you interacted more with others" show little sensitivity. The nurse must be careful not to give false reassurance and support. Although the purpose is encouragement, a statement such as "At least you still have your mother" may discount a client's true feelings.

When a client demonstrates a readiness to move on to the awareness phase, the nurse might explain the recognized grief reactions. Anticipatory guidance provides an important normalizing function for the client and family. Effective listening techniques, as well as communication of concern and understanding, also help the client move through the grieving process.

No topic that a dying client wishes to discuss should be avoided. The client is more likely to talk about death with a person who listens. The client may initially test the nurse by offering a statement that does not express true concerns. For example, the client may make an open-ended statement such as "My doctor talked with me today," hoping that the nurse will respond.

It is important to let the clients discuss their concerns. The nurse responds to questions as honestly and positively as possible. The nurse may use several strategies to support hope (see box). The strategies chosen depend on the clients' dimensions of hope (Dufault, Martocchio, 1985).

When a client's condition is terminal, the nurse should not encourage expressions of denial. However, the nurse can help the client develop a hopeful attitude. It is easy for the dying client to become depressed. If the nurse can promote feelings of hope,

---

Nursing Implications for Promoting Hope

AFFECTIVE DIMENSION

- Convey an empathetic understanding of clients' worries, fears, and doubts.
- Reduce the degree to which clients become immobilized by concerns.
- Build on client and family strengths of patience and courage.

COGNITIVE DIMENSION

- Clarify or modify hoping persons' reality perceptions.
- Offer information about the illnesses or treatments, correct misinformation, and share the experiences of others as a basis of comparison.

BEHAVIORAL DIMENSION

- Help clients use personal and family resources in relation to hope.
- Balance levels of independence, interdependence, and dependence when planning care.
- Enhance clients' self-esteem and capabilities; give praise and encouragement appropriately.

AFFILIATIVE DIMENSION

- Strengthen or foster relationships that provide hope.
- Help clients know that they are loved, cared for, and important to others.

TEMPORAL DIMENSION

- Attend to client's experiences.
- Use clients' insights from past experiences and apply them to the present.

CONTEXTUAL DIMENSION

- Provide the opportunity to communicate about life situations that influence hope.
- Encourage discussion about desired goals, reminiscing, reviewing values, and reflecting on the meaning of suffering, life, or death.

the client will be better able to participate in treatment. As death approaches the client will be better able to shift the focus of hope to coping with dying.

When all hope is lost, there may be premature psychological and then physical surrender to the environment. This depends on the client's perception of self-worth and effectiveness. The nurse supports hope by helping the client retain control, dignity, and self-esteem. This is done by focusing on the present and immediate future, by emphasizing remaining potentials and abilities, and by structuring life events to render a sense of predictability and continuity. The nurse looks for opportunities to foster accomplishments that cause satisfaction and anticipation. The nurse encourages the client and family to reminisce about previous joys and fulfillments.

Refusal to die or accept the feeling of helplessness is a motivator. Clients who remain confident and determined despite severe illness are better able to tolerate the side effects of treatment, make fewer demands on the staff, serve as models for other clients, and often live longer than predicted. By teaching clients and families the early signs of hopelessness and despair (such as asking few questions about treatment, avoiding discussions of the client's condition, refusing to eat, or ignoring efforts to maintain personal hygiene), the nurse can help the client assume healthier behaviors.

As the grieving client moves to the resolution or reorganization phase, the nurse can encourage discussion of the effects of the loss on the client's life and perceptions of the situation. The nurse may share with the client and family the signs of resolution. The nurse should encourage the client's efforts to loosen ties with the past and look ahead.

The nurse has limitations when attempting to provide appropriate interventions for grieving clients. The nurse may not have the time to address all of the needs of terminally ill clients. In this case, it is important to use other resources within the health care setting and community. When other professionals are needed, the nurse explores with the client and family alternatives in selecting resource persons, community agencies, or groups to enhance grief work. Self-help, bereavement, widow-to-widow, and parent groups are available in some communities. Signs of unresolved grief and pathological grieving may require referral to a psychologist, psychiatrist, or counselor.

Maintenance of Self-Esteem

Nursing interventions focus on promoting a sense of identity, dignity, and self-esteem (see Chapter 31). The nurse can help by listening, responding quickly and positively to requests, maintaining confidential-

ity, and providing comfort and support. The quality and quantity of the time spent with the client are important in creating a therapeutic environment for the grieving process. Davitz and Davitz (1980) have explored the characteristics of nurses who have "highly refined" empathy. They identified the relationship with the client as the core of nursing. Measures that provide comfort and support should be implemented in a caring, pleasant manner to reinforce the client's feelings of self-worth and dignity and to decrease the fear of rejection, isolation, and sense of hopelessness.

Self-esteem and dignity complement each other. Dignity is the ability to maintain self-concept. The disabilities of dying clients may threaten dignity. Care givers often take control of these clients' lives. Taking away the right to make decisions about care fosters hopelessness and feelings of despair, and clients may lose their wills to live. To maintain self-esteem, clients must believe that their opinions are valuable in decisions that affect their dying.

The nurse can promote self-esteem by giving attention to the client's appearance. Cleanliness, a lack of body odors, attractive clothing, and personal grooming (shaving or well-groomed hair) promote sense of worth. The nurse who manages the client's body functions must show an attitude of respect and helpfulness rather than encourage dependence or guilt.

Promotion of Return-to-Life Activities

As clients begin to accept their losses, it is important for the nurse to encourage a return to their normal lifestyles. If clients and families are able to express grief openly and progress through the grief process with support and understanding, resolution of grief is easier. Depending on the nature of the loss, many demands may be placed on family resources.

The nurse can help by encouraging clients to participate in decisions about relationships and resources for the future. The identification of usual lifestyle practices helps bring a sense of closure to the loss. For example, if a woman has begun to accept the loss from a mastectomy, the nurse introduces her to a member of Reach for Recovery, who explains breast prostheses, talks about clothing, and discusses ways to resume normal activities.

Care of Dying Clients and Their Families

Nursing care of the terminally ill client can be demanding and stressful. However, helping a dying person retain dignity is one of nursing's greatest rewards. A client may experience many symptoms for months before death occurs. The nurse can share the dying client's suffering and intervene in a way that improves the quality of life. A dying client must be

The Dying Person's Bill of Rights

- I have the right to be treated as a living human being until I die.
- I have the right to maintain a sense of hopefulness, however changing its focus may be.
- I have the right to be cared for by those who can maintain a sense of hopefulness, however changing this might be.
- I have the right to express my feelings and emotions about my approaching death in my own way.
- I have the right to participate in decisions concerning my care.
- I have the right to expect continuing medical and nursing attention even though "cure" goals must be changed to "comfort" goals.
- I have the right not to die alone.
- I have the right to be free from pain.
- I have the right to have my questions answered honestly.
- I have the right not to be deceived.
- I have the right to have help from and for my family in accepting my death.
- I have the right to die in peace and dignity.
- I have the right to retain my individuality and not be judged for my decisions, which may be contrary to beliefs of others.
- I have the right to discuss and enlarge my religious and/or spiritual experiences, whatever these may mean to others.
- I have the right to expect that the sanctity of the human body will be respected after death.
- I have the right to be cared for by caring, sensitive, knowledgeable people who will attempt to understand my needs and will be able to gain some satisfaction in helping me face my death.

From Barbus AJ: *Am J Nurs* 75(1):99, 1975.

cared for with respect and concern. The dying person's bill of rights (see box) ensures comprehensive and compassionate care.

PROMOTION OF COMFORT. Comfort for dying clients includes relief of psychobiological distress (Oncology Nursing Society, ANA, 1979). The nurse provides a variety of comfort measures for terminally ill clients (Table 28-3 on p. 876). Pain control is important because pain alters sleep, appetite, mobility, and psychological function. Fear of pain is common in cancer clients. However, research suggests that only 50% of cancer victims experience pain (Anderson, 1982). The sooner dying clients obtain pain relief, the more energy they have for maintaining quality life activities. Providing comfort for terminally ill clients also involves controlling the symptoms of disease or the therapies administered.

Personal hygiene is a routine part of keeping the terminally ill client comfortable. The client eventually depends on the nurse or family for basic needs. The client may be embarrassed by this dependence. When possible, clients make their own decisions about care.

MAINTENANCE OF INDEPENDENCE. An important choice for a dying client is choosing a location of care. There are options other than the acute-care hospital. Hospice care (see later section) allows comprehensive care in the home. The nurse should inform clients about these options.

Most dying clients gain satisfaction from being as self-sufficient as possible. Allowing the client to perform simple tasks such as washing, putting on eyeglasses, and eating maintains dignity and sense of worth. When a client becomes physically unable to perform self-care, the nurse encourages participation in decision making to give a sense of control. The nurse looks for nonverbal cues that suggest unwillingness to participate in care. The nurse should not force participation, particularly if physical limitations make it difficult. The family must also encourage the client to make decisions because they often have a tendency to take over. When care occurs in the home, normal routines can be reestablished to help create a sense of control.

PREVENTION OF LONELINESS AND ISOLATION. When the nurse is detached and avoids discussion of the situation, dying clients may experience overwhelming loneliness. It takes experience for a nurse to react positively to dying clients. Nurses are oriented to the cure of clients and may find it difficult to provide the necessary support for those who die. Death symbolizes failure for many health care providers. Furthermore, the process of dying may cause clients to be unpleasant. If conditions cause offensive odors, incontinence, confusion, or combativeness, nurses may avoid clients. In hospitals, dying persons are often confined to private rooms to avoid exposing others to suffering. The room may be dimly lit, the curtains may be drawn, and sounds are reduced. Without meaningful sensory stimulation, dying people probably feel abandoned and isolated.

To prevent loneliness and sensory deprivation the nurse intervenes to improve the quality of the environment. Dying clients should not be routinely placed in private rooms in out-of-the-way locations. Clients feel a sense of involvement when sharing a

TABLE 28-3 Promoting Comfort in the Terminally Ill Client

Characteristics or Causes	Nursing Implications
PAIN	
Pain can be acute or chronic.	Administer narcotic analgesics on regular schedule and not as needed (see Chapter 37).
Pain from progressive cancer is usually chronic and constant.	Use relaxation, guided imagery, distraction, and peripheral nerve stimulators to provide relief.
	Use combinations of analgesics or other therapies as client's needs change.
	Administer narcotics as ordered. (Oral route for narcotics is preferred, but rectal suppositories, injections, continuous intravenous infusions, and intrathecal infusions are available.)
Any source of physical irritation may worsen pain.	Minimize irritants through skin care, including daily baths, lubrication of skin, frequent repositioning, and dry and clean bed linens.
As client approaches death, mouth remains open, tongue becomes dry and edematous, and lips become dry and cracked.	Provide frequent oral care every 2 to 4 hours. Use soft toothbrushes or foam swabs for frequent mouth care. Apply light film of petroleum jelly to lips and tongue (see Chapter 33).
Blinking reflexes diminish near death, causing drying of cornea.	Remove crusts from eyelid margins and provide eye care. Reduce corneal drying with artificial tears.
NAUSEA AND VOMITING	
Nausea and vomiting result from disease process (e.g., gastric cancer), complications (e.g., bowel obstruction), or medications.	Confer with physician about changing medications when possible. Administer antiemetics before meals. Ask physician about providing relief from obstruction with bowel decompression with insertion of nasogastric tube. Provide mouth care and promptly clean up emesis.
FATIGUE	
Metabolic demands of cancerous tumor cause weakness and fatigue.	Set mutual goals with client after identifying valued or desired tasks, and conserve client's energy for only those tasks. Provide frequent rest periods in quiet environment. Time and pace nursing activities to conserve client's energy.
CONSTIPATION	
Narcotic medications and immobility slow peristalsis. Lack of bulk in diet or reduced fluid intake may occur with appetite changes.	Provide preventive care, including increasing fluid intake (e.g., bran, whole grain products, and fresh vegetables in diet) and encouraging exercise.
DIARRHEA	
Diarrhea results from disease process (e.g., colon cancer) and complications of treatment or medications.	Assess for fecal impaction. Confer with physician to change medication if possible. Provide low-residue diet (see Chapter 35).
URINARY INCONTINENCE	
Urinary incontinence results from progressive disease (e.g., involvement of spinal cord or reduced level of consciousness).	Protect skin from irritation or breakdown using absorbent pads and clean linen. Prepare for possible use of indwelling urinary or condom catheter.

*Data from Marino L: *Cancer nursing,* St Louis, 1981, Mosby–Year Book.

TABLE 28-3 Promoting Comfort in the Terminally Ill Client—cont'd	
Characteristics or Causes	Nursing Implications
INADEQUATE NUTRITION	
Nausea and vomiting can decrease appetite. Depression from grieving may cause anorexia.	Suggest that smaller portions and bland foods may be more palatable.* Allow home-cooked meals, which may be preferred by client and gives family chance to participate.
DEHYDRATION	
As disease progresses, client is less willing or able to maintain oral fluid intake. Certain forms of cancer cause obstruction to portions of gastrointestinal tract.	Provide relief of thirst by using ice chips, sips of fluids, or moist cloth to lips. Provide frequent mouth care.
INEFFECTIVE BREATHING PATTERNS	
Causes include disease progression involving lung tissue capacity, pneumonia, and pulmonary edema. Clients may also be severely anemic, causing reduced oxygen capacity.	Position client upright to improve breathing capacity. Administer supplemental oxygen as ordered. Administer bronchodilator as ordered. Administer narcotics as ordered to suppress cough and ease breathing and apprehension. Suction accumulated secretions from mouth and throat.

room and watching the nurse's activities. The client can then also share conversation and companionship with roommates and visitors. When the client dies, however, the nurse should give attention to the roommate, because watching a person die can be frightening.

Providing meaningful environmental stimulation comforts the client. Rooms in the hospital or home should be well lit and attractively decorated and should offer a stimulating view. Pictures, cherished objects, cards or letters from family members, and live plants console the client.

Perhaps most important in preventing loneliness is involvement with family members and friends. In the home, family and friends can more easily interact with the client. In a hospital or extended care facility, visitors should be allowed to remain with the dying client at any time. If the client shares a room, however, the nurse should be sure that visitors do not disturb the roommate. If several family members visit, a private room may be necessary. The dying client becomes particularly lonely at night and may feel more secure if someone stays at the bedside. The nurse should know how to contact family members if a visit is requested or the client's condition worsens.

The client must have someone who can share the dying experience. Nurses should not feel guilty if they cannot always provide this support. However, care may require long intervals of time with the client. The nurse should try to stay with dying clients when needed and show concern and compassion. To provide the care needed by the dying client, it may be necessary to ask for help from other nurses.

PROMOTION OF SPIRITUAL COMFORT. Providing spiritual comfort means much more than asking spiritual advisers to visit. The nurse must support the client in the expression of a philosophy of life. As death approaches, the client often seeks comfort by analyzing values and beliefs related to life and death. A dying client seeks to find purpose and meaning to life before surrendering to death (Conrad, 1985). A dying client often feels guilt if life is perceived as unfulfilled. Therefore the client often asks for forgiveness, either from the supreme being or family members. Additional spiritual needs are hope and love (Conrad, 1985). The nurse and family can assist in understanding and expressing hope. Love can best be expressed through kind, compassionate care.

The nurse or family can provide spiritual comfort by using therapeutic communication skills, expressing empathy, praying with the client, reading inspirational literature, and playing music. Prayer should not be used to avoid the client or the dying process and should only be offered at the request of the client or family. Reciting prayers or praying as a means to close a discussion does not address the client's feelings (Conrad, 1985).

The nurse must feel comfortable about personal spiritual beliefs and values before offering support.

The nurse should never impose personal beliefs or practices on clients or families. Attentive listening encourages clients to express feelings, clarify them, and accept death. When clients seek spiritual advisers but do not have their own, the nurse makes referrals (see Chapter 33).

SUPPORT FOR THE GRIEVING FAMILY. Family members must be supported through the dying and death of their loved one and, at the same time, be encouraged to provide support. In an institutional setting, families often have greater difficulty giving support. The nurse must recognize the value of family members as resources and assist them in working with the dying person (see teaching box).

In the home the family becomes closely involved in the client's care. A terminal illness places heavy demands on social and financial resources. The emotional strain often disrupts normal communication channels. The family may become afraid to interact with the client. Benoliel (1985) describes circumstances that make it difficult for families to cope with demands of terminal illness. These include a lengthy period of dying, symptoms difficult to control, un-

pleasant sights and smells, limited coping resources, and poor relationships with care givers; when a child is dying it may be even more difficult for the family to cope.

Acknowledging grief is the nurse's first step in developing a supportive relationship with the family. The family senses the nurse's concern and should be more willing to share feelings. When the client is in a hospital, the nurse can ease family anxieties and fears by explaining equipment used. Most families want to know where a tube or equipment is located in the body, whether it hurts, why is it needed, and when it will be removed (Johnson, 1986).

Before using family members as resources, the nurse must determine whether they want to be involved. Some do not. The nurse assesses the family's role as observer, comforter, or care giver. Their roles may change often.

HOSPICE CARE. A desire to change traditional care for the dying has led to hospice programs. A hospice program is family-centered care designed to help the terminally ill client be comfortable and maintain a satisfactory lifestyle through the process of dying. Most clients in hospice programs have 6 months or less to live. Hospice programs began in England and reached the United States and Canada in the 1970s.

There are several types of hospice programs. Acute-care hospitals and long-term care facilities often have separate units or designated beds for hospice care. A trained interdisciplinary team works with clients and families. The home care component of a hospice is operated by a hospital or separate home health care agency. In addition, independent hospices care only for the terminally ill. Pitorak (1985) describes the following components of hospice care:

1. Coordinated home care with available inpatient beds under hospital administration
2. Control of symptoms (physical, sociological, psychological, and spiritual)
3. Physician-directed services
4. Provision of an interdisciplinary care team of physicians, nurses, spiritual advisers, social workers, and counselors
5. Medical and nursing services available at all times
6. Client and family as the unit of care
7. Bereavement follow-up after a client's death
8. Use of trained volunteers as a part of the team
9. Acceptance into the program on the basis of health care needs rather than ability to pay

A hospice program emphasizes **palliative treatment**, which is the control of symptoms rather than curative treatment of disease (Aroskar, 1985). The client and family participate in care. Client care is coordinated between the home and inpatient setting.

Client Teaching for the Dying Client's Family

OBJECTIVE

- The family will be able to demonstrate basic client care measures.

TEACHING STRATEGIES

- Describe and demonstrate feeding techniques and selection of foods to facilitate ease of chewing and swallowing.
- Demonstrate bathing, mouth care, and other hygiene measures and allow family to perform return demonstration.
- Show video on simple transfer techniques to prevent injury to themselves and the client; help family to practice.
- Instruct family on need to enforce rest periods.
- Teach family to recognize signs and symptoms to expect as the client's condition worsens and information on whom to call in an emergency.
- Discuss ways to support the dying person and listen to needs and fears.
- Solicit questions from family and provide information as needed.

EVALUATION

- Family will perform client care independently.
- Observe the family and client interacting using effective communication skills.

Efforts are directed at keeping the client at home as much as possible. The family becomes the primary care giver, administering medication and treatment, and the interdisciplinary team provides psychological and physical resources needed for family support.

Care After Death

In most states the physician is responsible for certifying a death in the medical record. The time of death and a description of therapies or actions taken are described in the medical record. The physician may request permission from the family for an **autopsy.** Autopsies are required in circumstances of unusual death (for example, violent trauma or unexpected death in the home).

Recent federal legislation requires hospitals to formulate policies and procedures for the identification and referral of potential donors to procurement agencies or tissue banks (see box). Hospital policies are meant to ensure that families of appropriate potential donors are provided the option of organ, eye, or tissue donation. Discussions of donations should be performed in a sensitive and caring manner. A trained staff member, often a nurse, discusses donation with families or guardians, making certain that they understand that donation is an option and that it is all right not to donate.

The nurse may be the best person to care for the client's body after death because of the therapeutic nurse-client relationship; thus the nurse may be more sensitive to the need of caring for the client's body with dignity and sensitivity. After death the body undergoes a number of physical changes (Table 28-4 on p. 880). The body should be cared for as soon as possible after death to prevent tissue damage or disfigurement. If the family requests organ donation, appropriate measures must be taken immediately.

The nurse offers the family the opportunity to view the body. It may help to suggest that this is an opportunity to say "good-bye" to their loved one, especially if they were not present at the time of death. If the family hesitates, the nurse lets them think about it. If they decide not to view the body, the nurse accepts their decision without judgment. If the family decides to view the body, they are assured that they

---

Suggestions for Involving the Family in the Care of a Dying Client

- Assist in planning a visitation schedule for family members to prevent client and family from becoming fatigued.
- Allow young children to visit a dying parent when the client is able to communicate.
- Be willing to listen to family complaints about the client's care and feelings about the client.
- Help family members learn to interact with the dying person (e.g., using attentive listening, avoiding false reassurances, conducting conversations about normal family activities or problems).
- Allow family members to help with simple care measures such as feeding, bathing, and straightening bed linen. Recognize that family members are often more successful than nursing staff in persuading the client to eat.
- When the family becomes fatigued with care activities, relieve them from their duties so that they can acquire needed rest and support. Refer them to resources for meals and lodging.
- Support the act of grieving between client and family. Provide privacy when preferred. Do not discourage open expression of grief between family and client.
- Provide information daily with regard to the client's condition. Prepare the family for sudden changes in the client's appearance and behavior.
- Communicate news of impending death when the family is together, if possible. Remember that members can provide support for one another. Convey the news in a private area and be willing to stay with the family.
- As death nears, help the family stay in communication with the dying person through short visits, caring silence, touch, and telling the client of their love.
- After death, assist the family with decision making, such as selection of a mortician, transportation of family members, and collection of the client's belongings.

Tissues and Organs Used for Transplant

NONVITAL TISSUES	VITAL ORGANS*
- Corneas	- Heart
- Skin	- Liver
- Long bones	- Lungs
- Middle ear bones	- Kidneys
	- Pancreas

*These organs are recovered after a client is pronounced clinically dead or brain dead; circulatory and ventilatory support is maintained to perfuse the organs before removal.

TABLE 28-4 Physiological Changes after Death	
Change	Related Interventions
Stiffening of body (rigor mortis), developing 2 to 4 hr after death (involves contraction of skeletal and smooth muscle from lack of adenosine triphosphate)	Before rigor mortis develops, position body in normal anatomical alignment, close eyelids and mouth, and insert dentures in mouth.
Reduction in body temperature with loss of skin elasticity (algor mortis)	Remove tape and dressings gently to avoid tissue breakdown. Avoid pulling on skin or body parts.
Purple discoloration of skin (livor mortis) in dependent areas from breakdown of red blood cells	Elevate head to prevent discoloration.
Softening and liquifying of body tissues by bacterial fermentation	Store body in cool place in hospital morgue or other designated area.

will not be alone and that the nurse will be glad to accompany them or will request whomever they would like. The nurse spends as much time as possible assisting the grieving family and offers to contact other support services, such as social services and the spiritual adviser. The family now becomes the client.

Before the family views the body, the nurse prepares it and the room to minimize the stress of the experience (Table 28-4). The nurse removes supplies and equipment from sight. Tubes remaining in the body are removed, clamped, or cut to within 2.5 cm (1 in) of the skin and taped in place. Care of tubes and specimens depends on agency policy, as well as on whether an autopsy will be performed. Dirty linen and other clutter should be removed. A spray deodorizer eliminates unpleasant odors.

The nurse prepares the body by making it look as natural and comfortable as possible. If it is placed in a supine position with arms at the sides, palms down, or across the abdomen, a **mortician** can better prepare it for interment. The nurse places a small pillow or folded towel under the head to prevent discoloration from blood pooling. The eyelids usually remain closed if gently held down for a few seconds. If this does not work, a moistened cotton ball will hold them in place.

The nurse inserts the client's dentures to maintain normal facial features. A rolled-up towel under the chin keeps the mouth closed.

The nurse washes soiled body parts, dresses the body in a clean gown, combs or brushes the hair, and covers the body to the shoulders with clean linen. Most shroud kits contain absorbent pads placed under the perineal and rectal area to collect oozing feces or urine from relaxed sphincter muscles. The nurse removes jewelry and presents it and other valuables to the family. In some agencies, wedding bands may be left in place as long as they are taped securely to the finger.

After the body is prepared, the family is invited into the room. Generally, family members cope best if they are not alone. The nurse or another family member should be there to provide emotional support. The nurse can model loving acceptance of the body by calling it by name, gently stroking the head or holding the hand and saying, "Good-bye John, we'll really miss you," or whatever is appropriate to the situation. It is important not to rush the family while they spend time with the deceased.

After the family leaves, the nurse places tags containing name and other information on the deceased client's wrist and ankle or toe. The gown is removed, and the body is wrapped completely in a shroud, a large bag or rectangular piece of plastic or cotton material. Another identification tag is placed on the shroud. If a client had a transmissible infection, special labeling is used to alert those who move and store the remains. The body is then transported to the morgue, or the mortician picks it up from the client's room. Methods for transporting the body through hallways vary between institutions.

Nurses are also responsible for disposing of the deceased's personal belongings and noting this in the medical record. The nurse can check with the client's family about taking the belongings or ensure that they are transported with the deceased. If the family or friends have left, the nurse contacts a supervisor. No clothing, dentures, plants, gifts, hair pieces, or other personal items are discarded.

Caring for the Nurse

Nurses working with critically or terminally ill clients also experience grief. Grief is the natural response to loss, and each loss needs to be grieved. When nurses experience multiple losses and fail to adequately process them, they can experience bereavement overload. They experience frustration, anger, guilt, sadness, helplessness, anxiety, depression, and feelings of being overwhelmed. Self-care is criti-

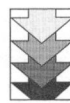

Sample Evaluation of Interventions for Dysfunctional Grieving

Goals	Evaluative Measures	Expected Outcomes
Client will resolve dysfunctional grief and will accept reality of loss.	Observe client discussing loss with significant other. Observe client's behaviors. Ask client to talk about feelings of loss.	Client will discuss feelings related to loss. Client will express sorrow and anger. Client will describe meaning of loss.
Client will gain sense of self-esteem.	Observe client's appearance and grooming habits. Observe client's willingness to interact with others.	Client will maintain neat, well-groomed appearance. Client will initiate discussion with nurse and family about future.
Client will return to routines of daily living.	Observe client's involvement in self-care activities. Ask client to discuss plans.	Client will resume self-care activities. Client will verbalize decisions about care.
Client will discuss plans to return to work or school or will make plans, as appropriate.	Evaluate client's level of participation in social activities with family.	Client will participate in more social activities.

cal to survival. Nurses need to do for themselves what they do for their clients and families. They need to mourn their losses. This is done on an individual basis and as part of a larger group caring for the client. Nurses need to develop personal support systems that allow time away from the care-giving setting, opportunities to share feelings in nonjudgmental, open relationships, and use of stress-management techniques that restore energy (see Chapter 30). Sometimes the institution provides opportunities for staff to get together for mutual support and for closure and grieving over the loss of a client. Nurses' roles in the care of the dying and bereaved are filled with experiences that bring grief and stress. They must attend to the need for relief from these demands. Unrelieved grief and stress can lead to diminished well-being and inability to care for others.

Evaluation

Although resolution of grief may require months or years, most clients are under a nurse's care only a short time. The nurse may become frustrated when, just as the client or family begins to express grief, the client leaves the health care institution or dies. Grieving is an individual process, and resolution of loss does not follow a set schedule. It is important for the client to discuss or share the experience with significant others. The goals established with the client and family become the bases for evaluation; for example, if one of the goals is to communicate love and caring to the family, the nurse would evaluate whether this has occurred in verbal or written form.

The nurse also observes the quality of interactions (see evaluation box).

The care of the dying client requires the nurse to evaluate the client's level of comfort with illness and quality of life. The success of the evaluation depends partly on the bond formed with the client. Unless the client trusts the nurse, expression of true feelings and concerns is unlikely. The client's level of comfort is evaluated on the basis of outcomes such as a reduction in pain, control of symptoms, maintenance of functioning body systems, accomplishment of unfinished tasks, and emotional comfort.

 SUMMARY

Categories of loss include loss of an aspect of self, an external object, a significant other, a known environment, and life. The nurse interacts daily with clients and families experiencing loss. Knowledge of the concepts and theories of loss, death, and the grieving process provides a framework for the nursing process. The nurse's responses and interactions with clients and families create the climate for openness in expressing grief. The nurse explores clients' strengths and support systems by listening, being available when needed, and conveying respect for values and beliefs. A trust relationship creates a therapeutic environment that encourages expression of grief and fosters dignity and self-esteem. Understanding promotes growth and paves the way for effective care of grieving or dying clients and their families.

Key Concepts

- The grieving process involves a set of emotional, cognitive, and behavioral responses to an actual or perceived loss.
- The purpose of grieving is to achieve more effective functioning.
- Individuals experience different aspects of the grieving process at different times.
- The phases of the grieving process vary among theories but progress from distress and shock to resolution and acceptance.
- Dying may lead to a grief response similar to that with other kinds of losses.
- A nurse's support of a client's hope can help relieve grieving associated with a loss.
- The individual's perception of a loss is influenced by many factors, including developmental stage, beliefs, roles, relationships, and socioeconomic status.
- During assessment the nurse considers behavioral characteristics that suggest the client's stage of grieving.
- Risk factors (e.g., physical health) indicate whether a person in grief will suffer psychological or physical illness during bereavement.
- Nursing diagnoses focus on the type of grief experienced by clients or health-related problems common to grieving clients.
- Therapeutic communication helps the nurse assist the grieving and the dying client in coping with loss.
- Nursing care of the grieving and dying client should promote sense of identity, dignity, and self-esteem.
- Nursing interventions to promote return-to-life activities assist the client in resolving grief and accepting the loss.
- Nursing care of the terminally ill client focuses on promoting comfort and improving the quality of remaining life.
- As death approaches, a client reviews and analyzes values and beliefs pertinent to the meaning of life and death.
- A nurse must assess whether family members are willing to be involved in a dying client's care before using them as resources.
- Care after death involves caring for the body with dignity and sensitivity.
- The evaluation of nursing care for the grieving and dying client is ongoing and is based on identifiable behavioral changes through the grieving process.
- The nurse's own loss history influences responses to client losses.
- Nurses who work with critically or terminally ill clients experience loss and grief.
- Nurses need to be aware of and mourn their own losses on an ongoing basis to avoid bereavement overload.

Key Terms

Anticipatory grief, p. 869

Autopsy, p. 879

Bereavement, p. 861

Dysfunctional grief, p. 871

Grief, p. 861

Grieving process, p. 862

Hope, p. 867

Maturational loss, p. 860

Mortician, p. 880

Mourning, p. 861

Palliative treatment, p. 878

Situational loss, p. 860

Critical Thinking Exercises

1. You are caring for a 16-year-old male accident victim, who lost his right leg in the accident. It has been 2 weeks since the accident, and you notice that he has become progressively withdrawn. He refuses to do physical therapy or anything for himself. You suspect that he is grieving but are not sure. Describe how you would approach the client and what you would assess.

2. Your 65-year-old client, Mrs. White, has been acting depressed. When you ask her what is happening, she tells you that she lost her husband of 50 years 6 months before. Her children have been telling her that she should sell her house and get on with her life. She says there must be something wrong with her because she "just can't forget" her husband. What would your response be and what would you teach her about the grieving process?

3. Mrs. Jones' husband is nearing the final phase of his terminal illness. Identify four needs that she may have and describe how you plan to address them.

4. You have been spending a lot of time with Mr. Charles; your instructor says you spend far too much time with him. His condition has progressively deteriorated, and you find yourself thinking about him all the time. You do not trust anyone else to get him the care you know he needs. Your instructor comments on your attachment to the client and asks you to reflect on what is influencing your response to the client. What might be some factors that would influence a nurse to become overly attached to a client and how would you recommend dealing with it?

5. Mr. Carlson's family has decided to take him home during the last days of his illness because they do not want him to die in the hospital. They realize that he requires total care. His wife is handicapped, and both children work full time. What would you need to teach the family and what will they need to consider before taking him home?

REFERENCES

Anderson J: Nursing management of the cancer patient in pain: a review of the literature, *Cancer Nurs* 5:33, 1982.

Aroskar MA: Access to hospice—ethical dimensions, *Nurs Clin North Am* 20:299, 1985.

Benoliel JQ: Loss and terminal illness, *Nurs Clin North Am* 20:439, 1985.

Conrad NL: Spiritual support for the dying, *Nurs Clin North Am* 20:415, 1985.

Davitz L, Davitz J: *Nurses' responses to patients' suffering,* New York, 1980, Springer.

DeSpelder LA, Strickland AL: *The last dance: encountering death and dying,* Mountain View, Calif, 1987, Mayfield.

Dufault K, Martocchio BC: Hope: its spheres and dimensions, *Nurs Clin North Am* 20:379, 1985.

Engel GL: Grief and grieving, *Am J Nurs* 64:93, 1964.

Gonda TA: Coping with dying and death, *Geriatrics* 26:71, 1971.

Hampe SO: Needs of the grieving spouse in a hospital setting, *Nurs Res* 24:113, 1975.

Johnson SH: 10 ways to help the family of a critically ill patient, *Nurs 86* 16:50, 1986.

Kim MJ, McFarland GK, McLane AM: *Pocket guide to nursing diagnoses,* St Louis, 1991, Mosby–Year Book.

Kübler-Ross E: *On death and dying,* New York, 1969, Macmillan.

Leavitt PF et al: The patient who is dying. In Lewis S et al, editors: *Manual of psychosocial nursing interventions: promoting mental health in medical-surgical settings,* Philadelphia, 1989, Saunders.

Lewis K: Grief in chronic illness and disability, *J Rehabil* 49:8, 1983.

Lewis S et al: *Manual of psychosocial nursing interventions: promoting mental health in medical-surgical settings,* Philadelphia, 1989, Saunders.

Martocchio BC: Grief and bereavement: healing through hurt, *Nurs Clin North Am* 20:327, 1985.

McGrory A: *A well model approach to care of the dying client,* New York, 1978, McGraw-Hill.

Oncology Nursing Society and the American Nurses Association: *Outcome standards for cancer nursing practice,* Kansas City, Mo, 1979, The Association.

Pitorak EF: Establishing a medicare-certified inpatient unit, *Nurs Clin North Am* 20:311, 1985.

Rando TA: *Grief, dying and death,* Champaign, Ill, 1984, Research Press.

Rando TA: *Loss and anticipatory grief,* Lexington, Mass, 1986, Lexington Books.

Raphael B: *The anatomy of bereavement,* New York, 1983, Basic Books.

Worden JW: *Grief counseling and grief therapy,* New York, 1982, Springer.

ADDITIONAL READINGS

Ames B: Art and a dying patient, *Am J Nurs* 80:1094, 1980.

Brown P: The concept of home: implications for care of the critically ill, *Crit Care Nurse* 9:97, 1989.

Bruss CR: Nursing diagnosis of hopelessness, *J Psychosoc Nurs* 26:29, 1988.

Buturusis B et al: Assessing health needs: the well elderly, *J Gerontol Nurs* 12(6):11, 1986.

Castles MR, Murray RB: *Dying in an institution: nurse patient perspectives,* New York, 1979, Appleton-Century-Crofts.

Ebersole P, Hess P: *Toward healthy aging: human needs and nursing responses,* ed 3, St Louis, 1990, Mosby–Year Book.

Engel GL: *Psychological development in health and disease,* Philadelphia, 1962, Saunders.

Evans MA, Esbenson M, Jaffe C: Expect the unexpected when you care for a dying patient, *Nurs 81* 11:55, 1981.

Fairbairn W: Synoposis of an object-relations theory of the personality, *Int J Psychoanal* 44:244, 1963.

Garritson SH: Ethical decision making patterns, *J Psychosoc Nurs* 26:22, 1988.

Groves J: Differentiating grief, mourning and bereavement, *Am J Psychiatry* 135:(7):875, 1978.

Herth KA: The relationship between level of hope and level of coping response and other variables in patients with cancer, *Oncol Nurs Forum* 16:67, 1989.

Kalish RA: *Death, grief, and caring relationships,* ed 2, Monterey, Calif, 1985, Brooks/Cole.

Lee R: Object loss and counseling the bereaved. In Fruehling J, editor: *Sourcebook on death and dying,* Chicago, Ill, 1982, Marquis.

Lindemann E: Symptomatology and management of acute grief. In Parad H, editor: *Crisis intervention,* New York, 1965, Family Association of America.

Marino L: *Cancer nursing,* St Louis, 1981, Mosby–Year Book.

Miles HS, Hays DR: Widowhood, *Am J Nurs* 75:280, 1975.

Moseley JR: Alterations in comfort, *Nurs Clin North Am* 20:427, 1985.

Mulhern RM: When there's no treatment left but the truth, *RN* 49:26, 1986.

Musgrave CF: The ethical and legal implications of hospice care: an international overview, *Cancer Nurs* 10:183, 1987.

O'Connor AP: Understanding the cancer patient's search for meaning, *Cancer Nurs* 13:167, 1990.

Perryman JP: Providing the option to donate, *Forum Newsl* 13:6, 1989.

Reed PG: Religiousness among terminally ill and healthy adults, *Res Nurs Health* 9:35, 1986.

Rothman DA, Rothman NL: *The professional nurse and the law,* Boston, 1977, Little, Brown.

Schowalter JE: Parent death and child bereavement. In Schoenberg B et al, editors: *Bereavement: its psychosocial aspects,* New York, 1975, Columbia University Press.

Smith S, Duell D: *Nursing skills and evaluation: a nursing process approach,* Los Altos, Calif, 1982, National Nursing Review.

Stickney SK, Gardner ER: Companions in suffering, *Am J Nurs* 84:1491, 1984.

Stockdale L, Hutzenbiler, T: How you can comfort a grieving family, *Nurs Life* 6:23, 1986.

Taylor PB, Gideon MD: Holding out hope to your dying patient, *Nurs 82* 12:42, 1982.

Tyner R: Elements of empathetic care for dying patients and their families, *Nurs Clin North Am* 20:393, 1985.

Wegmann JA: Hospice home death, hospital death, and coping abilities of widows, *Cancer Nurs* 10:148, 1987.

Werner-Beland JA: *Grief response of long term illness and disability,* Reston, Va, 1980, Reston.

Zach MV: Loneliness: a concept relevant to the care of dying persons, *Nurs Clin North Am* 20:403, 1985.

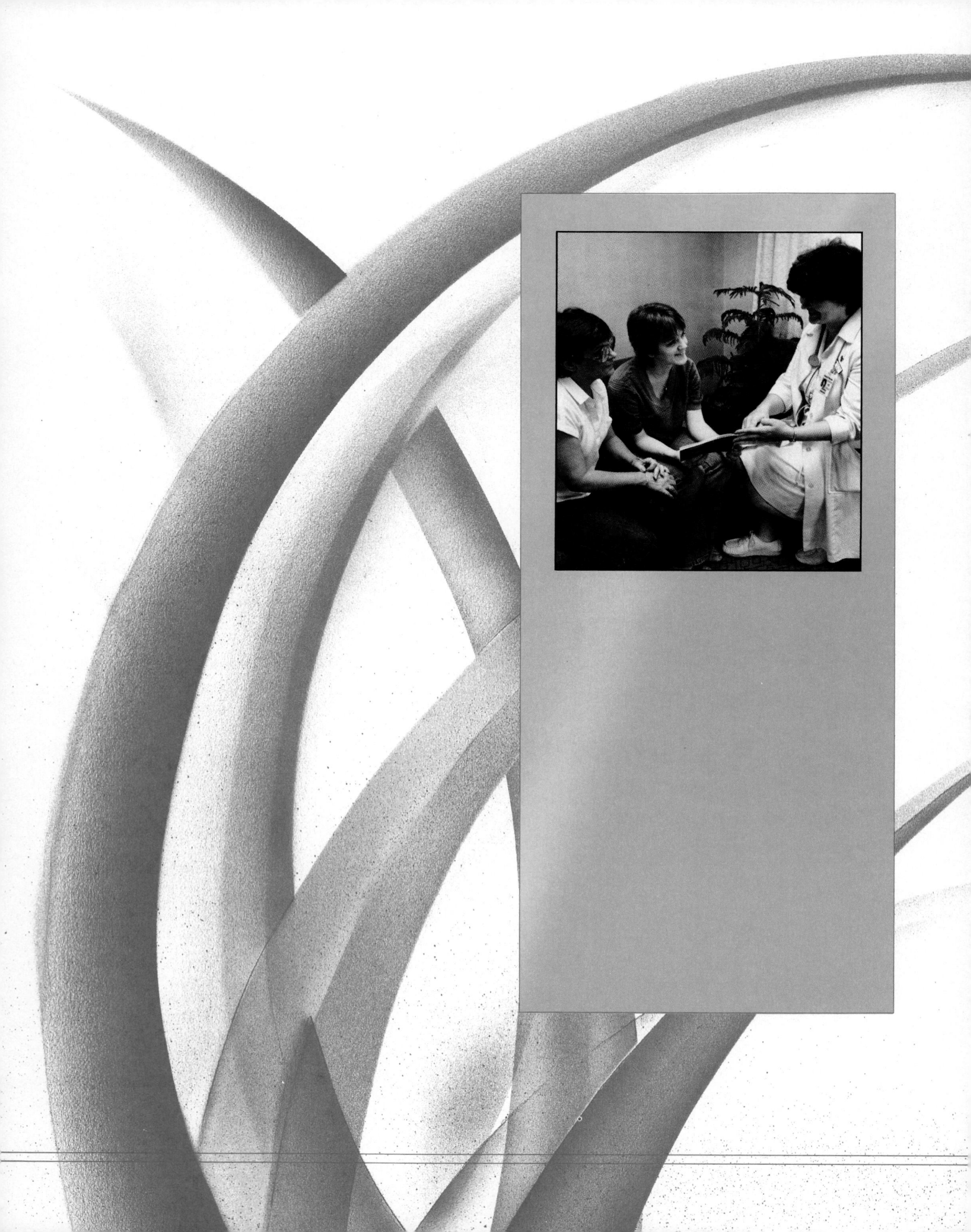

UNIT 6

Human Needs in Health and Illness

CHAPTER 29

Basic Human Needs

OBJECTIVES

Mastery of content in this chapter will enable the student to:

- Define the key terms listed.
- Discuss each component of Maslow's hierarchy of needs.
- Describe assessment techniques for identifying unmet needs.
- Identify actual or potential conditions that threaten fulfillment of a client's needs.
- Identify nursing diagnoses appropriate for unmet basic needs.
- Describe the basic nursing implications concerning unmet needs.
- Describe relationships among the different levels of needs.
- State factors that influence the individual need priorities.

CHAPTER OUTLINE

Physiological Needs
    Oxygen
    Fluids
    Nutrition
    Temperature
    Elimination
    Shelter
    Rest
    Sex
    Nursing diagnosis

Safety and Security Needs
    Physical safety
    Psychological safety

Love and Belonging Needs

Esteem and Self-Esteem Needs

Need for Self-Actualization

Application of Basic Needs Theory
    Relationships among needs
    Simultaneous meeting of needs
    Factors influencing need priorities

Basic human needs are matters such as food, water, safety, and love that are necessary for survival and health. Although each person has additional, unique needs, everyone has the same basic human needs. The extent to which basic needs are met determines a person's level of health and position on the health-illness continuum (see Chapter 2). Nurses are therefore concerned with ensuring that basic human needs are met.

Maslow's **hierarchy of basic human needs** is a theory that nurses can use to understand the relationships among basic human needs when providing care. Maslow has assigned priorities to basic needs. According to his theory, certain human needs are more basic than others; that is, some needs must be met before others. For example, a starving person is more likely to seek food than to engage in activities that increase self-esteem.

The hierarchy of human needs arranges the basic needs in five levels of priority (Fig. 29-1). The most basic, or first, level includes **physiological needs** such as air, water, and food. The second level includes **safety and security needs,** which involve physical and psychological security. The third level contains **love and belonging needs,** including friendship, social relationships, and sexual love. The fourth level encompasses **esteem and self-esteem needs,** which involve self-confidence, usefulness, achievement, and self-worth. The final level is the need for **self-actualization,** the state of fully achieving potential and having the ability to solve problems and cope realistically with life's situations.

Through life experiences an individual's basic human needs may be unmet, partially met, or wholly fulfilled. According to this theory, a person whose needs are all met is healthy, and a person with one or more unmet needs is at risk for illness or may be unhealthy in one or more of the human dimensions.

The hierarchy of needs is a theoretical model; that is, the priorities given to human needs are generally true of people but not necessarily true of all individuals. Thus the hierarchy of needs can still be applied to individuals who seem to have different priorities. When providing care to individuals with unmet needs, the nurse should always take into account their priorities, as well as other factors such as environment and social interactions that influence how well needs can be met.

Clients entering the health care system generally have unmet needs, or they may be unable to continue meeting their needs. A person brought to an emergency room experiencing cardiac arrest has an unmet need for air, the most basic physiological need. An older woman in a high-crime area may be concerned about physical safety and, while hospitalized, may have a need for psychological security from fear that her home will be burglarized. A widowed homemaker whose children have moved away may feel that she does not belong or is not loved. Nurses in all practice settings encounter clients whose needs might be unmet. Nursing care includes helping clients, and often the family, meet these needs.

The hierarchy of needs is a useful way for nurses to evaluate and understand the needs and behaviors of a client. Although one need may take priority over another (such as restoration of an adequate airway before education that will help the client adjust to an emotional conflict), the nurse simultaneously assesses needs on different levels. An example is helping a client meet the need for social belonging while also helping achieve adequate nutrition. The nurse assesses the client's needs and then considers how to use the nursing process and mutual goal setting to best help the client.

 PHYSIOLOGICAL NEEDS

Physiological needs have the highest priority in Maslow's hierarchy. An individual who has several unmet needs generally seeks first to fulfill physiological needs (Maslow, 1970). For example, a person who lacks food, safety, and love usually searches for food before seeking love.

Physiological needs are necessary or important for survival. Humans have eight such needs; they in-

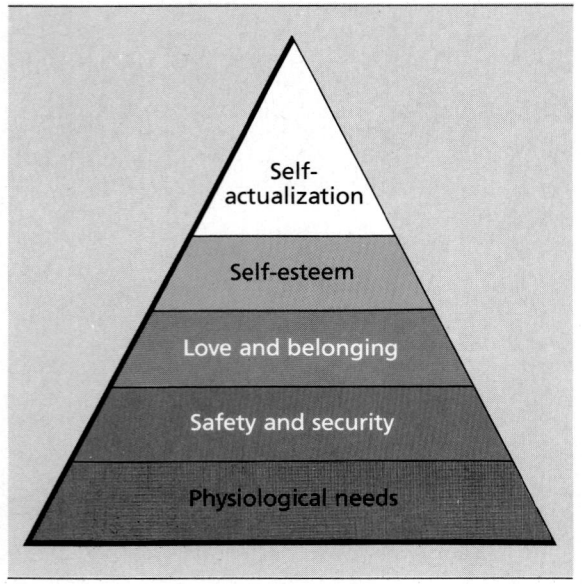

Fig. 29-1   Maslow's hierarchy of needs.

clude oxygen, fluid, nutrition, temperature, elimination, shelter, rest, and sex.

An infant requires someone to meet the needs for food, shelter, fluids, adequate temperature, and elimination. As the individual grows and progresses developmentally, the ability to satisfy physiological needs is increased. A 2-year-old who wants a drink of water usually knows where water is and how to get it. Although the child's efforts may not be very efficient, if the motivation is great enough, the child will meet the need. A healthy adult is usually able to meet physiological needs without assistance.

The very young, very old, poor, ill, and handicapped clients frequently depend on others for meeting basic physiological needs. The nurse often has a role in helping these clients meet those needs.

Oxygen

Oxygen is the most essential physiological need. The body depends on oxygen for moment-to-moment survival. Some tissues, such as skeletal muscle, can survive for a time without oxygen through **anaerobic metabolism,** a process by which these tissues provide their own energy in the absence of oxygen. In long-distance running, for example, the runner's skeletal muscles undergo anaerobic metabolism so that the available oxygen can be used by more vital organs such as the heart, brain, and lungs.

Tissues that carry out only **aerobic metabolism,** the process of providing energy in the presence of oxygen, depend totally on oxygen for survival. The brain, for example, cannot function without oxygen for longer than 4 to 5 minutes.

Oxygen must be adequately delivered from the environment to the lungs, the bloodstream, and finally the tissues. At any point in their lives, clients are at risk for not meeting their oxygen needs. The need can be acute, as with a cardiac arrest, or chronic, as with the disease emphysema.

Assessment

Nurses continually evaluate clients' oxygenation to determine whether this need is being met. This assessment is basically the same in chronic and acute situations (see Chapter 38). Clients may be confused or lethargic because the level of oxygen in their blood and tissues is decreased. When oxygen needs are unmet, people are often unable to lie flat because of air hunger and are forced to remain upright so that gravity can assist in lung expansion. Clients breathe quickly to deliver more oxygen to their lungs, and respirations are usually shallow. Frequently, this effort fatigues clients rather than meets the need for oxygenation. Other signs of inadequate oxygenation include nasal flaring and sternal, substernal, and suprasternal retractions. Clients appear to be struggling for air.

Clients with progressive, long-term decreases in tissue oxygen levels show **cyanosis,** a bluish discoloration of skin and mucous membranes caused by decreased oxygen in the blood. Cyanosis is a late sign of poor oxygenation, so the nurse should be aware of the earlier, more subtle indicators.

Nursing Implications

Oxygen has the highest priority of all physiological needs because many organs such as the brain and heart cannot survive without it. The nurse must be able to assess the need for oxygen and meet it. For example, the nursing diagnosis, *anxiety,* is supported by the defining characteristic of hyperventilation. During hyperventilation, there is a decrease in the intake of oxygen and an increase in the expiration of carbon dioxide. The person becomes more anxious and confused and may feel a tingling of the hands and feet, numbness around the lips, and dizziness. The nursing intervention is directed at controlling the imbalance of respiratory gases by having a client breathe into a paper bag, which will cause the client to re-breathe carbon dioxide and slow the respiratory rate. After the client has adequate oxygen, the nurse may use reassurance, teaching, and counseling to help control anxiety.

In other instances the nurse uses specific techniques to help the client meet oxygen needs. For example, a 50-year-old man has a long smoking history and a medical diagnosis of chronic obstructive pulmonary disease. Nursing assessment documents chronic breathlessness and a requirement of 1 L/min of oxygen every night administered through a nasal cannula. Using the nursing diagnosis of *impaired gas exchange,* the nurse develops a care plan so that the client has adequate opportunity to meet needs for hygiene, nutrition, and rest. The nurse also teaches the client to rest in a position that increases respiratory volume and thus the level of oxygen.

Nursing measures to meet oxygen needs range from emergency cardiopulmonary resuscitation for cardiac arrest to supportive measures such as administration of oxygen to clients with pulmonary disease during exercise. Chapter 38 discusses in detail measures necessary for meeting oxygen needs of clients.

Fluids

The human body requires a balance between intake and output of fluids (see Chapter 39). Fluids are taken in by mouth, or parenterally, and fluids leave the body from the intestines, lungs, skin, and kidneys. Clients of any age can have unmet fluid needs, but the very young and very old have the greatest risk. Severely ill, traumatized, or handicapped clients are also more likely to have unmet fluid needs.

Dehydration and edema indicate unmet fluid needs. **Dehydration** is the excessive loss of water from body tissues; it is accompanied by a disturbance of body electrolytes. Dehydration may result from excessive and prolonged fever, vomiting, diarrhea, trauma, or any condition that causes a rapid fluid loss. **Edema** is the abnormal accumulation of fluid in the interstitial spaces of tissues, pericardial sac, intrapleural space, peritoneal cavity, or joint capsules. Edema is also accompanied by a disturbance of electrolytes and may occur in a nutritional, cardiovascular, renal, malignant, traumatic, or other disorder that results in a rapid accumulation of fluids.

Assessment

The nurse examines clients for actual or potential fluid imbalance. Poor skin turgor, flushed dry skin, decreased tearing or salivation, a coated tongue, decreased urine output, confusion, and irritability indicate dehydration. Skin turgor is the normal elasticity of the skin, which becomes lax with dehydration; when grasped and raised between two fingers, the skin slowly returns to its former position.

The dehydrated client's skin is dry because the body transfers fluid to the circulation and vital organs. The skin may be flushed because of an elevated body temperature that can accompany dehydration. The tongue is coated and dry. A dehydrated person may cry but not have tears. **Oliguria,** a diminished ability of the kidneys to form and excrete urine, is frequently caused by dehydration. Because of the fluid and associated electrolyte imbalances, mental status is altered, and the client may be irritable and confused. In cases of severe dehydration the client may even be comatose.

Excessive body fluids most commonly manifest as edema. Edema may be caused by decreased serum protein levels; severe burns; altered functioning of the cardiovascular, renal, or hepatic system; or drugs. Edema is usually observed in lower body regions; when the person is standing, edema is seen in feet and legs. The client with edema may also have a daily weight gain, shortness of breath, or an increased heart rate (see Chapter 39).

Nursing Implications

The overall nursing goal for clients with unmet fluid needs is to restore body fluid and electrolyte balances. The nurse uses simple or complex measures to meet this goal. For example, during assessment the nurse documents diarrhea without vomiting and

arrives at the nursing diagnosis of *high risk for fluid volume deficit.* An appropriate nursing intervention is to increase the client's oral intake of fluids. If fluid loss is greater, as with a severe burn, the nursing diagnosis is *fluid volume deficit,* and nursing interventions are more complex and may include carrying out the physician's order for administration of intravenous fluids.

When the nursing assessment reveals findings consistent with *fluid volume excess,* nursing actions restrict the client's fluid intake and facilitate elimination of fluids from the body. Chapter 39 describes in detail the knowledge and techniques the nurse needs for restoring fluid, electrolyte, and acid-base balances.

Nutrition

The human body has an essential need for nutrients, although it can survive without food longer than without fluids. Like other physiological needs, nutritional needs may be unmet in a person of any age (see Chapter 35).

The body's metabolic processes control digestion, storage of nutrients, and elimination of waste products. Digestion and storage of nutrients are essential in meeting the body's nutritional demands.

After food is eaten, digestive processes break down nutrients into usable compounds such as glucose, amino acids, and fatty acids, which meet immediate nutritional needs. Glucose is a body sugar that satisfies immediate energy requirements. Nutrients not needed immediately are stored as glycogen, protein, and fat.

When a person skips a meal, eats insufficiently or sporadically, or fasts, the body uses its stored reserves to meet nutritional needs. Glycogen, stored in the liver and muscles, is used first because it is readily available and can be quickly converted to glucose. If the person still has not eaten when glycogen is depleted, the body begins to use stored protein and fat.

The body also needs vitamins and minerals to function with full efficiency. For example, deficiencies in vitamin C impair wound healing. Deficiencies in calcium and vitamin D retard bone growth and bone metabolism.

Assessment

To determine whether clients are meeting nutritional needs, the nurse considers body weight and many other factors. Clients with appropriate body weight may still have nutritional deficits. Nutritional assessment should include measurement of body muscle mass, laboratory data, and food intake patterns (see Chapter 35). Signs and symptoms indicating that clients are not meeting nutritional needs include failure to grow or gain weight, unplanned weight loss, fatigue, pallor, and recurring mouth and gum sores.

Nursing Implications

Clients require adequate nutrition to carry out activities of daily living, promote wound healing, and maintain wellness. In some cases the nurse takes a direct role in meeting clients' nutritional needs. For example, when caring for infants with the syndrome known as *failure to thrive* and a nursing diagnosis of *altered nutrition: less than body requirements*, the nurse and health care team assume total responsibility for nutrition.

Sometimes a nurse assists in meeting nutritional needs through teaching. An adult with *altered nutrition: more than body requirements* and recently diagnosed insulin-dependent diabetes mellitus, for example, needs to be taught to balance nutritional needs, insulin intake, and exercise habits.

To help clients meet their nutritional needs, the nurse must understand the digestive and metabolic processes of the body. The nurse may use various nutritional supplements and techniques to correct nutritional deficits. Chapter 35 discusses in detail nursing measures related to the nutritional needs of clients.

Temperature

The body can function normally within only a narrow temperature range, 37° C (98.6° F) ± 1° C. (Mountcastle, 1980). Body temperatures outside this range can result in injuries, permanent effects such as brain damage, or death.

The body can temporarily regulate temperature by certain mechanisms. For example, a person shivers when moving from a warm environment to one of 55° F. This adaptive response can temporarily increase body temperature. Chapter 19 discusses other responses to temperature imbalance.

Assessment

The body has a physiological response to extreme temperatures. Prolonged exposure to cold decreases the rate of metabolism and use of oxygen. If body temperature is lowered beyond the point at which the body can adapt, vital signs decrease, consciousness decreases, the person is more difficult to arouse, the skin is pale and cold, and urinary output decreases. A localized exposure to cold (for example, when hands are bare in winter) leads to frostbite (see Chapter 19). **Frostbite** is a traumatic effect of extreme cold on the skin and subcutaneous tissues and is first displayed as distinct pallor. Blood circulation in the area is impaired, leading to decreased oxygen in tissues. This may cause tissue death.

Prolonged exposure to heat increases the body's metabolic activity and increases tissue oxygen demand. Extreme or prolonged heat exposure can also have specific physiological effects. Local exposure to heat can result in first-, second-, or third-degree burns. Overexposure to the sun can lead to sunstroke, which is characterized by high fever, convulsions, and coma (see Chapter 19). Older persons living in poorly ventilated homes without air conditioning are at risk for heatstroke during prolonged hot weather. Symptoms are elevated body temperature, dehydration, and fluid and electrolyte imbalances. If this condition is untreated the person becomes disoriented and confused, enters a coma, and dies.

Nursing Implications

Nursing care for clients exposed to extreme heat or cold is directed at restoring normal body temperature. In addition, the nurse helps clients avoid exposure to heat or cold.

To treat frostbite, the nurse gently warms the affected area. The nurse does not rub the area in an attempt to increase circulation because this action can further damage skin and underlying tissues. A client with sunstroke needs emergency treatment to reduce body temperature. Nursing measures include a tepid sponge bath, fluid replacements, and medications.

Elimination

The elimination of waste materials is one of the body's metabolic processes. Waste products are eliminated by the lungs, skin, kidneys, and intestines.

The lungs primarily eliminate carbon dioxide, a gas formed during tissue metabolism. Most carbon dioxide is carried to the lungs by the venous system and excreted through breathing. If a client has difficulty eliminating this gas (for example, with acid-base imbalances that originate in the respiratory system), nursing measures are needed to prevent severe impairment or death (see Chapter 38).

The skin eliminates water and sodium, most noticeably as sweat. This also assists in temperature regulation because evaporation of sweat lowers body temperature. Sweat cannot always be seen, but the skin excretes water continuously, about 200 ml a day. A client with fever or prolonged exposure to hot, humid weather has an increased water loss from the skin. The nurse considers water loss from the skin when caring for a client with actual or potential dehydration.

The kidneys are the body's primary means of excreting excess body fluids, electrolytes, hydrogen ions, and acids. Urinary elimination normally depends on fluid intake and circulatory blood volume; if either is decreased, urinary output decreases. Urinary output is also changed in persons with kidney disease, which affects the quantity of urine and the content of waste products within the urine. Kidney disease can be life threatening (see Chapter 40).

The intestines eliminate solid waste products and some fluid from the body. The elimination of solid waste by bowel evacuation usually becomes a pattern at 30 to 36 months of age (see Chapter 41).

Assessment

A client whose urinary elimination needs are unmet may become incontinent or develop urinary tract infection. *Total incontinence* can occur because the person is unable to perceive the urge to void, as when waking from general anesthesia or after severe head injury or spinal cord injury. Total incontinence may also occur if an immobilized person is unable to reach a bedpan or obtain assistance.

Unmet urinary elimination needs also result in fluid and electrolyte imbalances. A *fluid volume deficit* such as that occurring with dehydration or shock may lead to an imbalance in waste products eliminated by the kidneys. An electrolyte imbalance may result from an acute or chronic kidney disorder.

A client's unmet needs for bowel elimination may lead to changes in the pattern of elimination or diet intake. Changes in bowel elimination patterns can result in the nursing diagnoses of *bowel incontinence, constipation,* and *diarrhea.* Altering the diet intake of fluids and foods can also change elimination patterns and needs.

Nursing Implications

Nursing care assists the client in meeting elimination needs. Nursing intervention may be simple, such as providing privacy or changing the diet, or complex, such as inserting a catheter or administering an enema. When helping clients meet urinary and bowel elimination needs, a nurse uses knowledge of anatomy and physiology, as well as specific skills and techniques. Chapters 40 and 41 describe in detail the knowledge and skills needed to meet urinary and bowel elimination needs of clients.

Shelter

All humans need shelter. Although most people have some kind of shelter, sometimes it is substandard and does not offer full protection. Disasters such as floods, fire, and tornadoes can render an entire community homeless. Disaster agencies such as the Red Cross and health care services such as Visiting Nurses Association, Public Health Nursing Clinics, and homeless shelters are resources in helping clients obtain permanent shelter.

Assessment

Often the nurse can identify environmental risk factors in a client's home that may indicate that shelter needs are not being meet. These include exposure to temperature extremes, as in a poorly insulated, drafty home or a poorly ventilated home without air conditioning. Others may involve physical safety of the home and its environment. A home with a leaky roof and an unprotected home in a high-crime neighborhood are inadequate shelters.

Clients with limited financial, social, and family resources are at risk for unmet shelter needs. Frequently, such clients are older or handicapped or have limited job skills. Often, they feel trapped in their environment because they are unaware of resources that can help them relocate.

When assessing whether a client is meeting shelter needs, the nurse identifies risk factors for illness or injury. Environments that are dirty may attract insects or rodents that can increase the risk for illness. If a home is poorly lit or cluttered, there is an increased risk of accidental injury. In addition, overcrowding and lack of cleanliness are predisposing factors to communicable diseases.

Nursing Implications

In many situations, it is unrealistic for a nurse to seek new shelter for a client and family. However, the nurse makes referrals to community agencies that can help. Community agencies can establish standards for rental housing and help a client pay utility bills or make home repairs. Such agencies can also help the client identify alternatives for shelter.

The nurse can help the client make changes within the home to make it healthier. For example, rails can be installed in a bathroom for a client who has difficulty ambulating and maneuvering. Health promotion often involves teaching clients about the relationship between home environment and health.

Rest

Every person has a basic physiological need for regular rest. The amount of sleep needed varies, depending on the person's quality of sleep, health status, activity patterns, lifestyle, and age.

A client with chronic disease requires more rest than a healthy person of the same age. Pregnancy, lactation, and health status changes such as surgery also increase the need for rest. Physical and emotional stress may also increase a client's need for rest. Rest and sleep often provide temporary relief from stress. However, rest can also be a nonproductive method for resolving stress; a client may depend on it as an escape.

Assessment

With insufficient sleep, a person's appearance and behavior change. Circles under the client's eyes and a disheveled appearance are signs of such change. The person may also have less energy, seem less motivated, be more irritable or withdrawn, stare into space, have difficulty concentrating, and be restless.

Nursing Implications

When possible, the nurse should plan care to fit the client's usual sleep-wake cycle. Any bedtime habits, such as walking, bathing, reading, or drinking milk, should be incorporated into the care plan.

Frequently rest patterns are changed by illness or pain. The nurse uses specific methods to promote comfort and relieve pain so that the client's need for rest can be anticipated and met (see Chapters 36 and 37). If the client is unable to sleep and rest because of other factors, such as lifestyle or chronic stress, the nurse directs care at resolving the cause while helping meet these needs.

Sex

Sex is considered by Maslow (1970) to be a basic physiological need that generally takes priority over higher-level needs. Sexual needs and the manner in which they are met are influenced by age, sociocultural background, ethics, values, self-esteem, and level of wellness.

Health professionals are giving increasing attention to sexuality as a component of health. Nurses take sexual needs into consideration as they become more knowledgeable about them. Sexuality involves more than physical sex. It may be emotional, social, and spiritual needs. Sexuality can be affected by illness, chronic conditions, and hospitalization.

Assessment

A client unable to meet sexual needs may, through behavior, indicate that these needs are unmet. Some clients seek alternatives that may not meet sexual needs or may lead to other conflicts, such as excessive sexual language, excessive masturbation, or exposure of sexual organs. Other clients flirt or redirect sexual need to physical exercise, overeating, or overwork.

Paralysis, mastectomy, and colostomy are physical conditions that can affect how people feel about sexuality and the ability to fulfill sexual needs because of a change in physical appearance. Their sexual behaviors, including activities other than those involving sexual organs, may require readjustment.

Clients experiencing depression, grief, or lifestyle changes are at risk for having unmet sexual needs. For some clients the meeting of sexual needs is only temporarily interrupted. For others, especially those with severe depression, sexual needs are unmet longer and may resolve only with counseling.

Nursing Implications

Nursing care designed to resolve *altered sexuality patterns* or *sexual dysfunction* must consider the client's age, maturity, developmental level, values, habits, level of health, sexual partner, and sexual practices. Not all nurses feel competent to discuss sexuality with clients, but it is important to recognize a client's inability to meet sexual needs so that another nurse, physician, or social worker can help. Chapter 32 discusses sexuality in detail.

Nursing Diagnosis

The nurse assesses specific physiological and other basic needs. From the assessment, nursing di-

Examples of Nursing Diagnoses Related to Unmet Needs

NANDA-APPROVED NURSING DIAGNOSES

Impaired gas exchange related to:
- Physiological change resulting from escaping gas
- Slow adaptation to a high-altitude climate

High risk for fluid volume deficit related to:
- Excessive water loss secondary to prolonged vomiting and diarrhea

Altered nutrition: less than body requirements related to:
- Lack of finances
- Poor access to grocery stores

Activity intolerance related to:
- Inadequate nutrition
- Lack of rest

High risk for injury related to:
- Inadequate safe housing
- Lack of protection from environmental elements

Ineffective individual coping related to:
- Feelings of loss and loneliness
- Loss of friends or loved one

agnoses are developed by clustering defining and relevant characteristics. The diagnoses box on p. 895 provides examples of nursing diagnoses for clients with unmet needs. Identification of related factors further specifies the diagnostic statement, thus individualizing it for each client.

 SAFETY AND SECURITY NEEDS

Next in priority after the client's physiological needs are needs for physical and psychological safety and security.

Physical Safety

An infant enters the world totally dependent on others for needs and physical safety. As the infant grows and develops, greater independence is gradually achieved. Adults are generally able to provide for their physical safety, but the ill and handicapped may need help.

Maintaining physical safety involves reducing or eliminating threats to body or life (see Chapter 42). The threat may be illness, accident, danger, or environmental exposure. When ill, a client may be vulnerable to complications such as infection and therefore depends on professionals in the health care system for protection.

Meeting physical safety needs sometimes takes precedence over meeting a physiological need. For example, a nurse may need to protect a disoriented client from falling out of bed before providing care to meet nutritional needs.

Assessment

When assessing the physical safety needs of a client, the nurse considers actual and potential threats. Clients with limited movement or total immobilization of an extremity are at risk for developing joint contractures, skin breakdown, and muscle atrophy (see Chapter 43). Clients taking medication are at risk for side effects. Clients with indwelling intravenous lines or Foley catheters are at risk for secondary infections.

Clients with acute or chronic illnesses, disability, or handicaps may need help meeting safety needs. The nurse assesses the total environment, whether it is the client's home or a hospital, to identify potential or actual threats.

Health problems in other dimensions may also present a safety risk to a client. Clients under emotional stress, for example, may behave in a manner that might threaten their safety. A socially isolated client may be unaware of environmental factors that threaten physical safety.

Nursing Implications

The early identification of defining characteristics to support the diagnosis of *high risk for injury* is perhaps the best way to select strategies that maintain the client's safety. For example, nurses teach parents about common risks to their children throughout the developmental stages (see Chapters 24, 25, and 42).

The nurse teaches clients receiving medication or therapy about side effects, interaction effects, and potential hazards of treatments, as well as the desired effects. The nurse individualizes education for clients and families to best assist in meeting their safety needs.

In addition, the nurse increases the client's physical safety in a health care setting by maintaining electric beds in the low position, with the side rails up and call light within easy reach. The hospital or home bedroom is uncluttered so that the client can easily move about without risk of injury. Last, frequent observation of the client maintains continual assessment of physiological and psychosocial status and complications or threats that can be reduced.

Psychological Safety

To be safe and secure psychologically, a person must understand what to expect from others, including family members and health care professionals. The person must also know what to expect from procedures, new experiences, and encounters within the environment. Everyone feels some threat to psychological safety with new and unfamiliar experiences. A student entering college may feel insecure, a person starting a new job may feel threatened by having to interact with unfamiliar people, and a client about to undergo a diagnostic test may be threatened by the technology involved. In such cases, people generally do not directly state that their psychological safety is threatened, but their conversation may indirectly reveal their feelings.

Assessment

Assessment of psychological safety is often difficult because the nurse may have to interpret the client's language and behaviors. Because a perceived threat causes stress, the client may act in various ways to adapt to the stress (see Chapter 30). The client's behavior may change radically. For example, an outgoing, active person may become withdrawn, or a previously cooperative client may suddenly refuse to participate in care. Most clients want to be active and cooperative, and a drastic change in behavior is a clue that some threat to psychological safety may be felt.

Nursing Implications

The nurse can use teaching methods for the nursing diagnoses of *ineffective individual* or *family coping* or *high risk for ineffective coping* to reduce a threat to psychological safety, particularly when the potential threat includes a change in role, a change in body image, or an invasive diagnostic or surgical procedure. Because people often fear the unknown or have unrealistic expectations about it, telling clients and their families what to expect greatly reduces anxiety and increases their participation in health care.

Healthy adults are generally able to meet physical and physiological safety needs without help from health care professionals. However, ill or handicapped people are more susceptible to threats to physical and emotional well-being, so the nurse intervenes to help protect them from harm.

 ## LOVE AND BELONGING NEEDS

The next priority after physiological and safety needs is the need for love and belonging. People generally need to feel that they are loved by their family and that they are accepted by peers and the community. This need generally arises after physiological and safety needs are met because only when individuals feel safe and secure do they have the time and energy to seek love and belonging and to share that love with others (Rogers, 1961).

Even a person who is generally able to meet needs for love and belonging is often unable to fulfill them when illness or injury occurs. It becomes even more difficult in the hospital. The client is forced to adapt to aspects of the health care delivery system such as organization, routines, environmental limitations, and visiting hours. As a result, there is little time or energy left to meet the needs for love and belonging with family or significant others.

Assessment

A client of any age in any health care setting may have difficulty meeting love and belonging needs. The ways in which these unmet needs are manifested depend on the client. The client's behavior may be similar to the adaptive behaviors of a person responding to stress.

Discussion with the family is important as the nurse compares the client's needs for love and belonging with fulfillment of these needs. The nurse may identify changes in the family or in a relationship with a family member that can provide insight into the client's needs for love and belonging.

Physical and behavioral changes may indicate that a client is unable to meet love and belonging needs. The client's appearance and hygiene habits may change. A normally well-groomed person may seem uncaring about appearance. The client may complain of physical ailments such as headaches or gastrointestinal problems when separated from family. Sleep and eating habits may also change.

Conversation often demonstrates that needs for love and belonging are not being met. A hospitalized client may speak often of family or friends expected to visit. In addition, a client who becomes anxious because family or friends have not yet visited may attempt to cope with unmet needs by insisting that it does not matter. A child separated from parents because of illness or injury may seem to adopt the nurse as a surrogate parent. A client may attempt to interact with the nurse as a close friend or may even become possessive about the amount of time spent with the nurse. All of these behaviors are manifestations of the normal need for love and affection.

If a person's need persists for a long period without being met, behavior may change in more noticeable ways. A usually mild-tempered person may become easily irritated. An outgoing person may withdraw from interaction with co-workers and friends. The person's work habits may change, leading to increased absenteeism or overcommitment to the job.

Nursing Implications

The nursing care plan for clients should include means by which needs for love and belonging can be met. For example, if the client is a young child who will be hospitalized for a long time, the care plan should include specific opportunities for the child and family to interact. In some cases, it may be important for the mother or father to remain overnight.

A client with the nursing diagnosis of *social isolation* caused by illness or injury cannot meet needs for love and belonging in the usual ways. If opportunities for social interaction are limited, the client may have a sense of not belonging and begin to withdraw. The nurse can take specific actions to help the client maintain social contacts and thus meet love and belonging needs. A hospitalized client may benefit from short social visits by members of the health care team. Resources in the community may help. For example, an older client can be helped to meet the need for contact through a senior citizens' center.

Finally, the nurse works with clients and families to adapt care plans to help clients meet their needs for love and belonging. The more actively involved clients are in developing care plans and the more control they have over the environment while receiving care, the easier it is for them to meet these needs.

ESTEEM AND SELF-ESTEEM NEEDS

People need a stable sense of self-esteem, as well as the feeling that they are held in regard by others. The need for self-esteem is linked to the desire for strength, achievement, adequacy, competence, confidence, and independence. People also need recognition or appreciation from others. When both of these needs are met, a person feels self-confident and useful. If needs for self-esteem and esteem of others are unfulfilled, a person may feel helpless and inferior (Maslow, 1970).

Assessment

A change in roles may threaten self-esteem. The change may be anticipated, such as retirement, or sudden, such as an injury. A change in independence and relationship with others occurs with role changes. A person who was formerly independent may become more dependent, and relationships with others may become strained. A person may become more dependent on family members, social agencies, or health care professionals and may begin to question usefulness and importance. The client may lose self-esteem. If no longer functioning in a former role, such as that of a worker, a person may feel that the esteem of others is lost as well.

Changes in body image, such as those caused by illness or injury, may also influence self-esteem. Body image changes include obvious changes such as the amputation of a leg and nonobservable changes such as a hysterectomy. Normal developmental changes such as puberty or menopause can change a person's image.

It is not the magnitude of a change in body image or role that affects self-esteem, but rather how the person perceives the self after the change. A person's sense of self-esteem and the esteem of others therefore depend on values and beliefs, support from others, and self-concept.

There are many indications of unmet needs for self-esteem or the esteem of others. A client who feels helpless or inferior may defer all decisions rather than express wishes. The client may become self-critical or seem unusually lethargic or apathetic about anything involving the self, including appearance. The person's general attitude may be summed up as a feeling of hopelessness. In some cases a client with low self-esteem may avoid or ignore opportunities for actions that could increase self-esteem because of the possibility of failure. The loss of self-esteem can thus become a self-fulfilling prophecy.

A client feeling the lack of esteem of other people may test others by making statements that call for their approval or praise. Conversely, the client may act in a way that prevents such approval if little self-esteem is present and the client is certain of failure.

Nursing Implications

Helping to resolve a *self-esteem disturbance* can begin with the first contact between client and nurse. From the beginning the nurse must convey respect for the client as an individual. Even though the client may have different beliefs and values, the nurse needs to accept, not judge, the client's values.

If clients' self-concepts are changed by illness or injury, nursing care involves improving self-concept and body image. Specific nursing actions depend on clients' support systems and personalities, the cause of altered self-concept, and available resources (see Chapter 31). If clients' levels of self-esteem are so low that they fail to care for themselves, the nurse may have to help meet other needs, such as those for nutrition and safety, while taking steps to increase self-esteem.

NEED FOR SELF-ACTUALIZATION

Self-actualization is the highest level of needs in Maslow's hierarchy of human needs. Theoretically, when people have met all the lower-level needs, it is by self-actualization that they achieve their fullest potential (Maslow, 1970).

Self-actualized people have multiple characteristics (see box). They have a mature multidimensional personality, frequently they are able to assume and complete multiple tasks, and they achieve fulfillment from the pleasure of a job well done. They do not totally depend on the opinions of others about appearance, quality of work, or problem-solving methods. Although they may have failings and doubts, they generally deal with them realistically.

Present needs, environment, and stressors depend on how well people meet their need for self-actualization. Self-actualization is possible when there is a balance among the clients' needs, stressors, and ability to adapt to changes of the body and environment.

Assessment

Illness, injury, loss of a loved one, change in role, and change in status can threaten or disturb self-ac-

---

Assessment Characteristics for Self-Actualization

- Solves own problems
- Assists others in problem solving
- Accepts suggestions of others
- Has broad interests in work and social topics
- Possesses good communication skills as a listener and communicator
- Manages stress and assists others in managing stress
- Enjoys privacy
- Seeks new experiences and knowledge
- Shows confidence in abilities and decisions
- Anticipates problems and successes
- Likes self

---

tualization. A loss of self-actualization occurs when a client can no longer achieve the fullest potential because of the limitations imposed by the illness or injury. This loss may result in behavioral changes. The client may feel frustrated because the illness prevents decision making, creativity, and independent problem solving. Instead, because of the illness, the client is forced to be more self-centered, more dependent on others, and motivated more by external factors.

Nursing Implications

The major focus for nursing care is to restore the client as much as possible to a self-actualized state. Nursing care is planned to encourage the client to make decisions when possible, particularly in regard to health care. Thus the nurse seeks the involvement of the client when planning and delivering nursing care.

Because the self-actualized person tends to be creative and highly individual in many ways, nursing care should include the opportunity to fulfill creative needs. The client should be encouraged to continue with specific projects, and if the client is hospitalized, time should be set aside for them. Frequently, hospital routines leave little free time for relaxing activities.

The client's need for privacy must be respected and met. When in good health the self-actualized person generally has a strong need for privacy. An illness, especially in a hospital setting, can greatly reduce privacy. Nurses can help meet this need by planning health care so that privacy will not be interrupted during specific times.

 ## APPLICATION OF BASIC NEEDS THEORY

Maslow's theory of human needs can provide a basis for nursing care of clients of all ages and in a variety of health settings. When the nurse applies this theory in practice, however, the focus is on the needs of the individual rather than rigid adherence to Maslow's hierarchy. Maslow's hierarchy is a generalization about the need priorities of most but not all people. In all cases, an emergency physiological need takes precedence over a higher-level need. With one client the need for self-esteem may be a higher priority than a long-term nutritional need, whereas for another client, this may be reversed. To provide the most effective care, the nurse needs to understand relationships among different needs for the individual. Furthermore, although the hierarchy of needs suggests that one need should be met before another, nursing care often addresses two or more at the same time.

Relationships Among Needs

In some nursing situations, it is unrealistic to expect a client's basic needs to be fulfilled in the fixed hierarchical order. For example, a client enters the health care system with a chronic respiratory infection. While providing care, the nurse learns that the client has not eaten adequately, slept well, or maintained social relationships since his wife died 2 years before. In this case the client has several unmet needs, including the physiological needs for nutrition and rest and needs for love and a sense of belonging. For the client, these separate needs are closely related. Nursing care in this situation would not simply be directed to helping the client meet the higher-priority needs for nutrition and rest because these needs in part occurred because the client was not meeting lower-priority needs. Nursing care focuses also on assisting this client through the grief process (see Chapter 28) so that, after grief and loneliness have been resolved, former eating and sleeping habits will be regained and thus these physiological needs will be met.

An opposite relationship among similar needs may be true of a different client. For example, a woman is receiving treatment for severe arthritis and often feels pain or discomfort during certain activities. Because of this, she has changed her habits and no longer visits family members and friends. The nurse realizes that the woman also has unmet needs for love and belonging. These two sets of needs are clearly related and the nurse provides care directed at meeting both. In this situation, however, the priority is to provide relief from pain, which will then allow the woman to return to former activities that meet the lower-priority needs.

For different individuals, needs on different levels may be related in different ways. Some people may give sexual need a higher priority than the need for love, whereas for others, sexual need is deferred until the need for love is met. Similarly, people with unmet needs for self-esteem may be unable to seek fulfillment of the need for love if their self-esteem is so low that they feel inferior and fear rejection. In these and many other ways, needs on different levels may be closely related for individuals. When assessing needs and planning care, the nurse must not assume that a lower-level need always takes priority. As with all other aspects of providing care, the nurse individualizes the nursing care plan to provide for unique needs and desires.

Simultaneous Meeting of Needs

The nurse provides care for clients with many needs because illness often disrupts the ability to meet needs on different levels. After identifying clients' specific needs, the nurse generally has to set priorities to help them meet these needs. However, setting priorities does not mean that the nurse provides care for only one need at a time. The nurse does not, for example, simply begin with the first need in the hierarchy and move up only after the first has been met. In emergency situations, of course, physiological needs take precedence, but even then the nurse is aware of other needs. Even in an emergency the nurse considers clients' higher-level needs.

A young man who is hospitalized with paraplegia resulting from a severed spinal cord, for example, needs assistance in meeting physiological needs. However, he may also have low self-esteem related to his condition. The nurse is faced with the challenge of simultaneously meeting his physiological needs and need for self-esteem because he may not eat properly or participate in physical care if he does not feel good about himself. The nurse should not offer the client false hope about future recovery. However, while planning care to meet physiological needs the nurse can include measures that will help restore self-esteem.

Factors Influencing Need Priorities

Ideally, nursing care can be directed at the simultaneous meeting of several needs. In practice, though, one need often takes precedence over another, and priorities must be determined so that care can be more focused and effective. Life-threatening situations always take priority, and unmet physiological needs that pose a threat to life certainly have a high priority. In other situations the nurse considers factors that influence the priority of needs for an individual.

A person's personality and mood affect the perception of and ability to meet a particular need. A depressed person may react negatively to a suggestion for an activity that could increase self-esteem, although in another mood the person might respond with enthusiasm. Thus when providing care to help meet several needs, the nurse can adjust the care plan to correspond most effectively to the client's personality and mood.

Some needs must be deferred until the client is in better health. A client recovering from an acute gastrointestinal infection should not be encouraged to resume physical activities related to needs for self-esteem until needs for physical safety and security have been met by achieving full health. Similarly, a diabetic client whose condition is unstable may have to defer other needs until nutritional needs related to insulin therapy are satisfied.

The client's perception of needs varies among socioeconomic and cultural groups (see Chapter 4). In addition, the client's perception of some needs, such as sexual needs, varies between the sexes and within different developmental levels. The nurse considers the client's perception of needs when planning care and does not impose personal perceptions about priorities.

The client's family structure can influence the way needs are satisfied (see Chapter 23). A mother may, for example, place the needs of an infant before her own, such as when she interrupts a meal or sleep to feed the child.

When setting need priorities, the nurse considers that basic needs are interrelated. Physiological functioning is closely related to body systems, environment, values, ethics, and culture. One need does not occur independently of others. For example, if nutritional needs are unmet for a long time, a person begins to show signs of malnutrition, the body deteriorates, weakness occurs, and the client is unable to recognize or meet the lower-priority needs of safety, love, and self-esteem. Needs are interrelated in unique ways for each person, and the nurse considers such relationships in planning care. Rather than simply following the hierarchy of the human needs theory, the nurse involves the client and family in planning so that need priorities are not neglected.

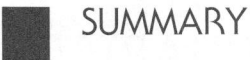

SUMMARY

Healthy adults are usually able to meet most of their basic needs. As an adult ages or becomes ill or handicapped, the risk of not being able to meet basic needs increases.

Maslow's theory proposes that a hierarchical relationship exists among different levels of human needs. A client entering the health care system may have one or more unmet needs at different levels. Nursing care addresses all client needs. Essential, life-sustaining needs generally take priority over others. The client's different needs may be interrelated in unique ways, and the nurse considers the client's priorities. Nursing care may be directed at meeting several needs simultaneously. The care plan is based on the nurse's assessment of the extent to which the client is meeting, and is able to meet, all needs.

Nursing involves providing care for the whole person. The nurse applies knowledge about the body systems and about the client's family, social system, emotions, values, ethics, and goals of health care. In this way the theory of human needs corresponds to nursing's holistic perspective by addressing the client's needs in the physiological, psychological, sociocultural, developmental, and spiritual dimensions. The basic needs theory is appropriate and applicable in community health, psychiatric, outpatient, and institutional settings, including critical-care units and rehabilitation centers. This theory can provide a basis for nursing care for clients of all ages and developmental stages, from the neonate to the geriatric client. The human needs theory is therefore a set of concepts important for the nurse's understanding of health and illness and the client's position on the health-illness continuum.

Key Concepts

- Basic human needs are the needs for things such as oxygen, food, water, safety, and love required to survive and be healthy.

- Some human needs are more necessary to survival than others and must be met first.

- Maslow's hierarchy is a theoretical representation of the levels of basic needs.

- The very young, very old, chronically ill, and handicapped are generally less able than others to meet needs without assistance.

- The highest priority is given to physiological needs, including oxygen, fluid, nutrition, temperature, elimination, shelter, rest, and sexuality.

- Oxygen is the most essential physiological need. A chronic or acute oxygen need can be identified by confusion, lethargy, rapid and shallow respirations, an inability to lie flat, nasal flaring, retractions, a decreased level of consciousness, and cyanosis.

- Fluid needs require a balance between the intake and output of fluids. Dehydration or edema indicates unmet fluid needs.

- Dehydration may result in flushed and dry skin, poor skin turgor, a coated tongue, dry mucous membranes, decreased saliva, decreased tears, and oliguria.

- Edema may result in the swelling of a dependent body part, weight gain, shortness of breath, increased heart rate, and smooth, shiny skin.

- Nutritional needs require an adequate intake of foods to allow the body to carry on metabolic processes. Unmet nutritional needs may be indicated by weight loss or failure to grow or gain weight, fatigue, pallor, and recurring sores in the mouth and gums.

- The body is able to function within only a small temperature range, 37° C (98.6° F) ± 1° C. Unmet temperature needs may result from exposure to cold or heat.

- Elimination needs involve the body's removal of excess fluids and wastes. The body meets these needs by elimination through the skin, lungs, kidneys, and intestines.

- The need for shelter is a physiological need. Unmet needs can be identified through assessment of the environment.

- Sleep and rest needs vary, depending on the individual's quality of sleep, age, health status, activity patterns, and lifestyle. Unmet needs may result in a decreased level of energy, disheveled appearance, irritability, decreased concentration, and restlessness.

- People have different needs related to sexuality at different times in life, and the manifestation of unmet sexual needs can take many forms.

- Safety and security needs include physical and psychological safety and the need to prevent complications.

- Clients in the health care system may be unable to meet their needs for love and belonging because of changes in relationships with others and the separation often imposed by illness.

- People need self-esteem and the esteem of others. Illness, role changes, and changes in body image may threaten the ability to meet these needs.

- The self-actualized person is autonomous, easily motivated, and not self-centered. The need for self-actualization can be threatened by changes that occur with illness or injury.
- To apply basic needs theory in practice, the nurse considers the relationships among the client's specific needs, sets priorities for meeting needs by considering the client's priorities, and when possible and necessary assists the client in simultaneously meeting needs on different levels.

Key Terms

Aerobic metabolism, p. 891

Anaerobic metabolism, p. 891

Basic human needs, p. 890

Cyanosis, p. 891

Dehydration, p. 892

Edema, p. 892

Esteem and self-esteem needs, p. 890

Frostbite, p. 893

Hierarchy of basic human needs, p. 890

Love and belonging needs, p. 890

Oliguria, p. 892

Physiological needs, p. 890

Safety and security needs, p. 890

Self-actualization, p. 890

Critical Thinking Exercises

1. When meeting clients' basic needs how do you establish priorities of care?
2. How do you determine when to meet psychosocial needs before physiological needs?
3. What information do you need to design a care plan to simultaneously meet several basic needs?

REFERENCES

Maslow AH: *Motivation and personality,* ed 2, New York, 1970, Harper & Row.

Mountcastle VR: *Medical physiology,* ed 14, St Louis, 1980, Mosby—Year Book.

Rogers C: *On becoming a person,* Boston, 1961, Houghton Mifflin.

ADDITIONAL READINGS

Maslow AH: *Toward a psychology of being,* ed 2, New York, 1968, Van Nostrand Reinhold.

Maslow AH: Toward a humanistic biology, *Am Psychol* 24:724, 1969.

CHAPTER 30

Adaptation to Stress

OBJECTIVES

Mastery of content in this chapter will enable the student to:

- Define the key terms listed.
- Discuss the limitations of homeostatic control.
- Discuss four models of stress as they relate to nursing practice.
- Describe how adaptation occurs in each of the five dimensions.
- Describe two forms of local physiological adaptation.
- Describe the three phases of the general adaptation syndrome.
- List and discuss behaviors that are responses to stress.
- List and discuss the most common ego-defense mechanisms that are responses to stress.
- Discuss the effects of prolonged stress on each of the five dimensions of a person's functioning.
- Describe stress-management techniques that nurses can help clients use.
- Discuss techniques of crisis intervention.
- Describe stress-management techniques that can benefit nurses themselves.

CHAPTER OUTLINE

Every person experiences forms of stress throughout life. Stress can provide the stimulus for change and growth, and in this respect, some stress can be positive. However, too much stress can result in poor judgment, physical illness, and inability to cope.

Various disciplines such as nursing, physiology, and sociology have attempted to define *stress* within the boundaries of that specific discipline. However, each group works in isolation from the other groups, leading to a disparity in the literature about stress. Stress is a phenomenon that affects the social, psychological, developmental, spiritual, and physiological dimensions. It involves the intellectual, behavioral, and metabolic responses to a stressor (Lindsay, Carrieri, 1986).

Claude Bernard, in 1867, was one of the first physiologists to recognize the consequences of stress. He proposed that changes in the internal and external environments disrupted the functioning of an organism and that it was essential for an organism to adapt to a stressor to survive. In 1920, Walter Cannon studied physiological responses to emotional arousal and emphasized the adaptive functions of the "fight-or-flight" reaction. Cannon also noted that these responses were the result of the influence of the emotional state on the body and that the subsequent responses were adaptive and physiological (Robinson, 1990).

In 1976, Hans Selye developed a biochemical model of stress known as the general adaptation syndrome (GAS), which described physiological events during a stress response. Selye also introduced the concept of **stressors,** which are internal or external stimuli that cause stress (Selye, 1976). Selye's classic research into stress and stressors has been important for health care professionals. Current research is focused on a variety of stress and stress-related concepts.

CONCEPTS OF STRESS

Stress and Stressors

Everyone experiences stress from time to time, and normally a person is able to adapt to long-term stress or cope with short-term stress until it passes. Stress can place heavy demands on a person, and if the person is unable to adapt, illness can result.

Stress is any situation in which a nonspecific demand requires an individual to respond or take action (Selye, 1976; Numerof, 1983; McNett, 1989; Lindsay, Carrieri, 1986). It involves physiological and psychological responses. Stress can lead to negative or counterproductive feelings or threaten emotional well-being. Stress can threaten the way a person normally perceives reality, solves problems, or thinks in general. It can threaten relationships and sense of belonging. In addition, stress can threaten a person's general outlook on life, attitude toward loved ones, job satisfaction, ability to problem solve, and health status (Kline-Leidy, 1990; Oberst et al, 1991; Bartoldus, Gillery, Sturges, 1989).

An individual's perception or experience of a major change initiates the stress response. The stimuli preceding or precipitating the change are called *stressors.* Stressors may be physiological, psychological, social, environmental, developmental, spiritual, or cultural and represent an unmet need. Stressors can generally be classified as *internal* or *external.* **Internal stressors** originate inside a person (for example, a fever, a condition such as pregnancy or menopause, or an emotion such as guilt). **External stressors** originate outside a person (for example, a marked change in environmental temperature, a change in family or social role, or peer pressure).

Physiological Adaptation

Physiological adaptation to stress is the body's ability to maintain a state of relative balance. This adaptive ability is a dynamic form of equilibrium in the body's internal environment. The internal environment constantly changes and the body's adaptive mechanisms continually function to adjust to these changes and thus to maintain equilibrium, or **homeostasis.**

Homeostasis is maintained by physiological mechanisms that control body functions and monitor body organs. For the most part, these mechanisms are controlled by the nervous and endocrine systems and do not involve conscious behavior. The body makes adjustments in heart rate, respiratory rate, blood pressure, temperature, fluid and electrolyte balances, hormone secretions, and level of consciousness—all directed at maintaining adaptation.

Mechanisms of Physiological Adaptation

When a person becomes aware of an unmet physiological need, such as food or warmth, deliberate actions can meet the need. For the most part, however, adaptation involves adjustments that the body makes automatically to maintain equilibrium. These homeostatic mechanisms are self-regulatory; in other words, they are automatic. In a person with an illness or injury, however, the mechanisms may not be able to maintain and sustain homeostasis.

Physiological mechanisms of adaptation function also through negative feedback, a process by which the controlling mechanism senses an abnormal state, such as lowered body temperature, and makes an adaptive response, such as initiating shivering to generate body heat. Three of the major mechanisms used in adapting to a stressor are controlled by the medulla oblongata, the reticular formation, and the pituitary gland.

MEDULLA OBLONGATA. The **medulla oblongata** controls vital functions necessary to survival. These include heart rate, blood pressure, and respiration. Impulses traveling to and from the medulla oblongata can increase or decrease these vital functions. For example, regulation of the heart beat is the result of sympathetic or parasympathetic nervous system impulses traveling from the medulla oblongata to the heart. The heart rate increases in response to impulses from sympathetic fibers and decreases with impulses from parasympathetic fibers.

RETICULAR FORMATION. The **reticular formation** is a small cluster of neurons in the brainstem and spinal cord. It also controls vital functions and continuously monitors the physiological status of the body through connections with sensory and motor tracts. For example, certain cells within the reticular formation can cause a sleeping person to regain consciousness or increase the level of consciousness when a need arises.

PITUITARY GLAND. The **pituitary gland,** a small gland attached to the hypothalamus, supplies hormones that control vital functions. The pituitary gland produces hormones necessary for adaptation to stress. In addition, the pituitary gland regulates the secretion of thyroid, gonadal, and parathyroid hormones. Hormone secretion, like other homeostatic mechanisms, is normally regulated by a feedback mechanism, which continuously monitors hormone levels in the blood. When hormone levels drop, the pituitary gland receives a message to increase hormone secretion. When hormone levels rise, the pituitary gland decreases hormone production.

Limitations of Physiological Mechanisms of Adaptation

Physiological mechanisms of adaptation work together through complex relationships in the nervous and endocrine systems and other body systems to maintain a relative constancy within the body. In a healthy person, these mechanisms affect physiological balance, and the body's needs are met. However, physiological mechanisms of adaptation can provide only short-term control over the body's equilibrium. They cannot adapt to long-term changes in hormone secretion or vital functions. Thus illness, injury, or prolonged stress can decrease the adaptive capacity. Decreased functioning can result in continued but inadequate homeostatic control or breakdown of the feedback mechanism that allows control. Either form of decreased function can result in further illness or death.

In severe stress situations, for example, the pituitary gland supplies the body with the necessary hormones. However, these hormones may be insufficient in quantity to provide the physiological energy necessary for coping. In this case the person's condition deteriorates, and functioning declines. The feedback mechanism of homeostatic control may break down because of organ abnormality.

Models of Stress

The origins and effects of stress can be examined in terms of medical and behavioral theoretical models. Stress models are used to identify the stressors for a particular individual and predict that person's responses to them. Each model emphasizes a different aspect of stress.

The nurse uses stress models to help a client cope with unhealthy, nonproductive responses to stressors. With modifications, these models can help the nurse individualize care plans.

Response-Based Model of Stress

The response-based model is concerned with specifying the particular response or pattern of responses that may indicate a stressor (Lyon, Werner, 1987). Selye's model of stress (1976) is a response-based model that defines stress as a nonspecific response of the body to any demand made on it. Stress is demonstrated by a specific physiological reaction, the GAS. Thus the response of a person to stress is purely physiological and is never modified to allow cognitive influences (McNett, 1989).

The response-based model does not allow individual differences in response patterns. This lack of flexibility may produce some difficulties for nurses because individual differences must be identified in the assessment phase.

Adaptation Model

The adaptation model proposes that four factors determine whether a situation is stressful (Mechanic, 1962). The ability to cope with stress, the first factor, usually depends on the person's experience with similar stressors, support systems, and overall perception of the stressor.

The second factor deals with the practices and norms of the person's peer group. If the peer group considers it normal to talk about a particular stressor, the client may respond by complaining or worrying about it. This response may help adaptation to the stress, or the client may respond in this way simply to conform to peer group behavior.

The third factor is the impact of the social environment in assisting an individual to adapt to a stressor. For example, a college freshman who may have a sexually transmitted disease may confide this fear to an upperclassman, who may then make a referral to a student health service. In this example the resources of the older student and the student health service offer the means of reducing the severity of the stressor.

The last factor involves the resources that can be used to deal with the stressor. In the example just given, the student needs a valid identification card to use the prepaid health benefits, and the health service is open 7 days a week from 9 AM to 9 PM. Both of these factors make the resource easily accessible to help the student cope with the stress.

The adaptation model is based on the understanding that people experience anxiety and increased stress when they are unprepared to cope with stressful situations. Using this model and appropriate interventions, nurses can help clients and families to reduce the effects of stress in all human dimensions.

Stimulus-Based Model

The stimulus-based model focuses on disturbing or disruptive characteristics within the environment. The classic research that identified stress as a stimulus has resulted in the development of the social readjustment scale, which measures the effects of major life events on illness (Holmes, Rahe, 1976). The stimulus-based model focuses on the following assumptions (McNett, 1989):

1. Life change events are normal, and they require the same type and duration of adjustment.
2. People are passive recipients of stress, and their perceptions of the event are irrelevant.
3. All people have a common threshold of stimulus, and illness results at any point after the threshold.

As with the response-based model, the stimulus-based model does not allow for individual differences in perception and response to stressors. Nurses may experience difficulty when attempting to use this model in stress management because of the lack of flexibility for individual needs.

Transaction-Based Model

The transaction-based model views the person and environment in a dynamic, reciprocal, interactive, relationship (Lazarus, Folkman, 1984). This model, developed by Lazarus and Folkman, views the stressor as an individual perceptual response rooted in psychological and cognitive processes. Stress originates from the relationship between the person and the environment. This model focuses on stress-related processes such as cognitive appraisal and coping (McNett, 1989).

Factors Influencing Response to Stressors

The response to any stressor depends on physiological functioning, personality, and behavioral characteristics, as well as the nature of the stressor. The nature of the stressor involves the following factors:

1. Intensity
2. Scope
3. Duration
4. Number and nature of other stressors

Each factor influences the response to a stressor. A person may perceive the intensity or magnitude of a stressor as minimal, moderate, or severe. The greater the magnitude of the stressor, the greater the stress response. Likewise, the scope of a stressor can be described as limited, medium, or extensive. The greater the scope of a stressor, the greater the response of the client to it (Lazarus, Folkman, 1984).

 ## ADAPTATION TO STRESSORS

Adaptation is the process by which the physiological or psychosocial dimensions change in response to stress. Because many stressors cannot be avoided, health care often focuses on a person's, family's, or community's adaptation to stress.

There are many forms of adaptation. Physiological adaptations make possible a physiological homeostasis. A similar process of adaptation, however, may occur in the psychosocial and other dimensions.

An adaptive response occurs when a stimulus from the internal or external environment causes a departure from the balanced state of the organism. **Adaptation** thus is an attempt to maintain optimal functioning. Adaptation involves reflexes, automatic body mechanisms for protection, coping mechanisms, and instincts (Selye, 1976; Lindsay, Carrieri, 1986). A stressor that stimulates adaptation may be short term, such as a fever, or long term, such as paralysis of a limb. To function optimally, a person must be able to respond to such stressors and adapt to the required demands or changes. Adaptation requires an active response from the whole person.

Like an individual, a family or group may need to adapt to a stressor. Family adaptation is the process by which a family maintains a balance so that it can fulfill its purposes and tasks, deal with stress, and promote the growth of individual members. For a family to adapt successfully, good communication skills, mutual respect for all family members, adequate resources for adaptation, and previous experience with stressors must exist (Fox, 1991; Haber, 1990).

Dimensions of Adaptation

Stress can affect the physical, emotional, intellectual, social, and spiritual dimensions. Adaptive resources exist in each of these dimensions. Therefore when assessing a client's adaptation to stress, a nurse must consider the total person.

Physical Dimension

Physiological adaptation is the process by which the body responds to a stressor to maintain functioning compatible with survival. Physiological adaptive responses are stimulated by demands in the internal environment, such as a fever or inflammation, or in the external environment, such as changes in altitude or ambient temperature. A physiological response to stress may be limited to a particular body area, or it may involve the entire body. The sections on local and general adaptation syndromes will discuss physiological adaptive responses in more detail.

Developmental Dimension

Each developmental stage involves particular tasks and thus potential stressors (see Unit 5). A young adult, for example, may have to adapt to stressors such as establishing a career and rearing children. At the same time, each developmental stage is characterized by potential adaptive resources by which an individual can respond to stress. For example, an older adult, because of greater past experience with certain stressors, may be better able to adapt than a young adult.

Emotional Dimension

Adaptation in the emotional dimension involves the use of normal psychological coping mechanisms to resolve stress. Because everyone has a different personality, every client copes with stress in a different way, although certain basic forms of psychological adaptation are common. Adaptive behavior is most successful when it leads to a sense of discovery and creativity. A person may not always be happy and content when adapting to stress, but the goal of adaptation is to live constructively.

Intellectual Dimension

A person's intellectual dimension includes not only development and education but also perceptions of other people and the world, problem-solving ability, communication patterns, and past coping strategies. Intellectual adaptive responses include gathering information, solving problems, and communicating with others to adjust.

Intellectual adaptation can be strongly influenced by emotions. If people are unable to adapt emotionally to the changes necessitated by illness, for example, they may be less able to adapt intellectually by learning more about their conditions. Similarly, success in emotional adaptation can lead to more effective intellectual adaptation. The nurse is often in a unique position to help clients adapt intellectually to stress.

Social Dimension

Everyone has social relationships with others, including a spouse, family members, co-workers, and peers. This network can be important in helping a person adapt to stressors. The social group may provide psychological support and can help direct a person to resources for coping with stress. For example, friends often can help a person adjust to the death of a loved one by encouraging the person to express feelings. In addition, organized social groups, such as Alcoholics Anonymous, can help people adapt to specific stresses in the social dimension.

A client's social dimension is often closely interrelated with other dimensions. For example, a client unable to cope emotionally with stress may withdraw from contact with people who can assist in adapting.

Spiritual Dimension

A person's spiritual dimension can include beliefs about a supreme being, a feeling of oneness with nature and the world as a whole, and a positive sense of life's meaning and purpose. These beliefs or attitudes can be a powerful resource for adapting to stress. Chapter 33 discusses ways that nurses can help a client meet spiritual needs and use spiritual strength to cope with the effects of illness and other stressors.

 ## RESPONSE TO STRESS

The total person is involved in responding and adapting to stresses. Most research into stress responses, however, focuses on psychological or emotional and physiological responses, even though these dimensions overlap and interact with the other dimensions.

Characteristics of the Stress Response

- Stress response is natural, protective, and adaptive.
- There are normal responses to stressors; stressors encountered in everyday circumstances increase catecholamine excretion, which causes an increase in heart rate and blood pressure.
- Physical and emotional stressors trigger similar responses (specificity versus nonspecificity). Magnitude and patterns may differ.
- There are limits in ability to compensate.
- Magnitude and duration of stressors may be so great that homeostatic mechanisms for adjustment fail, leading to death.
- Repeated exposure to stimuli results in adaptive changes; that is, tissue levels of the enzyme tyrosine hydrolase increase, which increases capacity for the body to produce norepinephrine and epinephrine.
- There are individual differences in response to same stressors.

From Lindsay AM, Carrieri VK: Stress response. In Lindsay AM, Carrieri VK, editors: *Pathological phenomenon in nursing: human response to illness*, Philadelphia, 1986, Saunders.

When stress occurs, a person uses physiological and psychological energy to respond and adapt. The amount of energy required and the effectiveness of the attempt to adapt depend on the intensity, scope, and duration of the stressor and the number of other stressors. The stress response is adaptive and protective, and the characteristics of this response are the result of integrated neuroendocrine response (see box).

Physiological Response

The classic research by Selye (1946, 1976) has identified the two physiological responses to stress: the **local adaptation syndrome (LAS)** and the **general adaptation syndrome (GAS)**. The LAS is a response of a body tissue, organ, or part to the stress of trauma, illness, or other physiological change. The GAS is a defense response of the whole body to stress.

LAS

The body produces many localized responses to stress. These include blood clotting, wound healing (see Chapter 48), accommodation of the eye to light, and response to pressure (see Chapter 44). All forms of the LAS share the following characteristics:

1. The response is localized; it does not involve entire body systems.
2. The response is adaptive, meaning that a stressor is necessary to stimulate it.
3. The response is short term. It does not persist indefinitely.
4. The response is restorative, meaning that the LAS assists in restoring homeostasis to the body region or part.

Two localized responses, the reflex pain response and the inflammatory response, are described here as examples of the LAS. Nurses encounter these responses in many health care settings.

REFLEX PAIN RESPONSE. The reflex pain response is a localized response of the central nervous system to pain (see Chapter 37). It is an adaptive response and protects tissue from further damage. The response involves a sensory receptor, a sensory nerve to the spinal cord, a connector neuron within the spinal cord, a motor nerve from the spinal cord, and an effector muscle. An example would be the unconscious, reflex removal of the hand from a hot surface.

INFLAMMATORY RESPONSE. The inflammatory response is stimulated by trauma or infection. This response localizes the inflammation, thus preventing its spread, and promotes healing. The inflammatory response may produce localized pain, swelling, heat, redness, and changes in functioning. It occurs in three phases. The first phase involves changes in cells and the circulatory system. Initially, narrowing of blood vessels occurs at the injury to control bleeding. Then histamine is released at the injury, increasing blood flow to the area and increasing the number of white blood cells to combat infection. Almost simultaneously kinins are released to increase capillary permeability to permit the flow of proteins, fluid, and leukocytes to the injury. At this point the localized blood flow decreases, keeping leukocytes in the area to fight infection.

The second phase is characterized by release of exudate from the wound. Exudate is a combination of fluid, cells, and other substances produced in the area of injury. The type and amount of exudate vary from injury to injury and from person to person. Exudate is usually released at the injury, which may be a cut, laceration, or surgical incision.

The last phase is repair of tissue by regeneration or scar formation. Regeneration replaces damaged cells with identical or similar cells. Scar formation replaces original tissue that is not functional. The inflammatory response alerts the nurse that the body is adapting to a local injury. During adaptation the inflammatory response protects the body from infection and promotes healing.

GAS

The GAS is a physiological response of the whole body to stress. It involves several body systems, primarily the autonomic nervous system and the endocrine system. Some textbooks refer to the GAS as the *neuroendocrine response*. The GAS consists of the alarm reaction, the resistance stage, and the exhaustion stage (Fig. 30-1).

ALARM REACTION. The alarm reaction involves the mobilization of the defense mechanisms of the body and mind to cope with the stressor. Hormone levels rise to increase blood volume and thereby prepare the person to act. Other hormones are released to increase blood glucose levels to make energy available for adaptation. Increased levels of other hormones—epinephrine and norepinephrine—result in an in-

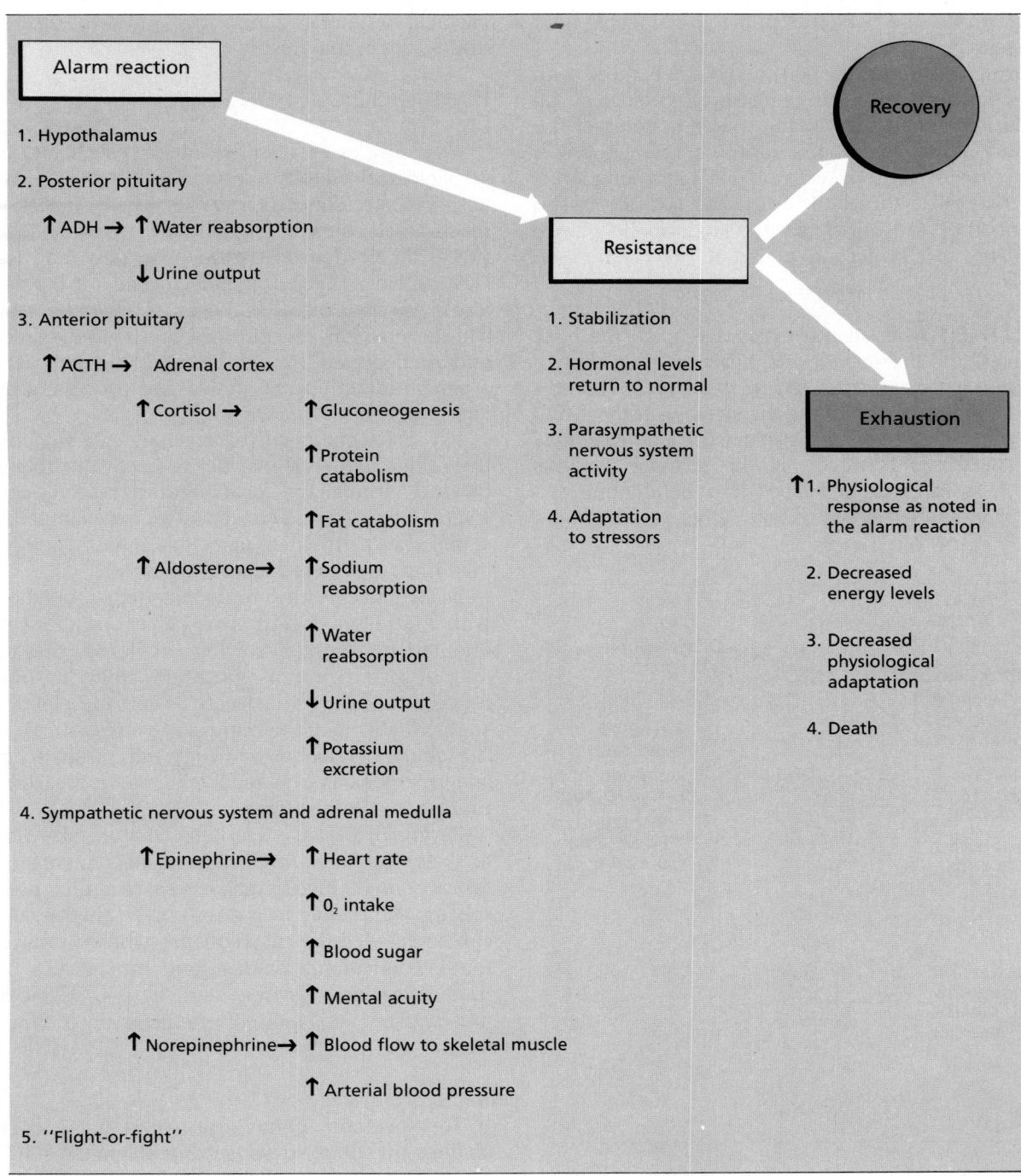

Fig. 30-1 General adaptation syndrome.

creased heart rate, increased blood flow to muscles, increased oxygen intake, and greater mental alertness.

This extensive hormonal activity prepares the person for the **flight-or-fight response**. Cardiac output, oxygen intake, and respiratory rate are increased; the pupils of the eyes are dilated to produce a greater visual field; and the heart rate is increased for more energy. Other changes occur to prepare the person to act (Fig. 30-2). With this increased mental energy and alertness, the person is prepared to flee or fight the stressor.

During the alarm reaction the person is faced with a specific stressor. The person's physiological response is extensive, involving major systems of the body, and it may last from a minute to many hours. If the stressor is extreme or remains for a long time, there may be a threat to life. If the stressor is still present after the initial alarm reaction, the person progresses to the second phase of the GAS, resistance.

RESISTANCE STAGE. In the resistance stage the body stabilizes, and hormone levels, heart rate, blood pressure, and cardiac output return to normal. The person is attempting to adapt to the stressor. If the stress can be resolved, the body repairs damage that may have occurred. However, if the stressor remains present, as in continued blood loss, debilitating disease, or long-term severe mental illness, and adapta-

tion is impossible, the person enters the third phase of the GAS, exhaustion.

EXHAUSTION STAGE. The exhaustion stage occurs when the body can no longer resist stress and when the energy necessary to maintain adaptation is depleted. The physiological response is intensified, but the person's energy level is compromised and adaptation to the stressor diminishes. The body is unable to defend itself against the impact of the stressor, physiological regulation diminishes, and if the stress continues, death may result.

Psychological Response

Exposure to a stressor results in psychological and physiological adaptive responses. As people are exposed to stressors, their ability to meet their basic needs is threatened. This threat, whether actual or perceived, produces frustration, anxiety, and tension (Kline-Leidy, 1990). Psychological adaptive behaviors assist the person's ability to cope with stressors. These behaviors are directed at stress management and are acquired through learning and experience as a person identifies acceptable and successful behaviors.

Psychological adaptive behaviors can be constructive or destructive. Constructive behaviors help an individual accept the challenge to resolve conflict. Even anxiety can be constructive; for example, it can signal that a threat is present so that a person can take measures to reduce its severity.

Destructive behaviors do not help a person cope with a stressor. Destructive behaviors affect reality orientation, problem-solving abilities, personality, and, in severe circumstances, the ability to function. Anxiety can also be destructive (for example, if a person is unable to act to remove the stressor). To some, the abuse of alcohol or drugs may seem to be an adaptive behavior; in reality, it may increase rather than decrease the stress.

Psychological adaptive behaviors are also referred to as *coping mechanisms.* Such mechanisms can be task oriented, involving the use of direct problem-solving techniques to cope with the threats, or they can be ego-defense mechanisms, whose purpose is to regulate emotional distress and thus give a person protection from anxiety and stress. Ego-defense mechanisms are indirect methods of coping with stress.

Task-Oriented Behaviors

Task-oriented behaviors involve using cognitive abilities to reduce stress, solve problems, resolve conflicts, and gratify needs (Stuart, Sundeen, 1991).

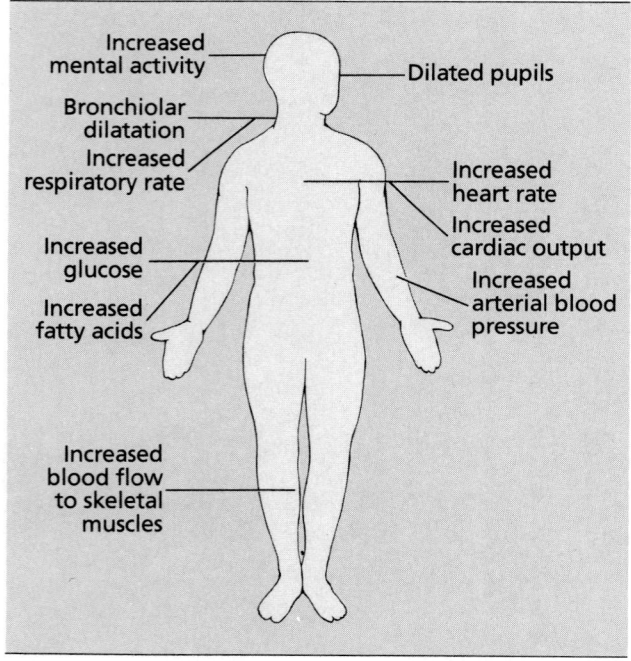

Fig. 30-2   Flight-or-fight response.

Task-oriented behaviors enable a person to cope realistically with the demands of a stressor. The three general types of task-oriented behavior are attack behavior, withdrawal behavior, and compromise (see box).

Ego-Defense Mechanisms

Ego-defense mechanisms, first described by Sigmund Freud, are unconscious behaviors that offer psychological protection from a stressful event. They are used by everyone and help protect against feelings of worthlessness and anxiety. Occasionally a defense mechanism can become distorted and is no longer able to assist the person in adapting to a stressor.

There are many ego-defense mechanisms (see box). They are frequently activated by short-term stressors and usually do not result in psychiatric disorders.

NURSING PROCESS AND ADAPTATION TO STRESS

Assessment

Each client has specific perceptions and responses to stress. A person's perception of a stressor is based on beliefs and norms, life experiences and patterns, environmental factors, family structure and function, developmental stage, past experiences with stress, and coping mechanisms.

Because nurses spend a great deal of time with clients and their families or friends, they are in a unique position to help clients cope with stress. Nurses also provide care for clients in various settings, and thus they are often able to assess reactions to stress. The nurse assesses for indicators of stress in all dimensions of adaptation.

Physiological Indicators

Physiological indicators of stress are objective and more readily identified (see box). These parameters can be commonly observed or measured. However, they are not always observed all the time in all clients experiencing stress, and they vary with individuals. Vital signs are usually elevated, and the client may appear restless and be unable to rest or concentrate.

Psychological Adaptive Behaviors

TASK-ORIENTED BEHAVIORS

- Attack behavior is acting to remove or overcome a stressor or to satisfy a need.
- Withdrawal behavior is removing the self physically or emotionally from the stressor.
- Compromise behavior is changing the usual method of operating, substituting goals, or omitting the satisfaction of needs to meet other needs or to avoid stress.

EXAMPLES OF EGO-DEFENSE MECHANISMS

- Compensation is making up for a deficiency in one aspect of self-image by strongly emphasizing a feature considered an asset.
- Conversion is unconsciously repressing an anxiety-producing emotional conflict and transforming it into nonorganic symptoms.
- Denial is avoiding emotional conflicts by refusing to consciously acknowledge anything that might cause intolerable emotional pain.
- Displacement is transferring emotions, ideas, or wishes from a stressful situation to a less anxiety-producing substitute.
- Identification is patterning behavior after that of another person and assuming that person's qualities, characteristics, and actions.
- Regression is coping with a stressor through actions and behaviors associated with an earlier developmental period.

Physiological Indicators of Stress

- Elevated blood pressure
- Increased muscle tension in neck, shoulders, back
- Elevated pulse and increased respiration
- Sweaty palms
- Cold hands and feet
- Slumped posture
- Fatigue
- Tension headache
- Upset stomach
- Higher-pitched voice
- Nausea, vomiting, and diarrhea
- Change in appetite
- Change in weight
- Change in urinary frequency
- Abnormal laboratory findings: elevated adrenocorticotropic hormone, cortisol, and catecholamine levels and hyperglycemia
- Restlessness: difficulty falling asleep or frequent awakening
- Dilated pupils

These indicators can appear at any stage of stress. The duration and intensity of the symptoms are directly related to the perceived duration and intensity of the stressor. Physiological indicators arise from a variety of systems. Therefore the assessment of stress involves collecting data from all systems.

The link between psychological stress and disease is frequently called the *mind-body interaction*. Research has shown that stress can affect illness and disease patterns. At the turn of the century, infectious diseases were the leading causes of death, but since then, antibiotics, improved living conditions, increased knowledge of nutrition, and better sanitation methods have lowered the death rate. Now the leading causes of death are diseases involving lifestyle stressors.

During any stage, there may be physical complaints such as nausea, vomiting, diarrhea, or headache. Physical appearance is changed; posture may be slumped, hygiene and grooming are poor, and style of dress differs. Prolonged stress has been linked with cardiovascular and gastrointestinal diseases. Some cancers and immunological disorders, as well as fatigue, burnout, and irritability, are associated with prolonged, unresolved stressors (Carr, Powers, 1986; Bargagliotti, Trygstad, 1987).

Mild stress situations do not usually produce chronic physiological damage, but moderate and severe stress can create a risk of medical illness or a worsening of a chronic illness (Kline-Leidy, 1990). **Mild stress situations** are stressors that everyone encounters regularly, such as oversleeping, traffic jams, a flat tire, or criticism from a superior. Such situations usually last a few minutes to a few hours. By themselves, these stressors are not significant risks for symptom development. However, multiple mild stressors over a short time can increase risk of illness (Holmes, Rahe, 1976).

Moderate stress situations last longer, from several hours to days. For example, an unresolved disagreement with a co-worker, work overload, new job expectations, and the prolonged absence of a family member are moderate stress situations.

Severe stress situations are chronic situations that may last several weeks to several years, such as continual marital disagreements, prolonged financial difficulties, and long-term physical illness. The more intense and longer the stress situation, the higher the health risk (Wheeler, 1989). The development of stress-related disease can be examined in terms of the health-illness continuum (Fig. 30-3). As a person's stress increases, stress behaviors increase gradually, which decreases energy and adaptive responses.

Identifying the mind-body interaction is crucial for predicting the risk of stress-related illness. A nurse can often consider the effects of a stressful lifestyle or event and assess the client's coping mechanisms.

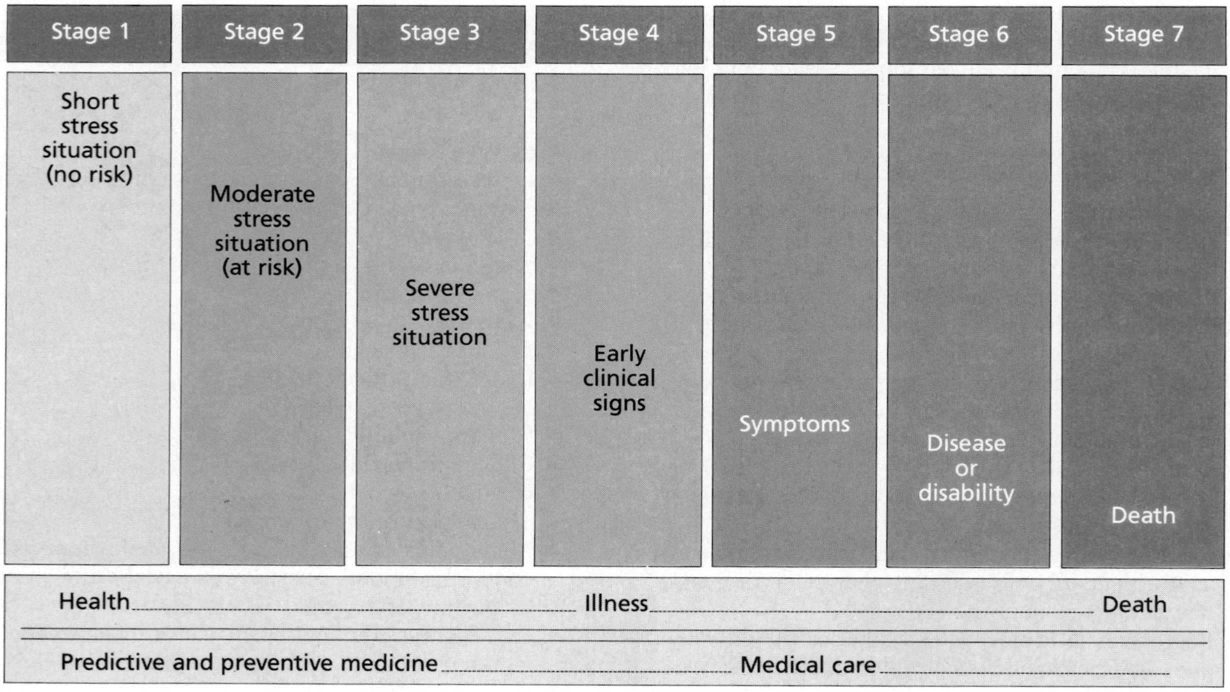

Fig. 30-3 Stages of illness development in stress-related diseases.

Developmental Indicators

Prolonged stress can affect the ability to complete developmental tasks. In any developmental stage a person normally encounters tasks and engages in behaviors characteristic of the stage. Prolonged stress can interrupt or impede passage through the stage. In extreme forms, prolonged stress can lead to maturational crises, which can generate stress.

Infants or young children generally encounter stressors at home. When nurtured in responsive, empathetic environments, they are able to develop healthy self-esteems and ultimately learn healthy adaptive coping responses (Wheeler, 1989). However, the absence of parental figures or their failure to provide the security needed to develop a sense of trust can be stressors. In later life, there may be chronic distrust, resulting in withdrawal and limited interpersonal relationships. If parents or the environment prevent children from developing a sense of autonomy, the children may experience stress, which is indicated by excessive dependence on others.

Preschool children normally develop by exploring their surroundings, exploring differences between boys and girls, and developing conscience. Children are ashamed when caught being "bad" and want to be told when they are "good." An indicator of stress at this stage may be passive, inactive behavior toward the environment.

School-age children normally develop a sense of adequacy. They begin to realize that accumulation of knowledge and mastery of skills can help them accomplish goals, and self-esteem develops through friendships and sharing with peers. At this stage, stress is indicated by the inability or unwillingness to develop friendships.

Adolescents normally develop a strong sense of identity but at the same time need to be accepted by peers. Adolescents with strong social support systems report an increased ability to problem solve and adjust to stressors, but adolescents without social support systems frequently report increased physical and behavioral symptoms (Yarcheski, Mahon, 1986). There are many stressors in this age group, including conflicts involving sexual drive and expected standards of behavior. Prolonged conflict may indicate indecision and confusion, rebellion, depression, or anxiety.

Young adults are in transition from youthful experiences to adult responsibilities. They must prepare for careers, for living alone, and perhaps for starting families. Conflicts may develop between work and family responsibilities. Stressors include conflicts between expectations and reality. Kolotylo, Parker, and Chapman (1990) studied the stress experience of 15 mothers whose newborns were admitted into neonatal intensive care units or intermediate-care units. The mothers reported frustrations over the expectation of healthy newborns and the reality of having very ill infants. Because of the conflict between expectation and reality, the mothers experienced feelings of helplessness, fear of the unknown, and alienation from the other mothers.

Middle adults are usually involved in family building, creating stable careers, and perhaps caring for older parents. They are generally able to control desires and in some cases substitute the needs of spouses, children, or parents for their needs. Stress can result, however, if they feel that too many responsibilities have been placed on them. A recent trend is looking at the impact of stressors of the family care giver's role. The middle years have been called the *sandwich generation* in which middle adults are frequently responsible for chronically ill parents while raising their own families. Because of the stressors involved, care givers have reported increases in fatigue, minor illnesses (for example, colds and influenza), depression, and dissatisfaction with family interaction (Musolf, 1991).

Older adults are commonly faced with adapting to changes in family and perhaps to the deaths of spouses. Older adults must also adjust to changes in physical appearance and physiological functioning. In addition, the stress of decreasing social interactions, as friends die or become unable to maintain contact, and retirement often brings more change. Prolonged fear and stress can be indicated in older adults by overdependence and worsening of preexisting chronic illness, which may cause further stress on family or social relationships (Riffle, 1989).

Psychosocial Indicators

Psychosocial changes are direct and sometimes obvious results of prolonged stress. Frequently a nurse can observe the emotional impact of stress through changes in behavior.

Stress affects emotional well-being in many ways (see box on p. 916). Because everyone's personality involves a complex relationship among many factors, the reaction to prolonged stress depends on support systems, prior experience with stressors, coping mechanisms, and the overall stress response. A change in behavior should alert a nurse, family member, or friend that the person needs help in adapting to stress. Ideally, coping problems should be anticipated and preventive measures taken, but often it is difficult to anticipate unique psychosocial reactions to stress.

Intellectual Indicators

Prolonged stress can manifest itself in the intellectual dimension and have observable indicators. A per-

---

Behavioral and Emotional Indicators of Stress

- Anxiety
- Depression
- Burnout
- Increased use of chemical substances
- Change in eating habits, sleep, and activity pattern
- Mental exhaustion
- Feelings of inadequacy
- Loss of self-esteem
- Increased irritability
- Loss of motivation
- Emotional outbursts and crying
- Decreased productivity and quality of job performance
- Tendency to make mistakes (i.e., poor judgment)
- Forgetfulness and blocking
- Diminished attention to detail
- Preoccupation (i.e., daydreaming or "spacing out")
- Inability to concentrate on tasks
- Increased absenteeism and illness
- Lethargy
- Loss of interest
- Proneness to accidents

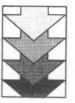

Examples of Nursing Diagnoses Related to Stress

NANDA-APPROVED NURSING DIAGNOSES

Anxiety related to:
- Change in health status
- Maturational or situational crisis

Altered growth and development related to:
- Separation from significant others
- Situational crisis (e.g., unplanned pregnancy)

Fatigue related to:
- Overwhelming psychological demands
- Excessive role demands

Hopelessness related to:
- Long-term stress
- Lost belief in values

Ineffective family coping: compromised or *disabled* or *ineffective individual coping* related to:
- Inadequate coping methods
- Prolonged stress (e.g., physiological, maturational, situational)

High risk for injury related to:
- Impaired problem-solving abilities

Sleep pattern disturbance related to:
- Maturational or situational crisis

---

son's ability to acquire new knowledge or skills is impaired. For example, a client with a chronic illness may have difficulty learning about the illness and treatment. As a result, stress is indicated by this inability.

Prolonged stress affects role performance, too. The client may have difficulty parenting, for example. The client may also be unable to continue employment and must give up the role of wage earner.

Stress can impede communication between the client and others. The family may be unable to resolve conflicts. In addition, the client's ability to effectively solve problems is reduced. As a result, increased dependence on others occurs.

Spiritual Indicators

People use spiritual resources to adapt to stress in many ways, but stress can also threaten a person in the spiritual dimension. Severe stress may result in anger at the supreme being, or the person may view the stressor as punishment. Stressors such as acute illness or the death of a loved one may threaten a person's meaning of life and can lead to spiritual depression. When providing care to a client who is affected spiritually, a nurse should not judge the appropriateness of religious feelings or practices but should assist the client in using spiritual resources to adapt.

Nursing Diagnosis

A review of assessment data provides the opportunity to cluster data that indicate a potential or actual

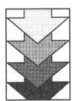

Nursing Diagnostic Process for Stress

Assessment Activities	Defining Characteristics	Nursing Diagnosis
Ask client about changes in energy level.	Client states need for additional rest. Client comments on inability to perform usual activities.	*Fatigue* related to overwhelming psychological demands and excessive role demands
Observe client's behavior.	Cries easily Appears listless Decreased ability to concentrate	
Ask client about level of health.	Client states increased occurrence of "cold," upset stomach, and diarrhea.	

stressor and the client's response. These data clusters ultimately result in the listing of examples of nursing diagnoses occurring from stress (see diagnoses box).

The nursing diagnosis should also identify the probable etiology for the problem. Incorrect identification of the cause of a nursing diagnosis can result in an inappropriate care plan and selected interventions.

Stress can result in multiple diagnostic statements. Examples selected here do not represent the entire list. Units 7 and 8 contain additional nursing diagnoses that occur when an individual has unmet physiological or environmental needs resulting from stress. Chapters 31 and 33 include nursing diagnoses associated with unmet self-concept and spiritual and sociocultural needs.

Identification of a nursing diagnostic label requires the presence of appropriate defining characteristics (see diagnostic process box). The diagnostic label must be supported by the defining characteristics in the data base.

 ## Planning

The formulation of nursing diagnoses initiates the formation of a care plan (see care plan). The care plan is individualized to the client's perception of the stressor and response to stress. The nurse and client develop realistic goals and interventions designed to assist the client with coping with the stressor. Whenever possible, a friend or family member should be involved in planning.

In most situations, stress-management plans are long term and are conducted in the client's home. Therefore the nurse must also know about the availability and cost of resources in the community.

Stress-management techniques are designed to match the client's actual and potential stressors. The general goals for clients who require stress management include the following:

1. Reduction in frequency of stress-inducing situations
2. Decreased physiological response to stress
3. Improved behavioral and emotional responses to stress

 ## Implementation

People are subjected to a variety of stressors every day. For some the stressors are minimal and do not threaten physical or emotional well-being. In other situations, multiple stressors can result in prolonged stress and the need for stress-management tech-

 ### Sample Nursing Care Plan for Fatigue

Nursing diagnosis: *Fatigue* related to overwhelming psychological and excessive role demands
Definition: Fatigue is an overwhelming sense of exhaustion and decreased capacity for physical and mental work regardless of adequate sleep (Kim, McFarland, McLane, 1991).

Goal	Expected Outcomes	Interventions	Rationale
Pattern of rest/activity that enables fulfillment of role demands will be established (5/2).	Client will reduce work schedule from 55 to 40 hours a week (3/30).	Formulate with client options for decreasing work demands.	Work partnerships are successful methods for reducing chance of role fatigue (Musolf, 1991).
	Client will establish 4-hour period per week for self (4/15).	Provide client with community resources for house cleaning and laundry services.	Increased use of community support services provides respite from task-oriented stressors, resulting in increased opportunities to meet individual needs (Riffle, 1989).
		Assist client in developing time-management schedule.	Time-management interventions are resourceful in reducing stressors. The client learns to control demands (Pender, 1987).
	Client will verbalize increased energy level (4-29).		

niques. When helping the client reduce stress, the nurse reduces stressful situations, decreases the physiological response to stress, and improves the behavioral and emotional responses to stress.

Reducing Stressful Situations

It is unrealistic to try to eliminate all stressors. However, the nurse can reduce some stressors and thereby provide the client with a greater sense of control. Pender (1987) identifies five methods to assist in reducing stressful situations.

HABITUATION. Each client has unique habits and routines that help accomplish day-to-day activities. According to Pender (1987), "Routines reduce the need for expenditure of physical and psychological energy, resist change, and thus serve as a stabilizing force." Illnesses, crises, or hospitalization disturbs a client's routine, thereby disturbing the pattern of living and resulting in greater energy expenditure.

During actual or potential stress an established routine is effective in supporting energy conservation. For example, a woman who has chosen to stay at home to raise children is now sending her youngest child to school. Although she anticipated this change, she is unable to obtain a job in her field. She verbalizes fear about being "unable to get anything done at home." In this situation the client's habits have been disrupted, and a new routine has not been developed. A plan that assists the client in developing a new routine consistent with her goals can reduce the stress.

CHANGE AVOIDANCE. Change avoidance is merely limiting unnecessary and avoidable changes. For example, a father of two school-age children is divorcing his wife and is experiencing stress-related symptoms. A college roommate is pressuring him to relocate. The man and his children are experiencing a change in family structure; therefore they should not consider a move.

Tension created by multiple changes increases the response to stress. The capacity for upsetting a client's well-being increases with each distressing change. Deliberately reducing or postponing changes that result in tension assists the client in dealing more constructively with unavoidable change.

Controlled or self-initiated changes provide a challenge for the client. The client is able to turn the challenge into personal growth such as increased coping strategies or increased self-confidence.

TIME BLOCKING. Time blocking is a technique in which an individual has a specific period of time to focus on and adapt to stressors. The major advantage of time blocking is that the client establishes a period of time to address specific goals or concerns and reduce the sense of time urgency. In addition, the client uses time and resources more effectively because the level of anxiety is reduced (Pender, 1987; Girdano, Everly, 1979).

TIME MANAGEMENT. Persons who use time efficiently generally experience less stress related to social, family, and job activities. For some clients, time-management techniques may include establishing an order of priorities for a list of tasks. This technique can be beneficial for clients unable to get anything done because there seems to be too much to do.

Another time-management technique is learning to say "no" to potential disruptions. Time management may also include scheduling appointments realistically to avoid rushing from task to task, meeting to meeting, or errand to errand.

Controlling the demands of others is essential for effective time management. Few people are able to meet all requests made by others. It is important to learn to recognize which requests can be realistically met, which are impossible to meet, and which are negotiable.

ENVIRONMENTAL MODIFICATION. Realistic changes in environment can reduce stressful situations. For example, job stress can be reduced by avoiding situations and people that produce stress. Changing factors in the home to reduce housework or provide safety measures reduces stress. Eliminating committee work or club memberships also helps.

When clients have realistic control over their environments, stress is mediated. After the minimal or moderate stressors are mediated the client is better able to resolve severe stressors.

Decreasing Physiological Response to Stress

In general, stress-management techniques involve health-enhancing habits that can reduce the impact of stress on physical and mental health. These are often commonsense approaches that provide a basis for low-stress living. General prerequisites for stress management include regular exercise, humor, good nutrition and diet, adequate rest, and relaxation techniques.

REGULAR EXERCISE. A regular exercise program improves muscle tone and posture, controls weight, reduces tension, and promotes relaxation. In addition, exercise reduces the risk of cardiovascular disease and improves cardiopulmonary functioning.

A client who has a history of chronic illness, who is at risk for developing an illness, or who is over the age of 35 should begin a physical exercise program only after discussing it with a physician. In general, for a fitness program to have positive physical effects, a person should exercise at least 3 times a week for 30 to 40 minutes.

Everyone should use warm-up exercises before vigorous exercise such as jogging, aerobic dancing, or tennis. Warm-up exercises stimulate blood flow to the muscles and increase flexibility. They reduce the risk of damage to the musculoskeletal system during exercise. Similarly, after vigorous exercise, a person should do cool-down exercises rather than stop abruptly. For example, after jogging or aerobic dancing a person should walk around at a moderate pace, gradually slowing down and stopping. Cool-down exercises allow the cardiovascular, pulmonary, musculoskeletal, and metabolic systems to gradually return to their resting states.

Exercise programs are effective in decreasing the severity of stress-related conditions such as hypertension, obesity, tension headaches, fatigue, mental exhaustion, irritability, and depression. Adults particularly need routine exercise plans because they are occupied with rearing children, developing careers, and establishing homes.

HUMOR. Humor as therapy has been popularized in the lay literature by Norman Cousins (1979). The ability to perceive fun and laugh alleviates stress (Robinson, 1978; Robinson, 1990). The physiological hypothesis is that laughter releases endorphins into the circulation, and feelings of stress are relieved. Simon (1990) notes that humor can influence an older adult's perception of health and morale; in turn the

ability to observe situational humor is related to successful aging (see research highlight).

In addition, humor has also been studied with a variety of students. In one study, Warner (1990) investigated the way that nursing students used humor to mediate stressors associated with clinical practicums. Humor allowed the students to regulate stressful emotions and alter a stressful person-environment relationship.

NUTRITION AND DIET. Nutrition and exercise are closely related. Food provides the fuel for activity and increased exercise, which improves circulation and the delivery of nutrients to body tissues.

Everyone is encouraged to maintain weight according to standard ranges for sex, age, and body build. In addition to avoiding overeating or undereating, a person should be aware of the nutritional quality of foods. Too much fat, caffeine, salt, or sugar can upset the body's metabolic functioning; deficiencies in vitamins, minerals, and nutrients can also cause metabolic problems. Poor dietary habits can worsen a stress response and make a person irritable, hyperactive, and anxious. This impairs the ability to meet personal, family, and job responsibilities. Nursing measures for helping a client meet nutritional needs are detailed in Chapter 35.

REST. An established, habitual pattern of sufficient rest and sleep is also important for managing stress. A person experiencing stress should be encouraged to allow time for rest and sleep. Sleep not only refreshes the body but also helps a person become mentally relaxed. A client may need specific help in learning to relax to fall asleep.

RELAXATION TECHNIQUES. Progressive relaxation with and without muscle tension and imagery reduce the physiological and emotional components of stress. Relaxation techniques are learned behaviors and require training and practice sessions (see Chapter 37). After the client becomes skilled at these techniques, tension is reduced and physiological parameters are changed (see box on p. 920).

Improved Behavioral and Emotional Responses to Stress

Behavioral and emotional responses to stress can be mediated by the use of support systems, crisis intervention, and enhancment of self-esteem.

SUPPORT SYSTEMS. The saying, "No man is an island," is of particular importance for stress management. A support system of family, friends, and colleagues who will listen and offer advice and emo-

---

 **Research Highlight**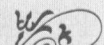

Simon examined the use of humor as a coping strategy and its relationship to perceived health, life satisfaction, and morale in older adults. Seventy-three noninstitutionalized older adults over 55 years of age were selected. Questionnaires were used to measure humor, perception of health, life satisfaction, and morale. The analysis demonstrated a positive relationship between humor and morale in older adults. The researcher concluded that the use of humor as a coping strategy increased successful adaptation to the aging process.

Simon JM: Humor and its relationship to perceived health, life satisfaction, and morale in older adults, *Issues Ment Health Nurs* 11:17, 1990.

Changes Resulting from Relaxation Techniques

- Lowered blood pressure (baseline)
- Lowered heart rate (baseline)
- Decreased cardiac dysrhythmias
- Decreased oxygen demands and oxygen consumption
- Decreased muscle tension
- Lowered metabolic rate
- Increased alpha brain waves, which occur when the client is awake, nonattentive, and relaxed
- Increased restfulness
- Improved concentration
- Improved ability to cope with stressors

---

tional support is beneficial to a person experiencing stress. Support systems can reduce stress reactions and promote physical and mental well-being. Nursing research has documented the correlation of positive social supports and the reduction of symptoms in chronic diseases. Traver and Kline-Leidy (1989) note a reduction in sensations of dyspnea and the frequency of asthmatic attacks in adults with chronic asthma who had strong family, social, and employer support. Kemp and Hatmaker (1989) studied social support and the stress response in high-risk pregnancy. Their results identified lower urine catecholamine (epinephrine and norepinephrine) levels in mothers with strong family support systems.

Nurses can use various methods to help clients build support systems, such as encouraging family to visit, making support groups available, encouraging involvement in church groups, and encouraging recreational activities. Nurses can use therapeutic communication skills to encourage clients to express their feelings and identify causes of stress. When stress is the result of confusion or wrong information, a nurse can use teaching techniques to help relieve clients' stress. If stress results from differences between expectations and realities, a nurse can help clients gain stronger self-concepts or body images. All of these methods help clients build stronger support systems. If stress is the result of social isolation, nursing strategies are aimed at helping clients develop new social networks.

CRISIS INTERVENTION. Crisis intervention is a therapeutic technique for helping a client resolve a partic-

ular, immediate stress problem. Crisis intervention does not involve an in-depth analysis of a situation but addresses the immediate, urgent need for stress reduction. The goal is to restore the person as quickly as possible to the precrisis level of functioning in all dimensions.

Crises occur when people encounter problems or stress situations with which they are unable to cope in usual ways. Behavior tends to be disorganized, and clients may make only abortive attempts at resolving the problems (Aguilera, 1989).

Clients and nurses are at risk for two types of crises, situational and developmental. A **situational crisis** arises suddenly in response to an external event or conflict involving a specific circumstance. Symptoms associated with situational crises are transient, and the episode is brief. Situational crises include giving birth, major role changes, acute physical illness, physical assault or rape, family changes such as remarriage or the death of a family member, and unexpected unemployment.

A **developmental crisis** occurs when a person is unable to complete the developmental tasks of a psychosocial stage and is therefore unable to continue developing. A developmental crisis can occur at any point in life if circumstances prevent a person from meeting the challenge of a particular stage.

After determining that a client is experiencing a crisis, the nurse plans and implements specific measures to help resolve it. Aguilera (1989) has developed an approach to intervention that can be used for both types of crises (Fig. 30-4). This approach enables the nurse to understand how a stressful event has led to a state of crisis. Resolution of the crisis depends on the person's realistic perceiption of the stressful event and use of adequate coping mechanisms. If the client is lacking in one or more of these areas, the nurse and client plan specific methods to restore equilibrium. If the crisis has arisen because perception of the event is distorted, the nurse helps the client perceive the stressful event realistically. If the crisis has arisen because of a lack of situational support or coping mechanisms, the nurse initiates measures to assist the client in these areas by maximizing available coping mechanisms and developing additional supports. The nurse then evaluates the extent to which the client is able to resolve the crisis with these means.

ENHANCING SELF-ESTEEM. Improvement in a client's self-esteem can assist in positive stress-reduction strategies (see Chapter 31). When clients identify their positive characteristics, they can focus attention on them instead of on the stressor. This increased positive self-awareness will result in behavior that reflects the client's positive characteristics (Pender, 1987).

Stress Management for Nurses

Rapid changes in society, health care technology, and health care knowledge, as well as changes in the nursing profession, can place stress on nurses. **Job stress** can result from a series of factors at work that interact with the worker to disrupt psychological or physiological balance and decision making (Numerof, Abrams, 1984).

Most nurses experience stress in their work environments. Stressors can be related to workload, client needs, on-the-job conflicts, and clients' families (Wolfgang, 1988; Numerof, Abrams, 1984; Bailey, 1989). In addition, intensive care and hospice nurses report more job stress resulting from the frequent client deaths on these particular divisions (Foxall, Zimmerman, Bene, 1990; Bailey, 1989). Rotation of shifts, floating to different units, and institutional policies increase nurses' perceptions of stress (Skipper, Jung, Coffey, 1990; Numerof, Abrams, 1984). Reaction to a job-related stressor depends on the nurse's personality, health status, previous experience with stress, and coping mechanisms.

Job stress frequently results in a condition called **burnout,** which is characterized by a decreased concern for the people with whom one is working. During burnout, the client experiences physical and emotional exhaustion. The job or profession no longer has any positive rewards. The client may also experience anger and apathy while on the job.

Nurses are at risk for job stress as a result of three factors. First, new graduates generally have high expectations that may not be met in the workplace, leading to frustration. Second, nurses usually work in close contact with others, specifically, clients and other health care professionals. Such continuous interaction can lead to conflicts and other stresses. Finally, the workplace itself increases the risk for job stresses. Most nurses work in institutional settings in which client and employee needs are often unmet. When these stressors become insurmountable, the employees' desire to change jobs becomes greater (Parasuraman, 1989). Therefore if the stressors can be reduced by the institution or employee, the turnover rate can be reduced.

Nurses can reduce stressors by using the same stress-management techniques that they teach clients. Those commonsense techniques improve physical and mental well-being, enabling nurses to cope more successfully with stressors. In addition, nurses should identify specific stressors in their workplaces

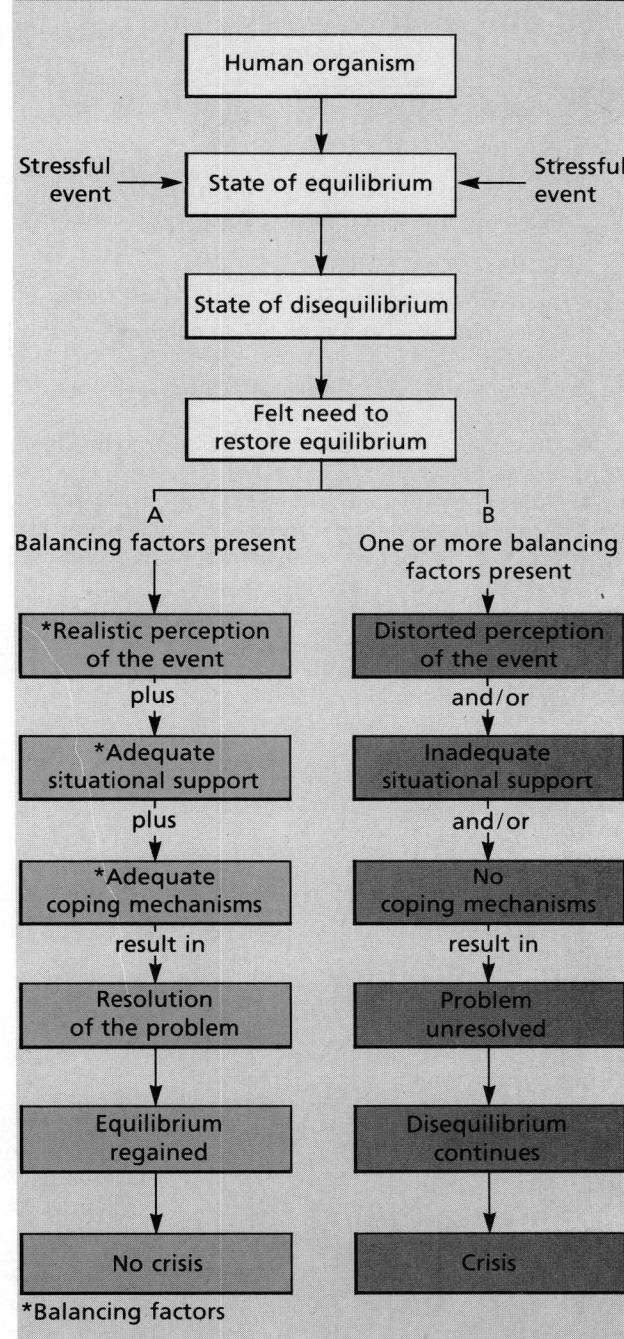

Fig. 30-4   Crisis intervention model.
From Aguilera DC: *Crisis intervention: theory and methodology,* ed 6, St Louis, 1989, Mosby–Year Book.

Client Teaching for Reducing Stress in the Workplace

OBJECTIVE

- Client will use a problem-solving method for defining, analyzing, and resolving stressors or conflicts.

TEACHING STRATEGIES

- Discuss with client the need to define overall needs, purposes, and goals. Help client define the problem.
- Teach client to analyze capabilities, constraints, and interest groups.
- Assist client in specifying an approach to problem solving.
- Teach client to state behavioral objectives, generate solutions, analyze alternatives, choose best alternative, implement and control action chosen, and evaluate its effectiveness.

EVALUATION

- Observe client using the problem-solving method for stress or conflict resolution.

Modified from Sundeen S et al: *Nurse-client interaction: implementing the nursing process*, ed 4, St Louis, 1989, Mosby–Year Book.

and if possible eliminate or minimize them. Finally, nurses can use problem solving to reduce stress and resolve conflict (see teaching box).

Evaluation

Because clients' perceptions of stress differ, their perceptions of stress reduction do, too. Therefore evaluation of nursing interventions directed at stress management must be individualized.

To evaluate interventions directed at stress management the nurse must obtain objective measures of reduced frequency of stressful situations, decreased physiological response to stress, and improved behavioral and emotional responses to stress.

Achievement of care goals can indicate the degree of stress reduction. The nurse evaluates the effectiveness of stress-management techniques through expected outcome measures (see evaluation box).

SUMMARY

Each person reacts to stress differently, according to perception of the stressor, personality, prior experi-

Sample Evaluation of Interventions for Fatigue

Goals	Evaluation Measures	Expected Outcomes
Pattern of rest and activity that enables fulfillment of role demands will be established (5/2).	Examine and review client's work schedule for last 2 weeks.	Client will reduce work schedule from 55 to 40 hours a week (3/30).
	Ask if client has been able to have 4 hours for self; evaluate whether this time is sufficient.	Client will establish a 4-hour period for self each week (4/15).
	Ask client to compare present and previous energy levels. Use visual analog in which 1 represents client's previous energy level.	Client will verbalize increased energy level (4/29).
		Client will report use of support system (3/10).
Behavioral and emotional responses to stress will improve (5/2).	Observe client's verbal and nonverbal cues about stress.	Client will state more positive attributes about self (3/10).
	Obtain information from family and friends about client's behavioral and emotional responses to stress.	Client will give more attention to hygiene and grooming (3/30).
		Excessive crying, anger, and aggression will be absent (4/15).

ence with stress, and use of coping mechanisms. Various models of stress help the nurse understand causes and responses to stress.

Prolonged stress can affect level of health, resulting in physical or mental illness. Stress-management techniques are directed at changing a person's reactions to stressors. Through the use of health-promotion and health-maintenance strategies, nurses can help clients manage stress successfully.

REFERENCES

Aguilera DC: *Crisis intervention: theory and methodology*, ed 6, St Louis, 1989, Mosby–Year Book.

Bargagliotti CA, Trygstad LN: Differences in stress and coping findings: a reflection of social realities or methodologies, *Nurs Res* 36:170, 1987.

Bartoldus E, Gillery B, Sturges PJ: Job-related stress and coping among home-care workers with elderly people, *Health Care Soc Work* 14:204, 1989.

Bailey FC: Stress in high dependency units, *Intensive Care Nurs* 5:134, 1989.

Carr JA, Powers MJ: Stressors associated with coronary bypass surgery, *Nurs Res* 35:243, 1986.

Cousins N: *Anatomy of an illnness*, New York, 1979, Bantam.

Fox P: Stress related to family change among vietnamese refugees, *J Community Health Nurs* 8(1):45, 1991.

Foxall MJ, Zimmerman L, Bene B: A comparison of frequency and sources of nursing job stress perceived by intensive care, hospice, and medical-surgical nurses, *J Adv Nurs* 15:77, 1990.

Girdano D, Everly G: *Controlling stress and tension*, Englewood Cliffs, NJ, 1979, Prentice-Hall.

Haber J: A family systems model for divorce and the loss of self, *Arch Psychiatr Nurs* 6(4):228, 1990.

Holmes T, Rahe R: The social readjustment scale, *J Psychosom Res* 12:213, 1976.

Kemp VH, Hatmaker DD: Stress and social support in high risk pregnancy, *Res Nurs Health* 12:331, 1989.

Kim MJ, McFarland GK, McLane AM: *Pocket guide to nursing diagnoses*, ed 4, St Louis, 1991, Mosby–Year Book.

Kline-Leidy N: A structural model of stress, psychosocial resources, and symptomatic experience in chronic physical illness, *Nurs Res* 39.30, 1990.

Kolotylo CJ, Parker NI, Chapman JS: Mother's perception of their neonates' in-hospital transfers from a neonatal intensive care unit, *JOGGN* 20(2):146, 1990.

Lazarus RS, Folkman S: *Stress appraisal and coping*, New York, 1984, Springer.

Lindsay AM, Carrieri VK: Stress response. In Lindsay AM, Carrieri VK, editors: *Pathological phenomenon in nursing: human response to illness*, Philadelphia, 1986, Saunders.

Lyon B, Werner J: Stress: ten years for practice-relevant research. In Fitzpatric J, Tauton, RL, editors: *Annual review of nursing research*, vol 5, New York, 1987, Springer.

McNett SC: Lazarus' theory of stress and coping. In Riegel B, Ehrenreich D, editors: *Psychological aspects of critical care nursing*, Rockville, Md, 1989, Aspen.

Mechanic D: *Students under stress*, Glencoe, Ill, 1962, Free Press.

Musolf JM: Easing the impact of the family caregiver's role, *Rehabil Nurs* 16(2):82, 1991.

Numerof RE: *Managing stress: a guide for health professionals*, Rockville, Md, 1983, Aspen.

Numerof RE, Abrams MN: Sources of stress among nurses: an empirical investigation, *J Human Stress* 10:88, 1984.

Oberst MT et al: Self-care burden, stress appraisal, and mood among persons receiving radiotherapy, *Cancer Nurs* 14(2):71, 1991.

Parasuraman S: Nursing turnover: an integrated model, *Res Nurs Health* 12:267, 1989.

Pender NJ: *Health promotion in nursing practice*, ed 2, Norwalk, Conn, 1987, Appleton & Lange.

Riffle KL: Stress: nurses dealing with family members, *J Gerontol Nurs* 15(7):18, 1989.

Robinson L: Stress and anxiety, *Nurs Clin North Am* 25(4):935, 1990.

Robinson V: Humor in nursing. In Carlson C, Blackwell B, editors: *Behavioral concepts and nursing intervention*, ed 2, Philadelphia, 1978, Lippincott.

Selye H: The general adaptation syndrome and the diseases of adaptation, *Clin Endocrinol* 6:117, 1946.

Selye H: *The stress of life*, ed 2, New York, 1976, McGraw-Hill.

Simon JM: Humor and its relationship to perceived health, life satisfaction, and morale in older adults, *Issues Ment Health Nurs* 11:17, 1990.

Skipper JK, Jung JD, Coffey LC: Nurses and shiftwork: effects on physical health and mental depression, *J Adv Nurs* 15:835, 1990.

Stuart GW, Sundeen SJ: *Principles and practice of psychiatric nursing*, ed 4, St Louis, 1991, Mosby–Year Book.

Traver GA, Kline-Leidy N: Asthma and stress, *J Adv Med Surg Nurs* 1(4):25, 1989.

Warner SL: Humor: a coping response for student nurses, *Arch Psychiatr Nurs* 5(1):10, 1990.

Wheeler K: Self-psychology's contributions to understanding stress and implications for nursing, *J Adv Med Surg Nurs* 1(4):1, 1989.

Wolfgang AP: Job stress in the health professions: a study of physicians, nurses, and pharmacists, *Hospital Top* 66(4):24, 1988.

Yarcheski A, Mahon NE: Perceived stress and symptom patterns in early adolescents: the role of mediating variables, *Res Nurs Health* 9:289, 1986.

ADDITIONAL READINGS

Caroselli-Dervan C: Modifying stress in cardiovascular patients: nursing intervention, *J Adv Med Surg Nurs* 1(4):11, 1989.

MacNeil JM, Weisz GM: Critical care nursing stress, *Heart Lung* 16:274, 1987.

Norbeck JS: Types and sources of social support for managing job stress in critical care nursing, *Nurs Res* 34:225, 1985.

Qamar SL: The stress-carative model of nursing practice, *Focus Crit Care* 13(6):15, 1986.

Roberts JG et al: Analysis of coping responses and adjustment: stability of conclusions, *Nurs Res* 36:94, 1987.

Selye H: The general adaptation syndrome and the diseases of adaptation, *Clin Endocrinol (Oxf)* 6:117, 1946.

Sund K, Ostwald SK: Dual-earner families' stress levels and personal and life-style–related variables, *Nurs Res* 34:357, 1985.

Thomas SP, Groër M: Relationship of demographic, life-style, and stress variables to blood pressure in adolescents, *Nurs Res* 35:169, 1986.

Wilson VS: Identification of stressors related to patients' psychologic responses to the surgical intensive care unit, *Heart Lung* 16:267, 1987.

CHAPTER 30 REVIEW

Key Concepts

- Physiological adaptive mechanisms are controlled by the medulla oblongata, reticular formation, and pituitary gland.

- Prolonged stress decreases the adaptive capacity of the body.

- Stress is physiological or psychological tension that can affect a person in any or all human dimensions.

- An individual may encounter stressors in the internal or external environment.

- Stressors necessitate change or adaptation so that a state of equilibrium can be maintained.

- A person's response to stress is influenced by the intensity, duration, and scope of the stressor and by the number of stressors present at one time.

- A person adapts to stress by using resources in the physical and developmental, emotional, intellectual, social, and spiritual dimensions.

- The two forms of physiological response to stress are the local adaptation syndrome and the general adaptation syndrome.

- The local adaptation syndrome involves several specific responses to stress, including the reflex pain response and the inflammatory response.

- The general adaptation syndrome involves a multisystem physiological response to stress.

- The three stages of the general adaption syndrome are the alarm reaction, the resistance stage, and the exhaustion stage.

- Psychological responses to stress include task-oriented behaviors and ego-defense mechanisms.

- Task-oriented behaviors include attack behavior, withdrawal, and compromise.

- Ego-defense mechanisms are unconscious behaviors that offer a person psychological protection from stressful feelings or events.

- Stress has an impact on the onset, course, and outcome of illness.

- Prolonged stress decreases the ability to adapt to the stress and affects the person in all five dimensions.

- People generally learn to use short- and long-term strategies to cope with stress.

- Stress-management techniques include health-enhancing habits, crisis intervention, and methods of reducing job stress.

Key Terms

Adaptation, p. 908

Burnout, p. 921

Coping mechanisms, p 912

Crises, p. 920

Crisis intervention, p. 920

Developmental crisis, p. 920

Ego-defense mechanisms, p. 913

External stressors, p. 906

Flight-or-fight response, p. 912

General adaptation syndrome (GAS), p. 910

Homeostasis, p. 906

Internal stressors, p. 906

Job stress, p. 921

Local adaptation syndrome (LAS), p. 910

Medulla oblongata, p. 907

Mild stress situations, p. 914

Moderate stress situations, p. 914

Physiological adaptation, p. 906

Pituitary gland, p. 907

Reticular formation, p. 907

Severe stress situations, p. 914

Situational crisis, p. 920

Stress, p. 906

Stressors, p. 906

Task-oriented behaviors, p. 912

Critical Thinking Exercises

1. Craig Johnson is 26 years old and has a high-level management position in an advertising firm. He states that he enjoys his job, but it has been "very stressful for the last month." He has noted increased gastrointestinal problems and headaches and reports an increase in alcohol consumption. What stategies can the nurse design to assist in reducing Mr. Johnson's response to stress.

2. Calvin Kleiger had a myocardial infarction yesterday. What are the important physiological responses to stress that can increase the risk for further cardiac damage? What nursing measures can reduce these stress responses?

3. During a home visit, you note that a young mother appears stressed and expresses difficulty in managing time and work demands. What time-management strategies would be appropriate to teach this client?

CHAPTER 31

Self-Concept

OBJECTIVES

Mastery of content in this chapter will enable the student to:
- Define the key terms listed.
- Discuss factors that influence each component of self-concept, including identity, body image, self-esteem, and roles.
- Describe the five processes of socialization.
- Identify stressors that affect each component of self-concept.
- Explain the processes that can lead to role conflict, role ambiguity, and role strain.
- Discuss identity confusion as a developmental aspect of adolescence and as a problem of self-concept.
- Describe development of self-concept, relating Erikson's psychosocial stages and cognitive stages.
- Discuss ways in which the nurse's self-concept and nursing activities can affect the client's self-concept.
- Describe behaviors or defining characteristics that may indicate identity confusion, disturbed body image, low self-esteem, and role conflict.
- List, for each component of self-concept, a common nursing diagnosis related to self-concept disturbance and related factors.
- Describe goals of care, specific nursing interventions, and outcome and evaluation measures for a client with self-concept disturbance.

CHAPTER OUTLINE

Self-concept represents a complex integration of conscious and unconscious feelings, attitudes, and perceptions about the total self, the body, a sense of worth, and roles. It reflects interpretations of past experiences, social interactions, and sensations. Self-concept is the identification of the self as a separate and distinct entity. Self-concept is based in part on how people believe that others see them (Cooley, 1956).

Self-concept is a person's subjective image of the self—the perception of physical, emotional, and social attributes or qualities. Self-concept is a frame of reference that affects the management of situations and relationships with others. This self-image may be accurate, and although aspects of it may undergo change, self-concept is slow to change (Yamamoto, 1972). In fact, self-concept is relatively stable even for a preadolescent (Marsh, 1990). Discrepancies between certain aspects of personality and self-concept may become sources of stress or conflict.

Self-concept is not the same as the self. The self includes the total subjective and objective qualities of a person as seen by the person and others. For example, the self includes appearance, values, ideas, knowledge, self-perception and the perceptions of others.

Self-concept is influenced by positive and negative factors. In fact, self-concept and perception of health are closely associated with each other. A client's belief in good health can enhance self-concept. Statements such as "I'm strong as an ox" or "I've never been sick a day in my life" indicate that a person's thoughts about health are positive and that these thoughts are important to self-perception. The nurse can build on positive views of health to further enhance the client's self-concept.

Hospitalization, illness, surgery, separation from family, and other negative factors can also affect self-concept. For example, amputation of an extremity results in altered body image. Adaptation includes integrating the bodily change into the physical concept of self (that is, body image). Chronic illness may affect the ability to provide financial support, thereby affecting self-worth and roles within the family. These changes also alter self-concept. In these cases, problems with self-concept is apparent. However, many changes may not be as apparent; therefore a nurse must understand the affect of stressors on self-concept and recognize behaviors that show that a client needs nursing interventions.

 ## OVERVIEW OF SELF-CONCEPT

The development and maintenance of self-concept constitute a complex process involving many variables. Self-concept, body image, and self-esteem are interrelated concepts.

Self-concept is the psychic representation or identity of an individual, the central core of "I" around which all perceptions and experiences are organized. Self-concept is a dynamic combination formulated over years and based on the following sources:

1. Reactions of others to the infant's or child's body and behavior
2. Ongoing perceptions of others' reactions to the self
3. Experiences with self and others
4. Personality structure
5. Perceptions of physiological and sensory stimuli that impinge on the self
6. Prior and new experiences
7. Present feelings about the physical, emotional, and social self
8. Expectations about the self

Self-concept gives a sense of continuity, wholeness, and consistency to a person. It has a high degree of stability and represents general positive or negative feelings toward the self. Self-concept is expressed through behavior, words, intellect, goals, attitudes, and values (Cooley, 1956; Coopersmith, 1967; Jacobsen, 1964; Murray, 1982).

A person has many self-perceptions based on perceived health status, gender, age, family roles and background, occupational and social roles, and use of leisure activity. Normally, these facets of the self, the "masks" worn when in different situations, are not too diverse or different from one other. A consistency remains even though a person feels differently about the self from time to time or is perceived in different ways by others. An ill person not only experiences negative feelings about the self but also may feel a lack of wholeness, a sense of distortion, and discontinuity because of pain, surgery, or disease or emotional illness.

Body image is a personal mental picture of an individual's body, including the external, internal, and postural images. These mental images are not necessarily consistent with the actual body structure or appearance. Body image includes attitudes, emotions, and personality reactions to the body as an object in space, with a distinct boundary and separate from all others and the general environment (Schilder, 1951). Body image develops gradually over several years as children learn about their bodies and their structures, functions, abilities, and limitations. Body image may change within a few hours, days, weeks, or months, depending on external stimuli on the body and actual changes in appearance, structure, or function. Other people's positive or negative responses may also create changes in body image (Fisher, Cleveland, 1968). For example, if the nurse shows acceptance of a mastectomy scar, the woman is assisted in reconstructing a more positive, whole view of herself. If a family member reacts with disgust, avoidance, or repugnance to a deformed or amputated limb, the individual may construct a negative or distorted body image that lacks a sense of a whole or unified being, or the individual may be more helpless than is warranted by the change.

Self-esteem is the evaluation that an individual customarily maintains of the self and conveys to others by verbal reports or overt behavioral expressions. This judgmental feeling includes approval or disapproval and indicates the extent to which an individual believes in personal capabilities, significance, value, success, and worth (Coopersmith, 1967). Self-esteem involves the acceptance of self because of basic worth and despite weaknesses, limitations, or deficiencies. A person who values the self and feels valued by others usually has a positive self-concept. A person who feels worthless, does not feel respected by others, and has no self-respect usually has negative self-concepts.

An ill person may feel inferior, less valued, unaccepted by others, and unacceptable to the self. A client may need considerable assistance in overcoming limitations, weaknesses, or deficiencies. The nurse avoids judgment or criticism while assisting, teaching, or supporting this client. The nurse's acceptance of a client as an individual with worth and dignity is crucial in helping the improvement of self-esteem.

COMPONENTS OF SELF-CONCEPT

Self-concept has four aspects: identity, body image, self-esteem, and roles. Each aspect develops after birth and reflects the changes taking place throughout the life span. Although these four components can be considered as separate aspects of self-concept, they overlap and are interrelated. Thus self-concept can be described in terms of a continuum from strong to weak or positive to negative, depending on the individual strengths of the four components.

Identity

Identity is derived from the Latin word *idem*, which means "the same." **Identity** involves the internal sense of individuality, unity, and sameness of a person over time and in various circumstances. Identity thus includes a level of consistency and continuity. It implies a consciousness of being distinct and separate from others, a sense of wholeness and maintenance of solidarity with the ideals of the social group while expressing individuality and uniqueness (Erikson, 1963).

Adolescence is a particularly crucial time for the development of the sense of self, or identity. During adolescence, many physical, emotional, cognitive, and social changes occur; extreme peer pressure exists, and preparation for future independence begins. When unable to meet personal and social expectations and define the self, the teenager experiences identity diffusion or identity confusion resulting from a sense of distortion, fragmentation, and unclear roles. An adolescent has a need to belong and be accepted by a peer group. The ability to form an identity is also related to cognitive development because a person must be able to label the self and perceive labeling by others. A person with a sense of identity will feel integrated rather than diffuse, fragmented, or out of touch with the self or others (Erikson, 1963).

During socialization, a child experiences the identification process and thereby learns culturally accepted behaviors and roles. A child identifies first with parenting figures and later with teachers, peers, and cultural heroes. To form an identity, a child must be able to bring together learned behaviors into a coherent, consistent, and unique whole (Erikson, 1963). This process is particularly characteristic of adolescence. The sense of identity continuously evolves and is influenced by circumstances throughout life. The achievement of identity is necessary for involvement in intimate relationships because identity is expressed in relationships with others.

Sexuality is a part of identity. Sexual identity is a person's image of the self as a man or woman and the meaning of this image. This image and its meaning depend on standards learned through socialization.

When behaving in ways that conform to self-concept, a person reinforces personal identity. However, when behaving in ways that contradict the self-concept, individuals may experience anxiety, apprehension, and identity conflict.

Body Image

Body image is the individual's psychological and mental images and experiences of the internal and external body. It includes feelings and attitudes toward the body. Body image is influenced by personal views of physical characteristics and physical abilities and by perceptions of others' views. Body image is an important factor in self-concept; however, self-concept also influences body image.

Body image is also affected by cognitive growth and physical development. Internal and external physical stimuli affect the mental images or concepts of a person's body. Normal developmental changes such as growth and aging have a more apparent effect on body image than on other aspects of self-concept. For example, a 2-year-old's body image is very different from an infant's because of the ability to walk. This change depends on physical maturation.

Somatic, kinesthetic, and behavioral stimuli also play a part in the development and maturation of body image. Somatic elements include neurological, metabolic, endocrine, and hormonal factors. Hormonal changes occur during adolescence and in later stages of life (for example, menopause) and influence body image. Aging involves a decrease in visual acuity, hearing, mobility, and perception; these changes may affect body image.

Kinesthetic elements include neuromuscular functions (for example, walking, dancing, or engaging in sports or gymnastics) and conscious recognition of the orientation of different parts of the body with respect to each other. They also include the rates of movement of different parts of the body (Schilder, 1951).

Behavioral elements include experiences related to cognitive, motor, and perceptual experiences and development. Topological stimuli are superficial sensations and physical characteristics of the body surface. Stimuli are particularly important during adolescence, when significant physical changes occur. During aging, stimuli are again important, as a person recognizes the physical signs of old age.

Cultural and societal attitudes and values influence body image. Youth, beauty, and wholeness are emphasized in American society, a fact apparent in television programs, movies, and advertisements. These attitudes and values affect people's perceptions of their physical bodies because body image is a combination of the ideal and the real.

Because body image depends only partly on the reality of the body, a person generally does not adapt quickly to changes in the physical body. As with total self-concept, physical changes may not be incorporated into a person's ideal body image. Studies have shown, for example, that people who have experienced significant weight loss do not readily perceive themselves as thin. A client who has a limb amputated may experience phantom limb syndrome. The limb can be "felt," and pain is perceived. Another example is normal aging. Older adults often report that they do not feel different, but when they look in the mirror, they are surprised by the wrinkled skin or the gray hair.

Self-Esteem

Like body image, self-esteem is based on many internal and external factors. **Self-esteem** is a sense of self-worth, an evaluation that an individual makes and maintains about the self. According to Erikson, young children begin to develop a sense of usefulness or industry by learning to act on their own initiative. Self-esteem is often related to individual evaluation of effectiveness at school, at work, within the family, and in other situations.

Society and family generally set the standards by which individuals evaluate themselves. Frame of reference, in other words, is an important determinant of people's comparisons of themselves to others. For example, a child who excels in science is comfortable among peers in a classroom, and self-esteem is high. However, if the same child is placed in a more difficult science class with new classmates, self-esteem may decrease somewhat until the child gains confidence and familiarity with the environment.

Self-evaluation is an ongoing mental process. Self-worth, or self-esteem, is a basic human need, according to Maslow's hierarchy (see Chapter 29). People have a need to feel competent and worthy of living. Self-esteem thus is involved in the enhancement and maintenance of self-concept. Level of self-esteem is an important factor in psychosocial development and motivations (Gibson, 1980).

Self-esteem can be understood in terms of the relationship of a person's self-concept and the ideal self, or ego ideal. The **ideal self** consists of the aspirations, goals, values, and standards of behavior that a person considers ideal and strives to attain. The ideal self originates in the preschool years and develops throughout life; it is influenced by societal norms and the expectations and demands of parents and significant others. In general, a person whose self-concept almost matches the ideal self has high self-esteem, whereas a person whose self-concepts varies widely from the ideal self has low self-esteem (Fig. 31-1). Studies have shown that a negative self-concept, or an extreme difference between ideal self and self-concept, is characteristic of many persons with mental illness.

Self-esteem also is influenced by the amount of control that people believe they have over life goals and successes. A person with high self-esteem tends to attribute personal qualities and efforts with success. A person with a low self-esteem tends to think that personal characteristics contribute to failure to reach goals. When successful, an individual with low self-esteem tends to attribute this to luck or others' help rather than personal ability (Marsh, 1990; Tenner, Hertzberger, 1987).

Roles

A **role** is a set of behaviors by which a person participates in social groups. Roles involve expectations

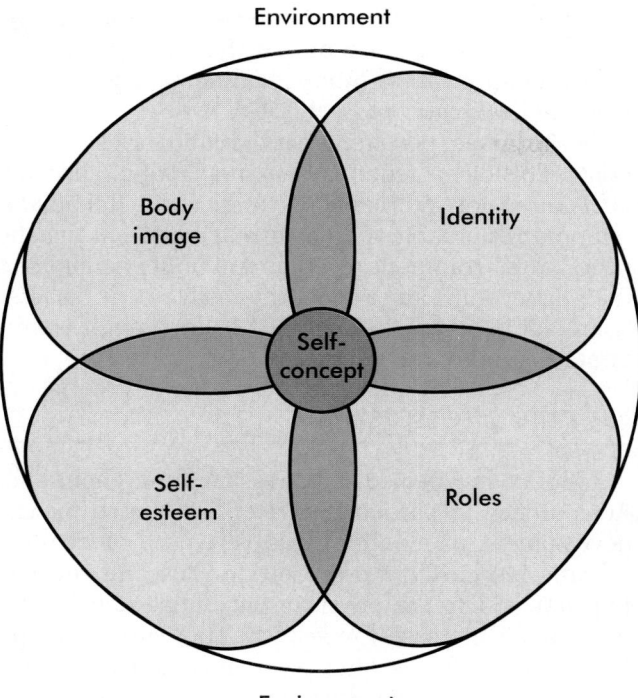

Environment

Body image

Identity

Self-concept

Self-esteem

Roles

Environment

Fig. 31-1 Interaction between self-concept and body image identity, role and self-esteem.

or standards of behavior that have been accepted by society or the social group, such as family or community. Behavior is based on patterns established through socialization. **Socialization** is the "acquisition of the requisite orientation for satisfactory functioning in a role" (Parsons, 1951). Socialization begins just after birth, when an infant responds to adults and adults respond to the infant's behaviors. Parsons (1951, 1972) considers the value-orientation patterns established in childhood to be a basic personality structure. The patterns are stable and change only minimally during adulthood. A child learns behaviors that are approved by society through the following methods:

1. **Reinforcement-extinction**. Certain behaviors become common or are avoided, depending on whether they are approved and reinforced or discouraged and punished.
2. **Inhibition**. A child learns to refrain from behaviors, even when motivated to engage in them because of reinforcement.
3. **Substitution**. A child replaces one behavior by another, which provides the same personal gratification.
4. **Imitation**. A child acquires knowledge, skills, or behaviors from members of the social or cultural group.

5. **Identification**. A child internalizes the beliefs, behavior, and values of role models into a personal, unique expression.

During socialization, a child generally develops the skills necessary for satisfactory functioning in many different roles. Unsuccessful socialization may lead to an inability to function acceptably according to society's values.

Brim and Wheeler (1966) differentiate between socialization of a child and an adult. An adult is more concerned with the actual behavior appropriate to roles than with learning the basic values implicit in roles. An adult is also expected to distinguish between ideal role expectations and realistic expectations. In addition, an adult experiences many roles and role expectations and increased role specificity. The adult is concerned about relationships with other persons. The success of various roles and relationships contributes to the sense of well-being or self-esteem. In contrast, a child learns about the personal physical self and the immediate environment. Only after becoming comfortable with the physical self and establishing trust in parents can a child begin to socialize with other children. A school-age child and an adolescent are influenced by this socialization as they develop and learn role behaviors.

Individuals learn behaviors appropriate to given roles through interactions with people who hold beliefs about appropriate behaviors and who reward or punish them on the basis of their beliefs. To function effectively in roles, people must know the expected behavior and values, must desire to conform to them, and must be able to meet the role requirements. Roles involve the following components (Biddle, Thomas, 1966):

1. The individual, or actor
2. The behavior, or action
3. The relationships between the individual and the behavior

Most individuals have more than one role. Common roles include mother or father, wife or husband, daughter or son, employee, friend, and boss. Each role involves meeting certain expectations of others. Fulfillment of these expectations leads to rewards. Failure to comply with them leads to disapproval.

 STRESSORS AFFECTING SELF-CONCEPT

A self-concept stressor is any real or perceived factor or change that threatens identity, body image, self-esteem, or role behavior. Stressors challenge the adaptive capacities of a person. Stress is not unique to any one age group or to any cultural or economic group (see Chapter 30). Selye (1956) states that stress is the normal wear-and-tear of life, not the specific result of any one action or typical response to any one thing. The normal process of maturation and development itself is a stressor. Changes that occur in physical, spiritual, emotional, sexual, familial, and sociocultural health are stressful. These internal and external factors affect equilibrium.

Different individuals react to the same situation with varying degrees of stress. A variety of responses to stress may be observed, including anxiety, frustration, anger, inability to adjust to a situation, difficulty with making decisions, and various physical or mental changes. Perception of stress is an important factor that influences the response to it. People do not have to understand a specific stressor to feel stress, as long as they perceive the stressor. All people learn patterns of behavior that usually provide the means for coping with or adapting to stressors, thus providing methods for coping with future stressors. However, some people are immobilized by perceived threats and require help from other people. Prolonged stress can deplete adaptive ability.

Stressors can affect any or all of the components of self-concept. Any change in health can be a stressor that affects self-concept. The nurse must understand the effect of health changes on clients and provide appropriate support and intervention. A physical change in the body leads to an altered body image, but identity and self-esteem may also be affected. Certain chronic illnesses alter roles, which may change identity and self-esteem. The following case study illustrates the interrelationship of the four components of self-concept:

A young man is injured in a diving accident and is paralyzed from the neck down, causing an altered body image. The man had been a construction worker but can no longer function in that job, resulting in an altered role. His self-esteem may be diminished because he can no longer support himself, and his identity as a self-supporting, active man will change. Because he no longer has the same self-concept and body image he had before the accident, a disparity between the prior self-concept and his present reality leads to stress and anxiety. His previous life experiences, sense of identity, unconscious use of defense mechanisms, mental coping strategies, and family and societal resources will influence his adaptation to this stressful change.

A crisis is an imbalance occurring when a person cannot overcome obstacles with usual methods of problem solving and adapting. Any crisis requires change and thus threatens self-concept. Some crises directly affect self-concept, identity, or body image. During self-concept crises, as with other kinds of crises, supportive resources are necessary to help a person learn new ways of coping with and responding to the event or situation and to maintain positive self-esteem and self-concept.

For example, becoming paralyzed involves a major crisis. This client requires help in adapting, and time is required for interventions to succeed. Rehabilitation and restoration of a positive self-concept usually occur after traumatic events. An understanding of the relationships among identity, body image, self-esteem, and roles is essential to the planning of appropriate nursing interventions.

Identity Stressors

Identity is affected by stressors throughout life. Adolescence in particular is a critical period for the development of identity. This is a time of change, causing insecurity and anxiety. Adolescents are trying to adjust to the physical, emotional, and mental changes of increasing maturity. They are preparing for a vocation, seeking economic independence, forming close relationships, and coping with emerging sexuality. Stressors may arise in any of these areas or as a result of conflicts among them (see Chapter 25).

An adult generally has a more stable identity and thus a more firmly developed self-image. Cultural and social, rather than personal, stressors may have more impact on an adult's identity. Cultural and social stressors may challenge values (see Chapter 26). For example, an adult may have to decide between career and marriage, cooperation and competition, or dependence and independence in a relationship (Stuart, Sundeen, 1991).

Menopause, retirement, decreasing physical abilities, and other factors associated with aging also affect identity. Identity, like body image, is closely related to appearance and ability. Changes in appearance and physical capabilities require adaptation. Another potential stressor during middle and later life involves achievement of life goals (see Chapters 26 and 27). Retirement may mean the loss of an important means of achievement and continued success. People may begin to question their identities and accomplishments. Physical and emotional isolation may add stress when significant others die. Finally, in older adulthood, despair rather than ego integrity may result (Erikson, 1963). In fact, depression is common in this population, and it is a diagnosis often missed by health care professionals (Reed, 1991).

Identity confusion, a form of altered self-concept in which people do not maintain a clear, consistent, and continuous consciousness of personal identity, may result at any stage of life if a person is unable to adapt to identity stressors. In extreme cases, an individual may experience **depersonalization,** a state in which inner and outer realities or the differences between the self and others are indistinguishable.

Body-Image Stressors

Changes in the appearance, structure, or function of a body part or feature will require change in body image. Changes in the appearance of the body, such as amputation or facial disfigurement, are obvious stressors affecting body image. Mastectomy, colostomy, or ileostomy also alters the appearance and function of the body, although the changes are not apparent when people are dressed. Body image stressors involving a change in function include renal disease and cardiac disease, in which the body no longer functions at an optimal level and people are physically limited. Even the "normal" body changes resulting from the developmental tasks of aging can affect body image. Pregnancy and significant weight gain or loss change body image. Stressors influencing body image can be related to injuries, diseases involving sensorimotor change, physical alterations from surgical intervention, or toxic or metabolic disorders that may slowly alter body function or require changes in areas such as diet and activity level.

The significance of changes in appearance or a loss of structure or function varies among individuals, families, and cultures. Paralysis caused by war injuries may be considered acceptable; these people may be treated as heroes and praised for bravery and strength, and governmental resources will be available for rehabilitation. However, people who have automobile accidents while drunk and suffer severe injuries and paralysis may receive a different response from society. Society is less likely to accept this situation, and financial resources may be more difficult to obtain.

The significance of a loss of function or structure or a change in appearance is affected by perception of the alteration because body image consists of ideal and real elements. For example, femininity is sometimes associated with the size of the breasts, and if a woman's body image incorporates this as the ideal, the loss of a breast by mastectomy may be a very significant alteration. Another consideration is the importance of the body to self-concept. The greater the importance of the body or a specific body part, the greater the threat felt from a change in body image.

Many people associate success with a specific body part or function. For example, athletes may consider their bodies and physical activities to be the focus of personal success. However, if they can never again participate in physical activities because of an accident, their adaption and rehabilitation are affected. They must revise long-accepted assumptions about themselves and alter their lifestyles, including sexual functioning. To regain positive self-concepts and self-esteem and to maintain good health, they must adapt to the body-image stressor.

After head and neck surgery, people generally participate less in social interaction (Dropkin, 1979). People who have had facial alterations may feel isolated, excluded, stigmatized, or helpless. This feeling of social isolation is often based in reality because people are afraid of embarrassing or offending individuals who are badly burned or "deformed," and thus they avoid contact with them. People with altered body images may fear rejection and isolation or may have experienced it.

Positive social changes with regard to illness and altered body image have occurred. The media more frequently present positive stories about persons who have had major body-altering surgery. For example, accounts of a Canadian runner who was struck by a car and paralyzed showed this young man in a realistic but positive light. Recovery after mastectomy and procedures for performing breast self-examination have been presented on television. Movies have documented the amazing rehabilitation of people after severe trauma. These stories provide role models for persons undergoing unusual stressors and for families, friends, and society. This social change may help eliminate much of the stigma associated with altered physical appearance or functioning, thereby reducing body-image stressors.

Self-help groups are available in most communities for persons who have had ostomies (United Ostomy Association), mastectomies (Reach to Recovery), or laryngectomies (Laryngectomy Club). Self-help groups assist people who are trying to lose weight, parents of children with spina bifida, and people with cancer. These groups provide a special kind of support. People who have experienced particular stressors and who have adapted to them can be instrumental in helping clients adapt to body-image changes. Such people can be special role models, and their families can help other families assist the clients in adapting.

Self-Esteem Stressors

Self-esteem is the sense of being respected, accepted, competent, and worthy. Self-esteem begins to develop in infancy, when perceived acceptance or rejection by parents is an important factor. A person with high self-esteem is generally happier and more able to cope with demands and stressors than a person with low self-esteem (Gibson, 1980). A person with low self-esteem tends to feel unloved and often experiences depression and anxiety. Self-esteem fluctuates with surrounding conditions, although a basic core of positive or negative feeling is maintained.

Many stressors affect the self-esteem of the infant, toddler, preschooler, or adolescent. Inability to meet parental expectations, harsh criticism, inconsistent punishment, sibling rivalry, or repeated defeats may reduce the level of self-worth. Stressors affecting the self-esteem of an adult include lessened ability compared with the spouse, friends, or work colleagues; failures in relationships; a divorce; and loss of a job.

Illness, surgery, or accidents that interrupt or change life patterns may also decrease feelings of self-worth. Chronic illnesses such as diabetes, arthritis, and cardiac dysfunction require changes in accepted and long-assumed behavioral patterns. When changes are slow and progressive, people have opportunities for anticipatory mourning, and adaptation occurs with the change. However, the more that chronic illness interferes with the ability to engage in activities contributing to feelings of worth or success, the more it affects self-esteem.

Self-evaluation is based on relationships with others and on activities. Individual definitions of success or failure influence whether a change is a self-concept stressor. Many people, for example, consider success at work to be important to a sense of achievement and worth. Chronic illness, surgery, or severe trauma may necessitate a career change and thus may be a self-esteem stressor.

Societal standards and the responses of families also affect the importance of a stressor and its impact on self-esteem. Dyk and Sutherland (1956), in a classic study of ostomy patients, found that a husband generally accepted his wife's colostomy more readily than a wife accepted her husband's, apparently because society expects men to be strong and healthy and thus able to work. The wife tended to view the colostomy as an indication that her husband was ill, in need of physical help, and unable to reenter the work force, even when the colostomy did not alter his ability to work.

Role Stressors

Throughout life, people undergo numerous role changes. Change within the same role and the adoption of new roles require the incorporation of new expectations and standards for behavior. Meleis (1975) identifies the developmental, situational, and health-illness categories of role transition. Normal changes associated with growth and maturation result in developmental transitions. Situational transitions occur when parents, spouses, or close friends die or people move, marry, divorce, or change jobs. A health-illness transition is a movement from a state of health or well-being to one of illness. Any of these transitions may threaten self-concept, resulting in role conflict, role ambiguity, or role strain.

Role Conflicts

Role conflict is a lack of compatible role expectations (Broadwell, 1983). When a person is required to simultaneously assume two or more roles that are inconsistent, contradictory, or mutually exclusive, role conflict may occur. For example, a middle-age woman with teenage children has to care for her older parents in her home. Conflicts may occur as she interacts with them simultaneously as care giver and as child. Negotiating a balance of time and energy between her children and parents may also create role conflict. The importance of each conflicting role influences the degree of conflict experienced. A major role is a significant frame of reference. It influences people's evaluations of other role situations. Role conflict usually involves situations in which an inconsistency between two or more expected and sanctioned behaviors exists and the major role does not eliminate this inconsistency.

There are four basic kinds of role conflict: interpersonal, interrole, person-role, and role overload. **Interpersonal conflict** occurs when one or more persons have opposing or incompatible expectations for an individual in a particular role. For example, a woman's friends and her mother may have very different expectations of how she should care for her children.

Interrole conflict occurs when pressures or expectations associated with one role oppose pressures or expectations associated with another. A man who works 10 to 12 hours a day may have problems if his wife expects him to be at home with the family. **Person-role conflict** occurs when role requirements violate an individual's values. For example, a nurse who values the preservation of life experiences conflict when faced with caring for a client who chooses to refuse life-support therapies.

Role overload occurs when an individual cannot decide with which pressures to comply because of an excessive number of demands and a conflict of priorities. Role overload is a complex type of conflict involving internal and external conflicts. People may be expected to comply with the role expectations of one or more persons. They attempt to establish priorities. However, if it is impossible to deny any of these pressures, role overload develops. The expectations of the various roles become overwhelming, and the person does not have the physical, intellectual, economic, emotional, and other resources to adapt to or perform them.

Role Ambiguity

Role ambiguity involves unclear role expectations and an inability to predict the reactions of others to behavior (Broadwell, 1983). When there are unclear expectations, people are unsure of what to do, how to do it, or both. Such a situation is often stressful and confusing. Role ambiguity is common in adolescence. Adolescents are pressured by parents, peers, and the media to assume adultlike roles. They may be expected to work; yet employment opportunities may be severely limited. Their parents may emphasize one set of expectations but not meet them themselves. For example, parents may demand that adolescents not drink alcoholic beverages and drive; yet they may observe their parents doing this same thing. Role ambiguity is also common in employment situations. In complex, rapidly changing, or highly specialized organizations, employees often become unsure of what is expected of them.

Role Strain

Role strain is a general term incorporating role conflict and role ambiguity. Role strain may be expressed as a feeling of frustration when a person feels inadequate or unsuited to a role. Role strain is often associated with gender role stereotypes (Stuart, Sundeen, 1991) (see Chapter 32). Women in positions typically held by men may be perceived by others as less competent, less objective, or less knowledgeable than their male counterparts. Thus they may feel that they must work harder and be better to compete. Men in typically female roles also encounter bias. In addition, femininity or masculinity may be questioned, resulting in further stress.

Chapter 2 describes the sick role as an aspect of illness behavior. This role involves the expectations of others and society, and thus role strain may occur with the sick role. A person is expected to seek health care, be ill only temporarily, acknowledge that illness is undesirable, and depend on health care providers. Role conflict may occur between any of these general societal expectations and the expectations of co-workers, family members, and others. For example, even though people with cardiac illness are expected to reduce their participation in physically stressful activities, friends may after a month or two expect them to again participate in such activities, producing additional stress.

The sick role may also involve role ambiguity. People are expected to be dependent and simultaneously participate actively so that they can get well and leave the sick role quickly. However, chronically ill people cannot do this. The sick role is supposed to be temporary; yet compliance with therapy may be necessary for the remainder of life.

Clients who bring work to the hospital, keep in close contact with business associates, and ask many questions may be considered "bad" clients by some health care workers; however, clients who will not help themselves, are too dependent, or do not resume social roles are considered "bad" clients, too. In addition, sick role behaviors and expectations are based on societal standards. The standards adopted by health care providers may change more quickly than those accepted by clients, resulting in role strain.

Self-concept can be altered by stressors affecting identity, body image, self-esteem, or roles. Examples of stressors that may affect self-concept and each of its components are described in the box on p. 936. Self-concept may also be affected by physical stressors, which can temporarily alter perceptions or levels of consciousness. Lack of oxygen, hyperventilation, biochemical imbalances, endocrine and metabolic disorders, and sensory deprivation, for example, alter people's perceptions of the world and themselves. Alcohol, drugs, radiotherapy, chemotherapy, and exposure to other toxic substances may also distort these perceptions or levels of consciousness.

These stressors can also affect health. If people are unable to adapt to such stressors, their health may be at risk, and if the resulting identity confusion, disturbed body image, low self-esteem, or role conflict, strain, or ambiguity is not relieved, illness may result (Fig. 31-2 on p. 936).

Psychosocial Theories

Although there are several theories of psychosocial development, the theories are consistent in that they represent multiple ways of viewing the development of self-concept. In each stage of psychosocial development, individuals face certain tasks that may lead to psychological problems if they are not positively completed. Through social and cultural reinforcement, individuals learn the relevance, cultural connotations, and emotional significance of concepts. Erikson's theory demonstrates the influence of society on the development of self-concept. For example, infants need to develop a sense of trust if they are to be psychologically healthy. Infants who learn through parental reinforcement to trust their worlds will feel secure as adults. Mistrust arises from uncertainty, frustration, discomfort, or physical harm. People who do not develop trust as infants may have difficulty with later psychosocial development (Erikson, 1963). If they become ill as adults, for example, they may experience physical and psychosocial vulnerabil-

Examples of Self-Concept Stressors

IDENTITY

- School entry (e.g., elementary, secondary, college)
- Developmental tasks of adolescence
- Peer pressure
- Parent-child conflicts
- Relationship concerns
- Sexual concerns
- Alcohol or drug abuse
- Death of spouse or family member
- Employer-employee conflicts
- Appearance changes in middle and older adulthood
- Burglary of home
- Rape
- Assault

BODY IMAGE

- Impaired sensory function (e.g., deafness, blindness, chronic pain)
- Altered motor and sensory-perceptive function after cerebrovascular accident (stroke)
- Alteration in or loss of body structure or function (e.g., hysterectomy, mastectomy, ileostomy, ileobladder, colostomy, tracheostomy)
- Arthritis, musculoskeletal disease
- Normal growth and developmental changes (e.g., puberty, pregnancy, menopause, aging)
- Anorexia nervosa
- Diabetes mellitus or insipidus
- Incontinence
- Dermatitis
- Obesity

SELF-ESTEEM

- Lack of advancement in job
- Loss of job
- Marital stress, separation, or divorce
- Doing less well than expected
- Repeated failures
- Unrealistically high aspirations for self
- Dependency on others
- Abuse or battering from parent or spouse
- Neglect by parents
- Victim of assault or rape
- Sexuality concerns, infertility
- Child having to assume adult responsibilities
- Unemployment in family
- Marital role conflict
- Conflict with employer or colleagues
- Incompatible role expectations
- Lack of preparation for role
- Unclear role expectations
- Inability to adequately perform and cope with multiple roles
- Societal attitudes of ageism
- Imposed social isolation
- Excessive competition in relationships with others
- Restriction of ability to perform role for which prepared

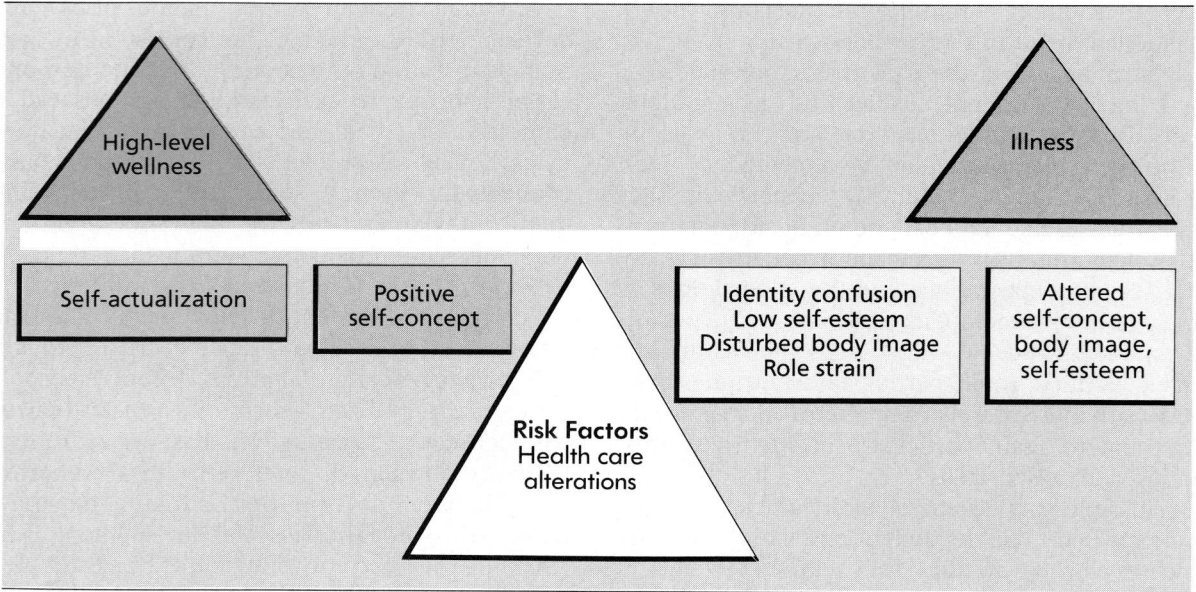

Fig. 31-2 Self-concept health-illness continuum.

ity and distrust the environment, especially a hospital environment. Because they have insecure self-concepts, they may have difficulty adapting to changes caused by illness or therapy.

Development of Self-Concept

Development of self-conflict is a lifelong process. Each stage of development has specific activities that assist the client in developing a positive self-image (see box).

Infant

At first, newborns can barely discriminate between their own pleasurable sensations and the objects from which the sensations are derived. Newborns have diffuse feelings of hunger, pain, rage, and comfort. They do not differentiate themselves from the environment. In other words, they do not have a clear sense of body boundaries. The external world is an extension of themselves. Only as perceptive and sensory functions mature do infants gradually learn about their bodies. Infants totally depend on adults to take care of their basic needs. When needs such as feeding and nurturance are met promptly and consistently, infants begin to develop trust in the world. Because infants view themselves as part of the primary care giver, positive experiences help them gain confidence in themselves (Haber et al, 1987). Babies gradually distinguish themselves from other objects as they are fed, diapered, and touched or bang their heads, bite their hands, and put objects in their mouths. The process of defining themselves begins when they act reflexively, such as when they suck or grasp an object. The act and the significance attributed to it by parents are important because they rein-

---

Positive Developmental Tasks Related to Self-Concept

INFANCY (0-1 YR)

- Learns to tolerate small frustrations
- Learns to trust
- Begins to distinguish self from environment
- Internalizes sensory images into body image

TODDLERHOOD (1-3 YR)

- Learns to be aware of and like body
- Learns mastery of motor and language skills and bowel training
- Develops beginning sense of autonomy and separateness
- Learns more socialization skills

PRESCHOOL YEARS (3-6 YR)

- Learns initiative
- Learns sex typing
- Identifies with parental models
- Increases motor and language skills
- Experiences growing self-awareness and control of feelings
- Receives positive feedback from others, which develops into positive self-appraisal

SCHOOL-AGE YEARS (6-12 YR)

- Develops sense of industry
- Has clear sex-role identification
- Learns peer interaction
- Develops academic skills
- Masters new skills so self-esteem increases
- Becomes aware of limitations and strengths

ADOLESCENCE (12-20 YR)

- Integrates changing body image
- Develops a positive sense of identity
- Defines sex roles and interacts with members of opposite sex
- Explores life goals

YOUNG ADULTHOOD (EARLY 20s TO MID 40s)

- Establishes functional patterns of employment, intimate relationships, and family
- Possesses stable self-definition
- Creates satisfying life roles

MIDDLE ADULTHOOD (MID 40s TO MID 60s)

- Adapts to changes in physical appearance and endurance
- Accepts loss of youth
- Reassesses or recommits to chosen life values
- Is content with age

OLDER ADULTHOOD (AFTER 60s)

- Successfully copes with reduction of physical and sensory abilities
- Accepts older appearance
- Possesses personal sense of wholeness and control

force behavior. Gradually, children experience visceral, visual, auditory, kinesthetic, and motor sensations (Anthony, 1968; Schilder, 1951).

Weaning, contact with others, and exploration of the environment also heighten self-awareness. As children approach their first birthdays, coordination of these sensory experiences is internalized into their motor body images. They are aware that some body parts give greater pleasure than other parts and that differences in sensation occur when their body or when another object is touched (Anthony, 1968; Murray, Zentner, 1985; Schilder, 1951).

Without adequate stimulation of the motor abilities and the senses, body image and self-concept development are impaired, as shown by studies of infants in premature incubators who lacked rocking, stroking, and cuddling (Kramer et al, 1975). Infants' initial experiences with their bodies, determined largely by maternal care and attitudes, are the bases for developing body images and later acceptance and management of the body and reactions to others (Murray, Zentner, 1985).

Toddler

As children move into the toddler stage (1 to 3 years of age), they are more mobile and able to interact with others. At this age, a major psychosocial task is the development of autonomy. Children move from total dependence to a greater sense of independence and separateness of themselves from others. Children at this age also tend to view others and themselves in terms of black and white (for example, "all good" or "all bad"). Before age 4, children begin to combine negative and positive aspects of themselves into unified wholes. They gain skills by feeding themselves and performing basic hygiene tasks. Toddlers learn to coordinate movements and imitate others. They learn control of their bodies through locomotion, toilet training, speech, and socialization skills.

Young children are not always aware of the whole body and might even consider distal parts such as hands and feet as something apart from themselves. In addition, other parts of themselves may be viewed as "permanent," so getting a haircut or flushing waste products down the toilet may cause stress because they were a part of the self. These children do not always know when they are ill, fatigued, too cold, or thirsty or have wet pants. Toddlers are simply aware of general feelings and are increasingly aware of others' reactions to themselves and their behavior. For example, when toddlers play with toys or interact happily with people, they feel good and in control. Similarly, if they cannot succeed or are punished excessively, they feel bad and shameful (Anthony, 1968).

Preschooler

The preschool years (3 to 5 years of age) help children realize their capabilities. Body boundaries, sense of self, and gender become more definite to them because of a developing sexual curiosity and awareness of differences from others of the same and opposite gender. Increased motor skills with precision of movement and maturing sense of balance, improved spatial orientation, maturing cognitive and language abilities, ongoing play activities, and relationship and identification with parents add to self-concept and body-image development (Anthony, 1968).

Learning about the body, where it begins and ends, what it looks like, and what it can do, are basic to self-concept and body-image formation. Growing self-awareness includes discovery of feelings; for example, preschoolers learn names for their feelings. They begin to learn how they affect others and how others respond to them. They also learn the rudiments of control over feelings and behavior. The concept of body is reflected in the way that children talk, move, draw pictures, and play. Children who have no frame of reference in relation to themselves experience increased anxiety and misperceptions of themselves and others.

Parental and cultural attitudes about appropriate behavior for boys and girls may contribute to body-image confusion, especially if behavior and appearance do not match the expectations of others. Children begin to test roles and imitate people as they identify with the same-sex parent or a family member.

Although children still feel small in relation to adults, they have established positive or negative views of themselves. They hear and experience emotions and pronouncements of others, especially parents, about themselves as people. They also hear about things and events around them. When these expressions are repeated many times, they begin to form a predictable pattern, so children internalize the views of others and begin to see them as part of themselves. They then behave to match these views. This view of the self begins as a judgment made by another. For example, Johnny's parents consider him to be mechanically inclined. This behavior was not a part of Johnny at birth, but as he develops, the perception becomes a part of him and he acts accordingly. Children learn to value what their parents value. Appraisal by a family member becomes self-appraisal. A positive self-concept is imperative for happiness and personality unity. Negative self-concepts cause children to feel defensive toward others and about themselves. Negative self-concept hinders adjustment to school, academic progress, peer relationships, and developmental tasks.

School-Age Child

Until children attend school, self-concept and body-image development are based primarily on parental attitudes. At school, others contribute to self-concept and body image.

As the child enters the school years, growth is steady, and more motor, social, and intellectual skills are acquired. The physique changes, and sexual identity strengthens. Children are a part of a new group—teachers, peers, and school-age society. Attention span increases, and reading allows expansion of self-concept through imagination into other roles, behaviors, and places. Games become a major portion of children's activities. Through games, children interact with peers, develop additional motor and intellectual skills, and thereby expand self-concept and body image. Self-esteem is altered as new skills are mastered or are not attained. As children learn and follow rules, they also learn about their acceptability to others, strengthening a positive self-concept. Games also expand understanding and awareness of other people and other places. Children express feelings through games, literature, drawing, and music. They express positive and realistic images of themselves through behavior movements, drawings, music, statements, and games. The nurse can use these to gain clues to children's self-concepts. With increased problem-solving abilities, a greater self-awareness of personal strengths and limitations develops. Self-concept and body image can change because the child is changing physically, emotionally, mentally, and socially. Although children cannot accurately name body organs, they are increasingly aware of their bodies and their abilities.

Adolescent

Puberty, with hormonal changes and growth spurts, is a critical period in the development of self-concept. Adolescence brings physical, emotional, and social upheaval. Throughout sexual maturation, new feelings, roles, and values must be integrated into the self. Rapid growth, noticed by the adolescent and others, is an important factor in body-image revision.

Adolescent girls and boys are sometimes said to be "all legs." They are often clumsy and awkward. Adolescents are forced to alter their mental pictures of themselves. Physical changes in size and appearance cause changes in self-perception and use of the body. Adolescents spend a great deal of time in front of the mirror for hygiene, grooming, and dressing. Age, maturation, gender, size, shape, and even the person's name are emphasized in behavior, music, dance, or sports, all normal ways for the adolescent to integrate a changing body image.

Development of self-concept and body image is closely related to identity formation (Erikson, 1963).

Early experiences have important effects. Positive experiences enable adolescents to feel good about themselves. Negative experiences may result in poor self-concept. Children who enter adolescence with negative feelings find this a difficult period.

Growth, appearance, and functional changes draw adolescents' attention to changing body parts, and they become more sensitive about it, causing a distorted view of themselves. They may overemphasize perceived health problems, such as a pointed nose, large ears, short stature, or large body frame, and consequently underevaluate themselves. The body acts as the basic source of acceptance or rejection from others. Adolescents are idealistic but may not be able to achieve "ideal" bodies. If adolescents do not feel accepted for themselves or their bodies, they may try to compensate through sports, vocational or academic success, religious commitments, use of alcohol or drugs, or a date or group of friends to enhance prestige. Thus identification with the same-sex parent, harmonious relationships with other adults, and the capability to strive for ideals and realistic goals are essential.

Adolescents begin to relate to the opposite sex in new ways and with increasing interest. They sample various behavioral roles as they establish a sense of identity, including who they are, what life means, and where they are going.

If adolescents have disabilities, peers and adults may react with fear, pity, revulsion, or curiosity. Adolescents may retain and later reflect on these impressions because people tend to perceive themselves as others perceive them. If these adolescents develop negative self-images, their motivations, behaviors, and eventual lifestyles may lack harmony and be out of step with social expectations.

Young Adult

Although physical growth has stopped by this stage, cognitive, social, and behavioral changes continue for the rest of life. Young adulthood (early 20s to mid 40s) is a period of choice; it is a period of settling in to responsibility, gaining stability in the establishment of employment, and establishing intimate relationships. A young adult must decide whether to have a family. Self-concept and body image become relatively stable. Self-expectations, the reactions of others, perceived abilities and limitations, values, attitudes, knowledge, and habits have been integrated into a functioning, adaptive, unified whole.

Young adults' search for self-definition is complicated by confusion in society about gender behavior, the meaning of maleness and femaleness, and the variety of roles and occupations from which to choose. The masculine and feminine role stereotypes that once characterized these roles are disappearing. Self-concept and body image are social creations, and approval and acceptance are given for normal appearance and proper behavior according to societal standards. Self-image continually influences and enlarges the world, mastery of interaction with it, and ability to respond to its experiences. Self-concept constantly evolves and can be identified in values, attitudes, and feelings about the self. Experiences with the body are interpreted in terms of feelings, earlier self-views, and group or cultural norms (Coopersmith, 1967; Schilder, 1951).

In young adults, close interdependence among body image and personality, self-concept, self-esteem, and identity exists. Therefore self-concept is an important determinant of behavior. A positive, realistic self-concept, mature body image, and mature behavior depend on meeting the changing demands of each previous developmental era. In particular, the time for development of dominant body parts such as the mouth in infancy, the limbs in preschool and school years, and the genitals at puberty are important eras. If each of these body zones and their functioning and related social expectations are not integrated into the total self-image, self-concept and body image will remain immature in some aspects. The immature self-image may interfere with securing adult satisfactions and may be evidenced by a personality disturbance. However, mature young adults can accept their bodies without undue preoccupation with appearance, function, or control of these functions so that they are free to focus on other experiences (Cleveland, Morton, 1967).

Middle Adult

Gradually occurring physical changes confront the middle adult and are mirrored in others. These changes may include additional fat deposits, baldness, gray hair, wrinkles, varicosities, prominent veins, tissue atrophy, and sagging tissue. This developmental stage, resulting from changing hormone production, causes appearance and self-concept changes about sexuality. Cultural values about youth, negative attitudes about age, and other life stresses cause people to view themselves and their bodies differently. People realize that they look older, and they feel older, as well. Work may be stressful if middle-age people feel that they have less stamina, endurance, and vigor to cope with the task at hand.

This decrease in energy level often is the result of a lower basal metabolic rate, decreasing muscle tone, and sensory changes. The illnesses or deaths of loved ones can create concerns about personal health. These concerns can become excessive, and thoughts of death become more frequent. The person can feel inferior to youth as the previous self-image of a strong and healthy body with boundless energy is replaced with a self-image reflecting the changes of aging.

Personality largely influences the intensity of these feelings and the symptoms of body-image changes. Difficulties in accepting the loss of youth are also caused by fear of the effects of menopause or the climacteric, folklore about sexuality, social and advertising pressures describing the virtues of youth, and emphasis on obsolescence.

The middle adult years are often the time for a reassessment of life experiences and a redefinition of the self in terms of life roles and values. This is sometimes called the *midlife crisis*. This re-evaluation might include career or marriage choices or basic purpose in life. Successful resolution involves the integration of new qualities into self-concept or acceptance and recommitment to past choices and values.

Most people gradually adjust to their slowly changing bodies and accept the changes as part of maturing. Emotionally mature people realize that they cannot return to youth and acknowledge that their own pasts and experiences are valid and valuable. Middle-age people who are content with their ages and have no desire to relive the youthful years exhibit a healthy self-concept.

Older Adult

Physical changes in older adults can be seen as gradual reductions of structure and function. Loss of muscle strength and tone occurs. Osteoporosis, which is a loss of bone density and mass, may increase the risk of fractures or a "dowagers" hump. This may be incorporated into the self-image of older adults as frail.

Loss of sensory acuity is a factor that influences older adults in interacting with the environment (see Chapter 45). The normal process of aging causes decreased visual acuity. Eyeglasses and good illumination are helpful in maintaining function.

Hearing loss can cause negative personality changes as older people realize that they no longer are aware of all that is happening or said. Suspiciousness, irritability, impatience, or withdrawal may develop because of impaired hearing. In addition, older adults may be afraid to admit the problem or may hesitate in seeking treatment, especially if they are unaware of the possibilities of help through the use of hearing aids or corrective surgery. Often, older adults view a hearing aid as another threat to body image, although it is now possible to obtain aids that are hardly noticeable. Yet to many older adults, eyeglasses are more socially acceptable because they are worn by all age groups, but a hearing aid is perceived as direct evidence of age. Adjustment to the use of a hearing aid may be difficult; if motivation is low, hearing aids may be rejected. Loss of skin tone with accompanying wrinkles and appearance may affect self-esteem and cause older persons to feel ugly in a society that values youth and beauty.

Sexual activity usually diminishes with age, even though ability to perform is still functional. Often, many older people do not engage in sexual activity because they lack partners (Butler, Lewis, 1976). Changes in body image may deter sexual activity because of anticipated or perceived rejection by a partner or because of feared inability to perform, even though most research indicates that no physical barriers exist.

Self-concept during older adulthood is influenced by experiences throughout the person's life. It is a time when many people reflect on their lives, reviewing successes and disappointments and thereby creating a unified sense of meaning about themselves and the world (see research highlight). Self-concept is also influenced by people's present perceived health status. Persons over the age of 60 tend to view health in a much more positive way than younger people. One reason for this may be that living to an old age without severe health problems is an indication of fairly good health (Cockerham, Sharp, Wilcox, 1983).

Threats to self-esteem are thought to be related to decreased social interaction, loss of control over the environment, and age stigmatization (Taft, 1985). The nurse can affect these areas. A successful, consistent sense of self is characterized by personal wholeness and satisfaction in most areas of life. Basic attitudes indicating a positive self-concept focus on gratefulness, personal control, and acceptance of self (Hamachek, 1990).

Family Effect on Self-Concept Development

Family plays a substantial role in creating and maintaining its members' self-concepts. It is particularly crucial because children learn from parents and siblings a basic sense of who they are and how they are expected to live. Self-worth is also instilled in children from parents, and aspects of personality are difficult to change later in life (Crouch, Straub, 1983).

Negative self-concepts may be created in children, even by well-meaning parents. Parents who are

---

 Research Highlight

The purpose of Reed's study was to look at the concept of "self-transcendence" among the oldest-old (80 to 97 years). Specifically, she attempted to identify components of self-transcendence that are important to emotional well-being. Self-transcendence is the expansion of one's boundaries (1) inwardly, by introspection, (2) outwardly, through concern about others, and (3) temporally, by tying together past and future perceptions to make the present time better.

The sample consisted of 55 older adults living independently with average-to-good health. The self-transcendence scale, the Center for Epidemiological Studies' depression scale, the Langner Scale of Mental Health Symptomology, and a short interview were used to collect information for the study.

Four dimensions of self-transcendence have been identified from the participants' responses, including generativity, introjectivity, temporal integration, and body transcendence. The generativity dimension represents helping others. Introjectivity involves inner growth and learning. Temporal integration refers to respondents' views of the past, present, and future. Body transcendence relates to coping abilities regarding physical changes resulting from aging or illness.

Results indicate that when these four patterns are positive, they help promote emotional well-being. Persons who show no depression indicate flexible attitudes toward bodily changes, inner-directed activities, and positive integration of the present and future. This research also supports the importance of Erikson's developmental stage of generativity. Nursing implications include assessment of perception of physical changes and encouragement of outward concern for others and inner self-development.

Reed P: Self-transcendence and mental health in oldest-old adults, *Nurs Res* 49(1):5, 1991.

---

harsh or inconsistent or have low self-esteem may have learned these patterns from their parents, thereby creating a cycle that may be difficult to break. To reverse clients' low self-esteem, the nurse may need to work with their families. Even if clients have little contact with their original families, the nurse should work with other family members or friends that have contact with the clients. Assessing the developmental stage of the clients may be important in determining family members who should be included in treatment (Crouch, Straub, 1983).

NURSE'S EFFECT ON CLIENT'S SELF-CONCEPT

Impact of Nurse's Self-Concept

Nurses may be the first persons, and thus role models, met by a client undergoing changes in self-concept. Nurses' acceptance of a client with an altered self-concept may be the factor that stimulates positive rehabilitation. In the case of a client whose physical appearance has changed and who must adapt to a new body image, the client and family may look to nurses and observe responses and reactions to the new situation. To be effective role models, nurses should acknowledge that they have a significant impact on the client. The feelings and expectations of nurses are communicated nonverbally and verbally to the client, family, friends, and other health care providers. Nursing plans formulated to help a client with an altered self-concept can be enhanced or defeated by nurses' unconsciously communicated values and feelings. Thus nurses should try to understand the following:

1. Personal feelings regarding health and illness
2. Personal reactions to stress, such as coping behaviors
3. Coping behaviors and defense behaviors in others
4. Perception of professional role
5. Nonverbal communication with client and family
6. Personal values and expectations about people
7. Ability to positively intervene on the behalf of another person who has different values without trying to change or judge the other person

Nurses can develop greater cognitive self-awareness by using a three-step approach involving the following (Haber, 1987):

1. Listening to themselves. This refers to conversations that people have with themselves. It also refers to paying attention to the meanings of the client's statements.
2. Listening to others. Positive and negative feedback is evaluated seriously before discarding or incorporating it into the self-concept.
3. Letting others listen to them. This step involves self-disclosure or being honest and open about personal strengths and challenges. It is not permission to involve clients with nurses' problems; rather, it is more of an openness to share appropriate aspects of the self to develop more self-awareness.

Nurses can also pay attention to "triggers," which are feelings that occur in response to a given situation. Often, these feeling might be considered an overreaction to the situation. Becoming aware of these triggers can assist nurses in understanding personal feelings and beliefs, thereby providing opportunities for deeper self-awareness. For example, if nurses react with disgust or revulsion to a client with acquired immunodeficiency syndrome (AIDS), they can use that feeling as a starting point for examination of personal values and beliefs (see Chapter 12).

Nurses cannot deny that they have feelings, ideas, values, and expectations and that they make judgments. When providing care, nurses act as persons who are separate and autonomous from others and who therefore have unique self-concepts, identities, self-esteem, body images, and behavior roles. Self-awareness and self-acceptance can promote understanding and acceptance of others. All people make decisions about themselves, the environment, and other people on the basis of personal frames of reference. As professionals, nurses must be prepared to work with other people who have their own frames of reference. Nurses must develop an awareness of their own reactions to various situations and stressors.

Nurses' reactions to illness are influenced by their own self-concepts and can have a significant impact on clients' self-concepts. Clients with low self-esteem, for example, may be particularly sensitive to the way that nurses involve them in therapy. If nurses lack self-confidence, they may be hesitant in making suggestions, thus inadvertently implying that clients might be unable to follow suggestions. They may insist that clients assume too much responsibility for their own care, thus frightening them. In either case, clients' self-esteem may be additionally threatened, rather than strengthened. If, however, the nurse demontrates confidence in clients' abilities and is self-confident, clients' self-worth will be reinforced.

A similar principle operates in regard to identity. Nurses who are secure in their own identities more readily accept and thus reinforce clients' identities. However, nurses who are unsure of their own identities may be unable to accept clients and may react as if clients should be something or someone else, thus threatening their identities.

Nurses also have a significant impact on body image. Clients who must adapt to changed body image caused by illness or surgery need support, as do their families. If nurses feel, for example, that ostomies or mastectomies are horrible things, they should not express that opinion to clients. Nurses should talk with people who have had more experience in the care and rehabilitation of such clients. Meeting people who have had such surgery and who have recuperated can increase knowledge. Nurses who feel insecure about their own body images will probably react more strongly to changes in clients' physical appearances and functioning. Inadvertently frowning or grimacing or avoiding clients are indications that nurses are unable to cope with stress in regard to such physical changes. The self-concept of incontinent clients, for example, can be threatened by the perception that others find the situation unpleasant. Thus nurses should be aware of these reactions, acknowledge them, and focus on clients instead of the unpleasant situation. Otherwise clients may perceive nurses' behaviors as isolation or rejection. Nurses should try to empathize. If nurses can imagine such feelings, they can imagine measures to ease embarrassment, frustration, anger, and denial.

A nurse who works with someone undergoing body-image changes plays a major role in helping the client adapt and cope. This role may not be easy, but it is rewarding to the client and nurse.

Impact of Nursing Activities

Everyone perceives some aspects of the human experience as stressful, frightening, frustrating, anger provoking, or saddening. The stressors associated with illness and its treatment affect an individual's self-concept in various ways. A client needs a safe, nonjudgmental, and supportive environment. Sultenfuss (1982) has specified the following messages a nurse should convey to the client to provide a therapeutic environment that does not threaten the client's self-concept:

1. Whatever the client communicates is normal and acceptable. If the nurse, while providing care, implies that the client's values are in any way unacceptable, the client's sense of identity or self-esteem may be threatened.
2. The client's communciation is not threatening or frightening to the nurse. For example, the nurse should not react with anger to the client's anger. Clients who are angry at themselves, their disease, or someone else may direct their anger at nurses, other health care providers, or even families. It is often difficult not to react and to recognize that the anger may be related to loss of control or to an inability to act as usual. Reactions revealing that the nurse is frightened or threatened can become stressors for the client's self-concept, as well.
3. The nurse will not reject or isolate the client because of anything communicated. The nurse assesses and evaluates personal actions and reactions. In addition, nurses must notice when other nurses or other health care personnel are avoiding a client. Isolation and rejection, real or imagined, will negatively affect the client's self-concept.

Many health care activities can adversely affect a client's self-concept unless the nurse takes action. A hospitalized client, for example, almost always experiences role changes and lowered self-esteem as a result of dependence on those providing care. In addition, physical examination of the client's body, drawing blood samples for laboratory analysis, and many other routine actions can threaten the client's body and privacy. Because such nursing activities are far from routine for most clients, as is the health care environment itself, the client often feels alienated and vulnerable, and these feelings affect self-concept.

However, the nurse can minimize these feelings and assist the client in maintaining a positive self-concept. Encouraging visits by family members, for example, helps the client maintain a usual role within the family. Discussing all procedures with the client and encouraging participation in the care plan are examples of ways in which a nurse can respect client identity. If the client feels merely like a body being manipulated by health care professionals, loss of self-esteem may occur. In general, the nurse assists the client in carrying on as usual as much as possible with activities and relationships that support self-concept. If self-concept depends on activities in which the client is no longer able to participate, the nurse can encourage adaptation to change through other kinds of activities that rebuild self-concept and a sense of normalcy.

The nurse's role and impact differ with each client. The primary role, perhaps, is as a caring person who is a role model. The nurse provides an example for the client and family. Acceptance of the client as a human being who has ideas, feelings, and values and who is worthy and whole despite illness or physical alterations is important. Feelings of insecurity, fears of rejection, or loss of self-worth can be lessened through sensitive, knowledgeable nursing care.

■ ALTERED SELF-CONCEPT AND THE NURSING PROCESS

Assessment

When assessing self-concept, the nurse obtains objective and subjective data to give a more realistic view of the client's strengths and challenges. Objective data include behaviors demonstrated by the client or verbal and nonverbal interactions between the client and others. Past records are another objective source of data that may include a history of coping through the use of alcohol or other chemicals. Assessment of resources in the client's community can be useful when developing a realistic plan of continued care for the client.

TABLE 31-1 Assessment for Characteristics of Self-Concept Disturbance

Sample Assessment Questions	Indications of Identity Confusion
Describe what is different about you since your illness (problem).	Verbalizes distortion and feeling mixed up: "I didn't feel like myself" or "I don't feel like the same person"
Explain how you felt before and after the abuse.	
How has your illness influenced your life?	Expresses lifestyle change related to illness
What changes have you made in your life because of your health problems?	
What do you expect of your life in the next few months? 2 years?	Expresses feelings of hopelessness, helplessness, or powerlessness in relation to self of life
How much do you feel you can change your situation?	
What areas of your life do you feel you have control over?	
What areas do you feel a loss of control?	
Tell me about the relationships you are involved in.	Expresses inability to be autonomous or intimate with another
If you could change any part of a relationship, how would you prefer it?	
How independent are you?	
How comfortable are you getting close to other people?	
Tell me about your living arrangements.	Expresses feelings of aloneness or alienation from others or is suspicious about others' behavior to self
Are your relationships with others satisfying to you?	
How trusting are you of others?	
How do you cope with problems or make decisions for your life?	Demonstrates inability to make decisions about self or own lifestyle or is unable to act on suggestions
To what extent do you carry out your decisions?	
How do you feel about your body?	Expresses feelings of depersonalization of being someone else, or expresses feeling that part of body does not belong to self
Do you ever feel out of touch with your body? Explain.	
How much alcohol do you consume?	Demonstrates self-destructive acts (e.g., alcohol or drug abuse, accident proneness)
Tell me about any street drugs you use.	*Other Behavioral Indicators*
Would you consider yourself absent minded or accident prone?	Does not answer to own name, calls self by an impersonal pronoun or by the name of an object
	Demonstrates some defense mechanisms in variety of situations
	Refuses to engage in self-care or activities of daily living (e.g., eating, sleeping, elimination)
	Demonstrates or expresses exaggerated emotional responses
What do you think about when you look in the mirror?	Verbalizes distorted sense of body: "I feel like I don't know myself when I look in the mirror," "I can't stand how I look," "I get so mad that I can't move like I used to"
How do you feel about the changes that have affected your body?	
How are you coping with your physical problems?	Expresses feelings of depression about physical deterioration
What feelings are you experiencing about these changes?	
How do you think others will act toward you as a result of this situation?	Expresses fear of rejection from others as a result of health problems
What has your family said about you and your situation?	
Who is available to give you support now?	
What are some other losses you are experiencing as a result of these health changes?	Expresses grief about body changes (e.g., weeping, anger, despair, sadness)
	Other Behavioral Indicators
	Perceives machines (e.g., oxygen, monitor) as part of self
	Is unable to distinguish self from others
	Does not participate in or has difficulty with self-care
	Refuses to look at or acknowledge changes in body structure, appearance, or function
	Refuses to participate in nursing or medical therapies or rehabilitative activities
	Is unable to or is inaccurate in estimating spatial relationship of body in bed, wheelchair, or environment
	Overexposes or conceals all or parts of body

Sample Assessment Questions	Indications of Identity Confusion
How do you feel about yourself as a person? How do you see yourself?	Verbalizes negative feelings: "I hate myself," "I wish I were dead—I'm good for nothing," "I can't do anything right" Expresses excessive criticism of self or others
How are you adjusting to the changes you have experienced? Tell me about how you are feeling about this surgery.	Expresses shame or guilt about changes in appearance, structure, or function
Can you share how others help you feel loved and cared for? How do you express caring feelings to others?	Expresses feelings of being unloved, unlovable, or unable to love
Tell me about how you coped with problems in the past.	Repeats stories about negative experiences or feelings about self
What do you fore see happening out of this situation?	Expresses expectation of a bad outcome of the situation
How will you work through this health problem?	Expresses excessive worry or fear about the situation
Name some qualities you like about yourself.	Minimizes strength or abilities, exaggerates limits or weaknesses
Name some challenges you would like to work on.	
Are you the kind of person who tends to see things through?	Expresses sense of self-defeat, fragility, inadequacy, and self-contempt
How do you respond when others give you feedback?	Disregards opinion of others and hesitates to offer own opinions
Would you say you communicate in a more passive, assertive, or aggressive way?	*Other Behavioral Indicators* Demonstrates regressive behavior
How would you judge the way you communicate with others?	Demonstrates lack of confidence in self-care, performance of activities of daily living, and management of body, role performance Demonstrates lack of eye contact with others, stooped posture, and change in personal hygiene habits Does not acknowledge encouragement, realistic praise, or positive reinforcement Is unable to communicate feelings, needs, or ideas Demonstrates anxiety, apathy, or irritability when asked to engage in self-care or role performance
What are your activities during the day? How do you feel about carrying out these responsibilities? What are the expectations of your spouse, mother, child, boss, and teacher for you? How do you feel about yourself as a result? How would you evaluate your work or school activities? How are you feeling about not being able to do this activity anymore?	Verbalizes feeling inadequate in performance: "I can't do budgeting as well as Mary," "I can't manage the house anymore," "They expect too much of me," He (spouse, child) never does his share of the work," "I don't get a chance to do the things I enjoy and that I used to do," and "I'm just a bad person"
What is different about your abilities since you developed your health problem?	Expresses dissatisfaction or frustration over inability to perform previous tasks or activities
Do you have confidence in the person who is helping you take care of your needs? Explain how this is a problem.	Expresses mistrust of care givers and their performance
What is it that you want out of your situation?	Expresses uselessness of efforts at expressing will and self-direction
What are some barriers that keep you from reaching your goals?	Expresses excessively high expectations of self in self-care, performance of activities of daily living, or other roles
How will you be able to manage at home?	*Other Behavioral Indicators* Demonstrates inability to relate effectively with family, friends, or care givers
What things are you going to need to know to be better able to take care of yourself?	Demonstrates excessive dependence on or independence from others in relation to health care, activities of daily living, or other roles Changes usual patterns of lifestyle or responsibility Demonstrates lack of initiative in activities or roles Demonstrates change in social involvement or relationships with others

Subjective data are gathered to determine the client's view of the self and life. Significant others' perceptions are a vital source of data. Assessment should focus on actual and potential self-concept stressors and their nature, number, and intensity. Obtaining knowledge about past coping behaviors reveals positive and harmful patterns. Present internal and external adaptive resources are also explored. Table 31-1 gives examples of characteristics that may be assessed with self-concept disturbance.

The collection of assessment data can be a healing experience for the client. Initial supportive responses by the nurse set the tone for a collaborative relationship in all areas of the nursing process.

 ## Nursing Diagnosis

After collecting information about the client, the nurse interprets the data. Clients with self-concept disturbances may have many nursing diagnoses per-

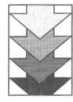 ## Examples of Nursing Diagnoses Related to Disturbance in Self-Concept

NANDA-APPROVED NURSING DIAGNOSES

Altered parenting related to:
- Identity confusion subsequent to earlier conflicts with own parents
- Lack of preparation for role

Altered role performance related to:
- Demands on time as result of entry into college
- Perceptions about ageist attitudes encountered in workplace
- Anxiety about abilities after myocardial infarction

Anxiety related to:
- Perception of midlife aging changes and implication for job security
- Marital role conflicts
- Concerns about sexuality

Body-image disturbance related to:
- Negative perception of self after hysterectomy
- Visual impairment

Dysfunctional grieving related to:
- Difficulty adjusting to 2 months unemployment
- Unresolved crisis of divorce

Fear related to:
- Feelings of powerlessness from recent home burglary
- Unresolved crisis of being assaulted

Impaired adjustment related to:
- Anxiety about body image (amputation)
- Fear of terminal illness (AIDS)

Impaired social interaction related to:
- Role ambiguity (widowhood)
- Depression resulting from recent admission to extended care facility

Impaired verbal communication related to:
- Low self-esteem
- Poor adjustment to hearing impairment

Ineffective individual coping related to:
- Low self-esteem
- Dysfunctional parent-child relationship
- Unclear role expectations

Parental role conflict related to:
- Feeling loss of control secondary to birth of child with congenital defect
- Anxiety about upcoming remarriage

Personal identity disturbance related to:
- Rapid loss of weight
- Value conflicts aroused by peer group
- Confusion about sexuality

High risk for violence: self-directed related to:
- Identity confusion in adolescence
- Inability to cope with multiple role expectations
- Low self-esteem after abuse from spouse

Powerlessness related to:
- Incompatible role expectations at home and work
- Feelings of low self-worth

Rape-trauma syndrome related to:
- Unresolved crisis of being assaulted sexually

Self-esteem disturbance related to:
- Job interview anxiety
- Perception of sexuality after infertility problems

Chronic low self-esteem related to:
- Negative self-talk
- Unrealistic parental expectations

Situational low self-esteem related to:
- Unresolved grief
- Lack of meaningful support system
- Role conflict with colleagues

Social isolation related to:
- Perception of disfigurement after accidental injury
- Low self-esteem after abuse from parents
- Marital role conflicts

Spiritual distress (distress of the human spirit) related to:
- Identity confusion in midlife
- Altered body image from accidental paralysis
- Alcohol and drug abuse

tinent to identity, body-image, self-esteem, or role-performance disturbance. The diagnoses box lists pertinent nursing diagnoses and related etiologies. The diagnostic label is validated by defining characteristics of behaviors, signs, symptoms, feelings, or beliefs. Examples of defining characteristics and possible related factors for two nursing diagnoses are presented in the diagnostic process box.

Planning

After determining the nursing diagnoses, the nurse, client, and family plan care directed at helping the client regain a healthy self-concept. The care plan should be based on short- and long-term goals of adaptation. For a client beginning to receive chemotherapy and experiencing body-image stressors, for example, short-term goals might include encouraging the client to describe the physical effects of the medication and express feelings about the illness and treatment. The long-term goal might be to help the

client adapt successfully to a new body image. Other health team members also have input into goals and interventions. It is important to establish with the client a priority for the problems. If the client's stay in the facility will be short, there may not be enough time to restructure body image. However, if the client has not resolved the problem by discharge, referral to a community resource is indicated. A list of community resources helpful to clients with self-concept difficulties is shown in the box.

Similarly, the nurse may not be the health professional most appropriate to address self-concept problems. For example, if the client is experiencing an extended period of depression or grief, a psychiatrist may need to evaluate the individual to determine whether an antidepressant medication is indicated.

After establishing goals, the nurse plans strategies to reduce the client's problems. Again, the client and significant others collaborate with the nurse in determining interventions. The care plan presents the goals, expected outcomes, and interventions for a client with a self-concept disorder. Interventions focus on helping the client adapt to the stressors that led to the self-concept disturbance and on supporting and reinforcing the development of coping methods (see care plan on p. 948).

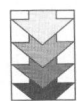

Sample Nursing Diagnostic Process for Disturbance in Self-Concept

Assessment Activities	Defining Characteristics	Nursing Diagnoses
Ask client to share how hysterectomy will make difference in her life.	Client communicates that she is no longer a woman and states she has been "neutered."	*Body-image disturbance* related to negative perception of self after hysterectomy
Observe congruency between client's verbal and nonverbal responses.	Jokes and smiles when talking about surgery but refuses to look at or touch incision area.	
Ask client what the diagnosis of AIDS means to him.	Client states he believes blood tests were mixed up and simply has bad case of "flu." Relates how close friend died a painful AIDS death alone.	*Impaired adjustment* related to fear of terminal illness (AIDS)
Question family regarding perception of client.	Family states client mentioned that he would "rather kill himself than die as his friend did."	

Community Resources*

- Support groups
  - Adult children of alcoholics
  - Groups for people with anorexia nervosa and associated disorders
  - Alcoholics Anonymous and AL-ANON
  - AIDS groups
  - Family groups for Alzheimer's disease
  - Compassionate friends (parents whose children have died)
  - Emotions Anomymous
  - Gay support groups
  - Narcotics Anonymous
  - National Alliance for the Mentally Ill
  - Ostomy groups
  - Overeaters Anonymous
  - Parents Anonymous
  - Parents without Partners and other single groups
  - Other self-help groups (men and women)
- Displaced homemakers
- University Counseling Centers
- Young Womens Christian Association (YWCA)

*Meetings are for people with similar problems for education, support, and growth.

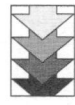

Sample Nursing Care Plan for Body-Image Disturbance

Nursing diagnosis: *Body-image disturbance* related to negative perception of self after hysterectomy
Definition: Body-image disturbance is a disruption in the way one perceives one's body image (Kim, McFarland, McLane, 1991).

Goals	Expected Outcomes	Interventions	Rationale
Clients will verbalize positive, realistic aspects of body image by discharge (projected 3/24).	Client will state one positive effect of surgery by 3/22.	Teach about physical and physiological effects of abdominal hysterectomy (3/19).	Providing clear information about aftereffects of hysterectomy will dispel misunderstandings and myths on results of surgery. It will also reinforce positive aspects of procedure. Including family members helps ensure reinforcement of information and support for client.
	Client will reframe and share values and beliefs regarding femininity by 3/23.	Encourage client to explore beliefs, perceptions, and values related to sexuality, femininity, and female roles. Begin twice a day on 3/20 (7-3, 3-11).	This gives client opportunity to redefine rigid concepts of gender and roles and reintegrate more positive self-image.
	Client will voice statements indicating some acceptance of physical self by 3/24.		
	Client will be able to look at incision by 3/24.		

When planning interventions, the nurse considers the client's present level of adaptation, which can be located on a continuum in each of the following areas (Bernstein, Cope, 1976):

1. Active coping ↔ Passive surrender
2. Leading and co-managing treatment ↔ Resisting treatment
3. Loving exchange ↔ Rage
4. Awareness ↔ Denial
5. Adaptive defenses % Maladaptive defenses

Planning should take into account the client's position on each continuum. For example, a client may perceive a situation as overwhelming and thus may passively surrender to circumstances rather than attempt to cope. The care plan should show acceptance, use open-ended questions and active listening, and provide understanding and support as the client explores self-concept and expresses feelings (for example, crying, anger, and depression). The client needs time to adapt to changes. The nurse must validate a client's strengths and provide resources and education to turn limitations into strengths. Client education should be actively planned, as well.

The nurse should plan for a therapeutic environment that supports the client through the stages of adaptation. Chapter 28 describes the stages of grieving. These stages also occur when a person is faced with the crisis of self-concept or body-image disturbances or changes. Sometimes a person appears to adapt to a change in the body but still does not emotionally accept it. A client may need a great deal of time to accept some changes.

A visit by a person who has experienced the same thing often helps the client. However, the timing of such a visit is important. If the client is still denying that the problem exists, the visit will not be constructive.

Implementation

The ability to establish a therapeutic relationship is critical to intervening with clients with self-concept problems. The first step in establishing a helping relationship is establishing rapport, or creating a sense of harmony by a warm, friendly manner, appropriate smile, and eye contact. The following behaviors are involved in establishing rapport:

1. Relate to clients as equals to eliminate social barriers, convey acceptance, and promote a sense of trust.
2. Find a common interest or experience for initiating conversation.
3. Establish a smooth, easy pattern of conversation.
4. Convey a keen, sympathetic interest in clients, give them full attention, listen carefully, and indicate that there is time to listen.
5. Adopt clients' terminology and conventions and meet them on their own ground as much as possible.

Trust is essential to any helping relationship. Trust is the firm belief on the part of clients in the honesty, integrity, reliability, and justice of the nurse. Thus a trusting relationship depends on the attitude, flexibility, consistency, maturity, and reliability of the nurse (Murray, 1982). Empathy, or feeling with clients, understanding behavior, and being motivated to act on clients' behalf are other essential characteristics for establishing a helping relationship. Empathy enables the nurse to sense clients' private worlds and feelings (Peplau, 1952). The following interventions are useful in assisting clients reintegrate positive self-concepts and realistic body images:

1. Determine clients' usual levels of coping and adaptation.
2. Establish rapport and trust.
3. Determine the families' ability to positively reinforce clients' perception of self.
4. Convey acceptance and empathy, establishing and maintaining a therapeutic nurse-client relationship.
5. Use therapeutic communication and effective interviewing techniques.
6. Encourage appropriate expression of anger.
7. Use interventions to help clients work through hopelessness, sadness, and grief.
8. Frequently give positive reinforcement to desired behavior and accomplishments, as appropriate.
9. Encourage understanding of behavior and feelings.
10. Present courses of action, ideas on others' coping mechanisms, and ways to change behavior to be more adaptive.
11. Build on previous client knowledge when teaching and finding "teachable moments" when clients are ready to learn. (An example of client teaching about self-concept can be seen in the box.)

Client Teaching for Avoiding Negative Thought Patterns

OBJECTIVE

- Client will make positive statements about self.

TEACHING STRATEGIES

- Discuss with client the interrelationship of thoughts, feelings, and behaviors and the reinforcement of family on these matters.
- Assist client in identifying patterns of negative self-talk (cognitive distortions) such as black-and-white thinking, thinking the worst, and jumping to conclusions.
  - Keep a daily dairy of negative thoughts and corresponding feelings. Graph feelings on a scale from 1 to 10.
  - Encourage supportive significant others to give client feedback when they note negative self-talk.
- Direct client to replace negative statements with positive affirmations when self-defeating thoughts are noted.
- Include family in education. Give them examples on reinforcing and supporting client's efforts.
- Educate family to understand negative patterns of self-talk ingrained in family system.

EVALUATION

- Observe client's appearance.
- Listen to what client says or read what client writes in diary about self.

---

12. Assist clients (and families) in identifying resources or support systems.
13. Reduce actual or perceived threats or hindrances as much as possible with clients and families.
14. Introduce changes gradually, one at a time if possible, to allow adequate time for adjustment and avoid further threats to self-concept.
15. Encourage clients to express self-affirmations ("I can").
16. Consult with other health care team members regularly and refer clients to community support groups as indicated.
17. Validate strengths, appropriate ideas and behavior, and choices in self-care and rehabilitation.
18. Summarize and reinforce progress in behavior or self-care activities, thus improving self-image as appropriate.

TABLE 31-2 Sequential Levels of Nursing Interventions for Self-Concept Disturbance

Principle	Rationale	Nursing Actions
LEVEL ONE **Goal: expand client's self-awareness**		
Establish open, trusting relationship.	This reduces threat that nurse poses to client and helps broaden and accept all aspects of personality.	Offer unconditional acceptance and listen. Encourage discussion of thoughts and feelings. Respond nonjudgmentally. Convey to individuals that they are valued people who are responsible for themselves and able to help themselves.
Work with resources client possesses.	Some resources, such as self-control and self-perception, are needed as foundations for later nursing care.	Confirm identity. Provide support measures to reduce anxiety. Approach client in undemanding way. Accept and attempt to clarify any verbal or nonverbal communication. Prevent client isolation. Help establish simple routine. Help set limits on inappropriate behavior. Orient client to reality. Reinforce appropriate behavior. Gradually increase activities and tasks that provide positive experiences. Assist in personal hygiene and grooming. Encourage client to care for self.
Maximize client's participation in therapeutic relationship.	Mutuality is necessary for client to assume ultimate responsibility for behavior and coping responses.	Gradually increase client's participation in decisions that affect care. Convey that client is responsible individual.
LEVEL TWO **Goal: encourage client's self-exploration**		
Show interest in and accept client's feelings and thoughts.	When nurse shows interest in and accepts client's feelings and thoughts, the nurse helps client to do so also.	Attend to and encourage client's expression of emotions, beliefs, behavior, and thoughts—verbally, nonverbally, symbolically, or directly. Use therapeutic communication skills and empathic responses. Note use of logical and illogical thinking and reported and observed emotional responses.
Help client clarify self-concept and relationships to others through self-disclosure.	Self-disclosure and understanding self-perceptions are prerequisites to bringing about future change; this may, in itself, reduce anxiety.	Elicit client's perceptions of strengths and weaknesses. Help describe ideal self. Identify self-criticisms. Help describe how client perceives relationships to other people and events.
Be aware and have control of your own feelings.	Self-awareness allows nurse to model authentic behavior.	Be open to your own feelings. Accept your positive and negative feelings. Practice therapeutic use of self: share your feelings with client, describe how another might have felt, and mirror your perception of client's feelings.
Respond empathically, not sympathetically, emphasizing that power to change lies with client.	Sympathy can reinforce client's self-pity; rather, nurse should communicate that client's life situation is subject to one's own control.	Use empathic responses and monitor yourself for feelings of sympathy or pity. Reaffirm that client is not helpless or powerless when dealing with problems. Convey verbally and behaviorally that client is responsible for behavior, including choice of maladaptive or adaptive coping responses. Discuss with client scope of choices, areas of strength, and coping resources available.

Modified from Stuart GW, Sundeen SJ: *Principles and practice of psychiatric nursing*, ed 4, St Louis, 1991, Mosby–Year Book.

Principle	Rationale	Nursing Actions
LEVEL THREE **Goal: assist client in self-evaluation**		
Help client to clearly define problem.	Only after problem is accurately defined can alternative choices be proposed.	Identify relevant stressors with client and ask for appraisal of them. Clarify that client's beliefs influence feelings and behaviors. Mutually identify faulty beliefs, misperceptions, distortions, illusions, and unrealistic goals. Mutually identify areas of strength. Place concepts of success and failure in proper perspective. Explore use of coping resources.
Explore client's adaptive and maladaptive coping responses to problem.	Examination of client's choices made during coping will help define successful and unsuccessful responses.	Describe how coping responses are chosen and have positive and negative consequences. Contrast adaptive and maladaptive responses. Mutually identify disadvantages of client's maladaptive coping responses. Mutually identify advantages or "payoffs" of client's maladaptive coping responses. Discuss how these payoffs have supported maladaptive response.
LEVEL FOUR **Goal: assist client in formulating realistic goals**		
Help client identify alternative solutions.	Only when all possible alternatives have been evaluated can change be effected.	Help client understand that one can only change oneself, not others. If client holds inconsistent perceptions, show that the following can change: Beliefs or ideals to bring them closer to reality, and environment to make it consistent with beliefs. If self-concept is not consistent with behavior, client can change the following: behavior to conform to self-concept, beliefs underlying self-concept to include behavior, and self-ideal. Mutually review use of coping resources.
Help client conceptualize realistic goals.	Goal setting that includes clear definition of expected change is necessary.	Encourage client to formulate personal (not nurse's) goals. Mutually discuss emotional and practical consequences of each goal. Help client define concrete change to be made. Encourage client to enter new experiences for growth potential. Use role rehearsal, role modeling, and role playing when appropriate.
LEVEL FIVE **Goal: assist client in becoming committed to decision and in achieving goals**		
Help client take necessary action to change maladaptive coping responses and maintain adaptive ones.	Ultimate objective in promoting client's insight is to replace maladaptive coping responses with more adaptive ones.	Provide opportunity for success. Reinforce strengths, skills, and healthy aspects of client's personality. Assist client in gaining assistance (e.g., vocational, financial, and social services). Use family and groups to enhance client's self-esteem. Allow client sufficient time to change. Provide appropriate amount of support and positive reinforcement to maintain progress.

19. Encourage mutual evaluation of progress.

20. Terminate the nurse-client relationship after working through feelings of separation and termination.

When providing care to clients experiencing stress that affects self-esteem and identity, the nurse includes activities in which clients will achieve success. Tasks should not be so difficult that the client cannot succeed. Ensuring a small success is better than risking a defeat at a larger task. Sequential tasks enable the client to build on each success, continuously reinforcing achievement.

The nurse should keep other nurses and other health care professionals up to date on the client's progress because they can be involved in offering support and reinforcement. If a health alteration is particularly severe, staff conferences are useful in helping the nurse handle personal feelings and emotions.

Interventions designed to help a client reach the long-term goal of adapting to changes in self-concept or attaining a positive self-concept are based on the premise that the client first develops insight and self-awareness concerning problems and stressors and then acts to solve the problems and cope with the stressors. This approach involves the following levels of intervention (Stuart, Sundeen, 1991):

1. Increased self-awareness
2. Self-exploration
3. Self-evaluation
4. Formulation of realistic goals
5. Commitment to goals and achievement through action

Each level includes specific nursing goals and actions. The nurse helps the client proceed step by step through these levels. The nursing actions should be individualized. If the alteration in self-concept is severe, the nurse should seek assistance from other professionals such as mental health nurses or should refer the client for specialized care. Table 31-2 describes in more detail the nursing interventions involved in each level. This table also demonstrates incorporation of interventions into the levels.

Evaluation

Evaluation determines client response to nursing therapies. Each goal includes objective evaluation criteria. Expected and unexpected responses are useful when restructuring the care plan. Frequent evaluation of client progress is recommended so that changes can be quickly instituted if necessary. The goals may be unrealistic or inappropriate as the client's condition changes or new information is learned. Planned interventions may be ineffective for this particular client, necessitating a modification of strategies.

The evaluation box presents evaluation measures for expected outcomes for one of the goals of care presented in the care plan. Desired outcomes for a client with a self-concept disturbance may include statements of self-acceptance, acceptance of change in appearance or function conveyed by significant others, social interaction, adequate self-care, acceptance of use of prosthetic devices, statements indicating understanding of healthy teaching, positive attitudes toward rehabilitation, movement toward independence, and return to preexisting roles at work or at home.

The early establishment of a therapeutic nurse-client relationship is essential so that the nurse can involve the client in evaluation. The nurse should continually evaluate the relationship with the client to determine whether effective communication methods have been used and whether the main verbal and nonverbal messages have met positive responses. The nurse should examine personal feelings and responses to the client and feelings conveyed by the client. Periodic meetings with a supervisor or clinical nurse specialist can help the nurse validate feelings and therapy approaches. The nurse's self-awareness serves as a basis for promoting the client's self-awareness.

The client's adaptation to major changes may take a year or longer, but the fact that this period is long does not signify maladaptation. The nurse should look for signs that the client has reduced some stres-

Sample Evaluation of Interventions for Body-Image Disturbance

Goal	Evaluative Measures	Expected Outcome
Client will verbalize positive, realistic aspects of body image by discharge.	Monitor client's communication with staff and family for gradual movement toward positive view of female body: "Being a woman doesn't just mean being able to have babies" or "I still am an attractive person." Observe nonverbal communication such as neutral-positive facial expressions when focused on abdominal incision. Note whether client verbalizes positive factual information presented in teaching session.	Client will reframe and share values and beliefs regarding femininity.

sors. Reorganization of self-concept takes time. It takes years for it to develop, and additional change and development also require time. Although change may be slow, care of the client with a self-concept disturbance can be rewarding.

Carrie B. is a 15-year-old client in the adolescent treatment program of a private psychiatric hospital. She dropped out of public school a year before and ran away from home. She supported herself "on the street" by prostitution and was also addicted to drugs and alcohol.

When Carrie first began interacting with her primary nurse, she had difficulty making decisions and believed she had no positive qualities. As the relationship and her treatment progressed, Carrie began to change maladaptive behaviors and thoughts to more functional ones. When Carrie wrote to her primary nurse a year later, she was doing well in public school, was planning to attend college, and had achieved over a year of sobriety. She then thanked the nurse for "helping me believe in myself."

SUMMARY

The self-concept is a complex, dynamic entity. Many health-related variables, including illness, injury, hospitalization, childbirth, aging, and surgery, can affect the components of self-concept—self-worth, body image, identity, and roles. Self-concept is a combination of the real and the ideal selves. The ideal self is based on social and cultural standards that an individual accepts and attempts to incorporate into the self-concept. A discrepancy between the real and the ideal self can be a source of stress. A positive self-concept is important to developmental and cognitive maturation throughout life, and numerous variables in each stage of life affect the self-concept.

When providing care for a client with a self-concept disturbance, the nurse depends on the severity, intensity, or suddenness of the change. Even an apparently minor loss of function, change in appearance, or role change can create a severe self-concept problem. A loss or change not apparent to others can also result in alteration of self-esteem or identity. The nurse's own self-concept and nursing actions can positively or negatively affect self-concept.

Everyone admitted to a hospital or seen by a health care provider should be assessed for stressors that may affect any component of self-concept. Although most people can adapt to stressful situations, a client may need assistance in learning to cope with a new situation. Using the nursing process, the nurse identifies self-concept stressors and plans and implements care to encourage the client's self-awareness, self-exploration, and self-evaluation, which lead to a formulation of realistic goals for coping with changes and then acting to achieve them.

Key Concepts

- Self-concept is physiologically, emotionally, and socially formed based on others' reactions to the person and then by the person's interpretations of others' reactions to the self and total life experiences.

- Self-concept is influenced by health, family experiences, social and occupational roles, and intellectual and leisure activities.

- The components of self-concept are identity, body image, self-esteem, and roles.

- Self-concept develops as a normal part of growth and maturation, and each developmental stage involves factors important to the development of a healthy, positive self-concept.

- Identity is a consistent and persistent sense of self as a person who is distinct from others.

- Body image is the mental picture of one's body, including external, internal, and postural aspects of the body, and is not necessarily consistent with actual structure or appearance.

- Body image includes the mental picture of the body, as well as attitudes, emotions, and personality reactions of the person toward the body as an object in space.

- Body image changes when the person experiences disease; a change in structure, function, or appearance; pain; or emotional illness.

- Body image is influenced by growth and development, cultural and societal values and attitudes, and individual perceptions of the body.

- Body-image stressors include changes in physical appearance, structure, or functioning caused by normal developmental changes or illness.

- Self-esteem depends on a person's self-ideal, or ego ideal, which is influenced by societal values, and on the person's behavior in the family, workplace, and other environments.

- Self-esteem stressors include developmental and relationship changes, illness (particularly chronic illness involving changes in normal activities), surgery, and accidents, as well as the responses of other individuals to changes resulting from these events.

- Roles are learned through socialization; they involve the expectations of others about how one should behave in particular positions (for example, family member or employee).

- Role stressors include role conflict, role ambiguity, and role strain, which may originate in unclear or conflicting role expectations and be aggravated by the effects of illness.

- Identity is particularly vulnerable during adolescence. Identity stressors during this time include the expectations of others to prepare for a career and independence, to cope with one's sexuality, and to make choices about relationships and roles; such stressors may lead to identity confusion or sense of depersonalization.

- The nurse's self-concept and nursing actions can affect a client's self-concept.

- A nursing assessment should include consideration of actual and potential self-concept stressors and observation for behaviors indicative of self-concept disturbance.

- Nursing diagnoses in regard to self-concept disturbance include changes in any or all of the four components of self-concept.

- Planning and implementing nursing interventions for self-concept disturbance involve expanding the client's self-awareness, encouraging self-exploration, aiding in self-evaluation, helping formulate goals in regard to adaptation, and assisting in acting to achieve goals.

Key Terms

Body image, p. 929

Depersonalization, p. 933

Ideal self, p. 930

Identification, p. 931

Identity, p. 929

Identity confusion, p. 932

Imitation, p. 931

Inhibition, p. 931

Interpersonal conflict, p. 934

Interrole conflict, p. 934

Person-role conflict, p. 934

Reinforcement-extinction, p. 931

Role, p. 930

Role ambiguity, p. 935

Role conflict, p. 934

Role overload, p. 934

Role strain, p. 935

Self-concept, p. 928

Self-esteem, p. 930

Socialization, p. 931

Substitution, p. 931

Critical Thinking Exercises

1. Your postpartum client is a 14-year-old, unmarried high school student who has delivered her first child. How would her development level have an impact on her new role as a mother, and how would her body image be affected?

2. You have developed a trusting relationship with a 72-year-old diabetic outpatient. He confides in you that he has not felt "whole" since his left foot was amputated last year. What principles would you use when responding to him?

3. At the AIDS clinic, you facilitate a support group for clients. A negative view of the self is common when a client first joins the group, but the client begins to be more positive after becoming a more active participant. What are two factors influencing self-esteem that might account for this change?

4. A 54-year-old businessman with a history of alcoholism is scheduled for a minor procedure on your surgical unit. You are assigned to assess him. Soon after you begin interviewing him, you notice yourself becoming disgusted and irritable with him for no apparent reason. To develop a therapeutic relationship with this man, what would be one of your first actions?

REFERENCES

Anthony EJ: The child's discovery of his body, *Phys Ther* 48:(6), 1103, 1968.

Bernstein NR, Cope O: *Emotional care of the facially burned and disfigured,* Boston, 1976, Little, Brown.

Biddle BJ, Thomas EJ, editors: *Role theory: concepts and research,* New York, 1966, Wiley.

Brim OG, Wheeler S: *Socialization after childhood: two essays,* New York, 1966, Wiley.

Broadwell DC: *Validation of a role conflict, role ambiguity, and role predictability instrument,* doctoral dissertation, Atlanta, 1983, Georgia State University.

Butler RN, Lewis MI: *Love and sex after sixty: a guide for men and women for their later years,* New York, 1976, Harper & Row.

Cleveland S, Morton R: Group behavior and body image, *Hum Relations* 15(1):77, 1967.

Cockerham WC, Sharp K, Wilcox JA: Aging and perceived health status, *J Gerontol* 38(3):349, 1983.

Cooley CH: *Human nature and the social order,* New York, 1956, Free Press.

Coopersmith S: *The antecedents of self-esteem,* San Francisco, 1967, Freeman.

Crouch MA, Straub V: Enhancement of self-esteem in adults, *Fam Community Health* 6(2):76, 1983.

Dropkin NJ: Compliance in postoperative head and neck patients, *Cancer Nurs* 2(5):379, 1979.

Dyk RB, Sutherland A: Adaptation of the spouse and other family members to the colostomy patient, *CA* 9:123, 1956.

Erikson EH: *Childhood and society,* New York, ed 2, 1963, Norton.

Fisher S, Cleveland S: *Body image and personality,* New York, 1968, Dover.

Gibson DE: Reminiscence, self-esteem, and self-other satisfaction in adult male alcoholics, *J Psychiatr Nurs* March 1980.

Haber J et al: Self awareness. In Haber J et al, editors: *Comprehensive psychiatric nursing,* New York, 1987, McGraw-Hill.

Hamachek D: Evaluating self concept and ego states in Erikson's last three psychosocial stages, *J Counsel Develop* 68:683, 1990.

Jacobsen E: *The self and the object world,* New York, 1964, International Universities Press.

Kim MJ, McFarland GK, McLane AM: *Pocket guide to nursing diagnoses,* ed 4, St Louis, 1991, Mosby–Year Book.

Kramer M et al: Extra tactile stimulation of the premature infant, *Nurs Res* 24(5):324, 1975.

Marsh H: A multidimensional, hierarchal model of self-concept: theoretical and empirical justification, *Educ Psychol Rev* 2(2):77, 1990.

Meleis A: Role insufficiency and role supplementation: a conceptual framework, *Nurs Res* 24:264, 1975.

Murray R: Model for psychiatric and mental health nursing. In Carlson C, Craft C, McGuire A, editors: *Nursing diagnoses,* Philadelphia, 1982, Saunders.

Murray R, Zentner J: *Nursing assessment and health promotion through the life span,* ed 3, Englewood Cliffs, NJ, 1985, Prentice-Hall.

Parsons T: Illness and the role of physician: a sociological perspective, *Am J Orthopsychiatry* 21:452, 1951.

Parsons T: Definitions of health and illness in light of American values and social structures. In Jaco EG, editor: *Patients, physicians, and illness,* 1972, ed 2, New York, Free Press.

Peplau H: *Interpersonal relations in nursing,* New York, 1952, Putnam.

Reed P: Self-transcendence and mental health in oldest-old adults, *Nurs Res* 40(1):5, 1991.

Schilder P: *Image and appearance of the human body,* New York, 1951, International Universities Press.

Selye H: *The stress of life,* New York, 1956, McGraw-Hill.

Stuart GW, Sundeen SJ: *Principles and practice of psychiatric nursing,* ed 4, St Louis, 1991, Mosby–Year Book.

Sultenfuss SR: Psychosocial issues and therapeutic intervention. In Broadwell DC, Jackson BS, editors: *Principles of ostomy care,* St Louis, 1982, Mosby–Year Book.

Taft LB: Self-esteem in later life: a nursing perspective, *ANS* 8(1):77, 1985.

Tenner H, Herzberger S: Depression, self-esteem, and the absence of self-protective attributional biases. *J Pers Soc Psychol* 52(1):72, 1987.

Yamamoto K: *The child and his image,* Boston, 1972, Houghton Mifflin.

ADDITIONAL READINGS

Archer SL: The status of identity: reflections on the need for intervention, *J Adolesc* 12:345, 1989.

Argyle M: *The psychology of interpersonal behavior,* Baltimore, 1967, Penguin.

Biddle BJ: *Role therapy: expectations, identities, and behaviors,* New York, 1979, Academic.

Blaesing S, Brockhuas J: The development of body image in the child, *Nurs Clin North Am* 7(4):597, 1982.

Boyd C: Testing a model of mother-daughter identification, *West J Nurs Res* 12(4):448, 1990.

Brundage DJ, Broadwell DC: Altered body image. In Phipps WJ et al, editors: *Medical-surgical nursing: concepts and clinical practice,* ed 4, St Louis, 1991, Mosby–Year Book.

Carpeninto L: *Handbook of nursing diagnosis*, Philadelphia, 1984, Lippincott.

Cornwell CJ, Schmitt MH: Perceived health status, self-esteem, and body image in women with rheumatoid arthritis or systemic lupus erythematosus, *Res Nurs Health* 13(2):99, 1990.

Coward DD: The lived experience of self-transcendence in women with advanced breast cancer, *Nurs Sci Q* 3(4):162, 1990.

Curbow B et al: Self-concept and cancer in adults: theoretical and methodological issues, *Soc Sci Med* 31(2):115, 1990.

Dempsey M: The development of body image in the adolescent, *Nurs Clin North Am* 7(4):609, 1972.

Dirksen SR: Theoretical modeling to predict subjective well-being, *West J Nurs Res* 12(5):629, 1990.

Duespohl T: *Nursing diagnosis manual for the well and ill client*, Philadelphia, 1986, Saunders.

Fink S: Crisis and motivation: a theoretical model, *Arch Phys Med Rehabil* 48(11):592, 1967.

Fisher S: Sex differences in body perception, *Psychol Monogr* 78:1, 1964.

Gilberts R: The evaluation of self-esteem, *Fam Community Health* 6:(2):29, 1983.

Gordon M: *Manual of nursing diagnosis: 1984-1985*, New York, 1985, McGraw-Hill.

Harris M: Helping the person with an altered self-image, *Geriatr Nurs* 7(2):90-92, 1986.

Hartley P: Body image and self-image in anorexia nervosa, *Br Rev Bulimia Anorexia Nervosa* 3(2):61, 1989.

Hockenberry Eaton MJ, Cotanch PH: Evaluation of a child's perceived self-competence during treatment for cancer, *J Pediatr Oncol Nurs* 6(3):55, 1989.

Janelli LM: Through the looking glass: body image perception among older adults, *Perspectives* 12(1):9, 1988.

Janelli LM: The impact of health status on body image in older women, *Rehabil Nurs* 13(4):178, 1988.

Jourard S: *The transparent self*, Princeton, NJ, 1964, Van Nostrand.

Jourard S, Secord P: Body cathexis and the ideal female figure, *J Abnorm Soc Psychol* 50:243, 1955.

Katchadourian HE, editor: *Human sexuality*, Berkeley, 1979, University of California Press.

Kersten L: Changes in self-concept during pulmonary rehabilitation. I. *Heart Lung* 19(5):456, 1990.

Kim M, McFarland G, McLane A, editors: *Classification of nursing diagnoses: proceedings of the seventh conference, (NANDA)*, St Louis, 1987, Mosby–Year Book.

Lisanti PA: Perceived body space and self-esteem in adult males with and without chronic low back pain, *Orthop Nurs* 8(3):49, 1989.

Maslow AH: *Motivation and personality*, New York, 1970, Harper & Row.

McFarland G, Wasli E: *Nursing diagnoses and process in psychiatric-mental health nursing*, Philadelphia, 1986, Lippincott.

Mearns J: Measuring self-acceptance: expectancy for success vs. self-esteem, *J Clin Psychol* 45(3):390, 1989.

Meisenhelder JB: Self-esteem: a closer look at clinical interventions, *Int J Nurs Stud* 22(2):127, 1985.

Miller S: Promoting self-esteem in the hospitalized adolescent: clinical interventions, *Issues Compr Pediatr Nurs* 10(3):187, 1987.

Molla PM: Self-concept in children with and without physical disability, *J Psychiatr Nurs* 19(6):22, 1981.

Morris C: Self-concept as altered by diagnosis of cancer, *Nurs Clin North Am* 20(4):611, 1985.

Murray R: Body image development in adulthood, *Nurs Clin North Am* 7(4):617, 1972.

Murray R: Principles of nursing intervention for the adult patient with body image changes, *Nurs Clin North Am* 7(4):697, 1972.

Murray R, Huelskoetter M, O'Driscoll D: *The nursing process in later maturity*, Englewood Cliffs, NJ, 1980, Prentice-Hall.

Norris J, Junes-Connell M: Self-esteem disturbance, *Nurs Clin North Am* 20(4):745, 1985.

Norris J, Junes-Connell M: Self-esteem disturbance: a clinical validation study, *Classification on nursing diagnoses: proceedings of the seventh conference (NANDA)*, St Louis, 1987, Mosby–Year Book.

Oldaker S: Identity confusion: nursing diagnosis for adolescents, *Nurs Clin North Am* 20(4):763, 1985.

Piaget J, Inhelder B: *The psychology of the child*, New York, 1969, Basic Books.

Robson PJ: Self-esteem: a psychiatric view, *Br J Psychiatry* 153:6, 1988.

Rubin R: Body image and self-esteem, *Nurs Outlook* 16(6):20, 1968.

Samonds RJ, Cammermeyer M: Perceptions of body image in subjects with multiple sclerosis: a pilot study, *J Neurosci Nurs* 21(3):190, 1989.

Sundeen SJ et al: *Nurse-client interaction: implementing the nursing process*, ed 3, St Louis, 1989, Mosby–Year Book.

Swanson B, Cronin-Stubbs O, Sheldon JA: The impact of psychosocial factors on adapting to physical disability: a review of the research literature, *Rehabil Nurs* 14(2):64, 1989.

Utz SW et al: Perceptions of body image and health status in persons with MVP, *Image J Nurs Sch* 22(1):18, 1990.

CHAPTER 32

Sexuality

OBJECTIVES

Mastery of content in this chapter will enable the student to:

- Define the key terms listed.
- Identify personal attitudes, beliefs, and biases related to sexuality.
- Discuss the nurse's role in maintaining or enhancing a client's sexual health.
- Define *sexuality* as a component of personality.
- Describe key concepts of sexual development during infancy, childhood, adolescence, and adulthood.
- Identify male and female genitalia and describe functions related to sexual stimulation and response and reproduction.
- Describe the sexual response cycle (Masters and Johnson model).
- Describe physical, therapeutic, and psychological issues affecting sexuality.
- Identify potential causes of sexual dysfunction.
- Assess a client's sexuality.
- Define appropriate nursing diagnoses on sexuality.
- Identify and describe nursing interventions to promote sexual health.
- Evaluate a client's sexual health.
- Identify sexual concerns outside the nurse's level of expertise, and identify potential referral resources.

CHAPTER OUTLINE

Concepts of Sexuality
Biological identity
Gender identity
Gender role
Sexual orientation
Variations in sexual expression
Sexual ethics

Attitudes Toward Sexuality
Factors influencing attitudes
Clients' sexual attitudes
Nurses' attitudes toward sexuality

Sexual Anatomy and Physiology
Female sex organs
Male sex organs

Sexual Development
Infancy
Toddlerhood and preschool
School-age years
Puberty and adolescence
Adulthood
Older adulthood

Sexual Response
Sexual response cycle
Aging and sexual response

Pregnancy and Sexuality

Issues Related to Sexuality
Contraception
Infertility
Abortion
Sexually transmitted diseases
Sexual abuse
Effects of illness on sexuality
Sexual dysfunction

Sexuality and the Nursing Process
Assessment
Nursing diagnosis
Planning
Implementation
Evaluation

Sex is a topic that was long considered taboo for proper adult conversation. Gradually, over the last 30 to 50 years, knowledge about sex and discussion of issues of sexuality have come to be recognized as important and necessary for human development. During the past 20 years, health care professionals have finally recognized the relevance of sexual health as a component of well-being. Even with this recognition, a lack of knowledge regarding human sexuality remains among many adults, including health care providers. More significantly, care givers lack comfort and confidence in addressing these issues.

Sexual issues should be included in health care as a component of overall wellness. Often, clients are reluctant to raise questions related to sexuality. Clients' concerns may include postpartum resumption of sexual intercourse, normalcy of development, and anxiety over the effects of antihypertensive medication on sexual function. The nurse must assume the responsibility of initiating discussion of relevant sexual topics within clients' current developmental and health status. Clients then may feel more comfortable and relate additional concerns. To address issues of sexuality in practice, the care giver must have the necessary knowledge base and skills in assessment and communication.

Because sexual issues are value laden, it is also critical that care givers recognize personal attitudes and beliefs. Religious teachings, culturally prescribed sex roles, beliefs about sexual orientation, and past and present social and environmental influences affect a client's values system. Health care professionals must acknowledge biases so that they can recognize interference in client interaction. Gaining knowledge and desensitization toward sexual issues may also broaden understanding of the vast range of normal sexual behavior. This enables health care providers to be nonjudgmental and more effective in working with clients.

 CONCEPTS OF SEXUALITY

Sexuality and sex are two different things. **Sexuality** is often described as the sense of being female or male. It has biological, psychological, social, and ethical components. Sexuality influences and is influenced by life experiences. The word *sex* has a more limited meaning. It usually describes the biological aspects of sexuality such as genital sexual activity. Sex may be used for pleasure and reproduction. As a result of life's changes or a choice, sexual activity may be absent from a person's life for brief or prolonged periods.

The process by which people come to know themselves as females or males is not clearly understood. Being born with female or male genitalia and subsequently learning female or male social roles seem to be key ingredients; yet this does not explain all variations of sexuality and sexual behavior. This diversity is more understandable when nurses remember that sexuality is intertwined with all aspects of self.

Biological Identity

Biological differences between men and women are determined at conception. Female fetuses receive two X chromosomes, one from each parent, and male fetuses receive an X chromosome from the mother and a Y chromosome from the father. Initially the genitalia of the fetus are undifferentiated. When the sex hormones begin to cue fetal tissues, the genitalia assume male or female characteristics. Hormones influence the individual again at puberty, during which girls develop cyclical menstrual cycles and female secondary sex characteristics and boys develop a relatively constant production of spermotozoa (sperm) and male secondary sex characteristics.

Gender Identity

Gender identity is the sense of being feminine or masculine. As soon as an infant is born (and perhaps sooner with use of amniocentesis or other antenatal testing) the parents and community label the child as *girl* or *boy*. Often the first words of the birth helper begin this process. After a label is attached to an infant, adults adjust their behavior to relate to a female or male baby. Different patterns of interaction influence the infant's developing sense of gender identity.

As children begin to explore and understand their own bodies, they combine this information with the way that society treats them to create images of themselves as girls or boys. By age 3, children are aware that they will remain girls and boys and that changes in outward appearance will not alter their gender. This recognition is part of the development of self-concept.

Gender Role

Much research and writing in the last decade has been produced on the origin of the **gender role**—the way that a person acts as female or male. Social learning theorists believe that society influences female and male behavior and is thus the primary source of femaleness or maleness. Because gender-role behavior is encouraged by parents, peers, and the media, differences among individuals' sexual behavior develop.

Environmental factors alone do not satisfactorily explain the differences and similarities between female and male sexual behavior. Some researchers believe that sex hormones influence the development of fetal brain tissue, contributing to the differences in female and male sexual behavior. Most likely, as with other human behaviors, sexual behavior is a combination of many interacting biological and environmental factors.

Cultural factors can be key elements in defining sex roles. Culture may tightly prescribe roles as feminine or masculine (for example, the role of breadwinner and home finance coordinator as masculine roles and child care provider and cook as feminine roles). Other cultural groups may be more flexible in role definition and encourage women or men to explore a variety of roles or behaviors without labeling the behavior as sex-linked. The women's movement of the 1970s did much to expand the North American cultural definition of appropriate feminine behavior (for example, primary breadwinner and mother). Ripple effects of this movement have also offered men a broader range of socially acceptable behavior, allowing them to openly express emotion and increase involvement in child care. These expanded options have created dilemmas. Conflicts may arise in juggling careers with childrearing responsibilities. Biological reproductive time frames and family attitudes may also cause conflict.

Sexual Orientation

Sexual orientation is the clear, persistent, erotic preference of a person for one sex or the other. Studies of human sexuality in the 1940s and 1950s developed a continuum between heterosexuality and homosexuality. Few, if any, individuals are totally confined to one end of the continuum throughout life. Most people cluster near the **heterosexual** end of the continuum, with a smaller percentage at the **homosexual** or **lesbian** end; however, some people are **bisexual** and feel comfortable having sexual relations with either sex. It is not unusual for an individual to have occasional erotic feelings toward someone of the same sex without acting on these feelings. Likewise, it is not uncommon to have a same-sex encounter during adolescence without settling at the homosexual end of the continuum.

The origins of sexual orientation are still not understood. Biological theories describe heterosexuality and homosexuality in genetic terms and thus as determined at conception. These theories attribute sexual orientation to the genetic composition of the individual. Psychological theories emphasize that early learning experiences and cognitive processes determine sexual orientation. Other theories acknowledge the influence of genetics and environment in the development of sexual-partner preference.

Variations in Sexual Expression

For some people the inner sense of sexual identity does not match the biological body. Such people are known as **transsexuals.** A man may think of himself as a woman in a man's body, or a woman may describe herself as a man trapped in a woman's body. Researchers do not clearly understand how this mismatch occurs. Transsexuals do not see their sexual identities as a matter of choice. Their identification of themselves as sexual and social females or males is as clear and persistent, often from early childhood.

Homosexuality and transvestism are separate phenomena. Society sometimes thinks of homosexual men as somehow feminized and wishing to be like women and of lesbians as desiring to be like men. This is an incorrect myth. Although there are some effeminate-behaving men and masculine-behaving women in the homosexual population, most homosexual men and women define themselves as satisfied with their gender and social role. They simply have a persistent desire for their own sex.

A **transvestite** is usually a heterosexual man who periodically dresses like a woman for psychological and sexual relief. Transvestites generally do this in private, and their behavior is sometimes kept secret even from the people closest to them.

Sexual Ethics

Because sexuality is linked to every aspect of living, any sexual decision involves personal, family, cultural, religious, and social standards of conduct. Ideas about ethical sexual conduct and emotions related to sexuality form the basis for sexual decision making. The spectrum of attitudes toward sexuality ranges from a traditional view of sex only within marriage to an attitude that allows individuals to determine what is right. Sexual decisions that transgress a person's ethical code may result in internal conflict.

Several general approaches to ethical sexual decision making are suggested by Masters, Johnson, and Kolodny (1982). In one approach, sexual decisions are based solely on religion. Another approach views any sexual act between consenting adults in private as moral. Some people believe that moral sexuality enhances personal growth and interpersonal relationships. Others believe that the morality of a sexual act must be decided on the basis of the situation in which it occurs. People will always differ in beliefs about sexual ethics. The split between conservative and liberal thinking concerning sexuality does not seem to be diminishing. The debate over sexuality-related issues such as abortion, contraception, sources of sex education, sexual variations, and premarital or extramarital intercourse continues. In the absence of a universally accepted moral code, each person must make sexual decisions and have the best interests of the individual and the community in mind.

 ## ATTITUDES TOWARD SEXUALITY

Each person learns a set of behaviors that represents femininity or masculinity. Individuals reveal themselves as females or males by their gestures, mannerisms, clothing, vocabulary, and patterns of sexual activity. Attitudes toward sexual feelings and behaviors change as people grow older. These changes may become more traditional or liberal because of societal changes, feedback from others, and involvement in religious or community groups.

Because wellness includes sexual health, sexuality should be part of a health care program. Yet sexual assessment and interventions are not always included in health care. The area of sexuality can be emotional for nurses and clients. Lack of information, conflicting value systems, anxiety, or guilt may invalidate the best intentions of nurses to promote sexual health. Clients may not discuss certain sexual concerns because they fear that nurses will be judgmental. Nurses may ignore clients' hints about sexual concerns because they are uncomfortable with sexuality. Words such as *masturbation, homosexuality, abortion,* and *orgasm* may have emotional connotations that can make people uncomfortable. On a more subtle level, the invasion of privacy, lack of regard for hospitalized clients' needs for time alone with sexual partners, or even the way nurses touch clients reflects attitudes toward sexuality.

Factors Influencing Attitudes

Biological factors and personality help shape attitudes and behaviors, but other powerful factors are involved. Sexual attitudes can result from religious beliefs, for example. Contemporary religious faiths view sexual values and behavior very differently (Hogan, 1982). In addition, people may publicly say they believe in a particular sexual value system but behave quite differently in private.

Society plays a powerful role in shaping sexual values and attitudes. Each social group has its own set of rules that guide the behavior of its members. These rules become an integral part of an individual's thinking. In the traditional, conservative value system, sex is considered to be a reproductive func-

tion, and masturbation and sexual variations may not be tolerated because they do not serve the reproductive role. Sexual behavior is often seen as binding the couple closer together in the reproductive role. Sex strengthens the monogamous, heterosexual partnership and becomes the ultimate expression of love between partners. This traditional view encompasses fixed roles for female and male sexual behavior.

A more individualistic morality became widespread in the 1960s and 1970s. Many people re-evaluated their moral codes and began to see sexuality as a mode of self-expression. Many women asserted their right to control pregnancy and the expression of their sexual feelings. This new morality emphasized ownership of one's own body and feelings, free choice, and self-actualization. The 1990s may see a return to a more conservative, monogamous expression of sexuality because of the increasing rate of diseases such as gonorrhea, chlamydia, human papilloma virus (HPV), and acquired immunodeficiency syndrome (AIDS).

Because of a belief in traditional gender-appropriate roles, clients may perceive the "nurse" as female and subservient. The historical image of the nurse is one of discipline, purity, and cleanliness. Because nurses had the right to touch hospitalized clients' bodies and carry out clients' personal hygiene, they were expected to suppress their own sexuality. Although these traditional attitudes have almost vanished from nursing practice, the bias may still be held by some clients. Moreover, as more males enter the nursing profession, clients and care providers may experience conflict in defining sex roles related to nursing practice.

Clients' Sexual Attitudes

All people have sexual value systems—personal beliefs and preferences concerning sexuality—acquired throughout life. These experiences make it easy for a client to deal with sexual concerns in a health care setting or are obstacles to expression. Some clients may be confused about their own sexual value systems and thus experience ambiguous or distressing feelings when they deal with their sexuality.

The most common concern is whether specific sexual attitudes, feelings, and actions are normal. Because society has not encouraged open talk about sexuality, such anxiety is understandable. Religion, society, the media, family, peers, and experience transmit messages about sexual normalcy.

Clients may be concerned about the effect of nursing interventions on their self-care abilities and sexual activities. In most hospitals, masturbation and sexual fantasy are the only sexual outlets available to clients who feel well enough to engage in them. Traditionally, strong societal and religious prohibitions exist against masturbation and fantasies, especially for women. The attitude of the nursing staff may also prevent these activities. Nurses who suggest fantasy or masturbation as part of an intervention may also bring the client into conflict with personal beliefs and prohibitions.

Nurses' Attitudes Toward Sexuality

Because health care professionals represent society and its diverse sexual attitudes and behaviors, diversity is understandable and expected among health care professionals. Nurses can deal with personal attitudes by accepting their existence, exploring their sources, and finding ways to work with them. Professional behavior does not have to compromise the personal sexual ethics of nurses or clients. Professional behavior must guarantee that clients receive the best health care possible without diminishing their self-worth.

Nurses may find it difficult to be nonjudgmental about a client's sexuality when the client's sexual orientation or values differ. Situations that seem strange or wrong to the nurse might seem normal and acceptable to the client. Attempting to change a client's sexual attitudes and behaviors ignores the fundamental differences in attitudes among people. Promotion of sex education and honest examination of sexual values and beliefs can help in reducing sexual bias. Such a process emphasizes the following (Hogan, 1980):

1. Awareness of beliefs, attitudes, and values about sexuality
2. Awareness of the effect of beliefs and attitudes on nursing practice
3. Knowledge of subject matter
4. Skill in assessment, intervention, and communication

Giving clients information about sexuality does not imply advocacy. Clients need accurate, honest information about the effects of illness on sexuality and the ways that it can contribute to wellness. Nurses need to provide this information so that biases do not interfere with care.

SEXUAL ANATOMY AND PHYSIOLOGY

Female Sex Organs

The female genitalia comprise the external and internal sex organs. The external sex organs, collectively called the *vulva*, include the mons veneris, la-

bia majora, labia minora, clitoris, and vaginal opening or introitus (Fig. 32-1). The vagina, uterus, fallopian tubes, and ovaries compose the internal sex organs (Fig. 32-2 on p. 964).

External Sex Organs

MONS VENERIS. The mons veneris (mons pubis) is a layer of fatty tissue that covers the pubic bone and is covered by pubic hair after puberty.

LABIA. The two labia majora are fatty folds of skin whose outer surfaces are covered with pubic hair and whose inner surfaces are smooth and hairless. The labia majora extend from the mons veneris and form the outer boundaries of the vulva. The labia majora covers and thereby protects the vaginal and urinary openings. They have sensory receptors that are sensitive to touch, pressure, pain, and temperature. The two labia minora, which are just inside the labia majora, are thin folds of pigmented skin that extend upward to form the clitoral hood. These inner folds possess many blood vessels and have many sensory nerve endings. Because of the number of blood vessels, the labia minora may display a significant color change during sexual arousal and are sometimes referred to as the *sex skin*.

CLITORIS. When the clitoral hood is pulled back, the glans of the clitoris is revealed. It looks like a smooth, shiny pea. The clitoris is composed primarily of erectile tissue, has many nerve endings, and is very sensitive to touch, pressure, and temperature. The clitoral hood also hides the clitoral shaft, which is com-

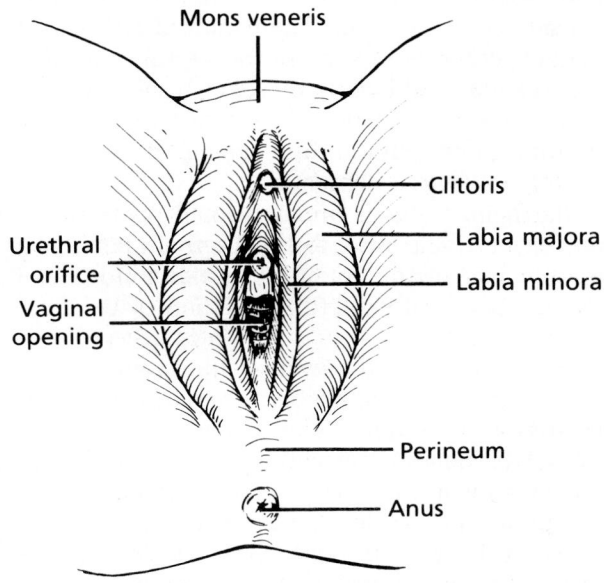

Fig. 32-1   External female genitalia.

Fig. 32-2 Internal female genitalia.

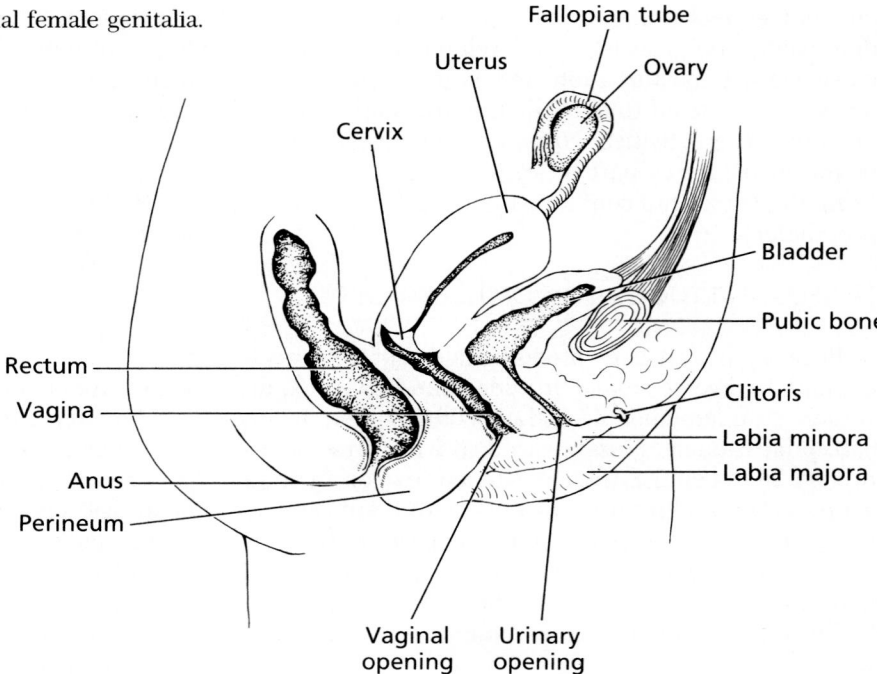

posed of two cylinders of fibrous tissue (corpora cavernosa) that branch internally like an inverted **V** into two long extensions, the crura. The crura attach to the bony pelvis. A third cylinder (corpus spongiosum) divides into two vestibular bulbs that flank the vaginal opening.

VESTIBULE. The area between the labia is called the *vestibule.* This area contains the urinary opening, the vaginal opening (or introitus), the openings of Bartholin's gland, and in some cases the openings of the paraurethral, or Skene's glands.

The urinary meatus lies midline in the vestibule between the clitoris and the vaginal opening. It is not considered a sex organ. The paraurethral, or Skene's, ducts open on both sides of the urethra, usually into the vestibule, although in some women they open just inside the meatus on the posterior wall of the urethra. The paraurethral gland may contribute slightly to vaginal lubrication.

Bartholin's glands are two small ducts that open on the vestibule next to the vaginal opening. They secrete a small amount of lubrication fluid. This fluid contributes minimally to lubrication of the introitus and vagina during sexual arousal; most of the lubrication comes from the walls of the vagina.

The vaginal opening or introitus is between the urethra and the anus. The hymen is a membranous fold of tissue that partially covers the introitus and has no known function. It usually remains intact until the first intercourse. At times the hymen in a virgin may be torn because of an athletic injury or, rarely, tampon insertion. Some women have intact hymens even after repeated intercourse, although this is rare.

Internal Sex Organs

VAGINA. The vagina is a thin-walled, muscular organ that tilts upward at a 45-degree angle toward the small of the back (Masters, Johnson, and Kolodny, 1982). The walls of the vagina consist of the following layers:

1. A thin outer serosa, which is part of the membrane that lines the body cavity and covers its organs
2. A middle layer of smooth, involuntary muscle that is continuous with the muscle of the uterus
3. An inner layer of moist mucous membrane called *mucosa*

The muscle layer is extremely distensible to allow sexual intercourse and childbirth. During sexual excitement, the mucosal layer sweats, with vasocongestion providing vaginal lubrication. The vagina serves as a passageway for menstrual flow, childbirth, and sexual pleasure.

UTERUS. The uterus is a thick-walled muscular organ located between the urinary bladder and rectum. It is about 7.6 cm (3 in) long and looks like a small pear turned upside down. The fallopian tubes enter the uterus on both sides near the top. The wide upper part of the uterus is known as the *body.* The bottom part, called the *cervix,* extends into the vagina. The external (vaginal) cervix is called the *ectocervix,* and the internal cervical canal is referred to as the *endocervix.* The junction of these areas is the site where squamous epithelium changes to columnar epithelial cells. Cells from this area are scraped and evaluated during a Papanicolaou (Pap) test (see Chapter 20) to assess for excessive precancerous or malignant growth.

The inner lining of the cervix contains many glands, which secrete varying amounts of mucus that plug the opening to the uterus. Changes in the cervical mucus indicate when ovulation is taking place. The mucus is more readily penetrable by sperm at the time of ovulation.

The uterus is composed of a thin external connective tissue layer called the *perimetrium,* the middle layer of smooth muscle called the *myometrium,* and the inner mucous membrane called the *endometrium.* Muscle fibers of the myometrial layer enlarge during pregnancy to allow fetal growth. Contractions of these intertwining muscles and pressure from the presenting part of the fetus cause cervical effacement and dilation. Uterine muscle contractions and bearing-down movements expel the fetus. Contraction of uterine muscles also occurs during orgasm.

Every month the endometrium thickens and prepares for possible implantation of a fertilized ovum. If no implantation occurs, the endometrium deteriorates and is discharged through the cervix and vagina during menstruation.

FALLOPIAN TUBES. The two fallopian tubes begin at the uterus and end in long, fingerlike fibriae near the ovaries. Fallopian tubes function as a conduit for the passage of egg and sperm so that fertilization can occur. Fertilization usually occurs in the upper part (ovarian portion) of one of the fallopian tubes.

OVARIES. There are two walnut-sized ovaries, one on each side of the uterus. They produce eggs that are released and transported through the fallopian tubes, and they secrete female hormones, including small amounts of androgen, directly into the bloodstream. The process of egg production begins in the female fetus and ends before birth. Every female is born with a total complement of ova. These eggs continue to undergo atresia (degeneration and resorption), so only about 400,000 remain at puberty. One egg undergoes maturation each month. The cycle continues until ovarian function ceases at menopause.

Breasts

The breasts are not a part of the external or internal sex organs but rather are considered **secondary sex characteristics** (physical characteristics other than genitals that distinguish females from males). The breasts are composed internally of fatty tissue and milk-producing glands. Variations in breast size are due mainly to the amount of adipose tissue around the milk glands. Breasts are often not symmetrical in size or shape. Visible changes occur during development (see Chapter 20).

Menstrual Cycle

Menstruation is the process by which the ovaries and uterus prepare for the development and implantation of a fertilized egg. This cycle lasts an average of 28 days. **Menarche,** the onset of a girl's first menstruation, usually occurs between 9 and 16 years of age. **Menopause,** the cessation of menstruation, usually takes place between 45 and 60.

The **menstrual cycle** is controlled through a feedback loop involving hormones of the hypothalamus, pituitary, and ovaries. The hormones produce changes in the ovaries and uterine endometrium (Fig. 32-3 on p. 966). The hypothalamus regulates the pituitary hormones through gonadotropin-releasing hormone (Gn-RH) at the beginning of the cycle. Gn-RH stimulates the pituitary to release large amounts of follicle-stimulating hormone (FSH) and small amounts of luteinizing hormone (LH). These hormones travel through the bloodstream and stimulate several ovarian primary follicles (immature eggs) to begin maturation. The ovaries produce increasing amounts of estrogen, which provides a negative feedback loop to the hypothalamus-pituitary level to inhibit further FSH production. This process is the follicular phase of the menstrual cycle.

A few days before ovulation, all but one follicle begins to regress. Affected by estrogen, the one follicle (occasionally more than one) grows rapidly and is known as the **Graafian follicle.** The estrogen influences the pituitary to increase production of LH, which surges about 24 hours before ovulation. **Ovulation** occurs about day 14 of an average 28-day cycle as the ovum ruptures from the Graafian follicle. The ova then is picked up by the fallopian tube and proceeds to the uterus during the next few days.

After ovulation the ruptured follicle becomes known as the **corpus luteum.** It produces large amounts of progesterone, peaking about 5 to 7 days after ovulation. The corpus luteum is maintained in part by continued circulating levels of LH. If pregnancy does not occur, LH levels decrease, and progesterone levels decrease about 10 to 11 days after ovulation. The luteal phase of the cycle ends as menstrual flow begins about 14 days after ovulation. The hormones that stimulate ovarian activities also cause uterine changes. The uterine phases of the menstrual cycle include the *proliferative* and *secretory*

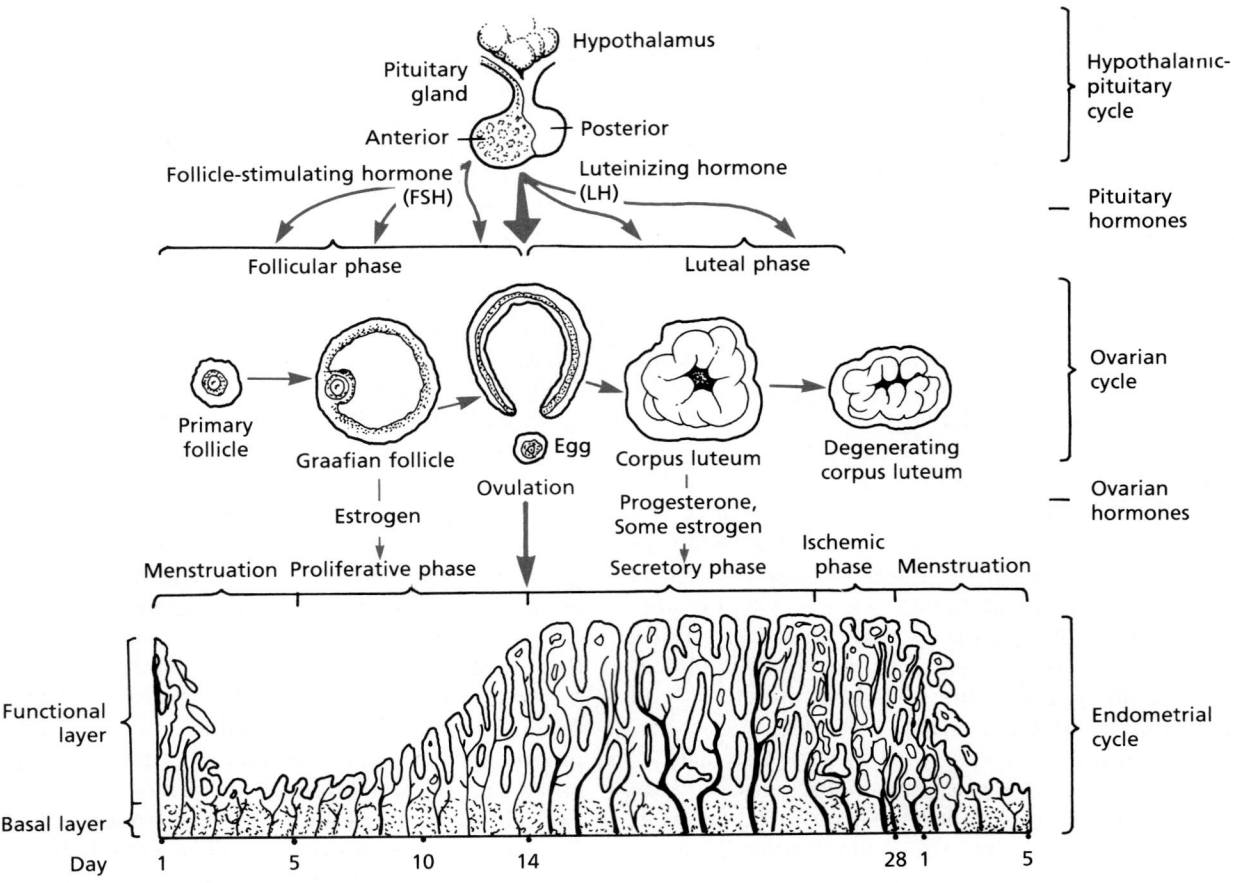

Fig. 32-3 Hormonal control of the menstrual cycle.
From Bobak IM, Jensen MD, Zalar M: *Maternity and gynecologic care,* ed 4, St Louis, 1989, Mosby–Year Book.

phases and *menstruation*. The proliferative phase is the period before ovulation. High levels of estrogen thicken the uterine endometrium. Cervical mucous becomes more clear and slippery and very stretchable. These qualities of the mucous peak at ovulation and produce an environment receptive to the entrance of sperm for fertilization. (Noting these changes in the quality of cervical mucus is a helpful aid in fertility awareness for planning or preventing conception.)

The secretory phase of the menstrual cycle occurs after ovulation. Under the influence of high levels of progesterone and estrogen, the endometrium continues to thicken to prepare to nourish a fertilized egg. If pregnancy does not occur, the endometrium begins to slough (shed) because of the decreased LH and progesterone. A new menstrual cycle begins with sloughing because the hypothalamus and pituitary repeat hormonal stimulation.

The average length of a complete menstrual cycle is 28 days. The length varies cycle to cycle. Normal cycle lengths may range from 21 to almost 40 days.

Menstrual flow consists of blood, mucus, and tissue particles. Average blood loss is about 3 ounces during menstrual flow lasting 3 to 7 days. Again, individuals vary from the average length and amount of blood loss from cycle to cycle.

PREMENSTRUAL SYMPTOMS. Many women experience symptoms at ovulation or during the postovulatory phase. Some symptoms are partly due to the effects of estrogen or progesterone and may include lower abdominal pain or discomfort at ovulation, breast fullness or tenderness, weight gain of about 3 pounds, fluid retention, irritability, and depression. For some women, these symptoms are more consistent and severe and cluster into the **premenstrual syndrome (PMS).** Although PMS is not a definite diagnosis and the physiological mechanisms are unclear, it is a documented disorder.

SEX DURING MENSTRUATION. There is no physiological reason for a woman to abstain from sexual activity during menstruation. The uterine contractions

Fig. 32-4 External and internal male genitalia.

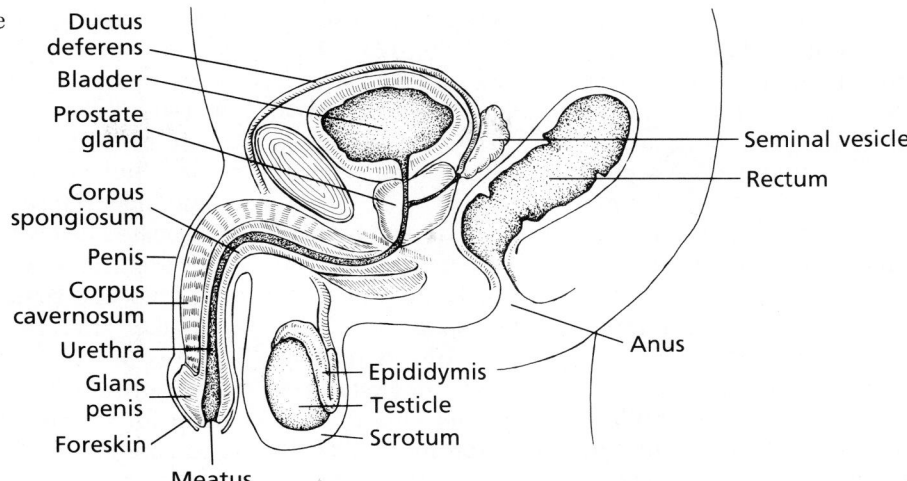

Ductus deferens
Bladder
Prostate gland
Corpus spongiosum
Penis
Corpus cavernosum
Urethra
Glans penis
Foreskin
Meatus
Seminal vesicle
Rectum
Anus
Epididymis
Testicle
Scrotum

that occur during orgasm may even ease the discomfort of pelvic congestion and cramping. However, excessive menstrual flow or physical discomfort may discourage a woman from sex while menstruating. Cultural attitudes or other factors may also inhibit sexual activity during menstruation. If a couple decides to abstain from genital sexual activity during menstruation, they can learn other ways of sharing intimacy until the woman is ready to resume sexual activity.

MENOPAUSE. One of the physiological responses to aging is the cessation of menstruation and fertility. Menopause takes place at around 45 to 60 years of age. The ovaries cease production of estrogen and progesterone, although low levels remain in the bloodstream from the continued activity of the adrenal glands. Each woman's body responds to menopause in its own way. For some women the only symptom is the disappearance of menstruation. Other women report headaches, hot flashes, insomnia, and changes in breast and vaginal tissue. Hot flushes or flashes occur when blood vessels rapidly dilate as a result of fluctuating hormone levels. The decrease in hormone levels also may affect the skin, breasts, and genitalia, causing the tissue to thin. The resulting decrease in the length and elasticity of the vagina and decrease in vaginal lubrication may make intercourse uncomfortable or painful.

Menopause should not interfere with a woman's sexual capacity, and many women continue to be sexually active. Some women find that the lack of concern about pregnancy enhances their enjoyment of sex. Physical discomfort during penetration can be eased with water-based lubricants. Water-based lubricants are necessary so that they can easily be removed with soap and water; if they are not removed,

they may provide a medium for bacterial growth and subsequent vaginitis and urethritis.

Male Sex Organs

The male sex organs produce sperm and hormones and provide a system for conveying sperm from the testicles to outside the body. The external genitalia are the penis and scrotum. The male internal sex organs include the testicles, which produce hormones and sperm; the epididymis and ductus deferens, a system of ducts that transport sperm; and the prostate gland, seminal vesicles, and Cowper's glands, whose secretions become part of the ejaculated semen (Fig. 32-4).

External Sex Organs

PENIS. The penis consists of the shaft, which is composed primarily of erectile tissue, and the glans, which has erectile and sensory tissue. The penile shaft comprises three parallel tubes: two corpora cavernosa, which lie side by side, and beneath them a single corpus spongiosum, which surrounds the urethra. All three fibrous tubes of the penile shaft are spongelike. The large vascular spaces between arteries and veins can become engorged with blood, causing the penis to become stiff and erect. The three tubes extend backward; each corpus cavernosum attaches to an arch of the pubic bone, and the corpus spongiosum extends into the urethral bulb.

The anterior end of the corpus spongiosum that fits over the corpora cavernosa is called the *glans.* The glans resembles an acorn. The area where the glans arises abruptly from the shaft is called the *corona,* meaning crown. The glans and especially the corona, which contains many nerve endings, are the most sensitive parts of the penis. If the male is uncircumcised, the skin of the shaft continues forward and forms a loose-fitting hood over the glans. This hood is the foreskin or prepuce. The undersurface of the glans is attached to the prepuce by a thin fold of skin, the frenulum, which is also very sensitive to touch. Circumcision is the removal of the foreskin.

SCROTUM. The scrotum is a thin, loose sac of skin that protects the two testicles. It is located at the base of the penis. The scrotum is divided into two compartments; each contains a testis, epididymis, and part of the ductus deferens. The scrotum is responsive to temperature changes; cold temperatures cause it to contract, pulling the testicles closer to the body. The temperature in the scrotum is slightly lower than body temperature so that spermatogenesis (formation of sperm) can occur.

Internal Sex Organs

The male internal sex organs are the testicles (or testes), a system of ducts (epididymis, ductus or vas deferens, and urethra), and some accessory organs (seminal vesicles, prostate gland, and bulbourethral glands). The left testicle usually hangs lower than the right. The testicles produce sperm and hormones. Sperm are produced in the seminiferous tubules inside each testicle. The hormones produced in the testicles are called *androgens*. Testosterone stimulates growth and development of the genital organs and contributes to growth and development of bones and muscles.

The sperm drain into the epididymis, a duct that lies just outside the testicle. Sperm take 2 to 4 weeks to travel from the epididymis to the ductus deferens. The ductus deferens is a long tube from each testicle that travels up and out of the scrotum. It curves around the urinary bladder and then turns downward and opens into the ampulla. The ampulla is a reservoir for sperm before they are discharged into the ejaculatory duct, which carries them through the prostate into the posterior urethra. The urethra continues from the bladder to the penis tip and carries urine or semen. These fluids are not carried simultaneously because of an internal bladder sphincter.

The seminal vesicles and prostate secrete seminal plasma. These secretions dilute and carry sperm and give ejaculate its characteristic odor. The seminal vesicles are glands secreting a portion of the ejaculate that contributes to the nutrition of the sperm. The prostate is about the size of a chestnut and is located beneath the bladder. The ejaculatory ducts and a portion of the urethra pass through it. In the prostate, prostatic secretions unite with the sperm and fluid from the seminal vesicles. This combined fluid is called *seminal fluid* and provides nutrients to the

sperm passing into the urethra. The seminal fluid also buffers vaginal acidity to aid fertility. Even when a male is not ejaculating, small amounts of prostatic secretions are discharged into the urethra and eliminated in the urine.

The bulbourethral glands are pea-sized structures sometimes referred to as the *Cowper's glands*. They are located below the prostate on both sides of the penile urethra. They secrete a clear, alkaline lubricating fluid that sometimes appears at the tip of the penis soon after sexual arousal. The function of this fluid is uncertain, but it is thought to neutralize the acidity of the urethra and make it a suitable environment for sperm. The fluid from this gland may contain sperm.

Male Climacteric

Men do not experience a true counterpart to female menopause. They do not experience the dramatic hormone changes or loss of fertility experienced by menopausal women. Men do experience changes in sexual response or the **climacteric.** At 90, a man may be capable of spermatogenesis. However, the delayed erectile and ejaculatory ability experienced at 50 or 60 may cause significant concerns about potency and masculinity.

As they age, men experience a gradual increase in the length of time it takes to achieve full erection. Older men maintain erections for longer periods than when younger, resulting in delayed ejaculation. The ejaculatory phase usually becomes shorter and less intense. The refractory period (time it takes to achieve another erection) is lengthened, and the penis returns to its flaccid state much more quickly than in men younger than 60.

The aging man may continue to have a satisfying sex life. The changes in delayed erection and ejaculation may bring about a more mutually satisfying sexual relationship between partners. Both partners may benefit from extended foreplay, which may increase vaginal lubrication and aid full erection.

 ## SEXUAL DEVELOPMENT

Infancy

At birth the infant is given a gender assignment of female or male. Rarely, infants are born with **ambiguous genitalia** and may be assigned a gender that seems consistent with external genitalia but is incongruous with internal sex organs and hormones. As discussed earlier, the self-perception of femaleness or maleness is not firmly established until about age 3. Obviously, for the least emotional trauma to the parents and child, the earlier that accurate gender can be assigned the better.

Infant genitalia are sensitive to touch from birth. With stimulation the male infant responds with penile erection and the female with vaginal lubrication. (Boys also experience spontaneous nocturnal erections without stimulation.) These behaviors and responses are not associated with erotic psychological contact as in puberty or adulthood but rather are normal learning behaviors in forming a sense of self. Parental response to these exploratory behaviors may set the tone for the child's sexual development, education, and comfort for dealing with sexuality in the home.

Parents should be encouraged to accept the infant's exploratory behavior as a positive step toward the development of a positive self-identity. Providing other forms of tactile stimulation through sucking, cuddling, and touching or stroking aids the infant in defining pleasant and comforting experiences through human interaction and from body contact. Touch and the human body begin to acquire a definition as "good."

Toddlerhood and Preschool

The child from age 1 to 5 or 6 continues to solidify the sense of gender identity and to differentiate socially defined, gender-appropriate behavior. This learning process occurs in the course of normal adult-child interactions from the toys given to the child, clothing worn, games played, and responses encouraged. The child also observes adult behavior, begins to imitate actions of the same-sex parent, and maintains or modifies behavior based on parental feedback.

Children reared in single-parent families need exposure to adults of both sexes. Particular attention should be given to the opposite-sex child of a single-parent or homosexual-parents household. Same-sex role modeling may occur through exposure to visitation periods in cases of divorce or through time with relatives, church, or community groups and organizations such as "Big Brothers" or "Big Sisters."

Body exploration continues at this age. Exploration may include self-stroking; genital manipulation; cuddling of dolls, pets or people; and other sensual experimentation. Concepts of pleasant and unpleasant are thus reinforced. During this stage the child may extend exploration to others as part of gaining a sense of autonomy and initiative (Erikson, 1963).

The child must begin to learn about socially acceptable behavior in an environment that is open to questioning about sex and that enhances self-worth. While learning that the body is good and that certain stimulation is pleasant, the child can also be taught the differences in private versus public behavior. Playmate sex games can be handled in a matter-of-fact manner. The parent can interpret the curiosity exhibited as an indication that the child is ready to learn the differences in and proper names for female and male genitalia.

Questions about where babies come from or sexual behavior the child observes should be addressed openly, honestly, and simply. If children wish more information than the answer provided, they should be encouraged to ask, and a more detailed response is given. Even if questions are not asked, learning opportunities should be offered through pointing out pregnant women or animal behavior at the zoo or through discussions of sexuality as a follow-up to stories or television programs that involve these topics.

School-Age Years

Children from 6 to 10 years of age, or prepuberty, expand their horizons from home to include school and the community. Education about and reinforcement of gender-appropriate behavior come from parents and teachers but more significantly from the peer group. North American society defines a broad range of behavior acceptable to girls and boys (for example, both sexes participate in cooking and woodworking activities). Parents should encourage socially acceptable behaviors without applying labels of feminine or masculine. Health care personnel must take their cues from the child, family, and community and should remain nonjudgmental in labeling behavior unless it is overtly gender inappropriate.

School-age children will likely continue self-stimulating behavior. Cultural and religious values become more strongly ingrained and must be respected. Parents and children can be informed that masturbation does not have any harmful physical or emotional effects. Explanations of times, places, and relationships appropriate for sexual expression should also be provided and should be given in the context of values and rationale on which these beliefs are based.

Children in this age group continue to have questions about sex and will assert their independence by testing the limits of appropriate behavior. Limit testing may be displayed by using dirty words or telling jokes with sexual connotations while watching adult reaction. Limit testing is an important part of developing a sense of independence from the family. The testing of sexual limits is also a means of identifying appropriate expressions of sexuality and an opportunity the parents should use to explore questions and concerns.

Children also have a desire and need for privacy. As children enter puberty, their bodies change, so the children experience increased modesty. Questions about sex may or may not be asked of parents, depending on communication patterns already established. Even in an open household, children may develop strange perceptions of sexual behavior because of misinformation and fantasies shared by peers. They may also learn that questions about sex cause uncomfortable responses from adults. This may limit their freedom in pursuing knowledge.

The child should receive accurate information from home and school about body changes during puberty. This timing allows the child to gain information and ask questions before they become personal concerns regarding normalcy and therefore too threatening to ask. The knowledge may also decrease the anxieties of puberty when an uninformed child may fear menstruation or nocturnal emission and view them as evidence of a dreadful disease. By the age of 10, many girls and some boys are already beginning some of the changes of puberty.

By early school age, the child should also be given information to guard against sexual abuse potential. Many schools are beginning to include this content in their curriculum. Parents should be encouraged to view this material to approve of the content and provide follow-up. Very young children can be taught the differences between good touch and bad touch and that certain body parts are not usually touched by adults except at bath time or during physical examination. Children should be told that if they feel uncomfortable about how they are touched, they should say *no* and tell a trusted adult about the incident. Other ways to limit the potential for abuse include teaching children that families should not keep secrets (other than birthday surprises or other time-limited events), that adults are not always right, and that all people should have control over their bodies and can decide who may hug them.

If abuse occurs, a child who knows the proper anatomical terms for genitalia will be able to accurately describe the incident. At these times the child should be assured that the adult abuser is the one who was wrong or did something bad and that the child is not responsible. Parental response can also be critical to how a child copes with the aftereffects of abuse. Parents should be encouraged to attempt controlled emotional expressions in front of the child and, as necessary, vent anger and frustration and find support with other adults.

Puberty and Adolescence

The onset of puberty in girls is usually signaled by the development of the breasts. After an initial growth of breast tissue, the nipple and areola increase in size. This process, which is in part controlled by heredity, may begin as early as 8 and may not be complete until the late teens. Rising levels of estrogen also begin to affect the genitals. The uterus begins to enlarge, and increased vaginal lubrication occurs, either spontaneously or as a result of sexual arousal. The vagina lengthens, and pubic and axillary hair appears. Menarche varies widely. It may occur as early as 8 or not until 16 or later. Although the menstrual cycle is initially irregular and ovulation may not occur at first, fertility should always be assumed unless proved otherwise.

Rising testosterone levels in boys during puberty are marked by an increase in size of the penis, testicles, prostate, and seminal vesicles. Boys and girls may experience orgasm before puberty, but ejaculation in boys does not occur until the sex organs begin to mature, around the age of 12 or 14. Ejaculation may first occur during sleep (nocturnal emission). This may be interpreted as an episode of bed-wetting and even in knowledgeable boys can be very embarrassing. About the time genital development takes place, pubic, facial, and body hair begin to grow. The voice changes as the larynx increases in size. This also occurs in girls, but in boys the more dramatic shifts or "cracking" of the voice may be a source of embarrassment. Boys must understand that, although they may not produce sperm with their first ejaculations, they will soon be fertile.

The emotional changes during puberty and adolescence are as dramatic as the physical ones. The adolescent confronts a powerful peer group with the almost constant anxiety concerning normalcy and acceptance. Same-sex peers remain influential in defining appropriate behavior, but the teenager must also deal with establishing a relationship with the opposite sex.

Adolescents are faced with many decisions and thus need accurate information on topics such as body changes, sexual relationships and activity, sexually transmitted diseases (STDs), and pregnancy. This factual information may come from home, school, books, or peers. Even with this information, adolescents may not integrate this knowledge into lifestyle. They have a present orientation and a sense of invulnerability. These characteristics may cause them to believe that pregnancy or disease cannot happen to them, and therefore precautions are not necessary. Health education must be provided within this developmental context.

More significant than the factual content is guidance in establishing a personal value or beliefs system to use as a framework for decision making. Much of this guidance has already been conveyed by parents. Values are expressed verbally and nonverbally as parents respond to infant self-exploratory behavior, preschool questioning about childbirth, family discussions of media topics such as rape, and parental public expression of affection. Attitudes of parents regarding gender-appropriate roles and behaviors also influence the adolescent's career and family choices and may also affect decisions regarding sexual activity and parenting (see research highlights).

School incidents such as a classmate's pregnancy, television and newspaper issues on abortion, or popular music can be used as bases for discussing family, religious, and personal values. This kind of discussion is difficult, even when two-way communication channels are well established. Parents must accept the responsibility to provide information, share their values, and promote sound decision-making styles, but they must be aware that the ultimate decision can only be made by the adolescent. Sexual issues that should be addressed from a knowledgeable and attitudinal standpoint include dating issues such as appropriate age, curfew, and dating activities; masturbation; emotional commitment in relationships; virginity versus premarital sexual behavior; contraception; teenage pregnancy and issues of adoption, abortion, or single parenthood; and risks of STDs. Ideally these discussions should be held in the context of mutual respect of beliefs to promote positive self-esteem.

This may be the age of identifying sexual orientation. Many adolescents have at least one homosexual experience with an individual or in a group. Adolescents may fear that this experience defines their total sexuality. This is not true; many individuals continue with a strictly heterosexual orientation after such experiences. However, some teens may recognize their preference as distinctly homosexual. This can be a frightening and confusing recognition for the adolescent and family and requires a great deal of support. Support may come from a variety of sources such as school counselors, spiritual advisers, family, and mental health professionals.

Adolescence may be the first time the child seeks health care without parental accompaniment. To be effective in interventions with this age group, the health care provider needs to establish an environment of trust and a willingness to listen. Issues of confidentiality must be clarified and respected. Nurses need to sort out personal values regarding teenage sexuality before they can be effective. Obtaining contraceptives or having an abortion without parental consent may be a legal issue in some states, but it is always an ethical issue. Those providing adolescent or reproductive health care must deal with the practitioners' ethical concerns, know about the legal concerns, and have an in-depth knowledge of adolescent development.

 Research Highlight

Howard and McCabe's study evaluated the effectiveness of a social influence model, a teen-taught sex education program in one Atlanta school system. Students in this program and other students from nonparticipating schools were interviewed, and rates of sexual activity were compared. Of the 387 eighth grade students who had not had sexual intercourse before the program, 20% of nonprogram and only 4% of students attending the program became sexually active by the end of eighth grade. By the end of ninth grade the rates were 39% and 24% respectively. This study has significant implications for teaching young teenagers about sexuality. Specifically incorporating peer teachers and dealing with issues of social peer pressure seems effective in helping postpone sexual activity.

Howard M, McCabe JB: Helping teenagers postpone sexual involvement, *Fam Plann Perspect* 22(1):21, 1990.

 Research Highlight

Casper's study assessed the effectiveness of family interaction in influencing four key behaviors in adolescent sexuality. The four key decision points were initiation of sexual activity; use of contraceptives; if pregnant, choice of abortion, adoption, or parenthood; and if decided to carry the baby, prenatal care received. Data were based on interviews with 1888 women ages 15 to 19. Results indicated that family interaction about pregnancy and risks of sexual behavior do not delay the age of first intercourse. The later age of first intercourse was correlated with higher socioeconomic status and maternal education. Family interaction about contraceptives increased the use of some form of birth control. Family interaction influenced adolescents to choose adoption or abortion over parenthood but was not associated with early prenatal care. Implications are present for teaching parents or teenagers about sexuality and the importance of including information on contraception and not just abstinence to influence teenage pregnancy rates.

Casper LM: Does family interaction prevent adolescent pregnancy? *Fam Plann Perspect* 22(3):109, 1990.

Adulthood

The adult has gained physical maturation but continues to explore and define emotional maturation in relationships. Young adults are traditionally viewed in roles of childbearing and childrearing. This model represents the vast majority of adults. Intimacy and sexuality are also issues for adults who choose to abstain from sex, remain single by choice or circumstance while desiring sexual activity, are again single after leaving a relationship, are homosexual, or are unable to bear children. For all individuals, sexuality should be defined and integrated into the self-image and sense of worth.

Sexual health has been defined as "the integration of the somatic, emotional, intellectual, and social aspects of sexual being, in ways that are positively enriching and that enhance personality, communication, and love" (World Health Organization, 1975). All adults can and should strive for sexual health regardless of their method of sexual expression. Although sexual activity is a basic need, it can be denied and channeled into other forms of intimacy. The single individual desiring sexual activity must make decisions about contraception, single parenthood, and risks of STDs. Gender roles and self-concept may need redefinition for women still single at 40 who desire motherhood. Self-worth can be maintained and nurturing roles fulfilled through community volunteer activities with children. The divorced individual may need to assume the added role of primary breadwinner while learning adult dating behavior. Homosexual adults confront the individual task of developing satisfactory intimate relationships while confronting community and possible career prejudice because of sexual orientation.

While developing intimate relationships, all sexually active adults must learn techniques of stimulation and sexual response that are satisfying to their partners. Some adults may only need permission to experiment with alternate behaviors or assurance that sexual expression other than penile-vaginal intercourse is normal. Religious teaching, family values, and attitudes influence acceptance of some forms of stimulation or may carry residual emotional effects that may be exhibited as guilt, anxiety, and sexual dysfunction.

Adults should also be encouraged to verbalize to their partners the types of stimuli and sexual or affectionate acts perceived as pleasant. To enhance sexual enjoyment, individuals should try to gather information about partner preferences. Mutual recognition of desires and preferences and negotiation of sexual practices provoke positive sexual expression.

Later in the adult years, the individual adjusts to social and emotional changes as children move out. Renewed intimacy may be possible or needed between partners. However, one spouse may experience a threat to self-image as the body ages and may attempt to regain youth through sexual relationships with a much younger partner. Couples can be helped to find novelty and new excitement in a long-standing, monogamous relationship through experimentation with sexual positions, techniques, and use of fantasy.

Physical changes occur in the course of aging. To prevent fears of performance, the reasons for these changes should be explained before they occur. Aging adults also need to adjust sexual action and response to chronic illness, medications, aches and pains, or other health concerns. The health care professional can again provide guidance on stimulation techniques to enhance sexual enjoyment.

Older Adulthood

The capacity for sexuality is lifelong. Theoretically people can engage in sex as far into old age as they choose. The best indicator for continued sexual satisfaction with aging is a regularly active sex life during adulthood and into later life. However, older people face health concerns and societal attitudes that may make it difficult for them to continue sexual activity. Although declining physical abilities may make intercourse painful or impossible, with sympathetic intervention they can experiment with and learn alternative ways of sexual expression. Decreasing vaginal lubrication may make a supplemental lubricant necessary. Decreases in the fat pads that surround the clitoris may make it hypersensitive even to clothing. Cushions and bolsters can be used to support the limbs and torso to ease the strain on the body during sexual activity. An erect penis is not necessary for sexual pleasure. If erectile capacity is diminished or absent, men can be encouraged to express their sexual feelings through touch. If erection is impossible or is delayed, the flaccid penis can also be used in touch to stimulate the partner.

The aging male may experience social and emotional concerns that affect sexual functioning. Masters and Johnson (1966) have identified the following general areas of concern: monotony in sexual relationships, career and financial concern, mental or physical fatigue, overindulgence in alcohol, illness, and fear of failure. Aging individuals, particularly women, face a concern over lack of sexual partners. The women may be widowed, and as age increases the number of available men decreases.

Perhaps the most difficult obstacle for older adults is the myth that sex is for the young. Some older people stop sexual activity because they feel that it is inappropriate. Hospitals, nursing homes, and other health care institutions may discourage sexual behavior among clients, although some nursing homes now give clients the opportunity and privacy to meet their needs for intimacy. Finding a partner may be a problem for some older persons. The older adults' needs to touch, be touched, and be sexual must not be left out of nursing care.

 ## SEXUAL RESPONSE

Sexual Response Cycle

Masters and Johnson (1966) have defined a **sexual response cycle** with the excitement, plateau, orgasm, and resolution phases. These phases are the result of vasocongestion and myotonia, which are the basic physiological responses of sexual arousal (Table 32-1). **Vasocongestion** is the pooling of blood in the genitals and female breasts during sexual arousal. In

---

TABLE 32-1   Comparison of Sexual Response Cycle in Women and Men

Women	Men
EXCITEMENT: GRADUAL INCREASE IN SEXUAL AROUSAL	
Vaginal lubrication: "sweating" of vaginal walls	Penile erection
Expansion of inner two thirds of vaginal barrel	Thickening and elevation of scrotum
Increased sensitivity and engorgement of clitoris and labia	Moderate elevation and enlargement of testicles
Nipple erection and increase in breast size	Nipple erection and tumescence
PLATEAU: HEIGHTENED RESPONSES OF EXCITEMENT PHASE	
Retraction of clitoris under clitoral hood	Increase in size of glans (tip) of penis
Formation of orgasmic platform: swelling of outer third of vagina and labia minora	Increase in intensity of glans color
Elevation of cervix and uterus: "tenting" effect	Elevation and 50% increase in size of testicles
"Sex skin": vivid color change in labia minora	Mucoid emission from Cowper's glands, possibly with sperm
Areolar and breast engorgement	Increase in muscle tension and breathing
Increase in muscle tension and breathing	Increase in heart rate, blood pressure, and respiratory rate
Increase in heart rate, blood pressure, and respiratory rate	
ORGASM: RELEASE OF POOLED BLOOD AND TENSION IN MUSCLES	
Involuntary contractions of orgasmic platform, uterus, rectal and urethral sphincters, and other muscle groups	Closing of internal urinary sphincter
Hyperventilation and increase in pulse rate	Sensation of ejaculatory inevitability
Peaking of heart rate, blood pressure, and respiratory rate	Contractions of ductus deferens, seminal vesicles, prostate, and ejaculatory duct
	Relaxation of external bladder sphincter
	Contractions of urethral and rectal sphincter muscles
	Peaking of heart rate, blood pressure, and respiratory rate
	Ejaculation: sperm mostly in first part
RESOLUTION: PHYSIOLOGICAL AND PSYCHOLOGICAL RETURN TO UNAROUSED STATE	
Gradual relaxation of vaginal walls	Loss of penile erection
Rapid color change of labia minora	Refractory period when continued stimulation is uncomfortable
Sweating	Sweating reaction
Gradual return to normal breathing, heart rate, blood pressure, and muscle tension	Descent of testicles
Often, ability to return to orgasm because women do not experience refractory period as often as men	Gradual return to normal of breathing, heart rate, blood pressure, and muscle tension

TABLE 32-2	Comparison of Sexual Response Cycle in Older Women and Men	
Older Women		**Older Men**

EXCITEMENT

Older Women	Older Men
Decrease in amount of vaginal lubrication	Longer period to attain erection, which can be maintained for long periods of time
Slower lubrication of vagina	Less enlargement of scrotum
Slower reaction of clitoris to stimulation	Less elevation of testes
Much less engorgement of labia majora	
Slight engorgement of labia minora	
Less enlargement of breasts	

PLATEAU

Older Women	Older Men
Reduction of orgasmic platform by half	Less likely to have intensity of color change of glans
Less expansive capacity of vaginal walls	Prolonged phase resulting from better ejaculatory control
Loss of consistency of sex skin	Penis becoming fully erect just before ejaculation
Reduced engorgement of areolae	

ORGASM

Older Women	Older Men
Less tension from muscle contraction	Elimination of feeling of ejaculatory inevitability
Less frequent rectal contractions	Fewer and less intense penile contractions
Shortened vaginal contraction phase	Less frequent rectal contractions
Shorter orgasm time	Decreased volume of semen

RESOLUTION

Older Women	Older Men
Vaginal changes returning quickly to prearousal state	Rapid loss of erection
Clitoral swelling lost	Greatly extended refractory period
Slower loss of nipple erection	Rapid descent of testicles

women this reaction leads to vaginal lubrication, **tumescence** (swelling) of the clitoris and the labia minora and majora, and engorgement of the outer third of the vagina. In men, vasocongestion leads to erection of the penis. **Myotonia,** or neuromuscular tension, gradually increases throughout the body during the excitement and plateau phases. It peaks during orgasm, resulting in involuntary contractions of the woman's vagina and the man's ductus deferens and urethra. Both genders experience contractions of the arm, leg, facial, and gluteal muscles. Carpopedal spasms, or spastic contractions of the muscles of the hands and feet, may occur. After orgasm, the body returns to prearousal levels.

The phases described by Masters and Johnson are not absolute. Although these phases vary in duration and intensity, the female and male response patterns are more similar than different. They are strongly influenced by psychological and environmental factors such as fatigue and alcohol intake, and the timing and intensity of these phases vary among individuals.

Aging and Sexual Response

There is no reason people cannot remain sexually active as long as they choose. This can most effectively be accomplished by maintaining regular sexual activity (sexual intercourse once or twice a week) throughout life. Particularly for the woman, regular intercourse helps maintain vaginal elasticity, prevent atrophy, and maintain the ability to lubricate. Nonetheless, the aging process does affect sexual behavior (Table 32-2).

 ## PREGNANCY AND SEXUALITY

As with menstruation, cultural attitudes and old wives' tales may inhibit sexual activity during pregnancy. Pregnancy does not present any physiological contraindication to intercourse. However, in some conditions or situations, intercourse may be contraindicated. These include bleeding, experiencing or being at risk for preterm labor, and rupture of membranes. Even in the presence of contraindications or maternal or paternal fears of miscarriage or fetal injury, the couple should be encouraged to continue expressions of sexual affection. These activities may include cuddling, kissing, hand holding, and massage. Cautions regarding noncoital sexual activity should be taken because often female orgasm should also be avoided when intercourse is contraindicated.

Women and men experience a variety of emotions with impending parenthood. Fear of injury may be a major concern limiting sexual activity. Conversely, some couples are relieved because they no longer fear an untimely pregnancy, so sexual desire is increased. During the first trimester, women may have a decreased interest in sex because of nausea, vomiting, and fatigue. Often an increased interest and responsivity during intercourse occurs in the second trimester because of a general sense of health and well-being. In addition, the pelvic and vulvar vasocongestion of pregnancy induces an almost constant state of semiarousal. Multiple orgasm may occur for the first time. During the third trimester, sexual intercourse often decreases, in part because of fatigue, size, position, and discomfort of pressure on the cervix from the penis and the fetal-presenting part. Couples who engage in intercourse after the second half of pregnancy should use positions that avoid having the woman flat on her back and placing uterine weight on the major blood vessels, which causes decreased maternal blood flow and therefore potential fetal hypoxia.

The nurse may need to inform couples that sexual intercourse or nipple stimulation may prompt labor to begin or accelerate. Semen contains some prostaglandins and may encourage uterine contractions. Breast stimulation induces the release of natural oxytocin, which also stimulates uterine contractions. For this reason, some health care providers may warn against intercourse late in pregnancy.

Changes in sexuality also continue after birth. Hormonal changes, particularly decreased estrogen, decrease the amount of vaginal lubrication and may necessitate the use of water-soluble lubricants. Fatigue caused by infant feedings and sleep interruption and general changes in household chores and routines may negatively influence sexual desire in both partners. Fear of pain because of vaginal or episiotomy discomfort can also deter sexual activity. Physiologically, the couple should refrain from sexual intercourse until bleeding has stopped and episiotomy and vaginal discomfort subside. This often occurs 2 to 3 weeks after birth. During this early period and even with breastfeeding, the couple must con-

sider contraceptives. The health care provider should discuss family planning options. Some women may remain disinterested in or have diminished sexual responses for 6 months or longer. Expressions of sexuality and affection should still be encouraged.

 ISSUES RELATED TO SEXUALITY

Potential fertility is an issue for premenopausal women having sexual intercourse. Often the concern is prevention of conception. At times the choice may be to not use contraception. In this case, the couple may experience anxiety until the next menstrual period occurs. For a smaller percentage of couples, the issue may be infertility when children are desired.

An additional issue for sexually active individuals is the practice of safe sex. Practicing safe sex has gained increasing recognition in the late 1980s as the fear of AIDS has arisen. The risks and consequences of STDs must always be considered.

Sexual intercourse and manipulation, although intended to provide pleasure for the participants, may be abusive in dysfunctional situations. Sexual abuse may include spouse abuse, rape, pedophilia (sexual activity with children), child pornography, and incest.

The nurse's major roles related to these issues are teaching and support. Nurses may also be involved in administering therapies and medications, providing assessment and evaluation of effectiveness, and providing public education regarding the facts, fiction, and importance of dealing with these issues in the family, school, and community.

Contraception

The ability to prevent a pregnancy or plan the time between pregnancies should be part of a client's health care plan. An unwanted pregnancy can affect health on many levels. The health of the parent, the child, and ultimately the community depends on adequate physical, emotional, and financial resources to care for the child. A client who is burdened with an unwanted child often enters the health care system with stress-related complaints. The unwanted child may suffer neglect or even abuse.

There are ways of preventing unwanted pregnancy. Each woman's right to choose if and when to become pregnant is generally acknowledged. It would seem a simple process then to control pregnancy with an appropriate method of **contraception.**

Yet the number of pregnancies among teenagers, abortions in all age groups, and unwanted children indicate that the decision to use contraceptives is much more complex.

Factors Influencing Use of Contraception

The nurse considers three major factors when exploring the reasons that clients do not use contraception effectively: the clients, their environments, and the appropriateness of the contraception technique (Fogel, Woods, 1981). The first factor involves clients' abilities to take meaningful action. For several reasons, clients might not act in their own best interests in using contraceptive techniques. Some clients truly do not believe that they can control conception and often view themselves as controlled by events or people outside of themselves. Clients may also fail to use contraceptive measures because of lack of knowledge about contraception or the potential danger of pregnancy to health or lifestyle. Shame, guilt, and denial can affect the ability to use contraception effectively. When using contraception, clients must acknowledge that sexual behavior is likely. This may be difficult for them to admit. If they have to deal with a pharmacist or health care provider to obtain contraceptives, the embarrassment or sense of personal risk may be too high for them to act.

Adolescents fail to use contraceptives for a variety of reasons, including lack of knowledge and issues of self-concept (for example, difficulty acknowledging themselves as sexually active or insecurity in the relationship). Reasons identified for not using contraceptives include lack of awareness that pregnancy could occur with first intercourse, lack of knowledge on availability of contraceptives, partner objection to use of contraceptives, fear of losing partner, unplanned intercourse, unavailability of contraceptives at the time of intercourse, perception that contraception is a woman's problem, and trust that the partner would take care of it (Zelnik, Kantner, 1979). Many of these issues relate to the adolescent's developmental level of establishing a sense of sexual self-concept, appropriate gender-role behavior related to sexual activity, egocentricity, orientation to the here and now, and a sense of invincibility and therefore risk-taking behavior. Characteristics of adolescents who use contraceptives effectively include high socioeconomic status, knowledge of a parent or sibling who uses contraceptives, older age, and personal experience or a close friend who has experienced a pregnancy scare (Flick, 1986).

A second factor influencing the effective use of contraception is the environment. The family, community, or religion may disapprove of or prohibit contraception. Clients may have been reared in family environments in which they were taught that sex for pleasure rather than procreation is wrong. Partners who do not know about contraception or do not cooperate in its use increase the risk of failure.

People learn about contraception from peers, health care providers, and public health agencies. Good contraception education requires a health care system and an educational system that can deliver such education to the community, but not all communities can afford or support that kind of education. Finally, the method of contraception must be appropriate for the client. The effectiveness of contraception is related to its safety, comfort, expense, availability, and ease of use. When discussing contraception with clients, the nurse should remember that each method has a theoretical effectiveness and an actual effectiveness. The former is based on the ideal circumstances under which the method could be used. The latter considers all personal and environmental factors and may be considerably lower if the client does not use the method regularly or properly.

The decision to use or not use a contraceptive method must be made by the client. The nurse can help the client clarify values (see Chapter 12) about contraception by providing accurate information. The discussion between nurse and client might include questions such as the following:

1. How does the method work?
2. What are the risks involved in using the method?
3. Are there contraindications that rule out particular methods?
4. How will it affect lovemaking?
5. Does the partner object to it?
6. Will it cause any discomfort?
7. Is it readily available, affordable, and easy to use?
8. Will either partner feel embarrassed using it?
9. Is the risk of pregnancy acceptable?
10. Are there other alternatives?

Biological Methods

For the purpose of this chapter, biological methods of contraception include any method not using chemical, mechanical, or surgical means to prevent pregnancy. The most effective means of preventing pregnancy is abstinence. This method is often overlooked when discussing options for pregnancy prevention with young, unmarried individuals (see research highlight). Because of the national campaigns promoting "say no" to smoking, alcohol, and drugs and the fear of AIDS, abstinence may become more common and socially acceptable for adolescents.

Coitus interruptus, or withdrawal, is a method of contraception often used by adolescents, but it is one

Research Highlight

Panzarine and Gould's study reports on 62 adolescent mothers' responses to nine questions on conception and birth control. Over half the questions were wrongly answered by 17 adolescents, even though all had borne at least one child and 46 were currently using some form of birth control. Increased age did not correlate with increased knowledge.

This study has implications regarding the lack of effectiveness of educating teens about pregnancy and contraceptive use. The need to include concrete, present-oriented teaching strategies with frequent reinforcement may be a more effective and age-appropriate method.

Panzarine S, Gould CL: Knowledge about contraceptive use and conception among a group of urban, black adolescent mothers, *J Obstet Gynecol Neonatal Nurs* 17(7):279, 1988.

of the least effective means of pregnancy prevention. Although the penis is withdrawn from the vagina before ejaculation, sperm are usually present in the preejaculation fluid discharged. A smaller but potential risk also is that sperm ejaculated just outside the vagina may still travel up the vagina and result in pregnancy. Douching immediately after intercourse is also an ineffective means of contraception sometimes used by adolescents. Sperm travel into the cervix far too rapidly for douching to wash away all possibility of pregnancy.

More scientific biological methods of contraception involve the timing of sexual intercourse to periods in the menstrual cycle when conception is least likely to occur. Contraceptive methods based on the menstrual cycle include the calendar method, the mucous method, and the basal body temperature method. Such methods are popular among clients who reject the idea of putting anything foreign into their bodies, who want a method with no side effects or health risks, or whose religious practices and beliefs prohibit the use of contraceptive agents. All three of the methods require that the client thoroughly understand the reproductive cycle of the body and be aware of its subtle signs and signals during the cycle.

Effective use of these methods requires consistent, accurate record keeping for 6 or more months before use as contraception and to determine least fertile days. All methods are not practical for women with irregular or recently established menstrual cycles. Last, these methods necessitate a degree of control

because intercourse must be postponed during fertile days. The degree of predictability and control does not correspond with certain lifestyles and therefore limits the individuals for whom these methods are appropriate.

The calendar method, also known as the *rhythm method,* calculates likely fertile days based on usual length of the menstrual cycle. One method recommends recording cycles for 8 months. Fertile days are calculated by subtracting 18 days from the length of the shortest cycle and 11 days from the longest cycle. These numbers then are the days one should avoid intercourse during each cycle. For example, with the shortest cycle of 27 days and longest cycle of 33 days (27 − 18 = 9 and 33 − 11 = 22), the woman would avoid intercourse from day 9 through day 22 of each menstrual cycle. To increase the effectiveness the woman should refrain from intercourse from the beginning of each cycle through the last calculated fertile day (Reeder, Martin, 1987).

More accurate methods of predicting ovulation are based on the body changes produced by hormones. One method requires the woman to record basal body temperature (BBT) the first thing each morning. Just after ovulation, body temperature rises 0.4° to 0.8° F because of the progesterone influence. The woman is no longer considered fertile after 2 to 3 full days of increased temperature. Because sperm survive several days, the individual may conceive if she has sexual intercourse 1, 2, or more days before the temperature rises. The effectiveness of the BBT method is also reduced when temperature fluctuates because of illness and schedule changes.

A method often combined with the BBT system monitors the quality of cervical mucus to predict ovulation. Just before ovulation the amount of mucus increases, and just after ovulation it becomes more clear, viscous (thick), and stringy or elastic. Days of wet, abundant, slippery, stretchable, clear cervical mucus are the most fertile. Use of spermicidal gels or creams, lubricants, douching, or checking mucus just after intercourse may affect the perceived quality of cervical mucus and decrease effectiveness of this contraceptive method.

Chemical Methods

One of the most effective methods of pregnancy prevention available is the oral contraceptive pill (OCP). The OCP combines various concentrations of estrogen and progestin. A progestin-only "mini-pill" is also available. OCPs suppress the release of FSH and LH, thereby preventing ovulation. The pills must be prescribed and may be contraindicated for women with histories of thrombophlebitis, liver disease, hypertension, and diabetes or for those who smoke and are over 35 years of age. The pills are costly and should be prescribed only under ongoing health supervision that includes an annual physical examination and Pap test.

Side effects of OCPs include weight gain, spotting between periods, headaches, nausea, breast tenderness, depression, and vaginal yeast infections. Side effects are mostly related to estrogen concentrations and may be minimized by adjusting the prescription to find the OCP with the proper combination of hormones. Serious reactions that should be promptly reported to the health care provider are severe chest pain, abdominal or leg pain, shortness of breath, severe headaches, blurred vision, and loss of vision.

The OCP is started on the fifth day of the menstrual cycle and is taken daily for 21 days. A menstrual period occurs usually within 2 or 3 days of stopping the hormones. Some packages of OCPs include an additional 7 pills containing an inert substance. This system provides a pill for every day and does not require the woman to count 7 days and remember to begin her next cycle of pills. OCPs should be taken at the same time every day to provide maximal effectiveness. If a pill is missed, the woman should take two doses the next day. When 2 or more pills are missed in one cycle, the woman should use another form of contraception (for example, condoms) for the remainder of that cycle.

Norplant is a new progestin-only contraceptive that is implanted under the skin of a woman's arm. The drug is continually released over a period of time (approximately 5 years) and suppresses ovulation as with oral hormones. The cost is initially high, but it is less than equivalent years of OCPs. The advantage is the ease with which the continuous effect is maintained without estrogen-related side effects. The disadvantages are related to the outpatient surgical procedure for implantation and removal and irregular or prolonged bleeding reported by some women.

Spermicidal creams and jellies used alone are not as effective as when combined with a barrier method of condom or diaphragm. The vaginal sponge combines the two approaches into one. Spermicidal products are sold over the counter and are relatively inexpensive. They act by providing a barrier at the cervical opening to prevent ejaculate from entering the uterus. A disadvantage is that the spermicide needs to be inserted into the vagina close to the time of intercourse and therefore may interrupt foreplay. Some women object to the contact with their genital area necessary to use these products, whereas others may object to the messiness. Dermal irritation may occur to the vagina or penis of some individuals.

The vaginal sponge is a sponge saturated with spermicide inserted into the vagina to provide a barrier. The sponge may be left in place for 24 to 30 hours and does not necessitate additional doses of spermicide for repeated intercourse during this period. The disadvantage of the sponge, which is different from other spermicides, is the risk of **toxic shock syndrome** (**TSS**). The risk of TSS can be decreased if women do not use the sponge while menstruating.

Mechanical Methods

Other forms of contraception, which ideally combine barrier and spermicide, are diaphragms and condoms. The diaphragm provides a barrier by covering the cervical os (opening). It must be fitted and prescribed by a health care provider. The diaphragm should be replaced yearly and must be refitted after a weight change of 10 pounds and after childbirth. Before each use the woman should check the diaphragm for tears and punctures.

The diaphragm should be used by placing spermicidal gel on the diaphragm, inserting the diaphragm over the cervix, and inserting additional spermicidal gel into the vagina. The process should take place 30 minutes or less before intercourse, and the diaphragm should be left in place 6 to 8 hours after intercourse but not more than 24 hours. The risk of TSS is present with this method. Potential disadvantages include the need for genital manipulation, which may be disagreeable, and the interruption of sexual spontaneity. Allergic reactions to the rubber of the diaphragm or the spermicide may occur. Effectiveness is less than that of OCPs but more than that of spermicide or a diaphragm alone. Diaphragms provide the added benefit of some protection against STDs.

The cervical cap is a barrier similar to the diaphragm. It fits only over the cervix. The advantages and disadvantages are the same as for the diaphragm. Fewer providers are trained in the more precise fitting necessary to effectively use this method.

The condom provides the most effective protection against STDs for men and women while providing a contraceptive alternative to abstinence. Condoms are latex sheaths that cover the penis and contain the ejaculate. The condom should be placed on the erect penis with a pocket or reservoir at the tip to collect the ejaculate. To prevent leakage, the base end of the condom should be held in place as the penis is removed from the vagina. Use with spermicide increases the effectiveness. Condoms can interfere with the spontaneity of sex. Condoms are the only readily available form of contraception used by men. With the increased awareness of STDs, sexually active women are beginning to carry condoms to ensure availability and protection during intercourse. Female condoms to line the vagina are available.

Intrauterine devices (IUDs) became less available in the late 1980s because of fear of litigation related to side effects. These products are addressed here because a progesterone-containing IUD is still available and some women may have other IUDs in place. The IUD is an object, which may contain hormones or copper, that is inserted into and retained in the uterus. It is thought that the IUD body causes endometrial inflammation, which prevents implantation. The IUD is inserted by health care personnel. The woman does not need to think about contraception other than to ensure that the IUD remains in place by periodically feeling inside the vagina for the placement of the string at the end of the device.

Surgical Methods

The two surgical methods of contraception are male and female sterilization. Sterilization has become more popular because of improved surgical methods and increased societal approval. It is the most effective contraception method other than abstinence. Newer surgical techniques can reverse surgical sterilization procedures. However, when choosing this method the client needs to understand the permanence of this decision.

Female sterilization or tubal ligation involves cutting the fallopian tubes. It is usually done with a laparoscope through a surgical incision in the abdominal wall, usually at the navel. The procedure involves only the fallopian tubes; no other part of the woman's sexual or hormonal system is affected.

In male sterilization, or vasectomy, the ductus deferens that carries the sperm away from the testicles is cut and tied. Using a local anesthetic, the surgeon makes an opening in the scrotal sac and removes a segment of the ductus deferens, tying off or cauterizing the ends to prevent them from rejoining.

Infertility

When one thinks of family planning, it is generally in terms of pregnancy prevention. One group with special needs that receives little public attention is adults who want to conceive but cannot.

Infertility is generally thought of as a female problem. In reality, an equal percentage of women and men have problems that contribute to difficulties bearing children. The evaluation of fertility must include both partners. Health care evaluation is usually recommended if pregnancy does not occur after 1 year of regular, unprotected intercourse. In couples over 30, this evaluation may be recommended if pregnancy does not occur in 6 months.

With advances in reproductive technology, the dilemmas that infertile couples face are multifaceted and can involve religious and ethical values and financial constraints. The decision to pursue adoption or medical assistance with fertilization or to adapt to the probability of remaining childless are options a couple must weigh.

Evaluation of potentially infertile couples includes physical examinations to determine general health, review of sexual activity, and understanding of the physiological concepts of conception. Specific procedures related to infertility include semen analysis for men, postcoital testing for mucus and sperm compatibility, endometrial biopsy, hysterosalpingogram (x-ray study) to evaluate uterine and tubal structures, and possibly laparoscopy.

Causes of infertility may be altered levels of sperm motility and lowered quantity or abnormal formation of sperm. The woman may have reduced tubal patency because of endometriosis or pelvic infections, abnormal uterine anatomy, or hormonal alterations that affect endometrial changes during the menstrual cycle or the quality of the cervical mucus. Depending on the causes of infertility, treatment may be hormonal to stimulate ovulation or surgical to restore tubal patency through microsurgery. Other available but controversial forms of treatment include artificial insemination using the husband's sperm or donor sperm, in vitro fertilization, and surrogate motherhood and embryo transfer.

The stress of fertility testing, the pain and continuing routine of therapies, and excessive cost produce a tense environment. Support groups are available for couples coping with these stressors. A percentage of couples remain infertile regardless of treatments used. These individuals need to work through a grief process for the loss of their potential children. Couples also need to be able to deal with the advice and misconceptions of friends and family. Support groups such as RESOLVE can assist. Contrary to community beliefs, recommendations such as "just relax" or "adopt a child and then you'll get pregnant" are not means of increasing fertility.

The decision to adopt or remain childless is one the couple must make based on values regarding family and parenthood. The number of children available for adoption has decreased because of improved contraceptive technology and increased abortions. Couples deciding on adoption may require support to decide to parent children who have physical handicaps or who are of multiple ethnic origin. Adoptions of South American, Korean, and European children have been a satisfying decision made by many couples. Support groups are available to assist these couples in continued integration of multiethnic families. North American infants are also available for adoption.

Abortion

Abortion is an issue that stimulates heated discussions of morality, women's rights to control their bodies, and the beginning of life. Abortions have been performed since ancient times. The increased safety and availability of abortions in the United States has improved since the 1973 Supreme Court decision, *Roe v Wade*. Abortions are also safer and less costly when performed in the early weeks of pregnancy. This is possible with improved pregnancy testing and more accurate early diagnosis. The availability of abortions, however, remains uncertain because of significant community opinions relating to the right to life. Various federal and state laws will be revised pending Supreme Court deliberation and advocacy by "pro-choice" and "pro-life" forces.

Rationales for abortion are varied and may include a decision to terminate an untimely pregnancy or a choice to abort a fetus that has a defect. Clients who decide to abort a pregnancy may experience guilt. The guilt may surface immediately after the procedure or may be more covert and manifest as sexual dysfunction or inappropriate perceptions (for example, a woman who later develops cervical cancer, viewing the condition as punishment for this wrongdoing). Some of these beliefs may be assessed before the procedures and should be evaluated by those counseling women experiencing unwanted pregnancies. The woman who has an abortion will experience a sense of loss and should be prepared for and supported through the necessary grief period. The male partner may also experience this loss and grief.

Health care providers must sort out personal values related to methods and rationale for abortion. Health care providers are entitled to personal opinions and should not be forced to participate in procedures or counseling contrary to personal beliefs and values. Nurses should choose specialties or places of employment so that their personal values are not compromised. Nurses must recognize that personal values should never prevent a client from obtaining needed health care and support.

Sexually Transmitted Diseases

Sexually transmitted diseases (STDs) have been a concern almost as long as individuals have engaged in sexual intercourse. These diseases spread more widely as individuals participate in intimate sexual contact at a young age and with multiple partners. An additional concern is the antibiotic resistance of some diseases (for example, syphilis and gonorrhea) over time.

A major problem in dealing with STDs is finding and treating the people who have them. Sometimes, people do not seek treatment because they are embarrassed. Some people may not even know that they are infected because symptoms are absent or go unnoticed. Because sexual behavior may include the whole body rather than just the genitalia, many parts of the body are potential sites for STD. The ears, mouth, throat, tongue, nose, and eyelids can be used for sexual pleasure. The entire surface of the skin can be thought of as having sexual potential. Although the perineum, anus, and rectum are rarely discussed in terms of sexual pleasuring, they are frequently included in sexual activity. Furthermore, any contact with another person's body fluids around the head or an open lesion on the skin, anus, or genitalia can transmit an STD.

Clients may hesitate to talk about their sexual behavior if they feel it is not "normal." Oral-genital sex, anal-genital sex, or any sexual behavior that embarrasses the client may hinder the detection of an STD. Specific STDs of the throat and intestine can thus go undetected at great cost to the client.

The most valuable tool the nurse can develop for providing care in areas of sexuality is communication skills. By questioning and talking with the client in a nonjudgmental manner that evokes trust, the nurse can pick up valuable clues about an STD that the client may have missed. The nurse can also begin to assess the client's attitudes toward sexuality and adjust the intervention to make it acceptable to the client's sexual value system.

Gonorrhea and Chlamydia

Gonorrhea has been known since the Middle Ages. Chlamydia has only been recognized more recently. Although they are separate diseases and require different antibiotic treatments, both have similar symptoms, consequences, and concerns.

Both responsible organisms are transmitted via intimate sexual contact. Usually the site of transmission is genital, but the diseases may also be transmitted through oral-genital and anal-genital sex. Symptoms occur in 90% of affected males within a few weeks of exposure. Symptoms are burning or itching on urination and a discharge of pus from the penis. Women with these diseases experience symptoms in only 25% to 30% of cases. These symptoms include burning on urination and vaginal discharge. With anal or oral transmission, the primary symptom is burning or soreness of the anus and rectum or throat, respectively. Left untreated, these diseases often progress through the reproductive organs, which may result in scarring of the tissue and permanent sterility.

Gonorrhea and chlamydia are diagnosed through a culture or "smear" from the affected organ. An antibiotic targeted to the specific organism is the treatment of choice. The individual should be considered capable of transmitting the disease until symptoms are resolved, the full course of medication is completed, and the health care provider indicates that the disease is cured. Clients must understand that all sexual contacts should be informed so that they may seek diagnosis and treatment. The client should clearly understand that reinfection is possible or likely at any time if the client again has sex with an infected partner.

Reproductive risks of gonorrhea and chlamydia must be considered. Male and female sterility are possible if the diseases are not adequately treated. Infants born to mothers with active gonorrhea are at risk for blindness. Routine newborn eye treatment with antibiotic ointment can prevent this infection. Chlamydia in mothers can result in pneumonia and eye infections in infants after birth. Treatment during pregnancy is easier than efforts to cure either disease in infants.

Pelvic Inflammatory Disease

Pelvic inflammatory disease (PID) is an infectious disorder causing inflammation, abscess, and scarring of ovaries, fallopian tubes, and other pelvic structures. The disorder is often caused by progressive unrecognized or untreated gonorrhea or chlamydia. PID usually produces pelvic pain, tenderness, and fever. A history of multiple sex partners, known exposure to an STD, use of an IUD, or recent procedures such as a D & C or abortion, accompanied by pelvic pain, should make the examiner suspicious of PID.

Treatment for PID includes vigorous antibiotic therapy, usually intravenous. Depending on the severity of symptoms, this treatment may be given in the hospital or through home nursing care. Severe cases of PID often necessitate surgery to remove abscesses, infected tubes, or ovaries and at times to perform a hysterectomy with removal of ovaries and tubes. This is a serious illness, requiring comprehensive, prolonged treatment. Sterility may result from residual scarring, even when surgery is unnecessary. The client may experience significant guilt and depression resulting from prior sexual activity, the disease, and possible subsequent sterility. The nurse provides education and emotional support in addition to the acute need for medication and physical care.

Syphilis

Syphilis has also been known for a long time. The organism is transmitted from an infected individual to a partner during intimate sexual contact. Usually the site of transmission is genital, but it may be oral or anal or even on fingers. Symptoms of the disease may take up to 3 months after exposure to become evident. The initial symptom is a small, painless lesion known as a *chancre*. The chancre occurs at the site of transmission and spontaneously heals in a few weeks to months.

Without treatment, syphilis advances to a more systemic secondary phase. Secondary syphilis exhibits influenza-like symptoms of fever, muscle aches, and sore throat. The hallmark feature is a generalized rash that may last for several months. Syphilis is curable with antibiotic treatment in the primary and secondary phase. Without treatment the infected individual is contagious to sex partners throughout this time.

If completely untreated, syphilis can advance to a nontreatable third phase. Tertiary syphilis includes central nervous system and cardiac effects. Although the organism is not transmittable at this phase, the damage is irreversible.

The fetus may contract syphilis in utero and be born with secondary syphilis. Routine prenatal care involves a blood test for syphilis so that appropriate prenatal treatment can be initiated. All clients should understand that antibiotics usually cure syphilis when taken for the full course of treatment. Sexual contact with an infected partner will always put the client at risk to again contract the disease.

Herpes Simplex Virus

The herpes simplex virus (HSV) is abundant in the environment. The specific organism of concern is HSV type II, the usual cause of genital herpes. As with the other diseases, sexual transmission may also occur at sites such as the mouth or anus. The common cold sore is usually caused by HSV type I, and it is not an STD. Cross infection can occur to produce genital HSV type I and oral HSV type II. For this reason, intimate sexual contact should be avoided with anyone with a lesion.

A herpetic lesion may occur a few days to weeks after exposure. Herpes appears as a small cluster of blisters that ulcerate and heal usually in several weeks. The lesions are quite painful. In addition to the local lesion, initial exposure to HSV often produces general influenza-like symptoms.

Herpes is not curable. The infected individual will experience recurrences of lesions throughout life. The disease does not progress but only recurs as blistery clusters that ulcerate and heal. Most individuals come to recognize early signs of tingling, pain, or itching at the area of infection. This precedes lesion development by several hours to days. Clients should be considered capable of transmitting the virus from the time that early symptoms appear until lesions are healed. During the intervening period, HSV cannot be transmitted.

Medications, such as acyclovir, are available to decrease the discomfort of lesions and decrease the frequency of recurrence. Generally, HSV should be considered a lifelong problem. Recurrences are more likely at times of illness and stress but may decrease in frequency over years.

If maternal genital lesions are present near term, the infant may contract HSV during birth. Herpes is a very serious and possibly fatal virus in the newborn. At term, the health care provider will check for genital lesions; if they are present, a cesarean delivery will be recommended.

Genital Warts

Venereal or genital warts, or condyloma acuminata, are caused by the human papilloma virus (HPV). The virus is spread through intimate sexual contact. The condition may be asymptomatic or cause a soft, flesh-color lesion at the area of sexual contact. HPV is the most common viral infection and possibly the most common of all STDs.

Genital warts may occur up to 6 months after exposure and can be difficult to treat. Treatment includes repeated application of medication such as podophyllum, or lesions may need to be removed through cryosurgery of lasers. HPV infections in women and possibly in men also have been linked to increased incidence of cancer.

In women, the Pap test often identifies atypical cervical cells or dysplasia (abnormal development) that require further investigation. Colposcopy is a procedure that allows examiners to view the cervix through magnification and identify and then biopsy suspicious areas. Often, no warts or lesions are seen until acetic acid is applied to highlight abnormal cellular growth. After identification of dysplasia the woman should have repeated Pap tests to observe for progression of cellular changes. In cases of severe dysplasia or early cancerous changes, the woman may need surgery to remove lesions, abnormal cells, or portions of the cervix.

Women who are sexually active, especially those with multiple partners, benefit greatly from regular Pap tests. Untreated cervical dysplasia may progress over several years to invasive cervical cancer. Aggressive surgical, chemotherapy, and radiation therapy are then necessary to attempt a cure.

Acquired Immunodeficiency Syndrome

AIDS or more specifically the human immunodeficiency virus (HIV) can be spread through sexual contact. Body fluids contain the virus in infected persons. No one knows exactly which fluids can transmit the disease. Transmission can occur with vaginal-penile intercourse, anal-genital intercourse, and oral-genital sex. Oral-oral transmission via intimate kissing may also be possible.

Transmission of HIV may produce AIDS. Some individuals may have no symptoms, whereas others may develop AIDS-related complex (ARC). AIDS may take as long as 7 to 10 years to present. Much remains to be learned about this virus, the disease, and those who have no symptoms or do not display the full range of symptoms. Symptoms of AIDS include persistent fever, diarrhea, swollen glands, fatigue, and weight loss. There is no cure for the disease, which is usually fatal. Treatments and vaccines are being investigated.

The HIV virus is also transmitted by the blood such as when intravenous drug users share needles. Individuals who practice high-risk sex behaviors, such as anal-genital intercourse, those who use IV drugs, and those have multiple sex partners should be considered at risk. Of increasing concern is the transmission of the virus in utero, resulting in increasing numers of children with AIDS.

Limiting Risks

Safe sex is a phrase used to describe responsible sexual practices aimed at minimizing STD transmission, particularly AIDS. Safe sex is responsible sex and includes knowing sex partners, having a relationship with open communication that enables the partners to discuss current health status and disease exposure, and using protective devices. Additional measures include limiting the number of sex partners, avoiding sexual contact with intravenous drug users, and using condoms properly. Condoms provide the barrier between body fluids only with sexual activity involving the penis. No protection would be provided for oral-genital contact, for example, and therefore these practices should be avoided. The only 100% effective method of avoiding contracting an STD is abstinence.

A controversial issue related to safe sex for adolescents is the placement of condom dispensers in public restrooms in places frequented by teenagers, particularly in schools. Those in favor of this program state that teenagers cannot be stopped from having sex; therefore adults should promote health through ensuring a means to minimize pregnancy and STDs. Those opposed believe that providing condoms implies approval for teenage sexual activity. The fact is that the rate of adolescent pregnancy and STD incidence continues to increase.

Discussion of limiting risks of STDs should be included with all sexually active clients. Middle-age and older adults may be engaged in relations with more than one partner and not realize the risk of

STDs. Assessment should be comprehensive and not based on stereotypes or assumptions.

Sexual Abuse

Sexual abuse occurs far more often than reported. The known cases of rape, incest, and child molestation probably only represent the tip of an iceberg. Incidents such as these have a traumatic effect on the victim and may cause psychological problems and later sexual dysfunction. Physical injury, STD, and pregnancy may be the result of sexual abuse. The covert nature of some forms of abuse is one rationale for assessing sexuality in all ages.

When abuse is recognized, support needs to be mobilized for the victims and families. All family members may require therapy in situations of incest to promote healthy interactions and relationships. Rape victims may need to work through the crises before feeling comfortable with intimate expressions of affection. Partners may need support in understanding this process and ways to assist the victims. Children who have been sexually molested need to understand that they are not at fault for the incident. The parents must understand the importance of their responses to the children's reactions and adaptation. Nurses may come in contact with clients confronting these stressors, so they should be aware of sources for referral and support in the community (for example, rape crisis centers and women's self-help centers) and refrain from applying personal values to the individuals and families.

Effects of Illness on Sexuality

Healthy sexuality involves all human dimensions, and illness can directly or indirectly influence any or all of these dimensions. Although illness and the healing process influence established living patterns, the idea that health is a matter of degree rather than a matter of illness or wellness may be a new one for the client. Viewing sexuality in terms of a continuum rather than as being present or absent may also be a new concept for the client. The nurse helps the client integrate the physical, psychological, and social systems during the course of the illness. The degree to which any nursing intervention involving sex is successful depends on the attitudes and beliefs of the nurse and client and their understanding of the effects of the illness and its treatment on sexual functioning.

Physiological and Psychological Changes and Illness

Sexual behavior depends on intact neural, vascular, and hormonal systems. The genitals and other soft body tissues that respond to sexual arousal require uninterrupted neural pathways and an adequate supply of blood. Hormones influence sexual moods and physiological functioning in sexual expression. Joints and muscles must bend and stretch as the body gives expression to sexual feelings. A change in any one of these systems can have a ripple effect on the others. To accommodate to changes in these systems, the client may have to learn new sexual behaviors. Changes in body functions and structures as a result of illness may not directly influence sexuality but may affect feelings of desirability and arousal. In this case the client's perception of the self as sexually capable and desirable is being influenced.

Chronic illness may interfere with sexuality because of the extended period of care and attention involved. A client or partner providing home care may have little energy left for sexual feelings or activity. For a client with a highly debilitating illness such as chronic lung disease, only very limited sexual activity may be possible. There are no therapies for reversing sexual impairment resulting from neurological or vascular disease (Unsain, Goodwin, Schuster, 1982). Diseases such as diabetes not only necessitate changes in daily habits but also may lead to reduced sexual desire. Vascular and neurological changes of diabetes may cause lack of or change in orgasmic response and erectile dysfunction. Spinal cord injuries may not only sever nerve pathways and remove genital sensation but also psychologically affect sexuality. Self-esteem is usually lowered with the accompanying change in body image, gender identity, and altered ability to perform sex-role behaviors (Weinberg, 1982). Chronic pain and limited range of movement present obstacles to sexual activity. To adjust to these limitations, the client must learn effective communication skills and be willing to experiment with new positions for sexual activity. The nurse has an essential role in easing these adjustments, particularly when the client's background does not encourage open discussion of sexual topics.

Cancer can also interfere with sexuality. Medical and surgical treatments alter body image. Alopecia (loss of hair), severe nausea, and fatigue from chemotherapy may temporarily remove all sexual desires. However, an individual with cancer or any terminal illness remains a sexual being. As stated above, altered expression of affection and sexual stimulation may need to be explored to adjust to pain and radiation effects. Even when death is imminent, the ill individual may wish to affirm life through intercourse. The client's spouse or partner will need to deal with grief and beliefs to respond sexually. The nurse acknowledges these desires as normal and healthy. The nurse may need to initiate discussion of these issues and support the partner in grief.

Effects of Medication on Sexuality

The effect of medications on sexual feelings and functioning is an enormously complex topic because of the number of medications in use and the individual responses to them. Medications can interfere with sexual desire and all phases of the sexual response cycle.

Antihypertensives such as methyldopa, propranolol, and clonidine often cause erectile dysfunction. Controversy exists as to whether the client should be told this when treatment is initiated; it could generate significant performance anxiety and a self-fulfilling prophecy. Methyldopa has been known to decrease **libido** (sexual drive). Thiazide diuretics, used to treat hypertension, also cause erectile dysfunction. Depression usually causes diminished desire. Antidepressant medication may produce an increased libido but may also cause delayed female orgasms and delayed or failed ejaculation. Chemotherapeutic agents, with the psychological effects caused by alopecia and nausea, may also result in decreased libido, impotence, amenorrhea (absence of menstruation), decreased spermatogenesis, and sterility. Young men interested in childbearing can freeze sperm before chemotherapy or radiation treatment. The sexual effects of all medications must be considered and included as appropriate teaching content.

Hospitalization

Clients tend to think that their situations are serious if hospitals are involved. The procedures of hospital health care may be beyond a client's capacity to understand. The need to have some power over life and the powerlessness of being hospitalized may become crucial issues. The client has left the home and its security and privacy and entered a more public and intrusive environment. The hospital room is open to the nurse at all times, and privacy is represented only by a cubicle curtain. Hospital clothing is scant. Even carrying out activities of personal hygiene may be beyond the client's ability. Often, sexual behavior and feelings may diminish or vanish.

Nurses can assist clients in learning to meet sexual needs in the hospital. Simply acknowledging the openness of the setting lets a client know that the nurse understands. Knocking or signaling before entering the client's space is a basic courtesy and provides a needed sense of privacy. The use of a do-not-disturb sign offers the client some feeling of control over the privacy of the environment.

Some hospitalized clients may act out sexually through use of obscene language, pinching or other suggestive contact with the nurse, or consistent nudity or exposure of genitals when the nurse enters the room. This behavior may be a means of exerting control over the clinical environment or an attempt to validate continued identity as a sexual being. It may also be a means of attracting needed attention or testing limits (Woods, 1984). Assessment and intervention to deal with persistent sexual acting out is a challenge that benefits from the psychiatric nurse specialist's expertise. Consistency in approach to the client and attention and reinforcement for desirable behavior are essential to minimize the problem.

Surgery not only changes body structures and functions but also influences body image (Dickman, Livingston, 1982). Surgical clients may experience loss of self-esteem and feelings of loss involving their masculinity or femininity (Lion, 1982). They may blame themselves for needing surgery and consider the surgical consequences a punishment. Alteration or removal of the internal or external genitalia can make conventional and accustomed sexual activities uncomfortable or impossible. The client is then faced with not only the loss or alteration of body parts but also the necessity of having to learn new sexual behaviors that may seem strange or repugnant. Prostatectomies, hysterectomies, mastectomies, and ostomies can create sexual problems for clients.

After a heart attack or heart surgery, clients often have a decline in sexual activity (Lion, 1982). This is true even after they are evaluated as fit and able to resume normal activities of daily living. These clients typically fear having another attack or dying while masturbating or having intercourse. The client's partner is often anxious about initiating sex because of fear of contributing to another attack. Such anxieties are cultivated through misunderstanding, misinformation, or lack of information (Shuman, Bohachick, 1987). Clear, accurate, and honest information is needed at every stage of rehabilitation.

Sexual Dysfunction

The causes of **sexual dysfunction** may be physiological or psychological. Sometimes the cause of a dysfunction cannot be identified or is a combination of several factors. About 10% to 20% of sexual dysfunctions are caused by physiological factors (Kolodny, Masters, Johnson, 1979). In another 15% of cases, physiological problems contribute to the sexual dysfunction but are not its sole cause (Masters, Johnson, Kolodny, 1982). In most instances a sexual assessment should include a complete physical examination to identify or rule out physiological conditions that might contribute to sexual dysfunction.

Psychological Factors

In many instances, sexual dysfunction can be traced to a lack of knowledge about sexuality, ignorance of sexual techniques, or general misinformation about sexuality. For example, unsatisfactory lovemaking can be the result of a lack of information about sexual anatomy. Some segments of society still place strong prohibitions on discussions of sexual behavior. Children may receive some information at home and in school, although sharing among peers may still be a major source of misinformation. Open discussion of sex, even between partners, traditionally has not been encouraged, and the result has been feelings of distance or alienation.

Another psychological factor is the destructive belief that the ability to perform sexually is inherently developed by the time a person reaches adulthood. Sexual performance is often perceived as instinctual and mysteriously understood when a person comes of age. Thus ignorance and silence about sexual matters prevail because a person who lacks knowledge about sexual function seldom realizes that the individual needs to be taught this information. Myths and outright misinformation about sexuality add to the problem of lack of knowledge for many individuals.

The psychological forces that prevent violation of sexual rules in many cultures are guilt and anxiety. When guilt and anxiety become associated with early sexual learning, the person develops a pattern of inhibited sexual response. For instance, a woman may be actively discouraged from sexual stimulation in early childhood. As an adult, she may find that she now has to learn to enjoy sexual stimulation and overcome negative feelings associated with her sexual self-concept.

Other sources of sexual anxiety, such as fear of failure, demand for performance, and rejection, can be destructive to sexual functioning. Anticipation of the inability to perform is a cause of erectile dysfunction and, perhaps to some extent, of orgasmic dysfunction. People who have experienced episodes of failure may have increased fears of its recurrence. Anticipatory anxiety related to sexual performance can start a self-defeating cycle of fear that escalates from a single failure into serious chronic dysfunction.

Fear of rejection by one's partner or an excessive need to please may also generate anxiety. To wish to give enjoyment and share pleasure with a partner is desirable and healthy. When this becomes a compulsive need to please, perform, serve, and not disappoint, the emotion becomes dysfunctional.

Poor communication is frequently associated with sexual dysfunction. A person with communication problems may be unable to discuss sex and thus may have limited knowledge and restrictive standards of acceptable sexual behavior. In this self-defeating cycle, partners perpetuate ignorance, lack of understanding, and misinformation about their sexual and emotional needs. To communicate effectively about sex, they must openly share information about their interests, desires, and wishes. Negotiation, compromise, and satisfaction result from effective communication patterns.

A history of sexual abuse usually has an impact on sexual functioning. Anger, guilt, and a need for control are emotional sequelae to abuse and often underlie the development of sexual problems, including inhibited desire and avoidance of sexual contact. Researchers have begun to examine the variables associated with molestation that contribute to adult sexual adjustment. These include the person's age at the time of molestation, the frequency and duration of molestation, and the negative feelings associated with molestation. These findings help explain variations in sexual functioning that exist among people with histories of abuse. Further investigation is needed to help nurses understand and effectively treat the population of abused persons who seek counseling for sexual difficulties (Livingston, McIntyre, Fogel, 1984). Tables 32-3 and 32-4 on pp. 986-987 summarize the most common female and male sexual dysfunctions, their possible causes, and intervention strategies.

Physiological Factors

Orgasmic dysfunction in women is seldom caused by physiological factors. However, diabetes, alcoholism (Livingston, McIntyre, Fogel, 1984), neurological problems, hormone deficiencies, and some pelvic disorders resulting from infections or surgery may impair or hinder orgasmic response. Vaginismus is most often caused by psychological factors, whereas dyspareunia is more likely the result of physical disorders such as infections, surgical scarring, diabetes, or use of drugs (for example, antihistamines, tranquilizers, and marijuana). Physiological causes for lack of sexual desire include hormone deficiencies, alcoholism, kidney failure, drug abuse, and severe chronic illness (Masters, Johnson, Kolodny, 1982).

Physiological factors that may cause erectile dysfunction in men include neurological disorders such as spinal cord injury or multiple sclerosis, vascular insufficiency problems, hormonal deficiencies, and genital infections or injuries. Diabetes and alcoholism are the two most common physiological causes of erectile dysfunction. Prescription medications and street drugs sometimes cause erection problems. Physiological problems rarely cause premature ejaculation, but delayed ejaculation is sometimes the result of neurological disorders. About 10% of cases of delayed ejaculation are due to drug abuse and alcoholism (Masters, Johnson, Kolodny, 1982).

TABLE 32-3 Common Female Sexual Dysfunctions

Description	Possible Causes	Interventions
Preorgasmic (primary) orgasmic dysfunction: impaired ability of woman to have orgasm	Religious prohibitions Restrictive learning environment Fear of losing control Poor communication with partner Inadequate clitoral stimulation Excessive drug or alcohol use Past negative sexual experiences	Provide information on sexual prohibitions and restrictions Teach sensate focus exercises* Suggest genital play Teach Kegel exercises† Suggest directed masturbation Encourage nondemand intercourse Initiate referral to sex therapist Initiate referral to preorgasmic support group
Secondary orgasmic dysfunction: impaired ability of woman to have orgasm currently but with history of ability to have orgasm	Low sexual interest Attitude toward partner Causes listed for primary orgasmic dysfunction	Discuss attitude toward partner Provide information on sexual prohibitions Teach sensate focus exercises* Suggest nondemand intercourse Suggest genital play Teach Kegel exercises† Suggest directed masturbation Encourage partner communication Initiate referral to sex therapist
Vaginismus: involuntary constriction of outer third of vagina, making vaginal penetration impossible	Religious prohibitions Sexual prohibitions Experience of sexual assault Painful intercourse Painful pelvic examinations Alcohol abuse Traumatic early experiences with sex Fear of pregnancy, venereal disease, or cancer	Legitimize existence of spasm Suggest use of vaginal dilators in graduated sizes Teach Kegel exercises† Encourage improvement of partner communication Initiate referral to sensitive, experienced health care provider
Dyspareunia: painful intercourse	Negative attitude toward partner Strong religious prohibitions Sexual prohibitions Genital sensitivity Physical problems (e.g., tears, infections, trauma, spasms, lack of lubrication) Roughness during intercourse Lack of arousal	Initiate referral to sensitive, experienced health care provider Treat physical problems Provide sufficient lubrication Discuss sexual attitudes Discuss comfortable positions
Lack of desire: loss of interest in being sexual	Strong negative emotions Illness Fatigue Drug or alcohol use Avoidance response because of feeling sexually pressured Unresolved anger or fear Depression History of sexual abuse or incest Pain associated with intercourse	Discuss attitude toward partner Provide information on sexual prohibitions and restrictions Teach sensate focus exercises* Teach Kegel exercises† Encourage genital play Encourage resolution of conflicts between partners Initiate referral to mental health professional or sex therapist

*Series of pleasurable touching exercises that are focused on sensual (not sexual) activities with partner.
†Exercises for pubococcygeus muscle to increase sensation and maintain muscle tone of pelvic floor.

TABLE 32-4   Common Male Sexual Dysfunctions

Description	Possible Causes	Intervention
Primary erectile dysfunction: inability of man to penetrate during sexual contact and to sustain an erection to point of penetration (Man may masturbate to ejaculation.)	Extreme religious prohibitions Traumatic initial failure Performance anxiety and fears	Relieve pressure of goal-oriented sexual performance Discuss sexual prohibitions and restrictions Provide accurate information Teach sensate focus exercises Reduce spectatoring Restrict intercourse Encourage female superior position with lubrication Encourage options to intercourse (e.g., manual stimulation, oral-genital sex) Initiate referral to sex therapist
Secondary erectile dysfunction: Inability of man to maintain or perhaps even experience erection but with a history of penetration at least one time (Man has experienced erectile failure during at least 25% of sexual opportunities.)	Interference with central nervous system caused by drugs, alcohol, stress, fatigue, diseases, or surgical procedures Performance anxiety Poor communication with partner Depression	Relieve pressure of goal-oriented sexual performance Discuss sexual prohibitions and restrictions Provide accurate information Teach sensate focus exercises Teach Kegel exercises Reduce spectatoring Initiate referral to urologist
Premature ejaculation: consistent premature ejaculation	Fast ejaculation patterning during adolescence Failure to attend to internal cues of approaching ejaculation Lack of sensual self-awareness Performance anxiety	Provide accurate information Encourage communication with partner Teach sensate focus exercises Teach Kegel exercises Explain stop-start technique Encourage different positions Teach retraining of ejaculatory response Relieve pressure of performance anxiety Suggest changing tempo of thrusting during intercourse Initiate referral to sex therapist
Delayed ejaculation: inability to ejaculate during penetration	Religious restrictions Fear of impregnating Lack of physical interest Active dislike for partner Past traumatic sexual event Infidelity Punishment for masturbation as child Excessive drug or alcohol use	Relieve pressure of goal-oriented sexual performance Discuss sexual prohibitions and restrictions Provide accurate information Teach sensate focus exercises Teach Kegel exercises Encourage communication with partner Initiate referral to mental health professional or sex therapist

The distinction between physiological and psychological causes of sexual dysfunction is not always clear. Physiological interventions sometimes clear up the problem. At other times, psychological concerns have been masked by a physiological condition. It is important to monitor the client's progress carefully, even when it seems that only a physiological condition is involved. An understanding of the possible psychological and physiological causes of sexual dysfunction is needed before the nurse can determine whether further assessment and intervention are necessary.

SEXUALITY AND THE NURSING PROCESS

Assessment

Ideally, sex is a natural, spontaneous act that passes easily through a number of recognizable physiological stages and culminates in satisfaction for both partners. After sexual activity, there should be a period of "afterglow" in which both partners experience a sense of warmth, well-being, and closeness. In reality, this sequence of events is often the exception rather than the rule, as demonstrated by the number of self-help sexual enhancement books available in bookstores. Nurses can expect to encounter clients who have problems with one or more of the stages of sexual behavior, including the feeling of wanting sex, the physiology and emotions of having sex, and the feelings experienced after sex. Clients may unconsciously provide the nurse with clues to their sexual problems. The nurse's role includes the promotion of sexual health as a component of overall wellness. The nurse can promote sexual health by helping clients gain insight into their problems and explore methods to deal with them effectively. The nurse must provide the opportunity for clients to discuss sex and can provide permission by initiating the topic at the time of assessment.

Many nurses are uncomfortable talking about sexuality with clients, but they can reduce their discomfort using several methods. First, nurses should build a sound knowledge base and understanding of healthy sexuality and the most common areas of sexual alteration or dysfunction. Nurses must understand how sexual orientation, culture, and religious beliefs influence sexuality. Second, nurses can assess their own comfort levels and limitations in discussing sexuality and sexual functioning (see Chapter 16). Finally, they can learn to recognize sexual problems that are outside the realm of their expertise and refer the client for help.

Factors Affecting Sexuality

Sexual desire is an appetite that waxes and wanes. Furthermore, appetites vary among individuals: some people want and enjoy sex every day, whereas others want sex only once a month, and still others have no sexual desire and are quite comfortable with that fact. Sexual desire becomes an issue if the client simply wants to feel sexual desire more often, if the client believes it is necessary to measure up to some cultural norm, or if a discrepancy in the sexual desires of partners causes conflict.

PHYSICAL FACTORS. A client may experience a decrease in sexual desire for physical reasons. Sexual activity may bring on pain or discomfort. Even imagining that sex could hurt can lessen sexual desire. Minor illness and fatigue are reasons a person may not feel sexual. Medications can affect sexual desire. Even the physician who prescribes a medication may be unable to predict the effects of a drug on sexual feelings and behavior. Poor body image, particularly when magnified by feelings of rejection or by body-altering surgery, can turn off a client sexually.

RELATIONSHIP FACTORS. Issues in a relationship can distract a person from wanting sex. Sexual appetite varies in an individual; sexual desire varies in a relationship. After the initial glow of the relationship has faded, couples often find that they are faced with major differences in their values or lifestyles. The degree to which they still feel close to each other and interact on an intimate level depends on their ability to negotiate and compromise. Thus communication skills play a crucial role when dealing with sexual desire in a relationship. Decreased interest in sexual activity can result just from the anxiety of having to tell a partner what sexual behavior is acceptable or pleasurable.

LIFESTYLE FACTORS. Lifestyle factors, such as the use or abuse of alcohol or the lack of time to devote to a relationship, can influence sexual desire. Traditionally associated with sexual behavior, particularly in advertisements, alcohol can induce a false sense of well-being or seductiveness in the initial stages of sex. However, ample evidence now shows that alcohol's negative effects on sexuality far outweigh the euphoria it may initially produce.

Finding the time for sexual activity is another lifestyle factor. Some clients do not know how to structure work and home time to include sexual behavior. Working parents, for example, may feel so overburdened that they perceive sexual advances from a partner as an additional demand on them. Such clients often describe their need to be alone to think and rest as more important than sex. Other individuals may not have sex partners.

SELF-ESTEEM FACTORS. The client's level of self-esteem can also lead to personal and emotional conflicts involving sexuality. The degree of sexual desire may depend on personal value and learned sexual skills. If sexual self-esteem has not been nurtured by developing a strong sense of a sexual self and by learning sexual skills, sexuality may cause negative feelings or lead to the suppression of sexual feelings. Sexual self-esteem can be lowered in many ways. Rape, incest, and physical or emotional abuse leave deep scars. Lowered sexual self-esteem can also result from lack of adequate sex education, negative role models, and attempts to live up to unrealistic personal or cultural expectations.

Sexual Health History

Every nursing history, whether taken in a clinic or hospital, should include a few sex-related questions to determine whether the client has any sexual concerns. These questions should be incorporated in the review of systems and addressed in a routine manner. The nurse must understand the reasons for the question and be able to provide this rationale to the client on request. Asking for information for the sake of curiosity is never appropriate. An opening statement such as "Sex is an important part of life and can be affected by our health status and vice versa. To better understand your health, it is useful to know . . ." is a good example to use. Other questions for adults follow:

1. How do you feel about the sexual part of your life?
2. Have you noticed any changes in the way you feel about yourself as a man, woman, husband, or wife?
3. How has your illness, medication, or impending surgery affected your sex life?
4. It is not unusual for people with your condition to be experiencing some sexual problems. Has that been a concern to you at all?

Questions that may be addressed to a child's parents include the following:

1. Have you noticed your child exploring his body, for example, touching his penis?
2. Has your child begun to ask questions about where babies come from?
3. Have you talked with your child about sex, pregnancy, and contraception?

Adolescents may best respond to a question such as the following:

1. Many adolescents have questions about STDs or whether their bodies are developing at the right rate. Do you have any questions about sex or other things?

It may be appropriate to explore physical, relationship, lifestyle, and self-esteem factors in more depth depending on other aspects of the assessment.

Some clients may be too embarrassed or do not know how to ask sexual questions directly. Thus they may be very subtle in asking for information. The nurse must be aware of cues that indicate a question or problem. Such cues might include the following (Siemens, Brandzel, 1982):

1. Talking about going home from the hospital and being afraid of their partner's thoughts or expectations of them
2. Asking direct easy questions and then seeming hesitant about the next question
3. Joking of a sexual nature
4. Asking questions that suggest concerns about achieving orgasms such as "When my episiotomy was repaired, could the doctor have sewn it up too tight?"
5. Making self-conscious comments such as, "Well, I'm just not as young as I used to be."
6. Using euphemisms such as, "I just want to be a good partner."
7. Looking down when asked a question about sexuality, blushing, and changing the topic
8. Asking questions about normal behavior such as, "Is it normal for a man not to ejaculate when he gets older?"

Observing and listening to clients' concerns about sexuality takes practice. The nurse clarifies and paraphrases or asks questions that will help clients be more direct about sexual concerns. If sexual concerns are identified, the nurse may wish to pursue a sexual health history in more detail. By including sexuality in the discussion, the nurse indicates that sexuality is an important component of health care and acknowledges the need for clients to discuss these concerns. When taking a sexual history, the nurse can use interview strategies to promote comfort (see Chapters 6 and 15).

A helpful guide for a brief sex history would include answers to the following questions (Annon, 1975):

1. What do clients see as their sexual concerns?
2. When did these sexual concerns begin and how have they changed over time?
3. What do the clients see as the cause of the concerns?
4. What sorts of treatment have clients sought to help alleviate this concern?
5. How would clients like this concern to be resolved, and what are their goals for treatment?

As indicated by age, sex, and review of systems, the history should include other aspects related to sexual assessment. The history should include concerns about STDs such as known exposure, genital discharge, and multiple partners. The adequacy of or need for contraception is an appropriate point of questioning for all men and premenopausal women who are sexually active.

Ascertaining whether clients are in abusive relationships is also relevant, particularly female clients. A question such as "Are you in a relationship in which someone is hurting you?" may open the door for a client to reveal present or previous abuse. An additional question such as "Has anyone ever forced you to have sex you did not wish to participate in?" may more specifically inform the client of the option to discuss concerns at the time of questioning or later during the contact with the health care provider.

A detailed assessment of long-standing sexual problems or concerns such as erectile dysfunction or vaginismus is outside the realm of general nursing practice. These clients should be referred to health providers specializing in areas of sex therapy. Often, however, the nurse may identify a sex concern related to medication, lack of knowledge, or fear of abnormality. Interventions aimed at these concerns are appropriate to nursing practice in any setting.

Physical Assessment

The physical examination is important in evaluating the cause of sexual concerns or problems and may be the best opportunity to teach the client about sexuality. The techniques of inspection and palpation are used in this examination (see Chapter 20). The nurse assesses the client's breasts and external and internal genitalia. The nurse has the opportunity to assess the client's reaction, answer questions, and provide information about the examination or anatomical and physiological structures.

The female client can learn to perform a breast self-examination during physical assessment (see research highlight). In addition, the nurse may choose to teach the client Kegel exercises (see teaching box). These exercises strengthen the pubococcygus muscle. Toning of the muscle decreases because of stretching during childbirth and loss of general elasticity during aging. Maintaining good tone help prevent bladder or rectal prolapse into the vagina (cystocele or rectocele), reduces problems with later urinary incontinence, and can enhance sexual enjoyment through and beyond menopause.

Male clients can learn to perform testicular self-examination during physical assessment. Knowledge of normal scrotal anatomical structures aids the client in detecting signs of testicular cancer.

Nursing Diagnosis

Altered sexuality patterns and *sexual dysfunction* are recognized as approved nursing diagnoses (Kim, McFarland, McLane, 1991) (see diagnoses box). The

---

| Client Teaching for Kegel Exercises | |

OBJECTIVE

- Client will demonstrate ability to tighten pubococcygeus muscle and will verbalize methods to assess correct procedures and increasing strength.

TEACHING STRATEGIES

- Explain method to identify proper muscle contraction by sitting on toilet with knees far apart and tighten muscles to stop the flow of urine.
- After muscle is identified, instruct client to contract muscle for a count of 3, hold and release for a count of 3 and repeat this 10 times. Client should do this about 5 times a day.
- Explain that within first week of exercises, client should assess if proper muscle contraction is occurring by placing 2 fingers in vagina to identify if tightening can be felt or asking partner to identify during sexual intercourse when muscle is tightened.

EVALUATION

- Ask client is she has identified pubococcygeous muscle via finger insertion or partner response.
- During vaginal bimanual examination, ask client to do exercises and assess muscle tone.

 Research Highlight

The purpose of Olson and Mitchell's study was to identify the influences on frequency of breast self-examination (BSE). Questionnaires were answered by 175 women, 20 to 89 years old, who had been taught BSE. BSE was performed significantly more frequently by women who were satisfied with their BSE ability and had received an explanation of the technique, which the women rated as helpful. The author encourages practitioners to provide BSE education that emphasizes explanation and demonstration of technique and provides for return demonstration.

Olson RL, Mitchell ES: Self-confidence as a critical factor in breast self-examination, *J Obstet Gynecol Neonatal Nurs* 18(6):476, 1989.

difference in diagnosing *sexual dysfunction* or *altered patterns of sexuality* depends on whether the client perceives problems in achieving sexual satisfaction or expresses concern regarding sexuality. When client concern is expressed, the diagnosis is *altered* sexuality patterns. When making diagnoses of sexual problems, the nurse must assess anatomical, physiological, sociocultural, ethical, and situational issues (see diagnostic process box).

Clustering of defining characteristics yields accurate nursing diagnoses. In addition to nursing diagnoses that pertain to sexual problems, the client may experience additional problems resulting from sexual dysfunction. For example altered body image may be a problem when a client is unable to perform sexually.

Based on the definition of sexuality, anything affecting physical, psychological, or emotional health or sociocultural or ethical attitudes and beliefs may have an impact on sexual functioning. These are areas for assessment, potential diagnosis of alterations or dysfunction, and intervention.

Examples of Nursing Diagnoses for Alterations in Sexual Health

---

NANDA-APPROVED NURSING DIAGNOSES

Altered sexuality patterns related to:
- Fear of pregnancy
- Effects of antihypertensives
- Marital conflicts or stressors
- Death of or separation from spouse

Sexual dysfunction related to:
- Spinal cord injury
- Chronic illness
- Pain
- Placement in a nursing home

Rape-trauma syndrome related to:
- Date rape
- Inability to discuss past rape experience

Body-image disturbance related to:
- Recent mastectomy or colostomy
- Sexual dysfunction
- Postpartum changes

Self-esteem disturbance related to:
- Perceived vulnerability after myocardial infarction
- Patterns of abuse as a child

Knowledge deficit related to:
- Sexual inexperience
- Age-related changes in sexual response

Decisional conflict related to:
- Premarital sexual activity
- Use of contraceptives

Planning

Goals for the client experiencing actual or potential alterations in sexual functioning include the following:

1. Obtaining knowledge of sexual development and functioning of women and men
2. Attaining or maintaining biologically and emotionally healthy sexual practices
3. Establishing or maintaining sexual satisfaction for self and partner if appropriate
4. Attaining, maintaining, or enhancing positive self-esteem with integration of cultural, religious, and ethical beliefs; past and present sexual practices; and situational realities

When planning interventions appropriate to the client's needs, the nurse must choose the appropriate

Sample Nursing Diagnostic Process for Altered Sexuality Patterns

---

Assessment Activities	Defining Characteristics	Nursing Diagnoses
Observe readiness to discuss sex using verbalization (e.g., "When can I return to life as normal?" or "There goes my love life") or behavior (e.g., exhibitionism). Ask client and spouse about previous level and method of sexual expression (e.g., frequency, initiator). Observe for affectionate behavior (e.g., touching, hand holding, kissing). In privacy, ask spouse about perceptions of recovery and return to full functioning. Observe for anxiety (e.g., hand wringing).	Client verbalizes concern that sexual activity may cause another myocardial infarction or death. Client's spouse exhibits reluctance to touch client. Verbalizes concern that client will need continuous care, attention, and protection.	*Altered sexuality patterns* related to fear of myocardial infarction or death during intercourse

diagnosis. The identified concern may be outside the realm of general nursing practice. Referrals may be necessary to physicians such as gynecologists or urologists for physical impediments to sexual functioning (for example, severe pelvic discomfort with intercourse or inability to obtain an erection). Sexual conflict in a marriage or trauma over past sexual assault or incest requires intensive treatment with mental health professionals or a sex therapist.

When planning interventions, the nurse should involve the client and, with permission, the sex partner. The client must wish to achieve the goals. Because of the interpersonal nature of sexuality, goals must be regularly reevaluated to determine whether they remain realistic and of mutual interest.

Any plan should include referrals to resources to promote achievement of goals after contact with the health care provider is discontinued. Many commu-

nity resource groups exist for self-help or peer support. The client experiencing diabetes, respiratory problems, cancer, and other physical problems may benefit from interaction with individuals with the same problem. They can share concerns and successes related to all aspects of coping with the disease, including sexual consequences. Self-help centers support women who experience abuse. Parents without partners and single adult groups appropriately deal with issues of sexuality such as STDs. Groups for older adults or community residents may be a source of help in confirming continuing sexual needs, issues of limited male partners, and raising concerns of safe sex for those again beginning sexual contact after widowhood. All plans should consider this type of community follow-up.

After a diagnosis is established and goals are set, expected outcomes should be established to serve as

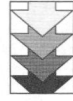 ## Sample Nursing Care Plan for Altered Sexuality Patterns

Nursing diagnosis: *Altered sexuality patterns* related to fear of MI or death with intercourse
Definition: Altered sexuality patterns is the state in which an individual expresses concern regarding his/her sexuality (Kim, McFarland, McLane, 1991).

Goals	Expected Outcomes	Interventions	Rationale
Client and spouse will resume intimate expression of affection by 2 wk after myocardial infarction.	Spouse will touch client by second visiting day. Client and spouse will progress to hand holding, hugging, or previous level of nonsexual affection by 2 wk.	Involve spouse in care; have spouse assist with bathing, shaving, and hair combing. Invite spouse to hug or kiss client goodbye. Schedule periods of ambulation to coincide with visiting hours (McCann, 1989).	Touch is basic form of communication and is basis of affection and sexual expression. Promoting intimacy while improving activity tolerance reinforces client's capacity.
Client and spouse will regain positive adult level interaction by 5 wk.	Client and spouse will speak in terms of their abilities in positive gender-appropriate terms by 5 wk. Spouse will describe fears of loss and proceed to acceptance of necessary lifestyle changes for heart health by 3 wk.	Guide client in imagery exercise to visualize self as healthy and performing daily routines and sexual function (McCann, 1989). Discuss grief-adaptation process and allow privacy and permission to share fears and tears. Refer to myocardial infarction support group for spouse and client. Provide weekly private opportunity for spouse to share concerns.	Client can verbalize fears and recognition that others experience same feelings. Support group provides contact with similar clients to provide evidence of progress.
Client will resume relationship by 8 wk.	Client and spouse will experiment with sensate pleasure exercises by 5 wk. Client and spouse will express satisfaction of sexual activity by 8 wk.	Discuss alternative sexual expression, (e.g., fondling, cuddling) as satisfying, not just as foreplay. Define realistic low-pressure expectation for gradual return to intercourse.	Sexual expression in continuum and sensate exercise provide low-stress, positive sexual experience (McCann, 1989).

guides during the course of care. For example, the nurse hoping to help a client achieve sexual satisfaction in light of diabetic vascular changes will need to identify steps to indicate progress. Outcomes such as discussion between client and spouse regarding satisfying behavior, satisfaction expressed after nonintercourse stimulation, and verbalization of possible delay in excitement or orgasm resulting from vascular changes indicate that interventions are proceeding as planned. When outcomes are not met by established dates, the nurse must evaluate interventions and goals to determine where modifications are necessary.

A sample care plan is provided in the box. Expression and recognition of the values and preferences of both partners are critical to achieving successful interventions. Goals will not be achieved if recommended interventions fail to match the client's sexuality (that is, gender identity, sex role, and partners' preference).

Implementation

Nursing interventions that address client alterations in sexual patterns or sexual dysfunction generally raise awareness, assist clarification of issues or concerns, and provide information. Nurses who have pursued specialized education in sexual functioning and counseling may provide more intensive sex therapy. Nurses should recognize when a client's needs exceed their expertise and provide appropriate referral. Most clients encountered in clinics or hospitals may benefit from the discussion and teaching provided by the nurse generalist.

The initial intervention often includes exploring present sexual practices with the client. The client should be encouraged to investigate and acknowledge social and ethical values and analyze the role of sexuality in self-concept. When there is significant discrepancy between values and past or present practices, the client may need referral for more intensive counseling.

Exploring and discussing values and levels of satisfaction and providing sex education require good communication skills. The environment and timing should be structured to provide privacy, uninterrupted time, and client comfort. For example, when discussing methods of contraception with a woman, the nurse provides comfortable chairs in an office rather than discussing this in the examination room when the client is only partially clothed.

Topics of education vary, depending on the defining characteristics and related factors (see teaching box). Education may provide guidelines for normal

Client Teaching for Resuming Sexual Activity After Myocardial Infarction

OBJECTIVE

- Client will identify factors related to activity intolerance and cardiovascular stressors during intercourse.

TEACHING STRATEGIES

- Provide privacy for client and spouse and sufficient time for uninterrupted discussion.
- Discuss MET needs for sexual intercourse as compared with other daily activities; excitement involves 3 to 4 METs and orgasm 4 to 6 METs, the equivalent of driving a car or briskly climbing 2 flights of stairs.*
- Discuss evidence of activity tolerance:
  - Heart rate increase of less than 20 beats/min
  - Heart rate returning to baseline within 3 min
  - Blood pressure increase of less than 40 mm Hg systolic or 20 mm Hg diastolic
  - Lack of angina, dizziness, shortness of breath †
  If during activities any of these appear, discontinue activity and call physician.
- Discuss environmental factors to decrease cardiovascular stress:
  - Room temperature: not too hot or cold
  - Refraining from food and alcohol for 3 hr before sexual activity
  - Position to decrease fatigue (Any position is possible; if discomfort is felt with usual position, couple may try client on bottom or side.)
  - Selection of a time of day when client feels rested (e.g. morning)*
- Provide opportunity within next 3 days to follow up on teaching and answer questions.
- In privacy, inform client of additional cardiac stress of sexual relations in new or extramarital relationship.

EVALUATION

- Client and spouse verbalize:
  - Evidence of activity tolerance
  - Signs and symptoms of intolerance
  - Methods to decrease environmental co-stressors
- If possible, follow up after discharge to evaluate satisfaction with sexual activity.

*Data from Whipple 1987; 1988.
†Data from Cohen JA: *Crit Care Nurs* 6(6):18, 1986.

development; for example, the nurse might talk to a toddler's mother regarding a new baby, a school-age child regarding appearance of pubic hair, or a 60-year-old man regarding delayed ejaculation. Details of physiological changes should be provided as a part

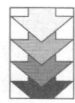

Sample Evaluation for Altered Sexuality Patterns

Goals	Evaluative Measures	Expected Outcomes
Client and spouse will resume intimate expression of affection.	Observe interaction between client and spouse.	Spouse will touch client. Client and spouse will progress in physical interaction.
Client and spouse will regain positive, adult-level interaction.	Observe client's nonverbal behavior (e.g., use of personal clothing, personal toiletries, and grooming aids). Listen to client's description of self, abilities, discharge plans, and interactions with visitors. Observe for signs of cheerfulness, description of self in positive terms, talk of future plans, and independent actions.	Client will describe self in terms of abilities and in positive gender-appropriate terms.
	Ask spouse in privacy about feelings about myocardial infarction and lifestyle and role changes required.	Spouse will describe fears of loss and proceed to acceptance of life with necessary lifestyle changes for heart health.
Client will resume sexual relationship.	Ask client and spouse about expression of intimacy and feelings related to these behaviors.	Client and spouse will experiment with sensate pleasure exercises.

of general health care. This also gives permission for clients to raise questions or concerns regarding personal functioning.

Major developmental crises (for example, puberty or climacteric or menopause) should prompt education about effects on sexuality. Situational crises such as a life change with pregnancy, illness, extreme financial stress, placement of a spouse in a nursing home, or loss and grief affect sexuality. The effect may last for days, months, or years or may even generate performance anxieties that lead to continued sexual dysfunction. If a client is prepared for possible changes in sexual functioning, performance anxieties may be minimized. The client feels comfortable raising concerns about sexuality as they occur when a professional relationship has been established.

Illness and surgery are situational stressors. Clients may experience major physical changes, effects of drugs or treatments, and the emotional stress of prognosis, future functioning, and separation and hospitalization. Sexuality, as a component of personality, may be affected by all components of illness. The nurse should never assume that sexual functioning is not a concern merely because of an individual's age or severity of prognosis. After concerns are assessed and identified, they can be addressed in the context of the individual's value system.

In response to identified concerns, the nurse may initiate discussion of methods of sexual stimulation, the sexual response cycle, or the use of creativity and fantasy in sexual relations. It may be appropriate to discuss sexual practices such as oral-genital sex or mutual masturbation as methods of expressing intimate affection when penile-vaginal intercourse is contraindicated. A partner experiencing joint pain may appreciate a discussion of various positions for intercourse. Use of fantasy or a sense of playfulness may add new romance or stimulation to a long-term relationship. A couple may need confirmation or assurance that the thoughts and acting out of non-harmful fantasy is normal and healthy.

Discussions of healthy sex should always include contraception when talking with clients of childbearing age. Men should not be excluded from discussions of contraception. The discussion may include desire for children, usual sexual practices, and acceptable methods of contraception. Factors that need to be considered when educating clients about contraceptives include scheduling or frequency of sex, comfort with genital touching, and comfort with interruption of sexual acts. All methods of contraception should be reviewed to provide necessary information for an informed client choice. The best method is the one that the client will use consistently.

All individuals having more than one sex partner or whose partner has other sexual experiences should learn more about safe-sex practices. As discussed earlier, information should be provided on STD transmission and symptoms, use of condoms, and risky sexual activities (for example, trauma from penile-anal sex). Safe sex may also consider the client's emotional risks within a relationship. Role play may be a useful educational tool so that the client can learn to say *no* or request that a partner use a condom.

When sexual dysfunctions are identified as ongoing premature ejaculation, vaginismus, or concerns over transsexual dressing, the nurse should provide appropriate referrals. Clients may still require support to follow through with a referral and reinforcement of explanations of procedures, treatments, or exercises. To be effective with any intervention, the nurse must be comfortable with sexuality and aware of personal values and biases. Referral may also be necessary when a client's values or needs conflict with those of the nurse.

Evaluation

Individuals have a right to understand their body functions and to predict developmental changes. Clients should understand development of the body, the manner of male and female sexual response, and changes that normally occur with aging and life stresses. Illness results in challenges to many bodily functions, and sexuality should be addressed as one area of concern. The sample evaluation box elaborates on the process of measuring actual versus expected outcomes.

Client or spouse verbalizations determine whether achievement of goals and outcomes has been achieved. Sexuality is felt more than observed, and sexual expression requires an intimacy not amenable to observation. Clients should be asked to verbalize concerns, share activities and satisfaction, and relate risk factors. The nurse can then observe for behavioral cues such as eye contact, posture, and extraneous hand movements that indicate comfort or suggest continued anxiety or concern. As outcomes are evaluated, the client, spouse, and nurse may need to modify expectations or establish more appropriate time frames to achieve the target goals. All people involved may need to be reminded of the individual nature of sexual expression and the multiple factors that affect perceptions and responses.

Sexual wellness is not an absolute. An individual must define what is acceptable and satisfying. The partner's level of sexual satisfaction must also be considered. To effectively resolve concerns, the client must also have positive self-esteem.

 ## SUMMARY

Sexuality is an integral component of personhood and therefore may have an impact on or be affected by health status. The nurse, as a provider of care and education, confronts issues of client sexuality. Cultural, religious, and ethical beliefs significantly influence the nurse's and client's sexual values and practices. These beliefs must be recognized and acknowledged and should never compromise meeting health care needs. The nurse should consistently assess and intervene to address a client's sexuality concerns. Areas beyond the scope of basic nursing practice must be clearly recognized, and the client should be referred to specialists, physicians, or therapists.

Sex will always remain a controversial issue because of ethical value systems. Facts of conception, development, contraception, and sexual disease transmission may be taught but cannot be totally separated from ethical issues. Issues such as appropriate age for first intercourse, homosexuality, and oral-genital sex will continue to polarize opinions and complicate care and education. With sensitivity and insight, the nurse can assist clients in assuming responsibility for decisions about sexuality, thus enhancing their total health.

CHAPTER 32 REVIEW

Key Concepts

- Sexuality is related to all dimensions of health; therefore sexual concerns or problems should be addressed as a part of nursing care.

- Sexuality is a component of personality and includes biological sex, gender identity, gender role, and sexual partner preference.

- Attitudes toward sexuality vary widely and are influenced by religious beliefs, society's values, the media, the family, and other factors.

- Nurses' attitudes toward sexuality also vary and may differ from clients'; nurses should be nonjudgmental about clients' sexual preferences and needs.

- The range of sexual behavior includes manual stimulation, oral-genital stimulation, anal stimulation, and coitus.

- The four-phase sexual response cycle is one way of understanding the physiological changes of sexual response during excitement, the plateau phase, orgasm, and resolution.

- Sexual development is a process beginning in infancy and involves some level of sexual behavior or growth in all developmental stages.

- The physiological sexual response changes with aging, but aging does not lead to diminished sexuality.

- Sexual health involves physical and psychosocial aspects and contributes to an individual's sense of self-worth and positive interpersonal relationships.

- Clients' problems involving sexuality include personal and emotional conflicts, the effects of illness on sexuality, and sexual dysfunction.

- Specific sexual dysfunctions result from psychological and physiological factors.

- Interventions for sexual dysfunctions depend on the condition and the client; interventions often include giving information, teaching specific exercises, and improving communication between partners.

- Concerns regarding acquired immunodeficiency syndrome and other sexually transmitted diseases should promote the use of condoms, but sexual transmission can only be prevented by abstinence.

- Choice and use of effective contraception methods are affected by sexual biases, comfort with touching genitalia, desire for future fertility, financial status, ability to plan sexual contact, and ability to communicate with sex partner regarding sensitive issues.

- A brief review of sexuality should be included in every nursing assessment of a client's level of wellness.

- Most nursing interventions to enhance a client's sexual health will involve providing information and education.

- Evaluation is primarily determined through observation of client and partner expressions of satisfaction in meeting personal goals for sexual functioning.

Key Terms

Ambiguous genitalia, p. 968

Bisexual, p. 961

Climacteric, p. 968

Coitus interruptus, p. 976

Contraception, p. 975

Corpus luteum, p. 965

Gender identity, p. 960

Gender role, p. 960

Graafian follicle, p. 965

Heterosexual, p. 961

Homosexual, p. 961

Lesbian, p. 961

Libido, p. 984

Menarche, p. 965

Menopause, p. 965

Menstrual cycle, p. 965

Menstruation, p. 965

Myotonia, p. 974

Ovulation, p. 965

Premenstrual syndrome (PMS), p. 966

Secondary sex characteristics, p. 965

Sex, p. 960

Sexual dysfunction, p. 984

Sexual orientation, p. 961

Sexual response cycle, p. 973

Sexuality, p. 960

Sexually transmitted diseases (STDs), p. 980

Toxic shock syndrome (TSS), p. 978

Transsexuals, p. 961

Transvestite, p. 961

Tumescence, p. 974

Vasocongestion, p. 973

Critical Thinking Exercises

1. Suzie is an 18-year-old student. She has had one elective abortion. Her current relationship is with her third sexual partner, and she is seeking a "good type of birth control." How would you counsel and educate Suzie about her options?

2. Mr. Burke is 60 years old and is hospitalized recovering from an acute myocardial infarction. He has been on antihypertensive medication for several years and will continue these after discharge. His rehabilitation has begun; however, Mr. Burke will only say "No problem, I'm just going to pick up where I left off." Mr. Burke persists in making off-color jokes, inappropriately touches nurses, and lies with his genitalia exposed. How do you plan for and address Mr. Burke's needs and the staff's comfort and entitled respect?

3. Mrs. Jackson has her 6-week check-up after the birth of her second child. Because of problems during pregnancy and work absence, she has lost her job. Since the birth, Mrs. Jackson has increased her consumption of alcohol and marijuana. Mrs. Jackson verbalizes concern over losing her husband because of her pregnant weight gain and loss of attractiveness. She shares a lack of desire in sexual intercourse, which her husband does not understand. What are five relevant points to begin counseling and support?

4. Mrs. Smith talks with you, an office nurse. She is 52 and has recently missed two menstrual periods. She is concerned also because her sexual response has lately been diminished. She appears depressed and shares that her youngest son has just left for college. What would you counsel her to expect at this developmental period and in the next 5 years as regards her sexuality?

5. John is 22 years old. He is scheduled to have back surgery and expresses some concern over possible neurological injuries. He shares his concern about possible effects on sexual functioning because he is engaged to be married in 6 months. As you explore his concerns, John reveals that at 14 he had a sexual encounter with a man and carries feelings of guilt and fear that he may really be a latent homosexual. What implications should this have for John's operation scheduled for tomorrow? What issues can you share with him? How do you proceed to refer John to appropriate counseling?

REFERENCES

Annon J: *The behavioral treatment of sexual problems, vol 1, Brief therapy*, Honolulu, 1975, Enabling Systems.

Dickman G, Livingston C: *Sex and the female ostomate*, Los Angeles, 1982, United Ostomy Association.

Erikson E: *Childhood and society*, New York, 1963, Norton.

Flick LH: Paths to adolescent parenthood: implications for prevention, *Public Health Rep* 101(2):132, 1986.

Fogel C, Woods NF: *Health care of women*, St Louis, 1981, Mosby–Year Book.

Hogan R: *Human sexuality: a nursing perspective*, New York, 1980, Appleton-Century-Crofts.

Hogan R: Influences of culture on sexuality, *Nurs Clin North Am* 17(3):365, 1982.

Kim MJ, McFarland GK, McLane AM: *Pocket guide to nursing diagnosis*, ed 4, St Louis, 1991, Mosby–Year Book.

Kolodny R, Masters W, Johnson V: *Textbook for sexual medicine*, Boston, 1979, Little, Brown.

Lion EM: *Human sexuality in nursing process*, New York, 1982, Wiley.

Livingston C, McIntyre M, Fogel C: Sexual dysfunction: etiology and treatment. In Woods NF, editor: *Human sexuality in health and illness*, ed 3, St Louis, 1984, Mosby–Year Book.

Masters W, Johnson V: *Human sexual response*, Boston, 1966, Little, Brown.

Masters W, Johnson V: *Human sexual inadequacy*, Boston, 1970, Little, Brown.

Masters W, Johnson V, Kolodny R: *Human sexuality*, Boston, 1982, Little, Brown.

McCann ME: Sexual healing after heart attacks, *Am J Nurs* 89(19):1133, 1989.

Reeder SJ, Martin LL: *Maternity nursing: family, newborn, and women's health*, ed 16, Philadelphia, 1987, Lippincott.

Shuman NA, Bohachick P: Nurse's attitudes toward sexual counseling, *DCCN* 6(2):75, 1987.

Siemens S, Brandzel R: *Sexuality: nursing assessment and intervention*, Philadelphia, 1982, Lippincott.

Unsain L, Goodwin M, Schuster E: Diabetes and sexual functioning, *Nurs Clin North Am* 17(3):387, 1982.

Weinberg JS: Human sexuality and spinal cord injury, *Nurs Clin North Am* 17(3):407, 1982.

Woods NF: *Human sexuality in health and illness*, ed 3, St Louis, 1984, Mosby–Year Book.

World Health Organization: *Education and treatment in human sexuality: the training of health professionals*, WHO Tech Rep Ser 572, Geneva, 1975, WHO.

Zelnik M, Kanter JF: Reasons for nonuse of contraception by sexually active women aged 15-19, *Fam Plann Perspect* 11(3):289, 1979.

ADDITIONAL READINGS

Allen DG, Whatley M: Nursing and men's health, some critical considerations, *Nurs Clin North Am* 21:1:3, 1986.

Boyle CA, Berkowitz GS, Kelsey JL: Epidemiology of premenstrual symptoms, *Am J Public Health* 77(3):349, 1987.

Brosnan CA: Long term results of an elementary sexuality program, *Pediatr Nurs* 13(2):130, 1987.

Brown MA, Zimmer PA: Personal and family impact of premenstrual symptoms, *J Obstet Gynecol Neonatal Nurse* 15(1):31, 1986.

Bunting S, Campbell JC: Feminism and nursing: historical perspectives, *ANS* 12(4):11, 1990.

Campbell JC, Alford P: The dark consequences of marital rape, *Am J Nurs* 89(7):946, 1989.

Casper LM: Does family interaction prevent adolescent pregnancy? *Fam Plann Perspect* 22(3):109, 1990.

Chapman J, Sughrue J: A model for sexual assessment and intervention, *Health Care Women Int* 8(11):87, 1987.

Cohen JA: Sexual counseling of the patient following myocardial infarction, *Crit Care Nurs* 6(6):18, 1986.

Davies K: Genital herpes: an overview, *J Obstet Gynecol Neonatal Nurs* 19(5):401, 1990.

Fischman SH et al: Changes in sexual relationships in postpartum couples, *J Obstet Gynecol Neonatal Nurs* 15(1):58, 1986.

Hatcher RA et al: *Contraceptive technology: 1986-1987*, ed 13, New York, 1986, Irvington.

Hosking R, Hiller G: Using nursing diagnosis in a cardiovascular clinical nurse specialist practice, *J Adv Med Surg Nurs* 1(3):33, 1989.

Howard M, McCabe JB: Helping teenagers postpone sexual involvement, *Fam Plann Perspect* 22(1):21, 1990.

Jain H, Shamoian CA, Mobarak A: Sexual disorders in the elderly, *Med Aspects Human Sexuality* (special issue) 21(3):14, 1987.

Katsin L: Chronic illness and sexuality, *Am J Nurs* 90(1):54, 1990.

Kisker EE: Teenagers talk about sex, pregnancy and contraception, *Fam Plann Perspect* 17(2):83, 1985.

Krajicek MJ: Developmental disability and human sexuality, *Nurs Clin North Am* 17(3):377, 1982.

Littlefield VM: *Health education for women*, Norwalk, Conn, 1986, Appleton-Century-Crofts.

Madaras L, Madaras A: *The what's happening to my body book for girls,* New York, 1983, Newmarket.

Madaras L, Saavedra D: *The what's happening to my body book for boys,* New York, 1984, Newmarket.

McCraken AL: Sexual practices by elders, *J Gerontol Nurs* 14(10):13, 1988.

Mims F, Swenson M: *Sexuality: a nursing perspective*, New York, 1980, McGraw-Hill.

Monier M, Laird M: Contraceptives: a look at the future, *Am J Nurs* 89(4):496, 1989.

Muscari ME: Obtaining the adolescent sexual history, *Pediatr Nurs* 13(5):307, 1987.

Olson RL, Mitchell ES: Self-confidence as a critical factor in breast self-examination, *J Obstet Gynecol Neonatal Nurs* 18(6):476, 1989.

Panzarine S, Gould CL: Knowledge about contraceptive use and conception among a group of urban black adolescent mothers, *J Obstet Gynecol Neonatal Nurs* 17(7):279, 1988.

Papadopoulos C: Sexual problems of the CAD patient, *Med Aspects Human Sexuality* 21(1):53, 1987.

Redeker NS: Health beliefs, health locus of control, and the frequency of practice of breast self-examination in women, *J Obstet Gynecol Neonatal Nurs* 18(1):45, 1989.

Rieve JE: Sexuality and the adult with acquired physical disability, *Nurs Clin North Am* 24(1):265, 1989.

Rondon N: KID-ABILITY: taking action against sexual abuse, *Child Today* 15(4):22, 1986.

Rosenberg E: *Growing up feeling good*, New York, 1987, Puffin.

Schuster EA, Unsain IC, Goodwin MH: Nursing practice in human sexuality, *Nurs Clin North Am* 17(3):345, 1982.

Shipes E, Lehr S: Sexuality and the male cancer patient, *Cancer Nurse* 5(5):375, 1982.

Talashek ML, Tichy AM, Epping H: Sexually transmitted diseases in the elderly: issues and recommendations, *J Gerontol Nurs* 16(4):11, 1990.

Tinkle MB: Genital human papillomavirus infection: a growing health risk, *J Obstet Gynecol Neonatal Nurs* 19(6):501, 1990.

Woods NF: Toward a holistic perspective of human sexuality: alterations in sexual health and nursing diagnosis, *Holistic Nurs Pract* 1(4):1, 1987.

CHAPTER 33

Spiritual Health

OBJECTIVES

Mastery of content in this chapter will enable the student to:

- Define the key terms listed.
- Discuss the relationship of spiritual health to physiological and psychosocial health.
- Contrast spiritual and religious aspects of health.
- Assess components of spiritual health.
- Describe a spiritually healthy person.
- Describe the signs of unmet spiritual needs.
- List interventions in the nursing plan for spiritual care.
- Evaluate attainment of spiritual health.
- Identify resources that can help clients attain spiritual health.

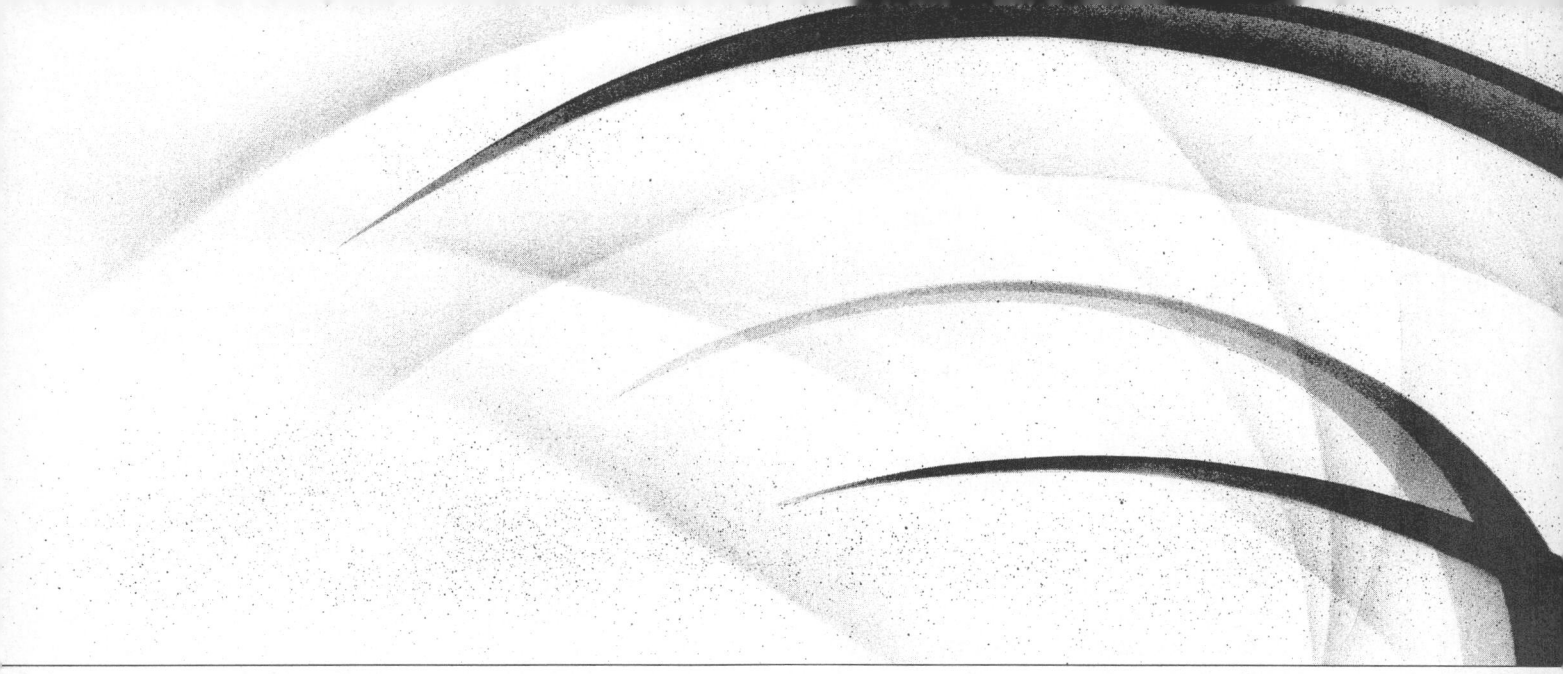

CHAPTER OUTLINE

uman nature has a spiritual component just as it has physiological, psychological, and sociocultural components. Living fully requires spiritual health, as well as mental and physical well-being. As with other dimensions of health, spiritual health is highly individualized and can change as other dimensions of health fluctuate. The ultimate state of health would seem to be a delicate balance of all dimensions—physical, psychological, sociocultural, and spiritual.

The spiritual dimensions of nursing care may be particularly significant for the client with a physical health problem. Physically unhealthy clients may not be able to manage their spiritual needs. The nurse giving holistic care determines all these needs, including those within the spiritual realm. Although physiological or sociocultural needs may take precedence, spiritual needs are sometimes of the most concern to the client and nurse.

Nurses' needs for information about applying standards of care in the spiritual realm have prompted authors and educators to address this topic in more depth. The North American Nursing Diagnosis Association (NANDA) classification of nursing diagnoses has included spiritual problems under the classification *spiritual distress* (Kim, McFarland, McLane, 1991). Several researchers have compiled descriptions of the beliefs and practices of different religions. With this understanding, nurses can better facilitate client participation in religious rituals and practices.

DEFINITION OF SPIRITUAL HEALTH

Spirituality, or the spiritual self, pervades a person's being and encompasses the human search for meaningful answers to questions about life, illness, and death. At the core is a person's deepest relationships with self, others, and a supreme being. Thus spirituality suggests vertical and horizontal relationships. In the vertical dimension, humans seek a relationship with the source of strength outside themselves, a supreme being. In the horizontal dimension, the individual expresses life values, belief systems, and relationships with self and others. A spiritually healthy person lives in conscious awareness of personal relationships in both dimensions.

Throughout life, an individual grows in spirituality, becoming increasingly aware of the meaning, purpose, and values of life. When assessing the client, the nurse should be aware that spiritual and faith development is represented by developmental tasks.

Horizontal spiritual development, which involves the cultivation of meaningful relationships with others and the emergence of a healthy self-concept, begins as children learn about themselves and their relationships with others. Self-esteem development begun in childhood continues into adolescence as people begin to redefine relationships in the attempt to further establish personal identity (see Chapter 31). The emergence of positive self-worth is crucial for healthy spirituality.

Many adults experience spiritual growth by entering into lifelong relationships. An ability to care meaningfully for others and the self is evidence of healthy spirituality. Older adults often turn to important relationships and the giving of themselves to others as spiritual tasks.

Relationships with supreme beings, or vertical spirituality, also develop as people grow. Children often begin with a concept of the supreme being as presented to them by their home or religious community. Adolescents often reconsider their childlike concept of the supreme being and, in the search for identity, may question many practices and values. This, too, is an important spiritual task.

As people mature, they often turn inward to enduring values and to a concept of the supreme being that has been sustaining and meaningful. A healthy spirituality in older people is one that gives peace and acceptance of self and that is often based on a lifelong relationship with the supreme being. Illness and loss can threaten and challenge the spiritual developmental process. A nurturing environment is necessary for optimal growth.

Faith, too, is a developmental process. **Faith** is defined by Studzinski (1986) as more than a set of beliefs but "a way of relating to self, others, and God and integrating our past, present, and future with God as center." Hanley (1985) describes the six stages of faith based on 400 interviews with persons of several religions and beliefs. The research identifies that some adults remain in early stages of spiritual development, whereas others develop a strong faith, which involves all life experiences.

The nurse must respond personally and flexibly to each client's state of faith. Some questions that Washkoviak (1989) suggests for an individual's consideration in achieving a degree of spiritual wellness include the following:

1. Do you feel you have lived and are currently living in accordance with your own personally identified value system?
2. Do you feel a sense of contentment with your life?
3. Do you have faith in your fellow human beings?

4. Do you feel loved by others?
5. Do you feel loved by your supreme being, power, or God when involved in a situation over which you can assert no control?
6. Are you able to express your own love for others?
7. Are you able to forgive others?
8. Are you able to accept the forgiveness of others, including your supreme being, power, or God?
9. Have you set realistic, yet challenging, life goals?

The goal of spiritual care is to help healthy or ill clients use faith for greater wellness and healing by living out these spiritual values and beliefs. The answers to Washkoviak's questions may provide some direction for insight and growth in the spiritual dimension.

RELATIONSHIP OF THE SPIRITUAL TO OTHER DIMENSIONS OF HEALTH

The interrelatedness of the physiological, psychological, sociocultural, and spiritual dimensions is demonstrated by the great number of clients with psychosomatic diseases. Unexpressed anger and resentment can cause diseases, and forms of spiritual distress such as guilt, vindictiveness, and lack of forgiveness can lead to illness.

Health care providers use a body-mind-spirit conceptual model of human nature; they are concerned with the moral, ethical, and spiritual dimensions of personality and character development. The nurse's goal in holistic health care is to help the client achieve a balanced, dynamic integration of body, mind, and spirit. Holistic health care includes meeting the client's physiological needs, promoting psychological development, fostering sociocultural relationships, and supporting the fulfillment of spiritual aspirations.

RELIGIOUS ASPECTS OF HEALTH

Everyone has a spiritual dimension. Many persons express their spirituality by participating in religious activities. **Religion** is a set of organized beliefs, rituals, and practices taken on by people to understand and worship a deity.

Religion can make sense of sickness. Using the Biblical book of Job, Sevensky (1981) illustrates how suffering can be seen as educational, purifying, sacrificial, and finally, as mysterious. Although rec-ognizing the potential misuse of religion in fostering guilt and negative attitudes toward sexuality and emotions, Sevensky reviews the resources available to a religious person. Some of these resources include prayer; support from a caring, religious community; and religious rituals such as forgiveness, communion, anointing with oil, and laying on of hands.

Information about religions and sects is available from a number of sources. General information about world religions helps illustrate the rich diversity in basic belief systems. Generalizations provide only a starting point, however, in determining the actual beliefs and practices of any individual. Such information is gathered through a more specific spiritual assessment. Nurses should keep in mind that the spiritual dimension of health care is not limited to the practices, beliefs, and teachings of organized religion. The nurse, however, may meet a client's spiritual needs by understanding and responding to religious concerns.

Beliefs about Health

Hindus believe that praying for health is the lowest form of prayer; thus they tend to dismiss or be unconcerned about bodily ills. The devotees of Buddhism have rich, multireligious influences from Confucianism, Christianity, and Shintoism. Some branches and sects of Buddhism emphasize differing practices. For example, the Theravada branch uses an intellectual approach, the Mahayana branch emphasizes involvement with humanity, and the Zen sect practices austerity. Followers of Hinduism and Buddhism usually accept modern medical science.

In Islam, the believer is considered a unique individual with an eternal soul. Moslems (Muslims) pray 5 times a day, facing Mecca. Older or more conservative Moslems may have a fatalistic view and may resist compliance with medical treatment.

Jewish persons believe in the sanctity of life. This basic principle overrides any conflicting beliefs and promotes acceptance of modern medical science. Observance of Sabbath regulations may conflict with scheduled therapeutic procedures.

Christians generally regard themselves as children of God, redeemed by Christ and destined for eternal life. They seek to discern the will of God in life and suffering, but their beliefs generally do not conflict with modern medical practice (Table 33-1 on p. 1004).

Health Crises

Hindus may view illness as the result of misuse of the body or as a consequence of sins committed in a

TABLE 33-1 Religious Beliefs about Health		
Religious	Health Care Beliefs	Response to Health Crises
Hinduism	Accepts modern medical science	Views illness as result of misuse of body
		Considers therapy as transitory benefit
Buddhism	Accepts modern medical science	May ask for Buddhist priest for counseling
		Asks family to be available for physical and emotional care
Islam	Is older and more conservative, has fatalistic view and may resist compliance with medical science	Uses faith healing and group prayer
		Submits to will of God
Judaism	Believes strongly in sanctity of life	Is obligated to seek medical care
	Has Sabbath regulations that may interfere with therapeutic procedures	Is supported by family and friends
Christianity	Seeks will of God in suffering but accepts modern medical science	Uses prayer, faith healing, laying on of hands, and sacraments

previous life. However, they generally do not oppose medical treatment but consider its benefits transitory. Buddhists may ask to have a Buddhist priest for counseling during illness. A family member usually remains with the sick person to care for physical and emotional needs.

Moslems use faith healing to provide psychological support rather than to treat the pathological condition. Family members are a great comfort to a Moslem, and Moslems consider group prayer strengthening. There is usually no priest. The person submits to Allah's will in health and in illness.

In Judaism, the belief in the sanctity of life obligates the sick to seek medical care. Various laws apply to the donation or transplantation of organs. Visiting the sick is considered a religious obligation for Jews.

Christians may want to receive communion from their minister or priest during illness; Roman Catholics may wish to receive several sacraments: reconciliation, the Eucharist, and Anointing of the Sick. Jehovah's Witnesses are generally opposed to blood transfusions. Christian Scientists do not usually seek health care, relying instead on God's power for healing. Some religious sects believe in faith healing and some in laying on of hands (Table 33-1).

Birth

No special birth ritual is required by Hinduism. Buddhist rites such as infant presentation, affirmation, confirmation, or ordination are performed in late childhood. According to Islamic doctrine, if abortion occurs after 130 days gestation, the fetus is treated as a fully developed human being. Ritual circumcision is required by Orthodox and Conservative Jews on

the eighth day after birth. Reform Jews favor ritual circumcision but do not consider it a religious imperative. Among Jewish people a fetus is buried, not discarded.

Various forms of baptism are practiced by Christians. Most Protestant denominations and Roman Catholics require infant baptism. Roman Catholics baptize aborted fetuses and stillborn infants. Baptists, Seventh-Day Adventists, Baha'i followers, and Mennonites do not practice infant baptism. The form of baptism differs from sect to sect. For example, sprinkling is sufficient for the Orthodox Presbyterians and Methodists, whereas the Pentecostals, Mormons, Baptists, and Church of Christ members require immersion (Table 33-2).

Death

To Hindus, death and rebirth are nearly synonymous. After death, certain rites are prescribed. The priest may tie a thread around the neck or wrist to indicate a blessing; he may pour water into the mouth. The family washes the body before it is cremated. The family of a Buddhist may wish to call a priest at the time of death; last rite chanting is often practiced at the bedside.

Before death the Islamic client confesses sins and asks for forgiveness of the family. After death the family washes the body, then turns the body toward Mecca. As with Hindus, only relatives and friends touch the body. No autopsy is performed unless required by law.

All Orthodox Jews and some Conservative Jews also oppose autopsy and cremation. Human remains sometimes must be cleansed by members of a ritual burial society, and burial is always carried out as

TABLE 33-2 Religious Practices Related to Life Events		
Religion	Birth	Death
Hinduism	No special ritual	Priest ties thread around neck or wrist and pours water into mouth. Only family touches and washes body before cremation.
Buddhism	Infant presentation, affirmation, confirmation, ordination	Buddhist priest is present. Last rite is chanted.
Islam	In case of abortion after 130 days gestation, fetus treated as fully developed human being	Before death, client confesses sins and asks forgiveness of family. Only family touches and washes body.
Judaism	Ritual circumcision Fetal burial	Jews oppose autopsy and cremation. Ritual cleansing of body is done by members of ritual burial society.
Christianity	Infant baptism required by Episcopalians and Roman Catholics Baptism of aborted fetus and stillborn infants by Roman Catholics	Last rites are optional for some Protestants and are mandatory for Eastern Orthodox Christians and Roman Catholics.

soon as possible. Because customs vary, the nurse should always consult the deceased's family to determine their preference.

Among Christians, no rituals are required before or after death by Christian Scientists, Church of Christ members, and Jehovah's Witnesses. Last rites are optional for Episcopalians and Lutherans but are mandatory for Eastern Orthodox Christians and Roman Catholics. Additional restrictions may be applicable to cremation, autopsy, and burial of amputated parts or burial in consecrated ground (Table 33-2).

Diet

Hindus have many dietary restrictions. Some sects are vegetarian, believing that meat and intoxicants are too stimulating to the senses. Some Buddhists also are vegetarians. Most members of the Buddhist religion practice moderation and do not use alcohol, tobacco, and drugs.

Eating pork is prohibited by Islam, and Ramadan, the ninth month of the Muhammadan or Muslim year (around June and July), is a period of daylight fasting. Many Orthodox, Conservative, and some Reform Jews strictly observe kosher dietary laws, which prohibit eating pork and shellfish and eating any meat with milk or milk products. Jews also have regulations about food preparation.

Many Christian traditions have no special dietary restrictions. Some groups, such as Seventh-Day Adventists, Baptists, and Mormons, prohibit the use of

TABLE 33-3 Religious Dietary Regulations Affecting Health Care	
Religion	Dietary Practices
Hinduism	Some sects are vegetarians, prohibiting meat and intoxicants.
Buddhism	Some are vegetarians; most do not use alcohol, tobacco, or drugs.
Islam	Eating pork is prohibited. Ramadan is period of daylight fasting with nighttime feasting.
Judaism	Some observe kosher dietary laws (prohibit eating pork, shellfish, and meat with milk or milk products; regulate food preparation).
Christianity	Some groups (Seventh-Day Adventists, Baptists, and Mormons) prohibit use of alcohol, coffee, tea, and tobacco. Roman Catholics fast and abstain from meat on Ash Wednesday and Food Friday. They fast for 1 hour before Communion.

alcohol, coffee, and tea; certain groups include tobacco with these prohibitions. Roman Catholics fast and abstain from meat on Ash Wednesday and Good Friday; some older Catholics continue to adhere to Friday abstinence. Armenian Catholics fast during Lent, and several branches of Christianity fast 1 to 6 hours before communion (Table 33-3).

SPIRITUAL HEALTH AND THE NURSING PROCESS

Assessment

Fish and Shelly (1978) define spiritual health as meaning and purpose in life and love and relatedness with other human beings. Brallier (1978) enumerates the progressive or cumulative characteristics of holistic health, including realization of human potential, affirmation of the uniqueness and unlimited potential of each person, and achievement of a balanced, dynamic integration of body, mind, and spirit.

Stoll (1979) suggests that, when making a spiritual assessment, the nurse include specific questions in the nursing history about the client's concept of a supreme being, the client's source of strength and hope, the significance of religious practices and rituals, and perceived relationships between spiritual beliefs and health. According to Lafferty (1979), positive spiritual health choices for clients seeking to improve quality of life include meditating and praying, engaging in value-oriented spiritual or religious discussions, reading a spiritual book or attending a religious or spiritual meeting, and developing a highly valued personal characteristic or eliminating a weak personal trait. These needs should be a part of the spiritual assessment.

Spiritual needs may be intensified in certain situations, such as birth, death, or a major health crisis; times of anxiety, apprehension, or fear; newly diagnosed serious or chronic disease; isolation; and psychiatric episodes. Spiritual assessment should be an extension of the psychosocial assessment and should be pursued to the extent that the nurse intends to use the information for planning client and family care.

Determining who or what sustains the client helps the nurse plan spiritual care. The answers to the following questions about spiritual health will influence nursing care:

1. Who is the client's supreme being? Governing principle? Money? Power? Another human being?
2. What is the client's relationship with a supreme being? One of fear or of love?
3. How does the client express this spiritual relationship? Are spiritual and religious practices part of this expression?
4. How does the client view the self? Positively or negatively? Worthy of the supreme being's love?
5. Does the client act authentically and relate openly?
6. Does the client assume responsibility for behavior and its consequences?
7. How effectively does the client relate to family and friends?
8. How effectively does the client relate to health care personnel? To other clients? To strangers?
9. Does the client see illness as a supreme being's punishment? Or as an indication of love?
10. Does the client view illness as threatening?
11. How have the client's diagnosis and therapy affected self-concept? Emotional state? Will to live? Cooperation with rehabilitation?

Spiritually healthy persons generally believe in a supreme being and view their ultimate welfare and peace in terms of their relationship to this being and the world at large. They are generally aware of their limitations as human beings but strive to act in accordance with their beliefs. They assume responsibilities with joy and cheerfulness.

As the nurse observes and analyzes the behaviors that demonstrate the client's level of spiritual health, it becomes obvious that the client's attitudes toward a supreme being, the self, and others demonstrate the value that the client places on spiritual health. Reactions to adversity, setbacks, delays in plans, aging, sickness, and suffering give clues to the client's spiritual values. As the nurse assesses the client's state of spiritual health, signs of unmet spiritual needs may emerge.

The client may express anger at the supreme being, a member of the spiritual care team, or the nurse. The client may question the meaning of life and suffering. Verbalizations about internal conflicts of beliefs and required treatment may indicate a spiritual need. For example, if a client believes that disease is a punishment for sinfulness, cooperation with therapy will aggravate guilt and prevent the restitution sought through suffering. If clients believe that eternal life follows temporal life, they may repudiate any attempt at treatment and rehabilitation.

Observation of the client's affect and attitude, behaviors, verbalizations, interpersonal relationships, and environment might give clues to spiritual needs. Young and Dowling (1987) indicate that among older adults, meaningful social networks support spiritual well-being. Their findings suggest that general engagement in social life increases participation in organized religious activity and in private devotions (see research highlight).

Spiritual assessment continues throughout all interactions with the client. The nurse determines whether the client's actions reflect professed views on the worth of human life and whether the client's spiritual values are reflected in interaction with visitors. The nurse notes the number of get-well cards that reflect appreciation of prayer and contain inspirational verse. The nurse also observes for open questioning about the reason for existence or suffering. In addition, the nurse determines whether the client seeks spiritual assistance or admits an inability to continue usual religious practices. Requests for prayers may indicate a spiritual value or need. The client may ask the nurse about the moral implications of certain procedures in relation to beliefs about human life.

The conceptual model of human nature in physiological, psychosocial, and spiritual dimensions offers an additional approach to assessing spiritual needs. From this model the following questions can be derived:

1. To what extent have the client's physical disability and the therapeutic regimen altered the ability to maintain relationships with the supreme being and others?

2. Are there moral or ethical implications of the diagnosis and treatment that conflict with the client's religious or spiritual values?
3. Do the etiology, diagnosis, and treatment of the disease conflict with the client's belief system?

Nursing Diagnosis

If the client's behavior is inconsistent with professed beliefs and values, a nursing diagnosis of *spiritual distress* may be indicated. NANDA has defined **spiritual distress** and suggested etiologies and defining characteristics (see diagnoses box). The client's

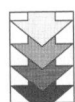

Spiritual Distress (Distress of the Human Spirit)

DEFINITION

- Disruption in the life principle that pervades a person's entire being and that integrates and transcends one's biological and psychosocial nature

RELATED FACTORS

- Separation from religious and cultural ties
- Challenged belief and value system (e.g., result of moral or ethical implications of therapy or result of intense suffering)

DEFINING CHARACTERISTICS

- Expresses concern with meaning of life and death and/or belief systems
- Anger toward God (as defined by the person)
- Questions meaning of suffering
- Verbalizes inner conflict about beliefs
- Verbalizes concern about relationship with deity
- Questions meaning of own existence
- Is unable to choose or chooses not to participate in usual religious practices
- Seeks spiritual assistance
- Questions moral and ethical implications of therapeutic regimen
- Displaces anger toward religious representatives
- Describes nightmares or sleep disturbances
- Display alteration in behavior or mood evidenced by anger, crying, withdrawal, preoccupation, anxiety, hostility, or apathy
- Regards illness as punishment
- Does not experience that God is forgiving
- Is unable to accept self
- Engages in self-blame
- Denies responsibilities for problems
- Describes somatic complaints

Research Highlight

The importance of social support in maintaining good health in older adulthood has been established. Young and Dowling, from the results of their research on 123 members of the American Association of Retired Persons (AARP) in El Paso, Texas, suggest that social networks also support spiritual well-being.

The purpose of Young and Dowling's study was to determine the factors in the lives of AARP members that account for differences in religious participation. The participants' average age was 71; 78% were women, and 98% were European Americans. The researchers had developed hypotheses about the influence of nine independent variables on two dependent variables (organized religious activity and private religious activity). The independent variables were general activities, interaction, living arrangements, religious preference, religious belief, spiritual experiences, health, income, and age.

Data analysis for participation in organized religious activity show that general involvement in social life, strength of religious convictions increased participation and that increasing age decreased participation in organized religious activities. All other variables were insignificant in influencing participation in organized religious activity. Being older and having poor health, strong religious convictions, and more interaction with family and friends were positively correlated with the level of nonorganized religious participation or private devotions.

Young G, Dowling W: Dimensions of religiosity in old age: accounting for variations in types of participation, *J Gerontol* 42(4):376, 1987.

From Kim MJ, McFarland GK, McLane AM: *Pocket guide to nursing diagnoses,* ed 4, St Louis, 1991, Mosby–Year Book.

answers to questions in the nursing history and the nurse's observations of the client's behaviors and interrelationships give clues to spiritual needs. However, clues must be validated and clarified before the nurse plans interventions. With spiritual care, the importance of the nurse's own spiritual aspirations, inspiration, and perception cannot be overemphasized. The nurse should attempt to provide for client's spiritual needs without substituting personal religious or spiritual values for those of the clients.

To be attuned to spiritual aspects of care, a nurse should be aware of a personal spiritual dimension and be comfortable discussing spiritual matters. In addition, the nurse's perception of clues to the client's spiritual needs requires sensitivity, active listening, and response to comments. Less than a third of clients' spiritual problems were recognized by a majority of oncology nurses, according to Highfield and Cason (1983).

The nurse seeks validation from the client about a diagnosis of *spiritual distress*. If the client concurs with the diagnosis, the nurse and the client plan interventions together. If there are doubts about the client's ability to recognize spiritual needs, consultation with the family may provide clarification. If the client and family deny the existence of a spiritual need, the nurse should accept their decision without question. The nurse may need to find out whether the client's minister, priest, or other spiritual adviser or a member of the pastoral care team has already recognized and ministered to the client's spiritual needs. Ideally, the health care team works together to identify and meet all the needs of a client, including spiritual needs (see diagnostic process box).

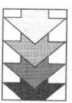

Sample Nursing Diagnostic Process for Spiritual Distress

Assessment Activities	Defining Characteristics	Nursing Diagnosis
Explore client's verbalization of relationship between health state and spiritual concerns. Observe for excessive sadness, expressions of guilt or hopelessness, callousness, or anger.	Verbalizing belief in unforgiving deity Viewing illness as punishment or vindication Confessing past faults	*Spiritual distress* related to need for forgiveness

Planning

If the client agrees with the diagnosis, the nurse and client plan steps to meet the spiritual need. The nurse uses the resources of the entire health care team to meet the client's needs.

Dickenson (1975) suggests that ministry and spiritual care are inherent in nursing. She identifies the following factors in the nurse-client relationship that demonstrate the nurse's commitment to the client's spiritual health: support, self-awareness and other-awareness, understanding, openness, and nonjudgmental acceptance. Several circumstances, however, may cause the nurse to be uncomfortable in providing spiritual care. One barrier may be the past role of spirituality or organized religion in the nurse's life.

An authoritarian upbringing may cause the nurse to rebel against the religious practices of childhood. The nurse may believe that religion or the spiritual dimension is a private matter for the client, although only 10% of critical-care nurses surveyed in Yancey's

 Research Highlight

Yancey assessed nurses' attitudes and practices on spiritual care. The sample population of 230 registered nurses, members of the American Association of Critical-Care Nurses, responded to a previously validated, two-part, mailed questionnaire, the Health Professional's Spiritual Role Scale. The first part of the scale measured attitudes toward spiritual care, and the second portion assessed frequency of performed spiritual practices.

A statistically significant relationship was found between attitudes and practices. Nurses who had higher scores on the attitude scale demonstrated more frequent performance of spiritual care practices. Among the variables—years of experience, level of educational preparation, and exposure to nursing theory—only the last showed a statistically significant correlation with attitude and practice.

About 90% affirmed that spiritual care is a responsibility of the health care professional. About 87% agreed that health care professionals are uncomfortable discussing spiritual matters with clients. Only 10% indicated that spiritual concerns are too personal to discuss, and 25% strongly disagreed and 46% disagreed to a lesser extent that health care professionals are too busy to give spiritual care. About 90% rejected the statement that spiritual well-being is not as important as physical well-being.

Yancey V: *Spiritual care: attitudes and practices of intensive care unit nurses,* unpublished master's thesis, St Louis, 1987, St Louis University.

study (1987) indicated that spiritual concerns were too personal to discuss (see research highlight). Some nurses may consider spiritual care only if and when time permits. The majority of the respondents in Yancey's study, however, disagreed that health care professionals are too busy to give spiritual care.

Some nurses feel unprepared to address the spiritual aspect of care with clients or have the misconception that spiritual needs should be left to the pastoral care department. Spirituality is interrelated with other dimensions of being human, and nurses should consider it when planning care (see care plan). By recognizing the important role of pastoral care in meeting spiritual needs, nurses, too, contribute in a vital way to the achievement of clients' spiritual health. In the spiritual dimension, as in other dimensions, the nurse assists clients toward states of well-being and fulfillment.

Implementation

When the nurse identifies the client's spiritual needs and arrives at a diagnosis of *spiritual distress,* plans should be made to meet this need. Resources included in the plan are nursing interventions, family involvement, and counseling by the clergy. Other possible sources for spiritual care are members of the pastoral care team and nurses' support groups.

Nursing Interventions

After defining clients' spiritual beliefs, the nurse supports and enhances these belief systems or finds someone able to do so. The nurse should not impose religious or spiritual beliefs on clients or their families and should never attempt to convert a client. The nurse's sincerity, patience, and awareness of the cli-

ent's spiritual distress encourage discussion about spiritual values. The nurse's own spirituality is a form of support in assisting the client to clarify beliefs about a supreme being, the spiritual dimension of life, and the meaning of suffering and pain. Soeken and Carson (1986) demonstrated that baccalaureate and graduate nursing students who scored higher on a Spiritual Well-Being Scale expressed more positive attitudes toward providing spiritual care.

A client's view of the self is another area for intervention. If the nurse consistently treats the client as a unique individual with significant value and unlimited potential, the client's self-concept will be enhanced. The nurse should consider the client's wishes when scheduling activities and should provide privacy and personal time. Reed (1987) learned that terminally ill hospitalized cancer clients, compared with the other two groups in the study, perceived in themselves more spirituality and noted an increasing spiritual perspective.

An individual at any point on the health-illness continuum has a need to be alone. The nurse may help a hospitalized client gain solitude through self-examination and redirection, a new perspective of a relationship with a belief system, a supreme being, and a more positive self-concept.

If clients ask the nurse to pray for them or with them, it is appropriate to do so. If nurses are not comfortable in this situation, they should be honest with clients and offer to locate other sources of support. Prayer can be offered aloud or in silence according to clients' wishes. In different religions, prayer has various purposes, including praise, petition, thanksgiving, and reparation for sin. Clients may want to praise the supreme being and offer thanks for blessings or to request health or freedom from pain. Cli-

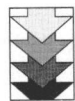

Sample Nursing Care Plan for Spiritual Distress

Nursing Diagnosis: *Spiritual distress* related to need for forgiveness
Definition: Spiritual distress is a disruption in the life principle that prevades a person's entire being and that integrates and transcends one's biological and psychosocial nature (Kim, McFarland, McLane, 1991).

Goals	Expected Outcomes	Interventions	Rationale
Client will experience sense of being forgiven or ability to forgive another.	Client will demonstrate acceptance of self and others. Client will express feeling of being reconciled wth supreme being.	Encourage client to verbalize feelings through use of responsive listening. Reinforce client's positive qualities. Facilitate client request for help from other spiritual resource.	Intrinsic and general forgiveness are restorative or health promoting. General and intrinsic forgivers are less blaming, angry, and self-defeating and feel that personal power is restored (Carson, 1989).

Client Teaching for Spiritual Distress

OBJECTIVE

- Client will recognize the need for reconciliation and willingly seek forgiveness from self and others.

TEACHING STRATEGIES

- Establish trusting interpersonal relationship to facilitate meaningful discussions with family.
- Involve appropriate spiritual care persons and resources.
- Use client's preferred meditational or devotional activities.

EVALUATION

- Observe client for increased sense of self-acceptance and serenity.

Research Highlight

To assess the therapeutic effect of intercessory prayer (IP), Byrd entered 393 clients into two groups, a prayer group and a control group. The client, staff, and physicians, as well as the investigator, did not know who was in each group throughout the study. Intercessors (persons offering prayers) were assigned to each client. IP was made outside the hospital and until the client was discharged; each intercessor was given the client's first name and asked to pray daily for a rapid recovery and for prevention of complications and death. No attempt was made to limit prayer among the control group.

Results showed that the prayer group experienced fewer incidences of congestive heart failure, required less diuretic and antibiotic therapy, suffered fewer episodes of pneumonia and cardiac arrest, and experienced intubation and ventilation less frequently. The IP group had an overall better outcome.

Byrd RC: Positive therapeutic effects of intercessory prayer in a coronary care unit population, *South Med J* 81(7):826, 1988.

ents should be allowed time to express these needs (see teaching box).

Involvement of Family and Friends

Relationships with others help sustain a person's belief system. The nurse should urge family and friends to visit the client and demonstrate their love and concern. In some cases, working with or through family or friends to provide spiritual care is the most effective way to meet this need. Members of parish or church groups may visit, or they can be encouraged to send cards and assurance of prayers for recovery. Positive therapeutic effects of intercessory prayer was reported by Byrd (1988), who studied its influence on clients in a coronary care unit (see research highlight).

Including family members in a prayer service is a thoughtful gesture if this is appropriate to the client's religion and family members are comfortable participating. Reading favorite religious passages or prayerbooks may be requested by the client and family. Encouraging clients to keep meaningful religious symbols nearby can be a source of consolation and spiritual support. Because a visit to the hospital chapel or attendance at services can be important to the hospitalized client and family, directions to the chapel should be included when orienting the client and family to the medical facility. Arrangements may need to be made with the pastoral care department for the client and family to receive the sacraments, especially Communion.

Role of the Clergy

Some hospitalized clients find a visit from a spiritual adviser consoling. If the spiritual adviser has known the client and family before the current health problem, the support offered can provide continuity. The spiritual adviser understands the religious belief system of the client and can focus on the potential spiritual growth resulting from illness and suffering. The spiritual adviser may pray with the client and family and perform religious rituals or administer sacraments.

The nurse should ask clients if they would like to have their spiritual adviser notified of their hospitalization. All spiritual advisers should be made welcome in nursing units. When requested by clients or families, the nurse should keep spiritual advisers informed of physiological, psychosocial, and spiritual concerns. This helps in providing holistic health care. The nurse shows respect for clients' spiritual values and needs by willingly cooperating with others giving spiritual care and by facilitating the administration of sacraments, rites, and rituals.

Providing privacy for the client and spiritual adviser is a thoughtful and sensitive gesture. If the nurse is unsure about the proper routine in a client's religion, asking the spiritual adviser, family, or client is appropriate. The nurse can adapt spiritual care to the client's religious tenets without sacrificing personal beliefs.

Other Resources

Other resources can assist in easing clients' spiritual health. Especially helpful are members of a hospital's pastoral care department, who can visit the client, administer sacraments or rites, and provide religious objects when requested. Taped meditations and televised religious services may also be available through the pastoral care department.

Pastoral care associates may serve also as counselors and consultants for nursing personnel. Discussion groups can help nurses recognize their own spiritual needs so that they can respect the client's right to do the same. Such groups can also focus on the responsible and appropriate application of the nursing process to spiritual needs.

 ## Evaluation

Attainment of spiritual health can be considered a lifelong goal. However, to evaluate the effectiveness of nursing interventions in this dimension of health, the nurse may compare the client's level of spiritual health with the behaviors and needs noted in the original assessment (see evaluation box). The following questions may help:

1. Is the client's belief system stronger?
2. Do the client's professed beliefs support and direct actions and words?
3. Does the client gain peace and strength from spiritual resources (such as prayer and visits from the spiritual adviser) to face the rigors of treatment, rehabilitation, or impending death?
4. Does the client seem more in control and have a clearer self-concept?
5. Is the client at ease in being alone? In having life's plans changed?
6. Is the client's behavior appropriate to the occasion?
7. Has reconciliation of any differences taken place between the client and others?
8. Are mutual respect and love obvious in the client's relationships with others?

It helps to consider the client's appearance and feelings when spiritual needs are met. The client should be experiencing emotions appropriate to the situation; developing a strong, realistic self-image; and experiencing warm, open interpersonal relationships. The client should also be maintaining a sense of mission in life and confidence and trust in a supreme being. A client whose spiritual needs are met

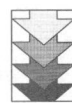 ### Sample Evaluation of Interventions for Spiritual Distress

Goal	Evaluative measures	Expected outcomes
Client will experience sense of being forgiven or ability to forgive another.	Explore client's verbalization of perception of self and family members. Ask client about recent changes in religious practices.	Client will demonstrate acceptance of self and others. Client will express feelings of being reconciled with supreme being.

may be peaceful, even while experiencing a severe illness.

If the client is comfortable in expressing spiritual needs to the nurse or in sharing beliefs and religious resources, the nurse can assume that the climate allows verbalization of these needs. The nurse considers whether the nursing care plan schedules time for quiet, prayer, a visit to the chapel, and attendance at services. Provision for spiritual health should be considered as important as plans for medical and nursing care of a physiological or psychological illness.

Thus evaluation of the attainment of spiritual health should include observation of the client's life situations and the nursing environment.

 ## SUMMARY

Nursing care that neglects the spiritual dimension cannot be holistic. To provide spiritual care, the nurse must understand spiritual health and be able to recognize the spiritually healthy person. As with other dimensions of care, the client's norm is identified first for comparison during assessment. If spiritual needs are identified in the assessment, plans are made to intervene appropriately. Nursing interventions are individualized according to the client's specific needs. The family's involvement and the ministrations of spiritual advisers are sought when indicated. Resources for facilitating a client's spiritual care and for providing support for nurses are used as necessary. The rewards of meeting spiritual needs include personal and professional fulfillment and enrichment.

Key Concepts

- A spiritually healthy person feels secure in a relationship with a supreme being or a system of beliefs and a presence with or in each person and in the world.
- To provide spiritual care in nursing, the nurse must understand spiritual health and be able to recognize the spiritually distressed person.
- Nurses should be aware of the client's general spiritual needs and facilitate the client's chosen practices.
- The spiritual dimension of care is not limited to the practices and dogma of organized religions.
- When making a spiritual assessment, the nurse includes questions about the client's concept of a supreme being, source of strength and hope, significance of religious practices and rituals, and perceived relationships between spiritual beliefs and health.
- The client's contradictory actions or attitudes may indicate spiritual distress.
- To be attuned to spiritual aspects of care, nurses should be aware of their own spiritual dimension and be comfortable in discussing spiritual matters.
- The nurse should use available resources such as family members, spiritual advisers, and other members of the health care team to help the client maintain or regain a state of spiritual health.

Key Terms

Faith, p. 1002
Religion, p. 1003

Spiritual distress, p. 1007
Spirituality, p. 1002

Critical Thinking Exercises

1. A nurse may help meet a client's spiritual needs by understanding and responding to religious concerns. List three religious practices a client may want to continue during hospitalization.

2. Mrs. Green has just been given the diagnosis of adult-onset diabetes mellitus. She is terribly upset about the long-term management of her condition. In assessing Mrs. Green's spiritual needs, what specific questions would you ask?

3. Certain life situations intensify spiritual distress. Describe four such situations. Select one of these situations and identify three interventions you could use to meet the client's spiritual needs.

4. You have an opportunity to visit with Mrs. Green (refer to 2) in the clinic 6 weeks after her hospitalization. How would you determine whether her spiritual needs were being met?

5. An older gentleman you are caring for tells you that he is afraid he will die and does not want to leave his devoted family members. How would you help this client through this crisis?

REFERENCES

Brallier LW: The nurse as holistic health practitioner, *Nurs Clin North Am* 13(4):643, 1978.

Byrd RC: Positive therapeutic effects of intercessory prayer in a coronary care unit population, *South Med J* 81(7):826, 1988.

Carson VB: *spiritual dimensions of nursing practice*, Philadelphia, 1989, Saunders.

Cox BJ, Waller L: *Communicating with the elderly*, St Louis, 1987, Catholic Health Association.

Dickenson SC: The search for spiritual meaning, *Am J Nurs* 75(10):1789, 1975.

Fish S, Shelly JA: *Spiritual care: the nurse's role*, Downers Grove, Ill, 1978, InterVarsity.

Hanley K: Fostering development in faith, *Hum Devel* 6(2):21, 1985.

Highfield MF, Cason C: Spiritual needs of patients: are they recognized? *Can Nurs* 6(3):187, 1983.

Kim MJ, McFarland GK, McLane AM: *Pocket guide to nursing diagnoses*, ed 4, St Louis, 1991, Mosby–Year Book.

Lafferty JA: Credo for wellness, *Health Educ* 10(5):10, 1979.

Reed PG: Spirituality and well-being in terminally ill hospitalized adults, *Res Nurs Health* 10:33, 1987.

Sevensky RL: Religion and illness: an outline of their relationship, *South Med J* 74(6):745, 1981.

Soeken KL, Carson VJ: Study measures nurses' attitudes about providing spiritual care, *Health Prog* 67(3):52, 1986.

Stoll R: Guidelines for spiritual assessment, *Am J Nurs* 79(9):1574, 1979.

Studzinski R: Adult faith is reward for long life, *Envoy* 15(2):4, 1986.

Washkoviak LF: Psychological, spiritual and social wellness. In Swinford PA, Webster JA, editors: *Promoting wellness: a nurse's handbook*, Rockville, Md, 1989, Aspen.

Yancey V: *Spiritual care: attitudes and practices of intensive care unit nurses*, unpublished master's thesis, St Louis, 1987, St Louis University.

Young G, Dowling W: Dimensions of religiosity in old age: accounting for variation in types of participation, *J Gerontol* 42(4):376, 1987.

ADDITIONAL READINGS

Burnard P: Spiritual distress and the nursing response: theoretical consideration and counselling skills, *J Adv Nurs* 12:377, 1987.

Buys SAM: Discussion series sensitizes nurses to patient's spiritual needs, *Hosp Prog* 62(10):44, 1981.

Ellis C: Course prepares nurses to meet patients' spiritual needs, *Health Prog* 67(3):76, 1986.

Hoyman HS: Models of human nature and their impact on health education, *Nurs Digest* 3(5):37, 1975.

Kasanof D, Levy J, Striffler RC: When religious belief affects therapy, *Patient Care* 8(19):99, 1974.

Kennison MM: Faith: an untapped health resource, *J Psychosoc Nurs Ment Health Serv* 25(10):28-30, 1987.

Kraft WF: Spiritual growth in adolescence and adulthood, *Hum Devel* 4(4):14, 1983.

Miller JF: Assessment of loneliness and spiritual well-being in chronically ill and healthy adults, *J Prof Nurs* 1(1):79, 1985.

Miller JF: Inspiring hope, *Am J Nurs* 85(1):22, 1985.

Nagai-Jacobson M, Burkhardt M: Spirituality: cornerstone of holistic health practice, *Holistic Nurs Pract* 3(3):18, 1989.

Newman M: *Theory development in nursing*, Philadelphia, 1979, Davis.

Peterson EA: The physical, the spiritual: can you meet all of your patient's needs? *J Gerontol Nurs* 11(10):23, 1985.

Piles CL: Providing spiritual care, *Nurs Educ* 15(1):36, 1990.

Pumphrey JB: Recognizing your patient's spiritual needs, *Nurs 77* 7(12):64, 1977.

Ruffing-Rahal MA: The spiritual dimension of well-being implications for the elderly, *Home Healthc Nurse* 2(2):12, 1984.

Shelly JA: *Spiritual care workbook: a companion to spiritual care: the nurse's role*, Downers Grove, Ill, 1978, InterVarsity.

Soeken KL, Carson VJ: Responding to the spiritual needs of the chronically ill, *Nurs Clin North Am* 22(3):601, 1987.

Stallwood J, Stoll R: Spiritual dimensions of nursing practice. In Beland I, Passos J, editors: *Clinical nursing: pathophysiological and psychosocial approaches*, ed 3, New York, 1975, Macmillan.

Stokes K: *Faith as a verb*, Mystic, Conn, 1989, Twenty-Third Publications.

Stuart E, Decro J, Mandle, C: Spirituality in health and healing: a clinical program, *Holistic Nurs Prac* 3(3):35, 1989.

Wheelock RD: Unmet patient needs, *Hosp Progr* 55(7):60, 1974.

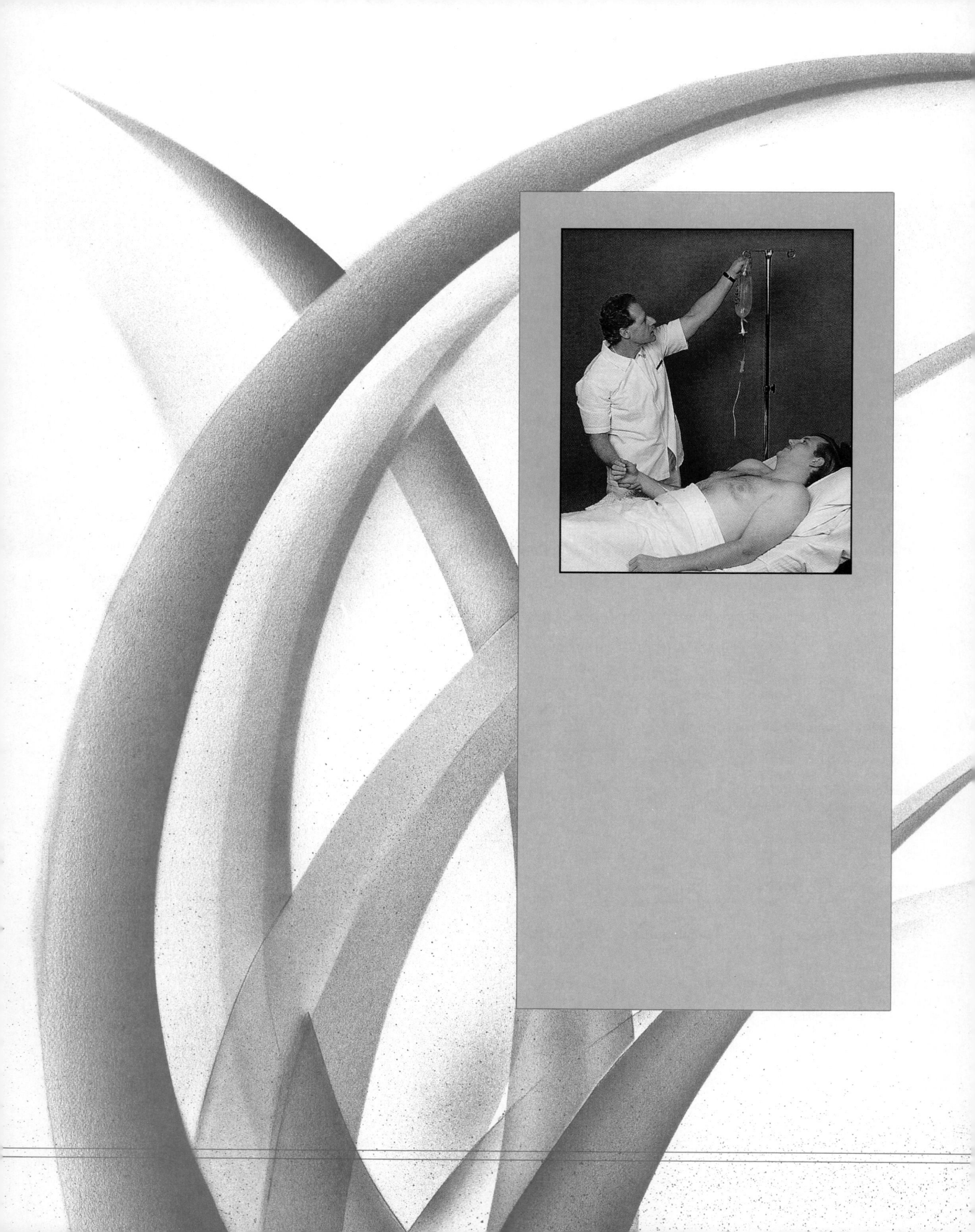

UNIT 7

Basic Physiological Needs

CHAPTER 34

Hygiene

OBJECTIVES

Mastery of content in this chapter will enable the student to:

- Define the key terms listed.
- Identify common skin problems and related interventions.
- Describe factors that influence personal hygienic practices.
- Discuss conditions that may put a client at risk for impaired skin integrity.
- Describe the types of bathing techniques used for various physical conditions.
- Develop a care plan based on client preferences and hygienic practices.
- Perform a complete bed bath and backrub.
- Discuss factors that influence the condition of the nails and feet.
- Explain the importance of foot care for the diabetic client.
- Describe the methods used for cleaning and cutting the nails.
- Discuss conditions that may put a client at risk for impaired oral mucous membranes.
- Discuss measures used to provide special oral hygiene.
- Assist with or provide oral hygiene.
- List common hair and scalp problems and their related interventions.
- Offer hygiene to meet the needs of clients requiring eye, ear, and nose care.
- Successfully make an occupied, unoccupied, and surgical hospital bed.

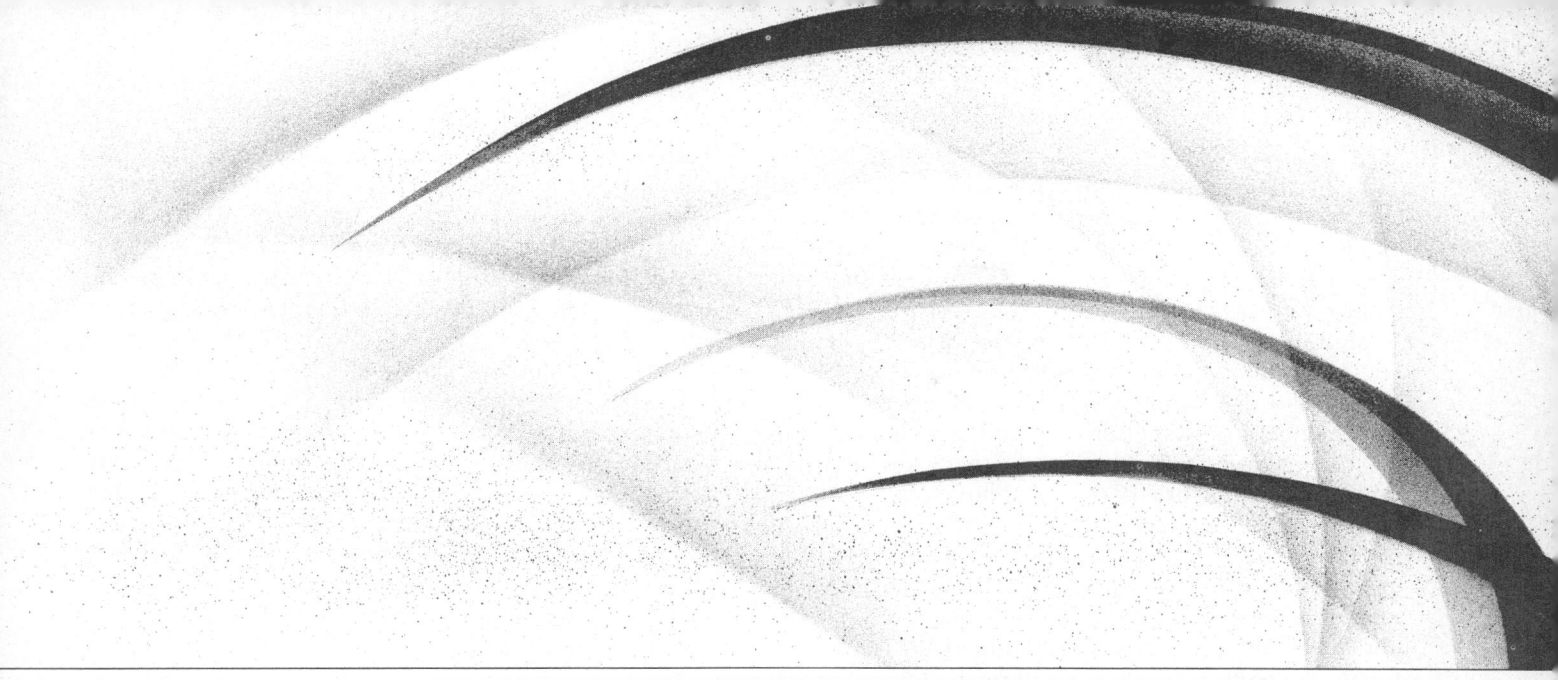

CHAPTER OUTLINE

Factors Influencing Hygienic Practice

    Body image
    Social practices
    Socioeconomic status
    Knowledge
    Cultural variables
    Personal preferences
    Physical condition

Types of Hygienic Care

Care of the Skin

    Assessment
    Nursing diagnosis
    Planning
    Implementation
    Evaluation

Care of the Feet and Nails

    Assessment
    Nursing diagnosis
    Planning
    Implementation
    Evaluation

Oral Hygiene

    Assessment

    Nursing diagnosis
    Planning
    Implementation
    Evaluation

Hair Care

    Assessment
    Nursing diagnosis
    Planning
    Implementation
    Evaluation

Care of the Eyes, Ears, and Nose

    Eyes
    Ears
    Nose
    Assessment
    Nursing diagnosis
    Planning
    Implementation
    Evaluation

Client's Room Environment

    Maintaining comfort
    Room equipment

Nurses work with a wide variety of clients who require assistance with personal hygiene or must learn proper hygienic techniques. **Hygiene** is the science of health. The self-care measures people use to maintain their health are personal hygiene.

Maintenance of personal hygiene is necessary for an individual's comfort, safety, and well-being. Whereas well people are capable of meeting their own hygienic needs, ill or physically challenged people may require the nurse's assistance to carry out routine hygienic practices. In addition, a variety of personal and sociocultural factors influences the client's hygienic practice. The nurse determines a client's ability to perform self-care and provides hygienic care according to the client's needs and preferences. While providing routine hygienic care, the nurse assesses the client's physical and emotional state. For example, complete assessment of the integument can be done during the client's bath.

Because hygienic care often requires close contact with the client, the nurse can use communication skills to promote the therapeutic relationship and to learn about the client's emotional needs (see Chapter 15). During hygienic care the nurse can also teach health promotion practices to the client. The nurse must also consider clients' specific physical limitations, beliefs, values, and habits. Unless the client's hygienic preferences significantly affect the client's health condition, they can usually be incorporated into the care plan. The nurse needs to preserve as much of the client's independence as possible, ensure privacy, and foster the client's physical well-being.

FACTORS INFLUENCING HYGIENIC PRACTICE

The manner in which a person performs personal hygiene can be influenced by a number of factors. Generally, people do not perform hygienic care in the same way, and the nurse can provide individualized care only after knowing the client's unique hygienic practices.

Body Image

The general appearance of clients may reflect the importance hygiene holds for them. Body images are people's subjective concept of their physical appearance. These images can change frequently. Body image affects the way in which hygiene is maintained. If clients are neatly groomed, the nurse considers details of grooming when planning care and consults

them before making decisions about how hygienic care is to be provided. Clients who appear unkempt or uninterested in hygiene may require education about the importance of hygiene. The nurse must not convey feelings of disapproval or revulsion when caring for clients whose hygienic practices are different from the nurse's.

Because the client's body image may change as a result of surgery or a physical ailment, the nurse must make an extra effort to promote hygiene. For example, a client who has undergone a colostomy may be concerned about the appearance of the stoma and fecal odors. In addition to helping the client keep the stomal area clean, the nurse can discuss ways to reduce or eliminate odors (see Chapter 41).

Social Practices

The social groups to which a client relates can influence personal hygienic practices. During childhood, children acquire the hygienic practices of their parents. Family customs, the number of people in the house, and the availability of hot or running water are just a few of the factors influencing hygienic care. Teenagers may become more concerned with hygienic practices as their interest in dating increases. Later in life, friends and work groups shape the expectations people have about their personal appearance and the care taken to maintain adequate hygiene.

Socioeconomic Status

A person's economic resources influence the type and extent of hygienic practices used. The nurse should determine whether the client can afford necessary hygienic supplies such as deodorant, shampoo, toothpaste, and cosmetics.

Knowledge

Knowledge about the importance of hygiene and its implications for well-being influences hygienic practices. However, knowledge alone is not enough. The person must also be motivated to maintain self-care. Often, learning about an illness or condition encourages the client to improve hygienic practices. For example, when diabetic clients are aware of the effect of diabetes on circulation to the feet, they are more likely to learn proper techniques for foot care.

Cultural Variables

A client's cultural beliefs and personal values influence hygienic care. People from diverse cultural backgrounds follow different self-care practices (see Chapter 4). In North America, for example, many people take daily showers or tub baths. In the Far East, cleanliness is viewed as essential to well-being. In European countries, however, it is not unusual to bathe completely only once a week. When caring for clients with different hygienic practices, the nurse avoids being judgmental.

Personal Preferences

Each client has individual desires and preferences on when to bathe, shave, and perform hair care. Clients select different hygienic products (for example, soap, shampoo, deodorant, and toothpaste) according to personal preferences or needs. Clients also have preferences regarding how hygiene is performed. For example, one man may prefer to shave before a bath, whereas another shaves after taking a shower. Client preferences should help the nurse develop a more individualized care plan. The nurse does not attempt to change a client's preferences unless the client's health is affected. For example, clients with diabetes must carefully keep their feet clean to avoid the risk of infection. The nurse must explain and reinforce good foot care if the client has repeated infections.

Physical Condition

People who suffer certain illnesses (for example, the late stages of cancer) or those who have undergone surgery often lack the physical energy or dexterity to perform personal hygiene. A client whose arm has been placed in a cast or who is in traction requires assistance in performing a complete bath. Serious cardiac, neurological, pulmonary, and metabolic conditions may exhaust or incapacitate clients and require the nurse to perform total hygienic care.

 TYPES OF HYGIENIC CARE

The nurse provides a variety of hygienic measures throughout a day and can often schedule other care measures around the times that hygiene is planned. The box describes the types of hygienic care commonly performed at certain times of day. However, these times may change because of factors affecting the nurse's organization and scheduling of care. These factors include client preferences and habits, the client's need for more hygiene (for example, soiling from a fever or infection), other scheduled activities or procedures, the nurse's other assignments, and the nurse-client staffing ratio.

Hygienic Care Schedule

EARLY MORNING CARE

- Nursing personnel on the night shift provide basic hygiene to clients getting ready for breakfast, scheduled tests, or early morning surgery. "AM care" includes offering a bedpan or urinal if the client is not ambulatory, washing the client's hands and face, and assisting with oral care.

MORNING OR AFTER-BREAKFAST CARE

- In care performed after breakfast, the nurse assists by offering a bedpan or urinal to clients confined to bed; providing a bath or shower; providing oral, foot, nail, and hair care; giving a backrub; changing the client's gown or pajamas; changing the bed linens; and straightening the client's bedside unit and room. This is often referred to as "complete AM care."

AFTERNOON CARE

- Hospitalized clients often undergo many exhausting diagnostic tests or procedures in the morning. In rehabilitation centers, clients may participate in physical therapy during the morning. Afternoon hygiene care includes washing the hands and face, assisting with oral care, offering a bedpan or urinal, and straightening bed linen.

EVENING OR HOUR-BEFORE-SLEEP CARE

- Before bedtime the nurse offers personal hygiene care that helps a client relax to promote sleep. "PM care" may include changing soiled bed linens, gowns, or pajamas; assisting the client in washing the face and hands; providing oral hygiene; giving a back massage; and offering the bedpan or urinal to nonambulatory clients.

 CARE OF THE SKIN

The skin is an active organ with the functions of protection, secretion, excretion, temperature regulation, and sensation (Table 34-1 on p. 1020). The skin has three primary layers: epidermis, dermis, and subcutaneous. The **epidermis** (outer layer) is composed of several thin layers of cells undergoing different stages of maturation. It shields underlying tissue against water loss and mechanical and chemical injury and prevents the entry of disease-producing microorganisms. The innermost layer of the epidermis generates new cells that migrate slowly toward the

TABLE 34-1 Function of the Skin and Implications for Care	
Function/Description	Implications for Care
PROTECTION	
Epidermis is relatively impermeable layer that prevents entrance of microorganisms. Although microorganisms reside on skin surface and in hair follicles, relative dryness of skin's surface inhibits bacterial growth. Sebum removes bacteria from hair follicles. Acidic pH of skin further retards bacterial growth.	Weakening of epidermis occurs by scraping or stripping its surface (e.g., use of dry razors, tape removal, or improper turning or positioning techniques). Excessive dryness causes cracks and breaks in skin and mucosa that allow bacteria to enter. Emollients soften skin and prevent moisture loss, soaking of skin improves moisture retention, and hydration of mucosa prevents dryness. However, constant exposure of skin to moisture causes maceration or softening, which interrupts dermal integrity and promotes ulcer formation and bacterial growth. Bed linen and clothing should be kept dry. Misuse of soap, detergents, cosmetics, deodorant, and depilatories can cause chemical irritation. Alkaline soaps neutralize protective acid condition of skin. Cleansing of skin removes excess oil, sweat, dead skin cells, and dirt that can promote bacterial growth.
SENSATION	
Skin contains sensory organs for touch, pain, heat, cold, and pressure.	Friction should be used judiciously to avoid loss of stratum corneum, which can result in development of pressure ulcers. Smoothing linen removes sources of mechanical irritation. Removing rings from fingers prevents nurse from accidentally injuring client's skin. Bath water should not be excessively hot or cold.
TEMPERATURE REGULATION	
Body temperature is controlled by radiation, evaporation, conduction, and convection.	Factors that interfere with heat loss can alter temperature control. Wet bed linen or gowns interfere with convection and conduction. Excess blankets or bed coverings can interfere with heat loss through radiation and conduction. Coverings can promote heat conservation.
EXCRETION AND SECRETION	
Sweat promotes heat loss by evaporation. Sebum lubricates skin and hair.	Perspiration and oil can harbor microorganisms. Bathing removes excess body secretions, although if excessive it can cause drying of skin.

epidermal surface or top layer (called the *stratum corneum*). These cells replace the dead cells that are continuously shed from the skin's outer surface. The epidermis also contains melanocytes, special cells that produce the melanin or dark pigment of the skin. Exposure to sunlight causes melanocytes to produce **melanin,** which gives some people a tan. Darker-skinned races have more active melanocytes, which produce more melanin. The distribution of pigmentation in dark-skinned people varies widely.

Bacteria commonly reside on the skin's outer surface. These resident bacteria (for example, *Corynebacterium* species) are normal flora (see Chapter 18) that do not cause disease but instead inhibit the multiplication of disease-causing microorganisms.

The **dermis** is a thicker skin layer containing bundles of collagen and elastic fibers to support the epidermis. Nerve fibers, blood vessels, sweat glands, sebaceous glands, and hair follicles course through the dermal layer. Sebaceous glands secrete **sebum,** an oily, odorous fluid, into the hair follicles. Sebum lu-

bricates the skin and hair to keep them supple and pliant. There are two types of sweat glands: eccrine and apocrine. The **eccrine glands** are distributed throughout the skin but are more abundant in the forehead, palms, and soles. Sweat excreted from the eccrine glands assists in temperature control through evaporation. The **apocrine glands** can be found in the axillary and genital areas. The bacterial decomposition of sweat from these glands is responsible for body odor. In the ears, ceruminous glands secrete **cerumen** into the external ear canal. This heavy, oily substance traps any foreign material entering the ear.

The subcutaneous tissue layer contains blood vessels, nerves, lymph, and loose connective tissue filled with fat cells. The fatty tissue serves as a heat insulator for the body. Subcutaneous tissue also provides support for upper skin layers, enabling it to withstand stresses and pressure without injury. Very little subcutaneous tissue can be found underlying the oral mucosa.

The skin exchanges oxygen, nutrients, and fluid with underlying blood vessels; synthesizes new cells; and eliminates dead, nonfunctioning cells. The cells of the integument require adequate nutrition and hydration to resist injury and disease. Adequate circulation is essential to maintain cell life. The skin often reflects a change in physical condition by alterations in color, thickness, texture, turgor, temperature, and hydration (see Chapter 20). As long as the skin remains intact and healthy, its physiological function remains optimal.

 ## Assessment

Nursing assessment continues throughout hygienic care. First, the nurse must determine whether the client can tolerate hygienic procedures, which can often be exhausting. An assessment will then guide the nurse in identifying the type of care required by the client.

Most assessment occurs as the nurse ministers to the client's hygienic needs. For example, during oral care, the condition of the teeth and mucosa can be observed. Hygienic care allows the nurse to make assessment findings for a variety of health care problems and thus helps set health care priorities.

Physical Assessment of the Skin

While assisting a client with personal hygiene, the nurse assesses all external body surfaces. Using the skills of inspection and palpation (see Chapter 20), the nurse looks for alterations in the integument, determines the client's need for ongoing hygiene, and notes changes of the integument in response to nursing and medical therapies.

The nurse determines the condition of the skin by observing its color, texture, thickness, turgor, temperature, and hydration. Chapter 20 describes in detail the techniques for assessing each of these characteristics. The box describes normal skin characteristics.

The nurse also assesses for skin problems influenced by hygienic measures (Table 34-2 on p. 1022). The nurse notes areas of dry skin as a result of too-frequent baths, excessive use of soap, or use of harsh alkaline soaps. Areas of skin **maceration** (softening) may have formed as a result of improper drying. The nurse observes for calloused areas on the feet or hands that might benefit from soaking and the application of lotion.

While inspecting the skin, the nurse notes the presence and condition of lesions (see Chapter 20). Certain types have implications for hygienic measures. When the nurse observes skin problems, it

---

Normal Skin Characteristics
■ Skin is intact and has no abrasions.
■ Skin feels warm when palpated.
■ Localized changes in texture can be palpated across skin's surface.
■ There is good turgor (elastic and firm), with skin generally smooth and soft.
■ Skin color varies from body part to body part.

helps to explain proper skin care to the client. For example, a rash on the skin often indicates an allergic reaction. The nurse teaches the client about the significance of the rash and the proper use of medications prescribed for the rash and cautions against use of over-the-counter drugs that may prove useless or even worsen the rash. Likewise, the nurse educates the client about avoiding use of irritants such as harsh soaps or cosmetics that can aggravate the condition.

Developmental Changes

Age influences the normal condition of the skin and the type of hygienic measures required. The neonate's skin is relatively immature. The epidermis and dermis are loosely bound together. The skin is extremely thin. Because any friction against the skin layers can cause bruising, the nurse must handle the neonate carefully during bathing. A break in the neonate's skin can easily lead to infection.

In a toddler the skin layers are more tightly bound together. The child thus has a greater resistance to infection and skin irritation. However, because of the child's more active play and the absence of established hygienic habits, greater attention is needed from parents and care givers to provide thorough hygiene and begin teaching good hygienic habits.

During adolescence the growth and maturation of the integument are increased. In girls, estrogen secretion causes the skin to become soft, smooth, and thicker in texture with increased vascularity. In boys, male hormones produce an increased thickness of the skin with some darkening in color. Sebaceous glands become more active, predisposing adolescents to **acne.** Eccrine and apocrine sweat glands become fully functional during puberty. Adolescents usually begin to use antiperspirants. More frequent bathing and shampooing also become necessary to reduce body odors. Sweating is usually more pronounced in boys. The growth of body hair increases during ado-

TABLE 34-2 Common Skin Problems

Characteristics	Implications	Interventions
DRY SKIN		
Flaky, rough texture on exposed areas such as hands, arms, legs, or face	Skin may become infected if epidermal layer is allowed to crack.	Have client bathe less frequently and rinse body of all soap because residue left on skin can cause irritation and breakdown. Add moisture to air through use of humidifier. Increase fluid intake when skin is dry. Use moisturizing lotion to aid healing. (Lotion forms protective barrier and helps maintain fluid within skin.) Use creams to clean skin that is dry or allergic to soaps and detergents.
ACNE		
Inflammatory, papulopustular skin eruption, usually involving bacterial breakdown of sebum; appearance on face, neck, shoulders, and back	Infected material within pustule can spread if area is squeezed or picked. Permanent scarring can result.	Wash hair and skin thoroughly each day with hot water and soap to remove oil. Use cosmetics sparingly because oily cosmetics or creams accumulate in pores and tend to make condition worse. Implement dietary restrictions, if necessary. (Foods that aggravate condition should be eliminated from diet.) Inform client that exposure to ultraviolet rays, either from sunshine or heat lamp, may help control acne. (Caution should be used to prevent burning of skin.) Use prescribed topical antibiotics for severe forms of acne.
HIRSUTISM		
Excessive growth of body and facial hair, especially in women	Hirsutism may cause negative body image by giving women a male appearance.	Use following to remove unwanted hair: depilatories (can cause infection, rashes, dermatitis), shaving (safest method), electrolysis (permanently removes hair by destroying hair follicles), tweezing (lasts only temporarily), bleaching of hair (lasts only temporarily).
SKIN RASHES		
Skin eruption that may result from overexposure to sun or moisture or from allergic reaction (may be flat or raised, localized or systemic, pruritic or nonpruritic)	If skin is continually scratched, inflammation and infection may occur. Rashes can also cause discomfort.	Wash area thoroughly and apply antiseptic spray or lotion to prevent further itching and aid in healing process. Apply warm or cold soaks to relieve inflammation, if indicated.

TABLE 34-2 Common Skin Problems—cont'd		
Characteristics	Implications	Interventions
CONTACT DERMATITIS		
Inflammation of skin characterized by abrupt onset with erythema, pruritus, pain, and appearance of scaly oozing lesions (seen on face, neck, hands, forearms, and genitalia)	Dermatitis is often difficult to eliminate because person is usually in continual contact with substance causing skin reaction. Substance may be hard to identify.	Avoid causative agents (e.g., cleansers and soaps).
ABRASION		
Scraping or rubbing away of epidermis that may result in localized bleeding and later weeping of serous fluid	Infection occurs easily because of loss of protective skin layer.	Be careful not to scratch client with jewelry or fingernails. Wash abrasions with mild soap and water. Observe dressing or bandage for retained moisture because it could increase risk of infection.

lescence as a result of hormonal changes. The body hair has a characteristic pattern of distribution, which the nurse can assess (see Chapter 20). Pubic and axillary hair develops in both sexes. Beard and mustache hair grows in boys as a result of testicular androgens. Some girls and women have increased androgen levels causing **hirsutism,** the growth of facial hair.

The condition of an adult's skin depends on hygienic practices and exposure to environmental irritants. Normally the skin is elastic, well hydrated, firm, and smooth. With age, the skin loses its resiliency and moisture, and sebaceous and sweat glands become less active. The epithelium thins and elastic collagen fibers shrink, making the skin fragile and subject to bruising and breaking. These changes warrant caution when turning and repositioning older adults. Typically the older person's skin is dry and wrinkled, which can be aggravated by the sun. Daily bathing and bathing with water that is too hot may cause the skin to become excessively dry.

Self-Care Ability

When a client becomes unable to bathe or perform personal skin care, the nurse provides the necessary assistance. To determine whether a client requires a bed bath instead of a tub bath or shower, the nurse should assess the client's balance, activity tolerance, muscle strength, and coordination. The degree of assistance needed by a client during bathing may also depend on vision, the ability to sit without support, hand grasp, attached equipment, and the range of motion of extremities. If a client's cognitive function is impaired, the nurse's help probably will be needed.

Risks for Skin Impairment

The nurse looks for certain conditions that place a client at risk for impaired skin integrity (see Chapter 44).

IMMOBILIZATION. A client who is unable to move freely as a result of illness or some external restraint is at risk for skin breakdown. The dependent body parts are exposed to pressure from underlying surfaces (for example, a mattress, a body cast, or a wrinkled layer of linen), reducing circulation to affected body parts. Chapter 44 describes how the impairment of circulation to dependent body parts can result in pressure ulcer formation. The nurse should be aware of clients who require assistance to turn and change positions. Localized redness and tenderness are early signs of pressure on dependent body parts and, if left untreated, can result in pressure ulcers.

REDUCED SENSATION. Many clients are unable to sense an injury to the skin's surface. Clients with paralysis, circulatory insufficiency, or local nerve damage do not receive normal transmission of nerve impulses when excessive heat or cold, pressure, friction, or chemical irritants are applied to the skin. During the bath, the nurse can easily assess the status of sensory nerve function by checking for pain,

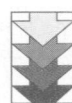

Examples of Nursing Diagnoses Related to Skin Integrity

NANDA-APPROVED NURSING DIAGNOSES

Impaired skin integrity related to:
- Pressure
- Immobilization
- Exposure to chemical irritants

High risk for impaired skin integrity related to:
- Immobilization
- Vascular insufficiency
- Inadequate nutritional intake

Altered peripheral tissue perfusion related to:
- Impaired arterial blood flow
- Impaired venous blood flow

Bathing/hygiene self-care deficit related to:
- Pain
- Forced immobilization
- Musculoskeletal weakness

Impaired tissue integrity related to:
- Altered circulation
- Nutritional deficit
- Mechanical irritation

Purposes of Bathing

CLEANSING THE SKIN

- Cleansing removes perspiration, some bacteria, sebum, and dead skin cells, which minimizes skin irritation and reduces the chance of infection.

STIMULATION OF CIRCULATION

- Good circulation is promoted through the use of warm water and gentle stroking of the extremities.

IMPROVED SELF-IMAGE

- Bathing promotes relaxation and a feeling of being refreshed and comfortable.

REDUCTION OF BODY ODORS

- Excessive secretion of sweat from apocrine glands located in the axillae and pubic areas causes unpleasant body odors. Bathing and use of antiperspirants minimize odors.

PROMOTION OF RANGE OF MOTION (ROM)

- Movement of the extremities during bathing maintains joint function.

Sample Nursing Diagnostic Process for Impaired Skin Integrity

Assessment Activities	Defining Characteristics	Nursing Diagnoses
Check to see if client is able to turn or move on own. Check for bowel or bladder incontinence. Ask if client is experiencing discomfort over bony prominences. Inspect skin surfaces for redness, irritation, dryness, excessive perspiration, lesions, or open wounds. Inspect lesions or wounds for color, size, location, drainage.	Disruption of skin surface (e.g., burn, blister, abrasion) Destruction of skin layers Erythema Pruritus	*High risk for impaired skin integrity* related to immobilization
Ask about preferred bathing supplies and routine. Assess amount of assistance needed. Note body odors. Determine whether client has visual or cognitive defects. Check to see if supplies are within client's reach.	Inability to wash body or body parts Inability to obtain or get to water source Inability to regulate flow of water	*Bathing/hygiene self-care deficit* related to cast on right lower extremity

tactile sensation, or temperature sensation (see Chapter 20).

NUTRITION AND HYDRATION ALTERATIONS. Adequate nutrients are essential for maintaining the normal integrity of the skin. Clients with limited caloric and protein intake have impaired tissue synthesis (see Chapter 35). The skin becomes thinner, less elastic, and smoother, with a subsequent loss of subcutaneous tissue, which can result in impaired or delayed tissue healing. Poor digestion and absorption of nutrients caused by inflammatory conditions of the bowel or bowel surgery, excessive protein metabolism caused by fever, burns, or surgery, and excessive loss of protein caused by blood loss, wound exudate, or burns place clients at risk for imbalances. A hospitalized client who is not permitted to eat is also a candidate for nutritional and hydration problems that can affect the integrity of the skin.

SECRETIONS AND EXCRETIONS ON THE SKIN. Moisture on the skin's surface is a medium for bacterial growth and can cause local irritation, soften epidermal cells, and contribute to skin maceration. Perspiration, urine, watery fecal material, and wound drainage can accumulate on the skin's surface, resulting in breakdown and infection. The nurse gives particular attention to body areas, such as under the woman's breasts, the perineal area, or under the arms, where moisture may collect and skin surfaces may rub against each other and cause friction.

VASCULAR INSUFFICIENCY. In peripheral vascular disease, the arterial blood supply to tissues is inadequate or venous return is impaired, causing decreased circulation to the extremities. Inadequate blood flow to the skin results in ischemia and breakdown. Clients with this disease have a high risk of infection because delivery of nutrients, oxygen, and white blood cells to injured tissues is inadequate.

EXTERNAL DEVICES. Often a client has some type of external device applied to or around the skin that can exert pressure or friction against the skin's surface. A cast, cloth restraint, bandage, dressing, or orthopedic brace can rub against the skin and cause breakdown. The nurse assesses all skin surfaces exposed to any external device.

 ## Nursing Diagnosis

The nurse's assessment reveals the condition of the client's skin and the client's need for and ability to maintain personal hygienic needs. Defining char-

acteristics direct the nurse to diagnose specifically the client's actual or potential health problems (see diagnoses box).

If the client has the potential for skin breakdown, the nurse plans preventive measures. The factors contributing to the problem determine the nurse's interventions (see diagnostic process box).

If the client has skin breakdown, the nurse must provide care that promotes healing of injured skin surfaces and prevents infection. The nurse also eliminates factors that may lead to further tissue injury.

 ## Planning

Providing skin care has many purposes other than maintaining cleanliness. A bath or shower helps the client relax, stimulates circulation to the skin, provides exercise through range of motion during bathing, improves self-image, and stimulates the rate and depth of respirations (see box). The interaction between nurse and client during bathing and skin care gives the nurse an opportunity to develop a meaningful relationship with the client.

Planning should focus on the methods of skin care that the nurse will deliver and on the variety of nursing care measures the nurse can perform as a client bathes. Teaching and providing emotional support and values clarification are just some of the types of interaction the nurse can include during hygiene.

The client's condition influences the plan for delivering hygiene. A seriously ill client usually needs a daily bath because body secretions accumulate and the client is unable to maintain cleanliness (see care plan on p. 1026). An older client at home may require a visit from the nurse to assist with a tub bath. If clients are normally inactive during the day and their skin tends to be dry, the nurse may need to bathe the client only twice a week. The nurse must plan for necessary assistance for clients who are weakened or possess poor muscle strength and coordination. For example, an obese client who has had difficulty getting out of a tub should have a tub chair, hand rails, or extra personnel available for help.

Timing is also important in planning hygienic care. Being interrupted in the middle of a bath to go to an x-ray examination can frustrate and embarrass a client. The nurse should try to plan hygienic care around tests and procedures the client must undergo. This can be difficult in a hospital because tests may not be scheduled for specific times.

Goals for clients receiving skin care include the following:
1. Skin will remain intact and free of body odors.
2. Range of motion will be maintained.

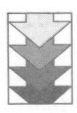

Nursing diagnosis: *High risk for impaired skin integrity* related to immobilization
Definition: High risk for impaired skin integrity is the state in which an individual's skin is at risk of being adversely altered (Kim, McFarland, McLane, 1991).

Goals	Expected Outcomes	Interventions	Rationale
Skin will remain intact during hospitalization.	Skin will be intact and without redness. Skin will be warm, soft, smooth, and well hydrated.	Bathe client daily.	Cleansing removes excess oil, sweat, dead skin cells, and dirt that promote bacterial growth.
Skin will be free of odors during hospitalization.	Drainage or secretions will be reduced or absent. Odors will be reduced or eliminated.	Dry skin thoroughly after each cleansing.	Excess moisture causes skin maceration, which promotes bacterial growth (NPUAP, 1989).
		Apply lotion to skin after bathing.	Emollients soften skin and prevent moisture loss.
		Turn regularly (at least every 2 hr).	Longer pressure is applied, greater the risk of skin breakdown. Pressure decreases or obliterates circulation, depriving tissue of oxygen and nutrients (Pires, Mueller, 1991).
		Give perineal care after each voiding and defecation.	Excessive secretion of sweat from apocrine glands in axillae and pubic areas causes unpleasant odors. Bathing minimizes odors. Secretions that accumulate on surface of skin around genitalia act as reservoir for infection.

Types of Therapeutic Baths

HOT WATER TUB BATH

- Immersion in hot water helps relieve muscle soreness and spasm. However, a danger of causing burns exists. Water temperature should be 45°-46° C (113°-114.8° F) for adults.

WARM WATER TUB BATH

- Bathing in warm water relieves muscle tension. Water temperature should be 43° C (109.4° F).

COOL WATER BATH

- Bathing in cool water can relieve tension or lower body temperature. Water temperature should be tepid (37° C [98.6° F]) rather than cold to avoid chilling and to promote slow cooling; this avoids temperature fluctuations. This type of bath is especially effective in reducing the body temperature of a small child with a fever (see Procedure 34-1).

SOAK

- Local application of water or a medicated solution can remove dead tissue or soften encrusted secretions. An aseptic technique is necessary when cleansing open or abraded areas of the skin. Soaks are also useful in reducing pain and swelling of inflamed or irritated skin surfaces (see Chapter 48).

SITZ BATH

- A sitz bath cleanses and reduces inflammation of the perineal and anal areas of a client who has undergone rectal or vaginal surgery or childbirth or who has local rectal irritation from hemorrhoids or fissures. Water temperature depends on the client's condition but should be 43°-45° C (109.4°-113° F). Cold sitz baths are more effective in relieving pain in the postpartum period.*

*Data from Ramler D, Roberts J: *JOGNN* 15:471, 1986.

3. Client will achieve a sense of comfort and well-being.
4. Client will participate in and understand methods of skin care.

Implementation

Bathing

Bathing a client is a part of total hygienic care. Baths can be categorized as cleansing or therapeutic. A physician's order is necessary for baths designed for therapeutic purposes (Procedure 34-1 on p. 1028). The order designates bath temperature (see box), the body part being treated (in the case of soaks), and any medicated solution used (for example, saline, sodium bicarbonate, or potassium permanganate).

The extent of the client's bath and the methods used for bathing depend on the client's physical capabilities and the degree of hygiene required. A complete bed bath is needed for clients who are totally dependent and require total hygienic care (Procedure 34-2 on p. 1029).

A **partial bed bath** consists of bathing only body parts that would cause discomfort or odor if left unbathed (for example, hands, face, perineal area, and axillae). Dependent clients in need of only partial hygiene or self-sufficient bedridden clients who are unable to reach all body parts receive a partial bed bath. Nurses need to assess carefully to determine that clients can sufficiently bathe other body parts on their own.

The tub bath or shower can be used to give a more thorough bath than a bed bath. Washing and rinsing all body parts are easier. Safety is of primary concern because the surface of a tub or shower stall is slippery. Clients vary in how much help they will need. Some tubs are specially designed for dependent clients. The nurse should follow the following guidelines when clients receive or take baths:

1. Provide privacy. Close the door or pull room curtains around the bathing area. While bathing the client, expose only the areas being bathed.
2. Maintain safety. Keep side rails up while away from the client's bedside. (This is particularly important for dependent or unconscious clients.) Place the call light in the client's reach if it is necessary to leave the room temporarily.
3. Maintain warmth. Keep the room warm because the client is partially uncovered and may be easily chilled. Control drafts; keep windows and bed curtains closed.
4. Promote the client's independence as much as possible during bathing activities. Offer assistance as needed.

Bathing an Infant

An infant can be bathed in much the same way as an adult, by a sponge bath or in a small tub. However, the nurse should take special precautions. Because an infant's temperature-control mechanisms are still immature, prolonged exposure of body parts may cause rapid cooling. When giving a sponge bath, the nurse keeps the infant covered as much as possible. When giving a tub bath, the nurse should work quickly and be sure the water temperature is warm enough to prevent chilling. Henningson et al (1981) note that bathing a newborn by immersion causes less heat loss and less crying.

The surface of an infant's skin has a pH of about 4.95 soon after birth (Whaley, Wong, 1991). This acidic covering helps prevent the growth of bacteria on the skin's surface. Thus plain water is preferred for bathing. Alkaline soaps such as Ivory and oils, powder, and lotion can alter the skin's pH and provide a medium for bacterial growth.

Care of the umbilical cord is a special consideration for the newborn. The umbilical stump is an excellent medium for bacterial growth. Thus sponge baths are given until the cord falls off and the skin heals. Immersion of the umbilicus in a tub of water before the skin heals can result in a serious infection. Triple dye is used by many institutions to prevent infection. The daily application of alcohol to the base of the cord aids drying. Normally, the umbilical stump falls off in 14 to 17 days (Wilson et al, 1985).

The nurse also gives special care to infants who have been circumcised. A small amount of bleeding normally occurs from the penis. The physician applies a sterile gauze dressing impregnated with petrolatum jelly around the circumcised area. The nurse may clean the penis periodically with moistened cotton balls until the dressing can be removed permanently (Whaley, Wong, 1991).

In hospitals where there is rooming-in of the infant and mother, the infant's bath is an excellent opportunity to involve the parents in the child's care. The parents can examine the infant's body parts and learn about normal variations in skin characteristics. A parent may worry about minor birth injuries unless the nurse explains how they occur and when they will disappear.

SPONGE BATH. Newborn infants are bathed after vital signs have stabilized. Nurses wear gloves when initially handling infants whose skin has become soiled from the blood of the mother. Initial washing only involves cleaning blood from the face and head. The **vernix caseosa,** a grayish-white, cheeselike substance covering the skin, may temporarily provide insulation and lubricating properties. The vernix caseosa dries and disappears within 24 to 48 hours.

Text continued on p. 1035.

Tepid Sponging

STEPS	RATIONALE
1. Assess client's body temperature and pulse.	Provides baseline for evaluating response to therapy. Sudden circulatory changes may alter pulse.
2. Explain to client that purpose of sponging with tepid water is to cool body slowly. Briefly describe steps of procedure.	Procedure can be uncomfortable because of cool applications. Anxiety over procedure can increase body temperature.
3. Prepare necessary equipment and supplies: a. Bath basin d. Washcloths b. Tepid water e. Waterproof pad (37° C or 98.6° F) f. Bath blanket c. Bath thermometer g. Thermometer	Tepid water prevents sudden heat loss and chilling.
4. Close room door or curtain.	Ensures privacy.
5. Wash hands. OPTION: Don gloves (if required by institution's policy/procedure).	Reduces transfer of microorganisms. Infections are caused by pathogenic microorganisms.
6. Place waterproof pads under client and remove gown.	Pads prevent soiling of bed linen. Removing gown provides access to all skin surfaces.
7. Keep the bath blanket over body parts not being sponged. Close the windows and door to prevent drafts.	Prevents chilling.
8. Check water temperature.	Prevents chilling.
9. Immerse washcloths in water and apply wet cloths under each axilla and over groin. If using tub, have client soak for 20-30 min.	Axillae and groin contain large superficial blood vessels. Application of washcloths promotes cooler temperature of body's core by conduction. Immersion provides more effective heat loss.
10. Gently sponge extremity for 5 min. Note client's response. Opposite extremity may be covered by cool washcloth. In tub, gently squeeze water over client's back and chest.	Prevents sudden temperature fall and minimizes risk of developing chills.
11. Dry extremity and reassess client's pulse and body temperature. Observe response to therapy.	Response to therapy is monitored to prevent sudden temperature change.
12. Continue sponging other extremities, back, and buttocks for 3-5 min each. Reassess temperature and pulse every 15 min.	Prevents sudden temperature fall and minimizes risk of developing chills.
13. Change water and reapply sponges to axillae and groin as needed.	Water temperature rises as result of exposure to client's warm body surface.
14. When body temperature falls to slightly above normal, discontinue procedure.	Prevents temperature drift to subnormal level. Follow institutional guidelines.
15. Dry extremities and body parts thoroughly. Cover client with light bath blanket or sheet.	Prevents chilling. Excessively heavy covering may increase body temperature.
16. Dispose of equipment and change bed linen if soiled. Wash hands.	Controls transmission of infection.
17. Measure client's body temperature and pulse.	Temperature indicates response to therapy. Dysrhythmias may be complication of therapy.
18. Record time procedure was started and terminated, vital sign changes, and client's response.	Recording communicates care provided in accurate and timely fashion.

STEPS	RATIONALE
1. Assess client's preferences for bathing practices, frequency of bathing, time of day preferred, type of hygiene products used.	Promotes participation and sense of comfort.
2. Consider client's condition and review orders for precautions concerning client's movement or positioning.	Prevents accidental injury to client during bathing activities.
3. Explain procedure and ask client for suggestions or ways to prepare supplies. If partial bath is to be performed, ask how much of bath client wishes to complete.	Promotes client cooperation and participation.
4. If shower or tub bath is to be done, schedule use of facilities if private bath unavailable.	Prevents unnecessary waiting that can cause fatigue.
5. Adjust room temperature and ventilation, and close room doors and windows. Close curtains around bed.	Prevents rapid loss of body heat during bathing. Ensures privacy.

6. Prepare necessary equipment and supplies:
  a. Two bath towels
  b. Two washcloths
  c. Washbasin (for complete or partial bed bath)
  d. Soap and soap dish
  e. Bath blanket or top spread (for complete or partial bed bath)
  f. Clean gown or pajamas
  g. Hygienic aids, such as skin lotion, deodorant, and powder
  h. Bedpan or urinal and toilet paper
  i. Linen hamper or laundry bag
  j. Disposable gloves
  k. Bed linen (optional)
	Separate towel and washcloth are used for client's face and for body to enhance feeling of cleanliness.
	
	Bath blanket maintains client's warmth during procedure.
	
	For client to use before bath.
	
	Prevents contact with potentially infected body secretions.

COMPLETE OR PARTIAL BED BATH

STEPS	RATIONALE
7. Offer client bedpan or urinal (see Chapter 40). Provide towel and washcloth for client.	Client will feel more comfortable after voiding. Prevents interruption of bath.
8. Wash hands. OPTION: Apply gloves if required by institution's policy or procedure.	Reduces transmission of microorganisms.
9. Lower side rail closest to you and assist client in assuming comfortable position maintaining body alignment.	Aids nurse's access to client. Maintains client comfort.
10. Bring client toward side closest to you. Place hospital bed in high position.	When you do not have to reach across bed, strain on back muscles is minimized.
11. Loosen top covers at foot of bed. Place bath blanket over top sheet. Fold and remove top sheet from under blanket. If possible, have client hold bath blanket while you withdraw sheet.	Removal of top linens prevents them from becoming soiled or moist during bath. Blanket provides warmth and privacy.
12. If top sheet is to be reused, fold it for replacement later. If not, dispose in laundry bag, taking care not to allow linen to contact your uniform.	Proper disposal prevents transmission of microorganisms.

Bathing a Client

STEPS	RATIONALE
13. Remove client's gown or pajamas while maintaining privacy. If extremity is injured or has reduced mobility, begin removal from unaffected side. If client has intravenous (IV) tube, remove gown from arm *without* IV first, and then lower IV container and slide gown covering affected arm over tubing and container. Rehang IV container and check flow rate (see illustrations).	Provides full exposure of body parts during bathing. Undressing unaffected side first allows easier manipulation of gown over body part with reduced ROM.
14. Pull side rail up. Fill washbasin two-thirds full, with water at 43°-46° C (110°-115° F). Have client place fingers in water to test temperature tolerance. OPTION: Place plastic container of bath lotion in bath water.	Raising side rail maintains safety as you leave bedside. Warm water promotes comfort and prevents chilling. Testing temperature prevents accidental burning of client's skin. Keeps lotion warm for application to skin.
15. Remove pillow if allowed and raise head of bed 30-45 degrees. Place bath towel under client's head.	Removal of pillow makes it easier to wash client's ears and neck. Placement of towel prevents soiling of bed linen.
16. Place bath towel over client's chest.	Prevents soiling of bath blanket.
17. Fold washcloth around fingers of your hand to form mitt (see illustration). Immerse mitt in water and wring thoroughly.	Mitt retains water and heat better than loosely held washcloth, keeps cold edges from brushing against client, prevents splashing.
18. Wash client's eyes with plain warm water. Use different section of mitt for each eye. Move mitt from inner to outer canthus (see illustration). Soak encrustations on eyelid for 2-3 min with damp cloth before attempting removal. Dry eye thoroughly but gently.	Soap irritates eyes. Use of separate sections of mitt reduces infection transmission. Bathing eye from inner to outer canthus prevents secretions from entering nasolacrimal duct. Pressure can cause internal injury.

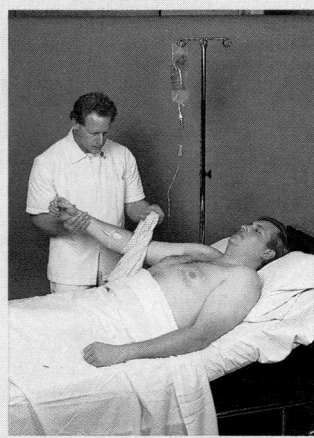 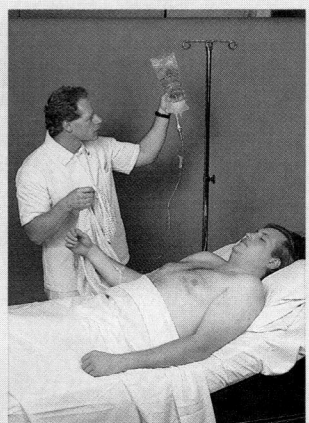 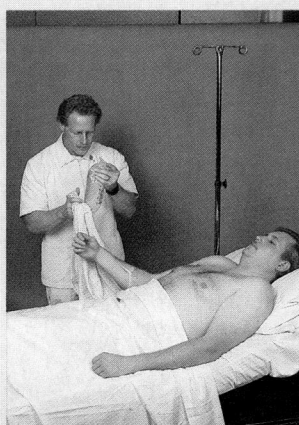 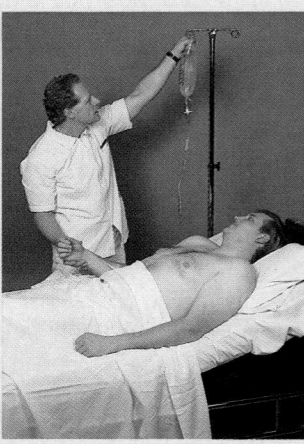

Step 13

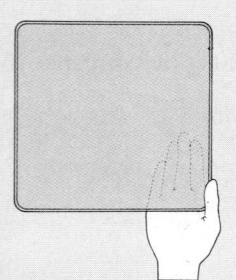 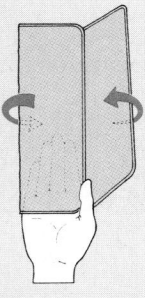 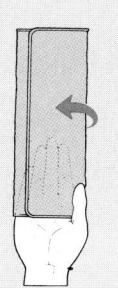 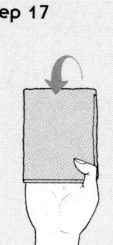

Step 17

Step 17 illustrations from Sorrentino SA: *Mosby's textbook for nursing assistants,* ed 3, St Louis, 1992, Mosby–Year Book.

STEPS	RATIONALE
19. Ask client about preference for using soap on face. Wash, rinse, and dry well forehead, cheeks, nose, neck, and ears. (Men may wish to shave at this point or after bath.)	Soap tends to dry face more quickly because it is exposed to air more than other body parts.
20. Remove bath blanket from over client's arm that is farthest from you. Place bath towel lengthwise under arm. OPTION: Raise side rail and move to other side to wash arm.	Bathing far side first prevents reaching over clean area.
21. Lower side rail if moved to opposite side. Bathe arm with soap and water using long, firm strokes from distal to proximal areas (fingers to axilla). Raise and support arm above head (if possible) while thoroughly washing axilla.	Soap lowers surface tension and facilitates removal of debris and bacteria when friction is applied during washing. Long, firm strokes stimulate circulation. Movement of arm exposes axilla and exercises joint's normal ROM.
22. Rinse and dry arm and axilla thoroughly. If client prefers, apply deodorant or talcum powder.	Excess moisture causes skin maceration or softening. Deodorant controls body odor.
23. Fold bath towel in half and lay it on bed beside client. Place basin on towel. Immerse client's hand in water. OPTION: Allow hand to soak for 3-5 min before washing hand and fingernails (Procedure 34-5). Remove basin and dry hand well.	Soaking softens cuticles and calluses of hand and loosens debris beneath nails. Soaking also enhances feeling of cleanliness. Thorough drying removes moisture from between fingers.
24. Repeat Steps 20-23 for other arm.	
25. Check temperature of bath water and change water if necessary.	Use of warm water maintains client's comfort.
26. Cover client's chest with bath towel and fold bath blanket down to umbilicus.	Prevents unnecessary exposure of body parts.
27. With one hand, lift edge of towel away from chest. With mitted hand, bathe chest using long, firm strokes. Take special care to wash skinfolds under female client's breasts, lifting breast if necessary. Keep chest covered between wash and rinse periods. Dry well.	Maintains warmth and privacy. Secretions and dirt collect easily in areas of tight skinfolds.

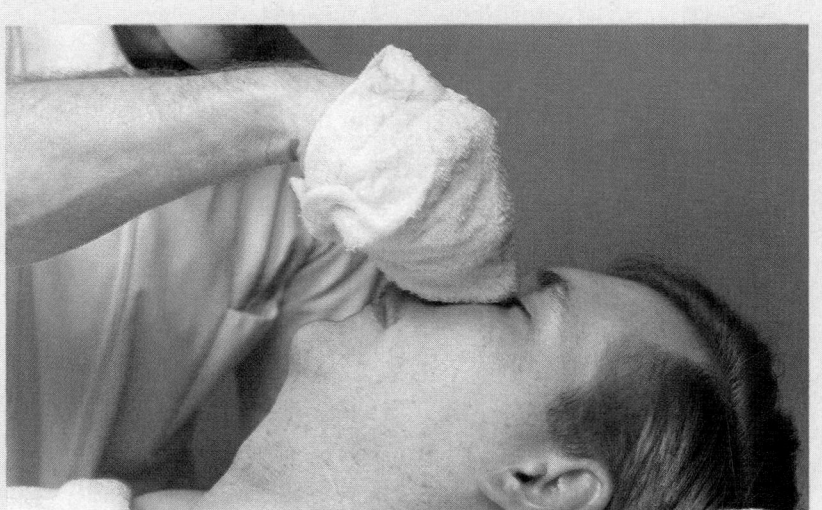

Step 18

Bathing a Client

STEPS	RATIONALE
28. Place bath towel lengthwise over chest and abdomen. (Two towels may be needed.) Fold blanket down to just above pubic region.	Prevents chilling and exposure of body parts.
29. With one hand, lift bath towel. With mitted hand, bathe abdomen, giving special attention to bathing umbilicus and abdominal folds. Stroke from side to side. Keep abdomen covered between washing and rinsing. Dry well.	Moisture and sediment that collect in skinfolds predispose client to skin maceration and irritation.
30. Apply clean gown or pajama top. If one extremity is injured or immobilized, always dress affected side first. (This step may be omitted until completion of bath; gown should not become soiled during remainder of bath.)	Maintains client's warmth and comfort. Dressing affected side first allows easier manipulation of gown over body part with reduced ROM.
31. Cover chest and abdomen with top of bath blanket. Expose far leg by folding blanket over toward midline. Be sure perineum is draped.	Prevents unnecessary exposure.
32. Bend client's leg at knee by positioning your arm under leg. While grasping client's heel, elevate leg from mattress slightly and slide bath towel lengthwise under leg.	Prevents soiling of bed linen. Support of joint and extremity during lifting prevents strain on musculoskeletal structures.
33. Ask client to hold foot still. Place bath basin on towel on bed and secure its position next to foot to be washed.	Sudden movement by client could cause spillage of bathwater. (This step is omitted if client is unable to hold leg in basin.)
34. With one hand supporting lower leg, raise it and slide basin under lifted foot. Make sure foot is firmly placed on bottom of basin. OPTION: Allow foot to soak while you wash leg (see illustration).	Proper positioning of foot prevents pressure from being applied from edge of basin against calf. Soaking softens calluses and rough skin. (NOTE: if client is unable to hold leg in basin, do not immerse; simply wash with washcloth.)
35. Unless contraindicated, use long, firm strokes in washing from ankle to knee and from knee to thigh. Dry well.	Promotes venous return. Long, firm strokes would not be used for client with blood clots.

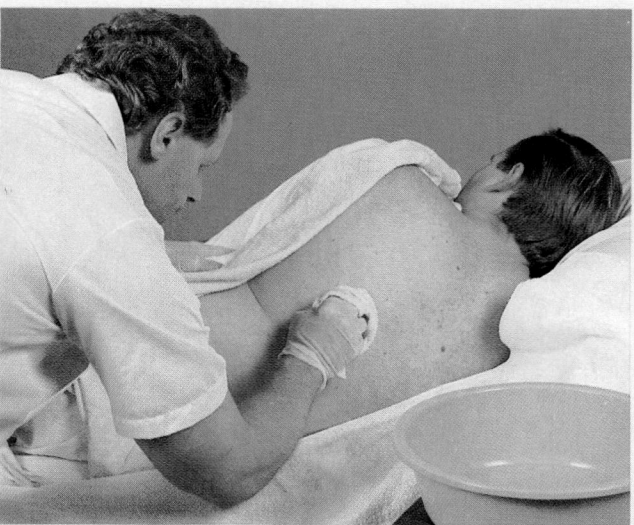

Step 34   Step 42

CONTINUED

STEPS	RATIONALE
36. Cleanse foot, making sure to bathe between toes. Cleanse and clip nails as needed (Procedure 34-5). Dry well. If skin is dry, apply lotion.	Secretions and moisture may be present between toes. Lotion helps to retain moisture and soften skin.
37. Repeat Steps 31-34 for other leg and foot.	
38. Cover client with bath blanket, raise side rail for client's safety, and change bathwater.	Drop in water temperature during bathing can cause chilling. Clean water reduces microorganism transmission.
39. Lower side rail. Assist client in assuming prone or side-lying position (as applicable). Place towel lengthwise along client's side.	Exposes back and buttocks for bathing.
40. Keep client draped by sliding bath blanket over shoulders and thighs.	Maintains warmth and prevents unnecessary exposure.
41. Apply disposable gloves (if not done in Step 2).	Prevents contact with microorganisms in body secretions.
42. Wash, rinse, and dry back from neck to buttocks using long, firm strokes (see illustration). Pay special attention to folds of buttocks and anus. Give backrub (Procedure 34-4).	Skinfolds near buttocks and anus may contain fecal secretions that harbor microorganisms.
43. Change bathwater and washcloth.	Prevents transfer of microorganisms from anal area to genitalia.
44. Assist client in assuming side-lying or supine position. Cover chest and upper extremities with towel and lower extremities with bath blanket. Expose only genitalia. (If client can help, covering entire body with bath blanket may be preferable.) Wash, rinse, and dry perineum (Procedure 34-3). Give special attention to skinfolds.	Maintains client's privacy. Clients capable of performing partial bath usually prefer to wash their own genitalia. Skinfolds are site for accumulation of secretions and moisture.
45. Dispose of gloves in receptacle.	Prevents transmission of microorganisms.
46. Apply any additional body lotion or oil as desired.	Moisturizing lotion prevents dry, chapped skin.
47. Assist client in dressing.	
48. Comb client's hair (see p. 1059). Women may want to apply makeup.	Maintains client's body image.
49. Make client's bed (Procedures 34-11 and 34-12).	Provides clean environment.
50. Remove soiled linen and place in dirty linen bag. Cleanse and replace bathing equipment. Replace call light and personal possessions. Leave room as clean and comfortable as possible.	Prevents transmission of infection. Clean environment promotes comfort. Keeping call light and articles of care within reach promotes safety.
51. Wash hands.	Reduces transmission of microorganisms.

TUB BATH OR SHOWER

STEPS	RATIONALE
52. Check tub or shower for cleanliness. Use cleansing techniques according to agency policy. Place rubber mat on tub or shower bottom. Place disposable bathmat or towel on floor in front of tub or shower.	Prevents transmission of infection. Mats prevent slipping and falling.
53. Collect all hygienic aids, toiletry items, and linen requested by client. Place within easy reach of tub or shower.	Prevents possible falls when client reaches for equipment.
54. Assist client to bathroom if necessary. Have client wear robe and slippers en route to bathroom.	Prevents accidental falls. Wearing robe and slippers prevents chilling.

Bathing a Client

STEPS	RATIONALE
55. Demonstrate to client how to use call signal for assistance when in hospital or extended care facility. NOTE: If safety is jeopardized, make arrangements for help during procedure.	Bathrooms are equipped with signaling devices in case client feels faint or weak or needs immediate assistance. Clients prefer privacy during bath if safety is not jeopardized.
56. Place "occupied" sign on bathroom door when in hospital or extended care facility.	Maintains privacy.
57. Fill bathtub halfway with warm water (43° C [109.4° F]). Ask client to test water, and adjust water temperature if it is too warm or too cold. Explain which faucet controls hot water. If client is taking shower, turn shower on and adjust water temperature before client enters shower stall.	Adjusting water temperature prevents accidental burns. Older clients and clients with neurological alterations (e.g., spinal cord injury) are at high risk for burns resulting from reduced sensation.
58. Instruct client to use safety bars when getting in and out of tub or shower.	Prevents slipping and falls.
59. Caution client against use of bath oil in tub water.	Oil causes tub surfaces to become slippery, predisposing client to accidental falls.
60. Instruct client not to remain in tub longer than 20 min. Check on client every 5 min.	Prolonged exposure to warm water may cause vasodilation and pooling of blood, leading to lightheadedness or dizziness.
61. Return to bathroom when client signals, and knock before entering.	Provides privacy.
62. For client who is unsteady, drain tub of water before client attempts to get out of it. Place bath towel over client's shoulders.	Prevents accidental falls. Client may become chilled as water drains.
63. Assist client in getting out of tub as needed and assist with drying.	Moisture may cause excessive softening of skin and promote spread of infection.
64. Assist client as needed in donning clean gown or pajamas, slippers, and robe. (In home, client may don regular clothing.)	Maintains warmth to prevent chilling.
65. Assist client to room and help client assume comfortable position in bed or chair.	Maintains relaxation gained from bathing.
66. Cleanse tub or shower according to agency policy. Remove soiled linen and place in dirty linen bag. Discard disposable equipment in proper receptacle. Place "unoccupied" sign on bathroom door. Return supplies to storage area.	Prevents transmission of infection through soiled linen and moisture.
67. Wash hands.	Reduces transfer of microorganisms.

EVALUATION OF BATH TECHNIQUES

STEPS	RATIONALE
68. Observe client's behavior and ask if fatigue or discomfort is felt.	Determines tolerance to bathing activities.
69. Note areas on skin that were previously soiled or reddened or showed early signs of breakdown.	Techniques used during bathing should leave skin clean and clear.
70. Record type of bath and client's tolerance of bathing. Also note condition of skin and any significant findings such as reddened skin areas or joint or muscle pain. Record level of assistance required by client.	Timely documentation maintains accuracy of client's record. Condition of skin documents response to therapy such as turning and positioning.

Supplies for the bath include a shirt, a diaper (disposable or plain cloth), safety pins if using cloth diapers, a soft washcloth, cotton balls, a towel, and facial tissue. Plain water is used for bathing to minimize skin irritation from soap or oils. A mild soap (for example, Ivory) should be used only for soiled areas such as around the anus. Optional supplies include alcohol for cleansing the umbilical cord and petrolatum jelly to prevent diaper rash.

The nurse prepares a basin with water at 38° to 40.5° C (100° to 105° F) so that it feels comfortably warm when tested on the inside of the nurse's forearm. To prevent cooling, the nurse washes the infant's face, eyes, ears, and scalp before removing the shirt and diaper. The towel may also be kept over the infant for warming.

The nurse cleanses the infant's eyes and ears with clean, moistened cotton balls or a washcloth. The eyes are gently wiped from the inner to the outer canthus, using a clean cotton ball with each stroke or turning the cloth so that only a clean part touches the eyes. While washing the face, the nurse inspects the nares for encrusted secretions. Cotton-tipped swabs should not be used to cleanse the nares or ears because an infant may move suddenly, causing the swab to break and damage the eardrum or mucous membranes. A rolled wisp of dampened cotton or the twisted end of the washcloth works well for cleansing the external ear canal and pinna.

The infant's scalp can be cleansed by wiping off any secretions with a washcloth. However, if shampooing is necessary, the nurse secures the baby's head with one hand and positions it over the bath basin. A mild soap is best for shampooing. The nurse rinses the scalp by pouring water from a small cup or container over the infant's head into the basin. Thorough drying is necessary to prevent evaporative heat loss.

The nurse then undresses the infant for the remainder of the bath. The towel is again used to drape areas not being washed. Keeping the infant covered may be difficult because infants often kick and twist. Because of the infant's sensitive skin, little rubbing should be done when cleansing. However, the nurse gives special attention to the folds in the neck, axillae, and creases at joints. For example, neck creases often collect regurgitated food, which may cause a rash. The umbilical cord should be cleansed with mild soap and water and dried thoroughly. Alcohol may be applied to the umbilicus to help dry it and to reduce chances of infection. Then the nurse dresses the infant in a shirt.

The nurse bathes the infant's buttocks and genitalia last. For a girl, it is important to retract the labia fully to remove the vernix caseosa after it has dried.

If the vernix caseosa is thick and adherent, the nurse may choose to remove it gradually during successive diaper changes to avoid causing unnecessary irritation during one bath. The vulva is cleansed from front to back to prevent the spread of microorganisms from the anal area to the urethra. This technique should be explained to the parents.

In male infants, the nurse washes carefully around the penis and scrotum. Noncircumcised infants should not have the foreskin retracted because it is often too tight. Later, after the foreskin loosens, the nurse should teach the parents to retract the foreskin, cleanse the area, and return the foreskin to its position. No special care is required around a circumcised penis. The nurse wipes off any blood with a clean cotton ball or washcloth. The original petrolatum jelly dressing remains in place for only a day.

The nurse bathes the buttocks last. Fecal material can be removed with facial tissue. Using mild soap helps ensure thorough cleansing of the anal area. After thorough drying, the application of a thin layer of petrolatum jelly or ointment helps retain skin moisture and prevents diaper rash.

After the bath the nurse applies a clean diaper, which should fit snugly around the thighs and abdomen to prevent leakage of urine. If the child is circumcised, the diaper should fit loosely to prevent friction against the penis. The diaper should always be below the umbilical site until it is completely healed. The nurse fastens the diaper with the back overlapping the front to permit full hip flexion.

TUB BATH. Infants can be given a tub bath after the umbilicus has healed. Supplies for the tub bath are the same as those for a sponge bath. Supplies should be within easy reach. The face, neck, ears, eyes, and scalp are washed before the infant is undressed and immersed in the tub. The nurse lowers infants slowly into the tub to avoid startling them. The child must always be held firmly with one hand. A child is never left unattended in the bathinette. Often infants enjoy the sensation of being immersed in water, and older infants may enjoy playing during the bath. Body creases are much easier to cleanse and rinse in a tub bath. After the bath, the nurse wraps the infant completely in a towel and gently pats the infant dry, paying special attention to body creases. Application of body lotion to dry, cracked areas of the skin is soothing and provides important tactile stimulation.

Perineal Care

Usually **perineal care** ("pericare") is part of the complete bed bath (Procedure 34-3 on p. 1036). Clients most in need of meticulous perineal care are those at greatest risk for acquiring an infection (for

Perineal Care

STEPS

RATIONALE

1. Identify clients at risk for developing infection of genitalia, urinary tract, or reproductive tract (e.g., presence of indwelling catheter, fecal incontinence, or surgical incision).

Secretions that accumulate on surface of skin around female and male genitalia act as reservoir for infection. Traumatized tissues provide route for introduction of infectious organisms.

2. Explain procedure and purpose to client.

Helps minimize anxiety during procedure that is often embarrassing to you and client.

3. Prepare necessary equipment and supplies:
   a. Washbasin
   b. Soap dish with soap
   c. Two or three washcloths
   d. Bath towel
   e. Bath blanket
   f. Waterproof pad or bedpan
   g. Toilet tissue
   h. Disposable gloves
   Additional supplies when pericare is given during times other than a bath:
   a. Cotton balls or swabs
   b. Solution bottle or container filled with warm water or prescribed rinsing solution
   c. Waterproof bag

Used when administering a bed bath.

Used for draping client.
Prevents soiling of bed linen.

Prevents contact with microorganisms in body secretions.

Used for cleansing menstruating women or around indwelling catheters.

For disposal of cotton balls.

4. Assemble supplies at bedside.

Ensures orderly procedure.

5. Wash hands

Reduces transmission of organisms.

6. Pull curtain around bed or close room door. Raise bed to comfortable working position.

Maintains client's privacy. Facilitates good body mechanics.

7. Lower side rail and assist client in assuming dorsal recumbent (female) or supine (male) position.

Provides easy access to genitalia.

8. Apply gloves.

Decreases contact with bodily secretions.

9. Position waterproof pad under client's buttocks or place bedpan under client.

Prevents bed linen from becoming wet.

10. Fold top bed linen down toward foot of bed and raise client's gown up above genital area.

Exposes perineal area for easy accessibility.

11. "Diamond" drape client by placing bath blanket with one corner between client's legs, one corner pointing toward each side of bed, and one corner over chest. Tuck side corners around legs and under hips (see illustrations).

Prevents unnecessary exposure of body parts and maintains client's warmth and comfort.

12. Raise side rail. Fill washbasin with water that is approximately 41°-43° C (105°-109.4° F).

Prevents client from accidentally falling. Proper water temperature prevents burns to perineum.

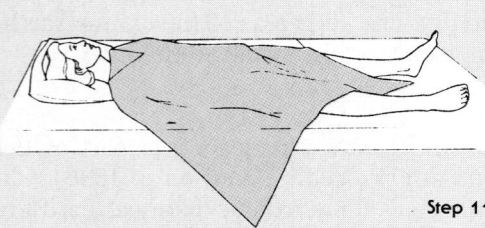

Step 11

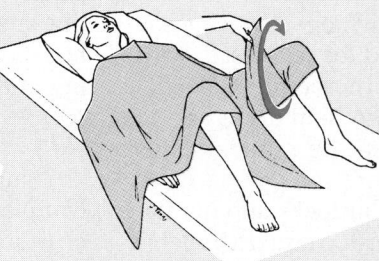

Illustrations from Sorrentino SA: *Mosby's textbook for nursing assistants*, ed 3, St Louis, 1992, Mosby–Year Book.

STEPS	RATIONALE
13. Place washbasin and toilet tissue on overbed table. Place washcloths in basin.	Equipment placed within reach prevents accidental spills.
14. Female perineal care:	
a. Lower side rail and help client flex her knees and spread legs apart (lithotomy position).	Provides full exposure of female genitalia.
b. Fold lower corner of bath blanket up between client's legs onto abdomen.	Keeping client draped until procedure begins minimizes anxiety.
c. Wash and dry client's upper thighs.	Buildup of perineal secretions can soil surrounding skin surfaces.
d. Wash labia majora. Then use nondominant hand to gently retract labia from thigh; with dominant hand, wash carefully in skinfolds. Wipe in direction from perineum to rectum. Repeat on opposite side, using separate section of washcloth. Rinse and dry area thoroughly.	Skinfolds may contain body secretions that harbor microorganisms. Wiping from perineum to rectum reduces chance of transmitting fecal organisms to urinary meatus.
e. Separate labia with nondominant hand to expose urethral meatus and vaginal orifice. With dominant hand, wash downward from pubic area toward rectum in one smooth stroke (see illustration). Use separate section of cloth for each stroke. Cleanse thoroughly around labia minora, clitoris, and vaginal orifice.	Cleansing method reduces transfer of microorganisms to urinary meatus. (For menstruating women or clients with indwelling urinary catheters, cleanse with cotton balls.)
f. If client is on bedpan, pour warm water over perineal area.	Rinsing removes soap and microorganisms more effectively than wiping.
g. Dry perineal area throughly.	Retained moisture harbors microorganisms.
h. Fold lower corner of bath blanket back between client's legs and over perineum. Ask client to lower legs and assume side-lying position for anal care (see Step 16).	Side-lying position provides access to anal area for cleansing.
15. Male perineal care:	
a. Lower side rail.	
b. Lower top corner of bath blanket below client's perineum. Gently raise penis and place bath towel underneath.	Towel prevents moisture from collecting in inguinal area.
c. Gently grasp shaft of penis. If client is uncircumcised, retract foreskin. If client has erection, defer procedure until later.	Gentle handling reduces chance of client having erection. Secretions capable of harboring microorganisms collect under foreskin.
d. Wash tip of penis at urethral meatus first. Using circular motion, cleanse from meatus outward and down the shaft. Discard washcloth and repeat with clean cloth until penis is clean. Rinse and dry gently (see illustration).	Direction of cleansing moves from area of least contamination to area of most contamination, preventing microorganisms from entering urethra.

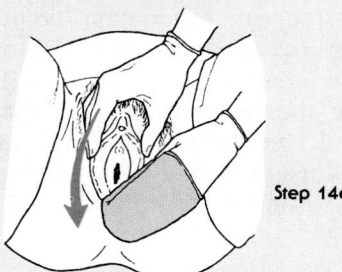

Step 14e

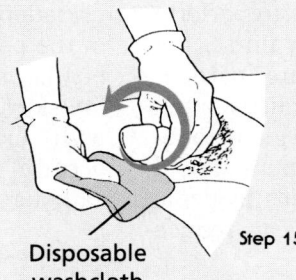

Disposable
washcloth

Step 15d

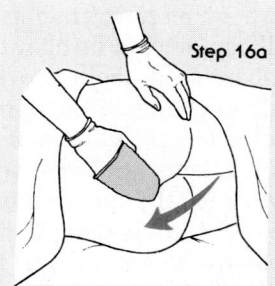

Step 16a

Perineal Care

STEPS	RATIONALE
e. Return foreskin to its natural position.	Tightening of foreskin around shaft of penis can cause local edema and discomfort.
f. Wash shaft of penis with gentle but firm downward strokes. Pay special attention to underlying surface of penis.	Vigorous massage of penis can lead to erection, which can cause embarrassment for client and you. Underlying surface of penis may have greater accumulation of secretions.
g. Rinse and dry penis thoroughly. Instruct client to spread legs slightly.	Abduction of legs provides easier access to scrotal tissues.
h. Gently cleanse scrotum. Lift it carefully and wash underlying surface of scrotum. Rinse and dry.	Pressure on scrotal tissues can be very painful to client. Secretions collect between skinfolds. Underlying surface of scrotum may develop pressure sores.
i. Fold bath blanket back over perineum and assist client in turning to side-lying position for anal care.	Draping promotes comfort and minimizes anxiety. Side-lying position provides access to anal area.
16. Anal care:	
a. Cleanse anal area by first wiping off fecal material with toilet tissue. Wash by wiping from genitalia toward anus with one stroke. Discard washcloth. Repeat with clean cloth until skin is clear of fecal material (see illustration on p. 1037).	Fecal material contains large numbers of microorganisms that can cause urinary tract infection, especially in women because vaginal opening and urinary meatus are in close proximity to anus.
b. Rinse area well and dry with bath towel.	Removes soap and microorganisms.
17. Remove disposable gloves and dispose in proper receptacle.	Moisture and body secretions on gloves can harbor microorganisms.
18. Assist client in assuming comfortable position and cover with sheet.	Client's comfort minimizes emotional stress of procedure.
19. Remove bath blanket and dispose of all soiled bed linen. Return unused equipment to storage area.	Reduces transmission of infection.
20. Raise side rail and lower bed to proper height. Return room to condition before procedure.	Prevents client from accidentally falling. Clean environment enhances client's comfort.
21. Wash hands.	Reduces transmission of infection.
22. Inspect surface of external genitalia and surrounding skin after cleansing.	Thick secretions may cover underlying skin lesions or areas of breakdown. Evaluation can determine need for additional therapy.
23. Record procedure and presence of any abnormal findings (e.g., discharge or condition of genitalia).	Ensures accurate and timely documentation of care.

example, clients who have in-dwelling urinary catheters), are recovering from rectal or genital surgery, or have undergone childbirth. A client able to perform self-care should be allowed to do so. Many nurses are embarrassed about providing perineal care, particularly to clients of the opposite sex. Male nurses often seek a female team member to provide hygiene to female clients, and vice versa. Embarrassment should not cause the nurse to overlook the client's hygienic needs. A professional, dignified attitude can reduce embarrassment and put the client at ease.

If a client performs self-care, various problems such as vaginal or urethral discharge, skin irritation, and unpleasant odors may go unnoticed. The nurse must be alert for complaints of burning during urination or localized soreness, excoriation, or pain in the perineum. The nurse also inspects the client's bed linen for signs of discharge. Clients most at risk for skin breakdown in the perineal area are those with urinary or fecal incontinence, rectal and perineal surgical dressings, and in-dwelling urinary catheters.

Backrub

A backrub or back massage usually follows the client's bath (Procedure 34-4). It promotes relaxation,

Administering a Backrub

STEPS	RATIONALE
1. Identify factors or conditions such as rib or vertebral fractures, burns, or open wounds that contraindicate backrub.	Massage of sensitive tissues might lead to further tissue injury. Due to age-related skin changes, massage is not recommended in routine skin care for older adult (Rousseau, 1988).
2. For clients with history of hypertension or dysrhythmias, assess pulse and blood pressure.	Massage may cause autonomic nervous system stimulation that induces changes in heart rate and blood pressure. Research has not shown consistent relationships between human touch and cardiac response of those being touched (Weiss, 1986).
3. Explain procedure and desired position to client.	Helps promote relaxation.
4. Prepare necessary equipment and supplies: a. Bath blanket b. Bath towel c. Skin application (lotion, alcohol, powder)	Lotion lubricates skin and prevents friction during massage. Alcohol cools skin but has drying effect. Powder reduces friction during massage.
5. Adjust bed to high, comfortable position.	Ensures proper body mechanics and prevents strain on back muscles.
6. Adjust light, temperature, and sound within room.	Environmental distractions can prevent client from relaxing.
7. Lower side rail and help client assume prone or side-lying (Sims') position with back toward you. Close curtain around bed.	Position makes it easier to apply necessary pressure to back muscles. Privacy promotes relaxation.
8. Expose client's back, shoulders, upper arms, and buttocks. Cover remainder of body with bath blanket. Lay towel alongside client's back.	Prevents unnecessary exposure of body parts and prevents excess lotion from touching linens.
9. Wash your hands in warm water. Warm lotion in your hands or by placing container under warm water. Place small amount of lotion in hands.	Cold causes muscle tension.
10. Explain to client that lotion will feel cool and wet.	Warning client reduces startled response.
11. Apply hands first to sacral area, massaging in circular motion. Stroke upward from buttocks to shoulders. Massage over scapulae with smooth, firm stroke. Continue in one smooth stroke to upper arms and laterally along sides of back down to iliac crests. Do not allow your hands to leave client's skin. Continue massage pattern for 3 min.	Gentle, firm pressure applied to all muscle groups promotes relaxation. Continuous contact with skin's surface is soothing and stimulates circulation to tissues.
12. Knead skin by grasping tissue between your thumb and fingers. Knead upward along one side of spine from buttocks to shoulders and around nape of neck. Knead or stroke downward toward sacrum. Repeat along other side of back.	Kneading increases circulation to muscles. Continuous motion is soothing and relieves muscle tension.
13. End massage with long stroking movements and tell client you are ending massage.	Long stroking is most soothing of massage movements.
14. If lying on side, ask client to turn to opposite side, and massage other hip.	

Administering a Backrub

STEPS	RATIONALE
15. Wipe excess lubricant from client's back with bath towel. Retie gown or assist with pajamas. Help client to comfortable position. Open curtain and raise side rails as needed.	Excess lotion can be irritant. Comfortable position enhances backrub's effects.
16. Dispose of soiled towel and wash hands.	Promotes infection control.
17. Ask client about comfort. Note any areas of muscle pain or tension.	Degree of relief gained depends on length of massage, client's ability to relax, and degree of discomfort before massage.
18. Reassess pulse and blood pressure.	Gentle back massage may increase heart rate and systolic blood pressure.
19. Record response to massage and condition of skin.	Describes response to therapy.

 Sample Evaluation of Interventions for Impaired Skin Integrity

Goals	Evaluative Measures	Expected Outcomes
Skin will remain intact and free of odors.	Inspect surfaces of skin after cleansing. Inspect existing lesions for cleanliness and reduction in drainage. Take time to note presence of obvious body odors.	Skin will be intact, warm, smooth, soft, and well hydrated. Areas of skin impairment will show signs of healing (e.g., reduced drainage, inflammation). Odors will be reduced or eliminated.
Joint ROM will be maintained.	Exercise joint through ROM during bathing of body part.	Joints will move within same ROM as client's baseline. Normal joints will move freely without discomfort.
Client will achieve sense of comfort and well-being.	Question client about sense of comfort. Observe client's body movements or gestures.	Client will verbalize less discomfort and will indicate sense of relaxation. Client will be calm. Body movements will be purposeful and relaxed. Client will express positive statements about well-being.
Client will participate in and understand methods of skin care.	Observe client's initiation of and assistance with bathing activities. Observe if client asks questions regarding self-care measures. Ask client to explain proper technique to follow in bathing.	Client will initiate hygiene measures or participate in bathing with nurse's assistance. Client will describe proper hygienic methods to maintain skin integrity.

relieves muscular tension, and stimulates skin circulation. During the backrub, the nurse can assess the condition of the client's skin.

An effective backrub takes 3 to 5 minutes. The nurse should first inquire whether the client would like a backrub because some clients dislike the physical contact. The nurse should also consult the client's medical record for any backrub contraindications before offering a massage to the client (Procedure 34-4).

Evaluation

During and at the completion of the client's bathing and skin care, the nurse evaluates the success of the interventions. For each goal established in the care plan, the nurse evaluates the accomplishment of expected outcomes. Evaluation involves physical assessment measures, as well as questions directed toward the client (see evaluation box).

CARE OF THE FEET AND NAILS

The feet and nails often require special attention to prevent infection, odors, and injury to tissues. Often, people are unaware of foot or nail problems until pain or discomfort occurs. Problems result from abuse or poor care of the feet and hands such as biting nails or trimming them improperly, exposure to harsh chemicals, and wearing poorly fitted shoes.

The feet are important to physical and emotional health. Foot pain can cause a person to walk differently, causing strain on different muscle groups. Many people must walk or stand comfortably to perform their jobs effectively.

Assessment

Physical Assessment

Assessment of the feet involves a thorough examination of all skin surfaces; the shape, size, and number of toes; the shape of the foot; and the condition of the toenails. The nurse inspects for lesions and notes whether areas of dryness, inflammation, or cracking are present. The areas between the toes should be carefully checked. The heels, soles, and sides of the feet are prone to irritation from poorly fitted shoes. The toes are normally straight and flat. The feet should be in straight alignment with the ankle and tibia. Table 34-3 on p. 1042 reviews common types of foot and nail problems.

The nurse assesses the client's gait. Painful feet disorders can cause limping or an unnatural gait. The nurse asks whether the client has discomfort of the feet and determines factors that aggravate the pain. Foot problems may result from bone or muscular alterations rather than skin disorders.

Clients with peripheral vascular disease, such as those with diabetes, should be assessed for the adequacy of circulation to the feet. Chapter 20 describes the signs of arterial and venous insufficiency. Palpation of the dorsalis pedis and posterior tibial pulses indicates whether adequate blood flow is reaching peripheral tissues. Edema and changes in skin color, texture, and temperature can indicate that the client is in need of special hygienic care.

If a client is also diabetic the nurse should also check for **neuropathy,** which is a degeneration of the peripheral nerves characterized by a loss in sensation. This is done by checking the client's sensation to light touch, pin prick, and temperature (see Chapter 20). The nails of the feet and hands are assessed using inspection and palpation.

A normal healthy nail is transparent, smooth, and convex with pink nail beds and translucent white tips. In African Americans, a brown or black pigmentation is normally present between the nail and nail base. The nail is surrounded by a cuticle, which slowly grows over the nail and must be regularly pushed back. The skin around the nail beds and cuticles should be smooth and without inflammation. The nurse asks women whether they frequently polish their nails and use polish remover because chemicals in these products cause excessive nail dryness. Disease can change the shape and curvature of nails (see Chapter 20). Inflammatory lesions of the nail bed cause the formation of thickened, horny nails, which can separate from the nail bed.

Developmental Factors

The nurse's assessment considers the special needs of older adults, who often are unable to maintain proper foot and nail care. Noting the presence of poor vision, hand tremors, obesity, or the inability to bend over reveals the level of assistance required by the older client. If foot or nail problems stay unresolved, an older adult can easily become disabled. The nurse also assesses common problems of older adulthood. Changes occur with years of continuous stress and the degenerative diseases that accompany older adulthood. A thorough nursing assessment should integrate these changes with the symptoms of chronic diseases and treatable conditions.

Older adults often have dry feet because of a decrease in sebaceous gland secretion, dehydration of epidermal cells, and poor condition of footwear. Fissures that result in itching commonly develop. Common foot problems of the older adult include heel pain; metatarsalgia (pain beneath the metatarsal head); hammer toes and clawtoes (flexion contractures); bunions, corns, and calluses; arthritis; loss of sensation; and nail pathological conditions (Osterman, Stuck, 1990). Fungal infections commonly occur under toenails, causing dirty yellow streaks or total discoloration. The nails can also become opaque, scaly, and hypertrophied.

If an older client has chronic foot problems, the nurse should assess the type of home remedies used.

TABLE 34-3 Common Foot and Nail Problems		
Characteristics	Implications	Interventions
CALLUS		
Thickened portion of epidermis consists of mass of horny, keratotic cells. Callus is usually flat, painless, and found on undersurface of foot or on palm of hand. Problem is caused by local friction or pressure.	Condition may cause discomfort when wearing tight shoes.	Nurse advises client to wear gloves when using tools or objects that may create friction on palmar surfaces. Nurse encourages client to wear comfortable shoes. Nurse soaks callus in warm water and Epsom salts to soften cell layers. Nurse uses pumice stone to remove callus after it softens. Applications of creams or lotions can reduce reformation.
CORNS		
Keratosis is caused by friction and pressure from shoes. It is seen mainly on toes, over bony prominence. Corn is usually cone shaped, round, and raised.	Conical shape compresses underlying dermis, making it thin and tender. Pain is aggravated when tight shoes are worn. Tissue can become attached to bone if allowed to grow. Client may suffer alteration in gait resulting from pain.	Surgical removal may be necessary, depending on severity of pain and size of corn. Nurse avoid use of oval corn pads, which increase pressure on toes and reduce circulation.
PLANTAR WARTS		
Fungating lesion appears on sole of foot and is caused by papilloma virus.	Warts may be contagious. They are painful and make walking difficult.	Treatment ordered by physician may include applications of salicylic acid, electrodesiccation (burning with electrical spark), or freezing with solid carbon dioxide.
ATHLETE'S FOOT (TINEA PEDIS)		
Athlete's foot is fungal infection of foot; scaliness and cracking of skin occurs between toes and on soles of feet. Small blister containing fluid may appear. Problem is apparently induced by wearing of constricting footwear.	Athlete's foot can spread to other body parts, especially hands. It is contagious and frequently recurs.	Feet should be well ventilated. Drying feet well after bathing and applying powder help prevent infection. Wearing of clean socks or stockings reduces incidence. Physician may order application of griseofulvin, miconazole, or tolnaftate.
INGROWN NAILS		
Toenail or fingernail grows inward into soft tissue around nail. Ingrown nail often results from improper nail trimming.	Ingrown nails can cause localized pain when pressure is applied.	Treatment is frequent hot soaks in antiseptic solution and removal of portion of nail that has grown into skin. Instruct client on proper nail-trimming techniques
RAM'S HORN NAILS		
Ram's horn nails are usually long curved nails.	Attempt by nurse to cut nails may result in damage to nail bed with risk of infection.	Nurse refers client to podiatrist.

TABLE 34-3   Common Foot and Nail Problems—cont'd

Characteristics	Implications	Interventions
PARONYCHIA		
Inflammation of tissue surrounding nail occurs after hangnail or other injury. It occurs in people who frequently have their hands in water and is common in diabetic clients.	Area can become infected.	Treatment is hot compresses or soaks and local application of antibiotic ointments. Paronychia can be prevented by careful manicuring.
FOOT ODORS		
Foot odors are result of excess perspiration promoting microorganism growth.	Condition may cause discomfort because of excess perspiration.	Frequent washing, use of foot deodorants and powders, and wearing clean footwear prevent or reduce problem.

Many over-the-counter preparations, such as those used to treat corns, can damage normal skin layers. Burns or ulcerations resulting from these products increase the risk of infection.

Footwear

The types of footwear worn can predispose clients to foot and nail problems. Children or young adults who frequently fail to wear socks may have excess perspiration that promotes fungal growth. Tight or poorly fitted shoes, socks, garters, or knee-high nylon stockings may cause certain skin lesions and interfere with circulation in the feet. The nurse also assesses whether clients wear clean footwear daily because repeated use of soiled footwear can lead to infection. Shoes should fit snugly, not tightly, and provide support for the arch of the foot. When the person stands, shoes should be at least ½ inch longer than the largest toe and wide enough to accommodate a weight-bearing foot. The widest part of the foot should match the widest part of the shoe (Graham, Morley, 1984).

Knowledge of Foot and Nail Care Practices

The nurse determines clients' knowledge about foot and nail care to assess educational needs. The nurse observes whether clients know how to cut nails or uses over-the-counter products for nail care and grooming. It is especially important to assess the knowledge of diabetic clients because they must inspect their feet daily. Because of vascular insufficiency and neuropathy, a diabetic is at risk for injury to the feet. Trauma to a diabetic's foot can easily lead to infection.

 ### Examples of Nursing Diagnoses Related to Foot and Nail Problems

> **NANDA-APPROVED NURSING DIAGNOSES**
>
> *Pain* related to:
> - Callus formation
> - Ingrown toenails
>
> *Impaired physical mobility* related to:
> - Painful foot lesion
>
> *Bathing/hygiene self-care deficit* related to:
> - Visual disturbance
> - Altered hand coordination
>
> *Impaired skin integrity* related to:
> - Impaired arterial perfusion
> - Improper nail-cutting practices
> - Friction of shoes
> - Injury to nails
>
> *High risk for impaired skin integrity* related to:
> - Impaired arterial perfusion
> - Poorly fitted footwear
>
> *High risk for infection* related to:
> - Broken or traumatized skin
>
> *Knowledge deficit about foot and nail care* related to:
> - Information misinterpretation
> - Lack of exposure to information

 ### Nursing Diagnosis

An assessment of the condition of a client's feet and nails reveals the presence of actual or potential health problems (see diagnoses box). The nature of a

Nail and Foot Care

STEPS	RATIONALE

1. Identify clients at risk for foot or nail problems, including the following:
   a. Older adults

   Changes in sensory and motor function with aging can impair self-care practices. Physiological changes of older adulthood alter condition of foot and nails.

   b. Clients with diabetes

   Vascular changes associated with diabetes can reduce blood flow to peripheral tissues.

   c. Clients with heart failure or renal disease

   These conditions can cause tissue edema and reduced blood flow to extremities.

   d. Clients who have had cerebrovascular accidents

   Residual paralysis or reduced sensation can cause abnormal walking patterns resulting in friction and pressure on feet.

2. Obtain physician's order for cutting nails if agency policy requires it.

   Client's skin may be accidentally cut. Certain clients are more at risk for infection, depending on medical condition.

3. Explain procedure to client, including fact that proper soaking requires several minutes.

   Client must be willing to place fingers and feet in basins for 10-20 min. Client may become anxious or fatigued.

4. Prepare necessary equipment and supplies:
   a. Washbasin
   b. Emesis basin
   c. Washcloth
   d. Bath or face towel
   e. Nail clippers
   f. Orange stick
   g. Emery board
   h. Body lotion
   i. Disposable bath mat
   j. Paper towels
   k. Disposable gloves (optional)

Step 15

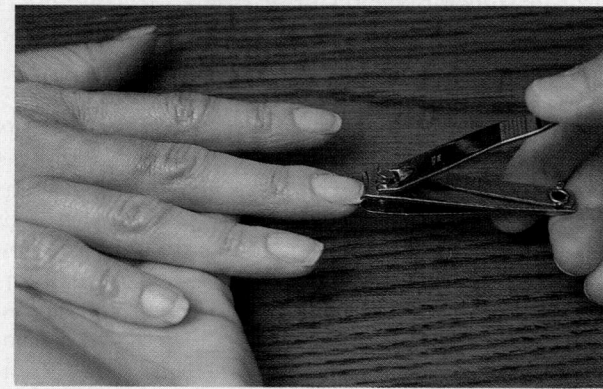

5. Wash hands. Arrange equipment on overbed table.

   Prevents delays. Reduces transmission of infection.

6. Pull curtain around bed or close room door (if desired).

   Maintaining client's privacy reduces anxiety.

7. Assist client to bedside chair if possible. Place disposable bath mat on floor under client's feet. Place call light within client's reach.

   Sitting in chair makes it easier to immerse feet in basin. Bath mat protects feet from exposure to soil or debris. Call light maintains safety of environment.

8. Fill wash basin with water at 43°-44° C (100°-110° F). Test temperature of water.

   Warm water softens nails and thickened epidermal cells, reduces inflammation of skin, and promotes local circulation. Proper water temperature prevents burns of skin.

9. Place basin on bath mat and help client place feet in basin.

   Clients with muscular weakness or tremors may have difficulty positioning feet.

10. Adjust overbed table to low position and place it over client's lap.

    Easy access prevents accidental spills.

11. Fill emesis basin with water at 43°-44° C (100°-110° F) and place basin on paper towels on overbed table.

    Warm water softens nails and thickened epidermal cells.

12. Instruct client to place fingers in emesis basin and place client's arms in comfortable position.

    Prolonged positioning can cause discomfort unless normal anatomical alignment is maintained.

STEPS	RATIONALE
13. Allow client's feet and fingernails to soak 10-20 min. Rewarm water in 10 min if needed.	Softening of corns, calluses, and cuticles ensures easy removal of dead cells and easy manipulation of cuticle.
14. Clean gently under fingernails with orange stick while fingers are immersed. Then remove emesis basin and dry fingers thoroughly.	Orange stick removes debris under nails that harbors microorganisms. Thorough drying impedes fungal growth and prevents maceration of tissues.
15. With nail clippers, clip fingernails straight across and even with tops of fingers (see illustration). Shape nails with emery board.	Cutting straight across prevents splitting of nail margins and formation of sharp nail spikes that can irritate lateral nail margins. Filing prevents cutting nail too close to nail bed.
16. Push cuticle back gently with orange stick.	Reduces incidence of inflamed cuticles.
17. Move overbed table away from client.	Provides easier access to feet.
18. Apply disposable gloves and scrub calloused areas of feet with washcloth.	Prevents transmission of fungal infection. Friction removes dead skin layers.
19. Clean gently under nails with orange stick. Remove feet from basin and dry them thoroughly.	Reduces chances of infection.
20. Clean and trim toenails using procedures in Steps 15-16.	
21. Apply lotion to feet and hands and then assist client back to bed and into comfortable position.	Lubricates dry skin by helping retain moisture.
22. Remove disposable gloves and dispose in receptacle. Clean and return equipment and supplies to proper place. Dispose of soiled linen in hamper. Wash hands.	Prevents transmission of infection.
23. Inspect nails and surrounding skin after soaking and nail trimming.	Evaluates condition of skin and allows you to note any rough nail edges remaining.
24. Record procedure and observations. Report breaks in skin.	Documents procedure and response. Abnormalities may pose risk of infection.

client's foot or nail problems directs the nurse to perform supportive or preventive nursing care.

 ## Planning

The nurse may provide foot and nail care during the bed bath or at a separate time in the day according to the client's preference. Many community health nurses visit clients at home solely to provide foot and nail care.

If a client's nails are extremely hard or if a client is unable to perform personal nail care, a podiatrist can provide nail care. The podiatrist is trained in the treatment of nail and foot problems. Goals for clients receiving nail and foot care include the following:

1. Skin and nail surfaces will remain intact and smooth.
2. Client will achieve sense of comfort and cleanliness.
3. Client will walk and bear weight normally.
4. Client will understand and perform methods for foot and nail care correctly.

 ## Implementation

Foot and nail care involves soaking to soften cuticles and layers of horny cells, thorough cleansing, drying, and proper trimming of nails. The nurse may provide the care in bed for an immobilized client or have the client sit in a chair (Procedure 34-5). The nurse must take time during the procedure to teach the client proper techniques for cleansing and nail trimming and provides tips on selecting proper footwear. By allowing the client to perform a part of foot and nail care, the nurse can stress principles related to promoting good circulation and preventing infection and tissue injury.

A diabetic client or one with peripheral vascular disease is at risk for foot and nail problems due to poor peripheral blood supply to the feet. In addition, sensation in the feet can become reduced. Trauma to a diabetic's foot can often go unnoticed. With a break in the skin, infection can easily develop as a result of poor circulation. The nurse can advise these clients to use the following guidelines:

1. Wash and soak the feet daily using lukewarm water. Thoroughly pat the feet dry, and dry well between the toes.
2. Do not cut corns or calluses or use commercial removers. Consult a physician or **podiatrist.**
3. If the feet tend to perspire, apply a bland foot powder. Wear shoes with porous uppers.
4. If dryness is noted along the feet or between the toes, apply lanolin, baby oil, or even corn oil and rub gently into the skin.
5. File the toenails straight across and square; do not use scissors or clippers. Consult a podiatrist as needed.
6. Do not use over-the-counter preparations to treat athlete's foot or ingrown toenails. Consult a physician or podiatrist.
7. Avoid wearing elastic stockings, knee-high hosiery, or constricting garters. Do not cross the legs. These impair circulation to the lower extremities.
8. Inspect the feet daily, including the tops and soles of the feet, the heels, and the area between the toes. Use a mirror to help inspect thoroughly.
9. Wear clean socks or stockings daily. Socks should be free of holes or darns that might cause pressure.
10. Do not walk barefoot.
11. Wear properly fitted shoes. The soles of shoes should be flexible and nonslipping. Lamb's wool can be used between toes that rub or overlap. Shoes should be sturdy, closed in, and not restrictive to the feet.
12. Exercise regularly to improve circulation to the lower extremities. Walk slowly and elevate, rotate, flex, and extend the feet at the ankles. Dangle the feet over the side of the bed 1 min, and then extend both legs and hold them parallel to the bed while lying supine for 1 min, and finally rest 1 min (Jordan, Nickerson, 1982).
13. Avoid applying hot-water bottles or heating pads to the feet. Use warm soaks or extra coverings instead.
14. Immediately wash minor cuts and dry them thoroughly. Only mild antiseptics (for example, neosporin ointment), should be applied to the skin. Avoid iodine or mercurochrome.
15. Contact a physician for treatment of cuts or lacerations.

 Evaluation

A client's response to nail and foot care is best evaluated over several days. If the client has any existing problems, it may take time for the alterations to improve. The nurse also instructs the client on ways to evaluate personal nail and foot care practices.

ORAL HYGIENE

The oral cavity is lined with mucous membrane continuous with the skin. The membrane is an epithelial tissue that lines and protects organs, secretes mucus to keep passageways of the digestive system moist and lubricated, and absorbs nutrients.

The oral, or **buccal,** cavity consists of the lips surrounding the opening of the mouth, the cheeks running along the side walls of the cavity, the tongue and its muscles, and the hard and soft palate forming the roof of the cavity. The oral mucosa is normally light pink and moist. The teeth are the organs of chewing, or **mastication.** A normal tooth consists of three parts: crown, neck, and root (Fig. 34-1). The periodontal membrane lies just below the gum margins and surrounds a tooth and holds it firmly in place. Healthy teeth appear white, smooth, shiny, and properly aligned.

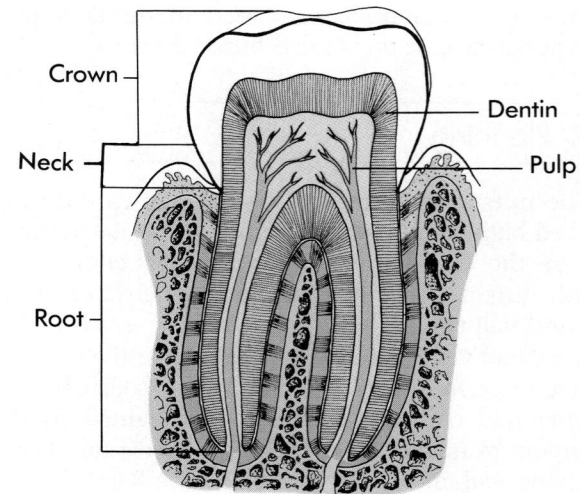

Fig. 34-1 A normal tooth.

Oral hygiene helps maintain the healthy state of the mouth, teeth, gums, and lips. Brushing cleanses the teeth of food particles, plaque, and bacteria; massages the gums; and relieves discomfort resulting from unpleasant odors and tastes. Flossing further helps remove plaque and tartar between teeth to reduce gum inflammation and infection. Complete oral hygiene gives a sense of well-being and thus can stimulate appetite.

The nurse's responsibilities in oral hygiene are maintenance and prevention. The nurse can help clients maintain good oral hygiene by teaching them correct techniques or by actually performing hygiene for weakened or disabled clients. Often the nurse must make referrals to a dentist for problems requiring special care. Education about common gum and tooth disorders and methods of prevention can motivate clients to follow good oral hygienic practices.

Assessment

Physical Assessment

Chapter 20 describes in detail the nurse's assessment of the client's lips, teeth, buccal mucosa, gums, palate, and tongue. The nurse inspects all of these areas carefully for color, hydration, texture, and lesions. Clients who do not follow regular oral-hygiene practices may have receding gum tissue, inflamed gums, discolored teeth (particularly along gum margins), dental caries, missing teeth, and halitosis. Localized pain is a common symptom of a gum disease and certain tooth disorders. An infection of the mouth may involve organisms such as *Treponema pallidum*, *Neisseria gonorrhoeae*, and Herpesvirus hominis.

Developmental Changes

Throughout a person's life span, physiological changes affect the condition and appearance of structures in the oral cavity (Table 34-4). As a person grows older, oral-hygiene practices change to further influence the teeth and mucosa. Age-related changes in the mouth, combined with chronic disease, physical disabilities, and prescribed medications that have side effects in the mouth, can result in poor oral care. Effects of inadequate care include dental caries and loss; periodontal disease; onset of systemic infections; and long-term effects on self-esteem, ability to eat, and the maintenance of relationships (Danielson, 1988). Assessment of a client's developmental level helps in determining the types of hygienic problems to expect.

TABLE 34-4 Physiological Development of the Mouth	
Developmental Level	Changes
Infant	Deciduous teeth begin to erupt at about 5 mo of age. Solid food can be taken in mouth at 5-6 mo. Chewing begins by 6-8 mo.
18 mo-6 yr	Twenty deciduous teeth are present. By age 6, "baby" teeth begin to fall out and are replaced by permanent teeth. By age 2, child can begin to brush teeth and learn hygienic practices from parents. Dental caries may become problem if dental hygiene is neglected.
6-12 yr	Deciduous teeth are replaced by permanent teeth. Permanent teeth are present by age 12 except second and third molars. Definite food preferences become apparent. Dental caries and irregularity in spacing of teeth are significant health problems.
12-18 yr	All permanent teeth are present. Dental hygienic practices tend to improve because of increased awareness of body image.
18-40 yr	Third molars appear. Good oral hygiene and nutrition practices are needed to avoid problems in later years.
Pregnancy	Changes in female sex hormones may exaggerate reaction to irritants in dental plaque, causing gingivitis and increased risk of severe periodontal disease.*
40-65 yr	Although loss of teeth, usually a result of periodontal disease, is declining, about half of people over age 55 have lost some or all of their teeth because of poor oral care. Root caries and oral cancer occur with higher frequency.
65 yr and over	Aging teeth become brittle, drier, and darker in color. Teeth become uneven, jagged, and fractured after years of crushing and grinding. Gums lose vascularity and tissue elasticity, causing dentures to fit poorly. Eating habits often change, and malnutrition may be a problem. Diminished taste sensitivity, thinning of mucosa, and decreased mass and strength of muscles of mastication also occur.

*Data from Deliefde B: *NZ Dent J* 80:41, 1984.

Hygienic Preferences and Practices

Because of the significant increase in the numbers of older adults and minorities, dental practice is facing new challenges. Data show a pattern of untreated dental caries in African and Mexican Americans and a prevalence of gingivitis in Spanish Americans (Ismail, Szpunar, 1990). Therefore it is important that the nurse assess the client's oral-hygiene practices to identify errors in technique, deficiencies in types of practices, and the client's knowledge level about dental care. Helpful questions include the following:

1. How often does the client brush the teeth?
2. What type of toothpaste or dentifrice is used?
3. Does the client have dentures? When and how are they cleansed?
4. Does the client use mouthwash or lemon-glycerin preparations?
5. Does the client floss? If so, how often?
6. When was the client's last dental visit? What were the results?
7. How often does the client visit a dentist?
8. Is water fluoridated?

Asking clients to demonstrate brushing and flossing techniques is useful when developing a teaching plan.

Risk Factors for Oral-Hygiene Problems

Certain clients are at risk for oral problems because of a lack of knowledge about oral hygiene, an inability to perform oral care, or an alteration in the integrity of teeth and mucosa resulting from disease or treatments (Table 34-5).

Common Oral Problems

It helps a nurse to be familiar with common oral problems. Each problem presents recognizable signs and symptoms and influences the type of hygiene teaching provided.

The two major types of problems are dental caries (cavities) and periodontal disease (**pyorrhea**). Dental caries is the most common oral problem of younger people. The development of cavities is a pathological process that involves the eventual destruction of the tooth enamel through decalcification. Decalcification is a result of an accumulation of mucin, carbohydrates, and lactic acid bacilli in the saliva normally found in the mouth, which forms a coating on the teeth called *plaque*. Plaque is transparent and adheres to the teeth, particularly near the base of the crown at the gum margins. The plaque prevents normal acid dilution and neutralization, preventing the dissolution of bacteria in the oral cavity. The acid eventually destroys the tooth enamel and in severe cases the pulp or inner spongy tissue of the tooth. A cavity first begins as a chalky white discoloration of the tooth. As the cavity advances, the tooth takes on a brown or black discoloration.

For people more than 35 years, the most common problem is pyorrhea. **Periodontal disease** is a long-term process involving infection and destruction of

---

TABLE 34-5 Risk Factors for Oral Problems

Type of Client	Risk Factors
Clients who are paralyzed, seriously ill, or have physical restrictions to upper extremities (e.g., cast or dressing)	Client lacks upper extremity strength or dexterity needed to perform oral hygiene
Unconscious, confused, combative, or depressed clients	Client is unable or unwilling to attend to personal hygiene needs
Diabetic clients	Client is prone to dryness of mouth, gingivitis, periodontal disease, and loss of teeth.
Clients who cannot take anything by mouth or are on fluid restrictions (see Chapter 39), have nasogastric tubes, receive continuous nasal oxygen, or are mouth-breathers	Client is prone to dehydration and drying of mucous membranes. Thick secretions develop on tongue and gums. Lips become cracked and reddened.
Clients undergoing radiation therapy	Radiation therapy causes soreness, mild erythema, swollen mucosa, dysphagia, dryness, taste changes, and possible oral infection.
Clients receiving chemotherapeutic drugs	Chemotherapeutic drugs cause ulcerations and inflammation of mucosa and possible oral infection.
Clients experiencing oral surgery, trauma to mouth, placement of oral endotracheal tubes or airways	Tissues in oral cavity become traumatized with swelling, ulcerations, inflammation, and possible bleeding.

the supporting teeth structures: the gingiva (gums), cementum, ligaments, and alveolar bone. Periodontal disease progresses in four stages (Levine, 1973):

1. Gingivitis or inflammation of the gums
2. Periodontitis
3. Acute necrotizing ulcerative gingivitis
4. Destruction of the tooth-supporting structures

Symptoms of periodontal disease include bleeding gums, swollen inflamed tissues, receding gumlines with the formation of gaps or pockets between the teeth and gums, and the eventual loss of teeth. If proper oral care is not maintained, dead bacteria, called *tartar,* can collect at the gumline. The tartar attacks the gums and fibers attached to the teeth, resulting in the loss of teeth. The best preventive measures are regular flossing and brushing.

Other oral problems include **stomatitis,** an inflammatory condition of the mouth resulting from contact with irritants such as tobacco or from vitamin deficiency, infection by bacteria, viruses, or fungi or use of chemotherapeutic drugs; **glossitis,** an inflammation of the tongue resulting from infectious disease or injury from a burn, bite, or other injury; and **gingivitis,** an inflammation of the gums usually resulting from poor oral hygiene or occurring as a sign of leukemia, vitamin deficiency, or diabetes mellitus.

Halitosis (bad breath) is a common problem of the oral cavity. It may be the result of poor oral hygiene, the ingestion of certain foods, or an infection or disease process. Proper oral hygiene can eliminate the odors unless the cause is a systemic condition such as liver disease or diabetes.

The nurse frequently encounters **cheilosis** in clients. The disorder involves cracking of the lips, especially at the angle of the mouth. Riboflavin deficiency, mouth breathing, and excess salivation may cause cheilosis. Lubrication of the lips helps retain moisture, and antifungal or antibacterial ointments discourage microorganism growth.

Oral malignancies appear as lumps or ulcers in or around the mouth. They are commonly found in clients with a history of pipe smoking or use of chewing tobacco. The most common site is at the base of the tongue. Early detection is vital to the success of treatment. Any sore in the mouth that does not heal should be brought to the attention of a dentist.

Nursing Diagnosis

Assessment may reveal actual or potential alterations in the integrity of mouth structures (see diagnoses box). Pertinent nursing diagnoses may reflect problems or complications resulting from alterations

Examples of Nursing Diagnoses Related to Oral-Hygiene Problems

NANDA-APPROVED NURSING DIAGNOSES

Altered oral mucous membrane related to:
- Oral trauma
- Restricted fluid intake
- Ineffective oral hygiene
- Trauma associated with chemotherapy or radiation therapy to head and neck

Pain related to:
- Gingivitis
- Loose teeth

Altered nutrition: less than body requirements related to:
- Ill-fitting dentures
- Gingivitis

Bathing/hygiene self-care deficit (oral) related to:
- Altered level of consciousness
- Upper extremity weakness

Body-image disturbance related to:
- Halitosis
- Absence of teeth

Knowledge deficit about oral-hygiene related to:
- Misunderstanding of hygienic practices

High risk for infection related to:
- Oral mucosa trauma

of the oral cavity. The nurse's findings may also reveal a client's need for assistance with hygienic care (see diagnostic process box on p. 1050).

Planning

Developing a care plan for clients in need of oral hygiene involves considering the client's personal preferences, emotional status, and physical capabilities. The nurse must establish a good relationship with the client to assist with oral-hygiene practices. Some clients are very sensitive about the condition of their mouths and are reluctant to let someone else care for them. In many cases, clients are also unaware that they are at risk for serious dental and periodontal disease and thus require extensive education (see care plan on p. 1050). Goals for clients in need of oral hygiene include the following:

1. Oral mucosa will be intact and well hydrated.
2. Client will be able to independently perform correct oral-hygiene care.
3. Client will achieve sense of comfort.
4. Client will understand oral-hygiene practices.

Sample Nursing Diagnostic Process for Oral Hygiene

Assessment Activities	Defining Characteristics	Nursing Diagnosis
Ask if client has pain, burning, irritation. Ask if client has had a change in tolerance to foods (hot or cold, acidic or highly seasoned). Ask if client has chewing difficulties. Check for proper-fitting dentures. Inspect oral cavity for redness, dryness, lesions, or ulcers and bleeding. Observe client's energy level. Note client's breath for mouth odor.	Coated tongue Xerostomia Stomatitis Oral lesions or ulcers Oral pain or discomfort Lack of or decreased salivation Halitosis Hyperemia	*Altered oral mucous membranes* related to radiation of oral cavity

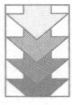

Sample Nursing Care Plan for Altered Oral Mucous Membranes

Nursing diagnosis: *Altered oral mucous membrane* related to radiation of oral cavity
Definition: Altered oral mucous membrane is the state in which an individual experiences disruptions in the tissue layers of the oral cavity (Kim, McFarland, McLane, 1991).

Goals	Expected Outcomes	Interventions	Rationale
Mucosa will be intact and well hydrated at time of discharge. Client will independently perform oral hygiene correctly by 9/12.	Mucosa, tongue, and lips will be pink, moist, and intact. Inflammation, crusts, lesions, and hard debris will remain absent. Infection will be absent. Client will verbalize comfort and feeling of oral cleanliness. Client will swallow and talk without discomfort.	Establish mouth-care regimen after meals and at bedtime: ■ Brush with soft toothbrush using horizontal strokes. ■ Rinse with warm salt or baking soda solution (½ tsp to 1 pt of water). ■ Floss with unwaxed dental floss 2 times a day. Avoid vigorous flossing near gumline.	Consistent brushing improves gingival tissue, removes debris, and results in plaque control (Kahn, 1986). Soft toothbrush with horizontal strokes helps protect delicate gingival tissue and prevent bleeding (Crosby, 1989). Rinsing dilutes oral acids, removes debris, and helps relieve dry mouth (xerostomia) that occurs with therapy-induced drop in saliva production (Greifzu, Radjeski, Winnick, 1990). Soda and salt solutions promote healing and aid in formation of granulation tissue. They act as astringent and may repress bacterial growth (Pettigrew, 1989). Systematic flossing removes decay-producing bacteria growing on tooth surfaces and near gumline (Kahn, 1986). Using unwaxed floss and avoiding vigorous flossing prevent bleeding (Greifzu, Radjesk, Winnick, 1990).

Implementation

Oral Hygiene

Good oral hygiene requires preventive and therapeutic measures. Proper care prevents oral disease and tooth destruction. Clients in hospitals or long-term care facilities often do not receive the aggressive care they need. Oral care must be provided on a regular daily basis. The frequency of hygienic measures depends on the condition of the client's oral cavity.

Brushing, flossing, and irrigation are necessary for proper cleansing. Clients also benefit from a proper diet, which excludes foods promoting plaque formation and tooth decay and promotes healthy periodontal structures. Clients of all ages should have a dental checkup at least every 6 months.

Diet

To prevent tooth decay, clients may have to change their eating habits, reducing the intake of carbohydrates, especially sweet snacks between meals. Sweet or starchy food adheres to tooth surfaces. After eating sweets, a client should brush within 30 minutes to reduce the action of plaque. Eating acid-containing fruits (for example, apples and fibrous foods such as fresh vegetables) also reduces plaque. The acidic quality of fruits eliminates bacteria that form on teeth. A well-balanced diet ensures the integrity of oral tissues.

For pregnant women, appropriate nutrients are essential for development of primary teeth in the fetus. The recommended amount of daily calcium intake is 1200 mg for the pregnant adult and 1600 mg for the pregnant adolescent (Neeson, May, 1986). Four to six cups of milk a day meet the calcium requirement.

Brushing

Thorough brushing of the teeth at least 4 times a day (after meals and at bedtime) is basic to an effective oral-hygiene program. A toothbrush should have a straight handle and a brush small enough to reach all areas of the mouth. An older adult with reduced dexterity and grip may require and enlarged toothbrush handle that provides an easier grip. This can be accomplished by piercing a soft rubber ball and pushing the brush handle through or by gluing a short piece of plastic tubing around the handle. An even, rounded brushing surface with soft, multitufted, nylon bristles is best. Rounded soft bristles stimulate the gums without causing abrasion and bleeding. All tooth surfaces—inner, outer, and chewing should be brushed thoroughly. Electric toothbrushes may be used, but the nurse must check for

any electrical hazards. Unflavored oral care sponges are used with clients unable to tolerate brushing because of oral trauma or bleeding tendencies.

A fluoride toothpaste is preferred for brushing teeth. Most toothpastes are pleasant tasting. Lemon-glycerin sponges can have harmful effects on teeth and mucosa. Glycerin has an astringent effect, drying and shrinking gums and mucous membranes. The lemon, if used extensively, changes the natural pH of the oral cavity, exhausts the salivary reflex through overstimulation, and can erode tooth enamel (Pettigrew, 1989). Because swabbing fails to cleanse teeth adequately, plaque accumulates around the base of the teeth. The glycerin provides nourishment for bacteria. A swab containing an aqueous solution of sorbitol, sodium, carboxymethylcellulose, and electrolytes has been shown effective in treating dry mouth. Moi-Stir is a salivary supplement that improves moisture and texture of the tongue and mucous membranes (Poland, 1987).

Whether a brush or sponge is used, thorough rinsing after brushing is important to remove dislodged food particles and excess toothpaste. Some people enjoy using mouthwash for its pleasant taste. Used over a long period, however, mouthwash dries mucosa.

When teaching clients about mouth care, the nurse reminds them not to share toothbrushes at home and not to drink directly from a bottle of mouthwash. Cross-contamination occurs easily. The use of disclosure tablets or drops to stain the plaque that collects at the gumline can be useful for showing clients how effectively they brush.

The amount of assistance needed by the client in brushing the teeth may vary. Many clients can perform their own oral care and should be encouraged to do so. The nurse observes the client to be sure proper techniques are used. Other clients need total assistance with hygiene.

Special Oral Hygiene

Some clients require special oral-hygiene methods because of their level of dependence on the nurse or the presence of oral mucosa problems.

UNCONSCIOUS CLIENTS. These clients are susceptible to drying of mucosa-thickened salivary secretions because they are unable to eat or drink, frequently breathe through the mouth, and often receive oxygen therapy. The unconscious client also cannot swallow salivary secretions that accumulate in the mouth. These secretions often contain gram-negative bacteria that can cause pneumonia if aspirated into the lungs. Therefore the nurse must protect the client from choking and aspirating. Procedure 34-6 on p. 1052 describes mouth care for debilitated clients.

Performing Mouth Care for the Unconscious or Debilitated Client

STEPS	RATIONALE
1. Assess for presence of gag reflex. Position client in Sims' or side-lying position with head turned well toward dependent side.	Reveals client's risk for aspiration. Allows secretions to drain from mouth instead of collecting in back of pharynx and prevents aspiration.
2. Explain procedure to client.	Unconscious client may retain ability to hear.
3. Prepare necessary equipment and supplies:	
a. Antiinfective solution (e.g., hydrogen peroxide diluted in equal parts of water)	Loosens encrustations and acts as antiinfective.
b. Sponge toothbrush or tongue blade wrapped in single layer of gauze; small toothbrush	Brush cleans teeth most effectively. Sponge or swab stimulates and cleans gums and mucosa.
c. Padded tongue blade	Keeps mouth open and teeth separated during procedure without traumatizing oral structures.
d. Face towel	
e. Emesis basin	
f. Paper towels	
g. Water glass with cool water	
h. Petrolatum jelly	Lubricates lips.
i. Portable suction machine (optional) with suction catheter	Removes retained oral secretions while oral cavity is cleansed.
j. Disposable gloves	Oral cavity contains highly infectious microorganisms.
4. Wash hands and apply disposable gloves.	Reduces transfer of miroorganisms.
5. Place paper towels on overbed table and arrange equipment. Turn on suction machine and connect tubing to suction catheter.	Prevents soiling of table top. Equipment prepared in advance ensures smooth, safe procedure.
6. Pull curtain around bed or close room door.	Provides privacy.
7. Raise bed to highest horizontal level; lower side rail.	Use of good body mechanics with bed in high position prevents injury to you and client.
8. Bring client close to side of bed and near you; be sure client's head is turned toward mattress.	Proper positioning of head prevents aspiration.
9. Place towel under client's face and emesis basin under chin.	Prevents soiling of bed linen.
10. Carefully retract client's upper and lower teeth with padded tongue blade by inserting blade quickly but gently between the back molars. Insert when client is relaxed, if possible.	Prevents client from biting down on fingers and provides access to oral cavity.
11. Clean mouth using brush or tongue blade moistened with peroxide and water. Have second nurse suction as secretions accumulate during cleansing. Clean chewing and inner tooth surfaces first (see illustration). Clean outer tooth surfaces. Swab roof of mouth and inside cheeks. Gently swab or brush tongue but avoid stimulating gag reflex (if present). Moisten clean swab or toothette with water to rinse. Repeat rinse several times. Suction any remaining secretions.	Brushing action removes food particles between teeth and along chewing surfaces. Swabbing helps remove secretions and encrustations from mucosa and moistens mucosa. Suction removes secretions and fluid that can collect in posterior pharynx. Repeated rinsing removes loose debris and peroxide that can be irritating to mucosa.
12. Apply thin layer of petrolatum jelly to lips (see illustration).	Lubricates lips to prevent drying and cracking.
13. Explain that procedure is completed.	Provides meaningful stimulation to unconscious or less responsive client.
14. Remove gloves and dispose in proper receptacle.	Prevents transmission of microorganisms.

STEPS	RATIONALE
15. Reposition client comfortably, raise side rail, and return bed to original position.	Maintains client's comfort and safety.
16. Clean equipment and return to its proper place. Place soiled linen in proper receptacle.	Proper disposal of soiled equipment prevents spread of infection.
17. Wash hands.	Reduces transmission of microorganisms.
18. Inspect oral cavity.	Determines efficacy of cleansing. After thick secretions are removed, underlying inflammation or lesions may be revealed.
19. Record procedure, including pertinent observation (e.g., bleeding gums, dry mucosa, ulcerations, or crusts on tongue) and report any unusual findings to nurse in charge or physician.	Documents response of client to nursing therapy. Bleeding may indicate more serious systemic problems. Lesions of oral cavity can be cancerous.

Step 12

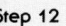

Step 11

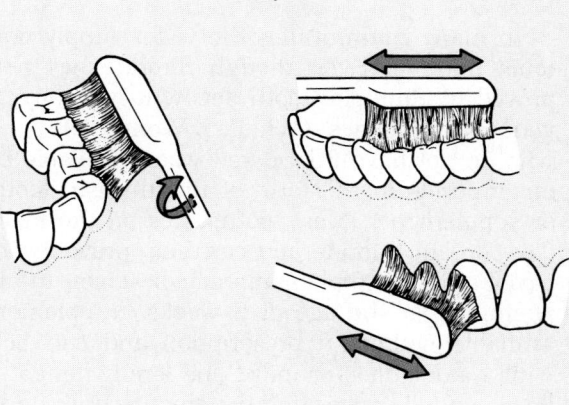

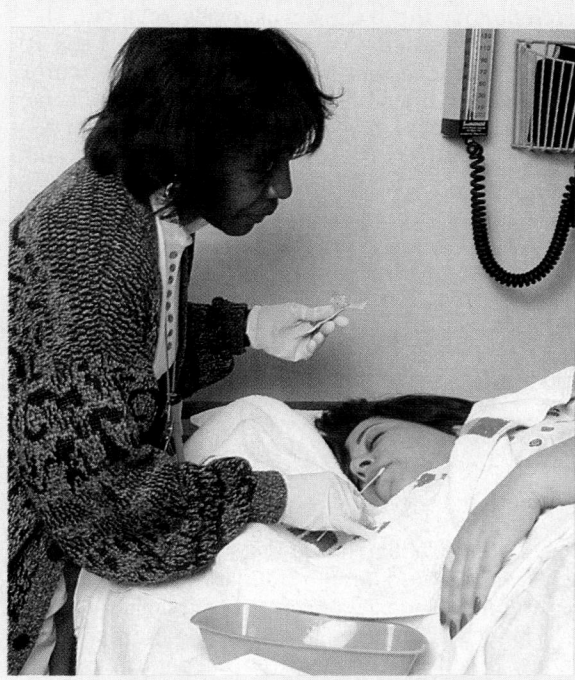

CONTINUED

CLIENTS AT RISK FOR STOMATITIS. Chemotherapy, radiation, and nasogastric tube intubation can cause stomatitis (see research highlights on p. 1054). Clients should rinse their mouths before and after each meal using a solution containing ½ to 1 tsp of salt or baking soda to 1 pt of water (Greifzu, Radjeski, Winnick, 1990). To remove thick mucus, they should use 1 tsp sodium bicarbonate solution to 1 pt of water (Wilson, 1986) or 1 part hydrogen peroxide to 4 parts normal saline (Greifzu, Radjeski, Winnick, 1990).

CLIENTS WITH DIABETES. Visits to the dentist are needed every 3 or 4 months. All tissues should be handled gently with a minimum of trauma. Clients should be taught to follow rigid cleansing schedules.

CLIENTS WITH ORAL INFECTIONS. The nurse notifies a physician when signs of an infection such as coated ulcerations or a red, dry, swollen tongue are seen. Yogurt (containing active cultures) with every meal is effective against yeast infections (Wilson, 1986). Liquid topical antibiotics can be applied to mucosal surfaces with a soft sponge or by having clients rinse the oral cavity with the medication. Clients who wear dentures must remove them before using topical antibiotics.

Research Highlight

Radiation therapy that involves the oral mucosa and salivary glands inevitably causes some degree of mucositis. Dudjak studied the effects of two oral care protocols on the physical condition of the mouth and the perception of comfort in clients receiving external radiation to the head and neck region. Fifteen patients were randomly assigned to one of two specific mouth care protocols: half-strength hydrogen peroxide or a solution of baking soda and water. Findings did not reveal a significant difference in the mean scores of the physical condition of the mouth; however, there was a significant difference in the mean scores of the perception of comfort. Results showed a preference for the hydrogen peroxide solution. The rate of oral infection was equal in both groups and at a lower incidence than suggested by the literature. The results of the study suggest that the systematic performance of oral care may be more effective in decreasing the effects of radiation than the type of oral agent used.

Dudjak LA: Mouth care for mucositis due to radiation therapy, *Cancer Nurs* 10(3):131, 1987.

Research Highlight

In a study similar to Dudjak's, Kenny compared the effect of two different oral care protocols in decreasing the incidence of stomatitis in clients receiving chemotherapy or chemotherapy and radiation therapy. Eighteen subjects were randomly assigned to one of two protocols. Protocols differed in the type of lip lubricant, toothette, and mouthwash used. No statistical difference was found in the incidence of stomatitis between the two groups. However, findings revealed that reinforcement of oral care instructions and regular nursing assessment of the oral cavity seemed to promote client compliance with the oral care regimen. These findings supported those of other researchers who claim that the systematic performance of oral care may be more effective in minimizing the destructive effects of chemotherapy and radiation therapy than the particular oral care regimen.

Kenny SA: Effect of two oral protocols on the incidence of stomatitis in hematology patients, *Cancer Nurs* 13(5/6):345, 1990.

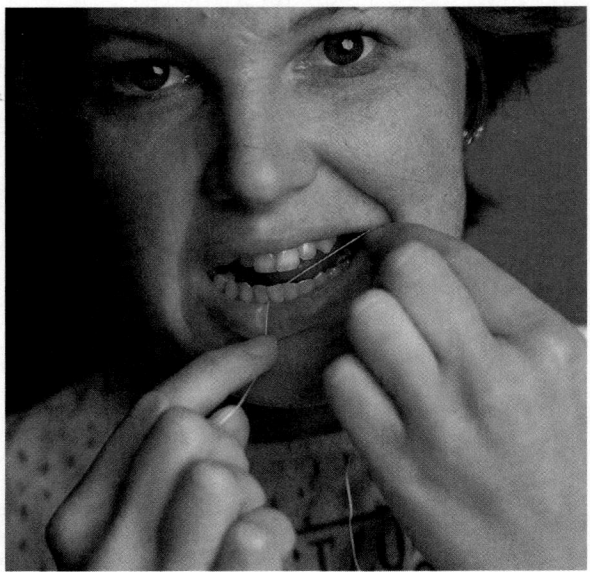

Fig. 34-2 Flossing.

Fluoride Use

In many communities the water supply now contains fluoride. Even though fluoride has not been proved to eliminate tooth decay, it is known to prevent dental caries (Whaley, Wong, 1991). People who do not have fluoridated water available can obtain fluoride in the form of mouthwash, toothpaste, or supplements. Most toothpastes on the market today contain fluoride and can help prevent tooth decay. Fluoride supplements can be given to children beginning at the age of 2 weeks. Supplements are available without a prescription and can be taken with water, juice, or milk. The family dentist should be consulted concerning the amount of fluoride to be given.

Excessive fluoridation can result in a discoloration of tooth enamel. Clients should be advised to watch for this condition. Parents should keep fluoride supplements out of the reach of children.

Flossing

Dental flossing is necessary for effective removal of plaque and tartar between teeth. Flossing involves insertion of waxed or unwaxed dental floss between all tooth surfaces, one at a time (Fig. 34-2). The seesaw motion used to pull floss between teeth removes plaque and tartar from tooth enamel. To prevent bleeding, clients receiving chemotherapy or radiation should use unwaxed floss and avoid vigorous flossing near the gumline. If toothpaste is applied to the teeth before flossing, the fluoride can come in direct con-

STEPS	RATIONALE
1. Ask client if dentures are loose fitting and if there is any gum or mucous membrane tenderness or irritation. After dentures are removed, inspect oral cavity and denture surfaces.	Ill-fitting dentures rub against gums and mucous membranes. Area of irritation may require special care.
2. Explain procedure and assure client that individual practice preferences will be used (when appropriate).	Promotes client understanding and cooperation.
3. Prepare necessary equipment and supplies:	
a. Soft-bristled toothbrush	Used to brush gums and tongue.
b. Denture toothbrush	
c. Emesis basin or sink	
d. Denture dentifrice or toothpaste	
e. Water glasses (for warm and cool water)	
f. Single 4 × 4 gauze	Used to remove dentures.
g. Washcloth	
h. Plastic denture cup	
i. Disposable gloves	Prevents contact with microorganisms in saliva.
4. Wash hands.	Reduces transmission of microorganisms.
5. Arrange supplies on bedside table or near sink.	Ensures smooth, organized procedure.
6. Pour emesis basin half full with tepid water or place washcloth in sink and run water until it is approximately 1-in deep.	Aids in distribution of dentifrice over denture surfaces. Cloth protects dentures against breakage. Hot water can cause warping or softening of dentures.
7. Apply disposable gloves.	Reduces transmission of infection.
8. Ask client to remove dentures and place them in emesis basin. If client is unable to remove dentures, grasp upper plate at front with thumb and index finger wrapped in gauze. Use steady, downward pull. Gently lift lower denture from jaw and rotate one side downward to remove from mouth. Place dentures in basin.	Gauze prevents accidental slipping while handling dentures. Rotating denture at angle reduces pulling of lips during removal.
9. Apply dentifrice to denture and brush surfaces of dentures (see illustrations). Hold dentures close to water. Hold brush horizontally and use back-and-forth motion to cleanse biting surfaces. Hold brush horizontally and use short strokes from top of denture to biting surfaces of teeth to clean outer tooth surface. Hold brush vertically and use short strokes to clean inner tooth surfaces. Hold brush horizontally and use back-and-forth motion to clean undersurface of dentures.	Prevents food and bacteria from collecting on denture surfaces and prevents odor and stain buildup. Holding dentures close to water reduces chance of breakage, because water will break fall if dentures slip.

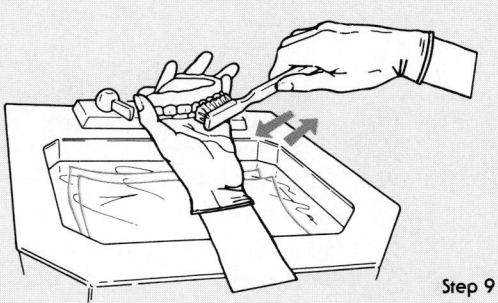

Step 9

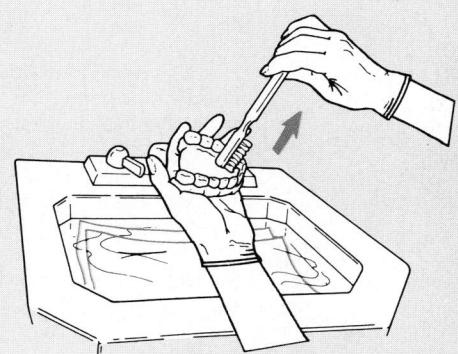

Illustrations from Sorrentino SA: *Mosby's textbook for nursing assistants*, ed 3, St Louis, 1992, Mosby—Year Book.

Cleaning Dentures

STEPS	RATIONALE
10. Rinse dentures thoroughly in tepid water.	Warm water dilutes and rinses dentifrice more effectively than cool water.
11. Return dentures to client or store in tepid water in denture cup.	Storage protects dentures from breakage. Tepid water keeps dentures well moistened to make eventual insertion easier. Plastic dentures become brittle and warp if not kept moist.
12. Empty emesis basin and add fresh cool water. Apply toothpaste to soft toothbrush, and gently brush gums, palate, and tongue.	Helps stimulate circulation to gums and removes residual film of debris on gums and mucosa.
13. Have client rinse mouth thoroughly.	Rinsing removes all food particles and secretions.
14. Reinsert dentures if client desires, or allow client to do so. Begin by gently inserting moistened upper denture. Have client use finger to press denture firmly in place, then insert moistened lower denture.	Bulkier upper denture easier to insert first when client has both upper and lower plates. Moistening lubricates denture for easier insertion. Applying gentle pressure to upper denture seals it against palate.
15. Dispose of gloves in proper receptacle. Clean and store supplies. Wash hands.	Controls spread of infection.
16. Ask client if dentures feel comfortable.	Cleansing removes sources of irritation.
17. Record procedure on flowsheet or nurses' notes.	Accurate and timely documentation maintains accuracy of client's record.

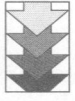 Sample Evaluation of Interventions for Oral Hygiene Problems

Goals	Evaluative Measures	Expected Outcomes
Oral mucosa will be intact and well hydrated.	Inspect condition of tongue, gums, and lining of cheeks. Observe condition of lips. Inspect tooth surfaces.	Mucosa will be moist and intact and will have uniform color. Tongue will be well hydrated. Lips will be smooth and hydrated. Teeth will be white, smooth, and shiny. Teeth will be free of food particles and plaque.
Client will independently perform oral-hygiene care correctly.	Observe client perform brushing, flossing, and denture care. Ask client to describe oral-hygiene techniques.	Oral-hygiene techniques will be properly demonstrated. Client will correctly describe steps to follow in brushing, flossing, or denture care.
Client will achieve sense of comfort.	Question client if discomfort is noted in oral cavity. Observe facial expression for discomfort.	Client will deny oral pain or irritation.
Client will understand oral-hygiene practices.	Ask client to explain purpose of regular oral hygiene.	Client will explain preventive measures against tooth decay and plaque.

tact with tooth surfaces, aiding in cavity prevention. Flossing once a day is sufficient. Because it is important to clean all tooth surfaces thoroughly, the nurse should not rush to complete flossing. Placing a mirror in front of the client helps the nurse demonstrate the proper methods for holding the floss and cleansing between the teeth. Flossing is most easily done immediately after brushing.

Denture Care

Clients should be encouraged to clean their own dentures as frequently as natural teeth to prevent gingival infection and irritation (Procedure 34-7). The nurse must assist with denture care if clients become disabled, incapacitated, or confused. Dentures are the client's personal property and should be handled with care because they can be easily broken. Dentures should be removed before going to bed to give the gums a rest and to prevent bacterial buildup and inflamed mucosa. They should be kept in water when they are not worn to prevent warping. The nurse always stores dentures in an enclosed, labeled cup during soaking or when the dentures are not being worn. The client is discouraged from wrapping dentures in facial or toilet tissue or placing them on meal trays because the dentures may be accidentally thrown away.

Evaluation

The beneficial outcomes of oral hygiene may not be seen for several days. Repeated cleansing is often needed to remove thick encrustations of the tongue and to restore the mucosa's hydration to normal. Likewise, it takes many weeks of rigorous hygiene to reduce the incidence of dental caries. The evaluation box outlines the evaluation of oral-hygiene care.

HAIR CARE

A person's appearance and feeling of well-being often depend on the way the hair looks and feels. Illness or disability may prevent a client from maintaining daily hair care. An immobilized client's hair soon becomes tangled. Dressings may leave sticky blood or antiseptic solutions on the hair. Brushing, combing, and shampooing are basic hygienic measures for all clients. Clients should be permitted to shave when their conditions allow.

Hair growth, distribution, and pattern can be indicators of general health status (see Chapter 20). Hormonal changes, emotional and physical stress, aging,

infection, and certain diseases or drugs can affect characteristics of the hair. The hair shaft is an inert structure. Any changes in its color or condition occur as a result of hormonal activity and nutrient supply to the follicle. Table 34-6 on p. 1058 describes common hair and scalp problems and nursing interventions.

Assessment

Physical Assessment

Before performing hair care, the nurse assesses the condition of the hair and scalp (see Chapter 20). Normally the hair is clean, shiny, and untangled, and the scalp is clear. The hair of black-skinned clients is usually thicker, drier, and curlier than lighter-skinned clients. The loss of hair (**alopecia**) can result from improper hair-care practices (Table 34-6) or the use of chemotherapy medications.

Developmental Changes

During life, changes in the growth, distribution, and condition of hair can influence the hygiene that a person requires (Table 34-7 on p. 1059).

Self-Care Ability

The nurse assesses a client's physical ability to care for hair. Painful conditions of the upper extremities such as arthritis, a weakened hand grip, fatigue, and physical encumbrances (for example, a cast or dressing) are just some of the conditions that impair a client's ability to perform hair care.

Hair-Care Practices

One way to assess a person's hair-care practices is by observing the appearance of the hair. Dull, tangled, dirty hair indicates improper care. Unkempt hair may be the result of lack of interest, depression, or physical inability to care for the hair.

By assessing a client's preferred hairstyle, the nurse can attempt to arrange the client's hair in the same manner. Asking the client to assist or teach the nurse how to style the hair correctly gives the client a greater sense of independence and helps the nurse avoid making a mistake that can damage hair.

The nurse also assesses the type of hair-care products a client prefers to use, as well as the time of day when hair care is usually performed. Assessment of shaving products is necessary with all clients.

Nursing Diagnosis

The problems most likely to be identified by the nurse after assessment of the hair and scalp center

TABLE 34-6 Hair and Scalp Problems

Characteristics	Implications	Interventions
DANDRUFF		
Scaling of scalp is accompanied by itching. In severe cases, dandruff is found on eyebrows.	Dandruff causes person embarrassment. If dandruff enters eyes, conjunctivis may develop.	Shampoo regularly with medicated shampoo. In severe cases, obtain physician's advice.
TICKS		
Small, gray-brown parasites burrow into skin and suck blood.	Ticks transmit several diseases to people. Most common are Rocky Mountain spotted fever, tularemia, and Lyme disease.	Do not pull ticks from skin because sucking apparatus remains and may become infected. Place a drop of oil or ether on tick or cover it with petrolatum jelly to ease removal. Oil suffocates tick.
PEDICULOSIS (LICE)		
Tiny, grayish-white parasite insects infest mammals.		
PEDICULOSIS CAPITIS (HEAD LICE)		
Parasite is found on scalp attached to hair strands. Eggs look like oval particles, similar to dandruff. Bites or pustules may be observed behind ears and at hairline.	Head lice are difficult to remove and may spread to furniture and other people if not treated.	Shampoo with Kwell shampoo and repeat 12-24 hr later. Change bed linens.
PEDICULOSIS CORPORIS (BODY LICE)		
Parasites tend to cling to clothing, so they may not be easily seen. Body lice suck blood and lay eggs on clothing and furniture.	Client itches constantly. Scratches seen on skin may become infected. Hemorrhagic spots may appear on skin where lice are sucking blood.	Bathe or shower thoroughly. After skin is dried, apply Kwell lotion. After 12-24 hr, take another bath or shower. Bag infested clothing or linen until laundered.
PEDICULOSIS PUBIS (CRAB LICE)		
Parasites are found in pubic hair. Crab lice are grayish white with red legs.	Lice may spread through bed linen, clothing, or furniture or between persons via sexual contact.	Shave hair off affected area. Cleanse as for body lice. If lice were sexually transmitted, notify partner.
HAIR LOSS (ALOPECIA)		
Alopecia occurs in all races. Balding patches are seen in periphery of hair line. Hair becomes brittle and broken. Condition is caused by use of hair curlers, hair picks, tight braiding, and use of hot comb.	Patches of uneven hair growth and loss alter client's appearance.	Stop hair-care practices that damage hair.

TABLE 34-7 Physiological Development of Hair Growth

Age	Condition of Hair
Infancy	Infants may have little or no scalp hair at birth. Scalp hair grows by first year. Fine body hair (lanugo) is present on forehead, cheeks, shoulders, and back.
Childhood	Scalp hair is lustrous, silky, strong, and elastic. Hair of black-skinned child is curlier and coarser.
Middle childhood to puberty	Androgenic hormones cause increase in thickening and darkening of scalp hair, growth of hair in axillae and pubic areas in both sexes, and growth of facial hair in boys.
Adolescence	Boys may acquire additional amounts of distribution of body hair, such as on chest. Increase in sebaceous gland activity causes hair to become oily.
Adulthood	Men with genetic tendency develop baldness.
Older adulthood	Axillary and pubic hair diminish in women. Scalp hair becomes thinner and depleted of melanin, causing gray coloring. Older women may develop chin and facial hair because of decreased estrogen production. Men may experience balding or receding hair line.

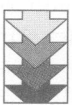 Examples of Nursing Diagnoses Related to Hair and Scalp Care

NANDA-APPROVED NURSING DIAGNOSES

Dressing/grooming self-care deficit related to:
- Altered level of consciousness
- Physical immobility or weakness

Impaired skin integrity related to:
- Scalp laceration
- Insect bite

Pain related to:
- Scalp lesion
- Accumulated secretions in hair

Body-image disturbance related to:
- Unkempt physical appearance

High risk for infection related to:
- Scalp laceration
- Insect bites

on comfort and grooming. If actual lesions or abnormalities involving the scalp are identified, nursing diagnoses focus on the integrity of the scalp (see diagnoses box).

 ## Planning

Good hair care practices must be done routinely to meet clients' hygienic needs. The nurse must remember that clients remain aware of their appearances at all times. Therefore an effective plan allows clients to initiate and participate in hygienic measures whenever possible.

Goals for clients in need of hair and scalp care include the following:
1. Hair and scalp will be clean and healthy.
2. Client will achieve a sense of comfort and self-esteem.
3. Client will participate in hair-care practices.

 ## Implementation

Brushing and Combing

Frequent brushing helps keep hair clean and distributes oil evenly along hair shafts. Combing merely styles the hair and prevents it from becoming tangled. Short-tooth combs are adequate for short hair, but large-tooth combs are preferred for curly hair. Combs with sharp, irregular teeth may scratch the scalp. The client able to perform self-care should be encouraged to maintain hair care daily. However, clients with limited mobility and poor coordination and those who are confused or seriously weakened by their illnesses require the nurse's help.

Long hair can easily become matted after a client has been confined to bed even for a short period. When lacerations or incisions involve the scalp, blood and topical medications can also cause tangling. Frequent brushing and combing keep long hair neatly groomed. However, braiding can help to avoid repeated tangles. The nurse should ask the client's permission to braid hair. If braids are made too tightly, balding patches can develop.

To brush hair properly the nurse parts the hair into two sections and then separates each section into two more sections. Parting allows for ease in brushing smaller sections of hair. The nurse brushes from the scalp toward the hair ends. If tangles are present, the nurse uses the fingers to separate a small lock of hair, grasps it firmly near the scalp, and combs the loose end of the lock. Anchoring the tangled hair prevents painful pulling of the scalp during combing. If the hair is excessively tangled, the nurse should comb out only a few sections at a time. Moistening the hair with water or alcohol often frees tangles for easier combing. The nurse never cuts the client's hair without written consent.

Clients who have curly hair usually comb their hair with a special comb that has long teeth spaced far apart. The open-toothed comb causes less pulling during combing. Wetting the client's hair with water before combing prevents trauma to the hair. To comb curly hair, the nurse starts at the client's neckline and slowly lifts and fluffs the hair outward until the forehead is reached. The nurse combs one side of the client's head at a time and then repeats on the other side.

Black-skinned clients have thick, coarse, curly hair that often becomes very dry and brittle. Thus the nurse should caution against use of hair-care practices that can damage hair. Daily braiding is more damaging than corn rows. The tight braids may cause balding patches. The use of petrolatum jelly and a hot comb for straightening hair may cause chronic inflammation and permanent scarring of the scalp. Application of hair straighteners with alkaline chemicals may cause the hair to become brittle.

Shampooing

Frequency of shampooing depends on a person's daily routine. The nurse should remind hospitalized clients that staying in bed, excess perspiration, or treatments that leave blood or solutions in the hair may require more frequent shampooing. For clients at home, the nurse's greatest challenge may be to find ways that the client can shampoo the hair without injury.

If clients are able to take showers or baths, the hair can usually be shampooed without difficulty. Shower chairs may be used for clients who are ambulatory but become tired or faint. Hand-held shower nozzles allow clients to wash their hair during a tub bath or shower. The hair of clients who are allowed to sit in a chair can usually be shampooed in front of a sink. If the client can sit only at the bedside, it is possible to shampoo the hair as the client leans forward over a washbasin. However, bending is limited or contraindicated in certain conditions (for example, eye surgery and total hip replacement surgery). In these situations, the nurse needs to teach the client the degree of bending allowed.

If a client is unable to sit but can be moved, the nurse may transfer the client to a stretcher for transportation to a sink or shower equipped with a hand-held nozzle. The nurse places a towel or small pillow under the client's head and neck, allowing the head to hang slightly over the stretcher's edge. Caution is needed with clients who have suffered neck injuries because hyperextension of the neck could cause further injury.

If the client is unable to sit in a chair or be transferred to a stretcher, shampooing must be done with the client in bed. After shampooing (Procedure 34-8), clients may like having their hair rolled on curlers or styled. Most health care centers have portable hair dryers. Dry shampoos that reduce the need to wet the client's hair are also available.

African Americans usually apply various types of oil preparations to the hair before or after shampooing. The hair and scalp have a natural tendency to be dry and require daily combing and gentle brushing. Oil prevents drying and subsequent breaking of hair at the follicles or ends. Grier (1976) recommends a solution of alcohol and mineral oil to remove old oils that adhere to the hair shaft. The alcohol is an antiseptic and cleansing agent. The mineral oil cleanses and lubricates the hair. The nurse confers with clients to determine the preferred type of oil preparation. Olive oil, baby oil, or Vasoline hair oil are commonly used. The application of an oil generally makes combing easier.

Normally, it is necessary for African Americans to shampoo their hair only once or twice a week or once a month. Water shampoos tend to make their hair curlier and harder to comb. A mild shampoo is preferred if they have had their hair straightened.

Shaving

Shaving of facial hair can be done after the bath or shampoo. Women may prefer to shave their legs or axillae during the bath. When assisting a client, the nurse should take care to avoid cutting the client with razor blades. Suicidal clients are not allowed to use razor blades. Clients prone to bleeding, such as those receiving anticoagulant medications (heparin or Coumadin) or high doses of aspirin, and those with bleeding disorders (hemophilia or leukemia) are instructed to use an electric razor. Before using an electric razor, the nurse checks for electrical hazards.

When a razor blade is used for shaving, the skin must be softened to prevent pulling, scraping, or cuts. For example, placing a warm washcloth over the male client's face for a few seconds, followed by the application of shaving cream or a lathering of mild soap, effectively softens the skin. If the male client is unable to shave his own face, the nurse may perform the shave. To avoid causing discomfort or razor cuts, the nurse holds the razor at a 45-degree angle to the skin and gently pulls the skin taut while using short, firm razor strokes in the direction the hair grows. Short downward strokes work best to remove hair over the upper lip. Often a client can explain the best way to move the razor. After the shave is completed, the nurse washes the client's face thor-

STEPS	RATIONALE
1. Determine if any risks exist that might contraindicate shampooing or positioning. Review physician's orders to determine if medicated shampoo is ordered.	Certain medical conditions (e.g., total hip replacement, cervical neck injuries, open incisions, tracheostomy) may place client at risk of injury because of positioning, exposure to moisture, or manipulation of scalp. For conditions such as lice or dandruff, special shampoos may be ordered.
2. Explain procedure to client.	Client may be anxious about positioning or risk of water entering eyes.
3. Prepare necessary equipment and supplies: a. Two bath towels b. Face towel or washcloth c. Shampoo (OPTIONAL: hair conditioner and cream rinse) d. Water pitcher e. Plastic shampoo trough f. Washbasin g. Bath blanket h. Waterproof pad i. Clean comb and brush j. Hair dryer k. Bottle of hydrogen peroxide (optional)	 Used to pour water over hair. Diverts water to basin to prevent soiling bed linen. Cleanses hair matted with blood.
4. Wash hands.	Reduces transmission of microorganisms.
5. Arrange equipment in convenient place and lower side rail.	Prevents interruptions.
6. Place waterproof pad under client's shoulders, neck, and head. Position client supine with head and shoulders at top edge of bed. Place plastic trough under head and washbasin at end of trough, being sure that trough spout extends beyond edge of mattress and runs into washbasin.	Prevents soiling of bed linen.

Step 7

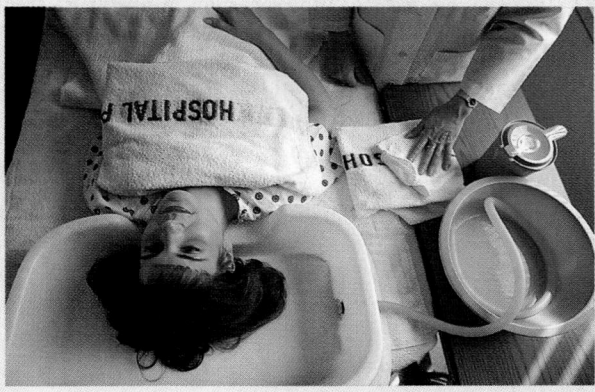

7. Place rolled towel under neck and bath towel across shoulders (see illustration).	Slight hyperextension of neck minimizes problem of water draining down back of neck.
8. Brush and comb hair.	Removing tangles results in more thorough cleansing.
9. Obtain water at about 43°-44° C (110° F) and fill pitcher. Check temperature by placing small amount of water on inner aspect of your forearm.	Prevents burns to face and scalp.
10. Ask client to hold face towel or washcloth over eyes.	Prevents shampoo or water from entering eyes.
11. With water pitcher, slowly pour water over hair until it is completely wet. Apply small amount of shampoo.	Water aids in distribution of shampoo suds over hair.

Shampooing Hair in Bed

STEPS	RATIONALE
12. Work upward with both hands. Start at hairline and work toward back of neck. Lift head slightly with one hand to wash back of head. Shampoo sides of head. Massage scalp by applying pressure with fingertips.	Systematic progression over hair and scalp ensures thorough cleansing. Massage increases scalp circulation. Use of fingernails during massage can cause scratching of scalp.
13. Rinse hair with water. Make sure water drains into basin. Repeat rinsing until hair is free of shampoo. To speed drainage from trough, press down on its spout.	Retained shampoo leaves dull finish on hair. Dried shampoo may cause scalp irritation.
14. Repeat Steps 11-13.	Ensures thorough cleansing.
15. Apply conditioner or rinse if requested and rinse hair thoroughly.	Conditioner prevents excess drying. Cream rinse makes combing and brushing easier.
16. Wrap head in bath towel. Dry face with cloth used to protect eyes. Dry off moisture along neck or shoulders.	Retained moisture may cause cooling and chills.
17. Dry hair and scalp. Use second towel if first becomes saturated.	
18. Comb hair to remove tangles and dry with dryer or remaining towel as quickly as possible.	Drying prevents chilling.
19. Assist client to comfortable position and complete styling of hair.	Promotes client's sense of well-being.
20. Return equipment to its proper place. Discard soiled linen in linen hamper. Wash hands.	Maintains cleanliness of environment and controls transmission of infection.
21. Ask client how hair feels.	Client will experience sense of cleanliness after shampooing.
22. Inspect condition of hair.	Shampooing should leave hair in clean condition.
23. Record procedure and pertinent findings related to condition of hair or scalp.	Documents client's response to therapy and condition of hair or scalp should further treatment be necessary.

oughly to remove soap and hair. After drying the face, the nurse assists in applying powder or an aftershave lotion to the client's face.

Mustache and Beard Care

Male clients with mustaches or beards require daily grooming. Keeping these clean is important because food particles can easily collect in the hair. If clients are unable to care for themselves, the nurse should trim, comb, or wash beards or mustaches when needed or on request. The nurse never shaves off a mustache or beard without the client's consent.

Evaluation

Evaluation of nursing care measures for the client's hair care are based on the expected outcomes and goals of care. The nurse uses evaluative measures, such as having the client demonstrate haircare practices or re-inspecting the condition of the hair and scalp, to determine the success of nursing interventions.

CARE OF THE EYES, EARS, AND NOSE

Special attention is given to the cleansing of the client's eyes, ears, and nose during the client's bath. However, clients may also have special problems that require cleansing of these organs throughout the day. Nursing care centers on preventing infection and maintaining the client's normal organ function.

Eyes

Normally no special care is required for the eyes because they are continually cleansed by tears and the eyelids and lashes prevent the entrance of foreign particles. A person needs only to remove any dried secretions that have collected on the inner canthus or the eyelashes. Unconscious clients are at risk for eye injury because the blink reflex may be absent. In these clients, excessive drainage frequently collects along eyelid margins. Special attention is also needed for clients who have had eye surgery or an eye infection that can result in increased discharge or drainage. The nurse often assists clients in the care of eyeglasses, contact lenses, or artificial eyes.

Ears

Hygiene of the ears has implications for hearing acuity when wax or foreign substances collect in the external ear canal and interfere with sound conduction. The nurse should be sensitive to any behavioral cues that might indicate a hearing impairment (see Chapter 45). When caring for a client with a hearing aid, the nurse instructs the client on proper cleansing and maintenance and communication techniques that promote hearing the spoken word.

Nose

The nose provides for the sense of smell but also controls the temperature and humidity of inhaled air and prevents the entrance of foreign particles into the respiratory system. The accumulation of encrusted secretions within the nares can impair olfactory sensation and breathing. Irritation of nasal mucosa can cause swelling, leading to obstruction of the nares. Typically, hygienic care of the nose is simple, but clients with nasogastric, enteral feeding, or endotracheal tubes that enter the nose may require special attention.

Assessment

Physical Assessment

Chapter 20 describes the techniques used to assess the condition and function of the eyes, ears, and nose. Normally the eyes are free of infection. The conjunctivae are clear, pink, and without inflammation. The eyelid margins are in close approximation with the eyeball, and the lashes are turned outward. The lid margins are without inflammation, drainage, or lesions. The eyebrows should be symmetrical.

Assessment of the external ear structures includes inspection of the auricle, external ear canal, and tym-

panic membrane. While performing hygienic measures, the nurse is most concerned with noting the presence of accumulated cerumen or drainage in the ear canal, local inflammation, or pain.

The nurse inspects the nares for signs of inflammation, discharge, lesions, edema, and deformity. The nasal mucosa is normally pink and clear and has no discharge. If clients have any form of tubing exiting the nose, the nurse should look at the nares surfaces that come in contact with the tubing for tissue sloughing, localized tenderness, inflammation, and even bleeding.

Use of Sensory Aids

If clients wear eyeglasses, contact lenses, artificial eyes, or hearing aids, the nurse assesses the client's knowledge, the methods used to care for the aids, and the presence of any problems caused by the aids.

Assessing Client's Use of Sensory Aids

EYEGLASSES
- Purpose for wearing glasses (e.g., reading, distance, or both)
- Methods used to clean glasses
- Presence of symptoms (e.g., blurred vision, photophobia, headaches, irritation)

CONTACT LENSES
- Type of lens worn
- Frequency and duration of time lenses are worn (including sleep time)
- Presence of symptoms (e.g., burning, excess tearing, redness, irritation, swelling, sensitivity to light)
- Techniques used by the client to cleanse, store, insert, and remove lenses
- Use of eyedrops or ointments
- Use of emergency identification bracelet or card that warns others to remove client's lenses in case of emergency

ARTIFICIAL EYE
- Method used to insert and remove eye
- Method for cleansing eye
- Presence of symptoms (e.g., drainage, inflammation, pain involving the orbit)

HEARING AID
- Type of aid worn
- Methods used to cleanse aid
- Client's ability to change battery and adjust hearing-aid volume

The box outlines factors to assess for clients using sensory aids. The nurse's findings have implications for client education.

Self-Care Ability

The nurse assesses a client's physical ability to perform eye, ear, and nose care, as well as care of any sensory aids. Clients who are unable to grasp small objects, who have limited mobility in the upper extremities, who have reduced vision, or who are seriously fatigued require assistance from the nurse.

Nursing Diagnosis

Assessment may reveal an actual alteration in the function of sensory organs, a problem in the client's ability to perform personal hygiene, or a deficit in the client's understanding of hygiene. The nursing diagnoses box lists common nursing diagnoses that the nurse may identify.

Planning

The client's personal preferences and habits are considered as the nurse plans hygienic care. The eyes, ears, and nose are sensitive to irritating or pain-

Examples of Nursing Diagnoses Related to Eye, Ear, and Nose Problems

---

NANDA-APPROVED NURSING DIAGNOSES

Bathing/hygiene self-care deficit related to:
- Physical limitations
- Visual impairment

Knowledge deficit about personal hygiene related to:
- Lack of exposure to information
- Information misinterpretation

Pain related to:
- Physical irritation of eye
- Inflammation of ear canal
- Mechanical irritation of nares

High risk for infection related to:
- Poor hygienic practices

Sensory/perceptual alterations (visual, auditory, or olfactory) related to:
- Obstruction in ear canal
- Nasal obstruction
- Inflammation of eyes or local eye infection

---

ful stimuli. Extra care must be taken to avoid injury to tissues. The goals of care for the client include the following:

1. Absence of infection
2. Normal sensory organ function
3. Understanding of methods used to care for the eyes, ears, and nose

Implementation

Basic Eye Care

Cleansing of the eyes is usually performed during the bath and involves washing with a clean washcloth moistened in water. The use of soap may cause burning and irritation and is usually omitted. The nurse wipes from the inner to the outer canthus of the eye to prevent secretions from draining into the lacrimal sac. A separate section of the washcloth is used each time to prevent the spread of infection. If a client has dried secretions that are not removed easily with wiping, the nurse may first place a damp cloth or cotton ball on the lid margins to loosen the secretions. Direct pressure should never be applied over the eyeball because it may cause serious injury.

The unconscious client may require more frequent eye care. Secretions may collect along the lid margins and inner canthus when the blink reflex is absent or when the eye does not close totally. It may be necessary to place an eye patch over the involved eye to prevent corneal drying and irritation. If necessary to prevent corneal drying, lubricating eyedrops may be administered according to the physician's orders.

CLEANSING GLASSES. Glasses are made of hardened glass or plastic that is impact resistant to prevent shattering. Nevertheless, because of the cost of glasses, the nurse uses care when cleaning glasses and should protect them from breakage or other damage when not worn. Glasses should be put in their case and in a drawer of the bedside table when not in use.

Warm water is sufficient for cleansing glass lenses. A soft tissue is best for drying to prevent scratching. Plastic lenses may scratch easily and require special cleaning solutions and drying tissues.

CONTACT LENS CARE. A contact lens is a thin, transparent, oval disk that fits directly over the cornea of the eye. The lens floats on the tear layer that lubricates the eye. Contact lenses are designed specifically to correct refractive errors of the eye or abnormalities in the cornea's shape. They are relatively easy to apply and remove. There are two major types of contact lenses: hard and soft.

Hard plastic lenses, introduced in the 1950s, are rigid, thick, durable, and optically precise. They are relatively easy to clean and handle. However, they can be uncomfortable and difficult to fit. In addition, the plastic lenses are not oxygen or gas permeable. The newer, more popular rigid gas-permeable lenses also provide clear vision but are more flexible and comfortable than the traditional hard lenses and allow oxygen through to the cornea. However, they are more likely to slip, causing blurred or distorted vision, or to pop out. They also are more readily scratched or chipped.

Soft contact lenses, introduced in the 1970s, are more comfortable because they are thinner, soft, and more pliable. Like rigid gas-permeable lenses, they are less likely to cause corneal epithelial damage because they are oxygen permeable. Soft lenses are more pliable and flimsy because they consist primarily of water, 38% to 70% by weight (Rakow, 1990). Therefore soft lenses easily tear and are thus less durable. Other disadvantages are that they absorb topical medications, can be sites for infection, may stimulate superficial corneal vascularization, can accumulate allergenic proteins, and can cause dry eyes (Harrison, 1989). There are several varieties of soft lenses: bifocal, multifocal, tinted (to enhance or alter eye color), toric (for astigmatism), and extended wear. Soft disposables, worn as daily or extended-wear lenses, are also available.

The normal eye needs oxygen and receives most of it through air and tears (OxyFlow, 1987). Although soft lenses and newer rigid lenses are gas permeable and allow oxygen to pass directly through the lens, all contact lenses still restrict the flow of oxygen to the eye's surface. Consequently, all lenses must be removed periodically to prevent ocular infection and corneal abrasions or ulcers (Stehr-Green et al, 1987). A major difference between the types of lenses is the length of time each can be safely worn. Rigid and daily wear soft lenses should be removed overnight and should not be worn more than 12 to 14 hours daily. It is not recommended that extended-wear soft lenses be left in place longer than 1 week (Egan, Bennett, Davis, 1988). Pain, tearing, discomfort, and redness of the conjunctiva may be symptomatic of lens overwear. The persistence of symptoms, even after lens removal, is abnormal, however, and may indicate serious ocular damage.

As contact lenses are worn by clients, they accumulate secretions and foreign matter. This material deteriorates and then irritates the eye, causing distorted vision and risk for infection. Once removed, contact lenses should be cleansed and thoroughly disinfected. A contact lens provides certain advantages over eyeglasses:

1. Improves clarity of vision
2. Is safer than eye glasses during certain physical activities
3. Smoothes optically irregular surfaces of the eye
4. Provides a more attractive appearance for the wearer

Clients who wear contact lenses generally care for their contact lenses themselves. An eye specialist instructs clients on the proper techniques to care for the lens. Often, the nurse is responsible for removing contacts in an emergency and for reinforcing techniques of proper lens care. The box lists some common guidelines for all contact lens wearers that the nurse can reinforce during hygienic care. Clients should also be aware of the symptoms of problems that may be related directly or indirectly to contact lens use (Table 34-8 on p. 1066).

The basic steps of contact lens care include cleansing to remove the accumulation of deposits from tear film, rinsing to remove lens debris after

---

Contact Lens Care

DO

- Wash and rinse hands thoroughly before handling a lens.
- Keep fingernails clean.
- Remove lenses from their storage case one at a time and place on the eye.
- Start with the same lens (left or right) each time of insertion.
- Use lens placement technique learned from eye specialist.
- Use proper lens care products.
- Wear lenses daily and follow the prescribed wearing schedule.
- Remove a lens if it becomes uncomfortable.
- Keep regular appointments with the eye specialist.
- Remove lenses during sunbathing, showering, or swimming.

DO NOT

- Use soaps that contain cream or perfume for cleansing lenses.
- Let fingernails touch lenses.
- Mix up lenses.
- Exceed prescribed wearing time.
- Use saliva to wet lenses.
- Use homemade saline solution or tap water to wet or clean lenses.
- Borrow or mix lens care solution.

TABLE 34-8 Common Problems for Contact Lens Wearers

Problem	Cause
Uncomfortable lens	Dirty or damaged lens
	Dust on eyelash entering eye
	Eye infection
	Decreased eye moisture (tears)
Redness of eye	Lens overwear
	Sensitivity to lens care solution
	Allergy
	Eye infection
Blurred vision	Dirty or damaged lens
	Mix up of left with right lens
	Corneal irritation
	Wearing lens inside out (soft lenses only)
Excess tearing	Corneal irritation
	Lens overwear
	Eye infection

Client Teaching for Maintaining and Improving Eyesight in Older Adults

OBJECTIVE

- The older adult will state methods for maintaining and improving eyesight.

TEACHING STRATEGIES

- Encourage regular eye examinations. Stress its importance in preserving sight and preventing blindness.
- Discuss vision changes that occur naturally with aging, including presbyopia, a need for increased illumination, a delayed adaptation to darkness, increased light scatter, increased glare sensitivity and glare recovery, disturbance in hue discrimination, mild reductions in total visual field, and slowed visual interpretive reaction.
- Identify major eye diseases associated with aging such as glaucoma and cataracts.
- Discuss signs and symptoms of eye diseases.
- Determine whether any health or hereditary factors make the client more likely to develop vision problems.
- Ascertain whether the client needs and is able to make changes in environment and lifestyle to accomodate vision changes.
- Review prescribed medications and any visual side effects. If client is taking medications for eye problems, review purpose, action, dosage, and proper administration technique.
- Correct misinformation and misconceptions.
- Demonstrate proper eyedrop administration technique if necessary.

EVALUATION

- Listen to client's statements for correct information about normal eye changes, diseases, and medications.
- Reappraise accuracy of information after correcting misinformation and misconceptions.
- Observe eyedrop administration technique.

cleaning, disinfecting to protect eyes from infection, and lubricating to replace water lost from lens and tears through evaporation. A variety of products is available for lens care, and each type of lens requires a different cleansing technique.

Some eye specialists also recommend periodic enzyme cleansing. The enzymes dissolve protein deposits on the lens surface. Some lenses can be cleansed with electrical heat disinfecting units.

Clients may require assistance with contact lens care, insertion, and removal. The nurse protects clients unable to care for their lenses properly. Prolonged wearing of contact lenses can cause serious corneal damage. Clients who become unconscious, who are restricted from moving their hands, or who lose clear judgment because of psychiatric illness, temporary mental confusion, or substance abuse should have their lenses removed immediately. Procedure 34-9 on p. 1068 describes one technique for the care of contact lenses. Lenses need not be reinserted in these clients' eyes until they are more capable of caring for the lenses themselves.

ARTIFICIAL EYES. Clients with artificial eyes have had an enucleation of an entire eyeball as a result of tumor growth, severe infection, or eye trauma. Some artificial eyes are permanently implanted. Others should be removed for routine cleaning. Clients with artificial eyes usually prefer to care for their own eyes. The nurse should respect the client's wishes and help by obtaining the necessary equipment.

For clients who are scheduled for surgery, are unconscious, or are unable to move their arms, head, or neck, the nurse assists with the removal and cleaning of artificial eyes. To remove an artificial eye, the nurse retracts the lower eyelid and exerts slight pressure just below the eye. This action causes the artificial eye to rise from the socket because the suction holding the eye in place has been broken. The nurse may also use a small, rubber-bulb syringe or medicine-dropper bulb to create a suction effect. The suction created by placing the bulb tip directly over the eye and squeezing lifts the eye from the socket.

The artificial eye is usually made of glass or plastic. Warm normal saline cleanses the prosthesis effectively. The nurse also cleanses the edges of the eye socket and surrounding tissues with soft gauze moistened in saline or clean tap water. Signs of infection should be reported immediately because bacteria can spread to the neighboring eye, underlying sinuses, or underlying brain tissue. To reinsert the eye, the nurse retracts the upper and lower lids and gently slips the eye into the socket, fitting it neatly under the upper eyelid. An artificial eye may be stored in a labeled container filled with tap water or saline.

PRESERVING VISION. All clients benefit from learning the following simple guidelines for their visual health:

1. Clients under the age of 40 should have an eye examination regularly every 3 to 5 years. Eye examination and routine testing for glaucoma are advised for all adults over age 40 every 2 years. (See teaching box for other strategies to preserve vision in older adults.)
2. Common symptoms of eye disorders include pain, photophobia, blurred vision, burning, itching, excess tearing, halos around lights, and floaters.
3. Clients should avoid home remedies for eye problems or injuries. Treatment for chemicals or dust that enters the eye includes flushing the eye continuously with tepid water for at least 10 minutes.
4. Clients should never try to remove foreign objects from the eye but should seek medical attention immediately.
5. Clients should wear eye goggles for protection when exposed to chemicals and dust.

Cleaning the Ears

The nurse cleanses the client's ears as a routine part of a bed bath. The clean end of a moistened washcloth, rotated gently into the ear canal, works best for cleaning. When cerumen is visible, gentle downward retraction at the entrance of the ear canal may cause the wax to loosen and slip out. The nurse instructs clients never to use sharp objects such as bobby pins or toothpicks to remove ear wax. The use of such objects can cause trauma to the ear canal and rupture of the tympanic membrane. Use of cotton-tipped applicators should also be avoided because they can cause wax to become impacted within the canal.

Children are the most common age group to have impacted cerumen. Excessive or impacted cerumen can usually be removed only by irrigation. The procedure first involves instilling 1 to 2 drops of mineral oil or other over-the-counter softeners (for example, Debrox) in the impacted ear twice daily for 4 to 5 days (Watkins, 1984). Then the instillation of approximately 250 ml of warm water (37° C or 98.6° F) into the external ear canal mechanically washes away loosened wax. Cold or hot water causes nausea or vomiting.

Children may sit or lie on their side with the affected ear up. The nurse places a small curved basin under the affected ear to catch the irrigating solution. A Water Pik (set on No. 2 setting) or a bulb irrigating syringe can be used to irrigate the ear canal. The tip of the syringe or Water Pick should not occlude the ear canal to avoid exerting pressure against the tympanic membrane. Gentle irrigation directed at the top of the canal loosens the cerumen from the sides of the ear canal. After the canal is clear, the nurse wipes off any moisture from the client's ear and inspects the canal for remaining cerumen.

HEARING AIDS. Chapter 45 discusses the need for and use of hearing aids. Hearing loss is a common health problem and an often forgotten disability that can affect the quality of a client's life. Although a large proportion of those suffering from a hearing loss admit to a hearing problem, only a small proportion own a hearing aid (Wilson, Wilson, 1988).

There are three popular types of hearing aids. An in-the-canal (ITC) aid is the newest, smallest, and least visible and fits entirely in the ear canal. It has cosmetic appeal, is easy to manipulate and place in the ear, does not interfere with the wearing of eyeglasses or telephone use, and can be worn during most physical exercise. However, it requires adequate ear diameter and depth for proper fit. It does not accomodate to progressive hearing loss, and it requires manual dexterity to operate, insert, remove, and change batteries. Also, cerumen tends to plug this model more than the others.

An in-the-ear (ITE or intraaural) aid (Fig. 34-3) fits into the external auditory ear and allows more fine tuning. It is more powerful and stronger and therefore is useful for a wider range of hearing loss than the ITC aid. It is also easy to position and adjust and does not interfere with eyeglass wearing. It is,

Text continued on p. 1073.

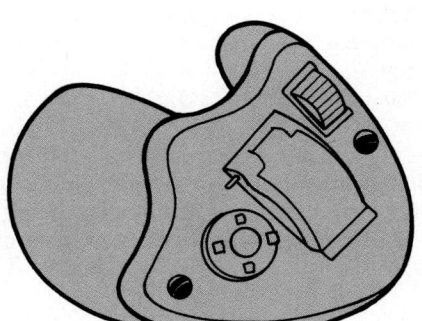

Fig. 34-3 In-the-ear hearing aid.

Taking Care of Contact Lenses

STEPS	RATIONALE
1. Assess client's ability to manipulate and hold contact lens.	Determines level of assistance required in care.
2. After lenses are removed, inspect eye for signs of corneal irritation.	Signs of corneal irritation may require client to refrain from contact use.
3. Prepare necessary equipment and supplies for lens removal:	
a. Contact lens storage container (see illustration)	Separate cups labeled *R* for right lens and *L* for left lens protect against lens breakage. (Certain lenses are stored dry, whereas others are stored in solution.)
b. Suction cup (optional)	Used to remove hard lenses from unconscious or debilitated client.
c. Sterile saline solution	Used to moisten cornea before lens removal.
d. Bath towel	
4. Prepare equipment and supplies for cleansing and insertion:	
a. Lenses in storage container	
b. Thermal disinfecting kit (optional)	Heats up to 80° C to sterilize soft lenses.
c. Surfactant cleaner	
d. Rinsing solution	
e. Sterile lens disinfectant and enzyme solution	Cleanses lens surfaces and reduces number of microorganisms present.
f. Sterile wetting solution for rigid lenses	Allows lens to glide easily over cornea during insertion.
g. Cotton ball or cotton-tipped applicator	Used to spread lens cleaner over surface of rigid contact lens.
h. Bath towel	
i. Emesis basin	
j. Glass of warm tap water	
5. Discuss procedure with client.	Client can assist in planning by explaining technique that may aid removal and insertion. Client may be anxious as nurse retracts eye lids and manipulates lenses.
6. Have client assume supine or sitting position in bed or chair.	Provides easy access while retracting eyelids and manipulating lens.
7. Remove soft lenses:	
a. Wash hands.	Reduces transmission of microorganisms.
b. Place towel just below client's face.	Catches lens if one accidentally falls from eye.
c. Add few drops of sterile saline to client's eye.	Lubricates eye to facilitate lens removal.
d. Tell client to look straight ahead.	Eases tipping of lens during removal.
e. Using middle finger, retract lower eyelid.	Exposes lower edge of lens.
f. With pad of index finger of same hand, slide lens off cornea onto white of eye.	Positions lens for easy grasping. Use of finger pad prevents injury to cornea and damage to lens.
g. Pull upper eyelid down gently with thumb of other hand and compress lens slightly between thumb and index finger.	Causes soft lens to double up. Air enters underneath lens to release suction.
h. Gently pinch lens and lift out.	Protects lens from damage. Prevents lens edges from sticking together.
i. If lens edges stick together, place lens in palm and soak thoroughly with sterile saline. Gently roll lens with index finger in back and forth motion. If gentle rubbing does not separate edges, soak lens in sterile solution.	Assists in returning lens to normal shape.

STEPS	RATIONALE
j. Clean and rinse lens (see Step 9). Place lens in proper storage case compartment: *R* for right lens and *L* for left lens. Be sure lens is centered.	Ensures that proper lens will be reinserted into correct eye. Proper storage prevents cracking or tearing.
k. Repeat Steps 7c-7j for other lens. Secure cover over storage case.	Proper storage prevents damage to lens.
l. Dispose of towel and wash hands.	Reduces transmission of infection.
8. Remove rigid lenses:	
a. Wash hands.	Reduces transmission of microorganisms.
b. Place towel just below client's face.	Catches lens if one accidentally falls from eye.
c. Be sure lens is positioned directly over cornea. If it is not, close eyelids, place index and middle fingers of one hand behind lens, gently but firmly massage lens back into place.	Correct position of lens allows easy removal from eye.
d. Place index finger on outer corner of eye and draw skin gently back toward ear (see illustration).	Tightens lids against eyeball.
e. Tell client to blink. Do not release pressure on lids until blink is completed.	Maneuver should cause lens to dislodge and pop out. Lid margins must clear top and bottom of lens until blink.
f. If lens fails to pop out, gently retract eyelid beyond edges of lens. Press lower eyelid gently against lower edge of lens.	Pressure causes upper edge of lens to tip forward.
g. Allow both eyelids to close slightly and grasp lens as it rises from eye.	Maneuver causes lens to slide off easily.
h. Cup lens in your hand.	Protects lens from breakage.
i. Cleanse and rinse lens (see Step 9). Place lens in proper storage case compartment: *R* for right lens and *L* for left lens. Center lens in storage case, convex side down.	Both lenses may not have the same prescription. Proper storage prevents cracking, tearing, or chipping.
j. Repeat Steps 8c-8i for other lens. Secure cover over storage case.	Proper storage prevents damage to lens.
k. Dispose of towel and wash hands.	Reduces spread of infection and keeps environment neat.
9. Cleanse and disinfect contact lenses:	
a. Wash hands.	Reduces transmission of microorganisms.
b. Assemble supplies at bedside.	Provides easy access to supplies.

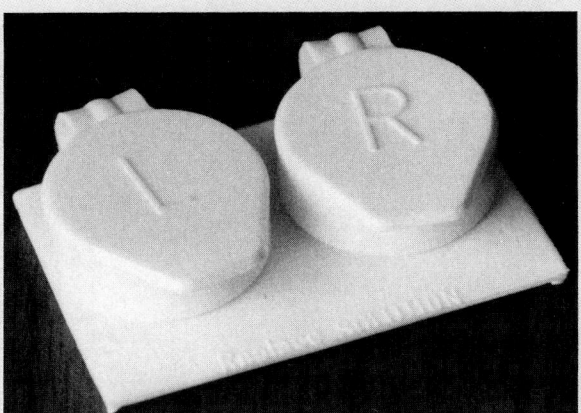

Step 3a

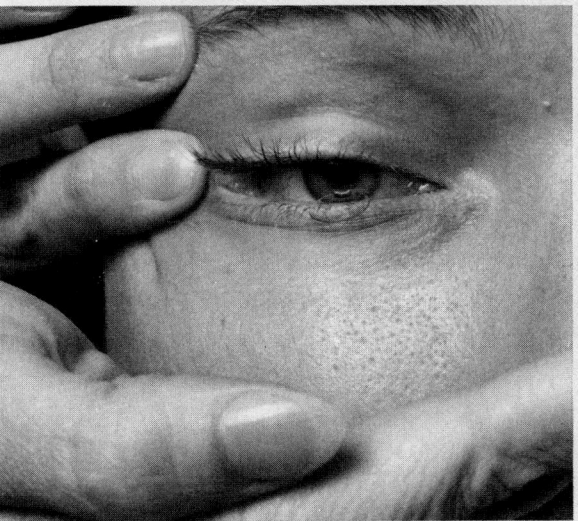

Step 8d

Taking Care of Contact Lenses

STEPS	RATIONALE
c. Place towel over work area.	Towel helps prevent lens breakage.
d. Open lens container carefully, taking care not to flip lens caps open suddenly.	Prevents lenses from being accidentally spilled or flipped out of case.
e. After removal of lens from eye, apply 1-2 drops of daily surfactant cleaner on lens in palm of your hand (use cleaner recommended by lens manufacturer or eye care practitioner).	Removes tear components, including mucus, lipid, and proteins that collect on lens.
f. Rub lens gently but thoroughly on both sides for 20-30 sec. Use index finger (soft lenses) or little finger or cotton tip applicator soaked with cleaner (rigid lenses) to clean inside lens. Be careful not to contact or scratch lens with fingernail.	It is easier to manipulate and clean lenses using fingertips. Cleanses all surfaces for microorganisms.
g. Holding lens over emesis basin, rinse thoroughly with manufacturer-recommended rinsing solution (soft lenses) or cold tap water (rigid lenses).	Removes debris and cleaning agent from lens surface.
h. Place lenses in storage case and fill with storage solution recommended by manufacturer or eye-care practitioner.	Disinfects lenses, removes residue, enhances wettability of lenses, and prevents scratches from dry case.
10. Insert rigid lenses:	
a. Wash hands thoroughly with mild noncosmetic soap. Rinse well. Dry with clean, lint-free towel or paper towel.	Lint or film on hands from soaps containing perfumes, deodorants, or complexion creams can be transferred to lenses and cause eye irritation.
b. Place towel over client's chest.	Towel will catch dropped lens and prevent breakage, scratching, or tearing.
c. Remove right lens from storage case; attempt to lift lens straight up (see illustration).	Sliding lens out of case can cause scratches on the surface.
d. Rinse with cold tap water.	Hot water causes lens to warp.
e. Wet lens on both sides using prescribed wetting solution.	Lubricates lens so that it slides easily over and adheres to cornea.
f. Place right lens concave side up on tip of index finger of dominant hand (see illustration).	Proper manipulation of lens ensures easy insertion. Inner surface of lens should face up so that it is applied against cornea.

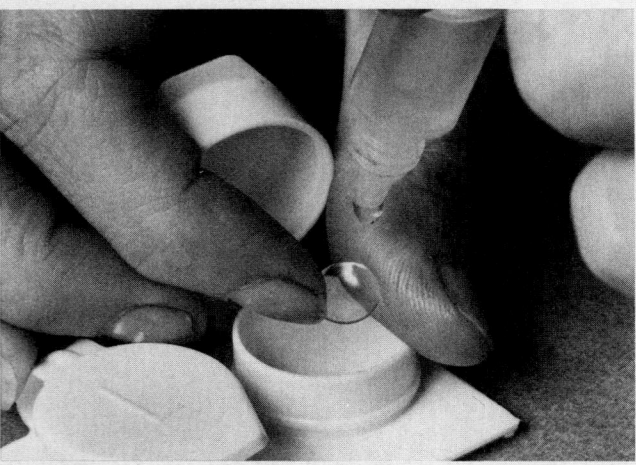

Step 10c

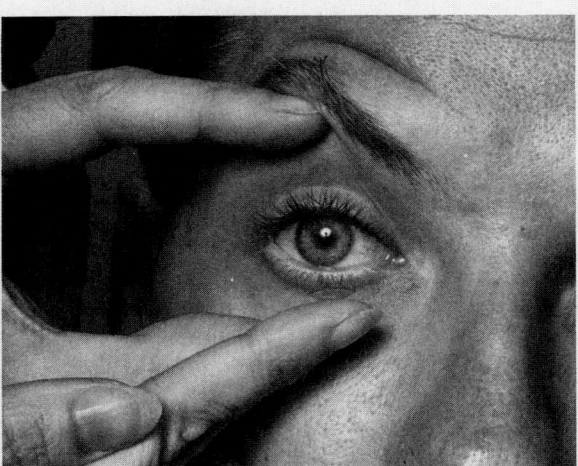

Step 10f

Taking Care of Contact Lenses

STEPS	RATIONALE
g. Instruct client to look straight ahead while retracting both upper and lower eyelids; place lens gently over center of cornea.	Hard lens is rigid and can be placed as client looks straight ahead. Retraction of lids promotes easy insertion between lid margins.
h. Ask client to close eyes briefly and avoid blinking.	Helps to secure position of lens.
i. Ask client to open eyes. Be sure lens is centered properly by asking client if vision is blurred.	If lens slips to side of cornea or into conjunctival sac, vision will blur.
j. Repeat Steps 10c-10i for left eye.	
k. Assist client to comfortable position.	Promotes client's comfort.
l. Discard soiled supplies, discard solution in storage case, rinse case thoroughly and allow to air dry, and wash hands.	Use of fresh solution daily prevents infection.

11. Insert soft lenses:

STEPS	RATIONALE
a. Wash hands with mild noncosmetic soap, rinse well, dry with clean lint-free or paper towel.	Lint or film left on hands from cosmetic or deodorant soaps can be transferred to lenses and irritate eye.
b. Place towel over client's chest.	Towel will catch dropped lens and prevent breakage, scratching, or tearing.
c. Remove right lens from storage case and rinse with recommended rinsing solution; inspect lens for foreign materials, tears, or other damage.	Removes disinfectant solution. Prevents irritation or damage to eye.
d. Check that lens is not inverted (inside out).	Soft lens is inverted if bowl has a lip; it is in proper position if curve is even from base to rim.
e. Using middle or index finger of opposite hand, retract upper lid until iris is exposed.	Soft lenses do not adhere as easily as hard lenses. Separating lids as much as possible allows room for lens to contact cornea without touching lids or lashes.
f. Use middle finger or hand holding lens to pull down lower lid.	
g. Tell client to look straight ahead and "through" lens and finger, gently place lens directly on cornea, and release lens slowly, starting with lower lid.	Ensures secure fit and comfort.
h. If lens is on sclera rather than cornea, tell client to slowly close eye and roll it toward lens.	Maneuver centers soft lens over cornea.
i. Tell client to blink a few times.	Ensures that lens is centered, free of trapped air, and comfortable.
j. Be sure lens is centered properly by asking client if vision is blurred.	If lens slips to side of cornea or into conjunctival sac, vision will blur.
k. If client's vision is blurred, retract eyelids, locate position of lens, ask client to look in direction opposite of lens and with your index finger, apply pressure to lower eyelid margin and position lens over cornea. Have client look slowly toward lens.	Repositions lens over center of cornea as client looks toward lens.
l. Repeat Steps 11c-11j for other eye.	
m. Assist client to comfortable position.	Promotes client's comfort.
n. Discard soiled supplies, discard solution in storage case, rinse case thoroughly and allow to air dry, and wash hands.	Prevents infection and maintains neat environment.

STEPS	RATIONALE
12. Ask client if lenses feel comfortable after reinsertion.	Determines whether debris is caught between lens and cornea.
13. Record or report any signs or symptoms of visual alterations noted during procedure.	May indicate eye injury or disease.
14. Record on nursing care plan or Kardex times of lens insertion and removal.	Determines safe period of time for insertion.

Care of a Behind-the-Ear Hearing Aid

STEPS	RATIONALE
1. Assess client's knowledge of and routines for cleansing and caring for hearing aid.	Determines client's understanding and need for health education. Adapts method of care to client's procedure.
2. Determine whether client can hear clearly with use of aid by talking slowly and clearly in normal voice tone.	Inability to hear may indicate faulty function of hearing aid.
3. Have client suggest any additional tips for care; explain that you are going to clean and replace hearing aid.	Client becomes uncomfortable when unable to hear clearly. Minimizes confusion and anxiety.
4. Assess whether hearing aid is working by removing from client's ear. Close battery case and turn volume slowly to high. Cup hand over earmold. If aid emits no sound, replace batteries and assess again.	Determines need for new battery. Feedback squeal will cause harsh whistling sound.
5. Check to be sure plastic connecting tube is not twisted or cracked.	Cracked or twisted tube prevents transmission of sound.
6. Check to see if earmold is cracked or has rough edges.	Can cause irritation to external ear canal.
7. Check for accumulation of cerumen around earmold and plugging of opening in mold.	Prevents clear sound reception and transmission.
8. Prepare necessary equipment and supplies: a. Emesis basin b. Mild soap and warm water c. Pipe cleaner (optional) d. Syringe needle (optional) e. Soft towel f. Wash cloth g. Storage case	Used to soak ear mold. Used to clean plastic connecting tube. Used to clean opening in ear mold.
9. Clean hearing aid: a. Wash hands. b. Assemble supplies at bedside table or sink area. c. Detach earmold from battery device. d. Add warm water and soap to emesis basin. Soak ear mold for several minutes. e. Wash ear canal with washcloth moistened in soap and water. Rinse and dry. f. If cerumen has built up in hole of earmold, carefully cleanse hole with tip of syringe needle. g. Rinse earmold thoroughly with clear water. h. Allow mold to dry thoroughly after wiping with soft towel. i. Cleanse connecting tube with pipe cleaner (optional). j. Reconnect ear mold to hearing aid device before inserting or storing hearing aid. k. Store hearing aid in storage case if client is about to bathe, walk in rain, use hair dryer, sit under sun lamp or heat, go to surgery or major procedure, go to sleep, or is diaphoretic.	Reduces transmission of microorganisms. Procedure can be performed without delays. Moisture entering battery and transmitter will cause permanent damage to aid. Soaking removes cerumen that can accumulate on mold. Removes cerumen and debris. Wax will prevent normal sound transmission. Soap may form residue that blocks opening in mold. Water droplets left in connecting tube could enter hearing aid and damage parts. Removes moisture and debris that can interfere with sound transmission and hearing aid function. Reassembly allows check of functioning. Protects hearing aid against damage and breakage.
10. Insert hearing aid: a. Check batteries (see Step 4); replace batteries as needed. b. Turn aid off and turn volume control down.	Necessary for proper sound amplification. Always change batteries over soft surface (e.g., towel or bed) to avoid breakage. Protects client from sudden exposure to sound.

STEPS	RATIONALE
c. Place earmold in external ear canal. Be sure that ear bore (hole) in mold is placed into canal first. Shape of mold indicates correct ear. Gently press and twist until mold feels snug.	Proper fit ensures optimal sound transmission.
d. Gently bring connecting tube up and over toward back of ear, avoiding kinking. Battery device fits around upper ear.	Ensures correct function of hearing aid device and maintains client's comfort.
e. Adjust volume gradually to comfortable level for talking to client in regular voice at a 1-1.25 m (3-4 ft) distance.	Gradual adjustment prevents exposing client to harsh squeal or feedback. Client should hear nurse comfortably.
f. Remove soiled equipment from bedside. Dispose of used supplies. Wash hands.	Maintains clean environment and reduces risk of infection.
11. Return to client to assess whether hearing is clear or hearing aid is producing inappropriate feedback sound.	If earmold is not securely in place, it will squeal or not function.
12. Document that aid is removed and stored if client is going to surgery or special procedure.	Protects from liability of loss of hearing aid.
13. Report difficulties client has in communicating to nursing staff.	Improves continuity of care in communication techniques for client.
14. Note on nursing Kardex that client uses hearing aid.	Alerts personnel to hearing impairment.

however, slightly more noticeable than the ITC aid and is not recommended for persons with moisture or skin problems in the ear canal.

A behind-the-ear (BTE or postaural) aid hooks around and behind the ear and is connected by a short, clear, hollow plastic tube to an ear mold inserted into the external auditory canal (Fig. 34-4). It also allows for fine-tuning adjustment. It is the largest of the three and is useful for clients with rapidly progressive hearing loss or manual dexterity difficulties or those who find partial ear occlusion intolerable. Disadvantages are that it is more visible (depending on hairstyle), may interfere with eyeglasses and telephone use, and is more difficult to keep in place during physical exercise. The care of a hearing aid involves routine cleaning, battery care, and proper insertion technique (Procedure 34-10).

Nose Care

The client can usually remove secretions from the nose by gently blowing into a soft tissue. This may be all the daily hygiene needed. The nurse cautions the client against harsh blowing that creates pressure capable of injuring the eardrum, nasal mucosa, and even sensitive eye structures. Bleeding from the nares is a key sign of harsh blowing, mucosal irritation, or dryness.

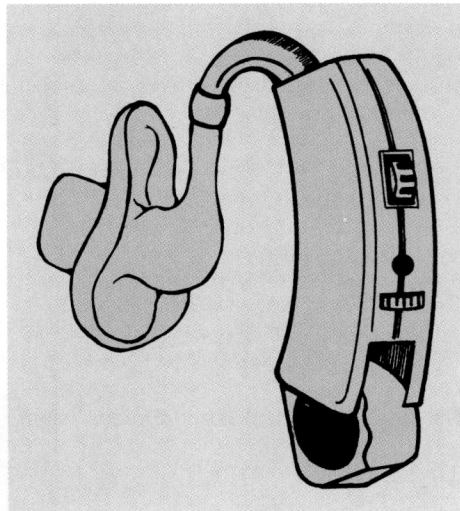

Fig. 34-4   Behind-the-ear hearing aid.

If the client cannot remove nasal secretions, the nurse assists by using a wet washcloth or a cotton-tipped applicator moistened in water or saline. The applicator should never be inserted beyond the length of the cotton tip. Excessive nasal secretions can also be removed by suctioning. Nasal suctioning is contraindicated in nasal or brain surgery.

When clients have feeding or suction tubes inserted through the nose, the nurse should change the tape anchoring the tube at least once a day (see Chapter 47). When the tape becomes moist from nasal secretions, the skin and mucosa can easily become macerated. The up-and-down movement of tubing causes tissue injury. The nurse should know how to tape tubing correctly to minimize tension or friction on the nares (see Chapter 47). When tissue injury occurs, it may be necessary to remove the tube and insert one through the other naris. The nurse should always cleanse the nares thoroughly around the tubing because secretions accumulate.

Evaluation

Evaluation of eye, ear, and nose care must be individualized on the basis of the client's existing sensory function. Hygienic care alone will not improve sensory function beyond a client's baseline level.

CLIENT'S ROOM ENVIRONMENT

Attempting to make clients' rooms as comfortable as their home environments is one of the nurse's pri-

orities. Clients with severe illnesses may be restricted to bed for many days. Likewise, clients immobilized by traction apparatus, casts, or monitoring equipment do not always enjoy the luxury of leaving their rooms as they wish. Clients hospitalized in semiprivate rooms must share the environment with other people. Chronically disabled persons living in nursing homes or skilled care facilities are often confined to rooms for long periods. Rooms should be comfortable, safe, and large enough to allow clients and visitors to move about freely. The nurse can control factors such as room temperature, ventilation, noise, and odors to create a more comfortable environment. Keeping rooms neat, clean, and orderly also contributes to a sense of well-being.

Maintaining Comfort

Providing a comfortable environment depends on age, severity of illness, and level of normal daily activity. Depending on the client's age and physical condition, room temperature should be between 20° and 23° C (68° and 74° F). Infants, older adults, and the acutely ill may need a warmer temperature. However, some critically ill clients benefit from cooler temperatures to lower the body's metabolic demands. A client who is physically active will usually be more comfortable in a cool room.

A good ventilation system keeps stale air and odors from lingering in the room. Because drafts may occur

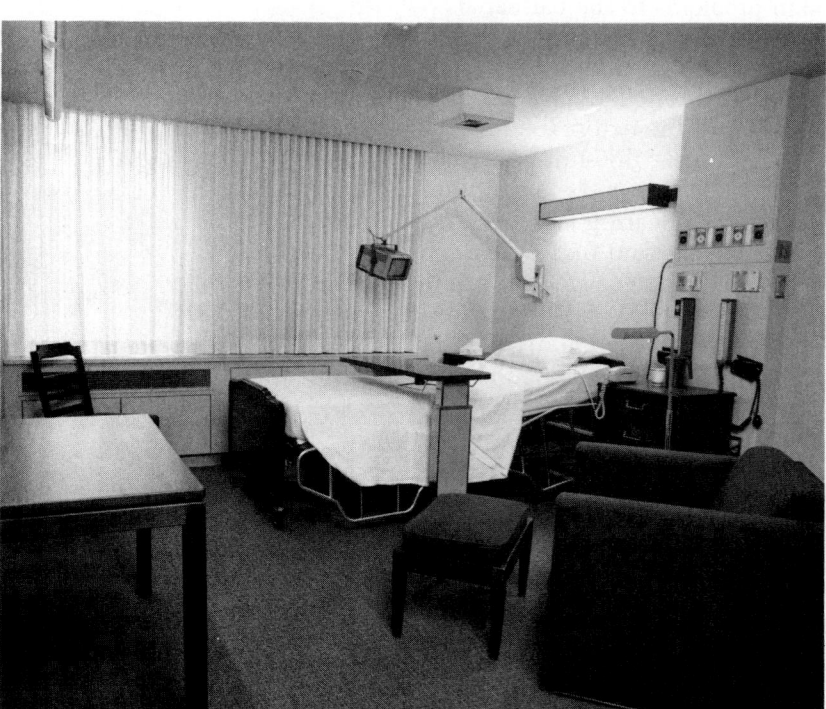

Fig. 34-5 A typical hospital room.

as the air moves about the room, the nurse must protect acutely ill clients, infants, and older adults by ensuring that they are adequately dressed and covered with lightweight blankets. Clients who complain of excess drafts, despite the nurse's interventions, may need to be moved to a different room.

Good ventilation also reduces lingering odors caused by draining wounds, vomitus, bowel movements, and the failure to empty bedpans and urinals promptly. Body and breath odors may also be offensive to some people. Room deodorizers help by eliminating many unpleasant odors. Nurses should always empty and rinse bedpans or urinals promptly after use. Thorough hygienic measures are the best way to control body or breath odors. Hospitals are now required to maintain no-smoking policies on client-care areas. The nurse should monitor visitors who attempt to smoke in clients' rooms. Only special orders by a physician will allow a client to smoke in a room. In such a situation, the client should have a private room.

Ill clients seem to be more sensitive to the noises commonly heard within a hospital environment: the clanging of metal equipment, wheelchairs or stretchers moving down halls, and loud talking and laughter at the nurse's station. The nurse should try to control the noise level by handling equipment properly, making sure that equipment is in proper working order, and controlling voice volume. The nurse also explains the source of any unfamiliar noises.

Proper lighting is necessary for the safety and comfort of the client and health care workers. A brightly lit room is usually stimulating. When clients attempt to fall asleep, the nurse reduces lighting levels. Room lighting can be adjusted by closing or opening drapes, regulating overbed and floor lights, and closing or opening room doors.

Controlling stimuli within the room environment helps promote the client's feeling of security. A comfortable environment enhances the client's ability to gain needed rest and sleep so that all energy can be directed to recovery.

Room Equipment

A typical hospital room (Fig. 34-5) contains certain basic pieces of furniture: overbed table, bedside stand, chairs, lights, and beds. Special equipment designed for comfort or positioning of clients includes footboards (Fig. 34-6), special mattresses, bed boards, and bed cradles (see box).

Overbed Table

The overbed table rolls on wheels and can be adjusted to various heights over the bed or a chair.

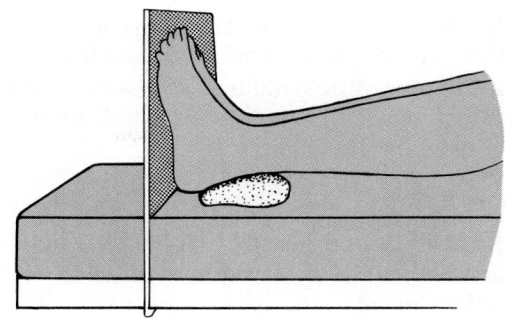

Fig. 34-6   Footboard.

Special Room Equipment

FOOTBOARD

■ A flat plastic or wood panel placed at the foot of the bed above the mattress level (Fig. 34-5) keeps the feet in the dorsiflexion position to prevent footdrop. A footboard also keeps bed covers up and off the client's feet.

FOOTBOOTS

■ Sheepskin or foam-lined boots made of smooth plastic or foam support each foot in dorsiflexion. They are preferred over footboards because they allow clients a variety of positions.

SPECIAL MATTRESSES AND BEDS

■ A variety of special mattresses, beds, and frames is available to support specific pressure-prone areas of the body and to provide client comfort (see Chapter 44). Flotation pads, egg-crate mattresses, and alternating air mattresses dispense pressure from the client's body weight over a large area and thus reduce the risk of pressure sores. Some beds and frames help to turn immobilized clients or maintain correct body alignment.

BED BOARD

■ A long wooden or Plexiglas board, the length of a regular bed mattress, is placed under a mattress to provide added support. Clients with back pain frequently use bed boards. The boards are rigid or hinged so that the foot or end of the bed can be elevated.

BED CRADLE

■ This curved, semicircular device made of metal can be placed over a portion of the client's body. The cradle keeps the top bed linens off the client's feet, legs, or abdomen. Bed cradles come in a variety of sizes.

Usually, two storage areas are under the table top. The table provides ideal working space for the nurse performing procedures and also serves as a surface to place meal trays, toiletry items, and objects frequently used by the client.

Bedside Stand

The bedside stand is used to store the client's personal articles and hygienic equipment such as a bath basin, extra towels, and an emesis basin. The telephone, water pitcher, and drinking cup are commonly found on a bedside table.

Chairs

Most hospital rooms contain a straight-back chair and a lounge chair with arms. The lounge chair is used by the client and visitors and is placed at the foot of the bed or beside it. Straight-back chairs are convenient when temporarily transferring the client from the bed (for example, during bedmaking). A straight-back chair is also more maneuverable than the larger lounge chair. Nurses often place clean linen on the chair or hang linen bags over the back.

Lights

Each room usually has an overbed light and ceiling lights. Some may also have a floor or table lamp. Movable lights that extend over the bed from the wall should be positioned for easy reach but moved aside when not in use to prevent clients or staff from bumping their heads. Gooseneck or special examination lights are portable standing lights used to provide extra illumination during bedside procedures.

A call light is at each bedside. When a client presses a button located on the side rail of the bed or at the end of an extension cord, a light goes on at the nurses' station or just outside the client's room. The call-light signal indicates that a client needs assistance. The nurse should respond as soon as possible. In addition to call lights, most hospitals have intercoms that allow clients to talk to a staff person at the nurses' station. Many hospitals also have emergency signal lights to call for assistance when clients are in trouble.

Beds

Beds should be designed for comfort, safety, and adaptability for changing positions. The typical hospital bed consists of a firm mattress on a metal frame that can be raised and lowered horizontally. The frame is divided into three sections, so the operator can raise and lower the head and foot of the bed, in addition to inclining the entire bed with the headboard up or down. Table 34-9 lists common bed positions. Most beds are powered by electrical motors, but some are run manually or by hydraulic power.

The position of a bed is usually changed by electrical controls on the side of the bed, at the foot of the bed, or in a bedside cable. Clients can thus raise or lower sections of the bed without expending much energy. Nurses instruct clients on the proper use of controls and caution them against raising the bed to a position that might cause harm. At its lowest level, a hospital bed is usually 65 to 70 cm (26 to 28 in) above the floor, whereas in the home, most beds are only 50 to 55 cm (20 to 22 in) high. The greater height of a hospital bed prevents undue musculoskeletal strain on the nurse and client. It is unnecessary for the nurse to reach across or bend down while caring for clients, and clients can move from the bed to a chair with minimal stress on their hips and knees. The client's bed should never be left in a high position when the client is unattended.

Beds contain a number of safety features. Locks on the wheels or casters are used when the bed is stationary to prevent movement during the performance of a procedure. Side rails, located on both sides of a bed, protect clients from falls, help clients position themselves, and provide upper extremity support as a client gets out of bed. Side rails are adjustable, metal frames that raise and lower by pushing or pulling a knob. The nurse never leaves the bedside when a side rail is lowered with the client in bed. Each bed also has a special removable headboard. This is important when the medical team must have easy access to the client's head during cardiopulmonary resuscitation.

Most beds have firm, water-repellent mattresses. A mattress should have an even surface for comfort. Most mattresses have handles on the sides to be used when the mattresses are removed or turned over.

BEDMAKING. Making a bed is a responsibility of the nurse. The nurse keeps the bed clean and comfortable. This requires frequent inspections to be sure that linen is clean, dry, and wrinkle free. The nurse usually makes a bed after the client's bath, while the client is bathing and showering, or when the client is out of the room for tests or procedures. Throughout the day, the nurse straightens linen that becomes loose or wrinkled. The bed linen should also be checked for food particles after meals and for wetness or soiling. Linen that becomes wet or soiled should be changed.

When changing the bed linen, the nurse follows principles of asepsis by keeping soiled linen away from the uniform. It is best to place soiled linen in special bags before discarding it in the hamper. To avoid air currents, which can spread microorganisms, the nurse never fans linen. Dirty linen should never be placed on the floor to prevent transmitting infection. If clean linen touches the floor, it is immediately discarded.

TABLE 34-9 Common Bed Positions

Position	Description	Uses
Fowler's	Head of bed raised to angle of 45 degrees or more; semisitting position	Is preferred while client eats Is used during nasogastric tube insertion and nasotracheal suction Promotes lung expansion
Semi-Fowler's	Head of bed raised approximately 30 degrees; inclination less than Fowler's position	Promotes lung expansion
Trendelenburg's	Entire bed frame tilted with head of bed down	Is used for postural drainage Facilitates venous return in clients with poor peripheral perfusion
Reverse Trendelenburg's	Entire bed frame tilted with foot of bed down	Is used infrequently Promotes gastric emptying Prevents esophageal reflux
Flat	Entire bed frame horizontally parallel with floor	Is used for clients with vertebral injuries and in cervical traction Is used for clients who are hypotensive Is generally preferred by clients for sleeping

The nurse must use proper body mechanics during bedmaking. The bed should be raised to a comfortable working height toward the nurse's center of gravity before changing linen so that the nurse does not have to bend or stretch over the mattress. When making an occupied bed, the nurse should also use the principles of body mechanics while turning and repositioning the client (see Chapter 43).

The client's privacy, comfort, and safety are all important when making a bed. Using side rails, keeping call lights within the client's reach, and maintaining the proper bed position help promote comfort and safety. After making a bed, the nurse always returns it to the lowest horizontal position to prevent falls.

Whenever possible, the nurse should make the bed while it is unoccupied (Procedure 34-11 on p. 1078). If the client is confined to bed, the nurse organizes bedmaking activities to conserve time and energy (Procedure 34-12 on p. 1083). When making an unoccupied bed, the nurse follows the same basic principles as those for making an occupied bed. However, the nurse loosens the bed linen on both sides, removes all soiled linen simultaneously, and positions the clean base and top linen on one side before going to the other side.

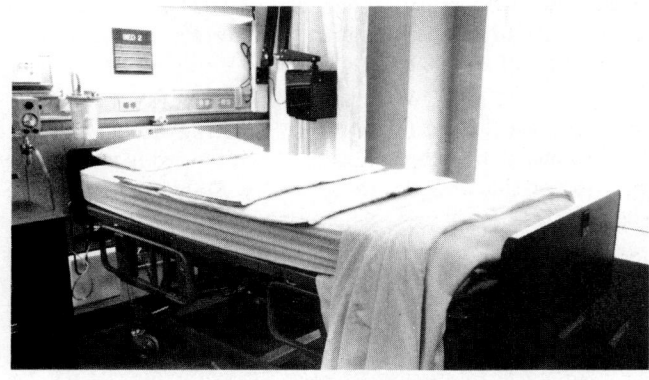

Fig. 34-7 Surgical or recovery bed.

An unoccupied bed can be open or closed. In an open bed, the top covers are folded back so that a client can easily get into bed (Fig. 34-7). In a closed bed, the top sheet, blanket, and bedspread are drawn up to the head of the mattress and under the pillows. A closed bed is prepared in a hospital room before a new client is admitted to that room.

A surgical, recovery, or postoperative bed is an open version of the unoccupied bed. The top bed linen is arranged for easy transfer from a stretcher to

Text continued on p. 1087.

Making a Conventional Unoccupied Bed

STEPS	RATIONALE
1. Assess potential for client being incontinent or having excess drainage on bed linen. Assess client's activity orders and physical mobility.	Determines need for protective waterproof pads or bath blankets on bed. Determines level of activity allowed, including whether client should be out of bed.
2. If client is in bed, explain that you wish to change bed while client is sitting up. Ask if client feels able to sit in chair. Assist client to chair if necessary.	Client should not feel inconvenienced by procedure. Client may feel anxious if uncomfortable or fatigued.
3. Prepare needed equipment and supplies: a. Linen bags	Collecting linen top to bottom in order of use makes it easier to make bed without delays.

b. Mattress pad (needs only be changed when soiled)
    c. Bottom sheet (flat or fitted)
    d. Drawsheet
	Used to help lift or move client and to protect bottom sheet from soiling.

e. Top sheet (flat or fitted at foot)
    f. Blanket
    g. Bedspread
    h. Waterproof pads or bath blankets (optional)
	Used to lay under client at points where drainage is expected. Reduces soiling of bed linen.

i. Pillow cases j. Bedside chair or table	Used to place linen on in order of use.
4. Wash hands.	Reduces transmission of microorganisms.
5. Assemble equipment and arrange it on bedside chair or table. Remove all unnecessary equipment, such as overbed table.	Provides orderly procedure and ensures client comfort. Placing linen on clean surface minimizes spread of infection.
6. Lower side rail on your side of bed and remove call light. Adjust bed height to comfortable working position.	Provides easy access to bed. Minimizes strain on back and muscles.
7. On your side, loosen linen, starting at top or bed. Move along sides and then down toward foot. Move to other side of bed, lower side rail, and loosen all linen.	Makes linen easier to remove.

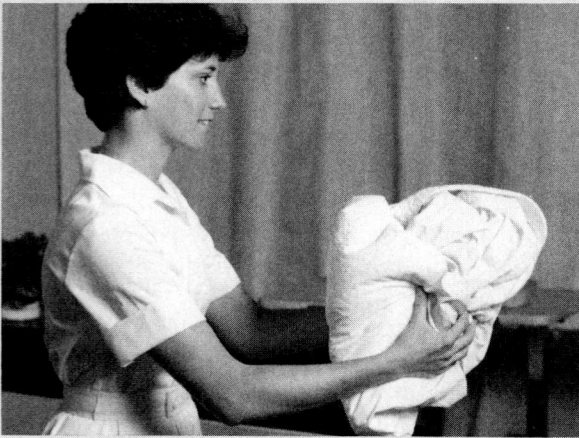

Step 8

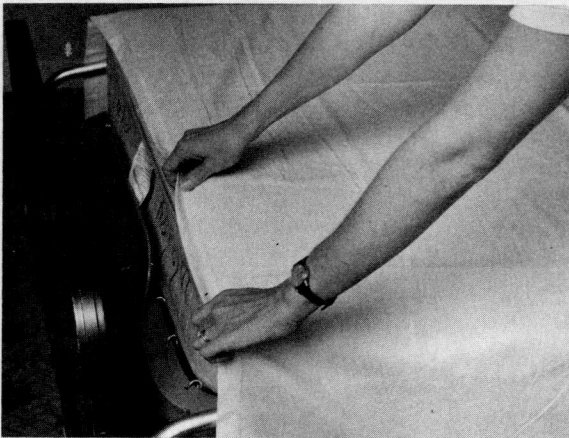

Step 14

STEPS	RATIONALE
8. Remove bedspread and blanket separately by folding each into ball or folded square and discarding into linen bag if they are not to be reused. Do not allow uniform to come in contact with soiled linen (see illustration). Avoid fanning or shaking linen.	Reduces transmission of microorganisms.
9. If spread or blanket is to be reused, fold each by grasping top edge with both hands, one hand at center, other hand at end. Fold top edge down, even with the bottom edge. Pick up spread at center and fold so that farthest side comes even with nearest side. Bring top and bottom edges together again. Place folded spread or blanket over back of chair.	Facilitates replacement and prevents wrinkling.
10. Remove soiled pillow cases by grasping closed end with one hand and slipping pillow out with other. Discard cases in linen bag and place pillows on table.	Pillows slide out easily, minimizing chance of contact with soiled linen.
11. Fold each piece of remaining bed linen into ball or folded square and discard into linen bag. Do not put linen on floor.	Attempting to fold all soiled linen at once creates bulky bundle that is difficult to discard and may easily come in contact with uniform.
12. Slide mattress toward head of bed. Wipe off any moisture on mattress with washcloth moistened in antiseptic solution; dry thoroughly.	If mattress slides toward foot of bed when head of bed is raised, it is difficult to tuck in linen. Reduces transmission of microorganisms.
13. Stand at side of bed where linen is placed. Spread mattress pad over mattress. Smooth out all wrinkles in pad.	Time is saved by making half of bed first and then moving to opposite side. Wrinkles or folds of linen are source of chronic irritation against client's skin.
14. If using flat sheet as bottom sheet, unfold bottom sheet lengthwise and place vertical center crease of sheet lengthwise along center of bed. Fold sheet's top layer over toward opposite side of bed. Smooth bottom layer of sheet across mattress on your side; bring edge over side of mattress. Allow it to hang 25 cm (10 in) over mattress edge. Hem of bottom edge of sheet should lie seam down, even with bottom edge of mattress (see illustration). Pull remaining top portion of sheet over top edge of mattress.	Method of unfolding linen saves time and energy. Making one side of bed at a time avoids excess movement. Proper placement of linen ensures that adequate length will be available to cover opposite side of bed. Keeping seam edge down eliminates source of irritation to client's skin. If bottom edge of sheet is not tucked in, it can later be changed without removing top linen.
15. While standing at head of the bed, miter top corner of bottom sheet: a. Face head of bed diagonally. Place hand that is away from head of bed under top corner of mattress near mattress edge and lift. b. With other hand, tuck top edge of bottom sheet smoothly under mattress so that side edges of sheet above and below mattress would meet if brought together. c. Face side of bed and pick up top edge of sheet approximately 45 cm (18 in) down from top of mattress (see illustration). d. Lift sheet and lay it on top of mattress to form neat, triangular fold, with lower base of triangle even with mattress side edge (see illustration on p. 1080).	Mitered corner is not loosened easily. 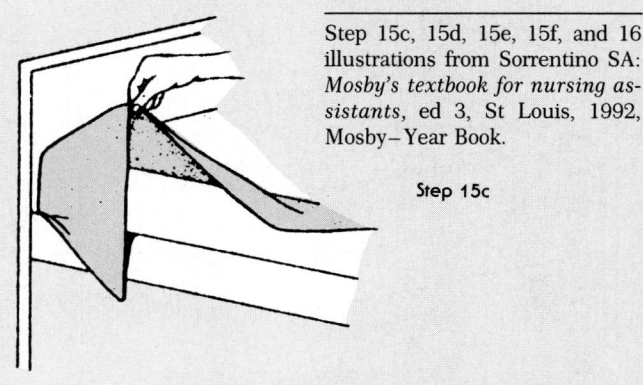 Step 15c, 15d, 15e, 15f, and 16 illustrations from Sorrentino SA: *Mosby's textbook for nursing assistants,* ed 3, St Louis, 1992, Mosby–Year Book. **Step 15c**

Making a Conventional Unoccupied Bed

STEPS	RATIONALE

e. Tuck lower edge of sheet, hanging free below mattress, under mattress. Tuck with your palms down. Do this without pulling triangular fold (see illustration).

f. Hold portion of sheet covering side edge of mattress in place with one hand. With other hand, pick up top of triangular linen fold and bring it down over side of mattress. Tuck this portion of sheet under mattress (see illustrations).

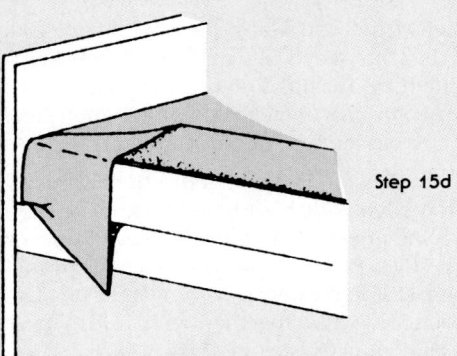

Step 15d

16. Tuck remaining portion of sheet under mattress. Keep linen smooth (see illustration).

Folds of linen can irritate client's skin.

17. OPTIONAL: Open draw-sheet so that it unfolds in half. Lay center fold lengthwise along middle of the bed. Fanfold top layer at center of bed. Smooth bottom layer of draw-sheet out over mattress. Tuck excess edge under mattress, keeping palms down.

Draw-sheet is used to lift and reposition client. Placement under client's torso distributes most of body weight over sheet. Tucking excess under mattress anchors sheet in place to prevent sliding and wrinkling.

18. Move to opposite side of bed.

One side of bed is completed before you move to other side.

19. Spread fanfolded bottom sheet smoothly over edge of mattress from head to foot of bed.

Wrinkles can cause irritation.

20. Miter top corner of bottom sheet (see Step 15). When tucking corner, be sure sheet is taut.

Taut sheet eliminates wrinkles and folds that can rub client's skin.

21. Facing side of bed, grasp remaining edge of bottom sheet, lean back, keeping your back straight, and pull as you tuck excess linen tightly under mattress. Proceed from head to foot of bed. (Avoid lifting mattress during tucking to ensure tight fit.)

Proper use of body mechanics while tucking linen prevents injury.

22. Smooth folded draw-sheet over bottom sheet. Grasp edge of drawsheet with palms down, lean back, and tuck sheet under mattress. Tuck first at middle, then at top, and then at bottom (see illustration).

Tucking first at top or bottom may pull sheet sideways, causing poor fit. Loose bedsheets reduce friction and help prevent pressure ulcers (Rousseau, 1988).

23. If needed, apply waterproof pad or bath blanket over draw-sheet.

Pad collects body secretions and drainage, protecting linen from becoming soiled.

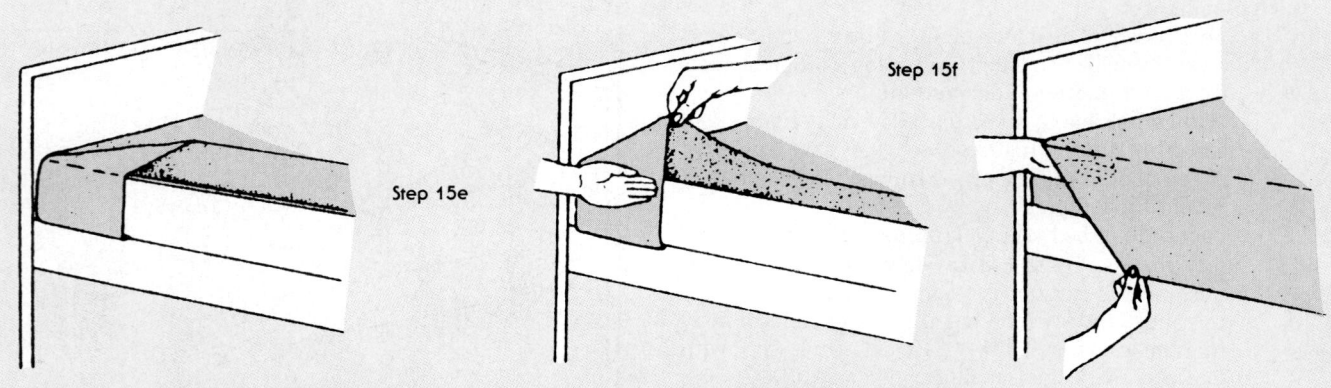

Step 15e   Step 15f

STEPS	RATIONALE
24. Move to side of bed where linen is located. Place top sheet over bed with vertical center fold lengthwise down middle of bed. Open sheet out from head to foot, being sure top edge of sheet is seam up and even with top edge of mattress. Spread excess sheet over bottom edge of mattress. (Do not fan top sheet over bed.)	Placement ensures equal distribution of sheet over bed. Positioning sheet with seam up prevents irritation of client's skin. Fanning creates air currents, which can spread microorganisms throughout room.
25. OPTIONAL: Make horizontal toe pleat: stand at foot of bed and form fold in sheet 5-10 cm (2-4 in) across bed. Pull sheet up from bottom to make fold. Fold should be approximately 15 cm (6 in) from bottom edge of mattress (see illustration on p. 1082).	Allows for free movement of client's feet and prevents friction against surface of toes.
26. Tuck in remaining portion of sheet on one side of foot of mattress (optional).	Anchors top sheet so that client can move freely.
27. Place blanket on bed, unfolding it so that crease runs lengthwise along middle of bed. Top edge should be parallel with edge of top sheet and 15-20 cm (6-8 in) down from mattress top edge. Bottom edge should hang over mattress. Spread blanket evenly over bed.	Blanket provides adequate warmth. Cuff will be formed with sheet folded over top edge of blanket and spread.
28. Place spread over bed according to Step 7. Be sure that top edge of spread extends about 2.5 cm (1 in) above blanket's edge. Then tuck top edge of spread over and under top edge of blanket.	Spread gives bed neat appearance and provides extra warmth.
29. Make cuff by running edge of top sheet down over top edge of blanket and spread.	Smooth cuff protects client's face from irritation.
30. Standing on one side at foot of bed, lift mattress corner slightly with one hand and with other hand tuck top sheet, blanket, and spread under mattress. Be sure you have not pulled out toe pleat of sheet so that linens are loose enough for client to move.	Pressure ulcers can develop on client's toes and heels if feet rub between tight-fitting bed sheets. Lifting mattress too high can loosen bottom linen.
31. Make modified mitered corner with top sheet, blanket and spread: pick up side edge of top sheet, blanket, and spread approximately 45 cm (18 in) up from foot of mattress. Lift linens to form triangular fold and lay it on bed. Tuck loose edge hanging down under side of mattress. Pick up triangular fold and bring it down over mattress, holding linen along side of mattress. Do not tuck tip of triangle (see illustration on p. 1082).	Modified mitered corner secures top linen but keeps even edge of top sheet, blanket, and spread draped over mattress.

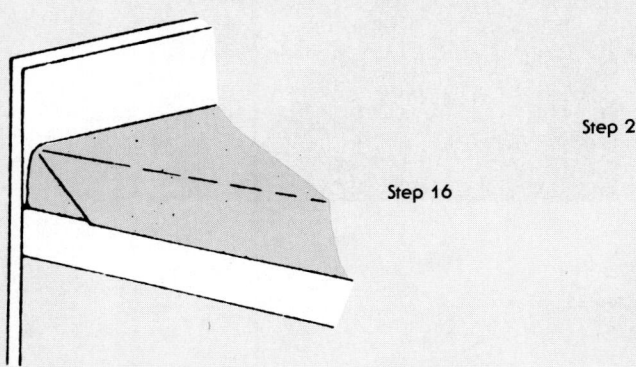

Step 16

Step 22

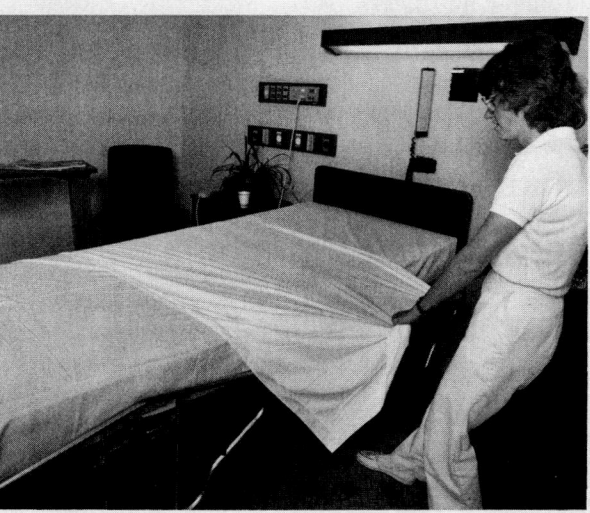

Making a Conventional Unoccupied Bed

STEPS	RATIONALE
32. Go to other side: spread sheet, blanket, and spread evenly. Fold top edge of spread over blanket and make cuff with top sheet (see Step 33). Make modified mitered corner at foot of bed (see Step 35).	Saves time and energy by completing one side of bed at time.
33. Apply clean pillowcase. With one hand, grasp pillowcase at center of closed end. Gather case, turning it inside out over hand holding it. With same hand, pick up middle of one end of pillow. Pull pillow case down over pillow with other hand. Be sure corners of case fit evenly over pillow.	Eases sliding of case smoothly over pillow.
34. Position pillows at center of head of bed.	Maintains neat appearance.
35. Place call light within client's reach and return bed to comfortable height.	Provides for client safety.
36. Fold back top covers to one side or fanfold them to bottom third of bed.	Eases client's return to bed.
37. Rearrange furniture and place personal items within easy reach.	Promotes sense of well-being.
38. Discard dirty linen in linen hamper or chute. Wash hands.	Prevents transmission of microorganisms.
39. Evaluate client's tolerance to sitting up in chair; compare heart rate to previous resting rate. Ask if client feels weak, dizzy, or fatigued; assess blood pressure if client complains of dizziness or weakness.	Client's inability to tolerate exertion, even low levels of exercise, may be reflected in changes in vital signs or subjective report of symptoms.
40. Assist client in returning to bed as necessary.	

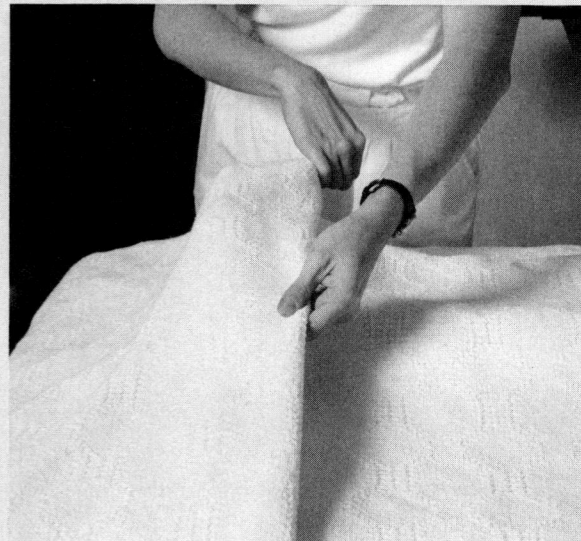

Step 25

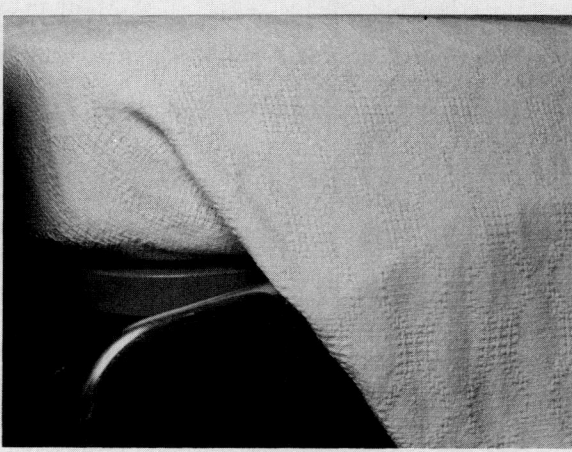

Step 31

STEPS	RATIONALE
1. Determine potential for client being incontinent or having excess drainage on bed linen.	Determines need for protective waterproof pads or extra bath blankets on bed.
2. Check chart for orders or specific precautions for movement and positioning.	Ensures client safety and use of proper body mechanics.
3. Explain procedure to client, noting that client will be asked to turn on side to roll over linen.	Minimizes anxiety and promotes client cooperation.
4. Prepare needed equipment and supplies:	
a. Linen bags	Collecting linen top to bottom in order of use makes it easier to make bed without delays.
b. Bath blanket	Provides warmth.
c. Mattress pad (needs only be changed when soiled)	
d. Bottom sheet (flat or fitted)	
e. Draw-sheet	Used to help lift or move client at points where drainage is expected. Reduces soiling of bed linen.
f. Top sheet (flat or fitted at foot)	
g. Blanket	
h. Bedspread	
i. Pillow cases	
j. Waterproof pads (optional)	Lay under client at points where drainage is expected. Reduces soiling of bed linen.
k. Bedside chair or table	
5. Wash hands.	Reduces transmission of microorganisms.
6. Assemble equipment and arrange it on bedside chair or table. Remove unnecessary equipment.	Assembling all equipment provides for smooth procedure and ensures comfort. Placing linen on clean surface minimizes spread of infection.
7. Draw room curtain around bed or close door.	Maintains client's privacy, thus promoting emotional and physical comfort.
8. Adjust bed height to comfortable working position. Lower side rail on your side of bed. Remove call light.	Minimizes strain on back. It is easier to remove and apply linen evenly to bed in flat position. Provides easy access to bed and linen.
9. Loosen top linen sheet at foot of bed.	Makes linen easier to remove.
10. Remove bedspread and blanket separately and place them in linen bag (if not to be reused). Do not allow linen to contact uniform. Do not fan or shake linen.	Reduces transmission of microorganisms.
11. If blanket and spread are to be reused, fold by bringing top and bottom edges together. Fold side farthest from your working side over onto nearer bottom edge. Bring top and bottom edges together again. Place folded linen over back of chair.	Folding method facilitates replacement and prevents wrinkles.
12. Cover client with bath blanket in following manner: unfold bath blanket over top sheet. Ask client to hold top edge of bath blanket. If client is unable to help, tuck top of bath blanket under shoulder. Grasp top sheet under bath blanket at client's shoulders and bring sheet down to foot of bed. Remove sheet and discard it in linen bag.	Provides warmth and keeps body parts covered during linen removal.
13. With assistance from another nurse, slide mattress toward head of bed.	If mattress slides toward foot of bed when head of bed is raised, it is difficult to tuck linen and is uncomfortable for client.

Making a Conventional Occupied Bed

STEPS	RATIONALE
14. Position client on side on far side of bed, facing away. Adjust pillow under head. Be sure side rail is up.	Moving client to side provides space for placement of clean linen. Side rail ensures client's safety.
15. Loosen bottom linens, moving from head to foot.	Prepares for removal of all bottom linen simultaneously.
16. With seam side down (facing the mattress), fanfold bottom sheet and draw sheet toward client: first draw-sheet, then bottom sheet. Tuck edges of linen just under buttocks, back, and shoulders. Do not fanfold mattress pad if it is to be reused (see illustration).	Provides maximum work space for placing clean linen. Later, when client turns to other side, soiled linen can be easily removed.
17. Wipe off any moisture on exposed mattress with towel and appropriate disinfectant.	Reduces transmission of microorganisms.
18. Apply clean linen to exposed half of bed:	
a. Place clean mattress pad on bed by folding it lengthwise with center crease in middle of bed. Fanfold top layer over mattress. (If pad is reused, simply smooth out any wrinkles.)	Applying linen over bed in successive layers minimizes energy and time used in bedmaking.
b. Unfold bottom sheet lengthwise so that center crease is situated lengthwise along center of bed. Fanfold sheet's (see illustraion) top layer toward center of bed alongside client. Smooth bottom layer of sheet over mattress and bring edge over your side of mattress. Allow sheet's edge to hang about 25 cm (10 in) over mattress edge. Lower hem of bottom sheet should lie seam down and even with bottom edge of mattress.	Proper positioning of linen on one side ensures that adequate linen will be available to cover opposite side of bed. Keeping seam edges down eliminates irritation to client's skin.
19. Miter bottom sheet at head of bed:	Mitered corner cannot be loosened easily even if client moves about frequently in bed.
a. Face head of bed diagonally. Place hand away from head of bed under top corner of mattress, near mattress edge, and lift.	
b. With other hand, tuck top edge of bottom sheet smoothly under mattress so that side edges of sheet above and below mattress would meet if brought together.	

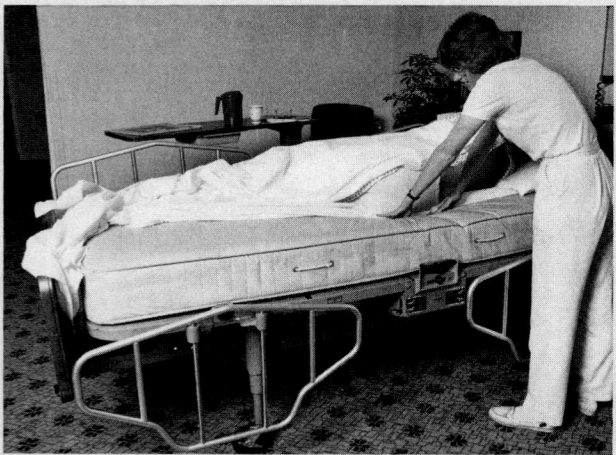

Step 16

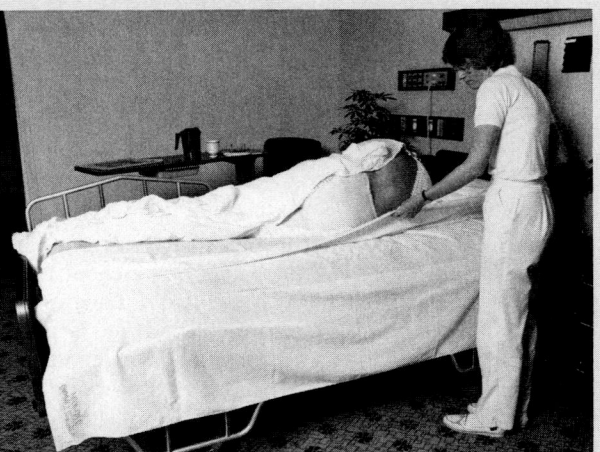

Step 18b

STEPS	RATIONALE
c. Face side of bed and pick up top edge of sheet at approximately 45 cm (18 in) from top of mattress.	
d. Lift sheet and lay it on top of mattress to form neat triangular fold, with lower base of triangle even with mattress side edge.	
e. Tuck lower edge of sheet, which is hanging free below mattress, under mattress. Tuck with palms down. Do this without pulling triangular fold.	
f. Hold portion of sheet covering side of mattress in place with one hand. With other hand, pick up top of triangular linen fold and bring it down over side of mattress. Tuck this portion under mattress.	
20. Tuck remaining portion of sheet under mattress, moving toward foot of bed. Keep linen smooth.	Folds of linen are source of irritation.
21. OPTIONAL: Open draw-sheet so that it unfolds in half. Lay center fold along middle of bed lengthwise and position sheet so that it will be under buttocks and torso. Fanfold top layer toward client with edge along back. Smooth bottom layer out over mattress and tuck excess edge under mattress (keep palms down).	Draw-sheet is used to lift and reposition client. Placement under client's torso distributes most of client's body weight over sheet.
22. Place waterproof pad over draw-sheet with center fold against client's side. Fanfold far half toward client.	Used to protect bed linen from soiling.
23. Raise side rail on working side and go to other side.	Maintains client's safety during turning.
24. Lower side rail. Assist client to roll slowly onto other side, over folds of linen.	Exposes opposite side of bed for removal of soiled linen and placement of clean linen.
25. Loosen edges of soiled linen from under mattress.	Makes linen easier to remove.
26. Remove soiled linen by folding it into bundle or square, with soiled side turned in. Discard it in linen bag.	Reduces transmission of microorganisms.
27. Spread clean, fanfolded linen smoothly over edge of mattress from head to foot of bed.	Smooth linen will not irritate client's skin.
28. Assist client in rolling back into supine position. Reposition pillow.	Maintains client's comfort.
29. Miter top corner of bottom sheet (see Step 20). When tucking corner, be sure sheet is smooth and free of wrinkles.	Wrinkles and folds can cause mechanical irritation to skin.
30. Facing side of bed, grasp remaining edge of bottom sheet. Lean back, keep back straight, and pull as you tuck excess linen under mattress. Proceed from head to foot of bed. (Avoid lifting mattress during tucking to ensure fit.)	Proper use of body mechanics while tucking linen prevents injury.
31. Smooth fanfolded draw-sheet out over bottom sheet. Grasp edge of sheet with palms down, lean back, and tuck sheet under mattress. Tuck from middle to top and then to bottom.	Tucking first at top or bottom may pull sheet sideways, causing poor fit.
32. Place top sheet over client with center fold lengthwise down middle of bed. Open sheet from head to foot and unfold it over client.	Sheet should be equally distributed over bed by correctly positioning center fold.

Making a Conventional Occupied Bed

STEPS	RATIONALE

33. Ask client to hold clean top sheet, or tuck sheet around client's shoulders. Remove bath blanket and discard it in linen bag (see illustration).

Sheet prevents exposure of body parts. Having client hold sheet encourages client participation in care.

34. Place blanket on bed, unfolding it so that crease runs lengthwise along middle of bed. Unfold blanket to cover client. Top edge should be parallel with edge of top sheet and 15-20 cm (6-8 in) from top sheet's edge.

Blanket should be placed to cover client completely and provide adequate warmth.

35. Place spread over bed according to Step 31. Be sure that top edge of spread extends about 2.5 cm (1 in) above blanket's edge. Tuck top edge of spread over and under top edge of blanket.

Gives bed neat appearance and provides extra warmth.

36. Make cuff by turning edge of top sheet down over top edge of blanket and spread.

Protects client's face from rubbing against blanket or spread.

37. Standing on one side at foot of bed, lift mattress corner slightly with one hand and tuck top linens under mattress. Top sheet and blanket are tucked under together. Be sure that linens are loose enough to allow movement of client's feet. (You may make horizontal toe pleat [Procedure 34-12, Step 29].)

Makes neat-appearing bed. Pressure ulcers can develop on client's toes and heels from feet rubbing between tight-fitting bed sheets.

38. Make modified mitered corner with top sheet, blanket, and spread:
  a. Pick up side edge of top sheet, blanket, and spread approximately 45 cm (18 in) from foot of mattress. Lift linens to form triangular fold and lay it on bed.
  b. Tuck lower edge of sheet, which is hanging free below mattress, under mattress. Do not pull triangular fold.
  c. Pick up triangular fold and bring it down over mattress while holding linen in place along side of mattress. Do not tuck tip of triangle.

Secures top linen but keeps even edge of blanket and top sheet draped over mattress.

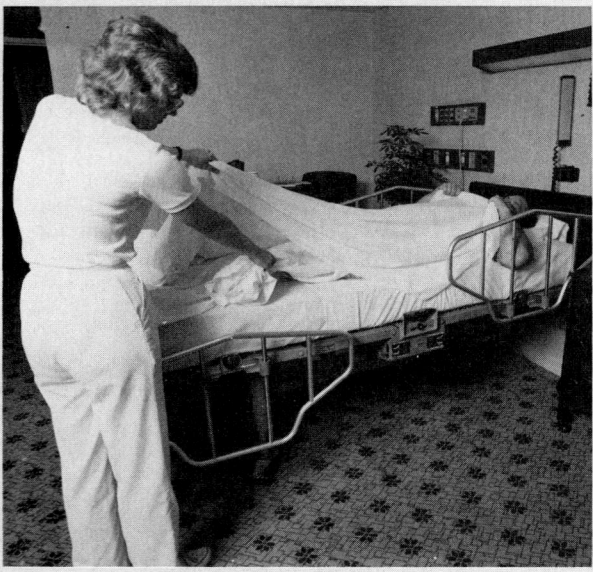

Step 33

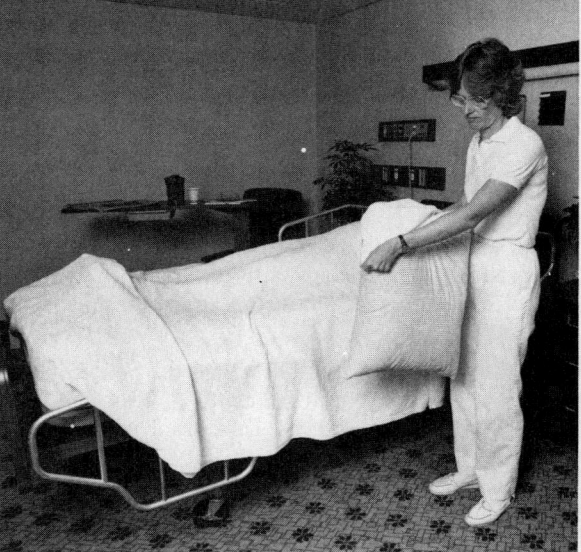

Step 40c

CONTINUED

STEPS	RATIONALE
39. Raise side rail. Make other side of bed; spread sheet, blanket, and bedspread out evenly. Fold top edge of spread over blanket and make cuff with top sheet (see Step 37); make modified mitered corner at foot of bed (see Step 38).	Side rail protects client from accidental falls.
40. Change pillowcase:	
a. Have client raise head. While supporting neck remove pillow. Allow client to lower head.	Support of neck muscles prevents injury during flexion and extension of neck.
b. Remove soiled case by grasping pillow at open end with one hand and pulling case over pillow with other hand. Discard case in linen bag.	Pillows slide out easily, thus minimizing contact with soiled linen.
c. Grasp clean pillowcase at center of closed end. Gather case, turning it inside out over hand holding it. With same hand pick up middle of one end of pillow. Pull pillowcase down over pillow with other hand (see illustration).	Eases sliding of pillowcase over pillow.
d. Be sure pillow corners fit evenly in corners of pillowcase. Place pillow under client's head.	Poorly fitting case constricts fluffing and expansion of pillow. Promotes comfort.
41. Place call light within client's reach and return bed to comfortable position.	Ensures safety and comfort.
42. Open room curtains. Rearrange furniture. Place personal items within easy reach on overbed table or bedside stand. Return bed to comfortable height.	Promotes sense of well-being.
43. Discard dirty linen in hamper or chute; wash hands.	Prevents transmission of microorganisms.

the bed. The top sheets and spread are not tucked or mitered at the corners. Instead, the top sheets are folded lengthwise or crosswise at the foot of the bed. If a client is returning from surgery, the nurse always makes a complete linen change. After a client is discharged, all bed linen is sent to the laundry, the mattress and bed are cleansed by housekeeping personnel, and new bed linen is applied.

LINENS. The nurse collects linens in order of their use. This makes it easier to make the bed without having to stop and search for specific linen pieces. It is also important to collect the client's personal linens such as bath towels and washcloths. The nurse should avoid bringing excess linen to the client's room because it can easily become contaminated. Linen should be collected in the following order: linen bag for soiled linen, mattress pad (optional), bottom sheet, cotton or plastic-backed draw-sheet, top sheet, blanket, bedspread, pillowcases, bath towels, hand towel, washcloths, hospital gown, and blanket.

Linens are pressed and folded to prevent the spread of microorganisms and to make bedmaking easier. Bed linens have a center crease that the nurse

places in the center of the bed from the head to the foot. The linens unfold easily to the sides, with creases often fitting over the mattress edge.

When soiled linen is removed, the side on which the client was lying is rolled inside. Soiled linen should never come in contact with the nurse's uniform. A complete linen change is not always necessary. The nurse may reuse the mattress pad, sheet, blanket, and bedspread for the same client if they are not wet or soiled.

 ## SUMMARY

Hygienic measures cover a variety of basic physical needs that clients are often unable to meet themselves. Promoting independence and participation in personal hygiene is a part of the nurse's role.

A nurse should be resourceful when delivering hygienic measures. The nurse takes time for therapeutic communication, teaching, and provision of emotional support. When clients need assistance, the nurse can conduct portions of a physical examination.

Key Concepts

- Hygiene is a personal matter, and the nurse considers all factors influencing personal hygiene routine.

- The nurse assumes responsibility for providing clients' daily hygienic needs if they are unable to care for themselves adequately.

- Providing hygienic care gives the nurse the opportunity to assess all external body surfaces and the client's emotional state.

- Assisting or providing the client with daily hygienic needs allows the nurse to use teaching and communication skills to develop a meaningful relationship with the client.

- The client's personal preferences must always be considered as the nurse plans the client's daily hygienic care.

- The nurse must maintain the client's privacy and comfort when providing daily care.

- During assessment of the skin and oral mucosa, the nurse observes characteristics most influenced by hygienic measures.

- Clients who are immobilized and poorly nourished and who have reduced sensation or peripheral circulation are at risk for altered skin integrity.

- Gloves should be worn by nurses during hygienic care when the risk of contacting body fluids is high.

- Techniques used during tepid sponging are designed to minimize the risk of a client chilling.

- Clients with diabetes require special consideration when a nurse provides nail and foot care.

- When administering oral care to unconscious clients, the nurse takes measures to prevent them from aspirating fluid into their lungs.

- Clients who wear contact lenses must learn proper self-care techniques to avoid corneal injury.

- The evaluation of hygienic care is based on the client's expression of a sense of comfort, relaxation, well-being, and an understanding of personal hygienic techniques.

Key Terms

Acne, p. 1021
Alopecia, p. 1057
Apocrine glands, p. 1020
Buccal, p. 1046
Cerumen, p. 1020
Cheilosis, p. 1049
Dermis, p. 1020
Eccrine glands, p. 1020
Epidermis, p. 1019
Gingivitis, p. 1049
Glossitis, p. 1049
Halitosis, p. 1049
Hirsutism, p. 1023
Hygiene, p. 1018
Maceration, p. 1021

Mastication, p. 1046
Melanin, p. 1020
Neuropathy, p. 1041
Oral hygiene, p. 1047
Partial bed bath, p. 1027
Perineal care, p. 1035
Periodontal disease, p. 1048
Plaque, p. 1048
Podiatrist, p. 1046
Pyorrhea, p. 1048
Sebum, p. 1020
Stomatitis, p. 1049
Stratum corneum, p. 1020
Vernix caseosa, p. 1027

Critical Thinking Exercises

1. You are assigned to care for a 77-year-old woman who has been hit by a car while crossing the street. She has been admitted for a fractured pelvis and fractures of her left femur and humerus. She is a non-English-speaking Russian-Jewish individual who recently immigrated.
   a. Identify the factors you need to consider when planning hygienic care for this person.
   b. What additional information would you need before implementing care for her?

2. Mr. Johannson is a 43-year-old insulin-dependent diabetic client who has been admitted for an infected ulcer on his right foot. Identify the physiological factors that put Mr. Johannson at risk for foot problems and correlate teaching interventions to these factors.

3. Mrs. Taylor, 83, has been admitted to the hospital for a total hip replacement for a fracture of the femoral neck of her right femur. Her past history reveals that she had a cerebrovascular accident 2 years before and has residual weakness on her left side. Given her age, past history, and current condition, discuss how you would intervene postoperatively to prevent skin breakdown. Discuss the reasons for your decisions.

REFERENCES

Crosby C: Method in mouth care, *Nurs Times* 85:38, 1989.

Danielson KH: Oral care and older adults, *J Gerontol Nurs* 14:6, 1988.

Egan D, Bennett E, Davis L: Soft lens care and handling, Bethesda Eye Institute and St Louis University School of Medicine, Department of Ophthalmology, St Louis, 1988, unpublished.

Graham S, Morley M: What "foot care" really means, *Am J Nurs* 84:889, 1984.

Greifzu S, Radjeski D, Winnick B: Oral care is part of cancer care, *RN* 53:43, 1990.

Grier ME: Hair care for the black patient, *Am J Nurs* 76:1781, 1976.

Harrison KW: Gas permeable lenses a growing trend, *J Ophthalmic Nurs Technol* 8:108, 1989.

Henningson A et al: Bathing or washing babies after birth? *Lancet* 2:1401, 1981.

Ismail AI, Szpunar SM: The prevalence of total tooth loss, dental caries, and periodontal disease among Mexican Americans, Cuban Americans, and Puerto Ricans: findings from HHANES 1982-1984, *AJPH* 80(suppl):66, 1990.

Jordan J, Nickerson D: Hygiene. In Guthrie D, Guthrie R, editors: *Nursing management of diabetes mellitus,* ed 2, St Louis, 1982, Mosby–Year Book.

Kahn R: Renewing the commitment to oral hygiene, *Geriatr Nurs* 7:244, 1986.

Kim MJ, McFarland GK, McLane AM: *Pocket guide to nursing diagnosis,* ed 4, St Louis, 1991, Mosby–Year Book.

Levine P: Safeguarding your patients against periodontal disease, *RN* 36:38, 1973.

National Pressure Ulcer Advisory Panel (NPUAP): Pressure ulcer incidence, economics, risk assessment: Concensus Development Conference Statement, *Decubitus* 2(2):24, 1989.

Neeson JD, May KA: *Comprehensive maternity nursing: nursing process and the childbearing family,* New York, 1986, Lippincott.

Osterman HM, Stuck RM: The aging foot, *Orthop Nurs* 9:43, 1990.

OxyFlow EW, *Rigid permeable contact lens: instructions for wearers,* Little Rock, Ark, 1987, PDC Contact Lens Network.

Pettigrew D: Investing in mouth care, *Geriatr Nurs* 10:22, 1989.

Pires M, Mueller A: Detection and management of early tissue pressure indications: a pictoral essay, *Progressions* 3(3):3, 1991.

Poland JM: Comparing Moi-Stir to lemon glycerine swabs, *Am J Nurs* 87:422, 1987.

Rakow PL: Where have all the dropouts gone? *J Ophthalmic Nurs Technol* 9:223, 1990.

Rousseau P: Pressure sores in the aged: a preventable problem? *Continuing Care* July 1988, p 37.

Stehr-Green JK et al: *Acanthamoeba* keratitis in soft contact lens wearers: a case control study, *JAMA* 258, 1987.

Watkins S: Clearing impacted ears, *Am J Nurs* 84:1107, 1984.

Weiss SJ: Psychophysiologic effects of care giver touch on incidence of cardiac dysrhythmias, *Heart Lung* 15(5):495, 1986.

Whaley LF, Wong DL: *Nursing care of infants and children,* ed 4, St Louis, 1991, Mosby–Year Book.

Wilson CB et al: When is umbilical cord separation delayed? *J Pediatr* 107:292, 1985.

Wilson D: Make mouth care a must for your patients, *RN* 49:39, 1986.

Wilson LA, Wilson KS: Hearing aids: who can benefit? What's new? One or two? *Postgrad Med* 83:249, 1988.

ADDITIONAL READINGS

Brinkmann KL: Why can't your patient hear you? *RN* 54:46, 1991.

Carden RC: The ins and outs of contact lenses, *RN* 48:48, 1985.

Centers for Disease Control: Recommendations for prevention of HIV transmission in health care settings, *MMWR* 36(suppl 25):3s, 1987.

Chenger P, Kovacik A: Dental hygiene during pregnancy: a review, *MCN* 23:342, 1987.

Davis M: Getting to the root of the problem: hair grooming techniques for black patients, *Nurs 77* 7:60, 1977.

Deliefde B: The dental care of pregnant women, *N Z Dent J* 80:41, 1984.

Dudjak LA: Mouth care for mucositis due to radiation therapy, *Cancer Nurs* 10:131, 1987.

Ebersole P, Hess P: *Toward healthy aging: human needs and nursing response,* ed 3, St Louis, 1986, Mosby–Year Book.

Egan D, Bennett E, Davis L: *Rigid lens care and handling,* Bethesda Eye Institute and St Louis University School of Medicine, Department of Ophthalmology, St Louis, 1988, unpublished.

Evanski PM, Reinherz RP: Easing the pain of common foot problems, *Patient Care* 25:38, 1991.

Forbes K, Stokes SA: Saving the diabetic foot, *Am J Nurs* 84:884, 1984.

Frantz RA, Kinney CK: Variables associated with skin dryness in the elderly, *Nurs Res* 35(2):98, 1986.

Gerali PS: Preventing blindness, *J Ophthalmic Nurs Technol* 10:181, 1990.

Harrell J, Damon J: Prediction of patient's needs for mouth care, *West J Nurs Res* 11:748, 1989.

Kenny SA: Effect of two oral care protocols on the incidence of stomatitis in hematology patients, *Cancer Nurs* 13:345, 1990.

Knight JJ: Hearing aids, *Practitioner* 231:1121, 1987.

Longman AJ, Dewalt EM: A guide for oral assessment, *Geriatr Nurs* 7:252, 1986.

Macmillan K: New goals for oral hygiene, *Can Nurse* 77(3):40, 1981.

Meckstroth RL: Improving quality and efficiency in oral hygiene, *J Gerontol Nurs* 15:38, 1989.

Michelson D: How to give a good back rub, *Am J Nurs* 78:1197, 1978.

Nurses' drug alert: Nicotine gum and dental work protection, *Am J Nurs* 85:171, 1985.

Palumbo MV: Hearing access 2000: increasing awareness of the hearing impaired, *J Gerontol Nurs* 16:26, 1990.

Rakow PL: Using soft toric lenses to solve RGP fitting problems, *J Ophthalmic Nurs Technol* 8:111, 1989.

Rakow PL: Maintaining a healthy eye, *J Ophthalmic Nurs Technol* 9:112, 1990.

Ramler D, Roberts J: A comparison of cold and warm sitz baths for relief of postpartum perineal pain, *JOGNN* 15:471, 1986.

Sorrentino SA: *Mosby's textbook for nursing assistants,* ed 3, St Louis, 1992, Mosby–Year Book.

Sykes J: Black skin problems, *Am J Nurs* 79:1092, 1979.

Thibodeau GA, Patton K: *Anatomy and physiology,* ed 2, St Louis, 1993, Mosby–Year Book.

CHAPTER 35

Nutrition

OBJECTIVES

Mastery of content in this chapter will enable the student to:

- Define the key terms listed.
- List the six categories of nutrients and explain why each is necessary for nutrition.
- Explain the importance of a balance between energy intake in foods and energy output.
- List the end products of carbohydrate, protein, and lipid metabolism.
- Explain the significance of saturated, unsaturated, and polyunsaturated lipids in nutrition.
- Describe the food guide pyramid and discuss its value in planning meals for good nutrition.
- Explain recommended daily allowances.
- List seven dietary guidelines for health promotion.
- Discuss the major areas of nutritional assessment.
- Identify three major nutritional problems and describe clients at risk for these problems.
- State the goals of enteral and total parenteral nutrition.
- Describe the procedure for initiating and maintaining tube feedings.
- Describe methods to avoid complications associated with tube feedings.
- Describe the procedure for initiating and maintaining total parenteral nutrition.
- Discuss the importance of diet counseling in evaluation and client teaching before discharge.

CHAPTER OUTLINE

Principles of Nutrition
    Water
    Carbohydrates
    Proteins
    Lipids
    Vitamins
    Minerals

Digestion

Absorption
    Metabolism
    Storage

Elimination

Foundations of an Adequate Diet
    Food guide pyramid
    Recommended daily allowances
    Other dietary guidelines
    Alternative food patterns

Developmental Variables in Nutrition
    Infants
    Toddlers and preschoolers
    School-age children
    Adolescents
    Young and middle adults
    Older adults

Nutrition and the Nursing Process
    Assessment
    Nursing diagnosis
    Planning
    Implementation
    Evaluation

The science of nutrition is relatively young, although nutritional support has always been a factor in the care of the ill. Because most other forms of treatments were lacking, early client care relied heavily on the preparation and administration of food to maintain the body's strength and fight disease.

The nurse's role in nutrition and diet therapy has changed over the years. Before World War II, nursing schools provided instruction in nutrition and diet therapy, laboratory courses in food preparation, and clinical experiences in the preparation and serving of therapeutic diets. The battlefield hospitals provided the surgical, pharmacological, and medical technologies necessary to save the lives of many victims. In addition, implementation of diets adequate in carbohydrates, fats, and proteins promoted wound healing and reduced the rate of complications in the soldiers recovering from war-related injuries.

After the war, knowledge about illness and trauma increased, changing the attitudes of people about hospitals. Hospitals were regarded as facilities for the restoration of health rather than placement facilities for the terminally ill.

Nursing curricula began to place greater emphasis on the impact of nutrition on health maintenance and health restoration. Nursing students were taught not only normal and therapeutic nutrition but also the role of the clinical dietitian in health care facilities. During the late 1960s and early 1970s, nursing curricula began to integrate nutrition content rather than having a single course.

Today, interest in health promotion and prevention of disease is increasing. This interest has also led to a greater awareness of the link between nutrition and the onset of acute and chronic illnesses. Research documented the link between food high in saturated fats, animal fats, and cholesterol with coronary artery disease. Foods high in grains and fiber are associated with reduced risk of colorectal cancers. High caffeine intake has been positively correlated with fibrocystic breast disease and certain cardiovascular symptoms. Finally, the specialty of critical care nursing and medicine has ongoing research on the impact of proteins on wound healing and the impact of excessive carbohydrates on weaning a person from a mechanical ventilator.

At present, diet therapy is recognized as an important adjunct to treatment. In some illnesses, such as non-insulin-dependent diabetes mellitus or mild hypertension, diet therapy may be the only therapy initiated. Other conditions, such as severe ulcerative colitis and Crohn's disease, require more invasive treatments (for example, total parenteral nutrition [TPN]). Other conditions such as prolonged infections, trauma, or head and neck surgeries require enteral feedings through a nasogastric or jejunostomy tube. The responsibility of meeting the client's nutritional needs should be shared among the nurse, dietitian, and physician.

PRINCIPLES OF NUTRITION

The body requires food to provide energy for organ function, body movement, and work; maintain body temperature; and provide raw materials for enzyme function, growth, replacement of cells, and repair. **Metabolism** refers to all the biochemical reactions within the body. It consists of anabolic reactions that build substances and body tissue and catabolic reactions that break down substances. Food is ingested, digested, and absorbed to produce the energy needed for these reactions.

People's energy requirements vary and are influenced by many factors. The energy requirement of an awake person at rest is called the **basal metabolic rate (BMR)**. The BMR is the energy needed at a person's lowest level of cellular function. Age, body size, body temperature, activity, environmental temperature, growth, sex, nutritional status, emotional state, and food intake affect individual energy requirements beyond the BMR.

When energy requirements are completely met by calorie intake in food, people maintain their activity levels without weight change. If the number of calories ingested exceeds the energy needs, people gain weight. When the calories ingested fail to meet energy requirements, people lose weight.

Nutrients are foods that contain the elements necessary for body function. The six categories of nutrients are water, carbohydrates, proteins, lipids, vitamins, and minerals. Energy needs are met by the metabolism of carbohydrates, proteins, and lipids. Water is needed because nutrients must be in solution for absorption, transportation, and excretion. Although vitamins and minerals do not provide energy, they are involved in the reactions that produce energy.

Foods are sometimes described according to the density of their nutrients. **Nutrient density** is the proportion of essential nutrients to the number of calories. Foods with the most nutrients in proportion to their total calories have high density. Foods with low nutrient density (for example, alcohol and refined sugar) provide an energy source but lack essential nutrients.

Water

Water is the most important nutrient because the function of cells depends on a fluid environment. Water composes 60% to 70% of total body weight. Lean people's bodies contain more water than obese people's bodies. Infants have the greatest percentage of total body weight as water, and older people have the least. As a result, they are most vulnerable to water deprivation or loss. Yet no one, when deprived of water, can survive for more than a few hours in a desert or a few days in the most protective environment. The ranges of daily fluid requirements for ages 3 days through adulthood are listed in Table 35-1.

Fluid needs are met by consumption of liquids and solid foods such as fresh fruits and vegetables and by water produced when food is oxidized during digestion. In a healthy individual the fluid intake from all sources equals the fluid output through elimination, respiration, and sweating (see Chapter 39). An ill person can have an increased need for fluid (for example, with a fever or hypermetabolic state). An ill person can also have a decreased need for fluid (for example, with cardiopulmonary or renal disease).

Carbohydrates

Carbohydrates are composed of carbon, hydrogen, and oxygen. The ratio of hydrogen to oxygen is the same as in water: two hydrogen ions for every oxygen ion. Carbohydrates are obtained primarily from plant foods. The only important source of animal carbohydrate is lactose (milk sugar). The carbohydrate content of the diet, as much as 90% of total caloric intake, tends to be greater in families with limited resources for food expenditure.

Carbohydrates are classified according to their sugar units, or **saccharides.** Monosaccharides such as glucose (dextrose) or fructose cannot be broken down into a more basic sugar unit. Disaccharides such as sucrose, lactose, and maltose are composed of two monosaccharides and water. Polysaccharides such as glycogen are composed of many sugar units. They are insoluble in water and are digested with varying degrees of completeness. **Glycogen** is synthesized from glucose and stored in the liver and muscles.

Plants store carbohydrate as **starch.** Starch is made up of granules enclosed by cell walls. When starch is cooked, the granules swell and burst their cellulose walls. Raw starch foods are more difficult to digest than the same foods after cooking because the freeing of the granules from the cellulose permits greater contact with digestive enzymes and more complete digestion. Starch digestion consists of several steps (Fig. 35-1). Dextrin is produced commercially and is used to increase the digestibility of foods such as baby foods, cereals, and toasted breads.

Some polysaccharides cannot be digested because humans do not have enzymes capable of breaking them down. Nevertheless, these polysaccharides have a role in human nutrition because they add fiber to the diet. **Fiber** is receiving increasing attention as a dietary factor in disease prevention and treatment. Examples of fiber are agar and pectin, which are used to form gels and as thickening agents; carrageen (Irish moss), which is used to increase the smoothness of ice creams and sauces; and lignin, a woody substance added to breads.

The metabolism of 1 g of carbohydrate produces 4 kilocalories (kcal), or 17 joules. Kilocalories and joules are units of measure for energy produced. Carbohydrate metabolism may produce three different results:

1. Catabolism into energy, carbon dioxide, and water

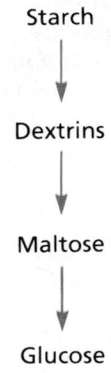

Fig. 35-1   Digestion of starch.

TABLE 35-1	Ranges of Daily Fluid Requirements		
Age	Fluid Requirements*	Age	Fluid Requirements*
3 days	80-100	6 yr	100-110
10 days	125-150	10 yr	90-100
3 mo	140-160	14 yr	50-60
6 mo	130-155	18 yr	40-50
9 mo	125-145	19-50 yr	50
1 yr	120-135		
2 yr	115-125		
4 yr	100-110		

*Per ml/kg/day.
Adapted from Behrman RE, Vaughan VC, editors: *Nelson's textbook of pediatrics,* ed 3, Philadelphia, 1987, Saunders.

2. Anabolism into glycogen for storage
3. Conversion into fat (adipose tissue) for storage

A recommended carbohydrate range (50 to 100 g) is 50% to 60% of total calories. Carbohydrates are the body's preferred energy source and are needed for the metabolism of lipids and protein sparing (replacing protein in meeting energy needs). A majority of carbohydrates should be derived from natural sugars and polysaccharides.

Proteins

Proteins are composed of hydrogen, oxygen, carbon, and nitrogen. Most proteins also contain sulfur and phosphorus. The atoms are arranged into amino acids linked into a chain to form proteins. Amino acids are the most important components of proteins. They are essential for synthesis (building) of body tissue in growth, maintenance, and repair. Protein can also be used as a source of energy.

Protein foods tend to be expensive. Protein intake is of particular importance during periods of rapid growth and after disease and injury.

Proteins are classified as simple, conjugated, or derived. Simple proteins are hydrolyzed (broken down) into amino acids or their derivatives. Albumin and globulin are simple proteins. The combination of a simple protein with a nonprotein substance produces a conjugated protein. Examples of conjugated proteins are mucoprotein, which is formed by the combination of a carbohydrate group and a simple protein, and lipoprotein, formed by a combination of a lipid and a simple protein. Derived proteins are formed during the hydrolysis of protein. For example, peptides and proteases occur during stages in the digestion of protein. Protein is metabolized to yield amino acids, nitrogen, and 4 kcal/g (17 joules). Amino acids are anabolized into tissues, hormones, and enzymes. Amino acids can also be converted to fat and stored as adipose tissue or catabolized into energy via **gluconeogenesis.**

The body cannot manufacture essential amino acids. Therefore the diet must provide them. Nonessential amino acids do not have to be present in the diet because the body can form them from the breakdown of other amino acids (see box). Incomplete proteins that combine to act as complete proteins are called *complementary proteins.* Grains and legumes are foods that contain complementary proteins. A complete protein contains all of the essential amino acids in sufficient quantity to support growth and maintain nitrogen balance. Complete proteins are also referred to as *high-biological value proteins.* Examples of foods containing complete or high-biological value proteins are meat, fish, poultry, milk, and eggs.

Essential and Nonessential Amino Acids

ESSENTIAL
- Histidine
- Isoleucine
- Leucine
- Lysine
- Methionine
- Phenylalanine
- Threonine
- Tryptophan
- Valine

NONESSENTIAL
- Alanine
- Arginine
- Asparagine
- Aspartic acid
- Citrulline
- Cysteine
- Cystine
- Glutamic acid
- Glutamine
- Glycine
- Hydroxyproline*
- Norleucine*
- Proline
- Serine
- Thyroxine*
- Tyrosine

*Whether these are true amino acids is questionable.

An incomplete protein does not contain all of the essential amino acids or does not have them in sufficient quantity to support growth and maintain nitrogen balance. Examples of foods containing incomplete proteins are cereals, legumes (beans, peas), and vegetables. The combination of one incomplete protein with another incomplete protein (which contains the missing amino acids or increases the amount of amino acids) in the same dish or meal supplies the essential amino acids (see box) to support growth and maintain nitrogen balance.

Incomplete proteins can also be made complete by the supplementation of synthetic amino acids. The addition of synthetic lysine to wheat is an example of amino acid supplementation.

Protein is the body's only source of nitrogen, and 16% of protein is nitrogen. The body is in **nitrogen balance** when the intake and output of nitrogen are equal. When the intake of nitrogen exceeds the output, the body is in positive nitrogen balance, as in growth, normal pregnancy, and wound healing. The nitrogen retained by the body is used for building, repair, and replacement of body tissues.

Negative nitrogen balance occurs when the body loses more nitrogen than it gains. The increased nitrogen loss is the result of body tissue destruction. Negative nitrogen balance is associated with infection, fever, starvation, injury, and prolonged immobilization.

Protein can be used to provide energy, but because of protein's essential role in growth, maintenance, and repair, it is important that protein be spared from energy production. Protein sparing is the provision of sufficient carbohydrate in the diet to meet the energy needs of the body to spare protein for its role in nitrogen balance and tissue building.

The required daily allowance for protein ranges from 13 g for infants under 6 months to 636 g for men 15 years or older (see Table 35-6). Pregnant women require 60 g and lactating women an additional 65 g. Their usual daily requirement is 55 to 50 g (Food and Nutrition Board, 1989).

Lipids

Lipid is a comprehensive term applied to compounds that are insoluble in water but soluble in organic solvents (for example, ethanol, ether, benzene, and acetone). Lipids include fats that are solid at room temperature and oils that are liquid at room temperature. Lipids are composed of carbon, hydrogen, and oxygen, but the proportion of each element differs from that of carbohydrate.

Lipids are classified as simple, compound, or derived. Simple lipids, such as monoglycerides, diglycerides, and triglycerides, are combinations of glycerol and fatty acids. A monoglyceride contains one fatty acid, a diglyceride contains two, and a triglyceride contains three. Compound lipids are simple lipids combined with a nonlipid substance, such as carbohydrate in glycolipids, phosphorus in phospholipids, and protein in lipoproteins. Derived lipids, such as cholesterol, steroid hormones, and the fat-soluble vitamins, are produced during the breakdown of simple or compound lipids.

Approximately 98% of the lipid in foods and 90% of the lipid in the human body are in the form of triglycerides. Triglycerides are termed *simple* when the three fatty acids that they contain are the same. A mixed triglyceride of two or three different fatty acids. High blood levels of triglycerides have been linked to **atherosclerosis** (hardening of the arteries).

Health care workers are also interested in the relationship between dietary intake of fatty acids and blood cholesterol levels. Increased blood cholesterol levels are associated with atherosclerosis, cerebrovascular accidents (stroke), and coronary occlusion.

Fatty acids can be saturated, unsaturated, or polyunsaturated. A saturated fatty acid contains as much hydrogen as it can hold. An unsaturated fatty acid can take up another hydrogen atom, and a polyunsaturated fatty acid can take up many more hydrogen atoms. Unsaturated and polyunsaturated fatty acids are oils. They have a low melting point and are liquid at room temperature. Hydrogenation is a process by which these oils are made more solid by the addition of hydrogen. The addition of hydrogen also makes them more saturated. Ingestion of saturated fatty acids appears to increase blood cholesterol levels. Ingestion of unsaturated fatty acids has a minimal effect on blood cholesterol, and polyunsaturated fatty acids appear to lower blood cholesterol levels.

Fatty acids are usually not purely saturated, unsaturated, or polyunsaturated. Most animal fats have high proportions of saturated fatty acids. Most vegetable fats have higher amounts of unsaturated and polyunsaturated fatty acids.

Linoleic acid is the only essential fatty acid. Because the body is unable to synthesize linoleic acid, it is dependent on an adequate dietary intake. Linoleic acid is a polyunsaturated fatty acid found in safflower, soybean, corn, cottonseed, and peanut oils.

Fat is the body's form of stored energy. The monoglycerides from the digested portion of lipids can be converted to glucose by gluconeogenesis. All body cells except red blood cells and central nervous system cells can oxidize fatty acids for energy. After a period of starvation, even the central nervous system can adapt to the use of amino acids and ketones as energy sources.

The metabolism of 1 g of lipid yields 9 kcal (38 joules), more than twice the energy provided by carbohydrates or proteins. Lipids account for 35% to 45% of the American diet. The American Heart Association (1988) and U.S. Department of Agriculture (USDA) and Department of Health and Human Services (USDHHS) (1990) recommend a daily lipid intake of 30% or less of total caloric intake. For example, a 2000-kcal diet should not contain over 600 kcal from fat (600 kcal ÷ 9 kcal/g of fat = 66 g of fat). Very low fat intakes can be dangerous to health. Overemphasis in young children, teenagers, and older adults can lead to growth failure, anorexic behavior, and malnutrition, respectively.

Vitamins

Vitamins are organic substances, present in minute amounts in foods, that are essential to normal metabolism. The body is unable to synthesize vitamins in the required amounts and depends on dietary intake. Although they are contained in many foods, vitamins are affected by processing, storage, and preparation. Vitamin content is usually highest in fresh foods that are used quickly after minimal exposure to heat, air, or water. Vitamins are classified as water and fat soluble.

Water-Soluble Vitamins

The water-soluble vitamins are vitamin C and vitamin B complex, which consists of eight different

TABLE 35-2 Water-Soluble Vitamins

Functions	Effects of Deficiency*	Effects of Excess	Sources
Vitamin C (Ascorbic Acid) Production of collagen; integrity of capillary walls; formation of red blood cells; metabolism of amino acids; reduction of iron salts; protection of other vitamins from oxidation	Scurvy, poor wound healing, bleeding gums, loose teeth, bruising	Kidney stones, scurvy on withdrawal, urinary tract infection	Citrus fruits, potatoes, cabbage, tomatoes, broccoli, strawberries, cantaloupe, green peppers
VITAMIN B COMPLEX **Vitamin B$_1$ (Thiamine)** Component of enzymes; carbohydrate oxidation; oxidative conversion of pyruvic acid and hence citric acid cycle	Beriberi (rare), polyneuritis, mental confusion, muscular weakness, ataxia, cardiac rhythm disturbances, cardiac enlargement	Rapid pulse, headaches, weakness, irritability, insomnia	Pork, fish, eggs, poultry, dried beans, whole grains, wheat germ, oatmeal, bread, pasta
Vitamin B$_2$ (Riboflavin) Metabolism of nutrients; growth; oxidation and reduction of fat, carbohydrates, proteins	Ariboflavinosis: cracks at mouth corners, scaly desquamation of skin around mouth, eye irritation, glossitis (shiny tongue), photophobia (light sensitivity)	Ulcer, elevated blood glucose level, increased uric acid levels in blood	Milk, whole grains, green vegetables, liver
Niacin Protein utilization; glycolysis; fat synthesis; tissue repair	Pellagra: weakness, anorexia, indigestion; severe pellagra: dermatitis, diarrhea, dementia	Ulcer, liver dysfunction, elevated blood glucose level, increased blood uric acid levels, diarrhea, nausea, flushing	Meats, dairy products, whole grains, cereals, tuna
Vitamin B$_6$ (Complex of Pyridoxine, Pyridoxal, Pyridoxamine) Metabolism of nutrients; synthesis of nonessential amino acids; conversion of tryptophan to niacin; proper function of blood and central nervous system cells	Anemia, irritability, skin lesions, cracks at corners of mouth	Bloating, depression, fatigue, headache, nerve damage, irritability	Whole grains, liver, fish, poultry, green beans, nuts, meats, potatoes
Folacin, Folic Acid, Folate Metabolism of some amino acids; maturation of red blood cells; synthesis of purines and pyrimidines, which are necessary for ribonucleic acid (RNA) and deoxyribonucleic acid (DNA)	Macrocytic anemia	Diarrhea, insomnia, irritability, masking of vitamin B$_{12}$ deficiency	Liver, green leafy vegetables, meat, fish, poultry, whole grains

*For normal ranges, see Table 35-7. Normal range for pantothenic acid is 4-7 mg/day, and for biotin, it is 30-100 µg/day.
From Grant JA, Kennedy-Caldwell C: *Nutritional support in nursing,* New York, 1988, Grune & Stratton; and Whitney EN, Cataldo CB, Rolfes SR: *Understanding normal and clinical nutrition,* St Paul, 1991, West.

TABLE 35-2	Water-Soluble Vitamins—cont'd		
Functions	Effects of Deficiency*	Effects of Excess	Sources
Vitamin B$_{12}$ (Cobralamin)			
Manufacture of enzymes essential to metabolism of nutrients, nucleic acid, folic acid; proper function of cells of bone marrow, gastrointestinal tract, and nervous system; formation of purines and thus RNA and DNA	Pernicious anemia and neurological disorders	None reported	Milk, eggs, cheese, meat, fish, poultry, foods of animal origin (Plant foods contain no vitamin B$_{12}$.)
Pantothenic Acid			
Metabolism of nutrients; synthesis of cholesterol and steroid hormones; activity of adrenal cortex	None known	Increased need for thiamin, occasional diarrhea, water retention	Meats, whole grain cereals, legumes
Biotin			
Synthesis of fatty acids; utilization of glucose; metabolism of protein; utilization of vitamin B$_{12}$ and folic acid	None known	None known	Liver, kidneys, dark green vegetables, egg yolk, green beans

vitamins. Water-soluble vitamins cannot be stored in the body and must be provided in the daily food intake. It was once assumed that, because water-soluble vitamins are not stored in the body, **hypervitaminosis** (condition caused by excessive intake of a vitamin) of these vitamins does not occur. However, recent studies of people who took megadoses of vitamin C, riboflavin (B$_2$), and niacin indicate that toxicity can occur. Vitamins are chemicals used as catalysts in biochemical reactions. When there is enough of any specific vitamin to meet the catalytic demands, the rest of the vitamin supply acts as a free chemical and may be toxic to the body. Table 35-2 lists the characteristics of water-soluble vitamins.

Fat-Soluble Vitamins

The fat-soluble vitamins—A, D, E, and K—can be stored in the body, and therefore daily intake is not needed. However, with the exception of vitamin D, these vitamins should be provided through dietary intake. Toxicity to some fat-soluble vitamins has been recognized for years. Toxicity is usually the result of megadoses of synthetic vitamins, but it has also been reported in people whose diet includes a large intake of fish liver.

Processing, storage, and preparation of foods have less effect on fat-soluble vitamin content, and many foods are fortified by the addition of vitamins A and D. The characteristics of fat-soluble vitamins are listed in Table 35-3 on p. 1100.

Minerals

Minerals are inorganic elements essential to the body because of their role as catalysts in biochemical reactions. Minerals are classified as macrominerals when the daily requirement is 100 mg or more and microminerals when less than 100 mg is needed daily. Because the required amount of microminerals is usually very small or a trace, microminerals are also referred to as *trace elements*. The characteristics of macrominerals are summarized in Table 35-4 on p. 1100.

In addition to the microminerals in Table 35-5 on p. 1101, arsenic, nickel, silicon, tin, vanadium, and possibly cadmium may play as yet unidentified roles in human nutrition. The toxic effects of arsenic and cadmium have been identified.

TABLE 35-3 Fat-Soluble Vitamins

Functions	Effects of Deficiency*	Effects of Excess	Sources
Vitamin A (Retinol, Retinal, Retinoic Acid)			
Growth and maintenance of epithelial tissue; maintenance of visual acuity in dim light; immune functions, especially antigen recognition	Night blindness, rough scaly skin, dry mucous membranes, decreased resistance to infection, faulty tooth and bone development	Nausea, vomiting, abdominal pain, and growth failure in children; weight loss in adults; megadoses: hair loss, bone swelling and tenderness, joint pain, hepatomegaly, splenomegaly, headache	Whole milk, whole milk products, eggs, green leafy vegetables, yellow fruits and vegetables, fish liver oil, liver
Vitamin D (Cholecalciferol, Ergosterol)			
Absorption and utilization of calcium in bone and tooth development	Rickets and delayed dentition in children, osteomalacia (softening of bones) in adults	Megadoses: loss of appetite, vomiting, growth failure, weight loss, increased calcium deposits in soft tissue, blood vessels, and kidneys	Sunlight, fortified milk, fortified margarines, fish liver oils
Vitamin E (Tocopherol)			
Protection of vitamins A and C and polyunsaturated fatty acids from oxidation; synthesis of heme	Increased hemolysis of red blood cells and macrocytic anemia in premature infants	Interference with utilization of vitamins A and K, prolonged prothrombin time, intestinal irritability, headache, fatigue, dizziness	Vegetable oils, green leafy vegetables, milk, eggs, meats, cereals
Vitamin K			
Prothrombin formation; blood clotting	Hemorrhagic disease of the newborn, prolonged clotting time in adults	Hyperbilirubinemia in infants, vomiting in adults	Green leafy vegetables, liver synthesis in gastrointestinal tract

*For normal ranges, see Table 35-7.
From Grant JA, Kennedy-Caldwell C: *Nutritional support in nursing*, New York, 1988, Grune & Stratton; and Whitney EN, Cataldo CB, Rolfes SR: *Understanding normal and clinical nutrition*, St Paul, 1991, West.

TABLE 35-4 Macrominerals

Functions	Effects of Deficiency*	Effects of Excess	Sources
Calcium			
Formation of teeth and bones; contraction of muscle fibers; transmission of nerve impulses; activation of enzymes; permeability of cell membranes; coagulation of blood; cardiac function	Tingling of fingers and area around mouth, muscle cramps, carpopedal (thumb or toe) spasm, tetany, convulsions, pathological fractures, stunted growth in children, bone loss in adults	Relaxed skeletal muscles, cardiac irregularities	Milk, milk products, leafy vegetables, fish and small edible bones
Magnesium			
Support of function of B vitamins; utilization of calcium, potassium, protein; maintenance of electrical activity in nerves and muscles	Neuromuscular irritability, confusion, hallucinations, growth failure	Lethargy, diarrhea	Whole grains, nuts, legumes, green vegetables

*For normal ranges, see Table 35-7.
From Grant JA, Kennedy-Caldwell C: *Nutritional support in nursing*, New York, 1988, Grune & Stratton; and Whitney EN, Cataldo CB, Rolfes SR: *Understanding normal and clinical nutrition*, St Paul, 1991, West.

TABLE 35-4 Macrominerals—cont'd

Functions	Effects of Deficiency*	Effects of Excess	Sources
Phosphorus			
Formation of bone and teeth; activation of B vitamins; transfer of energy in cells; promotion of muscle and nerve activity; metabolism of carbohydrates; regulation of acid-base balance; transmission of hereditary traits	Hemolytic anemia, defective white blood cell function, delayed clotting, bone pain, pathological fractures	Erosion of jaw, calcium loss	Pork, beef, dried peas and beans, milk and milk products

TABLE 35-5 Microminerals

Functions	Effects of Deficiency*	Effects of Excess	Sources
Copper			
Hemoglobin formation; synthesis of phospholipids; formation and activity of some enzymes; synthesis of prostaglandin	Abnormal blood cell development in infants, bone demineralization	Headache, dizziness, heartburn, weakness, nausea, vomiting, diarrhea, Wilson's disease	Liver, kidney, shellfish, nuts, raisins
Fluoride			
Formation of teeth; prevention of dental caries	Poor dental health	Mottling, pitting, and discoloration of tooth enamel	Fluoridated water, seafood, toothpaste, mouthwash
Iodine			
Basic component of thyroid hormones	Cretinism in infants, depressed thyroid activity	Toxic goiter	Iodized salt, seafood, food additives, dough oxidizers, dairy disinfectants, coloring agents
Iron			
Formation of hemoglobin; synthesis of vitamins, purines, and antibodies	Anemia, fatigue, weakness, lethargy, lowered immunity	Hemosiderosis, poisoning from accidental ingestion in infants and children: cramps, abdominal pain, nausea, vomiting, black stools, cirrhosis	Liver, lean meats, whole grains, enriched breads and cereals, green leafy vegetables
Zinc			
Connective tissue integrity; immune response; formation of enzymes and insulin	Impaired wound healing, decreased sensations of taste and smell, skin lesions, delayed growth	Anemia, fever, nausea, vomiting, diarrhea, muscle pain and weakness, decreased calcium absorption	Oysters, liver, meats, poultry, legumes, nuts

*For normal ranges, see Table 35-7. Normal range for copper is 1.5 to 3 mg/day, and for fluoride it is 1.5 to 4 mg/day.

From Grant JA, Kennedy-Caldwell C: *Nutritional support in nursing,* New York, 1988, Grune & Stratton; and Whitney EN, Cataldo CB, Rolfes SR: *Understanding normal and clinical nutrition,* St Paul, 1991, West.

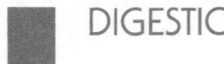

DIGESTION

The only nutrients that the body can use in their ingested forms are monosaccharides, water, vitamins, some minerals, and alcohol. Digestion consists of mechanical breakdown by chewing, churning, mixing with fluid, and chemical reactions by which food is reduced to its simplest form.

Enzymes are an essential component of the chemistry of digestion. **Enzymes** are proteinlike substances that act as catalysts to speed up chemical reactions. As catalysts, enzymes are not part of the end product of the reaction. Most enzymes have one specific function, although some enzymes are involved in several closely related reactions. Each enzyme functions best at a specific pH and is inactivated by major variations from that level. The secretions of the gastrointestinal tract have vastly different pH levels. For example, saliva is relatively neutral, gastric juice is highly acidic, and the secretions of the small intestine are alkaline.

The mechanical, chemical, and hormonal activities of digestion are interdependent. Enzyme activity depends on the mechanical breakdown of food to increase its surface area for chemical action. Hormones regulate the flow of digestive secretions needed for enzyme supply, and digestion may also be slowed or speeded by strong emotional states. The secretion of digestive juice and motility of the gastrointestinal tract are regulated by physical, chemical, and hormonal factors, and they are intricately bound to psychological, emotional, and nervous system alterations.

Digestion begins in the mouth, where food is mechanically broken down by chewing. The food is mixed with saliva, which contains ptyalin (salivary amylase), an enzyme that acts on cooked starch to begin its conversion to maltose. The longer food is chewed, the more starch digestion occurs in the mouth. Proteins and fats are broken down physically but remain unchanged chemically because enzymes in the mouth do not react with these nutrients. Chewing reduces food particles to a size suitable for swallowing, and saliva provides lubrication to further ease swallowing of the **bolus** (food ready to be swallowed).

Swallowed food enters the esophagus and is moved along by waves (**peristalsis**). At the cardiac sphincter, the upper opening of the stomach, the presence of the food mass causes the sphincter to relax and allow food to enter the stomach.

The stomach acts as a reservoir for food, and food remains in the stomach for varying periods, depending on the type of meal, gastric motility, and psychological influences. In the digestive sequence, carbo-hydrates are digested first, proteins second, and lipids last. Large meals and high fat intake decrease gastric motility and increase the length of time food remains in the stomach. Food remains in the stomach about 3 hours, with a range of 1 to 7 hours.

The activity of ptyalin continues in the stomach until hydrochloric acid decreases the pH enough to inactivate ptyalin. The stomach churns the food mass, mixing it with gastric secretions and causing further breakdown in the size of the food particles. The acid environment favors the action of pepsin. Pepsin is an enzyme that splits proteins into smaller polypeptides. Pancreatic and intestinal enzymes hydrolyse them into tripeptides, dipeptides, and amino acids. Lipase, an enzyme that functions best in an alkaline medium, is able to act on emulsified fats such as butter, egg yolk, milk, and cream at near-neutral pH levels. Lipase splits emulsified fats into fatty acids and glycerol.

Food leaves the stomach at the pyloric sphincter as an acidic, liquefied mass called **chyme.** Chyme flows into the duodenum and is quickly mixed with bile, intestinal juices, and pancreatic secretions. Bile emulsifies fat to permit enzyme action and holds fatty acids in solution.

Intestinal secretions contain seven enzymes: lipase for fat digestion, polypeptidase and dipeptidase for protein digestion, and amylase, sucrase, lactase, and maltase for carbohydrate digestion. Pancreatic juice contains five enzymes: amylase to digest starch, lipase to break down emulsified fats, and trypsin, chymotrypsin, and carboxypolypeptide to break down proteins.

Peristalsis continues in the small intestine, mixing the secretions with the chyme. The mixture becomes increasingly alkaline, inhibiting the action of the gastric enzymes and promoting the action of the duodenal secretions. The major portion of digestion occurs in the small intestine, producing glucose, fructose, and galactose from carbohydrates; amino acids from proteins; and fatty acids and glycerol from lipids.

ABSORPTION

The small intestine is also the site of absorption of simple nutrients. It is lined with numerous villi that project into the lumen and greatly increase the surface area available for absorption. Table 35-6 describes the means and route of absorption of major nutrients.

The intestinal contents continue to move by peristaltic action into the large intestine. Water is the only nutrient absorbed from the large intestine. Other nutrients remaining in the intestinal contents

TABLE 35-6 Intestinal Absorption of Some Major Nutrients

Nutrient	Form	Means of Absorption	Control Agent or Required Cofactor	Route
Carbohydrate	Monosaccharides (glucose and ga-lactose)	Competitive	—	Blood
		Selective	—	
		Active transport via sodium-potassium pump	Sodium	
Protein	Amino acids	Selective	—	Blood
	Some dipeptides	Carrier transport systems	Pyridoxine (pyridox-al phosphate)	Blood
	Whole protein (rare)	Pinocytosis (process by which cells absorb and digest nutrients)	—	Blood
Fat	Fatty acids	Fatty acid–bile complex (mi-celles)	Bile	Lymph
	Monoglyceride, dig-lyceride		—	Lymph
	Triglycerides (neu-tral fat)	Pinocytosis	—	Lymph
Vitamins	B_{12}	Carrier transport	Intrinsic factor	Blood
	A	Bile complex	Bile	Blood
	K	Bile complex	Bile	Large intestine to blood
Minerals	Sodium	Active transport via sodium pump	—	Blood
	Calcium	Active transport	Vitamin D	Blood
	Iron	Active transport	Ferritin mecha-nisms	Blood (as transfer-rin)
Water	Water	Osmosis	—	Blood, lymph, inter-stitial fluid

From Williams SR: *Nutrition and diet therapy,* ed 6, St Louis, 1989, Mosby–Year Book.

when they reach the large intestine are lost to the body and will be excreted as waste products. When intestinal motility is increased, as in diarrhea, the body loses nutrients that move through the small intestine too quickly for complete absorption.

Metabolism

Nutrients absorbed in the intestines, including water, are transported through the circulatory system to body tissues. Through metabolism the chemical changes of nutrients are converted into a number of substances required by the body. Carbohydrates, protein, and fat undergo metabolism to produce chemical energy and to maintain a balance between tissue buildup and breakdown. To carry out the body's work, the chemical energy produced by metabolism is converted to other types of energy by different tissues. Muscle contraction involves mechanical en-

ergy, nervous system function involves electrical energy, and the mechanisms of heat production involve thermal energy. All of these forms of energy originate in metabolism. The interrelationships of protein, carbohydrate, and fat metabolism are depicted in Fig. 35-2 on p. 1104.

The two basic types of metabolism are anabolism and catabolism. **Anabolism** is the production of more complex chemical substances by synthesis of nutrients. **Catabolism** is the breakdown of chemical substances into simpler substances. Although catabolism produces some energy, both processes require energy, which must be provided from food or stored energy sources.

Storage

Some but not all of the nutrients required by the body are stored in body tissues. The body's major

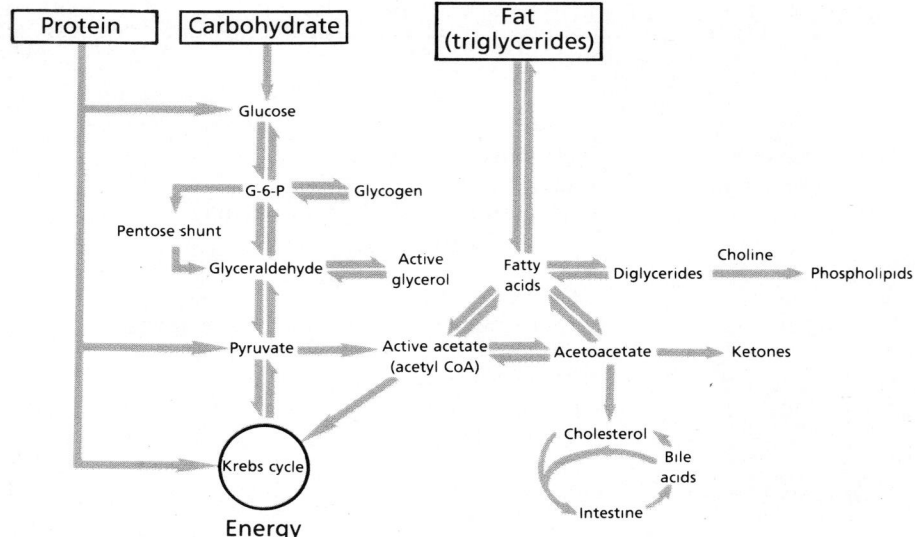

Fig. 35-2 Summary of metabolism of the nutrients. Note metabolic interrelationships of carbohydrate, protein, and fat.
From Williams SR: *Nutrition and diet therapy*, ed 6, St Louis, 1989, Mosby–Year Book.

form of stored energy is fat, which is stored as adipose tissue. Glycogen is stored in small reserves in liver and muscle tissue, and protein is stored in muscle mass. When the body's energy requirements exceed the energy supplied by ingested nutrients, stored energy is used. Conversely, unused energy is stored, principally in fat.

 ## ELIMINATION

The intestinal contents move through the various segments of the large intestine by peristalsis. As the material moves toward the rectum, water is absorbed into the mucosa. The longer the material stays in the large intestine, the more water is absorbed and the firmer the remaining solid material becomes. The end products of digestion include cellulose and similar fibrous substances that the body is unable to digest, sloughed cells from the intestinal walls, mucus, digestive secretions, water, and microorganisms.

 ## FOUNDATIONS OF AN ADEQUATE DIET

Food Guide Pyramid

The basic four food groups were introduced in 1956 as one of the earliest recommendations by the USDA. It was suggested that selecting foods from a wide variety of milk, meat, bread and cereal products, and fruits and vegetables would ensure the required amounts of needed nutrients.

In 1992 the food guide pyramid was designed as a guide for buying food and meal preparation (Fig. 35-3). This basic plan provides for diets ranging from 1600 to 1800 kcal/day (USDA, 1992). Additional foods to round out meals and meet energy requirements can be selected from enriched cereals, complex carbohydrates, and additional grains.

Recommended Daily Allowances

The Committee on Dietary Allowances of the Food and Nutrition Board of the National Academy of Sciences has published a list of **recommended daily allowances (RDAs)** since 1943. The RDAs are the level of intake of essential nutrients considered, in the judgment of the committee and on the basis of scientific knowledge, to be adequate to meet the nutritional needs of healthy people. The RDAs were originally designed as a guide for planning and securing food supplies for national defense during World War II. Now they are revised approximately every 5 years to incorporate changes and new knowledge based on current research (Table 35-7 on p. 1106).

In 1990, Congress passed the Nutrition Labeling and Education Act (NLEA) to require mandatory nutrition labeling for most FDA-regulated foods. It also requires the Food and Drug Administration (FDA) to issue voluntary nutrition guidelines to food retailers for providing nutrition information on certain vegeta-

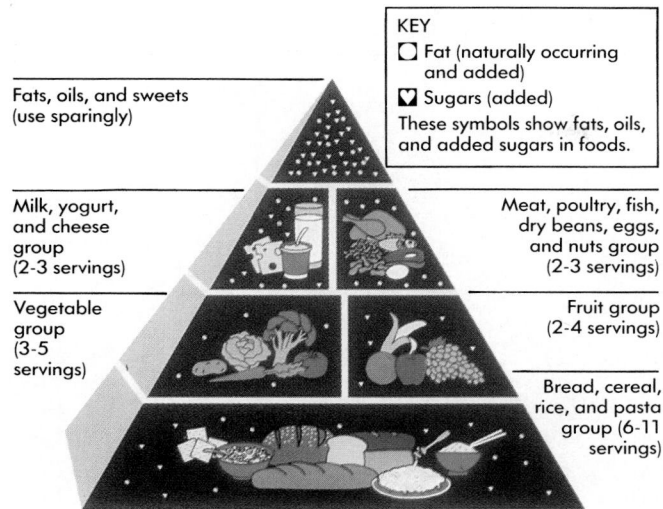

KEY
- ☐ Fat (naturally occurring and added)
- ☑ Sugars (added)

These symbols show fats, oils, and added sugars in foods.

Fats, oils, and sweets (use sparingly)

Milk, yogurt, and cheese group (2-3 servings)

Meat, poultry, fish, dry beans, eggs, and nuts group (2-3 servings)

Vegetable group (3-5 servings)

Fruit group (2-4 servings)

Bread, cereal, rice, and pasta group (6-11 servings)

Fig. 35-3 Food guide pyramid.
US Department of Agriculture: *USDA's food guide pyramid,* USDA Human Nutrition Information Pub No 249, Washington, DC, 1992, US Government Printing Office.

bles, fruits, and raw fish (Public Law 101-535, 1990). If retailers fail to comply substantially with the guidelines, the NLEA requires the FDA to issue mandatory requirements for these commodities.

A further proposal allows the use of health messages in the areas of fat and cancer, fat and heart disease, calcium and osteoporosis, and sodium and hypertension. In January 1991 the USDA announced that they would develop a mandatory nutrition labeling program for processed meat and poultry products and voluntary guidelines for fresh meat and poultry. The proposed nutrition label will clarify serving size, nutrient content, health claims, low-fat and low-cholesterol claims, and unclear terms such as *light* or *lite* to aid the consumer in understanding the actual nutritional content. The regulations were finalized by November 1992, and the industry has until November 1993 to redesign labels.

Other Dietary Guidelines

Before 1977, most public advice on dietary planning was based on the basic four food groups. In 1977 the Senate Select Committee on Nutrition and Human Needs formulated guidelines, which are designed to help avoid some of the nutrition-related problems identified by research studies. These guidelines—directed at the problems of obesity; excessive intake of fat, cholesterol, sugar, and salt; and inadequate intake of fiber—relate to heart disease, cancer, gastrointestinal disorders, diabetes mellitus, and other health problems.

1990 Dietary Guidelines

Eat a variety of foods.
- Choose fruits and vegetables.
- Choose whole grain and enriched breads, cereals, and other grain products.
- Choose milk, cheese, yogurt, and other milk products.
- Choose meat, poultry, fish, eggs, and dry peas and beans.

Maintain healthy weight.

Choose a diet low in fat, saturated fat, and cholesterol.
- Choose lean meat, fish, and poultry.
- Use dry peas and beans as protein sources.
- Use low-fat milk and milk products.
- Use egg yolk and organ meats moderately.
- Limit consumption of butter, cream, heavily hydrogenated fats and oils, and foods high in palm and coconut oil.
- Trim off excess fat on meats.
- Broil, bake, or boil rather than fry.

Choose a diet with plenty of vegetables, fruits, and grain products.
- Eat three or more servings of vegetables each day.
- Consume two or more servings of fruits daily.
- Eat six or more servings of grain products each day.

Use sugar in moderation.
- Use less sugar and eat fewer high-sugar foods.
- Avoid between-meal sweets.
- Avoid foods whose labels contain sucrose, glucose, and lactose.
- Select foods canned without syrup or with light syrup.

Use salt in moderation.
- Learn to enjoy unsalted food.
- Cook with only a small amount of added salt.
- Add little or no salt at the table.
- Limit intake of salty foods.
- Read food labels.
- Use new, lower-sodium products.

If you drink, do so in moderation.

Data from USDA and USDHHS: *Nutrition and your health: dietary guidelines for Americans,* USDA/DHHS Home and Garden Bull No. 232, Washington, DC, 1990, US Government Printing office.

The USDA and the USDHHS issued dietary guidelines in 1980. These guidelines consisted of seven categories and were revised in 1985 and in 1990 (see box).

In 1990, the USDHHS and Public Health Service (PHS), after a 4-year consensus process, published

TABLE 35-7 Recommended Dietary Allowances*

Category	Age (yr) or Condition	Weight† (kg)	Weight† (lb)	Height† (cm)	Height† (in)	kcal per day	Protein (g)	Fat-Soluble Vitamins Vitamin A (μg RE)‡	Vitamin D (μg)§	Vitamin E (mg α-TE)‖	Vitamin K (μg)
Infants	0.0-0.5	6	13	60	24	650	13	375	7.5	3	5
	0.5-1.0	9	20	71	28	850	14	375	10	4	10
Children	1-3	13	29	90	35	1300	16	400	10	6	15
	4-6	20	44	112	44	1800	24	500	10	7	20
	7-10	28	62	132	52	2000	28	700	10	7	30
Men	11-14	45	99	157	62	2500	45	1000	10	10	45
	15-18	66	145	176	69	3000	59	1000	10	10	65
	19-24	72	160	177	70	2900	58	1000	10	10	70
	25-50	79	174	176	70	2900	63	1000	5	10	80
	over 51	77	170	173	68	2300	63	1000	5	10	80
Women	11-14	46	101	157	62	2200	46	800	10	8	45
	15-18	55	120	163	64	2200	44	800	10	8	55
	19-24	58	128	164	65	2200	46	800	10	8	60
	25-50	63	138	163	64	2200	50	800	5	8	65
	Over 51	65	143	160	63	1900	50	800	5	8	65
Pregnant						2500	60	800	10	10	65
Lactating:	1st 6 mo					2700	65	1300	10	12	65
	2nd 6 mo					2700	62	1200	10	11	65

*The allowances, expressed as average daily intakes over time, are intended to provide for individual variations among most normal persons as they live in the United States under usual environmental stresses. Diets should be based on a variety of common foods to provide other nutrients for which human requirements have been less well defined.

†Weights and heights of Reference Adults are actual medians for the U.S. population of the designated age.

‡Retinol equivalents. 1 RE = 1 μg retinol or 6 μg β-carotene. See text for calculations of vitamin A activity of diets as retinol equivalents.

Healthy People 2000, National Health Promotion and Disease Prevention Objectives. The report defines national goals or objectives to be met in this decade to increase the proportion of Americans who live long, healthy lives.

All 21 nutrition-related goals for the year 2000 include baseline data. For example, one objective is to reduce the prevalence of overweight people to no more than 20% among people age 20 years and older, a decrease from the current baseline level of 26%. Other objectives are to reduce dietary fat intake to an average of 30% of total calories, down from the recent level of 36%, and to reduce saturated fat intake to less than 10%, down from the present 13%. Additional objectives include increasing intake of fruits, vegetables, and grain products and reducing sodium consumption.

The remaining challenge is to motivate consumers to put these dietary recommendations into practice. Health professionals (for example, nurses, registered dietitians, nutritionists, nutrition educators, physicians, teachers, and scientists) can play a key role in promoting healthy dietary habits.

Alternative Food Patterns

Long before recommended allowances and guidelines were issued, many people followed special patterns of food intake based on religion, cultural background, ethics, health beliefs, personal preference, or concern for the efficient use of land to produce food. Such special diets are not necessarily more or less nutritional than diets based on the basic four food groups or other nutritional guidelines because good nutrition depends on a balanced intake of all required nutrients. A common dietary pattern is the vegetarian diet.

Vegetarianism is the consumption of a diet consisting predominantly of plant foods. Vegetarians may be ovolactovegetarians, who avoid meat, fish, and poultry but eat eggs and milk, or lactovegetarians, who drink milk but avoid eggs. Vegans, or pure vegetarians, consume only plant foods, avoiding meat, poultry, and fish. The pure vegetarian diet is not recommended for infants and young children unless it is carefully planned (Jacobs, Dwyer, 1988).

	Water-Soluble Vitamins						Minerals						
Vitamin C (mg)	Thiamin (mg)	Riboflavin (mg)	Niacin (mg NE)¶	Vitamin B$_6$ (mg)	Folate (µg)	Vitamin B$_{12}$ (µg)	Calcium (mg)	Phosphorus (mg)	Magnesium (mg)	Iron (mg)	Zinc (mg)	Iodine (µg)	Selenium (µg) 35
30	0.3	0.4	5	0.3	25	0.3	400	300	40	6	5	40	10
35	0.4	0.5	6	0.6	35	0.5	400	500	60	10	5	50	15
40	0.7	0.8	9	1.0	50	0.7	400	800	80	10	10	70	20
45	0.9	1.1	12	1.1	75	1.0	800	800	120	10	10	90	20
45	1.0	1.2	13	1.4	100	1.4	800	800	170	10	10	120	20
50	1.3	1.5	17	1.7	150	2.0	120	1200	270	12	15	150	40
60	1.5	1.8	20	2.0	200	2.0	120	1200	400	12	15	150	50
60	1.5	1.7	29	2.0	200	2.0	120	1200	350	10	15	150	70
60	1.5	1.7	19	2.0	200	2.0	800	800	350	10	15	150	70
60	1.2	1.4	15	2.0	200	2.0	800	800	350	10	15	150	70
50	1.1	1.3	15	1.4	150	2.0	120	1200	280	15	12	150	45
60	1.1	1.3	15	1.5	180	2.0	120	1200	300	15	12	150	50
60	1.1	1.3	15	1.6	180	2.0	120	1200	280	15	12	150	55
60	1.1	1.3	15	1.6	180	2.0	80	800	280	15	12	150	55
60	1.0	1.3	13	1.6	180	2.0	80	800	280	10	12	150	55
70	1.5	1.6	17	2.2	400	2.2	120	1200	320	30	15	175	65
95	1.6	1.8	20	2.1	280	2.6	120	1200	355	15	19	200	75
90	1.6	1.7	20	2.1	260	2.6	120	1200	340	15	16	200	75

§As cholecalciferol. 10 µg cholecalciferol = 400 U of vitamin D.
‖α-Tocopherol equivalents. 1 mg d-α-tocopherol = 1 α-TE.
¶1 NE niacin equivalent = 1 mg of niacin of 60 mg of dietary tryptophan.
From Food and Nutrition Board, National Academy of Sciences—National Research Council: Recommended dietary allowances, Washington DC, 1989, The Council.

DEVELOPMENTAL VARIABLES IN NUTRITION

Infants

Infancy is marked by rapid growth and high energy requirements. The average birth weight of an American baby is 3.2 to 3.4 kg (7 to 7½ lb). The infant usually doubles birth weight at 4 to 5 months and triples it at 1 year. An energy intake of approximately 108 kcal/kg of body weight is needed in the first half of infancy and 98 kcal/kg in the second half (Food and Nutrition Board, 1989). A full-term newborn is able to digest and absorb simple carbohydrates, proteins, and a moderate amount of emulsified fat. Amylase, the starch-splitting enzyme, is not present until approximately 2½ or 3½ months. Infants need a high amount of fluid because a large portion of total body weight is water.

Breast-Fed Infants

Breast milk is the ideal food for infants. The current recommendation is that breast milk be the major source of nutrients for the first 4 to 6 months. Breast milk contains antibodies to protect against antigens in infant formulas and foods. As the infant grows, the gastrointestinal tract can fight against common bacteria and allergy-causing proteins.

Breast-feeding promotes bonding between mother and child. The lipid content of breast milk is better absorbed than that from other infant foods. Breast-feeding may prevent infant obesity and protect against hypercholesterolemia in later life. At the end of the nursing period, breast milk has a higher fat content that is thought to provide **satiety** (satisfied feeling of being full) and stop the infant from sucking. The high cholesterol level of breast milk is thought to foster the development of more efficient cholesterol metabolism.

Breast-fed infants need a source of vitamin C, fluoride, vitamin D, and iron. A vitamin C supplement can be given at 1 to 2 months. Fluoride should be given as a supplement in areas where the water supply is not fluoridated or if the infant does not drink enough fluoridated water to meet needs. Vitamin D is also given as a vitamin supplement. After 4 months,

TABLE 35-8 How to Feed Your Baby Step-By-Step

Food Group	Foods	Daily Servings	Suggested Serving Size	Feeding Tips
0-4 MO				
Milk	Breast milk or	8-12 or on demand		Nurse baby at least 5-10 min on each breast.
	Formula* 0-1 mo	6-8	2-5 oz	Six wet diapers a day is good sign.
	1-2 mo	5-7	3-6 oz	There is no need to force baby to finish bottle.
	2-3 mo	4-7	4-7 oz	
	3-4 mo	4-6	6-8 oz	Putting baby to bed with bottle could cause choking.
				Heating formula in microwave is not recommended.
4-6 MO				
Milk	Breast milk or	4-6		May need to start baby cereal (iron-fortified).
	Formula*	4-6	6-8 oz	
Grain	Baby cereal (iron-fortified)	2	1-2 tbsp	Feed only one new cereal each week.
				There is no need to add salt or sugar to cereal.
				Offer baby extra water.
				Use microwave with caution.
6-8 MO				
Milk	Breast milk or	3-5		Add strained fruits and vegetables at first. Add mashed or finely chopped fruits and cooked vegetables later on.
	Formula*	3-5	6-8 oz	
Grain	Baby cereal (iron-fortified)	2	2-4 tbsp	Feed only one new fruit or vegetable each week.
	Bread, bagel, or bun	Offer	½	
	Crackers		2 crackers	
Fruit-vegetable	Fruit or vegetables	4	2-3 tbsp	Take out of jar amount of food for one feeding. Refrigerate remaining food.
	Baby fruit juice	1	3 oz (from cup)	Try giving baby fruit juice in cup.
				Offer following foods only when baby has full set of teeth: apple chunks or slices, grapes, hot dogs, sausages, peanut butter, popcorn, nuts, seeds, round candies, hard chunks of uncooked vegetables. Inform parents that these foods can cause choking.
8-12 MO				
Milk	Breast milk,	3-4		Ask your doctor if baby is ready for whole milk.
	Formula,* or whole milk	3-4	6-8 oz	
	Cheese		½ oz	Add strained or finely chopped meats.
	Plain yogurt	Offer	½ cup	Feed only one new meat a week.
	Cottage cheese		¼ cup	Wait until baby's first birthday to feed egg whites. Some babies are sensitive to egg white. It is okay to give egg yolks.
Grain	Baby cereal (iron-fortified)	2	2-4 tbsp	
	Bread, bagel, or	2	½	
	Crackers		2 crackers	
Fruit-vegetable	Fruit or vegetables	4	3-4 tbsp	Be patient. Babies make messes when they feed themselves.
	Baby fruit juice	1	3 oz (from cup)	
Meat	Chicken, beef, pork	2	3-4 tbsp	Always test heated foods before serving them to baby.
	Cooked, dried beans, or egg yolks			

Every baby is very special. Do not worry if your baby eats a little more or less than this guide suggests. In fact, this is perfectly normal. The suggested serving sizes are only guidelines to help you get started.

*If you are bottle feeding, most doctors recommend iron-fortified formula. Ask your doctor which formula is best for your baby.

From National Dairy Council: *Feeding guide for the first two years*, Rosemont, Ill, 1990, The Council.

TABLE 35-8	How to Feed Your Baby Step-By-Step—cont'd			
Food Group	Foods	Daily Servings	Suggested Serving Size	Feeding Tips
12-24 MO				
Milk	Whole milk, yogurt	3	½ cup	Add whole milk now.
	Cheese		½ oz	Offer small portions and never force toddler to eat.
	Cottage cheese		¼ cup	
Grain	Cereal, pasta, or rice	4	¼ cup	"Food jags" are common now. Don't make big deal out of them.
	Bread, muffins, bagels, rolls		½	
	Crackers		2 crackers	Respect toddler's likes and dislikes. Offer rejected foods again.
Fruit-vegetable	All fruits and vegetables:	4		Make meals fun and interesting. Serve colorful foods that are crunchy, smooth, or warm.
	Cooked, juice		¼ cup	
	Whole		½ medium	
Meat	Fish, chicken, turkey, beef, pork	2	1 oz	Feed toddler at least three snacks every day.
	Cooked dried beans or peas		¼ cup	
	Eggs		1	

when the fetal store of iron is exhausted, the infant needs a dietary source of this nutrient. Premature infants need iron earlier and appear to absorb it better than full-term infants.

Bottle-Fed Infants

Bottle-fed infants are usually given 5% to 10% glucose or sterile water 4 hours after birth. Ingesting refined sugar at an early age may produce a desire later for sweet foods. The infant who handles the glucose feeding well progresses to diluted formula and then to full-strength formula. Infant formulas can also be fortified with vitamins and minerals to resemble human milk.

Neither undiluted whole milk nor skim milk should be used as a basis for infant formulas. Whole milk has excess protein and requires dilution, and skim milk does not contain linoleic acid and is too low in calories. Honey and corn syrup are potential sources of the botulism toxin and should not be used in the infant's diet. The toxin can be fatal in children under 1 year of age (Wardlaw, Insel, Seyler, 1992).

Introduction to Solid Food

The ability to swallow voluntarily is not fully developed until 10 to 12 weeks of age. Before that time, swallowing must be stimulated by sucking. The amount of saliva needed to ease swallowing solid food is not secreted until about 3 months of age. The **extrusion reflex** (pushing food out of the mouth with the tongue) is the dominant reflex until the infant is 4 months old. Enzymes to digest complex carbohydrates (for example, cereals) and taste sensation are not fully developed until 3 to 4 months of age.

Foods may be started gradually, beginning sometime between 4 and 6 months, depending on the infant's readiness. Indications of readiness include the following:

1. Infant doubling the birth weight
2. Infant's ability to consume 8 oz of formula and to become hungry in less than 4 hours
3. Infant's ability to sit up
4. Infant's ability to consume 32 oz a day and want more
5. 6 months of age

Table 35-8 presents a suggested sequence for introducing new foods (Whitney, Catallo, Rolfes, 1991). The addition of foods to an infant's diet should be governed by the infant's nutrient needs, the infant's physical readiness to handle different forms of foods, and the need to detect and control allergic reactions. With respect to nutrient needs, the earliest nutrient that needs supplementation is iron followed by vitamin C (Whitney, Catallo, Rolfes, 1991).

Toddlers and Preschoolers

The growth rate slows during toddler years (1 to 3). The toddler needs fewer calories but an increased amount of protein in relation to body weight. Toddlers are more interested in their environments and increasing motor skills than in food.

The toddler needs a minimum of two servings (16 oz) daily from the milk group to supply protein, calcium, riboflavin, and vitamins A and B$_{12}$. Fortified milk provides vitamin D and additional vitamin A. Whole milk should be used until the toddler reaches 2 years of age because of the linoleic acid in the milk fat. Half of the toddler's protein intake should consist of high-biological value proteins. Toddlers who consume more than 24 oz of milk daily instead of other foods may develop milk anemia. Lean red meats, as a part of the 1 to 3 oz of meat group foods, are a good source of iron. Whole grains, enriched cereals, and breads are also good sources. When meats are given to a toddler, the portions should be cut small to avoid the possibility of choking. Foods the size of toddlers' tracheas (for example, hotdogs and grapes) are dangerous for children at this age, unless they are cut in half.

The toddler should receive four servings daily from the fruit and vegetable group. One serving should be a good source of vitamin C. Green leafy vegetables and deep yellow fruits and vegetables should be served frequently. Toddlers like bite-sized raw vegetables but should not be given raw carrots because of the danger of choking.

The toddler's four servings from the bread and cereal group should include whole grain or enriched breads, cereals, and pastas. Infant cereals may continue to be used because of their higher iron content. Sugar-coated cereals and sugar on cereals should be avoided. Toddlers often prefer dry cereal. In addition to the basic four food groups, the toddler should have 1 to 2 tsp of margarine or butter for vitamin A.

Growth slows after 12 to 14 months, but energy and nutrient requirements are increased. Nutritious foods should be offered in small amounts. During the preschool years from ages 3 to 6, children gain an average of 2 kg (4½ lb) of body weight and 5 to 8 cm (2 to 3 inches) in height a year. At the end of the preschool period, the child's weight is double that at 1 year, and height is 1½ times that at 1 year. The average 6-year-old weighs 19 kg (42 lb) and stands 105 cm (42 inches) high.

Daily protein needs are increased to 24 g, half of which should be high-biological value proteins. Calcium and iron remain important. The child should be encouraged to eat fruits and vegetables for vitamins A and C. Interest in food continues to be overshadowed by interest in the enlarging environment and motor skills. Several small meals may be preferable to the traditional three.

Preschoolers need a minimum of 16 oz of milk daily, 1 to 3 oz from the meat group, four servings from the fruit and vegetable group (including a daily source of vitamin C and frequent servings of leafy green and deep yellow vegetables and fruits), four or more servings of whole grain or enriched foods from the bread and cereal group, and 1 to 2 tsp of margarine or butter.

School-Age Children

School-age children, 6 to 12 years old, grow at a slower and steadier rate, with a gradual decline in energy requirements per unit of body weight. The school-age child gains 3 to 5 kg (6½ to 11 lb) in weight and 6 cm (2½ inches) in height a year until puberty.

The appetites of school-age children are greater than those of younger children, and food intake is more varied. Recommended intake includes two servings from the milk group, 2 to 3 oz of meat group foods, four or more servings from the fruit and vegetable group (with a daily source of vitamin C and a source of vitamin A every other day), three to four servings from whole grain and enriched breads and cereals, and 1 to 2 tsp of margarine or butter.

Despite better appetites and more varied food intake, the diets of school-age children should be carefully assessed for adequate protein and vitamin A and C. Milk intake usually exceeds recommendations, but failure to eat a proper breakfast and unsupervised intake at school may result in an improper or inadequate diet.

Adolescents

During adolescence, physiological age is a better guide to nutritional needs than chronological age. Adolescence begins with the growth spurt of puberty at the end of childhood and ends with the completion of physical growth. Caloric needs are greatly increased to meet increased metabolic demands. Girls need approximately 2200 kcal/day; boys 2500 to 3000 kcal/day. Protein needs increase to a daily requirement of 45 to 59 g. Calcium is essential for the rapid bone growth of adolescence, and girls need a continuous source of iron to replace menstrual losses. Boys also need adequate iron for muscle development. Iodine supports increased thyroid activity, and B-complex vitamins support the heightened metabolic activity.

Adolescents' requirements from the basic groups include three or more servings from the milk group, two or more from the meat group, four or more from the vegetable-fruit group (with a daily source of vitamin C and a source of vitamin A every other day), four to six or more from the bread and cereal group (with emphasis on whole grains), and 1 to 2 tbsp of margarine or butter.

The adolescent's diet is influenced by many factors other than nutritional needs, including concern about body image and appearance, desire for independence, and fad diets. Nutritional deficiencies may occur in adolescent girls as a result of dieting and using oral contraceptives. The nutrients involved are folic acid, vitamin B_6, vitamin C, thiamine, riboflavin, and iron. The adolescent boy's diet may be inadequate in total calories, protein, iron, folic acid, B vitamins, and iodine.

Snacks provide approximately 25% of the teenager's total dietary intake (Whitney, Catallo, Rolfes, 1991). The irregular eating pattern of skipping meals or eating meals and the wrong choice of snacks contribute to obesity and nutrient deficits. Snack foods from the dairy and fruit-vegetable groups are good choices and contribute calcium, phosphorous, protein, zinc, vitamin A, vitamin C, and some of the B-complex vitamins.

Fast food eating is the "norm" but adds extra fat and calories and contributes to developing cardiovascular disease and weight-control problems. Table 35-9 on p. 1112 is a detailed listing of nutrients found in many items available in fast food restaurants.

Pregnant teenage girls must meet their own nutritional needs and the additional demands of the fetus. Pregnancy occurring within 4 years after menarche (which usually occurs at 10½ to 13 years in the United States) places mother and fetus at risk because of anatomical and physiological immaturity.

Most teenage girls do not want to gain weight. Counseling related to the nutritional needs of pregnancy may be very difficult, and suggestions are better than rigid directions. The diet of a pregnant adolescent is most often deficient in calcium, iron, and vitamins A and C.

Young and Middle Adults

The demands for most nutrients are reduced as the growth period ends. Mature adults need nutrients for energy, maintenance, and repair. Energy needs usually decline over the years. Obesity may become a problem because of decreased physical exercise, increased dining out, or the ability to afford more luxury foods.

Adult women who use oral contraceptives need extra folic acid, vitamin C, thiamin, riboflavin, vitamin B_6, and vitamin B_{12}. Iron and calcium intake are also necessary for all women.

Young and middle-age adults are subject to the same recommendations from the basic food groups: two or more servings from the milk group, four or more from the vegetable-fruit group (with a daily source of vitamin C and three to four weekly servings of sources of vitamin A), four or more from the whole grain or enriched bread and cereal group, and 1 to 2 tbsp of margarine or butter.

Pregnancy

Poor nutrition during pregnancy can cause low birth weight in infants and decreased chances of survival. Generally, the fetus' needs are met at the expense of the mother's. However, if nutrient sources are not available, both suffer. The nutritional status of the mother at the time of conception is important in terms of nutritional reserves and basic eating habits. Often significant aspects of fetal growth and development occur before pregnancy is even suspected.

The energy requirements of pregnancy are related to body weight and activity. A total weight gain of 10 to 15 kg (22 to 35 lb) is recommended. Inadequate weight gain and weight gain above 15 kg (35 lb) are not desirable. In the event of undesirable gains or losses, food intake should be evaluated. Pregnant women should be cautioned against fasting as a method of weight control, because fasting leads to **ketoacidosis,** which can be dangerous to the fetus.

Food intake in the first trimester should include balanced portions of essential nutrients with emphasis on quality. Protein intake throughout pregnancy is increased to 60 g (Food and Nutrition Board, 1989). High-risk mothers are advised to double their normal protein intake.

Calcium intake should be increased to 1200 mg/day. Calcium is needed for fetal tooth and bone development, muscle contraction, and blood clotting. Calcium intake is especially critical in the third trimester, when fetal bones are mineralized.

Pregnant women need more iron than can be supplied by even the most ideal diet. Iron needs are increased to 30 mg/day, and a supplement is usually given. Iron is needed to correct preexisting deficiencies and to provide for increased maternal blood volume, for fetal blood storage, and for blood loss during delivery.

Iodine needs are increased by 25 µg (15% to 17%) because of increased activity of the thyroid gland. Vitamin A is needed for cell development, epithelial tissue maintenance, and tooth and bone development. Requirements are increased to 800 retinol equivalents (REs).

Pregnancy also increases requirements for B vitamins, which are needed for enzyme production necessitated by increased metabolic activity. Folic acid intake is particularly important for DNA synthesis and the growth of red blood cells. Inadequate intake may lead to megaloblastic anemia, a type of anemia seen in women who have had many pregnancies.

TABLE 35-9 Reference Guide for Popular Fast Foods

Item	Serving Size	Calories*	Carbohydrates†	Protein†	Fat†	Sodium‡	Exchange*
ARBY'S							
Junior Roast Beef	3 oz	218	22	12	8	345	1½ starch, 1½ med. fat meat
Regular Roast Beef	5.2 oz	353	32	22	15	590	2 starch, 2 med. fat meat, 1 fat
Hot Ham 'n' Cheese Sandwich	5.7 oz	353	33	26	13	1655	2 starch, 3 med. fat meat
Potato cakes	3 oz	201	22	2	14	425	1½ starch, 3 fat§
Roasted chicken Boneless breast	5 oz	254	2	43	7	930	6 lean meat
BURGER KING							
Hamburger	1	275	29	15	12	509	2 starch, 2 med. fat meat
Cheeseburger	1	317	30	17	15	651	2 starch, 2 med. fat meat, 1 fat
Whopper	1	628	46	27	36	880	3 starch, 3 med. fat meat, 4 fat§
Chicken specialty sandwich	1	688	56	26	40	1423	4 starch, 2 med. fat meat, 5 fat§
Chicken Tenders	6 pc	204	10	20	10	636	1 starch, 2 med. fat meat
Onion Rings	1 serving	274	28	4	16	665	2 starch, 3 fat
French Fries	Regular	227	24	3	13	160	1½ starch, 2 fat
DAIRY QUEEN							
Single hamburger	1	360	33	21	16	630	2 starch, 2 med. fat meat, 1 fat
Hot dog	1	280	21	11	16	830	1½ starch, 1 med. fat meat, 2 fat
Fish fillet	1	430	45	20	18	674	3 starch, 2 med. fat meat, 1 fat
Chicken breast fillet	1	608	46	27	34	725	3 starch, 3 med. fat meat, 3 fat§
French fries	Regular	200	25	2	10	115	1½ starch, 2 fat
Onion rings	1 order	280	31	4	16	140	2 starch, 3 fat
Cone	Small	140	22	3	4	45	1½ starch, 1 fat
Chocolate sundae	Small	190	33	3	4	75	2 starch, 1 fat
Dilly Bar	1	210	21	3	13	50	1½ starch, 2 fat
DQ Sandwich	1	140	24	3	4	40	1½ starch, 1 fat
DOMINO'S PIZZA							
Cheese pizza	12" (2 slices)	340	52	18	6	660	3 starch, 1 med. fat meat, 1 vegetable
Pepperoni pizza	12"(2 slices)	380	48	20	12	880	3 starch, 2 med. fat meat, 1 vegetable
KENTUCKY FRIED CHICKEN							
Original Recipe chicken center breast	1 (107 g)	257	8	26	14	532	½ starch, 3 med. fat meat
Extra Crispy chicken center breast	1 (120 g)	353	15	27	21	842	1 starch, 3 med. fat meat, 1 fat

*1 serving.
†In g.
‡In mg.
§Note high fat content.
Med.. Medium; *NA*, not available.
From Franz M: *Fast food facts: nutritive and exchange values for fast food restaurants,* Minneapolis, 1984, International Diabetes Center.

TABLE 35-9 Reference Guide for Popular Fast Foods—cont'd

Item	Serving Size	Calories*	Carbohydrates†	Protein†	Fat†	Sodium‡	Exchange*
Mashed potatoes	1 (80 g)	59	12	2	trace	228	1 starch
Corn-on-the-cob	1 (143 g)	176	32	5	3	21	2 starch
Cole slaw	1 (79 g)	103	12	1	6	171	2 vegetable or 1 starch, 1 fat
LONG JOHN SILVERS							
Fish & fries	3 pc fish	853	64	43	48	2025	4 starch, 4 med. fat meat, 5 fat§
Tender chicken plank dinner with fries, slaw	4 pc chicken	1037	82	41	59	2433	5 starch, 4 med. fat meat, 1 vegetable, 7 fat
Shrimp, fish, chicken dinner with fries, slaw, 2 hushpuppies	1 pc Fish 2 shrimp 1 pc chicken	1022	87	34	60	2274	5 starch, 3 med. fat meat, 1 vegetable, 8 fat§
MCDONALD'S							
Hamburger	1 (100 g)	263	28	12	11	506	2 starch, 1 med. fat meat, 1 fat
Big Mac	1 (200 g)	570	39	25	35	979	2½ starch, 3 med. fat meat, 4 fat§
Filet-O-Fish	1 (143 g)	435	36	15	26	799	2½ starch, 1 med. fat meat, 4 fat§
Chicken McNuggets	1 (109 g)	323	15	19	20	512	1 starch, 2 med. fat meat, 2 fat
French fries	1 (68 g)	220	26	3	12	109	2 starch, 2 fat
Egg McMuffin	1 (138 g)	340	31	19	16	885	2 starch, 2 med. fat meat, 1 fat
PIZZA HUT							
Thin-n-Crispy pizza cheese	3 slices ½ 10" pizza	450	54	25	15	NA	3½ starch, 2 med. fat meat, 1 fat
Thick 'n Chewy pizza Cheese	3 slices ½ 10" pizza	560	71	34	14	NA	5 starch, 3 med. fat meat
TACO BELL							
Bean burrito	1	343	48	11	12	272	3 starch, 2 fat
Burrito Supreme	1	457	43	21	22	367	3 starch, 2 med. fat meat, 2 fat
Taco	1	186	14	15	8	79	1 starch, 2 lean meat
Tostado	1	179	25	9	6	101	1½ starch, 1 med. fat meat
WENDY'S							
Single hamburger patty on white bun	1 (127 g)	350	26	24	16	360	2 starch, 3 med. fat meat
Plain baked potato	1 (250 g)	250	52	6	2	60	3½ starch
Sour cream & chives potato	1 (310 g)	460	53	6	24	230	3½ starch, 5 fat§
Chili (regular)	1 (236 g)	240	24	19	8	990	1½, 2 med. fat meat
Taco salad	1 (398 g)	430	43	22	19	1260	3 starch, 2 med. fat meat, 2 fat
Chicken breast fillet on bun	1 (87 g)	320	31	25	10	500	2 starch, 3 lean meat
Garden spot salad bar:							
Lettuce, iceberg, or romaine	3 cup (165 g)	20	3	Trace	Trace	20	1 vegetable
Cole slaw	¼ cup	80	9	Trace	5	165	2 vegetable, 1 fat
Cottage cheese	½ cup	110	3	13	4	425	2 lean meat
American cheese	1 oz	90	trace	6	7	335	1 high fat meat
Sunflower seeds and raisins	1 oz	140	6	5	10	5	½ fruit, 1 high fat meat

Vitamin C requirements are increased by 10 mg to provide the intercellular cement in connective and vascular tissue and to enhance the absorption of iron. Vitamin D needs are increased by 5 μg (100%) because this vitamin promotes the absorption of calcium and phosphorus needed for tooth and bone development.

The pregnant woman should have four or more servings from the milk group; two or more (6 oz) from the meat group; five to seven from the vegetable-fruit group (including a citrus fruit and a potato daily and leafy green or dark yellow vegetables 3 to 4 times a week); four or more from the enriched or whole grain bread and cereal group; and at least 1 to 2 tbsp of margarine or butter daily.

Pregnant women should increase their fluid intake by drinking at least 8 glasses of water daily. They should avoid artificial sweetners, alcohol, excessive caffeine, and all drugs not specifically ordered. Adequate fluid intake can prevent constipation, commonly associated with pregnancy.

Lactation

The lactating woman needs 500 kcal above her prepregnancy requirement. The production of breast milk increases energy requirements. Protein requirements are increased to 65 g per day. The need for calcium remains the same as during pregnancy. Although the lactating woman requires less protein, folacin, and iron as compared to the pregnancy requirements, there is an increased need for vitamin A, C, niacin, riboflavin, iodine, and zinc over pregnancy needs. The need for vitamins D, E, B_6, B_{12}, and thiamine and for the minerals calcium, phosphorus, and magnesium is the same for the pregnant and the lactating woman, but the lactating woman requires approximately 100 ml more fluid for optimal milk production.

The increased calories from the basic food groups should be provided by leafy green vegetables, citrus fruits, whole grains, milk, meats, and poultry to provide vitamins A and C, niacin, riboflavin, and zinc. Daily intakes of the water-soluble vitamins (B and C) are needed to ensure adequate levels in breast milk. The woman should drink a quart of milk daily or its equivalent from the milk group. Fluid intake should total at least 3 quarts a day. Caffeine, alcohol, and drugs are excreted in breast milk and should not be used without a physician's supervision.

Older Adults

Adults 65 years and older have a decreased need for calories as the metabolic rate slows with age. Decreased activity of the thyroid gland reduces the need for iodine. Protein and calcium levels are often low, and foods from the meat and dairy groups need to be emphasized.

Numerous factors influence the nutritional status of the older adult. Income is probably the most important because a fixed income may reduce the amount of money used to buy food. Health is another important influence. The older adult may be on a therapeutic diet or have difficulty eating resulting from physical symptoms, lack of teeth, or dentures. Food shopping and preparation may be difficult because of physical disability or lack of transportation. Living alone decreases the interest and pleasure of preparing and eating meals.

Taste acuity normally declines with age, which may result from decreased zinc levels. The taste buds that recognize sweet and salt are the first to deteriorate, leaving bitter and sour as the dominant taste sensations. Dentures also increase bitter and sour taste sensations. A normal decline in gastric secretions results in less-efficient digestion.

The basic food group selections for older adults are the same as for younger adults, although the way that foods are prepared or the types of foods selected may need to be changed. Diets of older adults are typically low in protein foods and high in breads, cakes, and cereals. Meats may be avoided because of cost or because they are difficult to chew. Cheese, eggs, and peanut butter are useful in providing protein. Milk continues to be an important food, particularly for the older woman who needs adequate calcium to protect against osteoporosis (loss of calcium from bones). Whole grain cereals and breads should be encouraged. Cream soups and meat-based vegetable soups are good for the older adult with chewing problems. The diet of the older adult should contain choices from all food groups and may require vitamin supplements.

NUTRITION AND THE NURSING PROCESS

Nurses are in an excellent position to recognize signs of poor nutrition and to take steps to initiate change. Close daily contact with clients and their families enables nurses to make observations about their physical status, food intake, weight gain or loss, and responses to therapy. By using the four techniques of assessment, the nurse can identify actual or potential problems in nutritional status and implement appropriate nursing, medical, and nutritional therapies to reduce or reverse nutritional alterations.

Overweight and underweight clients are at risk for nutritional deficits because a 20% deviation from ideal body weight is considered a high-risk factor for diabetes, heart disease, and lowered resistance to disease. Gross increases or decreases in body weight may reduce the body's protein reserve.

 ## Assessment

Nurses make nutritional assessment part of daily nurse-client relationships. Because food and fluid are basic biological needs of all human beings, a nutritional assessment is essential. Nutritional assessment is particularly important for clients at risk for nutritional problems related to stress, illness, hospitalization, lifestyle habits, and other factors. The following nutritional assessment goals have been outlined by the American Society of Parenteral and Enteral Nutrition (ASPEN) (Forlaw, Grant, 1983):

1. Identify nutritional deficiencies adversely affecting health.
2. Obtain specific information to assist in planning and delivering nutritional care.
3. Evaluate the efficacy of nutritional care, modifying the nutritional care plan as needed to obtain the desired result.

The nutritional assessment consists of nursing and diet history, observation, anthropometry, and laboratory data. In addition, the assessment is individualized to determine clients at risk for nutritional alterations.

Nursing and Diet History

In addition to the general nursing history, the nurse obtains a more specific diet history to assess the client's actual or potential nutritional needs (Fig. 35-4). The diet history focuses on the client's habit-

---

Name _____ Date _____
Age _____ Hospital number _____
Family composition _____
Present weight _____ Usual weight _____
Height _____ Recent changes in weight _____
Number of meals per day _____ Number of snacks per day _____
Meals prepared by _____

Food preferences	Food allergies	Food aversions	Nonfavored but acceptable foods

List any foods that cause indigestion.
List any foods that cause diarrhea.
List any foods that cause flatulence (gas).
Any difficulty chewing or swallowing?
Dentures?
Usual bowel movements.
History of dietary problems.
History of diseases, surgical procedures, or weight problems.
Physical activity.

Appetite _____ Recent changes in appetite _____
Breakfast at _____ AM With _____
Usual breakfast _____ Serving size _____

Occasional breakfasts _____
Weekends _____ Holidays _____ Special _____
Eats lunch/dinner at _____ PM With _____
At home _____ At work _____
Usual lunch/dinner _____ Serving size _____

Occasional lunches/dinners _____
Weekend _____ Holiday _____ Special _____
Eats supper/dinner at _____ PM With _____
Usual supper/dinner _____ Serving size _____

Occasional supper/dinner _____
Weekends _____ Holidays _____ Special _____
Snacks _____ Time _____ Serving size _____

Fig. 35-4 Diet history.
From Bodinski LH: *The nurse's guide to diet therapy,* New York, 1982, Wiley.

ual intake of food and liquids, as well as information about preferences, allergies, problems, and other relevant areas (Fig. 35-4).

In addition, a detailed record can be kept of the client's food intake over 3 days, including a weekend day. This record allows the nurse to calculate the client's nutritional intake and to compare it with recommended allowances to determine whether the client's usual dietary habits are providing all nutrients in required amounts.

During the nursing history the nurse also gathers information about the client's activity level to determine the energy need and compare it with food intake.

FACTORS INFLUENCING DIETARY PATTERNS. A final area for the nurse to assess is a set of factors that influence the client's dietary pattern and nutritional status (see box). These factors include health status, cultural background, religion, socioeconomic status, personal preference, psychological factors, use of alcohol or drugs, and misinformation of beliefs about food values (Table 35-10).

Physical Assessment

As in other kinds of nursing assessment, the nurse observes the client for signs of actual or potential nutritional needs. Because improper nutrition affects all body systems, clues to malnutrition may be observed during physical assessment (see Chapter 20). When the general physical assessment of body systems is complete, the nurse can recheck pertinent areas to evaluate the client's nutritional status. The clinical signs of nutritional status (Table 35-11) provide guidelines for observation during physical assessment.

Factors Influencing Dietary Patterns

HEALTH STATUS

- A good appetite is a sign of health.
- Anorexia (lack of appetite) is usually a symptom of disease or can be a side effect of drugs.
- Nutritional support is an essential part of recovery from any medical treatment.

CULTURE AND RELIGION

- Cultural, ethnic, and religious patterns and restrictions concerning food must be taken into account.
- Special foods and diets should be given when appropriate.
- Older clients are more apt to cling to ethnic food habits. This tendency may be increased during illness.

SOCIOECONOMIC STATUS

- Food expenses are not fixed, and spending varies according to the amount of money available.
- Whether someone is around to prepare food determines the amount of convenience foods used.

PERSONAL PREFERENCE

- Individual likes and dislikes are perhaps the strongest influence on diet.
- Foods associated with pleasant memories tend to become favorite foods. Foods associated with unpleasant memories tend to be avoided.
- Luxury foods may be used as status symbols.
- Individual preferences must be considered when planning a therapeutic diet.

PSYCHOLOGICAL FACTORS

- Individual motivations to eat balanced meals and individual perceptions about diet are strong influences.
- Food has strong symbolic value for many people (e.g., milk symbolizing helplessness and meat symbolizing strength).

ALCOHOL AND DRUGS

- Excess alcohol or drug use contributes to nutritional deficiencies because money may be spent on alcohol instead of food, and alcohol may replace part of the diet and depress appetite.
- Excess alcohol can also affect gastrointestinal organs.
- Drugs that depress appetite can lower the intake of essential nutrients.
- Drugs can also deplete nutrient stores and lessen their absorption in the intestines.

MISINFORMATION AND FOOD FADS

- Food myths can be the result of cultural background, popular interest in natural foods, peer pressure, and a desire to control diet choices.
- Food fads often involve erroneous beliefs that certain foods are especially healthy (e.g., yogurt being more nutritional than milk, oysters increasing sexual potency, or honey being healthier than sugar).
- Nurses must be careful not to be condescending when teaching a client that foods may not have the qualities attributed to them.

TABLE 35-10   Examples of Food Fads and Myths

Food	Common Misinformation	Nutritional Facts
Honey	Thought to be healthier than sugar, curative for coughs or colds, better than sugar for digestion	Honey has no special curative powers and causes no significant differences in digestion.
Yogurt	Thought to ensure good health, more nutritious than milk	Yogurt is essentially equivalent to milk in nutritional qualities.
Citrus fruits	Thought to cause acid indigestion	Stomach acid production is unaffected.
Cabbage, onions	Thought to taint breast milk	Lactation requires specific nutrients, and breast milk is not tainted by any food.
Gelatin	Thought in large amounts to build strong nails	Gelatin is not necessary for nail formation, which depends on general nutrition, nail care, and other factors.
Oysters, raw egg, rare lean beef	Thought to increase fertility or sexual potency	No food affects sexual potency.
Raw milk	Thought to be more nutritious than pasteurized milk	Pasteurized milk may contain slightly less vitamin C but also includes vitamin D. Raw milk carries greater risk of contamination.

TABLE 35-11   Clinical Signs of Nutritional Status

Body Area	Signs of Good Nutrition	Signs of Poor Nutrition
General appearance	Alert; responsive	Listless, apathetic, cachetic, cachectic appearance
Weight	Weight normal for height, age, body build	Obesity or underweight appearance (special concern for underweight)
Posture	Erect posture; straight arms and legs	Sagging shoulders; sunken chest; humped back
Muscles	Well-developed, firm muscles; good tone; some fat under skin	Flaccid appearance; poor tone, underdeveloped tone; tenderness; edema; wasted appearance; inability to walk and properly
Nervous system control	Good attention span; lack of irritability or restlessness; normal reflexes; psychological stability	Inattention; irritability; confusion; burning and tingling of hands and feet (paresthesia); loss of position and vibratory sense; weakness and tenderness of muscles (may result in inability to walk); decrease or loss of ankle and knee reflexes; absent vibratory sense
Gastrointestinal function	Good appetite and digestion; normal regular elimination; no palpable organs or masses	Anorexia; indigestion; constipation or diarrhea; liver or spleen enlargement
Cardiovascular function	Normal heart rate and rhythm; lack of murmurs; normal blood pressure for age	Rapid heart rate (above 100 beats/min), enlarged heart; abnormal rhythm; elevated blood pressure
General vitality	Endurance; energy, good sleep habits; vigorous appearance	Ability to be easily fatigued; lack of energy; falling asleep easily, tired and apathetic appearance
Hair	Shiny, lustrous appearance; firmness; strands not easily plucked, healthy scalp	Stringy, dull, brittle, dry, thin, and sparse, depigmented appearance; strands that can be easily plucked

From Williams SR: Nutritional guidance in prenatal care. In Worthington-Roberts BS, Vermeersch JA, Williams SR: *Nutrition in pregnancy and lactation,* ed 4, St Louis, 1989, Mosby–Year Book; and Grant JA, Kennedy-Caldwell C: *Nutritional support in nursing,* New York, 1988, Grune & Stratton.

Continued.

TABLE 35-11	Clinical Signs of Nutritional Status—cont'd	
Body Area	Signs of Good Nutrition	Signs of Poor Nutrition
Skin (general)	Smooth and slightly moist skin with good color	Rough, dry, scaly, pale, pigmented, irritated appearance; bruises; petechiae; subcutaneous fat loss
Face and neck	Uniform color; smooth, pink, healthy appearance; lack of swelling	Greasy, discolored, scaly, swollen appearance; dark skin over cheeks and under eyes; lumpiness or flakiness of skin around nose and mouth
Lips	Smoothness; good color; moist (not chapped or swollen) appearance	Dry, scaly, swollen appearance; redness and swelling (cheilosis); angular lesions at corners of mouth; fissures or scars (stomatitis)
Mouth, oral membranes	Reddish pink mucous membranes in oral cavity	Swollen, boggy oral mucous membranes
Gums	Good pink color; healthy and red appearance; lack of swelling or bleeding	Spongy gums that bleed easily; marginal redness, inflamation; receding gums
Tongue	Good pink or deep reddish color; lack of swelling; smoothness, presence of surface papillae; lack of lesions	Swelling, scarlet and raw appearance; magenta color, beefiness (glossitis); hyperemic and hypertrophic papillae; atrophic papillae
Teeth	Lack of cavities and pain; bright, straight appearance; lack of crowding; well-shaped jaw; clean appearance with no discoloration	Unfilled caries; absent teeth; worn surfaces; mottled (fluorosis), malpositioned appearance
Eyes	Bright, clear, shiny appearance; lack of sores at corner of membranes; eyelids; moist and healthy pink color; prominent blood vessels or lack of mound of tissue or sclera; lack of fatigue circles beneath eyes	Pale eye membranes (pale conjunctivas); redness of membrane (conjunctival injection); dryness; signs of infection; Bitot's spots, redness and fissuring of eyelid corners (angular palpebritis); dryness of eye membrane (conjunctival xerosis); dull appearance of cornea (corneal xerosis); soft cornea (keratomalacia)
Neck (glands)	Lack of enlargement	Thyroid enlargement
Nails	Firm, pink appearance	Spoon shape (koilonychia); brittleness; ridges
Legs, feet	Lack of tenderness, weakness, or swelling; good color	Edema; tender calf; tingling; weakness
Skeleton	Lack of malformations	Bowlegs; knock-knees; chest deformity at diaphragm; prominent scapulae and ribs

ANTHROPOMETRY. Anthropometry is a system of measurement of the size and makeup of the body and specific body parts. Anthropometric measurements that aid in identifying nutritional problems include weight, height, wrist circumference, mid–upper arm circumference (MAC), and triceps skinfold (TSF).

Unless contraindicated, the client's height and weight measurements should be obtained on hospital admission or entry into an ambulatory care setting. A client should always be weighed at the same time each day, on the same scale, and with the same clothing or linen. The client's height and weight can be compared to the usual measurements and to standards for normal height-weight relationships.

Wrist circumference is used to estimate the client's body frame. A tape measure is used to measure the smallest portion of the wrist distal to the styloid process (Fig. 35-5). The nurse calculates the frame size (r-value) by dividing the wrist circumference into the client's height (height [cm] ÷ wrist circumference). The result is the calculated r-value. Body frame normal values include greater than 10.4 to 10.9 cm (small), 10.4 to 9.6 cm (medium), and less than 9.6 cm (large) (Shronts, 1989).

The MAC determines muscle wasting. The client should be sitting because measurements while the client is supine may decrease accuracy. If the client is bedridden, the measurement can be obtained with the client's arm placed across the chest. The client's nondominant arm is relaxed, and the circumference is measured at the midpoint of the arm, between the tip of the acromial process of the scapula and the olecron process of the ulna (Fig. 35-6). Measurement of the nondominant arm prevents false recordings secondary to increased muscle mass from activities of daily living or employment. Normal values are 28.3 cm (men) and 28.5 cm (women).

Skinfold measurements are used to determine fat content of subcutaneous tissue. TSF is the most common and easiest to measure. With the thumb and forefinger, pinch lengthwise a double fold of fat about 1 cm above midpoint of the MAC. With the other hand, place the teeth of calipers on either side of the fat fold (Fig. 35-7 on p. 1120). The average measurement is taken from three readings. Normal values include 12.5 cm (men) and 18.0 cm (women). Other anatomical areas for skinfold measurements include the biceps, scapula, and abdominal muscles.

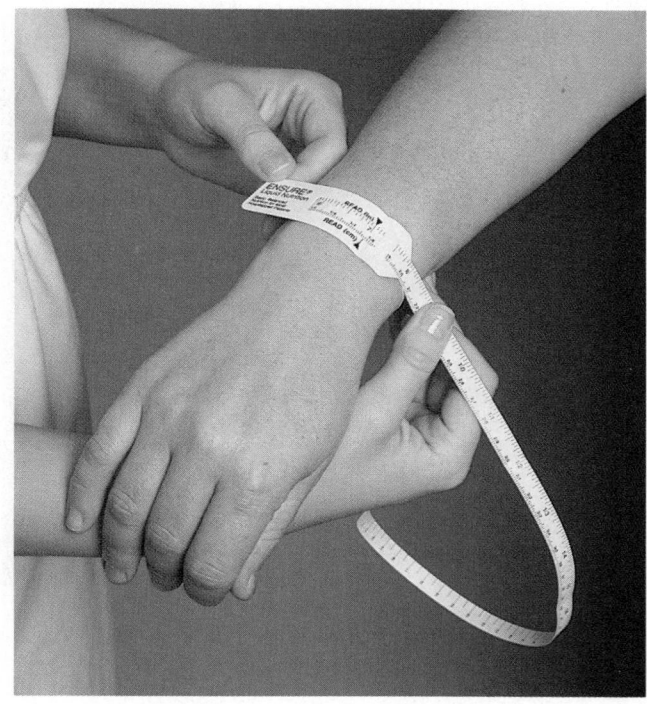

Fig. 35-5   Wrist circumference.

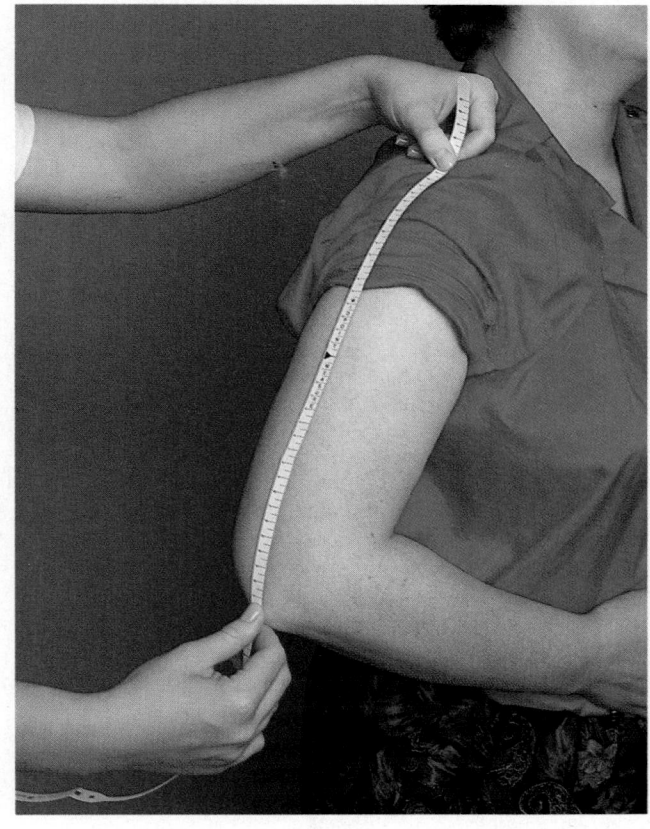

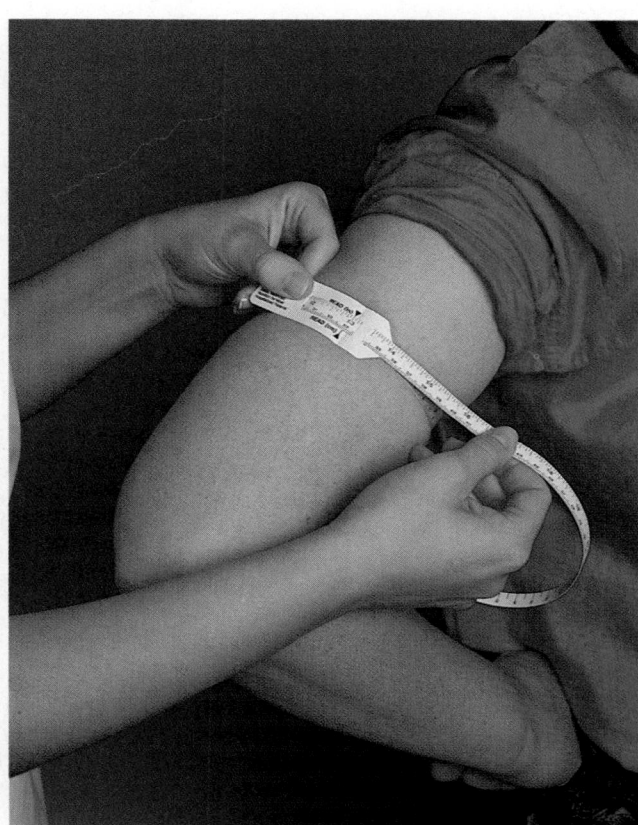

A

B

Fig. 35-6   **A,** Measurement at midpoint of arm, between the tip of the acromial process of the scapula and the olecron process. **B,** Mid–upper arm circumference.

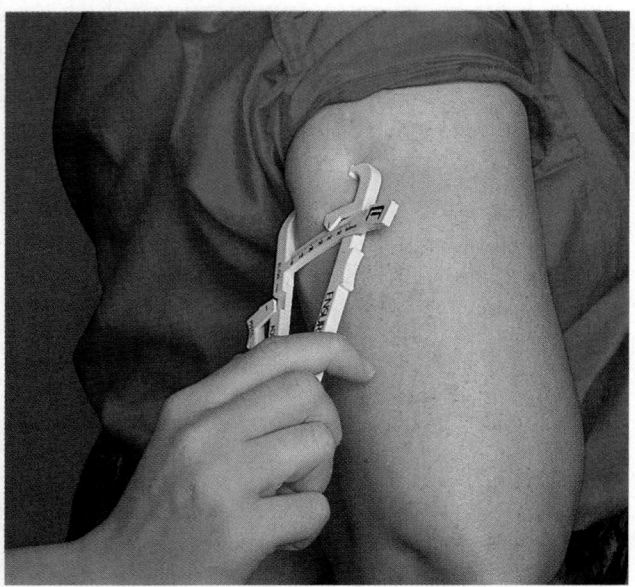

Fig. 35-7 Triceps skin fold.

The mid-arm muscle circumference (MAMC) is an estimation of skeletal mass. It is calculated from the MAC and TSF anthropometric measures. The formula is MAMC = MAC − (TSF × 3.14). The normal values include 25.3 cm (men) and 23.2 cm (women).

Laboratory Data

Laboratory values useful in nutritional assessment include the complete blood count, serum albumin level, transferrin level, and urinary concentrations of blood urea nitrogen and creatinine (Table 35-12). A low red blood cell count and depressed hemoglobin value indicate anemia. The hemoglobin and hematocrit values can also reflect the state of hydration. Serum levels of albumin and transferrin are used to identify protein-calorie malnutrition. Reduced levels of albumin and transferrin in adults also indicate a visceral protein deficit.

Urine specimens collected every 24 or 48 hours are helpful in assessing nutritional status. The blood

---

TABLE 35-12 Common Laboratory Tests to Evaluate Nutritional Status

Test	Purpose	Abnormal Findings
Serum album level (normal: 4-5.5 mg/100 ml)	Maintains serum protein levels Maintains fluid and electrolyte balance Determines prolonged protein wasting	Abnormal values may take up to 2 wks before they are reflected in blood studies. Abnormalities in liver and kidney diseases, stress, dehydration, and infection may be reflected. Level of 3.5 mg/100 ml indicates protein depletion.
Transferrin level (normal: 170-250 mg/100 ml)	Is more specific indicator of protein-calorie malnutrition than albumin (Blood protein binds with iron.)	Abnormal values respond quickly to changes in protein intake. Decrease in liver disease and chronic renal failure are reflected.
Total lymphocyte count (normal: >1800)	Reflects depression of immune system caused by impaired nutritional intake	Lymphocyte count is depleted in all immunosuppressed clients and clients with protein deficiency.
Hemoglobin level (normal: 12-15 g/100 ml)	Measures oxygen and iron-carrying capacity of blood	Decrease may indicate some form of anemia, or level can be lowered with blood loss.
Blood urea nitrogen level (normal: 10-20 mg/100 ml)	Measures breakdown of dietary protein Measures urea production in liver and excretion in kidneys	Level is elevated with excessive protein intake. Level is depressed with low protein intake. Level is elevated in liver and renal disease. Level is falsely elevated in hypovolemic dehydration.
Creatinine excretion in 24-hour urine (normal: 0.6-1.3 mg/100 ml for men and 0.5-1.0 mg/100ml for women)	Reflects total muscle mass Indirectly measures skeletal muscle mass depletion	Level is abnormally low in renal disease. Level is abnormally low in severe malnutrition and starvation.

urea nitrogen level is related to the use of exogenous protein and to nitrogen balance. Creatinine is used with height to indicate changes in lean tissue mass.

Clients at Risk for Nutritional Problems

Any client with a condition that interferes with the ability to ingest, digest, or absorb adequate nutrients should be considered at risk. Congenital anomalies and surgical revisions of the gastrointestinal tract interfere with normal function. Clients fed solely by the intravenous route for more than 10 days are at risk for nutritional deficiencies.

OBESITY. **Obesity** is a condition in which there is a 20% increase above ideal body weight. Obesity cuts across all socioeconomic levels and is a risk factor in most leading causes of death. American culture stresses slenderness, so excessive weight causes psychological problems, inconvenience, and unhappiness in addition to its impact on health.

To lose weight, a person must burn some of the body's store of fat. When insufficient calories are ingested to meet daily energy needs, the body is forced to burn its reserve stores for energy. A person may lose weight by reducing food intake or increasing energy needs through increased activity. Following dietary guidelines and reducing intake of fats and refined sugars should also reduce weight. A successful weight-control plan combines diet, behavior modification, and exercise.

ANOREXIA NERVOSA. **Anorexia nervosa** is a biopsychosocial disorder in which self-imposed starvation is used to establish identity and control, marked by denial of being underweight, hunger, and fatigue. It may be metabolic and possibly hereditary. Usually a problem in family dynamics is present. Early feeding patterns and attitudes toward food have also been implicated. The desirability of a slender figure in today's society is considered a potent factor.

The client with anorexia nervosa is usually a highly motivated adolescent girl. Extreme undernutrition leads to secondary endocrine disorders such as amenorrhea, delayed sexual development, and depressed organ function such as cardiac dysrhythmias that can be life threatening. The treatment of anorexia nervosa is a long-term combination of psychotherapy, behavior modification, and diet therapy.

BULIMIA. **Bulimia,** or the binge-purge syndrome, occurs in half of clients with anorexia nervosa, but not all bulimic clients have anorexia nervosa. The syndrome appears to develop with an abnormal craving for food accompanied by the desire to remain slender. The client gorges on food to satisfy the craving and then induces vomiting to prevent the digestion of food. The client may also use laxatives or enemas to increase gastric motility so that nutrients are not totally absorbed. The practice of secretly vomiting after eating usually starts with occasional binges and gradually becomes a daily activity and the preferred way of controlling weight. Frequent vomiting, laxative abuse, and overuse of enemas lead to electrolyte imbalances (hypokalemia being the most serious), esophageal lesions, dental caries, endocrine disturbances, and metabolic changes. Treatment includes dietary education, hospitalization, psychotherapy, drug therapy with phenytoin (Dilantin), group therapy, and behavioral modification.

POSTOPERATIVE CLIENTS. Surgery interferes with food intake. Preoperative preparation usually involves at least 8 hours of fasting. The resumption of food intake postoperatively varies with the client, surgical procedure, complications, and surgeon's protocol (see Chapter 47).

Clients who have had mouth and throat surgery must chew and swallow food in the presence of excision sites, sutures, or otherwise manipulated tissue. The ingestion of food causes discomfort, so clients are usually reluctant to eat or drink. Fluids are usually offered first. The use of a straw may help in some cases but is specifically contraindicated in others such as dental extractions, dental surgeries, and cleft palate repairs. Soft foods are sometimes easier to swallow than liquids. Hot fluids, tart juices, and fiber should be avoided after throat and mouth surgery. Milk, yogurt, sherbet, ice cream, ginger ale, and diluted fruit juices are usually allowed.

When surgery is performed on the stomach and intestines, an alternative method of food intake is usually prescribed to allow the suture line to heal and edema to subside. Nasogastric suction may also be used to prevent gastric and intestinal secretions from irritating the resected areas. When oral intake is restricted for a short period, fluids are usually given intravenously. Gastric surgery may limit the amount of food that can be ingested at any time. Intestinal surgery may interfere with absorption of nutrients, depending on the length of intestine involved and the location.

The diversion of intestinal wastes through the creation of artificial openings in the abdomen (**ileostomy** and **colostomy**) affects fluid loss and electrolyte balance. Clients with ileostomies also lose some of their ability to absorb vitamin B_{12}. Clients with ileostomies and colostomies have dietary concerns related to the consistency of the ostomy waste and control of odor.

IMMOBILIZED CLIENTS. Extended immobilization can result in deossification and osteoporosis of bones and in hypercalcemia (see Chapter 43). Hypercalcemia predisposes clients to kidney and bladder stones. It is a particular problem in children and adolescents because of their rapid bone growth. Early ambulation is the best way to prevent immobilization problems. When ambulation is not possible, adequate quantities of high-biological value proteins help prevent skin breakdown and infections, and high phosphorus intake in the early weeks of immobilization reduces blood calcium levels. Generous fluid intake also protects against kidney stones. Range of motion exercises for noninvolved joints provide some activity.

CANCER AND RADIOTHERAPY. Malignant cancer cells compete with normal cells for nutrients, increasing the metabolic needs of the client. Clients with cancer typically complain of anorexia and taste distortions, and treatment often causes nausea and vomiting. Nutritional support and the correction of nutritional deficits can enable clients to benefit from therapies previously denied them. Optimal nutrition improves cancer survival rates and the quality of life.

Although radiotherapy destroys the rapidly dividing neoplastic cells, it also destroys normal cells. Clients in good nutritional states can tolerate larger doses of radiation. Radiotherapy usually causes **anorexia** (lack or loss of appetite), nausea, and vomiting. Irradiation of the head and neck can lead to taste and smell distortions, decreased salivation, and **dysphagia** (difficulty swallowing). Irradiation of the abdomen and pelvis can result in **malabsorption** and diarrhea (Robuck, Fleetwood, 1992).

Nursing Diagnosis

The nursing assessment ends with the nurse clustering relevant data to determine whether actual or potential nutritional problems exist (see diagnoses box). A deficit may occur when one or more nutrients are not ingested, poorly digested, or incompletely absorbed. Specific diagnoses are related to the actual nutritional deficiency. The nursing diagnosis may also involve a general nutritional deficiency or problems that place the client at risk for nutritional deficiencies.

The nursing diagnostic statement is based on supporting diagnostic characteristics present in the assessment data base (see diagnostic process box). In addition, the suspected etiology of the diagnosis is stated. Identification of the cause further individualizes the nursing diagnostic statement and subsequent care plan.

Planning

Planning to maintain a proper nutritional status is better than having to correct deficits (see care plan). The identification of clients at risk for nutritional

Examples of Nursing Diagnoses Related to Altered Nutritional Status

NANDA-APPROVED NURSING DIAGNOSES

Altered nutrition: less than body requirements related to:
- Status of nothing by mouth
- Excessive dieting
- Anorexia
- Self-induced vomiting
- Alcoholism
- Excessive use of enemas or laxatives
- Food fads
- Alternative diet forms

Altered nutrition: more than body requirements related to:
- Excessive caloric intake

Altered nutrition: potential for more than body requirements related to:
- Dysfunctional eating patterns
- Closely spaced pregnancies

Feeding self-care deficit related to:
- Impaired mobility of both arms

Impaired swallowing related to:
- Surgical trauma
- Muscular weakness

Sample Nursing Diagnostic Process for Altered Nutritional Status

Assessment Activities	Defining Characteristics	Nursing Diagnosis
Ask client about planned or unplanned changes in weight.	Unplanned weight loss	*Altered nutrition: less than body requirements* related to decreased intake.
Weigh client.	Weight less than 20% of ideal body weight	
Ask client about food likes and dislikes.	Aversion to food	
Inspect client's oral mucosa.	Inflamed buccal mucosa	
Palpate abdomen.	Abdominal tenderness	

problems should result in a care plan that will prevent or minimize nutritional problems. Nutritional education and counseling are important for clients on regular diets to prevent disease and promote health. Clients on therapeutic diets who understand the rationale for the diets are more likely to be compliant. For this group of clients the care plan is based on one or more of the following goals:

1. Client will return to within 10% of ideal body weight.
2. Client will maintain fluid and electrolyte balance within normal limits.
3. No complications will result from therapies designed to assist clients to return to within 10% of ideal body weight.

In the health care setting and home, some clients with physiological conditions that cause more severe cases of malnutrition require total parenteral nutrition to meet fluid, electrolyte, and nutritional needs.

Total parenteral nutrition (TPN) is a nutritionally adequate hypertonic solution consisting of glucose, amino acids, lipids, minerals, and vitamins given through an indwelling peripheral or central intravenous catheter. Clients most at risk for requiring TPN suffer from severe trauma, febrile states, cancer, or severe **malnutrition** (any deficit of a necessary nutrient). The nursing care plan for clients receiving TPN is based on one or more of the following additional goals:

1. Clients will maintain positive nitrogen balances when illness prevents absorption of sufficient amounts of nutrients.
2. The delivery of essential nutrients for wound healing and restoration of body tissues will be increased.
3. Clients with severe physiological conditions affecting nutritional status will receive nutrients.
4. Clients' gastrointestinal tracts will heal.

Implementation

Ill or debilitated clients usually have poor appetites despite the efforts of dietitians, nurses, families, friends, and other support people. Nurses can help by displaying interest in clients' intakes, by under-

---

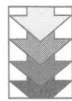 Sample Nursing Care Plan for Altered Nutrition: Less than Body Requirements

---

Nursing diagnosis: *Altered nutrition: less than body requirements* related to decreased intake
Definition: Altered nutrition: less than body requirements is the state in which an individual has decreased ability to voluntarily pass fluids and/or solids from the mouth to the stomach (Kim, McFarland, McLane, 1991).

Goal	Expected Outcomes	Interventions	Rationale
Client will return to within 10% of ideal body weight.	Client will gain 0.5-1.0 lb/wk (0.25-0.5 kg/wk).	Weigh client at 0800 daily with same scale.	Using same scale at same time increases consistency of measure.
		Obtain calorie and stool counts daily.	Measures provide more consistent documentation of total calories absorbed (Forlaw, Grant, 1983).
		Institute enteral feedings via small-bore feeding tube.	Clients with severe impairments in swallowing and nutritional deficiencies frequently need enteral feedings
	Client's gastrointestinal aspirate residuals will remain less than 75 ml.	Aspirate for gastrointestinal residuals twice a day.	Residuals less than 150 ml indicate greater absorption and reduce risk for aspiration (Petrosino, Christian, Becker, 1989).
	Serum electrolyte and blood chemistry tests will indicate improving nutritional status.	Obtain order for complete blood count with differential and blood chemistry tests 7-14 days after initiating nutritional support.	Certain chemistry levels (e.g., white blood cells and albumin) require 7-14 days to demonstrate improvement secondary to nutritional therapy (Forlaw, Grant, 1983).

standing the influences that reduce appetite, and by being willing to do everything possible to improve intake.

One of the most disruptive influences on intake is diagnostic testing. Some blood and radiographic studies require the client to fast. Therefore the client's breakfast is usually withheld until the client returns from the test or testing is completed.

Stress also influences intake. Clients who are worried about their families, finances, employment, or illnesses are unable to eat or to eat enough to compensate for the effect of stress on their metabolism.

Medications also affect intake and, in some cases, the utilization of nutrients. Medications can affect the sensations of taste or smell, and as a result, food is not as appetizing. In addition, medications can cause nausea or vomiting. The client is anorexic because of the nausea, or the nutrients are vomited before the client has properly digested them. Medications such as insulin and thyroid hormones can also affect metabolism.

Nurses design implementation measures around three general areas to promote nutrition. These areas include measures to stimulate the client's appetite, enteral nutritional therapies, and parenteral nutritional therapies.

Stimulating Appetite

A nurse can help stimulate the client's appetite through environmental adaptations, consultation with a diet therapist, special diets and food preferences, and client and family counseling.

ENVIRONMENT. Nurses are responsible for providing an environment conducive to eating. The client's room should be free of reminders of treatments. The environment should be free of odors. Mouth care should be provided when necessary to remove unpleasant tastes. The client needs to be positioned comfortably so that the meal can be more enjoyable. If the client has visitors or needs hygiene care before eating, sufficient time is given to permit anticipation and preparation for the meal.

DIET THERAPIST. After a meal, the client's intake is evaluated and charted. The nurse shares responsibility with the dietitian for food intake and works with the diet therapist. Sharing information about a client's concerns and response to diet therapy benefits the nurse, diet therapist, and client. The client's education about the therapeutic diet should be a shared responsibility. The dietitian is the expert in diet therapy, but the nurse can relate the dietary modification to the client's condition and explain how the diet contributes to the care plan.

SPECIAL DIETS. Nurses should be familiar with the special diets used in client care so that they can select appropriate between-meal liquids and snacks, monitor food brought in by visitors, and offer acceptable food supplements (Fig. 35-8). Numerous types of special diets are available to be used with food or as the only nutrient source. Examples of formulas are milk based, lactose free, high protein, and formulas with fiber and calories, which range from 1 to 2 kcal/ml of formula.

Hospital Diets. A regular hospital diet contains approximately 2500 kcal and consists of appropriate servings from a variety of food groups. In some hospitals the regular diet has been changed to reflect the dietary guidelines by decreasing lipids and increasing complex carbohydrates (Table 35-13). No particular food restrictions are in the regular diet, but foods that are difficult to digest and fried foods are usually kept to a minimum.

Diet Therapy in Disease Management

Good nutrition is important in health and illness, but the specific dietary intake pattern that results in good nutrition must often be modified for clients with particular diseases. Diet modifications are necessary to correspond with the body's ability to metabolize certain nutrients, correct nutritional deficiencies related to the disease, and eliminate foods that may be harmful.

GASTROINTESTINAL DISEASES. The treatment of **ulcerative colitis** may include a liquid diet in the acute stage, a low-residue diet during recovery, and thereafter a bland diet high in protein, calories, vitamins, and minerals and low in fat. During the chronic stage, adding fiber foods is often beneficial in creating bulk and reducing diarrhea. Vitamins and iron

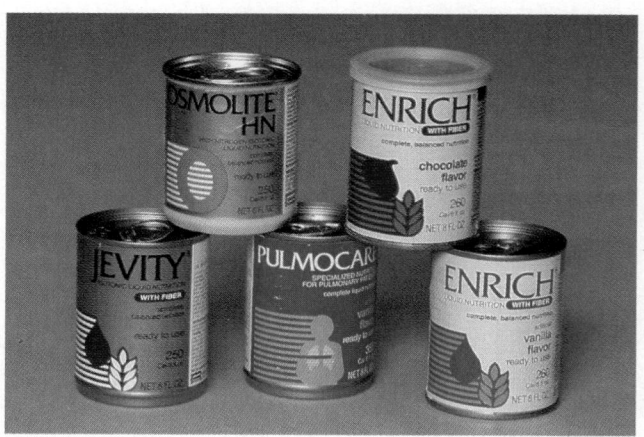

Fig. 35-8 Various diet supplements.

TABLE 35-13 Routine Therapeutic Diets			
Modification	Medical Indications	Rationale	Foods to Avoid
CLEAR LIQUID			
Eliminates all foods except clear liquids	Presurgical period	Empties gastrointestinal tract to prevent aspiration and possibly clean surgical site (no residue); prevents dehydration	All except clear liquids at room temperature
LIQUID			
Includes liquids at room temperature, including milk products	Postsurgical period	Increases calories and nutrients gradually, as tolerated	All except liquids at room temperature and milk products
SOFT			
Eases mechanical digestion	Problems with chewing, swallowing, poor digestive function; ulcerative colitis; Crohn's disease	Provides step between liquid to regular diet; provides more nutrition	Seeds, skins of fruits, fried foods, whole grains, raw fruit, vegetables, highly seasoned foods.
LOW RESIDUE			
Reduces fiber and cellulose	Diverticulitis, ulcerative colitis, Crohn's disease	Reduces physical irritation to mucosa	Raw fruits and vegetables (except bananas), raw plant fiber, whole grains, milk products (limited to 2 cups/day)
HIGH FIBER			
Is normal diet with increased fiber from raw fruits and vegetables	Diverticulosis	Promotes forward motion of indigestible wastes through colon	None (Use general guidelines.)
FAT CONTROLLED			
Reduces total fat and replaces saturated fats with monounsaturates and polyunsaturates; restricts cholesterol	Atherosclerosis, elevated cholesterol triglyceride level, coronary heart disease, obesity	Reverses and slows down conditions	Saturated (animal) fats, gravies, sauces, egg yolks, high-fat meats, whole milk
SODIUM RESTRICTED			
Restricts sodium intake: mild (2-3 g), moderate (1000 mg), strict (500 mg), severe (250 mg)	Hypertension, myocardial infarction, congestive heart failure	Reduces sodium levels to aid in reducing total fluid volume, thereby reducing blood pressure, workload on heart, and excess fluids	Highly salted foods, added salt at meal table (depends on level of restriction)
LIBERAL BLAND			
Eliminates foods that are chemical or mechanical irritants	Gastritis, gastrointestinal ulcers*	Reduces gastrointestinal irritation; improves food tolerance	Fried foods, strong spices, caffeine, alcohol, decaffeinated coffee

*Current treatment is often a regular diet omitting caffeine, decaffeinated coffee, highly seasoned foods, smoking, and alcohol.

*Adapted from Williams SR: *Nutrition and diet therapy,* ed 6, St Louis, 1989, Mosby–Year Book; and Whitney EN, Catallo CB, Rolfes SR: *Understanding normal and clinical nutrition,* ed 3, St Paul, Minn, 1991, West.

supplements are generally required because absorption is decreased.

The treatment of diarrhea may include a diet high in vitamins to counteract decreased absorption, low in residue, and high in calories if the client is emaciated. The treatment of **malabsorption syndrome,** including sprue and celiac disease, includes a gluten-free diet. Gluten is present in wheat, rye, barley, and oats.

The treatment of acute **enteritis** generally involves fasting initially, followed by a liquid diet and thereafter a bland diet. Acute **gastritis** is generally treated by a liquid diet initially, with a gradual transition to a low-residue diet and thereafter a bland diet. The treatment for chronic gastritis involves eliminating from the diet the foods or liquids that cause inflammation and thereafter permitting only easily digested foods.

The treatment of **diverticulitis** in which bowel perforation has not occurred includes a liquid or low-residue diet until the infection subsides. Afterward, a high-fiber diet is generally prescribed for chronic diverticulosis.

Peptic ulcers are better controlled with regular meals and medications such as cimetidine. This classification of drugs is antihistamine—H_2 receptors that blocks secretion of hydrochloric acid. Clients are also encouraged to avoid foods that increase stomach acidity such as those containing caffeine, decaffeinated coffee, and highly seasoned foods. Smoking and alcohol are not recommended.

CARDIOVASCULAR DISEASES. The general goals of dietary treatment of cardiovascular diseases include preventing stomach distention to avoid pressure against the heart, reducing the client's weight if needed, and lowering blood lipids to lessen the risk of atherosclerosis. The treatment of myocardial infarction includes a liquid diet for several days, progressing to a low-fat, low-sodium, high-carbohydrate soft diet during recovery. This is followed by a diet moderately low in fat and protein and high in carbohydrates. A diet high in cholesterol and saturated fat increases the risk of atherosclerosis and cardiovascular disease. Dietary therapy for treatment and prevention generally includes maintaining a recommended weight and a diet low in saturated fats, with less than 30% of total calories from fat and 300 mg of cholesterol. The treatment of hypertension includes weight reduction to normal if the client is overweight and a diet low in sodium and moderately low in fats.

Consistent with the Dietary Guidelines for Americans, the newly released National Cholesterol Education Program (NCEP) Report of the Expert Panel on Blood Cholesterol Levels in Children and Adolescents (NIH, 1991) recommends that all healthy children over 2 years of age and adolescents consume a diet that provides the following:

1. Less than 10% of total calories from saturated fatty acids
2. An average of no more than 30% of total calories from fat
3. Less than 300 mg/day dietary cholesterol

In addition to fat and cholesterol levels, a protein range of 10% to 20% and 50% to 60% carbohydrates is also recommended to lower cholesterol and lipid levels (NIH, 1991). Current research demonstrates that a 1% reduction in cholesterol level reduces the risk of heart disease by approximately 2% (Rifkind, 1988).

DIABETES. Adult-onset diabetes (non-insulin-dependent diabetes mellitus [NIDDM] or type II DM) can usually be controlled by diet therapy. Juvenile-onset diabetes (insulin-dependent diabetes mellitus [IDDM] or type I DM) requires insulin and dietary restrictions. In both cases the diet is individualized according to the client's age, build, weight, and activity level. Fats are moderately controlled, and complex carbohydrates make up a higher percentage of the diet than simple carbohydrates. Foods for dietary planning are classified in six exchange groups. Each item has about the same nutrient value as other foods in the same group. Meals are planned around balanced numbers of food exchanges, and foods may be exchanged within groups.

RENAL DISEASES. The dietary treatment of acute glomerulonephritis depends on individual tolerances but may begin with a limited liquid diet for a few days, gradually returning to a normal diet limited in protein. The diet for chronic glomerulonephritis is generally high in carbohydrates and fat and low in sodium, with protein amounts equal to normal plus the amount lost in urine.

The treatment of renal failure may begin with a diet of selected fruit juices or beverages containing carbohydrates and fats. A diet of protein, amino acids, and carbohydrates that is low in whole protein and sodium follows. Protein is decreased as renal function declines.

Dietary treatment for renal stones depends on the type of stones. For calcium phosphate stones the diet is low in calcium and high in acid ash. For uric acid stones the diet is low in purines. For calcium oxalate stones the diet avoids all foods high in calcium and oxalates.

PSYCHOSOCIAL EFFECTS OF SPECIAL DIETS. Foods have symbolic meanings for clients and are closely related to lifestyle, habits, cultural background, and other aspects of the individual. This causes many clients to have difficulty adjusting to special diets. Many clients had previously considered mealtime a pleasurable period distinct from routines or an interlude from work activities. The special diet, especially a bland diet, makes eating a dull affair. In addition, eating with others may have been a primary form of social interaction for the client, but now the client eats alone in a hospital room or at home and cannot eat the same foods as other family members. In such situations the nurse and other health care professionals should recognize the actual or potential psychosocial factors and make plans to counteract negative effects.

DISABILITIES. Clients with disabilities that interfere with independent food intake should be allowed to do as much as possible for themselves. The nurse should prepare the tray, cutting food into bitesized pieces, buttering bread, and pouring liquids. Special eating utensils should be used if they will contribute to client's independence. Some disabled clients may become tired from their efforts to feed themselves. Clients who stop eating may still be hungry and may need assistance to finish their meals. The results of self-feeding should be evaluated on the basis of food intake and not neatness. Success should be recognized and commended. Small, frequent meals may be best to achieve adequate nutrition. The nurse who finds a way to aid disabled clients in eating more independently should share this information by incorporating it into the care plan.

Client and Family Counseling

Clients discharged from a hospital with diet prescriptions often need dietary counseling to plan meals that meet specific diet requirements or general nutrition needs. Similarly, in other health care settings, clients with nutrition deficits or specific problems such as obesity may require assistance in menu planning and compliance with recommended diet therapies. The nurse's counseling role often includes families and information about community resources.

Meal planning must take into account the family's budget and differences in the preferences of family members. Specific foods are chosen on the basis of the dietary prescriptions or standard dietary guidelines such as the basic food groups. Meals should also provide a variety of foods and contrasting colors and consistencies. For families on limited budgets, substitutes can be used. For example, beans or cheese dishes can often replace meat in a meal, and evaporated or dry skim milk can be used for cooking. The method of preparation may also be modified when it is necessary to minimize certain substances. For example, baking rather than frying reduces fat intake, and lemon juice or spices can be used to replace salt in a low-sodium diet.

Planning menus a week in advance has several benefits. It helps ensure good nutrition or compliance with a specific diet and helps family members avoid impulse eating of less nutritional foods. Fruit and other nutritional items can be included in the plan for between-meal snacks. Careful advance planning can also help the family stay within the allotted budget because planned food buying is generally more economical. Last-minute shopping often includes more expensive processed and packaged foods. Often a simple tip can be of value in meal planning, such as advice to avoid grocery shopping when hungry, which can lead to spontaneous purchases of more expensive or less nutritional foods not included in meal plans.

Finally, the nurse can assist the client with referrals to community resources for assistance with dietary problems. Assistance in obtaining food is provided by several government programs such as food commodities; food stamps; the Women, Infant, Children (WIC) nutrition program; and school lunch programs. Private organizations such as Meals on Wheels provide assistance. Volunteer health agencies, such as the American Heart Association and the American Diabetes Association, provide nutrition consultation, diet information, and educational materials. Other community groups also offer planned menus and other nutritional guidelines. The American Dietetic Association, through its nutrition center, offers a wide range of materials. Detailed counseling can also be obtained from a registered or licensed dietitian.

Oral Feedings

ASSISTING CLIENTS WITH FEEDING. Being fed deprives clients of the independence they gained over their food intake as toddlers. At best, being fed is an unpleasant experience. Nurses can improve client feeding by carefully protecting clients' dignity and actively involving them in the process. Any material used to protect clothing should be referred to as a napkin, not a bib. The nurse should allow clients time to empty their mouths after every spoonful, attempting to match the speed of feeding to their readiness and asking frequently whether it is too fast or slow. The nurse should also allow clients to direct the order in which they wish to eat food items, and conversation about topics other than food should be an integral part of the process. The nurse who has several clients to feed should use ingenuity to prevent an assembly line approach, which is devastating to clients' self-esteem.

Enteral Nutrition

Enteral nutrition (EN) refers to nutrients given via the intestinal tract. This includes blended foods, modular formulas, and chemically defined elemental nutrients. The oral route is the preferred method of meeting nutritional needs if the client's gastrointestinal tract is functioning by providing safe, economical, nutritional support. For clients with eating difficulties, enteral nutrition may be supplied via nasogastric, jejunal, or gastrostomy tube (Robuck, Fleetwood, 1992). Problems with enteral feedings may be related to the following factors (Farley, 1988):

1. Negative attitudes by the client concerning tube feedings
2. Osmolality problems
3. Electrolyte imbalances
4. Gastrointestinal complications

Studies have demonstrated a beneficial effect in maintaining gastrointestinal function of enteral feedings over parenteral routes by better supporting the gastrointestinal barrier. Postoperative feeding by the enteral route can help reduce sepsis and enhance the immune response, and enteral nutrition is also preferable to TPN in protecting intestinal mucosal cells (Andressy, 1988; Randall, 1988).

Paige (1988) has successfully used EN through the **jejunostomy** (feeding tube placed directly into the jejunum) immediately after surgery to provide fluids, electrolytes, and nutritional support. Gastric ileus diminishes in this situation.

Nutrient content in EN formulas varies in specific components, and the delivery is readily adjusted to meet the client's needs. EN products enriched with the amino acid glutamine benefit intestinal mucosal cells and their function (Alverdy, 1989).

TUBE FEEDINGS. When the client is unable to ingest, chew, or swallow food but is still able to digest and absorb nutrients, a feeding tube is ordered. Feeding tubes can be inserted nasally into the stomach or small intestine or surgically into the stomach (**gastrostomy**).

Nursing research has investigated the problems associated with feeding tube placement, type of feeding instilled, rate of feeding, and complications associated with the tube feeding itself. Chapter 11 offers a brief synopsis of these problems as they are reported in the nursing research literature.

Until recently, large-bore rubber or plastic feeding tubes were used for nasogastric tube feedings. However the problems associated with these tubes—local irritation, pharyngitis, otitis, sinusitis, and esophageal sphincter incompetence—led to the development of the more pliable and flexible small-bore feeding tubes (Fig. 35-9) (Metheny, Spies, Eisenberg, 1988).

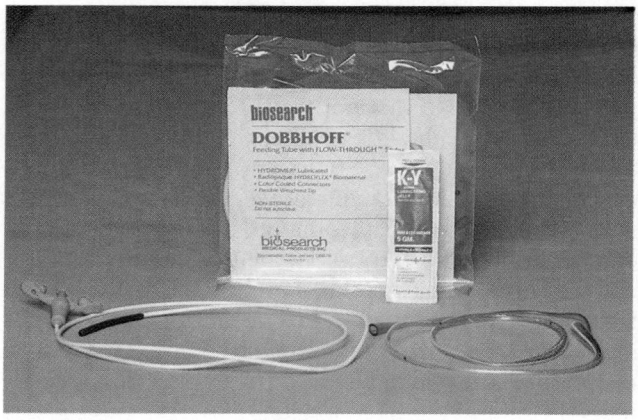

Fig. 35-9 Small-bore feeding tubes.

For the adult, most of these tubes are 8 to 12 Fr and 36 to 43 inches in length. They are manufactured with attached weights to assist introduction into the gastrointestinal tract and maintenance of the desired location (Grant, Kennedy-Caldwell, 1988).

Chapter 47 discusses the placement, management, irrigation, and removal of the large-bore nasogastric tube, which is frequently placed during abdominal surgery for gastric decompression and irrigation (see Procedure 47-3). This section and the procedure described focus solely on the small-bore nasogastric, gastric, and jejunostomy enteral feedings. Procedures 35-1 and 35-2 detail the complete procedure for inserting a small-bore nasogastric tube and initiating enteral feedings.

Verification of the placement of small-bore feeding tubes is difficult because of the size of the tubing. Historically, large-bore feeding tube placement has been verified by withdrawing gastric contents from the tube, injecting air through the nasogastric tube while auscultating the stomach for a gurgling or bubbling sound, or asking the client to speak (Metheny, Snively, 1983; Metheny, Spies, Eisenberg, 1988). These methods do not apply as readily to small-bore nasogastric tubes. A clinical study reported that over 50% of the attempts to aspirate even small volumes of fluid through small-bore feeding tubes were unsuccessful (Metheny, Spies, Eisenberg, 1988).

Because of the difficulty in withdrawing fluid from small-bore feeding tubes, nurses incorrectly rely on the auscultatory method to confirm nasogastric feeding tube placement. This method consists of insufflating 10 to 30 ml of air through the tube while auscultating the epigastrium or left upper quadrant for a gurgling or bubbling sound. Yet, many sources in the

STEPS	RATIONALE
1. Assess client for enteral tube feeding and intubation: impaired swallowing, head or neck surgery, decreased level of consciousness, abdominal surgeries, facial trauma.	Identifying clients who need tube feedings before they become nutritionally depleted facilitates preparation of care plan and promotes client education.
2. Assess client for appropriate route of administration:	
a. Close each nostril alternatively and ask client to breathe.	Evaluates nares for patency. Nares may be obstructed. Assessment determines which naris to use.
b. Assess for gag reflex.	Identifies ability to swallow and reduces risk of aspiration.
c. Review client's medical history: nose bleeds, nasal surgery, deviated septum.	Nurse may need to seek physician's order to change route of nutritional support.
3. Review physician's order for type of tube and enteral feeding schedule.	Procedure and enteral feedings require physician's order.
4. Wash hands.	Reduces transfer of microorganisms.
5. Assemble equipment at bedside:	Organizes procedure and limits client discomfort.
a. Small-bore nasogastric tube (8-12 Fr)	
b. Large syringe: 30-ml Luer-Lok or tip	Larger syringe (greater than 30 ml) may rupture small-bore tube.
c. pH test strips	Used to measure gastric acidity.
d. Hypoallergenic tape and tincture of benzoin	Tincture of benzoin increases adhesion of tape to nose.
e. Glass of water and straw	Client drinks to activate swallowing reflex. Water also activates lubricant for small-bore tube (see Step 11d).
f. Emesis basin	Nasogastric intubation may activate gag reflex and cause vomiting.
g. Tongue blade	Essential for testing gag reflex.
h. Penlight or flashlight	Used to visualize posterior pharynx for tube placement.
i. Towel	
j. Clean gloves	
k. Facial tissues	
l. Guidewire or stylet	Used to place soft, flexible feeding tube (e.g., Dobbhoff and Keofeed).
m. Safety pin and rubber band	
6. Explain procedure to client.	Ensures cooperation.
7. Stand on right side of bed if right handed (or on left side if left handed) and assist client to high Fowler's position with pillows behind head and shoulders. Place comatose clients in semi-Fowler's position	Allows easier manipulation of tube. Promotes ability to swallow.
8. Place bath towel over chest. Keep facial tissues within client's reach.	Prevents soiling of gown. Insertion through nasal passages may cause tearing.
9. Instruct client to relax and breathe normally.	Tube passes more easily when client is relaxed and breathing normally.
10. Determine length of tube to be inserted and mark with tape:	Determines approximate depth of insertion.
a. Traditional method: measure distance from tip of nose to earlobe to xiphoid process to sternum (see illustration on p. 1130).	Length provides distance from nose to stomach in 98% of clients. For duodenal or jejunal tubes, additional 20-30 cm is required (Grant, Kennedy-Caldwell, 1988).

Inserting a Small-Bore Nasogastric Tube for Enteral Feedings

STEPS	RATIONALE
b. Hanson method: first mark 50 cm point on tube, and then do traditional measurement. Tube insertion should be to midway point between 50 cm (20 in) and traditional mark.	
11. Prepare for intubation:	
a. Do not ice plastic tubes.	Tubes will become stiff and inflexible, causing trauma to mucous membranes.
b. Inject 10 ml of water from 30-ml Luer-Lok tip syringe into tube.	Aids in guidewire or stylet insertion.
c. Insert guideware or stylet into tube, making certain that it is securely positioned against weighted tip and that both Luer-Lok connections are snugly fitted together.	Promotes smooth passage of tube into gastrointestinal tract. Improperly positioned stylet can induce serious trauma.
d. Dip weighted tip of tube into glass of water.	Activates lubricant to facilitate passage of tube.
e. Cut 10-cm (4-in) piece of tape. Split one end lengthwise 5 cm (2 in).	Ensures timely anchoring of tube after its placement is verified.
12. Apply clean gloves.	Protects nurse from transmission of infection.
13. Insert tube through nostril to back of throat (posterior nasopharynx). Client may gag. Direct tube back and down toward ear.	Natural contours facilitate passage of tube.
14. Flex head toward chest after tube has passed through nasopharynx. Allow client to relax.	Closes off glottis and reduces risk of tube entering trachea. Allows client to "catch breath" (Grant, Kennedy-Caldwell, 1988).
15. Encourage client to swallow by giving small sips of water or ice chips when possible. Advance tube as client swallows. Rotate tube 180 degrees while inserting while emphasizing need to mouth breathe and swallow.	Facilitates passage of tube past oropharynx. Decreases friction. Mouth breathing and swallowing facilitate passage of tube and alleviates fears.
16. Advance tube each time client swallows until desired length has been passed.	Reduces discomfort and trauma.
a. Do not force tube. When resistance is met or client starts to gag, cough, choke, or become cyanotic, stop advancing tube and pull tube back. Check for position of tube in back of throat with tongue blade.	Tube may be coiled or kinked or in oropharynx or trachea.

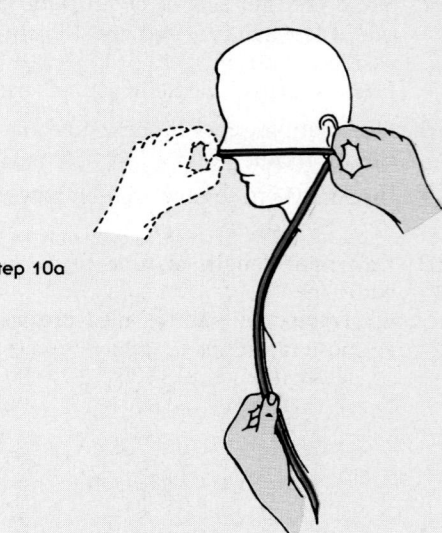

Step 10a

STEPS	RATIONALE
17. Check placement of tube:	Ensures proper position before initiating feedings.
a. Aspirate gastric contents with Luer-Lok syringe. (Insufflation of air into tube followed by auscultation of sound is no longer considered reliable in determining tube placement.)	Aspiration of contents provides measurement of pH of secretions and verification that tube is in gastrointestinal tract. (Sounds transmitted by insufflation may be transmitted from pleural space into upper abdomen, thus giving false impression of tube placement [Metheny, Spies, Eisenberg, 1988; Metheny et al, 1989].)
b. Measure pH of aspirate with color-coded pH paper with range of whole numbers from 1-11.	Gastric aspirates have decidedly acidic pH values; preferable value is 4 or less (Metheny et al, 1989).
c. Obtain x-ray film of tube placement (optional).	Determines correct tube placement. Physician's order is required.
18. Apply tincture of benzoin on tip of nose and tube. Allow to dry.	Helps tape adhere better.
19. Secure tube with tape and avoid pressure on naris.	Prevents trauma to nasal mucosa and permits mobility.
a. Take 10-cm (4-in) piece of tape that was split. Place intact end of tape over bridge of nose. Carefully wrap two ends around tube (see Step 32b, Procedure 47-3).	Secures tape to nose in manner that reduces pressure on nares.
b. Fasten end of tube to gown by looping rubber band around tube in slip knot. Pin rubber band to gown.	Reduces friction on nares in case client moves head. Pinning rubber band provides slack if client moves.
20. Position client on right side when possible until radiological confirmation of correct placement is verified.	Allows tube to pass into small intestine (duodenum or jejunum).
21. Leave stylet in place until correct position is ensured by x-ray study. Never attempt to reinsert partially or fully removed stylet while feeding tube is in place.	Guidewire or stylet may perforate gastrointestinal tract, especially esophagus or nearby tissue, and injure client.
22. Remain and talk with client.	Decreases anxiety.
23. Administer oral hygiene frequently (see Chapter 34). Cleanse tubing at nostril.	Promotes comfort and integrity of oral mucous membranes.
24. Remove gloves, dispose of equipment, and wash hands.	Reduces transmission of microorganisms.
25. Record type of tube placed, aspirate returned, and client tolerance.	Documents exact procedure.

literature report that "pseudoconfirmatory gurgling" can occur when the tube is elsewhere such as in the esophagus or lung (Miller, Tomlinson, Sahn, 1985; Muthuswamy, Patel, Rajendran, 1982). Metheny, Spies, and Eisenberg (1988) report that nurses were unable to discern gastric tube location by the auscultatory method. For example, nurses reported hearing air when the tube was in the esophagus, duodenum, jejunum, and stomach.

It is easier to aspirate fluid from some types of large-bore tubes. A laboratory study examining various large-bore feeding tube properties (for example, material and tube diameter) found that the polyurethane tubes were better than those made of silicone and that 10 and 12 Fr tubes were superior to 8 Fr tubes in terms of volume of fluid aspirated (Metheny, Eisenberg, McSweeney, 1988). However, physical properties of feeding tubes also need to be studied in a clinical setting because a number of variables were not addressed in this study.

It is generally accepted that the ability to speak is hindered by the inadvertent respiratory placement of a firm, large-bore feeding tube. However, a number of clients reported being able to speak when small-bore tubes entered the respiratory tract (Rombeau, Barot, 1981; McDanal, Wheeler, Ebert, 1983). Thus this method is not reliable to test for inadvertent respiratory placement of small-bore pliable tubes.

Initiating Enteral Tube Feedings

STEPS	RATIONALE
1. Assess client for enteral tube feedings: impaired swallowing, head or neck surgery, decreased level of consciousness.	Identify clients who need tube feedings before they become nutritionally depleted.
2. Verify physician's order.	Tube feedings must be ordered by physician. Order should include formula, route, amount, and frequency.
3. Place client in high-Fowler's position.	Reduces risk of pulmonary aspiration in case client vomits or regurgitates feeding.
4. Wash hands. Apply gloves.	Prevents transmission of blood-borne infection from gastric contents.
5. Assemble following equipment: a. Disposable gavage bag and tubing b. Asepto syringe (60-ml size)	Ensures prompt, efficient completion of feeding. Formula can be administered via syringe for bolus feedings. Syringe can also be used to verify placement of large-bore feeding tubes.
c. Prescribed formula and amount d. Infusion pump designed for feeding tubes. e. Disposable gloves	Pump is necessary to regulate continuous tube feedings. Prevents transmission of microorganisms.
6. Determine placement of feeding tube (see Procedure 35-1, Step 17): a. Aspirate gastric secretions and check gastric residual.	Verifies placement of tube in stomach. These measures have been proved effective and safe for large-bore tubes. Indicates whether gastric emptying is delayed, which means that 150 ml or more remain in stomach. Small-bore tubes may collapse on aspiration (Petrosino, Christian, Becker, 1989). Inability to satisfactorily measure gastric contents via aspiration interferes with ability to measure gastric retention.
b. Observe for abdominal distention.	Assessment for abdominal distention assists in recognizing delayed gastric emptying and reduces risk of regurgitation and pulmonary aspiration related to gastric distention (Petrosino, Christian, Becker, 1989).
7. Auscultate for bowel sounds.	Indicates presence of peristalsis and ability of gastrointestinal tract to digest nutrients.
8. Administer tube feeding. a. *Bolus or intermittent feeding:* (1) Pinch proximal end of feeding tube. (2) Attach syringe to end of tube and elevate 18 in above client's head. (3) Fill syringe with formula. Allow syringe to empty gradually, refilling until prescribed amount has been delivered to client. (4) For gavage feeding, fill bag and tubing with prescribed amount of formula. Attach tubing to end of feeding tube and raise bag 18 in above client's head. Regulate flow gradually. b. *Continuous-drip method:* (1) Hang gavage bag to IV pole.	 Prevents air from entering client's stomach. Gradual emptying reduces risk of diarrhea induced by bolus tube feedings. Method is designed to deliver prescribed rate of feeding that reduces risk of diarrhea. Clients who receive these feedings should have gastric residuals checked every 6-8 hr. Also decreases risk of feeding tube developing clogs that would occlude tube entirely (Petrosino, Christian, Becker, 1989).

STEPS	RATIONALE
(2) Connect end of bag tubing to proximal end of feeding tube.	
(3) Connect infusion pump and set rate.	
9. Administer additional water as ordered.	Ensures adequate hydration, which is supplement to tube-feeding formula (Haynes-Johnson, 1986).
10. Remove and dispose of gloves in proper receptacle. Wash hands.	Prevents transmission of microorganisms.
11. When tube feedings are not being administered, clamp proximal end of feeding tube.	Prevents air from entering the stomach between feedings.
12. Administer water via feeding tube as ordered with or between feedings.	Provides client with source of water to help maintain fluid and electrolyte balance.
13. Record amount and type of feeding in nurses' notes.	Documents administration of feeding.

CONTINUED

Little has been written on how the nurse should check for placement of small-bore nasointestinal feeding tubes. Nurses in practice frequently report using the auscultatory method, even though its reliability is in serious question.

Another study by Metheny, Spies, and Eisenberg (1986) examines nasoenteral feeding tube displacement. In this study, 92% of the subjects were fed with the small-bore feeding tubes, and a sizable number of these tubes were found by radiological examination to be spontaneously displaced. That is, the distal tips of the tubes dislocated upwardly in the gastrointestinal tract, whereas the proximal external portion of the feeding tube remained taped in place. Displacement was associated with risk factors such as coughing, vomiting, suctioning, and decreased level of consciousness.

Currently used bedside methods to test placement of small-bore feeding tubes are frequently ineffective. At present, the most reliable method is radiographical verification. This method is cost prohibitive. Therefore new methods to test placement must be explored. In the meantime, the nurse must have a high index of suspicion for tube displacement in clients at risk and use meticulous assessment skills.

In addition to the nasoenteral route, a gastrostomy or jejunostomy feeding tube is placed for EN. A **gastrostomy feeding tube** is a long, hollow, flexible tube inserted into the stomach through a surgical stoma inserted in the upper left abdominal quadrant.

Jejunal feedings, via jejunal feeding tube, are another method of EN. A **jejunal feeding tube** is a large-bore tube surgically inserted into the jejunum for the administration of liquified nutrition. Procedure 35-3 on p. 1134 details the procedure for gastrostomy and jejunostomy enteral feedings.

The solutions used for tube feedings must be nutritionally adequate, tolerated by the client, and appropriate to the area of the gastrointestinal tract to which they are delivered. A wide variety of commercial products is available for tube feedings. They are easy to prepare and offer standard nutritional content. The commercial preparations differ in osmolarity, digestibility, caloric density (ranging from 1 to 2 kcal/ml), lactose content, viscosity, and lipid content.

Clients may be maintained indefinitely on tube feedings, which can provide all the essential nutrients except fiber. Although cramping and diarrhea are commonly associated with tube feedings, these symptoms usually subside when the flow rate or concentration of the solution is reduced or a formula containing fiber is used.

TPN

Parenteral nutrition is a complex form of therapy designed to provide daily nutritional requirements by the intravenous route. The success of this form of nutrition depends on the dietary prescription, management of the intravenous catheter, dressing care, and complications resulting from the therapy itself (Grant, Kennedy-Caldwell, 1988).

Clients unable to ingest or digest enteral nutrition are candidates for TPN. TPN is contraindicated when clients' gastrointestinal tracts are functional

Administering Enteral Feedings via Gastrostomy or Jejunal Tube

STEPS	RATIONALE
1. Assess client's need for enteral tube feedings: impaired swallowing, decreased level of consciousness, head or neck surgery, facial trauma, surgery of upper alimentary canal.	Identifies clients who need tube feedings before they become nutritionally depleted.
a. Auscultate for bowel sounds before feeding.	Indicates presence of peristalsis and ability of gastrointestinal tract to digest nutrients.
b. Observe for abdominal distention.	Assessment for abdominal distention assists in recognizing delayed gastric emptying and reduces risk of regurgitation and pulmonary aspiration related to gastric distention (Petrosino, Christian, Becker, 1989).
c. While wearing gloves, assess gastrostomy or jejunostomy site for breakdown, irritation, drainage.	Infection, pressure from gastrostomy tube, or drainage of gastric secretions can cause skin breakdown.
2. Verify physician's order for formula, rate, route, and frequency.	Tube feedings must be ordered by physician.
3. Wash hands and apply clean gloves.	Reduces transmission of microorganisms.
4. Assemble equipment:	
a. Disposable gavage bag and tubing	Serves as container in which to place formula.
b. 60-ml catheter tip syringe	Formula can be administered via syringe for bolus feedings. Syringe is also used to check tube placement.
c. Stethoscope	Used to auscultate air entering stomach.
d. Formula	
e. Infusion pump (Use pump designed for tube feedings.)	Helps regulate flow of continuous feeding.
5. Prepare bag and tubing to administer formula:	
a. Connect tubing and bag.	Tubing must be free of contamination to prevent bacterial growth.
b. Fill bag and tubing with formula.	Prevents excess air from entering gastrointestinal tract.
6. Explain procedure to client.	Ensures cooperation and relaxation.
7. Place client in high-Fowler's position or elevate head of bed 30 degrees.	Helps prevent chance of aspiration.
8. Verify placement of tube:	
a. *Gastrostomy tube:*	
(1) Aspirate gastric secretions and check gastric residual.	Presence of gastric contents indicates that end of tube is in stomach. Gastric residual determines whether gastric emptying is delayed. Delayed emptying means that 150 ml or more remains in stomach from previous feeding.
(2) Auscultate over left upper quadrant with stethoscope and inject 10-20 ml of air into tube.	Air (i.e., whooshing or gurgling sound) can be heard entering stomach.
b. *Jejunostomy tube:*	
(1) Aspirate intestinal secretions and check for residual.	Presence of intestinal fluid indicates that end of tube is in jejunum. Large residual indicates slow small intestinal emptying.
9. Initiate feeding:	
a. *Gastrostomy tube:*	
(1) Bolus or intermittent feeding:	
■ Pinch proximal end of gastrostomy tube.	Prevents air from entering stomach.
■ Attach syringe to end of tube and elevate to 18 in above client's abdomen.	

STEPS	RATIONALE
■ Fill syringe with formula. Allow syringe to empty gradually, refilling until prescribed amount has been delivered to client.	Gradual emptying of tube feeding by gravity from syringe or gavage bag reduces risk of diarrhea induced by bolus tube feedings.
■ If gavage bag is used, attach bag to end of feeding tube and raise bag 18 in above client's abdomen. Fill bag with prescribed amount of formula, and allow bag to empty gradually over 30 min.	
(2) Continuous drip method:	Method is designed to deliver prescribed hourly rate of feeding and reduce risk of diarrhea. Clients who receive continuous drip feedings should have residuals checked every 4 hr.
■ Hang gavage bag to IV pole.	
■ Connect end of bag to proximal end of gastrostomy tube.	
■ Connect infusion pump and set rate.	
(3) When tube feedings are not being administered, clamp proximal end of gastrostomy tube.	Prevents air from entering stomach between feedings.
(4) Administer water via feeding tube as ordered with or between feedings.	Provides client with source of water to help maintain fluid and electrolyte balance.
(5) Rinse bag and tubing with warm water after all bolus feedings.	Clears old tube feedings and prevents bacteria growth.
(6) Advance tube feeding.	Tube feedings should be advanced gradually to prevent diarrhea and gastric intolerance of formula.
b. *Jejunal tube:*	
(1) Initiate continuous tube feeding (see Step 9a[2]).	Jejunal feedings are given continuously to ensure proper absorption.
(2) Advance tube feeding.	To provide maximum nutrition, formula needs to be increased to meet client's nutritional requirements.
10. Change exit site dressing as needed. Inspect exit site every shift. Skin around feeding tube should be cleansed daily with warm water and mild soap; small gauze dressing may be applied to exit site.	Leakage of intestinal drainage may cause irritation and excoriation.
11. Dispose of supplies and wash hands.	Reduces transmission of microorganisms.
12. Evaluate client's tolerance of tube feeding, and observe stoma site for skin integrity.	Tolerance of tube feeding is evaluated by checking amount of aspirate (residual) every 4 hr. Gastric and intestinal secretions can cause injury and necrosis at stoma site.
13. Record amount and type of feeding.	Documents amount and type of feeding administered to client.
14. Record client's response to tube feeding, patency of tube, and any untoward effects.	Documents client's reaction to therapy and identifies presence of adverse reactions (e.g., aspiration).
15. Report to oncoming nursing staff: type of feeding, status of gastrostomy or jejunostomy tube, client's tolerance, and adverse effects.	Provides new nursing personnel with status of gastric feeding. Allows new nursing staff to plan for next feeding.

within 7 to 10 days, when clients are well nourished, and when minimal stress and trauma are present. It is also of limited value for clients in untreatable disease states such as widely advanced metastatic malignancy. Last, it should not be used when the risks outweigh the benefits (Grant, Kennedy-Caldwell, 1988).

TPN solutions are hyperosmolar (that is, highly concentrated), and as a result, they are infused through central lines. The solution itself is tailored to the client's specific nutritional needs, with some common elements for all clients. A typical solution consists of approximately 25% dextrose and 3% to 4% protein, supplying close to 1000 kcal/L (Grant,

Kennedy-Caldwell, 1988). Electrolyte needs vary with the client's general status. TPN for pediatric clients may be administered by the peripheral route with a less concentrated dextrose solution (typically a 10% solution).

FAT EMULSIONS. Clients may also require nutritional supplements through fat emulsions. **Fat emulsions** provide supplemental calories to prevent essential fatty acid deficiencies (Atkins, Oakley, 1986). These nutrients can be administered through a separate peripheral line, through the central line by Y-connector tubing (see Chapter 39), or as additives to the TPN solution. The last option is based on research findings that fats (also called *lipids*) can be added to TPN solutions without causing incompatibility problems or compromising the solution's stability (Atkins, Oakley, 1986). Fat emulsions should be administered sterilely into a patent intravenous line. The emulsion should not be used if it appears oily or appears to have separated.

The recommended initial infusion rate for fat emulsions is 1 ml/min. Reactions to this emulsion can include dyspnea, cyanosis, allergy, nausea, vomiting, headache, chest pain, back pain, pressure over the eyes, and dizziness. The appearance of any of these symptoms warrants stopping the infusion and immediately notifying the physician. If the client tolerates the fat emulsion, the rate can gradually be increased as ordered by the physician.

INITIATING TPN. TPN requires a large-gauge intracatheter threaded into a central vein such as the jugular or subclavian or large peripheral vein. Nurses do not insert central catheters but assist in the procedure. The procedure is sterile and requires the following equipment:
1. Sterile drapes
2. Sterile gloves
3. Sterile Betadine swabs
4. Alcohol
5. Topical anesthetic (lidocaine)
6. Betadine ointment
7. Sterile 4 × 4 and 2 × 2 gauze pads or transparent dressing
8. Tape
9. Parenteral solution
10. Parenteral infusion tubing
11. Intracatheter needle
12. Sutures
13. In-line filter
14. Infusion pump

The nurse explains the procedure to the client and witnesses informed consent. The client is taught to perform the Valsalva maneuver, bearing down with mouth closed and holding a breath. This increases venous filling of the vein and reduces the risk of an air embolism during needle insertion. After the client has learned the technique satisfactorily, the catheter can be inserted.

The client is placed in Trendelenburg's position to dilate the central veins in the neck and shoulder. The physician drapes the venipuncture site with sterile barriers and cleanses the site with Betadine swabs followed by alcohol wipes. Lidocaine is injected for local anesthesia. The physician punctures the client's vein and looks for a nonpulsatile blood return. A pulsating blood return indicates that an artery, not the vein, was punctured. When the physician begins to thread the intracatheter through the needle, the nurse instructs the client to do the Valsalva maneuver.

After placement of the catheter, the needle is removed, and an intravenous infusion is connected to the hub of the catheter. The physician sutures the catheter in place and covers the site with a sterile dressing. A chest x-ray film is used to identify any complications such as accidental puncture of the lung or parietal pleura.

Clients receiving TPN should have their vital signs measured and their blood glucose levels monitored every 4 hours or as ordered by the physician. The nurse should be alert for changes and report any to the physician.

Medications or blood should not be given through the TPN line because this increases the risk of bacterial contamination. In a life-or-death situation the TPN line may be the only intravenous line available and may be used for emergency treatment.

Beginning an Infusion. Before beginning an infusion, the nurse compares the physician's order with the solution prepared by the pharmacy. The nurse connects the TPN infusion tubing to a filter and places the insertion spike in the solution. The tubing is filled with the solution and hung at the bedside. The nurse attaches the tubing to the infusion pump.

Infusion Flow Rate. Clients initially receive low doses of TPN solution, such as 1 L/24 hours, typically gradually increasing to 3 L/24 hours. The rate is included in the physician's orders.

Too-rapid administration of this hypertonic infusion can result in osmotic diuresis, dehydration, and death (see Chapter 39). Infusion pumps help regulate the flow. If an infusion falls behind schedule, the nurse should not attempt to catch up because a hyperosmotic reaction could result (Metheny, Snively, 1983).

MAINTAINING THE TPN SYSTEM. The infusion flow should be assessed every hour. All clients receiving TPN should be connected to infusion pumps. The nurse should also evaluate the catheter and infusion line for patency.

Preventing Infection. To prevent infection, the infusion tubing should be changed every 24 hours. It is best to change the tubing with the first new TPN solution administered each day. The procedure is the same as the procedure for changing intravenous infusion tubing (see Procedure 39-3), except that an in-line filter is added to trap bacteria. A 0.22 μm filter blocks all bacteria, including *Pseudomonas* species. In addition, the nurse observes the venipuncture site for infection (see Chapter 39).

The temperature of a client receiving TPN should be monitored every 4 hours. An increased temperature may be an early sign of line infection and should be reported. In addition, medications, blood, and blood products should not be administered through the TPN line because it increases the risk of bacterial contamination.

Preventing Complications. A chest x-ray film is used to document correct placement of the catheter in the superior vena cava, proximal to the right atrium (Munro-Black, 1984). The film can also show a pneumothorax, which may occur if the needle punctures the pleura during insertion. Pneumothorax assessment findings include chest pain, dyspnea, and coughing; the rapidity of onset and the degree of symptoms depend on the severity.

A second complication is the development of an air embolus during insertion of the catheter or changing of the tubing. This can be prevented by having the client do the Valsalva maneuver and placing the client in Trendelenburg's position.

Hyperglycemia is caused by a high concentration of dextrose in the TPN solution. Risk factors for hyperglycemia include increased secretion of adrenal hormones, increased age, and renal disease (Metheny, Snively, 1983). Hyperglycemia, which can cause dehydration, nausea, headache, and weakness, can also occur when the rate of infusion is too rapid. The risk of hyperglycemia can be reduced by giving the solution at the prescribed rate. If the solution falls behind schedule, the nurse should not increase the rate of flow unless ordered by the physician. Checking the client's urine for glucose and acetone every 4 to 6 hours can identify signs of glucose intolerance. Clients receiving TPN may be given insulin injections to increase the body's ability to metabolize the increased glucose. After the TPN has been discontinued, the insulin injections are discontinued.

Hypoglycemia can occur if TPN is abruptly discontinued. The high glucose concentration of the TPN solution stimulates the pancreas to secrete more insulin. The client may also be receiving supplemental insulin injections. If the TPN infusion is too slow or is abruptly discontinued, there is too little blood glucose and too much insulin, and hypoglycemia occurs. Symptoms include occipital headaches, cold clammy skin, dizziness, tachycardia, and tingling of the extremities and circumoral regions (Metheny, 1992). Hypoglycemia can be prevented by maintaining an accurate infusion rate and gradually reducing the TPN solution. The gradual reduction allows the pancreas time to adapt to the decreased glucose load. If the TPN solution must be discontinued abruptly, a 5% or 10% glucose in water solution usually provides enough glucose to prevent rebound hypoglycemia until the client's pancreatic insulin rate decreases in about 12 to 24 hours (Grant, 1980; Grant, Kennedy-Caldwell, 1988).

Fluid overload causes an increase in extracellular fluid volume. If severe, fluid overload can result in pulmonary edema and congestive heart failure. Signs and symptoms include shortness of breath, tachycardia, weak pulse, hypertension or hypotension, confusion, decreased urine output, crackles, and pitting edema. Fluid overload can be prevented by maintaining an accurate rate of infusion and monitoring central venous pressure. If signs of fluid overload occur, the nurse slows the infusion rate, notifies the physician, and remains with the client, continually assessing the client's status.

The major metabolic complications of TPN can be prevented by continually implementing seven nursing interventions (Table 35-14 on p. 1138). These interventions are designed for early identification and treatment of these complications.

 ## Evaluation

Nutritional evaluation must be ongoing to evaluate the results of nursing interventions. Care plans must be constantly updated to avoid continuing ineffective actions and to strengthen support of effective interventions. Adequate time should be allowed to test a nursing approach to a problem. A behavior change is as valid an indicator of success as changes in weight or laboratory results.

Nurses should establish outcomes for nursing actions and be alert for signs that goals are being met (see evaluation box on p. 1138). Whenever possible, the client should be an active participant in the planning and evaluation of care.

TABLE 35-14 Interventions for Preventing Metabolic Complications of TPN

Assessments/Interventions	Rationale
Weigh client daily.	Documents that client is maintaining or gaining weight and has proper fluid balance
Record intake and output.	Provides data base for ongoing fluid-balance assessment
If client is allowed oral intake, maintain calorie count of foods eaten.	Provides data needed to calculate TPN caloric requirement
Obtain urine to measure glucose and acetone levels every 4-6 hr.	Determines whether client is excreting glucose in urine and whether insulin supplement is needed
Obtain blood samples for measurement of iron, transferrin, and white blood cells.	Evaluates cellular nutritional status
Continually assess fluid and electrolyte status.	Prevents circulatory overload, dehydration, and electrolyte imbalance
Maintain infusion rate as ordered. Do not speed or slow infusion unless instructed by physician or severe complication occurs.	Prevents hyperglycemia, osmotic diuresis, hypoglycemia, and fluid overload

 Sample Evaluation of Interventions for Altered Nutritional Status

Goals	Evaluative Measures	Expected Outcomes
Client will return to within 10% of ideal body weight.	Weigh client.	Weight will show appropriate gain of 0.5-1.0 lb/wk (0.25-0.5 kg/wk).
	Observe client for signs of nutritional deficits.	Physical and laboratory indicators of nutritional deficits will be absent.
Client's fluid and electrolyte status will remain within normal limits.	Observe client for signs of dehydration or overhydration.	Signs of dehydration or overhydration will be absent.
	Palpate skin for loss of turgor.	Skin turgor will remain normal.
	Palpate skin for signs of edema.	Edema will be absent.
	Weigh client daily.	There will be no excessive weight loss or gain.
	Monitor electrolyte levels and observe for electrolyte imbalance.	Electrolyte levels will remain within normal limits.
Complications will be prevented.	Observe for signs of infection.*	Erythema, pain, and swelling will be absent at venipuncture site.
	Obtain blood glucose levels.*	Blood glucose levels will remain within normal range.

*Evaluative measures associated with TPN.

SUMMARY

Nurses must understand the functions of the basic nutrients and metabolism. An understanding of the guidelines for the selection of an adequate diet is essential so that nurses can teach clients about nutrients and answer questions related to diet. Nurses should also be alert to current research findings and their impact on dietary recommendations. They should be familiar with alternative food patterns and know how age and health status influence dietary needs.

Nurses must be able to assess the nutritional status of a client. They must also recognize that many divergent factors influence food intake and consider these factors when attempting to modify food intake.

Nurses must be able to identify clients at risk for nutritional problems and be aware of common nutritional conditions. They should be aware of the importance of their interactions with others in the area of food intake, be familiar with common hospital diets, and be able to assist clients at mealtime. Finally, nurses must evaluate their activities in the area of nutritional support to revise those that prove ineffective and continue those that are beneficial.

Key Concepts

- Nutrients needed by the body to carry out vital functions are water, carbohydrates, proteins, lipids, vitamins, and minerals.

- Body weight is maintained when food intake equals energy output.

- Carbohydrates are anabolized into glycogen and adipose tissue or catabolized into energy.

- Proteins are anabolized into tissue, hormones, or enzymes or catabolized into energy.

- Lipids may be anabolized into adipose tissue or catabolized into energy.

- Proteins are essential for growth, maintenance, and repair.

- The essential amino acids and the essential fatty acids must be supplied by dietary intake because the body is unable to synthesize them from other ingested substances.

- Through digestion, food is broken down into its simplest form for absorption. Digestion and absorption occur mainly in the small intestine.

- Recommended daily allowances, another basis for diet selection, were formulated for population groups, not individuals.

- Guidelines for dietary change advocate reduced intake of fat, saturated fat, salt, refined sugar, and cholesterol and increased intake of complex carbohydrates and fiber.

- Age affects the requirements for essential nutrients. Periods of rapid growth increase the need for protein, vitamins, and minerals.

- Because improper nutrition can affect all body systems, nutritional assessment includes a review of the total physical assessment.

- Nurses can improve food intake of clients by thoughtful attention to the preparation of the client and environment before meals are served.

- Disabled clients should be supported in their efforts to eat as independently as possible.

- Proper feeding techniques can protect the dependent client from loss of dignity and self-esteem.

- Special hospital diets alter the composition, texture, digestibility, and residue of foods to suit the client's particular needs.

- Tube feedings can be used for clients who are unable to ingest food but are able to digest and absorb foods.

- Enteral nutrition can help protect the intestinal mucosa and function and furnish nutrients in appropriate form and amount.

- Total parenteral nutrition supplies essential nutrients in appropriate amounts to support life through the introduction of a concentrated nutrient solution into a large central vein or the right atrium of the heart.

- Evaluation of the outcomes of nursing intervention in the area of nutritional support is essential to revise, update, or continue nursing activities.

Key Terms

Critical Thinking Exercises

1. Discuss the role of water- and fat-soluble vitamins with regard to function, needs, and client teaching regarding food source and amounts needed.

2. Mrs. Smith, age 45, is concerned about weight gain. How would you outline the minimum servings she needs to maintain a "healthy diet" and yet not gain weight?

3. Mrs. Lee is your 30-year-old client with a high intake of fat and sodium. She is concerned about her intake and asks you for information about the new dietary guidelines. How would you counsel Mrs. Lee?

4. The diet order for Jim, age 6 months, is "diet for age." What type of foods and how much would be a normal intake for a 6-month-old child of average weight and height?

5. The laboratory data on Joe, age 6, shows a hemoglobin level of 9 and serum albumin level of 3.4 g/100 ml. What assessment would you make regarding his nutritional status?

6. Mr. Miller has been placed on TPN after extensive gastrointestinal surgery. Identify appropriate nursing interventions for preventing metabolic complications.

REFERENCES

Alverdy JC: The GI tract as an immunologic organ, *Contemp Surg* 35:5a, 1989.

American Academy of Pediatrics, Committee on Nutrition, Forbes GB, Woodruff CW, editors: *Pediatric nutrition handbook,* ed 2, Elk Grove, Ill, 1985, The Academy.

American Heart Association: *Dietary treatment for hypercholesterolemia: handbook for counselors,* vol 70-2001, Dallas, 1988, The Association.

Andressy RM: Preserving the gut mucosal barrier and enhancing immune response, *Contemp Surg* 21:2A, 1988.

Atkins JM, Oakley CW: A nurse's guide to TPN, *RN* 6:20, 1986.

Department of Health and Human Services. *Healthy people 2000: national health promotion and disease prevention objectives,* DHHS Pub No (PHS) 91-50212, Washington, DC, 1990, US Government Printing Office.

Farley JM: Current trends in enteral feeding, *Crit Care Nurse* 8:(4):23, 1988.

Forlaw B, Grant P: *Introduction to nutritional and physical assessment of the adult client for the nurse,* Aspen, Colo, 1983, American Society for Parental and Enteral Nutrition (ASPEN).

Food and Nutrition Board: *Recommended dietary allowances,* ed 10, Washington DC, 1989, Nations Academy of Sciences.

Grant J: *Handbook of total parenteral nutrition,* Philadelphia, 1980, Saunders.

Grant JA, Kennedy-Caldwell C: *Nutritional support in nursing,* New York, 1988, Grune & Stratton.

Haynes-Johnson V: Tube feeding complications: causes, prevention, and therapy, *Nutr Support Serv* 6(3):17, 1986.

Jacobs C, Dwyer JT: Vegetarian children: appropriate and inappropriate diets, *Am J Clin Nutr* 48:811, 1988.

Kim MJ, McFarland GK, McLane AM: *Pocket guide to nursing diagnoses,* ed 4, St Louis, 1991, Mosby–Year Book.

McDanal J, Wheeler D, Ebert J: A complication of nasogastric intubation: pulmonary hemorrhage, *Anesthesiology* 59:356, 1983.

Metheny, NM: *Fluid and electroelyte balance: nursing considerations,* ed 2, Philadelphia, 1992, Lippincott.

Metheny NM, Snively WD Jr: *Nurse's handbook of fluid balance,* ed 4, Philadelphia, 1983, Lippincott.

Metheny NM, Eisenberg P, McSweeney M: Effect of feeding tube properties and three irrigants on clogging rates, *Nurs Res* 37(1):165, 1988.

Metheny NM, Spies M, Eisenberg P: Frequency of nasoenteral tube displacement and associated risk factors, *Res Nurs Health* 9(3):241, 1986.

Metheny NM, Spies M, Eisenberg P: Measures to test placement of nasogastric and nasointestinal feeding tubes: a review, *Nurs Res* 37:324, 1988.

Metheny N et al: Effectiveness of pH measurements in predicting feeding tube placement, *Nurs Res* 38:280, 1989.

Miller K, Tomlinson J, Sahn S: Pleuropulmonary complications of enteral tube feeding, *Chest* 88:203, 1985.

Munro-Black J: The ABC's of total parenteral nutrition, *Nurs 84* 14:50, 1984.

Muthuswamy P, Patel K, Rajendran R: Isocal pneumonia with respiratory failure, *Chest* 81:390, 1982.

National Institutes of Health: *National Cholesterol Education Program: report of the Expert Panel on Blood Cholesterol Levels in Children and Adolescents,* DHHS Pub No 91-2732, Washington, DC, 1991, US Government Printing Office.

Paige CP: Enteral feeding: NCJ for early and continued feeding, *Contemp Surg* 32:2a, 1988.

Petrosino BM, Christian BJ, Becker H: Implications of selected problems with nasoenteral tube feedings, *Crit Care Nurs Q* 12(3):1, 1989.

Public Law 101-535. *Nutrition Labeling And Education Act of 1990.* 103 STAT. 2353.21 USC 301, Nov 8, 1990.

Randall HT: Meeting protein and energy requirements in the postoperative period, *Contemp Surg* 2a:4, 1988.

Rifkind BM: Cholesterol lowering and reduced risk of coronary heart disease, *Pract Cardiol* 14:(suppl)3, 1988.

Robuck J, Fleetwood J: Nutrition support in the client with cancer, *Focus Crit Care Nurs* 19(2):129, 1992.

Rombeau J, Barot L: Enteral nutritional therapy, *Surg Clin North Am* 61:605, 1981.

Shronts EV: *Nutrition support dietetics core curriculum: 1989,* Silver Springs, Md, 1989, American Society for Parenteral and Enteral Nutrition.

US Department of Agriculture: *USDA's food guide pyramid,* USDA Human Nutrition Information Service Pub No 249, Washington, DC, 1992, US Government Printing Office.

US Department of Agriculture and US Department of Health and Human Services: *Nutrition and your health: dietary guidelines for Americans,* USDA/DHHS Home and Garden Bull No 232, Washington, DC, 1990, US Government Printing Office.

Wardlaw GM, Insel PM, Seyler MF: *Contemporary nutrition: issues and insights,* St Louis, 1992, Mosby–Year Book.

Whitney EN, Catallo CB, Rolfes SR: *Understanding normal and clinical nutrition,* ed 3, St Paul, Minn, 1991, West.

ADDITIONAL READINGS

Baker DJ: 10 years of TPN at home, *Am J Nurs* 84:1248, 1984.

Behrman RE, Vaughn VC, editors: *Nelson's textbook of pediatrics,* Philadelphia, 1987, Saunders.

Birdsall C: When is TPN safe? *Am J Nurs* 85:73, 1985.

Buergel N: Monitoring nutritional status in the clinical setting, *Nurs Clin North Am* 14:2, 1979.

Carr P: When the client needs TPN at home, *RN* 6:25, 1986.

Claggett M: Anorexia nervosa: a behavioral approach, *Am J Nurs* 80:8, 1980.

Food and Drug Administration, Department of Health and Human Services: *Federal Register* 55:5176, 1990.

Johnson S: A safer gastrostomy for the high-risk client, *RN* 3:29, 1986.

Keithley J: Proper nutritional assessment can prevent hospital malnutrition, *Nurs 79* 9:2, 1979.

Legislative Highlights: Update: the Nutrition Labeling and Education Act of 1990, *J Am Diet Assn* 91:1054, 1991.

Lucas A: Bulimia and vomiting syndrome, *Contemp Nutr* 6:4, 1981.

Moore MC: Do you still believe these myths about tube feeding? *RN* 5:51, 1987.

National Academy of Sciences: *Report on nutrition labeling: issues and directions for the 1990s,* Washington, DC, 1990, National Academy Press.

National Institutes of Health: *National Cholesterol Education Program: report of the Expert Panel on Population Strategies for Blood Cholesterol Reduction,* DHHS Pub No 90-3046. Washington, DC, 1990, US Government Printing Office.

National Research Council: *Estimated safe and adequate daily dietary intakes,* ed 10, Washington, DC, 1989, National Academy Press.

National Research Council Committee on Diet and Health of Food and Nutrition: *National Academy of Sciences Report: diet and health: implications for reducing chronic disease,* Washington, DC, 1989, National Academy Press.

Rose J: Nutritional problems in radiotherapy clients, *Am J Nurs* 78:6, 1978.

Rose J, editor: *Nutrition and killer diseases,* Park Ridge, NJ, 1982, Noyes.

Rudman D, Williams P: Megavitamins: use and misuse, *N Engl J Med* 309:8, 1983.

Surgeon General's report on nutrition and health: summary and recommendations, DHHS (PHS) Pub No 88-50211, Washington, DC, 1988, US Government Printing Office.

Thomas PR, editor: *Improving America's diet and health: from recommendations to action,* Washington, DC, 1991, National Academy Press.

Williams SR: Nutritional guidance in prenatal care. In Worthington-Roberts BS, Williams SR, Vermeersch JA: *Nutrition in pregnancy and lactation,* ed 4, St Louis, 1989, Mosby–Year Book.

CHAPTER 36

Sleep

OBJECTIVES

Mastery of content in this chapter will enable the student to:

- Define the key terms listed.
- Compare the characteristics of sleep and rest.
- Explain the effect the 24-hour sleep-wake cycle has on biological function.
- Discuss mechanisms that regulate sleep.
- Describe the stages of a normal sleep cycle.
- Explain the functions of sleep.
- Compare and contrast the sleep requirements of different age groups.
- Identify factors that normally promote and disrupt sleep.
- Discuss characteristics of common sleep disorders.
- Conduct a sleep history for a client.
- Identify nursing diagnoses appropriate for clients with sleep alterations.
- Identify nursing interventions designed to promote normal sleep cycles for clients of all ages.
- Describe ways to evaluate sleep therapies.

CHAPTER OUTLINE

Sleep and Rest
Promoting rest

Physiology of Sleep
Circadian rhythms
Sleep regulation
Stages of sleep

Functions of Sleep
Dreams
Normal sleep requirements and patterns

Factors Affecting Sleep
Physical illness
Drugs and substances
Lifestyle
Sleep patterns
Emotional stress

Environment
Exercise and fatigue
Caloric intake

Sleep Disorders
Insomnia
Sleep apnea
Narcolepsy
Sleep deprivation
Other sleep disorders

Nursing Process and Sleep
Assessment
Nursing diagnosis
Planning
Implementation
Evaluation

The need for sleep and rest is important in quality of life for all persons. All individuals need and receive different amounts and qualities of sleep and rest. Physical and emotional health depend on the ability to fulfill these basic human needs. Without rest and sleep, the ability to concentrate, make judgments, and participate in daily activities decrease, and irritability increases.

The theory that sleep is associated with healing suggests that achieving optimum sleep quality is important for the recovery of all health care clients. Nurses care for clients who often have preexisting sleep disturbances and for clients who develop sleep problems as a result of illness or hospitalization. Sleep problems may cause clients to seek health care, or problems may go unnoticed for years. Ill clients often require more sleep and rest than healthy clients. However, the nature of illness may prevent clients from gaining adequate rest and sleep. The environment of a hospital or long-term care facility and the activities of health care personnel may also make sleep difficult.

Identifying and treating sleep disturbances is an important goal for a nurse. To help a client gain needed rest and sleep, a nurse must understand the nature of sleep, the factors influencing it, and the client's sleep habits. Each client requires an individualized approach. Interventions can be effective in resolving short- and long-term sleep disturbances.

 SLEEP AND REST

People at rest feel mentally relaxed, free from anxiety, and physically calm. Rest does not imply inactivity, although everyone often thinks of it as settling down in comfortable chairs or lying in bed. People at rest are in a state of decreased mental and physical activity that leaves them feeling refreshed, rejuvenated, and ready to resume the activities of the day. All persons have their own habits for obtaining rest and can usually adjust to new environments or conditions that affect the ability to rest. Rest may be gained from reading a book, practicing a relaxation exercise (see Chapter 37), or taking a long walk.

Nurses frequently care for clients on bed rest. This treatment confines clients to bed to reduce physical and psychological demands on the body. Such people are not necessarily rested. They still may have emotional worries that prevent complete relaxation. Depending on others for care may cause such clients to feel stressed.

Sleep is a recurrent, altered state of consciousness that occurs for sustained periods, restoring energy and well-being. Sleep provides time for the repair and recovery of body systems for the next period of wakefulness. A sleeping person interacts less with the environment.

The rest and sleep habits of persons entering a hospital or other health care facility can easily be changed by illness or hospital routines. The extent of change depends on their physiological and psychological states and environment. The nurse must always be aware of clients' needs for rest. The lack of rest for long periods can cause illness or worsening of existing illness. The nurse can help clients learn the importance of rest and ways to promote it at home or in the health care environment.

Promoting Rest

Many factors affect the ability to gain adequate rest. In the home the nurse helps clients develop behaviors conducive to rest and relaxation. This may include controlling factors in the environment or changing certain lifestyle habits. For example, the home health care nurse frequently cares for clients with chronic debilitating disease. A simple care plan might include having clients set aside afternoons for rest. The nurse helps adjust medication schedules

---

Conditions for Proper Rest

PHYSICAL COMFORT
- Eliminate sources of physical irritation.
- Control sources of pain.
- Provide warmth.
- Maintain hygiene.
- Maintain proper anatomical alignment or positioning.
- Remove environmental distractions.
- Provide adequate ventilation.

FREEDOM FROM WORRY
- Make own decisions.
- Participate in personal health care.
- Have knowledge needed to understand health problems and implications.
- Practice restful activities regularly.
- Know that the environment is safe.

SUFFICIENT SLEEP
- Obtain average hours of sleep needed to avoid fatigue.
- Follow good sleep hygiene habits.

and instructs clients to regularly void before rest periods and ask friends not to call during a set time so that rest periods are uninterrupted. In a health care setting the nurse promotes rest by controlling clients' physical symptoms and altering stressful factors in the environment. This can be difficult on a busy nursing unit. Loud or unfamiliar noises, irritating lighting, loss of privacy, and frequency of therapeutic procedures can interfere with rest. For example, clients who are hospitalized for extensive diagnostic testing often have difficulty resting because of uncertainty about their future. A nurse can promote rest by allowing clients to determine the timing and methods of delivery of all basic care measures. Providing information about the purpose and routines of all procedures also helps. Giving clients' control over their health care minimizes uncertainty and anxiety. The box lists conditions needed to ensure proper rest.

PHYSIOLOGY OF SLEEP

Sleep is a set of complete physiological processes. It involves a sequence of states maintained by highly integrated central nervous system (CNS) activity associated with changes in the peripheral nervous, endocrine, cardiovascular, respiratory, and muscular systems (Hoch, Reynolds, 1986; Closs, 1988). Each sequence can be identified by specific behaviors, physiological responses, and patterns of brain activity. Instruments such as the electroencephalogram (EEG), which measures electrical activity in the cerebral cortex, the electromyogram (EMG), which measures muscle tone, and the electrooculogram (EOG), which measures eye movements, provide information about the physiological aspects of sleep.

Circadian Rhythms

Each person's life is a series of cyclical rhythms that influence and regulate physiological function and behavioral responses. The most familiar rhythm is the 24-hour, day-night cycle known as the *diurnal* or *circadian rhythm* (derived from Latin: *circa,* "about," and *dies,* "day"). Another rhythm is the woman's menstrual cycle, an **infradian rhythm** (longer than 24 hours). Biological cycles lasting less than 24 hours are called *ultradian rhythms.* Circadian rhythms influence the pattern of major biological and behavioral functions. The fluctuation and predictability of body temperature, heart rate, blood pressure, hormone and electrolyte secretions, sensory acuity, and mood depend on the 24-hour circadian cycle.

Circadian rhythms, including daily sleep-wake cycles are most affected by light and temperature. However, these **biological clocks** are also influenced by external factors such as social activities and work routines. All persons have biological clocks that synchronize their sleep cycles. Some people can fall asleep at 8 PM, whereas others go to bed at midnight or early in the morning. Different people also function best at different times of the day. Horne and Ostberg (1976) described two groups of people, morning and evening types. The morning person prefers to go to bed and get up early, performing best in the morning. The evening person prefers to go to bed and get up later, functioning best in the evenings.

Hospitals or extended-care facilities fail to adapt care to an individual's preference for sleep. If a person's sleep-wake cycle is altered significantly, a poor quality of sleep results. Reversals in the sleep-wake cycle such as sleeping during the day instead of the night (or vice versa for people who work nights) can indicate a serious illness. Anxiety, restlessness, irritability, and impaired judgment are common symptoms of reversal of the sleep cycle.

The biological rhythm of sleep frequently becomes synchronized with other body functions. Changes in body temperature, for example, correlate with sleep patterns. Normally, body temperature peaks in the afternoon, decreases gradually, and then drops sharply after a person falls asleep (see Chapter 19). When the sleep-wake cycle becomes disrupted (for example, by rotating job shifts), other physiological functions change, as well. The integrity of the sleep-wake cycle can influence the client's overall health.

Sleep Regulation

The control and regulation of sleep may depend on the interrelationship between two cerebral mechanisms that work against one another. Both intermittently activate and suppress the brain's higher centers to control sleep and wakefulness. One mechanism causes wakefulness, whereas the other causes sleep.

The **reticular activating system (RAS)** is located in the upper brainstem. It is believed to contain special cells that maintain alertness and wakefulness. The RAS receives visual sensory input and auditory, pain, and tactile stimuli. Activity from the cerebral cortex (for example, emotions or thought processes) also stimulates the RAS. Studies reported by Canavan (1984) and Chuman (1983) suggest that wakefulness results from neurons in the RAS releasing catecholamines such as norepinephrine.

Sleep may be produced by the release of serotonin from specialized cells in the raphe sleep system of

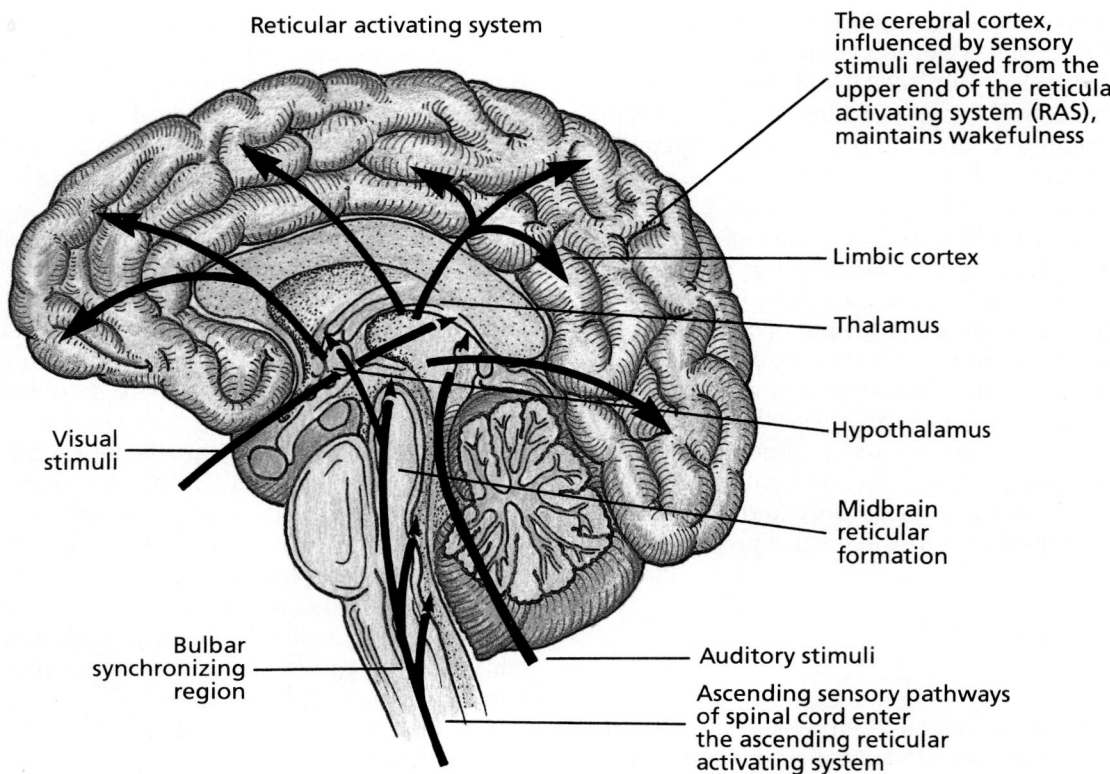

Fig. 36-1   RAS and BSR control sensory input, intermittently activating and suppressing the brain's higher centers to control sleep and wakefulness.

the pons and medial forebrain. This area of the brain is also called the *bulbar synchronizing region (BSR)*. Whether a person remains awake or falls asleep depends on a balance of impulses received from higher centers (for example, thoughts), peripheral sensory receptors (for example, sound or light stimuli), and the limbic system (emotions) (Fig. 36-1).

As people try to fall asleep, they close their eyes and assume relaxed positions. Stimuli to the RAS decline. If the room is dark and quiet, activation of the RAS further declines. At some point the BSR takes over, causing sleep.

Stages of Sleep

Studies with the EEG, EMG, and EOG show different levels of brain activity indicating different stages of sleep. Sleep involves two phases: nonrapid eye movement (**NREM sleep**) and rapid eye movement (**REM sleep**) (see box). During NREM a sleeper progresses through four stages during a typical sleep cycle. The quality of sleep from stage 1 through stage 4 becomes increasingly deep. Light sleep is characteristic of stages 1 and 2, and a person

is easily arousable. Stages 3 and 4 involve a deeper sleep called *slow-wave sleep*. REM sleep is the phase at the end of each sleep cycle. A person is usually difficult to arouse, and psychological restoration may occur at this time. The sleeping stages are highly individualized for each person. Many different factors promote or interfere with various stages of the sleep cycle. The nurse chooses therapies that foster sleep or attempts to eliminate factors that can disrupt it.

Sleep Cycle

Normally, in an adult the routine sleep pattern begins with a presleep period during which the person is aware only of a gradually developing drowsiness. This period normally lasts 10 to 30 minutes, but if a person has difficulty falling asleep, it may last an hour or more.

Once asleep, the person usually passes through four to six complete sleep cycles, each consisting of four stages of NREM sleep and a period of REM sleep. The cyclical pattern usually progresses from stage 1 through stage 4 of NREM, followed by a reversal from stage 4 to 3 to 2, ending with a period of

Stages of Sleep

STAGE 1: NREM

- Stage includes lightest level of sleep.
- Stage lasts few minutes.
- Decreased physiological activity begins with gradual fall in vital signs and metabolism.
- Person is easily aroused by sensory stimuli such as noise.
- Awakened, person feels as though daydreaming has occurred.

STAGE 2: NREM

- Stage 2 is period of sound sleep.
- Relaxation progresses.
- Arousal is still easy.
- Stage lasts 10 to 20 minutes.
- Body functions continue to slow.

STAGE 3: NREM

- Stage 3 involves initial stages of deep sleep.
- Sleeper is difficult to arouse and rarely moves.
- Muscles are completely relaxed.
- Vital signs decline but remain regular.
- Stage lasts 15 to 30 minutes.

STAGE 4: NREM

- Stage 4 is deepest stage of sleep.
- It is very difficult to arouse sleeper.
- If sleep loss has occurred, sleeper will spend considerable portion of night in this stage.
- Stage is responsible for restoring and resting body.
- Vital signs are significantly lower than during waking hours.
- Stage lasts approximately 15 to 30 minutes.
- Sleepwalking and enuresis may occur.

REM SLEEP

- REM stage is period of vivid, full-color dreaming. (Less vivid dreaming may occur in other stages.)
- Stage usually begins every 50 to 90 minutes after sleep has begun.
- It is typified by autonomic response of rapidly moving eyes, fluctuating heart and respiratory rates, and increased or fluctuating blood pressure.
- Loss of skeletal muscle tone occurs.
- Gastric secretions increase.
- This stage is responsible for mental restoration.
- It is very difficult to arouse sleeper.
- Duration of REM sleep increases with each cycle and averages 20 minutes.

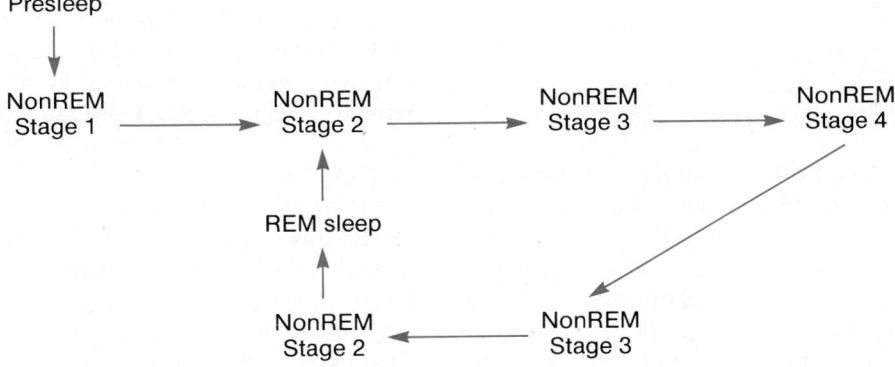

Fig. 36-2   Adult sleep cycle.

REM sleep (Fig. 36-2). A person usually reaches REM sleep within 90 minutes.

With each successive cycle, stages 3 and 4 shorten, and the period of REM lengthens. REM sleep may last 30 to 60 minutes during the last sleep cycle. If a person awakens from sleep during any stage, sleep begins again at stage 1.

Not all people progress consistently through the stages of sleep. For example, a sleeper may fluctuate for short intervals between NREM stages 2, 3, and 4 before entering REM stage. The amount of time spent in each stage varies (Fig. 36-3 on p. 1150). Shifts from stage to stage tend to accompany body movements, and shifts to light sleep tend to occur suddenly, whereas shifts to deep sleep tend to be gradual (Closs, 1988). The number of sleep cycles depends on the total amount of time that the client spent sleeping.

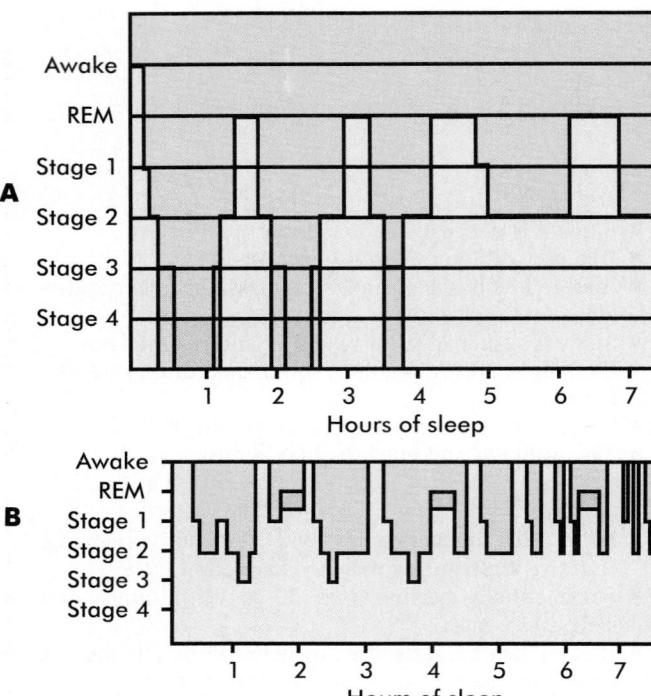

Fig. 36-3 Comparison of normal sleep patterns in a healthy young adult and older adult. **A,** The young adult has little awake time and moves through the sleep stages progressively. **B,** The older adult has frequent awakenings and more time spent in the lighter stages of sleep.
Redrawn from Emra KL, Herrera CO: *RN* 52:79, 1989; and Kavey NB, Anderson D: *RN* 49:16, 1986.

FUNCTIONS OF SLEEP

The purpose of sleep remains unclear, although it is believed to contribute to physiological and psychological restoration (Oswald, 1984). Traditionally, sleep is viewed as a time of restoration and preparation for the next period of wakefulness. During NREM sleep, biological functions slow. A healthy adult's normal heart rate throughout the day averages 70 to 80 beats per minute or less if the individual is in excellent physical condition. However, during sleep the heart rate falls to 60 beats per minute or less. This means that the heart beats 10 to 20 fewer times in each minute during sleep or 60 to 120 fewer times in each hour. Clearly, then, restful sleep is beneficial in preserving cardiac function.

Sleep is needed to routinely restore biological processes. During deep slow-wave (NREM stage 4) sleep the body releases human growth hormone for the repair and renewal of epithelial and specialized cells such as brain cells (Chuman 1983; Horne, 1983). However, Horne (1983) also argues that the usual role of growth hormone as a promoter of protein synthesis is limited because its release is unrelated to blood glucose levels and amino acids. Other studies have shown that protein synthesis and cell division for renewal of tissues such as the skin, bone marrow, gastric mucosa, or brain occur during rest and sleep (Oswald, 1984) NREM sleep may be especially important in children, who experience more stage 4 sleep.

The body conserves energy during sleep. The skeletal muscles relax progressively, and the absence of muscular contraction preserves chemical energy for cellular processes. Lowering of the basal metabolic rate further conserves the body's energy supply.

REM sleep appears to be important for psychological restoration. REM sleep is associated with changes in cerebral blood flow, increased cortical activity, increased oxygen consumption, and epinephrine release. This association may assist with memory storage, learning, and emotional adaptation (Chase, Weitzman, 1983; Greenberg et al, 1983). The brain filters stored information of the day's activities. The person who is asleep may be able to solve problems and gain new insights. Dreaming allows a person to clarify emotions and prepare the mind for the next day.

The benefits of sleep on behavior often go unnoticed until a person develops a problem resulting from sleep deprivation. A loss of REM sleep leads to feelings of confusion and suspicion. No clear cause-and-effect relationship exists between sleep deprivation and a specific body dysfunction (Webster, Thompson, 1986). However, various body functions (for example, reflexes, memory, and equilibrium) can be altered when prolonged sleep deprivation occurs.

Dreams

Dreams occur during NREM and REM sleep. The dreams of REM sleep are more vivid and elaborate. REM dreams progress in content throughout the night from dreams about current events to emotional dreams of childhood or the past. Personality can influence the quality of dreams; for example, a creative person usually has creative dreams, and a depressed person usually dreams of helplessness.

Most people dream about immediate concerns such as an argument with a spouse, plans for a wedding, or worries over work. Sometimes a person is unaware of fears represented in bizarre dreams. Psychologists attempt to analyze the symbolic nature of dreams. For example, an apple may represent a forbidden object, the sense of rushing to an unknown destination may represent an unresolved conflict, or a lion may symbolize rage. The ability to describe a dream and interpret its significance may help resolve personal concerns or fears.

The dreams of REM sleep are believed to be functionally important. Freud believed that dreams were a product of unconscious desires and released psychological tensions. Thus the nature and occurrence of dreams became a basis for psychotherapy.

Another theory suggests that dreams erase certain fantasies or nonsensical memories. Most dreams are forgotten. In fact, during REM sleep, consolidation of short-term memory is impaired. To remember a dream, a person must consciously think about it on awakening. People who recall dreams vividly usually awake just after a period of REM sleep. Some theorists therefore believe that people dream to forget. They discourage clients from attempting to remember dreams so that undesirable thought patterns are effectively forgotten. Other theorists believe that dreams consolidate memories for emotional and mental equilibrium.

Normal Sleep Requirements and Patterns

Sleep duration and quality vary widely among persons of all age groups. One person may gain adequate rest with 4 hours of sleep, whereas another requires 10 hours. Fig. 36-4 shows the change in the distribution of sleep stages during life.

Neonates

A neonate averages 16 hours of sleep a day, with a range of 10 to 23 hours. The infant born of an unmedicated mother enters the world in a state of wakefulness. Eyes are wide open and sucking is vigorous. After about an hour the newborn becomes quiet and less responsive to internal and external stimuli. A period of sleep lasting a few minutes up to 2 to 4 hours follows (Whaley, Wong, 1991). The infant then awakens again and often becomes overly responsive to stimuli. Hunger, pain, cold, or other stimuli frequently cause crying. For the first week the neonate sleeps almost constantly to recover from birth. Approximately 50% of this sleep is REM sleep, which stimulates the higher brain centers. This is essential for development because the neonate is not awake long enough for significant external stimulation. Table 36-1 on p. 1152 describes five distinct states of the newborn's sleep. The cycle of states varies based on the number of hours that the newborn sleeps.

Infants

Sleep patterns vary among infants. Active infants typically sleep less than quiet infants (Whaley,

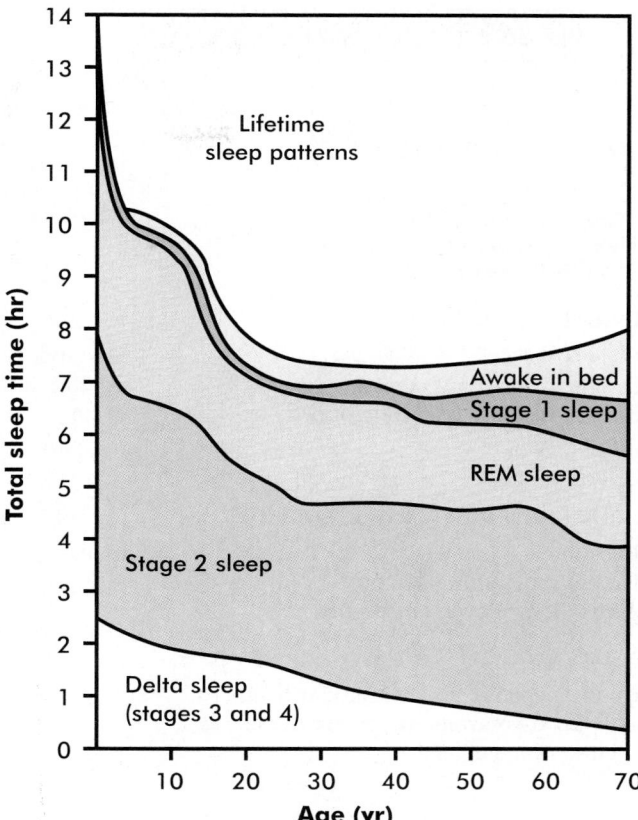

Fig. 36-4   Distribution of sleep stages over the life span. From Berman TM, Nino-Murcia G, Roehrs T: *Patient Care* 24:85, 1990.

Wong, 1991). Infants usually develop a nighttime pattern of sleep by 3 to 4 months of age. The infant may take several naps during the day but usually sleeps an average of 8 to 10 hours during the night. Awakening commonly occurs early in the morning, although it is not unusual for an infant to awaken during the night. If awakening during the night continues, the problem may be with diet because hunger frequently awakens the child. A breast-fed infant usually sleeps for shorter periods, with frequent waking, than a bottle-fed infant (Whaley, Wong, 1991). A large infant sleeps longer than a smaller one because of greater stomach capacity. An infant between 1 month and 1 year of age sleeps an average of 14 hours a day. REM sleep predominates.

Toddlers

By the age of 2, children usually sleep through the night and take daily naps. Total sleep averages 12 hours a day. Naps may be eliminated at 3 years. It is common for toddlers to awaken during the night. The percentage of REM sleep begins to fall because

TABLE 36-1 States of Sleep and Activity		
State and Behavior*	Duration	Implications for Parenting
REGULAR SLEEP		
Eyes are closed. Regular breathing occurs. There is no movement except for sudden bodily jerks.	4-5 hr/day, 10-20 min/sleep cycle	External stimuli do not arouse infants. Continue usual house noises. Parents should leave infant alone if sudden loud noise awakens infant and child cries.
IRREGULAR SLEEP		
Eyes are closed. Irregular breathing occurs. Slight muscular twitching of body occurs.	12-15 hr/day, 20-45 min/sleep cycle	External stimuli that did not arouse infant during regular sleep may minimally arouse the child. Periodic groaning or crying is usual; it should not be interpreted as an indication of pain or discomfort.
DROWSINESS		
Eyes may be open. Irregular breathing occurs. Active body movement occurs.	Variable	Most stimuli arouse infant. Parents should pick infant up rather than leave in crib.
ALERT INACTIVITY		
Infant responds to environment by active body movement and staring at close-range objects.	2-3 hr/day	Parents should satisfy infant's needs such as hunger. Parents should place infant in area of home where activity is continuous. Parents should place toys in crib or playpen. Parents should place objects within 17.5-20 cm (7-8 in) of infant's view.
WAKING AND CRYING		
Infant may begin with whimpering and slight body movement. Infant progresses to strong, angry crying and uncoordinated thrashing of extremities.	1-4 hr/day	Parents should remove intense internal or external stimuli. Stimuli that were effective during alert inactivity are usually ineffective. Parents should rock and swaddle infant to decrease crying.

*Some classifications divide the fifth state into two states: alert with activity and crying.

toddlers have access to a variety of meaningful external stimuli. As the brain matures there is less need for internal stimulation, so toddlers are often unwilling to go to bed at night. This may also be due to an expression of need for autonomy or fear of separation. Children prefer to stay awake and spend time with parents and siblings to satisfy the need to explore and be curious.

Preschoolers

An average preschooler sleeps about 12 hours a night and rarely takes naps (Whaley, Wong, 1991). The preschooler usually has difficulty relaxing or quieting down after long, active days. A preschooler also has problems with bedtime fears, waking during the night, or nightmares. Parents are most successful in getting a preschooler to bed by establishing a consistent bedtime ritual. A child should not be allowed to become manipulative by sleeping with parents or by staying up past a reasonable hour. When nightmares occur, parents should comfort the child in the child's own bed.

School-Age Children

The amount of sleep needed during the school years is highly individualized because of varying states of activity and levels of health. The school-age child usually does not require a nap. A 6-year-old averages 11 to 12 hours of sleep nightly, whereas an 11-year-old sleeps about 9 to 10 hours (Whaley, Wong, 1991). The 6- or 7-year-old can usually be persuaded to go to bed by encouraging quiet activities. The older child often resists sleeping because of an unawareness of fatigue or a need to be independent. A school-ager will be tired the following day if allowed to stay up later than usual. An older child may seek a later bedtime as a symbol of dominance over a younger child. Parents are usually successful in getting the older child to bed by using a firm, consistent approach. The older school-ager may be allowed to go to bed later, but such a privilege depends on going to bed promptly without complaints.

Adolescents

An adolescent's day is usually active and mentally and physically exhausting. Often the desire to spend time with peers prevents adolescents from realizing their need for sleep. Once bedtime approaches, however, the adolescent offers little resistance to sleep. An adolescent averages 8 to 9 hours of sleep a night. Because of staying up late, an adolescent frequently sleeps late in the mornings.

Young Adults

Healthy young adults require rest and sleep to participate in the busy activities that fill their days. However, it is common for busy lifestyles to interrupt sleep patterns. Most young adults average 6 to 8½ hours of sleep a night, but this can vary. It is unusual for young adults to take regular naps. Approximately 20% of sleep time is spent in REM sleep, which remains consistent throughout life. The stresses of jobs, family relationships, and social activities can often lead to the use of medication for sleep. Long-term use of such medications can disrupt sleep patterns and lead to other health problems.

Middle Adults

During adulthood the total time spent sleeping at night begins to decline. Also the amount of stage 4 sleep begins to fall, continuing throughout older age. Sleep disturbances are common; insomnia is particularly common because of the changes and stresses of middle age. Sleep disturbances can be caused by anxiety, depression, or certain physical ailments. Women experiencing menopausal symptoms may have insomnia. Members of this age group may rely on sleeping medications.

Older Adults

The total amount of sleep does not change as age increases. However, quality of sleep deteriorates

(Kales, Kales, 1974). REM sleep occurs cyclically at intervals of 90 minutes in all age groups, but episodes of REM sleep shorten. There is a progressive decrease in stages 3 and 4 NREM, and an older adult has almost no stage 4 sleep (Clapin-French, 1986). An older adult awakens more often during the night, and total wake time increases. It may also take more time for an older adult to fall asleep (Ross et al, 1986).

Hayter (1983) studied the sleep habits of 212 older persons ranging in age from 65 to 93 and found great variability among the sleep behaviors of different subjects. Subjects 85 and over reported more nap time than subjects 75 to 84 and all subjects under 85. The total time asleep for naps seems to increase progressively with age. The increased time spent napping increases total sleep time. Some nap more than once a day, but some older adults nap only occasionally during a week's time. By age 75, there was a definite increase in the amount of time spent in bed, both when nap time is included and excluded. Hayter (1983) also found a pattern of a gradually increasing need for rest and sleep with advancing age. The need for increased rest occurs earlier than the need for increased sleep.

The changes in an older person's sleep pattern are due to changes in the CNS that affect the regulation of sleep. Sensory impairment, common with aging, may reduce sensitivity to time cues that maintain circadian rhythms. An older adult's chronic illnesses may also impair the quality of sleep.

 ## FACTORS AFFECTING SLEEP

Factors that promote sleep in one person may hinder sleep in another. A single factor may not be the only cause for a sleep problem. Physiological, psychological, and environmental factors can alter the quality and quantity of sleep.

Physical Illness

Any illness that causes pain, physical discomfort (such as difficulty swallowing), anxiety, or depression can result in sleep problems. Persons with such alterations may have trouble falling or staying asleep. Illnesses also force clients to sleep in positions to which they are unaccustomed. Assuming an awkward position while in traction, for example, can interfere with sleep.

Respiratory disease often interferes with sleep. Clients with chronic lung disease such as emphysema are short of breath and frequently cannot sleep without two or three pillows to raise their heads. Asthma, bronchitis, and allergic rhinitis alter the rhythm of breathing and disturb sleep. A person with a common cold has nasal congestion, sinus drainage, and a sore throat, which impair breathing and the ability to relax.

Coronary heart disease is characterized by episodes of sudden chest pain and irregular heart rates. Clients with this disease are often afraid to go to sleep because they fear heart attacks at night. Heart attacks occur more often during REM sleep (Ross et al, 1986). Death from heart disorders most frequently occurs at night, between 5 and 6 AM, when REM sleep lasts longer.

Hypertension often causes early morning awakening and fatigue. Hypothyroidism decreases stage 4 sleep, whereas hyperthyroidism causes persons to take more time to fall asleep.

Nocturia, or urination during the night, disrupts sleep and the sleep cycle. This condition is most common in older people with reduced bladder tone or persons with cardiac disease, diabetes, urethritis, or prostatic disease. After a person awakens to urinate, returning to sleep may be difficult.

Older adults often experience "restless leg syndrome," which occurs during the presleep stage. People experience recurrent, rhythmical movements of the feet and legs. An itching sensation is felt deep in the muscles. Relief comes only from moving the legs, which prevents relaxation and subsequent sleep. Restless leg syndrome is a benign condition. In contrast, people who have severe leg cramps during the night may have a problem with arterial circulation.

Persons with peptic ulcer disease often awaken in the middle of the night. Gastric acid levels reach a peak in the stomach around 1 to 3 AM (McNeil et al, 1986), causing stomach pain.

Drugs and Substances

Various types of drugs affect the pattern and quality of sleep (see box). Medications prescribed for sleep often cause more problems than benefits. Young and middle adults may rely on sleeping medications to deal with lifestyle stressors. Older adults often take a variety of drugs to control or treat chronic illness, and the combined effects of several drugs can seriously disrupt sleep. L-Tryptophan, a protein found in foods such as milk, cheese, and meats, may help a person sleep.

Lifestyle

A person's daily routine may influence sleep patterns. An individual working a rotating shift (for example, 2 weeks of days followed by a week of nights) has difficulty adjusting to the altered sleep schedule. The body's internal clock might be set at 11 PM, but the work schedule forces sleep at 9 AM instead. The individual often can sleep only 3 or 4 hours because the body's clock perceives that it is time to be awake and active. Only after several weeks of working a night shift does a person's biological clock adjust. Other alterations in routine that can disrupt sleep patterns include performing unaccustomed heavy work, engaging in late-night social activities, and changing evening mealtime.

Sleep Patterns

The pattern and adequacy of sleep experienced each day affect a person's functioning. The most significant cause of daytime sleepiness is inadequate or abnormal sleep at night (Berman et al, 1990). Everyone has an increased sleep tendency from about 2 to 7 AM and to a lesser degree from 2 to 5 PM (Mitler et al, 1988). However, when sleep patterns are disrupted, the natural tendency to be sleeping at select times increases. A person who experiences temporary sleep deprivation as a result of an active social evening or lengthened work schedule usually feels sleepy the next day. Sleep deprivation may result in difficulty performing tasks and remaining attentive. Chronic lack of sleep is much more serious than temporary sleep deprivation and can cause serious alterations in the ability to perform daily functions. For example, single-vehicle accidents related to a driver falling asleep at the wheel occur most often between midnight and 4 AM, a period of normal sleepiness (Mitler et al, 1988).

Emotional Stress

Worry over personal problems or situations can disrupt sleep. Emotional stress causes a person to be tense and often leads to frustration when sleep does not come. Stress may also cause a person to try too hard to fall asleep, to awaken frequently during the sleep cycle, or to oversleep. Continued stress causes poor sleep habits.

Older clients frequently experience losses that lead to emotional stress. Retirement, physical impairment, death of a loved one, and loss of economic security are examples of situations that predispose older adults to anxiety and depression. With emotional stress, older adults experience delays in falling asleep, earlier appearance of REM sleep, frequent awakening, increased total bed time, feelings of sleeping poorly, and early awakening (Colling, 1983).

Environment

The environment has a significant influence on the ability to fall and remain asleep. Good ventilation is essential for restful sleep. The size, firmness, and position of the bed can affect the quality of sleep. Hospital beds are often harder than those at home. Schmidt-Kessen and Kendel (1973) observed that harder surfaces cause more body movement. If a person usually sleeps with another individual, sleeping alone can cause wakefulness.

Sound also influences sleep. The level of noise needed to awaken people depends on the stage of sleep (Webster, Thompson, 1986). Low noises are more likely to arouse a person from stage 1 sleep, whereas louder noises awaken people in stage 3 or 4 sleep. Some persons require silence to fall asleep, whereas others prefer noise such as soft music.

In hospitals, noise creates a problem for clients. Noise in hospitals is usually new or strange. Thus clients are prone to awaken. This problem is greatest the first night of hospitalization, when clients often experience increased total wake time, increased awakenings, and decreased REM sleep and total sleep time (Agnew et al, 1966). The level of noise in hospitals can be very loud. Normal conversation measures about 50 decibels. Seidlitz (1981) found that a wall-suction machine measured 67 decibels and a nurse opening a package of rubber gloves registered 86 decibels. People-induced noises (that is, nursing activities) are sources of increased sound levels. Intensive care units are sources for high noise levels. Close proximity of clients, noise from confused and ill clients, the ringing of alarm systems and telephones, and disturbances caused by emergencies make the environment unpleasant (see research highlight).

 Research Highlight

Hilton measured sound levels in client rooms to determine sources of noise and noise intensity. Twenty-five clients in six units (four intensive care units and two medical-surgical units) in three hospitals were included in the study. Microphones were placed near the head of each client. Sound levels were measured continuously for 24 hours.

A variety of equipment commonly found in hospitals creates excess noise. An intravenous controller-alarm created noise at 44 to 80 decibels, a cardiac monitor alarm at 44 to 78 decibels, a flushing toilet at 44 to 76 decibels, a voice over an intercom at 60 to 70 decibels, and paper ripping at 41 to 81 decibels. Sounds become noise at 35 to 40 decibels. Furthermore, sound above 50 decibels can enhance pain perception (Minckley, 1968).

Hilton found that sound can be reduced significantly by closing a client's room door. With doors closed, sound levels fall 6 to 18 decibels, depending on the source of noise. The researcher makes several recommendations for further reducing noise.

Hilton A: The hospital racket: how noisy is your unit? *Am J Nurs* 87:56, 1987.

Light levels may affect the ability to fall asleep. Some clients may prefer a dark room, whereas others, such as children, keep a soft light on at all times. Clients also may have trouble sleeping, depending on the temperature of a room. A room that is too warm or too cold causes a client to become restless. Sleeping at temperatures higher than 24° C causes poorer quality sleep (Schmidt-Kessen, Kendel, 1973).

Exercise and Fatigue

A person who is moderately fatigued usually achieves restful sleep, especially if the fatigue is the result of enjoyable work or exercise. Exercising 2 hours before bedtime allows the body to cool down and maintains a state of fatigue that promotes relaxation. However, excess fatigue resulting from exhausting or stressful work can make falling asleep difficult. This can be a common problem for school-agers and adolescents.

Caloric Intake

Weight loss or gain influences sleep patterns. When a person gains weight, sleep periods become longer with fewer interruptions. Weight loss can cause short and fragmented sleep. Certain sleep disorders may be the result of the semistarvation diets popular in a weight-conscious society.

 ## SLEEP DISORDERS

Sleep disorders are conditions that repeatedly cause a disruption in sleep patterns. They are common among clients. Research shows that most adults in the United States have significant sleep debts from cumulative sleep losses (Berman et al, 1990). Sleep disorders may cause clients to seek health care, or the effects of illness or hospitalization may create sleep disorders. The best way to diagnose sleep disorders is through the use of a nighttime **polysomnogram.** This involves use of the EEG, EMG, and EOG to monitor stages of sleep and wakefulness. Patterns of inadequate sleep can cause numerous problems for individuals.

Insomnia

Insomnia is a symptom of clients who have chronic difficulty falling asleep (initial insomnia), difficulty remaining asleep (intermittent insomnia), or inability to go back to sleep after awakening (terminal insomnia). The insomniac complains of insuffi-

cient quantity and quality of sleep. Frequently, however, the client gets more sleep than is realized. Insomnia may signal an underlying physical or psychological disorder.

Persons may experience insomnia only temporarily, usually as a result of situational stresses such as family or work problems, jet lag, illness, or loss of a loved one. The condition can develop at any age. Insomnia may recur, but between episodes the client is able to sleep well. A temporary case of insomnia can lead to a chronic problem. Removal of a stressful situation may not cure the sleep problem. As a result a person loses confidence in the ability to fall asleep and develops anxiety about sleeping well.

Insomnia is most commonly associated with poor sleep habits. If the condition continues, the fear of not being able to sleep can be enough to cause wakefulness. During the day, a person with chronic insomnia may feel sleepy, fatigued, depressed, and anxious.

Because there are many causes of insomnia, management involves several approaches. First, it is important to treat underlying emotional or medical problems. Treatment is also symptomatic, including improved sleep hygiene measures, biofeedback, cognitive techniques, and relaxation techniques. The exact cause of insomnia is unknown. In drug-dependence insomnia the client is unable to fall asleep because of excessive use of hypnotic medications. Such a client benefits from a gradual withdrawal of hypnotics.

Sleep Apnea

The easiest description of **sleep apnea** is the cessation of breathing for a time during sleep. **Apnea** is the cessation of airflow through the nose and mouth for at least 10 seconds (Block, 1980). There are three types: central, obstructive, and mixed.

The most common form, obstructive apnea, occurs when muscles or structures of the oral cavity or throat relax during sleep. The upper airway becomes blocked, and nasal airflow stops for as long as 30 seconds (Feierman, 1985). The person still attempts to breathe because chest and abdominal movement continue. During the apneic period, each successive diaphragmatic movement becomes stronger until the obstruction is relieved. Structural abnormalities such as a deviated septum, nasal polyps, or enlarged tonsils predispose a client to obstructive apnea. However, most clients with sleep apnea have anatomically normal airways (Berman et al, 1990).

Obstructive apnea causes a serious decline in arterial oxygen level (see Chapter 38). Clients are at risk for cardiac dysrhythmias, right heart failure, pulmonary hypertension, anginal attacks, stroke, and hypertension. Middle-age men tend to be more frequently affected, particularly when they have recently gained weight. The most frequent time of naturally occurring death is between 4 and 6 AM, and some researchers believe that sleep apneas are a cause (Berman et al, 1990).

Central apnea involves defects in the brain's respiratory-control center. The impulse to breathe temporarily fails, and nasal airflow and chest wall movement cease. The oxygen saturation of the blood falls slightly. The condition is seen in clients with brainstem injury, muscular dystrophy, and encephalitis. No treatment exists for central sleep apnea.

A person with sleep apnea typically snores at night. Cessation of breathing and then relief with marked snorting occurs. Near the end of each episode a brief arousal related to increased carbon dioxide levels occurs. The client rarely awakens. The client is also deprived of deep sleep periods. Complaints of excessive daytime sleepiness, sleep attacks, fatigue, morning headaches, and decreased sex drive are common. Treatment includes therapy for underlying cardiac or respiratory complications and emotional problems created by the disorder. Sleep hygiene and a weight-loss program can also help. One of the most effective therapies is use of a nasal continuous positive airway pressure (CPAP) device at night. CPAP requires a client to wear a mask over the nose. Room air is delivered through the mask at a high pressure. The air pressure keeps the tongue from dropping and occluding the airway, preventing its collapse. The CPAP device is portable and highly effective for obstructive apnea. In cases of severe sleep apnea the tonsils, uvula, or portions of the soft palate may be surgically removed. Success is variable.

Narcolepsy

Narcolepsy is a dysfunction of REM sleep processes and of mechanisms regulating alteration between sleep and awakened states. During the day a person may suddenly feel an overwhelming wave of sleepiness and fall asleep. REM sleep can occur within 15 minutes after sleep. **Cataplexy,** or sudden muscle weakness occurring during intense emotions such as anger, sadness, or laughter, may occur in the day. The client may lose muscle control and even fall to the floor. A person with narcolepsy may also have hallucinations that are like real dreams occurring just as the person falls asleep. The person may not know the difference between a dream and reality. Sleep paralysis, or the feeling of being unable to move or talk just before waking or falling asleep, is

another symptom. Recent studies show a genetic link for narcolepsy (Kales et al, 1987).

The greatest problem with narcolepsy is that the individual falls asleep at inappropriate times. Unless a person understands the disorder, a sleep attack can easily be mistaken for laziness, lack of interest in activities, or drunkenness. A client is treated with stimulants that increase wakefulness and reduce sleep attacks and medications that suppress REM sleep. Brief daytime naps no longer than 20 minutes help reduce narcoleptic attacks. Factors that increase a narcoleptic client's drowsiness (for example, alcohol or exhausting activities) should be avoided.

Sleep Deprivation

Although not a true sleep disorder, **sleep deprivation** is a problem many clients experience as a result of hospitalization, especially in intensive care units. Sleep deprivation involves decreases in the amount, quality, and consistency of sleep. When sleep becomes interrupted or fragmented, changes in the normal sequence of sleep stages occur, and cycles cannot be completed (Fisher, 1984). Gradually a cumulative sleep deprivation develops.

A person's response to sleep deprivation is highly variable. Clients may experience a variety of physiological and psychological symptoms (see box). The severity of symptoms is often related to the duration

---

Sleep Deprivation Symptoms

PHYSIOLOGICAL SYMPTOMS

- Hand tremors
- Decreased reflexes
- Slowed response time
- Reduction in word memory
- Decreased reasoning, judgment, and association
- Cardiac dysrhythmias
- Decreased auditory and visual alertness

PSYCHOLOGICAL SYMPTOMS

- Moods
- Disorientation
- Irritability
- Decreased motivation
- Fatigue
- Sleepiness
- Hyperactivity
- Agitation

1158 UNIT 7 Basic Physiological Needs

of sleep deprivation. Causes may include illness (for example, fever, difficulty breathing, or pain), sleep disorders, emotional stress, aging, medications, environmental disturbances (that is, frequent nursing care), and changes in sleep patterns such as shift work.

The most effective treatment for sleep deprivation is elimination or correction of factors that disrupt the sleep pattern. Nurses play an important role in treating sleep deprivation problems.

Other Sleep Disorders

Sleep problems common in children include **somnambulism** (sleepwalking), night terrors, nightmares, **nocturnal enuresis** (bedwetting), and tooth grinding (bruxism). When adults have these problems, it may indicate more serious disorders. Specific treatment for these disorders varies. However, in all cases, it is important to support clients and maintain their safety. For example, sleepwalkers are unaware of surroundings and are slow to react. Thus the risk of falls is great. A nurse should not startle sleepwalkers but instead gently awaken them and lead them back to bed.

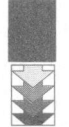 NURSING PROCESS AND SLEEP

Assessment

To promote a normal restful sleep for clients, the nurse assesses their sleep histories, including factors that normally influence sleep. If sleep is adequate the nursing history can be brief.

Sleep is a subjective experience. Only the client can report whether it is restful. If the client is satisfied with the amount of sleep received, it may be considered normal (Closs, 1988). If a client admits to or the nurse suspects a sleep problem a more detailed history is needed.

Sleep Assessment Tools

Most persons can provide a reasonably accurate estimate of their sleep patterns, particularly if any changes have occurred. One of the most effective subjective methods for assessing sleep quality is use of a visual analog scale (Closs, 1988). The nurse draws a straight horizontal line about 100 mm (4 inches) long. Opposing statements such as "best night's sleep" and "worst night's sleep" are at each end of the line. The middle represents an average night's sleep. Clients are asked to place marks on the horizontal line at points corresponding to their perceptions of the previous night's sleep. The distance of

the mark along the line can be measured in millimeters and offers a numerical value for satisfaction with sleep. The scale can be reused to show change over time.

The choice of sleep therapies for a client depends on the factors and conditions that normally promote sleep or cause a sleep problem. For example, if a client always reads before falling asleep, it makes sense to offer reading material at bedtime. Assessment is aimed at understanding the characteristics of any sleep problem and the client's usual sleep habits. Clapin-French (1986) strongly recommends the use of a sleep history, particularly in the care of older clients (see research highlight). Fig. 36-5 is one example of a sleep questionnaire used to assess a hospitalized client's sleep patterns. Often an institution does not have a special sleep assessment tool. In this case the nurse must define information important to assess. The nurse incorporates assessment data under existing categories on the assessment tool.

Sources for Sleep Assessment

The client is the best resource for describing a sleep problem. The client can also report the extent to which a sleep problem represents a change from normal. Often the client knows the cause for sleep problems, such as a noisy environment or worry over a relationship.

When caring for children, parents are often the best source of information. Parents are usually successful in learning why their children have trouble

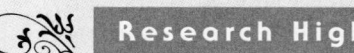 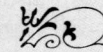

Older adults frequently experience sleep disturbances associated with age-related changes in physiological aspects of sleep. Clapin-French assessed the factors involved in changes in sleep patterns of older clients in long-term care facilities and evaluated the extent of the use of a nursing sleep history by nurses.

Of the 102 older adults studied, 71% received some type of sleep medication regularly. Significant shifts in sleep patterns after admission occurred in clients taking medication. However, only 54% had sleep histories conducted by nurses. Clients may receive inappropriately large amounts of sleep medications without adequate assessment of factors, promoting sleep problems. Detailed assessment of sleep patterns should be a routine part of a nursing history.

Clapin-French E: Sleep patterns of aged persons in long-term care facilities, *J Adv Nurs* 11:57, 1986.

THE SLEEP QUESTIONNAIRE

At home, what do you do at bedtime to help you sleep? _____
_____

Some of the statements may *appear* to be the same, but each is different and should be rated as such.*

A. I think I have difficulty with sleep
  a. in the hospital
  b. at home
B. I sleep more at home than in the hospital.
C. When I awaken in the hospital, I feel fatigued and groggy.
D. It takes me longer than 30 minutes to fall asleep in the hospital.
E. Since I've been in the hospital, I awaken frequently at night.
F. In the hospital, if I wake up in the middle of the night it takes me longer than 30 minutes to fall back to sleep.
G. It bothers me that I now go to bed at a different time than I would like.
H. It bothers me that I get up at a different time each morning.
I. Hospital staff awaken me while I'm sleeping.
J. I am awakened at night for treatments.
K. During the day, there is little time for rest.
L. At night I am awakened by noises.
M. At night I am awakened by light.
N. The mattress in the hospital bothers my sleep.
O. The pillow in the hospital bothers my sleep.
P. Having a roommate in the hospital affects my sleep.
Q. I sleep in a very warm room.
R. I have pain at night.
S. The medicines I take keep me awake.
T. My illness keeps me awake at night.

1. I drink coffee, tea, cola, or cocoa during the day.
2. I drink coffee, tea, cola, or cocoa around sleeping time.
3. I exercise during the day.
4. I exercise around sleeping time.
5. I smoke during the day.
6. I smoke around sleeping time.
7. I have unpleasant conversation during the day.
8. I have unpleasant conversation around sleeping time.
9. I have negative thoughts during the day.
10. I have negative thoughts around sleeping time.
11. I think about what happened during the day and at sleeping time plan for tomorrow.
12. I read during the day.
13. I read around sleeping time.
14. I eat around sleeping time.
15. I watch TV during the day.
16. I watch TV around sleeping time.
17. I have pleasant conversation during the day.
18. I have pleasant conversation around sleeping time.
19. I have positive thoughts during the day.
20. I have positive thoughts around sleeping time.
21. I drink alcohol around sleeping time.

*Response choices were: *Never, Rarely, Sometimes, Often, Very Often.*

Fig. 36-5   A sleep questionnaire can be used to assess sleep patterns. From McNeil BJ et al: *Am J Nurs* 86(1):26, 1986.

sleeping. Children often are able to relate fears or worries that inhibit their ability to fall asleep. If children frequently awaken in the middle of bad dreams, parents can identify the problem but perhaps do not understand the meanings of the dreams. Parents can also describe the typical behavior patterns that foster or impair sleep. For example, excessive stimulation from active play or visiting friends may predictably impair sleep. With chronic sleep problems, parents can relate the duration of the problem, its progression, and children's responses.

Information from clients' bed partners may reveal the nature of certain sleep disorders. Bed partners, for example, can report on the clients' patterns. Partners of clients with sleep apnea often complain that their sleep is disturbed by clients' snoring and restless movements. Often, partners must sleep in different beds or rooms. The nurse should ask bed partners whether the clients have pauses or interruptions of breathing or snoring during sleep. Some partners mention becoming fearful when clients apparently stop breathing and then struggle before airflow returns. Partners may also be able to describe the frequency of clients' apneic attacks.

Sleep History

Clients may report that they enjoy adequate sleep. In this situation the sleep history can be brief (see box). A determination of usual bedtime, normal bedtime rituals, and preferred environment for sleeping gives the nurse information for planning care conducive to sleep.

When suspecting a sleep problem, a nurse may assess the quality and characteristics of sleep. The categories of assessment chosen depend on the nature and severity of the sleep problem. For example, if early assessment reveals that the client's lifestyle has been hectic and excessive caffeine is consumed, it is unnecessary to start an extensive sleep-wake log. If

---

Components of a Sleep History

- Description of client's sleeping problem
- Normal sleep pattern
- Physical illness
- Current life events
- Emotional and mental status
- Bedtime rituals and environment
- Sleep-wake log
- Behaviors of sleep deprivation

---

therapies are ineffective in promoting sleep, the nurse may later conduct a reassessment to learn more about the problem.

DESCRIPTION OF SLEEPING PROBLEMS. When a client admits to or the nurse suspects a sleep problem, the nursing history must be detailed so that therapeutic care can be provided. Open-ended questions help a client to describe a problem more fully. A general description of a problem followed by more focused questions usually reveal specific characteristics that can be used in planning therapies.

To begin the nurse needs to understand the nature of the sleep problem, its signs and symptoms, its onset and duration, its severity, any predisposing factors or causes, and the overall effect on the client. Assessment questions might include the following:

1. *Nature of the problem:* Tell me what type of problem you have falling asleep. Tell me why you think your sleep is inadequate. Describe for me a typical night's sleep.
2. *Signs and symptoms:* Do you have difficulty falling asleep or re-awakening? Do you snore loudly or have you been told that you snore loudly? Do you have headaches when awakening? Does your child awaken from nightmares?
3. *Onset and duration:* When did you notice the problem? How long has this problem lasted?
4. *Severity:* How long does it take to fall asleep? How often during the week do you have trouble falling asleep? Tell me how many hours of sleep you got this week; compare that to normal.
5. *Predisposing factors:* Tell me what you do just before going to bed. Have you recently had any changes at work or at home?
6. *Effect on client:* How has the loss of sleep affected you? Ask a spouse or friend: Have you noticed any changes in behavior since the sleep problem started? Do you feel tired or irritable or have trouble concentrating?

Proper questioning helps the nurse determine the type of sleep disturbance and the nature of the problem. Table 36-2 gives examples of additional questions to ask when specific sleep disorders are suspected.

Normal Sleep Pattern

Normal sleep is difficult to define because individuals vary greatly. It is important, however, to have a client describe normal sleep to determine the significance of changes created by sleep disturbances. Knowing a client's normal sleep pattern allows a nurse to match sleeping conditions in a health care setting with those in the home. To determine the cli-

TABLE 36-2 Questions to Ask to Assess for Sleep Disorders

Assessment Questions	Rationale
INSOMNIA	
Do you fall asleep easily?	Determine nature and severity of insomnia. Help in selection of sleep therapies.
Do you fall asleep and have difficulty staying asleep?	
Do you awaken early from sleep?	
What causes you to awaken early?	
What do you do to prepare for sleep?	
What do you think about as you try to fall asleep?	
How often do you have trouble sleeping?	
SLEEP APNEA	
Do you snore loudly?	Reveal presence of sleep apnea and severity of condition.
Has anyone ever told you that you often stop breathing for a while and then start up again? (Spouse or friend may report this.)	
Do you feel fatigued and experience headaches after awakening?	
NARCOLEPSY	
Are you tired during the day?	Help diagnose narcolepsy and influence on daily activites.
Are you tired at special times?	
Are you tired for short periods?	
Do you fall asleep at inopportune times? (Friends or relatives may report this.)	
Do you have episodes of losing control or falling to the floor?	
Have you ever had the feeling of being unable to move or talk just before falling asleep?	

ent's normal sleep pattern the nurse asks the following questions:

1. What time do you usually go to sleep?
2. How quickly do you fall asleep?
3. What is the average number of hours you sleep during the night?
4. How many times do you awaken at night?
5. When do you typically awaken in the morning?
6. Do you rise once you awaken or do you stay in bed?

The nurse takes this data and compares them with the norm for the client's age. The nurse begins to assess for identifiable patterns such as insomnia.

Clients' sleep problems may show patterns drastically different from normal patterns, or they may be relatively minor. Hospitalized clients usually need or want more sleep as a result of illness, or they may require less sleep because they are less active. Clients may think that it is necessary to try to sleep longer than normal. These changes can disrupt sleep patterns and eventually make sleeping difficult.

PHYSICAL ILLNESS. The nurse determines whether the client has any preexisting health problems that might interfere with sleep. A history of psychiatric problems may make a difference. A manic depressive client sleeps more when depressed than when manic. A schizophrenic client may have fragmented sleep. Chronic diseases such as thyroid disease and painful disorders such as arthritis interfere with sleep, too. The nurse also assesses the client's medication history, including a description of over-the-counter and prescribed drugs. If a client takes medications to aid sleeping, the nurse determines the dosage. The nurse may also assess daily caffeine intake.

If the client has recently undergone surgery the nurse expects to assess a sleep disturbance. The effect on sleep depends on the severity of the surgery (Kavey, Anderson, 1986). Clients often awaken frequently during the first night after surgery and receive little deep or REM sleep. Depending on the type of surgery, it may take several days for a normal sleep cycle to return.

CURRENT LIFE EVENTS. The nurse learns whether the client is experiencing any changes in lifestyle. A person's occupation may offer a clue to the nature of a sleep problem. Changes in job responsibilities, rotating shifts, or long hours can contribute to a sleep disturbance. Questions about social activities, recent travel, or mealtime schedules help clarify the sleep assessment. The nurse tries to learn whether lifestyle activities are disrupting a client's normal sleep pattern. The nurse also asks about changes at work that may be affecting the ability to fall asleep at night.

EMOTIONAL AND MENTAL STATUS. If a client is anxious, excitable, or angry, mental preoccupations can seriously disrupt sleep. The client may be experiencing emotional stress related to illness or situational crises such as loss of job or a loved one. Thus the client's emotions may affect the ability to sleep. Clients with psychiatric disorders may need mild sedation for adequate rest. The nurse assesses the effectiveness of the medication and its effect on daytime function.

BEDTIME RITUALS. The nurse asks about the client's bedtime rituals. For example, the client may drink a glass of milk, take a sleeping pill, eat a snack, watch television, or exercise. The nurse assesses habits that are beneficial compared with those that disturb sleep. Not all clients are alike. Watching television may bore one person to sleep, whereas another individual may stay awake during a suspenseful movie.

Hospitalization often interferes with bedtime rituals. Restrictions caused by illness may prevent the client from eating, drinking, or exercising. A nurse learns about the effects of hospital routines on the person's ability to fall asleep.

The nurse should pay special attention to a child's bedtime rituals. The parents can report whether it is necessary, for example, to read the child a bedtime story, rock the child to sleep, or engage in quiet play.

BEDTIME ENVIRONMENT. The nurse asks the client to describe normal bedroom conditions. The bedroom may be dark or light. The door to the room may be open or closed. The client may listen to the radio or watch television. The nurse also observes the bed and mattress for type (for example, soft). The nurse also asks about types of noise that prevent the client from falling asleep. In addition, a child may require the company of a parent to fall asleep. The nurse may learn that changes in the home are necessary to promote sleep.

In a hospital the nurse needs to know the client's normal environment compared to the hospital room. There may be environmental distractions such as a roommate's television, an electronic monitor in the hallway, a noisy nurses' station, or another client who cries out at night. The nurse identifies factors that can be reduced or controlled.

SLEEP-WAKE LOG. If the cause of a sleep problem is unclear, a client and bed partner can keep a sleep-wake log for 2 weeks. The nurse should not rely only on the client's casual description of the problem. Descriptions of the worst sleeping nights may distort the real problem. A sleep-wake log is completed every morning to provide information on day-to-day variations in sleep-wake patterns over long periods. Entries into the log include physical activities, mealtimes, type and amount of intake (alcohol and caffeine), time and length of daytime naps, evening and bedtime rituals, the time the client tries to fall asleep, nighttime awakenings, and the time of morning awakening. A partner can help record the estimated times the client falls asleep or awakens. The log is helpful, but sometimes its completion can distract persons from sleeping. A client must be motivated to participate in the completion of a sleep-wake log. It is not a technique to use for acutely ill clients who have short hospital stays.

BEHAVIORS OF SLEEP DEPRIVATION. Some clients are unaware of their sleep problems. The nurse observes for behaviors such as irritability, disorientation (similar to a drunken state), and slurred speech. If sleep deprivation has lasted a long time, psychotic behavior such as delusions and paranoia may develop. For example, a client may report seeing strange objects or colors in the room. The client may act afraid when the nurse enters the room.

Clients with chronic sleep disorders usually have mild symptoms of sleep deprivation. Clients hospitalized in intensive care units for an extended time may show the "ICU syndrome" of sleep deprivation. Constant environmental stimuli within the ICU, such as

 **Research Highlight**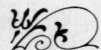

The purposes of Richards and Bairnsfather's descriptive study were to describe the first 3 nights of sleep of clients in a critical care unit (CCU) and to compare findings with matched normal subjects who slept in a laboratory. Ten male clients, 50 to 69 years old, who had cardiovascular disease were studied. Data describing the sleep of subjects were compared with data from 12 age- and sex-matched subjects who slept in a laboratory.

Subjects in the CCU demonstrated significant decreases in total sleep time, the percentage of stage 2 and REM sleep, and the percentage of time spent asleep in any stage (sleep efficiency index). There were wide variations in the night sleep patterns of the CCU subjects. When comparing subjects who normally slept during the day versus the night, the study revealed that day sleepers sleep 86 minutes less during the night in the CCU than the night sleepers. The sleep of day sleepers was also less efficient, with a decreased stage 1, 2, and REM sleep. However, day sleepers awoke fewer times and received more stage 3 sleep than night sleepers. A high percentage of day sleepers in the study could have led to overestimating disturbances in night sleep. Another finding from the study was a tendency for clients in the CCU to nap frequently during the day.

The implications for nursing practice reported from the study include development of alarm systems that do not disturb client sleep, designs of CCU rooms with observation windows so that doors can be closed, and schedule of care activities to allow uninterrupted sleep time. A limitation of the study was its small sample size.

Richards KC, Bairnsfather L: A description of night sleep patterns in the critical care unit, *Heart Lung* 18(1):35, 1988.

strange noises from equipment, the frequent monitoring and care given by nurses, and ever-present lights, confuse clients. Soon a client cannot tell the difference between night and day. Repeated environmental stimuli and the client's poor physical status lead to sleep deprivation (see research highlight).

 ## Nursing Diagnosis

Assessment reveals clusters of data that include defining characteristics for a sleep problem or problems that result from a sleep disturbance. If a sleep pattern disturbance is identified the nurse specifies the specific condition (see diagnoses box). By specifying the nature of a sleep disturbance, the nurse can design more effective interventions. For example, the nurse uses different therapies to help clients who are unable to fall asleep versus clients who have sleep attacks during the day. The diagnostic process box demonstrates how the identification of defining characteristics ensures an accurate nursing diagnosis.

Assessment should also identify the probable cause of the sleep disturbance such as a noisy environment or stress involving a marital relationship.

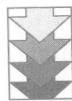 ## Examples of Nursing Diagnoses Related to Sleep Disturbances

---

NANDA-APPROVED NURSING DIAGNOSES

Sleep pattern disturbance (difficulty falling asleep) related to:
- Noisy environment
- Symptoms of chronic illness

Sleep pattern disturbance (frequent awakenings) related to:
- Concern over loss of job
- Barbiturate dependency

High risk for injury related to:
- Attacks of sleepwalking or narcolepsy

Ineffective family coping: compromised related to:
- Spouse's poor understanding of sleep problem

Self-esteem disturbance related to:
- Incidents of bed-wetting

Altered thought processes related to:
- Sleep deprivation

Fatigue related to:
- Chronic difficulty falling and staying asleep
- Altered sleep-wake pattern

 ## Sample Nursing Diagnostic Process for Sleep Disturbances

Assessment Activities	Defining Characteristics	Nursing Diagnoses
Ask client to explain nature of sleep problem.	Client reports difficulty in falling asleep, taking up to an hour. Client reports awakening 2-3 times nightly, with difficulty returning to sleep.	*Sleep pattern disturbance; difficulty falling and remaining asleep* related to worry over job loss
Observe client's behavior and ask bed partner if behavior changes have been noted.	Client admits to not feeling well-rested. Spouse describes episodes of client being lethargic and irritable.	
Determine if client has had recent lifestyle changes.	Spouse reports client recently lost job; has concern over finding new position.	
Ask client and spouse to describe nature of sleep problem.	Client reports feeling fatigued during the day with morning headaches. Spouse reports client snores loudly and often seems to stop breathing for several seconds.	*Ineffective family coping: compromised* related to spouse and client's poor understanding of sleep apnea
Ask client and spouse whether the sleep problem has affected their relationship.	Client admits to a decreased sexual drive, says spouse "doesn't understand." Spouse reports client is unwilling to talk about problem or seek help.	
Gather a sleep-wake log for a week.	Log indicates frequent sleep interruptions, spouse moved to different bedroom day 4.	

These causes become the focus of interventions for minimizing or eliminating the problem. For example, if a client is experiencing insomnia as a result of a noisy environment, the nurse could offer some basic recommendations for helping sleep such as controlling the noise of hospital equipment, reducing interruptions, or keeping doors closed. If the insomnia is related to worry over a threatened marital separation, the nurse's actions involve introduction of coping strategies and creation of an environment for sleep. If the probable cause or related factors are incorrectly defined, the client may not benefit from care.

Sleep problems may affect clients in other ways. For example, a nurse may find that a client with sleep apnea has problems with a spouse who is tired and frustrated over the client's snoring. In addition, the spouse is concerned that the client is breathing improperly and thus is in danger. The nursing diagnosis of *ineffective family coping* indicates that the nurse must provide support to the client and spouse so that they can understand sleep apnea and obtain the medical treatment needed.

Planning

After identifying each nursing diagnosis, the nurse develops a care plan (see box). An individualized care plan can be developed only after the nurse understands the client's current sleep pattern, the client's perception of a normal sleep pattern, and the factors disrupting sleep. Together the nurse and client develop realistic interventions to promote rest and sleep in the home or health care setting. The client's bed partner may have useful suggestions.

In a hospital the nurse plans treatments or routines so that the client will be able to rest. For example, in the intensive care unit, nurses check available electronic monitors to track trends in vital signs without awakening a client each hour. Other staff members should be aware of the care plan so that they can cluster activities at certain times to reduce awakenings.

The nature of a sleep disturbance determines whether referrals to additional health care providers are necessary. For example, if a sleep problem is related to a situational crisis or emotional problem, the nurse refers the client to a psychiatric clinical nurse specialist. When chronic insomnia is the problem, a referral to a sleep center can be beneficial. If the nurse works in a hospital and the client is to receive a referral for continued care, offering information about the sleep problem will be useful to the home health care nurse.

The success of sleep therapy depends on an approach that fits the client's lifestyle and the nature of any sleep disorder. The goals of any care plan for a client needing sleep or rest include the following:

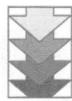

Sample Nursing Care Plan for Sleep Pattern Disturbance

Nursing diagnosis: *Sleep pattern disturbance (difficulty falling and remaining asleep)* related to worry over job loss
Definition: Sleep pattern disturbance is a disruption of sleep time that causes discomfort or interferes with desired lifestyle (Kim, McFarland, McLane, 1991).

Goals	Expected Outcomes	Interventions	Rationale
Client will report that regular sleep pattern is re-established within 1 month.	Client will fall asleep within 30 minutes of going to bed.	Remove any source of caffeine or alcohol from client's diet in evening.	Caffeine and alcohol act as stimulants, disrupting sleep patterns.
		Have client follow bedtime ritual: go to bed at same time each night, drink glass of milk beforehand.	Milk contains L-tryptophan, natural amino acid that induces sleep (Ross et al, 1986).
	Client will use relaxation therapies each night before bedtime.	Establish time before client goes to bed for quiet relaxation, soothing bath, meditation, or progressive relaxation exercises.	Effect of relaxation requires further study. Insomniacs may have increase in sympathetic tone, and relaxation may help reduce it (Berman et al, 1990).
	Client will report feeling of restfullness after awakening each morning.	Control sources of environmental noise and be sure that bedroom is darkened and well ventilated.	Loud noises can disrupt and interfere with rest.

1. Client obtains a sense of restfulness and renewed energy following sleep.
2. Client establishes a healthy sleep pattern.
3. Client understands factors that promote or disrupt sleep.
4. Client assumes self-care behaviors to eliminate factors contributing to sleep disturbance.

Implementation

Clients need adequate sleep and rest to recover from physical illness. Nursing care in an acute-care setting differs from that provided in a client's home. The primary differences are in the environment and the nurse's ability to support normal sleep habits. The client's age also influences the type of therapies most effective. Despite the cause or related factors for a sleep problem, the nurse performs specific interventions that promote normal sleep patterns.

Environmental Controls

All clients require a sleeping environment with a comfortable room temperature and proper ventilation, minimal sources of noise, a comfortable bed, and proper lighting. Infants sleep best when the room temperature is 18° to 21° C (65° to 69.8° F) at night. Cribs should be positioned away from open windows or drafts. The infant is covered with a light, warm blanket. Children and adults vary more in regards to comfortable room temperature. Some prefer to sleep without covers. Older adults often require extra blankets or covers. Many older clients sleep wearing socks.

It helps to eliminate sources of distracting noise so that a bedroom is as quiet as possible. Noise and other environmental and client factors can cause chronic fatigue (World Health Organization, 1980). Hilton (1987) has discovered that sound levels of talking staff and noise from equipment are higher than the level of sound that raises pain perception.

In a hospital the nurse can control noise in several ways (see box). In addition, nurses should make equipment manufacturers aware of the need for quiet in future product designs. At home, it may require the cooperation of people living with the client to reduce noise. For example, the volume of a television watched by family members in another room can be reduced. Some clients are used to sleeping with familiar inside noises, such as the hum of a fan.

A bed and mattress should provide support and comfortable firmness. Bed boards can be placed under mattresses to add support. The position of the bed in the room may make a difference for some clients.

Infants' beds must be safe. To reduce the chance of suffocation, pillows or the ends of loose blankets should not be placed in cribs. Loose-fitting plastic mattress covers should not be used because infants might pull them over their faces and suffocate. Infants are usually placed on their stomachs or sides to prevent suffocation or aspiration of stomach contents. The nurse places infants on their stomachs or sides until they are able to turn their heads side-to-side.

For any client prone to confusion or falls, the bed's side rails should be positioned up unless the client has a history of trying to crawl over the rails. In this situation, a client may be safer with the rails down. Many beds come equipped with an alarm that goes off when a client at risk for falling gets out of bed. A call light should also be placed within the client's reach so that the client may ask for help when needed.

Clients vary in regard to the amount of light that they prefer at night. Infants sleep best in softly lit rooms. Light should not shine directly on their eyes. Small table lamps in infants' rooms prevent total darkness. Older clients may sleep best with dimmed lights (see Chapter 27). This reduces the chance of confusion and prevents falls en route to the bathroom. If street lights shine through windows or if clients sleep during the day, heavy shades, drapes, or slatted blinds are helpful. Nurses should close curtains between clients in semiprivate rooms. Lights on a hospital nursing unit can be dimmed at night.

Control of Noise in the Hospital

- Close doors to a client's room (see research highlight on p. 1155).
- Reduce volume of nearby telephone and paging equipment.
- Wear rubber-soled shoes. Avoid wearing clogs.
- Turn off bedside equipment that is not in use (e.g., oxygen, suction equipment).
- Avoid abrupt loud noise such as flushing a toilet or moving a bed.
- Keep necessary conversations at low levels, particularly at night.
- Conduct discussions or nursing reports in a private, separate area away from client rooms.
- Turn off the television or radio unless client prefers soft music.

Promoting Bedtime Rituals

Bedtime rituals relax clients in preparation for sleep. It is always important for persons to go to sleep when they feel fatigued or sleepy. Going to bed while fully awake and thinking about other things can cause insomnia and interfere with the bed as a stimulus for sleep.

Newborns and infants sleep through so much of the day that a specific ritual is hardly necessary. However, quieting activities, such as holding them snugly in blankets, singing or talking softly, and gently rocking, help infants fall asleep.

A bedtime ritual (for example, same hour of sleep, snack, or quiet activity) used consistently helps young children avoid attempts to delay sleeping. Toddlers and preschoolers may be too excited and full of energy to go to bed. Parents are advised to ignore attention-seeking behaviors and reinforce patterns of preparing for bedtime. Reading stories, allowing children to sit in the parents' or nurse's lap while listening to music, or listening to a prayer are routines that can be associated with preparing for bed. Quiet activities such as coloring and reading work well with school-age children.

An adult should learn to avoid excessive physical or mental stimulation just before bedtime. Physical exercise can promote sleep if performed at least 2 hours before bedtime. Reading a light novel, watching a relaxing television program, or listening to music helps a person relax. A client should not try to finish office work or resolve family problems before bedtime. The bedroom should not be used as a place to work. The bedroom should always be associated with sleep.

Working toward a consistent time for sleep helps most clients gain a healthy sleep pattern and strengthens the rhythm of the sleep-wake cycle. Persons should also void before retiring so that they are not kept awake by a full bladder.

Relaxation exercises are a useful bedtime ritual. Slow, deep breathing for 1 or 2 minutes induces calm. Rhythmic contraction and relaxation of muscles (see Chapter 37) alleviates tension and prepares the body for rest (Hoch, Reynolds, 1986). Guided imagery, praying, meditation, and yoga may also promote sleep.

Promoting Comfort

People fall asleep only after feeling comfortable and relaxed. The nurse can use several measures to promote comfort (see box). Minor irritants can keep clients awake. Diapers should be changed before placing infants in bed. Soft cotton nightclothes keep infants or small children warm and comfortable.

Hospital beds tend to be harder than ones at home. A hard surface can cause more body move-

---

Comfort Measures For Promoting Sleep

- Administer analgesics or sedatives about 30 minutes before bedtime.
- Encourage clients to wear loose-fitting nightwear.
- Remove any irritants against the client's skin such as moist or wrinkled sheets or drainage tubing.
- Position and support body parts to protect pressure points and aid muscle relaxation.
- Offer a massage just before bedtime.
- Provide caps and socks for older clients and those prone to cold.
- Administer necessary hygiene measures.
- Keep bed linen clean and dry.
- Provide a comfortable mattress.
- Encourage client to void before going to sleep.

---

ment (Schmidt-Kessen, Kendel, 1973). Compared with beds at home, hospital beds also are often of a different height, length, or width. Keeping beds clean and dry and in a comfortable position may help clients relax. Some clients suffer painful illnesses requiring special comfort measures such as application of dry or moist heat, use of supportive dressings or splints, and proper positioning.

Providing for personal hygiene improves sense of comfort. A warm bath or shower before bedtime can be relaxing. Clients restricted to bed should be offered the opportunity to wash the face and hands. Toothbrushing and care of dentures also help to prepare the client for sleep.

Establishing Periods of Rest and Sleep

In a hospital or extended-care setting it is difficult to provide clients with the time needed to rest and sleep. However, the nurse plans care to avoid awakening clients for nonessential tasks. The nurse can help by scheduling assessments, treatments, procedures, and routines for times when clients are awake. For example, if a client's physical condition has been stable, the nurse should avoid awakening the client to check vital signs. Unless maintaining a drug's therapeutic blood level is essential, medications should be given during waking hours. The nurse should work with the radiology department and other support services to plan therapies at intervals that allow clients time for rest.

When the client's condition demands more frequent monitoring, the nurse can plan activities to allow extended rest periods. For example, if a client needs frequent dressing changes, is receiving intravenous therapy, and has drainage tubes from several sites, the nurse should not make a separate trip into the room to check each problem. Instead the nurse should use a single visit to change the dressing, regulate the intravenous system, and empty the drainage tubes. In the home, it may help to encourage clients to stay physically active during the day so that they are more likely to sleep at night. Increasing daytime activity lessens problems with falling asleep.

It is common for older adults to take short naps during the day. Hayter (1985) suggests that older clients take afternoon naps to restore the body physically. Hoch and Reynolds (1986) recommend that naps be taken at the same time each day to maintain a consistent schedule.

Controlling Physiological Disturbances

For clients with physical illness, the nurse can help control symptoms that disrupt sleep. For example, a client with respiratory abnormalities should sleep with two pillows or in a semisitting position to ease the effort to breathe. The client may benefit from taking prescribed bronchodilators before sleep to prevent airway obstruction. A client with a hiatal hernia also needs special care. After meals the client may experience a burning sensation as a result of gastric reflux. To prevent sleep disturbances, the client should eat a small meal several hours before bedtime and sleep in a semisitting position. Clients with pain, nausea, or other recurrent symptoms should receive any symptom-relieving medication at a time so that the drug's peak action takes effect at bedtime.

Stress Reduction

Sources of emotional stress can interfere with sleep. The inability to sleep can also make a person feel irritable and tense. When clients feel emotionally upset, they should be encouraged not to force sleep. Otherwise, insomnia frequently develops, and soon bedtime is associated with the inability to relax. A client who has difficulty falling asleep may find it helpful to get up and pursue a relaxing activity, such as reading or sewing, rather than stay in bed and think about sleep.

In a health care setting a nurse on the night shift should take time to sit and talk with clients unable to sleep. This helps the nurse determine the factors keeping clients awake. Explaining procedures or answering questions may give clients the peace of mind needed to fall asleep. Backrubs (see Chapter 37) can also be used to help clients relax more thoroughly. If a sedative is indicated, the nurse confers with the physician to be sure that the lowest dosage is used initially. Older adults can be vulnerable to the side effects of sedatives, hypnotics, or analgesics because the medications are metabolized slowly.

Children often have bedtime fears, awaken during the night, or have nightmares. Fears (for example, fear of the dark, strange noises or intruders) are usually normal for this age. After nightmares, parents should enter children's rooms immediately and talk to them briefly about fears to provide a cooling-down period. Children are comforted but left in their own beds. Their fears should not be used as excuses to delay bedtime.

Bedtime Snacks

Some persons enjoy bedtime snacks, whereas others cannot sleep after eating. A perfect snack includes a dairy product such as warm milk or cocoa that contains L-tryptophan. A full meal before bedtime can often cause gastrointestinal upset and interfere with the ability to fall asleep.

Nurses should discourage clients from drinking caffeine before bed. The stimulant can cause a person to stay awake or awaken throughout the night. Alcohol can interrupt sleep cycles and reduce the amount of deep sleep. Coffee, tea, colas, and alcohol act as diuretics and may cause a person to awaken in the night to void.

Infants require special measures to minimize nighttime awakenings for feeding. It is common for children to have a need for middle-of-the-night bottle- or breast-feeding. Whaley and Wong (1991) recommend offering the last feeding as late as possible. Eventually it may help to gradually reduce the amount of formula or duration of breast-feeding. Infants should not be given bottles in bed.

Administering Sleep Medications

Sleep medications can help a client if used correctly. However, long-term use of antianxiety, sedative, or hypnotic agents can disrupt sleep and lead to more serious problems. One group of drugs considered to be relatively safe are the benzodiazepines (Table 36-3 on p. 1168). These medications do not cause general CNS depression like **sedatives** or **hypnotics** do. The benzodiazepines create muscle relaxation, antianxiety, and hypnotic effects by stimulating receptors in the RAS to block stimulation of the limbic and cortical areas of the brain. Physicians prescribe this group of drugs because antianxiety effects occur at safe, nontoxic doses. The benzodiazepines are generally not available to children under 12 to 18 years, depending on the specific medication.

Pregnant clients should avoid benzodiazepines because their use is associated with risk of congenital anomalies. Nursing mothers should not receive the drugs because they are excreted in breast milk. Older adults are susceptible to side effects of any antianxiety or sedative agent because of physiological changes in metabolism. Short-acting benzodiaz-

TABLE 36-3   Pharmacology of Benzodiazepines

Generic Name	Trade Name	Onset of Action*	Dosage†	Indications
Flurazepam	Dalmane Apo-Flurazepam	15-45	15-30 at bedtime	Sleep disorder
Temazepam	Restoril	25-27	15-30 at bedtime	Sleep disorder
Triazolam	Halcion	15-30	0.25-0.5 at bedtime	Sleep disorder
Oxazepam	Serax Zapex	45-90	10-30 (3-4 times daily)	Anxiety
Lorazepam	Ativan Apo-Lorazepam	15-45	2-4 at bedtime	Anxiety
Alprazolam	Xanax	15-45	0.25-0.5 (3 times daily)	Anxiety

*Onset of oral administration in minutes.
†Oral dosage is in milligrams.

Client Teaching For Sleep Hygiene Habits

OBJECTIVE

- Client will follow proper sleep hygiene habits at home.

TEACHING STRATEGIES

- Instruct client to try to exercise daily (e.g., walking, swimming, bicycling), preferably in morning or afternoon and to avoid vigorous exercise in the evening.
- Caution client against sleeping long hours during weekends or holidays to prevent disturbance of normal sleep-wake cycle.
- Explain that bedroom should not be used for intensive studying, snacking, or other nonsleep activity.
- Explain that client should avoid worrisome thinking when going to bed and should use relaxation exercises.

EVALUATION

- Have client complete sleep-wake log for 1 week, and compare it with previous sleep-wake log.
- Ask client to complete visual analog scale for perceptions of quality of sleep.

---

epines such as oxazepam, lorazepam, temazepam, alprazolam, and triazolam are usually recommended (McKenry, Salerno, 1992). Initial doses should be small, and increments are added gradually, based on client response. If older clients are continent, ambulatory, and alert, excessive doses may cause incontinence, confusion, and impaired mobility.

The use of nonprescription sleeping medications is not advisable. Clients should learn the risks of such drugs, especially the long-term effects of sleep disruption. The nurse can help clients use behavioral measures instead of drugs to cure sleep problems.

Regular use of any sleep medication can lead to tolerance, and withdrawal can then cause rebound insomnia. All clients should understand the possible side effects of sleep medications. Routine medical monitoring of client response to the medication is important.

Client Teaching

To develop good sleep habits at home, clients and their bed partners should learn techniques that promote sleep and conditions that interfere with sleep (see teaching box). Parents of young children can also learn good sleep habits.

Clients benefit more from instructions based on information about their homes and lifestyles. For example, a suggestion to control noise at night is ineffective if the client lives near a busy airport. Any suggestions for relaxing bedtime activities should include activities that the client enjoys.

A client who takes sleep medications should know about risks and possible side effects. Nurses should caution clients against taking benzodiazepines with alcoholic beverages, opioid analgesics, or MAO and tricyclic antidepressants. CNS depression may result. The nurse also warns clients not to take more than the prescribed dose if the medication seems less effective.

Clients should also learn the effects of disease states on sleep. For example, a client with a hiatal hernia should learn to avoid eating large meals before bedtime. This prevents an irritating regurgitation of

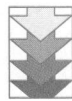

Sample Evaluation of Interventions for Sleep Disturbances

Goals	Evaluative Measures	Expected Outcomes
Client will report that regular sleep pattern is reestablished within 1 mo.	Observe client (in acute-care setting) 30-60 min after bedtime.	Client will fall asleep within 30 min of going to bed.
	Have client report on success in falling and staying asleep.	Client will use relaxation therapies each night before bed.
		Client will report feeling of restfullness after awakening each morning.
Client will experience fewer symptoms of sleep deprivation within 1 mo.	Have client describe behaviors at work or home during the day.	Client will describe fewer episodes of feeling irritable or depressed within 2 wk.
	Observe nonverbal expressions and behaviors.	Client will report being able to complete work-related responsibilities within 4 wk.

food into the esophagus that causes burning and keeps the person from being able to fall or stay asleep. Another important topic for client education is proper use of sleep medications. Clients should learn about alternative measures for promoting sleep (for example, relaxation and warm baths). A client should also be taught the hazards of sleeping medications to avoid side effects or drug-dependence insomnia.

Evaluation

Each client has a different need for sleep and rest. For this reason the evaluation of therapies designed to promote sleep and rest must be individualized. Clients in relatively good health may not need as much sleep or require as many adjustments to their sleep patterns as clients whose physical conditions are poor.

The nurse determines whether expected outcomes have been met (see evaluation box). Evaluative measures may be used shortly after a therapy has been tried (for example, observing whether a client falls asleep after reducing noise and darkening a room). Other evaluative measures may be used after a client awakens from sleep (for example, asking a client to describe the number of awakenings during the previous night). The client and bed partner can usually provide accurate evaluative information. Over longer periods, the nurse may use assessment tools such as the visual analog scale to determine whether sleep has progressively improved or changed.

The nurse also assesses the level of understanding that clients or family members gain after receiving instruction on sleep habits. Compliance with these practices may best be measured during a home visit, when the environment can be observed.

When expected outcomes are not met, the nurse revises nursing measures based on the client's needs or preferences. Finding an effective therapy depends on the client's sleep disturbance, age, and normal sleep pattern. The nurse documents the client's response to sleep therapies so that a continuum of care can be maintained. The nurse is effective in promoting rest and sleep if the goals of care are met.

SUMMARY

Each day a person needs sleep to protect and restore body functions. Normally the sleep-wake cycle follows a 24-hour rhythm coordinated with other physiological functions such as body temperature and hormonal secretions. Sleep is a rhythm within a rhythm. After falling asleep, a person passes through stages that help the body rest and recover.

All age groups have different sleep requirements and sleep habits. Age affects the type of sleep therapies used by the nurse. The nurse's care may differ in the home compared with measures used to promote sleep in a hospital or extended-care setting.

Many factors can promote or disrupt sleep, and a number of sleep disorders can cause specific problems. The nurse assesses the nature of any sleep pattern. The client's participation in the care plan ensures an individualized approach to sleep therapy.

CHAPTER 36 REVIEW

Key Concepts

- Rest is not inactivity but a feeling of physical calm and freedom from worry.
- Sleep is believed to provide physiological and psychological restoration.
- The 24-hour sleep-wake cycle is a circadian rhythm that influences physiological function and behavior.
- The control and regulation of sleep depends on a balance between central nervous system regulators.
- During a typical night's sleep a person passes through four to six complete sleep cycles. Each contains four NREM stages of sleep and a period of REM sleep.
- No specific number of hours of sleep is needed by each person to rest.
- Neonates, infants, and young children require more sleep than older children and adults.
- Symptoms of various diseases may disrupt sleep.
- Long-term use of sleeping pills may lead to difficulty in initiating and maintaining sleep.
- The hectic pace of a person's lifestyle, emotional and psychological stress, and alcohol ingestion disrupt the sleep pattern.
- An environment with a darkened room, reduced noise, comfortable bed, and good ventilation promotes sleep.
- The most common type of sleep disorder is insomnia, which is characterized by the inability to fall asleep, remain asleep during the night, or go back to sleep after awakening.
- If a client's sleep is adequate the nurse assesses the client's usual bedtime, normal bedtime ritual, and the preferred environment for sleeping.
- Only a client can report whether sleep is restful.
- When a client has a sleep problem, the nurse conducts a complete sleep history.
- Diagnosing sleep problems depends on identifying factors that impair sleep.
- When using environmental controls to promote sleep, the nurse should consider the client's home and normal lifestyle.
- Noise can disrupt sleep and enhance pain perception.
- A bedtime ritual of relaxing activities prepares a person physically and mentally for sleep.
- Pain or other symptom control is essential to promote the ability to sleep.
- One of the most important nursing interventions for promoting sleep is establishing periods for sleep and rest.

Key Terms

Apnea, p. 1156

Biological clocks, p. 1147

Bulbar synchronizing region (BSR), p. 1148

Cataplexy, p. 1157

Circadian rhythm, p. 1147

Hypnotics, p. 1167

Infradian rhythm, p. 1147

Insomnia, p. 1156

Narcolepsy, p. 1157

Nocturia, p. 1154

Nocturnal enuresis, p. 1158

NREM sleep, p. 1148

Polysomnogram, p. 1156

REM sleep, p. 1148

Reticular activating system (RAS), p. 1147

Sedatives, p. 1167

Sleep, p. 1146

Sleep apnea, p. 1156

Sleep deprivation, p. 1157

Somnambulism, p. 1158

Ultradian rhythms, p. 1147

Critical Thinking Exercises

1. Mrs. Wills visits the community health clinic for a routine visit. She is 78 years old. During a health history, she tells you that she normally gets only 7 hours of sleep and awakens as many as 3 times a night. Frequently, it may take her up to ½ hour to fall asleep. Mrs. Wills is concerned. What would you as the nurse tell her?

2. If a client has symptoms of insomnia, what type of sleep hygiene habits might you recommend?

3. When conducting an assessment of a client's sleep pattern, what information can be gathered from a bed partner?

4. Mr. John is a 55-year-old sheet-metal worker who works the evening shift. He typically drinks 3 to 4 beers before going to bed. He normally sleeps about 6 hours a night after he goes to bed around 1 AM. It is common for him to arise during the night to urinate. His favorite way to relax is reportedly watching television in bed. As the nurse, what would you assess regarding Mr. John's sleep history?

REFERENCES

Agnew HW et al: The first night effect: an EEG study of sleep, *Psychophysiology* 2:263, 1966.

Berman TM et al: Sleep disorders: take them seriously, *Patient Care* 24:85, 1990.

Block AJ: Respiratory disorders during sleep. I. *Heart Lung* 9:1011, 1980.

Canavan T: The psychobiology of sleep, *Nurs 84* 2:682, 1984.

Chase M, Weitzman ED, editors: *Sleep disorders: basic and clinical research,* New York, 1983, Spectrum.

Chuman MA: The neurological basis of sleep, *Heart Lung* 12:177, 1983.

Clapin-French E: Sleep patterns of aged persons in long-term care facilities, *J Adv Nurs* 11:57, 1986.

Closs SJ: Assessment of sleep in hospital patients: a review of methods, *J Adv Nurs* 13:501, 1988.

Colling J: Sleep disturbances in aging: a theoretical and empiric analysis, *ANS* 6:36, 1983.

Feierman JR: Disordered sleep, *Emerg Med* 17:160, 1985.

Fisher ME: ICU syndrome, *Crit Care Nurs* 4:39, 1984.

Greenberg R et al: Memory, emotion, and REM sleep, *J Abnorm Psychol* 92:378, 1983.

Hayter J: Sleep behavior of older persons, *Nurs Res* 32:242, 1983.

Hayter J: To nap or not to nap? *Geriatr Nurs* 6:104, 1985.

Hilton A: The hospital racket: how noisy is your unit? *Am J Nurs* 87:59, 1987.

Hoch C, Reynolds C III: Sleep disturbances and what to do about them, *Geriatr Nurs* 7:24, 1986.

Horne JA: Human sleep and tissue restitution: some qualifications and doubts, *Clin Sci* 65:569, 1983.

Horne JA, Ostberg O: A self-assessment questionnaire to determine morningness-eveningness in human circadian rhythms, *Int J Chronobiology* 4:97, 1976.

Kales A, Kales J: Sleep disorders: recent findings in the diagnostic and treatment of disturbed sleep, *N Engl J Med* 290:487, 1974.

Kales A et al: Sleep disorders: sleep apnea and narcolepsy, *Ann Intern Med* 106:434, 1987.

Kavey NB, Anderson D: Why every patient needs a good night's sleep, *RN* 49:16, 1986.

Kim MJ, McFarland GK, McLane AM: *Pocket guide to nursing diagnosis,* ed 4, St Louis, 1991, Mosby–Year Book.

McKenry LM, Salerno E: *Mosby's pharmacology in nursing,* ed 18, St Louis, 1992, Mosby–Year Book.

McNeil BJ et al: Sleep questionnaire, *Am J Nurs* 86(1):261, 1986.

Minckley BB: A study of noise and its relationship to patient discomfort in the recovery room, *Nurs Res* 17:247, 1968.

Mitler MM et al: Catastrophies, sleep and public policy: concensus report, *Sleep* 11:100, 1988.

Oswald I: Good, poor, and disordered sleep. In Priest RG, editor: *Sleep: an international monograph,* London 1984, Update Books.

Ross MS et al: When sleep won't come: helping our elderly clients, *Can Nurse* 82:14, 1986.

Schmidt-Kessen W, Kendel K: Einfluss der Raumtemperatur auf den Nachtschlaf, *Res Exp Med (Berl)* 160:220, 1973.

Seidlitz P: Excessive noise levels detrimental to patients, staff, *Hosp Prog* 62:54, 1981.

Webster RA, Thompson DR: Sleep in hospital, *J Adv Nurs* 11:447, 1986.

Whaley LF, Wong DL: *Nursing care of infants and children,* ed 4, St Louis, 1991, Mosby–Year Book.

World Health Organization: *Noise,* Geneva, 1980, The Organization.

ADDITIONAL READINGS

Brewer MJ: To sleep or not to sleep: the consequences of sleep deprivation, *Crit Care Nurs* 5:35, 1985.

Ebersole P, Hess P: *Toward healthy aging: human needs and nursing response,* ed 3, St Louis, 1990, Mosby–Year Book.

Fernsebner B: Sleep deprivation in patients, *AORN J* 37:35, 1983.

Hauri P: *Current concepts: the sleep disorders,* ed 2, Kalamazoo, Mich, 1982, Upjohn Co.

Hayter J: The rhythm of sleep, *Am J Nurs* 80:457, 1980.

Helton MC et al: The correlation between sleep deprivation and the intensive care unit syndrome, *Heart Lung* 9:464, 1980.

Littrell K, Schumann L: Sleep in the C.C.U.: the impossible dream? *Crit Care Nurs* 9(3):320, 1989.

Melnechuk T: The dream machine, *Psychol Today* 17:22, 1983.

Metzler DJ, Finesilver CA: When to worry if your patient can't sleep, *RN* 53:52, 1990.

Potempa K et al: Chronic fatigue, *Image J Nurs Sch* 18:165, 1986.

Reynolds CF III et al: Sleeping pills for the elderly: are they ever justified? *J Clin Psychiatry* 46:9, 1985.

Richards KC, Bairnsfather L: A description of night sleep patterns in the critical care unit, *Heart Lung* 18(1):35, 1988.

Schirmer MS: When sleep won't come, *J Gerontol Nurs* 9:16, 1983.

Simmons FB et al: The palatopharyngoplasty operation for snoring and sleep apnea: an interim report, *Otolaryngol Head Neck Surg* 92:375, 1984.

Synder-Halpern R: The effect of critical care unit noise on patient sleep cycles, *CCQ* 7:41, 1985.

Weaver TE, Millman RP: Broken sleep, *Am J Nurs* 86:146, 1986.

CHAPTER 37

Comfort

OBJECTIVES

Mastery of content in this chapter will enable the student to:
- Define the key terms listed.
- Discuss common misconceptions about pain.
- Identify components of the pain experience.
- Discuss the three phases of behavioral responses to pain.
- Explain the relationship of the gate-control theory to selected nursing therapies for pain relief.
- Perform an assessment of a client experiencing pain.
- Describe guidelines for individualizing pain therapies.
- Identify the techniques and rationales for selecting pain therapies.
- Explain common causes for undertreatment of pain with analgesics.
- Discuss the purpose and services of a hospice program.
- Provide nursing therapies that prevent or reduce a client's pain.

CHAPTER OUTLINE

Nature of Pain
    Prejudices and misconceptions

Physiology of Pain
    Reception
    Perception
    Reaction
    Matching physiological conditions with pain
        therapies

Acute and Chronic Pain

Factors Influencing Pain
    Age
    Sex
    Culture
    Meaning of pain

Attention
Anxiety
Fatigue
Previous experience
Coping style
Family and social support

Nursing Process and Pain
    Assessment
    Nursing diagnosis
    Planning
    Implementaion
    Evaluation

Everyone has experienced some type or degree of **pain.** Yet the concept of pain is difficult to communicate. It is the most common reason to seek health care. A person in pain feels distress or suffering and seeks relief. The nurse uses a variety of interventions to bring relief. However, the nurse cannot see or feel the client's pain. No two persons experience pain in the same way, and no two painful events create identical responses or feelings in a person. Pain is one of the most common problems faced by nurses. Yet it is a source of frustration and is often one of the most misunderstood problems the nurse confronts. The International Association for the Study of Pain (IASP) defined pain as "an unpleasant, subjective sensory and emotional experience associated with actual or potential tissue damage, or described in terms of such damage" (IASP, 1979). Pain can be a major factor inhibiting the ability and willingness to recover from illness.

Nurses care for clients in many settings and situations in which interventions are provided to promote comfort (for example, the home health nurse caring for a terminal cancer client, the school nurse delivering first aid to an injured child, a critical care nurse administering therapy for acute postoperative pain, and a clinic nurse suggesting therapies for chronic arthritic pain. The nurse has a responsibility to understand the experience of pain and to initiate measures that provide relief or help the client learn to cope.

 ## NATURE OF PAIN

Pain is much more than a single sensation caused by a specific stimulus. Pain is subjective and highly individualized, and the interpretation and meaning of pain involve psychosocial and cultural factors. The person experiencing pain is the only authority on it. According to McCaffery (1980), "Pain is whatever the experiencing person says it is, existing whenever he says it does." Pain cannot be objectively measured, such as with an x-ray examination or blood test. Although certain types of pain create predictable signs and symptoms, often the nurse can only assess pain by relying on the client's words and behavior. Only the client knows whether pain is present and what the experience is like. To help a client gain relief, the nurse must believe that the pain exists.

Pain is a protective physiological mechanism. A person with a sprained ankle avoids bearing full weight on the foot to prevent further injury. Pain is a warning that tissue damage has occurred. The client who is unable to feel sensations, such as one with a spinal cord tumor, is unaware of pain-inducing injuries.

Pain is a leading cause of disability. As the average life span increases, more people have chronic disease, in which pain is a common symptom. In addition, medical advances have resulted in diagnostic and therapeutic measures that are often uncomfortable. Nurses care daily for clients in pain. One of the earliest fears of any client with a diagnosed illness is the concern over the pain that might be experienced.

Prejudices and Misconceptions

Health care personnel often hold prejudices against clients in pain. Unless clients have objective signs of pain, a nurse may not believe that they are uncomfortable. The attitudes many nurses have about pain are caused in part by the traditional medical model of illness. This model suggests that physical problems result from physical causes. Thus pain is viewed as a physical response to organic dysfunction. When no obvious source of pain can be found, nurses may stereotype pain sufferers as complainers or difficult clients.

Taylor et al (1984) studied 268 registered nurses who worked in a variety of specialized and general medical-surgical units. Each nurse was asked to read a one-paragraph description of a hypothetical client, described as an acute or chronic pain sufferer. After reading the paragraph, each nurse estimated the suffering of the hypothetical client and rated the client on a series of personality and behavioral traits. The majority of nurses attributed significantly less suffering to the hypothetical clients in chronic pain than

---

Common Biases and Misconceptions about Pain

- Drug abusers and alcoholics overreact to discomforts.
- Clients with minor illnesses have less pain than those with severe physical alterations.
- Administering analgesics regularly will lead to drug dependence.
- The amount of tissue damage in an injury can accurately indicate pain intensity.
- Health care personnel are the best authorities on the nature of the client's pain.
- Psychogenic pain is not real.

those with acute pain. The nurses also believed that the hypothetical clients who had no signs of pathological conditions suffered less than those with pathological signs. The study also showed nurses to have negative attitudes toward clients having low-back pain.

The extent to which nurses make assumptions about clients in pain seriously limits their ability to offer pain relief. Unfortunately, all people are influenced by prejudices based on their culture, education, and experience. Too often, nurses allow misconceptions about pain (see box) to affect their willingness to intervene. Many nurses even avoid acknowledging a client's pain because of their own fear and denial.

To help a client gain comfort or relief, the nurse must view the experience through the client's eyes. Acknowledging personal prejudices or misconceptions also helps the nurse address the client's problem more professionally. Often a nurse who has personally experienced pain is better able to provide support (see research highlight). The nurse who becomes an active, knowledgeable observer of a client in pain will make a more objective analysis of the pain experience. The client makes the diagnosis that

Research Highlight

Holm et al studied the effect of nurses' personal pain experiences on the assessment of their clients' pain. In three Midwestern hospitals, 205 nurses were asked to complete three surveys: a sociodemographic questionnaire, a personal pain history questionnaire, and The Standard Measure of Inferences of Suffering Questionnaire. The Standard Measure of Inference of suffering measures the nurses' perceptions of physical pain and psychological distress. The 134 nurses responding to the survey represented nurses of widely varying ages and associate-degree, diploma, and baccalaureate graduates.

A major finding of the study was that assessment of a client's pain is significantly influenced by the intensity of a nurse's personal pain experience. Nurses who have experienced intense pain are generally more sympathetic to a client in pain. The researchers could not conclude whether a nurse's sympathy is directed at clients with specific conditions. The frequency of the nurses' personal pain experiences did not significantly influence their pain assessments.

Holm K et al: Effect of personal pain experience on pain assessment, *Image J Nurs Sch* 21(2):72, 1989.

pain is present, and the nurse works to apply techniques and skills that ultimately give relief.

PHYSIOLOGY OF PAIN

Pain is a complex mixture of physical, emotional, and behavioral reactions. To best understand the pain experience, it helps to describe its three physiological components: reception, perception, and reaction. A client in pain cannot discriminate among the components. However, understanding each component helps the nurse recognize factors that can cause pain, symptoms that accompany pain, and the rationale and actions of select therapies.

Reception

Nerve receptors in the skin and tissues respond to stimuli resulting from actual or potential tissue damage. **Noxious** (pain) stimuli may be thermal, mechanical, chemical, or electrical. Thermal stimuli result from skin contact with hot or cold substances. Pressure, friction, tension, and stretching are mechanical stimuli. Chemical stimuli originate from substances within the body, such as gastric enzymes, or from substances outside the body, such as caustic chemicals. An electrical current causes an electrical stimulus. Table 37-1 on p. 1178 summarizes the physical alterations that elicit pain-producing stimuli.

Not all tissues contain receptors that transmit pain signals. The brain and alveoli of the lung are examples of tissues insensitive to pain. Some receptors respond to only one type of pain stimulus, whereas others are also sensitive to temperature and pressure. The pain threshold is reached when a stimulus is intense enough to create a nerve impulse. Normally the physiological pain threshold does not differ among individuals, even those of different racial or cultural backgrounds (Guyton, 1985).

Nerve impulses resulting from the painful stimulus travel along afferent peripheral nerve fibers. Two types of peripheral nerve fibers conduct painful stimuli: the fast, myelinated A-delta fibers and the very small, slow, unmyelinated C fibers. The A fibers send pricking sensations that localize the source of pain and detect pain intensity. C fibers relay impulses of a deeper and diffuse nature. For example, after stepping on a nail, a person initially feels a sharp, localized pain, which is the result of A-fiber transmission. Within a few seconds pain becomes more diffuse and widespread until the whole foot aches because of C-fiber innervation.

TABLE 37-1	Examples of Physical Sources of Pain	
Type of Stimulus	Source	Pathophysiological Process
Mechanical	Alteration in body fluids	Edema distending body tissues
	Duct distention	Overstretching of duct's narrow lumen (e.g., passage of kidney stone through ureter)
	Space-occupying lesion (tumor)	Irritation of peripheral nerves by growth of lesion within confined space
Chemical	Perforated visceral organ	Chemical irritation by secretions on sensitive nerve endings (e.g., ruptured appendix, duodenal ulcer)
Thermal	Burn (heat or extreme cold)	Inflammation or loss of superficial layers of epidermis, causing increased sensitivity of nerve endings
Electrical	Burn	Skin layers burned with muscle and subcutaneous tissue injury, causing injury to nerve endings

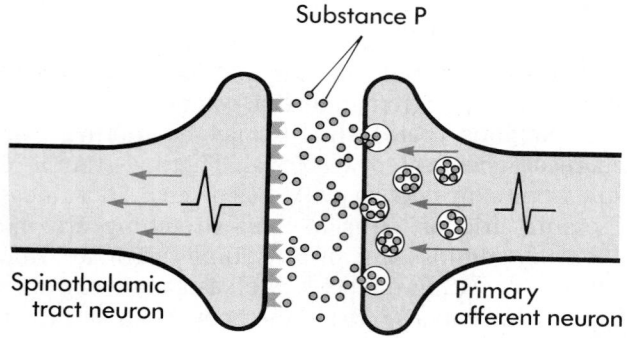

Fig. 37-1 Substance P and other neurotransmitters are released from primary afferent fibers that terminate in the dorsal horn of the spinal cord.
From Paice JA: *Oncol Nurs Forum* 18(5):843, 1991.

A and C fibers transmit impulses from peripheral projections to the end of the fiber in the dorsal horn of the spinal cord. Within the dorsal horn, **neurotransmitters** such as substance P are released, causing a synaptic transmission from the afferent (sensory) peripheral nerve to spinothalamic tract nerves (Paice, 1991). This allows the pain impulse to be transmitted further within the central nervous system (Fig. 37-1). Pain stimuli travel through nerve fibers in the spinothalamic tracts that cross to the opposite side of the spinal cord. Pain impulses then travel up the spinal cord. Fig. 37-2 shows the normal pain reception pathway. After the pain impulse ascends the spinal cord, information is transmitted quickly to higher centers in the brain, including the reticular formation, limbic system, thalamus, and sensory cortex.

A protective reflex response also occurs with pain reception (Fig. 37-3). A fibers send sensory impulses to the spinal cord, where they synapse with spinal motor neurons. The motor impulses travel via a reflex arc along efferent (motor) nerve fibers back to a peripheral muscle near the site of stimulation. Contraction of the muscle leads to a protective withdrawal from the source of pain. For example, when a person accidentally touches a hot iron, a burning sensation is felt, but the hand also reflexively withdraws from the iron's surface. When superficial fibers in the skin are stimulated, a person moves away from the pain source. If internal tissues such as muscle or mucous membranes become stimulated, tightening and guarding of muscles occur.

Pain reception requires an intact peripheral nervous system and spinal cord. Common factors that disrupt pain reception include trauma, drugs, tumor growth, and metabolic disorders.

Neuroregulators

Neuroregulators, or substances that affect the transmission of nerve stimuli, are divided into two groups: neurotransmitters and neuromodulators (see box on p. 1180). Neurotransmitters such as substance P send electrical impulses across the synaptic cleft between two nerve fibers. They are excitatory or inhibitory. Neuromodulators modify neuron activity without directly transferring a nerve signal through a synapse. They are believed to act indirectly by increasing and decreasing the effects of particular neurotransmitters (Whipple, 1987). Endorphins are an example of a neuromodulator.

Gate Control Theory of Pain

There have been several attempts to explain the complexity of pain in terms of the relationship of physiological, psychological, and cognitive variables. The gate control theory, proposed by Melzack and Wall (1965), is the most comprehensive. The theory

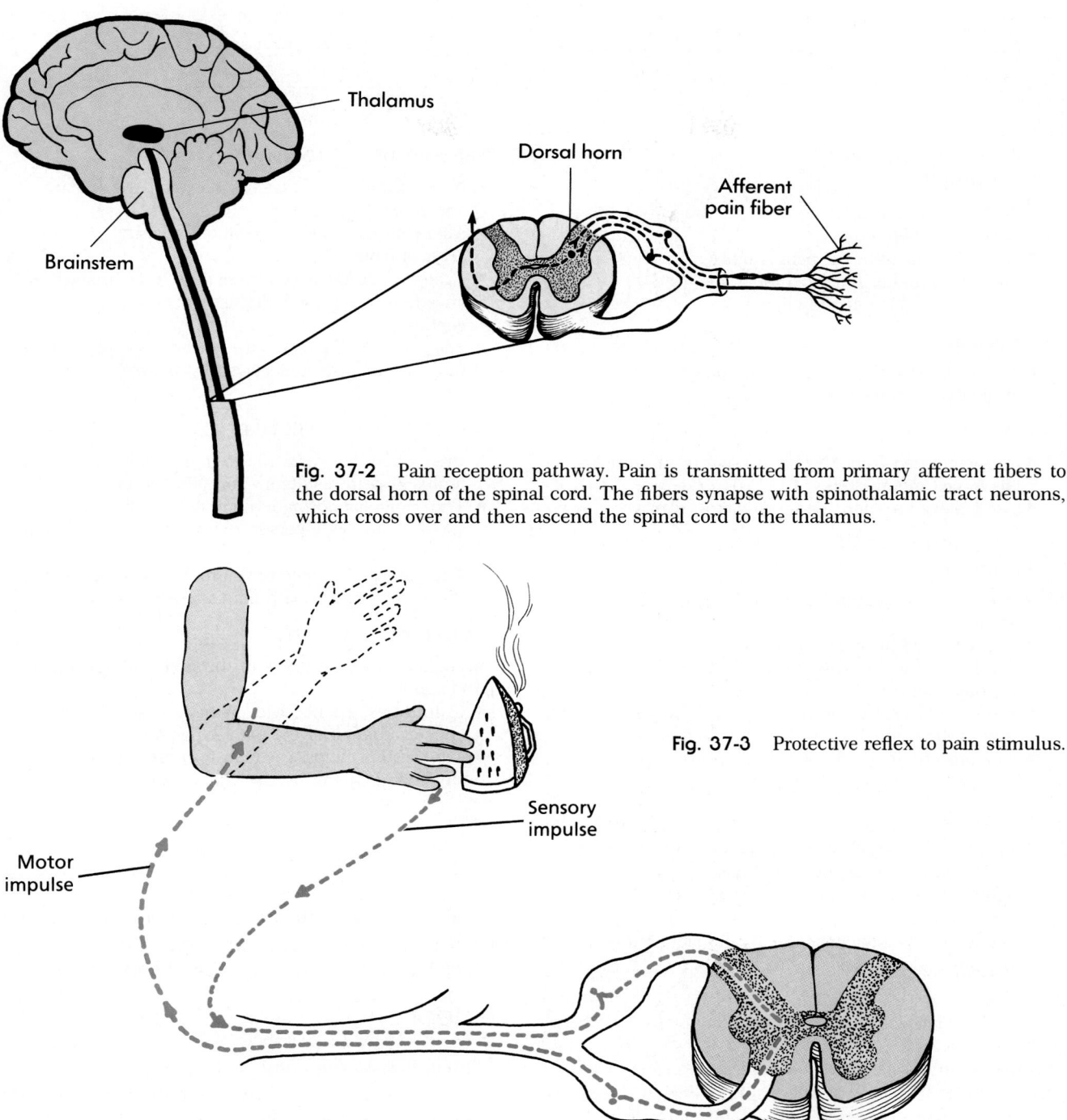

Fig. 37-2   Pain reception pathway. Pain is transmitted from primary afferent fibers to the dorsal horn of the spinal cord. The fibers synapse with spinothalamic tract neurons, which cross over and then ascend the spinal cord to the thalamus.

Fig. 37-3   Protective reflex to pain stimulus.

suggests that pain impulses can be regulated or even blocked by gating mechanisms along the central nervous system. The proposed location of the gates is in the dorsal horn of the spinal cord. Further findings have suggested that other gates exist (Melzack, Dennis, 1978). When gates are open, pain impulses flow freely. When gates are closed, pain impulses become blocked. Partial opening of the gates may also occur.

Small C fibers carry most potentially painful impulses. Excitation of C fibers inhibits gating mechanisms so that pain stimuli flow easily to cortical centers of the brain. Large A fibers pass through the same gating mechanisms. Whether the gates remain open or closed depends on whether competing passages from larger nerve fibers stimulate the gating mechanism. A bombardment of large-fiber sensory

Neurophysiology of Pain: Neuroregulators

NEUROTRANSMITTERS
Substance P

- Is found in the pain neurons of the dorsal horn (excitatory peptide)
- Is needed to transmit pain impulses from the periphery to higher brain centers
- Causes vasodilation and edema

Serotonin

- Is released from the brainstem and dorsal horn to inhibit pain transmission

Prostaglandins

- Are generated from the breakdown of phospholipids in cell membranes
- Are believed to increase sensitivity to pain

NEUROMODULATORS
Endorphins

- Are the body's natural supply of morphinelike substances
- Are activated by stress and pain
- Are located within the brain, spinal cord, and gastrointestinal tract
- Cause analgesia when they attach to opiate receptors in the brain
- Are present in higher levels in people who have less pain than others with a similar injury

Bradykinin

- Is released from plasma that leaks from surrounding blood vessels at the site of tissue injury
- Binds to receptors on peripheral nerves, increasing pain stimuli
- Binds to cells that cause the chain reaction producing prostaglandins

Interactional Systems of Pain Perception

SENSORY-DISCRIMINATIVE

- Nerve transmission occurs between the thalamus and sensory cortex.
- A person perceives the location, severity, and character of pain.
- Factors that lower consciousness (e.g., analgesics, anesthetics, cerebral disease) decrease pain perception.
- Factors that increase the awareness of stimuli (e.g., anxiety, sleep deprivation) increase pain perception.

MOTIVATIONAL-AFFECTIVE

- Interaction between the reticular formation and limbic system results in pain perception.
- The reticular formation creates a defensive response, causing a person to interrupt or avoid pain stimuli.
- The limbic system controls emotional response and the ability to cope with pain.

COGNITIVE-EVALUATIVE

- Higher cortical centers in the brain influence perception.
- Culture, experience with pain, and emotions influence evaluation of the pain experience.
- This system helps a person to interpret the intensity and quality of pain so that action can be taken.

The gate-control theory gives the nurse a conceptual basis for pain-relief measures. However, some studies have failed to support the theory.

Perception

Perception is the point at which a person experiences pain. Pain stimuli are transmitted up the spinal cord to the thalamus and midbrain. From the thalamus, fibers transmit the pain message to various areas of the brain, including the sensory cortex and association cortex (both in the parietal lobe), the frontal lobe, and the limbic system (Fields, 1987). After nerve transmission ends within the higher brain centers, a person actually perceives the sensation of pain.

There is an interaction of psychological and cognitive factors with neurophysiological ones in the perception of pain. Meinhart and McCaffery (1983) de-

impulses such as those from the pressure of a backrub or the heat of a warm compress closes the gates to pain stimuli. Transmission of pain impulses from the spinal cord to the cerebral cortex can be inhibited or facilitated, thus altering pain perception.

It is also believed that the reticular formation in the brainstem can send inhibitory signals to gating mechanisms. When there is excess sensory input (for example, with pain), the reticular formation can close gates. Some clients can be distracted from pain by removing the sensation of pain from their center of attention. Auditory or visual stimuli can distract clients and help make pain more tolerable.

TABLE 37-2 Physiological Reactions to Pain	
Response	Cause or Effect
SYMPATHETIC STIMULATION*	
Dilation of bronchial tubes and increased respiratory rate	Provides greater oxygen intake
Increased heart rate	Provides greater oxygen transport
Peripheral vasoconstriction (pallor, elevation in blood pressure)	Elevates blood pressure with shift of blood supply from periphery and viscera to skeletal muscles and brain
Increased blood glucose level	Provides additional energy
Diaphoresis	Controls body temperature during stress
Increased muscle tension	Prepares muscles for action
Dilation of pupils	Affords better vision
Decreased gastrointestinal motility	Frees energy for more immediate activity
PARASYMPATHETIC STIMULATION†	
Pallor	Causes blood supply to shift away from periphery
Muscle tension	Results from fatigue
Decreased heart rate and blood pressure	Results from vagal stimulation
Rapid, irregular breathing	Causes body defenses to fail under prolonged stress of pain
Nausea and vomiting	Causes return of gastrointestinal function
Weakness or exhaustion	Results from expenditure of physical energy

*Pain of low to moderate intensity and superficial pain.
†Severe or deep pain.

scribe three interactional systems of pain perception as sensory-discriminative, motivational-affective, and cognitive-evaluative (see box).

The gate-control theory suggests that gating mechanisms can also be altered by thoughts, feelings, and memories. The cerebral cortex and thalamus can influence whether pain impulses reach a person's consciousness. The realization that, in a sense, there is conscious control over pain perception helps explain the different ways people react and adjust to pain.

Reaction

The reaction to pain is the physiological and behavioral responses that occur after pain is perceived.

Physiological Responses

As pain impulses ascend the spinal cord toward the brainstem and thalamus, the autonomic nervous system becomes stimulated as part of the stress response. Pain of low to moderate intensity and superficial pain elicit the "flight-or-fight" reaction of the general adaptation syndrome (see Chapter 30). Stimulation of the sympathetic branch of the autonomic nervous system results in physiological responses (Table 37-2). If the pain is unrelenting, severe, or deep, typically originating from involvement of the visceral organs (such as with a myocardial infarction and colic from gallbladder or renal stones), the para-

sympathetic nervous system goes into action. Sustained physiological responses to pain could cause serious harm to an individual. Except in cases of severe traumatic pain, which may send a person into shock, most people reach a level of adaptation in which physical signs return to normal. Thus a client in pain will not always exhibit physical signs.

Behavioral Responses

Meinhart and McCaffery (1983) describe three phases of a pain experience: anticipation, sensation, and aftermath. The anticipation phase occurs before pain is perceived. A person knows that pain will occur. The anticipation phase is perhaps most important, becuase it can affect the other two. In situations of traumatic injury or unforeseen painful procedures a person will not anticipate pain.

Anticipation of pain often allows a person to learn about pain and its relief. With adequate instruction and support, clients learn to understand pain and control anxiety before it occurs. Nurses play an important role in helping clients during the anticipatory phase. With proper guidance, clients become aware of the unknown and thus cope with their discomfort. In situations in which clients are too fearful or anxious, anticipation of pain can heighten the perception of pain severity.

Sensation of pain occurs when pain is felt. The ways that people choose to react to discomfort vary widely. A person's **tolerance** of pain is the point at which there is an unwillingness to accept pain of greater severity or duration. The extent to which a person tolerates pain depends on attitudes, motivation, and values.

Pain threatens physical and psychological well-being. Clients may choose not to express pain, considering it a sign of weakness. Often clients believe that being a "good client" means not expressing pain to avoid bothering people around them. In addition, clients may not express pain because maintaining self-control is important in their culture. The client with high pain tolerance is able to endure periods of severe pain without assistance. Often a nurse must encourage such a client to accept pain-relieving measures so that activity or nutritional intake is not seriously curtailed.

In contrast, a client with low pain tolerance may seek relief before pain occurs. For example, a client may request an aspirin in anticipation of a headache. The client's ability to tolerate pain significantly influences the nurse's perceptions of degree of the discomfort. Often the nurse is willing to attend to the client whose pain tolerance is high. Yet it is unfair to ignore the needs of the client who cannot tolerate even minor pain.

Typical body movements and facial expressions that indicate pain include holding the painful part, bent posture, and grimaces. A client may cry or moan. Often a client expresses discomfort through restlessness and frequent requests to the nurse. The nurse soon learns to recognize patterns of behavior that reflect pain. However, lack of pain expression does not necessarily mean that the client is not expe-

riencing pain. Unless a client openly reacts to pain, it is difficult to determine the nature and extent of the discomfort. The nurse helps the client communicate the pain response effectively. Knowledge of the disease or illness helps the nurse anticipate the client's pain. For example, a ruptured intravertebral disk in a lower lumbar vertebra typically causes severe low-back pain and pain that radiates or extends down the leg. Table 37-3 summarizes common disorders that cause pain.

The aftermath phase of pain occurs when it is reduced or stopped. Even though the source of discomfort is controlled, a client may still require the nurse's attention. Pain is a crisis. After a painful experience clients may experience physical symptoms such as chills, nausea, vomiting, anger, or depression. If there are repeated episodes of pain, aftermath responses can become serious health problems. The nurse helps clients gain control and self-esteem to minimize fear over potential pain experiences.

Matching Physiological Conditions with Pain Therapies

It helps for the nurse to understand the effect of therapies on the human body. In the case of pain relief, several treatment options are available. Use of a combination of therapies may bring relief of pain, especially if several different physiological actions are used.

Nonsteroidal antiinflammatory drugs (NSAIDS) act by inhibiting the action of the enzyme that forms prostaglandin (Paice, 1991). With less prostaglandin released peripherally, the generation of pain stimuli is blocked. A reduction in pain sensitivity also occurs.

Neurotransmitters and opiate receptors are located in the dorsal horn of the spinal cord. Administration of opiates such as morphine results in the opiates binding to receptors and inhibiting the release of substance P. As a result, transmission of painful stimuli to the spinal cord is blocked. Opiates may be given orally, intramuscularly, or epidurally.

The administration of tricyclic antidepressants such as amitriptyline and imipramine creates an analgesic effect, as well as an antidepressant effect. The tricyclics inhibit the normal reuptake of serotonin at nerve terminals (Paice, 1991). With more serotonin present in nerve terminals, pain transmission is inhibited.

Spinothalamic nerve tracts are localized in a region of the spinal cord. Because of the nerve tract location, surgeons can **ablate,** or remove, the nerves and reduce pain isolated to one side of the body. The procedure is called a *cordotomy* and is generally used only in clients with a limited expected life span.

TABLE 37-3 Common Disorders That Cause Pain	
Disorder	Pain Characteristics
Kidney disease	Abdominal aching
Angina pectoris	Tenderness and pain in back area of costovertebral angle
	Crushing sensation in chest, often radiating down left shoulder and arm
Ruptured intravertebral disk	Low-back pain accompanied by pain radiating down leg
Gastric ulcer	Burning pain around umbilicus, referred pain in shoulder
Trigeminal neuralgia	Lightning-like or stabbing pain along distribution of trigeminal nerve, involving gums, lips, mouth, nose, and chin

ACUTE AND CHRONIC PAIN

Everyone experiences some level of pain throughout the day. Common examples include the ache of overexercised muscles, the burning discomfort from eye strain, and pressure from sitting in one position for too long. These minor discomforts rarely cause a person to seek health care.

The pain that nurses most often observe in clients includes three types: acute, chronic malignant, and chronic nonmalignant (National Institutes of Health, 1986; Engber, 1986). Acute pain follows acute injury, disease, or types of surgery and has a rapid onset, varying in intensity (mild to severe) and lasting for a brief time (Meinhart, McCaffery, 1983; NIH, 1986). The function of acute pain is to warn persons of impending injury or disease. Acute pain eventually resolves with or without treatment after a damaged area heals.

Clients in acute pain are frightened and anxious and expect relief quickly. The time sequence of acute pain usually results in a willingness by health team members to treat acute pain aggressively. However, conflict between nurse and client may arise if the nurse does not provide quick relief. Acute pain is self-limiting and the client therefore knows an end is in sight.

Acute pain seriously threatens a client's recovery and should be one of the nurse's priorities of care. For example, acute postoperative pain hampers the client's ability to become active and increases the risk of complications from immobility (see Chapter 43). Rehabilitation may be delayed and hospitalization may be prolonged if acute pain is not controlled. There cannot be physical or psychological progress as long as it persists because the client focuses all interests on pain relief. The nurse's efforts at teaching and motivating the client toward self-care will be useless. After pain is relieved, the client and health care team can direct full attention toward recovery.

Chronic pain is prolonged, varies in intensity, and usually lasts more than 6 months (McCaffery, 1986). Chronic pain caused by uncontrolled cancer or other progressive disorders is called *intractable pain (malignant pain)*. It can be prolonged until death.

Chronic nonmalignant pain results in persons whose tissue injury is nonprogressive or healed but whose pain is ongoing and often does not respond to treatment. Frequently the cause for nonmalignant pain is unknown. An injured area may have healed long ago. Yet pain persists. In chronic pain, endorphins often cease to function (Meinhart, McCaffery, 1983). An example of chronic nonmalignant pain is low-back pain.

Health care workers usually are willing to treat chronic malignant pain as aggressively as acute pain. In contrast, treatment for nonmalignant pain may not be as aggressive. If the cause of pain is unclear, care givers may question the severity of a client's discomfort. For clients with cancer, family members are often unwilling to administer needed narcotics for fear of causing side effects such as lethargy and drug dependence.

The client with chronic pain often has periods of **remissions** (partial or complete disappearance of symptoms) and **exacerbations** (increase in severity). The unpredictability of chronic pain frustrates the client, frequently leading to psychological depression. The pain becomes part of every aspect of life. Chronic pain is a major cause of psychological and physical disability, leading to problems such as loss of job, inability to perform simple daily activities, sexual dysfunction, and social isolation from family and friends.

The person with chronic pain often does not show overt symptoms. The individual does not adapt to the pain but seems to suffer more with time as physical and mental exhaustion occur. Chronic pain creates an insecurity of never knowing how one will feel from day to day. Symptoms of chronic pain include fatigue, insomnia, anorexia, weight loss, depression, hopelessness, and anger.

The life of a person with chronic pain can be tragic. Often the person consults many physicians and therefore accumulates various medications and therapies. However, taking several medications may result in undesirable side effects. Clients desperate for pain relief may fall prey to quackery (for example, special liniments, diets, or pain-relief devices). Alcohol abuse may become another alternative. Fortunately, pain clinics are available throughout the United States and Canada to help clients find more acceptable methods of pain control. Physicians and other health care providers understand pain better and offer therapies other than pharmacological remedies such as exercise and biofeedback.

Caring for the client with chronic pain is an unusual challenge. The nurse should not become frustrated when relief measures fail. Likewise, the nurse should not offer false hope for a cure. The nurse's primary goal may be to reduce the client's perception of pain.

FACTORS INFLUENCING PAIN

Because pain is complex, numerous factors influence an individual's pain experience (Fig. 37-4). The

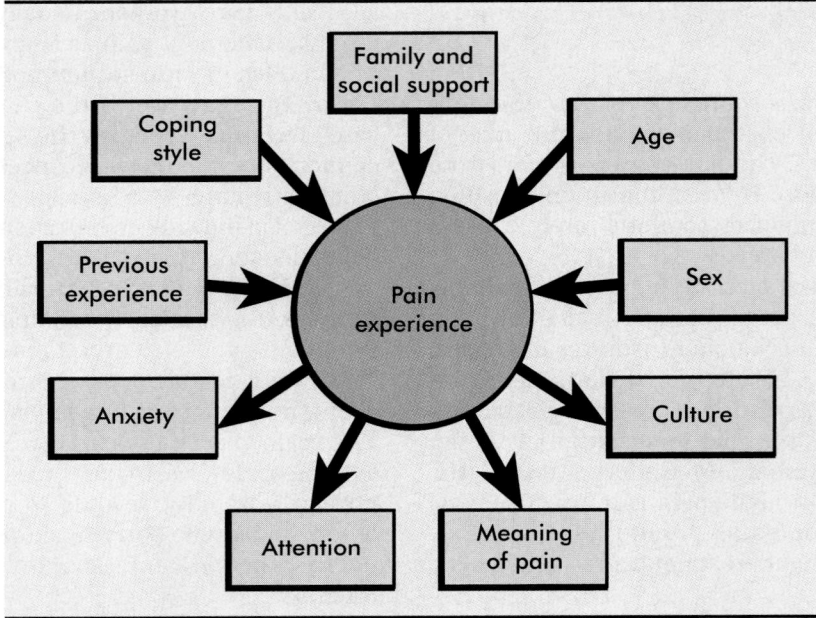

Fig. 37-4 Factors that influence the pain experience. From Gil K: *Anesthesiol Report* 2(2):246, 1990.

nurse considers all factors that affect the client in pain. This is necessary to obtain an accurate assessment of the client's pain and to select appropriate pain therapies.

Age

Age is an important variable that influences pain, particularly in children and older adults. Developmental differences found among these age groups can influence how children and the older adult react to the pain experience. Young children have difficulty understanding pain and the procedures nurses administer that may cause pain. Young children who have not developed full vocabularies also have difficulty verbally describing and expressing pain to parents or care givers. Cognitively, toddlers or preschoolers are unable to recall explanations about pain or associate pain as experiences that can occur in various situations.

A nurse must use simple but appropriate communication techniques to help children understand and describe pain. For example, asking children, "Tell me where you hurt" or "What helps to take away the hurt?" can help accurately assess pain. The nurse may also show a series of pictures depicting different facial expressions, such as smiling, frowning, or crying. Children may point to the picture that best describes how they feel.

Pain is not an inevitable part of aging. However, an older client can suffer serious impairment of functional status as a result of pain. Mobility, self-care activities, socialization outside the home, and activity tolerance can all be reduced. It is difficult for a client with cognitive impairment to recall pain experiences and provide detailed explanations.

The ability of older clients to interpret pain can be complicated by the presence of multiple diseases with vague symptoms that may affect similar parts of the body. When older clients have more than one source of pain, a nurse must gather detailed assessments. The manifestations of different diseases can cause an atypical presentation of painful conditions. In other words, different diseases can cause similar symptoms. For example, chest pain does not always indicate a myocardial infarction or heart attack. Instead, chest pain can be a symptom of arthritis of the spine, herpes zoster infection, and abdominal disorders (Zoob, 1978).

Herr and Mobily (1991) note that older clients may not report pain for the following reasons:
1. Older clients may believe that pain is something they must live with. Because care givers and children believe that pain is a natural result of aging, complaints are often ignored. This angers the older clients, who in turn decide not to report pain.
2. Older clients may deny pain because of fear of unknown consequences. They have considerable fear of the loss of independence. Admitting to pain can also lead to unpleasant and expensive diagnostic and therapeutic measures.

3. Older clients may choose not to admit having pain for fear of serious illness or death.
4. Older clients use different terminology to describe the pain experience. Terms such as *discomfort, ache,* or *hurt* are used instead to deny that pain exists.
5. Many older clients believe that it is not acceptable to show pain. Often older clients use a variety of mechanisms to distract attention from pain (McCaffery, Beebe, 1989).

Sex

Generally, men and women do not differ significantly in their responses to pain (Gil, 1990). It is doubtful whether gender by itself is a factor in the expression of pain. There are cultural influences on gender (for example, making it appropriate for a little boy to be brave and not cry, whereas a little girl in the same situation is allowed to cry). Pain tolerance has been the subject of research involving men and women. Burns et al (1989) studied postoperative narcotic requirements in clients undergoing abdominal surgery. Male clients required significantly more morphine than the female clients to achieve similar levels of pain relief.

Culture

Culture influences how people learn to react to and express pain. People respond to pain in different ways. The nurse must never assume to know how clients will respond. However, an understanding of cultural background, socioeconomic status, and personal attributes helps the nurse more accurately assess pain and its meaning for clients.

Many studies describe the influence of culture on the pain experience. Miller and Shuter (1982) found that European Americans expressed pain more often than African Americans. The same was true for clients over 40 years of age compared with younger clients. Several studies have shown that more educated and affluent clients respond quicker to symptoms and seek medical care for conditions that persons in lower social classes ignore. Expression of pain by children in different cultures also varies. For example, Eskimo children learn to laugh in response to pain, and Chinese children learn to respond favorably to surgery, whereas American children view hospitalization as traumatic (Ross, Ross, 1988). Nurses must learn that there are ways to respond to pain other than their own. Assessment of cultural influences on the way clients respond or react to pain assists in determining the significance of pain to clients and measures that will be effective in providing relief.

Meaning of Pain

The meaning that a person associates with pain affects the experience of pain. A person will perceive pain differently if it suggests a threat, loss, punishment, or challenge. For example, a woman in labor will perceive pain differently from a woman experiencing pain from a recent back injury. The degree and quality of pain perceived by a client are related to the meaning of pain. A client copes differently with pain, depending on its meaning.

Attention

The degree to which a client focuses on pain can influence pain perception. Increased attention has been associated with increased pain, whereas distraction has been associated with a diminished pain response (Gil, 1990). This concept is one that nurses apply in various pain-relief therapies such as relaxation, guided imagery, and massage. By focusing a client's attention and concentration on other stimuli, the nurse places pain on the periphery of awareness. Usually, this results in an increased tolerance for pain that lasts only during the time of distraction (McCaffery, 1986).

Anxiety

The relationship between pain and anxiety is complex. Anxiety often increases perception of pain, but pain may also cause feelings of anxiety. Autonomic arousal patterns are similar in pain and anxiety (Gil, 1990). It is difficult to separate the two sensations. Emotionally healthy persons are usually able to tolerate moderate or even severe pain better than those whose emotions are less stable. Research suggests that anxiety may be a major influence in how pain is perceived by cancer clients (Spiegel, Bloom, 1983; Twycross, Lack, 1983). Endorphins may cause differences in sensitivity to pain. In some persons, anxiety over pain may release endorphins.

Fatigue

Fatigue heightens perception of pain. This intensifies pain and decreases coping abilities. Pain is often experienced less after a restful sleep than at the end of a long day.

Previous Experience

Each person learns from painful experiences. Previous experience does not necessarily mean that a person will accept pain more easily in the future. If a person has had frequent episodes of pain without relief or bouts of severe pain, anxiety or even fear may recur. In contrast, if a person has had repeated experiences with the same type of pain but the pain has successfully been relieved, it becomes easier to interpret the pain sensation. As a result, the client is better prepared to take necessary actions in relieving the pain.

When a client has had no experience with pain, the first perception of it can impair the ability to cope with it. For example, after abdominal surgery, it is common for a client to experience severe incisional pain for several days. Unless the client is aware of this, the onset of pain may be viewed as a serious complication. Rather than participate actively in postoperative breathing exercises (see Chapter 47), the client may lie immobile in bed and maintain shallow breathing because of fear that something has gone wrong. The nurse should prepare the client with a clear explanation of the type of pain that will be experienced and methods to reduce it.

Coping Style

The experience of pain can be lonely. When clients experience pain in health care settings such as hospitals, the loneliness can be unbearable. Frequently, clients feel a loss of control and an inability to control their environments or the outcome of events. Coping style thus influences the ability to deal with pain.

Persons with internal loci of control perceive themselves as having personal control over their environments and the outcome of events, such as pain (Gil, 1990). In contrast, persons with external loci of control perceive other factors in their environments, such as nurses, as being responsible for the outcome of events. Individuals with an internal loci of control report less severe pain than those with external loci Schultheis et al, 1987). This concept is applied in the use of patient-controlled analgesia (PCA). Clients who are able to self-administer small doses of intravenous pain medication during an acute episode successfully achieve pain control more quickly than those who rely on nurses to administer intermittent doses of pain medications.

Pain may cause partial or total disability. Clients often find various ways to cope with the physical and psychological effects of pain. It is important to understand a client's coping resources during a painful experience. These resources, such as communicating with a supportive family, exercise, or singing, can be used in the nurse's care plan to support the client and offer a degree of pain relief.

Coping resources are more than just methods or techniques. A client may depend on the emotional support of a spouse, children, other family members, or friends. Although pain still exists, the presence of a loved one can minimize loneliness and fear. A client's religious beliefs can also provide comfort. Reading scriptures or saying a prayer gives many individuals an inner strength to cope more effectively with discomfort. Being actively involved in household chores or other work can be another mechanism for coping.

Family and Social Support

Another factor that can significantly affect pain response is the presence and attitudes of significant others. Persons of different sociocultural groups have different expectations of people to whom they complain about pain (Meinhart, McCaffery, 1983). People in pain often depend on family members for support, assistance, or protection. An absence of family or friends can often make the pain experience more stressful. The presence of parents is especially important for children experiencing pain.

 ## NURSING PROCESS AND PAIN

For the nurse to understand a client's pain and to provide appropriate therapies, there is a need for a systematic approach to pain management. The nursing process is a model for ensuring accurate analysis and management of pain.

 ## Assessment

Accurate pain assessment is critical for judging clients' progress, arriving at proper nursing diagnoses, and selecting appropriate therapies. Although pain assessment is one of the most common activities a nurse performs, it is one of the most difficult. The key to assessing pain is not ignoring the client. The nurse must explore the pain experience through the eyes of the client. Nurses cannot allow personal biases to prejudice assessment of pain (see research highlight). Viewing the pain from the client's perspective enables the nurse to make a more accurate assessment. It is important also to carefully interpret pain cues and remember that psychological and physical components of pain influence the reaction to it.

When assessing pain, the nurse must be sensitive to the client's level of discomfort. If pain is acute or severe, it is unlikely that the client can provide a detailed description of the entire experience. During an episode of acute pain the nurse primarily assesses how the client feels, determining physiological re-

A nurse's attitudes toward clients and the assessment of client suffering influences whether a client experiences acute or chronic pain. A study of 232 nurses representing eight different hospitals was conducted to determine the extent to which pain duration, psychological symptoms, and physical pathological condition influence a nurse's assessment and treatment choices. The nurses represented a variety of specialty areas and a range of educational and work experience. Each nurse completed a questionnaire containing vignettes of three types of hospital clients (those with low-back pain, headache, or joint pain). After reading the vignettes, nurses were asked to estimate the amount of pain they believed a client to be suffering. The nurses were also asked to complete a list of potential pain-relief actions that might be performed on behalf of the hypothetical clients.Finally, the nurses rated clients on personality and behavioral traits based on information from the vignettes.

Findings from the study revealed that nurses assessed significantly less pain in the hypothetical client when findings of physical pathological conditions were negative than when they were positive. In addition, nurses assessed significantly less pain in clients described as suffering from chronic pain than those suffering acute pain. In terms of attitudes assigned to clients, the client with chronic back pain was perceived less positively than clients with chronic joint or acute headache pain.

Among the choices of therapies on the questionnaire, nurses chose information-seeking or assessment actions (e.g., observing nonverbal behavior) most often.

Implications from the study suggest that nurses may treat acute and chronic pain sufferers quite differently regardless of the intensity of pain. Nurses must understand chronic pain. There is no reason to assume that an individual who has suffered from pain for a long time experiences less suffering than someone whose pain is acute and of short duration.

Taylor AG et al: Duration of pain, condition, and physical pathology as determinants of nurses' assessment of patients in pain, *Nurs Res* 33(1):4, 1984.

Possible Sources of Error in Pain Assessment

- Bias, which causes nurses to consistently overestimate or underestimate the pain that clients experience
- Vague or unclear assessment questions, which lead to unreliable assessment data
- Use of pain assessment tools that have not been proved reliable and valid with identical clients (A reliable assessment tool focuses only on pain cues that provide a reliable measure of relevant clinical changes.)
- Clients who do not always provide complete, pertinent, and accurate pain information
- Clients who may lack sufficient medical knowledge to be able to select information to help medical and nursing staff make decisions about the pain

pain, assessment should include level of function because it may not be possible to achieve complete pain relief. Numerous factors can cause errors in assessment (see box). The nurse should be aware of these factors and adapt assessment strategies to avoid error (Harrison, 1991). Some factors deal with the nature of the pain experience, and others deal with the types of assessment cues available for nurses and physicians.

Client's Expression of Pain

Many clients fail to report or discuss discomfort. In a study by Jacox and Stewart (1973), two thirds of the 72 clients studied were reluctant to discuss pain and tried instead to remain calm and silent. To complicate pain assessment, many nurses believe that clients will report pain if they have it. This is not always true.

Clients must trust a nurse and perceive the nurse's willingness to help before discussing pain experience openly. If clients sense that the nurse doubts that pain exists, they will share little information. The nurse must develop positive therapeutic relationships and give clients time to discuss pain. Attempting to find comfortable positions for clients before asking questions may help clients sense the nurse's interest. The nurse avoids aggravating pain with a lengthy assessment.

The nurse should learn the client's method of communicating discomfort. The nurse determines whether the client can communicate verbally or whether nonverbal behaviors will be the best source

sponses to pain and the location, severity, and quality of the pain. A more thorough pain assessment takes time and should be conducted when the client becomes more alert and attentive.

For clients with chronic pain, assessment may best be focused on affective and evaluative aspects of the pain experience and on its history and context (NIH, 1986). In the case of chronic nonmalignant

of information. If the client speaks a different language, pain assessment will be difficult. A family member or interpreter may be necessary to describe the client's feelings and sensations. Often a client in pain confides in only one person.

Classification of the Pain Experience

It can help to know the phase of pain clients are undergoing. The phase—anticipatory, sensation, or aftermath—influences not only clients' symptoms but also the types of therapies most likely to relieve pain. Clients likely to be in the anticipatory phase include those scheduled to undergo invasive diagnostic or therapeutic procedures or surgery and those with histories of recurring pain such as the anginal pain of myocardial ischemia. These clients may be anxious or fearful, or they may ask questions about upcoming pain.

Clients in the sensation phase generally demonstrate signs and symptoms of discomfort. Clients with traumatic injuries and clients who have had surgery are uncomfortable, so the nurse should not ask several detailed questions. Clients who are sensing pain, especially severe pain, want relief fast. After the pain has been relieved, the nurse must assess carefully for physical and psychological effects. Clients may later express apologies to the nurse for acting "improperly" during the pain experience.

The nurse assesses whether the client's pain is acute or chronic. If the pain is acute, a detailed assessment of pain characteristics is needed. With chronic pain the nurse determines whether it is intermittent, persistent, or of limited duration. After the phase or type of pain is assessed, findings direct the nurse to conduct further assessment for eventual determination of specific interventions.

Characteristics of Pain

The nature of the pain experience provides more detailed information for the nurse. Assessment data help establish medical and nursing diagnoses and determine pain relief therapies.

ONSET AND DURATION. The nurse asks questions to determine the onset, duration, and time sequence of pain. The nurse asks when the pain began, how long it has lasted, whether it occurs at the same time each day, and how frequently it recurs.

It may be easier to diagnose the nature of pain by identifying time factors. For example, certain types of headaches can be characterized by the time of day when they occur. The onset of sudden and severe pain is easier to assess than gradual, mild discomfort. An understanding of the time cycle of pain helps the nurse know when to intervene before the pain occurs or worsens (Table 37-4).

TABLE 37-4 Implications of Pain Assessment for Nursing Interventions	
Assessment Criteria	Nursing Interventions
Onset and duration	Administer analgesics so that peak action occurs when pain is most acute (e.g., during dressing change or exercise therapy).
Location	Position client off affected area. Apply local treatments (e.g., elastic bandage and splinting) directly over painful site.
Severity	Change or revise interventions, depending on success of one intervention.
Precipitating or aggravating factors	Avoid activities that cause or aggravate pain. Teach client or family to avoid same activities.
Relief measures	Use measures that client uses to relieve pain, as long as they are safe and appropriate.

LOCATION. To assess pain location the nurse asks the client to point to all areas of discomfort. To localize the pain more specifically, the nurse then has the client trace the area from the most severe point outward. This is difficult to do if pain is diffuse, involves several sites, or involves large segments of the body. Some assessment tools have figures of the body (Fig. 37-5) on which the nurse can draw the location of the pain. This can be useful as a baseline if the pain should change.

When recording pain location, the nurse uses anatomical landmarks and descriptive terminology. The statement "The pain is localized in the upper right abdominal quadrant" is more specific than "The client states the pain is in the abdomen." Knowing a client's disease or illness can help the nurse locate pain more easily. Pain, classified by location, may be superficial or cutaneous, deep or visceral, or referred or radiating (Table 37-5).

SEVERITY. The most subjective characteristic of pain may be its severity, or intensity. Clients are often asked to describe pain as mild, moderate, or severe. However, the meaning of these terms differs for the nurse and client. This type of information is also difficult to verify over time.

Descriptive scales are a more objective means of measuring pain severity (Fig. 37-6). A verbal descriptor scale (VDS) consists of a line with three- to five-word descriptors equally spaced along the line. The descriptors are ranked from "No pain" to "Unbearable pain." The word chosen by a client determines the

TABLE 37-5   Classification of Pain by Location

Definition	Characteristics	Examples
SUPERFICIAL OR CUTANEOUS		
Pain resulting from stimulation of skin	Pain is of short duration and is localized. It usually is sharp sensation.	Needlestick; small cut or laceration
DEEP VISCERAL		
Pain resulting from stimulation of internal organs	Pain is diffuse and may radiate in several directions. Duration varies but it usually lasts longer than superficial pain. Pain may be sharp, dull, or unique to organ involved.	Crushing sensation (e.g., angina pectoris); burning sensation (e.g., gastric ulcer)
REFERRED		
Common phenomenon in visceral pain because many organs themselves have no pain receptors; entrance of sensory neurons from affected organ into same spinal cord segment as neurons from areas where pain is felt; perception of pain in unaffected areas	Pain is felt in part of body separate from source of pain and may assume any characteristic.	Myocardial infarction, which may cause referred pain to jaw, left arm, and left shoulder; kidney stones, which may refer pain to groin
RADIATING		
Sensation of pain extending from initial site of injury to another body part	Pain feels as though it travels down or along body part. It may be intermittent or constant.	Low-back pain from ruptured intravertebral disk accompanied by pain radiating down leg from sciatic nerve irritation

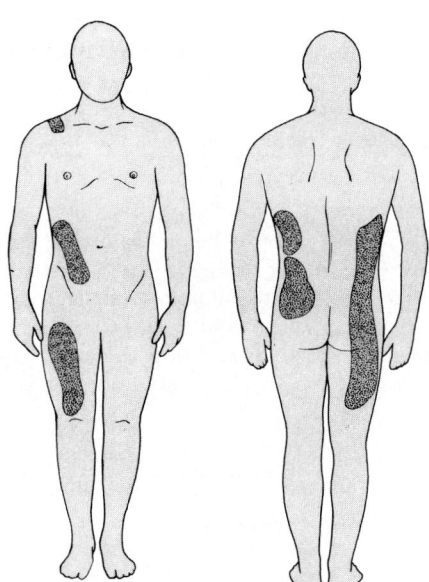

Fig. 37-5   Diagrammatic figures used to locate a client's pain.

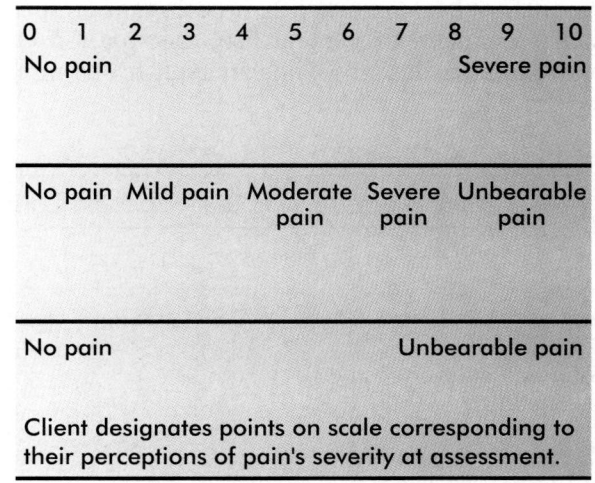

Fig. 37-6   Sample pain scales. **A,** Numerical. **B,** Verbal descriptive. **C,** Visual analog.

intensity of painful sensation. Numbers may also be used on scales instead of word descriptors. The VDS enables a client to choose a category for describing pain. The scale works best when assessing the intensity of pain before and after therapeutic interventions (McGuire, 1984).

A visual analog scale does not have labeled subdivisions. It consists of a straight line, representing a continuum of intensity, and has verbal descriptors at each end. This scale gives the client total freedom in identifying severity of pain. The visual analog scale may be a more sensitive measure of pain severity because clients mark at any point on the continuum rather than being forced to choose one word (McGuire, 1984).

A pain scale should be designed so that it is easy for the nurse to administer and is not time consuming for the client to complete. If the client can easily understand the scale, the description should be more accurate. Descriptive scales are useful not only in assessing the severity of pain but also in evaluating changes in condition. The nurse can use the scales after therapy or when symptoms become aggravated to judge whether the pain has decreased or increased.

The nurse does not use pain scales to compare one client with another. Although the scales lend relative objectivity to measurement, the severity of pain is too subjective to permit comparisons between individuals.

QUALITY. Another subjective characteristic of pain is its quality. Because there is no common or specific pain vocabulary in general use, the words a client may choose to describe pain can apply to any number of things. Often, a client describes pain as crushing, throbbing, sharp, or dull. A client's pain is often indescribable.

The nurse should not provide descriptive words for a client. Assessment is more accurate if a client can describe the sensation after open-ended questions. For example, the nurse might say, "Tell me what your pain feels like." The only time that the nurse offers to list descriptive terms is when the client cannot describe pain. Meinhart and McCaffery (1983) report that the qualities of pricking, burning, and aching are useful to describe pain initially. Later the client may choose more descriptive terms.

There is some consistency in the way people describe certain types of pain. The pain associated with a myocardial infarction is often described as *crushing* or *viselike*, whereas the pain of a surgical incision is often described as *sharp* and *stabbing*. When the client's descriptions fit the pattern forming in the nurse's assessment, a clearer analysis can be made of the nature and type of pain.

PAIN PATTERN. Various factors can affect the character of pain. It helps to assess specific events or conditions that precipitate or aggravate pain (Table 37-6). The nurse may ask the client to demonstrate actions that elicit painful response such as coughing or ambulating. Body functions or movement may cause variation in the character of pain (Adams, 1980). After the nurse identifies precipitating or aggravating factors, it is easier to plan interventions to avoid worsening the pain.

Relief Measures. It is useful to know whether a client has an effective way for relieving pain such as changing position, eating, or applying heat to the

TABLE 37-6   Patterns of Pain for Specific Conditions

Condition	Pain Pattern*
Angina pectoris (insufficient blood flow through coronary arteries)	Physical exertion, emotional stress, exposure to cold temperature, eating large meal
Ruptured intravertebral disk	Bending over or stretching, lifting objects
Gastric ulcer	Tension, going to work, coffee or liquor ingestion
Urinary tract infection	Micturition (urinating)
Gallbladder inflammation	Eating foods high in fat content
Appendicitis	Sudden jarring or vibration of bed while lying down
Pharyngitis (sore throat)	Swallowing, talking
Peripheral vascular disease (insufficient blood flow to extremities)	Exercise (walking or running)
External otitis (inflammation of outer ear canal)	Rubbing or scratching ear canal, excessive drying of skin
Pleuritis (inflammation of pleura)	Inhaling deeply and coughing

*Precipitating and aggravating factors.

painful site. The client's methods often work best for the nurse, too. Clients gain comfort from knowing that the nurse is willing to try their relief measures. In the home, the nurse must be sure that relief measures are safely being used. Assessment of relieving factors should also include identification of practitioners (for example, internist, orthopedist, chiropractor, or dentist whose services the client has sought. Clients with chronic pain are more likely to try alternative health care methods.

CONCOMITANT SYMPTOMS. Symptoms that often occur with pain include nausea, headache, dizziness, urination, constipation, and restlessness. Certain types of pain have predictable accompanying symptoms. For example, severe rectal pain often results in constipation. The pain of an inflamed gallbladder or kidney stone frequently causes nausea and vomiting. **Concomitant symptoms** may be as much a treatment priority as the pain itself.

Effects of Pain on the Client

By recognizing the effects of pain on a client, the nurse can identify the nature and existence of the pain.

PHYSICAL SIGNS AND SYMPTOMS. The physiological response to pain can reveal the existence and nature of pain and the potential threat to the client's welfare. When a client experiences discomfort, the nurse should assess vital signs and observe for autonomic nervous system involvement (see Table 37-2). Physiological signs can reveal pain in a client who tries not to complain or admit discomfort. There is no predictable level or extent of change in a client's condition that indicates pain.

The nurse should not confuse signs and symptoms of pain with other behavioral or pathological changes. For example, a client who is highly anxious also exhibits elevated heart and respiratory rates. A client who is seriously dehydrated has an increased pulse because of volume depletion. The nurse considers all signs and symptoms before determining that pain is the cause.

It helps to determine clients at greater risk for having pain. Health status indicates whether pain is an expected symptom. The client who has had surgery and the victim of serious trauma are just two examples of clients who probably experience acute pain.

If pain is unrelieved, the nurse looks for signs of physical exhaustion. Decreasing vital sign values indicate parasympathetic nerve response. The client becomes less responsive to stimuli within the environment. The nurse should measure vital signs more often if the client's condition deteriorates.

BEHAVIORAL EFFECTS. When a client has pain, the nurse assesses verbalization, vocal response, facial and body movements, and social interaction (see box). A verbal report of pain is a vital part of the total assessment. The client's verbalization of pain may depend on the nurse's willingness to listen or understand. Many clients cannot verbalize discomfort because of the inability to communicate. An infant, an unconscious client, a disoriented or confused person, an aphasic person, and a client who speaks a foreign language are unable to explain the pain experience. In these cases, it is especially important for the nurse to be alert for behaviors that indicate pain (see research highlight on p. 1192).

Groaning, grunting, and crying are examples of vocalizations used to express pain. Certain vocalizations may be involuntary and may occur without warning when acute pain occurs. For some clients, vocalizations are culturally acceptable ways to communicate.

Behavioral Indicators of Effects of Pain

VOCALIZATIONS

- Moaning
- Crying
- Screaming
- Gasping
- Grunting

FACIAL EXPRESSIONS

- Grimace
- Clenched teeth
- Wrinkled forehead
- Tightly closed or widely opened eyes or mouth
- Lip biting
- Tightened jaw

BODY MOVEMENT

- Restlessness
- Immobilization
- Muscle tension
- Increased hand and finger movements
- Pacing activities
- Rhythmic or rubbing motions
- Protective movement of body parts

SOCIAL INTERACTION

- Avoidance of conversation
- Focus only on activities for pain relief
- Avoidance of social contacts
- Reduced attention span

Research Highlight

Confused, disoriented, or nonverbal older clients frequently suffer from painful conditions. A sample of 26 clients from the Alzheimer's unit of a large midwestern nursing home was studied for behaviors that indicated pain. Each client's medical record confirmed the presence of a painful disorder such as cancer and degenerative joint disease. A pain assessment was performed on each client by a certified nurse practitioner. Most clients had no pain behaviors despite their diagnosis. Only three clients showed typical pain behaviors. Staff were also surveyed and were able to describe clients' pain behaviors. Clients who normally moaned and rocked became quiet and withdrawn when in pain. Clients who were friendly and outgoing became agitative and combative. Clients who were outgoing and easily involved in activities began to cry easily and withdraw when pain developed. This study showed the need for further research involving nonalert older clients.

Marzinski LR: The tragedy of dementia: clinically assessing pain in the confused, nonverbal elderly, *J Gerontol Nurs* 17(6):25-28, 1991.

Subtle facial expressions or body movements often reveal more about the character of pain than precise questioning. For example, the client may grimace or begin to toss and turn at regular intervals. The amount of restlessness or protective movement may increase as the assessment progresses. The client may also react more uncomfortably while assuming different positions.

Some nonverbal expressions characterize sources of pain. The client with chest pain often grabs or holds the chest. A child or adult with severe abdominal pain often assumes a fetal position. A client with a severe headache may squint or rub the temples. The nonverbal expression of pain may support or contradict other information about pain. If a woman in labor reports that her labor pains are occurring more frequently and if she begins to massage her abdomen more frequently, her report is confirmed. If a client complains of severe abdominal pain but continues to grasp the chest, a more detailed assessment may be necessary.

The nature of pain causes a person to attend to the discomfort and fight it or give in to the discomfort and withdraw socially. The extent to which a client interacts with the environment can provide a clue for the nurse about the intensity or nature of pain. Severe pain can seriously hamper a person's lifestyle.

INFLUENCE ON ACTIVITIES OF DAILY LIVING. Clients who live with daily pain experience changes in their ability to participate in routine activities. Assessment of these changes reveals the extent of the client's disability and adjustments necessary to help clients participate in self-care.

The nurse asks whether pain interferes with sleep. There may be difficulty falling asleep. Sleeping pills or other medications may be needed to induce sleep. The pain may awaken the client during the night, or the client may have insomnia as a result of the pain (see Chapter 36).

Depending on the location of pain, the client may have difficulty performing normal hygiene measures. The nurse determines whether the client can dress independently or shampoo hair. The pain may restrict mobility to the point that the client is no longer able to bathe in a bathtub. The client may have problems performing other activities of daily living. For example, a client with severe arthritis may find it painful to grasp eating utensils. The nurse determines the client's need for assistance with self-care activities. The nurse also considers the need for family members or friends to assist the client with basic hygiene.

Pain can impair the ability to maintain normal sexual relations. Conditions such as arthritis, degenerative diseases of the hip, and chronic back pain make it difficult for a person to assume usual positions during intercourse. When assessing the extent to which pain has affected sexual activity, the nurse determines the frequency of sexual relations before and after the onset of pain. It also helps to learn whether a client is physically unable to participate or if the desire for sexual intercourse has been reduced by the pain.

The ability of people to work can be seriously threatened by pain. The more physical activity required in a job, the greater the risk of discomfort when the pain is associated with musculoskeletal and certain visceral alterations. Pain related to emotional stress is probably increased in individuals whose jobs involve tension-laden decision making. The nurse assesses the work that clients do and their abilities to function in regular jobs. The daily chores of homemakers are assessed in the same manner as the duties involved in jobs outside the home. The nurse assesses whether it is necessary for clients to stop activity occasionally because of pain. Often the nurse can help clients select ways of minimizing or controlling the pain so that they can remain productive.

It is also important to include an assessment of the effect of pain on social activities. The pain may be so debilitating that the client becomes too exhausted to socialize. The nurse identifies the client's normal social activities, the extent to which they have been disrupted, and the clients wish to participate.

Neurological Status

A client's neurological function can easily influence the pain experience. Any factor that interrupts or influences normal pain reception or perception affects the client's awareness and response to pain. For example, a client who has a spinal cord injury, **peripheral neuropathy,** or a neurological disease such as multiple sclerosis or intracerebral lesions is less likely to sense pain compared with a client who has normal neurological function. Some therapies influence pain perception and response. Analgesics, sedatives, and anesthetics depress functions of the central nervous system. It is important for the nurse to conduct a neurological assessment (see Chapter 20) of a client at risk for being insensitive to pain. This client could suffer injury easily and thus requires preventive nursing care. For example, an overly sedated client would not be able to sense the discomfort of a tight cast or dressing.

Nursing Diagnosis

The development of an accurate nursing diagnosis for a client in pain results from thorough data collection and analysis (see diagnoses box). A nurse must not diagnose pain simply if it is presumed that a client will be uncomfortable. Too often a nurse may choose the diagnosis of *pain* simply because a client is about to have surgery or a specific disease condition implies pain.

An accurate diagnosis is made only after a complete assessment (see diagnostic process box on p. 1194). Clusters of defining characteristics reveal the nursing diagnosis best fitted to the client's condition and needs. The nursing diagnosis should focus on the specific nature of the pain to help the nurse identify the most useful types of interventions for alleviating pain and minimizing its effect on the client's lifestyle and function.

The nurse may make diagnoses other than *pain.* The extent to which pain affects a client's lifestyle and general state of health determines whether other nursing diagnoses are relevant. For example, the nurse's assessment may reveal that a client suffers pain of the hands and shoulders. As a result, the client is unable to remove or fasten necessary items of clothing. The client has the pain of crippling arthritis. The nursing diagnosis would be *grooming self-care deficit related to arthritic pain.* The client would have a nursing diagnosis of *chronic pain* to di-

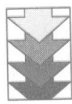

Examples of Nursing Diagnoses for Pain

NANDA-APPROVED NURSING DIAGNOSES

Anxiety related to:
- Unrelieved pain

Pain related to:
- Physical injury or trauma
- Reduced blood supply to tissues
- Natural childbirth processes

Chronic pain related to:
- Chronic physical disability
- Chronic psychosocial disability
- Inadequate pain control

Hopelessness related to:
- Chronic malignant pain

Ineffective individual coping related to:
- Chronic pain

Impaired physical mobility related to:
- Musculoskeletal pain
- Incisional pain

Risk for injury related to:
- Reduced pain reception

Self-care deficit related to:
- Musculoskeletal pain

Sexual dysfunction related to:
- Arthritic hip pain

Sleep pattern disturbance related to:
- Low-back pain

rect the nurse's interventions toward pain relief. The additional diagnosis of *self-care deficit* would lead the nurse to assist the client with alternative measures for performing self-care.

PLANNING

For each nursing diagnosis identified, the nurse develops a care plan for the client's needs (see care plan on p. 1194). Together the nurse and client discuss realistic expectations for pain-relief measures and the degree of pain relief to expect. Expected outcomes and goals are selected on the basis of the nursing diagnosis and client's condition. Appropriate therapies are chosen on the basis of the related factor contributing to the client's pain or health problem. For example, pain related to acute incisional pain responds to analgesics, whereas pain related to early labor contractions can be reduced with relaxation exercises.

A therapy that works for one client will not work for all. In the home, the nurse uses some of the remedies that the client has adopted. However, the nurse

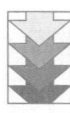

Sample Nursing Diagnostic Process for Pain and Chronic Pain

Assessment Activities	Defining Characteristics	Nursing Diagnoses
Have client describe character of pain.	Sharp, localized pain over lower abdominal incision, worsening during coughing and movement	*Pain* related to abdominal incision movement
Offer numerical descriptor scale to assess pain severity.	Pain rated 9 on scale of 1 to 10	
Observe client's movements.	Guards abdomen rigidly while turning and breathing deeply	
Observe client's facial expression.	Client grimaces and moans.	
Have client describe onset and duration of pain.	Pain first noticed 2 years ago in right hip while climbing path during hike. Physician diagnosed arthritis.	*Chronic pain* related to degenerative arthritic changes in hip
Ask client to describe character of pain.	Persistent, dull, sometimes burning ache that worsens during ambulation	
Observe client behaviors.	Client limps slightly after rising from sitting to standing position and hesitates to bear weight on right leg.	
Have client describe how pain has affected lifestyle.	Client enjoys birdwatching; hip pain prevents client from taking hikes; client feels confined to home.	

Sample Nursing Care Plan for Pain

Nursing diagnosis: *Pain* related to abdominal incision movement
Definition: Pain is the state in which an individual experiences and reports the presence of severe discomfort or an uncomfortable sensation (Kim, McFarland, McLane, 1991).

Goals	Expected Outcomes	Interventions	Rationale
Client will achieve control of pain within 24 hr after surgery.	Client will express relief during PCA infusion.	Explain to client purpose of patient-controlled analgesia device, method for initiating device, and expected response.	Client who has control over own pain achieves greater pain relief.
		Demonstrate and coach client through relaxation exercise.	Use of comfort measures aimed at distracting client may potentiate effect of analgesia.
	Client will initiate movement in bed without painful behavioral cues.	Position client anatomically on side with knees flexed and small pillow between legs.	Flexion of knees minimizes strain on abdominal muscles.
		Have colleague available to lift client in bed for repositioning; encourage client to ask for assistance.	Lifting of client prevents client from pulling self up in bed, aggravating abdominal pain.

cannot use therapies that are unsafe. It is often necessary for the client to understand that complete pain relief cannot be guaranteed but that it will be attempted.

When developing the care plan, the nurse selects priorities based on the client's level of pain and its effect on the client's condition. For acute, severe pain it is important to provide relief as soon as possible. Analgesics can provide relatively rapid relief and lessen the chance of pain worsening. After a client gains some relief from pain, the nurse plans other therapies such as relaxation or the application of heat to enhance the effect of analgesics.

A comprehensive plan includes a variety of resources for pain control. It is important to include the family in the care plan. The family may need to administer care in the home. In an acute-care setting the family must understand the nature and extent of the client's pain and the forms of therapy to be used. Family members who show a disinterest or prejudicial view toward pain can slow recovery. Additional resources available include nurse specialists, physical therapists, and occupational therapists. An oncology nurse specialist is very familiar with therapies most effective for chronic, malignant pain. Physical therapists can plan exercises that strengthen muscle groups and lessen pain in affected areas. Occupational therapists may devise splints to support painful body parts. When the nurse is caring for a client experiencing pain, client-centered goals might include the following:

1. Stating a sense of well-being and comfort
2. Maintaining the ability to perform self-care
3. Maintaining existing physical and psychosocial function
4. Explaining factors contributing to the pain experience

To establish an effective care plan, the nurse establishes a therapeutic relationship with the client and educates the client about pain.

Therapeutic Relationship

Clients in pain are highly vulnerable. Clients are not always convinced that someone is concerned with their welfare. Clients in pain need someone to trust. If the nurse is unable to establish a therapeutic relationship with clients, any resultant mistrust can heighten the awareness of pain. Unless clients have means to express concerns or fears about pain, their reactions to the pain may become inappropriate. Often, clients become angry or complain about the nurse's care when needs for pain relief are ignored.

The nurse can best help by seeing the client as a total person and conveying a sense of caring. Giving careful attention to the client's concerns during assessment is one way of building confidence in the nurse. Promptness in attending to the client's needs further establishes a strong therapeutic relationship. Making judgments about the validity of pain, bartering pain relief in return for "good" client behavior, and controlling sources of pain relief destroy the client's trust in the nurse.

A successful nurse-client relationship depends in part on the nurse's ability to respect the client's response to pain. Many nurses value firm self-control. However, a client may need to cry or moan or even become angry. The client should never feel ashamed or fearful that the nurse will not be accepting.

Education

Clients are better prepared to handle almost any situation when they understand it. The experience of pain is no exception. Teaching clients about the pain experience reduces anxiety and helps clients achieve a sense of control. For example, clients entering a clinic or hospital for the first time may know tests will be performed but do not understand them. As a result, they might fantasize about the experience. Fears are enhanced if friends have had unpleasant experiences in similar circumstances. Fear increases the perception of painful stimuli.

During the anticipatory phase of the pain experience, the nurse plans to teach clients about the procedures and associated discomfort. Price et al (1980) found that, when clients received instruction about an upcoming painful experience, they perceived the actual experience as less unpleasant. Clients changed the way that they evaluated the pain sensation and thus tolerated pain more effectively.

For some clients, early warning of pain can be a problem. The highly anxious or fearful client is often irrational and unable to learn from the nurse's explanations. Such clients tend to fantasize horrible events if they receive information too early about painful procedures. If clients seem unlikely to benefit from advance preparation, it is best to explain invasive procedures a short time before they occur. It is not always easy to know whether clients can accept impending unpleasant experiences. If clients are typically anxious or if previous teaching has not relieved anxiety, the nurse must use judgment in knowing when to tell clients about procedures.

Relevant play is a type of teaching that works well with children. Play reduces anxiety that might otherwise be created if the nurse tries to explain complicated procedures. For example, if a child is to have a laceration of the arm sutured, it helps to let the child put sutures into a doll's arm. Almost any procedure or situation can be acted out with dolls or other appropriate toys.

 ## Implementation

The nature of pain and the extent to which it affects physical and psychosocial well-being determine the choice of pain relief therapies. However, nurses can independently use pain-relief measures that complement those prescribed by a physician. Witt (1984) describes the following characteristics of ideal nursing interventions for chronic pain management:

1. Interventions should be within the scope of the average nurse's qualifications to use them effectively.
2. There should be no need for special equipment that may not be unavailable in the health care setting.
3. Therapies should not interfere with the client's medical treatments.
4. Nursing interventions should not be subject to a physician's approval or supervision and should not require the client's consent.

The nurse can play an important role in helping clients use techniques for acute and chronic pain relief. If there is doubt about a nursing therapy, the nurse must consult the client's physician. The least invasive or safest therapy should be tried first.

Guidelines for Individualizing Pain Therapy

When providing pain-relief measures, the nurse chooses therapies suited to the client's unique pain experience. McCaffery (1979) suggests nine useful guidelines for individualizing pain therapy (see box).

Measures that Alter Pain Reception

A basic nursing responsibility is protecting the client from harm. One simple way to promote comfort

---

Guidelines for Individualizing Pain Relief

- *Establish a relationship of mutual trust.* Always believe the client and try to convey concern. An adversarial relationship between nurse and client lessens the effectiveness of pain therapies.
- *Use different types of pain-relief measures.* Using more than one therapy has an additive effect in reducing pain. In addition, the character of pain may change throughout the day, requiring several different therapies.
- *Provide pain-relief measures before pain becomes severe.* It is easier to prevent severe pain than to relieve it after it exists. Giving an analgesic ½ hr before a client must walk or perform an activity is an example of controlling pain early.
- *Consider the client's ability or willingness to participate in pain-relief measures.* Some clients cannot actively assist with pain therapy because of fatigue, sedation, or altered levels of consciousness. However, there are variations of pain-relief measures that require little effort, such as relaxation exercises in bed or listening to music as a distraction.
- *Choose pain-relief measures on the basis of the client's behavior reflecting the severity of pain.* It would be poor judgment to administer a potent narcotic if a client has only mild pain. The nurse carefully assesses the client's comments and behavior before choosing pain therapy. Some clients acquire relief from severe pain after using only mild analgesics. Only the client can determine the potency of an effective therapy.

- *Use measures that the client believes are effective.* The client is the expert on pain. The client may have ideas about measures to use (e.g., rubbing lotion on a swollen finger) and times to use them that will make pain therapy successful.
- *If a therapy is ineffective at first, encourage the client to try it again before abandoning it.* Often anxiety or doubt prevents a therapy from relieving pain, or the measure may require adjustment or practice to become effective. The nurse should be patient and understanding in helping the client learn to use measures that do not afford immediate relief.
- *Keep an open mind about what may relieve pain.* New ways are often found to control pain. There is still much to be learned about the pain experience. Rejecting nonconventional therapies leads to mistrust. The nurse should be sure all therapies are safe.
- *Keep trying.* The nurse can easily become frustrated when efforts at pain relief fail. The nurse should *not* abandon the client when pain persists but reassesses the situation and considers alternative therapies.
- *Protect the client.* A pain therapy should not cause more distress than the pain itself. The nurse always observes the client's response to therapy. The nurse's aim is to relieve pain without disabling the client mentally, emotionally, or physically.
- *Educate the client about pain.* When possible, the nurse should explain the cause of the pain, times of occurrence, duration and quality, and ways to gain relief. Education promotes the prevention of pain.

is by removing or preventing painful stimuli (see box). This is especially important for clients who are immobilized or unable to sense discomfort.

Often, pain can be avoided by maintaining normal body function. For example, a client who is allowed to become constipated may suffer from distention and abdominal cramping. The nurse actively intervenes to ensure that the normal elimination process continues.

Pain can also be prevented by anticipating painful procedures or activities. Before performing procedures, the nurse considers the client's condition, aspects of the procedure that may be uncomfortable, and techniques to avoid causing pain. For example, for a client with knee pain caused by arthritis, the nurse knows that any extreme flexion of the knee causes much pain. Before walking the client to the bathroom the nurse makes sure that an elevated toilet seat is available. The client can then be seated and raise up with minimal discomfort.

It takes only simple consideration of the client's comfort and a little extra time to avoid pain-producing situations. Knowledge of factors that precipitate or aggravate pain helps the nurse prevent or minimize the client's discomfort. Learning proper lifting techniques and avoiding sudden turning movements help a client with a history of back pain avoid discomfort.

Cutaneous Stimulation

One way to prevent or reduce pain perception is through **cutaneous stimulation,** the stimulation of a person's skin to relieve pain. A massage, warm bath, application of liniment, hot and cold therapies, and transcutaneous electrical nerve stimulation (TENS) are simple ways to reduce pain perception. The specific way in which cutaneous stimulation works is unclear. One suggestion is that it causes release of endorphins, thus blocking the transmission of painful stimuli. Based on the gate-control theory, it is suggested that cutaneous stimulation activates large-diameter A-beta sensory nerve fibers, decreasing the transmission of painful stimuli through small-diameter A-delta and C fibers. Synaptic gates close to the transmission of pain impulses.

Cutaneous stimulation requires the nurse to touch the client. Work by Krieger (1975) suggests that therapeutic touch alone may result in a client's improved sense of well-being. Touch can communicate caring and thus help clients relax.

Cutaneous stimulation can provide effective, temporary pain relief. To enhance its effects, the nurse helps the client assume a comfortable position, eliminates environmental irritants such as noise and bright lights, and explains the purpose of therapy. Cutaneous stimulation should not be used directly on sensitive skin areas (for example burns, rashes, or bruises), incisions, inflamed areas, or underlying fractures.

Massage and backrub (see Chapter 34) are low-cost, safe ways to use cutaneous stimulation. Massage may lessen pain by promoting muscular relaxation. The nurse can use massage on one body part or several. It takes about 10 minutes to correctly massage a single body part. Procedure 37-1 on p. 1198 describes the techniques of massage.

Cold and heat applications (see Chapter 48) are routine measures that can be used in the home. The advantage is giving clients and families some control over pain symptoms and treatment. Ice bags, ice massage, warm and cold sitz baths, heating pads, and hot or cold compresses relieve pain and promote healing of injured tissues. The selection of heat versus cold therapies varies with clients' conditions. For example, moist heat relieves the early morning stiffness of arthritis, but cold applications reduce the acute pain and inflamed joints of the disease (Ceccio, 1990). When using any form of cold or heat application, the nurse must instruct the client to avoid injury to the skin. Clients can easily be burned by the incorrect use of heat applications. Especially at risk are clients with spinal cord or other neurological injury, older clients, and confused clients.

Ice massage and application of cold packs are two types of cold therapy that are particularly effective for pain relief. Ice massage involves use of a large ice cube or a small paper cup filled with water and frozen (water rises out of the cup as it freezes to create

---

Controlling Painful Stimuli in the Client's Environment

- Tighten and smooth wrinkled bed linen.
- Remove tubing on which client is lying.
- Loosen constricting bandages (unless specifically applied as a pressure dressing).
- Change wet dressings.
- Position client in anatomical alignment.
- Check temperature of hot or cold applications, including bath water.
- Lift client in bed—do not pull.
- Position client correctly on bed pan.
- Avoid exposing skin or mucous membranes to irritants (e.g., diarrheal stool, wound drainage).
- Prevent urinary retention by keeping Foley catheters patent and free flowing.
- Prevent constipation with fluids, diet, and exercise.

Using Massage Techniques

STEPS	RATIONALE
1. Assess the following:	
a. Condition of body part to be massaged	Massaging overly sensitive or damaged skin can cause further tissue injury.
b. Character of client's pain	Provides baseline to determine effectiveness of massage in relieving pain.
c. Contraindications to positioning (e.g., neck injury)	Massage of some body parts cannot be achieved without proper positioning and thus may be contraindicated.
2. Prepare following supplies:	
a. Skin lubricant (oil or lotion)	Eases movement of hands over client's skin.
b. Pillow (optional)	
3. Explain procedure: positioning, duration of massage, body parts to be massaged, and purpose.	Anticipation and understanding of procedure help client relax and cooperate.
4. Instruct client to tell you if massage becomes painful or feels especially good.	Avoids injury to client. Client is best judge of what therapy is effective in reducing pain or muscle tension.
5. Close door or pull curtains.	Ensures privacy.
6. Wash hands.	Reduces transmission of microorganisms.
7. Position height of bed to comfortable working level and lower side rail.	Promotes proper use of body mechanics. Makes access to client easy.
8. After determining area to be massaged, position body part appropriately:	
a. Hands: place arms on pillow with client sitting or supine.	Promotes venous return and supports arms comfortably.
b. Arms: same as Step 8a.	
c. Neck: Position client prone.	Provides easy access to neck muscles.
9. Drape client to expose only body parts to be massaged.	Promotes client's comfort, warmth, and privacy.
10. Apply lotion to hands and warm while rubbing hands together.	Prevents startling client and promotes comfort.
11. Massage each body part at least 10 min:	Improves likelihood that muscular relaxation and reduced perception of pain will occur.
a. Hands: make contact first with one hand and then other. Using both hands, slowly open client's palm, gliding your fingers over palmar surface. While supporting hand, use both thumbs to apply friction to palm. Use your thumbs in circular motion to stretch palm outward. Massage each finger outward. Massage each finger separately, using corkscrewlike motion from base of finger to tip. With your thumb and finger, knead each small muscle of client's fingers. Glide your hands smoothly from fingertips to wrists. Repeat for other hand.	Relaxes clenched muscles of fingers and palm.
b. Arms: use gliding stroke to massage from wrist to forearm. With thumb and forefinger of both hands, knead muscles from forearm to shoulder. Continue kneading biceps, deltoid, and triceps. Finish with gliding strokes from wrist to shoulder.	Thicker muscles require more kneading to cause relaxation.
c. Neck: support neck at hairline with one hand and massage up neck with gliding stroke. Knead muscles on one side of neck. Switch hands to support neck and knead other side of neck. Stretch neck slightly with one hand at top and other at bottom.	Movement of neck may interfere with ability to massage muscles fully. Relieves tension felt in deeper neck muscles.

STEPS	RATIONALE
12. During massages, note nonverbal cues indicating client's level of comfort.	Excess pressure to muscle groups or stretching of sensitive tissues may cause discomfort.
13. During massage, note which muscles are relaxed versus tight.	Tense muscles require more massage to achieve relaxation.
14. After massage, allow client to relax in assumed position. Give client time to relax or fall asleep.	Benefit of massage is increased by client remaining inactive. Stimulation of muscles reduces pain perception and promotes full relaxation.
15. Wash hands and store supplies.	Reduces transmission of microorganisms.
16. Record in nurses' notes: body part massaged, client's response to massage, and change in level of comfort.	Documents therapy and response. Provides information for choosing massage in future for pain relief.
17. Return to room 30 min later to evaluate client's level of comfort.	Determines degree of pain relief obtained.

CONTINUED

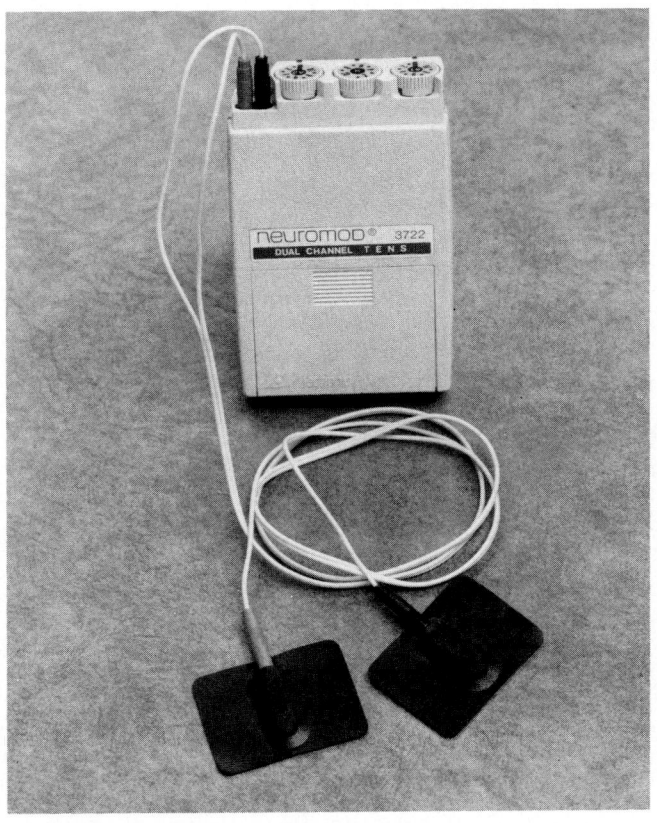

Fig. 37-7 TENS.

a smooth surface of ice for massage). The massage is simple. A nurse or the client can apply the ice with firm pressure to the skin, followed by a slow, steady, circular massage over the area. Cold may be applied near the pain site, on the opposite side of the body corresponding to the pain site, or on a site located between the brain and pain site (McCaffery, 1986). It takes about 5 to 10 minutes to use a cold application. Each client responds differently to the site of application that is most effective. However, application near the actual site of pain tends to work best. A client feels cold, burning, and aching sensations and numbness. When numbness occurs, the ice should be removed. Melzack et al (1980) found ice massage to be effective for tooth or mouth pain when ice was placed on the web of the hand between the thumb and index finger. This point on the hand is an acupuncture point that apparently influences nerve pathways to the face and head. Cold applications are also effective before invasive needle punctures such as intramuscular injections, bone marrow punctures, and lumbar punctures.

Transcutaneous electric nerve stimulation (TENS) involves stimulation of nerves beneath the skin with a mild electrical current passed through external electrodes. The therapy requires a physician's order. The TENS unit consists of a battery-powered transmitter, lead wires, and electrodes (Fig. 37-7). The electrodes are placed directly over or near the site of pain. Hair or skin preparations should be removed before attaching the electrodes. When a client feels pain, the transmitter is turned on. The TENS unit creates a buzzing or tingling sensation. The client may adjust the intensity and quality of skin stimulation. The tingling sensation can be applied as long as pain relief lasts. In a study conducted by Taylor et al (1983), clients who received TENS reported greater pain relief than clients who received narcotic analgesics. TENS is effective for postsurgical pain control and reduction of pain caused by postoperative procedures (for example, removing drains and cleaning and repacking surgical wounds) (Hargreaves, Lander, 1989).

Distraction

The reticular activating system inhibits painful stimuli if a person receives sufficient or excessive sensory input. With meaningful sensory stimuli, a person can ignore or become unaware of pain. Pleasurable stimuli also cause the release of endorphins to relieve pain. Persons who are bored or in isolation have only their pain to think about and thus perceive it more acutely. Distraction helps direct attention to something else. As a result, there is not a full awareness of pain. Distraction can often increase pain tolerance, but there is one disadvantage. If it works, health care personnel or family may question the existence or severity of pain. Distraction may work best for short, intense pain lasting a few minutes such as pain experienced by a client during a procedure or while waiting for an analgesic to work (Mayer, 1985).

The nurse assesses activities enjoyed by the client that may act as distractions. These might include singing, praying, describing photos or pictures aloud, listening to music, and playing games. Most distractions can be used in a hospital, home, or long-term care facility.

One effective distraction is music. Some institutions have music therapists. However, the nurse can use music creatively in many clinical situations. Clients generally prefer to perform (play an instrument or sing a song) or listen to music. Music that initially matches a person's mood is usually best (Baily, 1985). For example, a lonely person might initially enjoy playing a solo instrument or singing with another person. Selections might progress to songs by musical groups or even symphonic works. The box suggests ways to use music effectively.

Relaxation and Guided Imagery

Clients can alter affective-motivational and cognitive pain perception through relaxation and guided imagery. The ability to relax physically also promotes mental relaxation. Relaxation techniques provide clients with self-control when pain occurs, reversing the physical and emotional stress of pain. Clients who use relaxation techniques successfully experience several physiological and behavioral changes (see box). The nurse should obtain a physician's or-

---

Effects of Relaxation

- Decreased pulse, blood pressure, and respirations
- Decreased oxygen consumption
- Decreased muscle tension
- Decreased metabolic rate
- Heightened concentration on single idea
- Lack of attention to environmental stimuli
- No voluntary change of position

Adapted from Dimotto JW: *Am J Nurs* 84:754, 1984.

---

der for relaxation therapy if there is any legal uncertainty about the nurse's action or if the client's physical condition is unstable. Relaxation techniques include meditation, yoga, Zen, guided imagery, and progressive relaxation exercises.

Relaxation with or without guided imagery relieves tension headaches, labor pain, anticipated episodes of acute pain (for example, a needlestick), and chronic pain disorders. It may take five to ten training sessions before clients can effectively minimize pain (Carney, 1983). Relaxation training can be practiced indefinitely and usually has no side effects. Carney (1983) notes studies showing that 60% to 70% of clients with tension headache can reduce headache activity by at least 50% with relaxation.

Relaxation is mental and physical freedom from tension or stress. For effective relaxation, the client's participation and cooperation are needed. Relaxation techniques are taught only when the client is not in acute discomfort because the inability to concentrate makes the exercise ineffective. The nurse explains the technique in detail and notes that considerable practice is needed to achieve consistent pain reduction. The nurse describes common sensations the client may experience (for example, a decrease in temperature or numbness of a body part). The client should use these sensations as feedback.

The nurse is a coach, guiding the client slowly through steps of the exercise. The environment should be free of noises or other irritating stimuli. The client may sit in a comfortable chair or lie in bed (see box). A light sheet or blanket for warmth often helps the client feel more comfortable. The client may use guided imagery and relaxation exercises together or separately.

In **guided imagery** the client creates an image in the mind, concentrates on that image, and gradually becomes less aware of pain. The nurse coaches the client in forming the image and concentrating on the sensory experience. Initially the nurse asks the client

---

Using Music to Control Pain

- Match musical selections to a client's taste. Consider age and background.
- Use earphones to avoid annoying other clients or staff and help client to concentrate on music.
- If pain is acute, increase the volume of music. As pain decreases, reduce the volume.
- If background music is provided, select general types suited to the client's preferences.
- Have the client concentrate on the music and emphasize rhythm by tapping fingers or patting the thigh.
- Encourage clients to use music, particularly when it is enjoyed in the home.

Body Positions for Relaxation

SITTING

- Sit with entire back resting against back of chair.
- Place feet flat on floor.
- Keep legs separated.
- Hang arms at the side or rest on chair arms.
- Keep head aligned with spine.

LYING

- Keep legs separated with toes pointed slightly outward.
- Rest arms at sides without touching sides of body.
- Keep head aligned with spine.
- Use thin, small pillow under head.

---

to think of a pleasant scene or experience that promotes use of all senses. The client describes the image and the nurse records it so that it can be used during later exercises. The nurse uses specific information given by the client and does not make changes in the client's image. The following is an example of a portion of a guided imagery exercise:

Imagine yourself lying on a cool bed of grass with the sounds of rushing water from a nearby stream. It's a balmy day. You turn to see a patch of blue wildflowers in bloom and can smell their fragrance.

The nurse sits closely enough to the client to be heard but is not intrusive. The nurse's calm, soft voice helps the client focus more completely on the suggested image. While relaxing, the client focuses on the image, and it becomes unnecessary for the nurse to speak continuously. If the client shows signs of agitation, restlessness, or discomfort, the nurse should stop the exercise and begin later when the client is more at ease.

Progressive relaxation of the entire body takes about 15 minutes. The client pays attention to the body, noting areas of tension. Tense areas are replaced with warmth and relaxation. Some clients relax better with eyes closed. Soft background music can help.

Progressive relaxation exercise involves a combination of controlled breathing exercises and a series of contractions and relaxation of muscle groups. The client begins by breathing slowly and diaphragmatically, allowing the abdomen to rise slowly and the chest to expand fully. When the client establishes a regular breathing pattern, the nurse coaches the client to locate any area of muscular tension, think about how it feels, tense muscles fully, and then completely relax them. This creates the sensation of removing all discomfort and stress. Gradually the client can relax the muscles without first tensing them. When full relaxation is achieved, pain perception is lowered and anxiety toward the pain experience becomes minimal. The following is an example of how a nurse coaches a client:

Let's begin by finding as comfortable a position as possible. Arms at your side . . . legs uncrossed. . . . Move until you feel at ease. . . . Take a deep breath. Feel your stomach and chest slowly rise. . . . Relax. . . . Now breathe out slowly. . . slowly . . . and relax.

Count to 4, inhaling on 1 and 2, exhaling on 3 and 4. . . . Continue to breathe slowly. . . . Your body is beginning to relax. . . . Think "relax." . . . Feel the parts of your body. . . . Notice any tension in your muscles. . . . Continue to breathe slowly . . . and relax.

Concentrate on your face . . . your jaws . . . your neck. . . . Notice any tightness. . . . Breathe in warmth and relaxation. . . . Concentrate on any tension in your hands. . . . Notice how it feels. . . . Now make a fist—a tight fist! As you begin to exhale, relax your fist. . . . Good! Notice how your hand feels. . . . Think "relax." . . . Your hand feels warm . . . heavy or light. . . . Just relax more . . . and more. Now focus on your forearms. . . . Notice any tension. . . . Relax your arms. . . . Feel your body relaxing. . . . Let the feelings of relaxation spread from your fingers and hands through the muscles of your arms.

If the client becomes agitated or uncomfortable, the nurse stops the exercise. If the client seems to have difficulty relaxing only part of the body, the nurse slows the progression of the exercise and concentrates on the tensed body part. The client must also know from the beginning that the exercise can be stopped at any time. With practice the client can perform relaxation exercises independently.

Anticipatory Guidance

Modifying anxiety directly associated with pain relieves pain and adds to the effects of other pain-relief measures. Moderate anxiety may be useful when a client anticipates a painful experience. Clients can learn what is to be expected during a painful procedure or event. Knowledge about pain helps a client control anxiety and cognitively gain a level of pain relief.

The nurse gives clients information that prevents misinterpretation of the painful event and promotes understanding of what to expect. Information given to clients includes explanation of the following:
1. Occurrence, onset, and expected duration of pain
2. Quality, severity, and location of pain
3. Information on how the client's safety is ensured
4. Cause of the pain
5. Methods nurse and client take for pain relief
6. Expectations of the client during a procedure

An example of anticipatory guidance is preoperative teaching (see Chapter 47). Explanation of the incisional pain the client will feel and methods used to control it helps the client adapt postoperatively.

The nurse cannot say that the client will experience no pain. Anticipatory guidance gives an honest explanation of the pain experience. The nurse also gives instruction on pain-relief techniques so that the client will be prepared to cope with discomfort.

Biofeedback

Biofeedback is a behavioral therapy that involves giving individuals information about physiological responses (such as blood pressure or tension) and ways to exercise voluntary control over those responses (NIH, 1986). This therapy is especially effective for muscle tension and migraine headaches (see box). When headaches are treated, electrodes are attached externally over each temple. The electrodes measure skin tension in microvolts. A polygraph machine visibly records the tension level for the client to see. The client learns to achieve optimal relaxation, using feedback from the polygraph while lowering the actual level of tension experienced. The therapy takes several weeks to learn. Biofeedback can stop head-

---

Common Types of Headaches

MIGRAINE

- Migraine is vascular form of headache, caused by intracranial and subsequent vasodilation of cerebral arteries. Vasoactive substances like serotonin may precipitate headache. Client experiences severe, throbbing pain on one side of head, with nausea, vomiting, dizziness, and sensitivity to light and noise. Pain is concentrated around temple and behind ear. Attack may be triggered by foods or food preservatives.

CLUSTER HEADACHE

- Cluster headache is a vascular form of headache common in men. Client experiences severe, steady pain on one side of head, usually concentrated around or behind one eye. It is experienced in groups, up to several times a day for weeks or months at a time. It may be triggered by alcohol and foods containing preservatives.

TENSION HEADACHE

- Tension headache is a form of headache resulting from anxiety or excessive contractions of head and neck muscles. Client experiences mild to moderate steady pain at top, sides, and back of head, which can spread to neck. It may be triggered by tightening of face and scalp muscles resulting from teeth clenching, poor posture, fatigue, and stress.

---

aches and lessen the risk of development of future headaches.

Pharmacological Pain Therapy

Several pharmacological agents provide pain management. All require a physician's order. The nurse's judgment in the use of medications and management of clients receiving pharmacological therapies helps ensure the best pain relief possible.

ADMINISTERING ANALGESICS. Analgesics are the most common method of pain relief. However, nurses and physicians often have misconceptions about the dangers and effects of analgesics. Frequently, nurses and physicians undertreat clients because of incorrect pharmacological information, concerns about addiction, anxiety over errors in judgment while using a narcotic analgesic, and administration of less medication than was ordered. Rankin and Snider (1984) studied nurses' perceptions of pain suffered by cancer clients. The study showed that 89% of nurses believed that clients had adequate pain control. However, 67% assessed that the clients suffered moderate pain. Often nurses' uncertainty with correct administration of analgesics leads only to a reduction in pain, not relief.

There are four types of analgesics: (1) nonnarcotic analgesics (2) NSAIDS, (3) opioids, and (4) adjuvants or coanalgesics (see box). Nonnarcotic analgesics and NSAIDS provide relief for mild to moderate pain, such as the pain associated with rheumatoid arthritis, surgical and dental procedures, episiotomy, and low-back problems. Opioids are generally prescribed for severe pain such as malignant pain, whereas adjuvants may create **analgesia** (lack of pain) or relieve other signs and symptoms associated with pain such as depression and nausea.

Nurses must understand the drugs available for pain relief and their pharmacological effects. Pharmacological agents act at different levels of the nervous system to create pain relief. A drug may act at the peripheral receptor level or at the central nervous system level. The most common peripheral analgesics and NSAIDS act primarily on peripheral receptors to diminish transmission and reception of pain stimuli. All except acetaminophen inhibit the synthesis of prostaglandins at the site of injury.

Narcotic analgesics, when given orally or by injection, act on higher centers of the brain and spinal cord by binding with opiate receptors to modify perception of and reaction to pain. Morphine sulfate is a derivative of opium and has the following characteristic analgesic effects:

1. Raising the pain threshold, thereby reducing pain perception
2. Reducing anxiety and fear, which are components of the reaction to pain
3. Inducing sleep even in the presence of severe pain

The danger of morphine sulfate and other narcotic analgesics is the potential for depression of vital nervous system functions. Opiates cause respiratory depression by depressing the respiratory center within the brainstem. Clients also experience side effects such as nausea, vomiting, constipation, and altered mental processes. The following are characteristics of an ideal analgesic:

1. Rapid onset
2. Effective action over a prolonged time
3. Availability for all ages
4. Oral and parenteral use
5. Lack of severe side effects
6. Nonaddicting nature
7. Inexpensive cost

Sedatives, antianxiety agents, and muscle relaxants are adjuvants often prescribed to clients in

---

Examples of Analgesics

NONNARCOTIC ANALGESICS

- Acetaminophen (Tylenol, Datril)
- Acetylsalicylic acid (aspirin)
- Choline magnesium trisalicylate (Trilisate)

NSAIDS

- Ibuprofen (Motrin, Nuprin)
- Naproxen (Naprosyn)
- Naproxen sodium (Anaprox)
- Indomethacin (Indocin)
- Tolmetin (Tolectin)
- Piroxicam (Feldene)

NARCOTIC ANALGESICS

- Meperidine (Demerol)
- Methylmorphine (Codeine)
- Morphine sulfate (Morphine)
- Fentanyl (Sublimaze)
- Butorphanol (Stadol)
- Hydromorphone HCl (Dilaudid)

ADJUVANTS

- Amitriptyline (Elavil)
- Hydroxyzine (Vistaril)
- Caffeine
- Chlorpromazine (Thorazine)
- Diazepam (Valium)

---

chronic pain or clients who have other symptoms associated with pain. The drugs may be given alone or with other analgesics. Sedatives are the drugs most often prescribed to chronic pain sufferers (Brena, 1983). These drugs can cause drowsiness and impairment of coordination, judgment, and mental alertness. Misuse of sedatives and antianxiety agents is a serious health problem that can cause disabling illness behaviors.

Analgesics require careful assessment, application of pharmacological principles (see Chapter 21), and common sense. A person's response to an analgesic is highly individualized. A relatively mild nonnarcotic may prove as effective as a potent narcotic for some clients, or an orally administered analgesic may bring the same relief as an injectable form of analgesic. It is the nurse's responsibility to follow a few basic principles (see box on p. 1204).

The nurse should always know the comparative potencies of analgesics in oral and injectable form. For example, a physician may order meperidine 50 to

---

Nursing Principles for Administering Analgesics

Know the Client's Previous Response to Analgesics.

- Determine whether relief was obtained.
- Ask whether a nonnarcotic was as effective as a narcotic.
- Identify previous doses and routes of administration to avoid undertreatment.
- Determine whether the client has allergies.

Select Proper Medications When More Than One is Ordered.

- Use nonnarcotic analgesics or milder narcotics for mild to moderate pain.
- Know that nonnarcotics can be alternated with narcotics.
- In older adults, avoid combinations of narcotics.
- Remember that morphine and hydromorphone are the narcotics of choice for long-term management of severe pain.
- Know that injectable medications act quicker and can relieve severe, acute pain within 1 hour and that oral medication may take as long as 2 hours to relieve pain.
- Use a narcotic with a nonnarcotic analgesic for severe pain because such combinations treat pain peripherally and centrally.

- For chronic pain, give an oral drug for sustained relief.

Know the Accurate Dosage.

- Remember that doses at the upper end of normal are generally needed for severe pain.
- Adjust doses, as appropriate, for children and older clients.

Assess the Right Time and Interval for Administration.

- Administer analgesics as soon as pain occurs and before it increases in severity.
- Do not give analgesics only by ordered schedules. Remember that an around-the-clock administration schedule is usually best.
- Give analgesics before pain-producing procedures or activities.
- Know the average duration of action for a drug and the time of administration so that the peak effect occurs when pain is most intense.

---

100 mg intramuscularly or orally every 3 to 4 hours as necessary. This order leaves much to the judgment of the nurse and requires clarification. Such an order would create confusion. The nurse must select the best dose, route, and interval. The maximum dose of meperidine (100 mg) has about the same analgesic strength as 13 mg morphine intramuscularly (Heidrich, Perry, 1982). The lowest dose, 50 mg, by mouth is equal to the strength of two aspirin. If nurses on succeeding shifts choose different routes for the same doses the client will not receive the same level of analgesia, and pain control will be poor. Nurses must provide controlled, sustained pain relief.

PCA. Clients benefit from having control over pain therapy. When clients depend on nurses for analgesia, an erratic cycle of alternating pain and analgesia often occurs. The client feels pain and asks for a medication. The nurse may be unable to deliver the medication promptly. Within an hour after drug administration, analgesia finally occurs. Pain relief may last only ½ hour. The client may be sedated as long as an hour. Then, gradually, the client again feels discomfort, and the cycle begins again.

A drug delivery system called **patient-controlled analgesia (PCA)** allows clients to safely administer pain medications when they want them. The PCA is a portable pump (usually computerized) containing a chamber for a syringe. The pump delivers a small preset dose of medication either intravenously or subcutaneously. The analgesic of choice is morphine. To receive a dose the client pushes a button attached to the pump (Fig. 37-8). The system is designed to deliver no more than a specified number of doses every hour to avoid overdoses. For example, one PCA device delivers a dose as small as 1 ml or 1 mg of morphine sulfate every 6 minutes. Most pumps have locked safety systems that prevent tampering by clients or their family members. Even though a dose can be released only for a preset time, each time the client pushes the button a humming sound or small bell is activated. The bell acts as a placebo. The client believes that a dose is delivered with each ring. Benefits of PCA include the following:

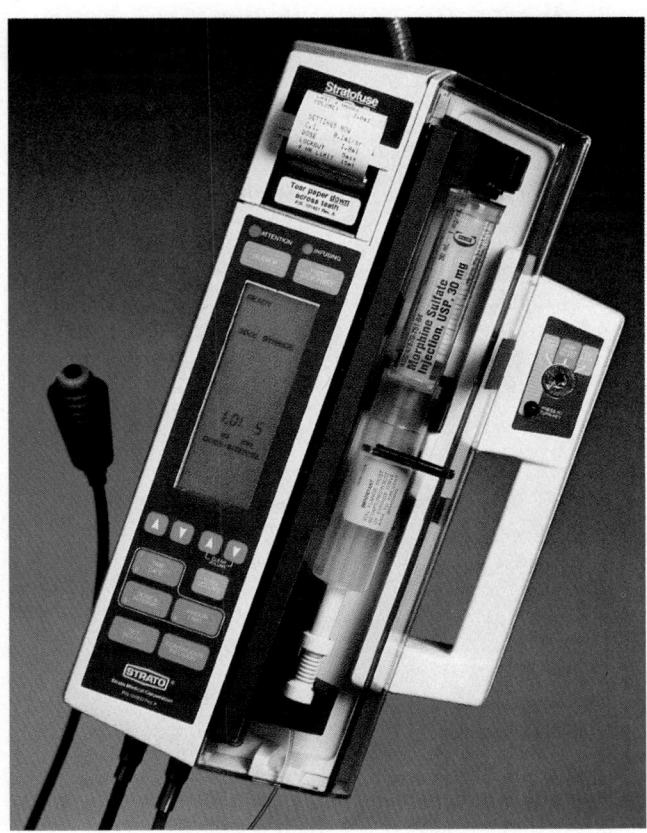

Fig. 37-8   Patient-controlled analgesic device.

1. Clients have control over their pain.
2. Pain relief does not depend on nurse availability.
3. Clients tend to take less medication, achieving a balance between the pain-relieving properties and the sedative effects.
4. Small doses of analgesics delivered at short intervals stabilize serum drug concentrations for sustained pain relief.

PCA has been found to be effective in controlling postoperative, traumatic, labor and delivery, and cancer pain. The nurse and physician assess the appropriateness of PCA for clients. Often, clients receive test doses of the drug before PCA is started. Vital signs serve as baselines in judging response to medication. Clients should be capable of handling the device and understanding correct use. The nurse explains the purpose of PCA therapy, operating instructions for the device, expected pain relief, precautions, and potential side effects (IV Nurses Society, 1990). Clients must know that the device prevents risk of overdose. Family members or friends should never operate the PCA device for clients. Clients should be

alert during explanation of the device. It also helps to demonstrate operation of the device. The nurse should not wait until immediately after surgery to instruct clients because they will be sedated. Even though clients control administration of analgesics, the nurse must routinely check that the PCA device operates correctly. The nurse also documents drug dosages and tracks any waste of narcotics.

LOCAL ANESTHETICS. Local anesthesia is the loss of sensation to a localized body part. Physicians use local anesthesia while suturing a wound, moving a body part in which the client is experiencing pain, delivering an infant, and performing some surgery. Local anesthesia has fewer risks than general anesthesia, which causes loss of consciousness and depression of vital functions.

Local anesthetics can be applied topically on skin and mucous membranes or injected to anesthetize a part of the body. Local anesthetics block the function of sensory, motor, and autonomic neurons supplying the affected area. Thus when the client temporarily loses sensation in a body part, motor and autonomic function is also lost. Smaller sensory nerve fibers are more sensitive to local anesthetics than large motor fibers. As a result, the client loses sensation before losing motor function, and conversely, motor activity returns before sensation.

Local anesthetics can cause side effects, depending on their absorption into the circulation. Itching or burning of the skin or a localized rash is common after topical applications. Application to vascular mucous membranes increases the chance of systemic effects such as a change in heart rate. Injection of anesthetics increases the risk of systemic side effects, depending on the amount of drug used and the area injected.

Table 37-7 on p. 1206 summarizes the types of local anesthesia by injection. Each produces a different level of anesthesia as a result of the amount of anesthetic used and location of the spinal nerve affected.

The nurse assists the physician during use of local anesthesia by providing emotional support to clients, watching for systemic side effects, and protecting clients from injury. Many clients are apprehensive about whether an anesthetic will prevent pain. The nurse explains application of the anesthetic and the sensations experienced. Injection of anesthetics can be painful if the physician does not first numb the injection site. The nurse prepares clients for such discomfort.

It is common for clients to fear paralysis because epidural and spinal injections come close to the spinal cord. The nurse explains the insertion sites and warns clients that they will temporarily lose motor

TABLE 37-7	Local Anesthesia Techniques		
Type	Area of Injection	Area Anesthetized	Indications for Use
Infiltration	In superficial area under skin or mucous membranes	Small peripheral nerves to area infiltrated	Small incisions of skin, insertion of sutures to close cuts or wounds, minor dental repairs
Peripheral nerve block	In area surrounding large peripheral nerve at point above bifurcation of nerve	Wider area than with infiltration, numbing entire body part (e.g., hand, upper gums, foot)	Major dental repairs, manipulation or reduction of extremity fractures, minor hand and foot surgery
Epidural or peridural nerve block	In lumbosacral region of spinal cord, around major nerve roots exiting base of spinal cord at site outside dura mater	Lower trunk and extremities	Delivery of newborn, major surgery to lower trunk and extremities (e.g., hemorrhoidectomy, appendectomy, vascular repair)
Spinal nerve block	Around major nerve root within subarachnoid space of spinal cord	Lower trunk and extremities	Major surgery to lower trunk and extremities, clients at risk with general anesthesia

and autonomic function (for example, bowel and bladder function).

Before the client receives an anesthetic, the nurse determines the history of allergies. To monitor systemic effects of local anesthetics, the nurse assesses blood pressure and pulse. Spinal anesthesia may also cause variations in respiratory rate.

After administration of a local anesthetic the nurse protects the client from injury until full sensory and motor function returns. Pain is a normal protective mechanism. Until a local anesthetic is absorbed and metabolized, the client must be careful in using an anesthetized body part. For example, after an injection into a joint, the nurse warns the client to avoid using the joint until function returns. For clients with topical anesthesia the nurse avoids applying heat or cold to numb areas. After spinal anesthesia the client stays in bed until sensory and motor function returns. The nurse assists the client during the first attempt at getting out of bed.

EPIDURAL ANALGESIA. The administration of medication into the spinal epidural space for acute and chronic pain management is becoming a common therapy. Initially used for the management of cancer pain, **epidural** infusions are now used to successfully treat acute pain after surgery and caesarean section (Turnage et al, 1990). The use of epidural analgesia permits control or reduction of severe pain without the sedative effects normally associated with narcotic administration. The therapy can be short or long term, depending on the client's condition and life expectancy. Short-term therapy is used for pain after surgery or caesarean section, whereas long-term therapy is appropriate for pain caused by cancer.

Epidural analgesia is administered into the spinal epidural space and the ventricles of the brain (Wilkie, 1990).Analgesics can also be introduced into the intrathecal route, the spinal subarachnoid space, creating the same effects as epidural analgesia. Each route requires a slightly different approach for placement of a small plastic catheter. A physician enters the epidural and subarachnoid spaces by inserting the catheter into the lumbar region (level L3 and L4). If the catheter is only temporary, it is connected to tubing positioned along the spine and over the client's shoulder. The entire catheter and tubing length is taped for stability and protection. The end of the catheter can then be placed on the client's chest for the nurse's access (Lonsway, 1988). Permanent catheters may be tunneled subcutaneously through the skin and exit at the client's side. The ventricular route involves surgical implantation of a small reservoir just underneath the scalp. The reservoir has a small, thin catheter that is threaded by a surgeon into the client's lateral ventricle (Fig 37-9). The medication is given through the reservoir.

Because of the location of the catheter, strict surgical aseptic technique (see Chapter 18) is needed to prevent a serious and potentially fatal infection. Physicians are notified immediately of any signs or symptoms of infection or pain at the insertion site. Thorough nursing care is needed during hygiene procedures to keep the catheter system clean and dry.

Nurses receive special training for the administration of epidural analgesia. Opiate narcotics such as

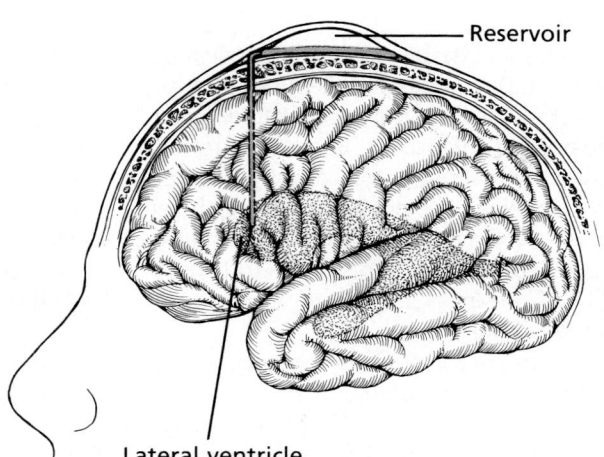

Reservoir

Lateral ventricle

Fig. 37-9 Ommaya reservoir.

TABLE 37-8 Nursing Care of Clients with Intraspinal Infusions

Goal	Actions
Prevent catheter displacement.	Limit client's activity.
	Secure catheter (if not connected to implanted reservoir) carefully to outside skin.
Maintain catheter function.	Check external dressing around catheter site for dampness or discharge. (Leak of cerebrospinal fluid may develop.)
Prevent infection.	Use strict aseptic technique when caring for catheter (see Chapter 18).
	Change tubing every 24 hours.
Prevent undesirable complications.	Monitor vital signs. (Hypotension, respiratory depression, and bradycardia indicate systemic absorption.)
	Assess for blurred vision, ringing in ears, pruritis (itching), and nausea and vomiting.
Maintain urinary and bowel function.	Monitor intake and output.
	Assess for bladder and bowel distention.

preservative-free morphine sulfate and fentanyl are two of the more common medications given. The opiates act like large doses of endorphins, blocking pain transmission. Frequently a local anesthetic such as bupivacaine is also administered. The anesthetic blocks pain conduction through local peripheral nerve fibers around the site of insertion. Bupivacaine also blocks the sympathetic nervous system, causing side effects such as hypotension, reduced intestinal peristalsis, and bladder dysfunction. Infusions may be given by a bolus, intermittently or continuously through established epidural catheters (see Chapter 21). Continuous infusions must be administered through electronic infusion devices for proper control (IV Nurses Society, 1990).

The nursing implications for managing epidural analgesia are numerous (Table 37-8). Monitoring of the medication's effects differs, depending on whether infusions are intermittent or continuous. Respiratory depression is the most serious side effect. When clients are started on epidural anesthesia, monitoring occurs as often as every 15 minutes. The client must receive thorough education about epidural analgesia in terms of the action of the medication and its advantages and disadvantages. A client on long-term therapy can be taught to safely administer infusions in the home with minimal ongoing intervention by the nurse.

PLACEBOS. Often a nurse's reassuring words seem to cause pain relief even though there are no direct physiological or chemical effects on a client. A **placebo** is any treatment that produces an effect because of its intent and not its physical or chemical properties (McCaffery, 1982). An inactive substance such as injectable normal saline or an oral preparation of sugar is often prescribed as if it were medica-

tion. The pharmacy can prepare placebos in the form of capsules or tablets to make them look the same as medications.

Considerable argument exists over how placebos relieve pain. Some researchers believe that placebos increase endorphin levels. Others believe that they create a psychological sense of pain relief, lowering pain perception. Regardless of the mode of action, when the placebo is administered correctly, the client is convinced that it will provide pain relief. The client's belief that a placebo is a real form of therapy may be the necessary factor in relieving pain.

The nurse requires a physician's order before administering a placebo. The placebo is not to be used as a form of punishment or as a test to prove whether the client is really in pain. The nurse may choose to give the placebo by telling the client that it is a medication or explaining its purpose and desired effect. The nurse may also choose not to give the placebo. It is important for nurses to consider their values related to the ethics of administering placebos.

The nurse enhances the chances of a placebo working by explaining that its intent is to relieve pain. It also helps to provide a quiet, comfortable environment that enables the client to relax. Trust in the nurse relieves doubts that the client might have about the therapy's benefit. The nurse administers the placebo as if it were an actual pain medication, assesses the client's pain carefully, and evaluates and records the placebo's effects.

Promoting Wellness

Pain can seriously disable and immobilize an individual. The effect of pain on physical mobility can alter self-care activities. Pain can also change self-esteem and desire to socialize with others. The nurse helps the client and family members find ways to cope with pain and maintain a functional lifestyle.

The nurse acts to minimize potential effects of immobilization (see Chapter 43) by practicing effective positioning techniques. Regular turning, range of motion exercise, and anatomical alignment of body parts prevent painful contractures from forming. When a client is mobile, the nurse ensures that painful body parts are protected. Elastic bandages, braces, splints, or even pillows can support injured parts during movement. If crutches or other assistive devices are required, the nurse makes sure that they are used properly. Otherwise, the client may be at risk for further injury or pain.

Painful disorders of the upper extremities create difficulty in eating, bathing, grooming, and dressing. The nurse may refer a client to an occupational therapist who can devise ways to maintain function, even when finger movement or grasp is impaired. Eating utensils, a comb and brush, and a toothbrush can be attached to extension devices. These devices have enlarged handles or splints that allow clients to pick up the items. Clothing fasteners made from Velcro tape make it easier for clients to remove or apply clothing. Shirts or blouses can be sewn so that garments can simply be pulled on or off over the head.

A warm bath can be relaxing. Personal cleanliness also promotes comfort. If chronic pain exists the nurse should encourage family members to help clients maintain hygiene practices in the home.

With fatigue, pain perception can increase. Procedures within a health care setting should be planned around rest periods. Clients with chronic discomfort should be encouraged to rest before social activities in the home.

A person with pain may avoid sexual activity for fear that it will cause or aggravate discomfort (see Chapter 32). However, the need for sexual warmth is not negated by pain (Cash, 1984). Clients can learn to express themselves sexually regardless of pain. A client whose movement is restricted by pain may not be able to assume the positions for intercourse. Alternative positions may be less uncomfortable and strenuous. Nurses should also caution clients about the fact that tranquilizers, muscle relaxants, and narcotics decrease libido and potency.

Surgical Measures for Pain Relief

When a client's pain persists despite medical treatment and it is clear that the pain is physical and not psychological, surgical therapies may give relief. A **posterior rhizotomy** involves surgically cutting the dorsal (posterior) roots of a spinal nerve. The resection involves the posterior root of the spinal cord. It is effective for relieving localized acute pain in the area supplied by the nerve root and deep visceral pain. The client loses sensation of pain but retains full motor function.

A **chordotomy** is more extensive and involves resection of the thoracic or cervical spinal cord at various levels. The procedure is used to treat intractable or unrelieved pain. The higher the focus of pain, the higher the site selected for a chordotomy. For example, pain in the thorax, upper extremities, and shoulders requires a high cervical chordotomy. The risks of the procedure are great because permanent paralysis may result from edema of the spinal cord or accidental resection of motor nerves. After the procedure the client has a permanent loss of pain and temperature sensation in the affected areas. If the surgery is uncomplicated, the senses of touch and position are retained.

Clients with Intractable Pain

Intractable pain cannot be permanently relieved. The pain can become so debilitating that a client assumes a dependent role. Chronic intractable pain encompasses a client's total existence. The client will try anything to gain relief. However, relief may never fully be obtained. Cleeland (1984) notes that one in three people with metastatic cancer reports pain that interferes with the quality of life. One of the greatest nursing challenges is to care for the client with intractable pain.

When therapy to control the spread of cancer fails, analgesic medications may be the only way to alleviate suffering. Administration of analgesics in treatment of cancer-related pain requires application of principles different from those used to treat acute pain. The World Health Organization (1986) recommends a three-step approach to managing cancer pain (Fig. 37-10). Basically, therapy begins with using nonopioids first and then progresses to strong opioids if pain persists. When a client with cancer first experiences pain, it is best to begin with a higher medication dosage than will be needed for relief. The physician can slowly decrease the dosage to the amount needed, thus providing the client with immediate pain relief. In addition, there is aggressive treatment of the side effects of analgesia such as nausea and constipation so that analgesia can be continued.

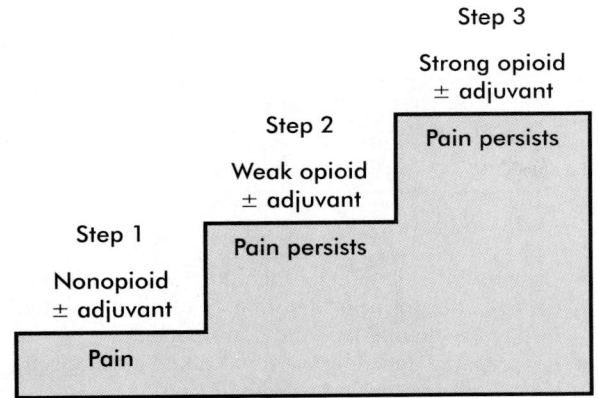

Fig. 37-10 WHO's analgesic ladder is a three-step approach to using drugs in cancer pain management. ± *adjuvant,* With or without adjuvant medications.
From World Health Organization: *Cancer pain relief and palliative care: report of a WHO Expert Committee,* WHO Tech Rep Series NO 804, Geneva, 1990, The Organization.

Often, opiates are underprescribed because physicians fear depression of the central nervous system. For example, most opiates such as codeine and morphine sulfate have a duration of action between 2 and 4 hours. However, standard prescriptions are for opiates to be given only every 4 hours. The client is needlessly exposed to unnecessary discomfort because the blood level of the drug is at its lowest point at the end of the fourth hour, before the next dose (Brena, 1983).

Studies show that drug dependence is low among clients with cancer-related pain. Administering the right drug and the required dose at the proper interval alleviates the fear of pain, protects the client from drug-seeking behavior, and reduces the incidence of dependence. It has also been shown that terminally ill clients with prolonged pain develop a tolerance to analgesics. As a result, clients require higher doses of analgesics to attain pain relief. Higher analgesic doses in clients who have become tolerant to narcotics are not lethal because clients also develop tolerance to life-threatening side effects (McCaffery, 1986).

For clients with cancer the aim of drug therapy is to anticipate and minimize pain rather than cure it. It is therefore necessary to give required doses on a regular basis. Prescribing analgesics on an as-needed basis for cancer clients is ineffective and causes more suffering. The cancer client must take an analgesic regularly, even when the pain, nausea, and other symptoms subside.

Some medications can provide pain relief. Epidural and intrathecal analgesia has been highly effective. In addition, new analgesics are being tested that have fewer side effects. Long-acting or controlled-release morphine sulfate has been very successful. Two of these medications are MS Contin and Roxanol SR. Pain relief can be obtained with MS Contin for 8 to 12 hours and with Roxanol SR for up to 6 hours (Wilkie, 1990).

Transdermal drug systems administer drugs such as fentanyl over predetermined rates up to 24 hours. This route is useful when clients are unable to take drugs orally. Self-adhesive patches release the medication slowly over time, achieving effective analgesia.

More traditional drug therapies include methadone and oral morphine sulfate. Methadone has the following advantages (Maxwell, 1980):

1. High oral potency
2. Long duration of action
3. Cumulative effect that maintains a steady analgesic level to prevent pain.
4. Relative lack of interference with a client's mood

After a client's methadone dosage becomes regulated, only two daily doses may be required. Opiate cocktails also achieve a significant level of pain relief for cancer clients. Brompton's mixture, Val-Streck elixir, and modified Brompton's mixtures do not interfere with mental alertness. Brompton's mixture includes a combination of drugs: morphine sulfate or methadone (narcotic analgesic), cocaine or an amphetamine (central nervous system stimulant that reduces sedation and respiratory depression caused by the narcotic), a phenothiazine (antipsychotic and antiemetic), and ethyl alcohol. The mixture often contains a fruit-flavored syrup to improve its taste. Brompton's mixture is easier to take than repeated injections. The client learns to adjust the dosage to ensure adequate pain relief. There is argument that Brompton's mixture is not as effective as morphine sulfate alone. However, its limited sedative effect offers an advantage.

Another popular measure for treatment of severe intractable cancer pain is morphine sulfate administered by continuous intravenous drip or intermittently by a PCA pump. Continuous intravenous drip provides improved, uniform pain control because lower doses of the drug are used. Thus there are fewer side effects. Although a client receives a continuous infusion of morphine sulfate, the total daily dose may be less than with conventional intramuscular injections. Candidates for continuous-drip therapy include clients with severe pain for which oral and intermittent parenteral narcotics provide minimal relief, clients with severe vomiting who are unable to take medications orally, clients with clotting disorders who cannot tolerate injections without bruising, and clients unable to swallow orally administered medications.

Continuous-drip morphine sulfate is given in the acute-care setting and in the home. In the hospital the drug is mixed in an intravenous solution of dextrose in water (D5W) or Ringer's lactate solution. The morphine sulfate is delivered by an infusion control pump to ensure a safe, accurate, and steady rate of infusion. The prescribed dosage of morphine sulfate depends on the severity of the client's pain, tolerance to the medication, and previous history of drug use. A typical mixture of morphine is 100 mg added to 500 ml of intravenous fluid. The higher the concentration of morphine sulfate, the smaller the amount of fluid the client receives. Each agency has guidelines for morphine sulfate dosage and infusion rates and the type of pump used.

When a client is first placed on continuous-drip morphine sulfate, the nurse must make careful, ongoing assessments. To prevent overdose and central nervous system depression, the nurse records baseline blood pressure and respiratory rate before infusion begins. After the infusion starts, the nurse monitors vital signs every 15 to 30 minutes for the first few hours until the client gains pain relief at a constant dosage. If blood pressure or respirations decrease, the rate is reduced according to the physician's order or agency policy. If the client shows signs of severe respiratory depression, the physician orders that the infusion be discontinued. The narcotic antagonist naloxone (Narcan) should be available to reverse respiratory depression.

In the home, clients may use ambulatory infusion pumps. The pumps are lightweight and compact (about the size of a transistor radio) and allow free movement. The pump is battery powered and worn in a pouch attached to a belt or harness. The bag of medication and intravenous fluid fits inside the pump. A dosage of morphine sulfate, delivered continuously over 24 hours, is usually slowly infused into a **central venous catheter.** These large catheters, inserted into the client's subclavian vein in the hospital, are relatively easy to maintain and can be left in place for an extended period. The client and family learn to manage the pump, observe for side effects, and maintain function of the central venous catheter (see box). Because the client is initially managed on morphine sulfate in the hospital before going home, the risk of side effects is not as great unless the client or family member increases drug doses. A home health care nurse makes routine visits to be sure that the client manages the pump correctly. The intravenous fluid bag and tubing are usually changed about once a week by the nurse. This maintains the sterility of the system.

The nurse uses all available pain-relief measures for the client with cancer. The nurse-client relation-

---

Tips for Managing Morphine Sulfate Administered via Ambulatory Infusion Pumps

- Observe for side effects, including sedation, hypotension, dizziness or fainting, nausea, vomiting, respiratory depression, and constipation.
- Be prepared to administer naloxone intramuscularly to reverse respiratory depression.
- Keep the central venous catheter patent. Maintain minimum pump flow rate. Irrigate catheter routinely with heparin flush.
- Prevent air from entering central venous catheter. Clamp catheter when infusion has stopped.
- Prevent infection at catheter site. Keep site clean with soap and water.

---

ship can help the client adapt to chronic pain. The client must feel that those responsible for managing the pain are competent and dependable.

Pain Clinics and Hospices

During the last decade, health professionals from the United States and Canada have recognized pain as a significant health problem. With an increased awareness of the multiple problems that pain can cause for clients, programs have been designed for pain management. Pain clinics offer several options. A comprehensive pain center can treat persons on inpatient and outpatient bases. Staff members representing all health care disciplines such as nursing, medicine, physical therapy, and dietetics work with clients to find the most effective pain-relief measures. A comprehensive clinic provides not only diverse therapy but also research into new treatments and training for professionals.

There are also syndrome-oriented and modality-oriented pain centers. A syndrome-oriented center cares for clients with only specific types of pain such as back pain or arthritis. Modality-oriented centers offer only specific types of treatment, such as biofeedback, acupuncture, or TENS.

Hospices are programs for care of the terminally ill. Hospice comes from the Latin word *hospes,* which means "a place to rest." Often, hospice programs are affiliated with hospitals. The programs help terminally ill clients continue to live at home in comfort and privacy with the help of a hospice health care team. Pain control is a priority for hospices. Clients receive the proper dosage and forms of analgesics

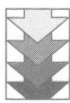

Sample Evaluation of Interventions for Pain

Goals	Evaluative Measures	Expected Outcomes
Client will achieve control of pain within 24 hr after surgery.	Have client report severity of pain on scale of 1 to 10, 2 hr after initiating PCA and at least every 4 hr thereafter.	Client will express relief during PCA infusion.
	Observe client's posture in bed, ease of position change, and facial expression.	Client will initiate movement in bed without painful behavior cues.
Client will perform self-care by discharge.	Observe client while dressing, eating, bathing, and grooming.	Client will independently perform self-care activities with or without self-care devices.
Client will use pain-relief measures in the home.	Ask client to demonstrate relaxation techniques.	Client will perform relaxation exercise.
	Have client explain analgesic dosage.	Client will explain prescribed analgesic regimen.

that provide pain relief. Under the guidance of hospice nurses, families learn to monitor clients' symptoms and become the primary care givers. A hospice client may become hospitalized in the event of a brief acute care crisis or family problem.

Evaluation

The client is the best resource for evaluating the effectiveness of pain-relief measures. The nurse must continually determine whether the character of the client's pain changes and whether individual therapies are effective. The family often is another valuable resource, particularly in the case of the client with cancer who may not be able to express discomfort during the latter stages of terminal illness. The nurse is successful in treating pain when the goals of care are met. The nurse uses evaluative criteria in determining the outcome of pain-relief therapies (see evaluation box).

If the nurse determines that a client continues to have discomfort after therapy, it may be necessary to try different or additional therapies. For example, if an analgesic provides only partial relief, the nurse may add relaxation exercises or guided-imagery exercises. The nurse may also consult with the physician about trying different analgesics.

The nurse also evaluates the client's perceptions of the effectiveness of therapy. The client may help decide the best times to attempt a treatment. For example, the client is the best judge of whether a therapy works better when anxiety and irritability are absent or when the pain is most severe.

The nurse also determines tolerance to therapy and the overall relief obtained. For example, if a nurse administers an analgesic, side effects from the medication and the client's reported pain relief must be assessed. Similarly, after turning a client, the nurse should return to determine whether the client is tolerating the new position and whether pain has subsided. If a therapy aggravates discomfort, the nurse stops it immediately and seeks an alternative.

The nurse and client should not become frustrated if a therapy does not act quickly. Time and patience are necessary to maximize the effectiveness of a therapy. The nurse considers factors that may be influencing the client's perceptions or reactions to pain. For example, a backrub may prove ineffective if the client has just learned the results of diagnostic tests and has had no opportunity to express concerns. The nurse evaluates the entire pain experience to determine therapies that are most effective and times that they should be administered.

 SUMMARY

The experience of pain is different for each person. The meaning that pain conveys, the threat to comfort, and the potential implications of serious illness make the experience highly subjective but very real. Pain is a problem faced in every health care setting. The nurse is most effective in providing comfort by understanding the nature of pain and the client's perceptions, eliminating personal prejudices about pain, and working closely with the client to find the best pain-relief measures.

Key Concepts

- Pain is largely a subjective experience.

- Pain is a protective mechanism that warns of tissue injury.

- A nurse's misconceptions about pain often result in doubt about the degree of the client's suffering and unwillingness to provide relief.

- Knowledge of the three components of the pain experience—reception, perception, and reaction—provides the nurse with guidelines for determining pain-relief measures.

- An interaction of psychological and cognitive factors affects pain perception.

- The pain experience is influenced by a variety of variables, including age, sex, culture, anxiety, meaning of pain, and previous experience.

- It is common for older clients not to report pain.

- The difference between acute and chronic pain involves duration of discomfort, physical signs and symptoms, and the client's perceptions regarding pain relief.

- Chronic pain can affect every aspect of life and lead to serious behavioral problems.

- The nurse does not collect a pain history when the client is experiencing severe discomfort.

- Pain scales are used to objectively evaluate the effectiveness of pain therapies.

- Pain can cause physical signs and symptoms similar to the signs and symptoms of certain disease processes.

- Clients waiting to undergo invasive tests may gain some pain relief by anticipatory guidance.

- To provide maximum pain relief the nurse develops a therapeutic relationship with the client and teaches the client about pain.

- The nurse individualizes pain therapy by collaborating closely with the client, using assessment findings, and trying a variety of therapies.

- Eliminating sources of painful stimuli is a basic nursing measure for promoting comfort.

- Proper administration of analgesics requires the nurse to know the client's response to the drugs, select the proper medication, and administer an accurate dose in a timely manner.

- Using a regular schedule for analgesic administration is more effective than an as-needed schedule in controlling pain.
- A patient-controlled analgesic device gives clients pain control with low risk of overdose.
- While caring for a client who receives local anesthesia, the nurse protects the client from injury.
- Nursing implications for administering epidural analgesia include preventing infection and monitoring closely for respiratory depression.
- The aim of therapy for cancer clients is to anticipate and prevent pain rather than treat it.
- Evaluation of the client's pain therapy requires consideration of the changing character of pain, response to therapy, and the client's perceptions of a therapy's effectiveness.

Key Terms

Critical Thinking Exercises

1. Sarah is 80 years old and has remained independent, living in a small apartment 2 blocks from her daughter. The nurse at the physician's office has seen Sarah regularly over the last 10 years. She notices Sarah to be less lively and regularly holding her hand over her abdomen. During examination, Sarah grimaces during abdominal palpation. When the nurse asks whether she has discomfort, Sarah says, "No, it just tickles." What should the nurse consider in further assessing Sarah for pain?

2. What is the best method for attempting to assess the severity of a client's pain?

3. It is 11 AM. Joe had surgery early in the morning and has just reached the nursing division. He is still somewhat sedated from anesthesia. No analgesics were given in the recovery room. Joe's surgical incision involves the right lower abdomen, and the dressing is saturated with drainage. The nurse observes Joe having difficulty turning over on his right side and grimacing while he moves. Joe's blood pressure and pulse have risen since he returned from the operating room. Describe appropriate pain therapies the nurse should use for Joe.

4. Tom suffers from chronic pain associated with metastatic cancer. His discomfort interferes with his ability to care for personal hygiene needs. Tom avoids talking with family and friends when his pain becomes severe. Morphine sulfate, 8 mg intramuscularly every 3 to 4 hours, has been ordered for Tom. What principles should the nurse follow in administering morphine sulfate? If the morphine sulfate proves ineffective, what options does the nurse have?

REFERENCES

Adams RD: Pain: general considerations. In Isselbacher KJ et al, editors: *Harrison's principles of internal medicine*, ed 9, New York, 1980, McGraw-Hill.

Baily LM: Music's soothing charms, *Am J Nurs* 85:1280, 1985.

Brena SF: In Brena SF, Chapman SL, editors: *Management of patients with chronic pain*, New York, 1983, SP Medical & Scientific.

Burns JW et al: The influence of patient characteristics on the requirements for postoperative analgesia, *Anaesthesia* 44:2, 1989.

Carney RM: Clinical applications of relaxation training, *Hosp Pract* 18(7):83, 1983.

Cash JT: Sexuality and chronic pain, *Am J Nurs* 84:1417, 1984.

Ceccio CM: Heat vs cold as treatment for arthritic pain, *RN* 53:83, 1990.

Cleeland CS: The impact of pain on the patient with cancer, *Cancer* 54(suppl):2635, 1984.

Engber E: Report on the NIH consensus development conference on pain, *J Pain Symptom Manage* 1:165, 1986.

Fields HL: *Pain*, New York, 1987, McGraw-Hill.

Gil K: Psychologic aspects of acute pain, *Anesthesiol Report* 2(2):246, 1990.

Guyton AC: *Anatomy and physiology*, New York, 1985, Saunders.

Hargreaves A, Lander J: Use of transcutaneous electrical nerve stimulation for postoperative pain, *Nurs Res* 38(3):159, 1989.

Harrison A: Assessing patients' pain: identifying reasons for error, *J Adv Nurs* 16:1018, 1991.

Heidrich G, Perry S: Helping the patient in pain, *Am J Nurs* 82:1828, 1982.

Herr KA, Mobily PR: Complexities of pain assessment in the elderly, *J Gerontol Nurs* 17(4):12, 1991.

International Association for the Study of Pain, Subcommittee on Taxonomy: Pain terms: a list with definitions and notes on usage, *Pain* 6:249, 1979.

Intravenous Nurses Society: Intravenous nursing standards of practice, *J IV Nurs*, S70-S71, suppl 1990.

Jacox AK, Stewart M: *Psychosocial contingencies of the pain experience*, Iowa City, 1973, University of Iowa College of Nursing.

Kim MJ, McFarland GK, McLane AM: *Pocket guide to nursing diagnoses*, ed 4, St Louis, 1991, Mosby–Year Book.

Krieger D: Therapeutic touch: the imprimatur of nursing, *Am J Nurs* 75:784, 1975.

Lonsway RA: Care of the patient with an epidural catheter: an infection-control challenge, *J IV Nurs* 11(1):52, 1988.

Maxwell MB: How to use methadone for the cancer patient's pain, *Am J Nurs* 80:1606, 1980.

Mayer DK: Non-pharmacologic management of pain in the person with cancer, *Adv Nurs* 10:325, 1985.

McCaffery M: *Nursing management of the patient with pain*, ed 2, Philadelphia, 1979, Lippincott.

McCaffery M: Understanding your client's pain, *Nurs 80* 10:26, 1980.

McCaffery M: Would you administer placebos for pain? These facts can help you decide, *Nurs 82* 12:22, 1982.

McCaffery M: *Pain: assessment and intervention in nursing practice*, course syllabus, St. Louis, 1986, Barnes Hospital.

McCaffery M, Beebe A: Pain in the elderly: special considerations. In McCaffery M, Beebe A: *Pain: clinical manual for nursing practice.* St Louis, 1989, Mosby–Year Book.

McGuire DB: The measurement of clinical pain, *Nurs Res* 33(3): 152, 1984.

Meinhart NT, McCaffery M: *Pain: a nursing approach to assessment and analysis,* Norwalk, Conn, 1983, Appleton-Century-Crofts.

Melzack R, Dennis FG: Neurophysiological foundations of pain. In Sternbach RA, editor: *The psychology of pain,* New York, 1978, Raven.

Melzack R, Wall PD: Pain mechanisms: a new theory, *Science* 150:971, 1965.

Melzack R et al: Relief of dental pain by ice massage of the hand, *Can Med Assoc J* 122:189, 1980.

Miller JF, Shuter R: An exploratory study of pain expression styles among blacks and whites, *Int J Intercult Rel* 6:281, 1982.

National Institutes of Health Consensus Develop Panel: New gains against pain, *Emerg Med* Nov 1986, p. 143.

Paice JA: Unraveling the mystery of pain, *Oncol Nurs Forum* 18(5):843, 1991.

Price DD et al: Psychophysical analysis of experimental factors that selectively influence the affective dimension of pain, *Pain* 8(2):137, 1980.

Rankin MA, Snider B: Nurse's perceptions of cancer patient's pain, *Cancer Nurs* 7:149, 1984.

Ross DM, Ross SA: *Childhood pain: current issues, research, and management,* Baltimore, 1988, Urban & Schwarzenberg.

Schultheis K et al: Preparation for stressful medical procedures and person × treatment interactions, *Clin Psych Rev* 7:329, 1987.

Spiegel D, Bloom J: Pain in metastatic breast cancer, *Cancer* 52(2):341-345, 1983.

Taylor AG et al: How effective is TENS for acute pain? *Am J Nurs* 83:1171, 1983.

Taylor AG et al: Duration of pain, condition, and physical pathology as determinants of nurses' assessment of patients in pain, *Nurs Res* 33:4, 1984.

Turnage G et al: Spinal opioids: a nursing perspective, *J Pain Symptom Manag* 5(3):154, 1990.

Twycross RG, Lack SA: *Symptom control in far advanced cancer: pain relief,* London, 1983, Pitman.

Whipple B: Methods of pain control: a review of research and literature, *J Nurs Sch Image* 19(3):142, 1987.

Wilkie DJ: Cancer pain management: state-of-the-art nursing care, *Nurs Clin North Am* 25(2):331, 1990.

Witt J: Relieving chronic pain, *Nurs Pract* 9:36, 1984.

World Health Organization: *Cancer pain relief,* Geneva, 1986, The Organization.

Zoob M: Differentiating the causes of chest pain, *Geriatrics* 33:95, 1978.

ADDITIONAL READINGS

Alberico JG: Breaking the chronic pain cycle, *Am J Nurs* 84:1222, 1984.

Barnett DC, Hair B: Use and effectiveness of transcutaneous electrical nerve stimulation in pain management, *J Neurosurg Nurs* 13:323, 1981.

Bast C, Hayes P: Patient-controlled analgesia, *Nurs 86* 16(1):25, 1986.

Bast C, Hayes P: PCA: a new way to spell pain relief, *RN* 49(8):18, 1986.

Boyer MW: Continuous drip morphine, *Am J Nurs* 82:603, 1982.

Cook JD: The therapeutic use of music: a literature review, *Nurs Forum* 20:253, 1981.

Cook JD: Music as an intervention in the oncology setting, *Cancer Nurs* 9:23, 1986.

Craig KD: Social modelling influences in pain. In Sternbach RA, editor: *The psychology of pain,* ed 2, New York, 1986, Raven.

Daake DR, Gueldner SH: Imager instruction and the control of postsurgical pain, *Appl Nurs Res* 2(3):114, 1989.

Daut RL, Cleeland CS: The prevalence and severity of pain in cancer, *Cancer* 50:1913, 1982.

Dimotto JW: Relaxation, *Am J Nurs* 84:754, 1984.

Hannon D et al: Pain: portable relief for terminal patients, *RN* 48:37, 1985.

Hauck SL: Pain: problem for the person with cancer, *Cancer Nurs* 9:66, 1986.

Holm K et al: Effect of personal pain experience on pain assessment, *Image J Nurs Sch* 21(2):72, 1989.

Kaido RF: Age and morphine analgesia in cancer patients with postoperative pain, *Clin Pharmacol Rev* 28:823, 1980.

Kanner RM, Portenoy RK: Are the people who need analgesics getting them? *Am J Nurs* 86:589, 1986.

Keller E, Bzdek VM: Effects of therapeutic touch on tension headache pain, *Nurs Res* 35:101, 1986.

LaFoy J, Geden EA: Postepisiotomy pain: warm versus cold sitz bath, *JOGNN* 18:399, 1989.

Locsin R: The effect of music on the pain of selected postoperative patients, *J Adv Nurs* 6:19, 1981.

Marks RM, Sachar EJ: Undertreatment of medical inpatients with narcotic analgesics, *Ann Intern Med* 78:173, 1973.

Marzinski LR: The tragedy of dementia: clinically assessing pain in the confused, nonverbal elderly, *J Gerontol Nurs* 17(6):25, 1991.

Mayer DK, Coyle N: Spinal relief of cancer pain, *Am J Nurs* 86:1050, 1986.

Melzack R: The McGill pain questionnaire: major properties and scoring methods, *Pain* 1:277, 1975.

Moore DE, Blacker HM: How effective is TENS for chronic pain? *Am J Nurs* 83:1175, 1983.

Moulin DE, Coyle N: Spinal relief of cancer pain, *Am J Nurs* 86:1050, 1986.

Proctor MR, Warfield CA: Biofeedback pain control, *Hosp Pract* 12:104, 1984.

Rahr V: Giving intrathecal drugs, *Am J Nurs* 86:829, 1986.

Timmermans G, Sternback RA: Human chronic pain and personality: a canonical correlation analysis. In Bonica JJ, Albe-Fessard D, editors: *Advances in pain research and therapy,* vol 1, New York, 1976, Raven.

Wells N: The effect of relaxation on postoperative muscle tension and pain, *Nurs Res* 31:236, 1982.

Williams DJ: Pushbutton pain relief puts the patient in control, *Am J Nurs* 85:1458, 1985.

Zahourek RP: Hypnosis in nursing practice. I. Emphasis on the "problem patient" who has pain, *J Psychosoc Nurs* 20:13, 1982.

CHAPTER 38

Oxygenation

OBJECTIVES

Mastery of content in this chapter will enable the student to:
- Define the key terms listed.
- Describe the gross structure and function of the cardiopulmonary system.
- Identify physiological processes in maintaining cardiac output, myocardial blood flow, and coronary artery circulation.
- Describe the electrical conduction system of the heart.
- Describe how cardiac output can be altered by preload, afterload, contractility, and heart rate.
- Identify physiological processes involved in ventilation, perfusion, and exchange of respiratory gases.
- Describe neural and chemical regulation of respiration.
- Explain the ways a client's level of health, age, lifestyle, and environment can affect tissue oxygenation.
- Identify causes and effects of disturbances in conduction, altered cardiac output, impaired valvular function, myocardial ischemia, and impaired tissue perfusion.
- Identify causes and effects of hyperventilation, hypoventilation, and hypoxemia.
- Perform a nursing assessment of the cardiopulmonary system.
- Develop nursing diagnoses for altered oxygenation.
- Describe nursing interventions to increase activity tolerance, maintain or promote lung expansion, promote mobilization of pulmonary secretions, maintain a patent airway, promote oxygenation, and restore cardiopulmonary function.
- Develop evaluation criteria for the nursing care plan for the client with altered oxygenation.

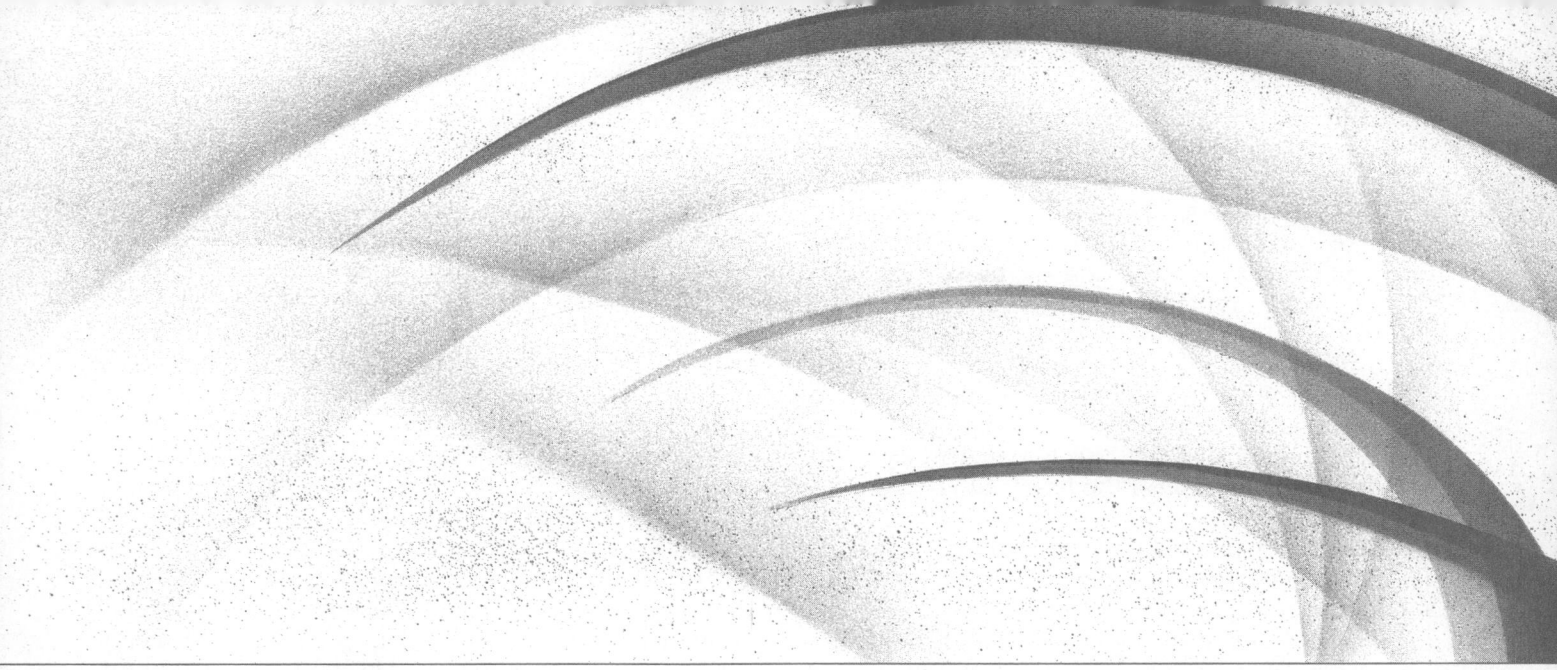

CHAPTER OUTLINE

Cardiovascular Physiology
   Structure and function
   Conduction system

Respiratory Physiology
   Structure and function
   Ventilation
   Perfusion
   Exchange of respiratory gases
   Regulation of respiration

Factors Affecting Oxygenation
   Physiological factors
   Developmental factors
   Behavioral factors
   Environmental factors

Alterations in Cardiac Functioning
   Disturbances in conduction
   Altered cardiac output
   Impaired valvular function
   Myocardial ischemia

Alterations in Respiratory Functioning
   Hyperventilation
   Hypoventilation
   Hypoxia

Nursing Process and Oxygenation
   Assessment
   Nursing diagnosis
   Planning
   Implementation
   Evaluation

Oxygen is a basic human need and is required to sustain life. The nurse often encounters clients who are unable to independently meet oxygen needs. To help clients meet their oxygen needs, the nurse must understand cardiac and respiratory physiology.

Cardiac physiology involves the delivery of oxygenated blood to the tissues and the delivery of deoxygenated blood to the pulmonary system. Once blood is delivered to the pulmonary circulation, the lungs oxygenate the blood, and this oxygenated blood is returned to the left side of the heart and then delivered to the tissues.

Respiratory physiology involves oxygenation of the body through the mechanisms of ventilation, perfusion, and transport of respiratory gases. In addition, neural and chemical regulators control fluctuations in respiratory rate and depth to meet tissue oxygen demands. Together, the cardiac and respiratory systems function to supply the body's oxygen demands.

 CARDIOVASCULAR PHYSIOLOGY

The function of the cardiac system is to deliver oxygen, nutrients, and other substances to the tissues and to remove the waste products of cellular metabolism. The objective is achieved through the cardiac pump, the circulatory vascular system, and the integration of other systems (for example, respiratory, digestive, and renal) (McCance, Huether, 1990).

Structure and Function

The heart pumps blood through the pulmonary circulation by way of the right ventricle and to the systemic circulation by way of the left ventricle. Both ventricles supply oxygen and nutrients to the tissues and remove wastes from the body (Fig. 38-1). The circulatory system is the route for the exchange of respiratory gases, nutrients, and waste products between the blood and the tissues.

Myocardial Pump

The pumping action of the heart is essential to maintain oxygen delivery. Diseases that decrease the pumping effectiveness of the heart, such as coronary artery disease and cardiomyopathic conditions, lessen the volume of blood ejected from the ventricles. Similar conditions that affect circulating blood volume (for example, hemorrhage and dehydration) decrease the available blood for the heart to eject from the ventricles.

The chambers of the heart fill during diastole and empty during systole. A client's blood pressure reading helps determine the effectiveness of the diastolic and systolic events of the cardiac cycle (see Chapter 19).

The myocardial fibers have contractile properties that enable the myocardial fiber to stretch during filling. In a healthy heart, this stretch is proportionally related to the strength of contraction. That is, as the myocardium stretches, the strength of the subsequent contraction also increases. This response is the Frank-Starling (Starling's) law of the heart.

In the diseased heart, Starling's law does not apply because the stretch of the myocardium is beyond physiological limits. The heart stretches or dilates, but the subsequent contractile response results in insufficient ventricular ejection (volume). The heart loses its ability to pump the blood forward, and blood begins to "back-up" in the pulmonary (left heart failure) or systemic circulation (right heart failure).

Myocardial Blood Flow

To maintain adequate blood flow to the pulmonary and systemic circulations, myocardial blood flow must sufficiently supply oxygen and nutrients to the myocardium itself.

The one-way flow of blood through the heart is ensured by the four heart valves (Fig. 38-2). During ventricular diastole the atrioventricular (mitral and tricuspid) valves open and blood flows from the higher pressure atria into the relaxed ventricles. After ventricular filling, the systolic phase begins. As the systolic intraventricular pressure rises, the atrioventricular valves close, preventing the back flow of blood into the atria, and ventricular contraction begins.

As the ventricles begin the systolic phase, ventricular pressure rises, causing the semilunar (aortic and pulmonic) valves to open. As the ventricles eject blood past these open valves, the intraventricular pressure falls and the semilunar valves close, thus preventing the back flow of blood into the ventricles.

Clients who have valvular diseases may have back flow or regurgitation of blood through the incompetent valve. This regurgitation causes a murmur that is heard on auscultation over the specific auscultation areas for each valve (see Chapter 20).

Coronary Artery Circulation

Blood flow through the atria and ventricles does not supply oxygen and nutrients to the myocardium itself. The coronary circulation is the branch of the systemic circulation that supplies oxygen and nutrients to and removal of waste from the myocardium

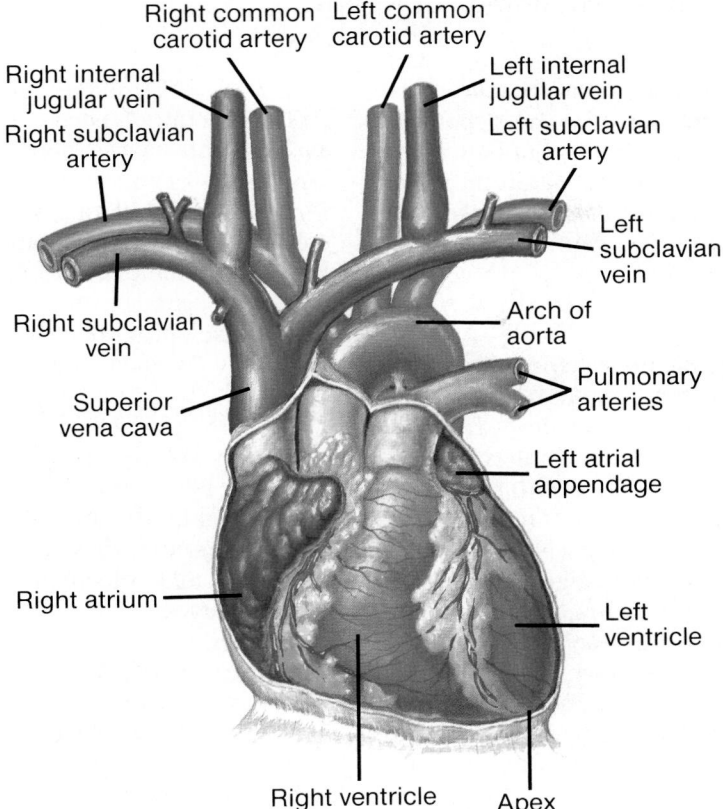

Fig. 38-1 Diagram showing serially connected pulmonary and systemic circulation. Right heart chambers propel unoxygenated blood through the pulmonary circulation; left heart chambers propel oxygenated blood through systemic circulation.
From Canobbio MM: *Cardiovascular disorders*, St Louis, 1990, Mosby–Year Book.

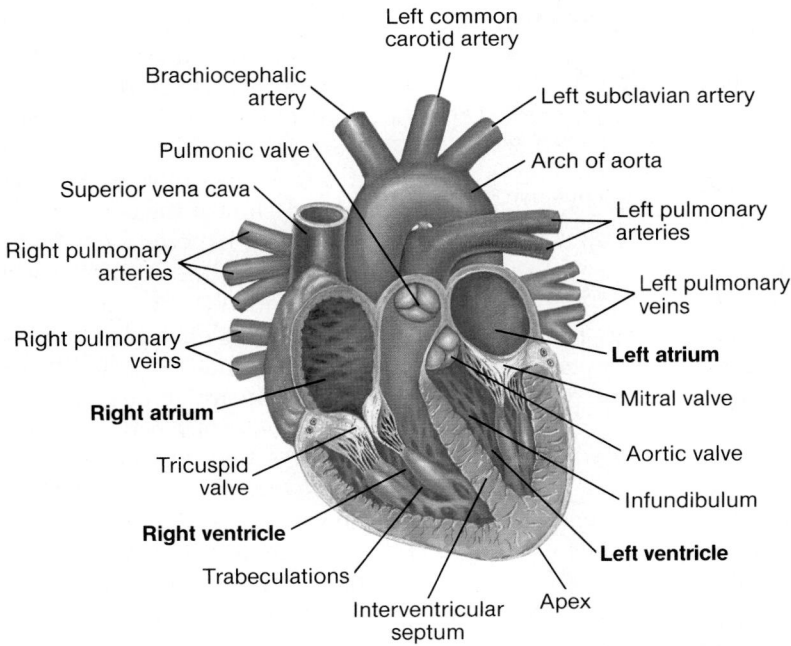

Fig. 38-2 Structures that direct blood flow through the heart. Arrows indicate path of blood through chambers, valves, and major vessels.
Adapted from Canobbio MM: *Cardiovascular disorders*, St Louis, 1990, Mosby–Year Book.

(see box). These arteries arise from the aorta just above and behind the aortic valve through openings called the *coronary ostia*. The most abundant blood supply feeds the left ventricular myocardium, which is more muscular and does most of the heart's work. The coronary arteries fill during ventricular diastole (McCance, Huether, 1990).

Systemic Circulation

The arteries and veins of the systemic circulation deliver nutrients and oxygen to and remove waste from the tissues. Oxygenated blood flows from the left ventricle by way of the aorta and into large systemic arteries. These arteries branch into smaller arteries and finally into arterioles. The arterioles branch further into the smallest vessels, the capillaries. At the capillary level, the exchange of respiratory gases, nutrients, and wastes occurs; the tissues are oxygenated; and nutrients are received. The waste products exit the capillary network by way of the venules that join to form veins. These veins form larger veins, which carry deoxygenated blood to the right heart to be returned to pulmonary circulation.

Coronary Arteries

RIGHT CORONARY ARTERY

Right atrium, anterior right ventricle
Supplies:
Posterior aspect of septum (90% of population)
Posterior papillary muscle
Sinus and AV nodes (80%-90% of population)
Inferior aspect of left ventricle

LEFT CORONARY ARTERIES
Left Anterior Descending (LAD)

Supplies: Anterior left ventricular wall
Anterior interventricular septum (septal branches supply conduction system, bundle of His, and bundle branches)
Anterior papillary muscle
Left ventricular apex

CIRCUMFLEX

Supplies: Left atrium
Posterior surfaces of left ventricle
Posterior aspects of septum

From Canobbio MM: *Cardiovascular disorders,* St Louis, 1990, Mosby–Year Book, p. 14.

Regulation of Blood Flow

The amount of blood ejected from the left ventricle each minute is the **cardiac output.** For a healthy 150-lb (70-kg) adult at rest, the cardiac output is 5 L/min. The circulating volume of blood changes according to the oxygen and metabolic needs of the body. For example, during exercise, pregnancy, and fever, the cardiac output increases, but during sleep, the cardiac output decreases. Cardiac output is represented by the following formula:

Cardiac output (CO) = Stroke volume (SV) × Heart rate (HR)

Stroke volume is the amount of blood ejected from the left ventricle with each contraction. It can be affected by the amount of blood in the left ventricle at the end of diastole (preload), the resistance to left ventricular ejection (afterload), and myocardial contractility.

Preload is essentially the end diastolic volume. As the ventricles fill, they stretch. According to the principles of the Frank-Starling law, the greater the stretch on the ventricle, the greater the contraction and the greater the stroke volume. In clinical situations, the preload and subsequent stroke volume can be manipulated by changing the amount of circulating blood volume. For example, in the client with hemorrhagic shock, fluid therapy and replacement of blood volume increases volume, thus increasing the preload and subsequent cardiac output. If volume is not replaced, preload decreases, as does subsequent cardiac output, and ultimately the venous return to the right atrium decreases. This decreased venous return further decreases preload and cardiac output.

Afterload is the resistance to left ventricular ejection. For the left side of the heart, afterload is the work the heart must overcome to fully eject blood from the left ventricle. The diastolic aortic pressure is a good clinical measure of afterload. In a client with an acute hypertensive crisis, the afterload is increased and the cardiac workload also increases. Afterload in this situation can be manipulated by decreasing systemic blood pressure.

Myocardial contractility also affects stroke volume and cardiac output. Poor contraction decreases the amount of blood ejected by the ventricles during each contraction. Myocardial contractility can be increased by drugs that increase the force of contraction, such as digitalis preparations, epinephrine, and sympathomimetic drugs (drugs that mimic the effects of the sympathetic nervous system).

Heart rate affects blood flow because of the interaction between rate and diastolic filling time. With a faster heart rate, particularly sustained rates greater than 160 beats/min, diastolic filling time decreases.

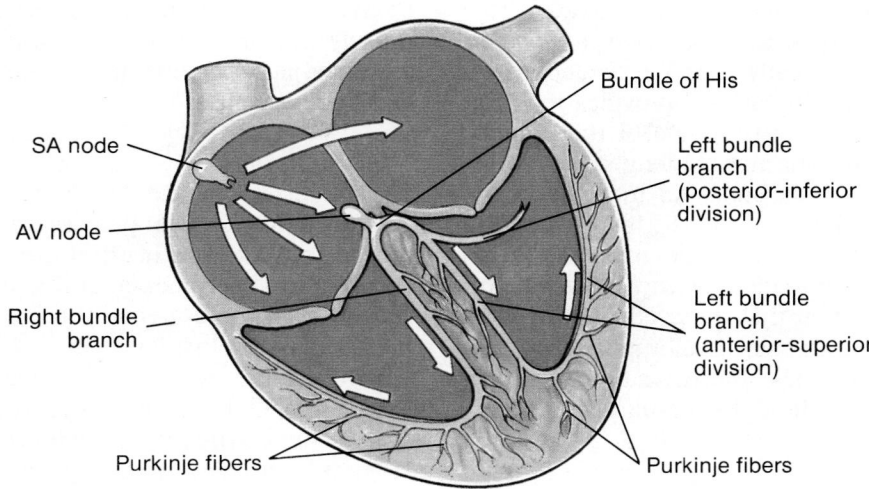

Fig. 38-3 Eletrical conduction system.
From Canobbio MM: *Cardiovascular disorders*, St Louis, 1990, Mosby–Year Book.

As filling time decreases, stroke volume and cardiac output decrease.

Conduction System

The rhythmic relaxation and contraction of the atria and ventricles depend on continuous, organized transmission of electrical impulses. These impulses are generated and transmitted by way of the conduction system (Fig. 38-3).

The heart's conduction system generates the necessary action potentials that conduct the impulses required to initiate the electrical chain of events resulting in the heart beat. The autonomic nervous system influences the rate of impulse generation as well as the speed of transmission through the conductive pathway and the strength of atrial and ventricular contractions. Sympathetic nerve fibers, which increase the rate of impulse generation and the speed of impulse transmission, innervate all parts of the atria and ventricles. Parasympathetic fibers from the vagus nerve, which decrease this rate, also innervate these parts as well as the sinoatrial and atrioventricular nodes (McCance, Huether, 1990).

The conduction system originates with the **sinoatrial (SA) node,** which is "the pacemaker of the heart." The SA node is in the right atrium next to the entrance of the superior vena cava (McCance, Huether, 1990). Impulses are initiated at the SA node at an intrinsic rate of 60 to 100 beats/min. The resting adult rate is approximately 75 beats/min.

The electrical impulses are then transmitted through the atria to the **atrioventricular (AV) node.**

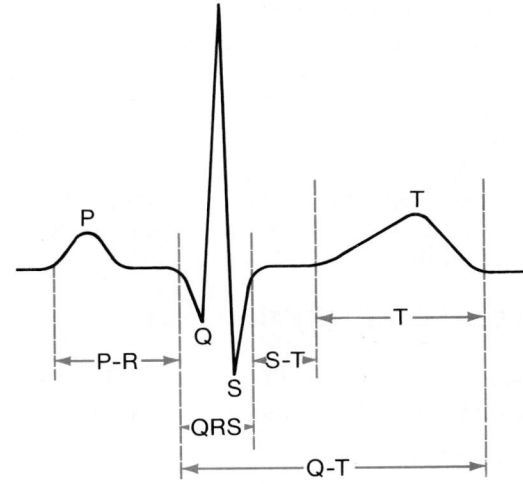

Fig. 38-4 Normal ECG waveform.
From Canobbio MM: *Cardiovascular disorders*, St Louis, 1990, Mosby–Year Book.

The AV node mediates impulses between the atria and the ventricles. It assists atrial emptying by delaying the impulse before transmitting it through the **bundle of His** and the ventricular **Purkinje network.**

The electrical activity of the conduction system is reflected by an **electrocardiogram (ECG).** An ECG monitors the regularity and path of the electrical impulse through the conduction system. The normal sequence on the ECG is called *normal sinus rhythm (NSR)* (Fig. 38-4).

A finding of NSR means that the impulse originated at the SA node and followed the normal sequence through the conduction system. The P-wave on the ECG indicates that the atria have received an electrical impulse. Normally, atrial contraction follows the P-wave. The PR interval provides information about the delay in transmission of the impulse through the AV node. The normal length for the PR interval is 0.12 to 0.20 seconds. An increase in the time indicates that there is a block in the impulse transmission though the AV node, whereas a decrease indicates the initiation of the electrical impulse from a source other that the SA node. The QRS complex is a sign that the electrical impulse has traveled through the ventricles, and normally the ventricles contract following the QRS complex.

RESPIRATORY PHYSIOLOGY

Most cells in the body obtain much of their energy from chemical reactions involving oxygen. Cells must also eliminate carbon dioxide. The exchange of respiratory gases occurs between the environmental air and the blood. There are three steps in the process of oxygenation: ventilation, perfusion, and diffusion (McCance, Huether, 1990). For the exchange of respiratory gases to occur, the organs, nerves, and muscles of respiration must be intact. In addition, the central nervous system must be able to regulate the cycle of inspiration and expiration.

Structure and Function

Respiration can be altered by conditions or diseases that occur in the pulmonary system, resulting

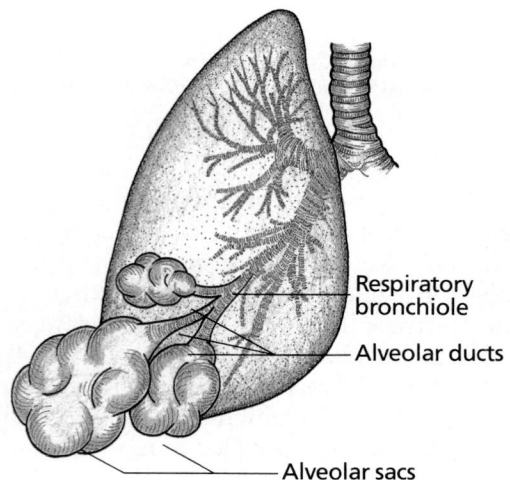

Fig. 38-5 Alveoli at the terminal end of the lower airway. From Gröer MW, Shekleton ME: *Basic pathophysiology: a conceptual approach*, ed 2, St Louis, 1989, Mosby–Year Book.

in changes of structure and function. The respiratory muscles, pleural space, lungs, and alveoli (Fig. 38-5) are essential for ventilation, perfusion, and exchange of respiratory gases (see box).

Ventilation

Ventilation is the process by which gases are moved into and out of the lungs. Adequate ventilation requires coordination of the muscular and elastic properties of the lung and thorax and intact innervation. The major inspiratory muscle is the diaphragm, which is innervated by the phrenic nerve. This nerve exits the spinal cord at the fourth cervical vertebra. Spinal cord disruption at the fourth cervical level can sever the phrenic cervical nerve and impair the diaphragm's function.

Work of Breathing

Breathing is the effort required to expand and contract the lungs. It is determined by the degree of compliance of lung tissue, resistance of the airway, presence of active expiration, and use of accessory muscles of respiration (Groër, Shekleton, 1989).

Compliance is the ability of the lungs and thorax to expand in response to increased intraalveolar pressure (Groër, Shekleton, 1989). Simply stated, it is the ability of the lungs to distend (Dettenmeier, 1992). Compliance is decreased in diseases such as pulmonary edema, interstitial fibrosis, and pleural fibrosis. In addition, congenital or traumatic structural abnormalities, such as kyphosis or fractured ribs, decrease compliance.

Airway resistance is the pressure difference between the mouth and the alveoli in relation to the rate of flow of inspired gas. Airway resistance can be increased by an airway obstruction (such as a foreign body), small airway disease (such as asthma), and tracheal edema. When resistance is increased, the amount of air traveling through the anatomical airways is decreased.

Active expiration is the use of muscle groups to contract the lungs. Expiration is normally a passive process that depends on elastic recoil properties and requires little or no muscle work. Elastic recoil is produced by elastic fibers in lung tissue and by surface tension in the fluid film lining the alveoli (Dettenmeier, 1992).

Accessory muscles of respiration can increase lung volume during inspiration. Clients with chronic obstructive pulmonary disease, especially emphysema, frequently use these muscles to increase lung volume. During assessment the nurse may observe the client's clavicles being elevated in the inspiratory phase of respiration.

Major Anatomical Structures of the Thorax and Their Functions

INSPIRATORY MUSCLES
Diaphragm

- Contraction causes the diaphragm to descend, creating a negative pleural pressure and increasing the vertical dimension of the lungs, which contributes to inflation of the lungs. The increase in vertical dimension and the decrease in intrapulmonary pressure (negative with respect to atmospheric pressure) causes air to enter the lungs.

External Intercostal

- Contraction elevates the anterior ends of the ribs, causing them to move upward and outward. This increases the anteroposterior dimension of the thorax.

Accessory Muscles

- Accessory muscles include the scalene, sternocleidomastoid, and trapezius muscles. Contraction elevates the first two ribs and the sternum.

EXPIRATORY MUSCLES
Internal Intercostal

- Contraction pulls ribs down and in, thereby decreasing the anteroposterior diameter of the thorax.

Abdominal Respiratory

- Abdominal respiratory muscles include the rectus, transverse abdominis, internal oblique, and external oblique muscles. Contraction depresses lower ribs, forces the diaphragm up, and decreases the vertical dimension of the thoracic cavity.

PLEURAL SPACE

- The pleural space is a potential space that is only a thin film of liquid lying between the outer layer of the lung (visceral pleura) and the inner layer of the chest cavity (parietal pleura). It permits a smooth, gliding movement of the lungs along the chest wall. Normally, air is not present in the pleural space.

LUNGS

Left (Two Lobes) and Right (Three Lobes)

- The lungs transfer oxygen from the atmosphere into the alveoli and carbon dioxide from the alveoli to the lungs to be excreted as a waste product. They also filter toxic material from circulation and metabolize compounds such as angiotensin I, bradykinin, and prostaglandins.

Alveoli

- Alveoli transfer oxygen and carbon dioxide to and from the blood through the alveolar membrane. These tiny air sacs expand during inspiration, greatly increasing the surface area over which exchange of gases occurs.

Decreased compliance, increased airway resistance, active expiration, or use of accessory muscles increases the work of breathing, resulting in an increased energy expenditure. To meet this expenditure, the body increases its metabolic rate. Consequently, the need for oxygen, as well as the elimination of carbon dioxide, is increased. This sequence is a vicious circle for a client with impaired ventilation and causes further deterioration of respiratory status.

Volumes

Normal volumes within the lungs are measured through pulmonary function testing. Some of these measurements are taken with a spirometer, which measures the volume of air entering or leaving the lungs. Variations in lung volumes may be associated with health states such as pregnancy, exercise, obesity, or obstructive and restrictive pathological conditions of the lung. The amount of surfactant, degree of compliance, and strength of respiratory muscles can affect pressures and volumes within the lungs.

Pressures

Gases are moved into and out of the lungs through pressure changes (Fig. 38-6 on p. 1224). Intrapleural pressure is negative to (less than) atmospheric pressure, which is 760 mm Hg at sea level. For air to flow into the lungs, intrapleural pressure must become more negative, setting up a pressure gradient between the atmosphere and alveoli, thus moving air into the lungs and alveoli.

Perfusion

The primary function of pulmonary circulation is to move blood to and from the alveolar-capillary

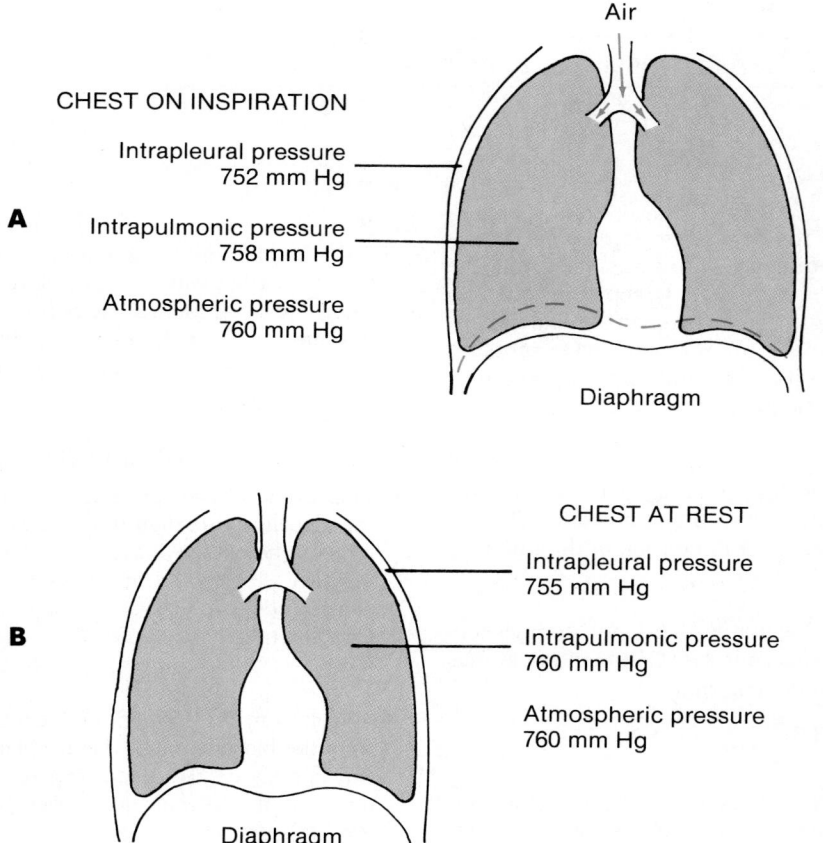

Fig. 38-6   **A,** Contraction of the diaphragm to increase vertical dimensions of the lungs. **B,** Relaxation of the diaphragm, decreasing vertical dimensions of the lungs. From Wade JF: *Comprehensive respiratory care*, ed 3, St Louis, 1982, Mosby–Year Book.

membrane so that gas exchange can occur. Pulmonary circulation is also a reservoir for blood so that the lung can increase its blood volume without large increases in pulmonary artery or venous pressures. Finally, this circulatory system filters blood to remove small thrombi before they reach the brain or other vital organs (West, 1979).

Pulmonary Circulation

Pulmonary circulation begins at the pulmonary artery, which receives mixed (poorly oxygenated) venous blood from the right ventricle. Blood flow through this system depends on the pumping ability of the right ventricle, which has an output of approximately 5 to 6 L/min. The flow continues from the pulmonary artery through the pulmonary arterioles to the pulmonary capillaries. At the capillary level, blood comes in contact with the alveolar–capillary membrane and the exchange of respiratory gases occurs. The oxygen-rich blood then circulates through the pulmonary venules and pulmonary veins and returns to the left atrium.

Distribution

Pressures within the pulmonary circulatory system are low in comparison to those in the systemic circulatory system. The normal pulmonary systolic arterial pressure is between 20 and 30 mm Hg, the diastolic pressure is less than 12 mm Hg, and the mean pressure is less than 20 mm Hg (Daily, Schroeder, 1989). Because of low pressure and low resistance, the walls of the pulmonary vessels are thinner than those in the systemic circulation and contain less smooth muscle. The lung accepts the total cardiac output from the right ventricle and, except in cases of alveolar hypoxia, does not direct blood flow from one region to another.

Exchange of Respiratory Gases

Respiratory gases are exchanged in the alveoli of the lungs and the capillaries of the body tissues. Oxygen is transferred from the lungs to the blood, and carbon dioxide is transferred from the blood to the alveoli to be exhaled as a waste product. At the tissue level, oxygen is transferred from the blood to tissues, and carbon dioxide is transferred from tissues to the blood to return to the alveoli and be exhaled. This transfer depends on the process of diffusion.

Diffusion

Diffusion is the movement of molecules from an area of higher concentration to an area of lower concentration. Diffusion of respiratory gases occurs at the alveolar–capillary membrane, and the rate of diffusion can be affected by thickness of the membrane.

Increased thickness of the membrane impedes diffusion because respiratory gases take longer to transfer across the thickened space. In clients with pulmonary edema, pulmonary infiltrate, or a pulmonary effusion, thickness of the respiratory membrane is increased. As a result, diffusion is slowed and the exchange of respiratory gases and subsequent delivery of oxygen to tissues are impaired.

The surface area of the membrane can be altered as a result of a chronic disease (such as emphysema), an acute disease (such as a pneumothorax), or a surgical process (such as a lobectomy). When fewer alveoli are functioning, the surface area is decreased.

Oxygen Transport

The oxygen transport system consists of the lungs and cardiovascular system. Delivery depends on the amount of oxygen entering the lungs (ventilation), blood flow to the lungs and tissues (perfusion), adequacy of diffusion, and capacity of the blood to carry oxygen. The capacity to carry oxygen is influenced by the amount of dissolved oxygen in the plasma, amount of hemoglobin, and tendency of hemoglobin to bind with oxygen (Ahrens, 1987, 1990).

Only a relatively small amount of required oxygen, about 3%, is dissolved in the plasma. Most oxygen is transported by hemoglobin, which serves as a carrier for oxygen and carbon dioxide. The hemoglobin molecule combines with oxygen to form oxyhemoglobin. Oxyhemoglobin is easily reversible, allowing hemoglobin and oxygen to dissociate, which frees oxygen to enter tissues.

Carbon Dioxide Transport

The transport of respiratory gases includes movement of carbon dioxide. Carbon dioxide diffuses into red blood cells and is rapidly hydrated into carbonic acid (H_2CO_3) because of the presence of carbonic anhydrase. The carbonic acid then dissociates into hydrogen (H^+) and bicarbonate (HCO_3^-) ions. The hydrogen ion is buffered by hemoglobin, and the HCO_3^- diffuses into the plasma (see Chapter 39). In addition, some of the carbon dioxide in red blood cells reacts with amino acid groups, forming carbamino compounds. This reaction can occur rapidly without the presence of an enzyme. Reduced hemoglobin (deoxyhemoglobin) can combine with carbon dioxide more easily than oxyhemoglobin, and therefore venous blood transports the majority of carbon dioxide.

Regulation of Respiration

The main purpose of respiratory regulation is to supply sufficient oxygen to meet the body's demands, such as during exercise, infection, or pregnancy. In addition, respiratory regulation promotes exhalation of metabolically produced carbon dioxide, which is a determinant of acid-base status (see Chapter 39).

There are two respiratory regulators: neural and chemical. Neural regulation includes the central nervous system control of respiratory rate, depth, and rhythm. Chemical regulation involves the influence of chemicals such as carbon dioxide and hydrogen ions on the rate and depth of respiration (see box).

Neural and Chemical Regulation of Respiration

NEURAL REGULATION

- Neural regulation maintains rhythm and depth of respiration as well as the balance between inspiration and expiration.

Cerebral Cortex

- Voluntary control of respiration delivers impulses to the respiratory motor neurons by way of the spinal cord. Voluntary control of respiration accommodates speaking, eating, and swimming.

Medulla Oblongata

- Automatic control of respiration occurs continuously.

CHEMICAL REGULATION

- Chemical regulation maintains appropriate rate and depth of respirations based on changes in the blood's carbon dioxide (CO_2), oxygen (O_2), and hydrogen ion (H^+) concentration.

Chemoreceptors

- Chemoreceptors are located in the medulla, aortic body, and carotid body. Changes in chemical content of O_2, CO_2, and H^+ stimulate chemoreceptors, which in turn stimulate neural regulators to adjust the rate and depth of ventilation to maintain normal arterial blood gas levels. Chemical regulation can occur during physical exercise and in some illnesses. It is a short-term adaptive mechanism.

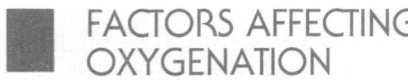

FACTORS AFFECTING OXYGENATION

Adequacy of circulation, ventilation, perfusion, and transport of respiratory gases to the tissues are influenced by four types of factors: (1) physiological, (2) developmental, (3) behavioral, and (4) environmental.

Physiological Factors

Any condition that affects cardiopulmonary functioning directly affects the body's ability to meet oxygen demands. The general classifications of cardiac disorders include disturbances in conduction, impaired valvular function, myocardial hypoxia, cardiomyopathic conditions, and peripheral tissue hypoxia. Respiratory disorders include hyperventilation, hypoventilation, and hypoxia.

Other physiological processes also affect a client's oxygenation (Table 38-1). These include alterations that affect the oxygen-carrying capacity of blood, such as the anemias; increases in the body's metabolic demands, such as during pregnancy or fever and infection; and alterations that affect the client's chest wall movement or the central nervous system.

TABLE 38-1   Physiological Processes Affecting Oxygenation

Process	Effect on Oxygenation
Anemia	Decreases oxygen-carrying capacity of blood
Toxic inhalant (e.g., carbon monoxide)	Decreases oxygen-carrying capacity of blood; carbon monoxide displaces oxygen from hemoglobin and decreases capacity of blood to carry oxygen
Airway obstruction	Limits inspired oxygen delivered to alveoli
High altitudes	Decreases inspiratory oxygen concentration because atmospheric oxygen concentration is lower
Fever	Increases metabolic rate and tissue oxygen demand
Deceased chest wall motion (e.g., from musculoskeletal impairments)	Prevents lowering of diaphragm and reduces anteroposterior diameter of thorax on inspiration, thereby reducing volume of inspired air

---

Decreased Oxygen-Carrying Capacity

As previously noted, hemoglobin carries 97% of the diffused oxygen to tissues. Thus any process that decreases or alters hemoglobin decreases the oxygen-carrying capacity of blood. Anemia and inhalation of toxic substances are two disorders that decrease oxygen-carrying capacity.

Anemia is characterized by below-normal levels of hemoglobin in the blood. Anemia reflects one or more of three basic processes: decreased hemoglobin production, increased red cell destruction, and blood loss. Clinical findings in clients with anemia include fatigue, decreased activity tolerance, increased breathlessness, pallor, and increased heart rate.

Carbon monoxide is the most common toxic inhalant decreasing the oxygen-carrying capacity of blood. A bond of the carbon monoxide molecule with the hemoglobin molecule is stronger than the bond between hemoglobin and oxygen. Because of the bond's strength, carbon monoxide is not easily dissociated from hemoglobin, making the hemoglobin unavailable for oxygen transport.

Decreased Inspired Oxygen Concentration

When the concentration of inspired oxygen declines, the oxygen-carrying capacity of the blood is decreased. Decreases in the fraction of inspired oxygen concentration (Fio_2) can be caused by an upper or lower airway obstruction (which limits delivery of inspired oxygen to alveoli), decreased environmental oxygen (as occurs at high altitudes), or decreased inspiration as the result of an incorrect oxygen concentration setting on respiratory therapy equipment.

Hypovolemia

Hypovolemia is a reduced circulating blood volume resulting from extracellular fluid losses that occurs with conditions such as shock and severe dehydration. If the fluid loss is significant, fluid available for circulation is diminished. The body tries to adapt by increasing the heart rate and peripheral vasoconstriction to increase the volume of blood returned to the heart and raise cardiac output.

Increased Metabolic Rate

Increases in metabolic activity of the body result in an increased oxygen demand. If the body systems are unable to meet this demand, the level of oxygenation declines.

An increased metabolic rate is a normal response of the body to pregnancy, wound healing, and exercise because the body is building tissue. Most people can meet the greater need for oxygen and do not display signs of oxygen deprivation.

When fever is present, metabolic demand, the tissues' need for oxygen, and carbon dioxide production increase. If the infection or febrile state persists, the metabolic rate remains high and the body begins to break down protein stores. As the body continues to break down protein, muscle wasting occurs and the client has decreased muscle mass. Respiratory muscles (for example, the diaphragm and intercostals) are also wasted, and the client may not be able to do the work of breathing and will eventually display signs and symptoms of hypoxemia.

During persistent fever, the body attempts to adapt to the increased carbon dioxide levels by increasing the rate and depth of respiration. This adaptive response enables the body to rid itself of excess carbon dioxide by "blowing off" the carbon dioxide during expiration. The increases in rate and depth of respiration also increase the work of breathing, and clients, particularily those with pulmonary diseases, are at risk for hypoxemia and hypercapnea.

Conditions Affecting Chest Wall Movement

Any condition that reduces chest wall movement can result in decreased ventilation. If the diaphragm cannot fully descend with breathing, the volume of inspired air decreases and less oxygen is delivered to the alveoli and subsequently to tissues.

PREGNANCY. As the fetus grows during pregnancy, the greater size of the uterus pushes abdominal contents upward against the diaphragm. During the last trimester of pregnancy the inspiratory capacity of a pregnant woman therefore declines. She may then experience shortness of breath on exertion and be easily fatigued.

OBESITY. Obese clients often have a heavy lower thorax and abdomen, which reduces lung volumes, particularly in the recumbent and supine positions. In some clients an obesity-hypoventilation syndrome develops in which oxygenation is decreased and carbon dioxide is retained, resulting in daytime sleepiness. The obese client is also susceptible to pneumonia after an upper respiratory tract infection because the lungs cannot fully expand and pulmonary secretions are not mobilized in the lower lobes.

MUSCULOSKELETAL ABNORMALITIES. Musculoskeletal impairments in the thoracic region reduce oxygenation. Such impairments may result from abnormal structural configurations, trauma, muscular diseases, and diseases of the central nervous system.

Abnormal Structural Configurations. Abnormal structural configurations impairing oxygenation include those that affect the rib cage, such as pectus excavatum, and those that affect the vertebral column, such as kyphosis. Pectus excavatum is a depression of the sternum that interferes with lung expansion. Kyphosis is an abnormal condition of the vertebral column characterized by increased convexity of the thoracic spine. This abnormality produces a structural barrier to lung expansion. The angle of curvature can progress with time, resulting in severe hypoventilation and hypoxemia.

Trauma. Trauma to the chest wall may also impede inspiration. The person with multiple rib fractures can develop a flail chest, a condition in which fractures cause instability in part of the chest wall and paradoxical breathing. In paradoxical breathing, the lung underlying the injured area contracts on inspiration and bulges on expiration. This asynchronous chest wall movement can result in hypoxia.

Chest wall or upper abdomen incisions may also decrease chest wall movement. The client may use shallow respirations to minimize chest wall movement to avoid pain. Narcotic analgesics may also depress the respiratory center, thus decreasing respiratory rate.

Muscle Diseases. Muscle diseases such as muscular dystrophy affect oxygenation of tissues. If muscular disease decreases the client's ability to expand and contract the chest, ventilation is impaired and atelectasis, hypercapnea, and hypoxemia can occur.

Nervous System Diseases. Myasthenia gravis, Guillain-Barré syndrome, and poliomyelitis are examples of nervous system diseases that can affect respiratory functioning and result in hypoventilation. Myasthenia gravis interferes with normal transmission of impulses from nerves to muscles. The disease involves the whole body, including muscles of respiration.

Guillain-Barré syndrome and poliomyelitis cause inflammation and paralysis of muscle groups. Guillain-Barré syndrome usually results in an ascending type of paralysis. If paralysis ascends to the thoracic region, respiratory muscles become paralyzed. Poliomyelitis may lead to general or local paralysis. As with Guillain-Barré syndrome, it may reverse, but poliomyelitis usually results in more residual paralysis.

Central Nervous System Alterations. Diseases or trauma involving the central nervous system, specifically the medulla oblongata and spinal cord, may result in impaired respiration. When the medulla oblongata is affected, neural regulation of respiration is damaged and abnormal breathing patterns may develop. Damage to the spinal cord can affect respiration in two ways. If the phrenic nerve is damaged, the diaphragm may not descend, thus reducing inspiratory lung volumes and causing hypoxemia. Spinal cord trauma below the fifth cervical vertebra usually leaves the phrenic nerve intact but damages nerves that innervate the intercostal muscles. This prevents the chest from expanding in the anteroposterior diameter.

INFLUENCES OF CHRONIC DISEASE. The level of oxygenation can be decreased as a direct consequence of chronic disease, as with cardiopulmonary disease. It can also be decreased as a secondary effect, as with anemia in a client with osteoarthritis.

Developmental Factors

The developmental stage of the client and the normal aging process can affect tissue oxygenation.

Premature Infants

Premature infants are at risk for hyaline membrane disease, which is thought to be caused by a surfactant deficiency. The surfactant-synthesizing ability of the lungs develops late in pregnancy and may therefore be lacking in preterm infants (Groër, Shekleton, 1989).

Infants and Toddlers

Infants and toddlers are at risk for upper respiratory tract infections as a result of frequent exposure to other children. In addition, during the teething process some infants develop nasal congestion, which encourages bacterial growth and increases the potential for respiratory tract infection. Upper respiratory tract infections are usually not dangerous, and infants or toddlers recover with little difficulty. However, airway obstructions can develop. Common airway infections are nasopharyngitis (for example, rhinoviruses, respiratory syncytial virus, and adenovirus), pharyngitis (for example, viral and beta-hemolytic streptococci), influenza, and tonsilitis. In addition, obstruction can occur with aspirated foreign objects, such as food, buttons, and candy.

School-Age Children and Adolescents

School-age children and adolescents are exposed to respiratory infections and respiratory risk factors such as smoking. A healthy child usually does not have adverse pulmonary effects from respiratory infections. A person who starts smoking in adolescence and continues to smoke into middle age, however, has an increased risk for cardiopulmonary disease (see Chapter 2).

Young and Middle-Age Adults

Young and middle-age adults are exposed to multiple cardiopulmonary risk factors: an unhealthy diet, lack of exercise, stress, and smoking. Reducing these modifiable risks may decrease the client's risk for cardiac or pulmonary diseases (see Chapter 2).

Older Adults

The cardiac and respiratory systems undergo changes throughout the aging process. The arterial system becomes less distensible due to atherosclerotic plaques, and the systemic blood pressure may rise. The connective tissue and bronchial tree undergo structural changes as the lungs lose elasticity. The alveoli are often enlarged, and the bronchial ducts are dilated (Groër, Shekleton, 1989).

Ventilation and transfer of respiratory gases decline with age. Osteoporotic changes of the thoracic cage and kyphosis of the vertebrae occur normally with aging. With these changes the lungs are unable to expand fully, leading to lower oxygenation levels.

Behavioral Factors

A person's behavior or lifestyle may directly or indirectly affect the body's ability to meet oxygen requirements. Lifestyle factors that influence respiratory functioning include nutrition, exercise, cigarette smoking, substance abuse, and stress.

Nutrition

Nutrition can affect cardiopulmonary function in several ways. First, severe obesity can decrease lung expansion because of the pressure of abdominal contents against the diaphragm and an increased oxygen demand on the body. Second, the malnourished client may experience respiratory muscle wasting, which results in decreased muscle strength and respiratory excursion. Third, muscle weakness may also decrease the ability to cough productively, putting the client at risk for the accumulation of pulmonary secretions. Fourth, high fat diets increase cholesterol and atherogenesis in the coronary arteries. Finally, obese and malnourished clients are at risk for anemia.

Exercise

Exercise increases the body's metabolic activity and thus oxygen demand. The respiratory rate and depth of respirations increase, enabling the person to inhale more oxygen and expire excess carbon dioxide.

A physical exercise program has many benefits (see Chapter 43). People who exercise regularly have a lower pulse rate and blood pressure, decreased cholesterol, increased blood flow, and greater oxygen extraction by working muscles. Fully conditioned people can increase oxygen consumption by 10% to 20% because of increased cardiac output.

Cigarette Smoking

Cigarette smoking is associated with a number of diseases, including heart disease, chronic obstructive lung disease, and lung cancer. The inhaled nicotine causes vasoconstriction of peripheral and coronary blood vessels. Cigarette smoking can worsen peripheral vascular and coronary artery diseases. The risk of lung cancer is 60 times greater for a person who smokes two packs of cigarettes a day than for someone who has never smoked. The mortality with lung cancer is high (greater than 70%), and it is frequently diagnosed only when it has reached an advanced stage (Groër, Shekleton, 1989).

Substance Abuse

Excessive use of alcohol and other drugs can impair tissue oxygenation in two ways. First, the person who chronically abuses substances often has a poor nutritional intake. With the resultant decrease in intake of iron-rich foods, hemoglobin production declines. Second, excessive use of alcohol and certain other drugs can depress the respiratory center in the central nervous system. The rate and depth of inspiration are reduced, decreasing the amount of oxygen inhaled.

Anxiety

A continuous state of severe anxiety increases the body's metabolic rate, and the body's oxygen demand also increases. The body responds to anxiety and other stresses by an increased rate and depth of respiration. Most people can adapt, but some, particularly those with chronic illnesses or acute life-threatening illnesses such as a myocardial infarction, cannot tolerate the oxygen demands associated with anxiety.

Environmental Factors

The environment can also influence oxygenation. The incidence of pulmonary disease is higher in smoggy, urban areas than in rural areas. In addition, the client's workplace may increase the risk for pulmonary disease. Occupational pollutants include asbestos, talcum powder, dust, and airborne fibers. For example, farm workers in dry regions of the southwestern United States are at risk for coccidioidomycosis, a fungal disease caused by inhalation of spores of the airborne bacterium *Coccidioides immitis*.

◼ ALTERATIONS IN FUNCTIONING

Alterations in cardiac functioning are caused by illnesses and conditions that affect cardiac rhythm, strength of contraction, blood flow through the chambers, myocardial blood flow, and peripheral circulation.

Disturbances in Conduction

Some disturbances in conduction are the result of electrical impulses that do not originate from the SA node. These rhythm disturbances are called *dysrhythmias,* meaning a deviation from the normal sinus heart rhythm (Table 38-2 on p. 1230). Dysrhythmias may occur as a primary conduction disturbance; as a response to ischemia, valvular abnormality, anxiety, and drug toxicity; as a result of caffeine, alcohol, or tobacco use; or as a complication of acid-base or electrolyte imbalance (see Chapter 39).

Dysrhythmias are classified by cardiac response and site of impulse origin (Table 38-2). Cardiac response can be either tachycardic (greater than 100 beats/min), bradycardic (less than 60 beats/min), premature (early beat), or blocked (delayed or absent beat).

Tachydysrhythmias and bradydysrhythmias can lower cardiac output and blood pressure. Tachydysrhythmias reduce cardiac output by decreasing diastolic filling time. Bradydysrhythmias lower cardiac output because of the decreased heart rate.

Some abnormal impulses originate above the ventricles, and these are referred to as *supraventricular dysrhythmias.* The abnormality on the waveform is observed in the configuration and placement of the P-wave. Because these impulses originate above the ventricles, ventricular conduction usually remains normal, and a normal QRS complex is observed.

Junctional dysrhythmias represent an abnormal site of impulse conduction above or below the AV node. The abnormality occurs with placement of the P-wave, which can occur before, during, or after the QRS complexes. In addition, the P-wave is inverted if visible. Because the beat originates above the ventricle, the QRS complex is usually normal.

Ventricular dysrhythmias represent an abnormal site of impulse conduction within the ventricles. The abnormality on the waveform is observed in the configuration and placement of the QRS complex.

Altered Cardiac Output

Failure of the myocardium to eject sufficient volume to the systemic and pulmonary circulations can result in decreased cardiac output and heart failure. Failure of the myocardial pump results from primary coronary artery disease, cardiomyopathic conditions, valvular disorders, and pulmonary disease.

Left-sided heart failure is an abnormal condition characterized by impaired functioning of the heart's

TABLE 38-2 Common Basic Cardiac Dysrhythmias

Rhythm Characteristics	Etiology	Clinical Significance	Management
SINUS TACHYCARDIA			
Regular rhythm, rate 100-180 beats/min (higher in infants), normal P-wave, normal QRS complex	Rate increase may be normal response to exercise, emotion, or stressors such as pain, fever, pump failure, hyperthyroidism, and certain drugs (e.g., caffeine, nitrates, atropine, epinephrine, isoproterenol, nicotine)	May have hemodynamic consequence in client with damaged heart that is unable to sustain increased workloads (increased myocardial oxygen consumption) brought on by persistent increases in heart rate	Correct underlying factors, remove offending drugs

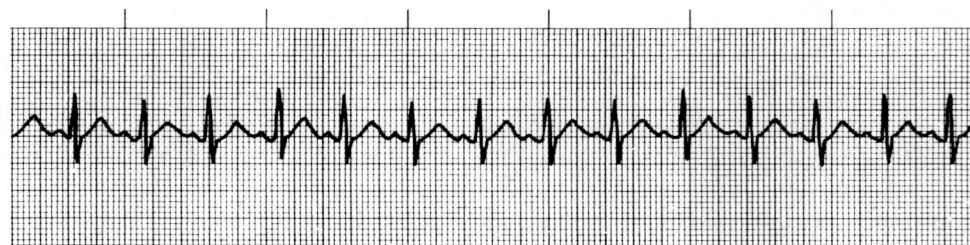

SINUS BRADYCARDIA			
Regular rhythm, rate less than 60 beats/min, normal P-wave, normal PR interval, normal QRS complex	Rate decrease may be normal response to sleep or in well-conditioned athlete; abnormal drops in rate may be caused by diminished blood flow to SA node, vagal stimulation, hypothyroidism, increased intracranial pressure, or pharmacological agents (e.g., digoxin, propranolol, quinidine, procainamide)	No clinical significance unless associated with signs of impaired cardiac output and symptoms of dizziness, syncope, chest pain	Correct underlying causes, administer atropine 0.5-1.0 mg IV, implant transvenous pacemaker

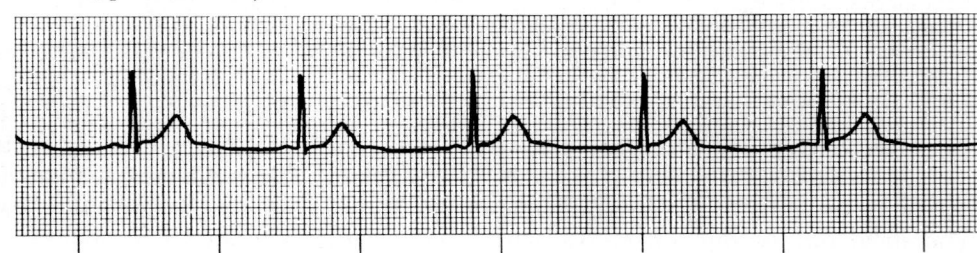

SINUS DYSRHYTHMIA			
Irregular rhythm; possibly phasic with respiration, slowing during inspiration and increasing with expiration; rate of 60-100 beats/min; normal P-wave; normal PR interval; normal QRS complex	Sinus rhythm with cyclic variation caused by vagal impulses that influence rhythm during respiration; occurs commonly in children, young adults, and older adults; usually disappears as heart rate increases	No clinical significance unless heart rate decreases and symptoms of dizziness with decreased rate	None indicated unless heart rate decreases and symptoms occur

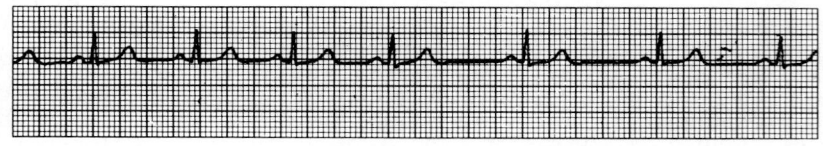

Adapted from Canobbio MM: *Cardiovascular disorders,* St Louis, 1990, Mosby–Year Book, pp. 64-67.

TABLE 38-2 Common Basic Cardiac Dysrhythmias—cont'd

Rhythm Characteristics	Etiology	Clinical Significance	Management

SUPRAVENTRICULAR TACHYCARDIA (SVT)

Sudden, rapid onset of tachycardia with stimulus originating above AV node; regular rhythm; rate 150-250 beats/min; P-wave uniform, possibly buried in preceding T-wave; PR interval variable, often difficult to measure; normal QRS complex	May begin and end spontaneously or be precipitated by excitement, fatigue, or caffeine, smoking, or alcohol use	Usually no significant impairment; client complains of palpitations and shortness of breath; if persistent or occurring in client with preexisting organic heart disease, may cause decrease in cardiac output and/or blood pressure resulting in pump failure or shock	Perform vagal stimulation with carotid sinus massage; decrease ventricular response with medication to block AV conduction: verapamil 5-10 mg IV push, propranolol slowly IV in 1 mg increments up to 4 mg [contraindicated in clients with heart failure], edrophonium, test dose 1 mg followed by 10 mg IV); perform cardioversion if resistant to preceding measures

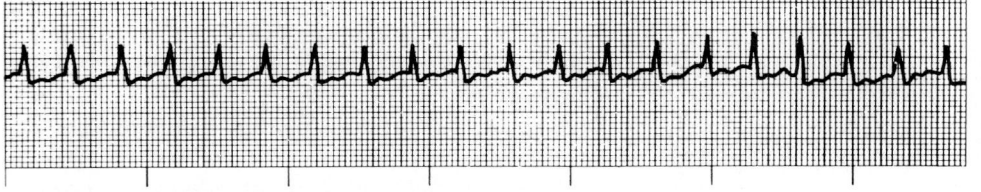

PREMATURE VENTRICULAR CONTRACTIONS (PVCs)

Irregular rhythm with ectopic beats followed by full compensatory pause; rate normal or increased depending on number of ectopic beats; P-wave absent in ectopic beat; PR interval absent; QRS complex widened and distorted; T-wave in opposition to R-wave	Caused by irritable focus within ventricle, commonly associated with myocardial infarction; other causes include hypoxia, hyopcalcemia, acidosis	PVCs occurring frequently (more than 6/min) or in pairs indicating increased ventricular irritability	Try to suppress PVCs; if PVCs frequent, administer IV bolus of lidocaine (50-100 mg) followed by continuous IV infusion; administer additional antiarrhythmic agents as needed

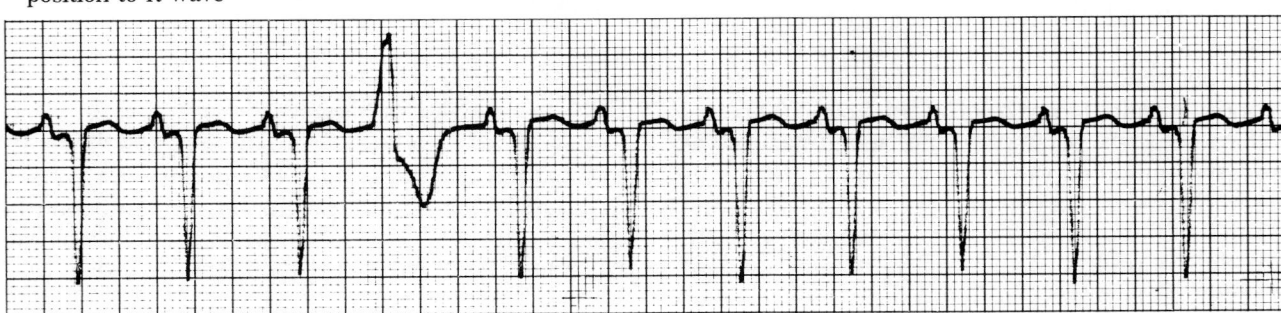

VENTRICULAR TACHYCARDIA

Rhythm slightly irregular, rate 100-200 beats/min, P-wave absent, PR interval absent, QRS complex wide and bizarre, >0.12 second	Caused by irritable ventricular foci firing repetitively, commonly caused by myocardial infarction	Often a forerunner of ventricular fibrillation; if condition persistent and rapid, causes decreased cardiac output because of decreased ventricular filling time	Most episodes terminate abruptly without treatment; administer lidocaine bolus 75-100 mg IV followed by continuous intravenous drip; perform defibrillation

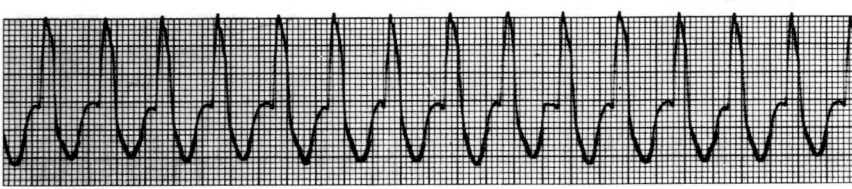

left side and by elevated pressure and congestion in pulmonary veins and capillaries. If failure of the left ventricle is significant, the amount of blood ejected from the left ventricle drops greatly. As a result, cardiac output also falls. Decreases in cardiac output can cause tissue hypoxia, which may result in decreased activity tolerance, breathlessness, dizziness, and confusion. As the left ventricle continues to fail, blood begins to "back up" in the pulmonary circulation, eventually causing pulmonary congestion. This results in crackles, hypoxia, dyspnea, cough, and paroxysmal nocturnal dyspnea (Canobbio, 1990).

Right-sided heart failure results from impaired functioning of the right ventricle characterized by venous congestion in the systemic circulation. Right-sided heart failure more commonly results from pulmonary disease or as a sequelae to left-sided failure. The primary pathological factor in right-sided failure is elevated pulmonary vascular resistance (PVR). As the PVR continues to rise, the right ventricle must generate more work, and the oxygen demand of the heart increases with the workload. As the failure continues, the amount of blood ejected from the right ventricle declines, and blood begins to "back up" in the systemic circulation. Clinically, the client has weight gain, distended neck veins, abdominal organ distention (for example, hepatomegaly and splenomegaly), and dependent peripheral edema.

Impaired Valvular Function

Valvular heart disease is an acquired or congenital disorder of a cardiac valve characterized by stenosis and obstructed blood flow or valvular degeneration and regurgitation of blood (Canobbio, 1990).

When stenosis occurs in the semilunar valves (aortic and pulmonic valves), the adjacent ventricles must work harder to move the ventricular volume beyond the stenotic valve. Over time the stenosis can cause the ventricle to hypertrophy (enlarge), and if the condition is untreated, left- or right-sided heart failure can occur. If stenosis occurs in the atrioventicular valves (mitral and tricuspid valves), the atrial pressure rises, causing the atria to hypertrophy.

When regurgitation occurs, there is a back flow of blood into an adjacent chamber. For example, in mitral regurgitation the mitral leaflets do not close completely. When the ventricle contracts, blood escapes back into the atria, causing a murmur, a "whooshing" sound (see Chapter 20).

Myocardial Ischemia

Myocardial ischemia results when the supply of blood to the myocardium from the coronary arteries

is insufficient to meet the oxygen demands of the organ. Two common manifestations of this ischemia are angina pectoris and myocardial infarction.

Angina pectoris is usually a transient imbalance between myocardial oxygen supply and demand. The condition results in chest pain. Anginal chest pain can be aching, sharp, tingling, or burning or feel like pressure. The location of the pain may be on the left side or substernal and may radiate to the left or both arms, jaw, neck, and back. In some clients, anginal pain may not radiate. The pain lasts from 3 to 15 minutes. Clients sometimes report that pain is precipitated by activities that increase myocardial oxygen demand (for example, exercise, anxiety, and stress). The pain is relieved with rest and coronary vasodilators, the most common being a nitroglycerine preparation.

Myocardial infarction results from sudden decreases in coronary blood flow or an increase in myocardial oxygen demand without adequate coronary perfusion. Infarction occurs because of ischemia and necrosis of myocardial tissue and is not reversible (Canobbio, 1990).

Chest pain associated with myocardial infarction is described as crushing, squeezing, or stabbing. The pain may be retrosternal and left precordial. If the pain radiates, it may move down the left arm and to the neck, jaws, teeth, epigastric area, and back. The pain occurs at rest or exertion. The pain lasts more than 30 minutes. It is unrelieved by rest, position change, or sublingual nitroglycerin administration.

 ## ALTERATIONS IN RESPIRATORY FUNCTIONING

Alterations in respiratory functioning are caused by illnesses and conditions that affect ventilation or oxygen transport. The three primary alterations are hyperventilation, hypoventilation, and hypoxia.

Hyperventilation

The goal of ventilation is to produce a normal arterial carbon dioxide tension ($Paco_2$) and maintain a normal arterial oxygen tension (Pao_2) (Dettenmeier, 1992). *Hyperventilation* and *hypoventilation* refer to alveolar ventilation and not to the client's respiratory rate.

Hyperventilation is a state of ventilation in excess of that required to eliminate the normal venous carbon dioxide produced by cellular metabolism. Hyperventilation can be induced by anxiety, infections, drugs, an acid-base imbalance, and hypoxia (such as with a pulmonary embolus or shock). Acute anxiety can lead to hyperventilation and result in loss of consciousness. Fever can occur in hyperventilation because of compensatory mechanisms within the body. For each degree Fahrenheit increase in body temperature, there is a 7% increase in the metabolic rate (Groër, Shekleton, 1989). Higher metabolic rates increase carbon dioxide production. This state leads to an increased respiratory rate and depth in clients without chronic obstructive pulmonary disease.

Hyperventilation may also be chemically induced. Salicylate poisoning causes excessive stimulation of the respiratory center because of the body's attempt to compensate for carbon dioxide excess. Amphetamines also increase ventilation, primarily by raising carbon dioxide production.

Hyperventilation can also occur as the body tries to compensate for metabolic acidosis. Ventilation increases to reduce the amount of carbon dioxide available to form carbonic acid (see Chapter 39).

Alveolar hyperventilation produces many signs and symptoms that can be assessed (see box). Hemoglobin does not release oxygen to tissues as readily, and tissue hypoxia results. As symptoms worsen, the client may become more agitated, which further increases the respiratory rate and can result in respiratory alkalosis.

Hypoventilation

Hypoventilation occurs when alveolar ventilation is inadequate to meet the body's oxygen demand or to eliminate sufficient carbon dioxide. As alveolar ventilation decreases, $Paco_2$ is elevated. Severe atelectasis can produce hypoventilation. **Atelectasis** is a collapse of the alveoli that prevents normal respiratory exchange of oxygen and carbon dioxide. As alveoli collapse, less of the lung can be ventilated and hypoventilation occurs.

In clients with chronic obstructive pulmonary disease, the inappropriate administration of oxygen can result in hypoventilation. These clients have adapted to a high carbon dioxide level, and their carbon dioxide–sensitive chemoreceptors are essentially not functioning. Their stimulus to breathe is a decreased Pao_2. If excessive oxygen is administered, the oxygen requirement is satisfied and the stimulus to breathe is negated. High concentrations of oxygen (for example, greater than 24% to 28% [1 to 3 L/min]) prevent the Pao_2 from falling and obliterate the stimulus to breathe, resulting in hypoventilation.

Hypoventilation may cause many signs and symptoms revealed through physical assessment (see box). If untreated, the client's status can rapidly decline. Convulsions, unconsciousness, and death can result.

The goals of treatment for hyperventilation and hypoventilation are to first treat the underlying cause while simultaneously restoring optimal ventilatory function, improving tissue oxygenation, and achieving acid-base balance (Gröer, Shekleton, 1989).

Hypoxia

Hypoxia is inadequate cellular oxygenation that results from a deficiency in the delivery or use of oxygen at the cellular level (Gröer, Shekleton, 1983). Hypoxia can be caused by (1) a decreased hemoglobin level and lowered oxygen-carrying capacity of the blood, (2) a diminished concentration of inspired oxygen such as may occur at high altitudes, (3) the inability of the tissues to extract oxygen from the blood such as with cyanide poisoning, (4) decreased diffusion of oxygen from the alveoli to the blood such as with pneumonia, (5) poor tissue perfusion with oxygenated blood such as with shock, and (6) impaired ventilation.

Signs and Symptoms of Alveolar Hyperventilation

- Tachycardia
- Shortness of breath
- Chest pain
- Dizziness
- Lightheadedness
- Decreased concentration
- Paresthesia
- Numbness (extremities, circumoral)
- Tinnitus
- Blurred vision
- Disorientation
- Tetany (carpopedal spasm)

Signs and Symptoms of Alveolar Hypoventilation

- Dizziness
- Headache (may be occipital only on awakening)
- Lethargy
- Disorientation
- Decreased ability to follow instructions
- Cardiac dysrhythmias
- Electrolyte imbalances
- Convulsions
- Coma
- Cardiac arrest

Signs and Symptoms of Hypoxia

- Restlessness
- Apprehension, anxiety
- Decreased ability to concentrate
- Decreased level of consciousness
- Increased fatigue
- Dizziness
- Behavioral changes
- Increased pulse rate

- Increased rate and depth of respiration
- Elevated blood pressure
- Cardiac dysrhythmias
- Pallor
- Cyanosis
- Clubbing
- Dyspnea

The clinical signs and symptoms of hypoxia include apprehension, restlessness, inability to concentrate, declining level of consciousness, dizziness, and behavioral changes (see box). The client with hypoxia is unable to lie down and appears fatigued and agitated. Changes in vital signs include an increased pulse rate and increased rate and depth of respiration. However, as the hypoxia worsens, the respiratory rate may decline as a result of fatigue. During early stages of hypoxia the blood pressure is elevated unless the condition is caused by shock. **Cyanosis,** a blue discoloration of the skin and mucous membranes caused by the presence of desaturated hemoglobin in capillaries, is a late sign of hypoxia. Central cyanosis observed in the tongue and soft palate, where blood flow is high, indicates hypoxemia. Peripheral cyanosis, as observed in the fingernail beds, may merely reflect stagnant blood flow (Luce, Tyler, Pierson, 1984). The nurse should observe other areas of the body besides the skin for signs of cyanosis, such as the conjunctivae, mouth, nail beds, and extremities. The presence or absence of cyanosis is not an absolute measure of oxygenation status.

Dyspnea is another clinical sign of hypoxia and manifests as shortness of breath or difficulty in breathing. It is the subjective sensation of difficult or uncomfortable breathing (Gift, 1990). Pathological dyspnea must be differentiated from physiological dyspnea, which is shortness of breath after exercise or excitement. Pathological breathlessness is a distressing sensation of not being able to catch a breath (Gröer, Shekleton, 1989).

Hypoxia is a life-threatening condition. Untreated, it can produce cardiac dysrhythmias that result in death. Hypoxia is managed by administration of oxygen and by treatment of the underlying cause, such as shock or pneumonia.

NURSING PROCESS AND OXYGENATION

Assessment

The nursing assessment of a client's cardiopulmonary functioning should include data collected from the following areas:
1. Nursing history of the client's normal and present cardiopulmonary function, past impairments in circulatory or respiratory functioning, and measures the client may use to optimize oxygenation
2. Physical examination
3. Review of laboratory and diagnostic test results, including sputum

Nursing History

The nursing history should focus on the client's ability to meet oxygen needs. The nursing history for cardiac function includes pain and characteristics of pain, dyspnea, fatigue, peripheral circulation, cardiac risk factors, and the presence of past or concurrent cardiac conditions. The nursing history for respiratory function includes presence of a cough, shortness of breath, wheezing, pain, environmental exposures, frequency of respiratory tract infections, pulmonary risk factors, past respiratory problems, and current medication use.

FATIGUE. Fatigue is a subjective sensation in which the client reports a loss of endurance. Fatigue in the client with cardiopulmonary alterations is often an early sign of a worsening of the chronic underlying process. To provide an objective measure of fatigue, the client may be asked to rate the fatigue on a scale of 1 to 10, with 10 correlating with the worst level of fatigue and 1 representing no fatigue.

DYSPNEA. The sensation of dyspnea can occur with other objective findings, for example, exaggerated respiratory effort, use of the accessory muscles during respiration, flaring of the nares, and an extreme increase in the rate and depth of respirations (Gröer, Shekleton, 1989). To provide an objective measure of dyspnea, the client may be asked to use a visual analog scale. This objective measure allows the nurse and client to determine if specific nursing interventions are having an effect on the client's dyspnea. The visual analog scale is a 100 mm vertical line with 0 equated with no dyspnea, and the 100 mm marker equated with breathlessness as bad as it can be. The use of a visual analog scale to evaluate a client's dyspnea in the clinical setting is valid and reliable (Gift, Plaut, Jacox, 1986; Gift, 1989).

Jansen-Bjerklie, Carrieri, and Hudes (1986) studied the sensation of dyspnea for four classifications of pulmonary diseases: emphysema-bronchitis, restrictive conditions, asthma, and vascular conditions (see research highlight).

The nursing history of dyspnea includes the circumstances under which it occurred, such as with exertion, stress, or respiratory tract infection. The nurse also determines whether the client's perception of dyspnea affects the ability to lie flat. **Orthopnea** is an abnormal condition in which the person must use multiple pillows when lying down or must sit to breathe. The presence of orthopnea is usually quantified, such as two- or three-pillow orthopnea. This means that the client perceives shortness of breath unless two or three pillows are used for sleeping.

COUGH. **Cough** is a sudden, audible expulsion of air from the lungs. The person breathes in, the glottis is partially closed, and the accessory muscles of expiration contract to expel the air forcibly. Coughing is a protective reflex to clear the trachea, bronchi, and lungs of irritants and secretions.

A cough is difficult to evaluate. Almost everyone has periods of coughing. Moreover, clients with a chronic cough tend to deny, underestimate, or minimize their coughing, often because they are so accustomed to it that they are unaware of how frequently it occurs.

Once the nurse determines that the client has a cough, it must be identified as productive or nonproductive and its frequency must be assessed. A **productive cough** is one that results in sputum. Sputum is material coughed up from the lungs that may be swallowed or expectorated through the mouth. It contains mucus, cellular debris, and microorganisms, and it may contain pus or blood. The nurse must collect data about the type and quantity of sputum (see box). The client should try to produce some sputum so that the nurse can inspect it for color, consistency, odor, and amount.

If **hemoptysis** (bloody sputum) is reported, the nurse should be certain that it is associated with coughing and bleeding from the upper respiratory tract or from the gastrointestinal tract (**hematemesis**). In addition, the hemoptysis should be described according to amount, color, and duration and whether it is mixed with sputum. When a client reports bloody or blood-tinged sputum, diagnostic tests, such as examination of sputum specimens, chest x-ray examinations, bronchoscopy, and other x-ray studies, should be performed.

Coughing is classified according to the time when the client most frequently coughs. Clients with chronic sinusitis may cough only in the early morning or immediately after rising from sleep. This clears the airway of mucus resulting from sinus drainage. Clients with chronic bronchitis generally produce sputum all day, although greater amounts are produced after rising from a semirecumbent or flat position. This is the result of the dependent accumulation of sputum in the airways and is associated with reduced mobility (see Chapter 43).

 Research Highlight

The purpose of this research was to compare recalled physical and emotional sensations during episodes of acute dyspnea for four types of pulmonary disease groups: emphysema-bronchitis, asthmatic, restrictive conditions, and vascular conditions. The study population consisted of 68 subjects. Researchers noted that the frequency of sensations were similar in all disease categories, but few significant differences were identified. However, the intensity of dyspnea had the greatest effect on the quality and frequency of the symptoms reported. Subjects with asthma reported the lowest mean score, and females reported the highest scores.

Janson-Bjerklie S, Carrieri VK, Hudes M: *Nurs Res* 35(3):154, 1986.

Sputum Characteristics

COLOR

- Clear
- White
- Yellow
- Green
- Brown
- Red
- Streaked with blood

QUALITY

- Same as usual
- Increased
- Decreased

CHANGES IN COLOR

- Same color throughout the day
- Clearing with coughing
- Progressively darker

CONSISTENCY

- Frothy
- Watery
- Tenacious, thick

ODOR

- None
- Foul

PRESENCE OF BLOOD

- Occasional
- Early morning
- Bright or dark red
- Blood-tinged

WHEEZING. Wheezing is characterized by a high-pitched musical sound. It is caused by high-velocity movement of air through a narrowed airway. Wheezing may be associated with asthma and acute bronchitis. Clients can usually describe when they wheeze and whether wheezing is present on inspiration or expiration. The nurse should also obtain information about any precipitating factors such as a respiratory infection, allergens, exercise, and stress.

PAIN. The presence of chest pain needs to be thoroughly evaluated with regard to location, duration, radiation, and frequency. Cardiac pain does not occur with respiratory variations. It is most often on the left side of the chest and may radiate. Pericardial pain resulting from an inflammation of the pericardial sac is usually nonradiating and may occur with inspiration.

Pleuritic chest pain is peripheral and may radiate to the scapular regions. It is worsened by inspiratory maneuvers, such as coughing, yawning, and sighing. Pleuritic pain is often caused from an inflammation or infection in the pleural space. Clients often describe pleuritic pain as knifelike. It lasts from a minute to hours and is always associated with inspiration.

Musculoskeletal pain may be present following exercise, rib trauma, and prolonged coughing episodes. This pain is also aggravated by inspiratory movements and may easily be confused with pleuritic chest pain.

ENVIRONMENTAL OR GEOGRAPHICAL EXPOSURES. Environmental exposure to many inhaled substances is closely linked with respiratory disease. The nurse should investigate exposures in the client's home and workplace. The most common environmental exposures in the home are cigarette smoke and radon. The nurse should determine whether a client who is a nonsmoker is passively exposed to smoke. Radon gas, a radioactive substance, enters homes through the ground. When homes are overinsulated, this gas is not able to escape into the atmosphere, and thus it becomes trapped in the home.

An employment history should be obtained to assess exposure to substances such as asbestos, coal, cotton fibers, fumes, or chemical inhalants. It is particularly important with middle-age and older adults who may have worked in places without regulations to protect workers from carcinogens. Dopico et al (1984) noted that the respiratory effects on workers exposed to grain dust was similar to those of smokers and that the effects of smoking and grain dust were additive but not synergistic. In addition, exposure to minimal dust resulted in an increased incidence of symptoms associated with chronic obstructive pulmonary disease (Churg et al, 1985).

Exposure to substances may occur during travel. Schistosomiasis infection can be acquired in Asia, Africa, the Caribbean, and South America. Coccidioidomycosis (valley fever) can be acquired, for example, in southwestern desert regions, at chicken farms, and in river valleys, such as the Ohio and Mississippi valleys (Smith, 1982).

RESPIRATORY INFECTIONS. A nursing history should contain information about the client's frequency and duration of respiratory tract infections. Although everyone occasionally experiences a cold, for some people it can result in bronchitis or pneumonia. The nurse also asks about any known exposure to tuberculosis and about the results of the tuberculin skin test.

Because the acquired immunodeficiency syndrome (AIDS) may initially be diagnosed after *Pneumocystis carinii* or *Mycobacterium pneumonia* infection is found, the nurse needs to assess the client for high-risk behaviors related to AIDS. Some of these risks include exposure to illicit intravenous drug use and multiple heterosexual and homosexual contacts (Bennett, 1986) (see Chapters 2 and 32).

RISK FACTORS. The nurse must also investigate familial and environmental risk factors. A family history of cancer, particularly lung cancer, or cardiovascular diseases should be noted. If the client's family has such a history, it is necessary to document which blood relatives have had the disease and their present level of health or age at time of death. Other family risk factors include the presence of infectious diseases, particularly tuberculosis. The nurse should determine who in the client's household has been infected and the status of treatment.

MEDICATIONS. The last component of the nursing history should describe medications the client is using. These include prescribed, over-the-counter, and illicit drugs and substances. Such medications may have adverse effects by themselves or because of interactions with other drugs. A person using a prescribed bronchodilator drug, for example, may decide that using an over-the-counter inhalant as well will be beneficial. This product may react with the prescribed medication by potentiating or decreasing the effect of the prescribed medication.

As with all medication, the nurse assesses clients' knowledge and ability to use the "five rights" of medication administration (see Chapter 21). Of particular importance is the nurse's assessment of clients' understanding of potential side effects of the medications. Clients should be able to recognize adverse reactions and be aware of the dangers in combining prescribed medications with over-the-counter drugs.

When clients are prescribed drugs for which toxic levels can be monitored by blood analyses, the nurse needs to review these laboratory values. Common drugs that can be monitored include theophylline preparations (theophylline levels), digitalis preparation (digitalis levels), and phenobarbital (phenobarbital levels). Toxic effects of these medications can impair cardiopulmonary functioning. Illicit drugs, particularly parenterally administered narcotics, are often diluted with talcum powder. Their injection can cause pulmonary disorders resulting from the irritant effect of talcum powder on lung tissues.

Physical Examination

The physical examination performed to assess the client's level of tissue oxygenation includes evalua-

tion of the entire cardiopulmonary system. Inspection, palpation, auscultation, and percussion techniques are used (see Chapter 20).

INSPECTION. Using inspection techniques, the nurse performs a head-to-toe observation of the client for skin and mucous membrane color, general appearance, level of consciousness, adequacy of systemic circulation, breathing patterns, and chest wall movement. (Tables 38-3 to 38-5). Any abnormalities should be investigated during palpation, percussion, and auscultation.

PALPATION. Palpation of the chest provides assessment data in several areas. It documents the type and amount of thoracic excursion, elicits any areas of

---

TABLE 38-3   Inspection of Cardiopulmonary Status

Abnormality	Cause
EYES	
Xanthelasma (yellow lipid lesions on eyelids)	Associated with hyperlipidemia
Corneal arcus (whitish opaque ring around junction of cornea and sclera)	Abnormal finding in young to middle adults associated with hyperlipidemia (normal finding in older adults with arcus senilius)
Pale conjunctivae	Associated with anemia
Cyanotic conjunctivae	Associated with hypoxemia
Petechiae on conjunctivae	Associated with fat embolus or bacterial endocarditis
SKIN	
Peripheral cyanosis	Vasoconstriction and diminished blood flow
Central cyanosis	Hypoxemia
Decreased skin turgor	Dehydration (normal finding in older adults as a result of decreased skin elasticity)
Dependent edema	Associated with right- and left-sided heart failure
Periorbital edema	Associated with kidney disease
FINGERTIPS AND NAIL BEDS	
Cyanosis	Decreased cardiac output or hypoxia
Splinter hemorrhages	Bacterial endocarditis
Clubbing	Chronic hypoxemia
MOUTH AND LIPS	
Cyanotic mucous membranes	Decreased oxygenation (hypoxia)
Pursed-lip breathing	Associated with chronic lung disease
NECK VEINS	
Distention	Associated with right-sided heart failure
NOSE	
Flaring nares	Air hunger, dyspnea
CHEST	
Retractions	Increased work of breathing, dyspnea
Asymmetry	Chest wall injury

From Dennison R: *Nurs 86* 16(4):34, 1986.

TABLE 38-4	Assessment of Breathing Patterns	
Pattern		**Causes**
Eupnea—normal respiratory rate; adult range of 12-20 breaths/min; normal tidal volume of 5-7 ml/kg body weight*		
Tachypnea—increased respiratory rate above client's normal rate; shallow respirations		Exercise, pregnancy, fever, pulmonary diseases, anxiety, neurological conditions, airway obstruction
Bradypnea—decreased respiratory rate below client's normal rate		Drug overdose, central nervous system dysfunction, airway obstruction
Kussmaul respiration—abnormally deep, very rapid sighing type of respiration; increased tidal volume and rate		Diabetic ketoacidosis
Ataxic respirations—uncoordinated respiratory patterns; no coordinated rate or depth of respiration		Central nervous system disorders
Cheyne-Stokes respiration—breathing pattern characterized by alternating periods of apnea and deep rapid breathing; cycle beginning with slow, shallow breaths that gradually increase to abnormal depth and rate; respiration gradually subsiding as breathing slows and becomes shallow		Congestive heart failure, bronchopneumonia, drug overdose, sleep, central nervous system damage

*From Luce JM, Tyler ML, Pierson DJ: *Intensive respiratory care*, Philadelphia, 1984, Saunders.

TABLE 38-5	Assessment of Abnormal Chest Wall Movement	
Abnormality		**Cause**
Retraction—visible sinking in soft tissues of chest between and around firmer tissue and cartilaginous and bony ribs; retractions having specific beginning point and worsening with need for increased inspiratory effort; possibly found at intercostal space, intraclavicular space, trachea, and substernally*		Any condition that causes increased inspiratory effort (e.g., airway obstruction, asthma, tracheobronchitis)
Paradoxical breathing—asynchronous breathing; chest contraction during inspiration and expansion during expiration		Flail chest
Increased anteroposterior diameter		Senile emphysema or chronic obstructive pulmonary disease

*Infants can experience sternal and substernal retractions with only slight inspiratory effort because of chest pliability.

tenderness, and can identify tactile fremitus, thrills, and heaves. With palpation the nurse can locate the cardiac point of maximal impulse. Palpation also allows the nurse to feel for abnormal masses or lumps in the axilla and breast tissue (see Chapter 20). Palpation of the extremities provides data about the peripheral circulation. The nurse obtains information about the presence and quality of peripheral pulses, skin temperature, color, and capillary refill (see Chapter 20).

PERCUSSION. With percussion, the nurse can detect the presence of abnormal fluid, air in the lungs, or diaphragmatic excursions (see Chapter 20).

AUSCULTATION. The use of auscultation enables the nurse to identify normal and abnormal heart and lung sounds (see Chapter 20). Auscultation of the cardiovascular system should include assessment for normal S_1 and S_2 sounds, the presence of abnormal S_3 and S_4, and murmurs and rubs. The examiner must identify location, radiation, intensity, pitch, and quality of a murmur. Auscultation is also used to identify a bruit over the carotid arteries, abdominal aorta, and femoral arteries.

Auscultation of lung sounds involves listening for the movement of air throughout all lung fields. Adventitious breath sounds occur with collapse of a lung region, fluid in lung field, or airway obstruction.

Auscultation also evaluates the response of a client to interventions for improving respiratory status.

Diagnostic Tests

TESTS TO DETERMINE ADEQUACY OF THE CARDIAC CONDUCTION SYSTEM. Tests used to determine the adequacy of the cardiac conduction system include electrocardiogram, Holter monitor, exercise stress test, and electrophysiological studies.

ELECTROCARDIOGRAM. The electrocardiogram (ECG) produces a graphic recording of the heart's electrical activity. The ECG commonly detects the abnormal transmission of impulses and the electrical position of the heart (the axis).

Holter Monitor. The **Holter monitor** is a portable device that records the heart's electrical activity and produces a continuous ECG over a specified period, such as 24 hours. The Holter monitor allows clients to continue with their normal activities while recording the heart's electrical activity. This device enables clinicians to determine if activities such as walking and straining at stool are associated with abnormal electrical activity.

Exercise Stress Test. The **exercise stress test** is used to evaluate the cardiac response to physical stress. It provides information on myocardial response to increased oxygen requirements and determines the adequacy of coronary blood flow. Heart rate, electrical activity, and cardiac recovery time are reflected in the ECG tracing (Canobbio, 1990). In addition, data about the client's blood pressure, presence of chest pain, changes in respiration, and color are monitored.

Electrophysiological Studies. An **electrophysiological (EP) study** is an invasive measure of electrical activity. An electrode catheter is inserted into the right atrium, usually via the femoral vein. Electrical stimulation is then delivered through the catheter. ECG monitors and computers record the heart's electrical response to the stimulus. This procedure provides more specific information about difficult to treat dysrhythmias.

TESTS TO DETERMINE MYOCARDIAL CONTRACTION AND BLOOD FLOW. Echocardiography, scintigraphy, cardiac catheterization and angiography are used to determine myocardial contraction and blood flow.

Echocardiography. **Echocardiography** is a noninvasive measure to evaluate the internal structures of the heart and heart wall motion. Sonar (radar) technology is used to measure ultrasonic waves and translate them into formed images. The echocardiogram graphically demonstrates overall cardiac performance.

Scintigraphy. **Scintigraphy,** or radionuclide angiography, is a noninvasive imaging technique that uses radioisotopes to evaluate cardiac structures, myocardial perfusion, and contractility (Canobbio, 1990).

Cardiac Catheterization and Angiography. **Cardiac catheterization** and **angiography** is an invasive procedure used to visualize cardiac chambers, valves, the great vessels, and coronary arteries. Pressure and volume determinants within the four chambers are also measured. This procedure requires the insertion of a catheter into the heart via a percutaneous venous puncture. A contrast material is injected through the catheter, and fluoroscopic pictures are obtained of the vessels. Both right- and left-sided catheterizations can be performed.

TESTS TO MEASURE ADEQUACY OF VENTILATION AND OXYGENATION. Pulmonary function tests, peak expiratory flow rates, arterial blood gas tests, oximetry, and complete blood counts are used to assess the adequacy of ventilation and oxygenation.

Pulmonary Function Tests. **Pulmonary function tests** determine the ability of the lungs to efficiently exchange oxygen and carbon dioxide. Basic ventilation studies are performed with a spirometer and recording device as the client breathes through a mouthpiece into a connecting tube. Measurements include tidal volume (TV), inspiratory reserve volume (IRV), residual volume (RV), and forced expiratory volume in 1 second (FEV_1).

Pulmonary function tests are usually performed in a pulmonary function laboratory. The nurse prepares the client by explaining the procedure. A nose clip prevents air from being inhaled or exhaled through the nose. The client breathes through a mouthpiece attached to a spirometer for measuring lung volume. The client is asked at certain times in the test to inhale or exhale as much air as possible. The nurse needs the client's cooperation to ensure accurate results.

Peak Expiratory Flow Rate. **Peak expiratory flow rate (PEFR)** is the point of highest flow during maximal expiration, and it reflects changes in large airway sizes. The measure is similar to and correlates well with the FEV_1 (Walsh, 1992). The peak expiratory flow meter is a handheld instrument that allows clients with chronic asthma to follow the degree of airway openness. Information about peak expiratory flow rate is essential assessment data for clients with asthma.

Arterial Blood Gas Tests. Arterial blood gas measurement is performed in conjunction with pulmonary function tests to determine the hydrogen ion concentration, partial pressure of carbon dioxide and oxygen concentration, and oxyhemoglobin saturation. Arterial blood gas tests provide information about diffusion of gas across the alveolar-capillary

Pulse Oximetry

STEPS	RATIONALE

1. Identify client who will benefit from pulse oximetry.

Identifies hypoxemia before signs and symptoms develop.

   a. Assess client's respiratory status: oxygen therapy, hemoglobin level.

   b. Review client's medical record for physician's order for pulse oximetry.

   c. Identify clients who may have oxygen desaturation with sleep, activity, suctioning.

Allows nurse to monitor trends in client's level of oxygen. Enables nurse to use objective criteria to adjust nursing intervention to optimize oxygen saturation.

2. Obtain equipment and place at bedside:

   a. Pulse oximeter

   b. Senser probe

Type of sensor	Client's weight*
(1) Adhesive neonatal	Less than 3 kg (6.6 lb); more than 40 kg (88 lb)
(2) Adhesive infant	From 1 kg (2.2 lb) to 20 kg (44 lb)
(3) Adhesive pediatric	From 10 kg (22 lb) to 50 kg (110 lb)
(4) Adhesive adult	More than 30 kg (66 lb)
(5) Adhesive adult nasal	More than 50 kg (110 lb)
(6) Finger clip	More than 40 kg (88 lb)

Ensures error-free data regarding oxygen saturation.

   c. Continuous printout (optional)

3. Explain purpose of procedure to client and family.

Ensures client and family understanding and increases compliance.

4. Wash hands.

Reduces transmission of microorganisms.

5. Select appropriate area on client to apply sensor based on peripheral circulation and extremity temperature.

Peripheral vasoconstriction alters oxygen saturation.

   a. Determine adequacy of peripheral circulation by assessing capillary refill (toe and finger sites).

   b. Do not use adhesive adult nasal sensor if client has large-bore nasogastric tube or nasoendotracheal tube (nose).

Prevents interference with oxygen saturation readings because of poor peripheral circulation and excessive equipment or dressings.

   c. Determine use of vasoactive drugs.

   d. Align photoelectron and light-emitting diode.

Permits transmission of light. Alignment ensures accurate oxygen saturation readings.

6. Prepare selected site:

   a. Remove nail polish.

   b. Remove artificial nails.

   c. Remove earrings.

   d. Wash selected site, wipe with alcohol, and air dry.

Body oils, nail polish, and artificial nails interfere with transmission of light through nail, tissue, venous and arterial blood, and skin pigmentation (Sonnesso, 1991).

7. Attach sensor probe to finger, bridge of nose, earlobe, toe.

8. Instruct client to breathe normally.

Prevents large fluctuations in minute ventilation and possible change in oxygen saturation.

9. Attach pulse oximeter sensor to client cable.

   a. Turn machine on.

   b. Listen for audible beep.

Senses with each pulse and indicates how well oximeter monitors pulse.

   c. Observe waveform for bar of light.

Light or waveform fluctuates with each pulsation and reflects pulse strength. Poor light on small waveform usually indicates that signal is too weak to give accurate oxygen saturation reading.

*From Sonnesso G: Nurs 91 21(8):60, 1991.

STEPS	RATIONALE
10. Ensure that alarm limits for *both* high and low oxygen saturation and high and low pulse are set according to physicians's order and *turned on*.	Manufacturers preset limits, and adjustments can be made according to client's underlying physical condition, therapy, and risks (Sonnesso, 1991). Provides an audible and visual signal that high or low limits have been exceeded.
11. Read saturation level as ordered and while performing nursing interventions.	Documents oxygen saturation levels at rest, with activity such as ambulation, during procedure such as suctioning, and with changes in physical condition.
12. Move a finger sensor every 4 hr and a spring-tension sensor every 2 hr.	Allows nurse to assess for and prevent impaired skin integrity caused by pressure from sensor.
13. Record in nurses' notes client's use of continuous pulse oximetry and record oxygen saturation.	Documents use of equipment for third-party payers, documents oxygen saturation.
14. Correlate oxygen saturation value with arterial blood gas measurements if available.	Documents reliability of oximeter.
15. Report oxygen saturation and respond to changes in therapy to oncoming shift.	Provides oncoming nurse with baseline information and response to therapy.

membrane and adequacy of tissue oxygenation (see Chapter 39).

Oximetry. Continuous measurements of capillary oxygen saturation are available with cutaneous **oximetry** (Procedure 38-1). Oxygen saturation (O_2 sat) is the percentage of hemogloblin saturated with oxygen. One of the most common is a finger oximeter. The nurse attaches a noninvasive sensor to the client's finger. The sensor monitors capillary blood oxygen saturation. Continuous monitoring of oxygen saturation is useful in assessing sleep disorders, exercise tolerance, and transient decreases in oxygen saturation.

Transcutaneous oximeter measurements have the advantages of being easy to use, noninvasive, and readily available (Whitney, 1990). Clients with poor tissue perfusion such as with shock, hypothermia, and peripheral vascular diseases may not have reliable oximetry measures.

Complete Blood Count. A complete blood count determines the number and type of red and white blood cells per mm^3 of blood. The nurse obtains a venous blood sample by using the venipuncture technique (see Chapter 39). Normal values for a complete blood count vary with age and gender.

The complete blood count also measures the hemoglobin level. Hemoglobin is contained within the red blood cells (erythrocytes). A deficiency in red blood cells decreases the blood's oxygen-carrying capacity because there are fewer hemoglobin molecules available to carry oxygen to tissues.

When the number of red blood cells is increased, such as with polycythemia in chronic lung conditions and cyanotic heart conditions, the oxygen-carrying capacity of the blood is increased. However, increased red blood cells increase blood viscosity and the client's risk for thrombus formation.

TESTS TO VISUALIZE STRUCTURES OF THE RESPIRATORY SYSTEM. Chest x-ray examination, bronchoscopy, and lung scan are used to visualize structures of the respiratory system.

Chest X-Ray Examination. A chest x-ray examination consists of a radiograph of the thorax that allows the physician and nurse to observe the lung fields for fluid (such as occurs with pneumonia), masses (as with lung cancer), fractures (as with rib and clavicular fractures), and other abnormal processes (such as tuberculosis).

Bronchoscopy. Bronchoscopy is visual examination of the trachea and bronchial tree. A narrow, flexible fiberoptic bronchoscope is used. Bronchoscopy is performed to obtain biopsy and fluid or sputum samples for examination. It can also remove mucus plugs or foreign bodies that have become lodged in the airways.

The client is maintained in a fasting state before bronchoscopy. The nurse also administers medications before the procedure. A sedative is usually administered, and atropine may be used occasionally to reduce oral secretions. The nurse continues to observe the client after the procedure for signs and symptoms of respiratory distress or hypoxia. Assessment of the client's gag/swallow reflex is obtained before beginning oral fluids.

Lung Scan. The most common lung scan is the computed tomogram (CT) scan. CT scanning combines x-ray and computer technology. X-ray beams pass through a section or plane of the thorax from different angles, and the computer calculates tissue absorption and displays a printout and scan picture of the tissues showing densities of various intrathoracic structures. A CT scan can identify abnormal masses by size and location but cannot identify tissue types, which requires a biopsy.

TESTS TO DETERMINE ABNORMAL CELLS OR INFECTION IN THE RESPIRATORY TRACT.

Tests to determine whether there are abnormal cells or infection in the respiratory tract include throat cultures, sputum specimens, skin testing, and thoracentesis.

Throat Cultures. A throat culture sample is obtained by swabbing the oropharynx and tonsillar regions with a sterile swab. The throat culture determines the presence of pathogenic microorganisms and the antibiotics to which they are most sensitive.

When obtaining a throat culture, the nurse inserts the swab into the pharyngeal region and passes it along reddened areas and areas of exudate. Some clients have an active gag reflex, making it difficult to obtain the specimen. The reflex may be less active if the client is sitting straight and leaning forward slightly. In addition, the client may be able to control gagging if informed that the procedure will take only a few seconds.

Sputum Specimens. Sputum specimens identify a specific microorganism and its drug resistance and sensitivities. This specimen is referred to as *sputum for culture and sensitivity* (C and S). A sputum specimen may also be obtained to identify the presence of the tubercle bacillus (TB). This sputum specimen is called *sputum for acid-fast bacillus* (AFB). The AFB specimen is obtained 3 consecutive days in the early morning. Finally, sputum specimens are obtained to identify abnormal cells. This is called *sputum for cytology* and involves a serial collection of three early morning sputum specimens. Cytological sputum examination is performed to identify lung cancers by cell type.

When sputum specimens are obtained, the nurse must ensure that the specimen consists of mucus deep from the bronchus and not saliva. The nurse should record the color, consistency, amount, and odor of the sputum and document that the specimen was sent to a specific laboratory for analysis on a specific date and time.

Skin Testing. Skin testing enables the clinician to determine the presence of bacterial, fungal, or viral pulmonary diseases. The antigen is injected intradermally (see Procedure 21-3). The antigen should be properly injected, the injection site should be circled, and the client should be instructed not to wash off the circle. This procedure enables the clinician to evaluate the response.

Positive results are based on the size of the induration. An induration is a palpable, elevated, hardened area around the client's injection site. It is caused from edema and inflammation from the antigen/antibody reaction. If induration is present, it is measured in millimeters. Reddened flat areas are not positive reactions and thus should not be measured.

Thoracentesis. Thoracentesis is surgical perforation of the chest wall and pleural space with a needle to aspirate fluid for diagnostic or therapeutic purposes or to remove a specimen for biopsy. The procedure is performed with aseptic technique using a local anesthetic. The client usually sits upright with the anterior thorax supported by pillows or an over-the-bed table (Figure 38-7).

Whether this procedure is painful depends on the client's tolerance to pain (see Chapter 35). The nurse can reduce the client's anxiety by explaining the procedure and telling the client what to expect. The client must understand the importance of holding the breath as requested and of not coughing during the procedure. Sudden movements of the thorax may result in the lung being punctured by the thoracentesis needle. The client is instructed to notify the physician before coughing or sneezing so that the needle can be withdrawn. After the procedure the nurse monitors the client for signs of pneumothorax (see Procedure 38-2).

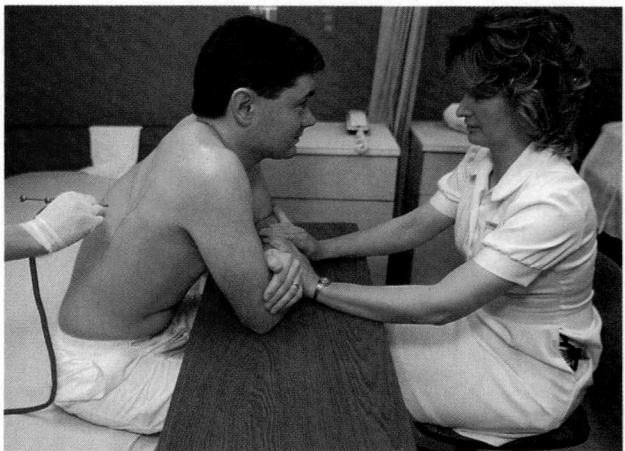

Fig. 38-7   Position for thoracentesis.
From Wilson SF, Thompson JM: *Respiratory disorders*, St Louis, 1990, Mosby–Year Book.

Nursing Diagnosis

Clients with an altered level of oxygenation can have nursing diagnoses that are primarily from a cardiovascular or pulmonary origin (see diagnosis box). Each nursing diagnosis should be based on specific defining characteristics and should include the related etiology. The diagnostic label is validated by the defining characteristics or signs and symptoms (see diagnostic process box).

Two recent nursing studies have validated nursing diagnoses resulting from pulmonary causes (McDonald, 1985; York, 1985). McDonald (1985) researched *ineffective airway clearance, ineffective breathing patterns,* and *impaired gas exchange.* The study validated a partial list of defining characteristics and identified 20 nursing interventions appropriate for the diagnostic categories. The second study attempted to validate defining characteristics associated with ineffective breathing patterns and ineffective airway clearance (York, 1985). In addition to identifying the most common defining characteristics for both categories, the researcher developed a model for validating other diagnostic classifications (York, 1985; York, Martin, 1986).

Planning

Clients with impaired oxygenation require a nursing care plan directed toward meeting the actual or potential oxygenation needs of the client (see care plan on p. 1244). The plan includes one or more of the following client-centered goals:

1. Client achieves improved activity tolerance.
2. Client maintains maintenance and promotion of lung expansion.
3. Client maintains mobilization of pulmonary secretions.
4. Client has a patent airway
5. Tissue oxygenation is maintained or promoted.
6. Client's cardiopulmonary function is restored.

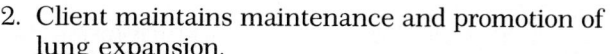

Examples of Nursing Diagnoses Related to Cardiopulmonary Dysfunction

NANDA-APPROVED NURSING DIAGNOSES

Ineffective airway clearance related to:
- Impaired cough
- Incisional pain
- Decreased level of consciousness

Impaired gas exchange related to:
- Decreased lung expansion
- Presence of pulmonary secretions
- Inadequate oxygen intake

Ineffective breathing pattern related to:
- Immobility
- Use of analgesics
- Neuromuscular damage
- Airway obstruction

Decreased cardiac output related to:
- Irregular cardiac rhythm
- Rapid heart rate

High risk for infection related to:
- Stasis of pulmonary secretions

Activity intolerance related to:
- Weakness
- Inadequate nutritional intake

Sample Nursing Diagnostic Process for Cardiopulmonary Dysfunction

Assessment Activities	Defining Characteristics	Nursing Diagnosis
Observe client while breathing.	Dyspnea Tachypnea Use of accessory muscles Nasal flaring Diaphoresis	*Ineffective airway clearance* related to thickened pulmonary secretions
Inspect client's skin and mucous membranes.	Cyanotic nail beds Circumoral cyanosis Pale mucous membranes	
Auscultate lung fields.	Lower lobe crackles Inspiratory wheezes throughout fields	
Observe cough and inspect sputum.	Poor cough Client tires trying to produce sputum Thick, yellow sputum	

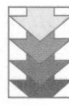

Sample Nursing Care Plan for Ineffective Airway Clearance

Nursing diagnosis: *Ineffective airway clearance* related to thickened pulmonary secretions
Definition: Ineffective airway clearance is the state in which an individual is unable to clear secretions or obstructions from the respiratory tract to maintain airway patency (Kim, McFarland, McLane, 1991).

Goal	Expected Outcomes	Interventions	Rationale
Pulmonary secretions will be removed.	Adventitious lung sounds will be absent within 48 hr.	Turn, cough, and deep breathe client every 2 hr.	Major complication of reduced mobility is retained secretions, which predisposes client to atelectasis and pneumonia (Dettenmeier, 1992).
		Perform postural drainage with percussion every 3 hr.	Postural drainage moves secretions from smaller to larger airways. Percussion provides additional mechanical force to loosen secretions adhered to walls of airways. Both techniques facilitate secretion removal (Dettenmeier, 1992).
	Client will maintain forceful, productive cough.	If client is unable to clear airway, suction for retained secretions.	Main indication for suctioning is when clients are unable to clear airways of mucus and adventitious lung sounds continue (Weilitz, 1991)
	Sputum will be clear, white, and frothy within 48 hr.	Increase fluid intake to 1000 ml within 24 hr.	Fluids and humidification help liquify secretions for easy removal (Feldman, 1982; Luce, Tyler, Pierson, 1984).
		Add high-humidity face mask.	Providing upper airway humidification prevents mucosal drying, keeps secretions moist, and maintains integrity of mucociliary clearance system (Shekleton, Nield, 1987).

The client's level of health, age, lifestyle, and environmental risks affect the level of tissue oxygenation. Clients with severe impairments in oxygenation frequently require nursing interventions directed toward all six goals.

Implementation

Nursing interventions for promoting and maintaining adequate oxygenation include independent nursing actions (such as positioning, coughing techniques, and preventive health behaviors) and interdependent or dependent interventions (such as oxygen therapy, lung inflation techniques, hydration, medications, and in some agencies, the use of chest physical therapy).

Improved Activity Tolerance

Nursing interventions for improving activity tolerance primarily include measures such as management of dyspnea, cardiopulmonary reconditioning, and respiratory muscle training.

DYSPNEA MANAGEMENT. Dyspnea is difficult to quantify and to treat. Treatment modalities need to be individualized for each client, and more than one therapy is usually implemented.

Ideally, the underlying process that causes or worsens dyspnea must be treated. After this initial phase, there are four additional therapies: pharmacological measures, oxygen therapy, physical techniques, and psychosocial techniques (Gift, 1990). Pharmacological agents may include bronchodilators, steroids, mucolytics, and antianxiety medications.

Oxygen therapy can reduce dyspnea associated with exercise. Physical techniques, such as cardiopulmonary reconditioning, breathing techniques, and cough control, can help to reduce dyspnea (DeVito, 1990). Relaxation techniques, biofeedback, and meditation are physiosocial measures that can lessen the sensation of dyspnea (Gift, 1990).

CARDIOPULMONARY RECONDITIONING. The major method of cardiopulmonary reconditioning is a structured rehabilitation program. **Cardiopulmonary rehabilitation** is actively assisting the client to achieve and maintain an optimal level of health through controlled physical exercise, nutrition counseling, relaxation and stress management techniques, prescribed medications and oxygen, and adherence to the program. Goals of rehabilitation are defined by the client and the rehabilitation team.

As physical reconditioning occurs, the client's complaints of dyspnea, chest pain, fatigue, and activity intolerance should decrease. Researchers noted the amount of anxiety, depression, and somatic concerns decreased as clients participated in cardiopulmonary rehabilitation. This occurred whether there was clinical improvement in the cardiopulmonary disease itself (Shenkman, 1985; Agle et al, 1973).

RESPIRATORY MUSCLE TRAINING. Respiratory muscle training improves muscle strength and endurance, resulting in improved activity tolerance. Respiratory muscle training may prevent respiratory failure in clients with chronic obstructive pulmonary disease (Kim, 1984).

One method for respiratory muscle training is the **incentive spirometer resistive breathing device (ISRBD).** Resistive breathing is achieved by placing a resistive breathing device into a volume-dependent incentive spirometer. Muscle training is achieved when the client uses the ISRBD on a scheduled routine, for example, twice a day for 15 minutes or four times a day for 15 minutes. Two studies investigated clients with chronic obstructive pulmonary disease and measured muscle training following use of the IRSBD (Larson, Kim, 1984; Larson et al, 1988). Subjects demonstrated a significant increase in respiratory muscle strength and sputum expectoration and a clinical improvement in exercise tolerance and performance of activities of daily living.

Maintenance or Promotion of Lung Expansion

Nursing interventions to maintain or promote lung expansion include noninvasive techniques such as positioning and breathing exercises. Lung expansion is also promoted by procedures using equipment such as incentive spirometers. In cases of pneumo-thorax and pleural effusions, reexpansion can also be achieved by invasive procedures such as insertion of a chest tube.

POSITIONING. In the healthy, completely mobile person, adequate ventilation and oxygenation are maintained by frequent changes of position during the activities of daily living. However, when a person's mobility is restricted as a result of illness or injury, there is a risk for respiratory impairment. Frequent changes of position are simple and cost-effective methods for reducing the risks of pulmonary complications such as stasis of pulmonary secretions and decreased chest wall expansion (see Chapter 43).

The most effective position for clients with cardiopulmonary diseases is high-Fowler's position. This position uses gravity to assist in lung expansion and to reduce pressure from the abdomen on the diaphragm. When the client uses this position, the nurse needs to ensure that the client does not slide down in bed, which could reduce lung expansion.

BREATHING EXERCISES. Breathing exercises include techniques to improve ventilation and oxygenation. The three basic techniques are deep breathing and coughing exercises, pursed-lip breathing, and diaphragmatic breathing. Deep breathing and coughing exercises are routine interventions for postoperative clients (see Chapter 47).

Pursed-lip breathing involves deep inspiration and prolonged expiration through pursed lips. This exercise keeps the alveoli from collapsing. While sitting up, the client is instructed to take a deep breath and to exhale slowly through pursed lips. Clients need to gain control of the exhalation phase so that exhalation is longer than inhalation (Dettenmeier, 1992). The client is usually able to perfect this technique by counting inhalation time and gradually increasing the count during exhalation.

Diaphragmatic breathing is more difficult and requires the client to relax intercostal and accessory respiratory muscles while taking deep inspirations. The client is taught to place one hand flat below the breastbone above the waist and the other hand 2 to 3 cm below the first hand. The client is asked to sniff, and with the sniff, the diaphragm will expand outward, causing the client's hand to move. Second, the client concentrates on expanding the diaphragm during controlled inspiration. The lower hand should move outward during expiration. The client observes for inward movement as the diaphragm ascends. These exercises are initially taught with the client in the supine position and are then practiced while the client sits and stands. The exercise is often used with the pursed-lip breathing technique.

Care of the Client with Chest Tubes

STEPS	RATIONALE
1. Assess client for decreased respiratory distress and chest pain, breath sounds over affected lung area, and stable vital signs.	Increase in respiratory distress and/or chest pain, decrease in breath sounds over the affected and nonaffected lungs, marked cyanosis, asymmetric chest movements, presence of subcutaneous emphysema around tube insertion site or neck, hypotension, tachycardia, and/or mediastinal shift are critical and indicate a severe change in client status, such as excessive blood loss or tension pneumothorax. Notify physician immediately.
2. Observe:	
a. Chest tube dressing	Ensures that dressing is patent and notes any drainage.
b. Tubing for kinks, dependent loops, or clots	Maintains a patent, freely draining system, preventing fluid accumulation in chest cavity.
c. Chest drainage system, which should be upright and below level of tube insertion	System must be in this position to function properly.
d. Water seal for fluctuations with client's inspiration and expiration	Fluid should rise in water seal with inspiration and fall with expiration, indicating that system is functioning properly (Erickson, 1981a; Carroll, 1986).
e. Bubbling in water-seal bottle or chamber (see Table 38-6)	When system is initially connected to client, bubbles are expected in chamber from air that was present in system and in client's intrapleural space (Farley, 1988). After a short period, bubbling will stop. Fluid will continue to fluctuate in water seal on inspiration and expiration until lung is reexpanded or system becomes occluded.
f. Type and amount of fluid drainage: Nurse should note color and amount of drainage, client's vital signs, and skin color.	Sudden gush of drainage may be retained blood and not active bleeding. Increase in drainage can be result of client position change (Farley, 1988).
(1) Less than 50-200 ml/hr immediately postoperative in mediastinal chest tube (Johanson et al, 1988); approximately 500 ml in first 24 hr; dark red drainage is expected early in postoperative period, turning serous with time.	Reexpansion of lungs forces drainage into tube. Coughing can also cause large gushes of drainage.
(2) Between 100-300 ml of fluid may drain in posterior chest tube during first 2 hr after insertion; rate will decrease after 2 hr, 500-1000 ml can be expected in first 24 hr; drainage will be grossly bloody during first several hours after surgery and then change to serous.	Excessive amounts and/or continued presence of frank, bloody drainage after first several hours of surgery should be reported to physician, along with client's vital signs and respiratory status.
g. Bubbling in the suction-control chamber (when suction is being used) (see Table 38-6)	Suction-control chamber has constant, gentle bubbling. Tubing to suction source should be free of obstruction, and suction source should be turned on to appropriate setting.
3. Provide two shodded hemostats for each chest tube. Shodded hemostats are usually attached to top of client's bed with adhesive tape or clamped to client's clothing during ambulation. Shodded hemostats have protective covering such as plastic over points. Covering prevents hemostat from penetrating chest tube.	Chest tubes are only clamped under specific circumstances:
	a. To assess air leak (see Table 38-6)
	b. To empty or change collection bottle or chamber (Farley, 1988); this procedure is performed only by physician or nurse who has received training in procedure
	c. To change disposable systems (Erickson, 1981b); have new system ready to be connected before clamping tube so that transfer can be rapid and drainage system reestablished
	d. To change a broken water-seal bottle in event that no sterile solution container is available

CONTINUED

STEPS	RATIONALE
	e. To assess if client is ready to have chest tube removed, which is done by physician's order (Farley, 1988); in this situation, nurse must monitor client for re-creation of pneumothorax (see Table 36-6)
4. Position the client:	Permits optimal drainage of fluid and/or air.
a. Semi-Fowler's to high Fowler's position to evacuate air (pneumothorax)	Air rises to highest point in chest. Pneumothorax tubes are usually placed on anterior aspect at midclavicular line, second or third intercostal space (Carroll, 1986).
b. High Fowler's position to drain fluid (hemothorax)	Permits optimal drainage of fluid. Posterior tubes are placed on midaxillary line, eighth or ninth intercostal space.
5. Maintain tube connection between chest and drainage tubes intact and taped.	Secures chest tube to drainage system and reduces risk of air leaks causing breaks in airtight system.
a. Water-seal vent must be without occlusion.	Permits displaced air to pass into atmosphere.
b. Suction-control chamber vent must be without occlusion when suction is used.	Provides safety factor of releasing excess negative pressure into atmosphere.
6. Coil excess tubing on mattress next to client. Secure with rubber band and safety pin or system's clamp.	Prevents excess tubing from hanging over edge of mattress in dependent loop. Drainage could collect in loop and occlude drainage system.
7. Adjust tubing to hang in straight line from top of mattress to drainage chamber. If chest tube is draining fluid, indicate time (e.g., 0900) that drainage was begun on drainage bottle's adhesive tape of bottle setup or on write-on surface of disposable commercial system.	Promotes drainage. Provides a baseline for continuous assessment of type and quality of drainage.
8. Strip or milk chest tube only if indicated:	Stripping is controversial and should be performed only if hospital policy permits and there is physician's order (Pierce, Piazza, Naftel, 1991; Johanson et al, 1988). Stripping creates high degree of negative pressure and has potential of pulling lung tissue or pleura into drainage holes of chest tube (Duncan, Erickson, 1982; Duncan, Erickson, Weigel, 1987).
a. Postoperative mediastinal chest tubes are manipulated if nursing assessment indicates obstruction of drainage secondary to clots or debris in tubing.	
b. Postoperative assessment is done every 15 min for the first 2 hr. This assessment interval then changes *based on client's status.*	
9. Wash hands.	Reduces transmission of infection.
10. Record in nurse' notes patency of chest tubes, presence of drainage, presence of fluctuations, client's vital signs, and level of comfort.	Documents accurate functioning of chest tubes and client's physical status.

The pulmonary results of these exercise patterns include decreased air trapping and reduced work of breathing (Luce, Tyler, Pierson, 1984). Diaphragmatic breathing is also useful for clients with pulmonary disease, for postoperative clients, and for women in labor to promote relaxation and provide pain control.

INCENTIVE SPIROMETRY. **Incentive spirometry** is a method of encouraging voluntary deep breathing by providing visual feedback to clients about inspiratory volume. Incentive spirometry is used to prevent or treat atelectasis and is particularly useful for postoperative clients (Luce, Tyler, Pierson, 1984). Postoperative complications are prevented by reinflating collapsed alveoli and removing secretions.

Flow-oriented incentive spirometers consist of one or more plastic chambers that contain freely moving colored balls. The client inhales briskly to elevate the balls and to keep them floating as long as possible. The goal is to keep the balls elevated for as long as possible to ensure a maximally sustained inhalation.

Even if a very slow inspiration does not elevate the balls, this breathing pattern alone may achieve greater lung expansion (Luce, Tyler, Pierson, 1984).

Volume-oriented incentive spirometry devices have a bellows that is raised to a predetermined volume by an inhaled breath (Fig. 38-8). An achievement light or counter is used in some devices. Some devices are constructed so that the light will not turn on unless the bellows is held at a minimum desired volume for a specified period to enhance lung expansion.

Incentive spirometry encourages clients to breathe to their normal inspiratory capacities. Because of postoperative pain, a postoperative inspiratory capacity one half to three fourths of the preoperative volume is acceptable (Luce, Tyler, Pierson, 1984).

CHEST TUBES. Chest tubes are inserted to remove air and fluids from the pleural space, to prevent air or fluid from reentering the pleural space, and to reestablish normal intrapleural and intrapulmonic pressures (Dettenmeier, 1992). A **chest tube** is a catheter inserted through the thorax to remove fluid or air and thus promote lung reexpansion. Chest tubes are used after chest surgery and chest trauma and for pneumothorax or hemothorax (Procedure 38-2 on p. 1247).

A **pneumothorax** is a collection of air or other gas in the pleural space. The gas causes the lung to collapse because it obliterates the negative intrapleural pressure and a counterpressure is exerted against the lung, which is then unable to expand. There are a variety of mechanisms for a pneumothorax. It may occur spontaneously or from chest trauma, such as a stabbing or automobile accident; from the rupture of an emphysematous vesicle on the surface of the lung; or from an invasive procedure, such as a thoracentesis or insertion of a subclavian intravenous line.

A client with a pneumothorax usually feels pain as atmospheric air irritates the parietal pleura. The pain may be sharp and pleuritic. Dyspnea is common and worsens as the size of the pneumothorax increases.

Hemothorax is an accumulation of blood and fluid in the pleural cavity between the parietal and visceral pleurae, usually as the result of trauma. It produces a counterpressure and prevents the lung from full expansion. A hemothorax can also be caused by rupture of small blood vessels from inflammatory processes, such as with pneumonia or tuberculosis. In addition to pain and dyspnea, signs and symptoms of shock can develop if blood loss is severe.

The one-bottle system is the simplest closed drainage system because the single bottle serves as a collector and a water seal (Fig. 38-9, *A*). During normal respiration, fluctuations in the water-seal tube are expected. The fluid should ascend with inspiration. A two-bottle system permits the liquid to flow into the collection bottle and air flows into the water-seal bottle (Fig. 38-9, *B*). Fluctuations in the water-seal tube are still anticipated. The advantage of the two-bottle system is that it permits more accurate measurement and observation of chest drainage (Erikson, 1981a).

A three-bottle system is used to evacuate any volume of air or fluid with controlled suction (Fig. 38-9,

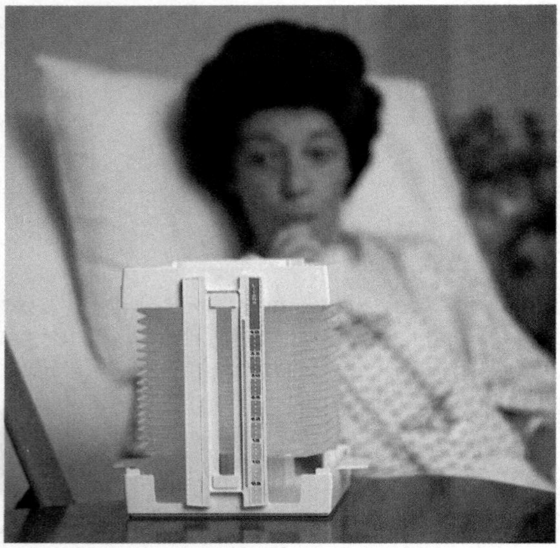

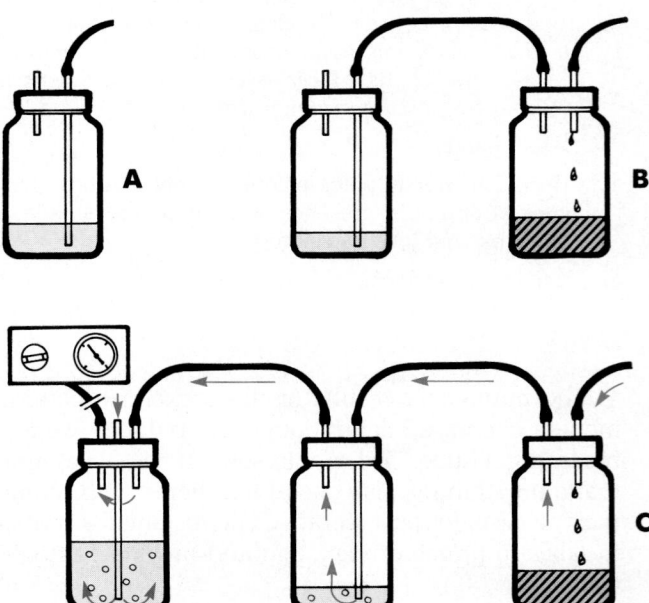

Fig. 38-9   Chest tube drainage. **A,** One-bottle system. **B,** Two-bottle system. **C,** Three-bottle system with suction.

Fig. 38-8   Volume-oriented spirometer.

C). The suction-control bottle contains a long tube, submerged under water, and two short tubes. The longer tube is submerged in water and vented to the atmosphere. One short tube connects bottles two and three. The second short tube is connected to an external suction source at a pressure that causes gentle, continuous bubbling in bottle three. Suction pressure, measured in centimeters of water, is equated with length of submersion in water of the long tube, as measured by centimeters. Usually −15 to −20 cm water, which requires the long tube to be submerged in 15 to 20 centimeters of water, is used for adults and a lesser amount for children (Erikson, 1981a). The disposable systems, such as a Pleur-Evac system, are a one-piece molded plastic unit that duplicates the three-bottle system (Fig. 38-10). The disposable units appear to be the system of choice because they are cost effective and some facilitate autotransfusion, a common practice in open-heart surgeries. Knowledge of the basics of chest tube management and troubleshooting maneuvers reduces client's side effects (Table 38-6).

Special Considerations. Clamping chest tubes is contraindicated when the client is ambulating. The nurse should handle the bottles carefully and maintain the drainage device below the client's chest. If the tubing disconnects from the bottles, the nurse should instruct the client to exhale as much as possible and to cough. This maneuver rids the pleural space of as much air as possible. The nurse needs to cleanse the tips of the tubing and reconnect them to the bottles.

Removal of chest tubes requires client preparation. A recent study investigated client's reported sensations during chest tube removal. The most frequent sensations reported included burning, pain, and a pulling sensation (Gift, Bolgiano, Cunningham, 1991).

Mobilization of Pulmonary Secretions

The ability of a client to mobilize pulmonary secretions may make the difference between a short-term illness and a long period of recovery involving complications. Nursing interventions that promote mobilization of pulmonary secretions include hydration, humidification, nebulization, and chest physiotherapy.

HYDRATION. Maintenance of adequate systemic hydration keeps mucociliary clearance normal. In clients with adequate hydration, pulmonary secretions are thin, white, watery, and easily removable with minimal coughing. Excessive coughing required to clear thick, tenacious secretions is fatiguing and leaves the client with little energy (Feldman, 1982).

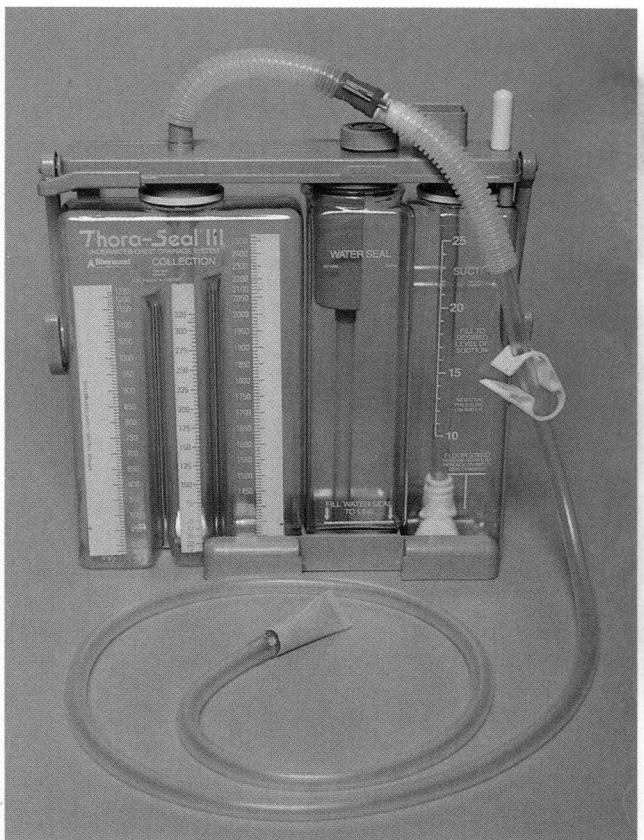

Fig. 38-10 Disposable, commercial chest drainage system.

Unless contraindicated, most clinicians recommend a fluid intake of 1500 to 2000 ml per day (Luce, Tyler, Pierson, 1984). Adequacy of hydration can be determined by the color, consistency, and ease of secretion expectoration.

HUMIDIFICATION. Humidification is the process of adding water to gas. Temperature is the most important factor affecting the amount of water vapor a gas can hold. The percent of water in the gas in relation to the gas' capacity for water is the relative humidity. Air or oxygen with a high relative humidity keeps the airways moist and loosens and mobilizes pulmonary secretions.

Humidification is necessary for clients receiving oxygen therapy. Oxygen delivered to the upper airways, as with a nasal catheter, nasal cannula, or face mask, can be humidified by bubbling it through water. Generally humidification is added when oxygen flow rates exceed 5 L/min.

Heating of humidifiers is impractical because condensed moisture fills the narrow tubing. There-

TABLE 38-6 Problem Solving with Chest Tubes	
Problem	Solution
Air leak is present.	Locate leak.
Continuous bubbling is seen in water-seal bottle/ chamber, indicating that leak is between client and water seal.	Tighten loose connections between client and water seal. Loose connections cause air to enter system. Leaks are corrected when constant bubbling stops.
Bubbling continues, indicating that air leak has not been corrected.	Cross-clamp chest tube close to client's chest. If bubbling stops, air leak is inside client's thorax (client centered) or at chest tube insertion site.* *Unclamp tube and notify physician immediately.* Reinforce chest dressing. Leaving chest tube clamped with client-centered leak can cause collapse of lung, mediastinal shift, and eventual collapse of other lung from buildup of air pressure within pleural cavity.
Bubbling continues, indicating that leak is not client centered.	In alternating fashion, gradually move clamps down drainage tubing away from client and toward suction-control chamber, moving one clamp at a time. When bubbling stops, leak is in section of tubing or connection that is between two clamps. Replace tubing or secure connection and release clamps.†
Bubbling continues, indicating that leak is not in tubing.	Leak is in drainage system. Change drainage system.*†
Tension pneumothorax is present.	Determine that chest tubes are not clamped, kinked, or occluded. Obstructed chest tubes trap air in intrapleural space when air leak originates within client.
Severe respiratory distress	Notify physician immediately.
Chest pain	Prepare immediately for another chest tube insertion; obtain a flutter (Heimlich) valve on large-gauge needle for short-term emergency release of air in intrapleural space; have emergency equipment (e.g., oxygen and code cart) near client.
Absence of breath sounds on affected side	
Hyperresonance on affected side	
Mediastinal shift to unaffected side	
Tracheal shift to unaffected side	
Hypotension	
Tachycardia	
Dependent loops of drainage tubing have trapped fluid.	Drain tubing contents into drainage bottle. Coil excess tubing on mattress and secure in place.
Water seal is disconnected.	Connect water seal and tape connection.
Water-seal bottle is broken.	Insert distal end of water-seal tube into sterile solution so that tip is 2 cm below surface level‡ and set up new water-seal bottle. If no sterile solution is available, double clamp chest tube while preparing new bottle.
Water-seal tube is no longer submerged in sterile fluid.	Add sterile solution to water-seal bottle until distal tip is 2 cm under surface level† or set water-seal bottle upright so that tip is submerged.

*Data from Paulau D, Jones S: *RN* Oct 1986.
†Data from Erickson R: *Nurs 81* 11(6):62, 1981.
‡Data from Carroll PF: *Nurs 86* 16(12):26; 1986.

fore the relative humidity of oxygen delivered to the upper airways is only 30% (Luce, Tyler, Pierson, 1984). Another method is the humidity tent. This is used for infants and children with illnesses such as croup and tracheitis. Children with these disorders require high humidity to liquefy secretions and help reduce fever. The nebulizer at the top of the humidity tent must remain filled with water to prevent nonhumidified air or oxygen from entering the tent. Air

in the humidity tent can become cool and fall below 20° C (68° F), causing the child to become chilled. Therefore the nurse monitors the child's body temperature as well as respiratory status. Children in humidity tents require frequent changes of clothing and bed linen to remain warm and dry.

When humidity is used, the nurse needs to ensure that the right solution is used for humidification and that the solution is changed according to agency procedures. Excess humidification and reservoirs used for humidity solutions are environments that support the growth of pathogens. Thus humidification can be a source for nosocomial infections in clients.

NEBULIZATION. **Nebulization** is a process of adding moisture or medications to inspired air by mixing particles of varying sizes with the air. A nebulizer uses the aerosol principle to suspend a maximum number of water drops or particles of the desired size in inspired air. The moisture added to the respiratory system through nebulization improves clearance of pulmonary secretions.

When the thin layer of fluid that supports the mucus layer over the cilia is allowed to dry, the cilia are damaged and cannot adequately clear the airway. Humidification through nebulization enhances mucociliary clearance, the body's natural mechanism for removing mucus and cellular debris from the respiratory tract. Therefore nebulization is often used for administration of bronchodilators and mucolytic agents.

The major types of nebulizers are the jet-aerosol nebulizer and the ultrasonic nebulizer. A jet-aerosol nebulizer uses gas under pressure, and the ultrasonic nebulizer uses high-frequency vibrations to break up the water or medication into fine drops or particles. When inspired with air or administered oxygen, the drops of particles are then deposited throughout the tracheobronchial tree.

CHEST PHYSIOTHERAPY. **Chest physiotherapy (CPT)** is a group of therapies used in combination to mobilize pulmonary secretions (see box). These therapies include postural drainage, chest percussion, and vibration. Chest physiotherapy should be followed by productive coughing. Suctioning is used if the client's ability to cough is inadequate. CPT also has multiple implications for a variety of lung diseases. Eid et al (1991) present a practical clinical synopsis of CPT maneuvers for a variety of clinical problems.

Chest percussion involves striking the chest wall over the area being drained. The hand is positioned so that the fingers and thumb touch and the hand is cupped (Fig. 38-11). Percussion on the surface of the chest wall sends waves of varying amplitude and frequency through the chest. The force of these waves can change the consistency of the sputum or dislodge it from airway walls (Luce, Tyler, Pierson, 1984). Chest percussion is performed by alternating hand motion against the chest wall (Fig. 38-12). Percussion is performed over a single layer of clothing and not over buttons, snaps, or zippers. The single layer of clothing prevents slapping the client's skin. Thicker material dampens the vibrations from percussion.

Guidelines for Chest Physiotherapy

Nursing care and selection of CPT skills are based on specific assessment findings. The following guidelines help the nurse in physical assessment and subsequent decision making:

- Know the client's normal range of vital signs: Conditions such as atelectasis and pneumonia requiring CPT can affect vital signs. The degree of change is related to the level of hypoxia, overall cardiopulmonary status, and tolerance to activity.
- Know the client's medications: Certain medications, particularly diuretics and antihypertensives, cause fluid and hemodynamic changes. These may decrease the client's tolerance to the positional changes of postural drainage. Steroid medications increase the client's risk of pathological rib fractures and often contraindicate rib shaking.
- Know the client's medical history: Certain conditions such as increased intracranial pressure, spinal cord injuries, and abdominal aneurysm resection contraindicate the positional changes of postural drainage. Thoracic trauma or surgery may also contraindicate percussion, vibration, and rib shaking.
- Know the client's level of cognitive function. Participation in controlled cough techniques requires the client to follow instructions. Congenital or acquired cognitive limitations may alter the client's ability to learn and participate in these techniques.
- Be aware of the client's exercise tolerance: CPT maneuvers are fatiguing. When the client is not used to physical activity, initial tolerance to the maneuvers may be decreased. However, with gradual increases in activity and planned CPT, client tolerance to the procedure improves.

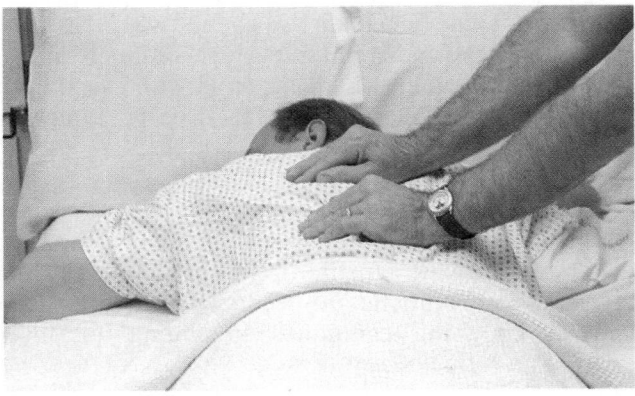

Fig. 38-11 Hand position for chest wall percussion during physiotherapy.

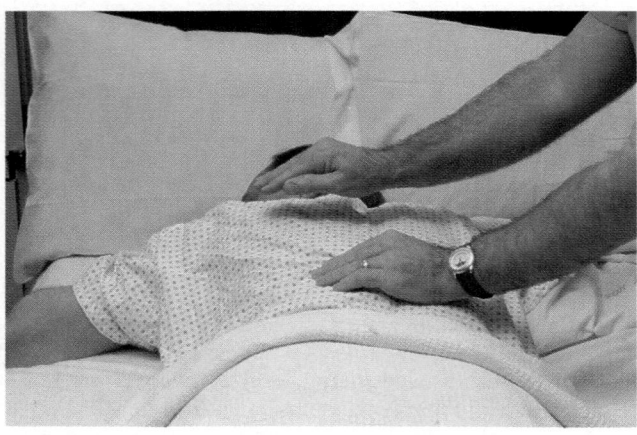

Fig. 38-12 Chest wall percussion, alternating hand motion against the client's chest wall.

Percussion is contraindicated in clients with bleeding disorders, osteoporosis, or fractured ribs. Caution should be taken to percuss the lung fields and not the scapular regions or trauma may occur to the skin and underlying musculoskeletal structures.

Vibration is a fine, shaking pressure applied to the chest wall only during exhalation. This technique is thought to increase the velocity and turbulence of exhaled air, facilitating secretion removal (Dettenmeier, 1992). Vibration increases the exhalation of trapped air and may shake mucus loose and induce a cough. Vibration is not recommended in infants and young children.

Postural drainage is the use of positioning techniques that draw secretions from specific segments of the lungs and bronchi into the trachea. Coughing or suctioning normally removes secretions from the trachea. The procedure for postural drainage can include most lung segments (Table 38-7). Because clients may not require postural drainage of all lung segments, the procedure is based on clinical assessment findings. For example, clients with left lower lobe atelectasis may require postural drainage of only the affected region, whereas a child with cystic fibrosis may require postural drainage of all lung segments.

Maintenance of a Patent Airway

The airway is patent when the trachea, bronchi, and large airways are free from obstructions. Three types of interventions are used to maintain a patent airway: coughing techniques, suctioning, and insertion of an artificial airway.

COUGHING TECHNIQUES. Coughing is effective for maintaining a patent airway. Coughing permits the client to remove secretions from both the upper and lower airways. The normal series of events in the cough mechanisms are deep inhalation, closure of the glottis, active contraction of the expiratory muscles, and glottis opening. Deep inhalation increases lung volume and airway diameter. Thus air can pass to partially obstructing mucus plugs or other foreign matter. Contraction of the expiratory muscles against the closed glottis allows a high intrathoracic pressure to develop. As a result, when the glottis is opened, a large flow of air is expelled at a high speed, providing momentum for mucus to move to the upper airway. After the cough the mucus can be expectorated or swallowed (Traver, 1982).

Various coughing techniques can be taught to different clients. (Chapter 47 details the technique of deep breathing and coughing for the postoperative client.) Other cough techniques are cascade, huff, and quad coughing.

With the cascade cough the client takes a slow, deep breath and holds it for 2 seconds, while contracting expiratory muscles. Then the client opens the mouth and performs a series of coughs throughout exhalation, thereby coughing at progressively lowered lung volumes. This technique promotes airway clearance and a patent airway in clients with large volumes of sputum.

With the huff cough the client, while exhaling, opens the glottis by saying the word "huff." The huff cough stimulates a natural cough reflex. This is generally effective only for clearing central airways, but with practice the client inhales more air and may be able to progress to the cascade cough.

The quad cough technique is used for clients without abdominal muscle control, such as those with spinal cord injuries. The client or nurse pushes inward and upward on the abdominal muscles toward the diaphragm while the client breathes with maximal expiratory effort, causing the cough (Luce, Tyler, Pierson, 1984).

The effectiveness of coughing is evaluated by sputum expectoration, the client's report of swallowed sputum, or clearing of adventitious sounds on auscultation. Clients with chronic pulmonary diseases, upper respiratory tract infections, and lower respiratory tract infections should be encouraged to cough at least every 2 hours when awake. Clients with a large amount of sputum should be encouraged to cough every hour while awake and every 2 to 3 hours while asleep until the acute phase of mucus production has ended.

SUCTIONING TECHNIQUES. When a client is unable to clear respiratory tract secretions with coughing, the nurse must use suctioning to clear the airways. The

TABLE 38-7 Positions for Postural Drainage

Lung Segment	Position of Client	Lung Segment	Position of Client
ADULT		Left lower lobe—lateral segment	Right side lying in Trendelenburg position
Bilateral	High Fowler's		
Apical segments Right upper lobe—anterior segment	Sitting on side of bed Supine with head elevated	Right lower lobe—lateral segment	Left side lying in Trendelenburg position
Left upper lobe—anterior segment	Supine with head elevated	Right lower lobe—posterior segment	Prone with right side of chest elevated in Trandelenburg position
Right upper lobe—posterior segment	Side lying with right side of chest elevated on pillows	Both lower lobes—posterior segment	Prone in Trendelenburg position
Left upper lobe—posterior segment	Side lying with left side of chest elevated on pillows	**CHILD** Bilateral—apical segments	Sitting on nurse's lap, leaning slightly forward flexed over pillow
Right middle lobe—anterior segment	Three-fourths supine position with dependent lung in Trendelenburg position	Bilateral—middle anterior segments	Sitting on nurse's lap, leaning against nurse
Right middle lobe—posterior segment	Prone with thorax and abdomen elevated	Bilateral lobes—anterior segments	Lying supine on nurse's lap, back supported with pillow
Both lower lobes—anterior segments	Supine in Trendelenburg		

three primary suctioning techniques are oropharyngeal and nasopharyngeal suctioning, orotracheal and nasotracheal suctioning, and suctioning an artificial airway.

These techniques are based on common principles. Because the oropharynx and trachea are considered sterile, sterile technique is required for suctioning. The mouth is considered clean, and therefore the suctioning of oral secretions should be performed after suctioning of the oropharynx and trachea. Each type of suctioning requires the use of a beaded-tip catheter with a ring of holes along the side of the catheter at the distal end. Frequency of suctioning is determined by continued client assessment. If secretions are identified by inspection or auscultation techniques, suctioning is required. Sputum is not produced continuously or every 1 or 2 hours but occurs as a response to a pathological condition. Therefore there is no rationale for routine suctioning of all clients every 1 to 2 hours.

Oropharyngeal and Nasopharyngeal Suctioning. The oropharynx extends behind the mouth from the soft palate above the level of the hyoid bone and contains the tonsils. The nasopharynx is located behind the nose and extends to the level of the soft palate. Oropharyngeal or nasopharyngeal suctioning is used when the client is able to cough effectively but is unable to clear secretions by expectorating or swallowing. The suction procedure is used after the client has coughed (Procedure 38-3). As the amount of pulmonary secretions is reduced and the client is less fatigued, the client may be able to expectorate or swallow the mucus. This type of suctioning is then no longer required.

OROTRACHEAL AND NASOTRACHEAL SUCTIONING. Orotracheal or nasotracheal suctioning is necessary when the client with pulmonary secretions is unable to cough and does not have an artificial airway present (see Procedure 38-3). A catheter is passed through the mouth or nose into the trachea. The nose is the preferred route because stimulation of the gag reflex is minimal. The procedure is similar to nasopharyngeal suctioning, but the catheter tip is moved farther into the client to suction the trachea. The entire procedure from catheter passage to its removal cannot take more than 15 seconds because oxygen does not reach the lungs during suctioning. Unless in respiratory distress, the client should be allowed to rest between passes of the catheter. If the client is using supplemental oxygen, the oxygen cannula or mask should be replaced during rest periods.

ARTIFICIAL AIRWAY. An artificial airway is an oral airway or an endotracheal, nasotracheal, or tracheostomy tube. Indications for an artificial airway include decreased level of consciousness, airway obstruction, mechanical ventilation, and removal of tracheal secretions.

Oral Airway. The oral airway, the simplest type of artificial airway, prevents obstruction of the trachea by displacement of the tongue into the oropharynx in the unconscious client (Fig. 38-13). The oral airway extends from the teeth to the oropharynx, maintaining the tongue in the normal position. The correct size airway must be used. If the airway is too small, the tongue is not held in the anterior portion of the mouth. If it is too large, it may force the tongue toward the epiglottis and obstruct the airway.

The artificial oral airway is inserted by turning the curve of the airway toward the cheek and placing it over the tongue into the oropharynx. When the airway is in the oropharynx, the nurse turns it so that the opening points downward. The correctly placed airway moves the tongue forward away from the oropharynx. The flange, the flat portion of the airway, should rest against the client's teeth.

If the nurse attempts to insert the oral airway with a curve toward the tongue, the client's natural airway can be further obstructed. Incorrect insertion merely forces the tongue back into the oropharynx.

Tracheal Airway. Artificial tracheal airways include endotracheal, nasotracheal, and tracheal tubes. These allow easy access to the client's trachea for deep tracheal suctioning. Because of the presence of the artificial airway, the client no longer has normal humidification of the tracheal mucosa. The nurse should ensure that humidity is being supplied to the airway through nebulization or with the oxygen-delivery system. This humidification is protective and helps removal of tracheal secretions. Removal of tra-

Text continued on p. 1259.

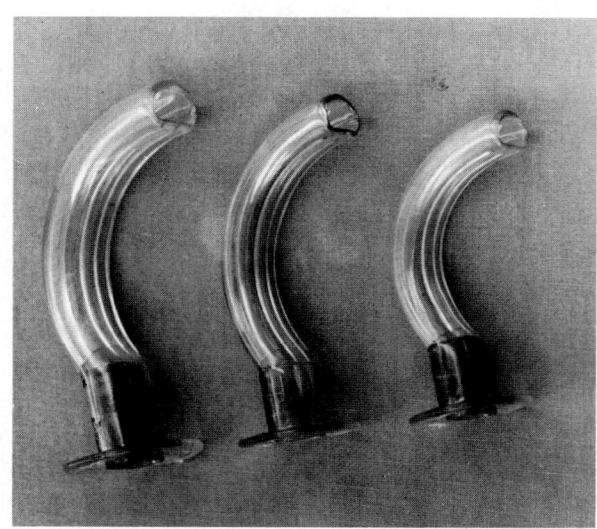

Fig. 38-13 Artificial oral airways.

STEPS	RATIONALE
1. Assess for signs and symptoms indicating presence of upper airway secretions: gurgling respirations, restlessness, vomitus in mouth, drooling.	Physical signs and symptoms result from decreased oxygen to tissues as well as pooling of secretions in upper airway.
2. Explain to client how procedure will help to clear airway and relieve some breathing problems. Explain that coughing, sneezing, or gagging is normal.	Explanation of procedure relieves client's anxiety.

3. Prepare necessary equipment and supplies:
  a. Portable or wall suction unit with connecting tubing with Y connector if needed
  b. Sterile catheter
  c. Yankauer catheter (oropharyngeal)
  d. Sterile water or normal saline, sterile basin
  e. Sterile gloves, nonsterile gloves (Yankauer only)
  f. Drape or towel
  g. Nasal or oral airway if indicated
	Ensures that procedure is completed quickly and efficiently.
	
	Cleans catheter.
	
	Protects linen and client's bedclothes.
	Ensures access to airway.

4. Close door or pull curtain.	Ensures privacy.

5. Properly position client:
  a. Place conscious client with functional gag reflex for oral suctioning in semi-Fowler's position with head turned to one side. Place such a client for nasal suctioning in semi-Fowler's position with neck hyperextended.
  b. Place unconscious client in side-lying position facing nurse.
	Gag reflex helps prevent aspiration of gastrointestinal contents. Positioning of head to one side or hyperextending neck promotes smooth insertion of catheter into oropharynx or nasopharynx, respectively.
	
	Prevents client's tongue from obstructing airway, promotes drainage of pulmonary secretions, and prevents aspiration of gastrointestinal contents.

6. Place towel on pillow or under client's chin.	Prevents soiling of bed linen or bedclothes from secretions. Secretions on towel can be discarded, thus reducing spread of bacteria.
7. Select proper suction pressure for client and type of suction unit. For wall suction units, this is 110-150 mm Hg in adults, 95-110 mm Hg in children, and 50-95 mm Hg in infants.	Provides safe but effective negative pressure according to client's age. Decreases possibility of damage to mucous membranes and hypoxemia.
8. Wash hands.	Reduces transmission of microorganisms.

9. Yankauer catheter:
  a. Apply nonsterile gloves.
  b. Connect one end of connecting tubing to suction machine and other to Yankauer suction catheter. Fill cup with water.
  c. Check that equipment is functioning properly by suctioning small amount of water from cup or basin.
  d. Remove oxygen mask, if present.
  e. Insert catheter into mouth along gum line to pharynx. Move catheter around mouth until secretions are cleared.
  f. Encourage client to cough. Replace oxygen mask.
 	
  g. Rinse catheter with water in cup or basin until connecting tubing is cleared of secretions. Turn off suction.
	Reduces transmission of microorganisms.
	Prepares suction apparatus.
	
	Ensures equipment function and lubricates catheter.
	
	Provides continuous suction. Care must be taken not to allow suction tip to invaginate oral mucosal surfaces.
	
	Moves secretions from lower airway into mouth and upper airway.
	Rinses catheter and reduces probability of transmission of microorganisms. Clean suction tubing enhances delivery of set suction pressure.

*Yankauer catheters, nasopharyngeal or nasotracheal suction, artificial airway

STEPS	RATIONALE

h. Reassess client's respiratory status.

Directs nurse to initiate or cease intervention.

i. Remove towel, place in laundry. Remove gloves and dispose in receptacle.

Reduces transmission of microorganisms.

j. Reposition client; Sims' position encourages drainage and should be used if client has decreased level of consciousness.

Facilitates drainage of oral secretions.

k. Discard remainder of water into appropriate receptacle.

Reduces transmission of microorganisms and maintains medical asepsis.

l. Rinse basin in warm soapy water and dry with paper towels. Discard disposable cup into appropriate receptacle.

m. Place catheter in clean dry area.

n. Wash hands.

Reduces transmission of microorganisms to other clients.

10. **Nasopharyngeal or nasotracheal suction:**

a. Turn suction device on and set vacuum regulator to appropriate negative pressure.

Excessive negative pressure damages nasal pharyngeal and tracheal mucosa and can reduce greater hypoxia.

b. If indicated, increase supplemental oxygen to 100% or as ordered by physician.

Reduces suction-induced hypoxemia. (The literature is inconclusive as to the necessity of hyperoxygenation.)

c. Connect one end of connecting tubing to suction machine and place other end in convenient location.

Prepares for connection of suction catheter to suction apparatus.

d. If using suction kit:

(1) Open package. If sterile drape is available, place it across client's chest or use towel.

Reduces transmission of microorganisms.

(2) Open suction catheter package. Do not allow suction catheter to touch any surface other than inside of its package.

Maintains medical asepsis.

(3) Unwrap or open sterile basin and place on bedside table. Be careful not to touch inside of basin. Fill with about 100 ml sterile normal saline.

Saline is used to clean tubing after each suction pass.

e. Open lubricant. Squeeze onto open sterile catheter package without touching package.

Prepares lubricant while maintaining sterility. Water-soluble lubricant is used to avoid lipoid aspiration pneumonia.

f. Apply sterile glove to each hand or apply nonsterile glove to nondominant hand and sterile glove to dominant hand.

Reduces transmission of microorganisms and allows nurse to maintain sterility of suction catheter.

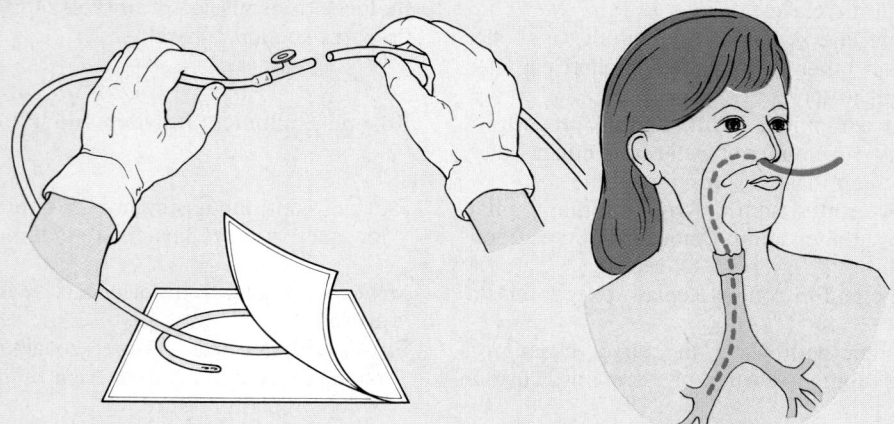

Step 10g

Step 10j

STEPS	RATIONALE
g. Pick up suction catheter with dominant hand without touching nonsterile surfaces. Pick up connecting tubing with nondominant hand. Secure catheter to tubing (see illustration).	Maintains catheter sterility. Connects catheter to suction.
h. Check that equipment is functioning properly by suctioning small amount of normal saline from basin.	Ensures equipment fuction. Lubricates internal catheter and tubing.
i. Coat distal 6-8 cm of catheter with water-soluble lubricant.	Lubricates catheter for easier insertion.
j. Remove oxygen-delivery device, if applicable, with nondominant hand. Without applying suction, gently but quickly insert catheter with dominant thumb and forefinger into naris using slight downward slant or through mouth when client breathes in. Do not force through naris (see illustration).	Application of suction pressure while introducing catheter into trachea increases risk of damage to mucosa, as well as increased risk of hypoxia due to removal of oxygen present in airways. Epiglottis is open on inspiration and facilitates insertion into trachea. Client should cough. If client gags or becomes nauseated, catheter is most likely in esophagus.
(1) *Pharyngeal suctioning:* In adults, insert catheter about 16 cm; in older children, 8-12 cm; in infants and young children, 4-8 cm. Rule of thumb is to insert catheter distance from tip of nose to base of ear lobe.	
{2) *Tracheal suctioning:* In adults, insert catheter 20-24 cm; in older children, 14-20; and in young children and infants, 8-14 cm.	
(3) *Positioning:* In some instances turning client's head to right helps nurse suction left mainstem bronchus; turning head to left helps nurse suction right mainstem bronchus.	
If resistance is felt after insertion of catheter for recommended distance, nurse has probably hit carina. Pull catheter back 1 cm before applying suction.	
k. Apply intermittent suction for up to 10 sec by placing and releasing nondominant thumb over vent of catheter and slowly withdraw catheter while rotating it back and forth between dominant thumb and forefinger. Encourage client to cough. Replace oxygen device, if applicable.	Prevents injury to mucosa. If catheter "grabs" mucosa, remove thumb to release suction. Suctioning longer than 10 sec can cause cardiopulmonary compromise.
l. Rinse catheter and connecting tubing with normal saline until cleared.	Removes secretions from catheter.
11. Artificial airway:	
a. Wash hands.	Reduces transmission of microorganisms.
b. Turn suction device on and set vacuum regulator to appropriate negative pressure (see Step 7).	Excessive negative pressure damages tracheal mucosa and can induce greater hypoxia.
c. Connect one end of connecting tubing to suction machine and place other end in convenient location.	Prepares suction apparatus.
d. If using sterile suction kit:	
(1) Open package. If sterile drape is available, place it across client's chest.	Prevents contamination of clothing.
(2) Open suction catheter package. Do not allow suction catheter to touch any nonsterile surface.	Prepares catheter and prevents transmission of microorganisms.

Suctioning

STEPS	RATIONALE
(3) Unwrap or open sterile basin and place on bedside table. Be careful not to touch inside basin. Fill with about 100 ml sterile normal saline.	Prepares catheter and prevents transmission of microorganisms.
e. If indicated, open lubricant. Squeeze onto sterile catheter package without touching package.	Prepares lubricant for use while maintaining sterility.
f. Apply one sterile glove to each hand or apply nonsterile glove to nondominant hand and sterile glove to dominant hand.	Reduces transmission of microorganisms and allows nurse to maintain sterility of suction catheter.
g. Pick up suction catheter with dominant hand without touching nonsterile surfaces. Pick up connecting tubing with nondominant hand. Secure catheter to tubing.	Maintains catheter sterility.
h. Check that equipment is functioning properly by suctioning small amount of saline from basin.	Ensures equipment function; lubricates catheter and tubing.
i. Coat distal 6-8 cm of catheter with water-soluble lubricant. In some situations, catheter is lubricated only with normal saline. Nursing assessment indicates need for lubrication.	Promotes easier catheter insertion. If lubricant is needed, it must be water soluble to prevent petroleum-based aspiration pneumonia. Excessive lubricant can adhere to artificial airway.
j. Remove oxygen- or humidity-delivery device with nondominant hand.	Exposes artificial airway.
k. Hyperinflate and/or oxygenate client before suctioning, using manual resuscitation (Ambu) bag or sigh mechanism on mechanical ventilator.	Decreases atelectasis caused by negative pressure. Preoxygenation converts large proportion of resident lung gas to 100% oxygen to offset amount used in metabolic consumption while ventilator or oxygenation is interrupted, as well as to offset volume lost out of suction catheter (Luce, Tyler, Pierson, 1984).
l. Without applying suction, gently but quickly insert catheter with dominant thumb and forefinger into artificial airway (best to time catheter insertion with inspiration).	Places catheter in tracheobronchial tree. Application of suction pressure while introducing catheter into trachea increases risk of damage to tracheal mucosa, as well as increased hypoxia due to removal of oxygen present in airways.
m. Insert catheter until resistance is met, then pull back 1 cm.	Stimulates cough and removes catheter from mucosal wall.
n. Apply intermittent suction by placing and releasing nondominant thumb over vent of catheter and slowly withdraw catheter while rotating it back and forth between dominant thumb and forefinger. Encourage client to cough.	Prevents injury to tracheal mucosal lining. If catheter "grabs" mucosa, remove thumb to release suction.
o. Replace oxygen-delivery service. Encourage client to deep breathe.	Reoxygenates and reexpands alveoli. Suctioning can cause hypoxemia and atelectasis.
p. Rinse catheter and connecting tubing with normal saline until clear. Use continuous suction.	Removes catheter secretions. Secretions left in tubing decrease suction and provide environment for microorganism growth.
q. Repeat Steps k-p as needed to clear secretions. Allow adequate time (at least 1 full min) between suction passes for ventilation and reoxygenation.	Clears airway of excessive secretions and promotes improved oxygenation.
r. Assess client's cardiopulmonary status between suction passes.	Suctioning can induce arrhythmias, hypoxia, and bronchospasm.
s. When artificial airway and tracheobronchial tree are sufficiently cleared of secretions, perform nasal and oral pharyngeal suctioning to clear upper airway of secretions. After this suctioning is performed, catheter is contaminated; do not reinsert into endotracheal or tracheostomy tube.	Removes upper airway secretions. Upper airway is considered clean, whereas lower airway is considered sterile. Therefore same catheter can be used to suction from sterile to clean areas but not from clean to sterile areas.

STEPS	RATIONALE
t. Disconnect catheter from connecting tubing. Roll catheter around fingers of dominant hand. Pull glove off inside out so that catheter remains in glove. Pull off other glove in same way. Discard into appropriate receptacle. Turn off suction device.	Reduces transmission of microorganisms.
u. Remove towel and place in laundry, or remove drape and discard in appropriate receptacle.	Reduces transmission of microorganisms.
v. Reposition client.	Promotes comfort. Sims' position encourages drainage and reduces risk of aspiration.
w. Discard remainder of normal saline into appropriate receptacle. If basin is disposable, discard into appropriate receptacle. If basin is reusable, place it in soiled utility room.	Reduces transmission of microorganisms.
x. Wash hands.	Reduces transmission of microorganisms.
12. Prepare equipment for next suctioning.	Provides ready access to suction equipment, especially if client is experiencing respiratory distress.
13. Observe client for absence of airway secretions, restlessness, oral secretions.	Indicates that secretions have been removed from oral and pharyngeal areas.
14. Record the amount, consistency, color, and odor of secretions and client's response to procedure; document client's presuctioning and postsuctioning respiratory status.	Documents that procedure was completed and client's status before and after.

cheal secretions must be aseptic, atraumatic, and effective.

Asepsis involves using a freshly opened sterile suction catheter that is handled with a sterile glove (see Chapter 18). Secretion removal should be as atraumatic as possible. To avoid trauma, suction should never be applied during insertion of the catheter but only during its withdrawal. The catheter is rotated and suction is applied intermittently during withdrawal.

Maintenance and Promotion of Oxygenation

Promotion of lung expansion, mobilization of secretions, and maintenance of a patent airway assist the client in meeting oxygenation needs. However, some clients also require oxygen therapy to keep a healthy level of tissue oxygenation.

GOALS OF OXYGEN THERAPY. The goal of oxygen therapy is to prevent or relieve hypoxia. Any client with impaired tissue oxygenation can benefit from controlled oxygen administration. Oxygen is not a substitute for other treatment, however, and should be used only when indicated. Oxygen should be

treated as a drug. It is expensive and has dangerous side effects. As with any drug, the dosage or concentration of oxygen should be continuously monitored. The nurse should routinely check the physician's orders to verify that the client is receiving the prescribed oxygen concentration. The five rights of medication administration also pertain to oxygen (see Chapter 20).

SAFETY PRECAUTIONS WITH OXYGEN THERAPY. Oxygen is a highly combustible gas. Although it will not spontaneously burn or cause an explosion, it can easily cause a fire to ignite in a client's room if it contacts a spark, such as from a cigarette or electrical equipment. Oxygen in high concentrations has a great combustion potential and fuels fire readily.

With increasing use of home oxygen therapy, clients and health care professionals must be aware of the dangerous combustible effects. Reports in the literature include information about incidents in the hospital settings, especially those associated with oxygen tents in the pediatric setting and cigarette smoking (Gjerde, Kraemer, 1980). A recent article noted a case in which there was a hazard with home oxygen therapy. A client using a portable oxygen source attempted to sharpen lawn mower blades on a home grinder. As soon as the blades touched the grindstone and created sparks, the client felt a burning sensation around and within his nasal passages. Although he quickly removed the oxygen cannula, he received first-degree burns to the face and cheeks from the blow torch effect produced by the cannula (McCauley, Boller, 1987).

The nurse should promote safety by using the following measures:

1. "No smoking" signs should be placed on the client's room door and over the bed. The client, visitors and roommates, and all personnel should be informed that smoking is not permitted in areas where oxygen is in use.
2. The nurse determines that all electrical equipment in the room is functioning correctly and is properly grounded (see Chapter 42). An electrical spark in the presence of oxygen can result in a serious fire.
3. The nurse should know the fire procedures and the location of the closest fire extinguisher.

SUPPLY OF OXYGEN. Oxygen is supplied to the client's bedside either by oxygen tanks or through a permanent wall-piped system. Oxygen tanks are transported on wide-based carriers that allow the tank to be placed upright at the client's bedside. Regulators are used to control the amount of oxygen delivered. One common type is an upright flow meter with a flow-adjustment valve at the top. A second type is a cylinder indicator with a flow-adjustment handle.

In the hospital or home, oxygen tanks are delivered with the regulator in place. In the hospital, connecting the regulator is usually done by the respiratory therapy department. Vendors are generally responsible for connecting the oxygen tank to the regulator for home use.

METHODS OF OXYGEN DELIVERY. Oxygen can be delivered to the client by nasal cannula, nasal catheter, face mask, or mechanical ventilator.

Nasal Cannula. A **nasal cannula** (Fig. 38-14) is a simple, comfortable device (Procedure 38-4). The two cannulae, about 1.5 cm (½ in) long, protrude from the center of a disposable tube and are inserted into the nares. Oxygen is delivered via the cannulae with a flow rate of up to 4 L/min. Higher flow rates dry airway mucosa and do not further increase inspired oxygen concentrations (Luce, Tyler, Pierson, 1984). The nurse must know what flow rate produces a given percentage of inspired oxygen concentration (Fio_2).

Nasal Catheter. Nasal catheters are used less frequently than nasal cannulae, but they are not obsolete. The procedure involves inserting an oxygen catheter into the nose to the nasopharynx. Because securing the catheter can cause pressure on the nostril, the catheter must be changed at least every 8 hours and inserted into the other nostril. For this reason the nasal catheter is often a less desirable method because the client may have pain when the catheter is passed into the nasopharynx and because trauma can occur to the nasal mucosa.

Transtracheal Oxygen. **Transtracheal oxygen** is a method of oxygen delivery for clients with chronic lung diseases in which a small, intravenous-size catheter is inserted directly into the trachea through a surgical tract in the lower neck. Oxygen is delivered directly into the trachea.

The transtracheal oxygen delivery system is more advantageous in clients needing continuous oxygen for several reasons. First, there is no oxygen lost to the atmosphere, which is the case with a nasal cannula. Therefore oxygen delivery is less expensive. Second, because oxygen travels directly into the trachea as opposed to through the nose to the posterior pharynx and into the trachea, clients achieve adequate oxygenation at lower flow rates. Third, clients are more likely to use oxygen as prescribed because of the mobility, comfort, and cosmetic improvement. Last, additional humidification is unnecessary because the nasopharynx, the area in most need of supplemental humidity, is bypassed (Spofford, Christopher, 1989).

Transtracheal oxygen is a potential source of danger to clients with chronic pulmonary disease who have a history of carbon dioxide retention. This therapy must be carefully monitored by nurses. These clients may require lower oxygen flow rates than predicted.

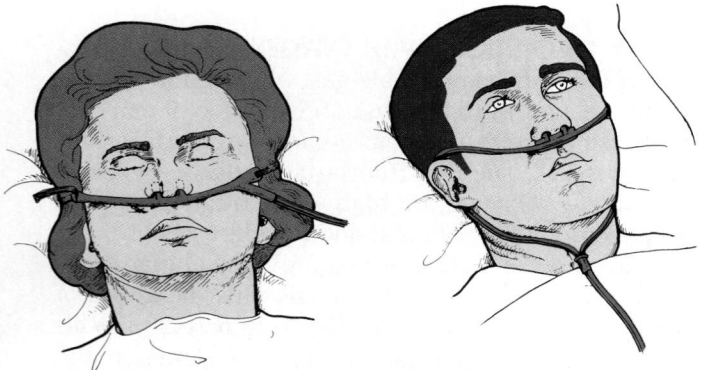

Fig. 38-14 Nasal cannula.
From Wade JF: *Comprehensive respiratory care*, ed 3, St Louis, 1983, Mosby–Year Book.

STEPS	RATIONALE
1. Inspect client for signs and symptoms associated with hypoxia and presence of airway secretions.	Left untreated, hypoxia can produce cardiac dysrhythmias and death. Presence of airway secretions decreases effectiveness of oxygen delivery.
2. Explain to client and family what procedure entails and purpose of oxygen therapy.	Decreases client's anxiety, which reduces oxygen consumption and increases client cooperation.
3. Assemble needed supplies and equipment: a. Nasal cannula b. Oxygen tubing c. Humidifier d. Sterile distilled water e. Oxygen source with flowmeter f. "No smoking" signs	Ensures that procedure is completed quickly and efficiently.
4. Wash hands.	Reduces transmission of infection.
5. Attach nasal cannula to oxygen tubing and attach to humidified oxygen source adjusted to prescribed flow rate.	Prevents drying of nasal and oral mucous membranes and airway secretions.
6. Place tips of cannula into client's nares.	Directs flow of oxygen into client's upper respiratory tract.
7. Adjust elastic headband or plastic slide until cannula fits snugly and comfortably.	Client is more likely to keep cannula in place if it fits comfortably.
8. Maintain sufficient slack on oxygen tubing and secure to client's clothes.	Allows client to turn head without dislodging cannula and reduces pressure on tips of nares.
9. Check the cannula every 8 hr.	Ensures patency of cannula and oxygen flow.
10. Keep humidification jar filled at all times.	Prevents inhalation of dehumidified oxygen.
11. Observe client's nares and superior surface of both ears for skin breakdown.	Oxygen therapy can cause drying of nasal mucosa. Pressure on ears from cannula tubing or elastic can cause skin irritation.
12. Check oxygen flow rate and physician's orders every 8 hr.	Ensures delivery of prescribed oxygen flow rate.
13. Wash hands.	Reduces transmission of microorganisms.
14. Inspect client for relief of symptoms associated with hypoxia.	Indicates that hypoxia is corrected or reduced.
15. Record in nurses' notes method of oxygen delivery, flow rate, patency of oxygen cannula, client response, and respiratory assessment.	Documents correct use of oxygen therapy and client's response.

Use of transtracheal oxygenation occurs in four steps. First is client evaluation and selection. Not all clients requiring oxygen therapy can use this method of delivery. Some clients do not wish to have the surgical procedure, which is done under local anesthesia. Other clients are unable to care for the transtracheal equipment. Therefore the nurse must completely assess the client and family to determine whether they can effectively and safely use transtracheal oxygen. The second phase begins with surgical insertion of the stent. The stent is a stoma-type access route directly into the trachea. Third is initiation of oxygen through a number 9 French catheter in to the stoma. Fourth, once the tracheal stoma is healed, the client must be taught to remove and irrigate the catheter at least three times a day with normal saline. Irrigation maintains catheter patency. The final oxygen flow rate, usually less than 4 L/min, is delivered through an 8 Fr catheter through the mature tract (Reinke, Hoffman, Wesmiller, 1992).

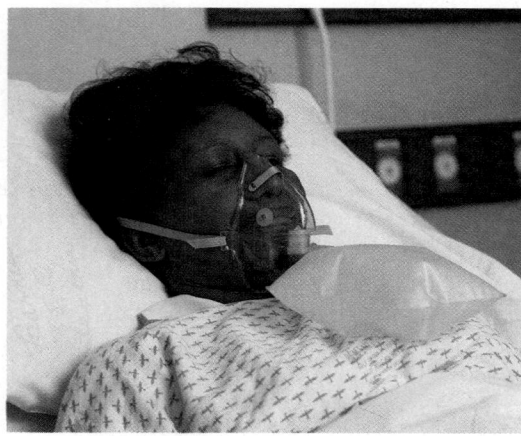

Fig. 38-15   Plastic face mask with reservoir bag.

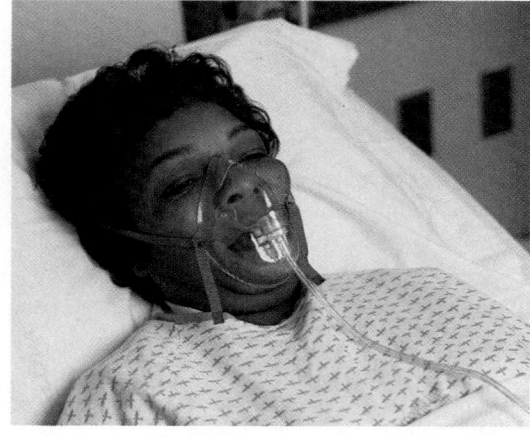

Fig. 38-17   Simple face mask.

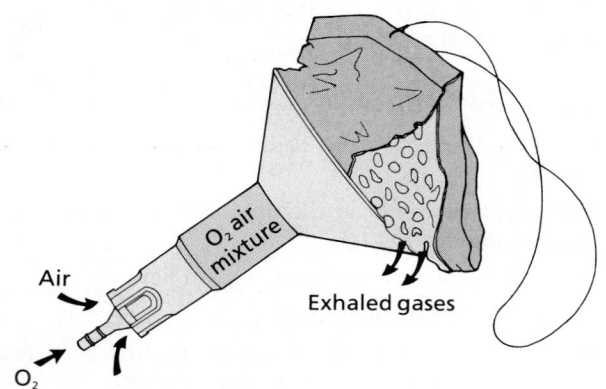

Fig. 38-16   Venturi mask.
Courtesy Puritan-Bennett Corp, Overland Park, Kansas.

Oxygen Masks. An oxygen mask is a device used to administer oxygen, humidity, or heated humidity. It is shaped to fit snugly over the mouth and nose and is secured in place with a strap. There are two primary types of oxygen masks: high and low concentration.

A plastic face mask with a reservoir bag (Fig. 38-15) and a Venturi mask (Fig. 38-16) are capable of delivering higher concentrations of oxygen. When used as a nonrebreather, the plastic face mask with a reservoir bag can deliver from 80% to 90% oxygen (70% when used as a rebreather) with a flow rate of 10 L/min. This oxygen mask maintains a high-concentration oxygen supply in the reservoir bag. The nurse should frequently inspect the bag to make sure it is inflated. If it is deflated, the client may be breathing large amounts of exhaled carbon dioxide.

The Venturi mask can be used to deliver oxygen concentrations of 24% to 28%, 30%, 35%, 40%, 45%, 55% with oxygen flow rates of 2 to 3, 4, 6, 8, 14 L/min, respectively, depending on which flow control meter is selected (Dettenmeier, 1992).

The simple face mask (Fig. 38-17) is used for short-term oxygen therapy. It fits loosely and delivers oxygen concentrations from 30% to 60%. The mask is contraindicated for clients with carbon dioxide retention because retention can be worsened.

Home Oxygen. When home oxygen is required, it is usually delivered by nasal cannula. When a cli-

TABLE 38-8   Home Oxygen Systems

Primary Use	Advantages	Disadvantages
COMPRESSED GAS CYLINDERS		
Intermittent therapy, such as for exercise or sleep only	100% oxygen, relatively inexpensive, no loss of gas during storage, relatively portable, delivery of up to 15 L/min	Bulky, possibly unsightly, frequent refilling necessary with continuous use
LIQUID OXYGEN SYSTEMS		
High liter flows and active patients	100% oxygen, conveniently portable, portable units refilled at home, delivery of up to 6 L/min	Usually weekly delivery necessary for refill, evaporates if not used, potential for frostbite at connections and if spilled
CONCENTRATORS		
Moderate liter flows and patients with limited mobility inside or outside home	Fixed monthly cost, minimal interruption of household by supplier, no refills of "main tank," most units with delivery of up to 4 or 5 L/min	Oxygen concentration decreases as liter flow increases (usually 85% to 90%), power supply necessary, electric bill increase of $15 to $20 a month, second system for portability necessary (usually gas cylinders)

From Dettenmeier PA: *Pulmonary nursing care,* St Louis, 1992, Mosby–Year Book.

ent has a permanent tracheostomy, however, a T-tube or tracheostomy collar is necessary. Three types of oxygen are used: compressed oxygen, liquid oxygen, and oxygen concentrators. The advantages and disadvantages (Table 38-8) of each type are assessed, along with the client's needs and community resources, before placing a certain delivery system in the home. In the home the major consideration is the oxygen-delivery source.

Clients requiring home oxygen need extensive teaching so that they are able to continue oxygen therapy efficiently and safely (Procedure 38-5). For this preparation, the nurse must coordinate efforts of the client, primary nurse, visiting nurse, and home oxygen equipment vendor. The nurse must also allow sufficient time for teaching so that the client is confident in maintaining the oxygen-delivery system.

Restoration of Cardiopulmonary Functioning

If a client's hypoxia is severe and prolonged, cardiac arrest may result. A cardiac arrest is a sudden cessation of cardiac output and circulation. When this occurs, oxygen is not delivered to tissues, carbon dioxide is not transported from tissues, tissue metabolism becomes anaerobic, and metabolic and respiratory acidosis occur. Permanent heart, brain, and other tissue damage occurs within 5 minutes.

Text continued on p. 1269.

Using Home Oxygen Equipment

STEPS	RATIONALE

1. Assess the following:

    a. Determine client's or family's ability to use oxygen equipment correctly while in hospital, if possible, or assess for appropriate use of equipment in home setting.

Physical or cognitive impairments may require instructing family member or significant other on how to operate home oxygen equipment. Candidates for home oxygen have $Pao_2 \leq 55$ mm Hg or oxygen saturation of 88% on room air or Pao_2 55-59 mm Hg or oxygen saturation of 86% to 89% with evidence of edema from right heart failure, cor pulmonale, or polycythemia (Herrick, Yeager, 1989).

    b. Assess client's or family's ability to observe for signs and symptoms of hypoxia: apprehension, anxiety, decreased ability to concentrate, decreased level of consciousness, increased fatigue, dizziness, behavioral changes, increased pulse, increased respiratory rate, pallor, and cyanosis.

Hypoxia can occur at home when client uses oxygen. It can be caused by worsening of client's physical problem or another underlying condition (e.g., change in respiratory status).

2. Explain procedure to client and family.

Reinforces education received in hospital. Enables client and family to ask questions.

3. Prepare needed equipment:

    a. Nasal cannula (see Procedure 38-4)

    b. Liberator and Stroller

        (1) Nasal cannula

        (2) Oxygen tubing

        (3) In-home oxygen supply (Liberator)

        (4) Portable system (Stroller)

Ensures that procedure is completed quickly and efficiently.

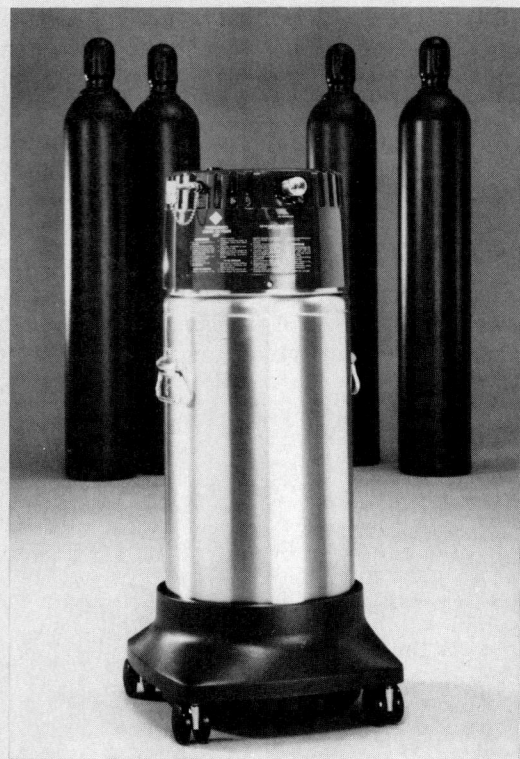

Step 6a

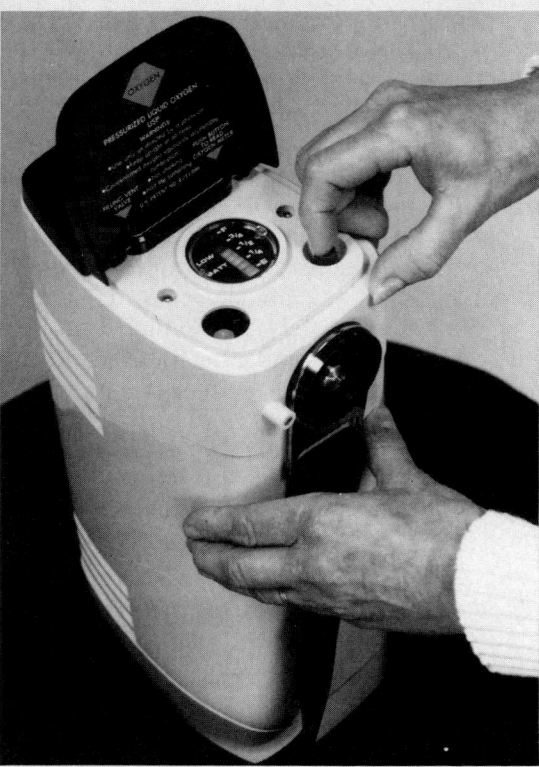

Step 6b

STEPS	RATIONALE
4. Wash hands.	Reduces transmission of infection.
5. Demonstrate steps for preparation and completion of oxygen therapy.	Teaches psychomotor skill and enables client to ask questions.
6. Prepare Liberator and Stroller for use:	
a. Place Liberator in clutter-free environment (see illustration).	30 L Liberator replaces 3½ compressed oxygen cylinders but requires sufficient space.
b. Check oxygen levels of both Liberator and Stroller by depressing button at lower right corner and reading dial (see illustration).	Ensures timely and effective use of remaining oxygen supply and allows time for refill.
c. When necessary, refill Stroller by turning bayonet coupling lock on Stroller 45 degrees. Insert female adapter (Stroller) to male adapter (Liberator) (see illustration).	Allows for secure connection between Liberator and Stroller to prevent leakage of oxygen into room air.
d. Select prescribed rate (see illustration).	Ensures delivery of prescribed amount of oxygen.
e. Lock flowmeter.	Prevents client from changing oxygen flow rate.
f. Connect nasal cannula and oxygen tubing to Stroller.	Connects oxygen source to delivery method.
g. Place Stroller on cart.	Allows client to ambulate freely without expending energy to carry Stroller.
7. Have client or family perform each step with guidance from nurse.	Allows nurse to correct errors in technique and discuss their implications.
8. Discuss signs and symptoms of respiratory tract infection: fever, increased sputum, change in sputum, foul sputum odor.	Respiratory tract infections increase oxygen demand and may affect oxygen transfer from lungs to blood.
9. Instruct client or family to notify physician if signs or symptoms of hypoxia or respiratory tract infections occur.	Can prevent severe exacerbation of client's pulmonary disease.
10. Wash hands.	Reduces transmission of infection.
11. Record teaching plan, information given to client, and validation of learning.	Provides written documentation for teaching plan for client and family. Documents client learning.

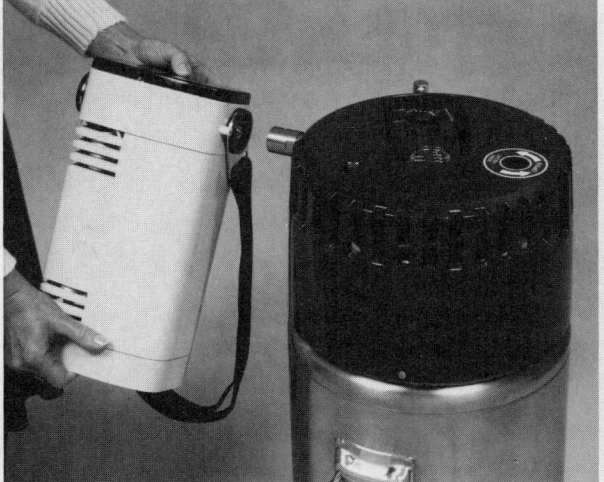

Step 6c

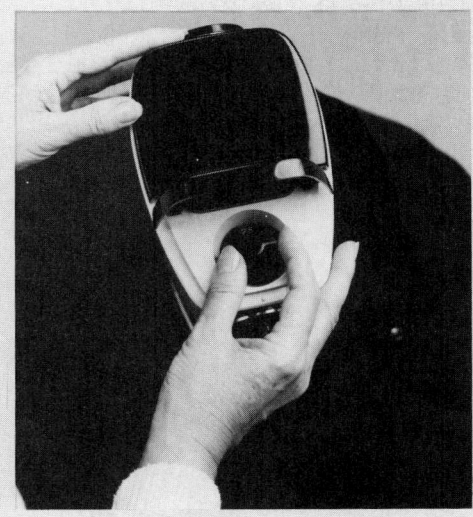

Step 6d

Cardiopulmonary Resuscitation

STEPS	RATIONALE

ONE NURSE

1. Assess for unresponsiveness, observe for spontaneous respirations, palpate carotid pulse; ask victim, "Are you OK?"

Prevents injury from attempted resuscitation of person who has not suffered a cardiac or respiratory arrest.

2. Call for help: in hospital setting, call a "code"; in community setting, call emergency phone number.

Activates mechanism for additional personnel.

3. Place victim supine on firm, flat surface or use backboard.

Facilitates external compression of heart. Heart is compressed between sternum and hard surface.

4. Kneel at victim's side.

Allows performance of rescue breathing and chest compressions without moving knees.

5. Open victim's airway:
  a. Head-tilt/chin-lift maneuver (adults and children): Place one hand on victim's forehead and apply firm, backward pressure with palm to tilt head back. Place fingers of other hand under bony part of lower jaw near chin and lift to bring chin forward and teeth almost to occlusion, thus supporting jaw and helping to tilt head back (see illustration). The fingers must not press deeply into the soft tissue under the chin. Thumb should not be used to lift chin.

This maneuver is more effective in opening airway than previously recommended head-tilt/neck-lift.
Removes tongue or epiglottis as airway obstruction.

  b. Jaw thrust maneuver (adults and children): Grasp angles of victim's lower jaw and lift with both hands, one on each side, displacing mandible forward while tilting head backward.

This technique without head-tilt is the safest first approach to opening airway of victim with suspected neck injury because it can usually be accomplished without extending neck.

6. Prepare for artificial respiration:
  a. For mouth-to-mouth resuscitation of adult, pinch victim's nose and occlude mouth. For infant, place your mouth over infant's nose and mouth.

Forms airtight seal and prevents air from escaping from nose.

  b. For Ambu bag resuscitation, use proper size face mask and apply it over victim's mouth and nose.

Forms airtight seal as bag is compressed and oxygen enters client.

7. Administer artificial respiration:
  a. For mouth-to-mouth resuscitation of adult, take a deep breath and seal lips around victim's mouth, creating air-tight seal. Give two slow breaths, followed by 10 to 12 breaths per min.

In most adults this volume of air is 800 ml and is sufficient to make chest rise. Adequate ventilation is indicated by observing chest rise and fall and hearing air escape during exhalation. Excess, rapid volume causes pharyngeal pressures to exceed esophageal opening pressures, allowing air to enter stomach.

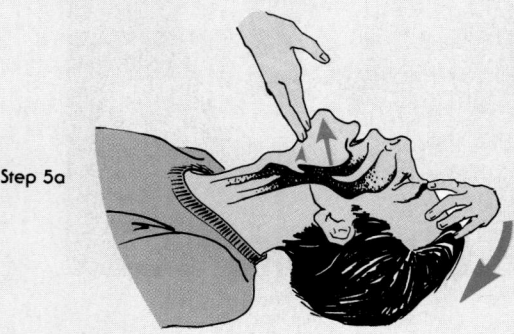

Step 5a

STEPS	RATIONALE

b. For mouth-to-mouth resuscitation of infant or child, administer two slow breaths, 1-1½ seconds per breath with pause between for rescuer to take a breath, followed by 20 breaths per min.

Since an infant's air passages are smaller with resistance to flow quite high, it is difficult to make recommendations about the force or volume of the rescue breaths. However, three factors should be remembered: (1) rescue breaths are the single most important maneuver in assisting a nonbreathing child, (2) an appropriate volume is one that makes the chest rise and fall, and (3) slow breaths provide an adequate volume at the lowest possible pressure, thereby reducing the risk of gastric distention.

c. For artificial respiration with an Ambu bag in an adult, compress the bag fully for two breaths.

d. For Ambu bag resuscitation in a child, use two small compressions of bag.

Prevents overinflation of child's lungs.

8. Observe for rise and fall of chest wall with each respiration. If lungs do not inflate, reposition head and neck and check for visible airway obstruction, such as vomitus.

Ensures artificial respirations are entering lungs.

9. Suction any secretions from airway. If suction is unavailable, turn victim's head to one side.

Prevents airway obstruction. Allows gravity to drain secretions.

10. Assess for presence of carotid pulse; pulse check should take 5-10 sec.
   a. Carotid pulse is most central and accessible artery in children over 1 yr. However, in an infant the short, shubby neck makes carotid difficult to palpate; brachial artery is recommended instead.

Carotid artery pulse will persist when more peripheral pulses are no longer palpable. Performing external cardiac compressions on a victim who has a pulse may result in serious medical complications.

11. If victim is pulseless, begin external cardiac compressions.
   Adult

   a. Proper hand position (see illustration):
      (1) Rescuer's hand locates lower margin of victim's rib cage on side next to rescuer.
      (2) Fingers are moved up rib cage to notch where ribs meet the lower sternum in center of lower part of chest.
      (3) Place heel of hand on lower half of sternum and place other hand on top of hand on sternum so that hands are parallel.

Properly performed external chest compressions can produce systolic blood pressure peaks of more than 100 mm Hg, but diastolic presure is low, with mean blood pressure in carotid arteries seldom exceeding 40 m Hg. Blood flow through carotid artery is only one fourth to one third of normal.

Results in maximum compression of heart between sternum and vetebrae. If compressions occur over xiphoid process, victim's liver can be lacerated.

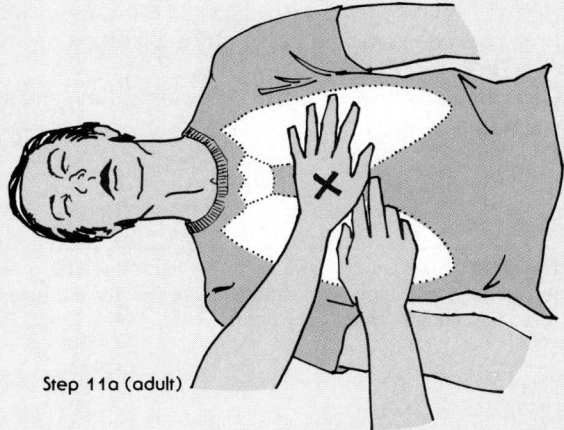

Step 11a (adult)

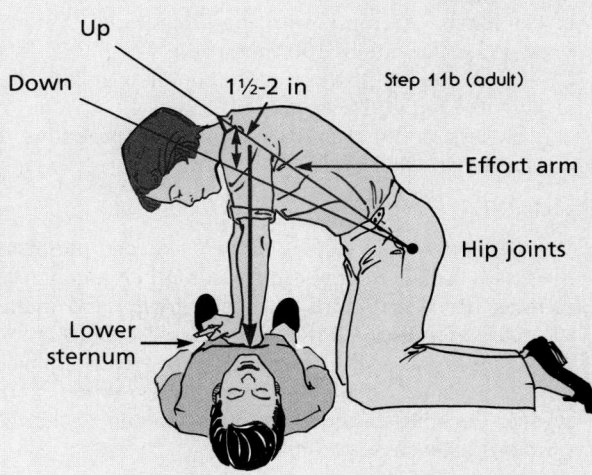

Up
Down
1½-2 in
Step 11b (adult)
Effort arm
Hip joints
Lower sternum

Cardiopulmonary Resuscitation

STEPS	RATIONALE

(4) Fingers may be extended or interlaced but should be kept off chest.

Reduces risk of rib fracture during compression.

a. Lock elbows, maintain arms straight and shoulders directly over hands on victim's sternum (see illustration):

Thrust for each compression is straight down on sternum.

(1) Compress chest 3.8-5.0 cm (1½-2 in)

(2) Compress chest 80-100 times/min. Perform 15 external compressions with mnemonic "one and, two and, three and . . ." to 15.

Increases blood flow with increased flow to brain and heart. Allows pause for ventilation in two-rescuer CPR.

b. Ventilate lungs with two slow rescue breaths as in Step 7a.

c. Reassess victim after four complete cycles (15 compressions, 2 ventilations each cycle).

Determines return of pulse and respiration and need to continue CPR.

Infant (1-12 mo)

a. Proper hand position:

Results in maximum compression.

(1) Draw imaginary line between nipples over breast bone (sternum).

(2) Place index finger of hand farthest from infant's head just under inframammary line where it intersects sternum.

Area of compression is one finger's width below this intersection at the location of middle and ring fingers.

b. Using two or three fingers, compress 1.3-2.5 cm (½-1 in) at least 100 times/min.

Promotes adequate cardiac output.

c. At end of every fifth compression, allow a pause for ventilation (1½ seconds).

Promotes adequate ventilation during CPR.

d. Reassess victim after ten cycles (5 compressions, 1 ventilation each cycle).

Determines return of pulse and respiration and need to continue CPR.

Child (1-7 yr)

a. Proper hand position:

Results in maximum compressions.

(1) Locate lower margin of victim's rib cage on side next to rescuer with middle and index fingers.

(2) Follow margin of rib cage with middle finger to notch where ribs and sternum meet.

(3) Place index finger next to middle finger.

(4) Place heel of hand next to point where index finger was located, with long axis of heel parallel to sternum.

(5) Rescuer's other hand maintains child's head position.

b. Compress sternum with one hand 2.5-3.8 cm (1-1½ in) at rate of 100 times/min.

Promotes adequate cardiac output.

c. At end of every fifth compression, allow a pause for a ventilation (1-1½ seconds).

Promotes adequate ventilation during CPR.

d. Reassess victim after 10 cycles (5 compressions, 1 ventilation each cycle).

Determines return of pulse and respiration and need to continue CPR.

TWO NURSES

12. One person is positioned at victim's side and performs external cardiac compression while other remains at victim's head, maintains an open airway, and monitors carotid pulse. Compression rate is 80-100/min. The compression-ventilation ratio is 5:1 with a pause for slow rescue breath (1-1½ seconds). When compressor becomes fatigued, rescuers should exchange positions as soon as possible.

Data from Emergency Cardiac Care Committee and Subcommittee, American Heart Association: Guideline for cardiopulmonary resuscitation and emergency cardiac care, *JAMA* 268:2171, 1992.

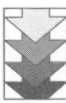 Sample Evaluation of Interventions for Ineffective Airway Clearance

Goals	Evaluative Measures	Expected Outcomes
Pulmonary secretions will be removed.	Auscultate all lung fields after coughing and postural drainage maneuvers.	Adventitious lung sounds will be absent within 48 hr.
	Observe client while coughing for amount of secretions, fatigue, dyspnea.	Client will maintain productive cough.
		Sputum will be clear, white, and frothy within 48 hr.
	Inspect sputum after cough and/or suctioning.	
Lung expansion will be improved.	Auscultate all lung fields after position change and coughing/suctioning.	Breath sounds will improve and adventitious lung sounds will be absent.
	Observe chest wall motion.	Chest wall motion will be symmetrical.
	Observe for dyspnea.	There will be no nasal flaring or use of accessory muscles.

CARDIOPULMONARY RESUSCITATION. Cardiac arrest is characterized by an absence of pulse and respiration and by dilated pupils. If the nurse determines that the client has cardiac arrest, **cardiopulmonary resuscitation (CPR)** must be initiated. CPR is a basic emergency procedure of artificial respiration and manual external cardiac massage (Procedure 38-6). CPR has three main goals—the ABCs of cardiopulmonary resuscitation: to establish an *a*irway, initiate *b*reathing, and maintain *c*irculation.

 Evaluation

Nursing interventions are evaluated by comparing the client's progress as a result of nursing therapies to the goals and desired outcomes of the nursing care plan. Each goal and category of interventions has objective evaluation criteria (see evaluation box).

When nursing measures directed to improve oxygenation are unsuccessful, the nurse must immediately modify the nursing care plan. New interventions are then developed. The nurse should not hesitate to notify the physician about a client's deteriorating oxygenation status. Prompt notification can avoid an emergency situation or even the need for cardiopulmonary resuscitation.

 SUMMARY

Clients with impaired oxygenation require planned nursing care that focuses on returning the client to a maximal level of wellness. Many nursing interventions can be used to promote lung expansion, mobilize secretions, maintain a patent airway, promote oxygenation, and restore cardiopulmonary functioning.

Nursing interventions are individualized to the client's level of health, age, lifestyle, and needs. Many nursing skills are used to help the client achieve a maximal level of oxygenation.

CHAPTER 38 REVIEW

Key Concepts

- The primary function of the heart is to deliver deoxygenated blood to the lungs for oxygenation and to deliver oxygen and nutrients to the tissues.
- Cardiac output is altered by preload, afterload, contractility, and heart rate.
- Cardiac dysrhythmias are classified by cardiac activity and site of impulse origin.
- The primary function of the lungs is to transfer oxygen from the atmosphere into the alveoli and to transfer carbon dioxide out of the body as a waste product.
- Ventilation is the process of providing adequate oxygenation from the alveoli to the blood.
- Compliance, or the ability of the lungs to expand and contract, depends on the function of musculoskeletal and neurological systems and on other physiological factors.
- The process of inspiration (active process) and expiration (passive process) is achieved with lung changes in pressures and lung volumes.
- Respiration is controlled by the central nervous system and by chemicals within the blood.
- Decreased hemoglobin levels alter the client's ability to transport oxygen.
- Impaired chest wall movement reduces the level of tissue oxygenation.
- Hyperventilation is a respiratory rate greater than that required to maintain normal levels of carbon dioxide.
- Hypoventilation causes carbon dioxide retention.
- Hypoxia occurs if the amount of oxygen delivered to tissues is too low.
- The nursing assessment includes information about the client's cough, dyspnea, fatigue, wheezing, chest pain, environmental exposures, respiratory infection, cardiopulmonary risk factors, use of medications, and physical functioning.
- Diagnostic and laboratory tests may be needed to complete the data base for a client with decreased oxygenation.
- Breathing exercises improve ventilation, oxygenation, and sensations of dyspnea.
- Nebulization delivers small drops of water or particles of medication to the airways.
- Chest physiotherapy includes postural drainage, percussion, and vibration to mobilize pulmonary secretions.
- Coughing and suctioning techniques are used to maintain a patent airway.
- Oxygen therapy is used to improve levels of tissue oxygenation and is delivered by nasal cannula, nasal catheter, or oxygen mask.
- Cardiac arrest requires the use of cardiopulmonary resuscitation.

Key Terms

Critical Thinking Exercises

1. Mr. Havens is 65 years old and has a history of congestive heart failure. In addition, he mentions poor activity tolerance. What data are important in determining the cardiac response to exercise? What criteria are used to determine when the exercise demand has exceeded cardiac workload capacity?

2. Your client experiences chest pain. State how you assess this pain. What are three important interventions for a client with chest pain?

3. You are caring for a client who had abdominal surgery 24 hours ago. This client has a 10-year history of chronic obstructive pulmonary disease. What are the important aspects of assessment and intervention necessary to maintain a patent airway?

4. You are at a shopping center when the gentleman ahead of you collapses in the mall. What do you do to maintain adequate cardiopulmonary function?

REFERENCES

Agle DP et al: Multidiscipline treatment of chronic pulmonary insufficiency, *Psychosom Med* 35:41, 1973.

Ahrens, TS: Concepts in the assessment of oxygenation, *Focus Crit Care* 14(1):36-44, 1987.

Ahrens TS: Svo₂ monitoring: is it being used appropriately? *Crit Care Nurse* 10(7):70, 1990.

Bennett JA: What we know about AIDS, *Am J Nurs* 86:1016, 1986.

Canobbio MM: *Cardiovascular disorders*, St Louis, 1990, Mosby Year Book.

Carroll PF: The ins and outs of chest drainage systems, *Nurs 86* 16(12):26, 1986.

Churg A et al: Small airways disease and mineral dust response, *Am Rev Resp Dis* 131:139, 1985.

Daily EK, Schroeder JS: *Techniques in bedside hemodynamic monitoring*, ed 4, St Louis, 1989, Mosby–Year Book.

Dettenmeier PA: *Pulmonary nursing care*. St Louis, 1992, Mosby–Year Book.

DeVito AJ: Dyspnea during hospitalizations for acute phase of illness as recalled by patients with chronic obstructive pulmonary disease, *Heart-Lung* 19(2):186, 1990.

Dopico GA et al: Epidemiologic study of clinical and physiologic parameters in grain handlers of Northern United States, *Am Rev Resp Dis* 130:759, 1984.

Duncan CR, Erickson RS: Pressures associated with chest tube stripping, *Heart Lung* 11(2):166, 1982.

Duncan CR, Erickson RS, Weigel RM: Effect of chest tube management on drainage after cardiac surgery, *Heart Lung* 16(1):1, 1987.

Eid N et al: Chest physiotherapy in review, *Resp Care* 36(4):270, 1991.

Emergency Cardiac Care Committee and Subcommittee, American Heart Association: Guidelines for cardiopulmonary resuscitation and emergency cardiac care, *JAMA* 268:2171, 1992.

Erickson R: Chest tubes: they're really not that complicated, *Nurs 81* 11(5):34, 1981a.

Erickson R: Solving chest tube problems, *Nurs 81* 11(6):62, 1981b.

Farley J: About chest tubes. *Nurs 88* 18(6):16, 1988.

Feldman J: Chronic obstructive pulmonary disease. In Traver GA, editor: *Respiratory nursing: the science and the art*, New York, 1982, Wiley.

Gift AG: Validation of a vertical visual analog scale as a measure of clinical dyspnea, *Rehab Nurs* 14:323, 1989.

Gift AG: Dyspnea, *Nurs Clin North Am,* 25(4):955, 1990.

Gift AG, Bolgiano CS, Cunningham J: Sensations during chest tube removal, *Heart Lung* 20(2):131, 1991.

Gift AG, Plaut SM, Jacox AK: Psychologic and physiologic factors related to dyspnea in subjects with chronic obstructive pulmonary disease, *Heart Lung* 15:595, 1986.

Gjerde GE, Kraemer R: An oxygen therapy fire, *Resp Care* 25:363, 1980.

Groër MW, Shekleton MS: *Basic pathophysiology: a holistic approach,* St Louis, 1989, Mosby–Year Book.

Herrick TW, Yeager H: Home oxygen therapy, *Ann Fam Pract* 32(2):157, 1989.

Jansen-Bjerklie S, Carrieri VK, Hudes M: The sensation of pulmonary dyspnea, *Nurs Res* 35(3):154, 1986.

Johanson BC et al: *Standards for critical care,* ed 3, St Louis, 1988, Mosby–Year Book.

Kim MJ: Respiratory muscle training, *Heart Lung* 13:333, 1984.

Kim MJ, McFarland GK, McLane AM: *Pocket guide to nursing diagnoses,* ed 4, St Louis, 1991, Mosby–Year Book.

Krauss 1985.

Larson M, Kim MJ: Respiratory muscle training with incentive spirometer resistive breathing device, *Heart Lung* 13:341, 1984.

Larson JL et al: Inspiratory muscle training with a pressure threshold breathing device in patients with chronic obstructive pulmonary disease, *Am Rev Resp Dis* 138(3):689, 1988.

Luce JM, Tyler ML, Pierson DJ: *Intensive respiratory care,* Philadelphia, 1984, Saunders.

McCance KL, Huether SE: *Pathophysiology: the biologic basis for disease in adults and children,* St Louis, 1990, Mosby–Year Book.

McCauley CS, Boller LR: The hazards of home oxygen therapy, *N Engl J Med* 316(2):107, 1987.

McDonald BR: Validation of three respiratory nursing diagnoses, *Nurs Clin North Am* 20(4):697, 1985.

Pierce JD, Piazza D, Naftel DC: Effects of two chest tube clearance protocols on drainage in patients after myocardial revascularization surgery, *Heart Lung* 20(2):125, 1991.

Reinke LF, Hoffman LA, Wesmiller SW: Transtracheal oxygen therapy: an alternative delivery approach, *Pers Respir Nurs* 3(3):3, 1992.

Shekleton ME, Nield M: Ineffective airway clearance related to artificial airway, *Nurs Clin North Am* 22(1):167, 1987.

Shenkman B: Factors contributing to attrition rates in a pulmonary rehabilitation program, *Heart Lung* 14(1):53, 1985.

Smith SJ: Clinical assessment of the pulmonary patient. In Traver GA, editor: *Respiratory nursing: the science and the art,* New York, 1982, Wiley.

Sonnesso G: Are you ready to use pulse oximetry? *Nurs 91* 21(8):60, 1991.

Spofford B, Christopher K: The clinician's guide for SCOOP transtracheal oxygen system, Englewood, Colo, 1989, Transtracheal Systems.

Traver GA: *Respiratory nursing: the science and the art,* New York, 1982, Wiley.

Walsh M: Peak expiratory flow-rate minitoring, *Perspect Respir Nurs* 3(1):1, 1992.

Weilitz P: *Pocket guide to respiratory care,* St Louis, 1991, Mosby–Year Book.

West JB: *Respiratory physiology, the essentials,* ed 2, Baltimore, 1979, Williams & Wilkins.

Whitney JD: The measurement of oxygen tension in tissues, *Nurs Res* 39(4):203, 1990.

York K: Clinical validation of two respiratory nursing diagnoses and their defining characteristics, *Nurs Clin North Am* 20(4):657, 1985.

York K, Martin PA: Clinical validation of respiratory nursing diagnoses: a model. In Hurley MH, editor: *Classification of nursing diagnoses: proceedings of the sixth conference (NANDA),* St Louis, 1986, Mosby–Year Book.

ADDITIONAL READINGS

Beck GJ, Schachter EN, Marinder LR: The relationship of respiratory symptoms and lung function loss in cotton textile workers, *Am Rev Resp Dis* 130:6, 1984.

Clinical News: Transtracheal oxygen: the nose knows the difference, *Am J Nurs* 87:421, 1987.

Dennison R: Cardiopulmonary assessment: how to do it better in 15 easy steps, *Nurs 86* 16(4):34, 1986.

Kerr JAC: Adherence and self-care, *Heart Lung* 14(1):24, 1985.

Perry AG, Potter PA: *Shock: comprehensive nursing management,* St Louis, 1983, Mosby–Year Book.

Perry AG, Potter PA: *Clinical nursing skills and techniques: basic, intermediate, and advanced,* St Louis, 1986, Mosby–Year Book.

Standards and guidelines for cardiopulmonary resuscitation (CPR) and emergency cardiac care, *JAMA* 255(21):2903, 1986.

Wade JF: *Respiratory nursing care,* ed 3, St Louis, 1982, Mosby–Year Book.

Weaver TE: New life for lungs . . . through incentive spirometers, *Nurs 81* 11(2):53, 1981.

Wilson SF, Thompson JM: *Respiratory disorders,* St Louis, 1990, Mosby–Year Book.

CHAPTER 39

Fluid, Electrolyte, and Acid-Base Balances

OBJECTIVES

Mastery of content in this chapter will enable the student to:

- Define the key terms listed.
- Describe the regulation of sodium, potassium, calcium, magnesium, chloride, bicarbonate, phosphate, and acid base.
- Describe the isotonic fluid imbalances of fluid volume excess and fluid volume deficit.
- Discuss the alterations in serum osmolality caused by water excess and deficit.
- Describe third-space syndrome.
- Discuss the variables affecting fluid, electrolyte, and acid-base balances.
- Compile a nursing history and complete a physical examination for fluid, electrolyte, and acid-base balances.
- Describe laboratory studies associated with fluid, electrolyte, and acid-base imbalances.
- Develop a nursing care plan for clients with fluid, electrolyte, and acid-base disturbances.
- Discuss the purpose of intravenous therapy.
- Describe the procedure for initiating and maintaining an intravenous line and calculating intravenous flow rate.
- Demonstrate how to change intravenous solutions, tubing, and dressings and to discontinue an infusion.
- Discuss the complications of intravenous therapy.
- Discuss the procedure for administering a blood transfusion and nursing actions for a transfusion reaction.

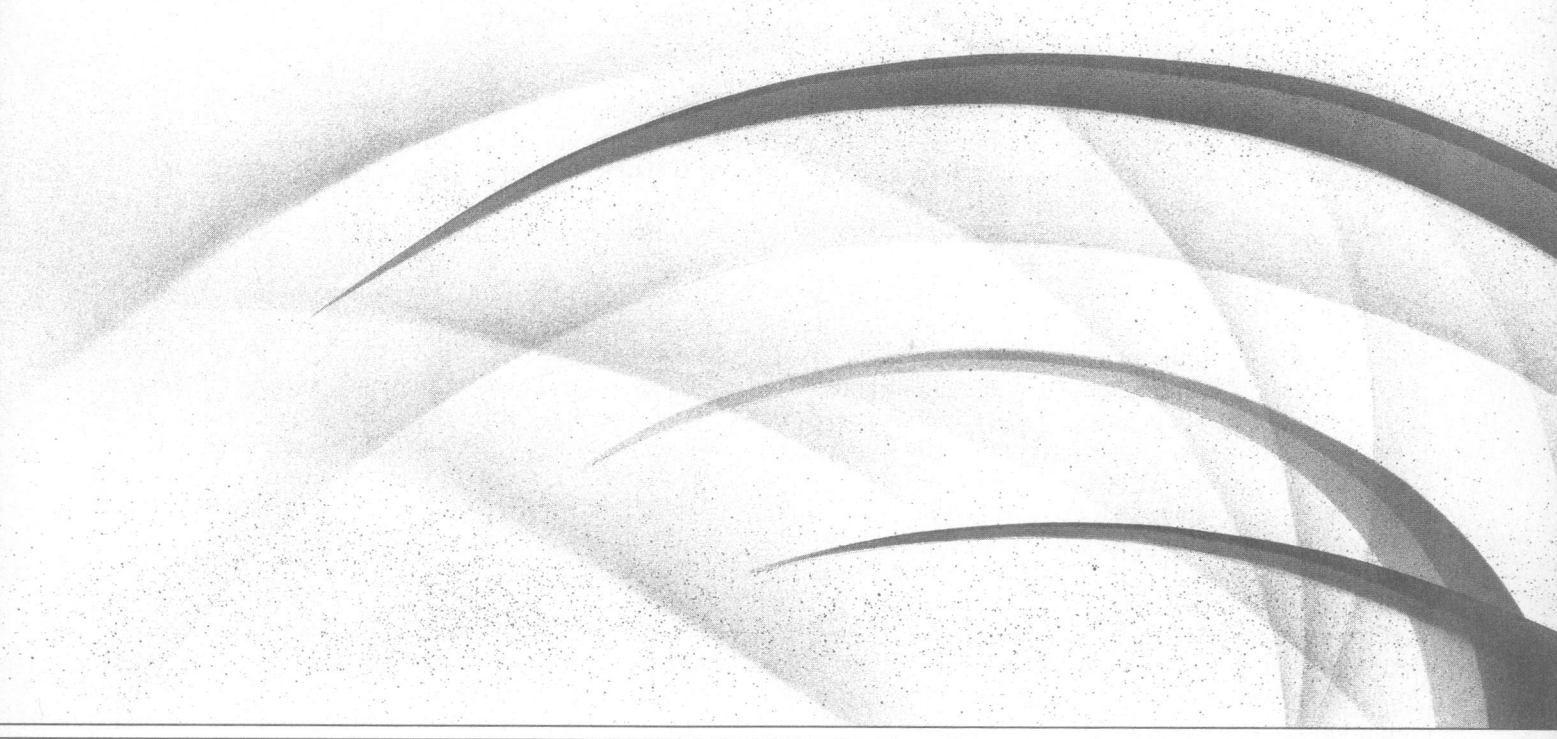

CHAPTER OUTLINE

Fluid and Electrolyte Balances
Distribution of body fluids
Composition of body fluids
Movement of body fluids
Regulation of body fluids
Regulation of electrolytes

Acid-Base Balance
Chemical regulation
Biological regulation
Physiological regulation

Disturbances in Fluid, Electrolyte, and Acid-Base Balances
Fluid disturbances
Electrolyte imbalances
Acid-base imbalances

Variables Affecting Fluid, Electrolyte, and Acid-Base Balances
Age
Body size
Environmental temperature
Lifestyle
Level of health

Nursing Process and Fluid, Electrolyte, and Acid-Base Imbalances
Assessment
Nursing diagnosis
Planning
Implementation
Evaluation

luid, electrolyte, and acid-base balances within the body are necessary to maintain health and function of all systems. These balances are maintained by the intake and output of water and electrolytes, their distribution in the body, and the regulation of renal and pulmonary function. Imbalances may result from many factors and are associated with illnesses. Therefore nursing care for many different kinds of clients includes assessment and correction of imbalances or maintenance of balance. Acid-base balance is necessary for physiological processes, and imbalances can alter respiration, metabolism, and central nervous system function.

A healthy, mobile, well-oriented adult can usually maintain normal fluid, electrolyte, and acid-base balances because of the body's adaptive mechanisms. However, the infant, the severely ill adult, the disoriented or immobile client, and the older adult are frequently unable to respond independently, and after time the body's adaptive capacities can no longer maintain balance.

 ## FLUID AND ELECTROLYTE BALANCES

Distribution of Body Fluids

Body fluids are distributed in two distinct compartments, one containing extracellular fluids and the other containing intracellular fluids.

Extracellular fluids include interstitial fluid and intravascular fluid. Interstitial fluid fills the spaces between most cells of the body and provides a substantial portion of the body's liquid environment. About 15% of body weight consists of interstitial fluids. Extracellular fluid is plasma, the watery, colorless, fluid portion of the lymph and blood in which the leukocytes, erythrocytes, and platelets are suspended. Plasma composes 5% of body weight.

Intracellular fluids are liquids within cell membranes containing dissolved substances or solutes essential to fluid and electrolyte balance and metabolism. Intracellular fluids constitute 40% of body weight. Many of the solutes in the intracellular fluid compartment are the same as those located in the extracellular fluid space. However, the proportion of the substances is different. For example, a larger proportion of potassium exists in intracellular fluids than in extracellular fluids.

Composition of Body Fluids

The fluids circulating throughout the body in extracellular and intracellular fluid spaces contain electrolytes, minerals, and cells.

An **electrolyte** is an element or compound that, when melted or dissolved in water or another solvent, dissociates into ions and is able to carry an electric current. Positively charged electrolytes are **cations.** Negatively charged electrolytes are **anions.** The concentration of each electrolyte differs in extracellular and intracellular fluids. However, the total number of anions and cations in each fluid compartment should be the same.

Electrolytes are commonly measured in milliequivalents per liter (mEq/L), which is a measure of chemical activity representing the amount of electrolyte that will react with a given amount of hydrogen (Chenevey, 1987). Electrolytes are vital to many body functions (for example, neuromuscular function and acid-base balance).

Minerals, which are ingested as compounds, are usually referred to by the name of a metal, nonmetal, radical, or phosphate rather than by the name of the compound of which they are a part. They are constituents of all body tissues and fluids and are important in maintaining physiological processes. Minerals also act as catalysts in nerve response, muscle contraction, and metabolism of nutrients in foods. In addition, they regulate electrolyte balance and hormone production and strengthen skeletal structures. Examples of minerals include iron and zinc.

Cells, which are also located in body fluids, are the functional basic units of all living tissue. Examples of cells within body fluids are the red blood cell (RBC) and the white blood cell (WBC).

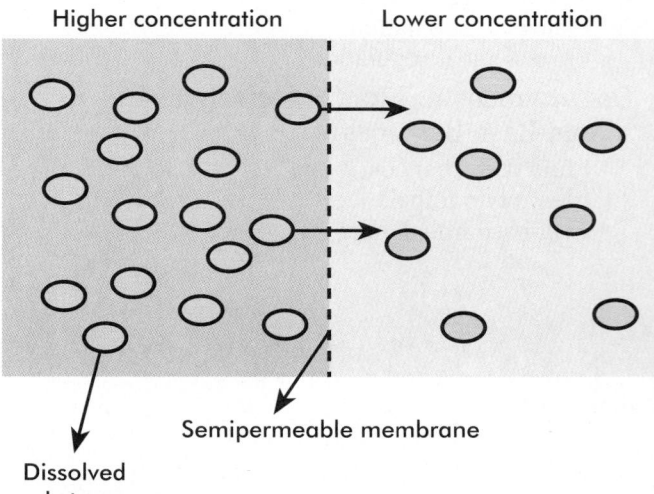

Fig. 39-1 Diffusion is the movement of molecules across a semipermeable membrane from an area of higher concentration to an area of lower concentration (along its concentration gradient).

Movement of Body Fluids

Body fluids are not static. Fluids and electrolytes shift from compartment to compartment to meet metabolic needs such as tissue oxygenation, response to illness, acid-base disturbances, and response to drug therapies. Body fluid and electrolyte movement occur by diffusion, osmosis, active transport, or filtration. In addition, movement of fluid components depends on cell membrane permeability (the ability of the membrane to allow fluids and electrolytes to pass through it).

Diffusion

Diffusion is a process in which solid, particulate matter such as sugar in a fluid moves from an area of higher concentration to an area of lower concentration, resulting in an even distribution of the particles in the fluid or across a cell membrane permeable to that substance (Fig. 39-1). Substances that are diffusing therefore move down their concentration gradients (Gröer, Shekleton, 1989).

Osmosis

Osmosis is the movement of a pure solvent, such as water, through a semipermeable membrane from a solution that has a lower solute concentration to one that has a higher solute concentration (Fig. 39-2). The membrane is permeable to the solvent, but it is impermeable to the solute, the particulate matter. The rate of osmosis depends on the concentrations of the solutes in the solutions, the temperature of the solutions, the electrical charges of the solutes, and the differences between the osmotic pressures exerted by the solutions. The concentration of a solution is measured in osmols, which reflect the amount of a substance in solution in the form of molecules, ions, or both.

Osmotic pressure is the drawing power for water and depends on the number of molecules in the solution. A solution with a high solute concentration has a high osmotic pressure and draws water into itself. Osmotic pressure is exerted through a semipermeable membrane and depends on the activity of the solute separated by the membrane. If the concentration of the solute is greater on one side of the semipermeable membrane, the rate of osmosis is quicker, and a more rapid transfer of solvent across the membrane occurs. This continues until an equilibrium is reached. The osmotic pressure of a solution is also called its *osmolality,* which is expressed in osmols, or milliosmols per kilogram (mOsm/kg), of the solution. The normal serum osmolality is 280 to 295 mOsm/kg.

A solution with the same osmolality as blood plasma is called *isotonic.* The intravenous (IV) administration of an isotonic solution prevents shifting of fluid and electrolytes from intracellular compartments. A **hypotonic** solution that has a lesser concentration of solutes than is normal in body fluids may be administered to a client to help promote movement of water into the cells. For example, half-normal saline (½ NS or 0.45% NaCl) may be ordered for clients recovering from ketoacidosis in which water moves into cells. Conversely, a **hypertonic** solution has a greater concentration of solutes than is normal in body fluids. IV administration of a hypertonic solution results in movement of water out of cells.

The osmotic pressure of the blood is affected by plasma proteins, especially albumin, a serum protein naturally produced by the body. Albumin exerts colloid osmotic or **oncotic pressure,** which tends to keep fluid in the capillaries. At the venous end of capillaries, this oncotic pressure and decreased venous hydrostatic pressure facilitates the movement of water and waste produces back into the capillaries.

Filtration

Filtration is the process by which water and diffusible substances move together in response to fluid pressure. This process is active in capillary beds, where pressure differences determine the movement of water, electrolytes, and other dissolved substances between the capillaries and interstitial fluid.

Hydrostatic pressure is the pressure exerted by a liquid in a column. Blood and fluid entering the capillaries do so at a pressure greater than interstitial pressure, so fluid and solutes move out of the capillaries. At the venous end of the capillary bed, hydro-

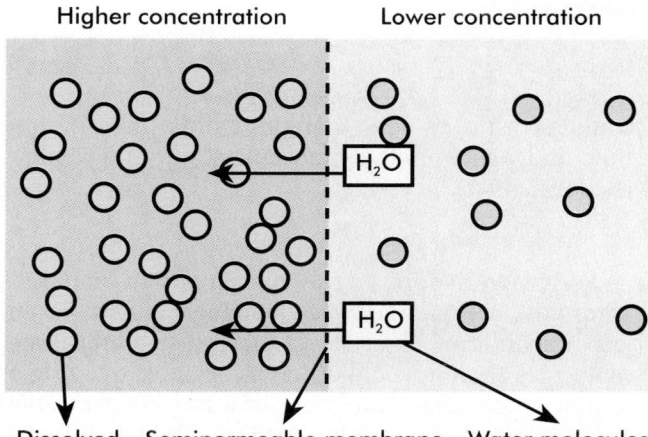

Higher concentration   Lower concentration

Dissolved   Semipermeable membrane   Water molecules
substances

Fig. 39-2 In osmosis, water molecules move from the less concentrated area to the more concentrated area in an effort to equalize the concentration of solutions on two sides of a membrane.

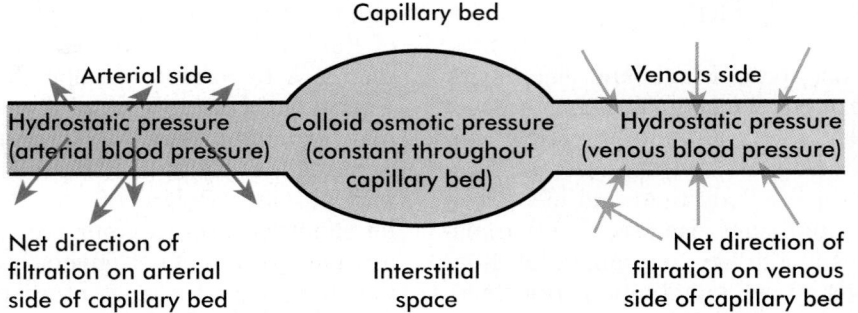

Fig. 39-3   An example of filtration pressure changes within a capillary bed. **A,** Arterial blood pressure exceeds colloid osmotic pressure, resulting in the movement of water and dissolved substances out of the capillary into the interstitial space. **B,** Venous blood pressure is less than colloid osmotic pressure, resulting in the movement of water and dissolved substances into the capillary.

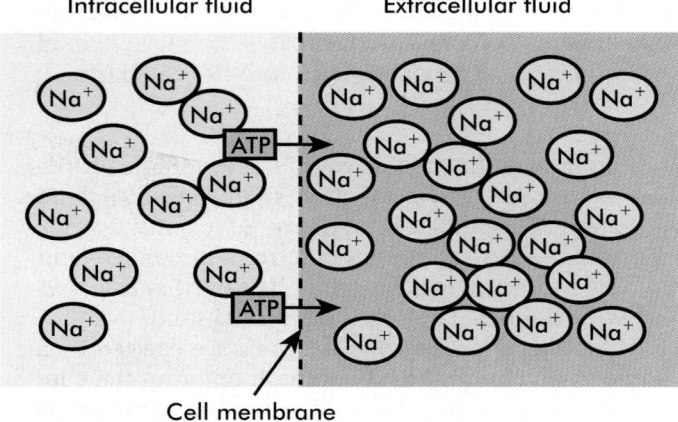

Fig. 39-4   An example of active transport. Energy (ATP) is used to move sodium molecules across a semipermeable membrane against sodium's concentration gradient (that is, from an area of lesser concentration to an area of greater concentration).

static pressure is less than interstitial pressure, so fluid and waste products move back into the capillaries. (Fig. 39-3).

Active Transport

Active transport is the movement of materials across the cell membrane by chemical activity or energy expenditure that allows the cell to admit larger molecules than it would otherwise be able to admit or to move molecules from areas of lesser concentration to areas of greater concentration. Unlike diffusion and osmosis, active transport requires metabolic activity and energy expenditure. Examples of active transport in the body are found in sodium and potassium pumps (Fig. 39-4). Sodium is pumped out of

the cell. Potassium is pumped in, against a concentration gradient.

Active transport is enhanced by carrier molecules within a cell that bind themselves to incoming molecules. For example, insulin binds itself to glucose and serves as a transport vehicle to permit entry of glucose into the cell. Active transport is the mechanism by which the cell absorbs glucose and other substances to carry out metabolic activities.

Regulation of Body Fluids

Fluid Intake

Fluid intake is regulated primarily through the thirst mechanism. The thirst-control center is located within the hypothalamus in the brain. Psychological factors, dry pharyngeal mucous membranes, and angiotensin I create a sensation of thirst (Gröer, Shekleton, 1989) (Fig. 39-5). Major physiological stimuli to the thirst center are increased plasma concentration and decreased blood volume. Receptor cells called *osmoreceptors* continually monitor osmolality. When too much fluid is lost, the osmoreceptors detect the loss and activate the thirst center. As a result the person feels thirsty and seeks water.

Water is also acquired from food intake, such as fruits, vegetables, and meat, and from the oxidation of food substances during digestion. As discussed in Chapter 35, water is one of the end products of the metabolism of carbohydrates, proteins, and fats. This quantity ranges between 150 and 250 ml/day, depending on a person's rate of metabolism (Guyton, 1986). Oral fluid intake requires an alert state. Infants, clients with neurological or psychological impairments, some older adults, and clients who are restrained are unable to perceive or respond to their

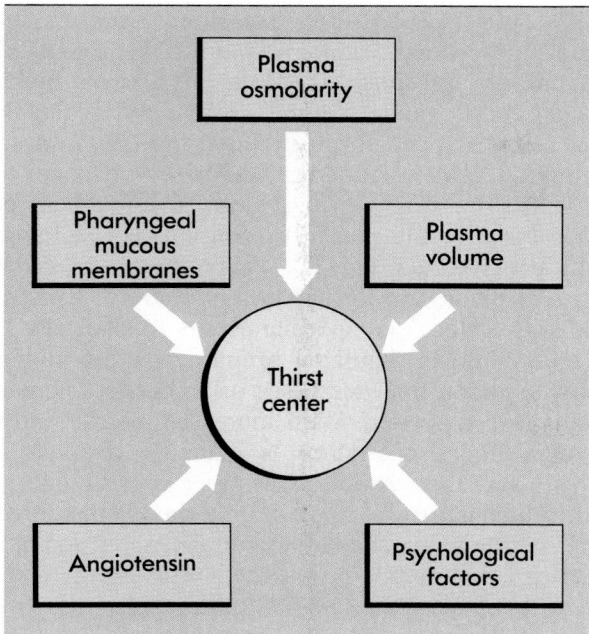

Fig. 39-5   Stimuli affecting the thirst mechanism.

TABLE 39-1 Average Daily Fluid Output in a 70-kg (187-lb) Adult	
Organ or System	Amount (ml)
Kidneys	1500
Skin	
Insensible loss	600-900
Sensible loss	0-5000
Lungs	400
Gastrointestinal tract	100
TOTAL*	2600-2900

*Excludes sensible loss.

thirst mechanisms. As a result, they are at risk for dehydration.

Fluid Output

Fluid output occurs through the kidneys and the gastrointestinal tract. Average daily fluid losses are summarized in Table 39-1.

The kidneys are the major regulatory organs of fluid balance. They receive about 170 L of plasma to filter each day and in the adult produce 1.5 L of urine to be excreted. Approximately 1 ml of urine per kilogram of body weight per hour (1 ml/kg/hr) is produced by all age groups (Metheny, 1992). The amount of urine produced by the kidneys is influenced by antidiuretic hormone (ADH) and aldosterone. These hormones affect water and sodium excretion and are stimulated by changes in blood volume.

Water loss from the skin is regulated primarily by the sympathetic nervous system, which activates the sweat glands. Stimulation of the sweat glands can result from muscular exercise, elevated environmental temperature, and increased metabolic activity (for example, fever).

Water loss from the skin can be a sensible or insensible loss. **Insensible water loss** is continuous and is not perceived by the person. The average insensible water loss is 600 ml/day (Metheny, 1992). **Sensible water loss** occurs through excessive perspiration and is perceived by the person. The amount of sensible perspiration is directly related to the amount

of exercise, environmental temperature, and metabolic activity. As these factors increase, so does the amount of sweat produced and water lost through the skin. Sensible water loss can range up to 1000 ml or more, depending on exercise and external and body temperatures (Metheny, 1992).

The lungs also produce an insensible water loss by expiring approximately 400 ml of water daily. This loss may increase in response to changes in respiratory rate and depth (for example, increased exercise or fever). In addition, devices for oxygen administration can increase insensible water loss from the lungs.

The average fluid loss from the gastrointestinal tract is approximately 100 ml/day. Vomiting or diarrhea increases fluid loss by preventing the normal absorption of water and electrolytes, which have been secreted for the digestive process.

Hormones

The major hormones affecting fluid and electrolyte balance are ADH and aldosterone. The stimulus for ADH secretion is an increase in blood osmolarity (concentration of solute per liter of solution), which indicates a state of water deficit. The hormone itself is released by the posterior pituitary gland. ADH decreases the production of urine by increasing the reabsorption of water by the kidney tubules. During transient periods of fluid volume deficit such as with vomiting and diarrhea or hemorrhage, the amount of ADH in the blood increases. As a result the water reabsorbed by the kidney tubules increases and is returned to the circulating blood volume. Urinary output declines in response to the hormone's action.

Aldosterone is a mineralocorticoid produced by the adrenal cortex that regulates sodium and potassium balance. The presence of aldosterone causes the kidney tubules to excrete potassium and reabsorb sodium, and as a result, water is also reabsorbed and returned to the blood volume. Fluid volume deficits such as those produced by hemorrhage or gastrointestinal losses can stimulate the secretion of aldosterone into the blood.

A third class of hormones, glucocorticoids, also affects water and electrolyte balance. Whereas normal glucocorticoid hormone secretion does not result in major fluid imbalances, excesses of the hormone in the circulation alter fluid and electrolyte balance. For example, a client with Cushing's syndrome retains sodium and water because of the action of excess glucocorticoids. Likewise, a client receiving steroid medications, such as cortisone or prednisone, retains sodium and water.

Regulation of Electrolytes

Cations

The major cations—sodium (Na^+), potassium (K^+), calcium (Ca^{++}), and magnesium (Mg^{++})—are located in the extracellular and intracellular fluid. Their actions affect neurochemical and neuromuscular transmissions, which influence muscular function, cardiac rhythm and contractility, mood and behavior, and gastrointestinal functioning, as well as other processes. Cations may be interchanged when one cation exits the cell and is replaced by another because cells tend to maintain electrical neutrality. Therefore one positively charged ion must be exchanged with another positively charged ion.

SODIUM REGULATION. Sodium is the most abundant cation in the extracellular fluid. Sodium ions are involved in maintaining water balance, transmitting nerve impulses, and contracting muscles. The normal extracellular concentration of sodium is 135 to 145 mEq/L.

Water goes where sodium goes in fluid and electrolyte balances. For example, if the kidneys retain sodium, they retain water also. Conversely, if the kidneys excrete sodium, they excrete water. The action of many drugs (for example, diuretics) is based on this principle.

Sodium is regulated by salt intake, aldosterone, and urinary output. The major sources of sodium are table salt, processed meats, snack foods, and canned vegetables. In individuals with normal renal function the excretion of urine sodium can be increased to keep the serum sodium level within normal limits. When sodium intake decreases or a person loses body fluids (for example, through burns or trauma), the body attempts to conserve sodium through the secretion of aldosterone. Aldosterone exerts its action on the kidney tubules to reabsorb sodium, thus returning sodium to the extracellular fluid.

POTASSIUM REGULATION. Potassium is the predominant intracellular cation regulating neuromuscular excitability and muscle contraction. Sources include whole grains, meat, legumes, fruits, and vegetables. Potassium is needed for glycogen formation, protein synthesis, and correction of acid-base imbalances.

Potassium assists in regulating the acid-base balance because the potassium ion can be exchanged with the hydrogen ion (H^+). Therefore in an acidotic state, a potassium ion is conserved and a hydrogen ion is excreted. The opposite occurs in alkalosis.

Potassium is regulated primarily by the kidneys. Any condition that decreases urine output decreases potassium excretion. With increased aldosterone secretion, more potassium is excreted through the urine, and the serum potassium level can fall. Another mechanism of regulation is the exchange with the sodium ion in the kidney tubule. When sodium is retained, potassium is excreted. The normal range for serum potassium is 3.5 to 5.3 mEq/L.

CALCIUM REGULATION. Calcium is the most abundant element in the body (Metheny, 1992). The body requires calcium for cell membrane integrity and structure, adequate cardiac conduction, blood coagulation, bone growth and formation, and muscle relaxation. Calcium is in the following forms in body fluids:

1. Ionized (4.5 mg/100 ml)
2. Nondiffusible, which is calcium complexed to protein anions (5 mg/100 ml)
3. Calcium salts such as calcium citrate and calcium phosphate (1 mg/100 ml)

The normal ionized serum calcium value is 4 to 5 mEq/L. Calcium in body fluid is a small percentage of the total body calcium. The major portion of calcium is in bones and teeth.

Calcium in extracellular fluid is regulated through the actions of the parathyroid and thyroid glands. Parathyroid hormone (PTH) controls the balance among bone calcium, gastrointestinal absorption of calcium, and kidney excretion of calcium. Thyrocalcitonin from the thyroid gland also has a minor role in determining serum calcium levels by inhibiting release of calcium from bones.

MAGNESIUM REGULATION. Magnesium is the second most important cation of the intracellular fluids and is essential for enzyme activities, neurochemical activities, and muscular excitability. Plasma concentrations of magnesium range from 1.5 to 2.5 mEq/L.

Magnesium is primarily excreted through renal mechanisms. Altered magnesium levels, hypomagnesemia and hypermagnesemia, are often associated with serious disease and produce symptoms reflecting altered neuromuscular and cardiovascular function (Metheny, 1992).

Anions

The major anions are chloride (Cl^-), bicarbonate (HCO_3^-), and phosphate ($PO_4^=$). Like cations, they are found in the extracellular and intracellular spaces. Anions affect fluid, electrolyte, and acid-base balances and functions.

CHLORIDE REGULATION. Chloride is found in extracellular and intracellular fluid. Chloride balance is maintained through dietary intake and renal excretion and reabsorption. The chloride ion balances cations within the extracellular fluid. If a negatively charged ion leaves the extracellular fluid and enters the intracellular fluid, a chloride ion will be exchanged and enter the extracellular fluid. The ion exchange maintains electrical neutrality. The processes regulating sodium, chloride, and bicarbonate ions are related, and any factor that affects one can affect the others. Therefore changes in serum chloride levels can affect fluid, electrolyte, and acid-base balances. One example of this is decreased serum chloride levels resulting in renal retention of bicarbonate (to maintain electrical neutrality), which results in metabolic alkalosis (Kokko, Tannen, 1990).

Chloride is regulated through the kidneys. The amount excreted is related to dietary intake. A person with normal kidneys who has a high chloride intake will excrete a higher amount of chloride in the urine. Normal serum chloride levels range from 100 to 106 mEq/L.

BICARBONATE REGULATION. Bicarbonate is the major chemical base buffer within the body. The bicarbonate ion is found in extracellular and intracellular fluid. The kidneys regulate bicarbonates. When the body needs to retain more base, the kidneys reabsorb greater quantities of bicarbonate and return it to the extracellular fluid. Normal arterial bicarbonate levels range between 22 and 26 mEq/L. In venous blood, bicarbonate is measured as carbon dioxide content, and the normal value for adults is 24 to 30 mEq/L. The bicarbonate ion is an essential component of the carbonic acid–bicarbonate buffering system essential to acid-base balance.

PHOSPHATE REGULATION. Phosphate is a buffer anion in intracellular and extracellular fluid. Phosphate and calcium help develop and maintain bones and teeth. Phosphate also promotes normal neuromuscular action, participates in carbohydrate metabolism, and assists in acid-base regulation.

Serum phosphate concentration is regulated by the kidneys, parathyroid hormone, and activated vitamin D (Gröer, Shekleton, 1989). Phosphate is normally absorbed through the gastrointestinal tract in a range of 3 to 12 mg/100 ml. Calcium and phosphate are inversely proportional. If one rises, the other falls. The normal serum phosphate level is 2.5 to 4.5 mg/100 ml.

ACID-BASE BALANCE

Acid-base balance exists when the net rate at which the body produces acids or bases equals the rate at which acids or bases are excreted. This balance results in a stable concentration of hydrogen ions in body fluids. The concentration of hydrogen ions in a body fluid is expressed as the pH value. The **pH** is a scale for measuring the acidity or alkalinity of a fluid. A pH value of 7 is neutral. Below 7 is acid, and above 7 is alkaline. An increase in the number of hydrogen ions in the bloodstream increases the acid component, thereby lowering the pH. Normal arterial pH values range from 7.35 to 7.45.

The human body has regulatory mechanisms for maintaining the acid-base balance and for adapting to short-term changes in hydrogen ion concentration. Such changes occur during physical exercise, moderate anxiety states, and minor gastrointestinal upsets. The body can make adjustments (compensate) for transient changes in pH. However, with severe trauma, uncontrolled diabetes mellitus, or shock, the body's normal compensatory mechanisms are unable to maintain the pH within a physiological range. In such cases, medical intervention is required.

The types of acid-base regulators within the body are chemical, biological, and physiological buffering systems. A **buffer** is a substance or group of substances that can absorb or release hydrogen ions to correct an acid-base imbalance.

Chemical Regulation

The largest chemical buffer in extracellular fluid is the carbonic acid–bicarbonate buffer system. The carbonic acid–bicarbonate buffer system responds immediately to acid-base imbalance, is an adaptive system, and has a relatively brief effect. This system can be expressed as the following equation:

$$CO_2 + H_2O \rightleftarrows H_2CO_3 \rightleftarrows H^+ + HCO_3^-$$

carbon dioxide water carbonic acid hydrogen bicarbonate

The carbonic acid–bicarbonate buffer system is the first buffering system to react to change in the pH of extracellular fluid, and it reacts within seconds. The excretion of carbon dioxide resulting from metabolism is controlled primarily by the lungs. The excretion of hydrogen and bicarbonate ions is controlled by the kidneys. The reaction of these substances buffers a strong acid or base to maintain a relatively constant pH (Fig. 39-6).

A second chemical buffering system involves the plasma proteins (albumin, fibrinogen, and prothrombin) and the gamma globulins, which constitute about 6% to 7% of blood plasma. These proteins can bind with or release hydrogen ions to correct acidosis or alkalosis. However, their capacity to maintain the acid-base balance of extracellular fluid is limited, and they cannot correct long-term imbalances.

Biological Regulation

Biological buffering occurs when hydrogen ions are absorbed or released by body cells. The hydrogen ion has a positive charge and must be exchanged with another positively charged ion, frequently potassium. In conditions with excessive acid, a hydrogen ion enters the cell, and a potassium ion leaves the cell and enters the extracellular fluid. The extracellular fluid is thus less acidic because fewer hydrogen ions are present. As a result of this exchange, however, people with acidosis are also hyperkalemic. After the acidosis is corrected, potassium reenters the cells, and potassium levels return to normal. This biological buffering occurs after chemical buffering and takes 2 to 4 hours.

A second type of biological buffer is the hemoglobin-oxyhemoglobin system. Carbon dioxide diffuses into the RBC and forms carbonic acid. The carbonic acid dissociates into hydrogen and bicarbonate ions. The hydrogen ions attach to the hemoglobin, and the bicarbonate ion becomes available for buffering by exchanging with extracellular chloride (Kokko, Tannen, 1990).

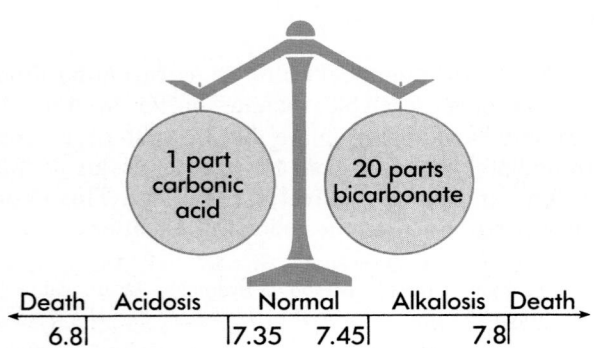

Fig. 39-6 Carbonic acid–bicarbonate ratio and pH.

Physiological Regulation

Lungs

The physiological buffers in the body are the lungs and the kidneys. The lungs can provide a rapid adaptation to an acid-base imbalance. In fact, they can act to return the pH to normal before the biological buffers can.

Ordinarily, hydrogen ions and carbon dioxide provide the stimulus for respiration. When the concentration of hydrogen ions is altered, the lungs react to correct the imbalance by altering the rate and depth of respiration. In alkalosis, the rate of respiration is reduced, and the person retains carbon dioxide. The carbon dioxide combines with water in the blood to form carbonic acid, which helps increase the acid component and balance the alkaline excess. If an excess in acid occurs, respiratory rate is increased, and the lungs excrete larger amounts of carbon dioxide (Gröer, Shekleton, 1989). Therefore less carbon dioxide is available to combine with water and create carbonic acid.

Kidneys

The kidneys can take from a few hours to several days to regulate acid-base abnormalities. They use three mechanisms to regulate hydrogen ion concentration. They can reabsorb bicarbonate during acid excess and excrete it during acid deficit. The kidneys use a phosphate ion ($PO_4^=$) to carry hydrogen ions by excreting phosphorous acid (H_3PO_4) and forming an acid base. The kidneys also convert ammonia (NH_3) to ammonium (NH_4) by attaching a hydrogen ion to ammonia.

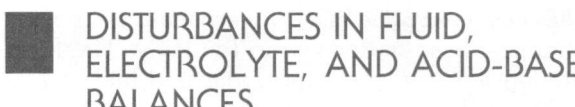

DISTURBANCES IN FLUID, ELECTROLYTE, AND ACID-BASE BALANCES

Disturbances in fluid, electrolyte, and acid-base balances seldom occur alone and can disrupt normal body processes. A client who loses body fluids through burns, illness, or trauma is at risk for electrolyte imbalances. In addition, untreated electrolyte imbalances (for example, potassium loss) result in acid-base disturbances.

Fluid Disturbances

The basic types of fluid imbalances are isotonic and osmolar. Isotonic deficit and excess exist when water and electrolytes are gained or lost in equal proportions. In contrast, osmolar imbalances are losses or excesses of only water so that the concentration (osmolality) of the serum is affected. Another type of imbalance, third-space syndrome, occurs when fluid is trapped in a space from which it is not easily exchanged with the extracellular fluid. Table 39-2 lists the causes and symptoms of common disturbances.

Isotonic Imbalances

Fluid volume deficit (FVD) results when water and electrolytes are lost in isotonic proportions. Unless other imbalances are present, serum electrolyte levels remain unchanged. Clients at risk include those with gastrointestinal losses of fluid and electrolytes such as from vomiting, gastric suction, diarrhea, or fistulas. A fistula is an abnormal opening from the gastrointestinal tract into the peritoneum, another organ, or the skin. The very young and old are quickly affected by these losses (Metheny, 1992). Other causes can include hemorrhage, diuretic administration, profuse sweating, fever, and decreased oral intake.

Fluid volume excess (FVE) results when water and sodium are retained in isotonic proportions, re-

---

TABLE 39-2 Fluid Disturbances

Causes	Signs and Symptoms
ISOTONIC IMBALANCES **Fluid volume deficit (FVD)**	
Losses from the gastrointestinal system such as from diarrhea, vomiting, or drainage from fistulas or tubes Loss of plasma or whole blood, such as with burns or hemorrhage Excessive perspiration Fever Decreased oral intake of fluids Use of diuretics	*Physical examination:* postural hypotension, tachycardia, dry skin and mucous membranes, poor skin turgor, rapid weight loss, collapsed veins, lethargy, oliguria, weak pulse *Laboratory findings:* urine specific gravity >1.025, increased hematocrit level >50%, and increased blood urea nitrogen (BUN) level >25 mg/100ml (hemoconcentration)
Fluid volume excess (FVE)	
Congestive heart failure Renal failure Cirrhosis Increased serum aldosterone and steroid levels Excessive sodium intake	*Physical examination:* rapid weight gain, edema (especially in dependent area), hypertension, polyuria, neck vein distention, increased venous pressure, crackles in lungs *Laboratory findings:* decreased hematocrit level <38% and decreased BUN level <10 mg/100ml (hemodilution)
THIRD-SPACE SYNDROME	
Portal hypertension Small bowel obstruction Peritonitis Burns	*Physical examination:* increased abdominal girth (with ascites and small bowel obstruction) *Laboratory findings:* decreased serum sodium level <135mEq/L and decreased albumin level <3.5 g/100ml (lost in trapped fluids)
OSMOLAR IMBALANCES **Hyperosmolar imbalance**	
Diabetes insipidus Interruption of neurologically driven thirst drive Diabetic ketoacidosis Osmotic diuresis Administration of hypertonic fluids	*Physical examination:* weight loss, dry and sticky mucous membranes, flushed and dry skin, thirst, elevated body temperature, irritability, convulsions, coma *Laboratory findings:* increased serum sodium level >145 mEq/L and increased serum osmolality >295 mOsm/kg
Hypoosmolar imbalance	
SIADH Excess water intake	*Physical examination:* decreased level of consciousness, convulsions, coma *Laboratory findings:* decreased serum sodium level <136 mEq/L and decreased serum osmolality <280 mOsm/kg

sulting in hypervolemia with unchanged levels of serum electrolytes. Clients at risk include those with congestive heart failure, renal failure, cirrhosis, increased serum levels of aldosterone and corticosteroids, and abnormal intake of salt (for example, in the too-rapid administration of IV fluids containing sodium) (Metheny, 1987).

Third-Space Syndrome

Third-space syndrome occurs when there is a loss of extracellular fluid into a body space, where it becomes trapped. The net result is a deficit in extracellular fluid volume. Conditions such as portal hypertension, small bowel obstruction, peritonitis, or burns can result in the shift of 5 to 10 L out of the extracellular fluid spaces, although the volume of third-space losses cannot be measured directly (Metheny, 1987). The client with a severe third-space loss experiences the effects of a FVD.

Osmolar Imbalances

Hyperosmolar imbalance (**dehydration**) occurs when there is a loss of water without a proportionate loss of electrolytes, especially sodium, or a gain in osmotically active substances. This results in an increased serum sodium level and osmolality (concentration) and intracellular dehydration.

Risk factors for dehydration include conditions that impair sufficient oral intake (for example, alterations in neurological function). Frail, infirm older clients are at great risk for developing dehydration because there is a marked decrease in intracellular fluid, decrease in renal concentrating ability, decrease in responsiveness to thirst, and increase in proportion of body fat, which limits the older client's

reserve in situations of water deficit (Aaronson, Seaman, 1989) (see research highlight).

A decrease in ADH secretion (diabetes insipidus) can lead to profound water losses. Other conditions that can cause a hyperosmolar imbalance are diabetic ketoacidosis or any condition associated with an osmotic diuresis and administration of hypertonic tube-feeding formulas or IV solutions that increase the number of solutes and the concentration of the blood. In these conditions, water moves out of the intracellular fluid to maintain extracellular fluid volume. Eventually cellular function is impaired, and circulatory collapse occurs (Metheny, 1987).

Hypoosmolar imbalance (water excess) occurs when there is an excess intake of water (psychogenic polydipsia) or excess ADH secretion. Surgery or injury to the brain can cause a syndrome of inappropriate secretion of ADH (SIADH). The overall effect is dilution of the extracellular fluid volume with osmosis of water into the cells (Gröer, Shekleton, 1989). Brain cells are particularly sensitive, and this process can lead to cerebral edema, which can cause decreased level of consciousness, coma, and even death.

Electrolyte Imbalances

Sodium Imbalances

Sodium excess and deficit share many characteristics with osmolar fluid disturbances. Hyponatremia is a less-than-normal concentration of sodium in the blood, which can take place when a net sodium loss or net water excess occurs (Table 39-3). Usually hyponatremia results in a decrease in the osmolality of plasma and extracellular fluid (Gröer, Shekleton, 1989).

When a sodium loss occurs, the body initially adapts by reducing water excretion to maintain serum osmolality at near-normal levels. As sodium loss continues, the body attempts to preserve the blood volume. As a result, the proportion of sodium in the extracellular fluid lessens. However, hyponatremia caused by sodium loss can result in vascular collapse and shock. When a pure sodium deficit occurs, there is a distinct loss of extracellular fluid volume, a condition different from hyponatremia associated with normal or increased extracellular fluid volume. Severe hyponatremia can result in neurological changes at a serum level of 120 mEq/L and in irreversible neurological alterations or death at 110 mEq/L. Any trend of decreasing serum sodium levels should be promptly reported to the client's physician.

Hypernatremia is a greater-than-normal concentration of sodium in the extracellular fluid, which can be caused by extreme water loss or overall sodium excess (Table 39-3). If the cause of hypernatremia is

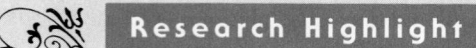
Research Highlight

Fifty-eight randomly chosen older clients residing in a continuing-care unit were followed for 2 years. The mean plasma osmolality of these clients was 302 (standard deviation 8) mOsm/kg, and only seven of the clients had a normal serum osmolality, supporting the belief that older adults are prone to hyperosmolar states. Clients with serum osmolality of greater than 307 mOsm/kg had a significantly reduced ($p = 0.025$) survival time; 15 of the 20 clients in this group died within 2 years ($p = 0.053$).

O'Neill P et al: Reduced survival with increasing plasma osmolality in elderly continuing-care patients, *Age Aging,* 19:68, 1990.

TABLE 39-3   Electrolyte Imbalances

Causes	Signs and Symptoms
HYPONATREMIA	
Kidney disease Adrenal insufficiency Gastrointestinal losses Increased sweating Use of diuretics, especially when combined with low-sodium diet Interruption of sodium-potassium pump with decreased cell potassium and decreased serum sodium Metabolic acidosis	*Physical examination:* apprehension, anxiety, personality change, postural hypotension, postural dizziness, abdominal cramping, nausea and vomiting, diarrhea, tachycardia, convulsions and coma, fingerprints remaining on sternum after palpation, and cold, clammy skin *Laboratory findings:* serum sodium level <135 mEq/L, serum osmolality <280 mOsm/kg, and urine specific gravity <1.010
HYPERNATREMIA	
Ingestion of large amounts of concentrated salt solutions Iatrogenic administration of hypertonic saline solution parenterally Excess aldosterone secretion	*Physical examination:* thirst, dry and flushed skin, dry tongue and mucous membranes, fever, agitation, convulsions, restlessness, excitability, and oliguria or anuria *Laboratory findings:* serum sodium levels >145 mEq/L, serum osmolality >295 mOsm/kg, and urine specific gravity >1.030 (if water loss is not caused by renal dysfunction)
HYPOKALEMIA	
Use of potassium-wasting diuretics Diarrhea, vomiting, or other gastrointestinal losses Alkalosis Cushing's syndrome or adrenal hormone–producing tumors Polyuria Extreme sweating Excessive use of potassium-free IV solutions	*Physical examination:* weakness and fatigue, muscle fatigue, decreased muscle tone, intestinal distention, decreased bowel sounds, heart block (severe hypokalemia), paresthesia, and weak, irregular pulse *Laboratory findings:* serum potassium level <4 mEq/L* and electrocardiogram (ECG) abnormalities (e.g., appearance of U wave, ventricular dysrhythmias) (likely when potassium level is <3.0 mEq/L*)
HYPERKALEMIA	
Renal failure Hypertonic dehydration Massive cellular damage such as from burns and trauma Iatrogenic administration of large amounts of potassium intravenously Adrenal insufficiency Acidosis Rapid infusion of stored blood Use of potassium-retaining diuretics	*Physical examination:* anxiety, irritability, dysrhythmias, hypotension, paresthesia, and weakness *Laboratory findings:* serum potassium level >5.3 mEq/L and ECG abnormalities (Bradycardia, heart block, dysrhythmias† usually appear with serum potassium level >7 mEq/L.‡)
HYPOCALCEMIA	
Rapid administration of blood transfusions containing citrate Hypoalbuminemia Hypoparathyroidism Vitamin D deficiency Neoplastic diseases Pancreatitis Rapid administration of citrated blood	*Physical examination:* numbness and tingling of fingers and circumoral region, hyperactive reflexes, positive Trousseau's sign (carpopedal spasm with hypoxia), positive Chvostek's sign (contraction of facial muscles when facial nerve is tapped), tetany, muscle cramps, and pathological fractures (chronic hypocalcemia) *Laboratory findings:* serum calcium level <4.3 mEq/L or 10 mg/100 ml and ECG changes

*Data from Groër MW: *Physiology and pathophysiology of the body fluids*, St Louis, 1981, Mosby–Year Book.
†Levels >8.5 mEq/L are frequently fatal as a result of cardiac arrest (Metheny, 1987).
‡Data from Metheny NM, *Overview of fluid and electrolyte problems: nursing considerations*, ed 2, Philadelphia, 1992, Lippincott.

Continued.

TABLE 39-3 Electrolyte Imbalances—cont'd	
Causes	Signs and Symptoms

HYPERCALCEMIA†

Hyperparathyroidism
Metastatic tumors of bone
Paget's disease (alteration in osteoclast and osteoblast activity in the bone)
Osteoporosis
Prolonged imobilization

Physical examination: decreased muscle tone, anorexia, nausea and vomiting, weakness and lethargy, low back pain (from kidney stones), decreased level of consciousness, and cardiac arrest
Laboratory findings: serum calcium level >5 mEq/L; roentgenographic examination showing generalized osteoporosis, widespread bone cavitation, radiopaque urinary stones; and elevated BUN level >25 mg/100ml and elevated creatinine level >1.5 mg/100ml caused by FVD or renal damage caused by urolithiasis

HYPOMAGNESEMIA*

Inadequate intake: malnutrition and alcoholism
Inadequate absorption: diarrhea, vomiting, nasogastric drainage, fistulas; excessive dietary calcium (competes with magnesium for transport sites); diseases of small intestine
Hypoparathyroidism
Excessive loss resulting from thiazide diuretics
Aldosterone excess
Polyuria

Physical examination: muscular tremors, hyperactive deep tendon reflexes, confusion and disorientation, dysrhythmias, and positive Chvostek's and Trousseau's sign
Laboratory findings: serum magnesium level >1.5 mEq/L‡; (also associated with hypocalcemia and hypokalemia‡)

HYPERMAGNESEMIA

Renal failure
Excess parenteral administration of magnesium

Physical examination: physical findings that are more frequent in acute elevations in magnesium levels: hypoactive deep tendon reflexes, decreased depth and rate of respirations, hypotension, and flushing
Laboratory findings: serum magnesium level >2.5 mEq/L

increased aldosterone secretion, sodium is retained and potassium is excreted. When hypernatremia occurs, the body attempts to conserve as much water as possible through renal reabsorption. Interstitial osmotic pressure increases, and fluid shifts from the cells into the extracellular fluid, causing the cells to shrink and interrupting most of the physiological cellular processes.

Potassium Imbalances

Hypokalemia is a condition in which an inadequate amount of potassium circulates in the extracellular fluid. When severe, hypokalemia can affect cardiac conduction by causing dangerous irregularities. Because the normal amount of potassium is so small, there is little tolerance for fluctuations in serum potassium levels.

Hypokalemia can result from several conditions (Table 39-3). The most common cause is the use of potassium-wasting diuretics such as thiazide and loop diuretics. This is a particular problem when clients are also receiving digitalis preparations because hypokalemia is the most common cause of digitalis toxicity. Hypokalemia is also observed in clients who are recovering from massive cellular injuries such as burns, crushing injuries, or massive trauma. Initially the extracellular fluid becomes hyperkalemic because of the release of potassium from the damaged cells, but if renal function is normal, the excess potassium is excreted by the client's kidneys.

Hyperkalemia is a greater-than-normal amount of potassium in the blood. Severe hyperkalemia produces marked cardiac conduction abnormalities such as ventricular dysrhythmia and cardiac arrest (Metheny, 1987). The primary cause of hyperkalemia is renal failure, but other illnesses also result in increased potassium (Table 39-3). Any decrease in renal function diminishes the amount of potassium the kidney can excrete.

Calcium Imbalances

Hypocalcemia represents a drop in serum and ionized calcium levels and can result from several illnesses, some of which directly affect the thyroid and parathyroid glands (Table 39-3). The signs and symptoms of hypocalcemia correlate directly to the physiological role of serum calcium in neuromuscular function.

Hypercalcemia is an increase in the total serum concentration of calcium and ionized calcium. Frequently, hypercalcemia is a symptom of an underlying disease resulting in excess bone resorption with release of calcium (Table 39-3).

Magnesium Imbalances

Hypomagnesemia occurs when the serum concentration level drops below 1.5 mEq/L. The causes of hypomagnesemia (Table 39-3) produce symptoms similar to hypocalcemia. Magnesium acts directly on the neuromuscular junction. Decreases in the serum magnesium concentration increase neuromuscular irritability (Metheny, 1987). Hypermagnesemia occurs when the serum concentration of magnesium rises above 2.5 mEq/L (Table 39-3). Hypermagnesemia diminishes the excitability of muscle cells.

Chloride Imbalances

Hypochloremia occurs when the serum chloride level falls below 100 mEq/L. Vomiting or prolonged and excessive nasogastric or fistula drainage can result in hypochloremia. A newborn can quickly develop hypochloremia as a result of diarrhea. Some diuretic medications also result in increased chloride excretion. When serum chloride levels fall, the body adapts by increased reabsorption of the bicarbonate ion, affecting acid-base balance, and metabolic alkalosis results.

Hyperchloremia occurs when the serum chloride level rises above 106 mEq/L, resulting in a decreased serum bicarbonate value. Hypochloremia and hyperchloremia rarely occur as single disease processes but are commonly associated with acid-base imbalance. No single set of symptoms is associated with these alterations.

Acid-Base Imbalances

The primary types of acid-base imbalance are respiratory acidosis, respiratory alkalosis, metabolic acidosis, and metabolic alkalosis (Table 39-4 on p. 1288).

Respiratory Acidosis

Respiratory acidosis is marked by an increased arterial carbon dioxide concentration ($Paco_2$), excess carbonic acid, and an increased hydrogen ion concentration (decreased pH). Respiratory acidosis is caused by hypoventilation or any condition that depresses ventilation (Table 39-4). Decreased ventilation may begin in the respiratory system (respiratory failure) or outside the respiratory system (drug overdose). In clients with respiratory acidosis the cerebrospinal fluid and brain cells become acidic, causing neurological changes. Hypoxemia (decreased oxygen levels) occurs because of respiratory depression, resulting in further neurological impairments (see Chapter 38). Electrolyte changes such as hyperkalemia may accompany acidosis.

Respiratory Alkalosis

Respiratory alkalosis is marked by decreased $Paco_2$ and decreased hydrogen ion concentration (increased pH). Respiratory alkalosis results from excessive exhalation of carbon dioxide, or hyperventilation (Table 39-4). Like respiratory acidosis, respiratory alkalosis can begin outside the respiratory system (anxiety) or within the respiratory system, such as in the initial phases of an asthmatic attack.

Metabolic Acidosis

Metabolic acidosis results from a rise in hydrogen ion concentration (decreased pH) in the extracellular fluid, caused by an increase in hydrogen ion levels or a decrease in bicarbonate levels (Gröer, 1981). Metabolic acidosis is caused by many conditions (Table 39-4). The types of metabolic acidosis, normochloremic and hyperchloremic, are classified according to the client's plasma chloride concentration.

Metabolic Alkalosis

Metabolic alkalosis is marked by heavy loss of acid from the body or by increased levels of bicarbonate. The most common cause is vomiting. Metabolic alkalosis may also result when a client with a gastric acid disturbance ingests large amounts of sodium bicarbonate. Other causes are listed in the Table 39-4.

 # VARIABLES AFFECTING FLUID, ELECTROLYTE, AND ACID-BASE BALANCES

Fluid, electrolyte, and acid-base status is neither a static nor single physiological entity. Many variables can change the distribution of body fluid and electrolytes. In some instances (for example, with normal changes during pregnancy and exercise), fluid and electrolyte alterations is a normal and expected response. In other situations, however, fluid, electrolyte,

TABLE 39-4   Acid-Base Imbalances

Causes	Signs and Symptoms
RESPIRATORY ACIDOSIS	
Pneumonia	*Physical examination:* confusion, dizziness, lethargy,
Respiratory failure	headache, dysrhythmias, abdominal cramps, warm and
Atelectasis (obstruction of small airways often caused by	flushed skin, muscular twitching, and convulsions
retained mucus)	*Laboratory findings;* arterial blood gas alterations: pH <
Drug overdose	7.35, partial pressure of carbon dioxide in arterial blood
Paralysis of respiratory muscles, various neurological alter-	($Paco_2$) >45 mm Hg, arterial partial pressure of oxygen
ations	(Pao_2) <80 mm Hg, and bicarbonate level normal (if
Traumatic injuries	uncompensated) or >26 mEq/L (if compensated)
Obesity	
Airway obstruction	
Head injuries	
Cerebrovascular accident (stroke)	
Drowning	
Cystic fibrosis	
RESPIRATORY ALKALOSIS	
Anxiety	*Physical examination:* headache, irritability, dizziness,
Fear	dysrhythmias, tachypnea, and numbness and tingling of
Anemia	extremities
Hypermetabolic states	*Laboratory findings:* arterial blood gas alterations: pH >
Disorders of the central nervous system (head injuries,	7.45, $Paco_2$ < 35 mm Hg, Pao_2 normal, and bicarbonate
infections)	level normal (if short lived or uncompensated) or <22
Use of drugs (aspirin overdose)	mEq/L (if compensated)
Asthma	
Pneumonia	
Inappropriate mechanical ventilator settings	
METABOLIC ACIDOSIS	
Starvation	*Physical examination:* headache, lethargy, confusion, dys-
Diabetic ketoacidosis	rhythmias, tachypnea with deep respirations, abdominal
Renal failure	cramps, and flushed skin
Shock	*Laboratory findings:* arterial blood gas alterations: pH <
Diarrhea	7.35, $Paco_2$ normal (if uncompensated) or <35 mm Hg
Use of drugs (methanol, ethanol, formic acid, paralde-	(if compensated), Pao_2 normal or increased (with rapid,
hyde, aspirin)	deep respirations), and bicarbonate level <22 mEq/L
Renal tubular acidosis	
METABOLIC ALKALOSIS	
Excessive vomiting	*Physical examination:* headache, irritability, lethargy, dys-
Prolonged gastric suctioning	rhythmias, abdominal cramps, numbness, tingling,
Hypokalemia or hypercalcemia	muscle cramps, tetany
Cushing's syndrome	*Laboratory findings:* arterial blood gas alterations: pH
Use of drugs (steroids, sodium bicarbonate, diuretics)	>7.45, $Paco_2$ normal (if uncompensated) or >45 mm
Hyperaldosteronism	Hg (if compensated), Pao_2 normal, and bicarbonate
	level >26 mEq/L

and acid-base imbalances can have severe conse-quences.

During assessment the nurse identifies altered fluid, electrolyte, and acid-base states. To assess cli-ents effectively, the nurse considers variables influ-encing fluid, electrolyte, and acid-base status, the way normal balance changes, and whether the change is a normal anticipated change or a conse-quence of a pathological process. The major factors that can affect fluid, electrolyte, and acid-base status include age, body size, environmental temperature, lifestyle, and level of health.

Age

Age affects distribution of body fluids and electrolytes. The major differences are observed in infants, older adults, and pregnant clients.

Fluid and electrolyte changes occur normally with developmental changes. However, when an illness is also present, the client may be unable to adapt adequately to these changes. Therefore the nurse needs to include the fluid changes associated with aging and development in nursing assessment.

Infants

Infants' proportions of total body water are greater than those of school-age children, adolescents, or adults. However, although infants have greater proportions of body water, they are not protected from fluid loss (for example, from diarrhea) because they ingest and excrete a relatively greater daily water volume than adults (Riddle, 1992). In fact, infants are at greater risk for FVD or hyperosmolar imbalances because their body water losses are proportionately greater per kilogram of body weight.

Children

In childhood illnesses, the regulatory and compensatory responses to imbalances are less stable and tend to operate within a more narrow range with less tolerance for large changes in balance. Children frequently respond to illness with fevers of higher temperature or longer duration than those of adults. Fever in childhood can increase the rate of insensible water loss (Metheny, 1987).

Adolescents

In adolescence, rapid and major changes occur in anatomical and physiological processes. The increased growth rate increases metabolic processes and, as a result, the amount of water produced as an end product of metabolism. Changes in fluid balance are greater in adolescent girls because of hormonal changes associated with the menstrual cycle.

Pregnant Women

The pregnant woman experiences several changes in fluid and electrolyte balance. Aldosterone secretion and excretion increase as a result of changes in reproductive hormones and the renin-angiotension system (Metheny, 1987). In some, the elevation can be 10 times normal, which may result in fluid retention.

As the fetus and uterus grow, reaching their preterm size, they exert pressure on the inferior vena cava. This pressure and the pressure of vascular congestion of the pelvis further increase vena caval pressure. These changes and the increased permeability of capillary walls may influence the capillary filtration pressure, resulting in dependent edema (Metheny, 1987). However, when the woman lies down, pressure on the vena cava is relieved, and after a time the edema disappears.

An increase of 45% to 50% in circulating blood volume occurs at the tenth week of pregnancy. At the end of pregnancy, before delivery of the infant, the average woman's body has 6.5 L of extra fluid. Of this amount, 3.5 L is from the fetus, placenta, and amniotic fluid. The other 3 L results from increases in blood volume, breast size, and uterine mass (Metheny, 1987).

Older Adults

The older client's risk of fluid and electrolyte imbalance may be closely associated with decreased renal function and a consequent lack of urine concentration. The older adult may also have chronic illness, such as diabetes mellitus, cardiovascular disorders, or cancer, that can impair fluid balance. In addition, the total amount of body water decreases approximately 6% with age (Robinson, 1987). Other risk factors that particularly affect the older adult are use of diuretics, often given for hypertension and congestive heart failure; overuse of laxatives and enemas; and colon-cleansing procedures used in preparation for diagnostic tests (Robinson, 1987). Common imbalances associated with aging include hyperosmolar fluid disturbance and hypernatremia (Tables 39-2 and 39-3). The nurse investigates these imbalances and other treatable causes when older adults suddenly develop changes in mental status. Other imbalances are hyperthermia and hypocalcemia, which result in osteoporosis.

Obtaining assessment data related to fluid and electrolyte disturbance requires modification when caring for an older client. For example, skin turgor is best tested over the forehead or sternum because skin elasticity remains most normal in these areas. Body temperature is decreased in the older client, so the client's baseline temperature must be known to detect elevations associated with hyperosmolar imbalances or hypernatremia. A sensitive indicator of fluid balance in the older adult is observation of the rate and degree of filling of small veins in the foot (Robinson, 1987). The older adult has decreased salivation, so mucous membrane moistness is assessed by inspecting the area under the tongue for a pool of saliva. Other elements of fluid balance assessment include using intake and output measurements and daily weight measurements so that trends can be detected despite the renal function changes.

Body Size

Body size has an effect on total body water. Because fat contains no water, the obese client has proportionately less body water. Women have more fat deposits, such as in the breasts and hips, than men. As a result, the total body water in women is less than in men of the same age.

Environmental Temperature

Fluid and electrolyte imbalances are associated with extremes in environmental temperature and relative humidity. The overall body response to environmental temperatures exceeding 28° to 30° C (82.4° to 86° F) is to increase sensible water loss by sweating, which cools the peripheral blood and helps reduce body temperature.

The healthy adult can sweat about 1 L/hr for 2 hours, losing about 5% of body weight without straining the cooling mechanism. However, after a body weight loss of 7% is exceeded, the cooling mechanism declines to conserve body water (Metheny, 1987).

The relative humidity of the environmental temperature also affects body water loss and body temperature regulation. The evaporation of sweat decreases at 60% humidity and ceases at 75% (Metheny, 1987).

The body responds with fluid changes to excessive environmental temperature. It increases peripheral vasodilation, which allows more blood to come to the surface for cooling. Sweating increases body fluid loss, which results in loss of sodium and chloride ions. The body also increases cardiac output and pulse rate. Finally, increased aldosterone secretion occurs, resulting in sodium retention and potassium excretion by the kidneys (Metheny, 1987). Each of these responses can affect overall fluid and electrolyte balance, and the nurse needs to assess the environment to determine actual or potential alterations in fluid and electrolyte balance.

Lifestyle

Lifestyle can have an indirect effect on fluid, electrolyte, and acid-base balance. Habits that can affect fluid balance include diet, stress, and exercise.

Diet

Dietary intake of fluids, salt, potassium, calcium, magnesium, and necessary carbohydrates, fats, and proteins helps maintain normal fluid, electrolyte, and acid-base status. When nutritional intake is inadequate, the body tries to preserve its protein stores by breaking down glycogen and fat stores. When excess free fatty acids are released, metabolic acidosis can occur because the liver converts free fatty acids to ketone, a strong acid. However, after those resources are depleted, the body begins to destroy protein stores. When serum protein levels drop below normal, hypoalbuminemia results. In hypoalbuminemia the serum colloid osmotic pressure is decreased, and fluid shifts from the circulating blood volume and enters the interstitial fluid spaces, resulting in edema.

Stress

The impact of stress on fluid and electrolyte balance can be understood in terms of the general adaptation syndrome (see Chapter 30). Stress increases aldosterone and glucocorticoid levels, leading to sodium and water retention. In addition, increased ADH secretion decreases urine output. The effect of the stress response is to increase fluid volume. As a result, cardiac output, blood pressure, and perfusion to the major organs are increased.

Exercise

Exercise results in increased sensible water loss through sweat. The client who exercises can respond to the thirst mechanism and help maintain fluid and electrolyte balance by increasing fluid intake. Athletes undergoing sustained vigorous exercise must have fluid loss replaced by a liquid that contains electrolytes. One such substance is Gatorade, which contains glucose, sodium, chloride, and potassium (see Table 39-7).

Level of Health

Generally, the better the client's health, the easier it is to tolerate fluid and electrolyte changes. One of the most important nursing functions is to recognize clients at risk for fluid and electrolyte disturbances. The client's overall level of health influences fluid, electrolyte, and acid-base status. Clients with chronic illness, concomitant depression of the immune system, and decreases in nutritional intake are at a greater risk for fluid, electrolyte and acid-base imbalance than healthier persons who have an acute gastrointestinal inflammation for 24 to 36 hours. In all cases the nurse must assess the actual or potential risk factors for fluid, electrolyte, and acid-base balances. In addition to the following categories of illness, fluid, electrolyte, and acid-base imbalances also occur with gastrointestinal disturbances and diseases of the endocrine system.

Surgery

Surgical procedures result in changes in fluid balance because of the body's stress response to surgical trauma during the second to fifth days after surgery. The more extensive the surgery, the greater the response of the body. Postoperative fluid imbalances result from increased secretion of aldosterone, gluco-corticoids, and ADH. Increases in aldosterone and glucocorticoid levels result in sodium and chloride retention and potassium excretion. An increase in the ADH level results in decreased urinary output. These hormonal increases and the activity of the sympathetic nervous system help maintain circulating blood volume and blood pressure after surgery.

After the immediate postoperative period, hormone secretion returns to normal levels, and excess sodium and water are excreted from the body. Postoperative fluid and electrolyte changes are normal and should be anticipated in surgical clients.

After surgery, clients can experience many acid-base alterations. For example, the client who is reluctant to breathe deeply and cough may develop respiratory acidosis because of retained $Paco_2$. The client with nasogastric suction may develop metabolic alkalosis with the loss of gastric acid.

Burns

In clients with severe second- or third-degree burns, body fluids are lost. The greater the body surface burned, the greater the fluid loss. The burned client loses body fluids by one of five routes. First, plasma leaves the intravascular space and becomes trapped as edema. This is also called the plasma-to-interstitial fluid shift. Along with the shifting of fluid, serum proteins are lost from extracellular fluids. Second, plasma and interstitial fluids are lost as burn exudate, a visible fluid loss on the burned surface and common with second-degree burns. Third, water vapor and heat are lost because burned skin can no longer serve as a barrier against such losses. This loss increases in proportion to the amount of skin burned. Fourth, blood leaks from damaged capillaries, contributing to an already decreased extracellular fluid volume. Last, sodium and water shift into the cells, again depleting extracellular fluid volume (Metheny, 1987).

The client may devleop metabolic acidosis after a burn as a result of the release of acids from the injured tissue. If the client has experienced an inhalation injury, respiratory acidosis may develop because of a decreased oxygen–carbon dioxide exchange (Metheny, 1987).

Cardiovascular Disorders

The failing heart has a diminished cardiac output. As a result, perfusion to the kidneys is decreased, and urinary output drops. The client retains sodium and water, and edema, circulatory overload, and pulmonary edema may result.

Fluid and electrolyte imbalances associated with heart failure can be controlled for a time with diuret-ics, cardiotonics, vasodilators, angiotensin-converting enzyme (ACE) inhibitors, and fluid and sodium restrictions. The goal of fluid reduction is to reduce the work of the left ventricle by relieving the excess extracellular fluid volume.

Respiratory Disorders

Many alterations in respiratory function predispose the client to respiratory acidosis because of interference with the elimination of carbon dioxide (for example, chronic obstructive lung diseases such as emphysema, pneumonia, and sedative overdose). As the carbon dioxide builds up in the bloodstream, the body's compensatory mechanisms (buffers, renal processes) can no longer adapt, which allows the arterial pH to decrease. Any condition which causes hyperventilation (for example, decreased arterial oxygen level, anxiety, or fever) can result in respiratory alkalosis that is often acute and of short duration after the precipitating cause is removed.

Renal Disorders

Failing kidneys alter fluid and electrolyte balance. There is an abnormal retention of sodium, chloride, potassium, and water in the extracellular fluid. The plasma levels of metabolic waste products such as BUN and creatinine are elevated because the kidneys are unable to filter and excrete the waste products of cellular metabolism. This elevation is toxic to cellular processes. Hydrogen ions are also retained when renal function is decreased, which results in metabolic acidosis. The usual renal compensatory mechanisms such as bicarbonate reabsorption are not available, so the body's ability to restore normal acid-base balance is limited.

The severity of fluid and electrolyte imbalance is proportional to the degree of renal failure. Occasionally, acute renal failure induced by shock or a decrease in extracellular fluid may be reversible. Although chronic renal failure is progressive, the client may be treated successfully with dietary control of protein and salt intake, diuretic medications, and fluid restrictions. Most clients with chronic renal failure eventually require dialysis to maintain fluid and electrolyte balance.

Cancer

The types of fluid and electrolyte imbalances that are observed in a client with cancer depend on the type and progression of the cancer. All electrolyte imbalances can occur in the client with cancer and are caused by anatomical distortion and functional impairment from tumor growth and tumor-caused metabolic and endocrine abnormality (Kopec, Groeger, 1988).

NURSING PROCESS AND FLUID, ELECTROLYTE, AND ACID-BASE IMBALANCES

Assessment

During assessment the nurse identifies potential and actual fluid, electrolyte, and acid-base imbalances. In addition, assessment helps the nurse determine the effectiveness of interventions. For example, if a diuretic medication is prescribed for a client with congestive heart failure, the nurse assessing the client expects to note a decrease in weight, an increase in 24-hour urine output, and a decrease in or absence of dependent edema.

The nurse also assesses fluid, electrolyte, and acid-base balances to detect adverse reactions to treatment. For example, if IV fluids are ordered for a client with progressive renal failure, the nurse may find, on the third day, that the 24-hour fluid intake exceeds renal output by four to one, that the client's weight is increased, and that dependent edema and abnormal lung sounds are present.

Finally, fluid, electrolyte, and acid-base assessment helps the nurse anticipate needs for nursing care. For example, a client with edema who is placed on diuretic therapy should have a care plan to anticipate needs such as an increased use of the bathroom, bedpan, or urinal or instruction for a salt-restricted diet.

Nursing History

To collect data about fluid, electrolyte, and acid-base status the nurse must understand fluid and acid-base regulation, electrolyte and acid-base imbalances, and volume disturbances. In addition, the nurse needs to know why and how some diseases, treatments, drug therapies, and diet changes alter fluid balance. This information assists the nurse in identifying clients at risk for fluid, electrolyte, and acid-base imbalances.

Clients with cardiovascular and renal diseases, severe burns or trauma, and endocrine disorders are at high risk for fluid, electrolyte, and acid-base disturbances. In addition, prolonged gastrointestinal upsets, particularly in the very young and very old, can result in these imbalances.

Certain treatments such as IV therapy and total parenteral nutrition (TPN) alter fluid balance. Prescribed drugs also increase the risk for fluid, electrolyte, and acid-base disturbances. For example, diuretic medications usually increase the risk for sodium and potassium loss. In turn, the sodium loss can result in osmolar fluid disturbances. Conversely,

administration of steroid preparations results in sodium retention and can cause FVE.

The nurse also collects the nursing history to identify risk factors increasing the chances of fluid, electrolyte, and acid-base imbalances (see box). Eventually all types of chronic diseases can cause these imbalances. Because the progression of these diseases is usually slow, imbalances can be controlled. When nurses care for clients with chronic illnesses, however, they often find that the disease processes are no longer stabilized and that imbalances are present.

Head injuries can result in cerebral edema. Occasionally, this edema creates pressure on the pituitary gland, and as a result, ADH secretion is changed. Two alterations can occur. Diabetes insipidus occurs when too little ADH is secreted and the client excretes large volumes of dilute urine with a low specific gravity. The second alteration is SIADH, in which there is continued secretion of ADH, which results in a gradual increase of extracellular fluid volume, hyponatremia, and hypoosmolality (Vokes, Rob-

---

Risk Factors for Fluid, Electrolyte, and Acid-Base Imbalances

- Age
  - Very young
  - Very old
- Chronic diseases
  - Cancer
  - Cardiovascular disease such as congestive heart failure
  - Endocrine disease such as Cushing's syndrome and diabetes mellitus
  - Malnutrition
  - Chronic pulmonary disease
  - Renal disease such as progressive renal failure
  - Decreased level of consciousness
- Trauma
  - Crushing injuries
  - Head injuries
- Burns
- Therapies
  - Diuretics
  - Steroids
  - IV therapy
  - TPN
- Gastrointestinal losses
- Gastroenteritis
- Nasogastric suctioning
- Fistulas

TABLE 39-5 Physical and Behavioral Nursing Assessment for Fluid, Electrolyte, and Acid-Base Imbalances

Assessment	Imbalance	Frequency
WEIGHT CHANGES		
2%-5% loss	Mild FVD	On admission and daily
6%-9% loss	Moderate FVD	
10%-14% loss	Severe FVD	
20% loss	Death	
2% gain	Mild FVE	
5% gain	Moderate FVE	
8% gain	Severe FVE	
HEAD (HEENT)		
History:		
Headache	Metabolic or respiratory acidosis, metabolic alkalosis	Every hr
Dizziness	Respiratory alkalosis or acidosis, hyponatremia	Every hr
Observation:		
Irritability	Metabolic or respiratory alkalosis, hyperosmolar imbalance, hypernatremia, hypokalemia	Every hr
Lethargy	Metabolic acidosis or alkalosis, respiratory acidosis, hypercalemia	Every hr
Palpation: Chvostek's sign	Hypocalcemia, hypomagnesemia	
Fontanels (infant)		
Inspection:		Every hr
Depressed	FVD	
Bulging	FVE	
Eyes		
Inspection:		Every hr
Sunken eyes, dry conjunctivae, or decreased or absent of tearing	FVD	
Periorbital edema or papilledema	FVE	
History: blurred vision	FVE	Every hr
Ears		
None		
Bridge of nose		
Palpation: pinched skin that remains raised	FVD	Every 4 hr
Throat and mouth		
Inspection:		
Sticky, dry mucous membranes	Hypernatremia, FVD	Every 4 hr
Dry cracked lips and decreased salivation		
Longitudinal furrows on tongue		
CARDIOVASCULAR SYSTEM		
Inspection:		Every hr
Flat neck veins	FVD	
Distended neck veins	FVE	

Data from Groer MW: *Physiology and pathophysiology of the body fluids*, St Louis, 1981, Mosby–Year Book; Keithley JK, Frauline KE: *Nurs 82* 12:44, 1982; Metheny NM: *NITA* 4:38, 1981; and Metheny NM: *Fluid and electrolyte balance: nursing considerations*, ed 2, Philadelphia 1992, Lippincott.

Continued.

TABLE 39-5 Physical and Behavioral Nursing Assessment for Fluid, Electrolyte, and Acid-Base Imbalances—cont'd		
Assessment	Imbalance	Frequency
Palpation:		
Dysrhythmias	Metabolic acidosis, respiratory alkalosis and acidosis, potassium imbalance, hypomagnesemia	
Increased pulse rate	Metabolic alkalosis, respiratory acidosis, FVD, hyponatremia, hypomagnesemia	
Decreased pulse rate	Metabolic alkalosis, hypokalemia	
Weak pulse	FVD, hypokalemia	
Decreased capillary filling	FVD	
Bounding pulse rate	FVE	
Auscultation:		
Blood pressure low with or without orthostatic changes	FVD, hyponatremia, hyperkalemia, hypermagnesemia	
Third heart sound	FVE	
ECG: cardiac dysrhythmias	Hypokalemia, metabolic acidosis, respiratory alkalosis and acidosis, hyperkalemia, hypomagnesemia	
RESPIRATORY SYSTEM		
Inspection:		Every hr
Increased rate	FVE, respiratory alkalosis, metabolic acidosis	
Dyspnea	FVE	
Auscultation: crackles	FVE	
GASTROINTESTINAL SYSTEM		
History:		
Anorexia	Metabolic acidosis	
Abdominal cramps	Metabolic acidosis	
Inspection:		Every 2 hr
Sunken abdomen	FVD	
Distended abdomen	Third-space syndrome	
Vomiting	FVD, hypercalcemia, hyponatremia	
Diarrhea	Hyponatremia	
Palpation: poor skin turgor	FVD	
Auscultation: hyperperistalsis with diarrhea or hypoperistalsis	FVD, hypokalemia	
RENAL SYSTEM		
Inspection:		Every 2 hr
Oliguria or anuria	FVD, FVE	
Diuresis (if kidneys normal)	FVE	
Increased urine specific gravity	FVD	
NEUROMUSCULAR SYSTEM		
Inspection:		Every hr
Numbness, tingling	Metabolic alkalosis, hypocalcemia, potassium imbalances	
Muscle cramps, tetany	Hypocalcemia, metabolic or respiratory alkalosis	
Coma	Hyperosmolar or hypoosmolar imbalances, hyponatremia	
Tremors	Respiratory acidosis, hypomagnesemia	

TABLE 39-5 Physical and Behavioral Nursing Assessment for Fluid, Electrolyte, and Acid-Base Imbalances—cont'd		
Assessment	Imbalance	Frequency
Disorientation	Hypomagnesemia, metabolic acidosis	
Palpation:		
Hypotonicity (decreased muscle tone)	Hypokalemia, hypercalcemia	
Hypertonicity (increased muscle tone)	Hypocalcemia, hypomagnesemia, metabolic alkalosis	
Percussion:		
Deep tendon reflexes decreased or absent	Hypercalcemia, hypermagnesemia	
Increased or hyperactive	Hypocalcemia, hypomagnesemia	
SKIN		
Body temperature		Every 1-2 hr
Increased	Hypernatremia, hyperosmolar imbalance, metabolic acidosis	
Decreased	FVD	
Body surface		
Inspection: Dry flushed skin	FVD, hypernatremia, metabolic acidosis	
Palpation: Poor skin turgor; cold clammy skin	FVD	
Extremities (dependent body parts: sacrum, back, legs)		
Inspection: Slow venous filling	FVD	
Palpation: edema (1+ to 4+)	FVE	

ertson, 1988). In addition, physical assessment and laboratory findings are consistent with fluid volume overload.

Burns can result in the loss of plasma through the burned skin surface. Thus a loss of fluid and electrolytes occurs.

Drug therapies increase the risk for fluid and electrolyte disturbances. Although all diuretic medications cause excretion of water, they can be potassium sparing such as spironolactone (Aldactone) or potassium wasting such as furosemide (Lasix).

Gastroenteritis and nasogastric suctioning result in loss of potassium and chloride ions. Hydrogen ions are also lost, causing a disturbance in acid-base balance.

Gastrointestinal fistulas can also result in a loss of potassium, resulting in increased risk for hypokalemia. The loss of potassium increases the risk for acid-base disturbances.

Physical Examination

Because fluid, electrolyte, and acid-base disturbances can affect all systems, the nurse must systematically identify any abnormalities during the physical examination (Table 39-5 on p. 1293).

Measuring Fluid Intake and Output

Measuring and recording all liquid intake and output during a 24-hour period helps complete the assessment data base for fluid, electrolyte, and acid-base balances. Intake includes all liquids taken orally, by feeding tube, and parenterally.

Oral intake includes all liquids taken by mouth, such as gelatin, ice cream, soup, juice, and water. Liquid intake also includes fluids given through nasogastric or jejunostomy feeding tubes, liquids given as IV fluids, and blood or its components. Liquid output includes urine, diarrhea, vomitus, gastric suction, and drainage from postsurgical tubes. Frequently the recording of such data is referred to as the I & O.

Generally, I & O are routinely measured for clients after surgery and clients whose conditions are unstable, who have fever, whose fluids are restricted, or who are receiving diuretic or IV therapy. The nurse neither needs nor should wait for a physician's order

Barnes Hospital		B-8
DAILY INTAKE AND OUTPUT RECORD		

17-4 Rev. 2/83

FROM 0700 / / TO 0700 / /   Addressograph Plate

INTAKE	OUTPUT

Coffee mug	- 180cc	ORDERS: (CIRCLE)	SOURCE KEY:
Ice tea container to clear line (without ice)	- 250cc		V = VOIDED
Ice cream container (melted)	- 30cc	NPO	C = CATHETER
Sherbet container (melted)	- 50cc	WATER	INC = INCONTINENT
Juice container	- 120cc	CLEAR FLUIDS	
Milk carton	- 240cc	FULL FLUIDS	
Paper cup (1/4 from brim)	- 240cc		
Soup bowl (broth)	- 180cc	AMT. DESIRED	
Gelatin container (melted)	- 100cc	CC	

SOURCE KEY:
VOM. = VOMITUS
LIQ. S. = LIQUID STOOL
HV. = HEMOVAC
L.T. = LEVIN TUBE
T.T. = T. TUBE
OTHER

RATE   GTTS/MIN.   CC/HR.

PARENTERAL			ORAL		URINE		OTHER	
TIME	SOLUTION IN BOTTLE	AMT. (CC) ABSORBED	KIND	AMT. (CC)	SOURCE	AMT. (CC)	SOURCE	AMT. (CC)
	KIND AMT. (CC)							
0700 0800			Juice	120				
0800 0900			Jello	100	V	200		
0900 1000			Maalox	30				
1000 1100			Soup	180				
1100 1200			Juice	120				
1200 1300			Jello	100	V	180		
1300 1400								
1400 1500								
8 HR. TOT.			8 HR. TOT. 650		8 HR. TOT. 380		8 HR. TOT.	
1500 1600								
1600 1700								
1700 1800								
1800 1900								
1900 2000								
2000 2100								
2100 2200								
2200 2300								
8 HR. TOT.			8 HR. TOT.		8 HR. TOT.		8 HR. TOT.	
2300 2400								
2400 0100								
0100 0200								
0200 0300								
0300 0400								
0400 0500								
0500 0600								
0600 0700								
8 HR. TOT.			8 HR. TOT.		8 HR. TOT.		8 HR. TOT.	
24 HR. TOT.			24 HR. TOT.		24 HR. TOT.		24 HR. TOT.	

Fig. 39-7   Eight-hour fluid intake and output record.
Courtesy Barnes Hospital, St Louis.

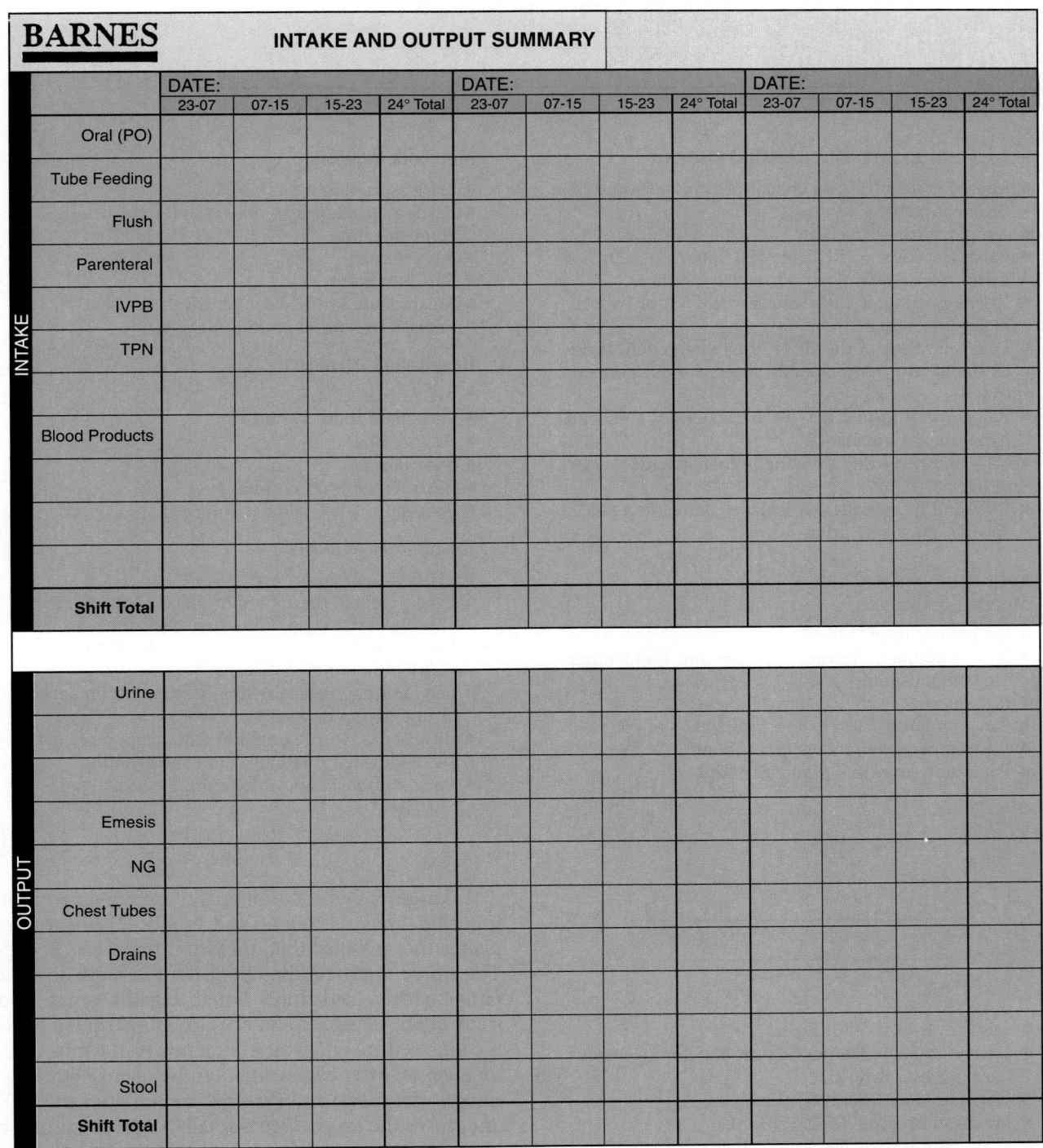

Fig. 39-8   Twenty-four hour intake and output record.
Courtesy Barnes Hospital, St Louis.

to begin I & O measurements. Clients with chronic cardiopulmonary or renal illnesses and those whose health status has declined also receive such measurements.

In the hospital, forms for recording I & O are attached to the bedside chart or room door. The records note the type of I & O and are broken down into at least 8-hour segments (Fig. 39-7). At the end of each 8-hour shift, I & O are totalled. These 24-hour totals are then recorded at midnight or 6 AM depending on policy. The 24-hour totals are included in the client's chart (Fig. 39-8).

Laboratory Data for Fluid, Electrolyte, and Acid-Base Imbalances

FLUID AND ELECTROLYTE IMBALANCES

- Altered concentrations of sodium, chloride, and bicarbonate ions
- Altered serum osmolality
- False elevation of RBC or WBC count because of hemoconcentration caused by dehydration
- False lowering of CBC values with FVE or hypoosmolar imbalance
- False elevation of the BUN level when client is dehydrated and extracellular fluid is hemoconcentrated
- False lowering of BUN level because of FVE and hypoosmolar imbalance
- Concentrated urine, causing higher specific gravity of urine
- FVE and hypoosmolar imbalance, causing a fall in specific gravity of urine

ACID-BASE IMBALANCES
Metabolic Alkalosis

- pH greater than 7.45
- $Paco_2$ normal or greater than 45 mm Hg if lungs are compensating
- Pao_2 normal
- Sao_2 normal
- Bicarbonate level greater than 26 mEq/L
- Potassium level less than 3.5 mEq/L

Metabolic Acidosis

- pH less than 7.35
- $Paco_2$ normal or less than 35 mm Hg if lungs are compensating
- Pao_2 normal
- Sao_2 normal
- Bicarbonate level below 22 mEq/L
- Potassium level above 5.3 mEq/L

Respiratory Alkalosis

- pH 7.45 or greater
- $Paco_2$ less than 35 mm Hg
- Pao_2 normal
- Sao_2 normal
- Bicarbonate level normal
- Potassium level below 3.5 mEq/L

Respiratory Acidosis

- pH less than 7.35
- $Paco_2$ greater than 45 mm Hg (unless client has chronic obstructive pulmonary disease)
- Pao_2 normal or below 80 mm Hg, depending on severity of underlying disease
- Sao_2 normal or below 95%, depending on severity of underlying disease
- Bicarbonate level normal in early respiratory acidosis or elevated if kidneys are compensating
- Potassium level above 5.3 mEq/L

Normal Laboratory Tests Values

- Calcium levels: 4-5 mEq/L
- Carbon dioxide content (bicarbonate in venous blood): 24-30 mEq/L
- Chloride level: 100-106 mEq/L
- Magnesium level: 1.5-2.5 mEq/L
- Phosphate level: 2.5-4.5 mEq/L
- Potassium level: 3.5-5.3 mEq/L
- Sodium level: 135-145 mEq/L
- Serum osmolality: 280-295 mOsm/kg
- Urine specific gravity: 1.003-1.030
- Arterial blood gas levels
  - pH: 7.35-7.45
  - $Paco_2$: 35-45 mm Hg
  - Pao_2: 80-100 mm Hg
  - Sao_2: 95%-99%
  - Bicarbonate level: 22-26 mEq/L

Taking I & O measurements is a procedure requiring help from the client and family. The nurse explains the reasons that measurements are needed. The nurse instructs the client not to empty any container with voided fluids but to ask the nurse to do so. A client using a toilet should be instructed to use a calibrated insert, which attaches to the rim of the toilet bowl. After each urination the client notifies the nurse, who measures, records, and empties the urine and rinses the insert. Occasionally, clients may also be instructed to measure and record their own output.

The output of a client who has an indwelling Foley catheter, drainage tube, or suction is recorded at the end of each nursing shift or even more frequently (for example, every hour) as the client's condition requires.

Clients occasionally receive a specific amount of a liquid medication every 1 to 2 hours. For example, antacids are commonly ordered in 30-ml doses every hour for clients who have or who are at risk for gastrointestinal bleeding. Over 24 hours, this hourly antacid can amount to a significant intake and should always be recorded on the I & O record.

Recording I & O is essential for obtaining an accurate data base. The nurse looks for trends over 24-, 48-, and 72-hour periods. This information helps maintain an ongoing evaluation of hydration status to prevent severe imbalances.

Laboratory Studies

Laboratory tests are performed to obtain further objective data about fluid, electrolyte, and acid-base balances (see box). These tests include serum electrolyte levels, complete blood count (CBC), BUN levels, blood creatinine levels, urine specific gravity, and arterial blood gas level. The nurse must be familiar with the normal values of common laboratory tests (see box).

Serum electrolyte levels are measured to determine the hydration status, the electrolyte concentration of the blood plasma, and the acid-base balance. Electrolytes frequently measured in venous blood include sodium, potassium, chloride, and bicarbonate ions and carbon dioxide combining power. The severity of the illness determines the frequency of the electrolyte measurements. Serum electrolytes are routinely measured when a client is admitted to the hospital. This provides baseline data for electrolyte status.

The CBC is a determination of the number and type of red and white blood cells per cubic millimeter of blood. Changes in the CBC, especially in the hematocrit, occur in response to dehydration or overhydration. Serious alterations in the CBC, such as anemia, can also affect oxygenation status.

Blood creatinine levels are useful in measuring kidney function. Creatinine is a normal by-product of muscle metabolism and is excreted at fairly constant levels, regardless of factors such as fluid intake, diet, and exercise.

The urine specific gravity test measures the urine's degree of concentration. The specific gravity can be measured at the bedside using a urinometer (see Chapter 40). Normally the urine specific gravity ranges between 1.003 and 1.030. Because water has a specific gravity of 1.000, urine with a lower specific gravity (1.003) is more dilute than urine with a higher specific gravity (1.030).

Arterial blood gas tests provide information on the status of acid-base balance and on the effectiveness of ventilatory function in providing normal oxygen–carbon dioxide exchange. The arterial pH tests measure the hydrogen ion concentration. A decreased pH is associated with acidosis, whereas an elevated pH is associated with alkalosis.

The Pa_{CO_2} measures the partial pressure of carbon dioxide in the arterial blood. Alveolar hypoventilation

results in an elevated Pa_{CO_2}, whereas hyperventilation is associated with a decreased Pa_{CO_2}. Regulation of carbon dioxide is the pulmonary component of acid-base balance, and changes in the Pa_{CO_2} may help explain an abnormal pH. Pa_{O_2} measures the partial pressure of oxygen in the arteries. This provides information concerning the ventilatory effectiveness of the lungs. Pa_{O_2} levels provide no direct information concerning acid-base balance. The oxygen saturation (Sa_{O_2}) measures the degree to which hemoglobin is saturated by oxygen.

The serum bicarbonate is another component of arterial blood gases. An elevated bicarbonate level is associated with alkalosis, either primary or as a compensation for respiratory acidosis. A decreased bicarbonate level is usually the result of metabolic acidosis. Bicarbonate levels reflect the renal portion of acid-base regulation. Using these results, the presence and severity of hypoxia and the type and severity of acid-base imbalances can be determined.

Nursing Diagnosis

Assessment reveals clusters of data indicating problems with fluid, electrolyte, acid-base balance, or other related problems (see diagnoses box). Nursing diagnoses have supporting defining characteristics, which are contained within the data base, and expected causes or related factors. Identification of ex-

Examples of Nursing Diagnoses Related To Fluid, Electrolyte, and Acid-Base Disturbances

NANDA-APPROVED NURSING DIAGNOSES

Actual or *potential fluid volume deficit* related to:
- Loss of plasma associated with burns
- Vomiting
- Failure of regulatory mechanisms

Fluid volume excess related to:
- Sodium retention
- Compromised regulatory mechanisms

Impaired tissue integrity related to:
- Edema

Impaired gas exchange related to:
- Altered oxygen supply
- Alveolar-capillary membrane changes
- Altered blood flow
- Altered oxygen-carrying capacity of blood

Decreased cardiac output related to:
- Dysrhythmias associated with electrolyte imbalance

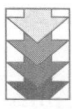 Sample Nursing Diagnostic Process for Fluid, Electrolyte, and Acid-Base Disturbances

Assessment Activities	Defining Characteristics	Nursing Diagnoses
Obtain daily weight measurements.	Client experiences sudden weight loss.	*Fluid volume deficit* related to loss of gastrointestinal fluids
Observe volume of urine output related to intake and specific gravity.	Decreased volume of output in comparison to intake; increased urine specific gravity is present.	
Palpate skin turgor.	Poor skin turgor noted.	
Ask if client is thirsty or weak.	Client verbalizes thirst and weakness.	
Inspect mucous membranes for degree of moisture.	Dry mucous membranes are noted.	
Observe for abnormal losses of fluids.	Client experiences severe vomiting.	
Observe client's orientation to person, place, and time.	Client is confused to place and time.	*Impaired gas exchange* related to alveolar-capillary membrane changes
Observe frequency and purposefulness of behavior.	Client is restless.	
Monitor $Paco_2$.	$Paco_2$ is 56 mm Hg.	
Observe amount and character of sputum.	Client has large amount of thick, creamy lung secretions.	

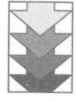 Sample Nursing Care Plan for Fluid Volume Deficit

Nursing diagnosis: *Fluid volume deficit* related to active loss of gastrointestinal fluid
Definition: Fluid volume deficit is the state in which an individual experiences vascular, cellular, or intracellular dehydration related to active loss (Kim, McFarland, McLane, 1991).

Goals	Expected Outcomes	Interventions	Rationale
Fluid balance will return to normal values within 48 hr.	Weight will stabilize by 1/25. Urine output will increase (>70 ml/hr) by 1/24. Specific gravity will decrease (<1.030) by 1/24. Client will have normal skin turgor by 1/24. Client will experience no thirst or weakness by 1/25. Client will have moist mucous membranes by 1/25. Client will experience no vomiting by 1/26.	Encourage intake of small amount of fluids containing electrolytes. Discourage intake of plain water.	Ingesting small volumes may prevent further vomiting. Presence of electrolytes prevents further depletion. Ingestion of plain water causes sodium content in stomach to increase as body attempts to make water isotonic to allow absorption.
		If vomiting occurs before absorption, more fluids and electrolytes are lost. Alter environment to lessen stimuli for vomiting (e.g., keep unpleasant odors to minimum).	This prevents triggering vomiting center in brain.
		Promote bed rest.	Sudden, quick movements may trigger vomiting.
		Measure amount of vomitus.	This allows precise replacement of lost fluid and electrolytes.
		Implement physician orders to provide parenteral fluids containing electrolytes during prolonged periods of vomiting.	These fluids will precisely replace losses.

Adapted from Metheny NM: *Fluid and electrolyte balance: nursing considerations*, Philadelphia, 1987, Lippincott.

pected causes further individualizes the nursing diagnostic statement and subsequent care plan (see diagnostic process box).

Planning

After identifying nursing diagnoses, the nurse develops a care plan (see care plan). The care plan is individualized according to the client's acute or chronic fluid, electrolyte, or acid-base imbalance. A client with a fluid, electrolyte, or acid-base imbalance requires a nursing care plan directed at meeting actual or potential fluid needs. The plan is based on one or more of the following goals:

1. Client's fluid, electrolyte, and acid-base balance are restored and maintained.

2. Causes of imbalance are identified and corrected.

3. Client has no complications from therapies needed to restore balance.

It is particularly important to include the client and family in this planning process. Fluid, electrolyte, and acid-base imbalances often result in subtle changes in behavior or status, and only the family may be familiar enough with the client's usual behavior to identify these changes in a timely manner. The client and family must know preventive measures, signs and symptoms to report, and measures that can be implemented if the imbalance occurs (see box). When medications, special diets, or oral or IV fluids are administered in the home, the client and family need careful teaching so that these interventions are performed safely. In the hospital, the

---

Case Study

ISOTONIC EXCESS

Mr. P. is 87 years old and has a history of heart failure. He has been unable to afford the cardiotonic and diuretic medications ordered to treat the heart failure. He is admitted to the hospital because of severe shortness of breath. He recalls that his shoes have been getting tighter and that he has gained 10 pounds over the last 2 weeks. During physical examination, the nurse notes bilateral jugular vein distension and crackles throughout all lung fields.

This example illustrates two important factors: (1) clients need resources (e.g., financial, psychosocial support, information), and (2) clients and significant others should be able to recognize signs and symptoms of worsening conditions. In this situation, if Mr. P. had recognized the significance of dependent edema and weight gain, the development of pulmonary edema might have been prevented.

HYPONATREMIA

Ms. K. is a 20-year-old woman who is admitted for dehydration possibly resulting from a pituitary dysfunction. She has undergone many diagnostic tests and is receiving 3000 to 4000 ml of IV fluids daily. The nurse notes that Ms. K.'s serum sodium has been gradually decreasing and is now 122 mEq/L. An examination of I & O records reveals that Ms. K. has oliguria and has received 5000 ml more fluid intake in relation to output over the last 3 days. The nurse reports these findings, and it is determined that Ms. K. is experiencing SIADH. The IV fluid rate is decreased, and the serum sodium corrects itself.

This example illustrates the importance of monitoring for trends (in this situation, the decreasing serum so

dium level and fluid retention) so that alterations can be detected early and treated promptly to prevent complications (e.g., a serum sodium level of 110 mEq/L can result in permanent brain damage).

RESPIRATORY ACIDOSIS

Mrs. D. is 68 years old and has smoked more than 1 pack of cigarettes per day for 48 years. She has had chronic obstructive lung disease for 6 years. She developed a productive cough and fever 3 days before. She believed that she could decrease the production of sputum by decreasing her daily intake of fluids. This resulted in a thick sputum that she cannot expectorate. The retained secretions result in a decreased exchange of oxygen and carbon dioxide across the alveolar-capillary membrane.

She is admitted to the hospital and arterial blood gases reveal the following: pH of 7.32, Pao_2 of 49 mm Hg, $Paco_2$ of 56 mm Hg, and bicarbonate level of 26 mEq/L. The decreased pH is associated with an acidotic state, and the elevated Pco_2 is the result of carbon dioxide retention by the lungs, causing acidosis. Decreased diffusion from the alveoli to the capillaries causes the markedly decreased Pao_2, resulting in cellular hypoxia. The bicarbonate level is normal because the renal buffering mechanism has not had time to respond.

In this situation, immediate medical and nursing care for Mrs. D. includes measures to remove the pulmonary secretions (see Chapter 38), provide support for her ventilatory efforts, and treat the respiratory infection. Before discharge, the nurse must teach Mrs. D. the occurrences that place her at risk for respiratory failure, ways to prevent them, and procedures to follow if they recur.

nurse anticipates these needs and initiates teaching before discharge so that the client and family are ready for these procedures. The home health care nurse continues the teaching and evaluates the effectiveness of the home interventions.

Implementation

Prevention of fluid, electrolyte, and acid-base imbalances is important. When imbalances occur, the nurse removes or treats the cause of the imbalance if possible. Other nursing interventions aim to correct fluid and electrolyte imbalances.

When volume is depleted, fluids and electrolytes can be replaced orally, with IV administration of fluids and blood components, or through TPN if the fluid deficit is caused by malnutrition. For clients with FVE, the nurse implements measures to reduce fluids, such as fluid intake restrictions, reduced sodium intake, and administration of diuretics.

Correcting Fluid and Electrolyte Imbalances

DAILY WEIGHING. All clients with fluid and electrolyte disturbances should be weighed daily. In this way, fluid retention can be detected early because 5 to 10 pounds of fluid is retained before edema appears (Metheny, 1987). Weight should be determined at the same time each day, and the same scale should be used. The client should also wear the same clothes, or if a bed scale is used, the same number of sheets should be on the scale with each daily weighing.

I & O MEASUREMENTS. In addition to providing assessment data, I & O records provide current information about fluid balance. These measurements can indicate whether excess fluid is excreted in the urine. Likewise, they can show whether the excretion of fluids through the kidneys has diminished.

ENTERAL REPLACEMENT OF FLUIDS. Fluids are replaced enterally via the oral route and tube feedings.

Oral. Unless contraindicated, oral replacement of fluids and electrolytes is appropriate as long as the client is not vomiting, is not experiencing a profound fluid loss, or does not have a mechanical obstruction in the gastrointestinal tract. Clients unable to tolerate solid foods may still be able to ingest fluids. Oral fluid replacement is easily implemented in the home and hospital. Mild illnesses such as viral diarrhea and respiratory tract infections, as well as fevers, may cause fluid and electrolyte disturbances. In addition, clients recovering from anesthesia or gastrointestinal surgery usually receive clear liquids first and then advance to a regular diet if they tolerate the liquids. When replacing fluids by mouth in a client with a FVE, the nurse should choose fluids with adequate calories and electrolyte content (Table 39-6), but if fluids are replaced through a feeding tube, the physician usually prescribes a nutritional supplement (see Chapter 35).

Tube Feedings. A feeding tube may be appropriate when the client's gastrointestinal tract is healthy but the client cannot ingest fluids (for example, after oral surgery or with impaired swallowing). All feeding tubes require a physician's order. Fluids can also be replaced through nasogastric, gastrostomy, or jejunostomy feeding tubes (see Chapter 35).

RESTRICTION OF FLUIDS. Clients who retain fluids and have FVE require restricted fluid intake. These

TABLE 39-6 Oral Fluids								
Solution	Calories (kcal/30ml)	HCO_3^- (mEq/L)	Na^+ (mEq/L)	Ca^{++} (mEq/L)	K^+ (mEq/L)	Mg^{++} (mEq/L)	Cl^- (mEq/L)	Predominant Carbohydrate
Water								
Pedialyte (oral electrolyte solution)	6.0	—	30.0	4.0	20.0	4.0	30.0	Dextrose
Lytren (oral electrolyte solution)	9.0 (isotonic)	—	30.0	4.0	25.0	4.0	25.0	Glucose
5% glucose in water	6.0	—	—	—	—	—	—	Glucose
10% glucose in water	12.0	—	—	—	—	—	—	Glucose
Pepsi-Cola	13.2	7.3	6.5	—	0.8	—	—	Sucrose
Coca-Cola	14.4	13.4	0.4	—	12.0	—	—	Sucrose
Ginger ale	10.0	3.6	3.5	—	—	—	—	Sucrose
Gatorade	5.5	—	23.0	—	3.0	—	17.0	Glucose, sucrose
Lemon-lime soda	9.6	—	7.5	0.3	0.2	—	—	—
Broth, beef (canned)	6.0	—	55.0	—	—	—	—	—
Tea, unsweetened	0.25	—	—	—	—	Trace	—	—

From Groër MW: *Physiology and pathophysiology of the body fluids,* St Louis, 1981, Mosby–Year Book.

clients have renal failure, congestive heart failure, cor pulmonale, or SIADH.

Fluid restriction is often difficult for clients, particularly if they are taking medications that dry the oral mucous membranes. The nurse should explain the reason that fluids are restricted. The client should also know how much fluid is permitted and that ice chips, gelatin, and ice cream are fluids.

Given this information, the client should help decide the amount of fluid with each meal, between meals, before bed, and with medications. Frequently clients on fluid restriction can swallow a number of pills with as little as 1 ounce (30 ml) of liquid.

A good rule of thumb for fluid restrictions is to allow half the allotted total oral fluids between 8 AM and 4 PM, the period when clients usually are more active and receive two meals and most of their oral medications. Then an additional two fifths of the allotted total fluid is permitted between 4 PM and 11 PM, permitting fluids with meals and evening visitors. Between the hours of 11 PM and 8 AM the remainder of the total fluid allotment is permitted. Because the client is usually asleep during this period, fluid needs decrease.

The nurse should also ensure that clients receive their favorite fluids (unless contraindicated). For example, if a client can have only 200 ml of fluid with breakfast and hates cranberry juice but likes apple or grape juice, the nurse should be sure that the diet kitchen has this information.

PARENTERAL REPLACEMENT OF FLUID AND ELECTROLYTES. Fluid and electrolytes may be replaced by infusion directly into the blood rather than intake through the digestive system. Parenteral replacement includes TPN, IV fluid and electrolyte therapy, and blood replacement.

With increasing risk to health care workers for transmission of the human immunodeficiency virus (HIV), the causative agent presently identified for acquired immunodeficiency syndrome (AIDS), and other infectious diseases, the principles of body fluid substance isolation must be practiced when administering parenteral fluids (see Chapter 18). The Centers for Disease Control (CDC) has issued guidelines pertaining to exposure to body substances (see box).

Vascular Access Devices. Vascular access devices are catheters, cannulas, or infusion ports designed for long-term repeated access to the vascular system (Fig. 39-9). These devices are safer than peripherally placed catheters and have improved mechanisms for delivering long-term IV therapy. Recently, peripherally inserted central catheters (PICC) have begun to be used for clients with poor peripheral venous access who need infusion therapy for only 1

Universal Precautions to Prevent Transmission of HIV as They Pertain to IV Therapy

- Gloves should be worn to reduce risk of exposure to blood, body fluids containing visible blood, and other fluids to which universal precautions apply.[*]
- Hands and other skin surfaces should be washed immediately and thoroughly if contaminated with blood or other body fluids. Hands should be washed immediately after gloves are removed.[†]
- To prevent needlestick injuries, needles should not be recapped, purposely bent or broken by hand, removed from disposable syringes, or otherwise manipulated by hand.[†]
- Used needles, syringes, and IV fluid equipment should be placed in puncture-resistant containers for disposal. The puncture-resistant containers should be located as close as practical to the use area.[†]
- Health care workers who have exudative lesions or weeping dermatitis should refrain from all direct care and from handling invasive equipment until the condition resolves.[†]
- Pregnant health care workers are not known to be at greater risk of contracting HIV infections than health care workers who are not pregnant. However, if a health care worker develops HIV infection during pregnancy, the infant is at risk of infection resulting from perinatal transmission. Because of this risk, pregnant health care workers should strictly adhere to precautions to minimize the risk of HIV transmission.[†]

[*]From Occupational Safety and Health Act: bloodborne pathogens, *Federal Registry* 56(235): 64175, 1991.
[†]From Centers for Disease Control: Recommendations for prevention of HIV transmission in health care settings, *MMWR* 36(suppl 25):3s, 1987.

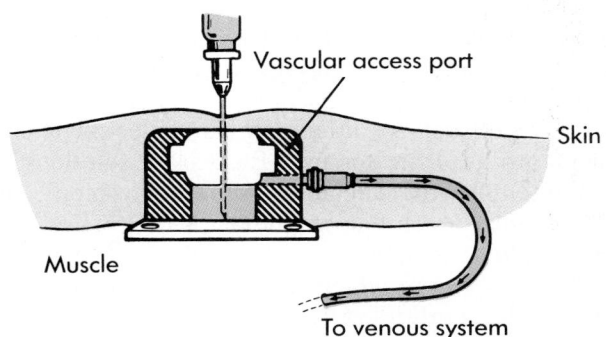

Vascular access port

Skin

Muscle

To venous system

Fig. 39-9 Examples of implantable vascular access devices.

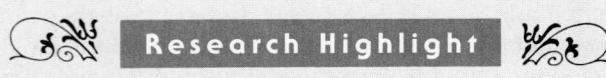

Research Highlight

Schulmeister's study compared the use of sterile gloves and the removal of povidone-iodine by alcohol to the use of no sterile gloves and alcohol followed by povidone-iodine. None of the 40 clients in either group experienced fever or septicemia (widespread infection carried through the bloodstream). Three clients in the gloved procedure group experienced irritation attributed to the removal of the povidone-iodine by the alcohol. The nongloved technique was more time efficient and cost effective ($3.50 versus $17.50).

Schulmeister L: A comparison of skin preparation procedures for accessing implanted ports, *NITA* 10(1):45, 1987.

week to 3 months (Silvestri, Masoorli, 1990). Increased use of central venous catheters and implanted infusion ports require nurses to be educated in the care of these devices (see research highlight).

TPN. TPN is a nutritionally adequate hypertonic solution consisting of glucose and other nutrients and electrolytes given through an indwelling peripheral or central IV catheter. Chapter 35 fully describes TPN administration.

IV Therapy. The goal of IV fluid administration is to correct or prevent fluid and electrolyte disturbances. For example, a client with third-degree burns over 40% of the body is critically ill and needs careful regulation of IV therapy because of continual changes in fluid and electrolyte balance. A client allowed to ingest nothing by mouth for 2 days after an appendectomy receives IV fluid replacement to prevent fluid and electrolyte imbalances. The infusion is discontinued with resumption of normal oral intake.

When IV fluid administration is required, the nurse must know the correct solution, equipment needed, and procedures required to initiate an infusion, regulate the fluid infusion rate; maintain the system; identify and correct problems; and discontinue the infusion.

Types of solutions. Many prepared electrolyte solutions are available for use. Electrolyte solutions fall into the following categories: isotonic, hypotonic, and hypertonic. A solution is isotonic if the total electrolyte content approximates 310 mEq/L. A hypotonic solution is one in which the total electrolyte content is below 250 mEq/L. A hypertonic solution has a total electrolyte content of 375 mEq/L or greater (Metheny, 1987).

In general, isotonic fluids are used for extracellular volume replacement (for example, FVD after prolonged vomiting). The decision to use a hypotonic or hypertonic solution is based on the specific electrolyte imbalance.

Certain additives are frequently instilled into IV solutions, most commonly vitamins and potassium chloride (KCl). The physician's order includes required additives, for example:

Bottle #1: 1000 ml—D5W with 20 mEq KCl and 1 ampule of multivitamins

Clients with normal kidneys who are receiving nothing by mouth should have potassium added to IV solutions. If the physician's order for such a client does not include potassium, the nurse should double-check the order. The body has no conservation mechanism for potassium, and even when the serum level falls, the kidneys continue to excrete potassium. If there is no potassium intake orally or parenterally, hypokalemia can quickly develop. The nurse collects and, if necessary, prepares the solution using the five rights of medication administration described in Chapter 21.

Equipment. Correct selection and preparation of equipment assist in safe and quick placement of an IV line. Because fluids are instilled into the bloodstream, sterile technique is necessary, and therefore the nurse must have all needed equipment organized and at the bedside. The nurse who must leave the bedside to obtain another piece of equipment must start the procedure again. Standard equipment includes IV solution and tubing, needle or catheter (Procedure 39-1, Step 6), antiseptic, tourniquet, gloves, and dressing. An armboard to restrict hand movement may also be used for some clients.

The arm board is used to reduce movement of the extremity with the IV infusion in place and to maintain the extremity in a flat position. Arm boards may be used if the IV insertion site is on the dorsal surface of the hand.

Other IV equipment includes solution containers, various types of tubing, and volume control devices. An injectable antibiotic medication such as ampicillin may be added to a small IV solution bag containing 50 to 100 ml and "piggybacked" into the main line to be administered over 30 to 60 minutes (see Chapter 21). The type and amount of solution depend on the medication added and the client's physiological status. For example, when ampicillin is administered parenterally, it must be infused within 1 hour after it is prepared. Otherwise the medication loses its potency. Different tubing types are used to administer a medication. A drug given rapidly needs to be infused with macrodrip tubing, which delivers large drops so that a rapid rate can be maintained. In addition, clients may require IV extension tubing to increase mobility or facilitate changes in position. **Volume control devices** are used with children, with clients with renal or cardiac failure, and with critically ill clients to prevent sudden, uncontrolled rapid infusion of large volumes. (Additional information on volume control devices is presented in the section on regulating the infusion flow rate.)

Initiating the intravenous line. After the equipment is collected at the bedside, the nurse prepares to place the IV line by assessing the client for the venipuncture site (Procedure 39-1 on p. 1306). A **venipuncture** is a technique in which a vein is punctured transcutaneously by a sharp, rigid stylet (for example, a butterfly needle or a metal needle) partially covered by a plastic catheter (over-the-needle catheter or ONC) or by a needle attached to a syringe. The general purposes of venipuncture are to collect a blood specimen, instill a medication, start an IV infusion, and inject a radiopaque or radioactive tracer for special examinations. Procedure 39-1 describes venipuncture for IV fluid infusion.

The nurse assessing clients for potential venipuncture sites should consider conditions, cautions, and contraindications that exclude certain sites. Because very young and old clients have fragile veins, the nurse should avoid sites that are easily moved or bumped such as the dorsal surface of the hand. It is often difficult to insert IV lines in clients who have had many venipunctures because their veins may be sclerosed with scar tissue. Obese clients present problems for venipuncture because of the difficulty in locating superficial veins. The veins of thin and emaciated clients' veins are also difficult to puncture. Although they may be visible, the veins are quite fragile, and as a result the nurse may puncture through entire veins instead of placing needles or catheters within them. When clients are severely dehydrated or have decreased extracellular fluid, such as with shock, the veins may collapse. The collapse results from decreased circulating blood volume. When veins collapse, venipuncture becomes extremely difficult, but it is also a lifesaving measure. For these difficult clients, venipuncture should be performed by someone with expertise. Some agencies have IV therapy teams whose members have special expertise in performing venipunctures and maintaining IV infusions.

Venipuncture is contraindicated in a site that has signs of infection, infiltration, or thrombosis (clotting). An infected site is red, tender, swollen, and possibly warm to the touch. Exudate may be present. An infected site is not used because of the danger of introducing bacteria from the skin surface into the bloodstream.

Common IV puncture sites include the hand and arm (Fig. 39-10, *A* and *B*). However, the superficial

Text continued on p. 1310.

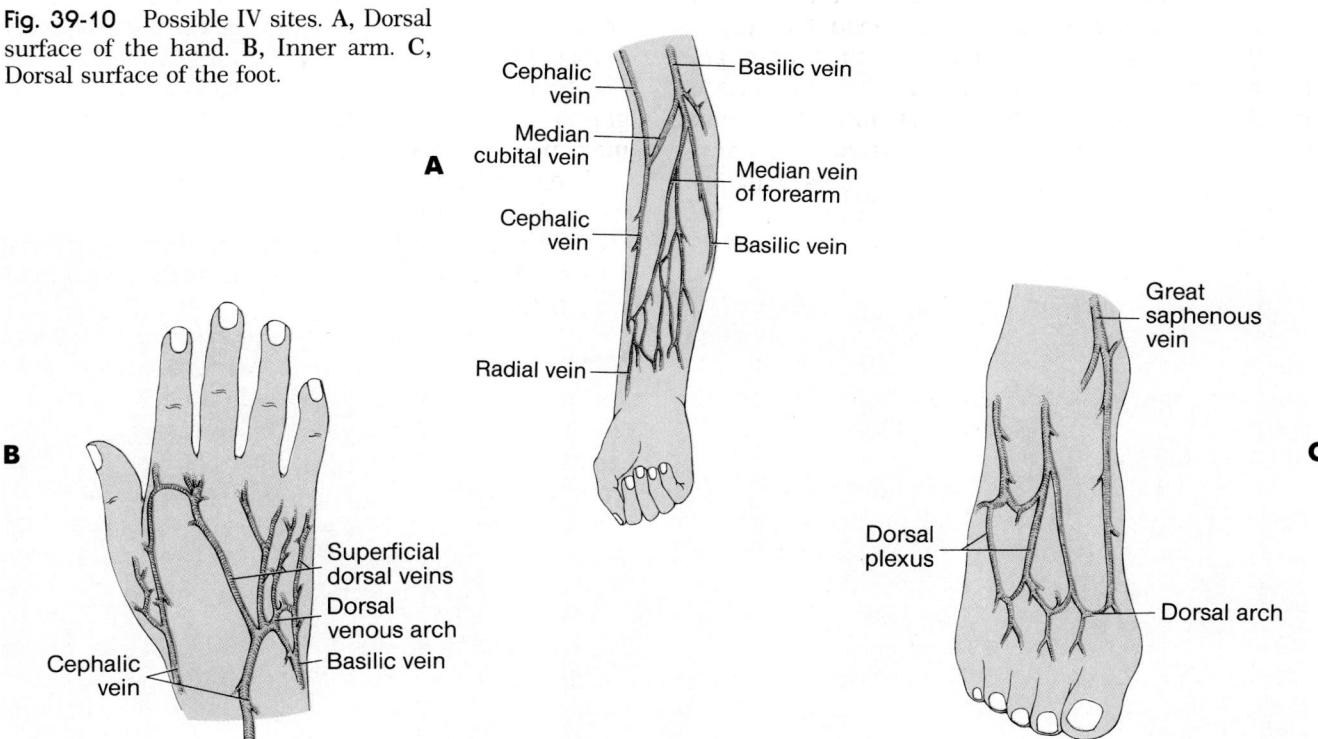

Fig. 39-10   Possible IV sites. **A,** Dorsal surface of the hand. **B,** Inner arm. **C,** Dorsal surface of the foot.

Venipuncture with an Over-the-Needle Plastic Catheter

STEPS	RATIONALE

1. Observe for signs and symptoms indicating fluid or electrolyte imbalances:
  a. Sunken eyes
  b. Periorbital edema
  c. Greater than 2% increase or decrease in body weight
  d. Dry mucous membranes
  e. Flattened or distended neck veins
  f. Change from baseline vital signs
  g. Irregular pulse rhythm
  h. Auscultation of crackles in lungs
  i. Poor skin turgor
  j. Increased or decreased bowel sounds
  k. Decreased urine output
  l. Behavioral changes
  m. Confusion
	Because fluid and electrolyte disturbances can affect every system in body, nurse must systematically assess client to identify abnormalities related to fluid or electrolyte imbalance. Daily weight measurements document fluid retention or loss. Change in body weight of 1 kg corresponds to 1 L of fluid retention or loss.

2. Review physician's fluid replacement orders.	Venipuncture before IV therapy is an invasive technique requiring a physician's order. IV fluids are medications and require an order.

3. Assemble necessary equipment for initiating IV line:
  a. Correct solution
  b. Proper needle for venipuncture (see Step 5 illustration)
  c. Infusion set (infants and children require a 60 drop/ml [gtt/ml] drip and often volume control device)
  d. IV tubing
  e. Alcohol and providone-iodine cleansing swabs
  f. Tourniquet
  g. Arm board
  h. Gauze or transparent dressing and povidone-iodine solution or ointment
  i. Tape
  j. Towel to place under client's hand
	Correct solution and preparation of equipment assist in safe and quick placement of IV line.

Step 5

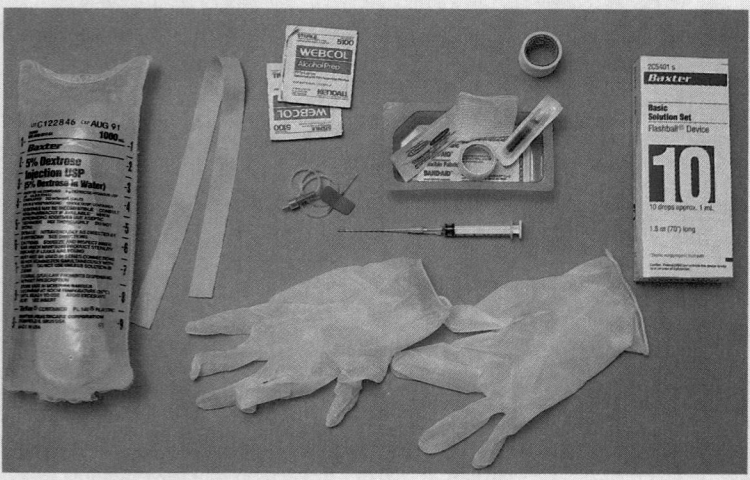

Step 11

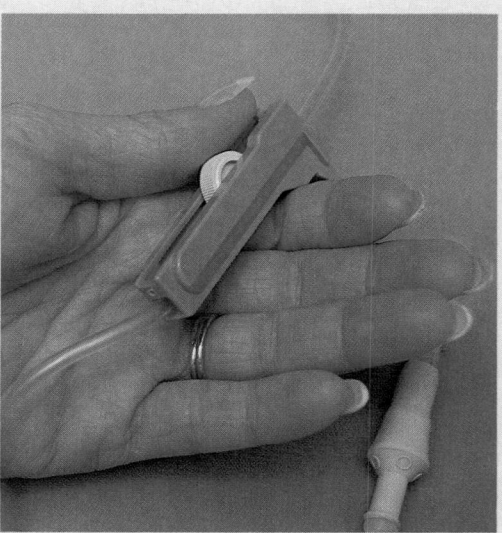

STEPS	RATIONALE
k. IV pole	
l. Disposable gloves	
4. Identify client and explain procedure.	Reduces anxiety and promotes cooperation.
5. Organize equipment on clutter-free bedside stand or overbed table (see illustration).	Reduces risk of contamination and accidents.
6. Identify accessible vein for placement of IV needle or catheter: a. Avoid bony prominences. b. Use most distal portion of vein first. c. Avoid placing IV line over client's wrist. d. Avoid placing IV line in dominant hand.	Promotes ease and placement of IV catheter and needle.
7. Wash hands.	Reduces transmission of microorganisms.
8. Open sterile packages using aseptic technique (see Chapter 18).	Maintains sterility of equipment and reduces spread of microorganisms.
9. Check solution, using five rights of drug administration. Make sure prescribed additives, such as potassium and vitamins, have been added.	IV solutions are medications and should be double-checked to reduce risk of error.
NOTE: When using bottled IV solution, remove metal cap and metal and rubber disks beneath cap.	Permits entry of infusion tubing into solution.
10. Open infusion set, maintaining sterility of both ends.	Prevents bacteria from entering infusion equipment and thus bloodstream.
11. Place roller clamp (see illustration) about 2-4 cm (1-2 in) below drip chamber, and move roller clamp to *off* position.	Close proximity of roller clamp to drip chamber allows more accurate regulation of flow rate. Prevents accidental spillage of fluid on client, nurse, bed, or floor.
12. Insert infusion set into fluid bag: a. Remove protective cover from IV bag without touching opening (see illustration).	Maintains sterility of solution.
b. Remove protector cap from tubing insertion spike, not touching spike, and insert spike into opening of IV bag (see illustration). Or insert spike into black rubber stopper of IV bottle.	Permits entry of infusion solution into tubing. Prevents contamination of solution from contaminated insertion spike.

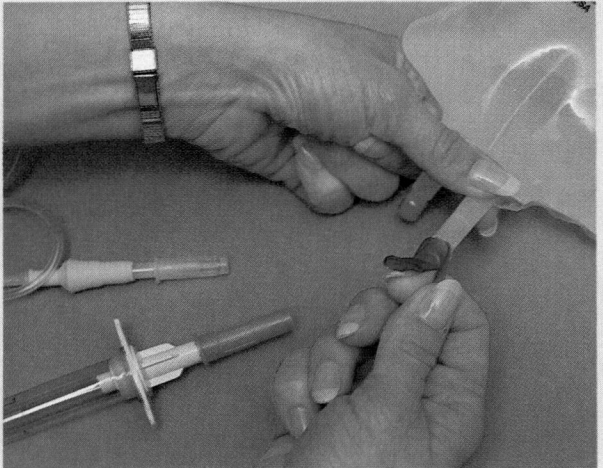

Step 12a

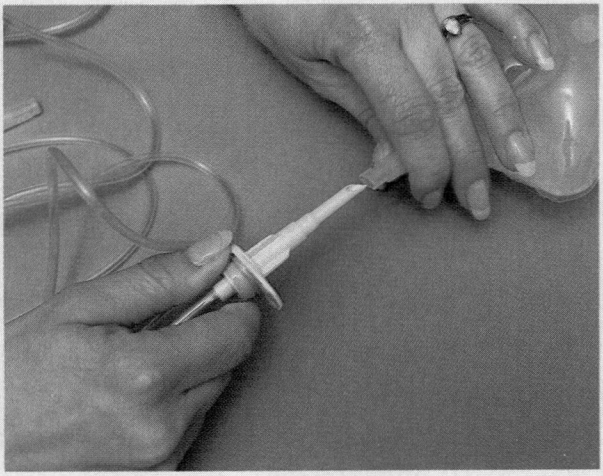

Step 12b

Venipuncture with an Over-the-Needle Plastic Catheter

STEPS	RATIONALE
13. Fill infusion tubing:	
a. Compress drip chamber and release.	Creates suction effect. Fluid enters drip chamber.
b. Remove needle protector and release roller clamp to allow fluid to travel from drip chamber through tubing to needle adapter. Return roller clamp to *off* position after tube is filled.	Removes air from tubing and permits it to fill with solution.
c. Be certain tubing is clear of air and air bubbles.	Large air bubbles can act as emboli.
d. Replace needle protector.	Maintains system sterility.
14. Select appropriate IV needle or ONC.	Needle or ONC is necessary to puncture vein and instill IV fluid.
15. Select distal site of vein to be used.	If sclerosing or damage to vein has occurred, proximal site of same vein is still usable.
16. If large amount of body hair is present at needle insertion site, clip it.	Reduces risk of contamination from bacteria on hair. Also assists in maintaining intactness of IV dressing and makes removal of adhesive tape less painful. Shaving may cause microabrasions and predisposes to infection (Roth, 1992).
17. If possible, place extremity in dependent position.	Permits venous dilation and visibility.
18. Place tourniquet 10-12 cm (5-6 in) above insertion site. Tourniquet should obstruct venous, not arterial, flow (see illustration). Check distal pulse.	Diminished arterial flow prevents venous filling.
19. Select well-dilated vein (see illustration). Methods to foster vein dilation include stroking extremity from proximal to distal, opening and closing fist, lightly tapping over vein, and applying warmth (Delaney, Lauer, 1988). NOTE: Be sure needle adapter end of infusion set is nearby and on sterile gauze or towel.	Increases venous dilation. Permits smooth, quick connection of infusion to needle after vein is punctured.
20. Apply disposable gloves.	Decreases exposure to HIV, hepatitis, and other blood-borne organisms.
21. Cleanse insertion site with firm, concentric, circular motion outward from insertion site using povidone-iodine solution. Allow to dry (see illustration). If client is allergic to iodine, use 70% alcohol for 30 sec.	Povidone-iodine is topical antiinfective that reduces skin surface bacteria. It must dry to be effective.
22. Perform venipuncture. Anchor vein by placing thumb over vein and by stretching skin against direction of insertion 2-3 in distal to site.	

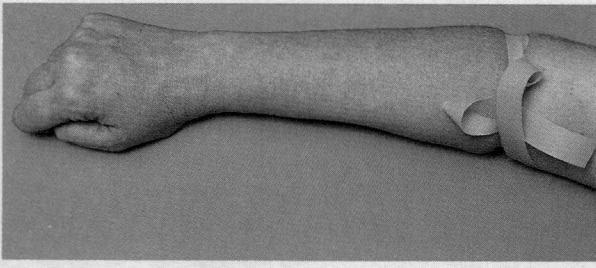

Step 18

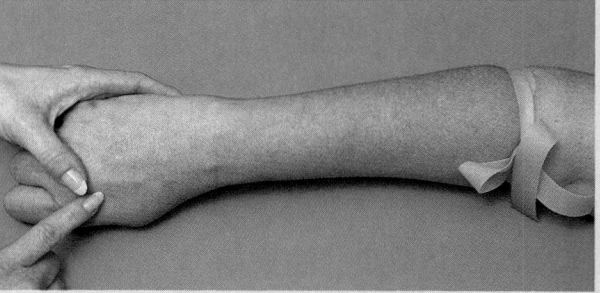

Step 19

STEPS	RATIONALE

a. *ONC:* insert bevel at 20- to 30-degree angle in direction of venous blood return distal to actual site of venipuncture.

Allows nurse to place needle parallel with vein. Thus when vein is punctured, risk of puncturing both sides is reduced.

b. *Butterfly needle:* place needle at 20- to 30-degree angle with bevel up, about 1 cm (½ in) distal to site of venipuncture.

23. Look for blood return through tubing of butterfly needle or flashback chamber on ONC, indicating that needle has entered vein. Lower needle until almost flush with skin. Advance catheter approximately ¼ in into vein and then loosen stylet (see illustration). Continue advancing flexible catheter or butterfly needle until hub rests at venipuncture site.

Increased venous pressure from tourniquet increases backflow of blood into catheter or tubing. Stylet helps puncture skin and advance catheter but must be removed to avoid puncture of vein.

24. Stabilizing catheter with one hand, release tourniquet and remove stylet from ONC.

Reduces backflow of blood.

25. Connect needle adapter of infusion to hub of ONC or needle. Do not touch point of entry of needle adapter or inside hub of ONC (see illustration on p. 1310).

Prompt connection of infusion set maintains patency of vein. Maintains sterility.

26. Release roller clamp to begin infusion at rate to maintain patency of IV line.

Permits venous flow and prevents clotting of vein and obstruction of flow of IV solution.

27. Secure IV catheter or needle:

a. Place narrow piece (½ in) of tape under hub of catheter with adhesive side up and cross tape over hub.

Prevents accidental removal of catheter from vein.

b. Place small amount of povidone-iodine solution or ointment at venipuncture site. Allow solution to dry.

Povidone-iodine solution or ointment is topical antiseptic germicide that reduces bacteria on skin and decreases risk of local or systemic infection. When transparent dressing is used, povidone-iodine solution is recommended; ointment interferes with adherence of dressing to skin.

c. Place second piece of narrow tape directly across catheter's hub.

Prevents accidental disconnection of IV infusion.

d. Place transparent dressing over venipuncture site, following manufacturer's directions (see illustration on p. 1310). (Alternate method, place 2 × 2 gauze dressing over venipuncture site and catheter hub. Do not cover connection between IV tubing and catheter hub. Secure it with two 1-in pieces of tape.)

Transparent dressing allows continual observation of venipuncture site. (Allows tubing changes without disturbing dressing.)

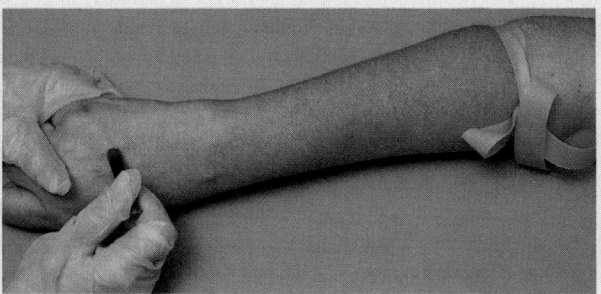

Step 21

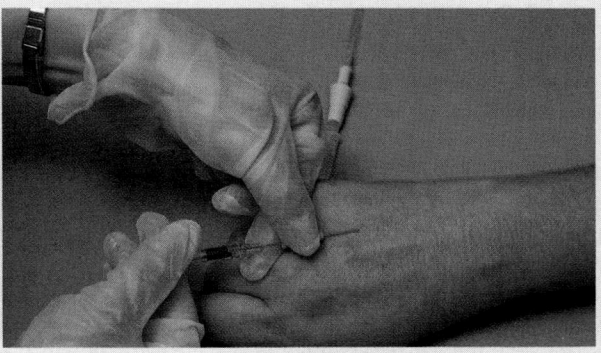

Step 23

Venipuncture with an Over-the-Needle Plastic Catheter

STEPS	RATIONALE
e. Secure infusion tubing to catheter with piece of 1-in tape.	Further stabilizes connection of infusion to catheter.
28. Write date, time of placement of IV line, size of needle, and nurse's initial and title on IV dressing.	Provides immediate data as to time of IV insertion and subsequent dressing changes.
29. Adjust flow rate to correct gtt/min.	Maintains correct rate of flow for IV solution.
30. Discard gloves and supplies and wash hands.	Reduces transmission of microorganisms.
31. Observe client every hr to determine response to fluid therapy: a. Correct amount of solution infused as prescribed b. Proper flow rate (gtt/min) c. Patency of IV catheter or needle d. Absence of infiltration, phlebitis, or inflammation	Provides continuous evaluation of type and amount of fluid delivered to client. Hourly inspection prevents accidental fluid overload or inadequate infusion rate.
32. Record in nurses' notes type of fluid, insertion site, flow rate, size and type of IV catheter or needle, and time infusion was begun. Note response to IV fluid, amount infused, and integrity and patency of IV system (whether infusing by gravity or by pump), according to agency policy.	Documents initiation of IV fluid therapy as ordered by physician. Follow-up documentation provides data about response to therapy.

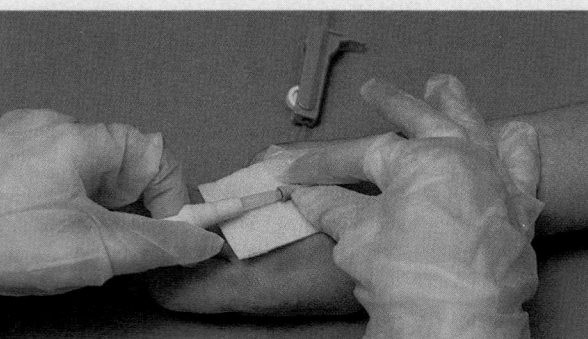

Step 25

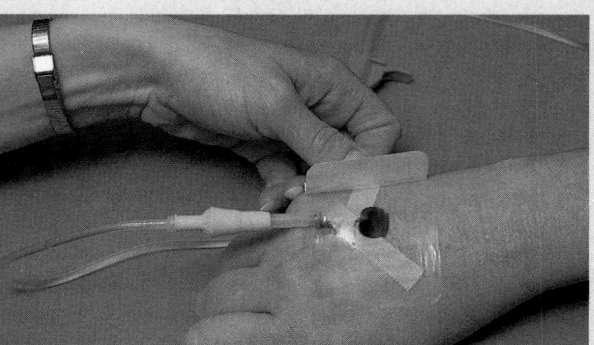

Step 27d

veins of the foot can be used if the client is not ambulatory. The use of the foot for an IV site is more common with pediatric clients but is generally avoided in the adult.

After completing the assessment for venipuncture sites, the nurse carefully explains the procedure to the client. The nurse should explain the reason the infusion was ordered, its expected results, and the nurse's expectations of the client (see teaching box).

The venipuncture and IV infusion procedure has many steps. Procedure 39-1 describes the steps for using an ONC, but the procedure is the same with a butterfly needle.

Large catheters placed into a central vein such as the subclavian vein are used to monitor central venous pressure and to deliver large volumes of fluids and TPN. Although these catheters are inserted by physicians, nurses are responsible for maintaining them.

Regulating the infusion flow rate. After the IV infusion is secured and the IV line is patent, the nurse must regulate the rate of infusion according to physician's orders (Procedure 39-2). An infusion rate that is too slow can lead to further cardiovascular and circulatory collapse in a client who is dehydrated, in shock, or critically ill. An infusion rate that is too

Client Teaching for IV Fluids

OBJECTIVE

- Client will verbalize appropriate procedures for co-operation and participation in administration of IV fluids.

TEACHING STRATEGIES

- Discuss the signs and symptoms of infiltration and phlebitis, including swelling, pain, and redness around the venipuncture site.
- Teach the importance of reporting the occurrence of these signs and symptoms to the nurse.
- Discuss the importance of the reason for not read-justing the flow rate or bending or lying on the IV tubing.
- Demonstrate how to avoid placing pressure on the venipuncture site, maintaining the extremity with the venipuncture site at an appropriate height, and avoiding dislodging the infusion catheter when changing positions, ambulating, or changing clothes.
- Demonstrate how to perform hygiene measures while ensuring that the IV site remains clean and dry.

EVALUATION

- Observe client during hygiene measures.
- Observe client changing positions, ambulating, and changing clothes.
- Quiz client concerning signs and symptoms that should be reported and methods to maintain correct flow rate.

Adapted from LaRocca J, Otto S: *Pocket guide to intravenous therapy,* St Louis, 1989, Mosby–Year Book.

rapid can result in fluid overload, which is particularly dangerous in some cardiovascular, renal, and neurological disorders. The nurse calculates the infusion rate to prevent too-slow or too-rapid administration of fluids.

Infusion pumps regulate the flow of IV fluids. They are designed to deliver a measured amount of fluid over a specified period of time or to deliver fluids based on the flow rate or drops per minute. Infusion pumps have an electronic eye that counts the number of drops flowing from an IV administration set. The electronic eye must be placed on the drip chamber below the origin of the drop and above the fluid level in the chamber.

The infusion pump's electronic eye monitors the drip rate. If the required number of drops per minute is not achieved, an alarm will sound. The alarm can be sounded if the IV bag is empty, the infusion tubing is kinked, or the vein is clotted. If the alarm sounds, the nurse investigates and corrects the cause of the drip rate problem. IV flow rates can be affected by the patency of the IV needle or catheter, infiltration, a knot or kink in the tubing, the height of the solution, and the position of the client's extremity.

Patency of the IV needle or catheter means that there are no clots at the tip of the needle or catheter and that the catheter or needle tip is not against the vein wall. The nurse can assess patency by lowering the IV bag below the level of the insertion site and observing for a blood return. If no blood return occurs and fluid does not flow easily from the drip chamber when the roller clamp is opened, a clot may be present at the catheter tip.

An infiltration may be present when the IV insertion site is cool, clammy, swollen, and in some cases painful. An **infiltration** occurs when the IV needle or catheter has become dislodged from the vein and is in the subcutaneous space. When an infiltration occurs, the IV line must be discontinued and a new line inserted.

A knot or kink in the tubing can decrease the flow rate. Occasionally the tubing is kinked under the IV dressing, which requires the nurse to open the dressing to locate the problem. Frequently the flow rate resumes after the tubing is straight. The client may also occlude the tubing by lying or sitting on it. The height of the IV bag can affect flow rates. Raising the bag may increase the rate because of gravity.

The extremity position can decrease flow rates, particularly with IV sites at the wrist or elbow. Occasionally the use of an arm board helps keep the joint extended. Sometimes, it is more comfortable for the client to have an infusion started in a new location rather than dealing with a site that causes problems. However, before discontinuing an infusion hampered by an extremity position, the nurse must be sure that the client has other accessible veins.

These influences on IV flow rates can occur with any client at any time. When caring for a client with an infusion, the nurse should assess the site and the infusion rate at least every hour.

Children, older adults, clients with severe head trauma, and clients susceptible to volume overload must be protected from sudden increases in infusion volumes. Sudden increases can occur accidentally. For example, a restless client may, with a sudden movement, loosen the roller clamp and increase the flow rate, or the flow rate may be accidentally increased if the client ambulates. A sudden increase in IV volume can result in serious illness or death. Volume control devices, such as a Volutrol or buret, can

Regulating IV Flow Rates

STEPS

RATIONALE

1. Observe patency of IV line and needle:

   For fluid to infuse at proper rate, IV line and needle must be free of kinks, knots, and clots.

   a. Open drip regulator and observe for rapid flow of fluid from IV solution into drip chamber, and then close drip regulator to prescribed rate.

   Rapid flow of fluid into drip chamber denotes patency of IV line. Closing drip to prescribed rate prevents fluid overload.

   b. If fluid does not flow, lower IV fluid bottle or bag below level of infusion site and observe for blood return.

   May indicate that needle is patent and in vein. Venous pressure is greater than pressure in IV tubing.

2. Check medical record for correct solution and additives. Usual order includes solution for 24 hr, usually divided into 2 or 3 L. Occasionally, IV order contains only 1 L to keep vein open (KVO). Record also shows time over which each liter is to infuse.

   IV fluids are medications. Five rights are followed to decrease chance of medication error.

3. Know drop factor in gtt/ml of infusion set:

Microdrip:	60 gtt/ml
Macrodrip (Metheny, 1987):	
Abbott Laboratory	15 gtt/ml
Travenol Laboratory	10 gtt/ml
McGaw Laboratory	15 gtt/ml

   Microdroppers, also called *minidrip,* universally deliver 60 gtt/ml. However, commercial parenteral administration sets for macrodrip exist. Nurse should know which company's infusion set that hospital uses.

4. Select one of following formulas to calculate flow rate (gtt/min) after determining ml/hr if necessary (Metheny, 1987):

   After hourly rate has been determined, formula will give correct flow rate in gtt/min.

   $$ml/hr = \frac{total\ volume\ (ml)}{hours\ of\ infusion}$$

   a. $\dfrac{ml/hr}{60\ min} = ml/min$

   Drop factor × ml/min = drops/min

   OR

   b. $\dfrac{ml/hr\ \times\ drop\ factor}{60\ min} = drops/min$

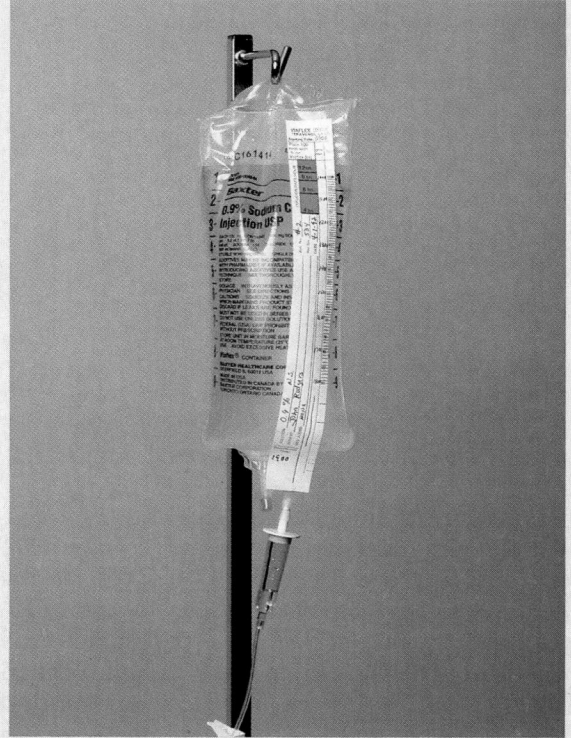

Step 7

STEPS	RATIONALE

5. If infusion pump or volume control device is used, place it at bedside.

Increases accuracy of fluid delivery rate.

6. Determine hourly rate by dividing volume by hours, for example:

$$\frac{1000 \text{ ml}}{8} = 125 \text{ ml/hr}$$

or if 4 L are ordered for 24 hr:

$$\frac{4000}{24} = 166.7 \text{ ml} = 167 \text{ ml/hr}$$

Provides for infusion of fluid at steady rate during prescribed period.

7. Place volume label vertically on IV bottle or bag next to volume markings. Mark adhesive tape based on hourly flow rate. For example, if entire volume of fluid is to be infused over 8, 10, or 12 hr, respective designations will be marked on tape (see illustration).

Gives nurse visual cue as to whether fluids are being administered over correct period.

8. After hourly rate has been determined, calculate min rate based on drop factor of infusion set. Minidrip or microdrip infusion set has drop factor of 60 gtt/ml. Regular drip or macrodrip infusion set used in this example has drop factor of 15 gtt/ml. Using formula, calculate minute flow rates: Bottle 1: 1000 ml with 20 mEq KCl   Microdrip:

$$\frac{125 \text{ ml} \times 60 \text{ gtt/ml}}{60 \text{ min}} = \frac{7500 \text{ gtt}}{60 \text{ min}} = 125 \text{ gtt/min}$$

Macrodrip:

$$\frac{125 \text{ ml} \times 15 \text{ gtt/ml}}{60 \text{ min}} = 31\text{-}32 \text{ gtt/min}$$

Allows nurse to calculate minute flow rate based on this formula:

$$\frac{\text{Total volume} \times \text{drop factor}}{\text{Infusion time in minutes}} = \text{gtt/min}$$

9. Time flow rate by counting drops in drip chamber for 1 min by watch, and then adjust roller clamp to increase or decrease rate of infusion (see illustration). Repeat until flow rate is accurate.

Ensures accurate rate of infusion. Determines whether fluids are being administered too slowly or fast.

10. Follow this procedure for infusion pump:
a. Place electronic eye on drip chamber below origin of drop and above fluid level in chamber (see illustration).

IV infusion pumps monitor fluids based on flow rate or gtt/min. Infusion pump has electronic eye that counts number of drops flowing from administration set.

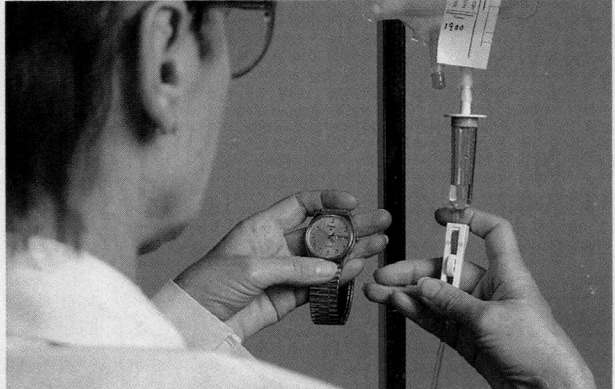

Step 9

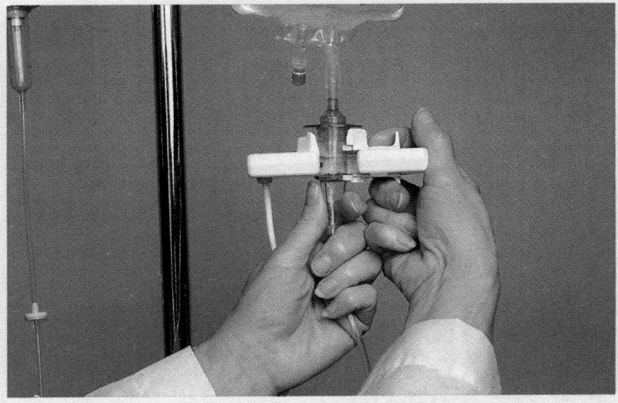

Step 10a

Regulating IV Flow Rates

STEPS	RATIONALE

b. Place IV infusion tubing with ridges of control box in direction of flow (i.e., portion of tubing nearest IV bag at top and portion of tubing nearest client at bottom). Required gtt/min or volume per hr is selected, door to control chamber is shut, power button is turned on, and start button is pressed.

Infusion pumps move fluid by compressing and milking tubing, thus propelling fluid through tubing.

c. Ensure that drip regulator on tubing is in *open* position while infusion pump is in use.

d. Monitor infusion rates at least hourly.

Infusion pumps are not infallible and do not replace frequent, accurate assessments.

e. Assess patency of IV system when alarm sounds.

Alarm indicates that electronic eye has not noted precise number of drips from drip chamber.

11. Follow this procedure for volume control device:

   a. Place volume control device between IV bag and insertion spike of infusion set (see illustration).

Reduces risk of sudden increases in fluid volume.

   b. Place 2 hr's worth of fluid into device.

Prevents IV line from running dry if nurse does not return in exactly 60 min. In addition, if accidental increase in flow rate occurs, client receives at most only 2 hr's fluid.

   c. Assess IV system at least hourly and add fluid to device. Regulate flow rate.

Maintains patency of IV system.

12. Observe client hourly to determine response to IV therapy and restoration of fluid and electrolyte balance. Also check IV site for signs of infiltration, inflammation, and phlebitis.

Signs and symptoms of dehydration or overhydration warrant changing rate of fluid infused. Signs of infiltration, inflammation, and phlebitis warrant changing IV site.

13. Record rate of infusion, gtt/min and ml/hr, in client's chart as required by agency policy.

Documents that prescribed IV flow is being delivered to client.

Step 11a

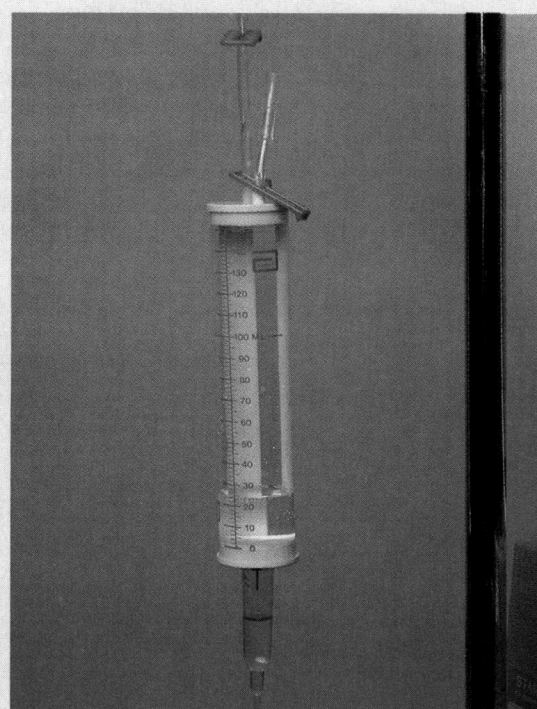

prevent sudden increases in volume (see Chapter 21).

The volume control device is placed between the IV bag and insertion spike of the infusion set or may be part of the infusion set. Most control devices can hold 150 ml. Nurses usually put 2 hours' worth of fluid in the buret. Therefore if the client is to have only 30 ml per hour, the nurse places 60 ml in the volume control device. If the nurse does not return to the client in exactly 1 hour, the IV line does not run dry. In addition, if an accidental increase in flow rate occurs, the client receives at most only 2 hours' allotment of fluid instead of 500 or 1000 ml.

Maintaining the system. After the IV line is in place and the flow rate is regulated, the nurse must maintain the system. The nurse provides comfort and assistance with hygiene measures, meals, and ambulation (see teaching box on p. 1311). IV catheters and drugs, especially those with potassium, can cause discomfort and burning sensations. Clients must be reassured that occasional discomfort is normal. Sometimes, discomfort is relieved by repositioning the extremity, but occasionally it is necessary to start a new IV line in a larger vein.

Because a client with an infusion in the arm finds it difficult to meet hygiene needs, the nurse should help with bathing and changing gowns. It helps to use gowns specifically made with snaps along the top sleeve seam to facilitate changing the gown without disturbing the venipuncture site. Gowns are changed by following six steps for maximal arm mobility and speed:

1. Remove the sleeve of the gown from the uninvolved arm (without IV).
2. Remove the sleeve of the gown from the involved arm (with IV).
3. Remove the IV bottle or bag from its stand and pass it and the tubing through the sleeve.
4. Place the IV bottle or bag and tubing through the sleeve of the clean gown and hang on its stand.
5. Place the involved arm through the gown sleeve.
6. Place the uninvolved arm through the gown sleeve.

The client with an arm or a hand infusion is able to walk, unless contraindicated. A walking IV pole, a standard IV pole with wheels, is needed. The nurse helps the client out of bed and places the pole next to the involved arm. The client is instructed to hold onto the pole with the involved hand and to push it while walking. The nurse assesses the equipment to make sure that the IV bag is at the proper height, that there is no tension on the tubing, and that the flow rate is correct. The nurse should instruct the client to report any blood in the tubing, a stoppage in the flow, or increased discomfort.

Because clients receiving IV therapy to restore a FVD may require frequent changing of solutions, the nurse should allow adequate time for this. Occasionally, clients require an IV infusion to deliver a drug every 4, 6, or 8 hours. An hourly infusion flow of about 10 to 15 ml/hr is used to KVO using a microdrip infusion set. A new solution bag or bottle should be hung at least once every 24 hours, even if the old bag is not empty, because the sterility of the solution cannot be guaranteed for longer than a day. When an IV solution container is changed, the nurse uses sterile technique and follows an organized procedure (Procedure 39-3 on p. 1316).

Technically, IV tubing can remain sterile for 48 hours. However, most institutions recommend that new sterile tubing be used every 24 hours. The procedure is much easier and more efficient if the nurse changes the infusion tubing when preparing to hang a new IV bag or bottle (Procedure 39-4 on p. 1318). To prevent entry of bacteria into the bloodstream, sterility must be maintained.

The dressing over the IV insertion site is changed according to hospital policy. Usually, gauze or transparent dressings are used (Procedure 39-4). Transparent dressings enable the nurse to continually assess venipuncture sites. The previously recommended practice of daily dressing changes has been reduced to every 48 to 72 hours when IV sites are changed (Maki, 1987). This practice is more cost effective and does not increase the risk of infection.

Complications of IV Therapy. The major complications of IV therapy are infiltration, phlebitis, fluid overload, bleeding, and infection. An infiltration occurs when IV fluids enter the subcutaneous space around the venipuncture site. This is manifested as swelling (from increased tissue fluid) and pallor (caused by decreased circulation) around the venipuncture site. Fluid may be flowing through the IV line at a decreased rate or may have stopped. Pain may also occur, usually resulting from edema, and increases in proportion to the amount of infiltration.

When infiltration occurs, infusion must be discontinued, and if necessary, the needle is reinserted into another extremity. To reduce discomfort caused by infiltration, the nurse raises the extremity, which promotes venous drainage and helps decrease edema, and wraps the extremity in a warm towel for 20 minutes, which increases circulation and reduces pain and edema.

Phlebitis is an inflammation of the vein caused by the catheter or by the chemical irritation of additives and drugs given intravenously. Signs and symptoms include pain, increased skin temperature over the vein, and in some instances redness traveling along the path of the vein. The IV line must be discontinued and a new line inserted in another vein. Warm,

Changing IV Solutions and Tubing

STEPS	RATIONALE

CHANGING IV SOLUTION

1. Identify client. Review physician's orders and have next solution prepared at least 1 hr before needed. If solution is prepared in pharmacy, be sure it has been delivered to floor. Check that solution is correct and properly labeled.

Ensures that correct client undergoes procedure. Prevents finding empty IV bag without having replacement. Checking prevents medication error. If order is written for KVO, change solution every 24 hr. Sterility of solution cannot be ensured longer than 24 hr (CDC, 1982).

2. Prepare to change solution when less than 50 ml remains in bottle or bag.

Prevents air from entering IV tubing and maintains patency of tubing and catheter or needle.

3. Be sure drip chamber is half full.

Provides IV fluid to vein while bag is being changed.

4. Wash hands.

Reduces transmission of microorganisms.

5. Prepare new solution for changing. If using plastic bag, remove protective cover from entry site. If using glass bottle, remove metal cap, metal disk, and rubber disk. Maintain sterility of entry site on bag or bottle.

Permits quick, smooth, and organized change from old to new solution.

6. Move roller clamp to reduce flow rate.

Prevents solution remaining in drip chamber from emptying while changing solutions.

7. Remove old solution from IV pole.

Brings work to nurse's eye level.

8. Quickly remove spike from old IV solution, and without touching tip, spike new solution bottle.

Reduces risk of solution in drip chamber (Step 3) running dry and maintains sterility.

9. Hang new bag or bottle of solution. Discard empty bag or bottle according to agency policy.

Allows gravity to assist with delivery of IV fluid into drip chamber.

10. Check for air in tubing.

Reduces risk of air embolus.

11. Make sure drip chamber contains solution.

Reduces risk of air entering IV tubing.

12. Regulate flow rate to prescribed rate.

Restores fluid balance and delivers IV fluid as ordered.

13. Observe IV system for patency, absence of infiltration phlebitis, and inflammation. Observe response to IV therapy.

Provides ongoing evaluation of response to IV therapy.

CHANGING IV TUBING

14. Determine when new infusion set is warranted:
    a. Hanging first solution of day
    b. Puncture of infusion tubing
    c. Contamination of tubing

    d. Occlusion of IV tubing (e.g., after infusion of packed RBCs, whole blood, or albumin)
    e. Date on tubing indicating that tubing has been in place 48 hr.

Changing tubing prevents infection. Procedure is simplified by changing tubing with new solution.
Punctured tubing results in leakage of fluid.
Contamination of tubing can allow entry of bacteria into bloodstream.
Whole blood or blood component products may occlude or partially occlude IV tubing.
CDC (1982) recommends changing tubing every 48 hr.

15. Assemble the following:
    a. Infusion tubing
    b. Sterile 2 × 2 gauze
    c. If new IV dressing must be applied:
       (1) Sterile 2 × 2 gauze or transparent dressing
       (2) Providone-iodine ointment or solution
       (3) Adhesive remover
       (4) Alcohol swabs
       (5) Strips of tape or polyurethrane film dressing
       (6) Disposable gloves

Enables nurse to efficiently and safely complete procedure.

STEPS	RATIONALE
16. Explain procedure to client.	Promotes cooperation and prevents sudden movement of extremity, which could dislodge needle or catheter.
17. Wash hands.	Reduces transmission of microorganisms.
18. Open new infusion set, keeping protective coverings over infusion spike and insertion site for butterfly needle or ONC.	Provides nurse with ready access to new infusion set and maintains sterility of infusion set.
19. Apply nonsterile disposable gloves.	Decreases risk of exposure to HIV, hepatitis, and other blood-borne bacteria.
20. Place sterile 2 × 2 gauze on bed near IV puncture site.	Provides sterile field for new sterile needle adapter before connection to IV needle or catheter.
21. If needle or catheter hub is not visible, remove IV dressing. Do not remove tape that secures needle or catheter to skin.	Needle hub must be accessible to provide smooth transition when removing old tubing and inserting new tubing.
22. Take new IV tubing and move roller clamp to *off* position.	Prevents spillage of solution after new bag or bottle is spiked.
23. Slow rate of infusion by regulating drip rate on old tubing.	Prevents complete infusion of solution remaining in tubing.
24. With old tubing in place, compress drip chamber and fill chamber.	Provides surplus in drip chamber so that there is sufficient fluid to maintain patency while changing tubing.
25. Discontinue old tubing from solution and hang drip chamber over IV pole.	Allows fluid to continue to flow through catheter while new tubing is prepared.
26. Place insertion spike of new tubing into old IV solution opening and hang solution on pole.	Permits flow of fluid from solution into new infusion tubing.
27. Compress and release drip chamber on new tubing.	Allows drip chamber to fill and promotes rapid, smooth flow of solution through new tubing.
28. Open roller clamp, remove protective cap from needle adapter, and flush tubing with solution.	Removes air from tubing and replaces it with fluid.
29. Place needle adapter of new IV tubing, with protective cap off, between sterile 2 × 2 gauze near IV site.	Will allow smooth, quick insertion of new tubing into needle hub while maintaining sterility of infusion tubing.
30. Turn roller clamp on old tubing to *off* position.	Prevents spillage of fluid as tubing is removed from needle hub.
31. Stabilize hub of IV catheter or needle, gently pull out old tubing, and quickly insert needle adapter of new tubing into hub.	Prevents accidental displacement of catheter or needle. Prevents clot formation in catheter or needle.
32. Open roller clamp on new tubing.	Permits solution to enter catheter or tubing.
33. Regulate IV drip according to physician's orders and monitor rate hourly.	Maintains infusion flow at prescribed rate.
34. If necessary, apply new dressing (Procedure 39-4).	Reduces risk of bacterial infection from skin.
35. Discard old tubing and gloves in container for contaminated materials, and wash hands.	Reduces transmission of microorganisms.
36. Evaluate flow rate and observe connection site for leakage.	Maintains prescribed rate of flow of IV therapy and determines whether fit is secure
37. Record changing of tubing and solution on client's record and place piece of tape with date and time below level of drip chamber. Record fluid infused on I & O form.	Documents procedure and records that measures to maintain sterility were carried out. Provides visual cue to all care providers of when IV tubing was changed.

Changing an IV Dressing

STEPS	RATIONALE
1. Assess need to change dressing:	
a. Determine when IV dressing was last changed. Many institutions require nurse to write date and time on dressing itself.	Provides information regarding length of time that present dressing has been in place. In addition, nurse is able to plan for dressing change.
b. Observe present dressing for moisture.	Moisture is medium for bacterial growth. Moisture on sterile dressing renders dressing contaminated.
c. Observe present dressing for intactness.	Nonadhering dressing increases risk of bacterial contamination to venipuncture site or displacement of catheter.
d. Observe IV system for proper functioning or complications: kinks in infusion tubing or IV catheter, infiltration, and inflammation.	Unexplained decrease in flow rate or pain and swelling at venipuncture site require nurse to investigate placement and patency of IV catheter.
2. Assemble necessary equipment:	Enables nurse to efficiently and safely complete procedure.
a. Sterile 2 × 2 gauze or transparent dressing	
b. Povidone-iodine ointment or solution	
c. Adhesive remover	
d. Alcohol swabs	
e. Strips of tape or polyurethane film dressing	
f. Disposable gloves	
3. Explain procedure to client. Explain that affected extremity must remain still for length of procedure.	Assists in obtaining client cooperation and gives time frame around which client can plan personal activities.
4. Wash hands.	Reduces transmission of microorganisms.
5. Apply disposable gloves.	Reduces risk of contact with HIV, hepatitis, and other blood-borne bacteria.
6. Remove transparent dressing in direction of client's hair growth, or remove tape and gauze from old dressing one layer at time. For both transparent and gauze dressings, leave tape that secures IV needle or catheter in place.	Prevents accidental displacement of catheter or needle, which can occur if catheter tubing becomes tangled between two layers of dressing.
7. If infiltration, phlebitis, or clot occurs or if ordered to do so by physician, discontinue IV infusion:	
a. Turn roller clamp to *off* position.	Prevents spillage of IV fluid on bed, client, nurse, or floor.
b. Place gauze or alcohol pad over venipuncture site and remove catheter or needle by pulling straight away from site.	Prevents damage to vein.
c. Apply pressure to site for 1 to 2 min.	Controls bleeding and hematoma formation.
8. If IV is infusing properly, remove tape securing needle or catheter. Stabilize needle or catheter with one hand.	Exposes venipuncture site. Prevents accidental displacement of catheter or needle.
9. Use adhesive remover to cleanse skin and remove adhesive residue.	Adhesive residue decreases ability of new tape to adhere tightly to skin.
10. Using circular motion from site outward, cleanse insertion site with povidone-iodine solution. Allow to dry for 30 sec.	Circular motion prevents cross-contamination from skin bacteria near venipuncture site. Povidone-iodine is topical antiinfective that reduces skin surface bacteria.
11. Replace strip of ½-in adhesive tape under catheter with adhesive side up to anchor catheter or needle.	Prevents accidental displacement of catheter or needle.
12. Place povidone-iodine ointment or solution on venipuncture site. Allow solution to dry. Place second piece of narrow tape directly across catheter.	Povidone-iodine solution or ointment is topical antiseptic germicide that reduces skin bacteria and reduces risk of local or systemic infection. When transparent dressing is used, povidone-iodine solution is recommended; ointment interferes with adherence of dressing to skin.

STEPS	RATIONALE
13. Place 2 × 2 gauze or transparent dressing over venipuncture site. If transparent dressing is selected, apply it in direction of hair growth (see manufacturer's directions).	Provides barrier against bacteria. Reduces discomfort when dressing is removed.
14. Anchor IV tubing with additional pieces of tape. (Do not cover transparent dressing.)	Prevents accidental displacement of needle or catheter or separation of tubing from needle adapter.
15. Place date and time of dressing change directly on dressing (following agency policy).	Documents dressing change.
16. Discard equipment in appropriate container, remove and dispose of gloves, and wash hands.	Reduces transmission of microorganisms.
17. Reassess functioning and patency of IV system in response to changing dressing.	Validates that IV is patent and functioning correctly.
18. Record in nurses' notes time dressing was changed, types of dressing used, patency of IV system, and observation of venipuncture site.	Documents that dressing was changed, description of IV system functioning, and venipuncture site free of infection.

moist heat on the site of phlebitis can offer some relief to the client. Phlebitis is potentially dangerous because blood clots (thrombophlebitis) can occur and in some cases may result in emboli.

Fluid overload occurs when the client has received too-rapid administration of solutions. Assessment findings are similar to those of FVE. The nurse should slow the rate of infusion, notify the physician, and be prepared to give diuretic medications. Prompt action is necessary to prevent worsening of the condition or even death.

Bleeding can occur around the venipuncture site during infusion. Bleeding is common in clients who have received heparin or who have a clotting disorder. If bleeding occurs around the venipuncture site and the catheter is within the vein, a pressure dressing may be applied over the site to control it. Bleeding from a vein is usually a slow, continuous seepage and is not fatal.

Infusion-related infections are caused by contamination of the IV system, venipuncture site, or the solution itself (Messner, Gorse, 1987). Clinical manifestations of these infections include purulent thrombophlebitis, cellulitis, and site infections, as evidenced by erythema, swelling, and pain at the venipuncture site.

Infusion-related infections can be reduced by four interventions. The nurse uses vigorous handwashing techniques to remove gram-negative organisms before applying gloves for the venipuncture procedure (Tomford, Hershey, McLakin, 1984). The nurse also changes KVO IV solutions at least every 24 hours. The nurse should also replace all peripheral venous catheters, including heparin locks, at least every 72 hours and preferably every 48 hours (CDC, 1987). In addition, the nurse maintains sterility of the IV system when changing tubing, solutions, and dressings (Axnick, Yarbrough, 1984).

Discontinuing IV Infusions. Discontinuing an infusion is necessary after the prescribed amount of fluids has been infused, when an infiltration occurs, if phlebitis is present, or if the infusion catheter or needle develops a clot at its tip. The nurse discontinuing an infusion first applies disposable gloves and removes the tape and dressing in the same manner as for the daily infusion dressing changes. The nurse then moves the roller clamp to the *off* position to prevent spillage of IV fluid. The nurse places a gauze or alcohol pad over the venipuncture site and, using the other hand, withdraws the catheter needle by pulling straight back from the puncture site. The nurse applies pressure to the site for 1 to 2 minutes to control bleeding and prevent hematoma formation. Clients who have received heparin require longer pressure because of the action of heparin on blood-clotting mechanisms. If needed, the nurse applies a sterile dressing over the venipuncture site. The nurse records the amount of fluid infused and the time of the discontinuation.

Blood Replacement. Blood replacement or transfusion is the IV administration of whole blood or a component such as plasma, packed RBCs, or platelets.

The following list includes objectives for blood transfusion:

1. To increase circulating blood volume after surgery, trauma, or hemorrhage
2. To increase the number of RBCs and to maintain hemoglobin levels in clients with severe anemia
3. To provide selected cellular components as replacement therapy (for example, plasma-clotting factors to help control bleeding in clients with hemophilia)

Blood Groups and Types. The most important grouping for transfusion is the ABO system, which includes the following groups: A, B, O, and AB. The determination of blood groups is based on the presence or absence of A and B red cell antigens. Individuals with A antigens, B antigens, or no antigens belong to groups A, B, and O, respectively. The person with A and B antigens have AB blood (Porth, 1986).

Agglutinins, or antibodies that work against the A and B antigens, are called *anti-A* and *anti-B agglutinins*. These agglutinins occur naturally (Patrick et al, 1986). Individuals with type A blood naturally produce anti-B agglutinins in their plasma. Similarly, type B individuals naturally produce anti-A agglutinins in their plasma. A type O individual naturally produces both agglutinins, which is why a person with type O blood is considered a universal donor. An AB type individual produces neither antibody, which is why type AB individuals can be universal recipients. If blood that is mismatched with the client's blood is transfused, a transfusion reaction occurs. The **transfusion reaction** is an antigen-antibody reaction and can range from a mild response to severe anaphylactic shock.

Another consideration when matching for blood transfusions is the Rh factor, an antigenic substance in the RBCs of most people. A person with the factor is Rh positive, whereas a person without it is Rh negative. If the blood given to an Rh-positive person is Rh negative, **hemolysis** (RBC destruction) and anemia occur. If an Rh-negative mother gives birth to an Rh-positive baby, the infant may be exposed to antibodies in the mother's Rh-negative blood and destruction of the infant's RBC's can result.

Autotransfusion. **Autotransfusion** is the collection, anticoagulation, filtration, and reinfusion of blood from an active bleeding site. Because the reinfused blood is the client's own, there are many advantages to autotransfusion. The risk of technical errors of blood typing and crossmatching is eliminated. Possible adverse effects associated with homologous blood transfusion are also eliminated. In addition, dependence on homologous blood banks is reduced, and possible exposure to serum hepatitis, HIV, and other blood-borne infections are eliminated.

When an elective surgical procedure is anticipated and transfusions are required, some individuals choose to give one or more units of their own blood in advance. This blood is stored and is available intraoperatively and postoperatively. This, too, is a type of autotransfusion.

Blood transfusions. Transfusing blood or blood components is a nursing procedure. The nurse is responsible for assessment before and during the transfusion and regulation of the transfusion (Procedure 39-5).

If the client has an IV line in place, the nurse should assess the venipuncture site for signs of infection or infiltration. The nurse should also determine whether the IV venipuncture was performed with an 18- or 19-gauge catheter. The large-gauge catheter promotes flow because the molecules of blood and its components are larger than the molecules of IV fluids. A large catheter also prevents hemolysis. The nurse should determine that the catheter is patent and functioning properly. Tubing for blood transfusion has an in-line filter and should be primed with 0.9% normal saline. Use of any other IV solution results in hemolysis.

Pretransfusion assessment also includes obtaining information from the client. The nurse asks whether the client knows the reason for the blood transfusion and whether the client has ever had a transfusion or a transfusion reaction. A client who has had a transfusion reaction is usually at no greater risk for a reaction with a subsequent transfusion. However, the client may be anxious about the transfusion, necessitating nursing intervention.

Pretransfusion assessment must include a baseline measurement of vital signs. These values must be recorded before the nurse gives any blood products because a change in vital signs can indicate a reaction.

When giving a transfusion, the nurse explains the procedure, asks the client to report any side effects, and makes sure the client has signed an informed consent. The nurse establishes the IV line, primes it with 0.9% normal saline, and hangs a solution container of 0.9% normal saline for use after the transfusion. The nurse then follows established procedures for obtaining blood products. With another registered nurse, the nurse checks the identity of the blood products, the client, and the compatibility of the blood to be infused against the client's blood. The infusion is begun slowly. The infusion is maintained, side effects are monitored, and the transfusion is recorded.

Clients with severe blood loss such as with a hemorrhage may receive rapid transfusions through a central venous pressure catheter. A blood-warming device is often necessary because the tip of the cen-

STEPS	RATIONALE
1. Explain procedure to client. Determine if there have been prior transfusions and note reactions, if any.	Clients who have had blood transfusion reactions in past may have greater fear of transfusion. Past occurrence of certain reactions may increase possibility of recurrence.
2. Ask client to report chills, headaches, itching, or rash immediately.	These are signs of transfusion reaction. Prompt reporting and discontinuation of transfusion can help minimize reaction.
3. Be sure client has signed consent forms.	Some agencies require clients to sign consent forms before receiving blood component transfusions.
4. Wash hands. Apply disposable gloves.	Reduces risk for transmission of HIV, hepatitis, and other blood-borne bacteria.
5. Establish IV line with large-gauge (#18 or #19) catheter. Refer to Procedure 39-1 for venipuncture technique.	Large-gauge catheters permit infusion of whole blood and prevent hemolysis.
6. Use infusion tubing that has in-line filter. Tubing should also be Y-type administration set (see illustration).	Filter removes debris and tiny clots from blood. Y-type set permits administration of additional products or volume expanders easily and immediate infusion of isotonic 0.9% sodium chloride solution after completion of isotonic infusion.
7. Hang solution container of 0.9% normal saline to be administered after blood infusion.	Prevents hemolysis of RBCs.
8. Follow agency protocol in obtaining blood products from blood bank. Request blood when you are ready to use it.	Whole blood or packed RBCs must remain in cold (1° to 6° C) environment.

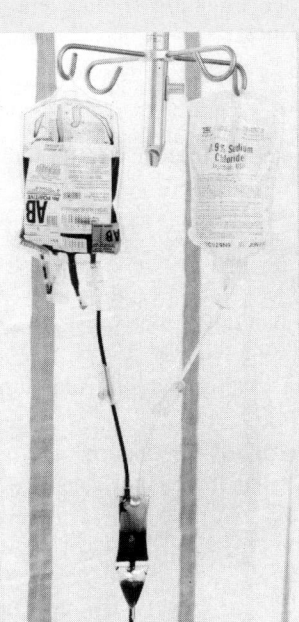

Step 6

Administering a Blood Transfusion

STEPS	RATIONALE
9. With another registered nurse, correctly identify blood product and client:	One nurse reads out loud while other nurse listens and double-checks information. Reduces risk of error.
a. Check compatibility tag attached to blood bag and information on bag itself.	Verifies that ABO group, Rh type, and unit number match.
b. For whole blood, check ABO group and Rh type, which is on client's chart.	Verifies that information matches that on compatibility tag and blood tag.
c. Double-check blood product with physician's order.	Verifies correct blood component.
d. Check expiration data on bag.	After 21 days, blood has only 70% to 80% of original number of cells and 23 mEq/L of potassium (Metheny, Snively, 1983).
e. Inspect blood for clots.	Anticoagulant citrate-phosphate-dextrose (CPD) is added to blood and permits preserved blood to be stored for 21 days. Another anticoagulant, citrate-phosphate-dextrose-adenine (CPD-A), allows storage for 35 days (Metheny, Snively, 1983). If clots are present, return blood to blood bank.
f. Ask client's name, and check arm band.	Verifies correct client. Do not administer blood to client without arm band. Identification name and number on wristband must be identical to those on blood compatibility tag.
10. Obtain baseline vital signs.	Verifies pretransfusion temperature, pulse rate, blood pressure, and respirations.
11. Begin transfusion:	
a. Prime infusion line with 0.9% normal saline.	Isotonic saline prevents hemolysis.
b. Begin transfusion slowly by first filling in-line filter.	If filter is not filled, transfusion will not infuse properly.
c. Adjust rate to 2 ml/min for first 15 min, and remain with client. If you suspect reaction, *stop* transfusion, flush line with normal saline, infuse normal saline slowly, and notify blood bank and physician.	Allows detection of reaction while infusing smallest possible volume of blood product. Flushing line prevents further infusion of blood product.
12. Monitor vital signs:	
a. Take vital signs every 5 min for first 15 min of transfusion and every hr thereafter.	Documents change in vital sign status that could indicate early warning of reaction.
b. Observe client for flushing, itching, dyspnea, hives, and rash.	May indicate early sign of reaction.
13. Maintain prescribed infusion rate using infusion pumps, if necessary.	Infusion pumps maintain prescribed rate.
14. Remove and dispose of gloves. Wash hands.	Reduces transmission of microorganisms.
15. Continually observe for adverse reactions.	Adverse reactions can occur at any point during transfusion (Table 39-8).
16. Record administration of blood or blood product.	Documents administration of blood component.
17. When infusion is completed, return blood bag and tubing to blood bank.	Provides material for analysis if reaction is later discovered.

tral venous pressure catheter lies in the superior vena cava, above the right atrium. Rapid administration of cold blood can result in cardiac dysrhythmias (LaRocca, Otto, 1989).

During blood infusion the client is at risk for a reaction, particularly during the first 15 minutes. Therefore the nurse should remain with the client and assess skin color and vital signs. The nurse will continue to monitor the client and obtain vital signs periodically during the transfusion as directed by agency policy (often every 15 minutes). The nurse will take vital signs when a reaction is suspected. The rate of a transfusion is usually specified in the physician's orders. Ideally a unit of whole blood or packed RBCs is transfused in 2 hours. However, a client with a low fluid tolerance can have a transfusion over 4 hours (Querin, Stahl, 1983).

Transfusion reactions. A **transfusion reaction** is a systemic response by the body to blood incompatible with that of the recipient. It is caused by RBC incompatibility or allergic sensitivity to the leukocytes, platelets, or plasma protein components of the transfused blood or to the potassium or citrate preservative in the blood. Blood transfusion can also result in disease transmission.

Several types of reactions can result from blood transfusions. General adverse reactions (Table 39-7 on p. 1324) range from immediate onset of fever, chills, and skin rash to hypotension, shock, and a delayed reaction that may not occur until several days or weeks after the transfusion.

A second category of reactions includes diseases transmitted by blood donors who have no symptoms of problems. Certain diseases transmitted through transfusions are malaria and hepatitis and HIV infection. Because all units of blood collected must undergo serological testing and HIV screening, the risk of acquiring blood-borne infections from transfusions is reduced.

Correct administration of blood and blood products reduces the risk of transfusion reactions. The nurse, although not actually a participant in the blood labeling process, is responsible for determining that the blood delivered to the nursing unit corresponds to the client's blood type listed in the medical record. Two nurses should check the blood against the client's identification number, blood group, and complete name. If even a minor discrepancy exists, the blood should not be given and the blood bank laboratory should be notified.

In addition to allergic reactions and the transmission of illnesses, certain risks (hyperkalemia, hypocalcemia, and circulatory overload) are associated with blood transfusions. Stored blood may cause hyperkalemia. Blood that is 1 day old has a plasma potassium content of approximately 7 mEq/L, and blood stored for 21 days has a plasma potassium content of 23 mEq/L (Metheny, Snively, 1983). The increase in potassium is related to the destruction of red blood cells. At the end of 21 days, 20% to 30% of cells are destroyed. Because the major intracellular cation is potassium, potassium enters the plasma as cells are destroyed. The potassium level of a client receiving several units of blood should be measured frequently. If the potassium level is elevated, measures to lower the serum level may be used, such as ion exchange resin for example, sodium polystyrene sulfonate [Kayexalate] or hemodialysis.

Clients receiving massive transfusions can develop hypocalcemia because of the action of the citrated blood as it combines with ionized calcium (Metheny, 1987). The preservative often added to blood, CPD contains more citrate than is needed to combine with calcium in the blood collected for the transfusion. Therefore when transfused blood is infused into the bloodstream, the preservative combines with the ionized calcium, and tetany can result. The risk of hypocalcemia increases with the number of blood transfusions the client receives.

Iron overload (hemosiderosis) can occur in clients who receive frequent transfusions. One milliliter of blood contains 1 mg of iron (Mountcastle, 1979). **Hemosiderosis** is an abnormal deposit of iron in a variety of tissues, usually in the form of hemosiderin, an iron-rich pigment that is a product of hemolysis. Clients at risk for hemosiderosis are those with illnesses involving chronic, extensive destruction of RBCs, such as anemias, thalassemia major, or splenic dysfunction.

Circulatory overload is a risk when a client receives massive whole blood or packed RBC transfusions for hemorrhagic shock or when a client with normal blood volume receives blood. Clients particularly at risk for circulatory overload are older adults and those with cardiopulmonary and renal failure diseases.

Transfusion reactions are life threatening, but prompt nursing intervention can maintain the client's physiological stability. In the event of a suspected reaction, the nurse should do the following:

1. Stop the transfusion immediately.
2. "Piggyback" 0.9% normal saline into the IV line. The nurse should not turn off the blood and turn on the 0.9% normal saline on the Y-tubing infusion set, which will merely infuse the blood in the tubing into the client. Even a small amount of mismatched blood can cause a major reaction.
3. Notify the physician.
4. Remain with the client, observe signs and symptoms, and monitor vital signs every 5 minutes.

TABLE 39-7   Adverse Reactions to Blood Transfusions

Description	Cause	Onset	Signs and Symptoms	Nursing Actions
FEBRILE NONHEMOLYTIC				
Is most common Usually occurs in previous transfusion recipients or multiparous clients	Antigen-antibody reaction to WBCs or platelets contained in blood product	Immediately or within 6 hr after transfusion	Fever (with or without chills), headache, nausea and vomiting, nonproductive cough, hypotension, chest pain, dyspnea	Stop transfusion. Keep vein open. Notify physician and blood bank. Take vital signs as necessary.
ALLERGIC URTICARIAL				
Is generally innocuous	Allergic reaction to plasma-soluble antigen contained in blood product	Any time during transfusion or within 1 hr after transfusion	Skin rash	Slow transfusion to KVO rate. Notify physician and blood bank.
DELAYED HEMOLYTIC				
Is more common than acute hemolytic reaction Is frequently missed Occurs in previous transfusion recipients or multiparous clients	Incompatibility of RBC antigens other than ABO group	Days to weeks after transfusion	Decreasing hemoglobin level, possible persistent low-grade fever	Notify physician and blood bank.
ACUTE HEMOLYTIC				
Can be life threatening	ABO group incompatibility	Usually during first 5 to 15 min, but any time during transfusion	*Mild form:* fever, chills, back pain, hypotension, nausea, vomiting, flushing, hematuria, oliguria *Severe form (in addition to above):* dyspnea, chest pain, anuria, shock, disseminated intravascular coagulation	Stop transfusion. Keep vein open. Notify physician and blood bank. Take vital signs as necessary. Assess for signs and symptoms of shock. Monitor I & O. Check for decreased urinary output. Start resuscitative measurements as necessary.
ANAPHYLACTIC				
Is extremely rare Can be life threatening	Idiosyncratic reaction in clients with immunoglobulin A (IgA) deficiency, sensitized to IgA through previous transfusion or pregnancy	Immediately (after transfusion of only few milliliters of blood)	Severe respiratory and cardiovascular collapse (with dyspnea, tachypnea, tachycardia, hypotension, cyanosis); severe gastrointestinal disturbances (with nausea, vomiting, diarrhea, cramping)	Stop transfusion. Keep vein open. Notify physician and blood bank. Take vital signs every 15 min (or as necessary). Start resuscitative measures as necessary.

From Querin JJ, Stahl LD: *Nurs 83* 13:34, 1983.

STEPS	RATIONALE
1. Collect following equipment and bring it to bedside:	Permits quick and efficient performance.
a. Heparinized 5-ml syringe	Prevents coagulation of arterial sample.
b. ⅝-in 20-gauge needle	Promotes atraumatic cannulization of artery.
c. Crushed ice for arterial blood sample	Decreases oxygen metabolism of sample.
d. Local anesthetic	Reduces local pain when more than one attempt is necessary and reduces likelihood of arterial spasm.
e. Topical skin antibacterial scrub and alcohol wipes	Reduces entry of surface bacteria into puncture site.
f. Air lock or cap for syringe	Prevents air from entering blood after sample has been obtained, thus altering results of blood gas analysis.
g. 2 × 2 gauze	Allows application of pressure after arterial puncture.
h. Disposable gloves	Reduces risk of exposure to HIV, hepatitis, and other blood-borne bacteria.
i. Tape	
2. Check client's identity. Explain procedure and client's responsibility.	Ensures that correct client undergoes procedure. Prevents hyperventilation due to anxiety and resulting temporary change in blood gases.
3. Palpate radial artery.	Radial artery is selected because it is superficially located, has collateral circulation, and is not adjacent to large vein.
Perform Allen's test:	Determines adequate collateral flow to hand.
a. Have client make tight fist.	Removes as much blood from hand as possible.
b. Apply direct pressure to radial and ulnar arteries.	Obstructs arterial blood flow to hand.
c. Have client open hand.	Fingers and hand should be pale and blanched, indicating lack of arterial blood flow.
d. Release pressure over ulnar artery; observe color of fingers, thumbs, and hand. Fingers and hand should flush within 15 sec. Flushing is positive Allen's test. If test is negative (no flushing), radial artery should be avoided. Check other hand.	If collateral circulation to hand is present through ulnar artery, hand and fingers flush. Ulnar artery can supply blood flow to hand if radial artery is damaged or becomes occluded during procedure.
4. Hyperextend client's wrist over rolled towel.	Maintains radial artery in superficial position.
5. Wash hands. Apply disposable gloves.	Reduces risk of exposure to HIV, hepatitis, and other blood-borne bacteria.
6. Cleanse site with circular motion using povidone-iodine followed by alcohol wipe.	Reduces risk of skin bacteria entering puncture site.
7. Apply local anesthetic. Xylocaine 2% is usually injected subcutaneously.	Anesthetic reduces pain and subsequent hyperventilation in some clients and decreases likelihood of arterial spasm.
8. Flush 3-ml syringe with small amount of heparin 1000 units/ml and then empty syringe, leaving heparin in needle and hub (Feldman-Malen, 1987).	Heparin in needle prevents clotting of blood sample. Excess heparin in syringe affects pH value of sample blood.
9. While palpating artery, insert needle at 45-degree angle while stabilizing client's artery with your free hand (see illustration on p. 1326).	Minimizes formation of hematoma at puncture site.
10. Observe for pulsating flow of blood into syringe.	Indicates puncture of artery.
11. Withdraw 2 ml of blood.	Provides sufficient amount for analysis.
12. Remove needle and syringe from artery. Expel any air in syringe. Cork syringe with air lock.	Prevents entry of air into syringe. If air enters syringe, blood must be discarded to avoid inaccurate blood gas results.
13. Rotate syringe so that blood mixes with heparin.	Prevents clotting of sample.
14. Submerge syringe in crushed ice	Reduces rate of oxygen metabolism of sampled blood.

STEPS	RATIONALE
15. Label specimen with client's name, body temperature, and (for client on oxygen therapy) inspired oxygen concentration.	Normally, 6% change in arterial Pao_2 occurs with each degree of centigrade of body temperature (Metheny, Snively, 1983). Measurement of oxygen concentration is important in evaluating effectiveness of oxygen therapy.
16. Have specimens transported to laboratory immediately.	Prevents alteration of blood gas values by cellular metabolism.
17. Apply pressure to puncture site by applying 2 × 2 gauze over site and holding for 5 min. Length of time may be increased for client receiving anticoagulants (see illustration).	Reduces risk of hematoma formation and damage to artery.
18. Apply tape over gauze if bleeding stops.	Prevents bleeding as extremity is moved.
19. Discard equipment in appropriate container, remove and dispose of gloves, and wash hands.	Reduces transmission of microorganisms.
20. Record in nurse' notes time of arterial blood gas test and extremity from which specimen was drawn.	Documents that arterial blood gas specimen was obtained.

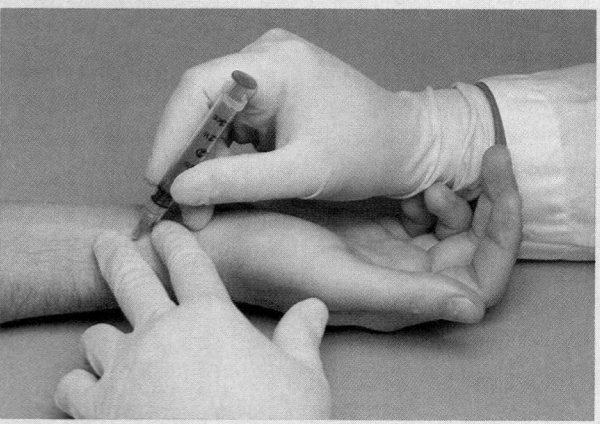

Step 9

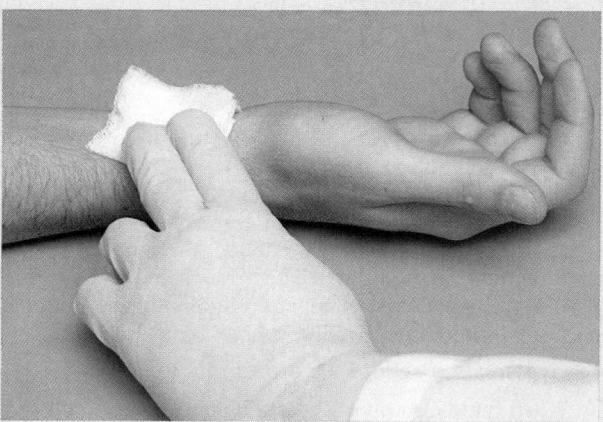

Step 17

5. Prepare to administer emergency drugs, such as antihistamines, vasopressors, fluids, and steroids.
6. Prepare for cardiopulmonary resuscitation. .
7. Obtain a urine specimen and send it to the laboratory.
8. Save the blood container and tubing for return to the laboratory.
9. Complete the necessary paperwork, such as reports about transfusion reactions and nurses' notes.

Although anaphylactic transfusion reactions are relatively rare, they can occur with any client. Correct administration of blood and blood products prevents reactions. When a client has a transfusion reaction, prompt nursing actions can decrease the severity of the response.

Correcting Acid-Base Imbalances

Nursing interventions to promote acid-base balance are performed to support prescribed medical therapies. Physicians often order a variety of drug therapies to correct acid-base imbalances. Because acid-base disturbances can be life threatening and require rapid correction, the nurse must maintain a functional IV line and frequently check the physician's orders for new medications or fluids. Prescribed drugs, such as insulin or sodium bicarbonate,

Sample Evaluation of Interventions for Fluid, Electrolyte, and Acid-Base Disturbances

Goals	Evaluation Measures	Expected Outcomes
Fluid and electrolyte balance will be restored and maintained.	Inspect the skin for edema or dry, scaly skin. Palpate for poor skin turgor, absence of edema, or weak pulse. Inspect oral cavity for dry, sticky mucous membranes, decreased saliva, and longitudinal furrows on tongue. Inspect for fluid and electrolyte imbalances such as weight loss or gain, Chvostek's sign, cardiac dysrhythmias, and anuria or oliguria. Auscultate for adventitious lung sounds and third heart sound. Obtain vital signs for tachycardia, bradycardia, hypotension, hypertension, and orthostatic hypotension. Obtain laboratory findings and observe for electrolyte imbalance.	Vital signs will return to baseline normal. Normal skin turgor will return. There will be no edema. Weight will be stable at baseline normal. Client will have clear breath sounds. Serum electrolyte level, arterial blood gas values, and blood chemistry results will be normal.
Causes of imbalance will be identified and corrected.	Observe for vomiting, diarrhea, and wound drainage. Observe for complications associated with fluid replacement. Obtain blood samples, and observe for electrolyte imbalance as evidenced by laboratory findings.	Client will experience no vomiting or diarrhea. Client will experience no fluid losses. Serum electrolyte levels will be normal.

and fluid and electrolyte replacement should be given promptly.

The nurse implements appropriate nursing measures to promote ventilation and oxygenation (see Chapter 38). This is particularly important for the client with respiratory acidosis. Stasis of pulmonary secretions and decreased lung expansion intensify the acidotic condition. Nursing interventions to mobilize pulmonary secretions and promote lung expansion can make the difference between life and death.

For clients with respiratory alkalosis resulting from anxiety, the nurse initiates nursing measures to reduce the anxiety after first correcting respiratory alkalosis. To correct respiratory alkalosis the nurse instructs the client to breathe into a paper bag so that the client rebreathes exhaled carbon dioxide. In this way, carbon dioxide combines with water to form carbonic acid, which increases blood acidity. After respiratory alkalosis is corrected, the symptoms disappear. At this point the nurse may be able to assist the client in determining the cause of anxiety and methods to control it. Some clients with repeated anxiety attacks need counseling, and the nurse should make an appropriate and prompt referral.

ARTERIAL BLOOD GASES. Clients with acid-base disturbances usually require repeated arterial blood gas analysis. This procedure requires the removal of blood from an artery to determine acid-base status and adequacy of ventilation and oxygenation. Arterial blood gas samples are drawn from a peripheral artery, such as the radial artery, or from an arterial line. In some agencies, nurses are responsible for radial artery punctures. Beginning nursing students do not draw arterial blood gas samples but frequently assist in the sampling process and care for the client after the procedure (Procedure 39-6).

Evaluation

The nurse evaluates the effectiveness of care provided to the client with alterations in fluid, electrolyte, or acid-base imbalances based on expected outcomes. The nurse uses inspection, palpation, percussion, and auscultation to determine the client's response to nursing interventions. Ongoing assessment enables the nurse to evalauate the response to therapy. Using evaluation data, the nurse determines whether the care goals have been or whether care plan requires modification.

Client care goals are developed using objective criteria to measure progress. The criteria in the evaluation box are examples of expected outcomes based on the specific goals of care.

SUMMARY

Clients with altered fluid and electrolyte status require nursing care plans designed to assist in restoring normal fluid volume and electrolyte concentrations. The nurse restores fluid balance through oral fluid replacement, administration of IV fluids, and maintenance of fluid restrictions. Electrolytes can be given orally or parenterally. The nurse also treats underlying illnesses that may cause fluid and electrolyte imbalances.

Acid-base imbalances may result from a number of underlying illnesses. With minor imbalances, the body compensates by chemical, biological, and physiological regulatory mechanisms. With more severe imbalances, however, medical and nursing interventions are required because acid-base imbalances are life threatening. Each type of imbalance creates clinical signs and symptoms assessed by the nurse. When providing care to clients with altered fluid, electrolyte, or acid-base balances, the nurse continually monitors for changes in the client's status and uses all components of the nursing process to maintain and restore balance.

REFERENCES

Aaronson L, Seaman L: Managing hypernatremia in fluid deficient elderly, *J Gerontol Nurs* 15(7):29, 1989.

Axnick KR, Yarbrough M: *Infection control: an integrated approach*, St Louis, 1984, Mosby–Year Book.

Centers for Disease Control: Guidelines for reducing intravascular infections, *Infect Control* 3(1) :52, 1982.

Centers for Disease Control: Recommendations for prevention of HIV transmission in health care settings, *MMWR* 36(suppl 25):3s, 1987.

Chenevey B: Overview of fluids and electrolytes, *Nurs Clin North Am* 22(4):749, 1987.

Delaney C, Lauer M: *Intravenous therapy: a guide to quality care*, Philadelphia, 1988, Lippincott.

Feldman-Malen J: The patient with chronic obstructive pulmonary disease. In Metheny N, editor: *Fluid and electrolyte imbalance: nursing considerations*, Philadephia, 1987, Lippincott.

Gröer, MW: *Physiology and pathophysiology of the body fluids*, St Louis, 1981, Mosby–Year Book.

Gröer M, Shekleton M: *Basic pathophysiology: a holistic approach*, ed 3, St Louis, 1989, Mosby–Year Book.

Guyton AC: *Textbook of medical physiology*, ed 7, Philadelphia, 1986, Saunders.

Kim MJ, McFarland GK, McLane AM: *Pocket guide to nursing diagnoses*, ed 4, St Louis, 1991, Mosby–Year Book.

Kokko J, Tannen R: *Fluids and electrolytes*, ed 2, Philadelphia, 1990, Saunders.

Kopec I, Groeger J: Life-threatening fluid and electrolyte abnormalities associated with cancer, *Crit Care Clin* 4(1):81, 1988.

LaRocca J, Otto S: *Pocket guide to intravenous therapy*, St Louis, 1989, Mosby–Year Book.

Maki D, Ringer M: Evaluation of dressing regimens for prevention of infection with peripheral intravenous catheters, *JAMA* 258(17):2396, 1987.

Messner RL, Gorse GJ: Nursing management of peripheral intravenous sites, *Focus Crit Care* 14(2):25, 1987.

Metheny NM, editor: *Fluid and electrolyte balance: nursing considerations*, Philadelphia, 1987, Lippincott.

Metheny NM, editor: *Fluid and electrolyte balance: nursing considerations*, ed 2, Philadelphia, 1992, Lippincott.

Metheny NM, Snively WD Jr: *Nurse's handbook of fluid balance*, ed 4, Philadelphia, 1983, Lippincott.

Mountcastle VC: *Medical physiology*, ed 14, St Louis, 1979, Occupational Safety and Health Act: bloodborne pathogens, *Federal Register Mosby–Year Book.*

Patrick ML et al: *Medical-surgical nursing: pathophysiological concepts*, Philadelphia, 1986, Lippincott.

Porth CM: *Pathophysiology: concepts of altered health status*, Philadelphia, 1986, Lippincott.

Querin J, Stahl L: Twelve simple sensible steps for successful blood transfusions, *Nurs 83* 13:34, 1983.

Riddle I: Fluid balance in infants and children, In Metheney N: *Fluid and electrolyte balance: nursing considerations*, ed 2, Philadephia, 1992, Lippincott.

Robinson S: Fluid balance in the elderly patient. In Metheny N: *Fluid and electrolyte balance: nursing considerations*, Philadelphia, 1987, Lippincott.

Roth D: Intravenous therapy. In Metheney N, editor: *Fluid and electrolyte balance: nursing considerations*, Philadelphia, 1992, Lippincott.

Silvestri A, Masoorli S: PICC lines: a new dimension in home health care, *J Home Health Care Practice* 2(4):1, 1990.

Tomford JW, Hershey CO, McLakin CE: Intravenous therapy team peripheral venous catheter-associated complications: a prospective controlled study, *Arch Intern Med* 144:1191, 1984.

Vokes T, Robertson G: Disorders of antidiuretic hormone, *Endocrinol Metab Clin North Am* 17(2):281, 1988.

ADDITIONAL READINGS

American Association of Blood Banks: Blood transfusions, *Am J Nurs* 89(4):486, 1989.

American Association of Blood Banks: The latest protocols for blood transfusions, *Nurs 86* 16(10):34, 1986.

Barta M: Correcting electrolyte imbalances, *RN* 50(2):30, 1987.

Bonato J: Blood transfusions: are they safe? *Crit Care Nurs* 9(7):40, 1980.

Bowman M et al: Effect of tube-feeding osmolality on serum sodium levels, *Crit Care Nurse* 9(1):22, 1989.

Byers P: Comparison of application factors among three brands of transparent semipermeable films for peripheral IVs, *NITA* 84:315, 1987.

Calloway C: When the problem involves magnesium, calcium, or phophate, *RN* 50(5):30, 1987.

Dennis EMP: An ambulatory infusion pump for pain control: a nursing approach for home care, *Cancer Nurs* 7:309, 1984.

Dickerson M: Protecting yourself from AIDS: infection control measures, *Crit Care Nurse* 9(10):26, 1989.

Dickerson R, Brown R: Hypomagnesia in hospitalized patients receiving nutritional support, *Heart Lung* 14(6):561, 1985.

Eisenberg P, Howard R, Gianino M: Improved long-term maintenance of central venous catheters with a new dressing technique, *J Intravenous Nurs* 13(5):279, 1990.

Feldstein A: Detect phlebitis and infiltration, *Nurs 86* 16:44, 1986.

Felver L, Pendarvis J: Electrolyte imbalances, *AORN J* 49(4):991, 1989.

Goodman MS, Weekham R: Venous access devices: an overview, *Oncol Nurs Forum* 11:16, 1984.

Hahn K: Monitoring a blood transfusion, *Nurs 89* 19:20, 1989.

Heitkemper M, Bon E: Fluid and electrolytes: assessment and interventions, *J Enterostom Ther* 15(1):18, 1988.

Horne M, Swearingen P: *Pocket guide to fluids and electrolytes*, St Louis, 1989, Mosby–Year Book.

Horne M, Heitz U, Swearingen P: *Fluid, electrolyte, and acid-base balance: a case study approach*, St Louis, 1991, Mosby–Year Book.

Howard M, Puri V, Paidiputy B: The effects of fluid resuscitation in the critically ill patient, *Heart Lung* 13:649, 1984.

Huzar J: Diabetes now: preventing acute complications, *RN* 52(8):34, 1989.

Innerarity S: Electrolyte emergencies in the critically ill renal patient, *Crit Care Nurs Clin North Am* 2(1):89, 1990.

Keyes JL: *Fluid, electrolyte, and acid-base regulation*, Belmont, Calif, 1985, Wadsworth.

Klass K: Troubleshooting central line complications, *Nurs 87* 17:58, 1987.

Lawson M et al: Comparision of transparent dressing to paper tape dressing over central venous catheter sites, *NITA* 9(1):40, 1986.

Levinsky N: Fluids and electrolytes; acidosis and alkalosis. In Wilson J et al, editors: *Harrison's principles of internal medicine*, ed 12, New York, 1991, McGraw-Hill.

Luce JM, Tyler ML, Pierson DJ: *Intensive respiratory care*, Philadelphia, 1984, Saunders.

Martin E et al: Autotransfusion systems (ATS), *Crit Care Nurse* 9(7):65, 1989.

Masoorli ST, Piercy S: A life-saving guide to blood products, *RN* 47:32, 1984.

Mathewson M: Intravenous therapy, *Crit Care Nurse* 9(2):21, 1989.

Maxwell M, Kleeman C, Narins R: *Clinical disorders of fluid and electrolyte metabolism*, ed 4, New York, 1987, McGraw-Hill.

McCance K, Huether S: *Pathophysiology: the biological basis for disease in adults and children*, St Louis, 1990, Mosby–Year Book.

McLaughlin M, Kassirer J: Rational treatment of acid base disorders, *Drugs* 39(6):841, 1990.

Mellema S, Poniatowski B: Geriatric IV therapy, *J Intravenous Nurs* 11(1):578, 1988.

Metheny N: Why worry about IV fluids? *Am J Nurs* 90(6):50, 1990.

Miller D: Tips on drawing blood through a heparin lock, *RN* 49:22, 1986.

Negon S: A smart way to secure an IV, *Am J Nurs* 89(5):687, 1989.

Nurses' Drug Alert: Hypomagnesemia in hospital patients with congestive heart failure, *Am J Nurs* 86(9):1046, 1986.

O'Neill P et al: Reduced survival with increasing plasma osmolality in elderly continuing-care patients, *Age Aging,* 19:68, 1990.

Pauley SY: Transfusing therapy for nurses, II. *NITA* 8:51, 1985.

Perez G, Oster J, Roger A: Acid-base disturbances in gastrointestinal disease, *Digest Dis Sci* 32(9):1033, 1987.

Runquist B, Aspina J, Hibbard L: A new approach for problem IV dressings, *RN* 47:49, 1984.

Schulmeister L: A comparison of skin preparation procedures for accessing implanted ports, *NITA* 10(1):45, 1987.

Sommers M: Rapid fluid resuscitation, *Nurs 90* 20(1): 52, 1990.

Toto K: When the patient has hypokalemia, *RN* 50(3):38, 1987.

Toto K: When the patient has hyperkalemia, *RN* 50(4):34, 1987.

Valle G, Lemberg L: Electrolyte imbalances in cardiovascular disease: the forgotten factor, *Heart Lung* 17(3):324, 1988.

Whaley LF, Wong DL: *Nursing care of infants and children*, ed 4, St Louis, 1991, Mosby–Year Book.

Whitney R: Comparing long-term central venous catheters, *Nurs 91* 21(4):70, 1991.

Winters V: Implantable vascular access devices, *Oncol Nurs Forum* 11(6):25, 1984.

Wiseman M: Setting standards for home IV therapy, *Am J Nurs* 85:421, 1985.

CHAPTER 39 REVIEW

Key Concepts

- Body fluids are distributed in extracellular and intracellular fluid compartments.
- Body fluids are composed of electrolytes, minerals, cells, and water.
- Body fluids are regulated through fluid intake, output, and hormonal regulation.
- Acid-base balance depends on the hydrogen ion concentration in the blood.
- The body's chemical buffering system is the first system to respond to acid-base abnormalities.
- Biological buffering occurs when hydrogen ions are absorbed or released by the cells to compensate for acid-base imbalances.
- Physiological buffering involves compensatory responses in the lung or kidneys.
- Volume disturbances include isotonic and osmolar fluid volume deficits and excesses.
- Chronic and severe acute illnesses increase the risk for fluid, electrolyte, and acid-base imbalances.
- Very young or old clients are at particularly greater risk for fluid, electrolyte, and acid-base imbalances.
- Assessment for fluid, electrolyte, and acid-base balances includes the nursing history, physical and behavioral assessment, measurements of intake and output, daily weighing, specific laboratory data such as complete blood count and measurement of serum electrolyte and BUN levels, specific gravity, and arterial blood gas levels.
- Fluid volume deficits can be corrected by oral or parenteral administration of fluid.
- Complications of intravenous therapy include infiltration, phlebitis, fluid overload, and bleeding at the infusion site.
- Blood transfusions replace fluid volume loss resulting from hemorrhage, treat anemia, and replace coagulation factors.
- Administration of blood or blood products requires the nurse to follow specific guidelines to prevent transfusion reactions.
- The risks of transfusion include transfusion reactions, hyperkalemia, hypocalcemia, circulatory overload, and blood-borne infections.
- Respiratory acidosis is characterized by increased carbon dioxide concentration, excess carbonic acid, and increased hydrogen ion concentration.
- Respiratory alkalosis is characterized by decreased carbon dioxide and hydrogen ion concentrations.
- Metabolic acidosis is characterized by a rise in hydrogen ion concentration.
- Metabolic alkalosis is characterized by a decrease in hydrogen ion concentration.
- The goals of therapy for acid-base imbalances are treatment of the underlying illness and restoration of the arterial pH to normal.

Key Terms

Active transport, p. 1278

Agglutinins, p. 1320

Anions, p. 1276

Autotransfusion, p. 1320

Buffer, p. 1281

Cations, p. 1276

Dehydration, p. 1284

Diffusion, p. 1277

Electrolyte, p. 1276

Extracellular fluids, p. 1276

Fluid volume deficit (FVD), p. 1283

Fluid volume excess (FVE), p. 1283

Hemolysis, p. 1320

Hemosiderosis, p. 1323

Hydrostatic pressure, p. 1277

Hypertonic, p. 1277

Hypotonic, p. 1277

Infiltration, p. 1311

Infusion pumps, p. 1311

Insensible water loss, p. 1279

Intracellular fluids, p. 1276

Isotonic, p. 1277

Metabolic acidosis, p. 1287

Metabolic alkalosis, p. 1287

Oncotic pressure, p. 1277

Osmolality, p. 1277

Osmoreceptors, p. 1278

Osmosis, p. 1277

Osmotic pressure, p. 1277

Patency, p. 1311

pH, p. 1281

Phlebitis, p. 1315

Respiratory acidosis, p. 1287

Respiratory alkalosis, p. 1287

Sensible water loss, p. 1279

Third-space syndrome, p. 1283

Transfusion reaction, p. 1323

Vascular access devices, p. 1303

Venipuncture, p. 1305

Volume control devices, p. 1305

Critical Thinking Exercises

1. Ms. Jay, 76 years old, has experienced vomiting and diarrhea for 2 days. Her son reports that she has been irritable and harder to "wake up" for the last 12 hours. On admission, laboratory data revealed that her serum osmolality was 325 mOsm/kg and that her serum sodium was 152 mEq/L. Based on this data, which alteration in fluid balance is Ms. Jay most likely to have? Considering her age, describe three specific methods to collect accurate assessment data related to fluid balance.

2. Mr. Mason is receiving intravenous fluids. He complains that his right arm hurts just above the IV insertion site. The nurse finds that the IV site is warmer than the surrounding skin and the vein is reddened. Based on these findings, which complication has Mr. Mason developed? What is the most appropriate nursing intervention?

3. After a blood transfusion is started, the client complains of back and chest pain. His blood pressure has dropped from 132/84 mm Hg to 98/40 mm Hg. What should the nurse do?

CHAPTER 40

Urinary Elimination

OBJECTIVES

Mastery of content in this chapter will enable the student to:
- Define the key terms listed.
- Explain the function of each organ in the urinary system.
- Describe the process of urination.
- Identify factors that commonly influence urinary elimination.
- Compare and contrast common alterations in urinary elimination.
- Obtain a nursing history for a client with urinary elimination problems.
- Identify nursing diagnoses appropriate for clients with alterations in urinary elimination.
- Obtain urine specimens.
- Describe characteristics of normal and abnormal urine.
- Describe the nursing implications of common diagnostic tests of the urinary system.
- Discuss nursing measures to promote normal micturition and reduce episodes of incontinence.
- Insert a urinary catheter.
- Discuss nursing measures to reduce urinary tract infection.
- Irrigate a urinary catheter.
- Identify two modalities of renal replacement therapy.
- Discuss organ system alterations in urinary system failure.
- Understand basic principles in selecting urinary catheters.

CHAPTER OUTLINE

ormal elimination of urinary wastes is a basic function most people take for granted. When the urinary system fails to function properly, virtually all organ systems can be affected. Clients with alterations in urinary elimination may also suffer emotionally from body image changes. The nurse provides understanding and a sensitivity to clients' needs. With older clients in particular, the nurse must know the reasons for problems and find acceptable solutions.

PHYSIOLOGY OF URINE ELIMINATION

Urinary elimination depends on the function of the kidneys, ureters, bladder, and urethra. Kidneys remove wastes from the blood to form urine. Ureters transport urine from the kidneys to the bladder. The bladder holds urine until the urge to urinate develops. Urine leaves the body through the urethra. All organs of the urinary system must be intact and functional for successful removal of urinary wastes (Fig. 40-1).

Kidneys

Kidneys are reddish-brown, bean-shaped organs that lie on either side of the vertebral column posterior to the peritoneum and against deep muscles of the back. The kidneys extend to the twelfth thoracic and third lumbar vertebrae. Normally the left kidney is 1.5 to 2 cm (6/10 to 8/10 in) higher than the right because of the anatomical position of the liver. Each measures approximately 12 cm by 7 cm (4¾ by 2¾ in) from the hilum to the cortex and weighs 120 to 150 g. An adrenal gland lies on the superior pole of each kidney but is not directly related to urinary elimination. Each kidney is covered by a tough capsule and surrounded by a cushion of fat.

Waste products of metabolism that collect in the blood are filtered in the kidneys. Blood reaches each kidney by the **renal** (kidney) artery that branches from the abdominal aorta. The renal artery enters the kidney at the hilum. Approximately 20% to 25% of the cardiac output circulates daily through the kidneys. Each kidney contains 1 million nephrons. The **nephron,** the functional unit of the kidney, is capable of forming urine. The nephron is composed of the glomerulus, Bowman's capsule, proximal convoluted tubule, loop of Henle, distal tubule, and collecting duct (Fig. 40-2).

Blood reaches nephrons through the afferent arterioles. A cluster of these blood vessels forms the capillary network of the **glomerulus,** which is the initial site of urine formation. The glomerular capillaries are porous and permit filtration of water and substances such as glucose, amino acids, urea, creatinine, and major electrolytes into Bowman's capsule. Protein does not normally filter through the glomerulus. Protein in the urine (**proteinuria**) is a sign of glomerular injury. The glomerulus filters approximately 125 ml of filtrate per minute.

Not all of the glomerular filtrate is excreted as urine. After the filtrate leaves the glomerulus, it passes through a system of tubules and collecting ducts, where water and substances such as glucose, amino acids, uric acid, and sodium and potassium ions are selectively reabsorbed back into the plasma. Other substances such as hydrogen ions, potassium ions (in the presence of aldosterone), and ammonia are secreted back into the tubules. About 99% of the filtrate is reabsorbed into the plasma, with the remaining 1% excreted as urine. Thus the kidneys play a key role in fluid and electrolyte balance (see Chapter 39). The normal adult 24-hour output of urine is about 1500 to 1600 ml. An output of 60 ml of urine per hour is generally normal. An output of less than 30 ml per hour may indicate renal alterations. The kidneys also produce several hormones vital to blood pressure regulation, production of red blood cells (RBCs), and bone mineralization.

The kidneys are responsible for maintaining a normal RBC volume. They produce **erythropoietin,** a hormone released primarily from specialized glomerular cells that sense decreased RBC oxygenation (local hypoxia). After it is released from the kidney, erythropoietin functions within the bone marrow to stimulate erythropoiesis (production and maturation of RBCs) by converting certain stem cells into erythroblasts (Richard, 1986). Erythropoietin also prolongs the life of mature RBCs. Clients with chronic alterations in kidney function cannot produce sufficient quantities of this hormone. Therefore they are prone to anemia. **Renin** is another hormone produced by the kidneys. Its major role is the regulation of blood flow in times of renal ischemia (decreased blood supply)(frequently referred to as *autoregulation*). Renin is synthesized and released from juxtaglomerular cells, which are located on the juxtaglomerular apparatus of the nephron (Fig. 40-3 on p. 1336).

Renin functions as an enzyme to convert angiotensin (a substance synthesized by the liver) into angiotensin I. As angiotensin I circulates through the lungs, it is converted to angiotensin II. Angiotensin II exerts its effect on vascular smooth muscle to cause vasoconstriction and stimulates aldosterone release from the adrenal cortex. The effect of both of these mechanisms is an increase in arterial blood pressure.

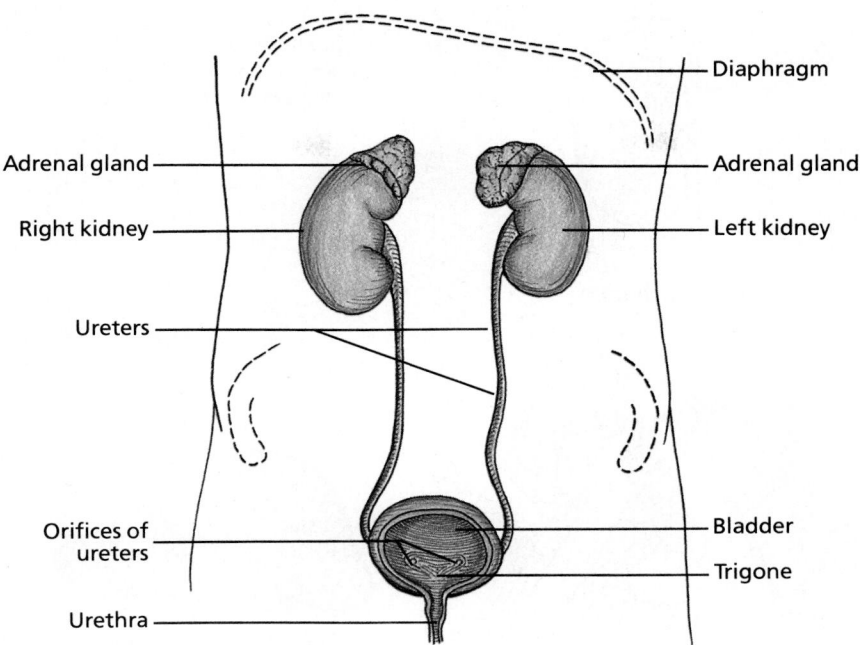

Fig. 40-1   Organs of the urinary system.

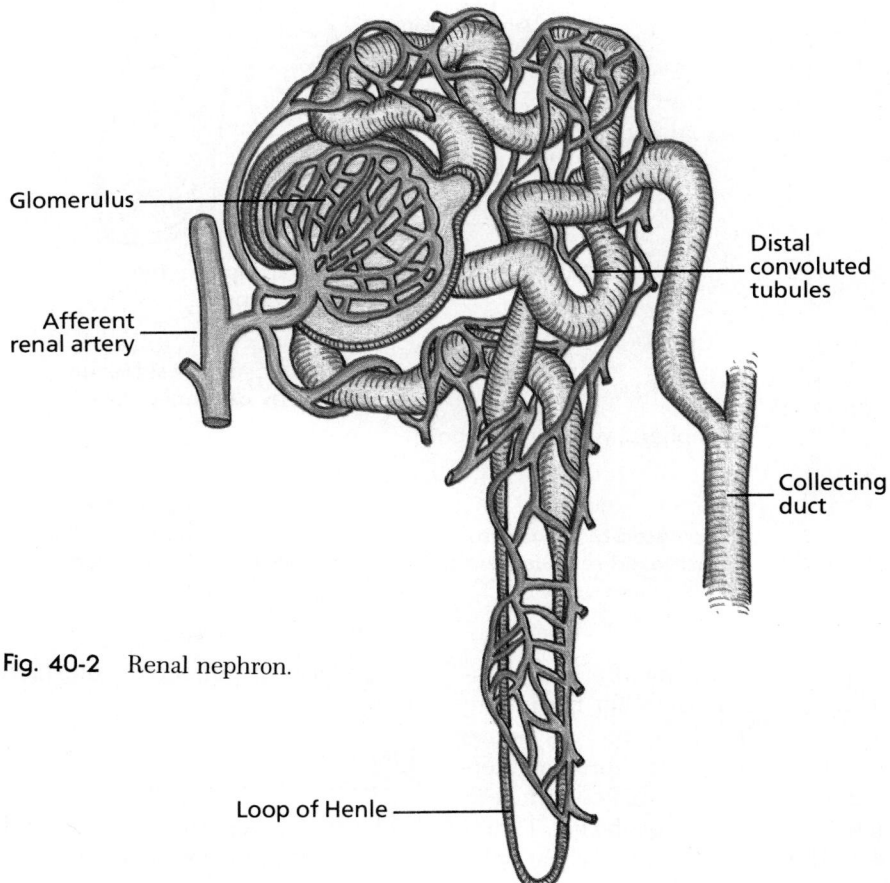

Fig. 40-2   Renal nephron.

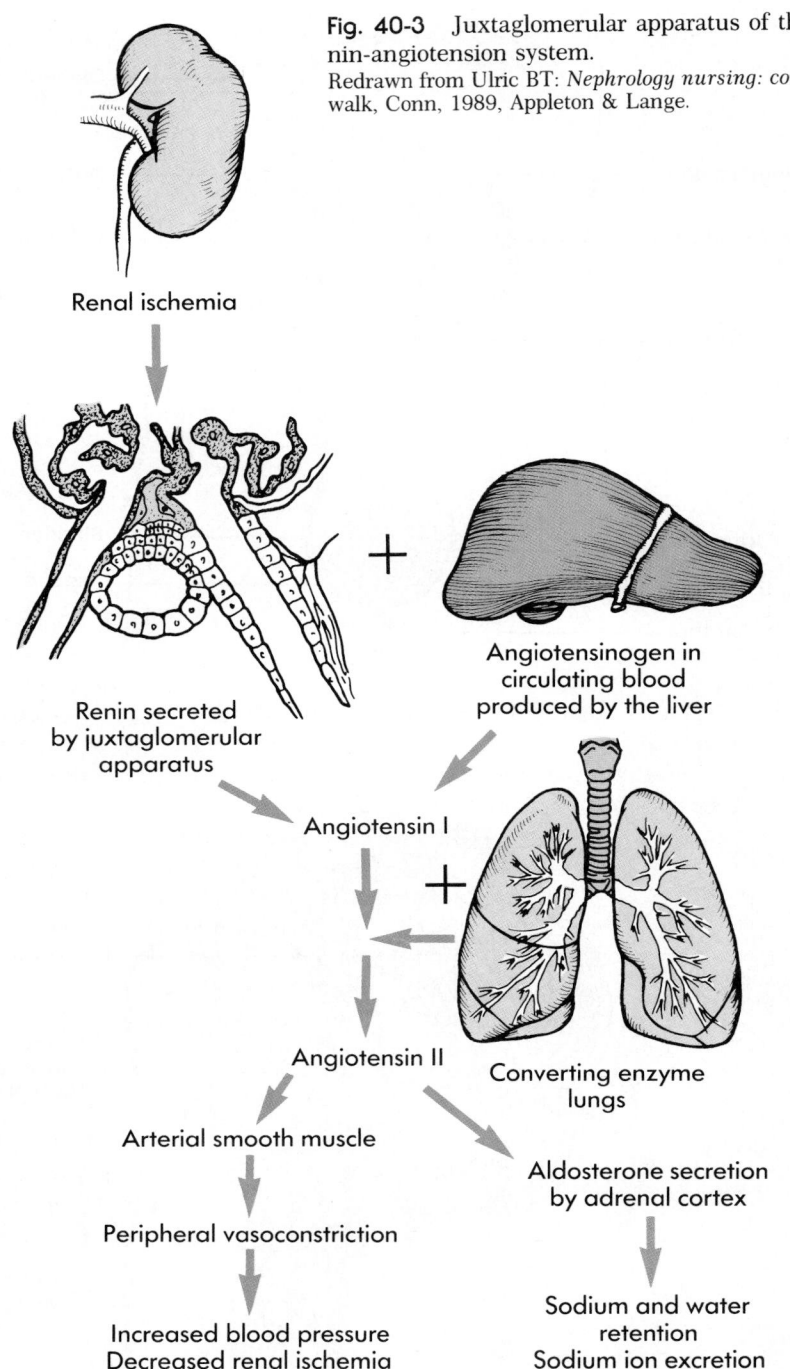

Fig. 40-3 Juxtaglomerular apparatus of the nephron and the renin-angiotension system.
Redrawn from Ulric BT: *Nephrology nursing: concepts and practices,* Norwalk, Conn, 1989, Appleton & Lange.

Renal ischemia

Renin secreted by juxtaglomerular apparatus

Angiotensinogen in circulating blood produced by the liver

Angiotensin I

Angiotensin II

Converting enzyme lungs

Arterial smooth muscle

Aldosterone secretion by adrenal cortex

Peripheral vasoconstriction

Sodium and water retention
Sodium ion excretion

Increased blood pressure
Decreased renal ischemia

The kidneys also play a role in calcium and phosphate regulation. They are responsible for producing a substance that converts vitamin D into its active form (see Chapter 39). Clients with chronic alterations in kidney function do not make sufficient quantities of the active vitamin D metabolite. Therefore they are prone to the development of renal bone disease resulting from the demineralization of bone secondary to impaired intestinal calcium absorption.

Ureters

Urine leaves the tubules and enters collecting ducts that transport it to the renal pelvis. A ureter joins each renal pelvis as the initial exit route for urinary wastes. Ureters are long, tubular structures measuring 25 to 30 cm (10 to 12 in) in length and 1.25 cm (½ in) in diameter in the adult. They extend retroperitoneally to enter the urinary bladder in the pelvic cavity at the ureterovesical junction. Urine draining from the ureters to the bladder is usually sterile.

Three layers of tissue form the wall of the ureter. The inner layer is a mucous membrane continuous with the lining of the renal tubules and urinary bladder. The middle layer consists of smooth muscle fibers that help transport urine through the ureters by peristaltic waves stimulated by distention with urine. An outer layer of fibrous connective tissue supports the ureters.

Peristaltic waves cause the urine to enter the bladder in spurts rather than steadily. To prevent the reflux of urine from the bladder into the ureters, a small valvelike mechanism exists at the ureterovesical junction (the juncture of the ureters with the bladder).

An obstruction within the ureters, such as a kidney stone (**renal calculus**), results in strong peristaltic waves that attempt to move the obstruction into the bladder. Simultaneously a reflex response causes the renal arterioles to constrict to reduce urine production in the kidney on the affected side.

Bladder

The urinary bladder is a hollow, distensible, muscular organ that is a reservoir for urine and the organ of excretion. When empty, the bladder lies in the pelvic cavity behind the symphysis pubis. In men the bladder lies against the rectum posteriorly, and in women it rests against the anterior wall of the uterus and vagina.

The bladder's shape changes as it becomes filled with urine. The walls of the bladder can expand. Normally it holds approximately 600 ml of urine. Pressure within the bladder is usually low, a factor that protects against infection.

When the bladder is full, it expands and extends above the symphysis pubis. A greatly distended bladder may reach the umbilicus. In a pregnant woman the fetus pushes against the bladder, causing a feeling of fullness and reducing the bladder's capacity.

The trigone (a smooth triangular area on the inner surface of the bladder) is at the base of the bladder. An opening exists at each of the trigone's three angles. Two are at the base of the trigone for the ureters, and one is at the apex for the urethra.

The wall of the bladder has four layers: the inner mucous coat, a submucous coat of connective tissue, a muscular coat, and an outer serous coat. The mus-

cular layer has bundles of muscle fibers that form the detrusor muscle. Parasympathetic nerve fibers stimulate the detrusor muscle during urination. The internal urethral sphincter, made of a ringlike band of muscle, is at the base of the bladder where it joins the urethra. The sphincter prevents escape of urine from the bladder and is under voluntary control.

Urethra

Urine travels from the bladder through the urethra and passes outside of the body through the urethral meatus. Normally the turbulent flow of urine through the urethra washes it free of bacteria. Mucous membrane lines the urethra, and urethral glands secrete mucus into the urethral canal. The mucus is believed to be bacteriostatic and forms a mucous plug to prevent entrance of bacteria. Thick layers of smooth muscle surround the urethra.

In women the urethra is approximately 4 to 6.5 cm (1½ to 2½ in) long. The external urethral sphincter, located about halfway down the urethra, permits voluntary flow of urine. The short length of the urethra in women provides an easy access for bacterial microorganisms. In men the urethra, which is a urinary canal and a passageway for cells and secretions from reproductive organs, is 20 cm (8 in) long. It has three sections: the prostatic urethra, the membranous urethra, and the penile urethra.

In a woman the urinary **meatus** (opening) is located between the labia minora, above the vagina and below the clitoris. In a male the meatus is located at the distal end of the penis.

Act of Urination

Urination, **micturition,** and *voiding* are all terms for the process by which urine is expelled from the urinary bladder. The bladder normally holds as much as 600 ml of urine. However, the desire to urinate can be sensed when the bladder contains only a small amount of urine (150 to 200 ml in an adult and 50 to 200 ml in a child). As the volume increases, the bladder walls stretch, sending sensory impulses to the micturition center in the sacral spinal cord. Parasympathetic impulses from the micturition center stimulate the detrusor muscle to contract rhythmically. The internal urethral sphincter also relaxes so that urine may enter the urethra, although voiding does not yet occur. As the bladder contracts, nerve impulses travel up the spinal cord to the midbrain and cerebral cortex. A person is thus conscious of the need to urinate. If the person chooses not to void, the external urinary sphincter remains contracted, and the micturition reflex is inhibited. However, when a person is ready to void, the external sphincter relaxes, the micturition reflex stimulates the detrusor muscle to contract, and urination occurs.

Damage to the spinal cord above the sacral region causes loss of voluntary control of urination, but the micturition reflex pathway may remain intact, allowing urination to occur reflexively. This condition is called a *reflex bladder.*

 ## FACTORS INFLUENCING URINATION

Numerous factors influence the volume and quantity of urine and the client's ability to urinate. Most important, disease processes can alter normal urinary elimination. These alterations can be acute (sudden cessation in urinary elimination of metabolic wastes) or chronic (slow, progressive development of renal dysfunction). Disease processes causing these disturbances are generally categorized as *prerenal, renal,* or *postrenal* in origin (see box). Prerenal alterations in urinary elimination involve factors that decrease circulating blood flow through the kidneys with subsequent decreased perfusion to renal tissue. In other words, the alterations are outside of the urinary system. The decrease in renal perfusion leads to **oliguria** (diminished capacity to form and pass urine) or, less commonly, **anuria** (inability to produce urine and to urinate). Renal alterations result from factors that cause injury directly to the glomeruli or renal tubules interfering with their normal filtering, reabsorptive, and secretory functions. Postrenal alterations result from obstruction to the urinary collecting system anywhere from the calyces (drainage structures within the kidney) to the urethral meatus (that is, outside of the kidney but within the urinary system). Urine is formed by the urinary system but cannot be eliminated by normal means. In addition to disease alterations, other factors should be considered when clients have symptoms related to urinary elimination.

Growth and Development

Infants and young children cannot concentrate urine and reabsorb water effectively. Their urine thus appears light yellow or watery. In relation to their small body size, infants and children excrete large volumes of urine. For example, a 6-month-old child who weighs 6 to 8 kg (10 to 16 pounds) excretes 400 to 500 ml of urine daily. The child weighs about 10% of an adult's weight but excretes 33% as much urine.

A child cannot control micturition voluntarily until age 18 to 24 months. A child must be able to recognize the feeling of bladder fullness, to hold urine for 1 to 2 hours, and to communicate the sense of urgency to an adult. The young child needs parents' understanding, patience, and consistency. A child may not gain full control of micturition until age 4 or 5. Boys are generally slower than girls. Daytime control of micturition is easier to accomplish than nighttime control and occurs earlier in the child's development, usually by 2 years of age.

The adult normally voids 1500 to 1600 ml of urine daily. The kidney concentrates urine, producing a normal amber-colored urine. A person does not void excessively during the night because of a reduction of renal blood flow during rest and because of the kidney's ability to concentrate urine.

Aging impairs micturition. Problems of mobility sometimes make it difficult for the older adult to reach a toilet in time. An older person may be too weak to rise from a toilet seat without assistance. Chronic neurological disease such as parkinsonism

---

Renal Conditions Causing Alterations in Urinary Elimination

PRERENAL CONDITIONS
- Decreased intravascular volume: dehydration, hemorrhage, burns, shock
- Altered peripheral vascular resistance: sepsis, anaphylactic (allergic) reactions
- Cardiac pump failure: congestive heart failure, myocardial infarction, hypertensive heart disease, valvular diseases, pericardial tamponade

RENAL CONDITIONS
- Use of nephrotoxic agents (e.g., gentamycin)
- Transfusion reactions
- Diseases of the glomeruli (e.g., glomenlonephritis)
- Neoplasms
- Systemic diseases (e.g., diabetes)
- Hereditary diseases (e.g., polycystic kidney diseases)
- Infections

POSTRENAL CONDITIONS
- Ureteral, bladder, or urethral obstruction: calculi, blood clots, tumors, stricture
- Prostatic hypertrophy
- Neurogenic bladder
- Pelvic tumors
- Retroperitoneal fibrosis

or cerebrovascular accident (stroke) impairs the sense of balance and makes it difficult for a man to stand while voiding. If an older person loses control of thought processes, the ability to control micturition is unpredictable. The person may lose the ability to sense a full bladder or be unable to recall the procedure for voiding.

Changes in kidney and bladder function also occur with aging. The glomerular filtration rate declines. The kidney's ability to concentrate urine also declines. Thus the older adult often experiences **nocturia** (excessive urination at night). The bladder loses its muscle tone and capacity to hold urine, resulting in increased **urinary frequency**. Because the bladder cannot contract as effectively, an older person often retains urine in the bladder after voiding (**residual urine**) (see Chapter 27). This increases the risk for bacterial growth and development of urinary tract infections (UTIs). Older men may also suffer from benign prostatic hypertrophy, which makes them prone to urinary retention and incontinence.

Sociocultural Factors

Cultural norms vary on the privacy of urination. North Americans expect toilet facilities to be private, whereas some European cultures accept communal toilet facilities. Social expectations (for example, school recesses) influence the time of urination.

The nurse's approach to a client's elimination needs must consider cultural and social habits. If a client prefers privacy, the nurse tries to prevent interruptions as the client voids. A client who is less sensitive to the need for privacy should be treated with understanding and acceptance.

Psychological Factors

Anxiety and emotional stress do not change the characteristics of urine but may cause a sense of urgency and increase frequency of urination. An anxious person may have the urge to void even after voiding only a few minutes earlier.

Anxiety may also prevent a person from being able to urinate completely. Emotional tension makes it difficult to relax abdominal and perineal muscles. If the external urethral sphincter is not completely relaxed, voiding may be incomplete, and urine is retained in the bladder.

Personal Habits

Privacy and adequate time to urinate are usually important to most people. Some people need distractions (for example, reading) to relax.

Muscle Tone

Weak abdominal and pelvic floor muscles impair bladder contraction and control of the external urethral sphincter. Poor control of micturition can result from muscle wasting caused by prolonged immobility, stretching of muscles during childbirth, menopausal muscle atrophy, and damage to muscles from trauma.

Continuous drainage of urine through an indwelling catheter causes loss of bladder tone or damage to uretheral sphincters. The bladder remains relatively empty when a client has an indwelling catheter in place, and thus it is never stretched to capacity. When a muscle is not stretched regularly, atrophy develops. When a catheter is removed, the client may have difficulty regaining urinary control.

Volume Status

The kidneys maintain a sensitive balance between retention and excretion of fluids (see Chapter 39). If fluids and the concentration of electrolytes and solutes are in equilibrium, an increase in fluid intake causes an increase in urine production. Ingested fluids increase the body's circulating plasma and thus increase the volume of glomerular filtrate and urine excreted.

This amount varies with food and fluid intake. The volume of urine formed at night is about half that formed during the day because intake and metabolism decline. Nocturia can be a sign of renal alteration. In a healthy person, the intake of water in food and fluids balances the output of water in urine, feces, and insensible losses in perspiration and respiration.

Ingestion of certain fluids directly affects urine production and excretion. Alcohol inhibits the release of antidiuretic hormone (ADH) and thus promotes urine formation. Coffee, tea, cocoa, and cola drinks that contain caffeine increase **diuresis** (increased formation and excretion of urine). Foods that contain a high fluid content, such as fruits and vegetables, may also increase urine production.

Febrile conditions influence urine production. The client who becomes diaphoretic loses a large amount of fluids through insensible water loss, which decreases urine production. However, the increased body metabolism associated with fever increases accumulation of body wastes. Although urine volume may be reduced, it is highly concentrated.

Disease Conditions

Several diseases can affect the ability to micturate. Any lesion of peripheral nerves leading to the bladder causes loss of bladder tone, reduced sensation of bladder fullness, and difficulty in controlling urination. For example, diabetes mellitus and multiple sclerosis cause neuropathic conditions that alter bladder function.

Diseases that slow or hinder physical activity interfere with the ability to void. Rheumatoid arthritis, degenerative joint disease, and parkinsonism are examples of conditions that make it difficult to reach and use toilet facilities. A client with rheumatoid arthritis often cannot sit on or rise from a toilet without an elevated seat.

Diseases that cause irreversible damage to the glomerulus or tubules result in permanent alterations in renal function. *Chronic* or *end-stage renal disease (ESRD)* are the terms used to describe the resulting decline in kidney function from these processes. The client with ESRD manifests numerous metabolic disturbances that require treatment for survival. These alterations are caused by the accumulation of nitrogenous waste products and various acid-base and biochemical derangements. The associated symptoms experienced by the client occur as a result of the **uremic syndrome** (the group of symptoms characterized by urinary constituents in the blood, altered regulatory functions [causing marked fluid and electrolyte abnormalities], nausea, vomiting, headache, coma, and convulsions). Treatment options include methods to correct these biochemical derangements. The problem may be managed conservatively (with dietary restrictions and medications). However, as continued deterioration in renal function or worsening of the uremic symptoms becomes evident, more aggressive treatment is indicated (see box). These treatments are known as **renal replacement therapies.** Dialysis and organ transplantation are the two methods of renal replacement. The two methods of dialysis are peritoneal and hemodialysis.

Peritoneal dialysis is an indirect method of cleansing the blood of waste products using the processes of osmosis and diffusion. The peritoneal capillary bed is a semipermeable membrane. Excess fluid and waste products are readily removed from the bloodstream when a sterile electrolyte solution (dialysate) is instilled into the peritoneal cavity by gravity via a surgically placed catheter. The dialysate is left in the cavity for a prescribed time interval and then is drained out by gravity.

Hemodialysis involves using a machine equipped with a semipermeable filtering membrane (artificial kidney) that removes accumulated waste products directly from the blood. In the dialysis machine, dialysate fluid is pumped through one side of the artificial kidney while the client's blood passes through the other side. The client's blood is simultaneously cleansed of waste products and returned through a specially placed vascular access device. Both dialysis modalities can be applied for a short or long time, and they require specialized equipment and trained nurses.

Organ transplantation is the replacement of the client's diseased kidneys with a healthy one from a living relative or cadaveric donor of compatible blood and tissue type. After the client (recipient) is deemed medically and psychosocially suitable, the organ is surgically implanted. Special medications (immunosuppressives) are administered to prevent the body from rejecting the transplanted organ. Unlike the other treatments, successful organ transplantation offers the client the potential for restoration of normal kidney function.

Surgical Procedures

The stress of surgery initially triggers the general adaptation syndrome (see Chapter 30). The posterior pituitary gland releases an increased amount of ADH, which increases water reabsorption and reduces urine output. The surgical client is often in an altered state of fluid balance before surgery, which aggravates the reduction in urine output. The stress response also elevates the level of aldosterone, resulting in reduction in urine output in an effort to increase circulatory fluid volume.

Anesthetic and narcotic analgesics slow the glomerular filtration rate, reducing urine output. These pharmacological agents also impair sensory and mo-

---

Indications for Dialysis

- Renal failure that can no longer be controlled by conservative management (i.e., dietary modifications and administration of medications to correct electrolyte abnormalities)
- A glomerular filtration rate (GFR) less than 5 ml/min
- Serum creatinine level greater than 10 mg/100 ml, blood urea nitrogen (BUN) level greater than 100 mg/100 ml
- Worsening of uremic syndrome associated with ESRD (i.e., nausea, vomiting, neurological changes, neuropathic conditions, pericarditis)
- Severe electrolyte or fluid abnormalities that cannot be controlled by simpler measures (e.g., hyperkalemia, pulmonary edema)

tor impulses traveling between the bladder, spinal cord, and brain. Clients recovering from anesthesia and deep analgesia are often unable to sense bladder fullness and are unable to initiate or inhibit micturition. Spinal anesthetics, in particular, create the risk of urinary retention because of an inability to sense the need to void.

Surgery of lower abdominal and pelvic structures can impair urination because of local trauma to surrounding tissues. The edema and inflammation associated with healing may obstruct the flow of urine from the bladder or urethra, interfere with relaxation of pelvic and sphincter muscles, or cause discomfort during voiding. After surgery involving the bladder and urethra, clients routinely need urinary catheters.

The surgical formation of a urinary diversion temporarily or permanently bypasses the bladder and urethra as the exit routes for urine. The client with a urinary diversion has a **stoma** (artificial opening) on the abdomen to drain urine.

Medications that Discolor Urine

YELLOW URINE

- Cascara
- Vitamin B_2
- Phenacetin

ORANGE URINE

- Azo-Gantrisin
- Sulfonamide
- Pyridium
- Warfarin Sodium (Coumadin)

PINK OR RED URINE

- Thorazine
- Ex-Lax
- Phenytoin (Dilantin)
- Phenacetin

GREEN OR BLUE-GREEN URINE

- Amitriptyline (Elavil)
- Vitamin B complex
- Methylene blue

BROWN OR BLACK URINE

- Injectable iron compounds
- Levodopa or L-dopa
- Nitrofurantoin
- Methyldopa
- Quinine
- Metronidazole

Medications

Diuretics prevent reabsorption of water and certain electrolytes to increase urine output. Urinary retention may be caused by use of anticholinergics (for example, atropine), antihistamines (for example, Sudafed), antihypertensives (for example, Aldomet), and beta-adrenergic blockers (for example, Inderal). Some medications change the color of urine (see box). Clients with alterations in kidney function require dosage adjustments in medications excreted by the kidneys.

Diagnostic Examination

Examination of the urinary system can influence micturition. Procedures such as an intravenous pyelogram or urogram require that the client not take fluids orally before the test. A restriction in fluid intake commonly lowers urine output. Diagnostic examinations (for example, cystoscopy) that involve direct visualization of urinary structures may cause localized edema of the urethral passageway and spasm of the bladder sphincter. The client often has urinary retention after such a procedure and may pass red or pink urine because of bleeding resulting from trauma to the urethral or bladder mucosa.

 ### ALTERATIONS IN URINARY ELIMINATION

The most common urinary problems encountered by the nurse involve disturbances in the act of micturition. These disturbances result from impaired bladder function, obstruction to urine outflow, or inability to voluntarily control micturition. Some clients may have permanent or temporary changes in the normal pathway of urinary excretion. The client with a urinary diversion has special problems because urine drains to the outside through a stoma.

Urinary Retention

Urinary retention is accumulation of urine in the bladder with inability of the bladder to empty fully. Urine collects in the bladder, stretching its walls and causing feelings of pressure, discomfort, tenderness over the symphysis pubis, restlessness, and diaphoresis (sweating).

Urine production slowly fills the bladder and prevents activation of stretch receptors. After it distends beyond a certain point, the bladder becomes unable to contract.

A key sign is absence of urine output over several hours and formation of bladder distention. The client under the influence of anesthetics or analgesics may feel only pressure, but the alert client has severe pain as the bladder distends beyond its normal capacity. In severe urinary retention the bladder may hold as much as 2000 to 3000 ml of urine.

As retention progesses, retention with overflow may develop. Pressure in the bladder builds to a point where the external urethral sphincter is unable to hold back urine. The sphincter temporarily opens to allow a small volume of urine (25 to 60 ml) to escape. As urine exits, the bladder pressure falls enough to allow the sphincter to regain control and close. With retention overflow the client voids small amounts of urine 2 or 3 times an hour with no real relief of distention or discomfort. Bladder spasms may occur with voiding.

Retention occurs as a result of urethral obstruction, surgical trauma, alterations in motor and sensory innervation of the bladder, medication side effects, and anxiety.

Lower UTIs

UTIs account for 40% of hospital-acquired (nosocomial) infections in the United States (Burgener, 1987). Bacteria in the urine (**bacteriuria**) may lead to the spread of organisms into the bloodstream and kidneys.

Microorganisms can enter the urinary tract through the urethral meatus or through the bloodstream. The ascending route through the urethra is more common. Bacteria inhabit the distal urethra, external genitalia, and vagina in women. Organisms enter the urethral meatus easily and travel up the inner mucosal lining to the bladder. Women are more susceptible to infection because of the proximity of the anus to the urethral meatus and because of the short urethra. In men, prostatic secretions contain an antibacterial substance that reduces UTI. Older adults and clients with progressive underlying disease or decreased immunity are also at increased risk.

In a healthy person with good bladder function, organisms are flushed out during voiding. However, bladder distention reduces blood flow to the mucosal and submucosal layer, and tissues become more susceptible to bacteria. Residual urine in the bladder is an ideal site for microorganism growth. The pH and chemical makeup of urine also affect the spread of organisms.

The most common cause of infection is the introduction of instruments into the urinary tract. For example, the introduction of a catheter through the urethra provides a direct route for microorganisms. With an indwelling bladder catheter, bacteria ascend along the outside of the catheter on the urethral wall or travel up the catheter's lumen. The catheter interferes with the normal voiding mechanism that acts as a defense against organisms entering the urethra. Local irritation to the urethra or bladder further predisposes tissues to bacterial invasion. UTIs acquired in health institutions also result from contaminated hands of personnel, irrigation fluids, and rectal thermometers.

Poor perineal hygiene is a common cause of UTI in women. Inadequate handwashing, failure to wipe from front to back after voiding or defecating, and frequent sexual intercourse predispose women to infection. In some young girls, **cystitis** (inflammation of the bladder and ureters) develops from exposure to ingredients in bubble baths or shampoo used in the bathtub (Rogers, 1985). Any interference with the free flow of urine can cause infection. A kinked or obstructed catheter and any condition resulting in urinary retention increases the risk of a bladder infection.

Clients with UTIs have pain or burning during urination (**dysuria**) as urine flows past inflamed tissues. Fever, chills, nausea and vomiting, and malaise develop as the infection worsens. An irritated bladder causes a frequent and urgent sensation of the need to void. Irritation to bladder and urethral mucosa results in blood-tinged urine (**hematuria**). The urine appears concentrated and cloudy because of the presence of white blood cells (WBCs) or bacteria. If infection spreads to the kidneys (**pyelonephritis**), flank pain, tenderness, low-grade fever, and chills are common.

Urinary Incontinence

Urinary incontinence is the loss of control over micturition. It may be temporary or permanent. The client cannot control the external urethral sphincter. Leakage of urine may be continuous or intermittent. The five types of incontinence are total, functional, stress, urge, and reflex (Table 40-1).

Incontinence should not be associated only with older adults and senile clients. It may develop in people of every age, although it is more common in adults. Incontinence can impair body image. Clothing becomes wet with urine, and the accompanying odor adds to embarrassment. Clients with this problem often avoid social activities.

Older adults have special problems with incontinence because of physical limitations and the environments in which they live (see research highlight). Older persons with restricted mobility have greater chances of being incontinent because of their inability to reach toilet facilities in time. Low-set chairs

TABLE 40-1   Types of Urinary Incontinence

	Description	Causes	Symptoms
TOTAL	Total uncontrolled and continuous loss of urine	Neuropathy of sensory nerves; trauma or disease of spinal nerves or urethral sphincter; fistula between bladder and vagina	Constant flow of urine at unpredictable times, nocturia, unawareness of bladder filling or incontinence
FUNCTIONAL	Involuntary, unpredictable passage of urine in client with intact urinary and nervous systems	Change in environment; sensory, cognitive, or mobility deficits	Strong urge to void that causes loss of urine before reaching appropriate receptacle
STRESS	Increased intraabdominal pressure that causes leakage of small amount of urine	Coughing, laughing, vomiting, or lifting with full bladder; obesity; full uterus in third trimester; incompetent bladder outlet; weak pelvic musculature	Dribbling of urine with increased intraabdominal pressure, urinary urgency and frequency
URGE	Involuntary passage of urine after strong sense of urgency to void	Decreased bladder capacity; irritation of bladder stretch receptors; alcohol or caffeine ingestion; increased fluid intake	Urinary urgency, abdominal frequency (more often than every 2 hr), bladder contracture or spasm, nocturia, voiding in small (less than 100 ml) or large (more than 550 ml) amounts
REFLEX OR OVERFLOW	Involuntary loss of urine occurring at somewhat predictable intervals when specific bladder volume is reached	Upper spinal cord injury or disease involving area above reflex arc, blocking cerebral awareness. Lower spinal cord injury blocking impulses to reflex arc	Unawareness of bladder filling, lack of urge to void, uninhibited bladder contraction or spasm at regular intervals

 **Research Highlight**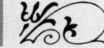

Kaltrieder et al examined the effectiveness of prompting and reinforcement techniques on the toileting habits of study participants. The study group consisted of 133 women age 65 or older. The women were divided into two groups. The treatment group ($n = 65$) received prompted toileting and social reinforcement from a group of nursing research assistants. The second group, the control group ($n = 68$), did not receive the prompting or reinforcement, and their needs were handled by the facilities' routine nursing personnel. About 72% of the women in the treatment group demonstrated a decreased incidence in incontinent episodes. This change was not noted in the control group. The findings from this study suggest that behavior therapy may be useful in decreasing incontinent episodes in cognitively alert clients or clients with severe incontinence problems because they are offered toileting opportunities more frequently and benefit from the social reinforcement obtained when continent.

Kaltrieder DL et al: Can reminders curb incontinence? *Geriatr Nurs* 11(1):17, 1990.

and beds raised well above the floor may be obstacles for older adults, who must get up to reach a toilet. Older clients who have difficulty undoing buttons or manipulating zippers face another obstacle. Older clients often lack the energy to walk very far at one time, and if there is only one toilet in the home, the distance may be too far for clients with urge incontinence.

Continued episodes of incontinence create the potential for skin breakdown. The acidic character of urine is irritating to skin. The immobilized client who has frequent incontinence is especially at risk for pressure ulcers (see Chapter 44).

Enuresis

Enuresis is repeated involuntary urination in children who have reached the age when voluntary control is possible. Usually this is around age 5 (Whaley, Wong, 1991).

Episodes occur more commonly at night (nocturnal enuresis), usually during deep sleep (see Chapter 24). Enuresis may occur during the day (diurnal enuresis) when the child is engaged in play and unaware of a full bladder. Some children are enuretic during a temper tantrum or dispute with a sibling or playmate.

With primary enuresis the child has never had a long dry or symptom-free period. Secondary or acquired enuresis occurs after a dry period of at least a year.

Theories explaining the cause of enuresis include heredity, delayed development, sibling rivalry, emotional trauma during toilet training, food allergies, and behavior problems. The condition tends to be more common in boys and in children of lower socioeconomic families.

Urinary Diversions

A urinary stoma to divert the flow of urine from the kidneys directly to the abdominal surface is done for several reasons (see box). Such a **urinary diversion** may be temporary or permanent. Fig. 40-4 illustrates several urinary diversions.

The ileal loop or conduit (one of the more common approaches to urinary diversion) involves separating a loop of intestinal ileum with its blood supply intact. The surgeon implants the ureters into the ileum, which is an outlet for urine drainage. The ileum is not a reservoir. The remaining ileum is reconnected to the rest of the digestive tract. The disadvantage is that, if urine outflow becomes obstructed, irreversible damage to the kidneys can occur secondary to chronic infections or hydronephrosis.

A **ureterostomy** involves bringing the end of one or both ureters to the abdominal surface. To avoid the need for two collecting devices, a transureter-oureterostomy connects the ureters and brings one out through the abdominal wall.

The client with a urinary diversion must wear a stomal pouch continuously because there is no sphincter control for regulation of urine flow. Local irritation and skin breakdown occur when urine comes in contact with the skin for long periods.

A urinary diversion poses threats to a client's body image. The client must wear an artificial device to collect urine and must learn to manage it. However,

---

Possible Indications for Urinary Diversions

- Cancer of the bladder, prostate, urethra, vagina, uterus, cervix
- Trauma
- Radiation injury to the bladder
- Vesicovaginal fistula
- Urethrovaginal fistula
- Neurogenic bladder
- Chronic cystitis

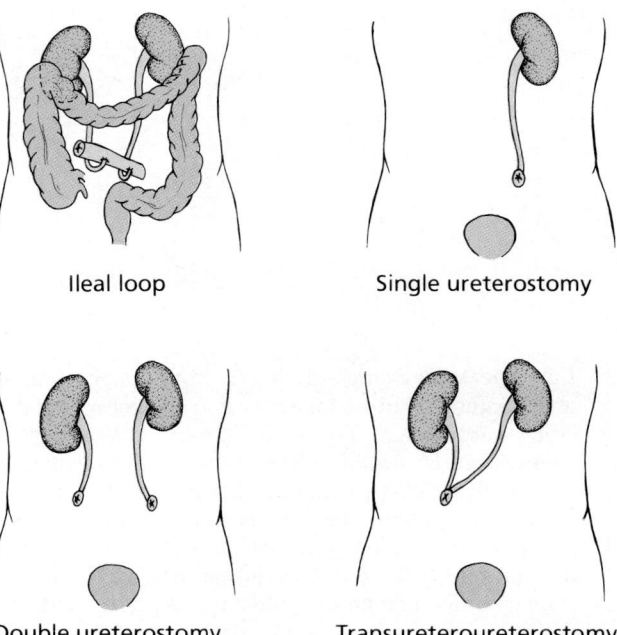

Ileal loop   Single ureterostomy

Double ureterostomy   Transureteroureterostomy

Fig. 40-4 Types of urinary diversions.

the client can wear normal clothing, engage in physical activity, travel, and have sexual relations.

A client with a urinary diversion should be referred to the enterostomal therapist (a nurse with specialized training in this area). This individual can serve as an invaluable resource to assist the client with matters pertaining to all aspects of care. The client should also be referred to the United Ostomy Association. This organization may be beneficial in providing information regarding support groups to enhance coping and adaptation to lifestyle and body-image changes.

 ## NURSING PROCESS AND URINARY PROBLEMS

 ## Assessment

To identify a urinary elimination problem and gather data for a care plan, the nurse obtains a nursing history, performs a physical assessment, assesses the client's urine, and reviews information from diagnostic tests and examinations.

Nursing History

The nursing history includes a review of the client's elimination patterns and symptoms of urinary alterations, as well as an assessment of other factors that may be affecting the ability to urinate normally.

PATTERN OF URINATION. The nurse asks the client about daily voiding patterns, including frequency and times of day, normal volume at each voiding, and recent changes. Frequency varies among individuals. The common times for urination are on awakening, after meals, and before bedtime. Most people void an average of 5 or more times a day. The client who voids frequently during the night may have renal disease. Information about the pattern of urination is necessary to establish a baseline of comparison.

SYMPTOMS OF URINARY ALTERATIONS. Certain symptoms specific to urinary alterations may occur in more than one type of disorder. During assessment the nurse asks the client about the symptoms listed in Table 40-2 on p. 1346. The nurse also assesses whether the client is aware of conditions or factors that precipitate or aggravate symptoms.

FACTORS AFFECTING URINATION. The nurse summarizes factors in the client's history that normally affect urination such as medication history. The name, amount, and frequency of prescription drugs should be noted. Over-the-counter drugs and exposure to cleaning solvents, pesticides, or other nephrotoxic agents are also important aspects of the history. Environmental barriers at home or a health care setting are also evaluated. The client may need an elevated toilet seat, grab bars, or a portable commode. The nurse observes for sensory restrictions such as clients with visual problems who may have trouble reaching toilet facilities. If the client has difficulty with hand coordination, the nurse assesses the type of clothing and ease in using clothing fasteners.

Past illness such as UTI or surgery that increases the risk for recurrent problems are important, as well. Chronic diseases (for example, multiple sclerosis) that impair bladder function require the nurse to consider preventive care measures. The nurse asks the client about the presence of urinary diversion. If the client has a urinary diversion, the nurse determines the rationale for its creation, type of diversion, and usual methods for management (type of appliance or pouch, type of skin barriers or applications, methods used to reduce skin irritation, frequency of appliance changes, and the type of nighttime drainage system). Personal habits also affect urination. If a client is hospitalized the nurse assesses the extent to which personal habits are altered. Privacy is often difficult to accomplish in a health care setting, particularly if a client must use a bedpan.

The nurse assesses for the presence of an indwelling catheter. A client recovering from major surgery or suffering critical illness or disability often has an indwelling catheter to aid urinary drainage and provide a measurement of urine output. The presence of a catheter places a client at risk for infection. A client's physical condition affects the frequency in which the nurse monitors fluid intake (see Chapter 39). Regular intake and output (I & O) measurements help assess a client's overall fluid balance. In addition, the nurse determines whether the client has a history of hereditary urinary elimination problems.

Physical Assessment

A physical examination (see Chapter 20) provides the nurse with data to determine the presence and severity of urinary elimination problems. The primary body organs reviewed include the skin, kidneys, bladder, and urethra.

SKIN. The nurse assesses skin integrity. Often, problems with urinary elimination are associated with fluid and electrolyte disturbances. The nurse assesses skin integrity, especially the skin's hydration status. Assessment of the oral mucosa also reveals whether the client's hydration is adequate.

TABLE 40-2	Common Symptoms of Urinary Alterations	
Symptoms	Description	Causes or Associated Factors
Urgency	Feeling of needing to void immediately	Full bladder, inflammation or irritation of bladder mucosa from infection, incompetent urethral sphincter, psychological stress
Dysuria	Painful or difficult urination	Bladder inflammation, trauma or inflammation of urethra
Frequency	Voiding at frequent intervals	Increased fluid intake, bladder inflammation, increased pressure on bladder (e.g., pregnancy, psychological stress)
Hesitancy	Difficulty initiating urination	Prostate enlargement, anxiety, urethral edema
Polyuria	Voiding of large amount of urine	Excess fluid intake, diabetes mellitus or insipidus, use of diuretics, postobstructive diuresis
Oliguria	Diminished urinary output in relation to fluid intake (usually less than 400 ml in 24 hr)	Dehydration, renal failure, UTI, increased ADH secretion (SIADH), congestive heart failure
Nocturia	Urination, particularly excessive, at night	Excess intake of fluids (especially coffee or alcohol before bedtime), renal disease, aging process
Dribbling	Leakage of urine despite voluntary control of micturition	Urine retention from incomplete bladder emptying, stress incontinence
Hematuria	Presence of blood in urine	Neoplasms of kidney, certain glomerular diseases, infections of kidneys or bladder, traumatic injury to urinary structure, calculi, blood dyscrasia
Retention	Accumulation of urine in bladder, with inability of bladder to empty	Urethral obstruction, bladder inflammation, decreased sensory activity, neurogenic bladder, prostate enlargement after anesthesia, side effects of certain medications (e.g., anticholinergics, antispasmodics, antidepressants).
Residual urine	Volume of urine remaining in bladder after voiding (volumes of 100 ml or more)	Inflammation or irritation of bladder mucosa from infection, neurogenic bladder, prostatic enlargement, trauma or inflammation or urethra

KIDNEYS. If the kidneys become infected or inflamed, flank pain typically develops. The nurse can assess for flank tenderness early in the disease by percussing the costovertebral angle (the angle formed by the spine and twelfth rib). Inflammation of the kidney results in pain during percussion. Auscultation is also performed to detect the presence of a renal artery bruit (sound resulting from turbulent blood flow through a narrowed artery).

Nurses with advanced examination skills learn to palpate the kidneys during abdominal examination. The position, shape, and size of the kidneys can reveal problems such as tumors.

BLADDER. Normally the bladder rests below the symphysis pubis and cannot be examined by the nurse. When distended, the bladder rises above the symphysis pubis at the midline of the abdomen and just below the umbilicus. During physical assessment the nurse may note a swelling or convex curvature of the lower abdomen. When distention is not visible, the nurse lightly palpates the lower abdomen. The bladder normally feels smooth and rounded. As the nurse applies light pressure to the bladder, the client may feel tenderness or even pain. Palpation may also cause the urge to urinate. Percussion of a full bladder yields a dull percussion note.

URETHRAL MEATUS. During the examination, a woman assumes a dorsal recumbent position to provide full exposure of the genitalia. While wearing gloves, the nurse retracts the labial folds to see the urethral meatus. Normally the meatus is pink and appears as a small slitlike opening below the clitoris and above the vaginal orifice. There is normally no discharge from the meatus. Drainage may indicate infection. The nurse notes its color and consistency. A clear, watery drainage is likely to be urine.

Women with vaginal infections are susceptible to UTIs because vaginal discharge may travel easily to the urethral meatus. Older women commonly have vaginitis as a result of hormonal deficiencies. The nurse inspects the vaginal orifice carefully and describes any drainage. Infection is indicated by reddened, inflamed vaginal mucosa.

A man's urethral meatus is normally a small opening at the tip of the penis. A **hypospadias** is a congenitally formed opening of the urethra on the undersurface of the penis. The nurse inspects the meatus for discharge, inflammation, and lesions. It may be necessary to retract the foreskin in uncircumcised men to see the meatus. Specimens of uretheral discharge should be obtained before the client voids.

Assessment of Urine

Assessment of urine involves measuring the client's fluid intake and urine output and observing characteristics of the client's urine.

INTAKE AND OUTPUT. The nurse assesses the client's average daily fluid intake. If a precise measurement of fluid intake is needed from the client who is at home, the nurse may ask the client to show a commonly used glass or cup on which the intake estimate is based.

In a health care setting the nurse measures a client's fluid intake when the physician orders I & O measurements (see Chapter 39). The nurse includes all sources, including oral intake, intravenous fluid infusions, tube feedings, and fluid instilled into nasogastric tubes.

Because it is often difficult for the client to estimate volumes of urine voided, the nurse must obtain measurements. A change in urine volume is a significant indicator of fluid alterations or kidney disease. While caring for the client, the nurse assesses volume by measuring (with plastic receptacles, bedpans or urinals, or a catheter bag) urinary output with each voiding. Special urimeters attach between indwelling catheters and drainage bags and are a convenient means of measuring urine volume on a regular basis (Fig. 40-5). A urimeter holds 100 to 200 ml of urine. After measuring urine from a urimeter, the nurse can drain the cylinder into the urinary drainage bag or into a receptacle for disposal. Urimeters are indicated when precise measurements of urine on an hourly basis are needed.

When urine from a drainage bag is measured, it is best to use a separate plastic graduate receptacle. Scales on the bags offer only an approximate volume. Each client should have a graduate receptacle isolated for exclusive use to prevent potential cross contamination.

The nurse reports any extreme increase or decrease in volume. A repeated hourly output of less

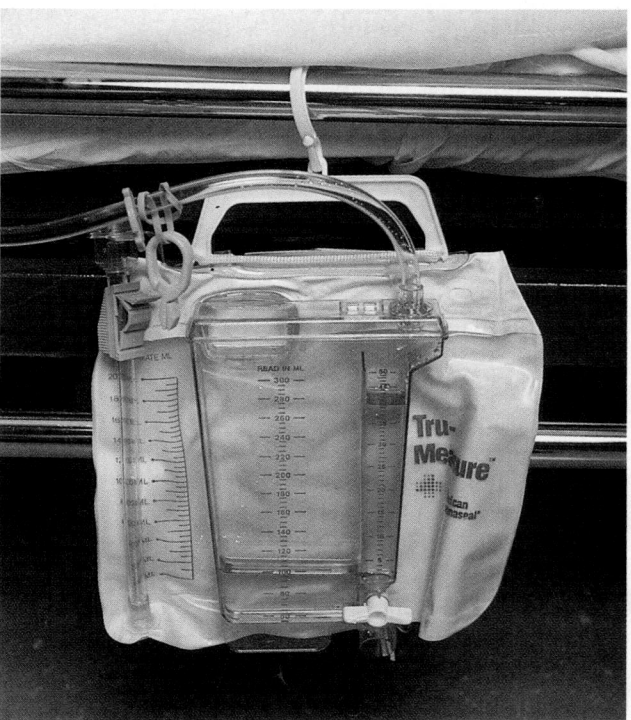

Fig. 40-5   Urimeter drainage bag.

than 30 ml is cause for concern. Similarly, high volumes of urine (**polyuria**), over 2000 ml daily, should be reported to a physician. The nurse can initiate an order to monitor I & O if necessary.

CHARACTERISTICS OF URINE. The nurse inspects the client's urine for color, clarity, and odor.

Color. Normal urine ranges from a pale, straw color to amber, depending on its concentration. Urine is usually more concentrated in the morning or with fluid volume deficits. As the person drinks more fluids, urine becomes less concentrated.

Bleeding from the kidneys or ureters causes urine to become dark red; bleeding from the bladder or urethra causes a bright red urine. Various medications also change urine color (see box on p. 1341). Beets, rhubarb, and blackberries may cause red urine. Special dyes used in intravenous diagnostic studies eventually discolor urine. Dark amber urine may be the result of high concentrations of bilirubin caused by liver dysfunction. Urine containing bilirubin (**bilirubinuria**) can be detected by the appearance of yellow foam when a specimen is shaken. The nurse reports any abnormal color or sediment to the physician, especially if the cause is unknown.

Clarity. Normal urine appears transparent at voiding. Urine that stands several minutes in a container becomes cloudy. Freshly voided urine in clients with renal disease may appear cloudy or foamy because of high protein concentrations. Urine also appears thick and cloudy as a result of bacteria.

Odor. Urine has a characteristic odor. The more concentrated the urine, the stronger the odor. Bacteria in the urine causes an ammonia odor, which is common in clients who are repeatedly incontinent. A sweet or fruity odor occurs from acetone or acetoacetic acid, by-products of incomplete fat metabolism, seen with diabetes mellitus or starvation.

URINE TESTING. The nurse is frequently responsible for collecting urine specimens for laboratory testing. The type of test determines the method of collection. All specimens are labeled with the client's name, date, and time of collection. Specimens should be transported to the laboratory in a timely fashion to ensure accuracy of test results. Agency infection-control policies dictate the adherence to universal isolation procedures by all personnel during specimen handling (see Chapter 18).

Specimen Collection. The nurse collects random, clean-voided or midstream, sterile, timed, and double-voided specimens.

Random Specimen. A random routine urine specimen can be collected with a client voiding naturally or through a Foley catheter or urinary diversion collection bag. The specimen should be clean but need not be sterile. Random specimens are used for urinalysis testing or measurements of specific gravity, pH, or glucose levels.

The client voids into a clean urine cup, urinal, or bedpan. Many clients are able to do this independently. However, mobility restrictions or poor vision may require the nurse to assist. It is easier to collect a specimen if the client drinks a glass of fluid 30 minutes before the procedure. A client should void before defecating so that feces do not contaminate the specimen. Female clients are also instructed not to place toilet tissue in the bedpan. Only 120 ml (4 oz) of urine is needed for accurate testing. After the specimen is collected the nurse places the lid tightly on the specimen container, washes off any urine that splashed on the outside of the container, places the container in a plastic bag, and sends the labeled specimen promptly to the laboratory.

Clean-Voided or Midstream Specimen. To obtain a specimen relatively free of the microorganisms growing in the lower urethra, the nurse instructs the client on the method for obtaining a clean-voided specimen (Procedure 40-1). This type of specimen is needed to test urine for culture and sensitivity. After appropriate cleansing of the external genitalia, a client begins the urinary stream allowing the initial portion to escape; then during the middle portion of voiding, the client collects the specimen. The initial stream of urine cleans or flushes the urethral orifice and meatus of resident bacteria. It is easiest for a client to obtain clean-voided specimens while using toilet facilities.

Sterile Specimen. Another method for collecting a urine specimen for culture is by obtaining it from an indwelling catheter. It is no longer recommended to catheterize a client just to obtain a specimen because the risk of causing an infection is high. A urine specimen is also not collected for culture from urine drainage bags unless it is the first urine drained into a new sterile bag. Bacteria grow rapidly in the drainage bags and would give a false measurement of bacteria.

For an indwelling retention catheter, the nurse uses a sterile syringe to withdraw urine. The nurse washes hands and applies nonsterile gloves to prevent transmission of microorganisms. A 3-ml syringe with a small-gauge needle (23- or 25-gauge) is best to prevent creation of a permanent hole in the catheter port. However, if blood is suspected in the urine, a large-bore needle prevents breakdown of RBCs. It is safe to insert a needle directly into the end of a self-sealing rubber catheter. Silastic, plastic, or silicone catheters are not self-sealing. Most urinary catheters have special ports to withdraw specimens (Fig. 40-6). First, the nurse clamps the tubing just below the site chosen for withdrawal, allowing fresh, uncontaminated urine to collect in the tube. The nurse then wipes the catheter or port with an antimicrobial swab. Inserting the needle at a 30-degree angle ensures entrance into the catheter lumen. While aspirating 3 to 5 ml of urine the nurse must be careful not to raise the tubing, which would cause urine to flow back into the bladder.

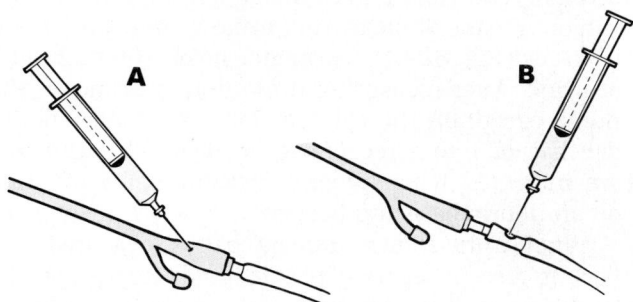

Fig. 40-6   Urine specimen collection from an indwelling catheter. **A,** Aspiration of a urine specimen from a catheter. **B,** Aspiration of a urine specimen from a collection port in the drainage tubing of an indwelling catheter.
Redrawn from McConnell EA: *Care of patients with urologic problems,* Philadelphia, 1983, Lippincott.

STEPS	RATIONALE
1. Assess client's mobility and balance in being able to use toilet facilities independently.	Determines level of assistance required by client.
2. Refer to medical record for indications of urinary infection.	Helps you understand purpose of specimen procedure for client.
3. Assess client's understanding of purpose of test and method of collection.	Information allows you to clarify misunderstandings and promotes client cooperation.
4. Prepare following equipment and supplies:	Agency policy may determine type of equipment to use. Adhere to universal isolation precautions.
a. Commercial kit for clean-voided urine (see illustration), sterile cotton balls, or 2 × 2 gauze pads	Used to clean, rinse, and dry perineum.
b. Antiseptic solution such as povidone-iodine	
c. Sterile water	Rinses antiseptic solution. Antiseptic solution can alter test results if allowed to enter specimen.
d. Sterile gloves	
e. Sterile specimen container	
f. Soap, towel, washcloth	
g. Bedpan (for nonambulating clients), specimen hat, bedside commode, or potty chair	Allows women to void in toilet seat in usual fashion. Children are more likely to use familiar facilities.
h. Completed specimen identification label	Completion of label and requisition before collecting specimen prevents confusing it with other specimens and ensures more rapid transport to laboratory.
5. Explain procedure to client:	
a. Reason midstream specimen is needed	Helps client provide specimen independently.
b. Way client and family member can assist	
c. Way to obtain specimen free of feces	Feces change characteristics of urine and may cause abnormal values.
6. Provide fluids to drink ½ hr before collecting specimen unless contraindicated (i.e., fluid restriction).	Improves likelihood of client being able to void.
7. Refer to agency procedures for specimen collection methods.	Agency policies may vary regarding proper way to collect or handle specimens.
8. Wash hands.	Reduces transfer of infection.
9. Provide privacy for client by closing bed curtain or closing door.	Privacy allows client to relax and produce specimen more quickly.

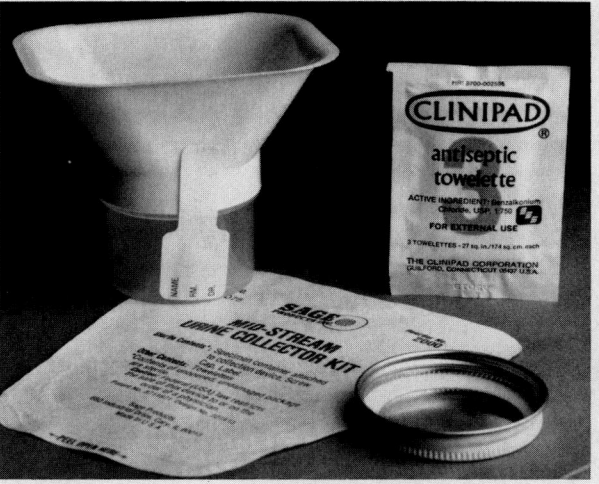

Collecting Midstream (Clean-Voided) Specimen

STEPS	RATIONALE
10. Give client or family member towel, washcloth, and soap to cleanse perineal area or assist client as needed to cleanse perineum.	Client prefers to wash own perineal area when possible.
11. Assist bedridden client onto bedpan.	Provides easy access to perineal areas to collect specimen.
12. Apply gloves (see Chapter 18).	Prevents introduction of microorganisms on your hands into specimen. Reduces risk of transmission of microorganisms to nurse.
13. Using surgical asepsis, open sterile kit or prepare sterile tray.	Sterile technique is essential to maintain sterility of equipment and specimen.
14. Pour antiseptic solution over cotton balls unless kit contains prepared gauze pads in antiseptic solution.	Cotton ball or gauze is used to cleanse perineum.
15. Open specimen container and place cap with sterile inside surface up and do not touch inside of container.	Contaminated specimen is most frequent reason for inaccurate reporting of urinary cultures and sensitivities.
16. Assist or allow client to independently cleanse perineum and collect specimen: a. *Male:*	
(1) Hold penis with one hand and, using circular motion and antiseptic swab, cleanse end of penis, moving from center to outside.	Cleanse from area of least contamination to area of greatest contamination to decrease bacterial levels.
(2) If agency procedure indicates, rinse area with sterile water and dry with cotton balls or gauze pad.	Prevents contamination of specimen with antiseptic solution.
(3) After client has initiated urine stream, pass specimen container into stream and collect 30-60 ml.	Initial urine flushes out microorganisms that normally accumulate at urinary meatus and prevents their collection in specimen.
b. *Female:*	
(1) Spread labia minora with thumb and forefinger of nondominant hand.	Provides access to urethral meatus.
(2) Cleanse area with cotton ball or gauze, moving from front (above urethral orifice) to back (toward anus). Repeat this movement 3 times (left side, right side, center), using separate cotton balls.	Prevents contamination of urinary meatus with fecal material.
(3) If agency procedure indicates, rinse area with sterile water, and dry with cotton.	Prevents contamination of specimen with antiseptic solution.
(4) While continuing to hold labia apart, client should initiate stream and after stream achieved, pass specimen container into stream and collect 30-60 ml.	Initial stream flushes out microorganisms that accumulate at urethral meatus.
17. Remove specimen container before flow of urine stops and before releasing labia or penis. Client finishes voiding into bedpan or toilet.	Prevents contamination of specimen with skin flora.
18. Replace cap securely on specimen container (touch only outside).	Retains sterility of inside of container and prevents spillage of urine.
19. Cleanse any urine from exterior surface of container, and place container in plastic specimen bag.	Prevents transfer of microorganisms to others.
20. Remove bedpan (if applicable) and assist client to comfortable position.	Promotes relaxing environment.
21. Label specimen and attach laboratory requisition.	Prevents inaccurate identification that could lead to errors in diagnosis or therapy.

STEPS	RATIONALE
22. Remove gloves, dispose in proper receptacle, and wash hands	Reduces transmission of infection.
23. Transport specimen to laboratory within 15 min or immediately refrigerate.	Bacteria grow quickly in urine, and specimen should be analyzed immediately to obtain correct results.
24. Record date and time urine specimen was obtained in nurses' notes.	Documents implementation of physician's order.

CONTINUED

After obtaining the specimen the nurse transfers the urine into a sterile container using sterile aseptic technique (see Chapter 18). The nurse removes the gloves, properly disposes of equipment, and washes hands to reduce the transfer of microorgansims to other clients and health care workers. The laboratory requisition should indicate the method of collection.

Timed Urine Specimens. Some tests of renal function and urine composition, such as measuring levels of adrenocortical steroids or hormones, creatinine clearance, or protein quantitation tests, require collection of urine over 2-, 12-, or 24-hour intervals.

The timed collection period begins after the client urinates. The nurse indicates the starting time on the gallon container and on the laboratory requisition, and discards the first sample (check agency policy). The client then collects all urine voided in the timed period.

Each voiding is collected in a clean container and immediately emptied into the larger gallon container. Some tests require the client to void at specific times. Each specimen must be free of feces or toilet tissue.

Any missed specimens will make test results inaccurate. The nurse should remind the client to void before defecating so that urine is not contaminated by feces. The collection jar usually contains a preservative or requires refrigeration. The laboratory should be consulted for instructions. The client should void the last specimen as close as possible to the end of the timed period.

Double-Voided Specimen. For accurate measurement of glucose and ketones (**glycosuria** and **ketonuria**) in the urine the specimen must be fresh. Urine that has been in the bladder for several hours does not reveal the amount of glucose and ketones at the time of testing. Ideally the client voids 30 to 45 minutes before the time a test specimen is required. The nurse discards the first specimen and then has the client drink at least 8 ounces of fluid. The client then voids a second or double-voided specimen for

testing. The second specimen accurately reflects the composition of urine recently filtered by the kidneys.

Urine Collection in Children. Specimen collection from infants and children is often difficult. Adolescents and school-age children are usually able to cooperate, although they may be embarrassed. Preschool children and toddlers have difficulty voiding on request. Offering a young child fluids 30 minutes before requesting a specimen may help. The nurse must use terms for urination that the child can understand. A young child may be reluctant to void in unfamiliar receptacles. A potty chair or bedpan placed under the toilet is usually effective. The nurse must use special collection devices for infants or toddlers who are not toilet trained. Clear, plastic, single-use bags with self-adhering material can be attached over the child's urethral meatus.

The nurse prepares an infant by first washing the genitalia, perineum, and surrounding skin with soap and water or an antiseptic. Thorough drying is necessary because the bag's adhesive does not stick to a moist, powdered, or oily surface. The nurse attaches the bag from back to front, first to the perineum and then toward the symphysis pubis. In girls the perineum should be gently stretched to ensure that the bag has a leak-proof fit. In boys the scrotum and penis fit inside the collection bag. A diaper is placed over the bag. The nurse checks the bag often and removes it as soon as urine is available. An active child can easily loosen the bag and cause a leak. For a clean-voided specimen the nurse uses a sterile collection bag. Specimens should not be obtained by squeezing urine from the diaper material.

Common Urine Tests. Urine tests include urinalysis, specific gravity, urine culture, and glucose and ketone tests.

Urinalysis. The laboratory performs a **urinalysis** on a specimen obtained by any of the previously described methods. Table 40-3 lists normal values for a urinalysis. The specimen should be examined as

TABLE 40-3   Routine Urinalysis Values

Measurement and Normal Value	Interpretation
pH (4.6-8.0)	pH helps indicate acid-base balance. Urine that stands for several hours becomes alkaline for bacterial invasion. Selected antibiotics (e.g., neomycin, streptomycin) are more effective against UTIs if pH is alkaline
Protein level (up to 10 mg/100 ml)	Normally protein is not present in urine. It is seen in renal disease because damage to glomerular membrane or tubules allows protein to enter urine. However, temporary presence of protein can occur after strenuous exercise, exposure to cold, psychological stress, or high dietary protein intake.
Glucose level (not normally present)	Diabetic clients have glucose in urine as result of inability of tubules to reabsorb high glucose concentrations (over 180 mg/100 ml). Ingestion of high concentrations of glucose may cause some to appear in urine of healthy persons.
Ketone level (not normally present)	Clients whose diabetes is poorly controlled experience breakdown of fatty acids. End product of fatty acid metabolism is ketones. Clients with dehydration, starvation, or excessive aspirin ingestion also have ketonuria.
Blood level (up to two RBCs)	Damage to glomerulus or tubules may cause RBCs to enter urine. Trauma or disease of lower urinary tract also causes hematuria. In women, blood in urine may indicate specimen collection during menstrual cycle.
Specific gravity (1.01-1.03)	Specific gravity measures concentration of particles in urine. High specific gravity reflects concentrated urine, and low specific gravity reflects diluted urine. Dehydration, reduced renal blood flow, and increase in ADH secretion elevate specific gravity. Overhydration and inadequate ADH secretion reduce specific gravity.
MICROSCOPIC EXAMINATION	
WBCs (0 to 8 per high-powered field)	Greater numbers may indicate infection within urinary tract.
Bacteria (normally not present)	Bacteria indicate infection within urinary tract.
Casts	Casts are cyclindrical bodies whose shape take on likeness of objects within renal tubule. There are several types, namely hyaline, WBCs, granular cells, and epithelial cells. Their presence in urine represents abnormal findings that indicate renal alterations.

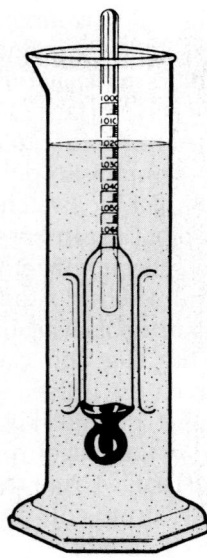

Fig. 40-7   Measurement of urine specific gravity using a urinometer.

soon as possible, preferably within 2 hours. It should be the first voided specimen in the morning to ensure a uniform concentration of constituents. For a quick screening the nurse can perform certain portions of the urinalysis with special reagent strips or tablets. The nurse dips the strips into the urine or applies droplets to tablets and then observes for a color change in the time interval designated on the package.

Specific Gravity. The **specific gravity** is the weight or degree of concentration of a substance compared with an equal volume of water. To measure specific gravity the nurse uses a urinometer and cylinder (Fig. 40-7). The urinometer has a specific gravity scale at the top and a weighted mercury bulb at the bottom. The nurse pours a urine specimen into a clean, dry cylinder. Next the nurse suspends and lightly twirls the weighted urinometer into the cylinder of urine. The concentration of dissolved substances in the urine determines the depth at which the urinometer will float.

With the urinometer at eye level the nurse reads the measurement at the base of the meniscus at the level of the urine. The specific gravity of a morning urine specimen voided by a fasting client reflects the kidney's maximum concentrating ability. A specific gravity below 1.010 reflects an inability of the kidneys to concentrate urine or an insufficient secretion of ADH. When the kidneys become diseased, they lose their ability to concentrate urine. Therefore the specific gravity becomes "fixed" at a low value (1.010). An elevated specific gravity can indicate dehydration. Radiopaque substances or high molecular weight substances in the urine (for example, protein or glucose) may cause a falsely high specific gravity.

If questions regarding the accuracy of specific gravity measurements arise, a urine osmolality test should be obtained. Although both tests measure urine concentration, the osmolality test is more accurate because it measures the total number of particles in a solution (see Chapter 39).

Urine Culture. A urine culture requires a sterile sample of urine. It takes approximately 48 hours before the laboratory can report findings of bacterial growth. If bacteria are present, an additional test for sensitivity determines which antibiotics are effective. If antibotics are ordered pending the results (sensitivities) of a urine culture, the culture should be obtained before administering the medication.

Glucose and Ketones Analysis. An accurate measurement of glucose and ketones always requires a double-voided specimen. Reagent strips contain chemicals that change color when exposed to glucose and ketone. The nurse dips a strip in a urine specimen and pulls it out. After a selected time period (10 to 15 seconds), the nurse compares the strip's color with that of the chart on the bottle. The color scale measures the quantity of glucose or ketone in urine (Fig. 40-8). The range on the color scale extends from negative, trace, 1+, 2+, to 3+. Urine glucose levels are no longer considered a reliable indicator for assessing a diabetic's level of control because of the variability in glucose secretion by the kidneys. Blood glucose monitoring is more accurate and can be done by the client after performing a simple fingerstick.

Diagnostic Examinations. The urinary system is one of the few organ systems amenable to accurate diagnostic study by radiographic techniques. The two approaches for visualization of urinary structures, direct and indirect techniques, can be quite simple or very complex, requiring extensive nursing intervention. These procedures are further subdivided into invasive or noninvasive categories.

Abdominal Roentgenogram. Abdominal roentgenogram, also referred to as *plain film, KUB,* or *flat*

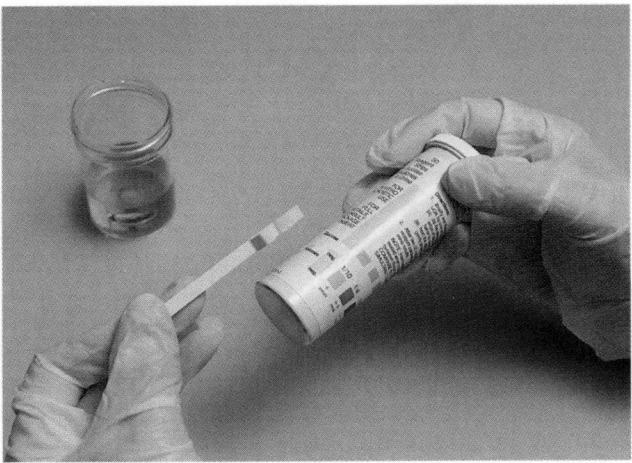

Fig. 40-8   Checking results on a glucose reagent strip.

plate, of the abdomen is commonly used to assess the gross structures of the urinary tract for abnormalities. It can be used to determine size, symmetry, shape, and location of the kidneys, ureters, and bladder structures. It is also useful in visualizing calculi (if they are calcified) or tumors in these organs. In addition, the ribs or other surrounding support structures can be assessed for fractures or abnormalities. This is important if the client has suffered some type of traumatic injury. The lack of positive findings on the roentgenogram does not rule out the possibility of abnormalities in the urinary tract. Additional diagnositic studies may be warranted.

The nursing implications for clients undergoing this procedure include explanation of the procedure and alleviation of client anxiety. No special bowel preparation is warranted unless the physician deems otherwise.

Intravenous Pyelogram. To view the entire urinary system, the physician orders the excretory urogram or intravenous pyelogram (IVP). This procedure visualizes the renal tissue and pelvis and outlines the ureters, bladder, and urethra. (The last two structures are better visualized by cystourethrogram.) Although this procedure is noninvasive, it requires that the client receive an intravenous injection of a radiopaque dye. Normally, the injected medium takes only a few minutes to circulate and be excreted. Because the kidneys and ureters lie behind the intestines, it is necessary that the client receive a bowel preparation to empty the intestines before the procedure. Procedures using barium should not be performed 2 to 3 days before an IVP because residual barium in the intestines will obscure the view (see Chapter 41).

During the IVP, x-ray studies are taken at specific intervals over 30 to 60 minutes as the dye concentrates. The client may also be asked to void during the procedure to measure bladder emptying. Diseases or disorders of the urinary tract that should be investigated by this means include renal artery occlusion, tumors, cysts or calculi, vesicoureteral reflux, and traumatic injuries.

Nursing implications before the test include recognizing clients at risk for alterations in renal function as a result of the intravenous injection of the contrast material. Any client with renal insufficiency is at risk. Older clients in particular are prone to the nephrotoxic effects of these substances because of their propensity for volume depletion during bowel preparation (see Chapter 39). Appropriate nursing assessment of volume status and its maintenance before this procedure is of utmost importance (see Chapter 41). Additional nursing implications follow:

1. Observe client sign informed consent.
2. Assess client for history of iodine allergy, which predicts allergies to the IVP dye.
3. Administer cathartic on evening before test.
4. Ensure that client takes nothing by mouth after midnight.
5. Explain that facial flushing is normal during dye injection and that client may feel dizzy or warm.
6. Explain that an intravenous infusion for dye injection is started before the test.
7. Explain that the test involves x-ray studies taken at several intervals and that client will void near the end of the test.

Not all agencies employ nurses in the radiology department. If a nurse is not present, the physician or radiology technician assumes these responsibilities. Implications during the test include the following:

1. Assess intravenous site for signs of infiltration of dye into tissues (for example, swelling, redness, and pain).
2. Observe for signs of allergic reaction to dye (for example, respiratory distress, fall in blood pressure, and hives).
3. Remind client of normal sensations caused by dye injection.

Nursing implications after the test include the following:

1. Ensure that client receives normal diet afterward.
2. Encourage fluid intake to minimize dehydration caused by fasting and to avoid the potential nephrotoxic effects of the contrast material.
3. Monitor I & O and promptly report alterations to physician.

Renal Scan. Radionuclide tests such as renal scans allow indirect visualization of urinary tract structures after an intravenous injection of radioac-

tive isotopes. There are several different radiopharmaceutical agents used during this procedure. Their selection depends on the physiological process to be investigated. The emissions from the radionuclides can be photographed by special cameras. The isotope can be detected without the need of bowel preparation. A very low dosage of radioisotope is used. Its half-life is short. Therefore no precautions against radioactive exposure are needed.

After a radionuclide is injected, it circulates through the kidney and is excreted. The renal scan measures radioactive concentrations while the client assumes a supine, prone, or sitting position. Except for the venipuncture, it is painless. The scanning procedure is completed in approximately 1 hour. Information pertaining to renal blood flow, anatomical structures, and their excretory function can be obtained from this procedure. The physician can diagnose abnormalities such as renal artery occlusion, urinary obstruction, and many other diseases of the kidney. This procedure is indicated for clients unable to receive IVP dyes. The nurse does not routinely give a sedative before the test unless the physician views the client as highly anxious. Nursing implications before the test include the following:

1. Observe client sign informed consent.
2. Explain that radioisotope is injected intravenously through an existing IV line or needle.
3. Explain that client will feel no discomfort but must lie still.
4. Explain that there is no risk of radioactive exposure.

Nursing implications during the test include the following:

1. Assist the client in changing positions during the test. (Technician may do this.)
2. Explain that the machine measuring the isotope uptake is similar to a Geiger counter.

A nursing implication after the test follows:

1. Instruct client to resume normal activities.

Computerized Axial Tomography. Computerized tomography (CT) is a computerized x-ray procedure used to obtain detailed images of structures within a selected plane of the body. The tomographic scanner is a large machine that contains specialized computers and x-ray detector systems that function concomitantly to photograph internal structures in thin, transverse cross sections. The computer, through a series of complex manipulations, is able to "reconstruct" the cross-sectional image as a recognizable photograph on the television monitor. With this procedure, it is possible to visualize abnormal pathological conditions such as tumors, obstructions, retroperitoneal masses, and lymph node enlargement. The CT scan can detect and characterize masses of less than 2 cm in size. Although this procedure is noninvasive, in some examinations, oral or intravenous contrast material is used to enhance the areas under study. If intravenous contrast is used, it may be necessary to administer an enema, especially if additional organs in the abdominal cavity will be examined. The nursing implications before, during, and after this test are the same as those listed under the IVP examination. However, the nurse explains that the client will be placed in a large machine, which may precipitate feelings of claustrophobia in susceptible individuals.

Renal Ultrasound. Ultrasonography is another procedure gaining widespread acceptance as a valuable noninvasive diagnostic tool in the assessment of urinary disorders. It makes use of high-frequency, inaudible sound waves that reflect off tissue. A conductive gel is applied to the skin and functions as a transmitter for sound waves. A transducer passed over the conductive gel emits a beam as it is also passed over body tissues of varying density. Some of the sound waves are reflected back to the transducer as echoes. The echoes are converted into electrical impulses that are displayed on an oscilloscope, presenting an image or photograph of the tissues being studied. The velocity of the sound waves varies with tissue density. The client is usually prone during the procedure but can be positioned in a sitting position. No biological hazards have been identified with energy or sound wave emissions from this procedure. Ultrasound is frequently used to identify gross renal structures and structural abnormalities of the kidneys or lower urinary tract and to assist with percutaneous biopsy. Abnormalities such as tumors or cysts in the kidney are easily identified with this procedure. If a Doppler is used with the transducer, examination of blood flow through the kidney can also be performed. This procedure is painless.

Nursing implications before the procedure involve explanation of the test and possibly encouraging the client to ingest oral fluids to cause bladder distention. No specific client care is indicated after the test.

Invasive Procedures. Invasive procedures include cystoscopy, biopsy, and arteriogram.

Cystoscopy. To view the interior of the bladder and urethra, the physician performs a cystoscopy. The cystoscope looks much like a urinary catheter, although it is not as flexible. It is inserted through the client's urethra. The instrument has an outer plastic or rubber sheath, an obturator that keeps the scope rigid during insertion, a telescope for viewing the bladder and urethra, and a channel for inserting catheters or special surgical instruments.

The procedure is painful during instrument insertion. Unless the client lies still, there is risk of bladder perforation. Local, spinal, or general anesthesia may be administered. Because the test requires insertion of a foreign object into a sterile cavity, the client receives large amounts of fluids (intravenously or orally) before and during the procedure to maintain a continuous urine flow and to flush out any bacteria. Antibiotics may also be administered intraveneously. During the test, urine and tissue specimens may be collected.

The physician usually performs the cystoscopy in a hospital cystoscopy room. Special cystoscopy tables minimize the stress and fatigue that clients may experience from maintaining one position for a prolonged time. Nursing implications before the test include the following:

1. Observe client sign informed consent.
2. Perform a bowel preparation or enema or administer a cathartic on the evening before the test.
3. If local anesthetic will be used, encourage intake of oral fluids.
4. If general anesthetic is to be used, ensure that client takes nothing by mouth after midnight.
5. Explain that insertion of the cystoscope is similar to insertion of urethral catheter.
6. Explain the importance of lying still during the test.
7. Explain that an intravenous line will be started to give fluids during the test.
8. Administer a sedative and analgesic per the physician's orders.

Nursing implications during the test include the following:

1. Assist client to assume a lithotomy position (see Chapter 20).
2. Prepare perineal area with antiseptic solution.
3. Explain (if client is awake) that insertion of cystoscope causes an urge to void.
4. Remind client to lie still.

Nursing implications after the test include the following:

1. Instruct the client to remain in bed as ordered.
2. Assess for signs of urinary retention and first voiding.
3. Observe characteristics of urine, noting bloody or cloudy urine.
4. Encourage increased fluid intake and monitor I & O.
5. Observe for fever, dysuria, or drop in blood pressure.
6. Administer medications to alleviate bladder spasms and/or lower back pain.

In addition to complete visual inspection of the bladder and urethra through the cystoscope, retrograde pyelography may also be performed. During this procedure, the physician passes a small catheter (4 to 6 French [Fr]) through the cystoscope into the bladder, which allows catheterization of the ureters and renal pelvis. Urine specimens are then collected separately from each ureter. Radiopaque dye can be instilled into the renal pelvis while serial x-rays are taken to examine the filling of the renal collecting system. X-ray examinations to visualize the bladder and urethra are also considered invasive studies. These examinations include retrograde cystograms, voiding cystourethrograms (VCUGs), and cystourethrograms. All of these studies involve the instillation of a radiopaque fluid into the bladder via a catheter (urethral or suprapubic). Serial x-ray films taken during these procedures provide information regarding abnormalities in bladder mucosa, demonstrate **vesicoureteral reflux** (backflow of urine from bladder to ureter), provide information regarding bladder function, and provide an assessment of the size and shape of the ureters. Nursing implications for this procedure would be the same as those for cystoscopy.

Renal Biopsy. A renal biopsy is performed to determine the nature, extent, and prognosis of renal disease. This procedure involves obtaining a piece of renal cortical tissue for examination with sophisticated microscopic techniques. The procedure can be performed by percutaneous (closed) or surgical (open) methods. The use of ultrasound examinations to localize the kidney has revolutionized the percutaneous approach. Tissue diagnosis allows differentiation between disease processes causing alterations in renal function. Therefore more specific treatment interventions can be applied. Nursing implications before this procedure include the following:

1. Observe client sign informed consent.
2. Explain procedure.
3. Obtain hematological studies (for example, complete blood count, bleeding time, prothrombin time, platelet count, and type and cross-match for possible blood transfusion) for evaluation.
4. Obtain urine specimens for routine analysis, culture, and sensitivity.
5. Instruct client in appropriate positioning (prone) with pillows placed under the abdomen to elevate the kidneys and breathing techniques (client may be asked to hold the breath when biopsy needle is introduced) during the procedure. Ask the client to hold the breath during inspiration to promote immobilization of the kidneys as the needle is inserted.
6. Administer a sedative to relieve anxiety.

Nursing implications during the test include the following:

1. Provide emotional support to the client.
2. Coach client about breathing and positioning.

3. Remind client of normal sensations caused by local administration of analgesics and biopsy instrument.

Nursing implications after the test include the following:

1. Observe color, amount, and character of urine, noting bloody urine.
2. Monitor vital signs, noting changes consistent with hemorrhagic shock (see Chapter 47).
3. Obtain hematological studies (complete blood count) after the biopsy.
4. Encourage client to consume fluids orally.
5. Instruct client to remain in bed for prescribed time (usually 24 hours).
6. Assess biopsy site for signs of bleeding and note complaints of pain.
7. Maintain pressure dressings on biopsy site.
8. Instruct client to refrain from strenous activity for at least 2 weeks.

Arteriogram (Angiogram). A renal angiogram is an invasive radiographic procedure that evaluates the renal arterial sytem. The arteriogram is most often used to examine the main renal artery or its segmental branches to detect any narrowing or occlusion. In addition, this procedure is useful in the evaluation of mass lesions (for example, neoplasms or cysts) to determine parity, collateral, or traumatic injury to blood vessels. The arteriogram is performed by placing a catheter into one of the femoral arteries and advancing it to the level of the renal arteries. Radiopaque contrast material is injected through the catheter while serial images are taken in rapid succession.

Venograms are most often performed to examine the excretory system and allow for sampling of renal vein blood to test for various renal hormonal levels (for example, renin and erythropoietin). During the venogram, a catheter is inserted into the femoral vein and advanced to the level of the renal veins.

Pretest nursing implications are similar to those denoted under the IVP procedure. In addition to those listed under the IVP procedure, nursing implications during the test include the following:

1. Monitor vital signs.
2. Administer intravenous mannitol during the injection of contrast material to promote diuresis and excretion of the contrast. This is especially important in clients who may be prone to its nephrotoxic effects (for example, older adults or individuals with renal insufficiency or a client with a single kidney).

Nursing implications after the test include the following:

1. Monitor vital signs hourly until stability is verified, and then advance intervals to every 2 hours and 4 hours respectively.

2. Ensure that the client maintains bed rest for 8 to 12 hours. (If a venogram was performed this time, interval may be less.)
3. Check pulse, assess the circulation in the cannulated extremity, and ensure that the extremity is kept in straight alignment.
4. Observe for bleeding, increased tenderness, and hematoma formation at the catheter insertion site for 24 hours.
5. Maintain a pressure dressing over the site for 24 hours.
6. Observe client for possible delayed reactions to the contrast material.
7. Monitor the client's I & O and report abnormalities in urine volume to the physician.

 ## Nursing Diagnosis

A thorough assessment of the client's urinary elimination function ensures the nurse's ability to make relevant and accurate nursing diagnoses. The diagnosis may be potential or actual, depending on risks and health alterations (see diagnoses box). The diagnosis may focus on a urinary elimination alteration or associated problems.

Identification of defining characteristics leads the nurse to select an appropriate diagnosis (see diagnostic process box on p. 1358). Specifying related factors for each diagnosis allows selection of individualized nursing interventions.

 ## Planning

The nurse plans therapeutic interventions for clients with urinary elimination problems, and preventive interventions may be required for clients with potential urinary problems (see care plan on p. 1358). The nurse plans therapies according to the severity of risks to the client.

It is important to consider the client's home environment and normal elimination routines when planning therapies. Reinforcement of good health habits that are already followed improves compliance with the care plan.

The client with actual or risks for alterations in urinary elimination learns to recognize signs of

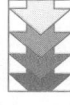 ## Examples of Nursing Diagnoses for Urinary Elimination

NANDA-APPROVED NURSING DIAGNOSES

Pain related to:
- Urethral inflammation
- Urinary retention

Toileting self-care deficit related to:
- Limited mobility of the lower extremities

Impaired skin integrity or *high risk for impaired skin integrity* related to:
- Incontinence of urine

Altered patterns of urinary elimination related to:
- Sensory motor impairment
- Traumatized urethral tissue

Body-image disturbance related to:
- Feelings about urinary diversion
- Feelings about frequent incontinence

Functional incontinence related to:
- Diuretic therapy
- Lack of established toileting regimen
- Mobility restrictions
- Unfamiliar toileting facilities

High risk for infection related to:
- Urethral catheter insertion
- Poor personal hygiene
- Inadequate primary defense mechanisms (skin breakdown)

Reflex incontinence related to:
- Neurological impairment
- Loss of voluntary control of micturition

Stress incontinence related to:
- Increased intraabdominal pressure
- Weak pelvic musculature

Total incontinence related to:
- Loss of voluntary control of micturition
- Presence of fistula
- Self-care limitations

Urge incontinence related to:
- Alcohol ingestion
- Irritation of bladder mucosa
- Decreased bladder capacity

Urinary retention related to:
- Weakened detrusor muscle
- Pain or anesthesia after surgery
- Fluid volume deficit
- Fluid volume excess
- Minimal activity

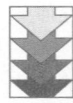

Nursing Diagnostic Process for Urinary Elimination

Assessment Activities	Defining Characteristics	Nursing Diagnosis
Ask client about sensations to void.	Sensation of bladder fullness or urge to void Sensation of pain during and after voiding.	*Urinary retention* related to inhibition of voiding reflex, weakened detrusor muscle, and pain after surgery
Ask client about presence of small, frequent dribbling. Palpate over symphysis pubis.	Reports of frequent dribbling in small amounts Palpable bladder Increased urge to void with palpation Possible dribbling with palpation	
Catheterize after client voids.	Residual volume greater than 150 ml present	

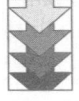

Sample Nursing Care Plan for Urinary Retention

Nursing diagnosis: *Urinary retention* related to weakened detrusor muscle
Definition: Urinary retention is the state in which an individual experiences incomplete emptying of the bladder (Kim, McFarland, McLane, 1991).

Goal	Expected Outcomes	Interventions	Rationale
Client will achieve complete bladder emptying after voiding by the fourth day after childbirth.	Bladder will not be distended after voiding. Client will deny feeling of bladder fullness after voiding. There will be less than 50 ml of residual urine.	Instruct client on use of Kegel exercises during non-voiding times. Have client use exercise with each voiding. Have client attempt voiding at regularly scheduled times. Have client use bladder compression (Credé method) during voiding.	Kegel exercises assist in strengthening muscles when pelvic nerves are intact and functional (Touch, 1988). Training bladder to empty regularly can reduce incidence of dribbling. Credé method helps stimulate micturition and bladder emptying.

change and to prevent serious problems. Alterations in urinary elimination pose a high risk to a client's overall state of health.

Planning care also involves an understanding of the client's need to control body function. Alterations in urinary elimination can be embarrassing, uncomfortable, and often frustrating. The nurse and client work together to establish ways of maintaining client involvement in nursing care and to maintain normal elimination patterns when possible. To promote normal urinary elimination, goals for the client include the following:

1. Understanding normal urinary elimination
2. Promoting normal micturition
3. Achieving complete bladder emptying
4. Preventing infection
5. Maintaining skin integrity
6. Gaining a sense of comfort

Associated problems require interventions that often have no direct effect on urinary elimination. Unless the nurse intervenes, however, associated problems are likely to continue. Problems involved with urinary elimination alterations are often interrelated and complex. The nurse must also anticipate problems that may develop as a result of therapy. For example, diagnosis of *high risk for infection* is appropriate when a client has an indwelling catheter.

Planning should also include preparations for discharge. The nurse determines any assistive devices that will be required and the client's educational needs. Teaching throughout the hospital stay is important. Theoretical concepts are continuously rein-

Client Teaching for Urinary Elimination Problems

OBJECTIVE

- Client will adhere to health practices to prevent UTI.

TEACHING STRATEGIES

- Instruct client or care giver about observations to make regarding urinary output.
- Inform clients about pertinent signs and symptoms of infections.
- Frequently remind clients about I & O measurements.
- Reinforce correct perineal hygiene measures.
- Determine client's knowledge of medications and provide instruction on medications that affect urination, color of urine, and urine volume.
- Instruct client and family to call physician if symptoms of dysuria develop after discharge from hospital or clinic.
- Instruct client and family regarding measures to prevent UTI.

EVALUATION

- Observe client perform I & O measurements.
- Observe client perform perineal hygiene.
- Ask client to describe the benefits of increased fluid intake.
- Determine whether client meets high-risk criteria for recurrence of UTI. Provide necessary follow-up care (see research highlight).

 Research Highlight

Fox' descriptive study examined factors observed to be associated with the development of UTI among college women. This study, which took place in an outpatient clinic, included 113 participants, 17 to 39 years old, with documented UTIs. A three-level symptom scale was developed as the testing instrument.

Commonly documented rationales for reasons that women have an increased incidence of UTIs were examined. These included frequency of sexual intercourse, diaphragm use, and voiding after sexual intercourse. These variables demonstrated no predictive value in recurrence of infection. However, stronger predictors were demonstrated among the following variables: (1) type of characteristics of the infection, (2) presence of the symptom of urgency, and (3) the finding of hematuria grossly or on microscopic examination of the urinalysis specimen. The researcher further reports that the 6-month risk of a second infection was 3 times higher among women with *all* of the aforementioned symptoms when compared with those without these symptoms. These data suggests that it is the characteristics of the bacteria causing the initial infection and the extent of symptoms during the infection that predict recurrence.

The nurse can use the information gathered from this study when performing client teaching. The nurse can assess whether clients report any of the symptoms of UTI that would place them at risk for recurrence of infection. The teaching material can then be tailored to include information geared toward the prevention of subsequent or recurrent infections.

Fox B: Recurring urinary tract infection: incidence and risk factors, *Am J Public Health* 80(3):331, 1990.

forced, and return demonstrations of important psychomotor and self-care skills are performed by the client. For example, a client being discharged with an indwelling catheter will need to perform catheter care, understand ways to empty the drainage bag, measure urine, and know signs and symptoms of urinary infection. The need for home health services should be explored, and appropriate referrals should be made. The nurse's role in planning these interventions will result in the client's smooth transition through each phase of the nursing process.

 ## Implementation

Client Education

Success of therapies aimed at eliminating or minimizing urinary elimination problems depends in part on successful client education (see teaching box). The nurse instructs clients on their specific elimination problems. For example, clients who practice poor hygiene benefit from learning about normal sterility of the urinary tract and ways to prevent infection. It may also be useful to discuss the basic mechanism for urine production and voiding for clients with elimination alterations. Knowledge of factors that promote normal urine production and voiding can also help. Clients learn the significance of symptoms of urinary alterations so that early preventive health care can be initiated (see research highlight).

The nurse can easily incorporate teaching during nursing care delivery. For example, if the nurse is attempting to increase the client's fluid intake, a good time to discuss benefits is while giving fluids with medications or meals. The nurse may be more successful in teaching about perineal hygiene while giving a bath or performing catheter care. Much of the information the nurse offers is practical. The nurse can easily include family members in informal discussions.

Promoting Normal Micturition

Many nursing measures have been designed to promote normal voiding in clients at risk for urination difficulties and in clients with established urination problems. The nurse can initiate many of these measures independently.

STIMULATING MICTURITION REFLEX. The client's ability to void depends on feeling the urge to urinate, being able to control the urethral sphincter, and being able to relax during voiding. The nurse can foster relaxation and stimulate the reflex to void by helping the client assume the normal position for voiding. A woman is better able to void in a squatting position. This position promotes contraction of the pelvic and intraabdominal muscles that assist in sphincter control and bladder contraction. If the client is unable to use toilet facilities, the nurse positions the client in a squatting position on a bedpan (see Chapter 41) or bedside commode. A man voids more easily in the standing position. At times, it may be necessary for one or more nurses to assist a man in standing. If the man cannot reach toilet facilities, he may stand at the bedside and void into a urinal, a metal or plastic receptacle for urine (Fig. 40-9).

Other measures that promote relaxation and the ability to void include sensory stimuli. The sound of running water helps many clients void through the power of suggestion. Stroking the inner aspect of the thigh may stimulate sensory nerves and promote the micturition reflex. Placing the client's hand in a pan of warm water often promotes voiding. It is also easier for a person to relax and void when sitting on a bedpan that has been warmed. The nurse can also pour warm water over the client's perineum and create the sensation to urinate. If urine output is to be measured, the nurse must first measure the volume of water to be poured over the perineal area. Offering the client a drink may also promote voiding.

MAINTAINING ELIMINATION HABITS. Many clients follow routines to promote normal voiding. In a hospital or long-term care facility the nurse's routines may conflict with those of clients. Integrating clients' habits into the care plan fosters normal voiding.

Clients usually require time to void. Asking clients to void quickly so that they can be transported to x-ray testing or requesting a urine specimen as soon as possible does not contribute to normal voiding habits. Clients should be given at least 30 minutes to provide a specimen. The nurse learns the times when clients normally void, such as on awakening or before meals, and offers the opportunity to use toilet facilities then. Also important is the need to respond to clients' urges to urinate. Delay in assisting clients to the bathroom may interfere with normal micturition.

Privacy is essential for normal voiding. If the client cannot reach the bathroom, the nurse makes sure that the bedside area is enclosed by a curtain. In the home the debilitated client may prefer using a bedside commode enclosed behind a partition or room divider. Some clients are embarrassed by the sound of voiding. Running water or flushing the toilet masks the sound. Often young children are unable to void in the presence of persons other than their parents.

If the client typically uses special measures to void, the nurse should encourage their continued use at home and, when possible, in the institution. The client may be able to relax and void more easily while reading or listening to music. Coffee or beer may also promote urination.

MAINTAINING ADEQUATE FLUID INTAKE. A simple method of promoting normal micturition is maintaining good fluid intake. A client with normal renal function who does not have heart disease or alterations requiring fluid restriction should drink 2000 to 2500 ml of fluid daily. However, an average daily intake of 1200 to 1500 ml of fluids is usually adequate.

When fluid intake is increased, the excreted urine flushes out solutes or particles that may collect in the urinary system. Because a client is usually unwilling to drink 2500 ml of water daily, the nurse should offer fluids that the client prefers. Vegetables and fruits also contain a high fluid content. At home it may help to set a schedule for drinking fluids (for example, with meals or medications). To prevent nocturia, fluids should be avoided 2 hours before bedtime.

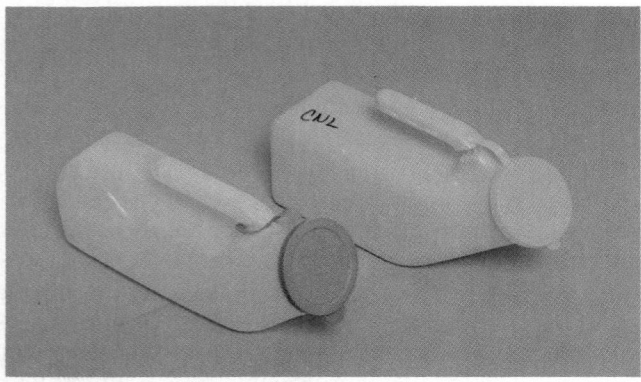

Fig. 40-9 Types of male urinals.

Promoting Complete Bladder Emptying

Under normal conditions, some of the client's urine remains in the bladder because urinary sphincters close. The sphincters provide more pressure than the pressure of urine in the bladder. Thus persons normally remain continent and dry. Urinary incontinence, however, occurs because pressure in the bladder is too great or because the sphincters are too weak. Urinary retention occurs from a strong or contracted sphincter that prevents normal bladder emptying.

Measures that promote micturition may help clients with incontinence or retention. Additional measures are used to promote and control bladder emptying so that clients gain a sense of elimination control (Table 40-4).

STRENGTHENING PELVIC FLOOR MUSCLES. Clients who have difficulty starting or stopping the urine stream may benefit from pelvic floor (Kegel) exercises (Table 40-5 on p. 1362). **Kegel exercises** improve the strength of pelvic floor muscles and consist of repetitive contractions of muscle groups (Kane et

al, 1984). A client begins these exercises during voiding to learn the technique. They are then practiced at nonvoiding times. Improvement is usually gradual. Clients should be alert and motivated to perform the exercises.

MEDICATIONS. Drug therapy given alone or with other therapies can help problems of incontinence and retention. There are two types of medications. One relaxes a spastic bladder and thereby increases bladder capacity. The other medication stimulates the bladder.

The bladder is innervated by the parasympathetic nervous system. When urine is present in the bladder, stress or urge incontinence may result from hyperactivity of the bladder muscle that suddenly increases intravesicular pressure. Uncontrolled bladder contractions may be caused by local bladder irritants such as calculi or infection. Drugs that depress the neurotransmitter acetylcholine, which stimulates the bladder, reduce incontinence caused by bladder irritation. Examples of these anticholinergic drugs include propantheline (Pro-Banthine) and oxybutynin

---

TABLE 40-4 Treatment Options for Incontinence

Primary Treatment	Other Treatments	Primary Treatment	Other Treatments
ACUTE INCONTINENCE		**STRESS INCONTINENCE**	
Management of acute illness	Catheter	Conditioning (Kegel) exercises	Estrogen
Appropriate toileting schedule		Surgery	Alpha-adrenergic agonists
Alteration of environment			Intravaginal electrical stimulation
Modification of drug regimen		Bladder neck suppression	Artificial sphincter
Adequate bowel care	Protective undergarments	**OVERFLOW INCONTINENCE**	
Treatment of UTI		Surgery	Indwelling catheter
Treatment of atrophic urethritis and vaginitis		Intermittent catheterization	
General supportive measures		**FUNCTIONAL INCONTINENCE**	
URGE INCONTINENCE		Habit training	Scheduled toileting
Anticholinergic drug therapy	Biofeedback		Incontinence undergarments
Bladder retraining			Environmental alterations
Treatment of associated UTI			Supportive measures
Treatment of associated vaginitis	Intravaginal electrical stimulation		Catheters: indwelling and external
			Skin care

From Orzeck S, Ouslander JG: *J Entero Ther* 14:24, 1987.

TABLE 40-5 Pelvic Floor Exercises

Exercise Steps	Rationale
EXERCISE I	
Instruct client to concentrate on pelvic muscles.	Assists client in feeling anterior muscles of pelvic floor.
Have client try to stop flow of urine during urination and then restart it. Practice with each voiding.	Teaches control technique.
EXERCISE II	
Have client assume sitting or standing position. Instruct client to tighten muscles around anus.	Assists client in feeling posterior muscles of pelvic floor.
EXERCISE III	
Have client tighten posterior muscles and then slowly contract anterior muscles while counting slowly to 4. Then have client relax muscles completely. Repeat exercise 4 times per hr while awake for 3 mo.	Improves pelvic muscle control, and aids relaxation of sphincters during voiding.
EXERCISE IV	
Instruct client to do situps.	Strengthens abdominal muscles for bladder control.

chloride (Ditropan). The anticholinergics can cause cardiac dysrhythmias and should be used with caution in clients with heart disease. Anticholinergics may also cause constipation and a dry mouth.

When the bladder empties, the detrusor muscle contracts in response to parasympathetic stimulation. Incomplete bladder emptying results from impaired innervation or weakness of the detrusor muscle. The client experiences retention and overflow incontinence. Cholinergic drugs increase contraction of the bladder and improve emptying. Bethanechol (Urecholine) stimulates parasympathetic nerves to increase bladder wall contraction and relax the sphincter. Bethanechol can be given by subcutaneous or oral routes. The nurse should administer the first dose 3 to 4 hours after the last voiding to be sure that the bladder contains urine. To gain the drug's peak effect, the nurse administers it shortly before micturition is attempted (15 to 30 minutes subcutaneously,

30 to 60 minutes orally). Cholinergic drugs may cause diarrhea as a side effect.

BLADDER RETRAINING. The goal of bladder retraining is to restore a normal pattern of voiding by inhibiting or stimulating voiding (Orzeck, Ouslander, 1987). This is useful in clients with a cerebrovascular accident, overdistention, a bladder injury, an indwelling urinary catheter, or an acute illness that caused incontinence. For bladder retraining to be successful, clients must be alert and physically able to follow a training program.

The nurse first assesses the client's pattern of urination (for example, frequency, time, habits, and volume). This information allows the nurse to plan a program that often takes 2 weeks or more to learn. The actual time for training depends on a client's condition. If an indwelling catheter has been inserted for 6 to 12 months, bladder capacity is greatly reduced, and permanent bladder wall changes may occur (Kristiansen et al, 1983). If the client has an underlying UTI, this should be treated at the same time. The following measures will help the incontinent client gain control over urination:

1. Learning exercises to strengthen the pelvic floor
2. Initiating a toileting schedule on awakening, every 2 hours during the day and evening, before getting into bed, and every 4 hours at night
3. Using methods to initiate voiding (for example, running water and stroking the inner thigh)
4. Using methods to relax to aid complete bladder emptying (for example, reading and deep breathing)
5. Never ignoring the urge to void
6. Taking fluids approximately 30 minutes before planned voiding times
7. Limiting fluids taken after supper to no more than 150 to 200 ml (5 to 7 ounces) and avoiding tea, coffee, alcohol, and other caffeine drinks
8. Taking prescribed diuretic medication or fluids that increase diuresis (such as tea or coffee) early in the morning
9. Progressively lengthening or shortening periods between voiding
10. Offering protective undergarments to contain urine and reduce the client's embarrassment (not diapers)
11. Following a weight-control program if obesity is a problem
12. Providing positive reinforcement when continence is maintained (see research highlight at right)

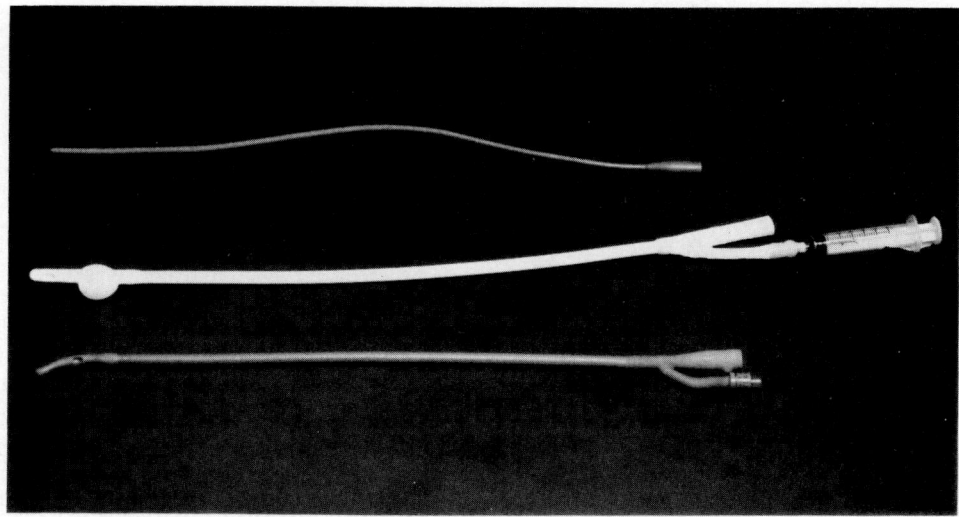

Fig. 40-10   Types of catheters. *Top:* straight catheter; *middle:* indwelling, double-lumen catheter with inflated balloon; *bottom:* Coudé catheter.

These guidelines help the client to establish a routine for voiding and control factors that might increase the number of incontinent episodes.

HABIT TRAINING. A client with functional incontinence may benefit from habit training, which helps clients improve voluntary control over urination. A flexible toileting schedule based on the client's pattern is established.

The nurse helps the client to the bathroom before incontinent episodes occur. Fluids and medications are timed to prevent interference with the toileting schedule. Clients with moderate or severe mental or physical function can benefit. Positive reinforcement to reward successful voiding and neutral interaction when accidental incontinence occurs help reinforce success.

CATHETERIZATION. **Catheterization** of the bladder involves introducing a rubber or plastic tube through the urethra and into the bladder. The catheter provides a continuous flow of urine in clients unable to control micturition or those with obstructions. It also provides a means of assessing hourly urine outputs in hemodynamically unstable clients. Because bladder catheterization carries the risk of UTI and trauma to the urethra, it is preferable to rely on other measures.

Types of Catheterization. Intermittent and indwelling retention catheterization are the two forms of catheter insertion. With the intermittent technique a straight single-use catheter (Fig. 40-10) is introduced long enough to drain the bladder (5 to 10 minutes). When the bladder is empty, the nurse immediately withdraws the catheter. Intermittent catheter-

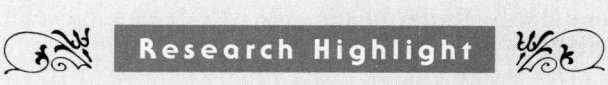

Research Highlight

This study by Palmer et al was conducted to identify nonurological risk factors for incontinence outcomes among nursing home clients 1 year after admission. This 1-year study involved 434 subjects over the age of 65. However, only 196 subjects remained throughout the study period. The majority of these participants were European American women with a mean age of 82 years.

The most frequent admitting diagnosis identified was dementia. Urinary incontinence was more frequently seen among subjects with dementia. Subjects with no detectable mental morbidity had the lowest incidence of incontinence. Urinary incontinence was also demonstrated more frequently among subjects with impaired ability to walk or transfer independently. Male subjects, although poorly represented in numbers by the end of the study period, exhibited a higher prevalence of incontinence than their female counterparts. The onset of urinary incontinence within the first 2 weeks of admission was seen as a major risk factor and correlated well with continued episodes of or progression to total incontinence.

This study defines risk factors and provides profiles of clients most likely to experience problems with incontinence. This information can be used to conduct further studies that target the development of appropriate nursing interventions to prevent or treat potentially vulnerable clients.

Palmer MH et al: Risk factors for urinary incontinence one year after nursing home admission, *Res Nurs Health* 14:405, 1991.

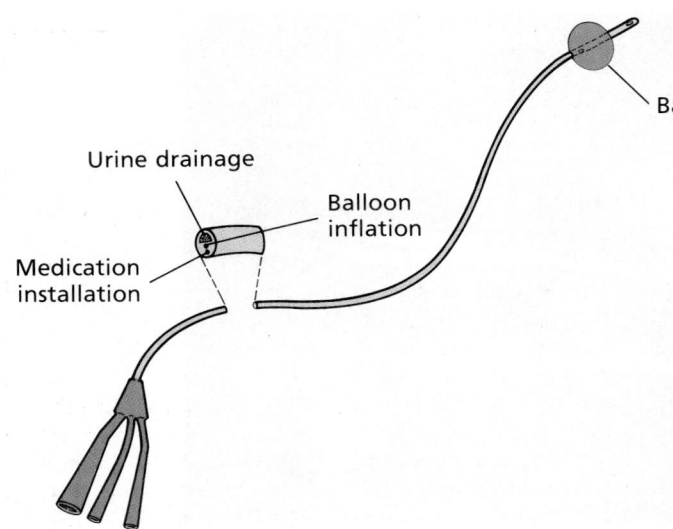

Fig. 40-11   Triple-lumen Foley catheter with balloon inflated.

ization can be repeated as necessary. An indwelling or Foley catheter remains in place for an extended period until a client is able to void completely and voluntarily. It may be necessary to change indwelling catheters periodically.

The straight single-use catheter (Fig. 40-10) has a single lumen with a small opening about 1.3 cm (½ in) from the tip. Urine drains from the tip, through the lumen, and to a receptacle. An indwelling Foley catheter has a small inflatable balloon that encircles the catheter just below the tip. When inflated, the balloon rests against the bladder outlet to anchor the catheter in place. The indwelling retention catheter also has two or three lumens within the body of the catheter (Fig. 40-11). One lumen drains urine through the catheter to a collecting tube. A second lumen carries sterile water to and from the balloon when it is inflated or deflated. A third (optional) lumen may be used to instill fluids or medications into the bladder. It is easy to determine the number of lumens by the number of drainage and injection ports at the catheter's end.

A third type of catheter has a curved tip. A Coudé catheter (Fig. 40-10) is used on male clients who may have enlarged prostates with obstructions along the urethra. The Coudé catheter is less traumatic during insertion because it is stiffer and easier to control than the straight-tip catheter.

Catheters come in many diameters to fit the size of a client's urethral canal. The Centers for Disease Control (CDC) suggests that nurses use as small a catheter as possible to provide good drainage and minimize urethral trauma (Wong, 1982). Paraurethral glands that bathe the urethra in its natural lubrication become blocked if a catheter lumen is too large. Suggestions on how to make appropriate decisions regarding catheter selection are provided (see box).

Indications for Catheterization. Catheterization may be indicated for many reasons. When catheterization time will be short and minimizing infection is a priority, the intermittent method is best. Intermittent catheterization is also preferred for persons with spinal cord injuries who have no bladder control. By intermittently draining the bladder on a routine basis, these clients have fewer infections. Indwelling catherization is used when long-term bladder emptying is necessary. Table 40-6 outlines specific indications for catheterization.

Catheter Insertion. Urethral catheterization requires a physician's order. The nurse must use strict aseptic technique (see Chapter 18). Organizing equipment before the procedure prevents interruptions. The steps for inserting indwelling and single-use straight catheters are basically the same. The difference lies in the procedure taken to inflate the indwelling catheter balloon and secure the catheter. While inserting an indwelling catheter the nurse has the opportunity to collect needed specimens. Procedure 40-2 on p. 1366 lists steps for performing female and male urethral catheterization.

Self-Catheterization. Some clients with chronic disorders such as spinal cord injury learn to perform self-catheterization. The client must be able to physically manipulate equipment and assume a position for successful catheterization. The nurse teaches the client the structures of the urinary tract, clean versus sterile technique, the importance of a limited fluid intake regimen, and the frequency of self-catheterization. Generally, the goal is to have clients perform self-catheterizations every 6 to 8 hours.

Closed Drainage Systems. After inserting an indwelling catheter, the nurse maintains a closed urinary drainage system to minimize the risk of infection. Urinary drainage bags are plastic and can hold about 1000 to 1500 ml of urine. The bag should hang on the bed frame without touching the floor when the bed is in its lowest position. A drainage bag should not be placed over or on the bed's side rails. The bag also fits on the frames of most wheelchairs. When the client ambulates, the nurse or client carries the bag below the client's waist. The nurse or

Guidelines for Appropriate Catheter Selection

■ Choose a catheter appropriate to the gender of the client. Women benefit from the use of shorter catheters (21 cm). These catheters are less prone to moving in and out of the urethra and thus introducing bacteria into the urinary tract.

■ The catheter size is determined by the size of the client's urethral canal. When the French system is used, the larger the gauge number, the larger the catheter. Generally, children require an 8 to 10 Fr. Women require a 14 to 16 Fr, and men usually require a 16 to 18 Fr.

■ The length of the catheterization period should dictate the type of material selected.

  □ Plastic catheters are only suitable for short-term use (1 week or less) because they are stiff and inflexible.

  □ Latex or rubber catheters are recommended for medium-term use (2 or 3 weeks).

  □ Pure silicone catheters are recommended for long-term use (2 to 3 months) because the material causes less encrustation at the urethral meatus. However, they are very expensive, and delamination of the coating can occur.

  □ Polyvinylchloride (PVC) catheters are also very expensive. They are suitable for intervals of 4 to 6 weeks. They soften at body temperature and conform to the urethra.

■ Determining the appropriate balloon size is also an important aspect of catheterization. Balloon sizes range from 3 ml (pediatric) to large postoperative volumes (75 ml). The 5-ml and the 30-ml sizes are the most common. The 5-ml volume is appropriate for standard catheterizations. This small volume allows optimal drainage of the catheter and does not interfere with bladder emptying. The 30-ml balloon catheter is usually reserved for use after prostatectomies as an aid in achieving postoperative hemostasis of the prostatic bed.

■ Only sterile water should be used to inflate the balloon. Normal saline crystallizes, thus causing incomplete deflation of the balloon on catheter removal. The practice of instilling additional sterile water into the balloon in a catheter that is leaking is also discouraged. This practice can cause overinflation of the balloon and distortions in the catheter tip, which can lead to bladder irritation.

TABLE 40-6   Indications for Catheterization

Intermittent Catheterization	Short-Term Indwelling Catheterization	Long-Term Indwelling Catheterization
Relief of discomfort of bladder distention, provision of decompression	Obstruction to urine outflow (e.g., prostate enlargement)	Severe urinary retention with recurrent episodes of UTI
Procurement of sterile urine specimen	Surgical repair of bladder, urethra, and surrounding structures	Skin rashes, ulcers, or wounds irritated by contact with urine
Assessment of residual urine when bladder empties incompletely	Prevention of urethral obstruction from blood clots	Terminal illness when bed linen changes are painful for client
Long-term management of clients with spinal cord injuries, neuromuscular degeneration, incompetent bladders	Measurement of output in critically ill or comatose clients	
	Continuous or intermittent bladder irrigations	

---

other health care personnel should *never* raise a drainage bag and tubing above the level of the client's bladder. Urine in the bag and tubing can become a medium for bacteria, and infection is likely to develop if urine flows back into the bladder.

Most drainage bags contain an antireflux valve to prevent urine from reentering the drainage tubing and contaminating the client's bladder. A spigot at the base of the bag provides a means for emptying the bag. The spigot should always be clamped, except during emptying, and tucked into the protective pouch at the bag's side. To keep the drainage system patent the nurse checks for kinks or bends in the tubing, avoids positioning the client on the drainage tubing, and observes for clots or sediment that may occlude the collecting tubing.

Text continued on p. 1373.

Inserting a Straight or Indwelling Catheter

STEPS	RATIONALE
1. Assess status of client:	
a. Time that client last voided	May indicate likelihood of bladder fullness.
b. Level of awareness or developmental stage	Reveals client's ability to cooperate during procedure.
c. Mobility and physical limitations (You can request additional nursing personnel to assist with procedure if necessary.)	Affects way that you will position client.
d. Client's age	Determines catheter size to use. No. 8-10 Fr is generally used for children and 14-16 for women. No. 12 may be considered for young women. No. 16-18 is used for men unless larger size is ordered by physician.
e. Distended bladder	Can indicate need to insert catheter if client is unable to void independently. Clients at risk for distension include women after childbirth, clients after surgery, and men with prostatic hypertrophy.
f. Pathological condition that may impair passage of catheter (e.g., enlarged prostate gland)	Obstruction prevents passage of catheter through urethra into bladder.
g. Allergies	Determines allergy to antiseptic, tape, or rubber.
h. Review of the physician's order for catheterization.	Catheterization requires physician's order. Physician may order catheterization after surgery or child birth if the client has not voided for 8 hr.
2. Prepare necessary equipment and supplies:	
a. Sterile gloves*	Procedure is considered sterile.
b. Sterile drapes, one fenestrated	
c. Lubricant*	Minimizes urethral trauma during insertion.
d. Antiseptic cleaning solution*	
e. Cotton balls or gauze squares	
f. Forceps	
g. Prefilled syringe with sterile water	Used to inflate balloon of indwelling catheter.
h. Catheters of correct size and type for procedure (intermittent or indwelling)	
i. Flashlight or gooseneck lamp	Helps in seeing woman's urinary meatus.
j. Bath blanket	Promotes privacy.
k. Waterproof absorbent pad	
l. Trash receptacle	
m. Disposable gloves, basin with warm water, soap, face cloth, and towel	Providing perineal hygiene before introducing catheter helps reduce risk of UTI. Provides opportunity to examine woman's urethral meatus or to retract foreskin of uncircumcised man.
n. Sterile drainage tubing and collection bag (may be preattached to catheter), tape, safety pin, elastic band	If indwelling catheter will be inserted, tape, elastic band, and pin help secure position of catheter, thus preventing trauma to external urethral sphincter.
o. Receptacle or basin (usually bottom of tray)	Provides area for urine to drain when straight or indwelling catheter is used.
p. Sterile specimen container	For sterile urine specimen to determine presence of bacteria.
3. Explain procedure to client. Also describe pressure sensation that will be felt during catheter insertion.	Reduces anxiety and promotes cooperation.
4. Arrange for extra nursing personnel to assist, if appropriate.	May be necessary to assist with positioning dependent client. Promotes use of correct body mechanics and safety.

*These items may be contained on catheterization tray or may need to be added after sterile field is established. This depends on whether disposable or nondisposable trays are used by institution. Check outer label on prepackaged container for contents.

STEPS	RATIONALE
5. Wash hands.	Reduces transmission of infection.
6. Raise bed to appropriate working height.	Promotes use of proper body mechanics.
7. Facing client, stand on left side of bed if right-handed (on right side if left-handed). Clear bedside table and arrange equipment.	Successful catheter insertion requires you to assume comfortable position with all equipment easily accessible.
8. Raise side rail on opposite side of bed.	Promotes client safety.
9. Close cubicle or room curtains.	Reduces client's embarrassment and aids in relaxation.
10. Place waterproof pad under client.	Prevents soiling of bed linen.
11. Position client: a. *Female:* assist to dorsal recumbent position (supine with knees flexed). Ask client to relax thighs so as to externally rotate them. (Legs may be supported with pillows.) Or position in side-lying (Sims') position with upper leg flexed at knee and hip if unable to be supine (optional). b. *Male:* assist to assume supine position with thighs slightly abducted.	Provides good view of perineal structures. Alternate position if client cannot abduct leg at hip joint (e.g., because of arthritic joints). Also, this position may be more comfortable for client. Support client with pillows, if necessary, to maintain position. Supine position prevents tensing of abdominal and pelvic muscles.
12. Drape client: a. *Female:* drape with bath blanket. Place blanket diamond fashion over client; one corner at neck, side corners over each arm and side, and last corner over perineum. Raise gown above hips. b. *Male:* drape upper trunk with bath blanket and cover lower extremities with bed sheets, exposing only genitalia.	Avoids unnecessary exposure of body parts and maintains comfort.
13. Apply disposable gloves. Wash perineal area with soap and water as needed; dry.	Presence of microorganisms near urethral meatus is reduced.
14. Position lamp to illuminate perineal area. (When using flashlight, have assistant hold it.)	Permits accurate identification and good view of urethral meatus.
15. Remove and dispose of gloves.	Prevents transmission of microorganisms.
16. Open catheterization kit and catheter (if packaged separately) according to directions, keeping bottom of container sterile.	Prevents transmission of microorganisms from table or work area to sterile supplies.
17. Apply sterile gloves (see Chapter 18).	Allows you to handle sterile supplies without contamination.
18. Organize supplies on sterile field. Open inner sterile package containing catheter. Pour sterile package of antiseptic solution in correct compartment containing sterile cotton balls. Open packet containing lubricant. Remove specimen container (cap should be loosely placed on top) and prefilled syringe from collection compartment of tray and set them aside on sterile field.	Maintains surgical asepsis and organizes work area. All activities requiring you to use both hands must be completed before cleansing urethral meatus.
19. When inserting indwelling catheter, test balloon by injecting fluid from prefilled syringe into balloon valve (see illustration on p. 1368). Balloon should inflate fully without leaking. Withdraw fluid and leave syringe on port of catheter.	Checks integrity of balloon. Balloon that leaks or inflates improperly is replaced.

CONTINUED

Inserting a Straight or Indwelling Catheter

STEPS

RATIONALE

20. Apply sterile drape:
   a. *Female:* allow top edge of drape to form cuff over both hands. Place drape down on bed between client's thighs. Slip cuffed edge just under buttocks, taking care not to touch contaminated surface with gloves. Pick up fenestrated sterile drape and allow it to unfold without touching unsterile object. Apply drape over perineum, exposing labia and being sure not to touch contaminated surface.
   b. *Male:* apply drape over thighs just below penis. Pick up fenestrated sterile drape. Allow it to unfold, and drape it over penis with fenestrated slit resting over penis.

Outer surface of drape covering your hands remains sterile until touched by buttocks. Sterile drape against sterile gloves is sterile. Maintains sterility of work surface.

21. Place sterile kit and its contents on sterile drape between client's thighs, and open urine specimen container, keeping top sterile.

Provides easy access to supplies during catheter insertion. Prepares container for transfers of urine.

22. Apply lubricant along sides of catheter tip:
   a. *Female:* 2.5-5 cm (1-2 in)
   b. *Males:* 7.5-12.5 cm (3-5 in)

Allows easy insertion of catheter tip through urethral meatus.

23. Cleanse urethral meatus:
   a. *Female:*
      (1) With nondominant hand, carefully retract labia to fully expose urethral meatus. Maintain position of nondominant hand throughout procedure.
      (2) With dominant hand, pick up cotton ball with forceps and clean perineal area, wiping front to back from clitoris toward anus. Use new clean cotton ball for each wipe: along near labial fold, along far labial fold, directly over meatus.
   b. *Male:*
      (1) If client is not circumcised, retract foreskin with nondominant hand. Grasp penis at shaft just below glans. Retract urethral meatus between thumb and forefinger. Maintain nondominant hand in this position throughout catheter insertion.

Provides full visualization of meatus. Full retraction prevents contamination of meatus during cleansing. Closure of labia during cleansing requires that procedure be repeated because area has become contaminated.

Cleansing reduces number of microorganisms at urethral meatus. Use of single cotton ball for each wipe prevents transfer of microorganisms. Preparation moves from area of least contamination to that of most contamination. Dominant hand remains sterile.

Minimizes chance of erection. (If erection develops, discontinue procedure.) Accidental release of foreskin or dropping of penis during cleansing requires process to be repeated because area has become contaminated.

Step 19

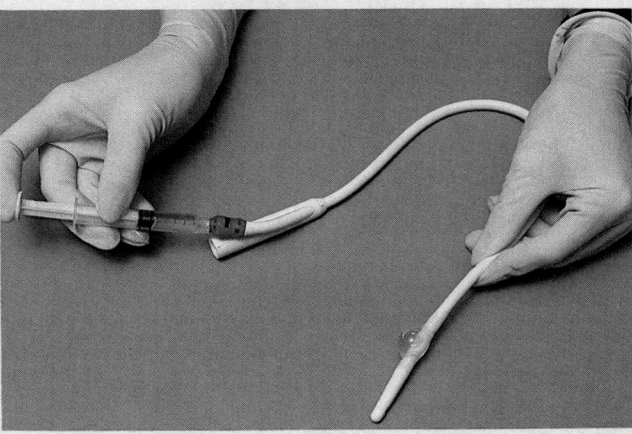

STEPS	RATIONALE
(2) With dominant hand pick up cotton ball with forceps and clean penis. Begin at meatus. Using circular motion, advance down toward base (shaft). Repeat this process 3 times, changing cotton ball each time.	Reduces number of microorganisms at meatus and moves from area of least to most contamination. Dominant hand remains sterile.
24. Pick up catheter with gloved dominant hand approximately 5 cm (2 in) from catheter tip. Hold end of catheter loosely coiled in palm of dominant hand. Place distal end of catheter in urine tray receptacle unless already attached to drainage bag.	Collection of urine prevents soiling of bed linen and allows accurate measurement of urinary output.
25. Insert catheter:	
a. *Female* (see illustration): grasp catheter in dominant hand with nondominant hand continuing to retract labia:	
(1) Ask client to take deep breath and slowly insert catheter through meatus. (If no urine appears, catheter may be in vagina. If catheter is in vagina, leave it in place; obtain and insert another catheter and remove first catheter.)	Relaxation of external sphincter aids in insertion of catheter. (Catheter in vagina is no longer sterile. Leaving first catheter in place helps prevent inserting second catheter in vagina.)
(2) Advance catheter approximately 5-7.5 cm (3 in) in adult, 2.5 cm (1 in) in child, or until urine flows out catheter's end. If inserting retention catheter, advance another 5 cm (2 in) after urine appears. Do not force catheter against resistance.	Female urethra is short. Appearance of urine indicates that catheter tip is in bladder or lower urethra. Further advancement of catheter ensures bladder placement. Balloon of retention catheter must be advanced into bladder. Forceful insertion may traumatize urethra.
(3) Release labia and hold catheter securely with nondominant hand.	Bladder or sphincter contraction may cause accidental expulsion of catheter.
b. *Male* (see illustration): lifting penis to position perpendicular to client's body and applying light traction upward:	Straightens urethral canal to ease catheter insertion.
(1) Ask client to bear down as if voiding and slowly insert catheter through meatus.	Relaxation of external sphincter aids in insertion of catheter.
(2) Advance catheter 17.5-22.5 cm (7-9 in) in adult, 5-7.5 cm (2-3 in) in young child, or until urine flows out catheter's end. If resistance is felt, withdraw catheter; do not force it through urethra. If inserting retention catheter, advance another 5 cm (2 in) after urine appears.	Adult male urethra is long. Appearance of urine indicates that catheter tip is in bladder or urethra. Resistance to catheter passage may be caused by strictures or enlarged prostate. Further advancement of catheter ensures proper placement. Ensures that balloon is advanced into bladder.

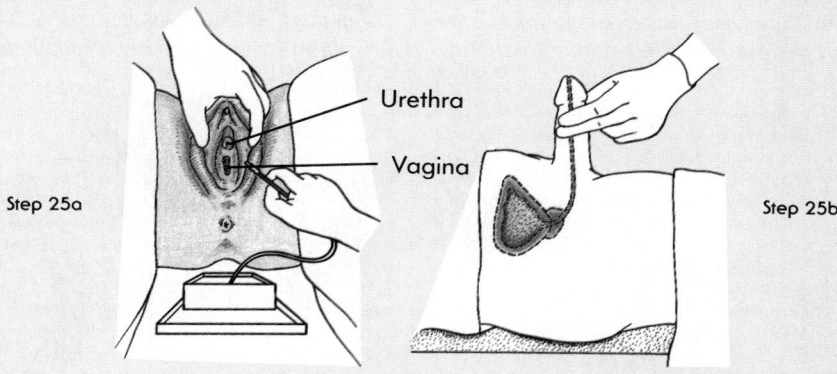

Urethra

Vagina

Step 25a   Step 25b

Inserting a Straight or Indwelling Catheter

STEPS	RATIONALE
(3) Release penis and hold catheter securely with dominant hand.	Bladder or sphincter contraction may cause accidental expulsion of catheter.
26. Collect urine specimen as needed: Fill specimen cup or jar to desired level (20-30 ml) by holding end of catheter in dominant hand over cup (or collect specimen from sterile drainage bag). With dominant hand, pinch catheter to stop urine flow temporarily, and then release catheter to allow remaining urine in bladder to drain into collection tray. Cover specimen cup and set it aside for labeling.	Allows sterile specimen to be obtained for culture analysis.
27. Allow bladder to empty fully, about 750-1000 ml (unless institution policy restricts maximal volume of urine to drain with each catheterization).	Retained urine may serve as reservoir for growth of microorganisms. Rapid emptying of large volume of urine may cause engorgement of pelvic blood vessels and hypovolemic shock.
28. Remove straight single-use catheter. Withdraw catheter slowly but smoothly until removed.	Minimizes client discomfort.
29. Inflate balloon of indwelling catheter:	
a. While holding catheter at urinary meatus with dominant hand, take end of catheter; place it between first two fingers of nondominant hand.	Catheter should be anchored while syringe is manipulated.
b. Take dominant hand and attach syringe to injection port at end of catheter. (In some sets, syringe is already connected.)	Port connects to lumen leading to inflatable balloon.
c. Slowly inject total amount of solution. If client complains of sudden pain, aspirate solution and advance catheter farther. Inject no more fluid than balloon size indicates.	Balloon within bladder is inflated. If balloon is malpositioned in urethra, pain occurs during inflation.
d. After inflating balloon fully, release catheter with nondominant hand and pull gently to feel resistance (see illustration). Then move catheter slightly back into bladder. Disconnect syringe.	Inflation of balloon anchors catheter tip in place above bladder outlet to prevent removal of catheter. Gentle pulling ensures proper placement and anchoring. Advancing catheter upward minimizes pressure on bladder neck.
30. Attach end of catheter to collecting tube of drainage system, unless already connected to bag. Place drainage bag in dependent position (see illustration). Do not place bag on side rails of bed.	Closed system for urine drainage is established. Dependent position of drainage bag promotes flow of urine away from bladder. Bags attached to side rails may be raised above level of bladder if rail is raised.
31. Tape catheter:	
a. *Female:* tape catheter to inside of thigh with strip of nonallergenic tape. Allow for slack so that movement of thigh does not create tension on catheter.	Anchoring of catheter minimizes trauma to urethra and meatus during movement. Catheter positioned over thigh prevents kinking. Nonallergenic tape prevents skin breakdown.

Step 29d

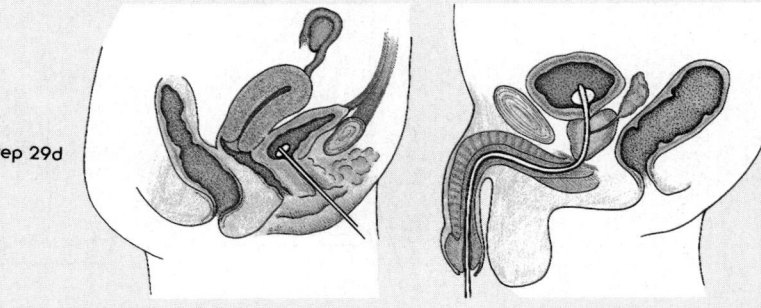

STEPS	RATIONALE
b. *Male:* tape catheter to top of thigh or lower abdomen (with penis directed toward abdomen). Allow some slack in catheter so that movement does not create tension on catheter.	Anchoring catheter to lower abdomen is thought to reduce pressure on urethra at junction of penis and scrotum, thus reducing possibility of tissue necrosis.
32. Be sure there are no obstructions or kinks in tubing. Place excess coil of tubing on bed and fasten it to bottom sheet with clip from drainage set or with rubber band and safety pin.	Patent tubing allows free drainage of urine by gravity and prevents backflow of urine into bladder.
33. Remove gloves and dispose of equipment, drapes, and urine in proper receptacles.	Prevents transmission of infection.
34. Assist client to comfortable position. While wearing clean gloves, wash and dry perineal area as needed.	Client's comfort and security are maintained.
35. Instruct client on ways to lie in bed with catheter: side-lying facing drainage system with catheter and tubing draped over lower thigh or side-lying facing away from system, catheter and tubing extending between legs.	Urine should drain freely without obstruction. Placing catheter under extremities can result in obstruction from compression of tubing from client's weight. When client is on one side facing away from system, catheter should not be placed over upper thigh; this forces urine to drain uphill.
36. Caution client against pulling on catheter.	Reduces trauma to urethral meatus.
37. Wash hands.	Reduces spread of infection.
38. Palpate bladder and ask if client is uncomfortable.	Determines whether distention is relieved.
39. Observe character and amount of urine in drainage system.	Determines whether urine is flowing adequately.
40. Report and record type and size of catheter inserted, amount of fluid used to inflate balloon, and characteristics and amount of urine.	Communicates pertinent information to all members of health care team.

CONTINUED

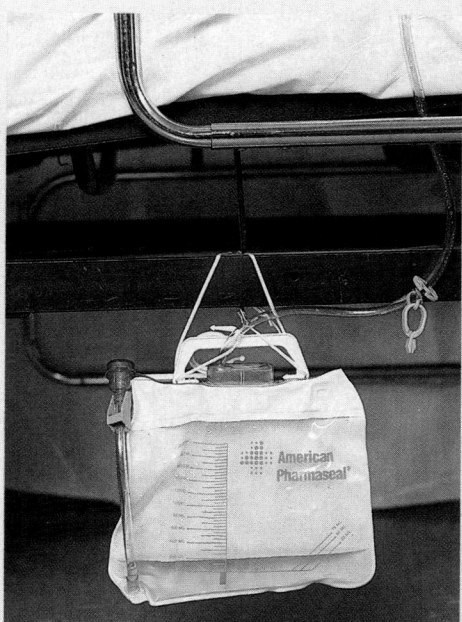

Step 30

Indwelling Catheter Care

STEPS	RATIONALE
1. Assess for episode of bowel incontinence or client's report of discomfort at catheter insertion site.	Accumulation of secretions or feces causes irritation to perineal tissues and acts as site for bacterial growth.

2. Prepare necessary equipment and supplies:
  a. Catheter care kit:
    (1) Gloves
    (2) Cotton balls or application swabs
    (3) Clean washcloth or towel
    (4) Warm water and soap
    (5) Antibiotic ointment (e.g., neomycin)
  b. Bath blanket
  c. Waterproof absorbent pad
	Ensures orderly procedure.
	
	Used to drape client.
	Prevents soiling of bed linen.

3. Explain procedure to client. Offer opportunity to perform self-care if able.	Reduces anxiety and promotes cooperation. Embarrassment may motivate client to perform own hygiene.
4. Provide privacy by closing door or bedside curtain.	Maintains client's self-esteem.
5. Wash hands.	Reduces transmission of infection.

6. Position client:
  a. *Female:* dorsal recumbent position
  b. *Male:* supine position
	Ensures easy access to perineal tissues.

7. Place waterproof pad under client.	Protects bed linen from soiling.
8. Drape bath blanket on bed clothes so that only perineal area is exposed.	Prevents unnecessary exposure of body parts.
9. Apply gloves.	
10. Remove anchor tapes to free catheter tubing.	

11. With nondominant hand:
  a. *Female:* gently retract labia to fully expose urethral meatus and catheter insertion site, maintaining position of hand throughout procedure.
  b. *Male:* retract foreskin if client is not circumcised and hold penis at shaft just below glans, maintaining position of hand throughout procedure.
	Provides full visualization of urethral meatus. Full retraction prevents contamination of meatus during cleansing. Accidental closure of labia or dropping of penis during cleansing requires process to be repeated.

12. Assess urethral meatus and surrounding tissues for inflammation, swelling, and discharge. Note amount, color, odor, and consistency of discharge. Ask client if burning or discomfort is felt.	Determines presence of local infection and status of hygiene.

13. Cleanse perineal tissue:
  a. *Female:* use clean cloth and soap and water, clean toward anus. Repeat process to cleanse labia minora, and then cleanse around urethral meatus moving down catheter. Be sure to cleanse each side. Dry area well.
  b. *Male:* while spreading urethral meatus, cleanse around catheter first, and then wipe in circular motion around meatus and glans.
	Cleansing reduces number of microorganisms at urethral meatus. Use of clean cloth prevents transfer of microorganisms. Cleansing moves from area of least to most contamination.

14. Reassess urethral meatus for discharge.	Determines whether cleansing is complete.
15. With towel, soap, and water, wipe in circular motion along length of catheter for 10 cm (4 in).	Reduces presence of secretions or drainage on outside catheter surface.
16. Apply antiseptic ointment at urethral meatus and along 2.5 cm (1 in) of catheter if ordered by physician.	Further reduces growth of microorganisms at insertion site.

STEPS	RATIONALE
17. Place client in safe, comfortable position.	Promotes comfort.
18. Remove gloves. Dispose of contaminated supplies and wash hands.	Prevents spread of infection.
19. Record and report condition of perineal tissues, time procedure was performed, client's response, and abnormalities noted.	Provides data to document procedure and informs staff of client's condition.

Routine Catheter Care. Clients with indwelling catheters have a number of special care needs. Nursing measures are directed at preventing infection and maintaining unobstructed flow of urine through the catheter drainage system.

Fluid Intake. All clients with catheters should have a daily intake of 2000 to 2500 ml if permitted. This can be met through oral ingestion or intravenous infusion. A high fluid intake produces a large volume of urine that flushes the bladder and keeps catheter tubing free of sediment.

Perineal Hygiene. Buildup of secretions or encrustation at the catheter insertion site is a source of infection. Nurses provide perineal hygiene (see Chapter 34) at least twice daily or as needed for a client with a retention catheter. Soap and water are effective in reducing the number of organisms around the urethra. The nurse must not accidentally advance the catheter up into the bladder during cleansing. Otherwise, bacteria may be introduced.

Catheter Care. In addition to routine perineal hygiene, many institutions recommend that clients with catheters receive special care 3 times a day and after defecation or bowel incontinence to help minimize discomfort and infection (Procedure 40-3).

Removal of Indwelling Catheter. When removing an indwelling catheter, the nurse promotes normal bladder function and prevents trauma to the urethra. Loss of muscle tone in the bladder is a common problem after prolonged catheterization. Bladder reconditioning, which can reduce the loss of bladder tone, requires a physician's order and is begun at least 10 hours before catheter removal (Williamson, 1982). The nurse clamps the indwelling catheter to allow urine to accumulate. The volume of urine stretches the bladder walls to stimulate muscle tone. Three hours later the nurse unclamps the catheter and allows urine to drain for 5 minutes. The process is repeated two more times. After the conditioning procedure the nurse removes the catheter. Clients who receive bladder conditioning are believed to be able to feel the urge to void sooner than those with no conditioning.

To remove a catheter the nurse requires a clean, disposable towel; a trash receptacle; and a sterile syringe the same size as the volume of solution within the catheter's inflated balloon. Disposable gloves are also recommended. The end of each catheter contains a label that denotes the volume of solution (5 to 30 ml) within a balloon.

The nurse positions the client in the same position as during catheterization. Some institutions recommend collecting a sterile urine specimen at this time or sending the catheter tip for culture and sensitivity tests. After removing the tape, the nurse places the towel between the woman's thighs or over the man's thighs. The nurse inserts the syringe into the injection port. Most ports are self-sealing and require that only the tip of the syringe be inserted. The nurse slowly withdraws all of the solution to deflate the balloon totally. If a portion of the solution remains, the partially inflated balloon will traumatize the urethral canal as the catheter is removed. After deflation the nurse explains that the client will feel a burning sensation as the catheter is withdrawn. The nurse then pulls the catheter out smoothly and slowly.

It is normal for the client to experience some dysuria, especially if the catheter has been in place several days or weeks. The catheter causes inflammation of the urethral canal. Until the bladder regains full tone, the client may also experience frequency of urination.

The nurse notes when the client first voids after catheter removal and assesses for bladder distention. If over 8 hours elapse, it may become necessary to reinsert the catheter. If the volume voided is small, residual urine may be in the bladder.

ALTERNATIVES TO URETHRAL CATHETERIZATION. To avoid the risks associated with catheters inserted

Applying a Condom Catheter

STEPS	RATIONALE
1. Assess status of client to determine need for condom catheter.	Client continuously incontinent of urine is at risk for skin breakdown.
2. Prepare necessary equipment and supplies:	
a. Rubber condom sheath (proper size)	
b. Strip of elastic tape and skin preparation (e.g., tincture of benzoin)	
c. Urinary collection bag with drainage tubing or leg bag and straps	Urinary leg bag allows client to remain mobile.
d. Basin with warm water and soap	
e. Towels and wash cloths	
f. Disposable gloves	Protects your hands; reduces client's risk of infection.
g. Bath blanket	
h. Razor (optional)	
3. Explain procedure to client.	Reduces anxiety and promotes cooperation.
4. Wash hands.	Reduces transmission of infection.
5. Provide privacy by closing door or bedside curtain.	Maintains client's self-esteem.
6. Assist client into supine position. Place bath blanket over upper torso. Fold sheets so that lower extremities are covered; only genitalia should be exposed.	Promotes client comfort and prevents unnecessary exposure of body parts.
7. Assess condition of penis.	Provides baseline to compare changes in condition of skin after condom application.
8. Apply disposable gloves. Provide perineal care (see Chapter 34) and dry thoroughly. Clip hair at base of penis.	Removes irritating secretions. Rubber sheath rolls onto dry skin more easily. Hair adheres to condom and pulls during condom removal.
9. Prepare urinary drainage collection bag and tubing or prepare leg bag for connection to condom, if necessary. Clamp off drainage exit ports. Secure collection bag to bed frame or client's leg; bring drainage tubing up through side rails onto bed.	Provides easy access to drainage equipment after condom is in place.
10. Apply skin preparation to penis and allow to dry (approximately 30-60 sec).	
11. With nondominant hand, grasp penis along shaft. With dominant hand, hold condom sheath at tip of penis and smoothly roll sheath onto penis.	Prepares penis for easy condom placement.
12. Allow 2.5-5 cm (1-2 in) of space between tip of glans penis and end of condom catheter.	Allows free passage of urine into collecting tubing when client passes urine.
13. Encircle penile shaft with strip of elastic adhesive. Strip should touch only condom sheath. Apply snugly but not tightly.	Condom must be secured so that it is snug and will stay on but not too tight to cause constriction of blood flow.
14. Connect drainage tubing to end of condom catheter. Be sure that condom is not twisted.	Allows urine to be collected and measured. Keeps client dry. Twisted condom obstructs urine flow.
15. Place excess coiling of tubing on bed and secure to bottom sheet.	Prevents looping of tubing and promotes free drainage of urine.
16. Place client in safe, comfortable position (lying down or sitting but not obstructing urine drainage).	Promotes client's comfort.
17. Remove gloves. Dispose of contaminated supplies and wash hands.	Prevents spread of infection.

STEPS	RATIONALE
18. Return in 30 to 60 min to observe for urinary drainage.	Determines whether normal voiding is occurring.
19. Regularly inspect skin on penile shaft for signs of breakdown or irritation.	Indicates whether condom or urine is causing irritation or whether adhesive is too restrictive.
20. Record and report time of catheter application, condition of skin, and voiding pattern.	Provides data to determine change in elimination status.

through the urethra, there are two alternatives for urinary drainage. Suprapubic catheterization involves surgical placement of a catheter through the abdominal wall above the symphysis pubis and into the urinary bladder. The physician performs the procedure under local or general anesthesia. The catheter is anchored in place with sutures, a commercially prepared body seal, or both. Urine drains into a urinary drainage bag. The suprapubic catheter is relatively painless and reduces the incidence of infection commonly seen with retention catheters. Clients with chronic incontinence or loss of bladder control benefit most from a suprapubic catheter. Women who have undergone a vaginal hysterectomy may also benefit temporarily from the insertion of a suprapubic catheter after surgery.

The suprapubic catheter can become blocked by sediment, clots, or the abdominal wall itself. Nurses must monitor the client's I & O carefully, observe for signs of kidney infection (for example, flank tenderness, chills, and fever), and monitor the appearance of urine. Spread of infection to the kidneys may indicate removal of the catheter. A suprapubic catheter must remain patent at all times. The nurse also administers skin care around the insertion site.

The second alternative to catheterization is the condom catheter (Procedure 40-4). It is suitable for incontinent or comatose men who still have complete and spontaneous bladder emptying. The condom is a soft, pliable, rubber sheath that slips over the penis. It may be worn at night only or continuously, depending on the client's needs. A strip of elastic tape fits around the top of the condom to secure it in place (Fig. 40-12). Some types of condoms are applied with skin paste. Care must be taken not to contract the band tightly, or blood supply to the penis will be impaired. Standard adhesive tape should never be used to secure a condom catheter because it does not expand with change in penis size and blood supply to the penis is impaired.

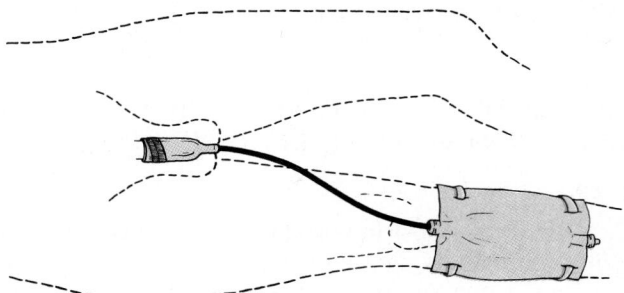

Fig. 40-12 Condom catheter with leg drainage bag.

The end of the condom fits into a plastic drainage tubing. A drainage bag can be attached to the side of the bed or strapped to the client's leg. The condom catheter itself poses little risk of infection. Infections with condom catheters usually result from buildup of secretions around the urethra, trauma to the urethral meatus, or buildup of pressure in the outflow tubing.

The nurse should change a condom catheter daily to check for skin irritation. With each catheter change the nurse cleans the urethral meatus and penis thoroughly. Twisting of the condom at the drainage tube attachment irritates the skin and obstructs urine outflow. The drainage tubing must be checked often for patency.

For a man with a retracted penis, maintaining the intactness of a conventional condom catheter may prove difficult. Special devices are available to help alleviate this problem (Fig. 40-13 on p. 1376). Manufacturers' guidelines for product application should be consulted.

In women, the most frequently used incontinent devices are diapers, pads, and protective clothing. There are few available options for women for continuous-wear external incontinence devices. The devices that are available have not eliminated concerns of wearability and effectiveness and the potential for

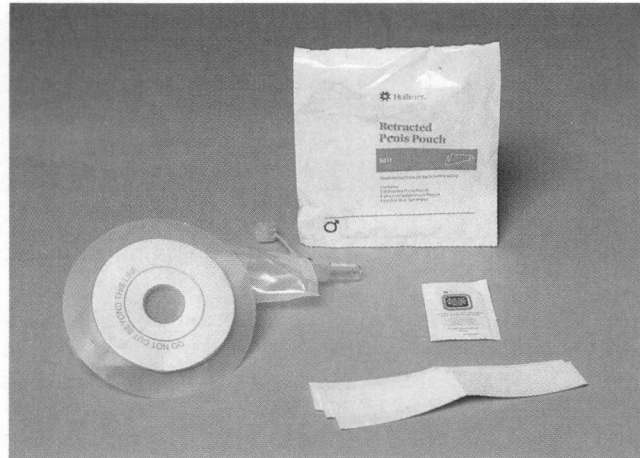

Fig. 40-13 Retracted penis-pouch external urinary device.

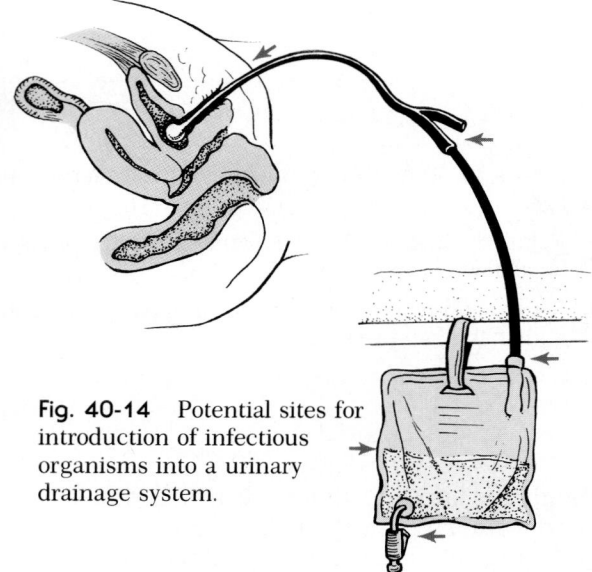

Fig. 40-14 Potential sites for introduction of infectious organisms into a urinary drainage system.

skin breakdown from adhesive products employed in their application (Pieper et al, 1989).

Prevention of Infection

One of the most important considerations for a client with urinary alterations is the need to prevent infection. Good perineal hygiene involving cleansing the urethral meatus after each voiding is essential. A daily intake of 2000 to 2500 ml dilutes urine and promotes regular micturition, which flushes the urethra of microorganisms.

Infection can develop in a catheterized client in many ways. Maintaining a closed urinary drainage system is important in infection control. A break in the system can lead to introduction of microorganisms. Sites at risk are at the site of catheter insertion, drainage bag, spigot, tube junction, and junction of tube and bag (Fig. 40-14). In addition, the nurse monitors the patency of the system to prevent pooling of urine within the tubing. Urine in the drainage bag is an excellent medium for microorganism growth. Bacteria can travel up drainage tubing to grow in pools of urine. If this urine flows back into the client's bladder, an infection will likely develop. Suggestions for ways to prevent infections in catheterized clients are provided (see box).

ACIDIFYING URINE. Acidic urine tends to inhibit growth of microorganisms. Meats, eggs, whole-grain breads, cranberries, prunes, and plums increase urine acidity. The foods metabolize into acid end products that eventually enter the urine. Cranberry juice increases urine acidity, whereas fruit juices such as orange or grapefruit juice produce alkaline urine. However, large volumes of juice must be taken to change urine pH. High doses of ascorbic acid may lower urine pH.

CATHETER IRRIGATIONS AND INSTILLATIONS. To maintain the patency of indwelling urinary catheters, it sometimes becomes necessary to irrigate or flush a catheter. Blood, pus, or sediment can collect within tubing and result in bladder distention and the buildup of stagnant urine. Instillation of a sterile solution ordered by the physician clears the tubing of accumulated material. For clients with bladder infections, a physician may order bladder irrigations to include instillation of antiseptic or antibiotic solutions to wash out the bladder or treat local infection. In both irrigations, sterile aseptic technique is followed.

Before performing an irrigation, the nurse assesses the catheter for blockage. If the amount of urine in the drainage bag is less than the client's intake or less than the output during the previous shift, blockage can be expected. If urine does not drain freely, the nurse milks the tubing. Milking is done by gently squeezing then releasing the drainage tube in an alternating fashion. The nurse should always milk from the client to the drainage bag so a clot or sediment will not be forced back into the catheter.

There is disagreement in the nursing literature about the most effective procedure for irrigations. Studies have shown higher or equal infection rates in clients receiving irrigation than those in which catheters were not irrigated (Dudley, Barriere, 1981; Gelmon, 1980). This was the case even with closed irrigation systems. Contamination of irrigating fluids and equipment and disconnection of the catheter system may be factors in causing infection.

Burgener (1987) recommends that a closed system be maintained during intermittent irrigations or instillations. The nurse uses a sterile 30- to 50-ml syringe with a 19- to 22-gauge, 1-inch needle to inject a prescribed solution into the catheter. This tech-

---

Tips for Preventing Infection in Catheterized Clients

- Follow good handwashing techniques (see Chapter 18).
- Do not allow the spigot on the drainage bag to touch a contaminated surface.
- Do not open the drainage system at connection points to obtain specimens or measure urine.
- If the drainage tubing becomes disconnected, do not touch the ends of the catheter or tubing. Wipe the ends of the tube with antimicrobial solution before reconnecting.
- Ensure that each client has a separate receptacle for measuring urine to prevent cross-contamination.
- Prevent pooling of urine and reflux of urine into the bladder.
    - Avoid raising the drainage bag above the level of the client's bladder.
    - If it becomes necessary to raise the bag during transfer of the client to a bed or stretcher, clamp the tubing.
    - Avoid allowing large loops of tubing to dangle from the bedside.
    - Before client exercises or ambulates, drain all urine from tubing into bag.
- Avoid prolonged clamping or kinking of the tubing (except during bladder conditioning).
- Empty the drainage bag at least every 8 hours. However if large outputs are noted, empty it more frequently.
- Remove the catheter as soon as possible after conferring with the physician.
- Tape the catheter to secure it in place, noting specific guidelines regarding the male client's taping procedures.
- Perform routine perineal hygiene per agency policy and after defecation or bowel incontinence.

---

nique is effective for irrigating a partially blocked catheter or for bladder instillations. Steps for using this closed system are in Procedure 40-5 on p. 1378.

A single intermittent irrigation is safer and less likely to introduce infections into the urinary tract. There are two additional methods for catheter irrigation. One is a closed bladder irrigation system (Procedure 40-5). This system provides for frequent intermittent or continuous irrigation without disruption of the sterile catheter system. It is used most often in clients who have had genitourinary surgery and are at risk for blood clots and mucous fragments occluding the catheter. The other system involves opening the closed drainage system to instill bladder irrigations (Procedure 40-5). This technique poses greater risk for causing infection. However, it may be needed when catheters become blocked and it is undesirable to change the catheter.

Maintenance of Skin Integrity

The normal acidity of urine is irritating to skin. When urine becomes alkaline, encrustation or precipitate collects on the skin, fostering breakdown. Continuous exposure of the perineal area or skin around an ostomy leads to gradual maceration and excoriation (see Chapter 44). Washing with mild soap and warm water is the best way to remove urine from skin. Body lotion keeps skin moisturized and provides a barrier to the urine. Clients who wet their clothing should receive partial baths and clean sets of clothes after voiding.

When the skin becomes irritated or inflamed, the physician may prescribe a cream or spray containing steroids (for example, Kenalog) to reduce inflammation. If fungal growth develops, the antifungal drug nystatin (Mycostatin), available in cream or powder, is effective.

The client with an ostomy has a special hygiene problem because urine drains continuously from the ostomy site. Often the drainage pouch or appliance becomes moist and slips from the skin. Continual oozing of urine around the stoma causes skin breakdown. Skin barriers provide a layer of protection between the client's skin and ostomy pouch. When urine leaks, it frequently covers the outer skin barrier. It also helps to select an appliance that fits snugly against the skin's surface around the stoma.

Promotion of Comfort

Clients with urinary alterations become uncomfortable as a result of the symptoms of urinary problems. Frequent or unpredictable voiding, dysuria, and painful distention are sources of discomfort.

The incontinent client gains comfort from having clean, dry clothing. When stress incontinence is the problem, a protective pad or sanitary belt offers protection against soiling. Wet clothing adheres to the skin and can cause rubbing and irritation.

Dysuria may be relieved by giving urinary analgesics that act on the urethral and bladder mucosa. Phenazopyridine helps relieve dysuria, burning, and itching. It comes with sulfonamide antibiotics in preparations such as Azo-Gantanol and Azo-Gantrisin. The sulfonamide provides additional antibacterial action. Clients taking drugs with phenazopyridine should be aware that their urine may appear orange. They must drink large amounts of fluids to prevent toxicity from the sulfonamides and to maintain optimal flow through the urinary system.

Closed and Open Catheter Irrigation

STEPS	RATIONALE
1. Assess physician's order for type of irrigation and irrigating solution to use.	Ensures proper selection of equipment.
2. Assess color of urine and presence of mucus or sediment.	Determines whether client is bleeding or sloughing tissue.
3. Determine type of catheter in place: a. Triple lumen (one lumen to inflate balloon, one to instill irrigation solution, one to allow outflow of urine) b. Double lumen (one lumen to inflate balloon, one to allow outflow of urine)	Indicates whether it is necessary to open system for irrigation.
4. Determine patency of drainage tubing.	Ensures that drainage tubing is not kinked, clamped incorrectly, or looped below bladder level.
5. Assess amount of urine in drainage bag.	Volume must be subtracted from that which drains into bag after irrigation to ensure that all irrigant returns.
6. Collect necessary equipment and supplies: a. Closed intermittent method: (1) Sterile irrigating solution at room temperature (2) Sterile graduated cup (3) Sterile 30- to 50-ml syringe (4) Sterile 19- to 22-gauge, 1-in needle (5) Antiseptic swab (6) Screw clamp (7) Bath blanket	Cold solution may cause bladder spasm. Used to instill irrigant into catheter. Temporarily occludes catheter as irrigant is instilled.
b. Closed continuous method: (1) Sterile irrigating solution, correct bag or solution at room temperature (2) Irrigation tubing with clamp (with or without Y-connector) (3) Metric container (4) IV pole (5) Antiseptic swab (6) Y connector (optional) (7) Bath blanket	Cold solution may cause bladder spasm. Clamp regulates irrigation flow rate. Y-connector allows IV bags to be connected to tubing. Used for measuring urine output in drainage bag. Connects irrigation tubing to double-lumen catheter.
c. Open method: (1) Disposable, sterile irrigation tray and set (2) Bulb syringe or 60-ml, piston-type syringe (3) Sterile collection basin (4) Waterproof drape (5) Sterile solution container (6) Antiseptic swabs (7) Sterile gloves (8) Ordered irrigating solution at room temperature (9) Tape (10) Bath blanket	Provides necessary force to dislodge clot. Cold solution may cause bladder spasm.
7. Explain procedure and purpose to client.	Helps client to relax and cooperate during procedure.
8. Wash hands.	Reduces transmission of infection.
9. Provide privacy by pulling curtains around bed and folding back covers so that catheter is exposed at junction where it connects to drainage tubing. Cover client's chest with bath blanket.	Promotes client comfort; shows respect for client while exposing area.

STEPS	RATIONALE
10. Assess lower abdomen for bladder distention.	Detects whether catheter is malfunctioning or blocking urinary drainage.
11. Position client in dorsal, recumbent, or supine position.	Promotes client comfort and provides easy access to catheter. Promotes flow of irrigating solution into bladder.
12. Closed intermittent irrigation:	
a. Prepare prescribed sterile irrigating solution in sterile graduated cup.	
b. Draw sterile solution into syringe using aseptic technique.	Ensures that irrigating fluid remains sterile.
c. Clamp indwelling retention catheter below soft injection port.	Occlusion of catheter provides resistance against which irrigant can be forcefully instilled into catheter.
d. Cleanse catheter injection port with antiseptic swab (same port used for specimen collections).	Reduces transmission of infection.
e. Insert needle of syringe through port at 30-degree angle.	Ensures that needle tip enters lumen of catheter.
f. Slowly inject fluid into catheter and bladder.	Slow, continuous pressure dislodges clots and sediment without traumatizing bladder wall.
g. Withdraw syringe, remove clamp, and allow solution to drain into urinary drainage bag. (OPTIONAL: keep tubing clamped to allow instilled fluid to remain in bladder.)	Allows drainage to flow by gravity.
13. Closed continuous irrigation:	
a. Using aseptic technique, insert tip of sterile irrigation tubing into bag containing irrigation solution.	Prevents entrance of microorganisms.
b. Close clamp on tubing and hang bag of solution on IV pole.	Prevents loss of irrigating solution.
c. Open clamp and allow solution to flow through tubing, keeping end of tubing sterile. Close clamp.	Removes air from tubing.
d. Wipe off irrigation port of triple-lumen catheter or attach sterile Y-connector to double-lumen catheter, and then connect to irrigation tubing.	Third lumen or Y-connector provides means for irrigating solution to enter bladder. System must remain sterile.
e. Be sure that drainage bag and tubing are securely connected to drainage port of triple-lumen catheter or other arm of Y-connector.	Ensures that urine and irrigating solution will drain from bladder.
f. For intermittent flow, clamp tubing on drainage system, open clamp on irrigation tubing, and allow prescribed amount of fluid to enter bladder (100 ml is normal for adult). Close irrigation tubing clamp, and then open drainage tubing clamp.	Fluid instills through catheter into bladder, flushing system. Fluid drains out after irrigation is completed.
g. For continuous irrigation (see illustration on p. 1380), calculate drip rate and adjust clamp on irrigation tubing accordingly. Be sure that clamp on drainage tubing is open and check volume of drainage in drainage bag.	Ensures continuous, even irrigation of catheter system. Prevents accumulation of solution in bladder, which may cause bladder distention and possible injury.
14. Open irrigation:	
a. Open sterile irrigation tray, establish sterile field, pour required amount of sterile solution into sterile container, and replace cap on large container of solution.	Adheres to principles of surgical asepsis.
b. Apply sterile gloves (see Chapter 18).	Reduces transmission of infection.
c. Position waterproof drape under catheter.	Prevents soiling bed linen.
d. Aspirate 30 ml of solution into irrigating syringe.	Prepares irrigant for instillation into catheter.

CONTINUED

Closed and Open Catheter Irrigation

STEPS	RATIONALE
e. Move sterile sollection basin close to client's thigh.	Prevents soiling of bed linen and prohibits reaching over sterile area.
f. Disconnect catheter from drainage tubing, allowing urine to flow into sterile collection basin. Cover open end of drainage tubing with sterile protective cap. Position this tubing so that it stays coiled on top of bed.	Maintains sterility of inner aspect of catheter lumen and drainage tubing and reduces potential of inducing pathogens into bladder.
g. Insert tip of syringe into lumen of catheter and gently instill solution.	Gentle instillation reduces incidence of bladder spasm but clears catheter of obstruction.
h. Withdraw syringe, lower catheter, and allow solution to drain into basin. Repeat instilling solution and draining several times until drainage is clear.	Allows drainage to flow by gravity. Provides for adequate flushing of catheter.
i. If solution does not return, have client turn onto side facing you. If changing position does not help, reinsert syringe and gently aspirate solution.	Change in position may move tip of catheter in bladder, increasing likelihood that fluid instilled will flow out.
j. After irrigation is complete, remove protector cap from drainage tube adapter, clean adapter with alcohol swab, and reinsert into lumen of catheter to reestablish closed drainage system.	Reduces entrance of microorganisms into system.
15. Reanchor catheter to client with tape.	Prevents trauma to urethral tissue.
16. Assist client into comfortable position.	Promotes relaxation and rest.
17. Lower bed to lowest position, side rails down if appropriate.	Promotes client safety.
18. Remove gloves. Dispose of contaminated supplies and wash hands.	Prevents spread of infection to other clients.
19. Calculate fluid used to irrigate bladder and catheter and subtract from volume drained.	Determines accurate urinary output.
20. Assess characteristics of output: viscosity, color, and presence of clots.	Evaluates response to therapy.
21. Record type and amount of solution used as irrigant, amount returned as drainage, and character of drainage.	Documents procedure and client's tolerance.

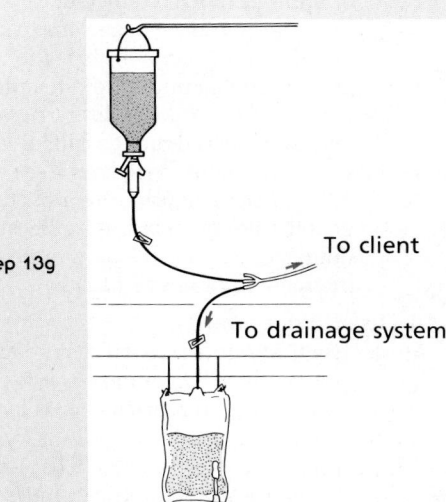

Step 13g

To client

To drainage system

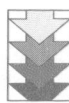

Sample Evaluation of Interventions for Urinary Retention

Goals	Evaluative Measures	Expected Outcomes
Client will achieve complete bladder emptying after voiding by the fourth day after childbirth.	Palpate bladder for distention after voiding. Ask client about sensations of bladder fullness after voiding. Use straight catheter for residual urine after each voiding.	Bladder will not be distended after voiding. Client will deny any sensation of fullness after voiding. There will be less than 50 ml of residual urine.
Client will understand normal urinary elimination.	Ask client to explain normal voiding. Ask client to describe factors that promote or impair urinary elimination. Observe client's toileting self-care habits.	Client will verbalize understanding of urinary elimination and follow appropriate health care practices promoting elimination.
Client will be free of infection.	Obtain urine sample for culture tests. Assess client for signs of dysuria, burning, or itching at urethral meatus and urgency or frequency. Observe characteristics of urine.	There will be no bacterial growth. Client will remain free of symptoms. Urine will be clear, amber, and without sediment.

If the client has local discomfort from an inflamed urethra, a warm sitz bath may provide pain relief. The warm water soothes inflamed tissues near the urethral meatus by improving blood supply. The client is often relaxed after a sitz bath, so voiding occurs easily. Pain of distention cannot be relieved unless the client is able to empty the bladder. Methods for stimulating micturition may be the only sources of pain relief.

Evaluation

To evaluate outcomes and responses to nursing care the nurse measures the effectiveness of all interventions. The optimal outcome is the client's ability to urinate voluntarily without symptoms (for example, urgency, dysuria, or frequency). The urine should be an amber color, clear, without abnormal constituents, and within the normal range of pH and specific gravity. The client should be able to identify factors that may influence normal voiding. The nurse also evaluates specific interventions designed to promote normal urinary function and prevent complications of urinary alterations (see evaluation box).

The nurse collects data related to the client's voiding pattern, exposure to risks for urinary tract alteration, and physical condition. Laboratory analysis of urine specimens and diagnostic review of urinary structures provide further information.

Nursing interventions promote normal urination and provide support to clients unable to maintain continence. Because of the urinary tract's vulnerability to infection, one of the nurse's primary concerns is infection control. The client with urinary alterations may also suffer embarrassment, social isolation, and depression. Whether the alteration is temporary (for example, catheterization) or long term (for example, ureterostomy), the nurse must maintain the client's privacy and dignity. The nurse also evaluates the client's need for additional support services (for example, home health care, physical therapy, and counseling) and initiates the referral.

As nurses become more comfortable with the roles of the client advocate and primary nurse, the provision of quality care delivery has become a paramount goal of the profession (Ulrich, 1989). To this end, nurses are actively involved in developing methods to systematically evaluate the nursing process. Nursing research is being conducted to validate nursing interventions. Quality improvement is evolving as a tool to evaluate nursing care delivery. The goal is to ensure the delivery of competent, state-of-the-art nursing care with positive outcomes for each client.

 SUMMARY

Normal elimination of urinary waste requires maintenance of urinary function. Nursing therapies promote or minimize factors that influence urinary function. Each client has a different pattern of elimination. The nurse must assess this pattern and design therapies to promote normal urinary elimination. When necessary, the nurse uses devices such as a condom or an indwelling catheter to assist the client with urine elimination.

Key Concepts

- The act of micturition or voiding is influenced by voluntary control from higher brain centers and involuntary control from the spinal cord.

- Symptoms common to urinary disturbances include urgency, dysuria, polyuria, oliguria, and difficulty in starting the urinary stream.

- When collected properly, a clean-voided urine specimen does not contain bacteria picked up from the urethral meatus.

- A client can better understand the importance of perineal hygiene by knowing that the urinary tract is normally sterile.

- Methods of promoting the micturition reflex assist clients in sensing the urge to urinate and controlling urethral sphincter relaxation.

- An increased fluid intake results in increased urine formation that flushes particles and solutes from the urinary system.

- An indwelling urinary catheter remains in the bladder for an extended period, making the risk of infection greater than with intermittent catheterization.

- Because urine drains almost continuously from a ureterostomy, there is a risk of skin breakdown around a stoma site.

- A primary function of the elimination process is fluid balance.

- Catheter irrigation becomes necessary when the catheter becomes occluded with sediment or blood clots.

- A catheter drainage system should be positioned to allow free drainage of urine by gravity.

- Condom catheters are applied snugly but not so tightly as to constrict blood flow.

- Incontinence is classifed as acute, urge, stress, overflow, and functional. Each type has specific nursing interventions.

- Specific guidelines for catheter selection should be followed so that the catheter does not cause harm during insertion procedures.

- Alterations in the urinary system can cause alterations in other organ systems.

Key Terms

Critical Thinking Exercises

1. An older man is admitted to your unit after having undergone a radical prostatectomy. He has an indwelling Foley catheter. Identify potential complications resulting from the indwelling catheter.

2. You are asked to obtain a clean-voided midstream urine specimen for culture and sensitivity tests from a client on your unit. What assessment data should be recorded in the nursing note regarding this specimen collection?

3. Mr. Ronald is a 23-year-old client who has been experiencing headaches and blurred vision for the past few weeks. He attributed these symptoms to intense studying during final examinations. However, Mr. Ronald also noticed that he had begun having to get up at night to urinate. When Mr. Ronald was examined by his physician he was noted to be hypertensive with a blood pressure of 190/128. What is the significance of Mr. Ronald's urinary frequency at night?

REFERENCES

Burgener S: Justification of closed intermittent urinary catheter irrigation/installation: a review of current research and practice, *J Adv Nurs* 12:229, 1987.

Dudley MN, Barriere SL: Antimicrobial irrigations in the prevention and treatment of catheter-related urinary tract infections, *Am J Hosp Pharm* 38(1):59, 1981.

Gelmon ML: Antibiotic irrigation and catheter-associated urinary tract infections, *Nephron* 25:259, 1980.

Kane RL et al: *Essentials of clinical geriatrics,* New York, 1984, McGraw-Hill.

Kim MJ, McFarland GK, McLane AM: *Pocket guide to nursing diagnoses,* ed 4, St Louis, 1991, Mosby–Year Book.

Kristiansen P et al: Long-term urethral catheter drainage and bladder capacity, *Neurol Urodyn* 2:134, 1983.

Orzeck S, Ouslander JG: Urinary incontinence: an overview of causes and treatment, *J Enterostom Ther* 14:20, 1987.

Pieper B et al: Inventing urine incontinence devices for women, *Image J Nurs Sch* 21(4):205, 1989.

Richard CJ, *Comprehensive nephrology nursing,* Boston, 1986, Little, Brown.

Rogers W: Shampoo urethritis (letter), *Am J Dis Child* 139:748, 1985.

Touch DCH: Pelvic floor musculature exercises in treatment of anatomical urinary stress incontinence, *Phys Ther* 68(5):652, 1988.

Ulrich BT: *Nephrology nursing: concepts and strategies,* Norwalk, Conn, 1989, Appleton & Lange.

Whaley LF, Wong DL: *Nursing care of infants and children,* ed 4, St Louis, 1991, Mosby–Year Book.

Williamson ML: Reducing post-catheterization bladder dysfunction by reconditioning, *Nurs Res* 31:28, 1982.

Wong ES: Guidelines for the prevention of catheter-associated urinary tract infections. In Centers for Disease Control: *Guidelines for the prevention and control of nosocomial infections,* Atlanta, 1982, The Centers.

ADDITIONAL READINGS

Alteresco V: Theoretical foundations for an approach to urinary incontinence, *J Enterostom Ther* 13:105, 1986.

Bates P: A troubleshooter's guide to indwelling catheters, *RN* 44:63, 1981.

Bello-Reuss E, Reuss L: Homeostatic and excretory functions of the kidney. In Klahr S, editor: *The kidney and body fluids in health and disease,* New York, 1983, Plenum.

Bielski M: Preventing infection in the catheterized patient, *Nurs Clin North Am* 15:703, 1980.

Brundage DJ: *Nursing management of renal problems,* ed 2, St Louis, 1980, Mosby–Year Book.

Crummey V: Ignorance can hurt, *Nurs Times* 85(21):66, 1989.

Daugirdas JT, Ing TS: *Handbook of dialysis,* Boston, 1988, Little, Brown.

Demmerle B, Bantol MA: Nursing care of the incontinent person, *Geriatr Nurs* 1:246, 1980.

Erickson PJ: Ostomies: the art of pouching, *Nurs Clin North Am* 22:311, 1987.

Fox B: Recurring urinary tract infections: incidence and risk factors, *Am J Public Health* 80(3):331, 1990.

Gibson LY: Bedwetting: a family recurrent nightmare, *MCN* 12(4), 1989.

Greengold BA, Ouslander JG: Bladder retraining, *J Gerontol Nurs* 12:31, 1986.

Harty JI, Catalona WJ: Management aspects of the genitourinary system. In Etheredge E, editor: *Management techniques in surgery,* New York, 1986, Wiley.

Kaltrieder DL et al: Can reminders curb incontinence? *Geriatr Nurs* 11(1):17, 1990.

Mandelstam D: Strengthening pelvic floor muscles, *Geriatr Nurs* 1:251, 1980.

McConnell EA: *Care of patients with urologic problems,* Philadelphia, 1983, Lippincott.

Nurses' drug alert: Urinary tract irritation from shampoo, *Am J Nurs* 86:66, 1986.

Pagana KD, Pagana TJ: *Diagnostic testing and nursing implications: a case study approach,* ed. 3, St Louis, 1990, Mosby–Year Book.

Palmer MH et al: Risk factors for urinary incontinence one year after nursing-home admission, *Res Nurs Health* 14:405, 1991.

Petillo MH: The patient with a urinary stoma, *Nurs Clin North Am* 22:263, 1987.

Rees-Williams C et al: Making sense of urinary catheters, *Nurs Times* 84(40):46, 1988.

Robb SS: Urinary incontinence verification in elderly men, *Nurs Res* 34:278, 1985.

Sampselle C et al: Pelvic muscle strength in childbearing women, *Nurs Res* 38(3):134, 1989.

Wilde MH: Living with a Foley, *Am J Nurs* 86:1121, 1986.

CHAPTER 41

Bowel Elimination

OBJECTIVES

Mastery of content in this chapter will enable the student to:
- Define the key terms listed.
- Discuss the role of gastrointestinal organs in digestion and elimination.
- Describe four functions of the large intestine.
- Explain the physiological aspects of normal defecation.
- Discuss psychological and physiological factors that influence the elimination process.
- Describe common physiological alterations in elimination.
- Assess a client's elimination pattern.
- Perform a guaiac test for occult blood.
- List nursing diagnoses related to alterations in elimination.
- Describe nursing implications for common diagnostic examinations of the gastrointestinal tract.
- Administer an enema.
- List nursing measures that promote normal elimination.
- Discuss the relationship between the structure and function of bowel diversions and nursing care required.

CHAPTER OUTLINE

Normal Digestion and Elimination
    Mouth
    Esophagus
    Stomach
    Small intestine
    Large intestine

Factors Affecting Elimination
    Age
    Diet
    Fluid intake
    Physical activity
    Psychological factors
    Personal habits
    Position during defecation
    Pain
    Pregnancy
    Surgery and anesthesia
    Medications
    Diagnostic tests

Common Bowel Elimination Problems
    Constipation
    Impaction
    Diarrhea
    Incontinence
    Flatulence
    Hemorrhoids

Bowel Diversions

Nursing Process and Bowel Elimination
    Assessment
    Nursing diagnosis
    Planning
    Implementation
    Evaluation

Regular elimination of bowel waste products is essential for normal body functioning. Alterations in elimination can cause problems with the gastrointestinal and other body systems. Because bowel function depends on the balance of several factors, elimination patterns and habits vary among individuals. However, there is increased evidence that frequent, high-volume, normal feces is consistent with a lower incidence of colorectal cancer (Robinson, Weigley, 1989).

Clients often need assistance from the nurse to maintain normal elimination habits. Illness can prevent them from following their bowel management programs. They might become physically unable to use normal toilet facilities. The home environment might present obstacles for clients with altered mobility, requiring changes in bathroom fixtures.

To manage a client's elimination problems, the nurse must understand normal elimination and factors that promote or impede elimination. Supportive nursing care respects the client's privacy and emotional needs. Measures designed to promote normal elimination should also minimize discomfort.

 ## NORMAL DIGESTION AND ELIMINATION

The gastrointestinal (GI) tract is a series of hollow mucous membrane–lined muscular organs. The purposes of these organs are to absorb fluid and nutrients, prepare food for absorption and use by the body's cells, and provide for temporary storage of feces (Fig. 41-1). The volume of fluids absorbed by the GI tract is high, making fluid balance a key function of the GI system. In addition to ingested fluids and foods, the GI tract also receives many secretions from organs such as the gallbladder and the pancreas (Table 41-1). A disorder that seriously impairs normal absorption or secretion of GI fluids causes fluid imbalance.

Mouth

The GI tract mechanically and chemically breaks down nutrients into a suitable size and form. All digestive organs work together to ensure that the mass, or **bolus,** of food reaches the areas of nutrient absorption safely and effectively. Mechanical and chemical digestion begin in the mouth. The teeth **masticate** (chew) food, breaking it down to a suitable size for swallowing. Salivary secretions contain enzymes, such as ptyalin, that initiate digestion of certain food elements. Saliva dilutes and softens the bolus of food in the mouth for easier swallowing.

TABLE 41-1 Gastrointestinal Tract Fluid Balance		
Item	Ingested and Secreted (ml)	Absorbed (ml)
Food and drink	1500	
Saliva	1500	
Gastric juice	3000	
Pancreatic juice	2000	
Bile	500	
Small intestine fluid		5850
Colon		2500
Feces		150
TOTAL	8500	8500

Esophagus

As food enters the upper esophagus, it passes through the upper esophageal sphincter, which is a circular muscle that prevents air from entering the esophagus and food from **refluxing** (moving backward) into the throat. The bolus of food travels approximately 25 cm (10 in) down the esophagus. Food is pushed along by slow peristaltic waves produced by alternating contractions of smooth muscle. As a portion of the esophagus contracts behind the food bolus, the circular muscle in front of the bolus relaxes. A peristaltic wave propels food toward the next wave (Fig. 41-2). **Peristalsis** moves food throughout the length of the GI tract.

In 15 seconds the bolus of food moves down the esophagus and reaches the lower esophageal sphincter. The lower esophageal sphincter lies between the esophagus and stomach, and a pressure difference exists at the lower end of the esophagus (Tortora, 1989). The lower esophageal pressure is 10 to 40 mm Hg, whereas pressure within the stomach is 5 to 10 mm Hg. The pressure gradient normally prevents reflux of stomach contents back into the esophagus. Factors influencing lower sphincter pressure include antacids, which minimize reflux, and fatty foods and nicotine, which increase reflux.

Stomach

In the stomach, food is temporarily stored and mechanically and chemically broken down for digestion and absorption (see Chapter 35). The stomach secretes hydrochloric acid (HCl), mucus, the enzyme pepsin, and intrinsic factor. The concentration of HCl influences stomach acidity and the body's acid-base balance (see Chapter 39). For every HCl mole-

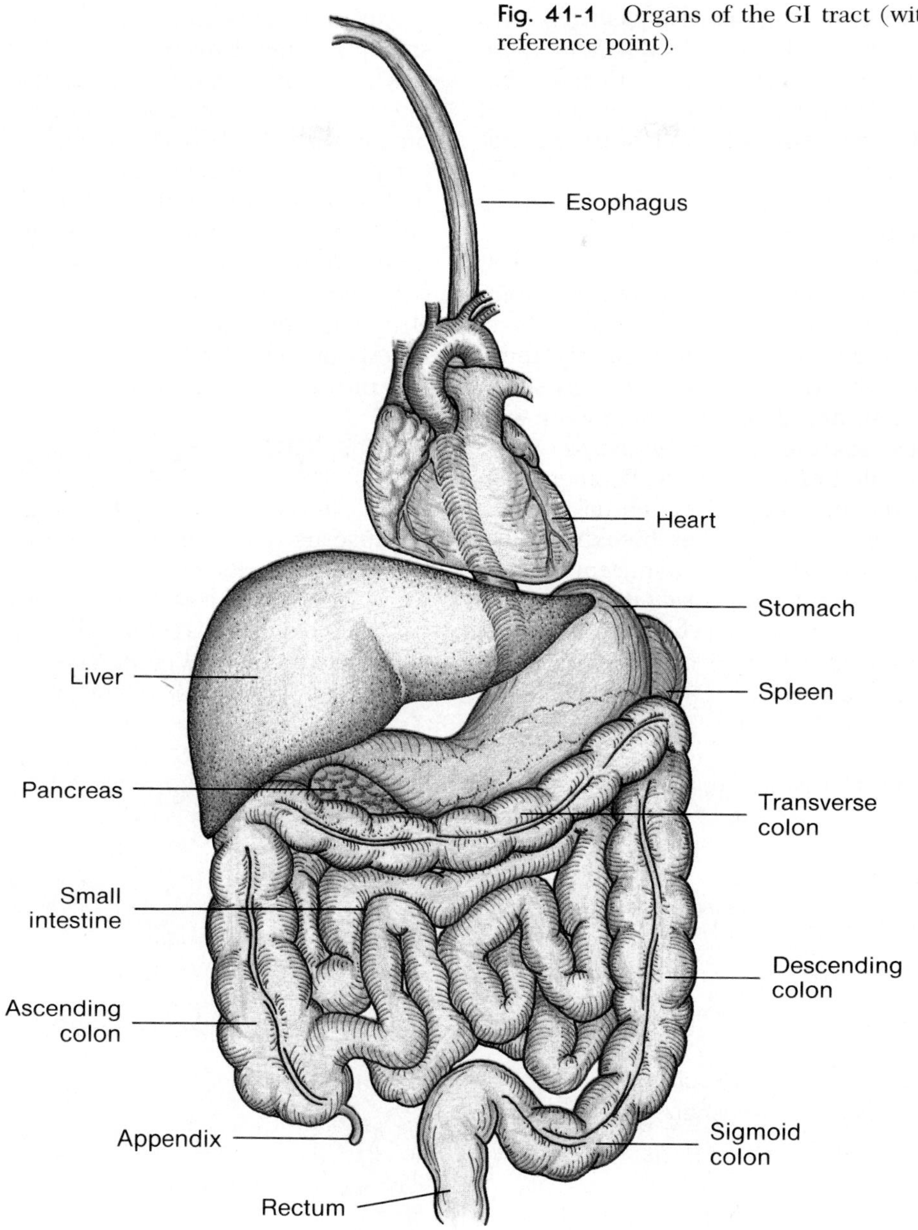

Fig. 41-1 Organs of the GI tract (with the heart as a reference point).

Esophagus

Heart

Liver

Stomach

Spleen

Pancreas

Transverse colon

Small intestine

Ascending colon

Descending colon

Appendix

Sigmoid colon

Rectum

cule secreted into the stomach, a bicarbonate molecule enters the blood plasma. HCl helps mix and break down food in the stomach. Mucus protects the stomach mucosa from acidity and enzyme activity. Pepsin digests proteins, although not much digestion occurs in the stomach. Intrinsic factor is the essential component needed for vitamin B_{12} absorption in the intestine and subsequent normal red blood cell formation. Lack of this intrinsic factor results in pernicious anemia.

Before food leaves the stomach, it is changed into a semifluid material called **chyme**. Chyme is more easily digested and absorbed than solid food. Clients who have portions of their stomachs removed or who

Segmentation

Peristalsis

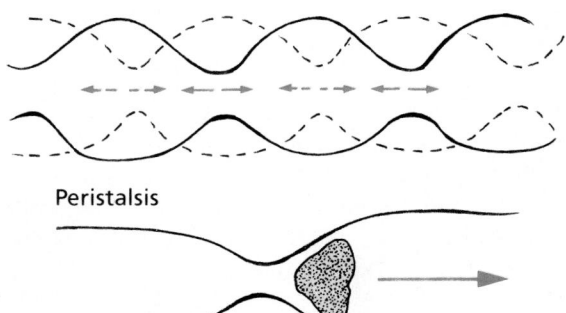

Fig. 41-2 Segmented and peristaltic waves.

have rapid stomach emptying (as with gastritis) have serious digestive problems because food is not broken down into chyme. Food enters the small intestine before being adequately broken down to a semifluid form. Absorption is less efficient, and nutritional alterations can develop.

Small Intestine

During normal digestion, chyme leaves the stomach and enters the small intestine. The small intestine is a tube about 2.5 cm (1 in) in diameter and 6 m (20 ft) in length. It contains three divisions: duodenum, jejunum, and ileum. Chyme mixes with digestive enzymes (such as bile and amylase) while traveling through the small intestine. Segmentation (alternating contraction and relaxation of smooth muscle) churns the chyme, further breaking down food for digestion (Fig. 41-2). As chyme mixes, forward peristaltic movement temporarily ceases to permit absorption. Chyme travels slowly down the small intestine to allow absorption.

Most nutrients and electrolytes are absorbed in the small intestine. Enzymes from the pancreas (such as amylase) and bile from the gallbladder are released into the duodenum. The intestine breaks down fats, proteins, and carbohydrates into basic elements (see Chapter 35). Nutrients are almost entirely absorbed by the duodenum and jejunum. The ileum absorbs certain vitamins, iron, and bile salts. If its function is impaired, the digestive process is greatly altered. For example, inflammation, surgical resection, or obstruction can disrupt peristalsis, reduce the area of absorption, or block passage of chyme. Electrolyte and nutrient deficiencies then develop.

Large Intestine

The lower GI tract is the large intestine (**colon**) because its diameter is larger than the small intestine. However, its length of 1.5 to 1.8 m (5 to 6 ft) is much shorter. The large intestine is divided into the cecum, colon, and rectum (Fig. 41-3). It is the primary organ of bowel elimination.

Fig. 41-3   Divisions of the large intestine.

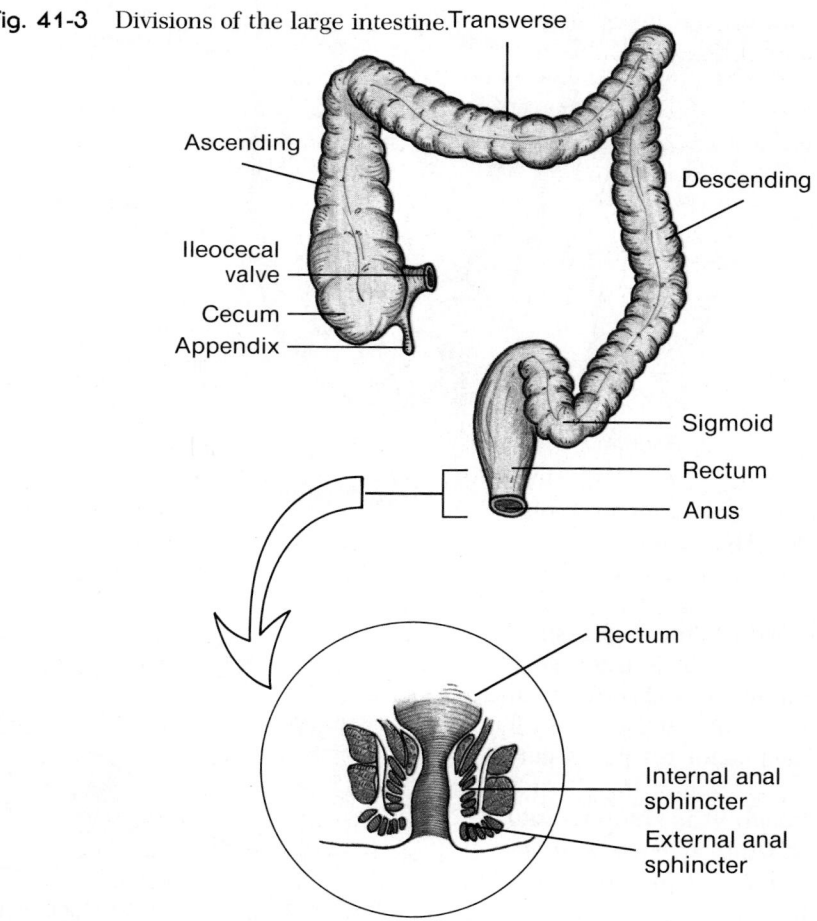

Transverse

Ascending

Descending

Ileocecal valve

Cecum

Appendix

Sigmoid

Rectum

Anus

Rectum

Internal anal sphincter

External anal sphincter

Cecum

Unabsorbed chyme enters the large intestine at the cecum through the ileocecal valve, which is a circular muscle layer that prevents colon contents from **regurgitating** (returning to the small intestine).

Colon

Although watery chyme enters the colon, the volume of water lessens as chyme moves along it. The colon is divided into the ascending, transverse, descending, and sigmoid colons. The colon is made of muscular tissue, which allows it to accommodate and thus eliminate large quantities of waste.

The colon has four interrelated functions: absorption, protection, secretion, and elimination. A large volume of water and significant amounts of sodium and chloride are absorbed by the colon daily. As food passes through the colon, **haustral contractions** occur. These are similar to segmental contractions of the small intestine but last longer—up to 5 min. The contractions produce large sacs in the colon's wall, providing a large surface area for absorption.

As much as 2.5 L of water can be absorbed by the colon in 24 hours. On the average, 55 mEq of sodium and 23 mEq of chloride are absorbed daily. The amount of water absorbed from chyme depends on the speed at which colonic contents move. Chyme is normally a soft, formed mass. If the speed of peristaltic contractions is abnormally fast, there is less time for water to be absorbed and the stool will be watery. If peristaltic contractions slow down, water continues to be absorbed, and a hard mass of stool forms, resulting in constipation.

The colon protects itself by releasing a supply of mucus. Mucus is normally clear to opaque with a stringy consistency. Mucus lubricates the colon, preventing trauma to its inner walls. Lubrication is especially important near the distal end of the colon, where contents become drier and harder.

The secretory function of the colon aids in electrolyte balance. Bicarbonate is secreted in exchange for chloride. About 4 to 9 mEq of potassium is released each day by the large intestine. Serious alterations in colon function can cause electrolyte imbalance.

Finally, the colon removes waste products and gas (**flatus**). Flatus results from air swallowing, diffusion of gas from the bloodstream into the intestine, and bacterial action on nonabsorbable carbohydrates. Fermentation of carbohydrates (such as in cabbage and onions) produces intestinal gas, which can stimulate peristalsis. An adult normally forms 400 to 700 ml of flatus daily.

Slow peristaltic contractions move contents through the colon. Intestinal content is the main stimulus for contraction. Waste products and gas exert pressure against the walls of the colon. The muscle layer stretches, stimulating the reflex that initiates contraction.

Mass peristaltic movements push undigested food toward the rectum. These movements are unlike the frequent peristaltic waves in the small intestine (usually heard during auscultation) in that they occur only 3 or 4 times daily.

When these mass peristaltic movements occur, large segments of the colon contract as a result of gastrocolic and duodenocolic reflex responses. These occur when the stomach or duodenum is filled with food. Filling initiates nerve impulses that stimulate the colon's muscular walls. Mass peristalsis is strongest during the hour after mealtime.

Rectum

Waste products that reach the sigmoid portion of the colon are called *feces*. The sigmoid stores feces until just before defecation.

The rectum is the final division of the GI tract. Its length varies according to age:

Infant	2.5 to 3.8 cm (1 to 1.5 in)
Toddler	5 cm (2 in)
Preschooler	7.5 cm (3 in)
School-ager	10 cm (4 in)
Adult	15 to 20 cm (6 to 8 in)

Normally the rectum is empty of feces until defecation. It contains vertical and transverse folds of tissue. Each vertical fold contains an artery and veins. If the veins become distended from pressure during the straining of defecation, hemorrhoids form. Hemorrhoids can make defecation painful.

When the fecal mass or gas moves into the rectum to distend its walls, **defecation** begins. The process involves involuntary and voluntary control. The internal sphincter is a smooth muscle innervated by the autonomic nervous system. As the rectum distends, sensory nerves are stimulated and carry impulses that cause the internal sphincter to relax, allowing more feces to enter the rectum. At the same time, impulses travel to the brain to create awareness of the need to defecate.

As the internal sphincter relaxes, so does the external sphincter. The person who is toilet trained can voluntarily control the external sphincter. If the time for defecation is not right, constriction of the levator ani muscles closes the anus and defecation is delayed. At the time of defecation, the external sphincter relaxes. Pressure can be exerted to expel feces through an increase in intraabdominal pressure or a Valsalva maneuver. A **Valsalva maneuver** is voluntary contraction of abdominal muscles during forced expiration with a closed glottis (holding one's breath while straining). Relaxation of the levator ani muscle allows feces to be expelled. If the act of defecation is voluntarily stopped, feces remain in the rectum until the defecation reflex is restimulated. Defecation can be promoted by flexing the thigh muscles, which puts pressure on the abdomen, and sitting, which increases pressure down on the rectum.

 ## FACTORS AFFECTING ELIMINATION

Many factors influence the process of bowel elimination (Table 41-2). Knowledge of these factors lets the nurse anticipate measures required to maintain a normal elimination pattern. Also, an understanding of the effects of these factors on normal elimination provides guidelines for reversing their effects.

Age

Developmental changes that affect elimination occur throughout life. An infant has a small stomach capacity and less secretion of digestive enzymes. Some foods such as complex starches are tolerated poorly. Food passes quickly through an infant's intestinal tract because of rapid peristalsis. The infant is unable to control defecation because of a lack of neuromuscular development. This development usually does not take place until 2 to 3 years of age.

During adolescence, there is rapid growth of the large intestine. The secretion of HCl increases, particularly in boys. Adolescents typically eat more.

Older adults often experience changes in the GI system that impair digestion and elimination. Many lose their teeth and thus the ability to chew food thoroughly. Food enters the digestive tract only partially chewed and cannot be digested because the amount of digestive enzymes in saliva and the volume of gastric acids decreases with aging. The in-ability to digest fat-containing foods reflects a loss of the enzyme lipase.

Hospitalized older adults are at particular risk of altered bowel function. One study indicated a 91% incidence of diarrhea or constipation in a population of 33 hospitalized persons with a mean age of 76 years (Ross, 1990).

In addition, peristaltic action declines, and esophageal emptying slows. Sluggish emptying of the esophagus can cause discomfort in the epigastric section of the abdomen. Absorptive properties of the intestinal mucosa change, causing protein, vitamin, and mineral deficiencies. Older adults also lose muscle tone in the perineal floor and anal sphincter. Although the integrity of the external sphincter may remain intact, older adults may have difficulty controlling bowel evacuation. Because of slowing of nerve impulses, some are less aware of the need to defecate and are likely to become constipated.

Diet

Regular daily food intake helps maintain a regular pattern of peristalsis in the colon. The food that a person eats influences elimination. **Fiber,** the undigestible residue in the diet, provides the bulk in fecal material. Bulk-forming foods absorb fluids, thereby increasing stool mass. The bowel walls are stretched, creating peristalsis and initiating the defecation reflex. An infant's immature bowel cannot usually tolerate fiber-containing foods until several months of age. By stimulating peristalsis, bulk foods pass quickly through the intestines, keeping the stool soft. The following foods contain a higher amount of fiber:
1. Raw fruits (apples, oranges)
2. Cooked fruits (prunes, apricots)
3. Greens (spinach, kale, cabbage)
4. Raw vegetables (celery, zucchini)
5. Whole grains (cereal, breads)

TABLE 41-2 Factors Affecting Elimination

Factors Promoting Elimination	Factors Impairing Elimination
Stress-free environment	Emotional stress (anxiety or depression)
Ability to follow personal bowel habits, privacy	Failure to heed defecation reflex, lack of time or privacy
High-fiber diet	High-carbohydrate, high-fat diet
Normal fluid intake (fruit juices, warm liquids)	Reduced fluid intake
Exercise (walking)	Immobility or inactivity
Ability to assume squatting position	Inability to squat because of immobility, advanced age, musculoskeletal deformities, pain, advanced pregnancy; pain during defecation
Properly administered laxatives and cathartics	Use of narcotic analgesics, antibiotics, and general anesthetics and over use of cathartics

Convenience foods such as pizza, pot pies, and sugar-coated cereals tend to be low in fiber. They are popular for people who have active lifestyles or who live alone (such as older adults).

Ingestion of a high-fiber diet improves the likelihood of a normal elimination pattern if other factors are normal. Gas-producing foods such as onions, cauliflower, and beans also stimulate peristalsis. The gas formed distends intestinal walls, increasing colon motility. Some spicy foods can increase peristalsis but can also cause indigestion and watery stools.

Some foods, such as milk and milk products, are difficult or impossible for some people to digest. This is caused by a **lactose intolerance.** Lactose, a simple form of sugar found in milk, is normally broken down by the enzyme lactase. The inability to digest lactose results from a failure to produce lactase. Intolerance to specific foods may result in diarrhea, gaseous distention, and cramping. Management involves simple avoidance of lactose-containing products.

Fluid Intake

An inadequate intake of fluids or disturbances causing loss of fluid (such as vomiting) affect the character of feces. Fluid liquefies intestinal contents, easing their passage through the colon. Reduced fluid intake slows passage of food through the intestine. An adult should drink 6 to 8 glasses (1400 to 2000 ml) of fluid daily. Hot beverages and fruit juices soften stool and increase peristalsis. A large ingestion of milk may slow peristalsis in some persons and cause constipation.

Physical Activity

Physical activity promotes peristalsis, whereas immobilization depresses colonic motility. Early ambulation after illness is encouraged to promote maintenance of normal elimination.

Maintaining tone of skeletal muscles used during defecation is important. Weakened abdominal and pelvic floor muscles impair the ability to increase intraabdominal pressure and to control the external sphincter. Muscle tone may be weakened or lost as a result of long-term illness or neurological disease that impairs nerve transmission.

Psychological Factors

The function of almost all body systems can be impaired by prolonged emotional stress (see Chapter 30). If an individual becomes anxious, afraid, or angry, the stress response initiates impulses from the parasympathetic division of the autonomic nervous system. This response allows the body to restore defenses. The digestive process is accelerated, and peristalsis is increased to provide nutrients needed for defense. Side effects of increased peristalsis are diarrhea and gaseous distention. If a person becomes depressed, the autonomic nervous system slows impulses and peristalsis can decrease. A number of diseases of the GI tract may be associated with stress. These include ulcerative **colitis,** gastric ulcers, and **Crohn's disease.** Repeated research endeavors have failed to prove the myth that clients with such diseases have underlying psychopathological conditions. Anxiety and depression may be a result of such chronic problems (Cooke, 1991).

A child's elimination pattern can be upset by the method of toilet training. Forcing a child to learn toilet training before nervous and muscular systems are developed is a waste of time. Punishing children for accidents makes toilet training stressful.

Personal Habits

Personal elimination habits influence bowel function. Most people benefit from being able to use their own toilet facilities at a time that is most effective and convenient for them. A busy work schedule may disrupt habits and result in alterations such as constipation. A person should learn the best time for elimination. The **gastrocolic reflex** is most easily stimulated to cause defecation after breakfast.

Hospitalized clients can rarely maintain privacy during defecation. Bathroom facilities are often shared with a roommate whose hygienic habits might be quite different. The client's illness often limits physical activity and requires the use of a bedpan or bedside commode. The sights, sounds, and odors associated with sharing toilet facilities or using bedpans are often embarrassing. Embarrassment prompts clients to ignore the urge to defecate, which can begin a vicious cycle of discomfort.

Position During Defecation

Squatting is the normal position during defecation. Modern toilets are designed to facilitate this posture, allowing the person to lean forward, exert intraabdominal pressure, and contract the thigh muscles. However, an older client or one with joint disease such as arthritis may be unable to rise from a low toilet seat. Attachments that raise the seat enable the client to get off the toilet without assistance. Clients who use such attachments, as well as short people, might require a footstool for proper hip flexion.

For the client immobilized in bed, defecation is often difficult. In a supine position, it is impossible to contract the muscles used during defecation. Assisting the client to a more normal sitting position on a bedpan enhances the ability to defecate.

Pain

Normally the act of defecation is painless. However, a number of conditions, including hemorrhoids, rectal surgery, abdominal surgery, and childbirth can result in discomfort. In these instances the client often suppresses the urge to defecate to avoid pain. Constipation is a common problem for clients with pain during defecation.

Pregnancy

As pregnancy advances and the size of the fetus increases, pressure is exerted on the rectum. A temporary obstruction created by the fetus impairs passage of feces. Constipation is a common problem during the last trimester. A pregnant woman's frequent straining during defecation can result in formation of permanent hemorrhoids.

Surgery and Anesthesia

General anesthetic agents used during surgery cause temporary cessation of peristalsis (see Chapter 47). Inhaled anesthetic agents block parasympathetic impulses to the intestinal musculature. The anesthetic's action slows or stops peristaltic waves. The client who receives local or regional anesthesia is less at risk for elimination alterations because bowel activity is affected minimally or not at all.

Surgery that involves direct manipulation of the bowel temporarily stops peristalsis. This condition, called *paralytic ileus,* usually lasts about 24 to 48 hours. If the client remains inactive or is unable to eat after surgery, return of normal bowel function may be further delayed.

Medications

Medications are available for promoting defecation. **Laxatives** and **cathartics** soften the stool and promote peristalsis. When used correctly, laxatives and cathartics safely maintain normal elimination patterns. However, chronic use of cathartics causes the large intestine to lose muscle tone and become less responsive to stimulation by laxatives. Laxative overuse can also cause serious diarrhea that can lead to dehydration and electrolyte depletion. Mineral oil, a common laxative, decreases fat-soluble vitamin absorption. Laxatives can influence the efficacy of other medications by altering the **transit time** (that

is, the time the medication remains in the GI tract for proper absorption).

Medications such as dicyclomine HCl (Bentyl) suppress peristalsis and treat diarrhea. Several medications have side effects that can impair elimination. Narcotic analgesics depress peristalsis in the GI tract. Opiates commonly cause constipation. Anticholinergic drugs, such as atropine or glycopyrrolate (Robinul), inhibit gastric acid secretion and depress GI motility. Although useful in treating hyperactive bowel disorders, anticholinergics can cause constipation. Many antibiotics produce diarrhea by disrupting the normal bacterial flora in the GI tract. If the diarrhea and associated abdominal cramping become severe, the client might need to change medications.

Diagnostic Tests

Diagnostic examinations involving visualization of GI structures often require that portions of the bowel be empty of contents. A client is not allowed to eat or drink after midnight of the day preceding examinations such as a barium enema, endoscopy of the lower GI tract, or an upper GI (UGI) series. In the case of a barium enema or endoscopy, the client usually receives cathartics and an enema. Such emptying of the bowel can interfere with elimination until normal eating is resumed.

Barium examination procedures pose an additional problem. Barium hardens if allowed to stay in the GI tract. This can lead to constipation or bowel impaction. A client should receive a cathartic to promote elimination of barium. Failure to evacuate all barium might require that the client receive a cleansing enema.

 ## COMMON BOWEL ELIMINATION PROBLEMS

The nurse might care for clients who have or are at risk for having elimination problems because of emotional stress (anxiety or depression), physiological changes in the GI tract, surgical alteration of intestinal structures, other prescribed therapy, or disorders impairing defecation.

Constipation

Constipation is a symptom, not a disease. It is a decrease in frequency of bowel movements, accompanied by prolonged or difficult passage of hard, dry stools. Straining during defecation is an associated sign. When intestinal motility slows, the fecal mass becomes exposed over time to the intestinal walls and most of the fecal water content is absorbed. Little water is left to soften and lubricate stool. Passage of a dry stool may cause rectal pain.

Each person has an individual defecation pattern that the nurse must assess. If daily records start to suggest a decrease in the frequency of defecation there is cause for concern. Older adults tend to report more problems with constipation if they are unable to have daily bowel movements. The causes of constipation are summarized in the box.

Constipation is a significant hazard to health. Straining during defecation causes problems to the client with recent abdominal or rectal surgery. The effort to pass a stool can cause sutures to separate, reopening the wound. In addition, clients with histories of cardiovascular disease, diseases causing elevated intraocular pressure (glaucoma), and increased intracranial pressure should prevent constipation and avoid using the Valsalva maneuver (see Chapter 19). Exhaling through the mouth during straining avoids a Valsalva maneuver.

Impaction

Fecal **impaction** results from unrelieved constipation. It is a collection of hardened feces, wedged in the rectum, that cannot be expelled. In cases of severe impaction, the mass can extend up into the sigmoid colon. Clients who are debilitated, confused, or unconscious are most at risk for impaction. They are too weak or unaware of the need to defecate.

An obvious sign of impaction is the inability to pass a stool for several days, despite a repeated urge to defecate. When a continuous oozing of diarrheal stool suddenly develops, impaction should be suspected. The liquid portion of feces located higher in the colon seeps around the impacted mass. Loss of appetite (anorexia), abdominal distention and cramping, and rectal pain may accompany the condition. The nurse who suspects an impaction can gently perform a digital examination of the rectum and palpate the impacted mass. Some institutions require a physician's order for a nurse to perform a rectal examination because of the risk of causing vagal stimulation that slows heart rate. Another danger with digital examination is bowel perforation, especially with older adults and clients with neoplastic colon diseases.

Diarrhea

Diarrhea is an increase in the number of stools and the passage of liquid, unformed feces. It is a symptom of disorders affecting digestion, absorption, and secretion in the GI tract. Intestinal contents pass

---

Common Causes of Constipation

- Irregular bowel habits and ignoring the urge to defecate can cause constipation.
- Clients who have a low-fiber diet high in animal fats (e.g., meats, diary products, eggs) and refined sugars (rich desserts) often have constipation problems. Also, low fluid intake slows peristalsis.
- Lengthy bed rest or lack of regular exercise causes constipation.
- Heavy laxative use causes loss of normal defecation reflex. In addition, the lower colon is completely emptied, requiring time to refill with bulk.
- Tranquilizers, opiates, anticholinergics, and iron can cause constipation.
- Older adults experience slowed peristalsis, loss of abdominal muscle elasticity, and reduced intestinal mucous secretion. Older adults often live alone and eat low-fiber foods.
- Constipation is also caused by GI abnormalities such as bowel obstruction, paralytic ileus, and diverticulitis.
- Neurological conditions that block nerve impulses to the colon (e.g., spinal cord injury, tumor) can cause constipation.

---

through the small intestine and colon too quickly to allow the usual absorption of fluid. Irritation within the colon can result in an increased mucus secretion. As a result, feces become watery, so the client may be unable to control the urge to defecate.

It is often difficult to assess diarrhea in infants. An infant who is bottle-fed may have one firm stool every second day, whereas a breast-fed baby may pass five to eight small, soft stools daily. The mother or nurse should note any sudden increase in number of stools, any reduction in fecal consistency with an increase in fluid content, and a tendency for feces to be greenish.

Excess loss of colonic fluid can result in serious fluid and electrolyte imbalance. Infants and older adults are particularly susceptible to associated complications (see Chapter 39). Because repeated passage of diarrheal stools also exposes the skin of the perineum and buttocks to irritating intestinal contents, meticulous skin care is needed to prevent skin breakdown (see Chapters 34 and 44). The client might experience abdominal cramping, nausea, and vomiting, depending on the severity of the diarrhea.

Many conditions cause diarrhea (Table 41-3). The aims of treatment are to remove precipitating condi-

TABLE 41-3	Conditions That Cause Diarrhea
Condition	Physiological Effects
Emotional stress (anxiety)	Increased intestinal motility
Intestinal infection (streptococcal or staphylococcal enteritis)	Inflammation of intestinal mucosa, increased mucus secretion in colon
Food allergies	Reduced digestion of food elements
Food intolerance (greasy foods, coffee, alcohol, spicy foods)	Increased intestinal motility, increased mucus secretion in colon
Medications	
Iron	Irritation of intestinal mucosa
Antibiotics	Suprainfection allowing overgrowth of normal flora, inflammation and irritation of mucosa
Laxatives (short term)	Increased intestinal motility
Colon disease (colitis, Crohn's disease)	Inflammation and ulceration of intestinal walls, reduced absorption of fluids, increased intestinal motility
Surgical alterations	
Gastrectomy	Loss of reservoir function of stomach, improper absorption because food is moved into duodenum too quickly
Colon resection	Reduced size of colon, reduced amount of absorptive surface

tions and to slow peristalsis. Any irritation to the intestinal mucosa must be eliminated.

Incontinence

Fecal **incontinence** is the inability to control passage of feces and gas from the anus. Physical conditions that impair anal sphincter function or control can cause incontinence. Conditions that create frequent, loose, large-volume, watery stools also predispose to incontinence.

Mental disorders such as schizophrenia, severe depression, or anxiety and dementia can prevent the client from being aware of the need to defecate.

Incontinence can harm a client's body image (see Chapter 31). In many situations the client is mentally alert but physically unable to avoid defecation. The embarrassment of soiling the clothes can lead to social isolation. The client must depend on the nurse for a basic need. Clients with mental or sensory alter-

ations often are unaware that they have passed a stool. The nurse must understand and support the client even though repeated cleaning of an incontinent client can become frustrating.

Like diarrhea, incontinence predisposes the skin to breakdown (see Chapters 34 and 43). The nurse must check often to be sure anal and perineal regions are clean and dry.

Flatulence

As gas accumulates in the lumen of the intestines, the bowel wall stretches and distends (**flatulence**). It is a common cause of abdominal fullness, pain, and cramping. Normally, intestinal gas escapes through the mouth (belching) or the anus (passing of flatus). However, if there is a reduction in intestinal motility resulting from opiates, general anesthetics, abdominal surgery, or immobilization, flatulence can become severe enough to cause abdominal distention. In addition, accumulation of gas forces the diaphragm up and reduces lung expansion, and shortness of breath can occur.

A person normally produces several hundred milliliters of it. Swallowed air makes up over 75% of intestinal gas. Bacterial decomposition of food in the colon releases methane gas. Carbon dioxide is a product of fermentation in the bowel. Any factor that causes gas (for example, ingestion of onions, beans, and cauliflower) increases intestinal flatulence.

Hemorrhoids

Hemorrhoids are dilated, engorged veins in the lining of the rectum. They are either external or internal. External hemorrhoids are clearly visible as protrusions of skin. If the underlying vein is hardened, there can be a purplish discoloration. Internal hemorrhoids have an outer mucous membrane. Increased venous pressure from straining at defecation, pregnancy, congestive heart failure, and chronic liver disease can cause hemorrhoids.

Hemorrhoids bleed easily when stretched. Passage of a hard stool commonly causes bleeding. The hemorrhoids become inflamed and tender, and clients might complain of itching and burning. Because pain worsens during defecation, the urge to defecate might be ignored, resulting in constipation.

 BOWEL DIVERSIONS

Certain diseases cause conditions that prevent normal passage of feces through the rectum. This creates the need for a temporary or permanent artificial opening (**stoma**) in the abdominal wall. Surgical openings are formed in the ileum (**ileostomy**) or colon (**colostomy**) (Fig. 41-4). Ends of the intestines are then brought through the opening to create the stoma. The stoma is covered with a plastic pouch or bag to collect fecal material.

The location of the ostomy determines the consistency of stool. An ileostomy bypasses the entire large intestine. As a result, stools are frequent and liquid. The same is true for a colostomy of the ascending colon. A colostomy of the transverse colon generally results in a more solid, formed stool. The sigmoid colostomy emits near-normal stool. The location of a colostomy is determined by the client's medical problem and general condition. There are three types of colostomy construction:

1. Loop colostomy
2. End colostomy
3. Double-barrel colostomy

A loop colostomy is usually performed in a medical emergency when closure of the colostomy is anticipated. The surgeon pulls a loop of bowel onto the abdomen. A communicating wall remains between the proximal and distal bowel. A plastic rod or rubber catheter is temporarily placed under the bowel loop to keep it from slipping back (Fig. 41-5, *A*, on p. 1398). The surgeon then opens the bowel and sutures it to the skin of the abdomen. The loop ostomy has two openings through the stoma. The proximal end drains stool while the distal portion drains mucous. Within 7 to 10 days the plastic rod is removed.

The end colostomy consists of one stoma formed from the proximal end of the bowel with the distal portion of the GI tract removed. For many clients, end colostomies are a result of surgical treatment of colorectal cancer. In such cases the rectum might also be removed.

The double-barrel colostomy consists of two distinct stomas: the proximal functioning stoma and the distal nonfunctioning stoma. Unlike the loop colostomy, the bowel is severed in a double-barrel colostomy (Fig. 41-5, *B*).

Ostomies that emit frequent liquids stools (for example, ileostomy) create a management challenge. A bag or pouch must always be worn. Regular defecation cannot be achieved because of a continuous oozing of stool. The bag must be emptied, washed, and replaced throughout the day. Skin care is vital to prevent exposure to fecal irritants.

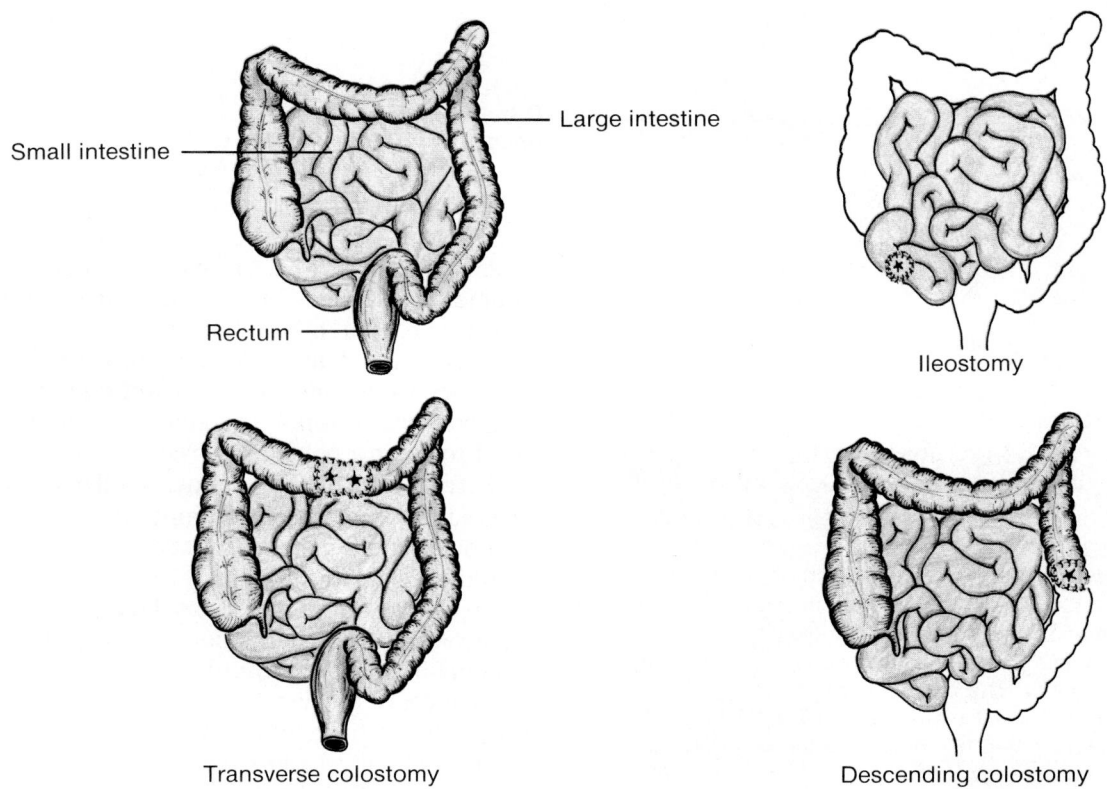

Fig. 41-4 Normal intestines and three types of ostomies. Shaded areas indicate excised tissue.

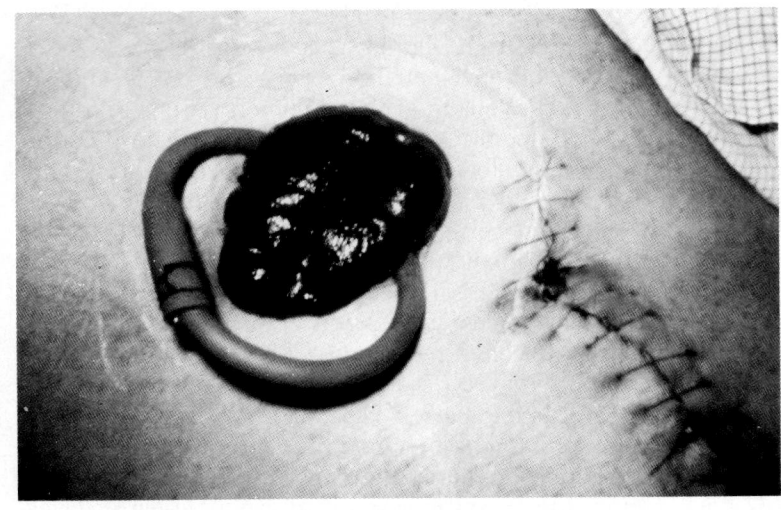

A

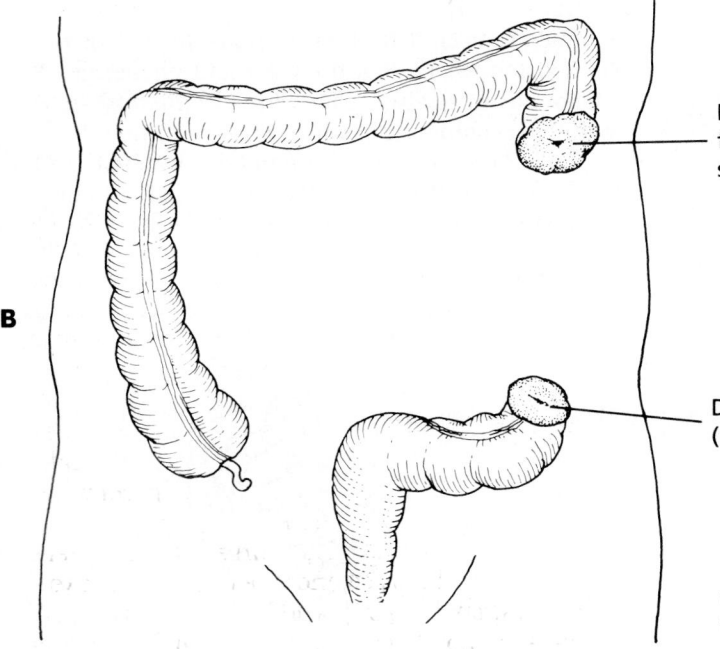

B

Proximal
functioning
stoma

Distal stoma
(mucous fistula)

Fig. 41-5   A, A transverse loop colostomy supported with a flexible red rubber catheter. **B,** Double-barrel colostomy in the descending colon.
From Broadwell DC, Jackson BS: *Principles of ostomy care,* St Louis, 1982, Mosby–Year Book.

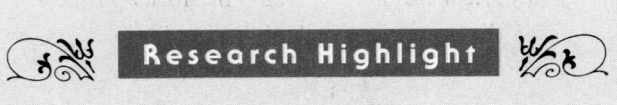

Research Highlight

A new two-piece system consisting of an adhesive base plate and a soft, pliable, carbon-filtered plug was tested on 53 clients. Fecal continence and the noiseless, odorless passage of flatus was accomplished in 90% of clients. The mean wear time of the plug was 8 hours, with an overall range of 5 to 24 hours. Use of bowel irrigation before application correlated positively with the length of wear.

Burcharth F et al: The colostomy plug: a new disposable device for a continent colostomy, *Lancet* 82(8515):1062, 1986.

A colostomy in the transverse or sigmoid colon is simpler to manage. The client wears a pouch at all times even though bowel movements may occur only once or twice daily. Selected foods can be eaten at prescribed intervals so that bowel movements occur at a convenient time. Therefore the client might not need to wear a pouch. A physician might order routine irrigations of the ostomy, similar to an enema. This allows the person to empty the bowel regularly and eliminate a pouch. Irrigations are not performed as routinely as in the past.

An ostomy causes serious body image changes, particularly if it is permanent. Clients often perceive a stoma as a form of mutilation. Even though clothing conceals the ostomy, the client feels different. Many clients have difficulty maintaining or initiating normal sexual relations (see Chapter 31). An important factor in the client's reactions is the character of fecal secretions and the ability to control them. Foul odors, spillage, or leakage of liquid stools and inabil-

Research Highlight

In a multicenter trial, 100 clients with established colostomies attempted to achieve continence through use of a new disposable colostomy plug. Forty-one of the 46 clients who completed the study expressed a desire to continue using the plug. Of these, 29 continue to use the plug daily. A number of clients dropped out of the study in the early stages because of leakage. Clients who irrigated the colostomy retained the plug an average of 16½ hours, twice as long as those who did not irrigate.

Clague MM, Heald RJ: Achievement of stomal continence in one third of colostomies by use of a disposable plug, *Surg Gynecol Obstet* 170(5):390, 1990.

ity to regulate bowel movements give the client a loss of self-esteem.

Since the late 1980s, some progress has been made toward the development and successful use of an ostomy plug, which can provide continence for up to 28 hours (Bellan, 1990) (see research highlights). In the future, surgery may provide continence for select colectomy clients. In a procedure called an *ileoanal pull-through,* the colon is removed and the ileum is anastomosed or connected to an intact anal sphincter (Corman, 1989; Dalton-Loehner, Connor, 1989). Not every colectomy client is a candidate for this procedure. Selection criteria require close coordination between the client and surgeon.

NURSING PROCESS AND BOWEL ELIMINATION

 ### Assessment

To assess bowel elimination pattern and determine abnormalities, the nurse takes a nursing history, does a physical assessment of the abdomen, inspects fecal characteristics, and reviews pertinent test results.

Nursing History

The nursing history provides a review of the client's usual bowel pattern and habits. What a client describes as "normal" may be different from factors and conditions that tend to promote normal elimination. Identifying normal and abnormal patterns and habits allows the nurse to determine the client's problems. Much of the nursing history can be organized around the factors that affect elimination. The

nurse then applies this knowledge through questions to determine the presence and extent of GI alterations. A typical nursing history of a client's elimination status includes the following:

1. Determination of the usual elimination pattern. Frequency and time of day are included.
2. Identification of routines followed to promote normal elimination. Examples are drinking hot liquids, using laxatives, eating specific foods, or taking time to defecate during a certain part of the day.
3. Description of any recent change in elimination pattern. This information is perhaps the most significant because elimination patterns are variable and the client can best detect change. If there were changes in the client's last bowel movement, the nurse asks the client to be very specific in describing the change and perhaps suggest a cause.
4. Client's description of usual characteristics of stool. The nurse determines whether the stool is usually watery or formed or soft or hard, as well as the typical color. The client also describes the stool's shape.
5. Diet history. The nurse determines the client's dietary preferences for a day. The nurse measures servings of fruits, vegetables, cereals, and breads. The nurse also determines whether mealtimes are regular or irregular and whether certain foods are eaten infrequently.
6. Description of daily fluid intake. This includes the type and amount of fluid. The client might have to estimate the amount using common household measurements.
7. History of exercise. The nurse asks the client to describe the type and amount of daily exercise. Simply asking whether the client exercises is not adequate because it leaves the judgment solely to the client. For example, a client who walks back and forth in an office may perceive this as adequate exercise. Therefore the nurse asks for a specific description of exercise patterns.
8. Assessment of the use of artificial aids at home. The nurse assesses whether the client uses enemas, laxatives, or special foods before having a bowel movement. If so, the nurse asks the freqency with which the client uses them.
9. History of surgery or illnesses affecting the GI tract. This information can often help explain symptoms. In addition, it provides an idea of the client's potential for maintaining or restoring a normal elimination pattern.

10. Presence and status of bowel diversions. If the client has an ostomy, the nurse assesses frequency of fecal drainage, character of feces, appearance and condition of the stoma (color, swelling, and irritation), type of appliance used, and methods used to maintain the ostomy's function.

11. Medication history. The nurse asks whether the client takes medications (such as laxatives, antacids, iron supplements, and analgesics) that might alter defecation or fecal characteristics.

12. Emotional state. The client's emotions can significantly alter frequency of defecation. During assessment, observation of the client's emotions, tone of voice, and mannerisms can reveal significant behaviors that indicate stress.

13. Social history. If the client is not independent in bowel management, the nurse determines who assists the client and how.

Physical Assessment

The nurse conducts a physical assessment (see Chapter 20) of body systems and functions likely to be influenced in the presence of elimination problems.

MOUTH. An assessment includes inspection of the client's teeth, tongue, and gums. Poor dentition or poorly fitting dentures influence the ability to chew (see Chapter 20).

ABDOMEN. The nurse inspects all four abdominal quadrants for contour, shape, symmetry, and skin color. Inspection also includes noting masses, peristaltic waves, scars, venous patterns, stomas, and lesions. Normally, peristaltic waves are not visible. However, observable peristalsis can be a sign of intestinal obstruction.

Abdominal distention appears as an overall outward protuberance of the abdomen. Intestinal gas, large tumors, or fluid in the peritoneal cavity may cause distention. A distended abdomen feels tight, and the skin appears taut as if stretched. Daily measurement of the abdomen's girth using a tape measure reveals whether distention is increasing. Measurements should be taken over the same anatomical landmarks (for example, umbilicus) to provide an accurate chronological measurement. If masses are present, they appear as localized bulges or protuberances.

The nurse auscultates the abdomen with the stethoscope to assess bowel sounds in each quadrant (see Chapter 20). While auscultating, the nurse notes the character and frequency of bowel sounds. An increase in pitch or a "tinkling" sound may be heard with abdominal distention. Absent or hypoactive sounds occur with paralytic ileus, such as after abdominal surgery. High-pitched and hyperactive bowel sounds occur with small intestine obstruction and inflammatory disorders.

The nurse palpates the abdomen for masses or areas of tenderness (see Chapter 20). It is important for the client to relax. Tensing abdominal muscles interferes with palpating underlying organs or masses. Palpation of a tender or sensitive area causes a guarding or voluntary tightening of abdominal muscles. Tenderness may be a sign of local injury or inflammation of tissues. If the nurse locates an unusual mass, deep palpation may be necessary for further examination. A mass may indicate a tumor.

Percussion detects lesions, fluid, or gas within the abdomen. Familiarity with the five percussion notes (see Chapter 20) also permits identification of underlying abdominal structures. Gas or flatulence creates a tympanic note. Masses, tumors, and fluid are dull to percussion.

RECTUM. The nurse inspects the area around the anus for lesions, discolorations, inflammation, and hemorrhoids. Abnormalities should be carefully recorded. To examine the rectum the nurse uses gentle palpation. After applying a clean disposable glove, the nurse lubricates the index finger with a lubricant. The nurse then asks the client to bear down and as the client does so, the nurse passes the index finger through the relaxed anal sphincter toward the client's umbilicus. The sphincter usually constricts around the nurse's finger. The nurse should methodically palpate all sides of the client's rectal wall for nodules or irregularities in texture. The rectal mucosa is normally smooth and soft. Pushing the index finger forcefully against the rectal wall or extending the finger too far may cause discomfort. Vigorous stimulation should be avoided to prevent triggering a vagal nerve reflex that can lower the client's heart rate. Manual rectal examinations are generally contraindicated in a client who might be hypervagal, such as one who has recently had a myocardial infarction.

The findings of an abdominal assessment might give clues about the nature of GI alterations. For example, abdominal distention and auscultation of hyperactive bowel sounds suggest gaseous formation, presence of an obstruction, or inflammation of the bowel. The nurse's assessment then focuses on other factors or conditions.

TABLE 41-4 Fecal Characteristics			
Characteristic	Normal	Abnormal	Cause
Color	Infant: yellow; adult: brown	White or clay	Absence of bile
		Black or tarry (melena)	Iron ingestion or upper GI bleeding
		Red	Lower GI bleeding, hemorrhoids
		Pale with fat	Malabsorption of fat
Odor	Pungent; affected by food type	Noxious change	Blood in feces or infection
Consistency	Soft, formed	Liquid	Diarrhea, reduced absorption
		Hard	Constipation
Frequency	Varies: infant 4 to 6 times daily (breast-fed) or 1 to 3 times daily (bottle fed); adult daily or 2 to 3 times a week	Infant more than 6 times daily or less than once every 1-2 days; adult more than 3 times a day or less than once a week	Hypomotility or hypermotility
Amount	150 g per day (adult)		
Shape	Resembles diameter of rectum	Narrow, pencil shaped	Obstruction, rapid peristalsis
Constituents	Undigested food, dead bacteria, fat, bile pigment, cells lining intestinal mucosa, water	Blood, pus, foreign bodies, mucus, worms	Internal bleeding, infection, swallowed objects, irritation, inflammation

Fecal Characteristics

Inspection of fecal characteristics (Table 41-4) reveals information about the nature of elimination alterations. Several factors can influence each characteristic. A key to assessment is knowing whether there have been any recent changes. The client can best provide this information.

Laboratory and Diagnostic Tests

Laboratory and diagnostic examinations yield useful information concerning elimination problems. Laboratory analysis of fecal contents can detect pathological conditions such as tumors, hemorrhage, and infection.

FECAL SPECIMENS. The nurse is directly responsible for ensuring that specimens are accurately obtained, properly labeled in appropriate containers, and transported to the laboratory on time. Institutions provide special containers for fecal specimens. Some tests require specimens to be placed in chemical preservatives.

Medical aseptic technique should be used during collection of stool specimens (see Chapter 20). Because about 25% of the solid portion of a stool is bacteria from the colon, the nurse should wear disposable gloves when handling specimens.

Handwashing is necessary for anyone who might come in contact with the specimen. Often the client can obtain the specimen if properly instructed. The nurse explains that feces cannot be mixed with urine or water. For this reason the client must defecate into a clean, dry bedpan or special container placed under the toilet seat.

Tests performed by the laboratory for occult (microscopic) blood in the stool (Procedure 41-1) and stool cultures require only a small sample. The nurse collects about an inch of formed stool or 15 to 30 ml of liquid diarrheal stool. To avoid contact with feces while transferring solid specimens to a container, the nurse should wear gloves and use a wooden tongue depressor. The nurse must pour liquid specimens carefully into the proper container. Tests for measuring the output of fecal fat requires a 3- to 5-day collection of stool. All fecal material must be saved throughout the test period.

After obtaining a specimen, the nurse labels and tightly seals the container and completes laboratory requisition forms. The nurse then records specimen collections in the client's medical record. It is important to avoid delays in sending specimens to the laboratory. Some tests such as measurement for ova and parasites require the stool to be warm. When stool specimens are allowed to stand at room temperature, bacteriological changes that alter test results can occur.

Guaiac Test. A common laboratory test that can be done at home or at the client's bedside is the **guaiac test,** which measures microscopic amounts of blood in the feces. Small amounts of blood are normally lost daily in the feces from minor abrasions of nasopharyngeal and oral surfaces. Quantities of blood

Measuring Occult Blood in Stool

STEPS	RATIONALE
1. Assess client's medical history for bleeding or GI disorder.	Routine screening can be instituted by nurse.
2. Assess type of medications client receives. Note drugs that can cause GI mucosal bleeding.	Anticoagulants increase risk of bleeding in GI tract, even from minor trauma to mucosa. Long-term use of steroids, nonsteroidal antiinflammatory drugs (NSAIDS), and acetylsalicylic acid can irritate mucosa.
3. Refer to physician's order for medication or dietary modifications/restrictions before test. Such restrictions include pretest avoidance of partially cooked red meat, broccoli, turnips, horseradish, and uncooked cantaloupe.	These foods can give false positive results. Iron supplements and supplemental vitamins should be avoided because they can provide false negative results (Eastwood, Avundu, 1988). Rare meats can cause same results.

4. Prepare necessary equipment and supplies:
   a. Paper towel
   b. Hemoccult test supplies (see illustration):
     (1) Cardboard Hemoccult slide
     (2) Wooden applicator
     (3) Hemoccult developing solution
   c. Disposable gloves

Step 4b

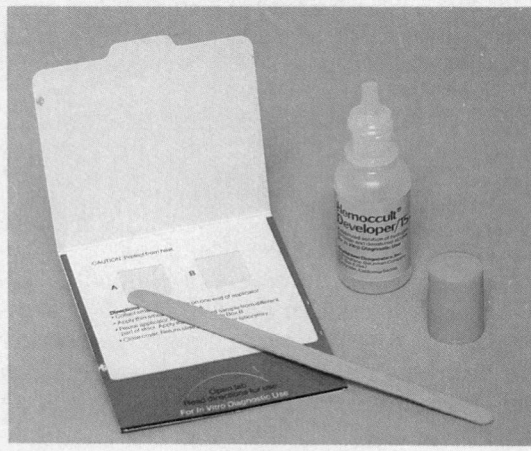

STEPS	RATIONALE
5. Explain purpose of test and ways that client can assist.	Client's understanding of test's purpose provides cooperation and minimizes anxiety.
6. Be sure that dietary or medication restrictions were followed.	Ensures accurate test results.
7. Wash hands.	Reduces transmission of infection.
8. Apply clean disposable gloves.	Reduces transmission of microorganisms from fecal specimen to your hands.
9. Obtain uncontaminated stool specimen.	Specimen is obtained in clean, dry container and not contaminated with urine, water, or toilet tissue.
10. Use tip of wooden applicator to obtain small portion of feces.	Small specimen is sufficient for measuring blood content in feces.
11. Perform Hemoccult slide test:	
a. Open flap of slide and apply thin smear of stool on paper in first box (see illustration).	Guaiac paper inside box is sensitive to fecal blood content.
b. Obtain second fecal specimen from different portion of stool and apply thinly to slide's second box (see illustration).	Findings of occult blood are more conclusive for GI bleeding when entire specimen contains blood.
c. Close slide cover and turn slide over to reverse side. Open cardboard flap and apply 2 drops of Hemoccult developing solution on each box of guaiac paper (see illustration).	Developing solution penetrates underlying fecal specimen. Blood is indicated by change in color of guaiac paper.

STEPS	RATIONALE
d. Read results of test after 30-60 sec (see illustration). Note color changes.	Bluish discoloration indicates occult blood (guaiac positive). No change in color indicates negative results.
e. Dispose of test slide in proper receptacle.	Reduces transfer of microorganisms.
12. Wrap wooden applicator in paper towel, remove gloves, and dispose in proper receptacle.	Feces contain large numbers of microorganisms.
13. Wash hands.	Reduces spread of infection.
14. Record results of test in nurses' notes and note unusual fecal characteristics.	All test results should be documented promptly. Findings may indicate need for further diagnosis.

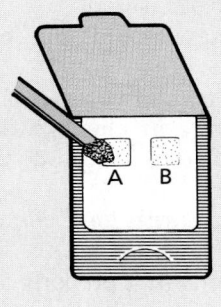

Step 11a

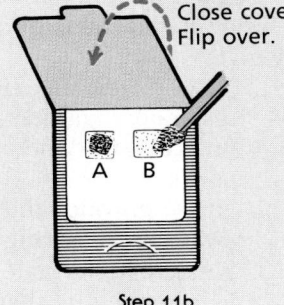

Close cover.
Flip over.

Step 11b

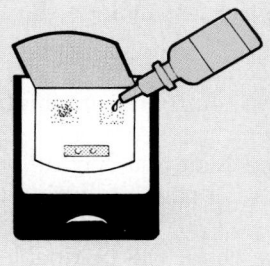

Step 11c

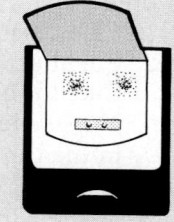

Step 11d

Screening for Colon Cancer

RISK FACTORS

- Age: over 50
- Family history: colon polyps or colorectal cancer
- History of inflammatory bowel disease (colitis, Crohn's disease)
- Living in urban area
- Diet: high intake of fats, low fiber intake

WARNING SIGNS

- Change in bowel habits
- Rectal bleeding

SCREENING TESTS

- Digital rectal examination every year after age 40
- Guaiac test for occult blood every year after 50
- Proctoscopy every 3-5 years after age 50, after two annual negative examinations

---

greater than 50 ml arising from the upper GI tract can be seen as **melena.** Guaiac tests help reveal visually undetectable blood. It is a useful diagnostic screening test for colon cancer (see box).

Clients who are receiving anticoagulants or who have a bleeding disorder or a GI disorder known to cause bleeding (for example, intestinal tumors, bowel inflammation, or ulcerations) should be guaiac tested. The most common guaiac test is the Hemoccult slide test (Procedure 41-1).

DIAGNOSTIC EXAMINATIONS. A client may have a diagnostic test as an outpatient or inpatient. Visualization of GI structures may be by direct or indirect approach.

Direct Visualization. Instruments introduced through the mouth (upper GI viewing) or the rectum (lower GI viewing) allow the physician to inspect the integrity of mucosa, blood vessels, and organ parts. A **fiberoptic endoscope** is an optical instrument with a lens viewer, a long flexible tube, and a light source at the end. It allows viewing of structures at the tip of the tube and insertion of special instruments for biopsy. The tube is flexible to minimize trauma and discomfort to the client.

Proctoscopes and sigmoidoscopes are rigid, tube-shaped instruments with attached light sources. The proctoscope looks like a speculum with a light. These instruments are less flexible than fiberoptic scopes and more capable of causing discomfort.

UGI **endoscopy** or **gastroscopy** allows visualization of the esophagus, stomach, and duodenum. The physician inspects for tumors, vascular changes, mucosal inflammation, ulcers, hernias, and obstructions. A gastroscope enables the physician to remove tissue specimens (or **biopsy**), remove abnormal tissue growth (**polyps**), and coagulate sources of bleeding. Nursing implications before the test include the following:

1. Client signs informed consent.
2. Client takes nothing by mouth after midnight.
3. Client removes dentures.
4. Nurse explains that the client may feel fullness in the throat and a sense of gagging during the test.
5. Nurse explains that the client will be unable to speak as the endoscope enters the esophagus.
6. Nurse positions the client in the left Sims' or left lateral position.
7. Nurse gives a sedative and an anticholinergic as prescribed.

Nursing implications during the test include the following:

1. Nurse describes steps of the test to the client.
2. Nurse places tissue specimens in a properly labeled container that is sealed tightly.
3. Nurse has emergency equipment available in case of respiratory complications.

Nursing implications afterward include the following:

1. Because the client's throat is anesthetized, the nurse instructs the client to avoid eating or drinking until the gag reflex returns (2 to 4 hours). To check for the gag reflex the nurse places a tongue blade at the back of the client's tongue.
2. Nurse explains that hoarseness and a sore throat are normal for several days; cool fluids and normal saline gargling relieve soreness.
3. Nurse observes for bleeding, fever, abdominal pain, difficulty with swallowing, and difficulty breathing.

Sigmoidoscopy allows visualization of the anus, rectum, and sigmoid colon. Proctoscopy allows visualization of the anus and rectum. Both tests enable the physician to collect tissue specimens and coagulate sources of bleeding. Nursing implications before the test include the following:

1. Client signs an informed consent.
2. Client receives an enema the night before and the morning of the test; laxatives are optional.
3. Client may be allowed a light breakfast.
4. Nurse explains that the client will feel discomfort and the urge to defecate as the instruments are inserted.
5. During the test the physician uses air to distend the bowel for better visualization; nurse explains that the client will feel "gas pains."
6. Nurse positions the client in a knee-chest position face down; Sims' position on the left side is acceptable.
7. Nurse drapes the client to avoid unnecessary exposure and minimize embarrassment.

Nursing implications during the test include the following:

1. Nurse keeps the client draped and observes for respiratory distress (especially in clients with lung disease who cannot tolerate a head-down position).
2. Nurse provides the physician with long cotton swabs for removing mucus.
3. Nurse places tissue specimens in a properly labeled container that is sealed tightly.

Nursing implications after the test include the following:

1. Nurse observes for rectal bleeding, rectal or abdominal pain, and fever.
2. Nurse cautions the client to observe for blood in stools and to report any bleeding.

Indirect Visualization. When direct visualization is impossible (as with deeper GI structures), the physician relies on indirect x-ray examination. The client ingests a **contrast medium** or has the medium given as an enema. One of the most common media is barium, a white, chalky, radiopaque substance that the client drinks like a milkshake. It is used in UGI studies and barium enemas. Contrast media usually contain a flavoring agent for better taste.

UGI study is an x-ray study of an ingested contrast medium that allows the physician to visualize the lower esophagus, stomach, and duodenum. The physician notes ulcerations, inflammation, tumors, and anatomical malposition of organs. The patency of organs and the pyloric valve are also observed. Nursing implications before the test include the following:

1. Client signs an informed consent.
2. Client takes nothing by mouth after midnight.
3. Nurse explains that the test might take several hours and requires frequent position changes; nurse explains that discomfort is minimal except for lying on a hard examination table.
4. Nurse explains that barium has a chalky taste (some preparations contain artificial flavoring).

A nursing implication during the test follows:

1. The test is done in the radiology department; a technician explains the steps of the test.

Nursing implications afterward include the following:

1. Client can resume eating after the test.
2. Client must expel the barium to avoid bowel impaction; nurse instructs the client to increase fluid intake (at least 2 L after the test). The physician may order a mild laxative or enema. Stools are lightly colored until the barium is expelled.

Small bowel follow-through (continuation of UGI) allows the physician to examine the small intestine. The flow of barium through the intestine may suggest motility problems. A barium enema allows indirect visualization of the lower colon to reveal location of tumors, polyps, and **diverticula**. The physician can also detect positional abnormalities. Nursing implications before the test include the following:

1. Client signs informed consent.
2. Bowel preparation varies; client may receive any of the following the evening before the test:
   a. Clear liquids for lunch and supper
   b. One glass of water 8 to 10 hours before the test
   c. Stimulant cathartics
   d. An enema
3. On the day of the test the client receives additional cathartic by suppository.
4. Nurse explains the purpose of extensive bowel preparation.
5. Nurse explains that a lengthy procedure might cause fatigue.
6. Nurse observes the results of enemas and cathartics to ensure that the bowel is empty before the test.
7. Nurse explains that the client might feel cramping and fullness after the barium is instilled.
8. Nurse explains that the client will be instructed to change positions often (supine, prone, and side-lying).

A nursing implication during the test follows:

1. Client expels barium after first set of x-ray films (30 minutes); a repeat film is taken to check for barium retention.

Nursing implications after the test include the following:

1. Client may resume eating after the test.
2. Nurse instructs the client to increase intake of oral fluids to promote barium evacuation and to counteract dehydrating effects of the cathartics.
3. Nurse instructs the client to observe stools for barium; the physician might order a mild cathartic.

Nursing Diagnosis

The nurse's assessment of the client's bowel function reveals data that may indicate an actual or potential elimination problem or a problem resulting from elimination alterations (see diagnoses box). Associated problems, such as body-image changes or skin breakdown, require interventions unrelated to bowel function impairment. However, in some instances the nurse must direct as much attention to the elimination problem as to the associated problem.

The nurse's ability to identify the correct diagnosis depends not only on the thoroughness of assessment but also on recognition of defining characteristics and factors that can impair elimination (see diagnostic process box on p. 1406). The nurse determines the client's risk and institutes measures to ensure maintenance of normal bowel function.

Planning

The care plan should incorporate the client's elimination habits or routines as much as possible. If the habits caused the elimination problem, the nurse helps the client learn new ones. Defecation patterns vary among individuals. For this reason, the nurse

Examples of Nursing Diagnoses Related to Bowel Elimination Problems

NANDA-APPROVED NURSING DIAGNOSES

Constipation related to:
- Immobility
- Lack of privacy
- Less-than-adequate fluid intake

Diarrhea related to:
- Stress and anxiety
- Dietary intake

Bowel incontinence related to:
- Neuromuscular involvement
- Depression, severe anxiety

Pain related to:
- Hemorrhoidal inflammation

Toileting self-care deficit related to:
- Decreased strength and endurance
- Intolerance to activity

Actual or high risk for impaired skin integrity related to:
- Fecal incontinence

Body-image disturbance related to:
- Presence of ostomy
- Fecal incontinence

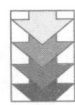

Sample Nursing Diagnostic Process for Bowel Elimination Problems

Assessment Activities	Defining Characteristics	Nursing Diagnoses
Ask client about usual bowel routine, including ease of bowel movement, frequency, time of day, and stool consistency.	Straining at stool Change from daily stool to once every 3 days	*Constipation* related to inadequate dietary intake of fiber and limited fluid intake
Ask client about dietary intake of fiber, fruit, and vegetables.	Describes small, marblelike, hard stools 24-hr dietary reivew reveals diet of cheese, beef, fried potatoes, no fruits and vegetables	
Palpate lower abdomen.	Abdominal tenderness in left lower quadrant Palpable mass in left lower quadrant	
Obtain fluid intake status, including types and amount.	Client drinks 2 cups of coffee, 1 soda/day, rarely drinks water or juice	

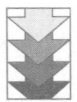

Sample Nursing Care Plan for Constipation

Nursing diagnosis: *Constipation* related to improper dietary habits
Definition: Constipation is the state in which an individual experiences a change in normal bowel habits characterized by a decrease in frequency and/or passage of hard, dry stools (Kim, McFarland, McLane, 1991).

Goals	Expected Outcomes	Interventions	Rationale
Client will understand and ingest food and fluid intake required to promote soft, formed stools by 2/20.	Client will decribe dietary sources high in fiber by 2/18. Client will explain the normal fluid intake to promote defecation by 2/19. Client will prepare 24-hr menu, including high-fiber foods and fluids by 2/20. Client will drink 1400-2000 ml daily.	Instruct client on preferred foods that stimulate persistalsis (wheat, bread, apples, lettuce, celery, apricots). Administer 8 6-oz glasses of fluids (prefers orange and grape juice) daily.	High-fiber foods increase peristalsis and help propel intestinal content through GI tract by increasing stool mass and fluid content (Brown, Everett, 1990). Adequate fluid intake helps keep fecal material soft (Swartz, 1989).
Client will return to regular defecation habits by 2/20.	Client will defecate routinely after meals by 2/20. Client will respond appropriately to each urge to defecate by 2/19. Client will report bowel movement of normal consistency by 2/20.	Encourage client to take time to defecate 30-60 min after breakfast. Obtain verbal commitment from client to attempt to defecate within 5 min after sensing urge to defecate.	Gastrocolic reflex is most sensitive in morning and after meals (Goldfinger, 1991). Behavioral contracts between client and nurse have demonstrated success for behavioral modification (Gilpatrick, 1989).

and client must work together closely to plan effective interventions (see care plan).

When clients are disabled or debilitated by illness, it is necessary to include the family in the care plan. Often family members have the same ineffective elimination habits as the client. Thus client and family teaching is an important part of the care plan. Other health team members such as dietitians and enterostomal therapists can be valuable resources.

The goals of care for clients with elimination problems include the following:

1. Understanding normal elimination

2. Attaining regular defecation habits
3. Understanding and maintaining proper fluid and food intake
4. Achieving a regular exercise program
5. Achieving comfort
6. Maintaining skin integrity
7. Maintaining self-concept

Implementation

Success of the nurse's interventions depends on improving the client's and family members' understanding of bowel elimination. In the home, hospital, or long-term care facility, clients capable of learning can be taught effective bowel habits.

The nurse should teach the client and family about proper diet, adequate fluid intake, and factors that stimulate or slow peristalsis, such as emotional stress. This often can best be done during the client's mealtime. The client should also learn the importance of establishing regular bowel routines and regular exercise and taking appropriate measures when elimination problems develop. When complications develop from elimination problems, the nurse can teach the client and family members to give proper skin care, administer enemas, and monitor drug effects.

The special needs of ostomy clients often require extensive education. Clients learn the skills needed to apply stomal appliances, irrigate colostomies (when appropriate), and administer skin care.

Promotion of Regular Bowel Habits

One of the most important habits a nurse can teach regarding bowel habits is to take time for defecation. Ignoring the urge to defecate and not taking time to defecate completely are common causes of constipation. To establish regular bowel habits, a client must know when the urge to defecate normally occurs.

The nurse advises the client to begin establishing a routine during a time when defecation is most likely to occur, usually an hour after a meal. If attempts are made to defecate during the time when mass colonic peristalsis occurs, the chances of success are great. If a client is restricted to bed or requires assistance in ambulating, the nurse should offer a bedpan or help the client reach the bathroom. The nurse must be prompt in assisting before the urge disappears or the client is incontinent.

Many clients have established rituals for defecation. In a hospital or long-term care facility, the nurse should make certain that treatment routines do not interfere with these schedules. It is also important to provide privacy. When clients forced to use a bedpan share rooms with other persons, the nurse should pull the curtain around the area so that clients can relax, knowing that interruptions will not occur. The call light should always be placed within clients' reach. Bathroom doors should be closed, although the nurse may stand close in case clients need assistance.

Promotion of Normal Defecation

To help clients evacuate bowel contents normally and without discomfort, a number of interventions can stimulate the defecation reflex, affect the character of feces, or increase peristalsis.

SQUATTING POSITION. The nurse might need to assist clients who have difficulty squatting because of muscular weakness and mobility problems. Regular toilets are too low for clients unable to lower themselves to a squatting position because of joint- or muscle-wasting diseases. Clients can purchase elevated toilet seats for the home. With such a seat, less effort is needed to sit or stand. In orthopedic and rehabilitation units in a health care center, toilet seats are elevated.

POSITIONING ON BEDPAN. Clients restricted to bed must use bedpans for defecation. Women use bedpans to pass both urine and feces, whereas men use bedpans only for defecation. Sitting on a bedpan can be extremely uncomfortable. The nurse should help position clients comfortably.

Two types of bedpans are available (Fig. 41-6). The regular bedpan, made of metal or hard plastic, has a curved smooth upper end and a sharp-edged lower end and is about 5 cm (2 in) deep. A fracture pan, designed for clients with body or leg casts, has a shallow upper end about 1.3 cm (½ in) deep. The upper end of the pan fits under the buttocks toward the sacrum, with the lower end just under the upper

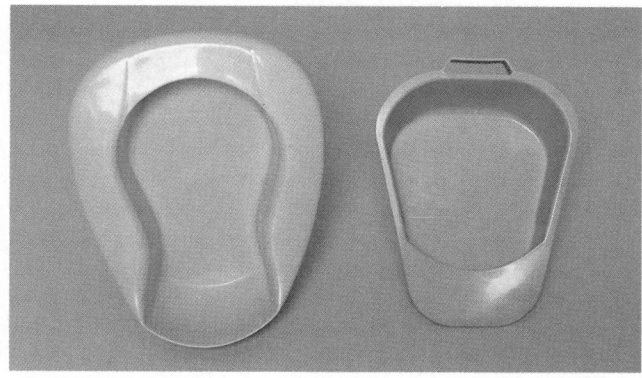

Fig. 41-6   Types of bedpans. *From left,* regular bedpan and fracture bedpan.

thighs. The pan should be high enough so that feces enter the pan. A metal bedpan should be warmed with water first, then dried.

When positioning a client, it is important to prevent muscle strain and discomfort. A client should never be placed on a bedpan and then left with the bed flat unless activity restrictions demand it. If the bed is flat, the hips remain hyperextended. It may be necessary to have the bed flat when placing the client on the bedpan. After the client is on it, the nurse raises the head of the bed 30 degrees. Raising the client to a 90-degree angle makes positioning difficult. In a sitting position, the client must rise straight up while using the strength of the arms as the nurse positions the pan. Most clients are too weak to accomplish this. Clients who have had abdominal surgery are hesitant to exert strain on suture lines. Furthermore, the nurse risks injury in trying to lift the client onto the bedpan.

Fig. 41-7 shows proper and improper positions on bedpans. The best method is to be sure the client is positioned high in bed. The nurse raises the client's head about 30 degrees, to prevent hyperextension of the back and provide support to the upper torso as the client raises the hips by bending the knees and lifting the hips upward. The nurse places a hand palm under the client's sacrum, resting the elbow on the mattress and using it as a lever to help in lifting, while slipping the pan under the client.

If the client is immobile or it is unsafe to allow the client to exert such effort, the client can roll onto the bedpan by using the following steps:

1. Lower the head of the bed flat and assist the client to roll onto one side, backside toward you.
2. Apply powder lightly to back and buttocks to prevent skin from sticking to the pan.

3. Place the bedpan firmly against the buttocks, down into the mattress with the open rim toward the client's feet (Fig. 41-8).
4. Keeping the hand against the bedpan, place the other around the client's far hip. Ask the client to roll back onto the pan, flat in bed. Do not shove the pan under the client.
5. With the client positioned comfortably, raise the head of the bed 30 degrees.
6. Place a rolled towel or small pillow under the lumbar curve of the client's back for added comfort.
7. Raise the knee gatch or ask the client to bend the knees to assume a squatting position. Do not raise the knee gatch if contraindicated.

The nurse should maintain the privacy of a client using a bedpan. The call light and a supply of toilet paper should be within easy reach. When the client finishes, the nurse responds to the call signal immediately and removes the pan. The client might require assistance with wiping. To remove the pan the nurse asks the client to roll off to the side or raise the hips. The nurse holds the pan steady to avoid spilling. The nurse should avoid pulling or shoving the pan from under the client's hips because this can pull the client's skin and cause tissue injury. After the pan is removed, the nurse, while wearing gloves, cleans the anal and perineal areas.

After assessing the stool, the nurse should immediately empty the bedpan's contents into the toilet or in a special receptacle in the utility room. A spray faucet attached to most toilets allows the nurse to rinse the bedpan thoroughly. The client uses the same bedpan each time. The nurse should chart the characteristics of the feces.

The nurse should offer the bedpan often. Clients may accidentally soil bedclothes if forced to wait. Many clients try to avoid using a bedpan because it is embarrassing and uncomfortable. They may try to

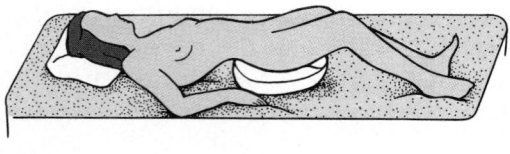
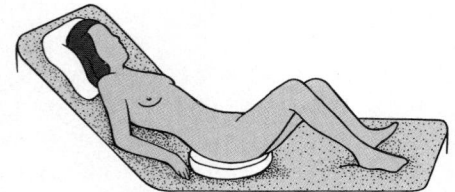

Fig. 41-7 Positions on a bedpan. *Top,* Improper positioning of client. *Bottom,* Proper position reduces client's back strain.

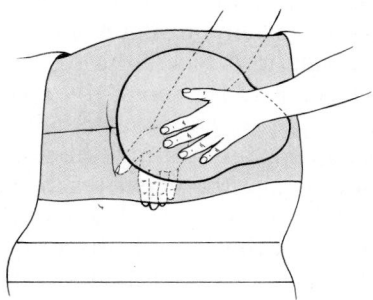

Fig. 41-8 Positioning an immobilized client on a bedpan.

get to the bathroom even though their conditions prohibit ambulation. The nurse must warn clients about the risk of falls or accidents.

CATHARTICS AND LAXATIVES. Often a client is unable to defecate normally because of pain, constipation, or impaction. Cathartics and laxatives have the short-term action of emptying the bowel. They are also used in bowel evacuation for clients undergoing GI tests and abdominal surgery. Although the terms *cathartic* and *laxative* are often used interchangeably, cathartics have a stronger effect on the intestines. Five types of laxatives and cathartics are available. The drug classes are based on the method by which the agent promotes defecation (Table 41-5 on p. 1410).

Cathartics and laxatives are available in oral, tablet, and powder suppository dosage forms (see Chapter 21). The same medication can sometimes be classified as a cathartic or a laxative, depending on the amount used. Although the oral route is more commonly used, cathartics that come prepared as suppositories are more effective because of their stimulant effect on the rectal mucosa. Cathartic suppositories such as bisacodyl (Dulcolax) can act within 30 minutes. The nurse should insert the suppository shortly before the client's usual time to defecate or immediately after a meal.

The nurse teaches clients about the potential harmful effects of repeated use of laxatives. The client should understand that laxatives and cathartics are not meant for long-term maintenance of bowel function.

ANTIDIARRHEAL AGENTS. For clients with diarrhea, frequent passage of liquid stools becomes a problem. The most effective antidiarrheal agents are opiates such as codeine phosphate, opium tincture (Paregoric), and diphenoxylate (Lomotil). Antidiarrheal opiate agents decrease intestinal muscle tone to slow passage of feces. Opiates inhibit peristaltic waves that move feces forward, but they also increase segmental contractions that mix intestinal contents. As a result, more water is absorbed by the intestinal walls. Antidiarrheal agents should be used with caution because opiates are habit forming.

Another drug effective against diarrhea is bismuth subsalicylate (Pepto-Bismol). The drug is a bismuth salt, believed to work by absorbing toxins (for example, bacteria) that cause diarrhea.

ENEMAS. An **enema** is instillation of a solution into the rectum and sigmoid colon. The primary reason for an enema is to promote defecation by stimulating peristalsis. The volume of fluid instilled breaks up the fecal mass, stretches the rectal wall, and initiates the defecation reflex. Enemas are also given as a vehicle for drugs that exert a local effect on rectal mucosa.

The most common use for an enema is temporary relief of constipation. Other indications include removing impacted feces; emptying the bowel before diagnostic tests, surgery, or childbirth; and beginning a program of bowel training.

Clients should be discouraged from relying on enemas to maintain bowel regularity. Enemas do not treat the cause of constipation. As with laxative abuse, frequent use of enemas inhibits normal defecation reflexes.

Types of Enemas. There are several types of enemas. Cleansing enemas promote the complete evacuation of feces from the colon. They act by stimulating peristalsis through the infusion of a large volume of solution or through local irritation of the colon's mucosa. Suggested maximum volumes follow:

Infant	150 to 250 ml
Toddler	250 to 350 ml
School-ager	300 to 500 ml
Adolescent	500 to 750 ml
Adult	750 to 1000 ml

Cleansing enemas include tap water, normal saline, soapsuds solution, and low-volume hypertonic saline. Each solution exerts a different osmotic effect (see Chapter 39), influencing the movement of fluids between the colon and interstitial spaces beyond the intestinal wall. Infants and children can tolerate only normal saline because they are at risk for fluid imbalance.

Tap water is hypotonic and exerts a lower osmotic pressure than fluid in interstitial spaces. After infusion into the colon, tap water escapes from the bowel lumen into interstitial spaces. The net movement of water is low. The infused volume stimulates defecation before large amounts of water leave the bowel. Tap water enemas should not be repeated because water toxicity or circulatory overload can develop if large amounts of water are absorbed.

Physiologically normal saline is the safest solution to use because it exerts the same osmotic pressure as fluids in interstitial spaces surrounding the bowel. The volume of infused saline stimulates peristalsis. Giving saline enemas does not create the danger of excess fluid absorption. If prepared saline is not available at home, 500 ml (1 pint) of tap water mixed with 1 teaspoon of table salt can be substituted.

Hypertonic solutions infused into the bowel exert osmotic pressure that pulls fluids out of interstitial spaces. The colon fills with fluid, and the resultant distention promotes defecation. Clients unable to tol-

TABLE 41-5   Common Types of Laxatives and Cathartics

Agent/Brand Name	Action	Indications	Risks
BULK FORMING			
Methylcellulose (Cologel, Hydrolose) Psyllium (Metamucil, Naturacil)	High-fiber content absorbs water and increases solid intestinal bulk. Agents stretch intestinal wall to stimulate peristalsis.	Agents are least irritating, most natural, and safest cathartics. Agents are drugs of choice for chronic constipation (e.g., pregnancy, low-residue diet). Agents may also be used to relieve mild, watery diarrhea.	Agents can cause obstruction if not mixed with at least 240 ml of water or juice and swallowed quickly. Caution is used with bulk-forming laxatives that also contain stimulants. Agents are not used in clients for whom large fluid intake is contraindicated.
EMOLLIENT OR WETTING			
Docusate sodium (Colace, Disonate) Docusate calcium (Surfak) Docusate potassium (Dialose)	Stool softeners are detergents that lower surface tension of feces, allowing water and fat to penetrate. They may increase secretion of water by intestine.	Agents are used for short-term therapy to relieve straining on defecation (e.g., hemorrhoids, perianal surgery, pregnancy, recovery from myocardial infarction).	Agents are of little value for treatment of chronic constipation.
SALINE			
Magnesium citrate or citrate of magnesia (Citroma) Magnesium hydroxide (Milk of Magnesia) Sodium phosphate (Fleet Phospho-Soda, Fleet Enema)	Agents contain salt preparation not absorbed by intestines. Osmotic effect increases pressure in bowel to act as stimulant for peristalsis. Agents may also lubricate feces.	Agents are used only for acute emptying of bowel (e.g., endoscopic examination, suspected poisoning, acute constipation).	Agents are not used in long-term management of constipation. Agents are not used in clients with kidney dysfunction (toxic buildup of magnesium). Phosphate salts are not used for clients on fluid restriction.
STIMULANT CATHARTICS			
Bisacodyl (Dulcolax) Castor oil (Neoloid, Purge) Casanthranol (Dialose Plus, Peri-Colace) Danthron (Modane Bulk) Phenolphthalein (Doxidan, Correctol, Ex-Lax)	Agents irritate intestinal mucosa to increase motility. Agents decrease absorption in small bowel and colon. Phenolphthalein and danthron may cause pink or red urine.	Agents may be used to prepare bowel for diagnostic procedures.	Agents may cause severe cramping. Agents are not for long-term use. Chronic use may cause fluid and electrolyte imbalances. Agents are avoided during pregnancy and lactation.
LUBRICANTS			
Mineral oil (Haley's MO, Petrogalar Plain)	Agents coat fecal contents, allowing easier passage of stool. Agents reduce water absorption in colon.	Agents are used to prevent straining on defecation (e.g., hemorrhoids, perianal surgery).	Agents decrease absorption of fat-soluble vitamins (A, D, E, and K). Agents can cause dangerous form of pneumonia if aspirated into lungs.

erate large volumes of fluid benefit most from this type of enema, which is, by design, low volume. Contraindications for this type of enema are clients who are dehydrated and young infants. A hypertonic solution of 120 to 180 ml (4 to 6 oz) is usually effective. The commercially prepared Fleet's Enema is the most commonly used.

Soapsuds may be added to tap water or saline to create the effect of intestinal irritation. Only pure castile soap is safe. Harsh soaps or detergents can cause serious bowel inflammation. The recommended ratio of soap to solution is 5 ml (1 teaspoon) of castile soap to 1000 ml of warm water or saline.

A physician may order a high or low cleansing enema. The terms *high* and *low* refer to the height from which and hence the pressure with which the fluid is delivered. High enemas are given to cleanse the entire colon. Fluid is delivered at a high pressure by raising the enema container to a high level. During administration of a regular enema, the enema can or bag is held 30 in (12 cm) above the client's hips. With a high enema the bag or can will be raised to 30 to 45 cm (12 to 18 in) or slightly higher. The client is asked to turn from the left lateral to the dorsal recumbent, over to the right lateral position. The position change ensures that fluid reaches the large intestine. With a low enema the nurse holds the can 7.5 cm (3 in) or less above the client's hips. A low enema cleans only the rectum and sigmoid colon.

Oil-retention enemas lubricate the rectum and colon. The feces absorb the oil and become softer and easier to pass. To enhance action of the oil, the client retains the enema for several hours if possible.

Carminative enemas provide relief from gaseous distention. They improve the ability to pass flatus. An example of a carminative enema is MGW solution, which contains 30 ml of magnesium, 60 ml of glycerin, and 90 ml of water.

A return-flow enema, or Harris flush, is a mild colonic irrigation that helps expel flatus. The nurse first administers a small amount (100 to 200 ml) of mild enema solution into the client's rectum and colon. Then the nurse lowers the enema container to allow the solution to flow back through the rectal tube and into the container. Repeating this process several times aids in reducing flatus and promoting peristalsis.

Medicated enemas contain drugs. An example is sodium polystyrene sulfonate (Kayexalate), used to treat clients with dangerously high serum potassium levels. This drug contains a resin that exchanges sodium ions for potassium ions in the large intestine. Another medicated enema is neomycin solution, an antibiotic used to reduce bacteria in the colon before bowel surgery.

Enema Administration. The nurse administers enemas in commercially packaged, disposable units or with reusable equipment prepared before use. Sterile technique is unnecessary because the colon normally contains bacteria. However, the nurse wears gloves to prevent the transmission of fecal microorganisms.

The nurse should explain the procedure, including the position to assume, precautions to take to avoid discomfort, and the length of time necessary to retain the solution before defecation. If the client is to receive the enema at home, the nurse explains the procedure to a family member.

Often the physician orders "enemas till clear." This means that the enema is repeated until the client passes fluid that is clear and contains no fecal material. It may be necessary to give as many as three enemas, but the nurse should caution the client against using more than three. Excess enema use seriously depletes fluids and electrolytes. If the enema fails to return a clear solution after three times (check agency policy) or if the client seems to not be tolerating the rigors of repeated enemas, the physician should be notified.

When an enema is given to a child, it helps to have a parent assist. The child should understand each step of the procedure and be able to see the equipment beforehand.

Giving an enema to a client who is unable to contract the external sphincter can pose difficulties. The nurse gives the enema with the client positioned on the bedpan. Giving the enema with the client sitting on the toilet is unsafe because the curved rectal tubing can abrade the rectal wall. Procedure 41-2 on p. 1412 outlines the steps for an enema administration.

DIGITAL REMOVAL OF STOOL. For clients with an impaction, the fecal mass may be too large to be passed voluntarily. If enemas fail, the nurse must break up the fecal mass with the fingers and remove it in sections. The procedure can be very uncomfortable for the client. Excess rectal manipulation may cause irritation to the mucosa, bleeding, and stimulation of the vagus nerve, which results in a reflex slowing of the heart rate. Because of the procedure's potential complications, a physician's order is necessary for the nurse to remove a fecal impaction.

The steps for removing stool digitally follow:

1. Explain the procedure and help the client lie on the side with knees flexed and back toward you.
2. Drape the trunk and lower extremities with a bath blanket and place a waterproof pad under the buttocks. Keep a bedpan next to the client.

Administering a Cleansing Enema

STEPS	RATIONALE
1. Assess status of client; last bowel movement, normal bowel patterns, presence of hemorrhoids, mobility, external sphincter control.	Determines presence of factors that indicate need for enema and that influence method of administration.
2. Review physician's order for enema.	Determines number of enemas client will require and type of enema to be given (e.g., oil retention, carminative, medicated).
3. Collect appropriate equipment:	Organizes nurse's activities, thereby increasing efficiency.
a. **Enema bag administration:**	
(1) Enema container	Depends on type of enema to be administered.
(2) Tubing and clamp, if not already attached to container, as in disposable set	

(3) Appropriately sized rectal tube
      Adult: #22 = #30 Fr
      Child: #12 = #18 Fr
	Rectal tubing should be small enough to fit diameter of anus and large enough to prevent leakage of solution from around tube.

(4) Ordered correct volume of solution warmed to 40.5°-43° C (105°-109° F) for adult and 37° C (98.6° F) for child	You must be aware of how much fluid client can safely tolerate. Hot water can burn intestinal mucosa; cold water can cause abdominal cramping and is difficult to retain.
(5) Bath thermometer	Used to measure temperature of solution.
(6) Lubricating jelly	Reduces friction and irritation to rectal mucosa.
(7) Waterproof pad	
(8) Bath blanket	
(9) Toilet tissue	
(10) Bedpan, plus either commode chair or access to toilet	
(11) Disposable gloves	Protects hands and reduces spread of microorganisms.
(12) Wash cloths, towel, and basin	Used to cleanse client after procedure, depending on client's level of mobility.
(13) Intravenous pole	Used to hang solution container.
b. **Prepackaged enema:**	
(1) Prepackaged disposable bottle with rectal tip	Contains solution and smooth tip for insertion.
(2) Disposable gloves	
(3) Lubricating jelly	
(4) Waterproof pad	
(5) Bath blanket	
(6) Toilet tissue	
(7) Bedpan or commode	
(8) Washcloth, towel, and basin	
4. Correctly identify client and explain procedure.	Reduces anxiety and promotes cooperation.
5. Assemble enema bag with appropriate solution and rectal tube.	
6. Wash hands.	Reduces transmission of infection.
7. Provide privacy by closing curtains around bed or closing door to room.	Reduces embarrassment for the client.
8. Raise bed to appropriate working height, and raise side rail on opposite side.	Promotes use of good body mechanics and client safety.
9. Assist client into Sims' position with right knee flexed. Children may also be placed in dorsal recumbent position. Position clients with poor sphincter control on bedpan in comfortable dorsal recumbent position.	Allows enema solution to flow downward by gravity along natural curve of sigmoid colon and rectum, thus improving retention of solution. (Clients with poor sphincter control cannot retain all enema solution.)
10. Place waterproof pad under client's hips and buttocks.	Prevents soiling of linen.

STEPS	RATIONALE
11. Cover client with bath blanket, exposing only rectal area.	Provides warmth, reduces exposure of body parts, and allows client to feel more relaxed and comfortable.
12. Place bedpan or commode in easily accessible position. If client will be expelling contents in toilet, ensure that toilet is free.	Ensures access in case client is unable to retain enema solution.
13. Put on disposable gloves.	Prevents transmission of microorganisms from feces.
14. Administer enema using prepackaged disposable container:	
a. Remove plastic cap from rectal tip. Tip is already lubricated, but more jelly can be applied as needed.	Lubrication provides for smooth insertion of rectal tube without causing rectal irritation or trauma.
b. Gently separate buttocks and locate rectum. Instruct client to relax by breathing out slowly through mouth.	Breathing out promotes relaxation of external anal sphincter.
c. Insert tip of bottle gently into rectum. Advance tip 7.5-10 cm (3-4 in) in adult, 5-7.5 cm (2-3 in) in child, or 2.5-3.75 cm (1-1.5 in) in infants.	Prevents trauma to rectal mucosa.
d. Squeeze bottle until all solution has entered rectum and colon. (Most bottles contain about 250 ml of solution.)	Hypertonic solutions require only small volumes to stimulate defecation.
15. Administer enema using enema bag:	
a. Add warmed solution to enema bag. (Warm tap water as it flows from faucet. Place saline container in basin of hot water before adding it to enema bag.) Check temperature of solution with bath thermometer or by pouring small amount of solution over inner wrist.	Hot water can burn intestinal mucosa. Cold water can cause abdominal cramping and is difficult to retain.
b. Raise container, release clamp, and allow solution to flow long enough to fill tubing.	Removes air from tubing.
c. Reclamp tubing.	Prevents further loss of solution.
d. Lubricate 7.5 = 10 cm (3-4 in) of tip of rectal tube with lubricating jelly.	Allows smooth insertion of rectal tube without risk of irritation of trauma to mucosa.
e. Gently separate buttocks and locate rectum. Instruct client to relax by breathing out slowly through mouth.	Breathing out promotes relaxation of external anal sphincter.
f. Insert tip of rectal tube slowly by pointing tip in direction of umbilicus. Length of insertion is 7.5-10 cm (3-4 in) for adult, 5-7.5 cm (2-3 in) for child, and 2.5-3.75 cm (1-1.5 in) for infant.	Prevents trauma to rectal mucosa from accidental lodging of tube against rectal wall. Insertion beyond proper limit can cause bowel perforation.
g. Hold tubing in rectum constantly until end of fluid instillation.	Bowel contraction can cause expulsion of rectal tube.
h. Open regulating clamp and allow solution to enter slowly with container at client's hip level.	Rapid infusion can stimulate evacuation of rectal tube.
i. Raise height of enema container slowly to appropriate level above anus: 30-45 cm (12-18 in) for high enema, 30 cm (12 in) for low enema, 7.5 cm (3 in) for infant. Infusion time varies with volume of solution administered (e.g., 1L in 10 min) and with client's ability to withstand given infusion rate.	Allows continuous, slow infusion of solution. Raising container too high causes rapid infusion and possible painful distention of colon. High pressure can cause rupture of bowel in infants.
j. Lower container or clamp tubing if client complains of cramping or if fluid escapes around rectal tube.	Temporary cessation of infusion prevents cramping. Cramping may prevent client from retaining all fluid, altering effectiveness of enema.
k. Clamp tubing after all solution is infused.	Prevents entrance of air into rectum.

Administering a Cleansing Enema

STEPS	RATIONALE
16. Place layers of toilet tissue around tube at anus and gently withdraw rectal tube.	Provides for client comfort and cleanliness.
17. Explain to client that feeling of distention is normal. Ask client to retain solution for 5-10 min or as long as possible while lying quietly in bed. (For infant or young child, gently hold buttocks together for few min.)	Solution distends the bowel. Length of retention varies with type of enema and client's ability to contact anal sphincter. Longer retention promotes more effective stimulation of peristalsis and defecation.
18. Discard enema container and tubing in proper receptacle or rinse out thoroughly with warm soap and water if container is to be reused.	Controls transmission and growth of microorganisms.
19. Remove gloves by pulling them inside out and discarding in trash can.	Prevents transmission of microorganisms.
20. Assist client to bathroom or help position client on bedpan.	Normal squatting position promotes defecation.
21. Observe character of feces and solution (caution client against flushing toilet before inspection).	When enemas are ordered "until clear," it is essential to observe contents of solution passed.
22. Assist client as needed to wash anal area with warm soap and water.	Fecal content can irritate skin. Hygiene promotes comfort.
23. Wash hands.	Reduces transmission of infection.
24. Inspect character of stool and fluid passed.	Determines whether stool is evacuated or fluid is retained.
25. Record pertinent information, including type and volume of enema given and color, amount, and consistency of fecal return.	Communicates pertinent information to all members of health care team. Prompt recording improves documentation of treatment results.

3. Apply disposable gloves and lubricate the index finger of your dominant hand with lubricating jelly.

4. Gently insert the gloved index finger into the rectum and advance the finger slowly along the rectal wall toward the umbilicus.

5. Gently loosen the fecal mass by massaging around it. Work the finger into the hardened mass.

6. Work the feces downward toward the end of the rectum. Remove small pieces at a time and discard into bedpan.

7. Reassess the client's heart rate and look for signs of fatigue. Stop the procedure if the heart rate drops significantly or the rhythm changes.

8. Continue to clean feces and allow the client to rest at intervals.

9. Once completed, offer a washcloth and towel to wash and dry the buttocks and anal area. Assist as needed.

10. Remove bedpan and dispose of feces. Remove gloves by turning them inside out, then discard.

11. Assist client to toilet or clean bedpan if urge to defecate develops.

12. Wash hands. Record results of disimpaction by describing fecal characteristics.

13. The procedure may be followed by enemas or cathartics.

BOWEL TRAINING. The client with incontinence is unable to maintain bowel control. A **bowel training** program can help some clients achieve normal defecation, especially those who still have some neuromuscular control. The training program involves setting up a daily routine. By attempting to defecate at the same time each day and using measures that promote defecation, the client gains control of bowel reflexes. The program requires time, patience, and consistency. The physician determines the client's physical readiness and ability to benefit from bowel training. A successful program includes the following:

1. Assessing the normal elimination pattern and recording times when the client is incontinent
2. Choosing a time in the client's pattern to initiate defecation-control measures
3. Giving stool softeners orally every day or a cathartic suppository at least half an hour before the selected defecation time (Lower colon must be free of stool so that suppository contacts intestinal mucosa.)
4. Offering a hot drink or fruit juice (or whatever fluids normally stimulate peristalsis for the client) before the defecation time
5. Assisting the client to the toilet at the designated time
6. Providing privacy and setting a time limit for defecation (15 to 20 minutes)
7. Instructing the client to lean forward at the hips while sitting on the toilet, to apply manual pressure with the hands over the abdomen, and to bear down but not strain to stimulate colon emptying
8. Not criticizing or conveying frustration if the client is unable to defecate
9. Providing regular meals with adequate fluids and fiber
10. Maintaining normal exercise within the client's physical ability

The client will require positive reinforcement and encouragement. It often takes several days to weeks before training is successful.

Care of Ostomies

Clients who have temporary or permanent bowel diversions face unique health care problems. Their patterns of bowel elimination differ from those of clients with intact colons. They must wear pouches or appliances to collect stool emitted from the stomas. Some clients learn to irrigate their ostomies to establish regular bowel elimination routines. Clients with ostomies must also follow good health practices such as maintaining proper dietary habits and exercising regularly to maintain normal elimination patterns.

POUCHING OSTOMIES. An ostomy requires a pouch to collect fecal material. An effective pouching system protects the skin, contains fecal material, remains odor free, and is comfortable and inconspicuous. A person wearing a pouch should feel secure in participating in any activity.

Many pouching systems are available. To ensure that a pouch fits well and meets the client's needs, the nurse considers the type of ostomy, size and contour of the abdomen, condition of the skin around the stoma, physical activities of the client, client's personal preference, and cost of equipment. An **enterostomal therapist (ET)** is a nurse trained to care for ostomy clients. The staff nurse collaborates with the ET to be sure the correct pouching system is used.

A pouching system consists of a pouch and skin barrier. Pouches come in one- and two-piece systems that are disposable or reusable. Skin barriers include wafers, pastes, powders, and liquid film that are applied to the skin around the stoma. A good skin barrier protects the skin and prevents irritation from repeated removal of the pouch. Procedure 41-3 describes steps for applying one type of pouch system.

IRRIGATING A COLOSTOMY. To establish a pattern of regular defecation, clients with descending and sigmoid colostomies often irrigate their ostomy. The muscular quality of the colon allows it to be safely irrigated with a relatively large volume of water. The irrigation acts like an enema, distending the bowel and stimulating peristalsis. Fluid is instilled into the colon via the stoma. Elimination thus occurs at a time chosen by the client. The irrigation also cleans the colon of gas and odor. Gentle irrigation is performed to reduce the risk of bowel perforation.

Surgical creation of a colostomy can seriously change a person's body image. Regaining control of fecal elimination through irrigation helps emotional adjustment. The client can also gain freedom without the need to wear a stomal pouch continuously.

The physician recommends when to begin irrigations and their frequency. Eventually, clients develop their own schedules. However, it is usually necessary to perform the procedure the same way every day or every other day. Some clients have physical or mental limitations that make colostomy irrigations unwise (see box). Young children and infants should not re-

---

Contraindications to Colostomy Irrigation

- Ascending colostomies
- Temporary colostomies
- Disease in remaining colon (diverticulosis, inflammatory disease)
- Infant or child
- Physical limitations (arthritis, paralysis)
- Mental limitations (confusion, dementia, retardation)
- Inadequate sanitary facilities
- Stomal abnormalities (prolapse, hernia)

Pouching a Colostomy or Ileostomy

STEPS	RATIONALE
1. Assess condition of existing bag for leakage and note appearance of underlying stoma and surgical incision. Question client about discomfort at or around stoma.	Determines need to change bag. Leakage of contents causes skin irritation. Stoma and peristoma sutures should be inspected daily to note early signs of complications.
2. Note amount of drainage from stoma.	Pouches should be emptied when half full to avoid premature leakage. Liquid output, common in postoperative phase, causes appliance to melt down and wear out sooner. Copious output also increases deterioration of appliance. Ileostomy output is more corrosive to appliance and skin and requires more durable equipment.
3. Assess skin around stoma, noting scars, folds, or protuberance of skin.	Determines site for pouch placement and size of underlying skin barrier. Allow 1½-2 in (3.75-5 cm) of skin barrier on all sides of stoma to ensure secure seal.
4. Determine client's knowledge and understanding of ostomy.	Reveals client's level of acceptance of ostomy and assists in determining extent to which client should be allowed to participate in care.
5. Collect appropriate equipment:	
a. Skin barriers (Stomahesive, Hollihesive, karaya paste or powder)	Maintains skin integrity.
b. Ostomy bag (see illustration)	Contains stool, can be emptied from bottom without removal, is odor proof, and can be cut to fit changing stoma sizes. Pouch should be drainable to avoid frequent changes; therefore it needs clamp.

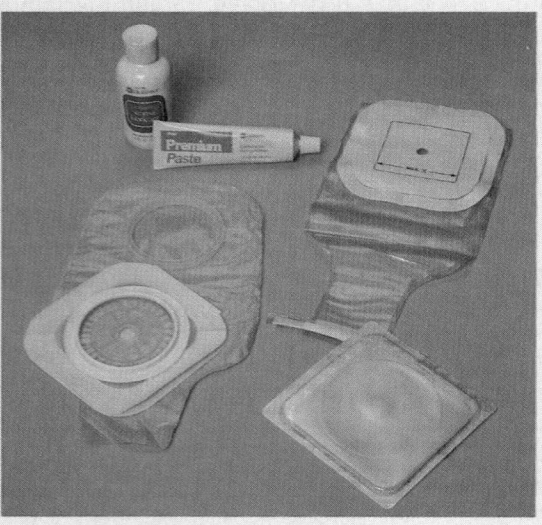

Step 5b

STEPS	RATIONALE
c. Clamp	Reinforces pouch to skin barrier.
d. Hypoallergenic tape	Prevents skin irritation.
e. Washcloth, towel, wash basin with warm water	
f. Skin cleanser (Sween or Bard) or mild soap	
g. Disposable gloves	Prevents contact with microorganisms in feces.
6. Select optimum time to change pouch (e.g., when client is comfortable, between meals, or before administration of medications that may affect bowel function).	Signs and smells of ostomy may reduce appetite. Changing pouch goes smoother when ostomy is least likely to function.
7. Explain procedure (if client is unfamiliar with technique); otherwise allow client to organize steps for pouch change. Be sure client observes procedure.	Encourages client's participation in care. Ultimately client must assume self-care.

STEPS	RATIONALE
8. Position client supine or sitting for pouch application; if able to stand, help client assume standing position.	When client is lying or standing, there are fewer wrinkles in skin and pouch.
9. Wash hands and apply gloves.	Reduces transmission of infection.
10. Close room curtains or door.	Provides privacy.
11. If pouch is full, remove clamp and empty contents through bottom into bedpan.	Prevents spillage on skin.
12. Remove old appliance as one piece.	Reduces trauma; jerking can cause skin tears.
13. Wash skin gently with skin cleanser or with regular soap and water. Remove secretions from skin.	Secretions act as irritant to skin. Bacteria in fecal secretions can enter incisional area (new colostomy) and cause infection.
14. Rinse soap off thoroughly. Blot dry.	Use of any soap could result in film or residue being left behind. These residues can result in chemical reactions or burns and can cause premature leakage because of interference with pouch adhesion. Blot dry gently to avoid trauma to stoma, which normally bleeds easily.
15. If blood appears after washing, reassure client that small amount is normal. Clarify what is abnormal.	Minimizes anxiety. Bowel has rich vascular supply. Client must be able to recognize complications.
16. Observe condition of skin and stoma. Encourage client to make these observations daily.	Allows for early monitoring of complications. Stoma is at risk for necrosis during first postoperative week. Necrosis is evidenced by dark color, dry appearance, failure to bleed, and sloughing. Client observation aids in acceptance and adjustment; client also develops habit of observing for skin-stomal problems, which are more easily correctable if detected and reported early.

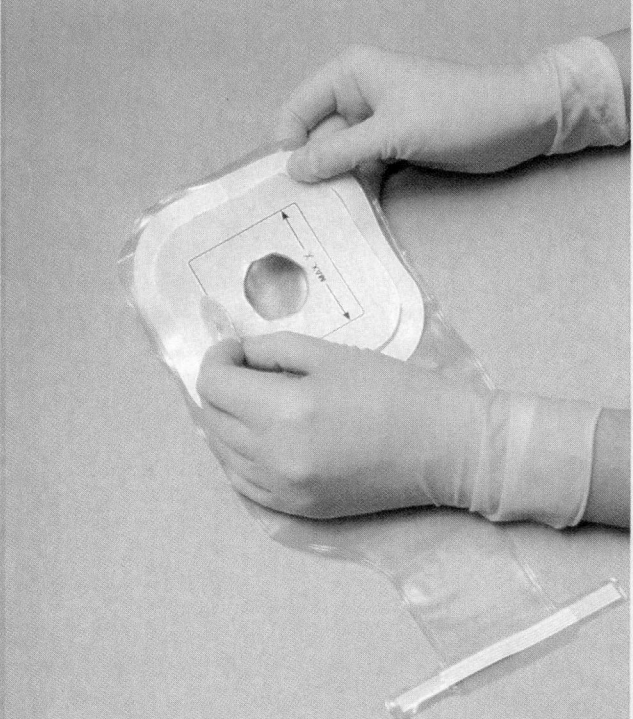

Step 20

CONTINUED

Pouching a Colostomy or Ileostomy

STEPS	RATIONALE
17. If abdominal crease is present or if contour is irregular, fill in with paste-type barrier.	Provides smooth surface for application of skin barrier and pouch's faceplate.
18. Allow paste to dry for 1-2 min.	Prevents alcohol burns to skin.
19. If abdominal contour is flat or after paste has dried, prepare skin barrier using skin sealant or karaya paste. Cut hole in barrier slightly larger than stoma, up to ¹⁄₁₆ in. Cut radial slits from center of hole. Cut rounded corners on edges of skin barrier.	Close fit of barrier around stoma prevents contact of skin with effluent. Barrier cut too tight loosens from peristalsis of stoma. Slits allow barrier opening to expand if stoma becomes edematous. Rounded corners adhere better to skin.
20. Prepare ostomy pouch; cut hole in center of faceplate ¹⁄₈ in larger than hole in barrier (see illustration on p. 1417).	Avoids risk of paper cut of stoma and ensures better seal with barrier.
21. Remove paper backing from pouch faceplate (see illustration) and apply to shiny, noncovered side of barrier.	Reduces risk of wrinkling if water is applied to skin before pouch is attached; gives better leakproof seal.
22. Remove backing from barrier and apply it and pouch (see illustration) as unit to skin. Smooth out from center. Hold in place for 1-3 min. Apply in position that facilitates emptying.	Creates wrinkle-free, secure seal onto skin.
23. Apply hypoallergenic tape as needed to edges of faceplate over skin barrier.	Adds extra reinforcement.

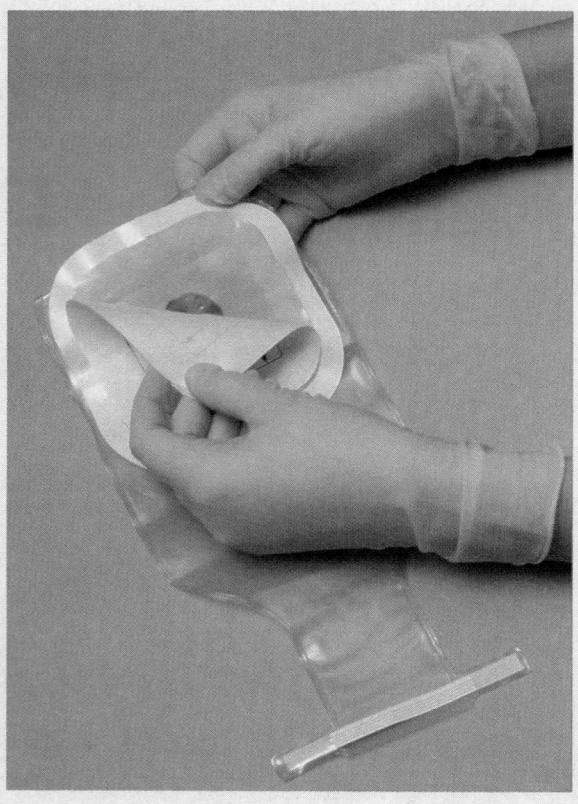

Step 21

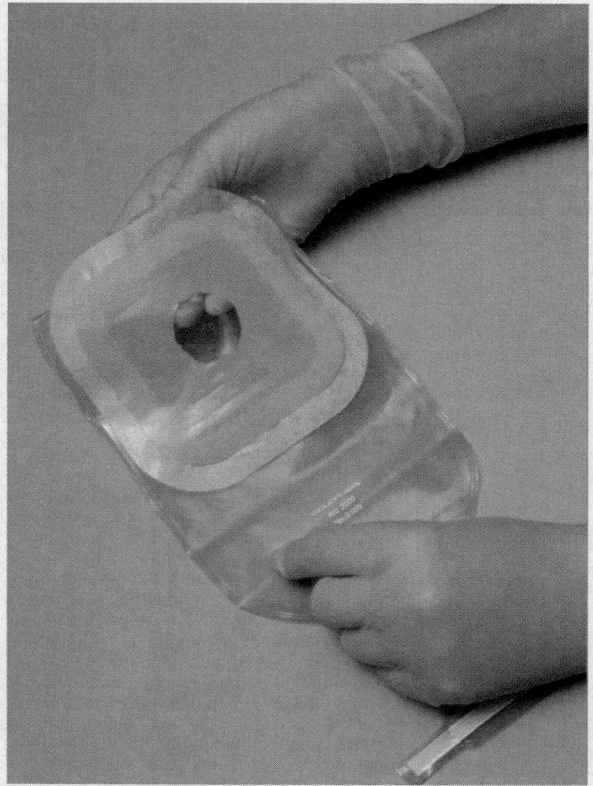

Step 22

STEPS	RATIONALE
24. Fold bottom edges of pouch over to fit clamp. Secure clamp.	Prevents leakage of pouch contents.
25. Dispose of old appliance in plastic bag and dispose in trash chute. (Be sure this is not reusable appliance because they should be washed and reused several times.)	Avoids odors lingering in room, which is unpleasant to client and staff.
26. Remove soiled gloves and dispose in proper receptacle.	Reduces transmission of infection.
27. Wash hands.	Reduces transmission of infection.
28. Assist client to comfortable position if necessary.	Ensures client comfort.
29. Record pertinent information: type of pouch and skin barrier, amount and appearance of feces, and condition of stoma and surrounding skin.	Documents care and provides data for later determining change in client's condition.

ceive colostomy irrigations. Infants are at risk for bowel perforation. Young children often cannot sit still for the procedure.

Clients may find irrigation a problem. The procedure is time consuming (45 to 60 minutes), and clients may be unwilling to interrupt their lifestyles. For many, irrigation is unpleasant. The nurse's emotional support can help clients make a choice. Alternate methods of ostomy management are available such as dietary control or laxative use. If a client initially decides against irrigations, the decision can be changed later. Procedure 41-4 on p. 1420 outlines the steps for an ostomy irrigation.

Maintenance of Proper Fluid and Food Intake

In choosing a diet for promoting normal elimination, the nurse should consider the frequency of defecation, characteristics of feces, and types of foods that impair or promote defecation. The client with frequent constipation or impaction requires an increased intake of high-fiber foods and more fluids. However, the client should realize that diet therapy provides only long-term relief of elimination problems and may not give immediate relief from problems such as constipation.

When diarrhea is a problem, the nurse can recommend foods with a low fiber content and discourage foods that typically cause gastric upset or abdominal cramping. The client with diarrhea is susceptible to potassium loss from heavy loss of GI contents. Fruits and vegetables contain potassium but are not ideal because they have a high fiber content. Better foods are baked chicken, seafood, pork, veal, and evaporated and dry nonfat instant milk. Supplements may be ordered by the physician, but they are extremely irritating to gastric mucosa.

Diarrhea caused by illness can be debilitating. If the client cannot tolerate foods or liquids orally, intravenous therapy (with potassium supplements) is necessary. The client returns to a normal diet slowly, often beginning with fluids. Excessively hot or cold fluids stimulate peristalsis, causing abdominal cramps and further diarrhea. As the tolerance to liquids improves, solid foods are ordered.

Diet therapy is important for clients with ostomies. During the first weeks after surgery, many physicians recommend low-fiber diets, particularly for ileostomy clients because the small bowel requires time to adapt to the diversion. Low-fiber foods include bread, noodles, rice, cream cheese, eggs (not fried), strained fruit juices, lean meats, fish, and poultry. As ostomies heal, clients can eat almost any food. High-fiber foods such as fresh fruits and vegetables help ensure a more solid stool needed to achieve success at irrigation. Blockage must be avoided. The stoma's surgical construction can affect the likelihood of blockage. Ileostomy clients should eat slowly and chew food completely. Drinking 10 to 12 glasses of water daily also prevents blockage. High-fiber foods that may cause problems include stringy meats, mushrooms, popcorn, wild fruits such as cherries, and some seafoods such as shrimp and crab. Ostomy

Irrigating a Colostomy

STEPS	RATIONALE
1. Assess frequency of defecation and character of stool.	Unrelieved constipation characterized by hardened feces can indicate need to irrigate colon.
2. Assess time when client normally irrigates ostomy. With a new ostomy, confer with physician for order.	Maintains established routine for bowel emptying.
3. Assess client's understanding of procedure and ability to perform techniques.	Determines level of client participation.
4. Collect appropriate equipment:	Organizes activities, thereby increasing efficiency.
a. Graduated container	
b. Tubing with regulatory clamp	Provides control of fluid instillation into colon.
c. Catheter with cone (see illustration)	Because stoma has no sphincters, there is no way for client to willfully retain solution. Therefore it is given via cone or tube with a backflow device to prevent premature loss of solution.
d. Irrigation sleeve, with or without belt	Directs flow of irrigating fluid from stoma into toilet.
e. Water-soluble lubricant	Makes insertion of cone into stoma easier. Water-soluble lubricants will not harm plastic equipment.
f. Clamps 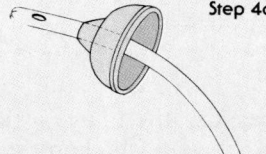 Step 4c	May use to close both top and bottom of sleeve, allowing ambulation after solution has returned and while awaiting final results.
g. New appliance	Will need new pouch when irrigation completed.
h. Disposable gloves	
i. Bedpan (optional)	
j. Washcloth, towel, wash basin	
k. Intravenous pole	
l. Liquid cleanser	
5. Prepare client by explaining procedure.	Allays client fears by explaining stoma is not painful. Ensures cooperation.
6. Choose proper time for irrigation, about 1 hr after meal.	Coordinates irrigation during normal time of duodenocolic reflex.
7. Assist client with positioning. If ambulatory, have client sit on chair in front of toilet; if confined to bed rest, have client lie on side.	Allows for directing sleeve into toilet for drainage of fecal contents and irrigant.
8. Wash hands and apply gloves.	Reduces transmission of infection.
9. Close bathroom door or room curtains.	Provides privacy.
10. Remove appliance and cleanse skin as normally done in changing enterostomy pouch.	Allows access to stoma.
11. Apply irrigation sleeve. Roll up so that bottom just touches water in toilet. (For client confined to bed, clip bottom of drain sleeve.)	Directs flow of stool into toilet. Rolling up sleeve prevents it from stopping up plumbing when commode is flushed. Also keeps end of sleeve clean.
12. Fill graduated container with required solution (usually 500-1000 ml tepid water). Hang on intravenous pole so that bottom of container is level with client's shoulder.	500-1000 ml is sufficient to distend colon and trigger effective emptying. Cold water results in syncope, and hot water could damage stoma or intestine. Height of bag creates pressure gradient for fluid to enter colon.
13. Attach cone to irrigating tube. Allow enough fluid to run through entire length of tube.	Flushes air out of tube. Air is expelled from tubing because it causes air lock and will not let solution flow.
14. Apply lubricant to cone.	Prevents trauma to stoma.
15. Insert cone through top of irrigation sleeve.	Ensures containment of stool within sleeve.

STEPS	RATIONALE
16. Insert cone gently but firmly into stoma (see illustration). Stoma should be dilated before first irrigation with gloved, lubricated finger to determine direction of bowel lumen.	Stoma is easily injured. Inserting tube toward direction of bowel facilitates introduction of solution.
17. Begin flow of solution and readjust position of cone as necessary (see illustration).	To get sufficient distention, solution must not leak around cone. Client or you may need to redirect direction of cone and slowly increase firmness against stoma until solution flows in easily and leakage around cone ceases.
18. Adjust flow of solution by raising or lowering irrigating container. To aid in this, bottom of irrigator bag should be hung 18 in above stoma.	Too-rapid administration results in cramping and inability to hold sufficient volume for adequate results.
19. Administer 500-1000 ml of solution slowly over 15 min, pausing when client cramps but not removing cone until above amount is given.	Usually 500-1000 ml is required to empty colon. Pauses prevent premature leakage of solution because cone replaces sphincter.
20. When solution runs in, clamp tubing and remove cone, making sure sleeve fits around hand. Should obtain small gush of fluid, then returns in spurts.	Clamping tubing prevents return of results into irrigator. Sleeve should be placed properly to avoid gush of solution over top of sleeve. If colon was distended sufficiently, contracting of bowel musculature results in return of solution in intermittent spurts.
21. Clamp top of sleeve.	Prevents leakage at top.
22. When most of solution has returned (15-20 min), rinse sleeve with water, fold end up, fasten it to top, and have client ambulate (unless restricted to bed).	Allows ambulation. Prevents leakage. Entire procedure takes about 1 hr, and client may become tired of sitting.

Step 17

Step 16 illustration from Broadwell DC, Jackson BS: *Principles of ostomy care,* St Louis, 1982, Mosby–Year Book; redrawn from Craig J: *Clin Symp* no 30, vol 5, 1978. Step 17 illustration from Broadwell DC, Jackson BS: *Principles of ostomy care,* St Louis, 1982, Mosby–Year Book.

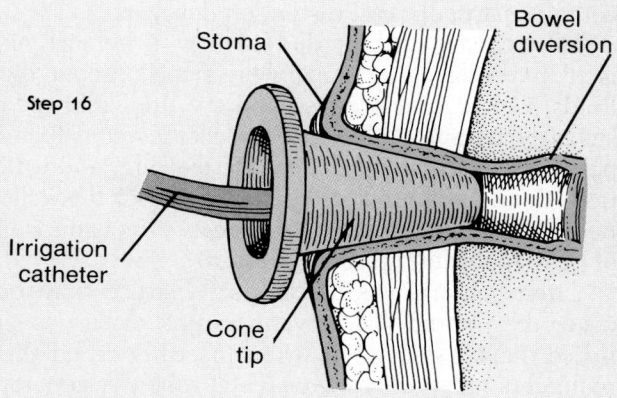

Step 16 — Stoma, Bowel diversion, Irrigation catheter, Cone tip

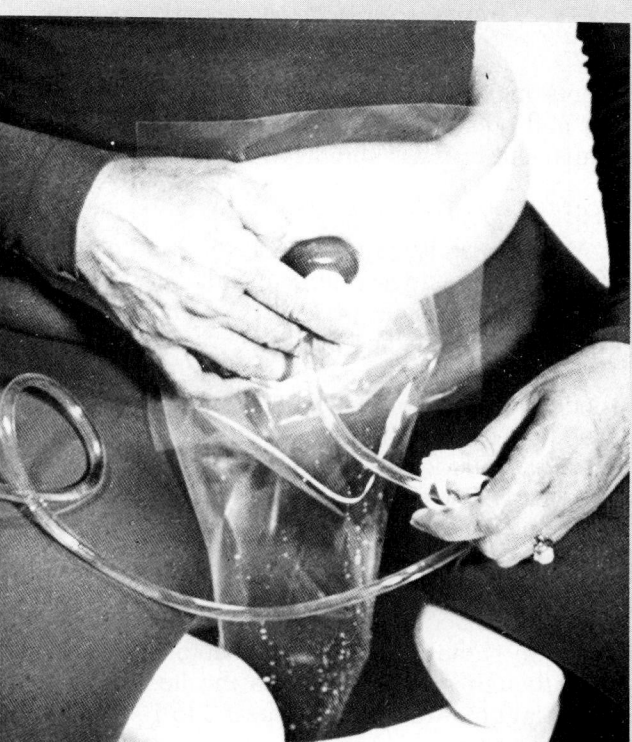

Irrigating a Colostomy

STEPS	RATIONALE
23. When all of feces have returned, rinse sleeve out with water and special liquid cleanser and remove. Then wash sleeve out with soap and water, rinse, and air dry.	Prevents sleeve from deteriorating, permitting reuse. Controls odor.
24. Apply new pouch according to procedure (see Procedure 41-3).	Avoids leakage and skin problems.
25. Dispose of equipment no longer needed. Remove gloves by turning them inside out and dispose in receptacle.	Reduces transmission of microorganisms.
26. Wash hands.	Prevents cross contamination.
27. Inspect volume and character of fecal material and fluid that returns after irrigation.	Determines whether irrigant is retained (serious fluid imbalances can occur if retained). Character and amount of stool reveal success of cleaning bowel.
28. Note client's response during irrigant infusion. Ask if client feels cramping or abdominal pain.	Reveals client's tolerance of irrigation.
29. Palpate and auscultate abdomen after return of irrigant.	Evaluates for potential complication of bowel perforation.
30. Assist client to comfortable position.	Ensures client comfort.
31. Record pertinent information, including character of feces and tolerance to procedure.	Communicates pertinent information to members of health care team.

clients may benefit from avoiding foods that cause gas and odor, including broccoli, cauliflower, dried beans, and brussels sprouts.

Promotion of Regular Exercise

A daily exercise program helps prevent elimination problems. Walking, riding a stationary bicycle, or swimming stimulates peristalsis. Clients who are sedentary at work are most in need of regular exercise.

For a client temporarily immobilized, the nurse should attempt ambulation as soon as possible. If the condition permits, the nurse assists a postoperative client in walking to a chair on the evening of the day of surgery. The client should walk farther each day.

Some clients have difficulty passing stool because of weak abdominal and pelvic floor muscles. Exercises help bedridden clients using a bedpan. The client can practice the exercises as follows:

1. Lie supine; tighten the abdominal muscles as though pushing them to the floor. Hold them tight to three; relax. Repeat 5 to 10 times as tolerated.

2. Flex and contract the thigh muscles by raising one knee slowly toward the chest. Repeat for each leg at least 5 times and increase frequency as tolerated.

Promotion of Comfort

Many clients have discomfort from alterations in elimination. Pain results when hemorrhoidal tissues are directly irritated. Flatulence can also create discomfort, particularly if distention develops.

The primary goal for the client with hemorrhoids is to have soft-formed, painless stools. Proper diet, fluids, and regular exercise improve the likelihood of stools being soft. If the client becomes constipated, passage of hard stools may cause bleeding and irritation. Local heat provides temporary relief to swollen hemorrhoids. A sitz bath is the most effective means of heat application (see Chapter 48).

Often hemorrhoids become so enlarged that they cover the rectum. To prevent trauma to tissues the nurse must use caution when inserting rectal thermometers, suppositories, or rectal tubes. A generous amount of lubricating jelly reduces friction when inserting an object past a hemorrhoid. Often the client is better able to insert an object safely into the rectum. The nurse should never attempt to force an object into the rectum without full view of the anus. When hemorrhoids cause chronic pain, surgical removal is the best treatment.

To relieve the discomfort of flatulence, the nurse should use measures that reduce flatus or promote its escape. Air swallowing increases flatus. The client can reduce the amount of air swallowed by not drinking carbonated beverages, not using straws for drinking, and not chewing gum or hard candies. When flatulence becomes severe as a result of reduced peristalsis, a nasogastric tube is often used.

When flatulence results in abdominal cramping, ambulation promotes passage of flatus. Having the client walk down the hall may be enough to stimulate peristalsis and relieve gas. When conservative measures fail, flatulence can be relieved by insertion of a rectal tube. The client assumes a side-lying position while the nurse inserts the tube in the same manner as for an enema (Procedure 41-2). Because fluid is not instilled into the bowel, the nurse can advance the tube deeper to reach areas where flatus has accumulated (15 cm or 6 in in an adult, 5 to 10 cm or 2 to 4 in in a child).

After inserting the tube the nurse instructs the client to lie quietly in bed. To prevent the tube from being dislodged, the nurse may tape it to one of the buttocks. A gauze dressing or waterproof pad placed around the open end of the rectal tube will catch liquid fecal material.

Continual use of rectal tubes can cause irritation and eventual **excoriation** of the anus and rectal mucosa. A rectal tube should not remain in place longer than 30 minutes. The physician determines the frequency with which the tube can be inserted. If flatulence persists, the nurse should notify the physician.

The return-flow enema is another means used to expel flatus. The alternating instillation and drainage of fluid into and out of the colon and rectum stimulates passage of flatus.

Maintenance of Skin Integrity

The client with diarrhea or fecal incontinence is at risk for skin breakdown when fecal contents remain on the skin. The same problem exists for the client with an ostomy that drains liquid stool (see teaching box). Liquid stool is usually acidic and contains digestive enzymes. Irritation from repeated wiping with toilet tissue aggravates skin breakdown. Bathing the skin after soiling helps but may result in more breakdown unless the skin is thoroughly dried.

Client Teaching for Stomal Care

OBJECTIVE

- Client will demonstrate the correct procedure for stomal care.

TEACHING STRATEGIES

- Instruct client to avoid using alcohol in cleansing around the stoma. Alcohol dilates capillaries and can cause bleeding of the stomal margin.
- Demonstrate how to wash around the stoma with water and a mild soap or with a commercial preparation, such as Peri Wash. Pat the skin dry but do not rub.
- Instruct client not to use cold cream on skin because it prevents the pouch from adhering to the skin.
- Explain to the client that peroxide is an irritant and should not be used.
- Instruct the client that if a yeast infection occurs, thorough cleansing, followed by patting the area dry, and applying Kenalog spray or Mycostatin usually resolves the infection.
- Show the client how to inspect the stoma daily and observe a stoma that is moist, shiny, and dark pink to red.
- Teach client to observe for and report excessive bleeding, edema or, abnormal discharge or color to the nurse or physician.

EVALUATION

- Client will correctly state skin care procedures.
- Client will correctly perform stoma skin care procedure.

The nurse should instruct the client on cleansing the anal area with mild soap and water after each passage of stool. When a client with an ostomy removes the pouch covering the stoma, the surrounding skin should be thoroughly cleaned.

When caring for a debilitated, incontinent client who is unable to ask for assistance, the nurse should check often for defecation. The anal areas can be protected with petrolatum jelly, zinc oxide, or another ointment that holds moisture in the skin, preventing drying and cracking. Yeast infections of the skin can develop easily. Several powdered antifungal agents are effective against yeast. Baby powder or cornstarch should not be used because they have no medical properties and they frequently cake on the skin and become difficult to remove.

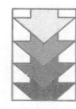

Sample Evaluation of Interventions for Constipation

Goals	Evaluative Measures	Expected Outcomes
Client will understand and ingest fluid and food intake required to promote soft, formed stools.	Evaluate meal plan created by client or family member. Measure client's fluid intake. Observe character of stools. Record frequency of defecation.	Meal plan will include foods that are suited to client's elimination needs and that promote normal defecation. Client will have a minimum intake of 1400-2000 ml daily. Client will attain a regular schedule of defecation, passing soft-formed stools without excess straining.
Client will understand normal elimination.	Ask client to describe factors that affect elimination. Ask client to discuss factors in hostory that may cause elimination problems.	Client will explain effects of diet, fluids, exercise, stress, medications, and personal habits on elimination.
Client will achieve regular exercise program.	Observe client initiate active exercises daily. Ask client to describe benefits of regular exercise.	Client will ambulate down halls or report activities (e.g., daily walking, swimming). Client will explain that regular exercise stimulates intestinal peristalsis.
Client will achieve comfort.	Ask client if discomfort is experienced, such as during defecation. Inspect anal area. Palpate abdomen.	Client will not have burning or pain during defecation. Tissue will be intact, without evidence of bleeding or inflamation. Abdomen will be flat, soft, without distention.

Promotion of Self-Concept

When a client has a bowel elimination problem, a threat to self-concept may be experienced. Frequent incontinence, foul odorous stools, and an ostomy appliance are just a few factors that may cause a client to perceive a change in body image. The result could be a client who avoids socializing with others or who is unwilling to assume responsibility for self-care. The client with an ostomy often sees a stoma as a form of mutilation. This client may thus have difficulty maintaining or initiating sexual relations with a partner. The nurse can play an important role in restoring a client's self-concept through the following interventions:

1. Give the client an opportunity to discuss concerns or fears about elimination problems.
2. Provide the client and family with information to understand and manage the elimination problem.
3. Give positive feedback when the client attempts self-care measures.
4. Help the client manage the condition but do not expect the client to like it.
5. Provide privacy during care.
6. Show acceptance and understanding.

Often, a client with an elimination problem goes through a process similar to grieving (see Chapter 28). The nurse's support is essential to help the client return to a more normal lifestyle.

 ## Evaluation

The effectiveness of care depends on success in meeting the expected outcomes of care (see evaluation box). Optimally, the client will be able to regularly defecate soft-formed, painless stools. The client will also gain information needed to establish a normal elimination pattern and to demonstrate ongoing success measured at specific intervals over an extended period of time. The client will be able to accomplish normal defecation by manipulating natural components of daily living such as diet, fluid intake, and exercise. The client will have minimal reliance on artificial means of defecation such as enemas and laxative use. The client will be comfortable with the ostomy protocol and identify it as one that can be practiced indefinitely.

 SUMMARY

Normal elimination of fecal wastes requires maintenance of gastrointestinal function. Each client has a different defecation pattern and presents risks for alterations in elimination. The nurse provides therapies that promote or minimize factors affecting peristalsis or the absorption and secretion of intestinal contents. Care usually involves educating clients about daily activities or habits that affect defecation.

Clients become dependent on the nurse when the ability to control body functions is lost. The nurse's approach with clients who have elimination problems must be sensitive and understanding.

REFERENCES

Bellan A: Coloplast-update on the conseal plug, *Ostomy Internat* 11(2):15, 1990.

Brown MK, Everett I: Gentler bowel fitness with fiber, *Geriatr Nurs* 11(1):26, 1990.

Cooke DM: Inflammatory bowel disease: primary health care management of ulcerative colitis and Crohn's disease, *Nurse Pract* 16(8):27, 1991.

Corman ML: *Colon and rectal surgery*, ed 2, Philadelphia, 1989, Lippincott.

Dalton-Loehner D, Connor P: Beyond ileostomy: surgery for a normal life, *RN* 52:29, 1989.

Eastwood A, Avundu KC: *Manual of gastroenterology: diagnosis and therapy*, Boston, 1988, Little, Brown.

Gilpatrick DM: Moving clients towards wellness: behavioral change, *Clin Nurse Spec* 3(1):25, 1989.

Goldfinger SE: Constipation: the hard facts. I. *Harvard Health Letter* 16(4):1, 1991.

Kim MJ, McFarland GK, McLane AM: *Pocket guide to nursing diagnoses*, ed 4, St Louis, 1991, Mosby–Year Book.

Robinson C, Weigley E: *Basic nutrition and diet therapy*, ed 6, New York, 1989, Macmillan.

Ross D: Constipation among hospitalized elders, *Orthop Nurs* 9(3):73, 1990.

Swartz ML: Citrucel (methylcellulose/bulk-forming laxative), *Gastroenterol Nurse* 12(1):50, 1989.

Tortora GJ: *Principles of human anatomy*, ed 5, New York, 1989, Harper & Row.

ADDITIONAL READINGS

Alterescu V: The ostomy, *Am J Nurs* 85:1241, 1985.

Alterescu V: The ostomy: what do you teach the patient? *Am J Nurs* 85:1250, 1985.

Alterescu V: Theoretical foundations for an approach to fecal incontinence, *J Entero Ther* 13:44, 1986.

Alterescu KB: Colostomy, *Nurs Clin North Am* 22:281, 1987.

Aman RA: Treating the patient, not the constipation, *Am J Nurs* 80:1634, 1980.

American Cancer Society: *Guidelines for the cancer-related checkup: recommendations and rationale*, 30:18, 1980.

Benedict P, Haddad A: Post-op teaching for the colostomy patient, *RN* 52:85, 1989.

Bitterman RA: Getting the bowels under control, *Emerg Med* 19:69, 1987.

Broadwell DC, Jackson BS: *Principles of ostomy care*, St Louis, 1982, Mosby–Year Book.

Burcharth F et al: The colostomy plug: a new disposable device for a continent colostomy, *Lancet* 2(8515):1062, 1986.

Burggraf V, Donlan B: Assessing the elderly, *Am J Nurse* 85:872, 1985.

Cleague MB, Heald RJ: Achievement of stomal continence in one-third of colostomies by use of a disposable plug, *Surg Gynecol Obstet* 170(5):390, 1990.

Davis A et al: Bowel management: a quality assurance approach to upgrading programs, *J Gerontol Nurs* 12:13, 1986.

Dolinger R: How radiation complicates stoma care, *RN* 49:32, 1986.

Erickson PJ: Ostomies: the art of pouching, *Nurs Clin North Am* 22:311, 1987.

Gershenson DM, Smith DB: *Enteric diversions in ostomy care and the cancer patient*, Orlando, Fla, 1986, Grune & Stratton.

Guyton AC: *Human physiology and mechanisms of disease*, ed 3, Philadelphia, 1982, Saunders.

Maresca JG, Stringari S: Assessment and management of acute diarrheal illness in adults, *Nurs Pract* 11(11):15, 1986.

Pagana K, Pagana TJ: *Diagnostic testing and nursing implications*, ed 2, St Louis, 1986, Mosby–Year Book.

Smith DB: The ostomy, how is it managed? *Am J Nurs* 85:1246, 1985.

Tedesco FJ: Laxative use in constipation, *Am J Gastroenterol* 80:303, 1985.

Thibodeau GA, Patton K: *Anatomy and physiology*, ed 2, St Louis, 1993, Mosby–Year Book.

Whaley LF, Wong DL: *Nursing care of infants and children*, ed 4, St Louis, 1991, Mosby–Year Book.

Wright BA, Statts DO: The geriatric implications of fecal impaction, *Nurse Pract* 11(10):53, 1986.

CHAPTER 41 REVIEW

Key Concepts

- A primary function of the elimination process is fluid balance.
- Mechanical breakdown of food elements, gastrointestinal motility, and selective absorption and secretion of substances by the large intestine influence the character of feces.
- Mass peristalsis in the large intestine is strongest an hour after mealtime.
- Food high in fiber content and an increased fluid intake keep feces soft.
- Regular use of laxatives can lead to constipation.
- Vagal stimulation, which slows the heart rate, may occur during straining while defecating, taking rectal temperatures, and enemas.
- The greatest danger from diarrhea is development of fluid and electrolyte imbalance.
- The location of an ostomy influences consistency of the stool.
- Assessment of elimination patterns should focus on bowel habits, factors that normally influence defecation, recent changes in elimination, and a physical examination.
- A guaiac test is recommended for clients who take anticoagulants, who have a bleeding disorder or gastrointestinal disorder causing bleeding, or who are at risk for colon cancer.
- Indirect and direct visualization of the lower gastrointestinal tract requires cleansing of the bowel before the procedure.
- The nurse should consider frequency of defecation, fecal characteristics, and effect of foods on gastrointestinal function when selecting a diet promoting normal elimination.
- Proper positioning on a bedpan allows the client to assume a position similar to squatting without experiencing muscle strain.
- Cathartics or laxatives should be administered shortly before the usual time of defecation.
- Proper administration of an enema is the slow instillation of a warm solution in the proper volume.
- Irrigation of an ostomy follows the same principles as an enema administration except a special irrigating tube is needed and the client cannot control passage of feces.
- Dangers during digital removal of stool include traumatizing the rectal mucosa and promoting vagal stimulation.
- Skin breakdown can occur after repeated exposure to liquid stool.

Key Terms

Biopsy, p. 1404

Bolus, p. 1388

Bowel training, p. 1414

Cathartics, p. 1394

Chyme, p. 1389

Colitis, p. 1393

Colon, p. 1390

Colostomy, p. 1397

Constipation, p. 1394

Contrast medium, p. 1404

Crohn's disease, p. 1393

Defecation, p. 1391

Diarrhea, p. 1395

Diverticula, p. 1405

Endoscopy, p. 1404

Enema, p. 1409

Enterostomal therapist (ET), p. 1415

Excoriation, p. 1423

Feces, p. 1391

Fiber, p. 1392

Fiberoptic endoscope, p. 1403

Flatulence, p. 1390

Flatus, p. 1391

Gastrocolic reflex, p. 1393

Gastroscopy, p. 1404

Guaiac test, p. 1401

Haustral contractions, p. 1391

Hemorrhoids, p. 1390

Ileostomy, p. 1397

Impaction, p. 1395

Incontinence, p. 1396

Lactose intolerance, p. 1393

Laxatives, p. 1394

Masticate, p. 1388

Melena, p. 1403

Paralytic ileus, p. 1394

Peristalsis, p. 1388

Polyps, p. 1404

Refluxing, p. 1388

Regurgitating, p. 1391

Stoma, p. 1397

Transit time, p. 1394

Valsalva maneuver, p. 1391

Critical Thinking Exercises

1. A 24-year-old man with a history of good health is admitted to your unit after a motor vehicle accident. Bed rest has been prescribed for the next 2 weeks. What type of plan would you design to prevent him from becoming constipated during this period of immobility?

2. You are asked to provide an outpatient client with material and instructions for three stool quaiac tests. Identify and explain four important points of information you would want to include in your instructions.

3. An older woman with a new, permanent colostomy is about to be discharged from your unit to her daughter's home. The skin around her stoma has no breakdown. She and her daughter realize the importance of maintaining this skin integrity. How would you go about advising them?

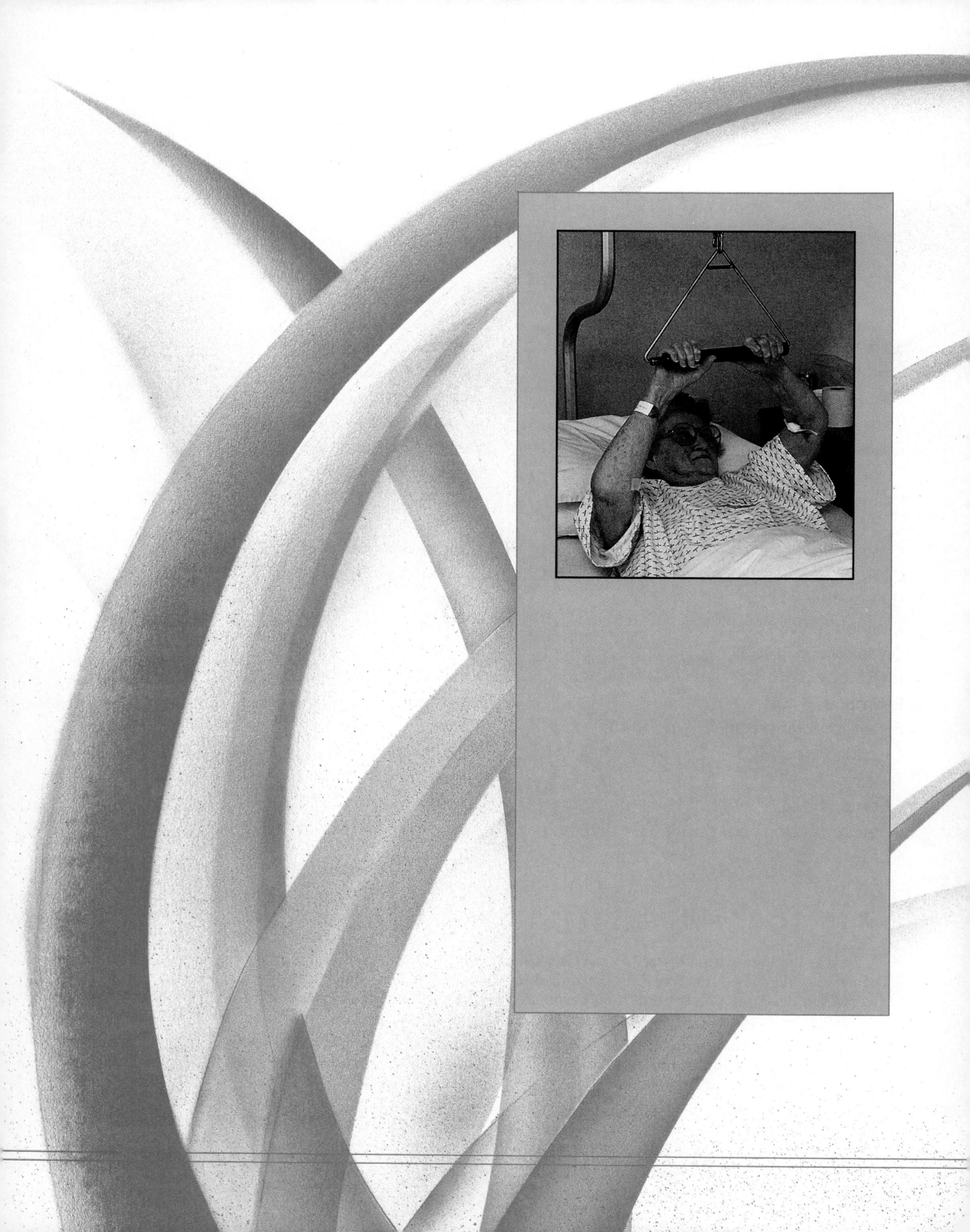

UNIT 8

Providing a Safe Environment

CHAPTER 42

Safety

OBJECTIVES

Mastery of content in this chapter will enable the student to:

- Define the key terms listed.
- Describe how unmet basic physiological needs of oxygen, fluids, nutrition, and temperature can threaten a client's safety.
- Discuss methods to reduce physical hazards.
- Describe current methods to reduce the transmission of pathogens and parasites.
- Describe present methods of pollution control.
- Discuss the specific risks to safety related to developmental age.
- Describe the four categories of risks in a health care agency.
- State nursing diagnoses associated with risks to safety.
- Develop a care plan for clients whose safety is threatened.
- Describe nursing interventions specific to the client's age for reducing risk of falls, fires, poisonings, and electrical hazards.
- Describe methods to evaluate interventions designed to maintain or promote safety.

CHAPTER OUTLINE

Environmental Safety
    Basic needs
    Reduction of physical hazards
    Reduction of transmission of pathogens
    Pollution control

Nursing Process and Safety
    Assessment
    Nursing diagnosis
    Planning
    Implementation
    Evaluation

Nursing care directed at health maintenance and illness prevention involves promoting the client's safety in the community or within the health care environment and is just as essential as meeting other physiological and psychosocial needs. Protection and safety are basic to survival, and these needs continue throughout life.

Defined broadly, an *environment* is all of the many physical and psychosocial factors that influence or affect the life and survival of the client. A safe health care environment reduces the length of treatment or hospitalization, the frequency of treatment-related accidents, the number of work-related injuries to personnel, and the overall cost of health care services. In addition, a safe health care environment allows staff members to function at their optimal levels.

Safety in the home reduces the risk of accidents and illnesses and the subsequent need for health care service. Safety is positively correlated to health promotion. The greater the safety in a home, the greater the level of health promotion in that home.

ENVIRONMENTAL SAFETY

A safe environment is one in which basic needs are achieved, physical hazards are reduced, transmission of pathogens and parasites is reduced, sanitation is maintained, and pollution is controlled.

Basic Needs

Meeting basic human needs is necessary for achieving safety and security needs (see Chapter 29). Frequently, certain physiological needs, including oxygen, optimum humidity, nutrition, and optimum temperature, influence a person's safety.

Oxygen

The nurse must be aware of factors in a client's environment that decrease the amount of available oxygen. One of the most common environmental hazards in the home is an improperly functioning furnace. A furnace that is not operating properly or is not properly vented introduces carbon monoxide into the environment. **Carbon monoxide** is a colorless, odorless, poisonous gas produced by the combustion of carbon or organic fuels. Carbon monoxide binds strongly with hemoglobin, preventing the formation of oxyhemoglobin and thus reducing the supply of oxygen delivered to tissues (see Chapter 38). A client who moves to a new residence or who has an older furnace should be encouraged to have the furnace inspected. This inspection is usually performed free

of charge or for a nominal fee. Public buildings such as schools, hospitals, and businesses are required by municipal codes to have periodic furnace inspections to reduce the risk of carbon monoxide poisoning.

Humidity

The relative humidity of the air in the environment may affect the client's health and safety. **Relative humidity** is the amount of water vapor in the air compared with the maximum amount of water vapor that the air could contain at the same temperature. The comfort zone for humidity varies from person to person, but most people are comfortable when the humidity is between 60% and 70%.

When the relative humidity is high, the skin's moisture evaporates slowly. Thus during hot, humid weather, people feel uncomfortably hot and sticky. If the relative humidity is low, the skin's moisture evaporates quickly. This is why people feel cooler and more comfortable when the temperature is 32.2° C (90° F) with a relative humidity of 30% than when the temperature is 32.2° C (90° F) with a relative humidity of 85%.

Increasing the environmental humidity can have therapeutic benefits. Children and adults with upper respiratory tract infections usually experience improvement in their symptoms when a humidifier is placed in the room while they sleep. The humidifier increases the relative humidity of the inhaled air, which helps liquefy secretions and improve breathing.

Nutrition

Meeting nutritional needs adequately and safely requires environmental controls and knowledge. In the home the client needs a refrigerator and a freezer compartment to keep perishable foods fresh. An adequate, clean water supply is needed to wash fresh produce and dishes. Provisions for garbage collection are necessary to maintain sanitary conditions.

Foods that are inadequately prepared or stored increase the client's risk for **food poisoning** (an illness resulting from the ingestion of a food contaminated by toxic substances or by bacteria containing toxins). Symptoms of food poisoning can occur immediately or up to a week after ingestion of the toxic food (Kuhn, 1985). Assessments for suspected food poisoning include obtaining a client's history, gathering gastrointestinal (GI) and central nervous system (CNS) data, observing for a fever, and analyzing laboratory samples of feces for leukocytes, blood, and *Vibrio* organisms, which are comma-shaped organisms (Kuhn, 1985). Accurate assessment data are crucial in isolating the type of organism present. In addition, the Centers for Disease Control (CDC) needs to be contacted when specific toxins, such as botulism from home-preserved foods or preserved fish or salmonella from undercooked poultry, fish, and pork or contaminated milk, water, ice cream, and eggs, are isolated.

Temperature

The comfort zone for environmental temperature varies among individuals, but the usual comfort range is between 18.3° and 23.9° C (65° and 75° F). Temperature extremes that frequently occur during the winter and summer affect not only comfort and productivity but also safety.

Exposure to severe cold for prolonged periods causes frostbite and hypothermia. **Hypothermia** occurs when the core body temperature is 35° C (95° F) or below. The client experiences confusion and a declining level of consciousness, which can result in coma. Shivering is present in the early stages, and trembling may occur on one side of the body or in one extremity. Ultimately the client's vital signs decline, and death ensues.

Older adults, children, and clients with spinal cord injuries (for example, paraplegia and quadriplegia) are at higher risk for hypothermia. Chronic or acute illness increases susceptibility to hypothermia. Similarly, the ingestion of alcohol interferes with temperature regulation and increases the risk for hypothermia.

Exposure to extreme heat can result in heatstroke or heat exhaustion. In either case the body's electrolyte balance is changed, the core body temperature rises, and brain damage results. With heat exhaustion the client has sudden changes in mental status, GI distress, and elevated rectal temperature up to 41.1° C (105° F). **Heatstroke** is a life-threatening condition with severe changes in mental status, including coma, abnormal fluid and electrolyte status, hyperpyrexia, and rectal temperatures in excess of 41.1° C (105° F) (Posey, Caruso, 1986). The chronically ill, older adults, infants, and the poor are at greatest risk for injury from extreme heat (see Chapter 19).

Reduction of Physical Hazards

Physical hazards in the environment may threaten client safety. These hazards can result in a physical injury. Injuries are the leading cause of death for clients up to 45 years of age (National Center for Health Statistics, 1988). In 1987 the lost work days due to injuries were greater than the lost work days resulting from heart disease, cancer, and stroke (CDC, 1989). Many physical hazards can be minimized through adequate lighting, reduction of obsta-

cles, control of bathroom hazards, and security measures.

Ensuring Adequate Lighting

Adequate lighting reduces physical hazards by illuminating areas in which the client moves and works. Outside the home, lighting brightens walkways from the street to the house, from the garage to the house, and on the stairs to the front or back door. Inside the house the halls, staircases, and individual rooms should be adequately lighted so that residents can safely carry out activities of daily living. Nightlights in dark halls, bathrooms, and rooms of children and older adults help maintain safety by reducing the risk of falls. A night-light in a guest room can help orient an overnight guest who needs to get up in the middle of the night. Adequate lighting also helps protect the home and its inhabitants from crime. Welllighted garages, walkways, and doorways discourage intruders from entering the premises or hiding in shadows.

Decreasing Obstacles

Injuries in the home frequently result from objects on the stairs and floor, wet spots on the floor, and clutter on places such as bedside tables, closet shelves, the top of the refrigerator, and bookshelves. The risk of injury from obstacles is greatest for older adults. Injury can be the result of an illness, normal changes associated with aging, and medications (Tideiksaar, 1989).

To reduce the risk of injury, all obstacles should be removed from halls and other heavily traveled areas. Necessary objects such as clocks, glasses, tissues, or medications should remain on bedside tables within reach of the client but out of the reach of children in the home. Care should also be taken to ensure that end tables are secure and have stable, straight legs. Nonessential materials such as books, needlework, and newspapers should not be routinely placed on end tables.

If small area rugs are used, they should be secured with a nonslip pad or skid-resistant adhesive strips. Area rugs and runners should not be used on stairs. Any carpeting on the stairs should be secured with carpet tacks.

Controlling Bathroom Hazards

Accidents happen frequently in the bathroom from scalds, burns, and accidental poisoning. Care should be taken to lower the thermostat setting on the water heater to reduce the risk of burns and scalds. Secure, easily seen grab bars and nonslip colored adhesive tape on the bottom of the tub are useful in reducing accidental falls in the bathtub (Tideiksaar, 1989).

Medication in the medicine cabinet should be clearly marked and out of the reach of children, and excess or out-of-date medication should be discarded.

Securing the Home

Clients need to take precautions to secure their homes from intruders, who are a threat to physical and mental safety. When assessing the client's home for safety, the nurse should evaluate the presence and quality of locks on doors and windows. Adequate exterior lighting can also reduce the risk of break-ins.

For the client who is relocating, it might help to inquire about the crime rate in the proposed location. Statistics about crime rates can be obtained from the local police department and home insurance companies.

Reduction of Transmission of Pathogens

A **pathogen** is any microorganism capable of producing an illness. A **parasite** is an organism living in or on another organism and obtaining nourishment from it. Pathogens and parasites can be found in water, food, humans and other animals, and insects.

In a health care setting, effective and efficient methods are used for the control of pathogen transmission, including medical and surgical asepsis (see Chapter 18). The transmission of pathogens from person to person can be reduced and in some cases prevented by immunization. **Immunization** is the process by which resistance to an infectious disease is produced or augmented. Immunity is acquired after the oral administration or injection of an **antigen,** which causes production of an antibody within the body. The body is then immune to the effects of the intended pathogens.

The rising number of cases of acquired immunodeficiency syndrome (AIDS) and other sexually transmitted diseases is increasing the public's awareness of pathogen transmission. Safe sexual practices through the correct use of condoms and a decrease in casual sexual activities reduce risk for STDs.

The human immunodeficiency virus (HIV), the pathogen that causes AIDS, is also transmitted through intravenous (IV) drug abuse. Drug abusers frequently share syringes and needles, which increases the risk of acquiring AIDS. HIV is blood borne. Thus it is transmitted through contaminated syringes and needles (CDC, 1987). In the community, the risk factors for acquiring HIV and other blood-borne pathogens can be reduced or eliminated by modifying certain illness-causing behaviors (see Chapter 32).

Food Sanitation

Improperly processed or contaminated food can cause illness and death through transmission of pathogens and parasites. Commercially processed and packaged foods are subject to **Food and Drug Administration** (FDA) regulations and usually contain a minimal amount of contaminants. The FDA is a federal agency responsible for the enforcement of federal regulations regarding the manufacture, processing, and distribution of food, drugs, and cosmetics to protect consumers against the sale of impure or dangerous substances.

Insect and Rodent Control

Control of fleas and ticks on domestic animals and in the environment reduces the incidence of bites, skin irritations, and disease transmission. Tick bites are the mode of transmission for Rocky Mountain spotted fever and Lyme disease.

Rodents also transmit pathogens. A rat or mouse can transmit rat-bite fever, which in the United States is caused by the *Streptobacillus moniliformis* organism and in the Far East by the *Spirillum minus* organism. Although both of these organisms are sensitive to penicillin, the best approach to controlling rat-bite fever is prevention, which is achieved by reducing the rodent population through proper disposal of garbage.

Disposal of Human Wastes

The transmission of pathogens is also controlled by adequate disposal of human waste through proper construction and repair of sewers and drains. Without a satisfactory sewer and waste system, the population is at risk for illnesses transmitted by human feces (for example, typhoid fever and hepatitis).

Pollution Control

A healthy environment is free of pollution. A **pollutant** is a harmful chemical or waste material discharged into the water or air. People commonly think of pollution only in terms of air or water pollution, but noise can also be a form of pollution that presents health risks.

Air pollution is the contamination of the atmosphere. Prolonged exposure to air pollution increases the risk of pulmonary disease. In urban areas, industrial waste and vehicle exhaust are common contributors to air pollution. In the home, school, or workplace, cigarette smoke is the primary cause of air pollution. Environmental pollution can also be caused by improper disposal of radioactive and bioactive waste products such as dioxin.

Water pollution is the contamination of lakes, rivers, and streams, usually by industrial pollutants. Water-treatment facilities filter harmful contaminants from the water, but these systems often contain flaws. If water exiting the treatment facility becomes contaminated, the public is notified to boil water used for drinking and cooking. Flooding frequently causes damage to water-treatment stations and also requires the boiling of drinking and cooking water.

Noise pollution occurs when the noise level in an environment becomes uncomfortable to the inhabitants of the environment. Noise levels are measured in units of sound intensity called *decibels*. Noise level tolerances vary from individual to individual and are influenced by health status. A high noise level can produce hearing loss over time. If the noise level is maintained or the person does not use earplugs, complete deafness can result.

A health care agency such as an intensive care unit can also be polluted by noise. The sounds of machines, people talking, and intercoms can create increased noise levels. Even when the noise level is not high enough to affect hearing acuity, it may produce a syndrome called *sensory overload*. **Sensory overload** is a marked increase in the intensity of auditory and visual stimuli. It disrupts processing of information and problem solving and increases anxiety, paranoia, hallucinations, depression, and unrealistic feelings (see Chapter 45) (Lindenmuth, Breu, Malooley, 1981).

Pollution impairs the level of health of all those exposed to the pollutants. A nurse assessing a client's environment may be the first to recognize the potential threat to the client.

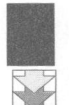

NURSING PROCESS AND SAFETY

Assessment

Nurses provide care to clients and their families in their homes or communities. Clients who are ill, illiterate, poor, or older often require help to achieve a safe environment. To do this the nurse needs to understand what contributes to a safe environment in the home or health care agency and then thoroughly assesses the environment for threats to safety.

Community

RISKS AT DEVELOPMENTAL STAGES. Threats to safety within the community are influenced by developmental stage, lifestyle habits, mobility status, sensory impairments, and safety awareness.

Infant, Toddler, and Preschooler. Home accidents kill, disfigure, and permanently disable thousands of children each year. Children younger than 5 are at greatest risk for death. Two conclusions can be drawn about the underlying causes or precipitating factors in childhood accidents (Roy, 1982). First, accidents involving children are largely preventable, but frequently parents need to be shown the specific dangers by nurses and other health care professionals. Second, as the infant grows, accident potential increases. The newborn's accident potential is influenced by people or external agents, but growth and the acquisition of new motor skills place the active child at risk for injuries (Table 42-1 on p. 1436). Accident prevention thus requires health education for parents and removal of dangers whenever possible.

School-Age Child. When a child enters school, the environment expands to include the school, transportation to and from school, school friends, and after-school activities. Each of these is a potential threat to the child's safety. Injuries can be minor, such as falling and bruising the knee, or major, such as being hit in the head by a baseball. Through discussions and examples, parents, teachers, and nurses instruct the child to safely cross the street, choose the proper foods to eat, brush teeth, and perform other hygiene measures.

Because school-age children are participating in more activities outside their home and neighborhood environments, they are at greater risk of injury from strangers. Therefore the child should be warned repeatedly not to accept candy, food, gifts, or rides from strangers. In addition, a child needs to know what to do if a stranger approaches. Frequently neighborhoods have a "block home" or "safe house." In these homes the owner ensures that an adult is home during the times when children are walking to and from school. If a stranger approaches a child, the child can run to that home, and the adult will protect the child and call the proper authorities. Nurses can work with school systems or neighborhoods to initiate such a system to protect children.

Sports safety is stressed in school sports, but parents and health professionals can reinforce these safety tips by insisting that children wear protective gear while participating in sports in the home. For example, schools provide hard batting helmets for baseball games, and parents should also provide this equipment when children are playing baseball in their own backyards.

Bicycle safety is an important issue for nurses and parents. CNS injury is the primary cause of death in 90% of childhood fatalities from bicycle or pedestrian collision with a motor vehicle (US Preventive Ser-

TABLE 42-1 Motor Development Changes that Increase Risk of Injury in Infants and Toddlers		
Age	**Motor Development**	**Hazard**
1 mo	Baby can hold head midline and parallel to body but is unable to hold head erect.	If not supported, infant's head flops forward or backward.
2 mo	Grasp reflex is present; infant grasps and holds object for few moments or longer.	Child can grasp electrical cords and other dangerous items on floor.
3 mo	Child may begin to roll from back to abdomen and bears weight on forearms.	There is increased risk of falling off bed, changing table, and counter.
4 mo	Increased grasping ability is present. Child explores new objects with mouth.	Infant is able to pick up small objects, which usually are placed immediately into mouth.
	Child possesses increased ability to roll from abdomen and from side to side and to move in rocking motion.	There is increased risk of falling from surfaces.
5 mo	Ability of locomotion increases by rocking, rolling, and twisting.	Infant is able to purposefully move toward objects that may be dangerous.
	Child is able to grasp bottle but should not be left unattended.	Risk of choking on contents increases. Drinking from bottle in supine position can increase risk of ear infections and dental caries in baby and permanent teeth.
	Ability to grasp small objects increases.	There is increased risk of choking on small objects.
6 mo	Infant creeps by propelling self on abdomen, steering with arms and legs.	Child is able to move to potential dangers, such as electrical outlets and household cleaners.
7 mo	Child may be crawling and is able to sit alone for short periods of time.	Infant can move rapidly from one spot to another.
8 mo	Infant may be able to pull self to standing position and can sit unsupported.	Child can easily fall unless helped back to sitting or lying position.
9 mo	Child begins to crawl up stairs and can stand and move by using furniture for support. (Walking may occur any time after 8 mo.)	Infant can lose balance and fall down stairs, can lose balance with wobbly furniture, and can bruise self on sharp corners of tables and bookcases.
10 mo	Infant climbs up and tries to climb down from chairs and is able to change from prone to sitting position.	Child may fall from chair and is unable to judge distances or limits.
11 mo	Interest in feeding self begins.	Unless foods are cut into small pieces, choking may result.
12 mo	Child may climb out of crib.	There is increased risk of falling out of crib or playpen.
	Infant takes cover off plastic screwtop containers.	Child can open and possibly taste harmful substances.*
15 mo	Child walks with help but cannot walk around corners or stop suddenly without losing balance.	Infant loses sense of balance and easily falls.*
18 mo	Child runs clumsily and falls often.	Child may injure head from severe falls.
	Infant moves furniture and climbs on it.	Infant may pull furniture over on self or fall off furniture.
24 mo	Child is able to turn door knobs.	Child can independently open closed door and may ingest harmful products stored in cabinet, closet, or bathroom. Child may wander to backyard swimming pool.*

Data from Whaley LF, Wong DL: *Nursing care of infants and children*, ed 4, St. Louis, 1991, Mosby–Year Book.
*Data from US Preventive Services Task Force: *Ann Family Pract* 42(1):136, 1990

vices Task Force, 1990). Recent studies have demonstrated that the risk of head injuries to bicyclists could be reduced by 80% if bicyclists would wear proper safety helmets (Thompson, Rivara, Thompson, 1988).

Adolescent. As children enter adolescence, they develop greater independence and begin to develop a sense of identity and their own values. In addition, adolescents begin to separate emotionally from their families, and peer groups begin to have a stronger influence.

The struggle toward identity may cause the teenager to experience shyness, fear, and anxiety, with resulting dysfunction at home, at school, or within the peer group. Psychoactive substances, such as drugs and alcohol, may make the world more bearable for the troubled teenager (see Chapter 46). Unfortunately, substances used for this purpose put the adolescent at a high risk for continued alcohol or drug abuse (Rice, Kibbee, 1983; Acee, Smith, 1987; Lowenstein, Hunt, 1990).

Young men between the ages of 15 and 24 are at the greatest risk for drowning, and drowning is the second leading cause of death among adolescents (US Preventive Services Task Force, 1990). Drowning accidents most frequently occur in lakes, rivers, or ponds. These accidents also increase in frequency when alcohol and drugs that affect the CNS are used (Wintermute et al, 1988).

When adolescents learn to drive, their environment expands and so does their potential for injury. The young driver must be taught and expected to comply with rules and regulations regarding use of a car. In addition, 85% of the population lives in states with mandatory seat belt laws (Lowenstein, Hunt 1990). Common rules include proper use of seat belts, abstinence from alcohol, not riding in a car when the driver is under the influence of alcohol or drugs, and setting a time to be home with the car.

Because adolescence is a time when mature sexual physical characteristics develop, adolescents also begin to have physical relationships with other adolescents. They need prompt, correct instruction about abstinence or safe sexual practices and birth control. They also need counseling about peer pressure. Specifically, the nurse determines how teenagers handle constant pressure to participate in sexual or drug-related activities. Many school health programs have instituted the DARE (Drug Abuse Resistance Education) program. This program provides realistic alternatives to peer pressure by providing education and role-playing and increasing self-esteem. Strategies learned in the DARE program can be applied to other areas such as cheating and sexual practices.

Adult. The threats to an adult's safety are frequently related to lifestyle habits. For example, the client who uses alcohol excessively is at greater risk for motor-vehicle accidents (CDC, 1991). The long-term smoker has a greater risk of cardiovascular or pulmonary disease as a result of the inhalation of smoke into the lungs and the effect of nicotine on the circulatory system. Likewise, the adult experiencing a high level of stress is more likely to have an accident or illnesses such as headaches, GI disorders, and infections (see Chapter 26).

Older Adult. Falls are the leading cause of death by injury among older adults (Lowenstein, Hunt, 1990; Urton, 1991). Of all fatal home falls, 70% are experienced by adults over 65 years of age (US Pre-

ventive Services Task Force, 1990). Older clients are more likely to fall in the bedroom, bathroom, and kitchen. These falls most often occur while transferring from beds, chairs, and toilets; getting into or out of bathtubs; tripping over carpet edges or doorway thresholds; slipping on wet surfaces; and descending stairs (Tideiskaar, 1989). The physiological changes that occur during the aging process increase the client's risks for falls (see box). Some of these changes, such as slowed response time and sensory impairments, can increase the older client's risk for automobile accidents and burns.

OTHER RISK FACTORS. Other risk factors include lifestyle, mobility, sensory impairments, and safety awareness.

Lifestyle. Lifestyle can increase safety risks. At greater risk of injury are people who drive or operate machinery while under the influence of chemical substances, who work at inherently dangerous jobs, and who are risk-takers or daredevils. In addition,

---

Physiological Changes that Increase the Risk of Falls

- Arthritic changes affecting range of motion, balance, and weight bearing
- Decreased circulation in the brain, causing dizziness and fainting
- Mechanical obstruction of vertebral arteries to the brain, caused by crushed osteoporotic vertebrae
- Decreased auditory acuity
- Decreased night vision, color vision, and visual acuity
- Orthostatic hypotension
- Loss of sense of position
- Diminished space perception
- Decreased muscle mass, strength, and coordination or hemiparesis or hemiparalysis
- Decreased ability to balance
- Osteoporosis and increased stress on weight-bearing areas, resulting in an unsteady gait and susceptibility to fractures
- Decreased muscle activity necessary for adequate venous return
- Decreased capacity of blood vessels
- Slowed nervous system response
- Changes in metabolism, which affect the rate of drug metabolism and the systemic effects of medications

Modified from Tideiksarr R: *Geriatr Nurs* 116:280, 1989; and Witte NS: *Am J Nurs* 79:1950, 1979.

people experiencing stress, anxiety, fatigue, or alcohol or drug withdrawal or taking prescribed medications may be more accident prone. Because of these factors, clients may be too preoccupied to notice the source of potential accidents such as cluttered stairs or a stop sign.

Mobility. A client with impaired mobility has many kinds of safety risks. First, immobilization itself can predispose the person to other physiological and emotional hazards, which in turn can further restrict mobility and independence (see Chapter 43). A client with impaired mobility is at risk for injury when entering motor vehicles and buildings that are not equipped for the handicapped.

Sensory Impairments. Clients with visual, hearing, or communication impairments, such as aphasia, illiteracy, or language barriers, are at greater risk for injury in the community. Such clients may not be able to perceive a potential danger or express needs for assistance (see Chapter 45).

Safety Awareness. Some clients are unaware of safety precautions, such as keeping medicine away from children or reading the expiration date on food products. A complete nursing assessment should help the nurse identify the client's level of knowledge regarding home safety so that deficiencies can be corrected with an individualized nursing care plan.

Health Care Agency

The basic types of risks to a client's safety within the health care environment are falls, client-inherent accidents, procedure-related accidents, and equipment-related accidents. The nurse learns to recognize factors associated with these four potential problem areas and to take steps to prevent or minimize accidents in the agency.

High-Risk Conditions Leading to Falls in Hospitals

HIGH-RISK CONDITIONS

- Neurological disorders
- Parkinsonism
- Brain tumor
- Seizure disorder
- Cerebrovascular accident
- Head injury
- Spinal cord injury
- Multiple sclerosis
- Mental status deterioration
- Confusion
- Disorientation
- Depression
- Mental retardation
- Dementia, organic brain syndrome, Alzheimer's disease

PHARMACOLOGICAL AGENTS

- Tranquilizers
- Sedatives
- Anesthesia
- Diuretics
- Antidysrhythmics

DEBILITATING DISEASE

- Anemia
- Pulmonary disease
- Coronary artery disease

DEBILITATING DISEASE—CONT'D

- Cushing's syndrome
- Diabetes mellitus
- Cancer (especially metastatic cancer)

DIFFICULTIES WITH GAIT OR LOCOMOTION

- Use of walker, cane, crutches, or wheelchair
- Prosthesis
- Dizziness
- Hemiparesis, hemiparalysis

DEBILITATION

- Hospital-acquired: bowel preparation, invasive procedures, postoperative status
- Natural: restrictive pain, diminished caloric intake, prolonged bed rest

SENSORY DEFICITS

- Blindness, cataracts
- Eye patches
- Hearing loss
- Hemiplegia
- Paraplegia
- Quadriplegia
- Decreased space perception
- Language barrier

Modified from Rubenstein LZ et al: *Ann Intern Med* 113:308, 1990; Gehlsen GM, Whaley MH: *Arch Phys Med Rehabil* 71:739, 1990; and Lynn FH: *Am J Nurs* 80:1098, 1980.

An accident necessitates the filing of an **incident report,** a confidential document that completely describes any client accident occurring on the premises of a health care agency (see Chapter 14). It documents the accident, any reactions by or effects on the client, and treatment performed for the client. In addition to completing the incident report, the nurse must document the accident in the client's medical record and describe its effects on the client's health status.

Falls. Falls account for 29% to 89% of all incidents reported in hospitals (Whedon, Sheed, 1989). About 10% to 20% of falls in hospitals, extended care facilities, and nursing homes result in serious injury, and 2% to 6% of those who fall have a fracture (Rubenstein et al, 1990). Falls result from slipping or sliding, knees buckling under, fainting, or tripping over tubes, equipment, or furniture. A client can fall from the bed, wheelchair, toilet, or commode or can fall while walking. The occurrence of falls increases during the evening and night. Risk factors include age, degree of physical or mental debility, psychomotor status, and use of medications (see box).

Jankin, Reynolds, and Swiech (1986) have investigated client falls in acute, long-term, and home settings (see research highlight). Reduction in the risks and frequency of falls reduces complications, length of stay, and the client's ultimate limits of independence. In addition, the hospital-based Risk Assessment Tool for falls has been developed and modified for use in hospitals (Brians, 1991). This instrument is a two-part checklist that identifies clients' potential for falling. The instruments are easily used and incorporated within the nursing assessment (see box on p. 1440 at bottom).

When delivering nursing care in the home, the nurse must also assess this environment for risk of falls (see box). Assessment and subsequent prevention of falls reduce the chance for further physical impairments to the client. In addition, family members and friends are also protected from injury. The prevention of injury to the primary care giver in the home also reduces future hospitalization of the client.

Client-Inherent Accidents. **Client-inherent accidents** are accidents other than falls in which the client is the primary factor. Examples of client-inherent accidents are self-inflicted cuts, injuries, and burns; ingestion or injection of foreign substances; self-mutilation or fire setting; and pinching fingers in drawers or doors.

The nurse must file a complete and accurate incident report for client-inherent injuries. A thorough report describing the incident and the client's physical and behavioral status is necessary for studying risk factors within the agency that require preventive action and for protecting the institution and health care professionals from any subsequent lawsuits (see Chapter 14).

Procedure-Related Accidents. A procedure-related accident occurs during therapy. They include medication and fluid administration errors, improper application of external devices, and accidents related to improper performance of procedures, such as dressing changes.

The nurse can prevent many procedure-related accidents. For example, correct administration of medications, using the "five rights" described in Chapter 21, helps prevent medication errors. In addition, proper administration of IV fluids prevents fluid overload or deficit (see Chapter 39). Also, injury from the introduction of pathogens is reduced when surgical asepsis is used for sterile dressing changes (see Chapter 18) or invasive procedures, such as insertion of a Foley catheter (see Chapter 40). Finally, correct use of body mechanics and transfer techniques reduces the risk of injuries from transfer procedures (see Chapter 43).

Equipment-Related Accidents. **Equipment-related accidents** result from the malfunction, disrepair, or misuse of equipment or from an electrical hazard. To avoid injury, the nurse should not operate

---

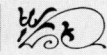

Research Highlight

Jankin, Reynolds, and Swiech conducted a chart review on two groups of clients. Clients 60 years of age and older who fell during hospitalization ($N = 331$) were compared with a random sample of clients 60 years of age and older who were hospitalized during the same period but did not fall ($N = 300$). For both groups, 2 days of hospital record review was sampled. In the fall group, record review included admission day and the day preceding the fall. For the group of clients who did not fall, their admission day and a random hospital day were reviewed.

The study identified seven statistically significant variables that increased the risk of injury. The significant variables included general weakness, decreased mobility of lower extremities, sleeplessness, incontinence, confusion, depression, and substance abuse. Many of these variables have also been supported by other nursing research studies (Innes, Thurman, 1983; Nickens, 1985; Perry, 1982).

Jankin JK, Reynolds BA, Swiech K: Patient falls in the acute care setting: identifying risk factors, *Nurs Res* 35:214, 1986.

Checklist for Electrical Hazards

- Loose control knobs
- Ungrounded equipment
- Frayed cords or cords improperly taped to floor
- Circuits overloaded by too many appliances in one area
- Improperly functioning equipment
- Use of extension cords
- Tangled or cluttered cords
- Use of electrical appliances near sink, bathtub, shower, or damp areas

From Top D: *Insuring electrical safety in the critical care setting,* New York, 1987, American Journal of Nursing Co. Educational Services Division.

monitoring or therapy equipment without instruction.

A checklist should be used to assess potential electrical hazards to reduce the risk of electrical fires, electrocution, or injury from improperly wired equipment (see box at left).

 Nursing Diagnosis

Nursing diagnoses identify risks to the client's safety based on the data provided by the nursing assessment. Assessment reveals clusters of data that indicate when a client has an actual or potential risk to safety (see diagnoses box). General categories involve threats related to poisoning, inhalants, pollutants, or trauma.

The nursing diagnostic statement identifies the expected cause (for example, impaired vision, sub-

---

Home Assessment for Falls

HOME EXTERIOR

- Are sidewalks uneven?
- Are steps in good repair?
- Do steps have handrails?
- Are handrails securely fastened?
- Is there adequate lighting?
- Can client sit down and get up from outdoor furniture easily?

HOME INTERIOR

- Are lights bright enough to compensate for limited vision?
- Are there enough night-lights to improve vision during darkness?
- Do area rugs have secure rubber backings?
- Are rooms uncluttered to permit mobility?
- Do chairs and stools provide sufficient support for sitting down and getting up?
- Is temperature within a comfortable range (65° to 75° F)?
- Do thresholds impair mobility?

Stairs

- Are stairways well lighted?
- Are steps in good repair?
- Are step edges clearly marked with colored tape?
- Are handrails available on both sides of stairways?
- Are handrails securely fastened to walls?

Kitchen

- If there is a gas stove, is the pilot light in good repair?
- Are chairs of proper height for ease in sitting down and getting up?
- Are storage areas easily reached?
- Are floors slippery?
- Is there adequate light?
- Are mats nonskid?

Bathroom

- Is there a mat or skidproof strips in the bathtub or shower?
- Do the bathtub and toilet have grab bars nearby?
- Will the client need an elevated toilet seat to get on and off easily?
- Is the medicine cabinet well lighted?

Bedroom

- Are the bed and chairs of adequate height to allow for getting on and off easily?
- Are rugs and carpets nonskid or well anchored to the floor?
- Are night-lights available?
- Are light switches accessible?
- Is there adequate lighting?

From Tideiksaar R: *Home Healthc Nurse* 4(2):21, 1986; and Tideiksaar R: *Geriatr Nurs* 11(6):280, 1989.

stance abuse, or side effects of prescribed medications). While developing the nursing diagnostic statement, the nurse must ensure that the appropriate defining characteristics are present in the assessment data base (see diagnostic process box).

Planning

The nurse plans therapeutic interventions for clients with actual or potential risks to safety (see care plan on p. 1442). The nurse plans therapies according to severity of risks to the client, and the plan is individualized according to developmental stage, level of health, and client and family lifestyle.

It is important to consider the client's home when planning therapies to maintain or improve level of safety. Reinforcement of good health habits improves compliance with the care plan.

Planning care also involves an understanding of the client's need to maintain independence. The nurse and the client work together to establish ways of maintaining client involvement in nursing care and to create a safe environment in the hospital and home.

Implementation

Nursing interventions are directed at maintaining the client's safety in the home and the health care agency. Because most nursing measures are applicable in both environments, the interventions are presented in two sections: developmental considerations and environmental protection. The first category of

interventions includes those specifically for reducing risks for each developmental age group. Environmental interventions are developed to modify the environment so that present or potential hazards are eliminated or minimized.

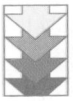

Examples of Nursing Diagnoses for Safety Risks

NANDA-APPROVED NURSING DIAGNOSES

High risk for poisoning related to:
- Improperly prepared or stored foods
- Accessibility of medications, household cleaners, or poisonous plants to children
- Impaired vision

High risk for suffocating related to:
- Use of outdated or broken infant cribs or playpens
- Improperly vented furnace

High risk for trauma related to:
- Cluttered home environment
- High-crime area
- Improper or inadequate lighting

Altered thought processes related to:
- Substance abuse
- Side effects of prescribed medications
- Sensory overload

Impaired home maintenance management related to:
- Limited financial resources
- Physical inability to maintain surroundings

Knowledge deficit related to:
- Unfamiliarity with child-care safety
- Environmental safety

High risk for altered body temperature related to:
- Exposure to temperature extremes

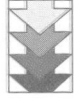

Sample Nursing Diagnostic Process for Safety Risks

Assessment Activities	Defining Characteristics	Nursing Diagnosis
Observe client's mobility in the home.	Client has uncoordinated gait and complains of muscle fatigue.	*High risk for injury* related to poorly lighted and cluttered home environment
	Client frequently bumps into furniture.	
Ask client about visual acuity.	Client reports difficulty with night vision and seeing objects in poorly lighted areas.	
Observe client's home for hazards and obstacles.	Home has poorly lighted, narrow hallways.	
	End tables are unsteady and cluttered.	
	Rugs on floors are not secured.	

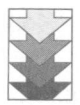

Nursing diagnosis: *High risk* for injury related to poorly lighted and cluttered home environment
Definition: High risk for injury is the state in which an individual is at risk for injury as a result of environmental conditions interacting with the individual's adaptive and defensive resource (Kim, McFarland, McLane, 1991).

Goal	Expected Outcome	Interventions	Rationale
Client will be able to state and change potential risks for injury in home in 72 hr.	Client will list hazards within home by end of third teaching session.	Give three 20-min teaching sessions on identifying and avoiding hazards or falls and injuries, and increasing safety.	Counseling and teaching sessions increase client's awareness of hazards (US Preventive Services Task Force, 1990).
	After 3 mo, client will modify hazards by 50%.	Complete home assessment (nurse and client) to identify potential risk to safety.	Thorough review of potential hazards can increase client's knowledge of risk preventions (Tideiksaar, 1989; Urton, 1991).
	After 6 mo, client will modify 100% of hazards.	Secure safety bars on bathtub and shower area.	Grab bars and nonslick surfaces reduce risk of falls (Tideiksaar, 1989).
		Place at least 75-watt bulbs in all fixtures.	Improving lighting changes environmental hazards and reduces risk of falling (Tideiksaar, 1989).

Client Teaching for Preventing Accidents in the Home*

OBJECTIVE

- Parents will discuss child-proofing measures for home.

TEACHING STRATEGIES

- Discuss with parents child-proofing of home, which becomes necessary when the child begins to be mobile while learning to scoot, crawl, pull up to standing positions, and move around while holding onto the furniture, at about 6 months of age.
- Tell parents that young children, particularly infants and toddlers, learn about their environment by putting everything into their mouths and by touching and smelling.
- Inform parents that child-proofing is securing or removing anything from the home that could hurt child or that a child could hurt. Tell parents to place out of reach all cleaning fluids, paint, matches, guns, sharp tools, plastic bags, poisonous houseplants, insecticides, petroleum products (e.g., gasoline, charcoal, lighter fluid), household cleaning products (e.g., dishwasher detergent, bleach, ammonia), and electrical cords that child could chew or use to pull objects (e.g., lamps, coffee pots) onto the child. "Out of reach" for the toddler and preschooler may mean locking cabinet doors and placing objects out of sight because the child can easily move chairs and climb to places that were secure for the infant.

- Instruct parents that, in the bathroom, cosmetics, mouthwash, soap, razors and blades, deodorizers, hair dryers, and electric curlers must be out of reach.
- Tell parents that all electrical outlets not in place should have plug guards.
- Instruct parents to flush any unused prescription drugs down the toilet and to keep medications in safety-capped bottles and a locked box, drawer, or cabinet.
- Tell parents that child should not be allowed access to mother's purse because of potentially harmful substances (e.g., cosmetics, coins, medications).
- Inform parents that small objects (e.g., buttons, coins, beads, nuts, popcorn, parts of toys, such as wheels) must be safely stored.
- Encourage parents to use gates to prevent child access to stairs and parts of home that are unsafe.
- Inform parents to protect child from fireplaces, freestanding heaters, and floor furnaces by using safety screens or other devices.
- Instruct parents to keep syrup of Ipecac and directions for its administration in locked medicine cabinet in case of poisoning and to post the telephone number for the Poison Control Center at the phone.

EVALUATION

- Ask parents to describe measures they have already taken to child-proof their homes and additional ones they will implement.

*Developed by Janice Rumfelt, Assistant Professor, School of Nursing, Southern Illinois University at Edwardsville.

Developmental Considerations

INFANT, TODDLER, AND PRESCHOOLER. Infants and preschoolers depend on adults to protect them from injury. Growing children are curious and completely trusting of their environment and do not perceive themselves to be in danger.

Nurses are frequently in a position to educate parents or guardians about reducing risks of injuries for young children (see teaching box). Nurses working in prenatal clinics can easily incorporate safety into the care plan of the childbearing family. Community health nurses can assess the home and show parents how to promote safety in their homes (Table 42-2 on p. 1444). The nurse can teach the child and the parents about safety (Figs. 42-1 and 42-2).

SCHOOL-AGE CHILD. School-age children increasingly explore their environment. They have friends outside their immediate neighborhood, they may walk to school, and they become more active in school, church, and community activities. All of these activities help the child develop social skill and independence, but they also increase the risk of injury, such as from falls from playground equipment and sports injuries. The school-ager begins to align some activities with those of the adult, learning from parents, teachers, and often television heroes. This patterning of behavior and activities is not necessarily a threat to the child, except when the child imitates an adult behavior that presents safety risks (for example, operating an electric saw). Some nursing interventions help guide the parent to provide for the safety of the school-age child (Table 42-2).

Approximately 20% of school-age children are also at risk for depression (Rhyne et al, 1986). Loss and impaired parent-child relationships are primary causes. Children commonly exhibit depression through apathy and changes in appetite, sleeping, and activity levels. Prompt recognition results in prompt intervention in the form of family or individual counseling or support groups.

ADOLESCENT. When children approach their adolescent years, much of their time is spent away from home and with their peer group. During adolescence, young people learn to drive. Risks to the adolescent's safety therefore involve many factors outside the home environment. Adults serve as role models for adolescents and through example and education can help adolescents minimize risks to their safety. The box lists measures by which nurses and parents can help the adolescent prevent accidents.

Adolescents' adjustment to responsibilities and changes in their bodies may result in mood swings, withdrawal, or even depression. In addition, this age group has a high incidence of suicide because of de-

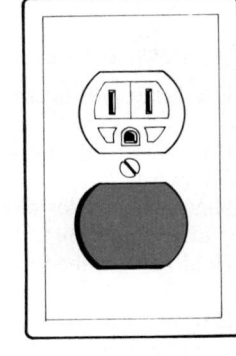

Fig. 42-1 Safety covers for electrical outlets.

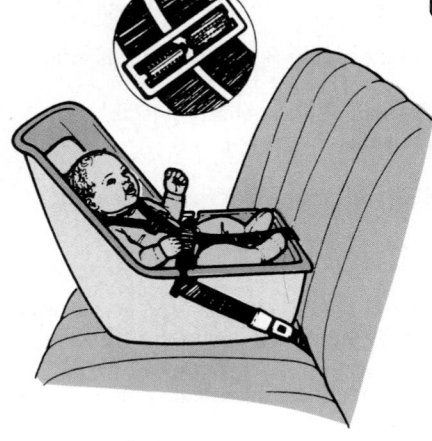

Fig. 42-2 Infant car seat.
From Whaley LF, Wong DL: *Nursing care of infants and children*, ed 4, St Louis, 1991, Mosby–Year Book.

Measures for Adolescents to Prevent Accidents

- Enroll teenagers in driver's education courses and make practice drives with them in good and bad weather. Teach them to handle a motor vehicle in a skid. Teach them to adhere to driving regulations and speed limits.
- Teach them to wear seat belts while driving or while riding as passengers.
- Instruct them not to drive after using psychoactive drugs or enter an automobile when the driver has been using such drugs.
- Form a contract with teenagers that stipulates that if they drink at a party, they can call home for a ride with no questions asked.
- Help teenagers develop safe eating, sleeping, and relaxation habits.
- Inform them of the dangers of psychoactive drugs.
- Recognize changes in adolescents' behavior and mood.
- Listen to adolescents.
- Do not try to be a buddy. Remain a parent.

TABLE 42-2 Nursing Interventions to Promote Safety*

Intervention	Rationale

INFANTS, TODDLERS, AND PRESCHOOLERS

Intervention	Rationale
Use large, soft toys without plastic eyes, nose, or mouth.	Small parts can be dislodged by baby, and accidental aspiration can occur.
If playpen with mesh sides is used, do not leave one side down.	Baby's head can become wedged between playpen pad and lowered mesh side, and asphyxiation can occur.
Never leave sides of crib down or turn away from baby on changing table.	Child can suddenly roll and fall from crib or changing table.
Hold baby at feeding time; do not prop bottle.	This increases bonding with parent and reduces risk of choking.
If formula is used, be sure to read instructions. Most formulas must be diluted with water.	Using undiluted formula can cause fluid and electrolyte imbalances in newborn.
Discontinue use of infant seat at 3 mo or earlier if infant is very mobile.	At 3 mo, active infants may be able to propel themselves out of seat and fall.
Baby-proof house for small objects, sharp objects, and toxic and poisonous substances.	Babies explore their world with their hands and mouth, and ingestion of small objects can result in choking. Toxic and poisonous substances require prompt action.
Cover electrical outlets with protective covers (see Fig. 42-1).	Electrical wall outlets are at baby's eye level and stimulate curiosity. Crawling baby will frequently attempt to play with electrical wall plates regardless of number of toys available.
Use guardrails at top and bottom of stairs and at doorway of rooms considered off-limits to crawling or walking toddler.	This prevents child from falling down stairs or being exposed to rooms with unguarded dangers.
Never leave baby unattended in infant seat, walker, stroller, or high chair.	Active child can easily slide out of these devices and fall.
Never leave baby or child unattended in bath or wading pool.	Accidental drowning may occur.
Never attach pacifier to child with string around neck.	String can easily become tangled, and strangulation can result.
Restrain child in back seat of automobile. Child under 4 should be in approved car seat (see Fig. 42-2). Older children should be restrained with seat belt.	In event of sudden stop or auto accident, unrestrained child is bounced against hard, sharp surfaces of the vehicle's interior, and injuries result.
Plastic bags, such as those for storing fruit or dry cleaning, should be removed from home.	If child places these items over head, air supply decreases, and child suffocates.
Install on doors strong dead-bolt locks well beyond toddler's reach, even when child is standing on chair.	This prevents child from leaving home without parents' knowledge, reducing danger of child getting lost, freezing to death, falling into swimming pool, or being abducted.
Use the words *no* and *don't* to convey that object or action increases child's risk of injury, such as playing with matches.	Improperly using these words renders them meaningless to child.
Teach child to swim at early age, but always provide supervision.	Child is able to enjoy the water safely. Child who knows how to swim can still encounter difficulty in water and needs supervision.
Teach child to cross street and to walk in parking lots.	This provides child with self-protection against dangers from automobiles.
Teach child not to talk to or accept anything from stranger and to notify parents or responsible adult if approached by stranger.	This reduces risk of injury or abduction by stranger. Reporting stranger's presence helps law-enforcement personnel investigate and remove threat.
Do not allow child to run with sucker or popsicle in mouth.	Child may fall and stick from sucker or popsicle can cause puncture injury or foreign body in airway.
Impress on child not to eat anything found on street or in grass.	Substance may be poisonous and can cause severe illness.
Use back burners on stoves and get into habit of turning pot handles toward wall.	This reduces risk of child pulling down pot of hot liquid and being burned.
Remove doors from unused refrigerators and freezers, and instruct child not to hide in these items.	Door may latch and on older models cannot be released from inside; as result, asphyxiation can occur.

*Data from Whaley LF, Wong DL: *Nursing care of infants and children*, ed 4, St Louis, 1991, Mosby–Year Book.

TABLE 42-2 Nursing Interventions to Promote Safety*—cont'd

Intervention	Rationale

SCHOOL-AGE CHILD†

Teach child the safe use of equipment for play and work activities.

Teach child to ride bicycle safely and responsibilities that go with bicycling.

Teach child to wear protective helmet and knee and elbow pads when roller skating.
Never allow child to operate appliances while alone.

If parent chooses to have firearms in house, teach parent to keep them unloaded, locked up, and out of reach.

OLDER ADULT
Stairs

Install treads with uniform depth of 9 in and 9-in risers (vertical face of steps).
Install uniform-textured or plain-colored surfaces on each tread, and mark edge of tread with contrasting color.

Ensure proper lighting of each tread. Block sun or light bulb glare with translucent shades or screens or use lower wattage bulbs.
Ensure adequate head room so that users do not have to duck to use stairs.
Remove protruding objects from staircase walls.

Keep outdoor walkways and stairs in good condition (free of holes, cracks, and splinters) and well lighted.

Handrails

Install smooth but slip-resistant handrails at least 2 in from wall.
Secure handrail firmly so that user's weight is supported, especially at bottom and top of stairway.

Install guard rails in bathroom near toilet and bathtub.

Floor Coverings

Secure all carpeting, mats, and tile; place nonskid backing under area rugs.

Child needs to learn that some equipment is for play and other equipment is for work and that improper use can result in injury.
If bicycling is prohibited on sidewalks, child must learn to obey traffic signals and ride with traffic patterns or identify safe locations for bicycle riding.
When roller skating, child often falls; protective devices reduce risk of serious injury.
If electrical mishap occurs, no one would be available to help child.
This prevents injury from accidental discharge or improper use.

If stairs are of uniform size, older client need not continually adjust vision.
Uniform textures or color helps to decrease vertigo. Marking edge of tread provides obvious visual clue to end of stair.
Older client's vision is unable to adjust quickly to changes in lighting.

Sudden changes in head position may result in dizziness.

Decreased peripheral vision may prevent client from seeing object.
Decreased visual acuity can prevent older client from seeing structural defect.

Distance allows client to grasp handrail firmly for support.

Older client has greatest risk of falling at top and bottom of stairs because center of gravity is being shifted and balance is unstable.
This enables older clients to have support while rising from sitting to standing position.

Sudden slip may cause dizziness and inability of older client to regain balance. Decrease in muscle strength may decrease client's ability to adjust to slip and prevent fall.

†In addition to those appropriate for the school-age child.

---

pression, poor body image, or feelings of decreased self-worth. Suicide has devastating effects on the family because family members are left with feelings of loss, anger, inadequacy, and pain. Nurses can provide emotional support to these families and refer them to counselors and support groups such as Survivors of Suicide (Hoffman, 1987).

ADULT. Risks to young and middle-age adults frequently result from lifestyle factors such as child rearing, high-stress states, inadequate nutrition, excessive alcohol intake, and substance abuse. Adults need to be taught that their safety is threatened and as a result their lifestyle needs to be modified.

Stress-management centers (see Chapter 30) and health-promotion activities (see Chapter 2) have been incorporated into many community service programs and hospitals. In addition, neighborhood centers, community clinics, and outpatient clinics are equipped to assist the adult in modifying lifestyle

---

Steps Older People Can Take to Prevent Accidents

PREVENTING AUTOMOBILE ACCIDENTS

- See your physician if you suspect that you have a hearing problem.
- Leave your car window partially open to help you hear warning signals.
- Set the air conditioner or heater and the radio low so that their noise does not mask outside sounds.
- Place mirrors on both sides of the car, and use them and a wide rear-view mirror when you change lanes or pass other vehicles.
- Stop frequently to stretch your muscles and rest your eyes.
- Schedule regular eye examinations to check for vision changes or health problems that may affect your vision.
- Follow the physician's recommendations, if any, about limiting when and where you drive.
- Before driving, give yourself time to adjust to new lenses, especially bifocals or trifocals.
- Wear good-quality sunglasses to reduce glare. Wear them only during the day.
- Keep the windshield and all windows clean inside and out. Replace worn wiper blades. Keep headlights, tail lights, and turn signals clean to maintain maximum lighting.
- If you take medication, know its long- and short-term effects on your driving ability.
- Do not smoke while driving at night. Smoking impairs vision.
- Do not drive when you have been drinking.
- Enroll in a driver training course through your state motor-vehicle department.
- Take circuitous routes to avoid freeways.

PREVENTING BURNS

- Do not smoke in bed or when sleepy.
- When cooking, do not wear loose-fitting clothing (e.g., bathrobes, nightgowns, pajamas).
- Learn to use a microwave oven.
- Set thermostats for water heater or faucets so that water does not become too hot.
- Install a smoke detector and portable fire extinguisher in the kitchen.
- Change smoke detector batteries on April 1 and October 1.
- Keep access to outside doors unobstructed.
- Identify emergency exits in public buildings.
- Wear clothing that is nonflammable or treated with a permanent flame-retardant finish. Fabrics of animal hair, wool, or silk are less flammable than synthetic fabrics.
- Use several electrical outlets to avoid overloading.

From Cooper S: *Geriatr Nurs* 2:287, 1981.

---

habits that present risks to health (for example, smoking, overeating, lack of exercise, and alcoholism).

OLDER ADULT. Most injuries to the older adult involve falls, auto accidents, and burns. Advancing age and the concurrent physiological changes in vision, hearing, mobility, circulation, and the ability to make quick judgments may predispose some older adults to falls and other accidents. In addition, many medications make falls more likely (Rubenstein et al, 1990). Nursing interventions designed to reduce the risk of falls compensate for the physiological changes of aging (Table 42-2 and box at left).

Older people are more likely to have automobile accidents because of three specific physiological changes. First, changes in visual acuity and depth perception prevent the client from quickly observing situations in which an accident is likely to occur. Second, decreased hearing acuity alters older clients' abilities to hear emergency vehicle sirens or car and truck horns. Third, because of decreased nervous system response, older people may be unable to react as quickly as they once could to avoid an accident (Ebersole, Hess, 1990) (see box at left).

Pedestrian accidents can also be reduced by persuading older adults to wear reflectors on garments when walking at night, stand on the sidewalk and not in the street when waiting to cross a street, always cross at corners and not in the middle of the block (particularly if the street is a major one), cross with the traffic light and not against it, and look left, right, and left again before entering the street or crosswalk.

Burns and scalds are also more apt to occur with older people, whose risk is increased by several factors. Older people may forget and leave hot water running or become confused when turning the dials on a stove. Impaired visual acuity and sense of smell increase the danger that older people may not detect smoke or gas fumes (Cooper, 1981). Nursing measures developed for preventing burns are designed to minimize the risk from impaired vision and hearing (see box).

Environmental Considerations

GENERAL PREVENTIVE MEASURES. Nurses can contribute to a safer environment by helping the client meet basic physiological and psychosocial needs. Nurses use effective and efficient methods to control pathogen transmission. These include **medical asepsis,** the use of handwashing and environmental cleanliness to reduce the number of pathogens, and **surgical asepsis,** the removal or destruction of disease-causing organisms or infected material (see Chapter 18). Pathogen transmission from person to person can be reduced or prevented by immunization. In the home, awareness of methods of food handling helps reduce the risk of pathogen and parasite transmission through contaminated food.

SPECIFIC SAFETY CONCERNS. Specific safety concerns include falls, fires, poisoning, electrical hazards, and radiation.

Falls. Modifications in the home or health care environment can easily reduce the risk of falls. A heavy or debilitated client in a bed or wheelchair or on a toilet should be properly secured or supported. Excess furniture and equipment should be removed, and clients should wear rubber-soled shoes or slippers for walking or transferring from one device to another. Clients need to be instructed to inspect canes, walkers, and crutches to be sure that the rubber tip is intact.

Safeguards can be implemented or taught to the family to minimize the client's risk of falls (see boxes below and on p. 1448 and Figs. 42-3 and 42-4). In addition, confused, disoriented, very young, or very old clients may require the use of restraints and side rails to protect them from falling out of bed.

RESTRAINTS. A **restraint** is any one of numerous devices used to immobilize a client or an extremity. Physical restraints are any manual method or mechanical device, material, or equipment attached or

adjacent to a client's body that the client cannot easily remove and that restricts freedom of movement or normal access to one's body. The Omnibus Budget Reconciliation Act (OBRA) of 1987 defines clients' rights and choices regarding restraint. Under these guidelines, reasons for use of physical restraint are clearly stated. These include the following (Health Care Financing Administration, 1990):

1. Use of restraints is part of the medical treatment.
2. All less-restrictive interventions are first tried.
3. Other disciplines are used.
4. Supporting documentation is provided.

When the use of restraints is the only intervention available to maintain the client's safety, the client

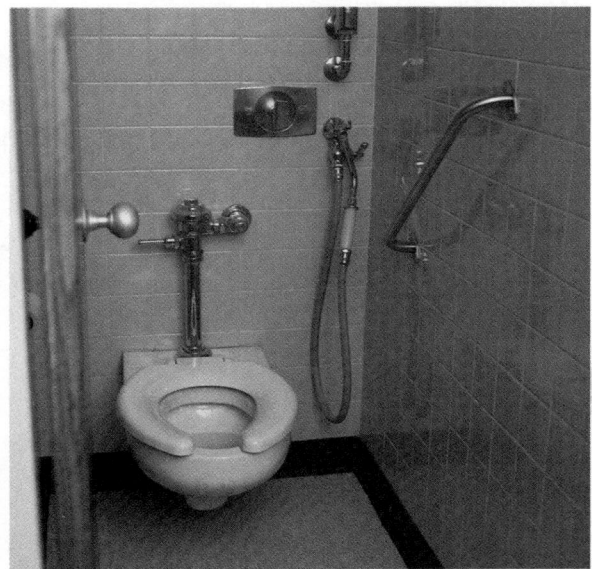

Fig. 42-3   Safety bars around toilets and showers.

Measures to Prevent Falls in the Health Care Agency

- Assess clients at risk for falling (see box on p. 1448).
- Assign clients at risk rooms near the nurses' station.
- Alert all health care personnel to client's increased risk of falling by using a Kardex notation or a sign on the door or over the bed.
- Use night-light in room.
- Reinforce to client and family the need for assistance when ambulating or getting up.
- Keep side rails up.
- Keep call lights easily accessible; answer them promptly.
- Keep client's personal items within easy reach.
- Maintain client's scheduled toileting routine.
- Reassess during each shift the client's risk of falling.
- Observe client frequently.
- Use restraints or sitters properly.

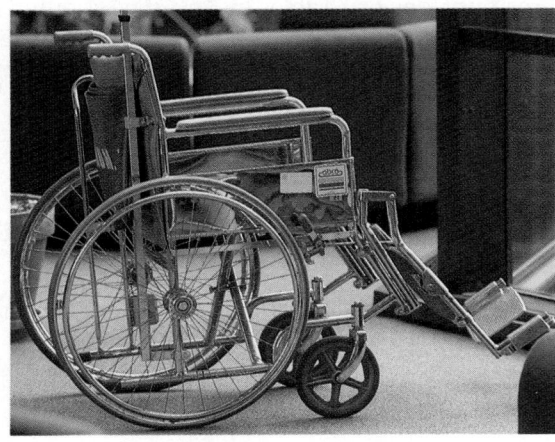

Fig. 42-4   Safety lock on wheelchairs.

Risk for Falls Assessment Tools

TOOL 1: RISK ASSESSMENT TOOL FOR FALLS

Directions: Place a check mark in front of elements that apply to your client. The decision of whether a client is at risk for falls is based on your nursing judgment. Guideline: A client who has a checkmark in front of an element with an asterisk (*) or four or more of the other elements would be identified as at risk for falls.

General Data

___ Age over 60
___ History of falls before admission*
___ Postoperative/admitted for operation
___ Smoker

Physical Condition

___ Dizziness/imbalance
___ Unsteady gait
___ Diseases/other problems affecting weight-bearing joints
___ Weakness
___ Paresis
___ Seizure disorder
___ Impairment of vision
___ Impairment of hearing
___ Diarrhea
___ Urinary frequency

Mental Status

___ Confusion/disorientation*
___ Impaired memory of judgment
___ Inability to understand or follow directions

Medications

___ Diuretics or diuretic effects
___ Hypotensive or CNS suppressants (e.g., narcotic, sedative, psychotropic, hypnotic, tranquilizer, antihypertensive, antidepressant)
___ Medication that increases GI motility (e.g., laxative, enema)

Ambulatory Devices Used

___ Cane
___ Crutches
___ Walker
___ Wheelchair
___ Geriatric (Geri) chair
___ Braces

TOOL 2: REASSESSMENT IS SAFE "KARE" (RISK) TOOL

Directions: Place a check in front of any element that applies to your client. A client who has a check mark in front of any of the first four elements would be identified as at risk for falls. In addition, when a high-risk client has a check mark in front of the element "Use of a wheelchair," the client is considered to be at greater risk for falls.

___ Unsteady gait/dizziness/imbalance
___ Impaired memory or judgment
___ Weakness
___ History of falls
___ Use of a wheelchair

From Brians LK et al: *Rehabil Nurs* 16(2):67, 1991.

---

and family must be prepared for the adjustment to the restraint device (Table 42-3). As with other procedures, the nurse must follow specific guidelines when using restraints (Procedure 42-1 on p. 1450). The overall objectives for restraints follow:

1. To reduce the risk of the client falling out of bed or from a chair or wheelchair
2. To prevent interruption of therapy such as traction, IV infusions, nasogastric tube feeding, or Foley catheter
3. To prevent the confused or combative client from removing any life-support equipment that is needed
4. To reduce the risk of injury to others by the client

When used correctly, restraints benefit the client. For legal purposes the nurse must be familiar with agency policy and procedures for the appropriate use of restraints. Most institutions require a physician's order. When making an independent judgment to apply restraints, the nurse documents the assessment of the client's activity and behavior, the conclusions about the client's status, the nursing action, and the fact that the action was explained to the client and family. In addition, the nurses' notes specify the type of restraint selected and body part where the restraints were applied.

Establishing a Restraint-Free Environment for Client Safety . Careful planning and education enable nursing staff to provide a safe environment without the

TABLE 42-3   Guidelines for the Use of Restraints

Guideline	Rationale
Restraint should be selected to reduce client's movement only as much as necessary.	Overrestraining client so that activities are unduly restricted can worsen hazards of immobility.
If restraint is necessary, nurse should carefully explain to client and family type of restraint and reasons for its use.	Restraint can increase confusion or hostility in client and family. Explanation of restraint can reduce or even prevent some of these negative perceptions.
Restraint should not worsen client's health problem.	Restraints that are too tight can impair circulation to distal extremities.
Restraint should not interfere with treatment.	Restraints placed over IV sites can impede flow of fluid into circulation. Restraints attached to fractured or dislocated extremities can impair healing.
Bony prominences should be padded before applying restraint.	Padding reduces risk of injury to skin from pressure.
Restraints should be changed when they become soiled or damp.	Soiled or damp restraints increase risk of skin breakdown.
Restraints should be secured in such manner that they cannot be undone by client.	When client is able to undo restraints, purpose of restraint is negated.
Restraint applied to client in bed should be attached to bed frame (see Step 9 illustration in Procedure 42-1), not side rails.	Release of side rails while restraint remains attached can result in injury to client's musculoskeletal system.
Restraints should be removed every 2 hr. Client should not be left unattended.	Removal provides oppotunity to assess skin integrity and provide skin care, often by massaging areas on which restraints were applied. Previously restrained client who is left unattended can cause self-injury or can injure others.
Circulation checks should be performed frequently (up to every hr) when extremity restraints are used.	Checks reduce risk of vascular extremity injury from poor distal circulation resulting from tightening of restraint.

use of restraints. Inherent to this plan are organizational strategies to schedule breaks and lunches to optimize the number of nurses available at any time. Second, a policy to answer call lights in a timely manner reduces clients' risk of falling because they attempt to get out of bed on their own (Haley, Nagy, Roberts, 1991; Brower, 1991).

Third, reduction of environmental risks (for example, improving poor lighting, strengthening unsteady furniture, attaching stabilizer bars to wheelchairs, and placing stop signs on restricted areas) reduces the need for restraints (Cutchins, 1991). Finally, designing therapeutic interventions reduces the risk of accidents and incidents.

Side Rails. Chapter 43 discusses side rails as a device for increasing the client's mobility and stability when in bed or when moving from bed to chair. Side rails also help prevent the unconscious client from falling out of bed or from a stretcher (Fig. 42-5). However, the use of side rails for a disoriented client may cause only more confusion and further injury. Frequently a confused client who is determined to

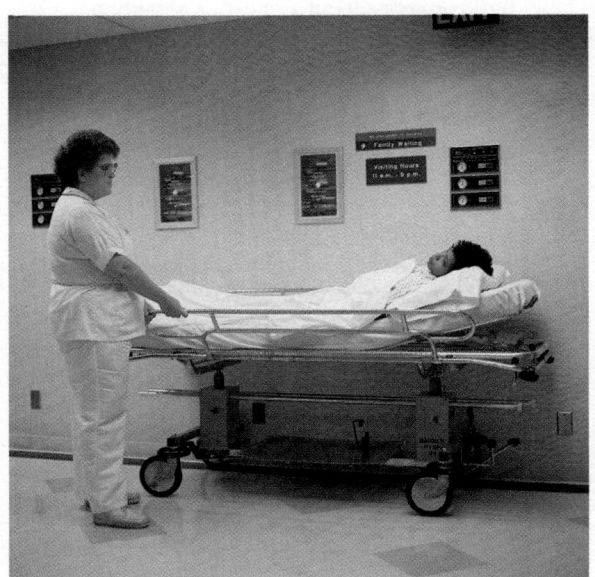

Fig. 42-5 Side rails in the up position on a stretcher.

Applying Restraints

STEPS

RATIONALE

1. Identify client whose safety is maintained by use of restraints: confused or disoriented client, client requiring immobilization of extremity, child requiring immobilization of elbow joint to prevent dislodgment of therapeutic equipment.

Physical restraints are used to reduce risk of client falling out of bed, chair, or wheelchair; prevent interruption of therapy (e.g., traction, IV infusions, nasogastric tube feedings); prevent confused or combative client from injuring self by removing Foley catheters, surgical drains, or life support equipment; and reduce risk of injury to others by client.

2. Check physician's order and assess type of restraint needed.

Aids in determining type of restraint to use. Physician's order protects nurse from liability.

3. Explain carefully to client and family reasons restraint is necessary, type of restraint selected, and anticipated duration of restraint.

Restraints can increase confusion or combativeness in client. In addition, family may express anger about restraint. Explanation and reinforcement can reduce or even prevent some of these negative perceptions.

4. Prepare following equipment:
   a. Proper restraint
   b. Padding

Ensures organized procedure.

Protects circulation to distal portion of extremity if wrist or ankle restraints are selected.

5. Wash hands.

Reduces transmission of microorganisms.

6. Pad bony prominences before applying restraint.

Decreases injury to underlying skin.

7. Apply selected restraint. Review manufacturer's directions to apply restraints listed in Steps 7a-7f.
   a. Jacket restraint: vestlike garment that usually crosses in back of client but may also cross in front (see Fig. 43-19).

   Restrains client while lying or reclining in bed and while sitting in chair or wheelchair. Is useful in home care but should not be used unless other methods to maintain safety have failed.

   b. Belt restraint: Device that secures client on stretcher (see illustration). Avoid placing belt too tightly across client's chest or abdomen.

   Restrains center of gravity and prevents client from rolling off stretcher or sitting up while on stretcher.

   c. Extremity restraints (ankle or wrist restraint): restraint designed to immobilize one or all extremities. Commercially available limb restraints are composed of sheepskin and foam pad that comes in contact with skin. *Modification* of commercial restraint can be devised by making clove hitch restraint, strip of cloth that does not tighten if client pulls against it. Clove hitch is made in two steps. Make figure eight with strip of cloth, and then pick up loops (see illustrations). Before attaching restraint to client's limbs, place gauze or padding around extremity to be restrained and then place loops of clove hitch directly over padded surface (see illustration).

   Maintains immobilization of extremity to protect client from injury from fall or accidental removal of therapeutic device (e.g., IV tube or Foley catheter).

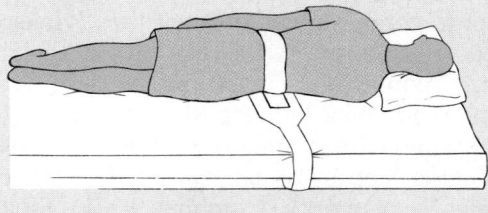

Step 7b

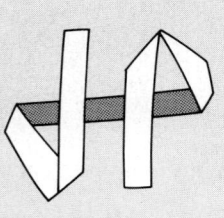
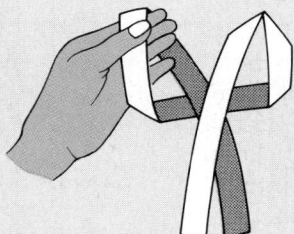
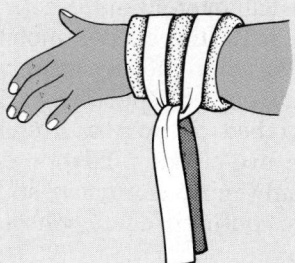

Step 7c

CONTINUED

STEPS	RATIONALE
d. Mitten restraint: thumbless mitten devices (see illustration) to restrain client's hands.	Prevents clients from dislodging invasive equipment, removing dressings, or scratching.
e. Elbow restraint: piece of fabric with slots in which tongue blades are placed so that elbow joint remains rigid (see illustration).	Used with infants and children to prevent elbow flexion.
f. Mummy restraint: blanket or sheet opened on bed or crib, with one corner folded toward center. Child is placed on blanket with shoulders at fold with feet toward opposite corner. With child's right arm straight down against the body, right side of blanket is pulled firmly across right shoulder and chest and secured beneath left side of body. Left arm is placed straight against side, and left side of blanket is brought across shoulder and chest and locked beneath child's body on right side. Lower corner is folded and brought over body and tucked or fastened securely with safety pins (Whaley, Wong, 1991).	Maintains short-term restraint of small child or infant for examination or treatment involving head and neck. Mummy device effectively controls movement of child's torso and extremities.

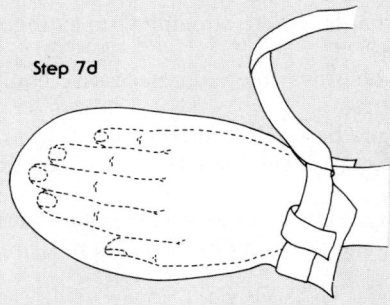

Step 7d

STEPS	RATIONALE
8. Secure restraints so that they cannot be undone by client.	When client is able to undo restraints, purpose of restraint is negated.
9. Attach restraints applied to client in bed or on stretcher to bed frame (see illustration), not side rails.	Release of side rails while restraint remains attached can result in injury to client's musculoskeletal system.
10. Wash hands.	Reduces transmission of microorganisms.
11. Completely remove restraints at least every 2 hr for 30 min. Client should not be left unattended.	Provides opportunity to assess skin integrity and provide skin care. Areas on which restraints were applied are often massaged.
12. Assess adequacy of restraint and presence of any potential injury to musculoskeletal system every 2 hr. Observe color of extremity and palpate pulses below extremity.	Enables nurse to routinely observe musculoskeletal system and prevent complications from restraint device.
13. Observe for correct application of restraint every 2 hr.	Incorrect application of restraints can result in injury to client's musculoskeletal system from falls or muscle strains.
14. Record in nurses' notes nursing assessment before and after restraints are used and each time they are checked, focusing on client's safety and level of orientation, type of restraint selected, and response to restraint.	Documents that client's physical safety was at risk and that specific restraint was warranted.

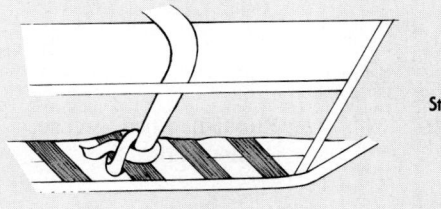

Step 7e

Step 9

Fire-Containment Guidelines

- Know the telephone number for reporting a fire and be sure the number is attached to all telephones.
- Know the agency's or unit's fire drill or fire evacuation routine.
- Know location of fire alarms.
- Post accurate, easy-to-follow routes to fire exits.
- Know where fire extinguishers are, how to use them, and which type of extinguisher to use for a specific fire (Table 42-6).
- Report a fire before attempting to extinguish it, regardless of its size.
- Keep hallways free of unnecessary equipment or furniture.
- Keep fire hoses clear at all times.
- Periodically check the efficiency of fire extinguishers.
- Post signs on the outside of elevators warning people to take the stairs in the event of a fire.

get out of bed attempts to climb over the side rail or climbs out at the foot of the bed. Either attempt usually results in a fall. Thus for the confused client, a jacket restraint is often used with elevated side rails.

Fires. The home and hospital are always at risk for fires. Accidental home fires typically result from smoking in bed, careless extinguishing of cigarette butts in trash cans, grease fires, or electrical fires resulting from faulty wiring or appliances. Institutional fires typically result from a client smoking in bed or from an electrical or anesthetic-related fire.

The interventions described here are directed toward fires occurring in health care agencies, but the same principles apply for fires in the home. It is important to have a plan of action in the event of fire (see box).

If a fire occurs in a health care agency, the nurse protects clients from injury, reports the location of the fire, and contains the fire. On observing a fire, the nurse should immediately report its exact location. The nurse may then attempt to extinguish the fire if there is no immediate threat to clients.

When hospital or institutional fires occur, all personnel are mobilized to evacuate clients. Clients who

TABLE 42-4 Types of Fire Extinguishers and Their Uses

Type	Class of Fire	How to Use	Precautions
Carbon dioxide	Grease, electrical	Direct carbon dioxide into flame, cutting off fire's oxygen supply.	
Soda and acid (water extinguisher)	Paper and rubbish, wood	Turn canister upside down, mixing soda and acid. Carbon dioxide is then produced, releasing water extinguisher under pressure. To stop flow, turn canister right side up.	Ineffective against grease and electrical fires because it causes grease to spatter, spreading fire, and because water conducts electricity
Dry chemical	Rubbish, electrical	Pull pin or press lever on extinguisher, blanketing fire with foam and cutting off fire's oxygen supply.	Ineffective against grease because it causes grease to spatter, spreading fire
Water pump	Rubbish, wood	Pump handle while pointing nozzle toward fire.	Ineffective against grease and electrical fires because grease can spatter, spreading fire, and because water conducts electricity
Antifreeze or water	Rubbish, wood, grease, anesthetics	Pull pin and handle of extinguisher and direct extinguisher toward fire.	Ineffective against electrical fires because water conducts electricity

are close to the fire, regardless of its size, are at risk of injury and should be moved to another area. If a client is receiving oxygen but not life support, the nurse discontinues the oxygen, which is combustible and can fuel an existing fire. If the client is on life support, the nurse may need to maintain the client's respiratory status manually with an Ambu bag (see Chapter 38) until the client is moved away from the threat of fire. Ambulatory clients can be directed to walk by themselves to a safe area and in some cases may be able to assist in moving clients in wheelchairs. Bedridden clients are generally moved from the scene of a fire by a stretcher, their bed, or a wheelchair. If none of these methods is appropriate, clients must be carried from the area. If a client must be carried, the nurse should be careful not to overextend physical limits for lifting because injury to the nurse can result in further injury to the client. If fire department personnel are on the scene, they can help evacuate the clients.

One helpful acronym for priorities in a fire is *RACE:* rescue, alarm, confine, and extinguish. Rescue and remove all clients from immediate danger. Use the alarm procedure to report the location of the fire. After clients are out of danger and the fire has been reported, personnel must take measures to contain or extinguish the fire (for example, closing doors and windows, turning off oxygen and electrical equipment, and using a fire extinguisher).

The three basic types of fires for which extinguishers are used are paper and rubbish (type A), grease and anesthetic gas (type B), and electrical (type C). The appropriate extinguisher must be used for each type (Table 42-4).

Poisoning. A **poison** is any substance that impairs health or destroys life when ingested, inhaled, or absorbed by the body. Specific antidotes or treatments are available for only some types of poisons. The capacity of body tissue to recover from the poison determines the reversibility of the effect. Poisons can impair the respiratory, circulatory, central nervous, hepatic, GI, and renal systems of the body.

Accidental poisonings are a greater risk for the toddler, preschooler, and young school-age child. The nurse can help parents reduce the risk of accidental poisoning by storing medications in child-resistant containers (US Preventive Services Task Force, 1990). Children's accidental poisonings have also been reduced by limiting the number of tablets in each container. Controlled trials using warning labels such as "Mr. Yuk" stickers do not deter children from playing with hazardous substances. In addition, these stickers do not reduce the risk of accidental poisonings commonly related to suicide attempts or

drug experimentation (Vernberg, Culver-Dickinson, Spyker, 1984; Fergusson et al, 1982; US Preventive Services Task Force, 1990).

Older clients are also at risk for poisoning because diminished eyesight may cause an accidental ingestion of toxic substances. The impaired memory of some older adults may result in accidental overdose of prescribed medications.

In the home the two major sources of poisons are plants and household cleaners. Experts recommend that, when poisoning is suspected, the nurse or family member call a **poison control center,** a facility that provides information regarding all aspects of intoxication, treatment, and referrals. The nurse should teach parents that calling such a center for information before attempting home remedies can save their child's life. Procedure 42-2 on p. 1454 lists accepted interventions for accidental poisonings that the nurse may teach to a parent or guardian.

Electrical Hazards. Much of the equipment used in health care settings is electrical and must be well maintained in a safe condition to prevent electrical hazards. All electrical equipment in the health care agency should be grounded (Top, 1987). The electri-

---

Prevention of Electrical Hazards

- Use only grounded equipment.
- Check electrical equipment for frayed cords or visible signs of damage before use.
- Avoid overloading outlets.
- If extension cords must be used, make sure they are taped to the ground with electrical tape to prevent people from tripping over the cord and pulling out the plug.
- Never pull a plug using the cord. Pull a plug by gripping it firmly and pulling it straight out of the wall socket.
- Send equipment that has been dropped to the biomedical department before reuse.
- Report any shocks experienced while using equipment.
- Believe a client who reports a tingling sensation or shocks from the equipment, and have the equipment evaluated for stray current. If possible, unplug equipment until evaluation takes place.
- If you do not understand how to operate a piece of equipment, ask for assistance.

Modified from Cooper KC: *Focus Crit Care* 10:17, 1983.

Intervening in Accidental Poisonings

STEPS	RATIONALE
1. Identify type and amount of substance ingested.	This information will help to determine correct type and amount of antidote needed for victim.
2. Call poison control center before attempting any intervention.	Poison control centers have all information needed to treat poisoned client or to offer referral to treatment centers. Majority of families have access to poison control centers (Woolf et al, 1987).
3. If instructed to induce vomiting: a. Infants (0-12 mo): under direction of physician. b. Children (1-12 yr): administer 1 tbsp (15 ml) of Ipecac. c. Adults: administer 2 tbsp (30 ml) of Ipecac.	Households should keep syrup of Ipecac in easily accessible place (Woolf et al, 1987). Ipecac causes vomiting and emptying of stomach rather than gagging or retching. Poison control experts recommend these dosages and do not advise inducing vomiting with substances other than Ipecac (Aronow et al, 1985). Vomiting should only be induced under physician's instruction and should not be induced only with ingestion of gasoline or other caustic poisons.
4. Give oral fluids to assist vomiting: a. Children (1-12 yr): 5-15 ml/kg, up to 8 oz of water b. Adults: 16 oz of water	Assists in emptying of stomach and avoids further gagging and retching.
5. If requested to do so, save vomitus and deliver to poison control center.	Laboratory analysis can determine further treatment.
6. Place victim with head turned to side.	Reduces risk of aspiration.
7. *Never* induce vomiting for following substances: lye, household cleaners, grease or petroleum products, furniture polish.	Vomiting can increase area of internal burns (in case of lye) and risk of aspiration.
8. *Never* induce vomiting in unconscious victim.	Vomiting increases risk of aspiration.
9. If instructed by poison control center to take client to emergency department, call ambulance.	Ambulance personnel will be able to provide emergency measures if needed. In addition, parent or guardian may be too upset to drive safely.

cal plug of grounded equipment has three prongs. The rounded, longer prong is the ground. Theoretically the ground prong carries any stray electrical current back to the ground, hence its name. The other two prongs carry the power to the piece of electrical equipment (Cooper, 1983).

Improperly grounded or malfunctioning electrical equipment increases the risk of electrical injury and fire. The use of a prevention checklist when assessing the environment can reduce such injuries in the health care agency and home (see box on p. 1453).

If a client receives an electrical shock, the nurse should immediately determine whether the client has a pulse. If the client has no pulse, cardiopulmonary resuscitation (CPR) should be initiated and emergency personnel should be notified (see Chapter 38). If the client has a pulse and remains alert and oriented, the nurse should quickly obtain vital signs and assess the skin for signs of thermal injury. The cli-

ent's physician must be notified. If an electrical shock occurs in the home, the nurse follows the same procedure but has the client go to the emergency room and then notify the client's physician.

Radiation. Radiation is a health hazard in the hospital environment and the community. In the hospital, particularly in large medical centers, radiation hazards can develop in the nuclear medicine diagnostic centers and the research laboratories.

Hospitals and medical centers have guidelines on the care of clients who have radiation implants. These clients are isolated to one room, and nursing and medical personnel follow strict guidelines to reduce their own and other clients' risks of exposure.

Hospital laboratories require personnel to attend a course on radiation hazards and to pass a test regarding these hazards. In addition, researchers and laboratory workers must follow strict policies when using radioactive substances. Failure to follow these guide-

Sample Evaluation of Interventions for High Risk for Injury

Goals	Evaluative Measures	Expected Outcomes
Client will be able to change potential risks for injury in the home in 72 hr.	Observe home environment after intervention. Ask client to state potential hazards.	Modifiable hazards in the home will be reduced by 100%. Client will list hazards within the home.
Client will acquire knowledge related to potential threats to personal safety in 2 wk.	Inspect client's safe use of home appliances, medications, and health care equipment. Inspect client's home for removal of hazards.	Client will correctly use medication, equipment, or treatments. Home will be free of hazards.
Potential for injury will be reduced in 72 hr.	Observe client for side effects or adverse reactions to medications. Inspect client's skin and musculoskeletal system for injury. Inspect equipment.	Side effects or adverse effects will be absent. Skin and tissues will be intact. Musculoskeletal system will be free of injury. Electrical grounding and functioning will be correct.
Risk of accidental poisoning will be reduced in 72 hr.	Observe client's self-medication. Inspect environment for potential poisonings.	Client will correctly administer medication. Poisonous substances will not be within easy access and will be securely sealed and marked as poisons. Syrup of Ipecac will be in the home. Client will know how to use Ipecac. Phone number of poison control center will be posted.

lines can result in loss of research funds, loss of research space, and loss of employment.

The community is at risk for radiation exposure because of incorrect disposal and transportation of radioactive waste products. Community health agencies and the Environmental Protection Agency (EPA) establish specific, strict guidelines for the disposal of radioactive waste. If a radioactive leak occurs, these agencies institute measures to prevent exposure of surrounding neighborhoods, to clean up radioactive leaks as quickly as possible, and to ensure that injured parties receive prompt medical care.

Evaluation

The interventions for reducing the threats to a client's safety are evaluated by comparing the responses to nursing therapies for outcome criteria established during planning (see evaluation box).

To evaluate the outcomes of care, the nurse measures the effectiveness of interventions. The optimal outcomes are the clients' ability to maintain a safe environment, to have a safe environment created by families or nurses, and to remain uninjured.

The nurse also evaluates specific interventions designed to promote safety and to teach the client and family to reduce threats to safety. Using the nursing process, the nurse collects data related to the client's safety, exposure to safety risks, and physical condition. Nursing interventions promote safety and provide support to clients unable to independently maintain their own safety needs. The nurse also evaluates the client's and family's need for additional support services (for example, home health care, physical therapy, and counseling) and initiates the referral.

 SUMMARY

A safe environment is essential to maintaining and restoring health. Nurses working in a health care setting or community-based agency are the client's first line of defense against falls, environmental hazards, medication errors, poisoning, and other injuries.

Clients' risks for injury increase with declining health status, decreases in mobility, and reduced functioning of special senses. In addition, clients at opposite ends of the life span, very young clients and older clients, have greater risks to their safety.

The nursing process is used to reduce the risk of injury through specific nursing interventions and client education. The nurse promotes a safe environment by removing threats to safety and by teaching clients and families about hazards in their homes.

CHAPTER 42 REVIEW

Key Concepts

- A safe health care environment reduces length of treatment or hospitalization, frequency of treatment-related accidents, potential for lawsuits, number of work-related injuries to personnel, and overall cost of health service.

- In the community a safe environment is one in which basic needs are achievable, physical hazards are reduced, transmission of pathogens and parasites is reduced, pollution is controlled, and sanitation is maintained.

- Factors that reduce the amount of available atmospheric oxygen include an improperly functioning furnace and high carbon monoxide levels from automobile exhaust and cigarette smoke.

- Prolonged exposure to extremely hot or cold environmental temperatures can reduce the client's level of health or even cause death.

- Reduction of physical hazards in the environment includes providing adequate lighting, decreasing clutter, and securing the home.

- The transmission of pathogens and parasites is reduced through medical and surgical asepsis, immunization, food sanitation, insect and rodent control, and appropriate disposal of human wastes.

- Children under 5 years of age are at greatest risk for home accidents that may result in severe injury and death.

- The school-age child is at risk for injury while at home and at school and while traveling to and from school.

- Adolescents are at risk for injury from auto accidents and substance abuse.

- Threats to an adult's safety are frequently associated with poor lifestyle habits.

- Risks of injury for older clients are directly related to the physiological changes of the aging process.

- Risks to client safety within a health care agency include falls and client-inherent, procedure-related, and equipment-related accidents.

- Nursing interventions for promoting safety are individualized for developmental stage, lifestyle, and environment.

- Nursing interventions are developed to modify the environment for protection from falls, fires, poisonings, and electrical hazards.

- The nursing care plan to promote safety is continually evaluated to identify new or continued risks to the client.

Key Terms

Air pollution, p. 1434

Antigen, p. 1434

Carbon monoxide, p. 1432

Client-inherent accidents, p. 1439

Decibels, p. 1435

Equipment-related accidents, p. 1439

Food and Drug Administration (FDA), p. 1434

Food poisoning, p. 1432

Heatstroke, p. 1433

Hypothermia, p. 1433

Immunization, p. 1434

Incident report, p. 1439

Medical asepsis, p. 1446

Noise pollution, p. 1435

Parasite, p. 1434

Pathogen, p. 1434

Poison, p. 1453

Poison control center, p. 1453

Pollutant, p. 1434

Procedure-related accident, p. 1439

Relative humidity, p. 1432

Restraint, p. 1447

Sensory overload, p. 1435

Surgical asepsis, p. 1446

Water pollution, p. 1435

Critical Thinking Exercises

1. You are assigned to provide home visits to a client with Alzheimer's disease. During a visit, his wife comments that her husband is "wandering around" during the night more often than in the past and that she is worried for his safety. What safety measures are necessary in the home to promote this client's safety?

2. During a home visit for a family with twin 2-year-old boys, you assess that medications are placed in the cabinets with dishes and glasses and that household cleaners are placed under the kitchen sink. How do you approach the parents about the potential threat of poisoning? What interventions are appropriate?

3. During your clinical rotation, you care for a confused client. What assessment data are necessary to justify using restraints? Likewise, what assessment data are necessary to justify not using restraints?

REFERENCES

Acee AM, Smith D: Crack, *Am J Nurs* 87:614, 1987.

Aronow R et al: Comments from AAPCC to U.S. Food and Drug Administration on poison treatment drug products, *Vet Hum Toxicol* 28:343, 1985.

Brians LK et al: *Rehabil Nurs* 16(2):67, 1991.

Brower HT: The alternatives to restraints, *J Gerontol Nurs* 17(2):18, 1991.

Centers for Disease Control: Recommendations for prevention of HIV transmission in health care settings, *MMWR* 36(suppl 25):35, 1987.

Centers for Disease Control: Years of potential life lost before age 65: United States, 1987, *MMWR* 38:27, 1989.

Centers for Disease Control: Safety-belt use among drivers involved in alcohol-related fatal motor vehicle crashes: United States, 1982, 1989, *MMWR* 40(24):417, 1991.

Cooper KL: Electrical safety: the electrically sensitive ICU patient, *Focus Crit Care* 10:17, 1983.

Cooper S: Common concern: accidents and older adults, *Geriatr Nurs* 2:287, 1981.

Cutchins CH: Blueprint for restraint-free care, *Am J Nurs* 91:36, 1991.

Ebersole P, Hess P: *Toward healthy aging: human needs and nursing process*, ed 3, St Louis, 1990, Mosby–Year Book.

Fergusson DM et al: A controlled field trial of a poisoning prevention program, *Pediatrics* 69:515, 1982.

Haley B, Nagy M, Roberts S: Care versus control: the key to unlocking physical restraints, *Chart* 88(4):5, 1991.

Health Care Financing Administration: *Federal Register* 54(21):1, 1990.

Hoffman Y: Surviving a child's suicide, *Am J Nurs* 87:955, 1987.

Innes EM, Thurman WG: Evaluation of patient falls, *QRB* 9(2):30, 1983.

Jankin JK, Reynolds BA, Swiech K: Patient falls in the acute care setting: identifying risk factors, *Nurs Res* 35:215, 1986.

Kim MJ, McFarland GK, McLane AM: *Pocket guide to nursing diagnoses*, ed 4, St Louis, 1991, Mosby–Year Book.

Kuhn PJ: What kind of food poisoning is it? *RN* 48:39, 1985.

Lindenmuth JE, Breu CS, Malooley JA: Sensory overload, *Am J Nurs* 80:1465, 1981.

Lowenstein SR, Hunt D: Injury prevention in primary care (editorial), *Ann Inter Med* 113(4):261, 1990.

National Center for Health Statistics: *Health United States, 1987*, DHHS publication no (PHS) 88-1232, Washington, DC, Public Health Service, US Government Printing Office.

Nickens H: Intrinsic factors in falling among the elderly, *J Intern Med* 145:1089, 1985.

Perry BC: Falls among the elderly: a review of the methods and conclusions of epidemiologic studies, *Am Geriatr Soc* 30:367, 1982.

Posey VM, Caruso CC: Life threatening heat-related emergencies, *Dimens Crit Care Nurs* 5(4):216, 1986.

Rhyne MC et al: Children at risk for depression, *Am J Nurs* 86:1374, 1986.

Rice MA, Kibbee PE: Review: identifying the adolescent substance abuser, *MCN* 8:139, 1983.

Roy G: Home accidents: developmental risks, *Community Outlook*, Aug 11, 1982 p 212.

Rubenstein LZ et al: The value of assessing falls in an elderly population, *Ann Intern Med* 113(4):308, 1990.

Thompson RS, Rivara FP, Thompson DC: Prevention of head injury by bicycle helmets: a field study of efficacy (abstract), *Am J Dis Child* 142:386, 1988.

Tideiksaar R: Home safe home: practical tips for fall-proofing, *Geriatr Nurs* 11(6):280, 1989.

Top D: *Insuring electrical safety in the critical care setting*, New York, 1987, American Journal of Nursing Co Educational Services Division.

US Preventive Services Task Force: Counseling to prevent household and environmental injuries, *Am Family Physician* 42(1):136, 1990.

Urton MM: A community home inspection approach to preventing falls among the elderly, *Public Health Rep* 106(2):192, 1991.

Vernberg K, Culver-Dickinson P, Spyker DA: The deterrent effect of poisoning-warning stickers, *Am J Dis Child* 138:1018, 1984.

Whaley LF, Wong DL: *Nursing care of infants and children*, ed 4, St Louis, 1991, Mosby–Year Book.

Whedon MB, Sheed P: Prediction and prevention of patient falls, *Image J Nurs Sch* 21(2):108, 1989.

Wintermute GJ et al: The epidemiology of drowning in adulthood: implications for prevention, *Am J Prev Med* 4:343, 1988.

Woolf A et al: Prevention of childhood poisoning: efficacy of an educational program carried out in an emergency clinic, *Pediatrics* 80:359, 1987.

ADDITIONAL READINGS

Baptiste MS, Feck G: Preventing tap water burns, *Am J Public Health* 70:727, 1980.

Brians LK et al: The development of the RISK tool for fall prevention, *Rehabil Nurs* 16(2):67, 1991.

Davidson M, Grant E: Accidental hypothermia: a community hospital perspective, *Postgrad Med* 70:42, 1981.

Doyle JT: You swallowed your what? *RN* 48:40, 1985.

Evans LK, Strumpf NE: Myths about elder restraint. *Image J Nurs Sch* 22(2):124, 1990.

Ferguson D, Beck C: H.A.L.F.: a tool to assess elderly abuse within the family, *Geriatr Nurs* 4:30, 1983.

Fife DD et al: A risk/falls program: code orange for success, *Nurs Manag* 15(11):50, 1984.

Ford AH: Use of automobile restraining devices for infants, *Nurs Res* 29:281, 1980.

Gehlsen GM, Whaley MH: Falls in the elderly. II, Balance, strength, and flexibility, *Arch Phys Med Rehabil* 71:739, 1990.

Gray-Victrey M: Education to prevent falls, *Geriatr Nurs* 5:179, 1984.

Hernandez M, Miller J: How to reduce falls, *Geriatr Nurs* 7(2):97, 1986.

Innes EM: Maintaining fall prevention, *QRB* 11:217, 1985.

Jones MK: Fire, *Am J Nurs* 84(11):1368, 1984.

Lynn FH: Incidents: Need they be accidents, *Am J Nurs* 80:1098, 1980.

Morse JM, McHutchion E: Releasing restraints: providing safe care for the elderly, *Res Nurs Health* 14:187, 1991.

Riffle KL: Falls: kinds, causes and prevention, *Geriatr Nurs* 3:165, 1982.

Rivara FP, Berger LR: Consumer product hazards: setting priorities for research and regulatory action, *Am J Public Health* 70:701, 1980.

Strumpf NE, Evans LK: Physical restraint of the hospitalized elderly: perceptions of patients and nurses, *Nurs Res* 37(3):132, 1988.

Tideiksaar R: Geriatric falls in the home, *Home Healthc Nurse* 4(2):21, 1986.

Witte NS: Why the elderly fall, *Am J Nurs* 75:1950, 1979.

CHAPTER 43

Mobility and Immobility

OBJECTIVES

Mastery of content in this chapter will enable the student to:

- Define the key terms listed.
- Describe the roles of the skeleton, skeletal muscles, and nervous system in regulation of movement.
- Discuss physiological and pathological influences on body alignment and joint mobility.
- Identify changes in physiological and psychosocial function associated with immobility.
- Assess for impaired body alignment and mobility.
- State correct nursing diagnoses for impaired body alignment and mobility.
- Write nursing care plans for impaired body alignment and mobility.
- Describe the procedures for assisting a client to move up in bed, repositioning a helpless client, assisting a client to a sitting position, and transferring a client from a bed to a chair or a bed to a stretcher.
- Describe complete range of motion exercises.
- Describe crutch safety.
- Evaluate the nursing plan for maintaining body alignment and mobility.

CHAPTER OUTLINE

Clinical nursing requires the nurse to incorporate knowledge and skills into practice. One component of knowledge and skill is *body mechanics,* a broad term used to describe coordinated efforts of the musculoskeletal and nervous systems.

Body mechanics includes knowing how and why certain muscle groups are used. To use proper body mechanics the nurse needs to understand the regulation of movement, including how coordinated body motion involves integrated functioning of the skeletal system, skeletal muscle, and nervous system. In addition, certain muscle groups are used primarily for movement and others primarily for posture.

Mobility serves many purposes, such as expression of an emotion with a nonverbal gesture, self-defense, satisfaction of basic needs, the activities of daily living, and recreational activities. To maintain optimal physical mobility, the nervous, muscular, and skeletal systems of the body must be intact and functioning.

 ## OVERVIEW OF BODY MECHANICS

Body mechanics is the coordinated effort of the musculoskeletal and nervous systems to maintain balance, posture, and body alignment during lifting, bending, moving, and performing activities of daily living. Use of proper body mechanics reduces risk of injury to the musculoskeletal system. Proper mechanics also facilitates body movement, which allows physical mobility without muscle strain and excessive use of muscle energy.

Body Alignment

Body alignment refers to the positioning of the joints, tendons, ligaments, and muscles while in the standing, sitting, and lying positions. Correct body alignment reduces strain on musculoskeletal structures, maintains adequate muscle tone, and contributes to balance.

Body Balance

Body balance is achieved when the **center of gravity** is balanced over a wide, stable base of support and a vertical line falls from the center of gravity through the base of support. When the body is improperly balanced, the center of gravity is displaced, increasing the force of gravity and the possibility of falling.

Body balance is also enhanced by posture. The nurse maintains proper body alignment and posture by using two simple techniques. First, the base of support can easily be widened by separating the feet to a comfortable distance. Second, balance is increased when the center of gravity is moved over and closer to the base of support. This is achieved by bending the knees and flexing the hips until the person is squatting and still maintaining proper back alignment by keeping the trunk erect (Stamps, 1989).

Coordinated Body Movement

Weight is the force exerted on a body by gravity. When an object is lifted, the lifter must overcome the object's weight and know its center of gravity. In symmetrical objects the center of gravity is located at the exact center of the object. Because people are not geometrically perfect, their centers of gravity are usually at 55% to 57% of standing height and are located in the midline. The force of weight is always directed downward, which is why an unbalanced object falls. Clients who are unsteady fall because, as their centers of gravity become unbalanced, the gravitational force of their weight eventually causes them to fall. Therefore the nurse needs to design nursing interventions that protect such clients from falling and ensure their safety (see Chapter 42).

Friction is a force that occurs in a direction to oppose movement. As the nurse turns, transfers, or moves a client up in bed, friction must be overcome. A nurse can reduce friction by following some basic principles. The greater the surface area of the object to be moved, the greater the friction. If a client is unable to assist in moving up in bed, the client's arms should be placed across the chest. This decreases surface area and reduces friction.

A passive or immobilized client produces greater friction to movement. Thus whenever possible, the nurse should use some of the client's strength and mobility when lifting, transferring, or moving the client up in bed. This can be done by explaining the procedure and telling the client when to move. The client can then participate, and friction is decreased.

Friction can also be reduced by lifting rather than pushing a client. Lifting has an upward component and decreases the pressure between the client and the bed or chair. The use of a pull sheet reduces friction because the client is more easily moved along the bed's surface.

 ## REGULATION OF MOVEMENT

Coordinated body movement involves integrated functioning of the skeletal system, skeletal muscle, and nervous system. Because these three systems cooperate so closely in mechanical support of the body, they can be considered as a single functional unit.

Skeletal System

The skeleton is the body's supporting framework and comprises four types of bones: long, short, flat, and irregular. **Long bones** contribute to height (for example, the femur, fibula, and tibia in the leg) and length (for example, the phalanges of the fingers and toes). **Short bones** occur in clusters and, when combined with ligaments and cartilage, permit movement of the extremities. Two examples of short bones are the carpal bones in the foot and the patella in the knee. **Flat bones** provide structural contour, such as bones in the skull and the ribs in the thorax. **Irregular bones** make up the vertebral column and some bones of the skull, such as the mandible.

The skeleton provides attachments for muscles and ligaments. These attachments allow movement of parts of the skeleton, such as opening and closing the mouth or extending an arm or a leg. The skeleton also protects vital organs. For example, the skull protects the brain, and the ribs protect the heart and lungs. Bones assist in regulation of calcium balance. Bones can store calcium and release it into the circulation as needed. Clients with altered calcium regulation and metabolism are at risk for developing osteoporosis and **pathological fractures** (fractures caused by weakened bone tissue), which can occur in all bones but are most common in the ribs and weight-bearing bones. In addition, the internal structure of bones contains bone marrow, participates in red blood cell (RBC) production, and acts as a reservoir for blood. Clients with altered bone marrow function or diminished RBC production are usually weakened and fatigue easily, which decreases mobility and places clients at risk of falling.

Characteristics of Bone

The characteristics of bone include firmness, rigidity, and elasticity. Firmness results from inorganic salts, such as calcium and phosphate, that are laid down in the bone matrix. Firmness is related to the bone's rigidity, which is necessary to keep long bones straight, and enables bones to withstand weight bearing. In addition, bones have a degree of elasticity and skeletal flexibility that changes with age. For example, the newborn has a large amount of cartilage and is highly flexible but is unable to support weight. The toddler's bones are more pliable than those of an older person and are better able to withstand falls.

Joints

Joints are the connections between bones. Each joint is classified according to its structure and de-

gree of mobility. There are four classifications of joints: synostotic, cartilaginous, fibrous, and synovial.

The **synostotic joint** occurs when bones are jointed by bones. No movement is associated with this type of joint, and the bony tissue that forms between the bones provides strength and stability. The classic example of this type of joint is the sacrum, in which vertebrae are joined (Fig. 43-1, *A*, on p. 1464).

The **cartilaginous joint** or synchondrodial joint, has little movement but is elastic and uses cartilage to unite body surfaces. Cartilaginous joints are found when bones are exposed to constant pressure, such as the costosternal joints between the sternum and ribs (Fig. 43-1, *B*).

The **fibrous joint,** or syndesmodial joint, has a tough layer of fibrous connective tissue that binds bones firmly together. Because of the flexibility of connective tissue, some movement of the joint is permitted. For example, the connective tissue between the tibia and fibula joins the bones in a fibrous joint at their distal ends, where they provide a socket for the upper part of the talar bones of the foot (Strand, 1978). Together these bones and connective tissues form the ankle joint, which permits plantar and dorsal flexion of the foot (Fig. 43-1, *C*).

The **synovial joint,** or true joint, is a freely movable joint in which contiguous bony surfaces are covered by articular cartilage and connected by ligaments lined with a synovial membrane. Joining of the humeral radius and ulna by cartilage and ligaments forms a pivotal joint (Fig. 43-1, *D*). Other types of synovial joints are ball-and-socket joints, such as the hip joint, and hinge joints, such as interphalangeal joints of fingers.

Ligaments

Ligaments are white, shiny, flexible bands of fibrous tissue binding joints together and connecting bones and cartilages. Ligaments are elastic and aid joint flexibility and support (Fig. 43-2 on p. 1464). In addition, some ligaments have a protective function. For example, ligaments between the vertebral bodies, nonelastic ligaments, and the ligamentum flavum prevent damage to the spinal cord during movement of the back.

Tendons

Tendons are white, glistening, fibrous bands of tissue that connect muscle to bone. Tendons are strong, flexible, and inelastic and occur in various lengths and thicknesses. The Achilles tendon (tendo calcaneus) is the thickest and strongest tendon in the body. It begins near the middle of the posterior of the leg and attaches the gastrocnemius and soleus muscles in the calf to the calcaneal bone in the back of the foot (Fig. 43-3 on p. 1465).

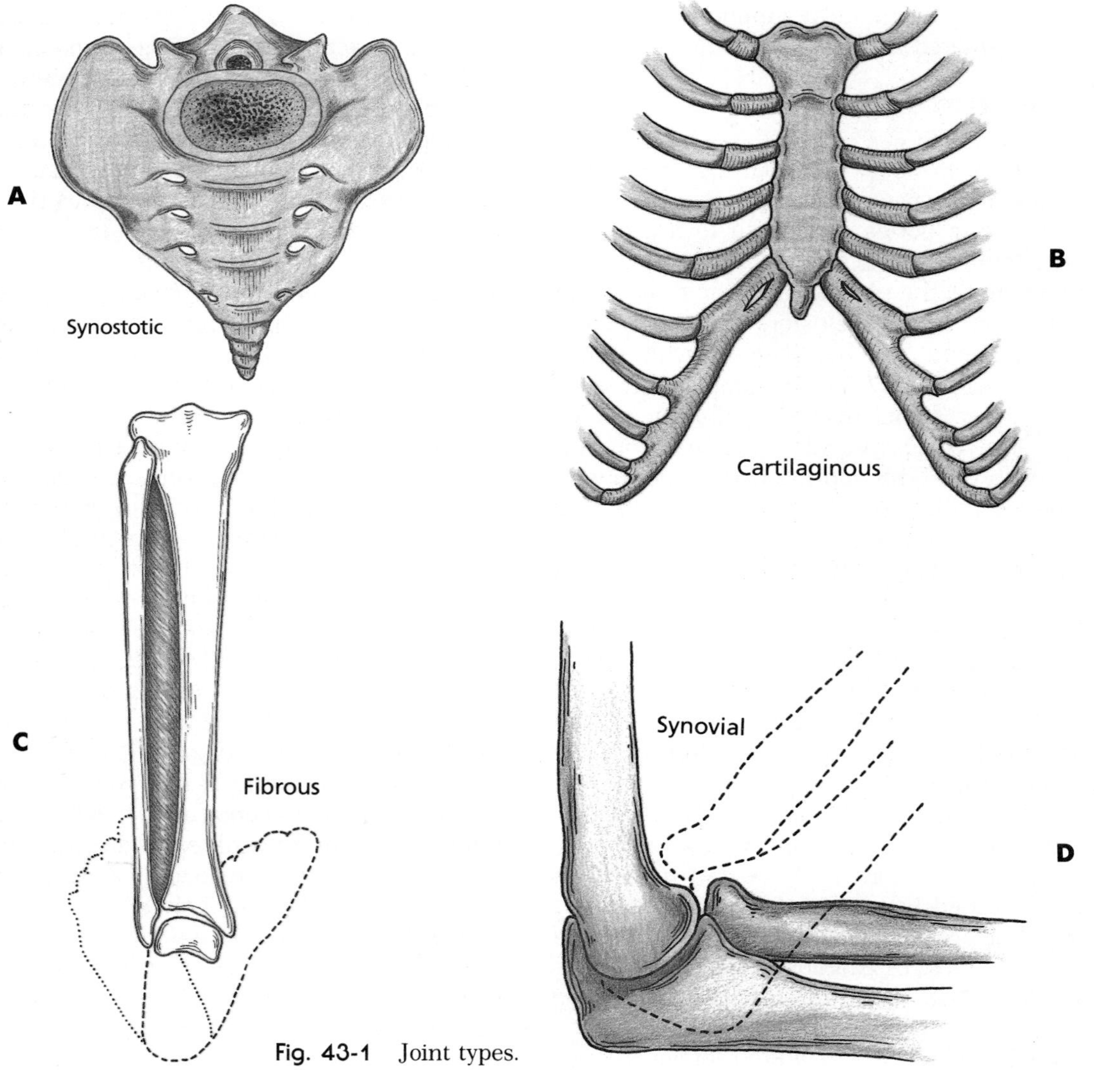

A

Synostotic

B

Cartilaginous

C

Fibrous

Fig. 43-1   Joint types.

Synovial

D

Fig. 43-2   Ligaments of the hip joint.

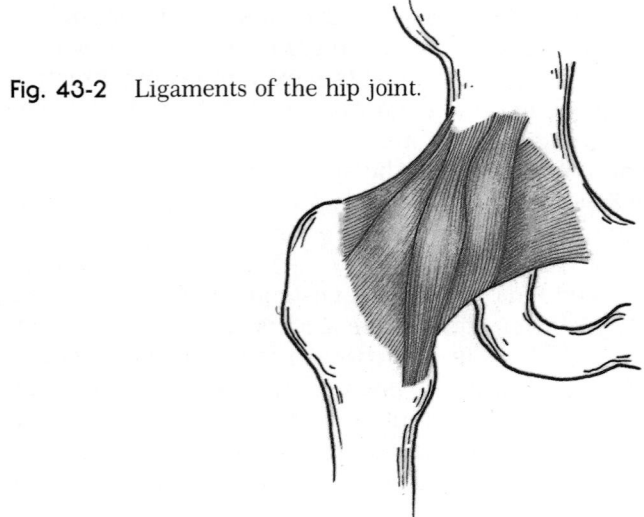

Cartilage

Cartilage is nonvascular, supporting connective tissue located chiefly in the joints and thorax, trachea, larynx, nose, and ear. The fetus has a large amount of temporary cartilage, which is replaced by bone developed during infancy. Permanent cartilage is unossified except in advanced age and diseases such as osteoarthritis.

Joints, ligaments, tendons, and cartilage permit strength and flexibility of the skeleton. Strength enables the skeletal system to support the body. A person's flexibility is demonstrated through range of motion (ROM). However, strength and flexibility do not result entirely from these four structures. Adequate skeletal muscle is also necessary.

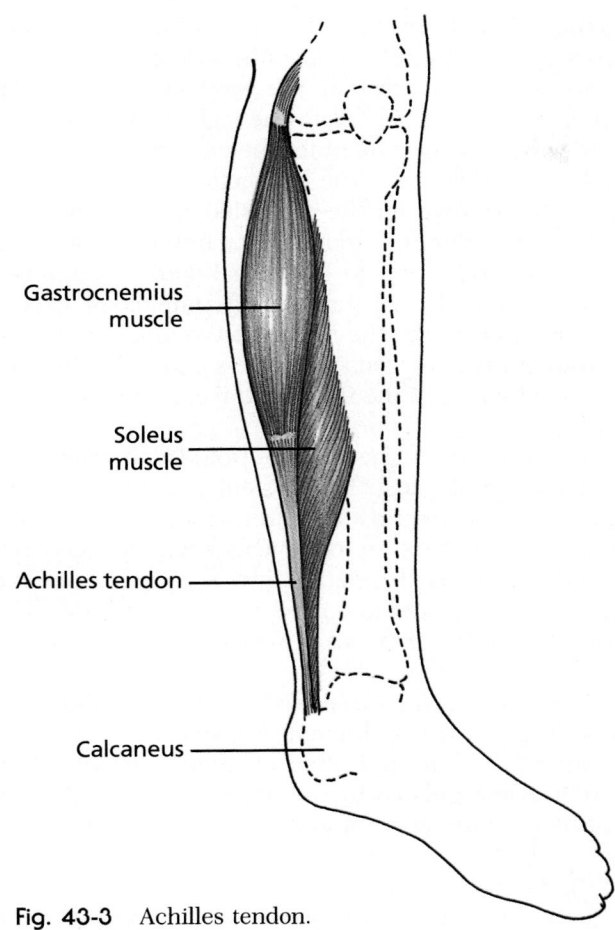

Gastrocnemius
muscle

Soleus
muscle

Achilles tendon

Calcaneus

Fig. 43-3   Achilles tendon.

Skeletal Muscle

Movement of bones and joints involves active processes that must be carefully integrated to achieve coordination. Skeletal muscles, because of their ability to contract and relax, are the working elements of movement. Contractile elements of the skeletal muscle are enhanced by anatomical structure and attachment to the skeleton.

Muscle contraction is stimulated by an electrochemical impulse that travels from the nerve to the muscle across the myoneural junction. The electrochemical impulse causes the thin, actin-containing filaments to shorten, thus contracting the muscle. Removal of the stimulus results in muscle relaxation.

There are two types of muscle contractions: isotonic and isometric. In **isotonic contraction**, increased muscle tension results in muscle shortening. **Isometric contraction** causes an increase in muscle tension or muscle work but no shortening or active movement of the muscle. Voluntary movement is a combination of isotonic and isometric contractions.

For example, when the nurse lifts a client up in bed, the client's weight causes increased tension in the muscles of the nurse's arms until the tension (isometric) is equal to the weight to be lifted and the weight of the lower arm. When this equilibrium is reached, continued stimulation to the muscles results in muscle shortening (isotonic) and bending of the elbow (active movement), and the client is lifted off the bed.

Although isometric contractions do not result in muscle shortening, energy expenditure is increased. This type of muscle work is comparable to having a car in neutral with the driver continually depressing the accelerator and racing the engine. The driver is not going anywhere but expends a large amount of energy. The nurse must recognize the energy expenditure associated with isometric exercises because they may be contraindicated in cardiopulmonary and other illnesses.

Each skeletal muscle is capable of isometric and isotonic contractions. Some skeletal muscles are concerned primarily with movement, whereas others are concerned primarily with posture.

Muscles Concerned with Movement

Muscles concerned primarily with movement are located near the skeletal region where movement is caused by leverage. Leverage occurs when specific bones, such as the humerus, ulna, and radius, and the associated joints, such as the elbow joint, act together as a lever. Thus the force applied to one end of the bone to lift a weight at another point tends to rotate the bone in the direction opposite that of the applied force. Muscles that attach to bones of leverage provide necessary strength to move the object.

Leverage is characteristic of movements of the upper extremities. Arm muscles are parallel to one another and extend the full length of the bones. The long parallel muscles provide strength and work together with the bones and joints to enable lifting an object with the arms.

Muscles Concerned with Posture

Muscles associated primarily with maintaining posture are short and featherlike in appearance because they converge obliquely at a common tendon. Muscles of the lower extremities, trunk, neck, and back are concerned primarily with **posture** (the position of the body in relation to the surrounding space). These muscle groups work together to stabilize and support body weight standing or sitting. These muscles allow an individual to maintain a sitting or standing posture.

MUSCLE REGULATION OF POSTURE AND MOVEMENT. Posture and movement can be reflections of personality and mood. For example, a person with a dramatic personality gestures with the hands, and a person who is fatigued or depressed may slouch.

Posture and movement also depend on the skeleton and the shape and development of skeletal muscles. Coordination and regulation of different muscle groups depend on muscle tone and activity of antagonistic, synergistic, and antigravity muscles.

Muscle Tone. **Muscle tone,** or tonus, is the normal state of balanced muscle tension. Tension is achieved by alternate contraction and relaxation, without active movement, of neighboring fibers of a specific muscle group. Muscle tone enables a body part to be maintained in a functioning position without muscle fatigue. In addition, muscle tone promotes venous return to the heart, as is the case with leg muscles.

Muscle tone is maintained through continual use of muscles. Activities of daily living require muscle action and help maintain muscle tone. As a result of immobility or prolonged bed rest, activity level and muscle tone decrease.

Muscle Groups. The antagonistic, synergistic, and antigravity muscle groups are coordinated by the nervous system and work together to maintain posture and initiate movement.

Antagonistic muscles work together to bring about movement at the joint. During movement, the active mover muscle contracts, and its antagonist relaxes. For example, when flexing the arm, the active biceps brachii contracts, and its antagonist, the triceps brachii, relaxes. During extension of the arm, the active triceps brachii contracts, and the new antagonist, the biceps brachii, relaxes.

Synergistic muscles contract together to accomplish the same movement. When the arm is flexed, the strength of contraction of the biceps brachii is increased by contraction of the synergistic muscle, the brachialis. Thus with synergistic muscle activity, there are two active movers, the biceps brachii and the brachialis, that contract while the antagonistic muscle, the triceps brachii, relaxes.

Antigravity muscles are specifically involved with stabilization of joints. These muscles continuously oppose the effect of gravity on the body and permit the person to maintain an upright or sitting posture. In an adult the antigravity muscles are the extensors of the leg, gluteus maximus, quadriceps femoris, soleus muscles, and muscles of the back.

Nervous System

Movement and posture are regulated by the nervous system. The major voluntary motor area, located in the cerebral cortex, is the precentral gyrus or motor strip. A majority of motor fibers descend from the motor strip and cross at the level of the medulla. Thus the motor fibers from the right motor strip initiate voluntary movement for the left side of the body, and motor fibers from the left motor strip initiate voluntary movement for the right side of the body.

During voluntary movement, impulses descend from the motor strip to the spinal cord. An impulse exits the spinal cord through efferent motor nerves and travels through the nerves to the muscles, where movement occurs. This impulse is controlled by synapses, which keep the impulse traveling in one direction.

Transmission of the impulse from the nervous system to the musculoskeletal system is an electrochemical event and requires a neurotransmitter. Basically, **neurotransmitters** are chemicals such as acetylcholine that transfer the electric impulse from the nerve across the myoneural junction to the muscle. The neurotransmitter reaches a muscle and stimulates it, causing movement.

Movement can be impaired by disorders that alter neurotransmitter production, transfer from the nerve to the muscle, or activation of muscle activity. Posture is also regulated by the nervous system. Posture requires coordination of proprioception and balance.

Proprioception

Proprioception is the sensation achieved through stimuli from within the body regarding spatial position and muscular activity. Proprioception in the body is monitored by proprioceptors, which are any nerve endings located in muscles, tendons, and joints.

As a person carries out activities of daily living, proprioceptors are continuously monitoring muscle activity and body position. For example, the proprioceptors on the soles of the foot contribute to correct posture while standing or walking. In standing, there is continuous pressure on the bottom of the feet. The proprioceptors monitor the pressure, communicating this information through the nervous system to the antigravity muscles. The standing person remains upright until deciding to change position. As a person walks, the proprioceptors on the bottom of the feet monitor pressure changes. Thus when the bottom of the moving foot comes in contact with the walking surface, the individual automatically moves the stationary foot forward. The proprioceptors allow people to walk without having to watch their feet.

Balance

When standing, running, lifting, or performing activities of daily living, a person must have adequate balance. Balance is assisted through control by the nervous system, specifically by the cerebellum and the inner ear. The major function of the cerebellum is to coordinate voluntary movement, particularly highly skilled movements such as those required in golf and skiing (Strand, 1978). In addition, the cerebellum assists in balance, such as permitting a person to stand on one foot with eyes closed (Romberg test of cerebellar function [see Chapter 20]).

Within the inner ear are semicircular canals, three fluid-filled structures that assist in maintaining balance. Fluid within the canals has a certain inertia, and when the head is suddenly rotated in one direction, the fluid remains stationary for a moment while the canals turn with the head. This allows a person to change position suddenly without losing balance.

 ## PRINCIPLES OF BODY MECHANICS

Proper body mechanics is important to the nurse and client. It affects their levels of wellness. Correct body mechanics is necessary for health promotion and prevention of disability.

Principles of Body Mechanics

- The wider the base of support, the greater the stability of the nurse.
- The lower the center of gravity, the greater the stability of the nurse.
- The equilibrium of an object is maintained as long as the line of gravity passes through its base of support.
- The stronger the muscle group, the greater amount of work that can be safely done by it.
- Facing the direction of movement prevents abnormal twisting of the spine.
- Dividing balanced activity between arms and legs reduces the risk of back injury.
- Leverage, rolling, turning, or pivoting requires less work than lifting.
- When friction is reduced between the object to be moved and the surface on which it is moved, less force is required to move it.
- Reducing the force of work reduces the risk of injury.
- Maintaining good body mechanics reduces fatigue of the muscle groups.
- Alternating periods of rest and activity help reduce fatigue.

Adapted from McAbee RR: *AAOHN J* 36(5):221, 1988; and Marchette L, Marchette R: *Orthop Nurs* 4(6):25, 1985.

The nurse uses a variety of muscle groups for each nursing activity, such as walking during nursing rounds, administering medications, lifting and transferring clients, and moving objects. The physical forces of weight and friction can influence body movement. Correctly used, these forces increase the nurse's efficiency. Incorrect use can impair the nurse's ability to lift, transfer, and position clients (Owen, Garg, 1991). The nurse also incorporates knowledge of physiological and pathological influences on mobility and body alignment. The box lists principles of body mechanics that are useful in a variety of settings.

 ## PATHOLOGICAL INFLUENCES ON BODY ALIGNMENT AND MOBILITY

Many pathological conditions affect body alignment and mobility. Although a complete description of each is beyond the scope of this chapter, tables and summaries provide baseline information about these pathological influences, four of which are presented here: postural abnormalities, impaired muscle development, damage to the central nervous system, and direct trauma to the musculoskeletal system.

Postural Abnormalities

Congenital or acquired postural abnormalities affect the efficiency of the musculoskeletal system, as well as body alignment, balance, and appearance. During physical assessment, the nurse observes body alignment and ROM (see Chapter 20). Postural abnormalities can impair alignment, mobility, or both.

Knowledge about the characteristics, causes, and treatment of common postural abnormalities (Table 43-1) is used first to improve the client's body alignment during lifting, transfer, and positioning. Because some postural abnormalities limit ROM in some joints, the nurse maintains maximum ROM in unaffected joints. Finally, the nurse designs nursing interventions to strengthen affected muscle and joint groups, improve the client's posture, and adequately use affected and unaffected muscle groups.

Impaired Muscle Development

Inadequate development of skeletal muscles affects body alignment, balance, and mobility. Muscular dystrophies are the most common developmental impairments of skeletal muscles. These are a group of genetically transmitted diseases characterized by progressive pathological changes in the skeletal muscles, resulting in muscle wasting and weakness (Gröer, Shekleton, 1989).

TABLE 43-1 Postural Abnormalities

Abnormality	Description	Cause	Treatment
Torticollis	Inclining of head to affected side, in which sternocleidomastoid muscle is contracted	Congenital or acquired condition	Surgery, heat, support, or immobilization, depending on cause and severity
Lordosis	Exaggeration of anterior convex curve of lumbar spine	Congenital condition Temporary condition (e.g., pregnancy)	Spine-stretching exercises (based on cause)
Kyphosis	Increased convexity in curvature of thoracic spine	Congenital condition Rickets Tuberculosis of spine	Spine-stretching exercises, sleeping without pillows, using bed board, bracing, spinal fusion (based on cause and severity)
Kypholordosis	Combination of kyphosis and lordosis	Congenital condition	Similar to methods used in kyphosis or lordosis (based on cause)
Scoliosis	Lateral curvature of spine, unequal heights of hips and shoulders	Congenital condition Poliomyelitis Spastic paralysis Unequal leg length	Immobilization and surgery (based on cause and severity)
Kyphoscoliosis	Abnormal anteroposterior and lateral curvature of spine	Congenital condition Poliomyelitis Cor pulmonale	Immobilization and surgery (based on cause and severity)
Congenital hip dysplasia	Hip instability with limited abduction of hips and, occasionally, adduction contractures (Head of femur does not articulate with acetabulum because of abnormal shallowness of acetabulum.)	Congenital condition (more common with breech deliveries)	Maintenance of continuous abduction of thigh so that head of femur presses into center of acetabulum Abduction splints, casting, surgery
Knock-knee (genu valgum)	Legs curved inward so that knees knock together as person walks	Congenital condition Rickets	Knee braces, surgery if not corrected by growth
Bowlegs (genu varum)	One or both legs bent outward at knee, which is normal until 2 to 3 years of age	Congenital condition Rickets	Slowing rate of curving if not corrected by growth With rickets, increase of vitamin D, calcium, and phosphorus intake to normal ranges
Clubfoot	95%: medial deviation and plantar flexion of foot (equinovarus) 5%: lateral deviation and dorsiflexion (calcaneovalgus)	Congenital condition	Casts, splints such as Denis-Browne splint, and surgery (based on degree and rigidity of deformity)
Footdrop	Plantar flexion, inability to invert foot because of peroneal nerve damage	Congenital condition Trauma Improper position of immobilized client	None (cannot be corrected) Prevention through physical therapy
Pigeon-toes	Internal rotation of forefoot or entire foot, common in infants	Congenital condition Habit	Growth, wearing reversed shoes

Data from McCance KL, Huether SE: *Pathophysiology: the biologic basis for disease in adults and children,* St Louis, 1990, Mosby–Year Book.

Damage to the Central Nervous System

Damage to any component of the central nervous system that regulates voluntary movement results in impaired body alignment and mobility. The motor strip in the cerebrum can be damaged by trauma from a head injury, ischemia from a cerebrovascular accident (stroke), or bacterial infection from meningitis. Motor impairment is directly related to the amount of destruction of the motor strip. For example, in the case of a person with a right-sided cerebral hemorrhage with complete necrosis, destruction of the right motor strip and left-sided hemiplegia are consequences. However, a person with a right-sided head injury will have cerebral edema and damage (but not destruction) of the motor strip, and with extensive physical therapy, voluntary movement may gradually return to the left side.

Because voluntary motor fibers descend from the motor strip in the cerebrum down the spinal cord, trauma to the spinal cord also impairs mobility. The most common trauma is transection of the spinal cord in which motor fibers are cut. This can cause a complete bilateral loss of voluntary motor control below the level of the trauma. Spinal cord trauma frequently results from diving or automobile accidents or gunshot or knife wounds to the neck and back.

Direct Trauma to the Musculoskeletal System

Direct trauma to the musculoskeletal system can result in bruises, contusions, sprains, and fractures. A **fracture** is a disruption of bone tissue continuity. Fractures most commonly result from direct external trauma, but they can also occur as a consequence of some deformity of the bone (for example, pathological fractures of osteoporosis, Paget's disease, and osteogenesis imperfecta).

As the fracture heals, bone begins to repair. The fractured bone initiates a cellular process that results in bone formation. Young children are able to form new bone more easily than adults and, as a result, have few complications after a bone fracture. Treatment includes positioning the fractured bone in proper alignment and immobilizing it to promote healing and restore function. Immobilization results in some muscle atrophy, loss of tone, and joint stiffness.

Acquired or congenital conditions that affect the structure of the musculoskeletal or nervous system impair body alignment or joint mobility. Impairment can be temporary or permanent. Regardless of duration of the impairment, the nursing care plan includes interventions that maintain the present level of alignment and joint mobility and that increase the client's level of motor function.

 IMPAIRED MOBILITY

Mobility serves many purposes such as expression of emotion, self-defense, attainment of basic needs, activities of daily living, and recreational activities. In addition, mobility assists in maintaining the body's normal physiological activities (Greenleaf, 1984). To maintain optimal physical mobility, the nervous, muscular, and skeletal systems of the body must be intact and functioning.

When a body part or the entire body is immobilized for a time, secondary disabilities may develop in one or more body systems (Rubin, 1988b; Reddy, 1986; Holm, 1989). The severity of the disabilities increases as the degree of immobility, the length of immobilization, and the severity of the illness increase (Heebink, 1981; Tyler, 1984; Winslow, 1985).

Mobility and Immobility

Mobility is a person's ability to move about freely. Mobility is often essential to the client's perception of health (Rubin, 1988a, 1988b; Tompkins, 1980). Complete, unrestricted mobility requires voluntary motor and complete sensory control of all body regions. Nurses in most health care settings care for clients at any point of the mobility-immobility continuum. Clients with complete mobility have an opportunity to achieve needs and goals independently. In addition, these clients have physiological and psychological benefits from their mobility.

A partial loss of mobility may be temporary (for example, the result of a fracture) or permanent (for example, the result of paralysis). In some cases the restriction of mobility is beneficial for the clients recovery (for example, a casted extremity).

The hazards associated with partial mobility depend on the degree and duration of immobilization (Rubin, 1988b; Greenleaf, 1984). The resulting hazards are usually temporary and resolve shortly after complete mobility is restored (Greenleaf, 1984). The client with a severely limited mobility is at risk for the hazards of immobilization. Nursing care and education is directed toward minimizing these hazards because it is easier to prevent the complications than 'o treat or cure them (Reddy, 1986).

Four conditions may result in immobility. Physical inactivity, such as bed rest, is manifested by reduction in body movement. Physical restriction or limitation of movement (for example, cast or traction) is manifested by imposed reduction of movement. Restriction in body position changes and posture result in a loss of the body's ability to adapt to such changes. Sensory deprivation also causes reduction in stimuli that cause movement and is manifested by even greater physical inactivity. The degree of the client's immobility depends on the extent these conditions are present (Gröer, Shekleton, 1989).

Bed Rest

Bed rest is an intervention in which the client is restricted to bed for therapeutic reasons. Bed rest has different meanings among nurses, physicians, and other health care professionals. The general objectives of bed rest include the following:

1. Reducing physical activity and the oxygen needs of the body
2. Reducing pain, including post-operative pain, and the need for large doses of analgesics
3. Allowing ill or debilitated clients to rest and regain strength
4. Allowing exhausted clients the opportunity for uninterrupted rest

Bed rest has physiological and psychological benefits only if the client finds it restful and if the client can freely move and change positions. Clients who are resistant to bed rest may actually expend more energy in fighting bed rest than they would if allowed to move from bed to chair (Greenleaf, 1984).

Clients with a wide variety of conditions are placed on bed rest. The duration of bed rest depends on the illness or injury and the client's prior state of health.

Immobility

Immobility occurs when the individual is confined to a position and is unable to move or change positions independently. Effects of immobility are systemic and functional. No body system is immune to the effects of immobility. Healthy people who are exposed to periods of immobility or prolonged bed rest suffer physiological and psychological effects (Deitrick et al, 1948; Greenleaf, Kozlowski, 1982). These effects can be gradual or immediate. The greater the extent and the longer the duration of immobility, the more pronounced the consequences.

Physiological Effects

Each body system is at risk for impairments resulting from immobility. The severity of the impairment depends on the client's age and overall health and the degree of immobility. Older clients with chronic illnesses develop pronounced effects of immobility more quickly than younger clients (Reddy, 1986).

METABOLIC CHANGES. Immobility disrupts normal metabolic functioning, including metabolic rate; metabolism of carbohydrates, fats, and proteins; fluid and electrolyte imbalances; calcium imbalance; and gastrointestinal disturbances.

Decreased mobility results in a decrease in basal metabolic rate (BMR). BMR falls in response to the decreased energy requirement of the body cells, which is directly related to cellular oxygen demands (Greenleaf, 1984; Gröer, Shekleton, 1989). However, in the presence of an infectious process, immobilized clients may have an increased BMR as a result of the fever or wound healing. Fever and repair of wounds increase cellular oxygen requirements (McCance, Huether, 1990).

As bed rest continues, pancreatic activity decreases and the body's ability to tolerate glucose also decreases. The client's insulin production loses its ability to lower serum glucose levels. These effects can be seen in 3 days but can reverse 7 days after resuming activity (Rubin, 1988b).

Because proteins are metabolized, nitrogen is produced as an end product. Nitrogen balance provides a reliable indicator of protein use by the body. A **negative nitrogen balance** (Fig. 43-4) exists when the excretion of nitrogen from the breakdown of protein exceeds protein intake (Gröer, Shekleton, 1989). This protein is not available for building and repairing body tissues. During periods of immobility, urinary excretion of nitrogen increases, increasing the risk of a negative nitrogen balance. The urinary excretion of nitrogen increases about the fifth or sixth day of immobilization (Natlow, 1983; Norton, McLaren, Exon-Smith, 1981; Gröer, Shekleton, 1989). Decreased mobility results in changes in fat stores. There is an increase in the percentage of body fat. This results from the loss of lean body mass as a result of protein breakdown (Greenleaf, Kozlowski, 1982).

Because the client is in a recumbent position, there are major shifts in blood volume (see section on cardiovascular changes). There is an immediate diuretic response during the first day of bed rest. The client loses an average of 600 ml of fluid (Rubin, 1988b; Greenleaf, Kozlowski, 1982). In addition, there is an increase in urinary excretion of calcium, chloride, and sodium (Greenleaf, Kozlowski, 1982).

Urinary excretion of calcium is increased through **bone resorption.** Immobility causes the release of calcium into the circulation. Normally the kidneys can excrete the excess calcium. However, if the kidneys are unable to respond appropriately, hypercalcemia results (Rubin, 1988b; Holm, 1989).

Impairments in gastrointestinal functioning vary and result from decreased gastrointestinal motility. Constipation is a common symptom. Diarrhea is fre-

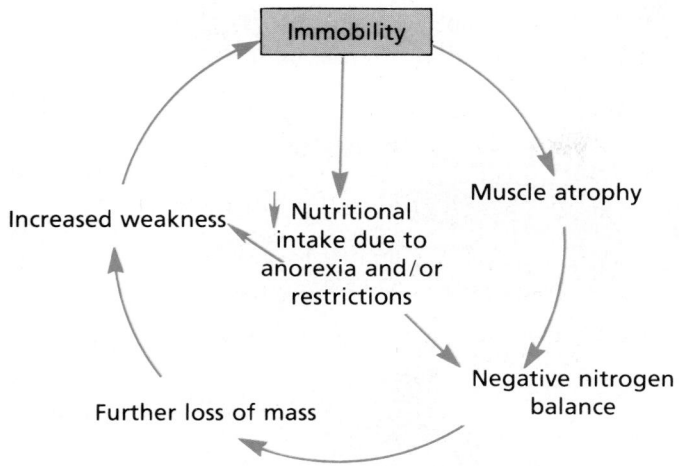

Fig. 43-4 Factors contributing to negative nitrogen balance associated with immobility.
From Gröer MW, Shekleton ME: *Basic pathophysiology: a conceptual approach,* ed 3, St Louis, 1989, Mosby–Year Book.

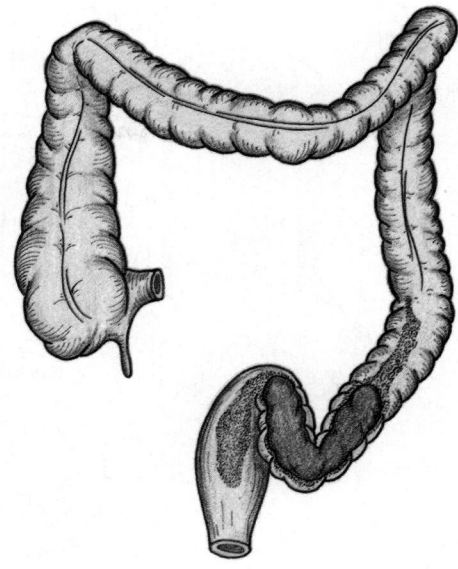

Fig. 43-5 Fecal impaction with liquid stool passing around the impaction.

quently the result of a fecal impaction (Fig 43-5). The nurse must be aware that this finding is not normal diarrhea, but rather liquid stool passing around the area of impaction. Left untreated, fecal impaction can result in a mechanical bowel obstruction that may partially or completely occlude the intestinal lumen, blocking normal propulsion of liquid and gas. The resulting fluid in the intestine produces distention and increases intraluminal pressure. Over time, intestinal function becomes depressed, dehydration occurs, absorption ceases, and fluid and electrolyte disturbances worsen.

RESPIRATORY CHANGES. When a client assumes a recumbent position, the lungs shift position 90 degrees. This shift in position and body fluids as well as the abdominal contents pushing against the diaphragm cause a decrease in long volume (Rubin, 1988b).

A majority of respiratory problems occurring with immobility are caused by decreased hemoglobin, decreased lung expansion, generalized muscle weakness, and stasis of secretions. Decreased hemoglobin values can result from the disease process causing reduced mobility or from restricted mobility. Hemoglobin is the carrier that transports oxygenated blood to tissues. When the oxygen-carrying capacity is reduced, there is a reduction in oxygen delivery to the tissues. Initially the body tries to adapt by increasing pulse and respiratory rates, but this is a short-term adaptive response and ultimately increases cardiac workload.

Immobilization decreases lung expansion. Any changes in a client's position changes the distribution of ventilation and blood flow through the lung. As a result the dependent lung is better oxygenated (West, 1985). The exception to this principle occurs when the client has a pathological condition of the lung. In addition, all lung volumes, except tidal volumes, are reduced during immobilization (Beckett et al, 1986; Convertino, Goldwater, Sandler, 1986).

The limited physical activity and the metabolic changes lead to weakened and decreased respiratory muscles. As a result, the work of breathing increases (Tyler, 1984). At some point, there is a proportional decline in the client's ability to cough productively. Ultimately the distribution of mucus in the bronchi increases, particularly when the client is in the supine, prone, or lateral position (Fig 43-6 on p. 1472). Mucus accumulates in the dependent regions of the airways (Fig. 43-7 on p. 1472). Because mucus is an excellent medium for bacterial growth, hypostatic bronchopneumonia may result.

CARDIOVASCULAR CHANGES. The cardiovascular system is also affected by immobilization. The three major changes are orthostatic hypotension, increased cardiac workload, and thrombus formation.

The occurrence of orthostatic hypotension is well documented in the client on bed rest, but it also occurs in clients experiencing prolonged immobility in the sitting position (Greenleaf, 1986). **Orthostatic hypotension** is a drop of 15 mm Hg or more in blood pressure when the client rises from a lying or sitting position to a standing position. In the immobilized client, decreased circulating fluid volume, pooling of

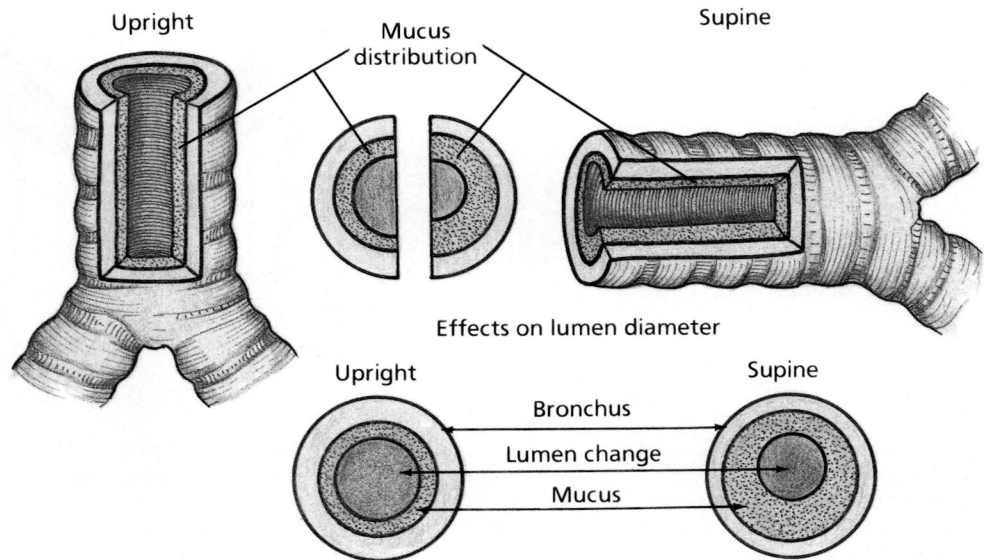

Mucus distribution

Upright · Supine

Effects on lumen diameter

Upright · Supine

Bronchus
Lumen change
Mucus

Fig. 43-6   Effect of recumbency and gravity on distribution of respiratory tract and diameter of bronchiolar lumen.
From Groër MW, Shekleton ME: *Basic pathophysiology: a conceptual approach*, ed 2, St Louis, 1989, Mosby–Year Book.

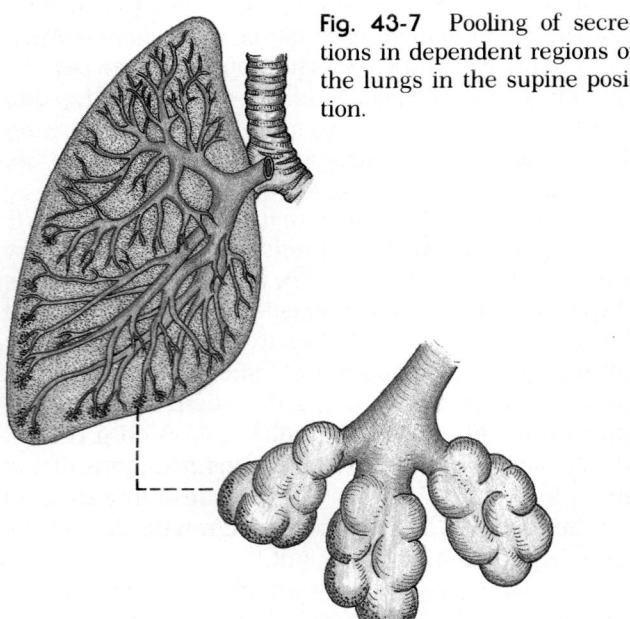

Fig. 43-7   Pooling of secretions in dependent regions of the lungs in the supine position.

blood in the lower extremities, and decreased autonomic response occur. These factors result in decreased venous return, followed by a decrease in cardiac output, which is reflected by a decline in blood pressure (Winslow, 1985; McCance, Huether, 1990).

Increased cardiac workload is demonstrated by rate changes. Prolonged bed rest increases resting heart rate 4 to 15 beats/min. When the immobilized client is asked to do physical activity, such as with ROM exercises or activities of daily living, the increase in rate is more pronounced (Winslow, 1985). As the workload of the heart increases, its oxygen consumption does, too. The heart therefore works harder and less efficiently during periods of prolonged rest. As immobilization increases, cardiac output falls, further decreasing cardiac efficiency and increasing workload.

Clients are also at risk for thrombus formation. A **thrombus** is an accumulation of platelets, fibrin, clotting factors, and the cellular elements of the blood attached to the interior wall of a vein or artery, sometimes occluding the lumen of the vessel (Fig. 43-8). Thrombi form for a variety of reasons. Because of hypovolemia, the hematocrit is increased, and the circulating blood is more viscous (Greenleaf, Kozlowski, 1982). After 8 days of bed rest, more procoagulants are found, and thromboplastin time shortens (Rubin, 1988b). Weight of the legs on the bed also compresses the blood vessels of the calves, causing vessel wall injury and stasis of blood (Gröer, Shekleton, 1989; Rubin, 1988b). Finally, fibrinolytic activity increases, suggesting that the liver produces increased amounts of fibrinogen (Rubin, 1988b).

MUSCULOSKELETAL CHANGES. The effects of immobility on the musculoskeletal system can include permanent impairment of mobility. Restricted mobility affects the client's muscles through loss of endur-

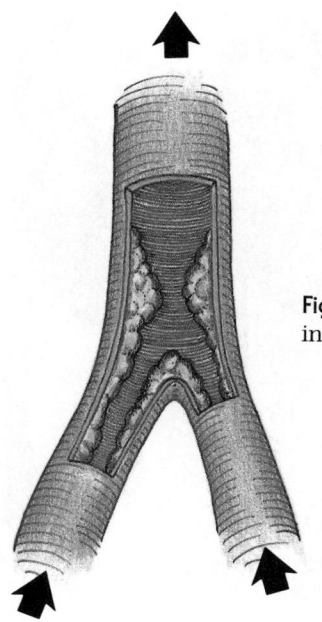

Fig. 43-8 Thrombus formation in a vessel.

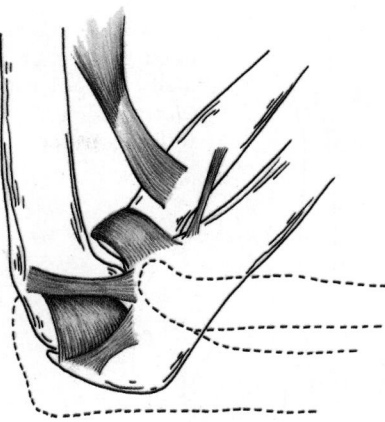

Fig. 43-9 Contracture of the elbow resulting in permanent flexion of the joint. Normally the elbow is able to extend to a 90-degree angle (*dotted line*) and to a 180-degree angle (not illustrated).

ance, decreased muscle mass, atrophy, and decreased stability. Other effects of restricted mobility affecting the skeletal system are impaired calcium metabolism and impaired joint mobility.

Muscle Effects. Reduced muscle endurance for physical activity results from changes in the muscles and altered cardiovascular functioning. As cardiac workload increases, muscle endurance decreases due to a reduced ability of the cardiopulmonary system to meet the tissue's oxygen needs (Winslow, 1985).

Because of protein breakdown, the client loses lean body mass, which is composed partially of muscle. Therefore the reduced muscle mass is unable to sustain activity without increased fatigue. The muscle mass is decreased from metabolic causes and disuse. As immobility continues and the muscles are not exercised, there is continued decrease in mass.

Muscle atrophy resulting from immobility is observable and measurable. As muscle atrophies, the size of the muscle decreases (Booth, 1982). Antigravity muscles in the legs appear to be the most affected, lending support to the theory that the normal stresses of gravity are important in maintaining function, development, and therefore mobility (Gröer, Shekleton, 1989).

Decreased stability results from loss of endurance, decreased muscle mass, atrophy, and actual joint abnormalities. Therefore these clients are unable to move steadily, and their risk for falling increases.

Skeletal Effects. Immobilization causes two skeletal changes: impaired calcium metabolism and joint abnormalities. Because immobilization results in

bone resorption, the bone tissue is less dense, and osteoporosis results (Greenleaf, Kozlowski, 1982; Holm, 1989). When osteoporosis occurs, the client is at risk for pathological fractures. Immobilization and non-weight-bearing activities increase the rate of bone resorption. Bone resorption also causes calcium to be released in the blood, and hypercalcemia results.

Immobility can lead to joint contractures. A **joint contracture** is an abnormal and usually permanent condition characterized by flexion and fixation of the joint. It is caused by disuse, atrophy, and shortening of the muscle fibers. When a contracture occurs, the joint cannot maintain full ROM. Unfortunately, contracture usually leaves the joint in a nonfunctional position (Lehmkuhl et al, 1990). (Fig. 43-9).

One common and debilitating contracture is footdrop (Fig. 43-10 on p. 1474). When **footdrop** occurs, the foot is permanently fixed in plantar flexion. Ambulation is difficult with the foot in this position.

Joint mobility can also be altered by inflammation, degeneration, or articular disruption. **Arthritis** is an inflammation of the joints characterized by swelling and pain. It can result from a direct inflammatory reaction in the joint tissue such as gouty arthritis, an infectious process such as septic arthritis, or an immune-mediated inflammatory process such as rheumatoid arthritis.

Joint degeneration is demonstrated by changes in articular cartilage combined with changes at the articular bone ends (Gröer, Shekleton, 1989). Synovial and cartilaginous joints are equally affected, and degenerative changes commonly affect weight-bearing joints. Although degenerative joint disease is not caused by inflammation, it is frequently termed *osteoarthritis*.

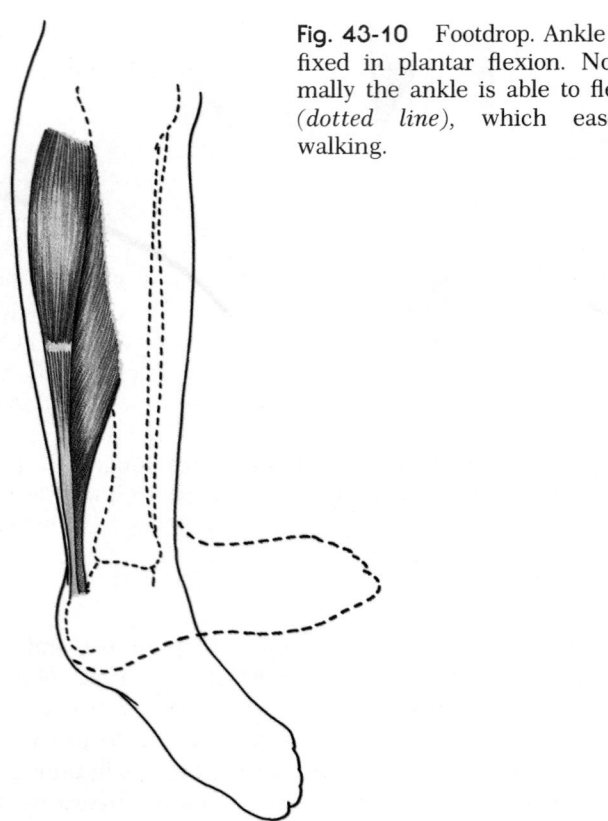

Fig. 43-10 Footdrop. Ankle is fixed in plantar flexion. Normally the ankle is able to flex (*dotted line*), which eases walking.

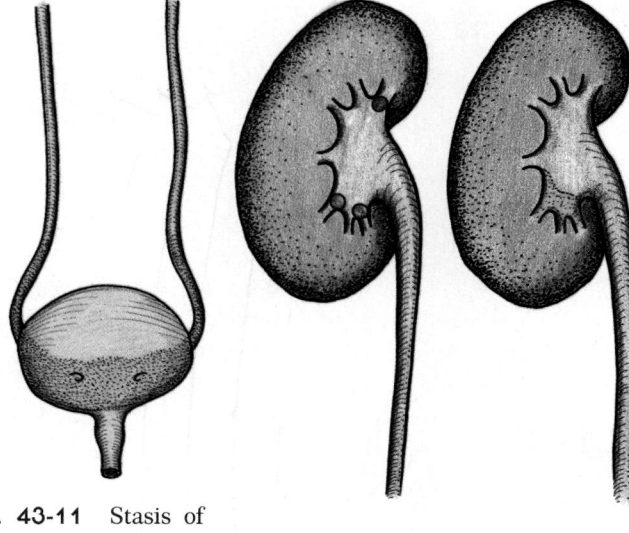

Fig. 43-11 Stasis of urine with reflux to ureters.

Fig. 43-12 Types of renal calculi in the renal pelvis.

INTEGUMENTARY CHANGES. The skin is affected by immobility but also by the resulting impaired metabolism, the loss of lean body mass, and negative nitrogen balance (Greenleaf, 1984; Gröer, Shekleton, 1989). Thus a break in the skin's integrity is difficult to heal in the immobilized client. An older client has a greater risk for developing pressure ulcers (Reddy, 1986; Pajk et al, 1986).

A **pressure ulcer,** or decubitus ulcer, is a localized area of tissue necrosis that develops when soft tissue is compressed between a bony prominence and an external surface for a prolonged period. Usually the ulcer forms over a bony prominence (National Pressure Ulcer Advisory Panel, 1989). **Ischemia** develops when pressure on the skin is greater than the pressure inside the small peripheral blood vessels supplying blood to the skin (Knight, 1988). Impairments in skin integrity have significant impact on level of wellness, nursing care, and length of hospital stay (see Chapter 44).

URINARY ELIMINATION CHANGES. The client's urinary elimination is altered by immobility. In the upright position, urine flows out of the renal pelvis and into the ureter and bladder because of gravitational forces. When the client is recumbent or flat, the kidneys and the ureters move toward a more level plane. Urine formed by the kidney must enter the bladder against gravity. Because the peristaltic contractions of the ureters are insufficient to overcome gravity, the renal pelvis may fill before urine enters the ureters (Fig. 43-11). This condition is called **urinary stasis** and increases the risk of urinary tract infection and renal calculi (see Chapter 40).

Renal calculi are calcium stones that lodge in the renal pelvis and pass through the ureters (Fig. 43-12). Immobilized clients are at risk for calculi because of altered calcium metabolism and the resulting hypercalcemia (Greenleaf, 1986; Holm, 1989).

During the initial period of immobility, urine volume is increased secondary to fluid shifts and a natural diuresis (Dietrick et al, 1948; Greenleaf 1986). As the period of immobility continues, fluid intake can diminish, and other causes, such as fever, increase risk for dehydration. As a result, urinary output declines on or about the fifth or sixth day. The urine that is produced is usually highly concentrated.

This concentrated urine increases the risk for calculi formation and infection. Poor perineal care after bowel movements, particularly in women, increases the risk of urinary tract contamination by *Escherichia coli* bacteria. Another cause of urinary tract infections in immobilized clients is the use of an indwelling urinary catheter.

Psychosocial Effects

Immobilization may lead to emotional, intellectual, sensory, and sociocultural responses. Changes in emotional status usually occur gradually. However, the older adult may be more susceptible to these changes, so the nurse may observe them earlier. The most common emotional changes are depression, behavioral changes, changes in the sleep-wake cycle, and impaired coping.

 DEVELOPMENTAL CHANGES

Throughout life, the body's appearance and functioning undergo change. The greatest impact is observed in childhood and old age.

Infants

The newborn infant's spine is flexed and lacks the anteroposterior curves of the adult. The first spinal curve occurs when the infant extends the neck from the prone position. As growth and stability increase, the thoracic spine straightens, and the lumbar spinal curve appears, which allows sitting and standing. The infant's musculoskeletal system is flexible. The extremities are flexed and joints have complete ROM. As the newborn matures, the musculoskeletal system becomes stronger, and the infant is able to resist movement and reach out and grasp objects (see Chapter 24). As the baby grows, musculoskeletal development permits support of weight for standing and walking. Posture is awkward because the head and upper trunk are carried forward. Because body weight is not evenly distributed along a line of gravity, posture is off balance, and falls occur often.

Toddlers

The toddler's posture—slightly swaybacked with a protruding abdomen—is awkward. As the child walks, the legs and feet are usually far apart and the feet are slightly everted. Toward the end of toddlerhood, posture appears less awkward, curves in the cervical and lumbar vertebrae are accentuated, and foot eversion disappears.

Preschool and School-Age Children

By the third year the body is slimmer, taller, and better balanced. Abdominal protrusion is decreased, the feet are not as far apart, and arms and legs have increased in length. The child also appears more coordinated. From the third year through beginning adolescence the musculoskeletal system continues to develop. Long bones in the arms and legs grow. Muscles, ligaments, and tendons become stronger, resulting in improved posture and increased muscle strength. Greater coordination enables the child to perform tasks that require fine motor skills (see Chapter 25).

Adolescents

Adolescence stage is usually initiated by a tremendous growth spurt (see Chapter 25). Growth is frequently uneven. As a result, the adolescent may appear awkward and uncoordinated. Adolescent girls usually grow and develop earlier than boys. Hips widen, and fat is deposited in the upper arms, thighs, and buttocks. The boy's changes in shape are usually the result of long-bone growth and increased muscle mass. Legs become longer and hips narrower. Muscular development increases in the chest, arms, shoulders, and upper legs.

Adults

An adult who has correct posture and body alignment feels good, looks good, and generally appears self-confident. The healthy adult also has the necessary musculoskeletal development and coordination to carry out activities of daily living (see Chapter 26). Normal changes in posture and body alignment in adulthood occur mainly in pregnant women. These changes result from the body's adaptive response to weight gain and the growing fetus. The center of gravity shifts toward the anterior. The pregnant woman leans back and is slightly swaybacked. She may complain of backache.

Older Adults

The aging process can result in musculoskeletal changes (see Chapter 27). Degenerative joint changes may decrease ROM. Skeletal muscle mass and strength may be reduced. Changes in the structure of the bone matrix may result in fragile, brittle bones (Hudson, 1983).

Older adults may walk more slowly and appear less coordinated. They may also take smaller steps, keeping the feet closer together, which decreases the base of support. Thus body balance is unstable, and they are at greater risk for falls and injuries.

 NURSING PROCESS FOR IMPAIRED BODY ALIGNMENT AND MOBILITY

Based on data collected during assessment, the nurse determines the client's care plan. When assessing mobility status, the nurse also evaluates the client's ability to perform activities of daily living.

Assessment

Nursing assessment is presented in two sections, mobility and immobility. Both areas are usually assessed during the complete physical examination.

Mobility

Assessment of client mobility focuses on range of motion, gait, exercise and activity tolerance, and body alignment.

RANGE OF MOTION. Range of motion (ROM) is the maximum amount of movement possible at a joint in one of the three planes of the body: sagittal, frontal, and transverse (Fig. 43-13). The sagittal plane is a line that passes through the body from front to back, dividing the body into a left and a right side. The frontal plane passes through the body from side to side and divides the body into front and back. The transverse plane is a horizontal line that divides the body into upper and lower portions.

Joint mobility in each of the planes is limited by ligaments, muscles, and construction of the joint. However, some joint movements are specific to each plane. In the sagittal plane, movements are flexion and extension (fingers and elbows) and hyperextension (hip). In the frontal plane, movements are abduction and adduction (arms and legs) and eversion and inversion (feet). In the transverse plane, movements are pronation and supination (hands), internal

and external rotation (knees), and dorsiflexion and plantar flexion (feet).

When assessing ROM, the nurse asks questions and makes observations to collect data about joint stiffness, swelling, pain, limited movement, and unequal movement. Clients whose joint mobility is restricted because of illness, disability, or trauma require exercise of joints to reduce the hazards of immobility. These exercises, performed by the nurse, are called *passive ROM exercises*. The nurse takes each affected joint through its complete *ROM* (Table 43-2 on p. 1478).

GAIT. Gait is the manner or style of walking, including rhythm, cadence, and speed. Assessing a client's gait allows the nurse to draw conclusions about balance, posture, safety, and ability to walk without assistance.

Initially the nurse observes the overall appearance of the walking client. Normally, the adult posture is well aligned. The actual activity of walking takes place in a four-phase sequence: heel strike, stance, push-off, and swing (Daniels, Worthingham, 1977). During heel strike, the foot is about at a right angle to the leg. The knee is extended but not locked and ready for slight flexion as the body weight is shifted forward into the stance phase. During stance, the trunk is maintained in a vertical position with the head and neck properly aligned. At push-off, there is plantar flexion of the foot and hyperextension of the metatarsophalangeal joints of the toes. During swing, the foot easily clears the floor with good alignment. Rhythm of movement is unchanged and remains coordinated.

EXERCISE AND ACTIVITY TOLERANCE. Exercise is physical activity for conditioning the body, improving health, and maintaining fitness. It can also be used as therapy for correcting a deformity or restoring the overall body to a maximal state of health. When a person exercises, physiological changes occur in body systems (see box).

Assessment of the client's energy level includes the physiological effects of exercise and activity tolerance. **Activity tolerance** is the kind and amount of exercise or work that a person is able to perform. Assessment of activity tolerance is necessary when planning activity such as walking, ROM exercises, or activities of daily living for clients with acute or chronic illness. In addition, knowledge of the client's activity tolerance is needed to plan other nursing therapies.

Activity tolerance assessment includes data from physiological, emotional, and developmental domains (see box). These assessments provide baseline data

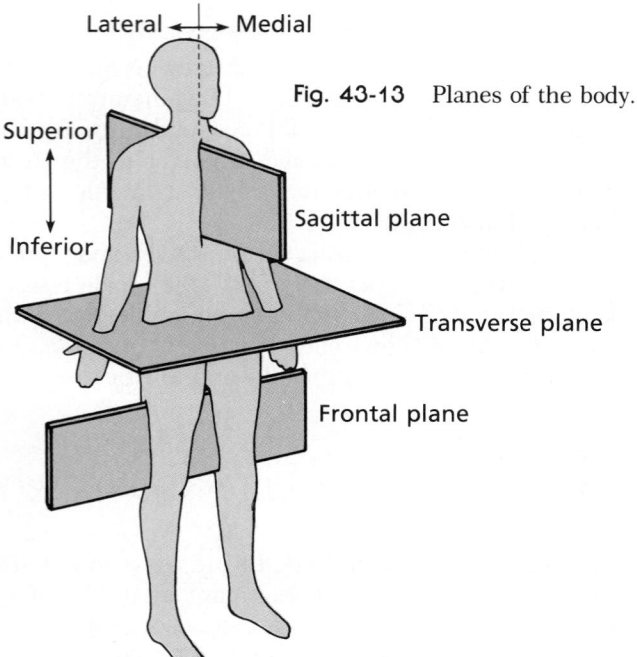

Fig. 43-13   Planes of the body.

about the client's activity patterns and tolerance (Gordon, 1976). In addition, this assessment is applicable in all clinical settings and is quickly completed by the nurse.

The client who experiences changes in physiological function during exercise such as dyspnea or chest pain will not tolerate activity as well as the client who does not. Likewise, the weak or debilitated client is unable to sustain activity because the greater energy needed to complete the activity creates fatigue and generalized weakness.

People who are depressed, worried, or anxious are frequently unable to tolerate exercise. Depressed clients are usually not motivated to participate. Clients who are worried or anxious fatigue easily because they expend a great deal of energy in worry and anxiety. Thus they may experience physical and emotional exhaustion.

Developmental changes also affect activity tolerance. As the infant enters the toddler stage, the activity level increases and the need for sleep declines. The child entering nursery school, preschool, or primary grades expends mental energy in learning and may require more rest after school or before strenuous play. The adolescent going through puberty may require more rest because much of the body's energy is expended for growth and hormone changes.

Effects of Exercise

CARDIOVASCULAR SYSTEM

- Increased cardiac output
- Improved myocardial contraction, thus strengthening cardiac muscle
- Decreased resting heart rate
- Improved venous return

PULMONARY SYSTEM

- Increased respiratory rate and depth followed by quicker return-to-rest rate
- Improved alveolar ventilation
- Decreased work of breathing
- Improved diaphragmatic excursion

METABOLIC SYSTEM

- Increased basal metabolic rate
- Increased use of glucose and fatty acids
- Increased triglyceride breakdown
- Increased gastric motility
- Increased production of body heat

MUSCULOSKELETAL SYSTEM

- Improved muscle tone
- Increased joint mobility
- Improved muscle tolerance to exercise
- Possible increase in muscle mass
- Reduced bone loss

ACTIVITY TOLERANCE

- Improved tolerance
- Decreased fatigue

PSYCHOSOCIAL FACTORS

- Improved tolerance to stress
- Reports of "feeling better"
- Reports of decrease in illness (e.g., colds and influenza viruses)

Adapted from Gröer MW, Shekleton ME: *Basic pathophysiology: a conceptual approach,* ed 3, St Louis, 1989, Mosby–Year Book; and McCance KL, Huether SE: *Pathophysiology: the biologic basis for disease in adults and children,* St Louis, 1990, Mosby–Year Book.

Factors Influencing Activity Tolerance

PHYSIOLOGICAL FACTORS

- Frequency of illness or surgery during past 12 mo
- Types of illnesses or surgery during past 12 mo
- Cardiopulmonary status (e.g., dyspnea, chest pain)
- Musculoskeletal status (e.g., decreased muscle mass)
- Sleep patterns
- Presence of pain, pain control
- Vital signs
- Exercise activity and pattern
- Abnormality in laboratory studies, such as decreased arterial oxygen concentration, decreased hemoglobin level, abnormal electrolyte levels

EMOTIONAL FACTORS

- Mood: depression, anxiety
- Motivation
- Chemical addictions (e.g., drugs, alcohol, nicotine)
- Self-image

DEVELOPMENTAL FACTORS

- Age
- Sex
- Pregnancy
- Change in muscle mass because of developmental changes
- Changes in skeletal system because of developmental changes

Physiological data from Gröer MW, Shekleton ME: *Basic pathophysiology: a conceptual approach,* ed 3, St Louis, 1989, Mosby–Year Book.

TABLE 43-2   Range of Motion Exercises

Body Part	Type of Joint	Type of Movement	Range (degrees)	Primary Muscles
Neck, cervical spine	Pivotal	Flexion: bring chin to rest on chest	45	Sternocleidomastoid
		Extension: return head to erect position	45	Trapezius
		Hyperextension: bend head back as far as possible	10	Trapezius
		Lateral flexion: tilt head as far as possible toward each shoulder	40-45	Sternocleidomastoid
		Rotation: turn head as far as possible in circular movement	180	Sternocleidomastoid, trapezius
Shoulder	Ball and socket	Flexion: raise arm from side position forward to position above head	180	Coracobrachialis, biceps brachii, deltoid, pectoralis major
		Extension: return arm to position at side of body	180	Latissimus dorsi, teres major, triceps brachii
		Hyperextension: move arm behind body, keeping elbow straight	45-60	Latissimus dorsi, teres major, deltoid
		Abduction: raise arm to side to position above head with palm away from head	180	Deltoid, supraspinatus
		Adduction: lower arm sideways and across body as far as possible	320	Pectoralis major
		Internal rotation: with elbow flexed, rotate shoulder by moving arm until thumb is turned inward and toward back	90	Pectoralis major, latissimus dorsi, teres major, subscapularis
		External rotation: with elbow flexed, move arm until thumb is upward and lateral to head	90	Infraspinatus, teres major, deltoid
		Circumduction: move arm in full circle (Circumduction is combination of all movements of ball-and-socket joint.)	360	Deltoid, coracobrachialis, latissimus dorsi, teres major

TABLE 43-2 Range of Motion Exercises—cont'd

Body Part	Type of Joint	Type of Movement	Range (degrees)	Primary Muscles
Elbow	Hinge	Flexion: bend elbow so that lower arm moves toward its shoulder joint and hand is level with shoulder	150	Biceps brachii, brachialis, brachioradialis
		Extension: straighten elbow by lowering hand	150	Triceps brachii
Forearm	Pivotal	Supination: turn lower arm and hand so that palm is up	70-90	Supinator, biceps brachii
		Pronation: turn lower arm so that palm is down	70-90	Pronator teres, pronator quadratus
Wrist	Condyloid	Flexion: move palm toward inner aspect of forearm	80-90	Flexor carpi ulnaris, flexor carpi radialis
		Extension: move fingers so that fingers, hands, and forearm are in same plane	80-90	Extensor carpi ulnaris, extensor carpi radialis brevis, extensor carpi radialis longus
		Hyperextension: bring dorsal surface of hand back as far as possible	89-90	Extensor carpi radialis brevis, extensor carpi radialis longus, extensor carpi ulnaris
		Abduction (radial flexion): bend wrist medially toward thumb	Up to 30	Flexor carpi radialis, extensor carpi radialis brevis, extensor carpi radialis longus
		Adduction (ulnar flexion): bend wrist laterally toward fifth finger	30-50	Flexor carpi ulnaris, extensor carpi ulnaris
Fingers	Condyloid hinge	Flexion: make fist	90	Lumbricales, interosseus volaris, interosseus dorsalis
		Extension: straighten fingers	90	Extensor digiti quinti proprius, extensor digitorum communis, extensor indicis proprius
		Hyperextension: bend fingers back as far as possible	30-60	
		Abduction: spread fingers apart	30	Interosseus dorsalis
		Adduction: bring fingers together	30	Interosseus volaris
Thumb	Saddle	Flexion: move thumb across palmar surface of hand	90	Flexor pollicis brevis
		Extension: move thumb straight away from hand	90	Extensor pollicis longus, extensor pollicis brevis
		Abduction: extend thumb laterally (usually done when placing fingers in abduction and adduction)	30	Abductor pollicis brevis
		Adduction: move thumb back toward hand	30	Adductor pollicis obliquus, adductor pollicis transversus
		Opposition: touch thumb to each finger of same hand		Opponeus pollicis, opponeus digiti minimi

Continued.

TABLE 43-2 Range of Motion Exercises—cont'd

Body Part	Type of Joint	Type of Movement	Range (degrees)	Primary Muscles
Hip	Ball and socket	Flexion: move leg forward and up	90-120	Psoas major, iliacus, iliopsoas, sartorius
		Extension: move back beside other leg	90-120	Gluteus maximus, semitendinosus, semimembranosus
		Hyperextension: move leg behind body	30-50	Gluteus maximus, semitendinosus, semimembranosus
		Abduction: move leg laterally away from body	30-50	Gluteus medius, gluteus minimus
		Adduction: move leg back toward medial position and beyond if possible	30-50	Adductor longus, adductor brevis, adductor magnus
		Internal rotation: turn foot and leg toward other leg	90	Gluteus medius, gluteus minimus, tensor fasciae latae
		External rotation: turn foot and leg away from other leg	90	Obturatorius internus, obturatorius externus
		Circumduction: move leg in circle		Psoas major, gluteus maximus, gluteus medius, adductor magnus
Knee	Hinge	Flexion: bring heel back toward back of thigh	120-130	Biceps femoris, semitendinosus, semimembranosus, sartorius
		Extension: return leg to the floor	120-130	Rectus femoris, vastus lateralis, vastus medialis, vastus intermedius
Ankle	Hinge	Dorsal flexion: move foot so that toes are pointed upward	20-30	Tibialis anterior
		Plantar flexion: move foot so that toes are pointed downward	45-50	Gastrocnemius, soleus

TABLE 43-2	Range of Motion Exercises—cont'd			
Body Part	Type of Joint	Type of Movement	Range (degrees)	Primary Muscles
Foot	Gliding	Inversion: turn sole of foot medially	10 or less	Tibialis anterior, tibialis posterior
		Eversion: turn sole of foot laterally	10 or less	Peroneus longus, peroneus brevis
Toes	Condyloid	Flexion: curl toes downward	30-60	Flexor digitorum, lumbricalis pedis, flexor hallucis brevis
		Extension: straighten toes	30-60	Extensor digitorum longus, extensor digitorum brevis, extensor hallucis longus
		Abduction: spread toes apart	15 or less	Abductor hallucis, interosseus dorsalis
		Adduction: bring toes together	15 or less	Adductor hallucis, interosseus plantaris

A pregnant woman has fluctuations in her energy tolerance. During the first trimester she may have increased fatigue. Hormonal changes and fetal development use body energy, and the woman may be unable or unmotivated to carry out physical activities. The second trimester of pregnancy usually results in a return of activity tolerance to the prepregnancy state. In fact, some women feel their activity tolerance is greater during this period. During the last trimester, fetal development consumes a great deal of the mother's energy. In addition, because of the size and location of the fetus, the pregnant woman's ability to take a deep breath is decreased and less oxygen is available for physical activities.

As the person grows older, activity tolerance changes. Muscle mass is reduced, posture changes, and the composition of bones is altered. The individual may still exercise but will do it at a reduced intensity.

There is an overall improvement of physiological functioning as a result of exercise. All systems become stronger and function more efficiently. In nursing, certain interventions are directed at exercise. However, nurses often care for clients whose mobility is restricted and, as a result, must develop nursing therapies designed to reduce the hazards of immobility.

BODY ALIGNMENT. Assessment of body alignment can be carried out with the client standing, sitting, or lying down. This assessment has the following objectives:

1. Determining normal physiological changes in body alignment resulting from growth and development
2. Identifying deviations in body alignment caused by poor posture
3. Providing opportunities for clients to observe their posture
4. Identifying learning needs of clients for maintaining correct body alignment
5. Identifying trauma, muscle damage, or nerve dysfunction
6. Obtaining information concerning other factors that contribute to poor alignment, such as fatigue, malnutrition, and psychological problems

The first step in assessing body alignment is to put clients at ease so that unnatural or rigid positions are not assumed. When the body alignment of an immobilized or unconscious client is assessed, pillows and positioning supports should be removed from the bed and the client placed in the supine position.

Standing. The nurse should focus assessment of body alignment for the standing client on the following points:

1. The head is erect and midline.
2. When observed posteriorly, the shoulders and hips are straight and parallel.
3. When observed posteriorly, the vertebral column is straight.
4. When the client is observed laterally, the head is erect and the spinal curves are aligned in a reversed **S** pattern. The cervical vertebrae are anteriorly convex, the thoracic vertebrae are

posteriorly convex, and the lumbar vertebrae are anteriorly convex.

5. When observed laterally, the abdomen is comfortably tucked in and the knees and ankles are slightly flexed. The person appears comfortable and does not seem conscious of the flexion of knees or ankles.
6. The client's arms are comfortably at the sides.
7. Feet are placed slightly apart to achieve a base of support, and the toes are pointed forward.
8. When the client is viewed anteriorly, the center of gravity is in the midline, and the line of gravity is from the middle of the forehead to a midpoint between the feet. Laterally the line of gravity runs vertically from the middle of the skull to the posterior third of the foot (Fig. 43-14).

Sitting. The nurse assesses alignment of the sitting client by the following observations:

1. The head is erect, and the neck and vertebral column are in straight alignment.
2. The body weight is evenly distributed on the buttocks and thighs.
3. The thighs are parallel and in a horizontal plane.
4. Both feet are supported on the floor (Fig. 43-15). With clients of short stature, a footstool is used and the ankles are comfortably flexed.
5. A 2- to 4-cm (1- to 2-in) space is maintained between the edge of the seat and the popliteal space on the posterior surface of the knee. This space ensures that there is no pressure on the popliteal artery or nerve to decrease circulation or impair nerve function.
6. The client's forearms are supported on the armrest, in the lap, or on a table in front of the chair.

It is particularly important to assess alignment when sitting if the client has muscle weakness, muscle paralysis, or nerve damage. Because of these alterations, the client has diminished sensation in the affected area and is unable to perceive pressure or decreased circulation. Proper alignment while sitting reduces the risk of musculoskeletal system damage in such a client.

Lying. People who are conscious have voluntary muscle control and normal perception of pressure. As a result, they usually assume the position of comfort when lying down. Because their range of motion, sensation, and circulation are within normal limits, they change positions when they perceive muscle strain and decreased circulation.

Assessment of body alignment while lying requires that the client be placed in the lateral position with all but one pillow and all positioning supports removed from the bed (Fig. 43-16). The body should be supported by an adequate mattress. The vertebrae should be in straight alignment without observable

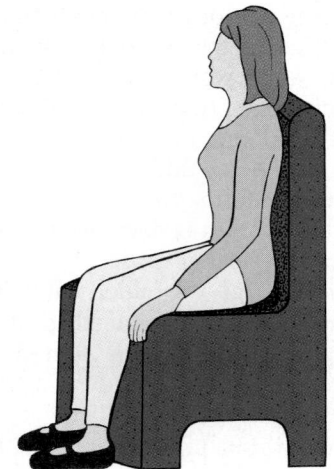

Fig. 43-15 Correct body alignment when sitting.

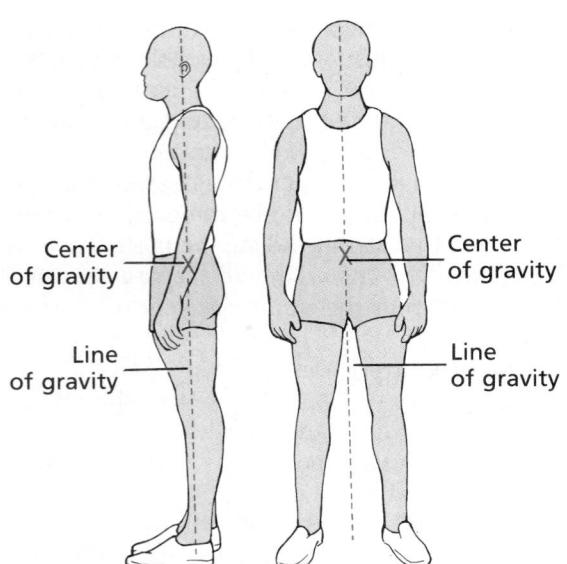

Fig. 43-14 Correct body alignment when standing.

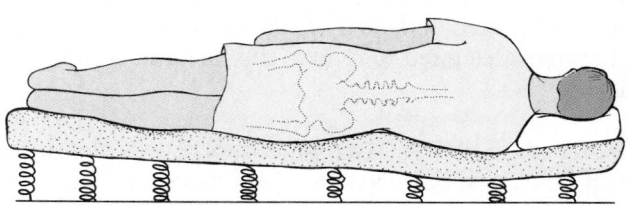

Fig. 43-16 Correct body alignment when lying down.

curves. This assessment provides baseline data concerning the client's body alignment.

Conditions that create a risk of damage to the musculoskeletal system when lying down include clients with impaired mobility, such as those in traction or with arthritis; clients with decreased sensation, such as those with hemiparesis resulting from a stroke; clients with impaired circulation, such as those with diabetes; and clients with lack of voluntary muscle control, such as those with spinal cord injuries.

When assessment indicates that a client is at risk for damage to the musculoskeletal system while lying down, interventions are directed at maintaining proper body alignment while positioning the client (see later section).

Immobility

The nurse assesses the immobilized client for hazards of immobility by performing a head-to-toe physical assessment (see Chapter 20). In addition, the nursing assessment should focus on certain physiological areas, as well as the client's psychosocial and developmental dimensions.

PHYSIOLOGICAL FACTORS. The physiological hazards of immobility that may be identified during a nursing assessment are summarized in Table 43-3.

Metabolic System. When assessing metabolic functioning, the nurse uses anthropometric measurements to evaluate muscle atrophy, uses intake and output records and laboratory data to evaluate fluid and electrolyte status and serum protein levels, assesses wound healing to evaluate alterations in the exchange of nutrients, and assesses the client's food intake and elimination patterns to determine altered gastrointestinal functioning.

Anthropometric measurements include height, weight, mid–upper arm circumference, and triceps skinfold measurements. Ideally, this assessment should be done early in the period of immobilization and should be repeated at 3-week intervals. A decrease in mid–upper arm circumference, measured in centimeters, or triceps skinfold, measured in millimeters, indicates a decline in muscle mass (Blackburn et al, 1977). This decline, along with decreased serum protein levels and decreased white cell count, can indicate that more protein is breaking down than building up. As a result, the client may be at risk for severe negative nitrogen balance. Measurements of the mid–upper arm circumference and triceps skinfold provide baseline information about subcutaneous fat, which may be lost during immobilization (see Chapter 35).

Intake and output measurements assist the nurse in determining whether a fluid imbalance exists. De-

---

TABLE 43-3   Physiological Hazards of Immobility

System	Assessment Techniques	Abnormal Findings
Metabolic	Inspection	Slowed wound healing, abnormal laboratory data
	Inspection	Muscle atrophy
	Anthropometric measurements (mid–upper arm circumference, triceps skinfold measurement)	Decreased amount of subcutaneous fat
	Palpation	Generalized edema resulting from hypoalbuminemia
Respiratory	Inspection	Asymmetrical chest wall movement, dyspnea
	Auscultation	Crackles, wheezes, increased respiratory rate
Cardiovascular	Auscultation	Orthostatic hypotension
	Auscultation, palpation	Increased heart rate, third heart sound, weak peripheral pulses, peripheral edema
Musculoskeletal	Inspection, palpation	Erythema, increased diameter in calf or thigh
	Palpation	Decreased ROM, joint contracture
	Inspection	Activity intolerance, muscle atrophy, joint contracture
Skin	Inspection, palpation	Break in skin integrity
Elimination	Inspection	Decreased urine output, cloudy or concentrated urine, decreased frequency of bowel movements
	Palpation	Distended bladder and abdomen
	Auscultation	Decreased bowel sounds

hydration and edema can increase the rate of skin breakdown in an immobilized client. Laboratory measurement of serum electrolyte levels can also indicate an electrolyte imbalance (see Chapter 39).

If an immobilized client has a wound, the rate of healing indicates how well nutrients are being delivered to tissues (see Chapter 48). Normal progression of healing indicates that metabolic needs of injured tissues are being met.

Anorexia occurs commonly in immobilized clients. The client's food intake should be assessed before the tray is removed to determine the amount eaten. Nutritional imbalances can be avoided if the nurse assesses the client's dietary patterns and food preferences early in immobilization (see Chapter 35).

Respiratory System. A respiratory assessment should be performed at least every 2 hours for clients with restricted activity. The nurse inspects chest wall movements during the full inspiratory-expiratory cycle. If a client has an atelectatic area, chest movement may be asymmetrical. In addition, the nurse auscultates the entire lung region to identify diminished breath sounds, crackles, or wheezes. Auscultation should focus on the dependent lung fields because pulmonary secretions tend to collect in these lower regions. A complete respiratory assessment identifies the presence of secretions and can be used to determine nursing interventions necessary for optimal respiratory function.

Cardiovascular System. Cardiovascular nursing assessment of the immobilized client includes blood pressure monitoring, evaluation of apical and peripheral pulses, and observation for signs of venous stasis (for example, edema and poor wound healing). Because of the risk for orthostatic hypotension, the client's blood pressure should be measured, particularly when changing from a lying (recumbent) to a sitting or standing position. In this way, the ability to tolerate postural changes can be assessed before the client leaves the safety of the bed.

The nurse also assesses the apical and peripheral pulses. Recumbency increases cardiac workload and results in an increased pulse rate. In some clients, particularly older adults, the heart may not tolerate the increased workload, and a form of cardiac failure may develop. A third heart sound, heard at the apex, can be an early indication of congestive heart failure. Monitoring peripheral pulses allows the nurse to evaluate the heart's ability to pump blood. The absence of a peripheral pulse in the lower extremities, particularly one that was previously present, should be documented and reported to the client's physician.

Edema may indicate the heart's inability to handle the increased workload. Because edema moves to dependent body regions, assessment of the immobilized client should include the sacrum, legs, and feet. If the heart is unable to tolerate the increased workload, peripheral body regions, such as the hands, feet, nose, and earlobes, will be colder than central body regions.

Finally, the nurse assesses the venous system because deep vein thrombosis is a hazard of restricted mobility. A dislodged thrombus, called an *embolus*, may travel through the circulatory system to the lungs or brain and impair circulation. Emboli to the lungs or brain pose a threat to life.

To assess for a deep vein thrombosis, the nurse removes the client's elastic stockings every 8 hours and observe the calves for redness, warmth, and tenderness. In addition, calf circumference should be measured daily. To do this the nurse marks a point on each calf 10 cm from the midpatella. The circumference is measured each day using the mark for placement of the tape measure. One-sided increases in calf diameter can be an early indication of thrombosis. Because deep vein thrombosis can also occur in the thigh, thigh measurements should be taken daily if the client is prone to thrombosis. In many clients, deep vein thrombosis can be prevented by active exercise and elastic stockings.

Musculoskeletal System. Major musculoskeletal abnormalities that may be identified during nursing assessment include decreased muscle tone, loss of muscle mass, and contractures. The anthropometric measurements described previously may indicate losses in muscle tone and muscle mass.

Assessment of ROM is important as a baseline against which later measurements can be compared to evaluate whether a loss in joint mobility has occurred. ROM is measured with a goniometer (see Chapter 20 and Table 43-1).

Disuse osteoporosis cannot be identified by physical assessment. However, postmenopausal women and persons with increased serum and urine calcium levels probably have a greater risk for bone demineralization. The risk of disuse osteoporosis should be considered when planning nursing interventions. For example, rib percussion and vibration (see Chapter 38) should be done cautiously with a client with probable disuse osteoporosis because of the risk of rib fracture.

Integumentary System. The nurse must continually assess the client's skin for signs of breakdown. The skin should be observed each time that the client is turned or hygiene measures are performed. At the minimum, assessment should occur every 2 hours (see Chapter 44).

Elimination System. The client's elimination status should be evaluated on each shift, and total intake and output should be evaluated every 24 hours.

The nurse should determine that the client is receiving the correct amount and type of fluids orally or parenterally (see Chapter 40).

Inadequate intake and output or fluid and electrolyte imbalances can increase the risk for renal system impairment, ranging from recurrent infections to kidney failure. Dehydration can also increase the risk for skin breakdown, thrombi formation, respiratory infections, and constipation. Such physical complications can decrease the overall level of mobility and increase duration and cost of care.

Assessment of elimination status should also include the frequency and consistency of bowel movements (see Chapter 41). Accurate assessment enables the nurse to intervene before constipation and fecal impaction occur.

PSYCHOSOCIAL FACTORS. Changes in the client's psychosocial status usually occur slowly and are often overlooked by health care personnel. The nurse should observe for changes in emotional status. The nurse should observe for several days before concluding that depression is the problem. Everyone becomes depressed at some time, especially hospitalized and immobilized clients, but not all depression requires nursing intervention. If the depression is caused by boredom or isolation, it can be alleviated by increasing bedside activities and occupational therapy.

The nurse also observes for behavioral changes, such as the cooperative client who becomes argumentative or the modest client who begins to expose genitalia repeatedly. The nurse should try to determine the reasons for such alterations to identify specific nursing therapies.

Unexplained changes in the sleep-wake cycle must be identified and corrected. Most can be prevented or minimized, such as those occurring because of nursing activities, a noisy environment, or discomfort. They may also occur because of medications such as analgesics, sleeping pills, or cardiovascular drugs (see Chapter 36).

Finally, the nurse should observe for changes in the client's use of normal coping mechanisms to adapt to immobilization (see Chapters 30 and 31). Decreasing coping ability may cause the client to become disoriented, confused, or depressed or to experience other behavioral changes.

Because psychosocial changes usually occur gradually, the nurse should observe the client's behavior on a daily basis. If behavioral changes occur, the nurse should determine the causes and evaluate the changes as short or long term. Identifying the cause helps the nurse design appropriate nursing interventions.

Developmental Factors

Assessment of the immobilized client should include developmental considerations to ensure that the client's needs are identified. The nurse determines whether the young child can meet developmental tasks and is progressing normally. The child's development may regress or be slowed because of immobilization. By identifying a child's overall developmental needs, the nurse can design nursing therapies to maintain normal development. The nurse may also need to assure the parents that developmental delays are usually temporary.

Developmental assessment is also important with the older client. Nursing assessment enables the nurse to determine the older client's ability to meet needs independently and to adapt to developmental changes such as declining physical functioning and altered family and peer relationships. A decline in developmental functioning needs prompt investigation to determine why the change occurred and what can be done to return to an optimal level of function as soon as possible.

Nursing Diagnosis

Nursing diagnoses identifying actual or potential alterations in body alignment and mobility are based on data collected during assessment. Analysis reveals clusters of data that indicate the presence or potential for a problem (see diagnoses box on p. 1486).

Body alignment and mobility are interrelated. A person with poor body alignment may have reduced mobility. When identifying nursing diagnoses, the nurse designs nursing strategies that reduce or prevent hazards associated with poor body alignment or impaired mobility.

Alterations in body alignment can result from developmental changes, postural abnormalities, abnormalities in bone formation, impaired muscle development, damage to the central nervous system, and direct trauma to the musculoskeletal system. Assessment data should contain appropriate defining characteristics to support the diagnostic label (see diagnostic process box on p. 1486).

Often, the physiological dimension is the only focus of nursing care for clients with impaired mobility. Thus the psychosocial and developmental dimensions are neglected. Yet they are important to health. For example, during immobilization, social interaction and stimuli are decreased. Ultimately the client may become isolated, withdrawn, and bored. Such clients may frequently use the nurse's call bell to request minor physical attention, when their real need is greater socialization.

Examples of Nursing Diagnoses Related to Improper Body Mechanics and Impaired Mobility

NANDA-APPROVED NURSING DIAGNOSES

Activity intolerance related to:
- Poor body alignment
- Decreased mobility

High risk for injury related to:
- Improper body mechanics
- Improper positioning
- Improper transfer techniques

Impaired physical mobility related to:
- Reduced ROM
- Bed rest
- Decreased strength

Ineffective airway clearance related to:
- Stasis of pulmonary secretions
- Improper body positioning

Ineffective breathing pattern related to:
- Decreased lung expansion
- Accumulation of pulmonary secretions
- Improper body positioning

Impaired gas exchange related to:
- Asymmetrical breathing patterns
- Decreased lung expansion
- Accumulation of pulmonary secretions

Actual or *high risk for impaired skin integrity* related to:
- Restricted mobility
- Pressure on skin's surface
- Shearing force

Altered patterns of urinary elimination related to:
- Restricted mobility
- High risk for infection
- Urinary retention

High risk for infection related to:
- Stasis of pulmonary secretions
- Impaired skin integrity
- Stasis of urine

Total incontinence related to:
- Altered elimination patterns
- Restricted mobility
- Infrequent offering of bed pan or urinal by nurses

High risk for fluid volume deficit related to:
- Decreased fluid intake

Ineffective individual coping related to:
- Reduced activity level
- Social isolation

Sleep pattern disturbance related to:
- Restricted mobility
- Discomfort

Sample Nursing Diagnostic Process for Impaired Physical Mobility and High Risk for Injury

Assessment Activities	Defining Characteristics	Nursing Diagnoses
Measure ROM during exercises of extremities.	Limited range of motion with left shoulder Reluctance to attempt movement with left shoulder Impaired coordination while attempting to perform ROM with left shoulder	*Impaired physical mobility* related to left shoulder pain
Ask client about perception of pain.	Client complains of sharp pain in shoulder	
Ask client about endurance and activity tolerance.	Client reports decreased muscle strength in left shoulder	
Inspect client's skin for degree of intactness around casted extremity.	Broken skin over areas of cast	*High risk for injury* related to pressure from cast
Observe client's gait and ability to move independently.	Decreased ability to independently change body position	

Planning

The nurse plans therapeutic interventions for clients with actual or potential risks to body alignment and mobility. The nurse plans therapies according to severity of risks to the client, and the plan is individualized according to the client's developmental stage, level of health, and lifestyle.

It is important to consider the client's home environment when planning therapies to maintain or improve body alignment and mobility. Planning care also involves an understanding of the client's need to maintain motor function and independence. The nurse and client work together to establish ways of maintaining client involvement in nursing care and to maintain optimal body alignment and mobility whether the client is in the hospital or home.

Clients at risk for hazards associated with improper body alignment and impaired mobility require a care plan directed at meeting their special needs. Clients at risk for hazards of immobility require a care plan toward actual or potential positioning and mobility needs (see care plan). The care plan is based on one or more of the following client goals:

1. Maintaining proper body alignment
2. Regaining proper body alignment or optimal level of body alignment
3. Reducing injuries to the skin and musculoskeletal systems resulting from improper body mechanics or alignment

4. Achieving full or optimal ROM
5. Preventing contractures
6. Maintaining a patent airway
7. Achieving optimal lung expansion and gas exchange
8. Mobilizing airway secretions
9. Maintaining cardiovascular function
10. Increasing activity tolerance
11. Achieving normal elimination patterns
12. Maintaining normal sleep-wake patterns
13. Achieving socialization
14. Achieving independent completion of self-care activities
15. Achieving physical and mental stimulation

Maintaining body alignment is especially important in clients with actual or potential limitations in mobility. For example, a comatose client should be positioned with pillows and the position changed at least every 2 hours to reduce the risk of poor alignment and future injury to the skin and musculoskeletal system.

Implementation

Body Alignment

To maintain proper body alignment the nurse correctly lifts the client, uses proper positioning techniques, and safely transfers clients from a bed to a chair or a bed to a stretcher. Procedures described in

Sample Nursing Care Plan for Impaired Physical Mobility

Nursing diagnosis: *Impaired physical mobility* related to left shoulder pain
Definition: Impaired physical mobility is the state in which an individual experiences a limitation of ability for independent physical mobility (Kim, McFarland, McLane, 1991).

Goal	Expected Outcomes	Interventions	Rationale
Client will regain normal ROM (180 degrees flexion and extension) of left shoulder within 4 mo.	Client will maintain present ROM in upper extremity joints.	Offer analgesic 30 min before ROM exercises.	Action of analgesic will peak as client begins exercises.
	Client will perform self-care activities using left arm within 2 days.	Teach client specific ROM exercises to left shoulder and arm.	Teaching provides client with opportunity and knowledge to maintain and increase ROM. (Lehmkuhl et al, 1990)
	Client will follow regular exercise program by discharge.	Schedule active exercises between meals and hygiene.	This promotes frequent exercise to affected joints and reduces risk of contracture development (Lehmkuhl et al, 1990).

Proper Lifting

STEPS	RATIONALE
1. Assess position of weight, height of object, body position, and maximum weight.	Determines whether you are able to do it yourself or require help (Stamps, 1989).
2. Lift object correctly from below center of gravity:	
a. Come close to object to be moved.	Moves center of gravity closer to object.
b. Enlarge your base of support by placing feet slightly apart.	Maintains better body balance, thus reducing risk of falling.
c. Lower your center of gravity to object to be lifted.	Increases body balance and enables muscle groups to work together in synchronized manner.
d. Maintain proper alignment of head and neck with vertebrae, keeping trunk straight.	Reduces risk of injury to lumbar vertebrae and muscle groups (Owen, Garg, 1991).
3. Lift object correctly from shelf above center of gravity:	
a. Use safe, stable step stool. Do not stand on top stair.	Raises center of gravity closer to object.
b. Stand as close to shelf as possible.	Increases body balance during the lift.
c. Quickly transfer weight of object from shelf to arms and over base of support.	Reduces danger of falling by moving lifted object close to center of gravity over base support.

this section incorporate principles of body mechanics needed to maintain or restore body alignment.

LIFTING TECHNIQUES. The rate of injuries in occupational settings has increased in recent years, and more than half are back injuries that are the direct result of improper lifting and bending techniques (Owen, 1980; Owen, Garg, 1991). The most common back injury is strain on the lumbar muscle group, which includes the muscles around the lumbar vertebrae (Owen, Garg, 1991). Muscle injury to these areas affects the ability to bend forward, backward, and side to side. In addition, the ability to rotate the hips and lower back is decreased.

The nurse is at risk for injury to lumbar muscles in lifting, transferring, or positioning the immobilized client. Before lifting, the nurse should assess ability to lift the client or object by determining the following basic lifting criteria:

1. Position of weight. The weight to be lifted should be as close to the lifter as possible. Positioning the object in such a manner uses the lifting force of the nurse because the object is in the same plane (Stamps, 1989).
2. Height of the object. The best height for lifting vertically is slightly above the level of the middle finger of a person with the arm hanging at the side (Owen, 1980; Owen, Garg, 1991).
3. Body position. When the lifter's body position varies with different lifting tasks, the following

general rule is applicable to most lifting situations: the body is positioned with the trunk erect so that multiple muscle groups work together in a synchronized manner.

4. Maximum weight. Each nurse should know the maximum weight that is safe to carry—safe for the nurse and the client. An object is too heavy if its weight is 35% or more of a person's body weight. Therefore a nurse who weighs 130 lb (59.1kg) should not try to lift an immobilized 100-lb (45.5-kg) person. Although the nurse may be able to do it, there is a risk of dropping the client or causing injury to the nurse's back.

When lifting, the nurse should follow a procedure designed to protect the musculoskeletal system (Procedure 43-1).

Lifting an object from a high shelf increases risks because it is more difficult to maintain body balance. To reach an object overhead, people often stand on tiptoe with their feet together, thereby decreasing their base of support, elevating their center of gravity, and ultimately decreasing their balance.

POSITIONING TECHNIQUES. Clients with impaired nervous, skeletal, or muscular system functioning and increased weakness and fatigability often require help from the nurse to attain proper body alignment while in bed or sitting. Several devices are available for the nurse to maintain good body alignment for clients while they are being positioned (Table 43-4).

TABLE 43-4   Devices Used for Proper Positioning

Device	Uses
Pillow	Provides support of body or extremity; elevates body part; splints incisional area to reduce postoperative pain during activity or coughing and deep breathing
Footboard or Posey footguard	Maintains feet in dorsiflexion
Trochanter roll (Fig. 43-17)	Prevents external rotation of legs when client is in supine position
Sandbag	Provides support and shape to body contours; immobilizes extremity; maintains specific body alignment
Hand roll	Maintains thumb slightly adducted and in opposition to fingers; maintains fingers in slightly flexed position
Hand-wrist splint	Are individually molded for client to maintain proper alignment of thumb; are slightly adducted in opposition to fingers; maintains wrist in slight dorsal flexion
Trapeze bar	Enables client to raise trunk from bed; enables client to transfer from bed to wheelchair; allows client to perform exercises that strengthen upper arms
Side rail	Allows weak client to roll from side to side or to sit up in bed
Bed board	Provides additional support to mattress and improves vertebral alignment

Pillows are readily available in hospitals or extended care facilities. However, when the client is at home, the supply may be limited. Before using a pillow, the nurse should determine whether it is the proper size. A thick pillow under the client's head increases cervical flexion. A thin pillow under body prominences may be inadequate to protect skin and tissue from damage caused by pressure. When additional pillows are unavailable or if they are an improper size, the nurse can fold sheets, blankets, or towels.

A footboard is placed perpendicular to the mattress, parallel to and touching the plantar surfaces of the client's feet (see Fig. 34-6). The **footboard** prevents footdrop by maintaining the feet in dorsiflexion. After placing it on the bed, the nurse needs to determine that it is correctly placed, with the client's feet placed firmly against the board. A Posey footguard is a device that uses foam structures to maintain the client's feet in the dorsiflexed position.

The **trochanter roll** prevents external rotation of the legs when the client is in a supine position. To form a trochanter roll, a cotton bath blanket is folded lengthwise to a width that will extend from the greater trochanter of the femur to the lower border of the popliteal space (Fig. 43-17). The blanket is placed under the buttocks and then rolled counterclockwise until the thigh is in the neutral position or in inward rotation. When correct alignment of the hip is achieved, the patella faces directly upward.

Sandbags are sand-filled plastic tubes that can be shaped to body contours. Sandbags can be used in place of or in addition to trochanter rolls. They immobilize an extremity or maintain body alignment.

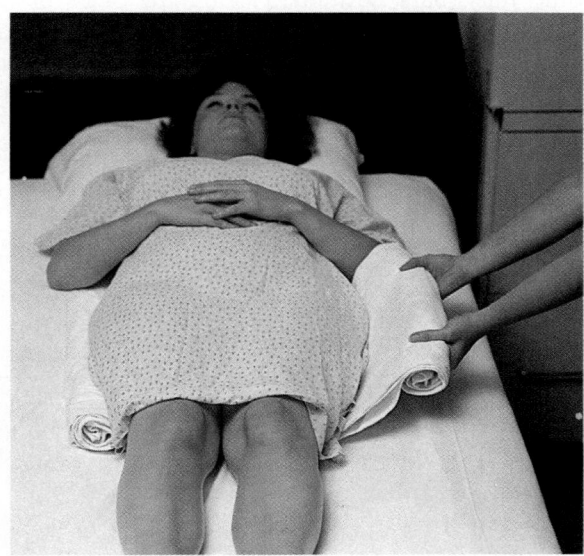

Fig. 43-17   Trochanter roll.

Hand rolls maintain the thumb in slight adduction and in opposition to the fingers. A hand roll maintains the hand, thumb, and fingers in a functional position. Hand rolls can be made by folding a washcloth in half, rolling it lengthwise, and securing it with tape. The roll is placed against the palmar surface of the client's hand. The nurse evaluates the hand roll to make sure that the hand is indeed in a functional position. If washcloths are in short supply, a roll of Kerlix can be used.

Hand-wrist splints are individually molded for the client to maintain proper alignment of the thumb (slight adduction) and the wrist (slight dorsiflexion). These splints should be used only by the client for whom the splint was made.

The **trapeze bar** is a triangular device that descends from a securely fastened overhead bar that is attached to the bed frame. It allows the client to pull with upper extremities to raise the trunk off the bed, to assist in transfer from bed to wheelchair, or to perform upper arm exercises (Fig. 43-18).

Restraints are devices used for immobilization, especially of confused or disoriented clients. A common jacket restraint is the Posey jacket (Fig. 43-19). When placing the jacket on the client, the nurse laps one side over the other on the client's back. The ties are placed under the loop on the jacket and secured to the bed, chair, or wheelchair frame. Restraints should *never* be tied to side rails because the client may be injured if a side rail is lowered with the restraint in place (see Chapter 42).

Side rails, bars positioned along the sides of the bed, ensure client safety (see Chapter 42) and are also useful for increasing mobility. In addition, they allow the weak client to roll from side to side or sit up in bed.

Bed boards are plywood boards placed under the entire mattress. They are useful for increasing back support and alignment, especially with a soft mattress.

Although each procedure for positioning has specific guidelines, there are some universal steps the nurse should follow for clients who require positioning assistance (Procedure 43-2).

Following the guidelines reduces the risk of injury to the musculoskeletal system when the client is sitting or lying. When joints are unsupported, their alignment is impaired. Likewise, if joints are not positioned in a slightly flexed position, their mobility is decreased. During positioning, the nurse also assesses for pressure points. When actual or potential pressure areas exist, nursing interventions involve removal of the pressure, thus decreasing the risk for development of pressure ulcers (see Chapter 44) and further trauma to the musculoskeletal system.

Supported Fowler's Position. In the supported Fowler's position, the head of the bed is elevated 45 to 60 degrees and the client's knees are slightly elevated without pressure to restrict circulation in the lower legs. The angle of head and knee elevation and the length of time that the client should remain in the Fowler's position are influenced by the client's illness and overall condition. Supports must permit flexion of the hips and knees and proper alignment of the normal curves in the cervical, thoracic, and lumbar vertebrae. The following are common trouble areas for the client in the Fowler's position:

1. Increased cervical flexion because the pillow at the head is too thick and the head thrusts forward

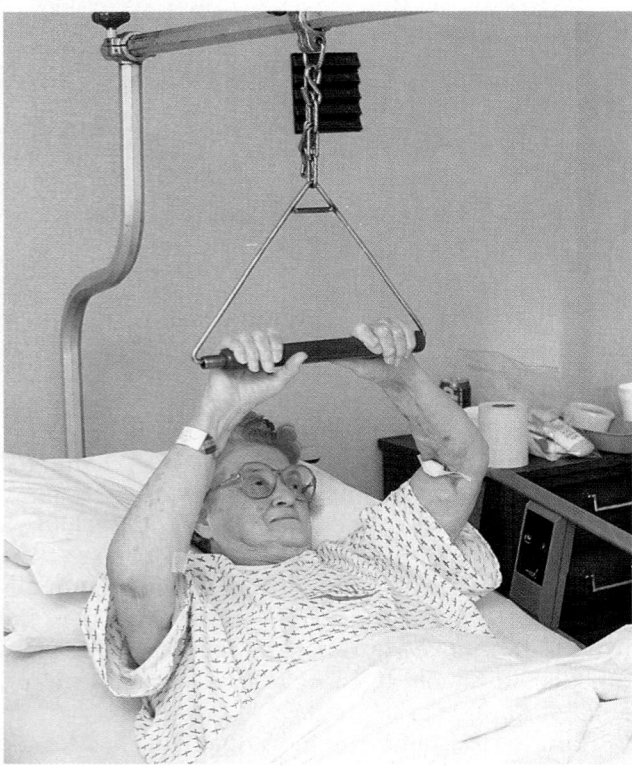

Fig. 43-18   Client using a trapeze bar.

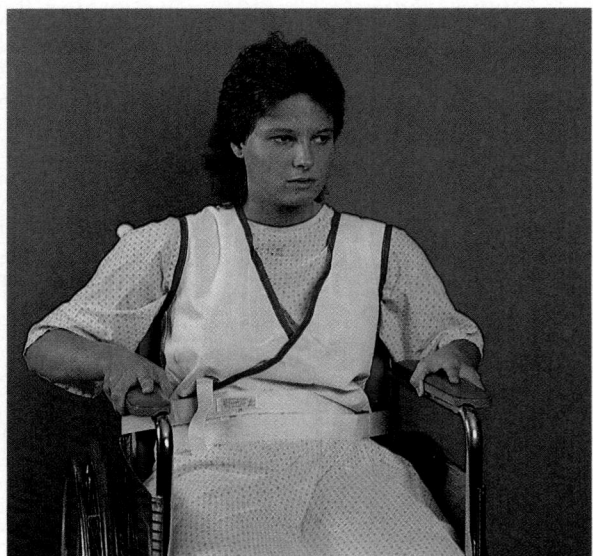

Fig. 43-19   Client restrained with Posey jacket looped through wheelchair arms.

STEPS	RATIONALE
1. Assess client's body alignment and comfort level while client is lying down.	Provides baseline data concerning client's body alignment and comfort level.
2. Prepare following equipment and supplies: a. Pillows e. Hand rolls b. Footboard f. Restraints c. Trochanter rolls g. Side rails d. Sandbags	Provides easy access to equipment necessary for proper positioning.
3. Raise level of bed to comfortable working height and remove pillows and devices used in previous position.	Raises level of work toward nurse's center of gravity, reduces interference from bedding during positioning procedure (Owen, Garg, 1991).
4. Obtain help as needed.	Provides for safety.
5. Explain procedure to client.	Helps decrease anxiety and increase cooperation.
6. Wash hands.	Reduces transmission of infection.
7. Provide for client privacy.	Ensuring client's mental comfort is important.
8. Put bed in flat position and move client to head of bed.	Provides easy access to client and allows nursing personnel to reposition client without working against gravity. Allows room for proper positioning. Helps maintain proper body alignment.
9. Position client in supported Fowler's position: a. Elevate head of bed 45-60 degrees.	Increases comfort, improves ventilation, and increases opportunity to socialize or relax.
b. Rest head against mattress or on small pillow.	Prevents cervical flexion contractures.
c. Use pillows to support arms and hand if client does not have voluntary control or use of hands and arms.	Prevents shoulder dislocation from effect of downward gravitational pull of unsupported arms, promotes circulation by preventing venous pooling, and prevents flexion contractures of arms and wrists.
d. Position pillow at lower back.	Supports lumbar vertebrae and decreases flexion of vertebrae.
e. Place small pillow or roll under thigh.	Prevents hyperextension of knee and occlusion of popliteal artery from pressure from body weight.
f. Place small pillow or roll under ankles.	Prevents prolonged pressure on heels from mattress.
g. Place footboard at bottom of client's feet (see illustration).	Maintains dorsal flexion and prevents footdrop.

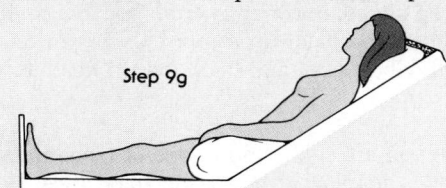

Step 9g

STEPS	RATIONALE
10. Position hemiplegic client in supported Fowler's position:	
a. Elevate head of bed 45-60 degrees.	Increases comfort, improves ventilation, and increases opportunity to relax.
b. Sit client up as straight as possible.	Counteracts tendency to slump toward affected side. Improves ventilation, cardiac output; decreases intracranial pressure. Improves ability to swallow and helps prevent aspiration of food, liquids, or gastric secretions.
c. Position head with chin slightly forward.	Reduces risk of joint dislocation.
d. Provide support for involved arm and hand on overbed table in front of client; place arm away from client's side and support elbow with pillow.	Paralyzed muscles do not automatically resist pull of gravity as they do normally. As a result, shoulder subluxation, pain, or edema may occur.

Positioning Clients in Bed

STEPS	RATIONALE
e. Position *flaccid* hand in normal resting position with wrist slightly extended, arches of hand maintained, and fingers partially flexed; OPTION: use one section of rubber ball cut in half.	Maintains hand in functional position. Prevents contractures (Lehmkuhl et al, 1990).
f. Position *spastic* hand with wrist in neutral position or slightly extended; fingers should be extended with palm down or may be left in relaxed position with palm up.	Maintains hand in functional position. Inhibits flexor spasticity (Lehmkuhl et al, 1990).
g. Flex knees and hips by using pillow or folded blanket under knees.	Ensures proper alignment. Prevents prolonged hyperextension, which could impair joint mobility.
h. Support feet in dorsiflexion with soft pillow or footboard.	Prevents footdrop. Stimulation of ball of foot by hard surface has tendency to increase muscle tone in client with extensor spasticity of lower extremity.

11. Position client in supine position:

a. Place client on back with head of bed flat.	Necessary for positioning in supine position.
b. Place small rolled towel under lumbar area of back.	Provides support for lumbar spine.
c. Place pillow under upper shoulders, neck, and head.	Maintains correct alignment and prevents flexion contractures of cervical vertebrae.
d. Place trochanter rolls or sandbags parallel to lateral surface of thighs.	Reduces external rotation of hip.
e. Place small pillow or roll under ankle to elevate heels.	Reduces pressure on heels, helping prevent pressure ulcers.
f. Place footboard or soft pillows against bottom of feet.	Maintains feet in dorsiflexion. Prevents footdrop.
g. Place pillows under pronated forearms, maintaining upper arms parallel to client's body (see illustration).	Reduces internal rotation of shoulder and prevents extension of elbows. Maintains correct body alignment.
h. Place hand rolls in hand.	Reduces extension of fingers and abduction of thumb. Maintains thumb slightly adducted and in opposition.

12. Position hemiplegic client in supine position:

a. Place head of bed flat.	Necessary for positioning in supine position.
b. Place folded towel or pillow under shoulder of affected side.	Decreases possibility of pain, joint contracture, or subluxation. Maintains mobility in muscles around shoulder to permit movement patterns.
c. Keep affected arm away from body with elbow extended and palm up. OPTION: place arm out to side with elbow bent and hand toward head to bed.	Maintains mobility in arm, joints, and muscles around shoulder to permit normal movement patterns. (Counteracts limitation of ability of arm to rotate outward at shoulder [external rotation]. External rotation must be present to raise arm overhead without pain.)
d. Position affected hand in one of recommended positions for flaccid or spastic hand (see Steps 12e and 12f).	Maintains hand in functional position.

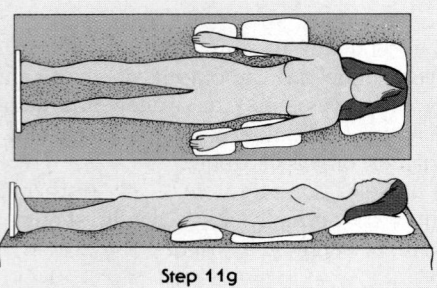

Step 11g

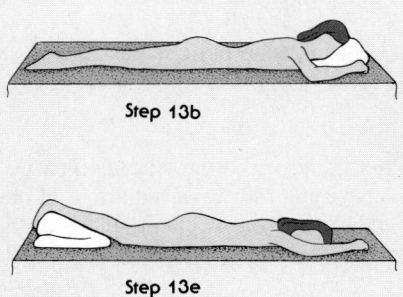

Step 13b

Step 13e

STEPS	RATIONALE
e. Place folded towel under hip of involved side.	Diminishes effect of spasticity in entire leg by controlling hip position.
f. Flex affected knee 30 degrees by supporting it on pillow or folded blanket.	Slight flexion breaks up abnormal extension pattern of leg. Extensor spasticity is most severe when client is supine.
g. Support feet with soft pillows at right angle to leg.	Maintains foot in dorsiflexion and prevents footdrop. Soft pillows prevent stimulation to ball of foot by hard surface, which has tendency to increase muscle tone in client with extensor spasticity of lower extremity.
13. Position client in prone position:	
a. Roll client over arm positioned close to body with elbow straight and hand under hip. Position on abdomen in center of bed with bed flat.	Positions client so that alignment can be maintained.
b. Turn client's head to one side and support with small pillow (see illustration).	Reduces flexion or hyperextension of cervical vertebrae.
c. Place small pillow under abdomen below level of diaphragm.	Reduces pressure on breasts of some women. Decreases hyperextension of lumbar vertebrae and strain on lower back. Improves breathing by reducing mattress pressure on diaphragm.
d. Support arms in flexed position level at shoulders.	Maintains proper body alignment. Support reduces risk of joint dislocation.
e. Support lower legs with pillow to elevate toes (see illustration).	Prevents footdrop. Reduces external rotation of legs. Reduces mattress pressure on toes.
14. Position hemiplegic client in prone position:	
a. With head of bed flat, move client toward unaffected side.	Ensures proper client alignment in center of bed when rolled onto abdomen.
b. Roll client onto unaffected side.	
c. Place pillow against abdomen.	Prevents sagging of abdomen when client is rolled over. Decreases hyperextension of lumbar vertebrae and strain on lower back.
d. Roll client onto abdomen by positioning involved arm close to client's body with elbow straight and hand under hip. Roll client carefully over arm.	Prevents injury to affected side.
e. Turn head toward involved side.	Promotes development of neck and trunk extension, which is necessary for standing and walking.
f. Position involved arm out to side with elbow bent and hand toward head of bed, fingers extended if possible.	Counteracts limitation of arm's ability to rotate outward at shoulder (external rotation). External rotation must be present to raise arm over head without pain.
g. Flex both knees slightly by placing pillow under both legs from knees to ankles.	Prevents prolonged hyperextension, which could impair joint mobility.
h. Keep feet at right angles to legs by using pillow high enough to keep toes off mattress.	Maintains feet in dorsiflexion.
15. Position client in lateral (side-lying) position:	
a. Lower head of bed completely or as low as client can tolerate.	Provides position of comfort for client and removes pressure from bony prominences on back.
b. Position client to side of bed.	Provides room for client to turn to side.
c. Turn client onto side:	
(1) To turn helpless client onto side, flex client's knee that will not be next to mattress. Place one hand on client's hip and one hand on shoulder.	Prevents injury to joints as client is rolled to side. Leverage on hip makes turning easy.
(2) Roll client onto side.	Rolling client toward you causes less trauma to tissues.
d. Place pillow under client's head and neck.	Maintains alignment. Reduces lateral neck flexion. Decreases strain on sternocleidomastoid muscle.

Positioning Clients in Bed

STEPS	RATIONALE
e. Bring shoulder blade forward.	Prevents weight from resting directly on shoulder joint.
f. Position both arms in slightly flexed position. Uppermost arm is supported by pillow level with shoulder.	Decreases internal rotation and adduction of shoulder. Protects joint. Ventilation is improved because chest can expand more easily.
g. Place tuck-back pillow behind client's back. (Make tuck-back pillow by folding pillow lengthwise. Smooth area is slightly tucked under back.)	Provides support to maintain client on side.
h. Place pillow under semiflexed upper leg level at hip from groin to foot (see illustration).	Prevents hyperextension of leg. Maintains leg in proper alignment. Prevents pressure on bony prominence.
i. Place sandbag parallel to plantar surface of dependent foot.	Maintains dorsiflexion of the foot. Prevents footdrop.
16. Position client in Sims' (semiprone) position:	
a. Place head of bed flat.	Provides for proper body alignment while client is lying.
b. Place client in supine position.	Prepares client for Sims' position.
c. Position client in lateral position lying partially on abdomen.	Client is rolled only partially on abdomen.
d. Place small pillow under head.	Maintains proper alignment and prevents lateral neck flexion.
e. Place pillow under flexed upper arm, supporting arm level with shoulder. Support other arm on mattress.	Prevents internal rotation of shoulder. Maintains proper alignment.
f. Place pillow under flexed upper legs, supporting leg level with hip (see illustration).	Prevents internal rotation of hip and adduction of leg. Prevents hyperextension of leg. Reduces mattress pressure on knees and ankles.
g. Place sandbags parallel to plantar surface of foot.	Maintains foot in dorsiflexion. Prevents footdrop.
17. Wash hands.	Reduces transmission of infection.
18. Lower bed.	Provides for client safety.
19. Observe body alignment position, level of comfort, and potential pressure points.	Determines effectiveness of positioning, maintenance of body alignment, and protection from pressure. Reduces risk of musculoskeletal injury related to improper positioning.
20. Record procedure in nurses' notes, including position assumed, frequency of turning, condition of skin, joint movement, use of supports or splints, client's ability to assist with repositioning, number of staff needed to complete procedure, and client comfort.	Documents effectiveness of nursing care. Provides for consistency among nursing staff.

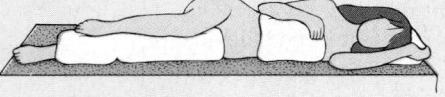

Step 15h

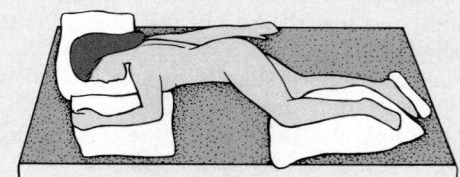

Step 16f

2. Extension of knees, allowing the client to slide to the foot of the bed
3. Pressure on the posterior aspect of the knee, decreasing circulation to the feet
4. External rotation of hips
5. Arms hanging unsupported at the client's sides
6. Unsupported feet
7. Unprotected pressure points at the sacrum and heels

Supine Position. The supine position, in which the client rests on the back, is also called the *dorsal recumbent position*. In the supine position the relationship of body parts is essentially the same as in good standing alignment except that the body is in the horizontal plane. Pillows, trochanter rolls, and hand rolls or arm splints are used to increase comfort and reduce injury to the skin or musculoskeletal system.

The mattress should be firm enough to support the cervical, thoracic, and lumbar vertebrae. Shoulders are supported and the elbows are slightly flexed to control shoulder rotation. A foot support is used to prevent footdrop and maintain proper alignment. The following are some common trouble areas for the supine position:

1. Pillow at the head too thick, increasing cervical flexion
2. Head flat on the mattress
3. Shoulders unsupported and internally rotated
4. Elbows extended
5. Thumb not in opposition to the fingers
6. Hips externally rotated
7. Unsupported feet
8. Unprotected pressure points at the occiput region of the head, lumbar vertebrae, elbows, and heels

Prone Position. The client in the prone position is lying face down. The pillow under the head should be thin enough to prevent cervical flexion or extension and maintain alignment of the lumbar spine. Placing a pillow under the lower leg permits dorsiflexion of the ankles and some knee flexion, which promotes relaxation. If a pillow is unavailable, the ankles should be in dorsiflexion over the end of the mattress. The nurse should assess for and correct any of the following potential trouble points:

1. Neck hyperextension
2. Hyperextension of the lumbar spine
3. Plantar flexion of the ankles
4. Unprotected pressure points at the chin, elbows, hips, knees, and toes

Side-Lying Position. In the side-lying (or lateral) position the client is resting on the side, with the major portion of body weight on the dependent hip and shoulder. Trunk alignment should be the same as in standing. For example, the structural curves of the spine should be maintained, the head should be supported in line with the midline of the trunk, and rotation of the spine should be avoided. The following trouble points are common in the side-lying position:

1. Lateral flexion of the neck
2. Spinal curves out of normal alignment
3. Shoulder and hip joints internally rotated, adducted, or unsupported
4. Lack of support for the feet
5. Lack of protection for pressure points at the ear, ilium, knees, and ankles

Sims' Position. The Sims' position differs from the side-lying position in the distribution of the client's weight. In the Sims' position the weight is placed on the anterior ilium, humerus, and clavicle. Trouble points common in the Sims' position include the following:

1. Lateral flexion of the neck
2. Internal rotation, adduction, or lack of support to the shoulders and hips
3. Lack of support for the feet
4. Lack of protection for pressure points at the ilium, humerus, clavicle, knees, and ankles

TRANSFER TECHNIQUES. Nurses often provide care for immobilized clients whose position must be changed, who must be moved up in bed, or who must be transferred from a bed to a chair or a bed to a stretcher. Proper body mechanics enables the nurse to move, lift, or transfer clients safely and also protects the nurse from injury to the musculoskeletal system. Although nurses use many transfer techniques, the following general guidelines should be followed in any transfer procedure:

1. Raising the side rail on the side of the bed opposite the nurse to prevent the client from falling out of bed
2. Elevating the level of the bed to a comfortable height
3. Assessing the client's mobility and strength to determine assistance the client can offer during transfer
4. Determing the need for assistance
5. Explaining the procedure and describing what is expected of the client
6. Assessing for correct body alignment and pressure areas after each transfer

The nurse who is attempting transfer or moving techniques for the first time should request help to reduce the risk of injury to client and nurse. The nurse should also recognize personal strength and its limits. Moving a completely immobilized client alone is difficult and dangerous.

Moving Clients. Clients require various levels of assistance to move up in bed, more to the side-lying position, or sit up at the side of the bed. For example, a young, healthy woman may need only a little support as she sits at the side of the bed for the first time after childbirth, whereas an older man may need help from one or more nurses to do the same task 1 day after an appendectomy.

To determine what the client is able to do alone and how many people are needed to help move the client in bed, the nurse assesses the client to determine whether the illness contradicts exertion (for example, cardiovascular disease). Next, the nurse determines whether the client comprehends what is expected. For example, a client recently medicated for postoperative pain may be too lethargic to understand instruction, so to ensure safety, two nurses are needed to move the client in bed. The nurse then determines the comfort level of the client. The nurse also evaluates personal strength and knowledge of the procedure. Finally the nurse determines whether the client is too heavy or immobile for the nurse to complete the procedure alone. In doubtful cases the nurse should always request assistance from another person. Procedures 43-3 and 43-4 describe the steps commonly used in moving clients in bed and transferring them to a sitting position at the side of the bed.

Transferring a Client from a Bed to a Chair.

Transfer of a client from bed to chair by one nurse requires assistance from the client and should not be attempted with a client who cannot help (Procedure 43-4). The nurse explains the procedure to the client before the transfer. The environment is also prepared by moving obstacles out of the way. The chair is placed next to the bed with the chair back in the same plane as the head of the bed. Placement of the chair allows the nurse to pivot with the client and to transfer the client's weight quickly.

A safe transfer is the first priority. The nurse who is doubtful about personal strength or the client's ability to help should request assistance. The client should sit and dangle the feet at the side of the bed for a minute before standing. Then the client should stand at the side of the bed for another minute so that the client can quickly be lowered back into it in case of dizziness or fainting.

Transferring a Client From a Bed to a Stretcher.

An immobilized client who must be transferred from bed to stretcher or bed to bed requires a three-person carry (Procedure 43-4). This technique is best implemented when personnel who are doing the lifting are similar in height. If their centers of gravity are within the same plane, they can lift as a team.

Caution is used when the client has spinal cord trauma. If the client must be moved, the three-person carry is used and spinal alignment is maintained during the transfer.

The client should be prepared for the transfer and asked to help when possible by, for example, folding the arms over the chest. The environment should be free from obstacles, and unnecessary equipment should be removed from the bed. The stretcher should be placed at a right angle to the bed so that the lifters can pivot toward the stretcher and transfer the client quickly.

As with all procedures, safety is the priority. Safety is increased in the three-person carry if the lifters

work together. Therefore one person should assume the leadership role.

Joint Mobility

To ensure adequate joint mobility the nurse can teach the client about ROM exercises. When the client does not have voluntary motor control, the nurse institutes passive ROM exercises. Joint mobility is also increased by walking. Occasionally clients need to use mechanical devices such as crutches to help them walk.

ROM EXERCISES. Clients with restricted mobility are unable to perform some or all ROM exercises independently. This limitation can be identified in clients in whom one extremity has limited movement or in completely immobilized clients. When caring for clients with actual or potential impaired mobility, the nurse designs interventions directed at maintaining maximum joint mobility. One such nursing intervention is ROM exercises.

To ensure that clients routinely receive these exercises, the nurse should schedule them at specific times, perhaps with another nursing activity, such as during the client's bath. This enables the nurse to systematically assess and improve the client's ROM. In addition, bathing or receiving a bed bath usually requires that extremities and joints are put through complete ROM.

ROM exercises may be active (the client is able to move all joints through their ROM unassisted), passive (the client is unable to move independently and the nurse moves each joint through its ROM), or somewhere in between. With a weak client, for example, the nurse may merely provide support while the client performs most of the movement, or the client may be able to move some joints actively while the nurse passively moves others. The nurse first assesses the client's ability to engage in active ROM exercises and the need for assistance from the nurse. In general, exercises should be as active as health and mobility allow. Contractures may develop in joints not moved periodically through their full ROM.

Unless contraindicated, the care plan should include moving the client's extremities through the full ROM possible. Passive ROM exercises should begin as soon as the client's ability to move the extremity or joint is lost. Movements are carried out slowly and smoothly and should not cause pain. The nurse should never force a joint beyond its capacity. Each movement should be repeated 5 times during the session.

When performing passive ROM exercises, the nurse stands at the side of the bed closest to the joint being exercised. If an extremity is to be moved or

Text continued on p. 1502.

STEPS	RATIONALE
1. Assess client's comfort level, activity tolerance, muscle strength, and mobility.	Provides baseline data to determine client's ability to assist in moving.
2. Raise level of bed to comfortable working height.	Raises level of work toward your center of gravity.
3. Remove pillows and devices used in previous position.	Reduces interference from bedding.
4. Get extra help as needed.	Provides for safety.
5. Explain procedure to client and provide for client privacy.	Decreases client anxiety and increases cooperation. Ensures client's mental comfort.
6. Wash hands.	Reduces transmission of infection.
7. Put bed in flat position with wheels on bed locked.	Provides easy access to client and allows you to reposition client without having to work against gravity.
8. Move helpless client up in bed (one nurse):	
a. Place client on back with head of bed flat. Stand on one side of bed.	Enables you to assess body alignment. Reduces gravitational pull on client's upper body.
b. Place pillow at head of bed.	Prevents striking client's head against bed.
c. Begin at client's feet. Face foot of bed at 45-degree angle. Place feet apart with foot nearest head of bed behind other foot (forward-backward stance). Flex knees and hips as needed to bring your arms level with client's legs. Shift your weight from front to back leg and slide client's legs diagonally toward head of bed.	Positioning is begun at client's legs because they are lighter and easier to move. Facing direction of movement ensures proper balance. Shifting your weight reduces force needed to move load. Diagonal motion permits pull in direction of force. Flexing knees lowers your center of gravity and uses thigh muscles rather than back muscles.
d. Move parallel to client's hips. Flex knees and hips as needed to bring your arms level with client's hips.	Maintains your proper body alignment. Brings you closest to object to be moved and lowers center of gravity. Uses thigh muscles rather than back muscles.
e. Slide client's hips diagonally toward head of bed.	Aligns client's hips and feet.
f. Move parallel to client's head and shoulders. Flex knees and hips as needed to bring arms level with client's body.	Maintains your proper body alignment. Brings you closer to object to be moved. Lowers your center of gravity. Uses thigh muscles rather than back muscles.
g. Slide your arm closest to head of bed under client's neck, with your hand reaching under and supporting shoulder.	Supports client's head and neck, maintaining proper alignment and preventing injury during movement.
h. Place your other arm under client's upper back.	Supports client's body weight and reduces friction.
i. Slide client's trunk, shoulders, head, and neck diagonally toward head of bed.	Realigns client's body on one side of bed.
j. Elevate side rail. Move to other side of bed and lower side rail.	Protects client from falling out of bed.
k. Repeat procedure, switching sides until client reaches desired height in bed.	
l. Center client in middle of bed, moving body in same three sections.	Maintains proper body alignment. Provides ample room for turning, positioning, or other nursing activities.
m. Raise side rails.	Provides for client safety.
9. Assist client to move up in bed (one or two nurses):	
a. Place client on back with head of bed flat.	Enables you to assess body alignment. Reduces gravitational pull on client's upper body.
b. Place pillow at head of bed.	Prevents striking client's head against bed.
c. Face head of bed.	
(1) If two nurses assist client, each nurse should have one arm under client's shoulders and one arm under client's thighs.	Facing direction of movement prevents twisting your body while moving client.

STEPS	RATIONALE
(2) *Alternate position:* Position one nurse at client's upper body. Nurse's arm nearest head of bed should be under client's head and opposite shoulder. Other arm should be under client's closest arm and shoulder. Position other nurse at client's lower torso. This nurse's arms should be under client's lower back and torso.	Prevents trauma to client's musculoskeletal system by supporting shoulder and hip joints and evenly distributing weight.
d. Place feet apart with foot nearest head of bed behind other foot (forward-backward stance).	Wide base of support increases your balance. Forward-backward stance enables you to shift body weight as client is moved up in bed, thereby reducing force needed to move load.
e. Ask client to flex knees with feet flat on bed.	Enables client to use femoral muscles during movement.
f. Instruct client to flex neck, tilting chin toward chest.	Prevents hyperextension of neck.
g. Instruct client to assist moving by pushing with feet on bed surface.	Reduces friction. Increases client mobility. Decreases your workload.
h. Flex your knees and hips, bringing your forearms closer to level of bed.	Increases balance and strength by bringing your center of gravity closer to client—the "object" to be moved. Uses thigh muscles instead of back muscles.
i. Instruct client to push with heels and elevate trunk while breathing out, thus moving toward head of bed on count of 3.	Prepares client for move. Reinforces client's assistance in moving up in bed. Increases client cooperation. Breathing out avoids Valsalva maneuver.
j. On count of 3, rock and shift your weight from front to back leg. At same time, client pushes with heels and elevates trunk.	Rocking enables you to improve balance and overcome inertia. Shifting your weight counteracts client's weight and reduces force needed to move load. Client's assistance reduces friction and your workload.
10. Realign client in supported Fowler's, supine, prone, lateral, or Sims' position.	Maintains client's proper body alignment, preventing injury to skin and musculoskeletal system.
11. Wash hands.	Reduces transmission of infection.
12. Lower bed.	Provides for client safety.
13. Observe client's body alignment, position, level of comfort, and potential pressure points.	Maintains support to musculoskeletal system and reduces risk of injury related to improper movement or positioning.
14. Record procedure in nurses' notes, including position assumed, frequency of turning, condition of skin, joint movement, use of supports or splints, and client's ability to assist with moving and positioning.	Documents effectiveness of nursing care. Provides for consistency among nursing staff.

STEPS	RATIONALE
1. Assess client's muscle strength, joint mobility, presence of paralysis or paresis, orthostatic hypotension, activity tolerance, level of consciousness, level of comfort, and ability to follow instructions.	Determines client's physiological and cognitive level for participating in transfer technique.
2. Prepare needed equipment and supplies: 　a. Transfer belt (if needed)	Reduces risk of injury. Should be used with all clients who require moderate-to-maximal assistance or have high risk of falling or injury. Researach (Owen, Garg, 1991) demonstrated that transfer belt was more readily and correctly used than mechanical devices.
b. Wheelchair (Position chair at 45-degree angle to bed; lock brakes; remove footrests; lock bed brakes.) 　c. Stretcher (position at 90-degree angle to bed; lock brakes on stretcher; lock brakes on bed.)	Position of wheelchair or stretcher facilitates quick transfer from bed to wheelchair or bed to stretcher.
3. Explain procedure to client. Close door or curtain.	Promotes client cooperation and understanding of procedure and benefits of mobilization. Ensures privacy.
4. Wash hands.	Reduces transfer of infection.
5. Assist client to sitting position in bed: 　a. Place client in supine position.	Enables continual assessment of client's body alignment and administration of additional care, such as suctioning or hygiene needs.
b. Remove pillows from bed.	Decreases interference while sitting client up in bed.
c. Face head of bed.	Reduces twisting of your body when moving client.
d. Place feet apart with foot nearer bed behind other foot.	Improves your balance and allows transfer of body weight as client is moved to sitting position.
e. Place hand that is farther from client under shoulders, supporting head and cervical vertebrae.	Maintains alignment of head and cervical vertebrae and allows for even lifting of client's upper trunk.
f. Place other hand on bed surface.	Provides support and balance.
g. Raise client to sitting position by shifting your weight from front leg to back leg.	Improves your balance, overcomes inertia, and transfers weight in direction in which client is moved.
h. Push against bed using arm that was placed on bed surface.	Divides activity of raising client to sitting position between your arms and legs and protects back from strain. By bracing one hand against mattress and pushing against it as client is lifted, part of weight that would be lifted by your back muscles is transferred through arms onto mattress (Stamps, 1989).
6. Assist client to sitting position on side of bed: 　a. Place client in side-lying position, facing you on side of bed on which client will be sitting.	Prepares client to move to side of bed and protects client from falling.
b. Raise head of bed to highest level client is able to tolerate.	Decreases amount of work needed by client and nurse to raise client to sitting position.

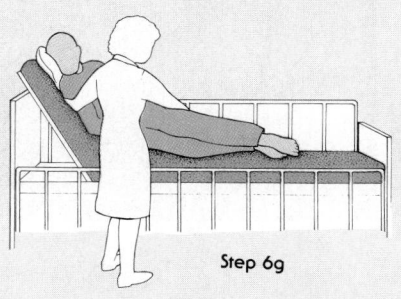

Step 6g

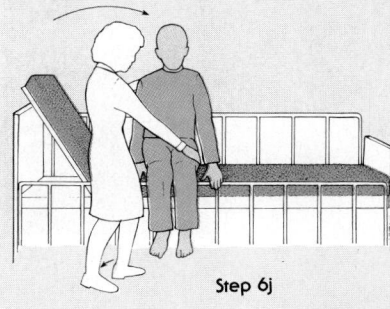

Step 6j

Transfer Techniques

STEPS	RATIONALE
c. Stand opposite client's hips.	Places your center of gravity nearer client.
d. Turn on diagonal so that you are facing client and far corner of foot of bed.	Reduces twisting of your body because nurse is facing direction of movement.
e. Place feet apart with foot closer to head of bed in front of other foot.	Increases balance and allows you to transfer weight as client is brought to sitting position at side of bed.
f. Place arm nearer head of bed under client's shoulders, supporting the head and neck.	Maintains alignment of head and neck as you bring client to sitting position.
g. Place other arm over client's thighs (see illustration on p. 1499).	Supports hip and prevents client from falling backward during procedure.
h. Move client's lower legs and feet over side of bed.	Decreases friction and resistance.
i. Pivot toward your rear leg, allowing client's upper legs to swing downward.	Allows gravity to lower client's legs.
j. At same time, shift your weight to your rear leg and elevate client (see illustration on p. 1499).	Allows you to transfer weight in direction of motion.
k. Remain in front of client until balance is regained.	Reduces risk of falling.
l. Lower level of bed until client's feet touch floor.	Supports client's feet in dorsal flexion and allows client to easily stand at side of bed.
7. Transfer client from bed to chair:	
a. Assist client to sitting position on side of bed. Have chair in position at 45-degree angle to bed.	Positions chair within easy access for transfer.
b. Apply transfer belt if necessary.	Allows you to maintain stability of client during transfer and reduces risk of falling.

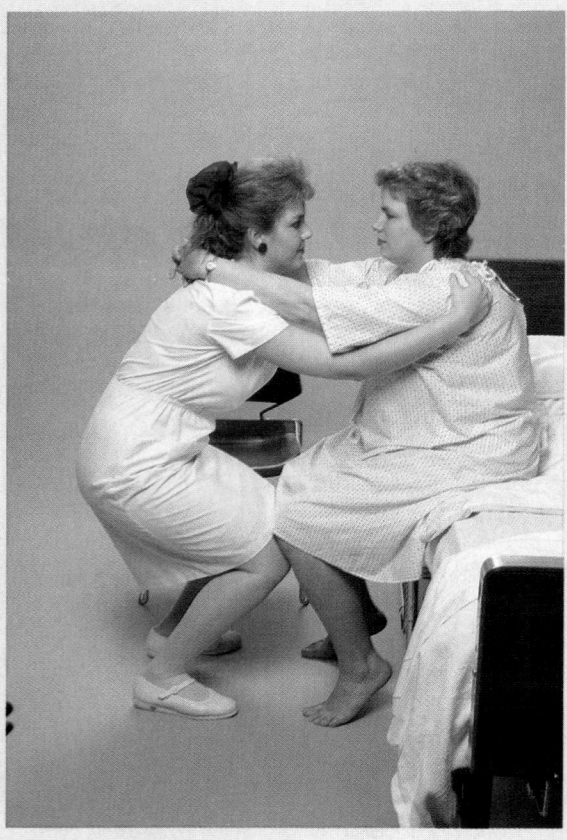

Step 7f

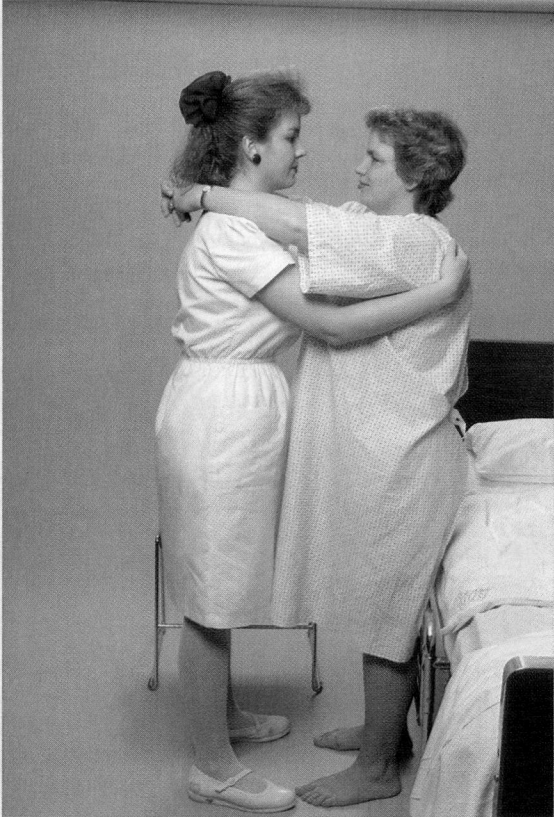

Step 7g

CONTINUED

STEPS	RATIONALE
c. Ensure that client has stable, nonskid shoes.	Decreases risk of slipping during transfer.
d. Spread your feet apart.	Ensures balance with wide base of support.
e. Flex your hips and knees, aligning your knees with client's.	Lowers your center of gravity to object to be raised and allows stabilization of knees when client stands.
f. Grasp transfer belt from underneath or reach through client's axillae and place hands on client's scapulae (see illustration).	Reduces pressure on axillae and maintains client stability.
g. Rock client up to standing on count of 3 while straightening your hips and legs, keeping knees slightly flexed (see illustration).	Gives client's body momentum and requires less muscular effort to lift client. Uses correct body mechanics to raise client to standing position.
h. Maintain stability of weak or paralyzed leg with knee.	Ability to stand can often be maintained in paralyzed or weak limb with support of knee to stabilize.
i. Pivot on foot that is farther from chair (see illustration).	Maintains support of client while allowing adequate space for client to move.
j. Instruct client to use arm rests on chair for support.	Increases client stability.
k. Flex your hips and knees while lowering client into chair (see illustration).	Prevents injury resulting from poor body mechanics.
l. Assess client for proper alignment for sitting position.	Prevents injury to client from poor body alignment.

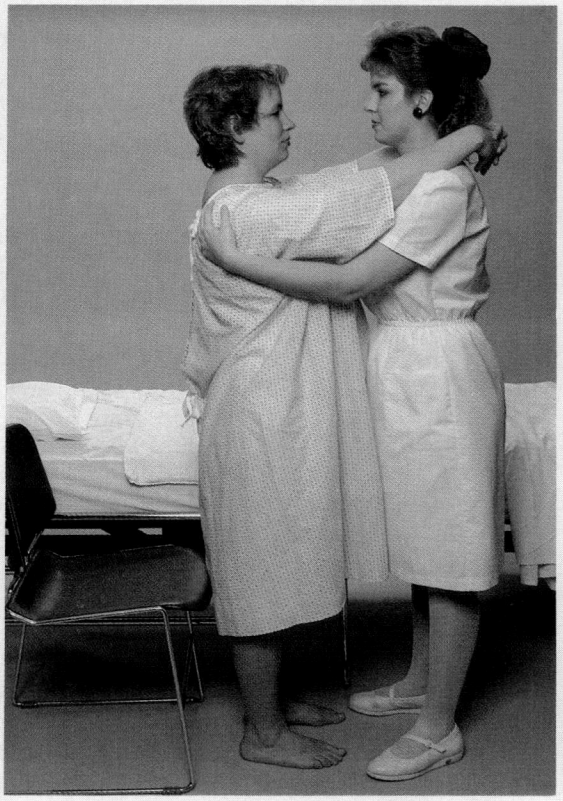

Step 7i

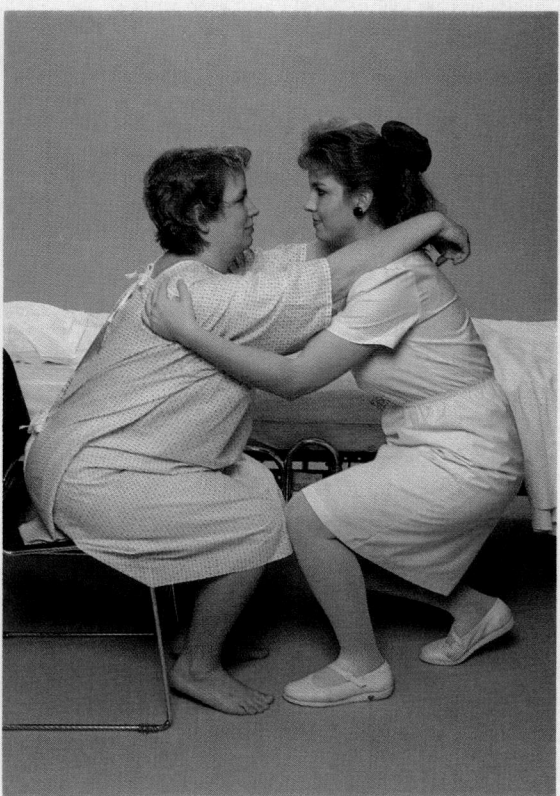

Step 7k

Transfer Techniques

STEPS	RATIONALE

8. Perform three-person carry:

a. Three nurses of nearly equal height stand side by side facing side of client's bed.

Prevents twisting of bodies. Client's alignment is maintained.

b. Each person assumes responsibility for one of three areas: head and shoulders, hips, and thighs and ankles.

Distributes client's body weight.

c. Each assumes wide base of support with foot that is closer to stretcher in front, knees slightly flexed.

Increases balance and lowers lifters' center of gravity.

d. Lifters' arms are placed under client's head and shoulders, hips, and thighs and lower legs, with their fingers securely around other side of client's body (see illustration).

Distributes client's weight over lifters' forearms.

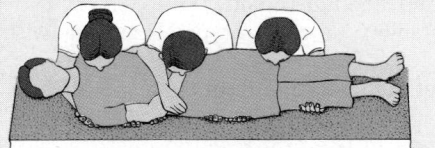

Step 8d

e. Lifters roll client toward their chests.

Moves workload over lifters' base of support.

f. On count of 3, client is lifted and held against nurses' chests.

Enables lifters to work together and safely lift client.

g. On second count of 3, nurses step back and pivot toward stretcher, moving forward if needed.

Transfers weight toward stretcher.

h. Nurses gently lower client onto center of stretcher by flexing their knees and hips until their elbows are level with edge of stretcher.

Maintains alignment during transfer.

i. Nurses assess client's body alignment, place safety straps across client, and raise side rails.

Reduces risk of injury from poor alignment or falling.

9. Position client in selected position.

Reduces risk of injury to musculoskeletal system from improper positioning.

10. Wash hands.

Reduces transmission of infection.

11. Observe client to determine response to transfer. Observe for correct body alignment and presence of pressure points.

Reduces risk of injury from subsequent transfers and positioning.

12. Record procedure in nurses' notes.

Documents effectiveness of nursing care. Provides for consistency among nursing staff.

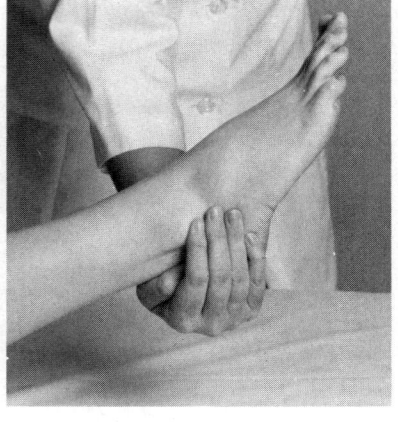

Fig. 43-20 Using a cupped hand to support a joint.

lifted, the nurse places a cupped hand under the joint to support it (Fig. 43-20), supports the joint by holding the adjacent distal and proximal areas (Fig. 43-21), or supports the joint with one hand and cradles the distal portion of the extremity with the remaining arm (Fig. 43-22).

The following sections describe specific movements for major joints in the body. Table 43-2 details ROM for each area and illustrates motion of each joint.

Neck. ROM for the neck is permitted by the flexibility of the cervical vertebrae and the pivotal connection between the head and neck. Unless contrain-

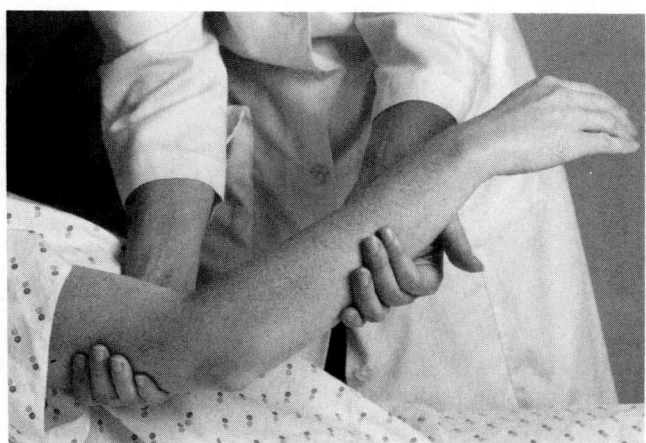

Fig. 43-21 Supporting the joint by holding the distal and proximal areas adjacent to the joint.

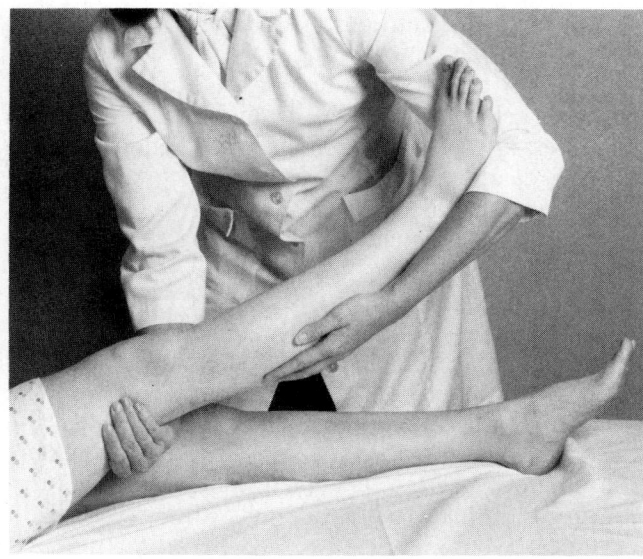

Fig. 43-22 Cradling the distal portion of an extremity.

dicated because of spinal surgery, spinal cord trauma, or other central nervous system trauma, ROM exercises should be performed by clients with limited neck mobility. When flexion contracture of the neck occurs, the client's neck is permanently flexed with the chin close to or actually touching the chest. Ultimately, the client's body alignment is altered, the visual field is changed, and the level of independent functioning is decreased.

Shoulder. One feature of the shoulder that sets it apart from other joints in the body is that the strongest muscle controlling it, the deltoid, is in complete elongation in the normal position. No other muscle exerts its full strength when in complete elongation. Thus exercising the shoulder effectively increases the power of the deltoid and ROM. To accomplish this, the shoulder must first be abducted.

The goal of action in the shoulder is full ROM. Shoulder movements include flexion, extension, hyperextension, abduction, adduction, internal and external rotation, and circumduction. The full ROM must be maintained or regained to avoid pain.

When caring for a client with limited mobility of the shoulder, the nurse should design interventions to place and support the shoulder in the adducted position. This can be achieved with slings when the client is standing or sitting or pillows when the client is in bed. Correctly positioning the shoulder prevents pain, joint dislocation, and further changes in body alignment.

Elbow. The elbow functions optimally at an angle of about 90 degrees. An elbow fixed in full extension is disabling and limits the client's independence.

Forearm. Most functions of the hand are best carried out with the forearm in moderate pronation.

When the forearm is fixed in a position of full supination, the client's use of the hand is limited. For optimal functioning the forearm must be able to rotate from supination to pronation.

Wrist. The primary function of the wrist is to place the hand in slight dorsal flexion, the position of functioning. Therefore full ROM is not as great a priority as maintaining the wrist in a functional position. When the wrist is fixed in even a slightly flexed position, grasp is weakened. In the immobilized client the functional position of the wrist can be achieved by using hand rolls and splints.

Fingers and Thumb. The ROM in fingers and the thumb enables the client to perform activities of daily living and activities requiring fine motor skills such as carpentry, needlework, drawing, and painting. The functional position of the fingers and thumb is slight flexion of the thumb in opposition to the fingers. In clients with restricted mobility, hand rolls help maintain this position.

Hip. Because the lower extremities are concerned chiefly with locomotion and weight bearing, stability of the hip joint may be more important than its mobility. For example, if one hip has no mobility but is fixed in a neutral position and fully extended, it is possible to walk without a significant limp.

However, contractures often fix the hip in positions of deformity. Excessive abduction makes the affected leg appear too long, whereas excessive adduction makes the affected leg appear too short. In either case the client has limited locomotion and walks with an obvious limp. Flexion contractures result in lordosis when the person is standing. Internal and external rotation contractures cause an abnormal and unbalanced gait.

Knee. A primary function of the knee is stability, which is achieved by ROM, ligaments, and muscles. However, knees cannot remain stable under weight-bearing conditions unless there is adequate quadriceps power to maintain the knee in full extension. ROM exercises should include pulling the knee into full extension.

An immobile knee joint can result in serious disability. The degree of disability depends on the position in which the knee is stiffened. If the knee is fixed in full extension, the person must sit with the leg thrust out in front. When the knee is flexed, the person limps while walking. The greater the flexion, the greater the limp. Complete flexion contractures prevent the person from walking without a walker or crutches.

Ankle and Foot. During walking, movement of the ankle joint is minimal. However, the joint must be stabilized and able to bear weight, or the person will fall. If joint mobility is diminished, the nurse should maintain the joint in a position in which walking can be carried out with a forward rolling motion from the heel onto the forefoot.

When the person relaxes as in sleep or coma, the foot relaxes and assumes a position of plantar flexion. This results from relaxation of the gastrocnemius and soleus muscles, which maintain dorsiflexion. If the foot remains in plantar flexion without support, these two muscles shorten and the dorsiflexion muscles try to compensate by overstretching. As a result the foot becomes fixed in plantar flexion (footdrop), which impairs the ability to walk.

Inversion and eversion must also be avoided to allow the foot to rest flat on the floor (Table 41-3). The foot must be flat to allow weight bearing and proper walking.

Toes. Excessive flexion of the toes results in a clawing. When this is a permanent deformity, the foot is unable to rest flat on the floor and the client is unable to walk properly. Flexion contractures are the most common foot deformity associated with reduced joint mobility.

Adequate ROM gives the necessary mobility to carry out activities of daily living and exercise and engage in relaxing activities. In addition, adequate ROM in the lower extremities allows walking.

Walking

In the normal walking posture the head is erect; the cervical, thoracic, and lumbar vertebrae are aligned; the hips and knees have appropriate flexion; and the arms swing freely with the legs. Illness or trauma can reduce activity tolerance, so assistance in walking is required. In addition, temporary or permanent damage to the musculoskeletal and nervous systems may necessitate use of a mechanical device for walking.

ASSISTING A PATIENT TO WALK.. Like other procedures, assisting the client to walk requires preparation. The nurse assesses the client's activity tolerance, strength, presence of pain, coordination, and balance to determine the amount of assistance needed.

The nurse explains how far the client should try to walk, who is going to help, when the walk will take place, and why walking is important. In addition, the nurse and client determine how much independence the client can assume.

The nurse also checks the environment to be sure that there are no obstacles in the client's path. Chairs, over-the-bed tables, and wheelchairs are cleared out of the way so that the client has ample room to walk safely.

Before starting, rest points should be established in case activity tolerance is less than estimated or the client becomes dizzy. For example, a chair might be placed in the hall for the client to rest if needed.

To prevent orthostatic hypotension, the client should be assisted to a position of sitting at the side of the bed and should rest for 1 to 2 minutes before standing. Likewise, after standing, the client should remain stationary for 1 to 2 minutes before moving. The client's balance must stabilize before walking. Thus the nurse can quickly ease a dizzy client back to bed. The longer the period of immobility, the greater the risk of hypotension when the client stands.

The nurse should provide support at the waist so that the client's center of gravity remains midline. This can be achieved when the nurse places both hands at the client's waist or uses a walking belt. A **walking belt** is a leather belt that encircles the waist and has handles attached for the nurse to hold. While walking, the client should not lean to one side because this alters the center of gravity, distorts balance, and increases the risk of falling.

The client who at any point appears unsteady or complains of dizziness should be returned to a close bed or chair. If the client faints or begins to fall, the nurse should assume a wide base of support with one foot in front of the other, thus supporting the body weight. Then the nurse gently lowers the client to the floor, protecting the head. Although lowering a client to the floor is not difficult, the student should practice this technique with a friend or classmate before attempting it in a clinical setting.

Clients with **hemiplegia** (one-sided paralysis) or **hemiparesis** (one-sided weakness) often need assistance to walk. The nurse always stands on the client's affected side and supports the client by holding one arm around the client's waist and the other arm around the inferior aspect of the client's upper arm so that the nurse's hand is under the client's axilla. Providing support by holding the client's arm is incorrect because the nurse cannot easily support the weight to lower the client to the floor if the client faints or falls. In addition, if the client falls with the nurse holding an arm, a shoulder joint may be dislocated.

A nurse who does not have a lot of strength and who is unable to ambulate a client alone should request help. The two-nurse method helps distribute the client's weight evenly. The two nurses stand on either side of the client. Each nurse's near arm is around the client's waist, and the other arm is around the inferior aspect of the client's arm so that both nurses' hands are supporting the client's axillae.

A second method requires that the nurses and client be of similar height. The nurses stand on either side of the client with their near arms slipped under the client's arms toward the back. The nurses then grasp each other's arms. The client's arms are placed over the nurses' shoulders, and the nurses stabilize the client's hands with their hands. This technique is effective with weaker, heavy clients.

USING ASSISTIVE DEVICES FOR WALKING

Walkers are extremely light, movable devices, waist high, made of metal tubing. They have four widely placed, sturdy legs. The client holds the upper bars, takes a step, moves the walker forward, and takes another step (Fig. 43-23).

Canes are light, easily movable devices, waist high, made of wood or metal. The most common types of canes are the single straight-legged cane and the quad cane (Fig. 43-24). The straight-legged cane is more common and is used to support and balance a client with decreased leg strength. The cane should be kept on the stronger side of the body. For maximum support when walking, the client places the cane forward 15 to 25 cm (6 to 10 in), keeping body weight on both legs. The weaker leg is moved forward to the cane so that the body weight is divided between the cane and the stronger leg. The stronger leg is advanced past the cane so that the weaker leg and the body weight are supported by the cane and weaker leg. To walk, the client continually repeats these steps. The client is taught that two points of

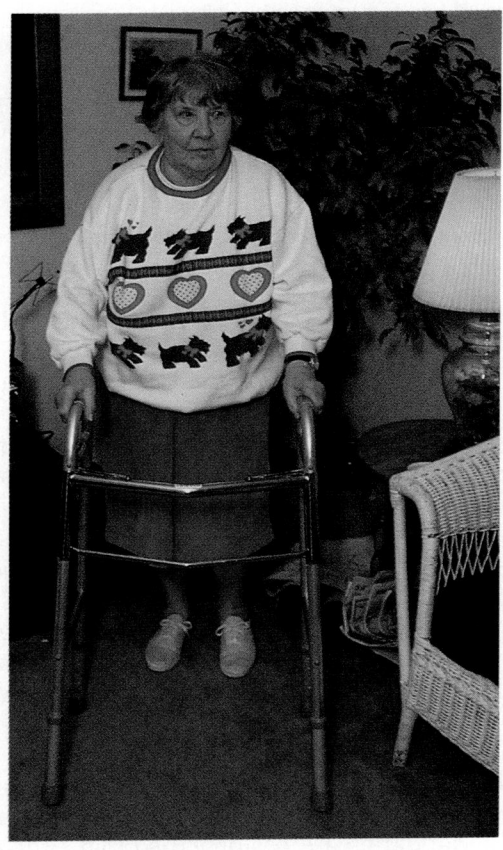

Fig. 43-23 Client using a walker.

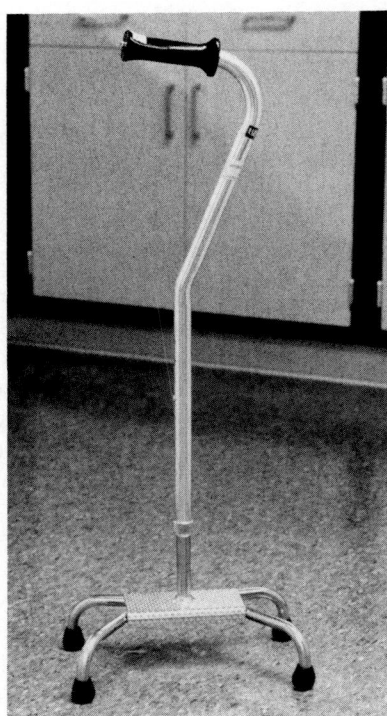

Fig. 43-24 Quad cane.

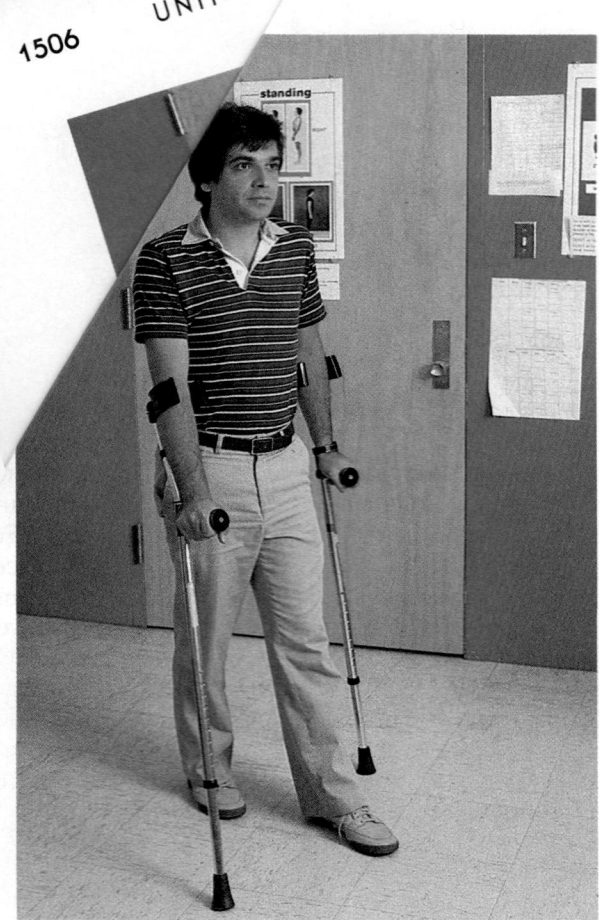

Fig. 43-25 Double adjustable Lofstrand or forearm crutches.

Client Teaching for Crutch Safety	

OBJECTIVE

- Client will state and demonstrate safe crutch walking.

TEACHING STRATEGIES

- Teach client with axillary crutches about the dangers of pressure on the axillae, which occurs when leaning on the crutches to support body weight.
- Explain why client must use crutches that fit properly and were measured for client.
- Show client to routinely inspect crutch tips. Rubber tips should be securely attached to the crutches. When tips are worn, they should be replaced. Rubber crutch tips increase surface friction and help prevent slipping.
- Explain that crutch tips should remain dry. Water decreases surface friction and increases the risk of slipping.
- Show client how to dry the crutch tips if they become wet.
- Show client how to inspect the structure of the crutches. Cracks in a wooden crutch decrease its ability to support weight. Bends in aluminum crutches can alter body alignment.
- Provide client with a list of medical supply companies in the community for obtaining repairs, new rubber tips, handgrips, and crutch pads.
- Instruct client to have spare crutches and tips readily available.

EVALUATION

- Client states and demonstrates principles of crutch safety.

support, such as both feet or one foot and cane, are present at all times.

The quad cane provides the greater support and is used when there is partial or complete leg paralysis or hemiplegia. The same three steps used with the straight-legged cane are taught to the client.

Crutches are often needed to increase mobility. Their use may be temporary, such as after ligament damage to the knee. Crutches may be needed permanently (for example, by the client with paralysis of the lower extremities). A crutch is a wooden or metal staff. There are two types of crutches, the double adjustable Lofstrand or forearm crutch (Fig. 43-25) and the axillary wooden crutch (used in Figs. 43-26 through 43-35). The forearm crutch has a handgrip and a metal band that fits around the forearm. Both the metal band and the handgrip are adjusted to fit the client's height. The axillary crutch has a padded curved surface at the top, which fits under the axilla. A handgrip in the form of a crossbar is held at the level of the palms to support the body. Crutches must

be measured for the appropriate length, and clients must be taught to use their crutches safely, achieve a stable gait, ascend and descend stairs, and rise from a sitting position.

Measuring for Crutches. The axillary crutch is more commonly used. When preparing the client for crutches, the nurse must also teach crutch safety (see teaching box) and correctly measure the client for crutches. Measurements include the client's height, the angle of elbow flexion, and distance between the crutch pad and axilla. When crutches are fitted, their length should be from 3 to 4 finger widths below the axilla to a point 15 cm (6 in) lateral to the client's heel (Sine et al, 1981) (Fig. 43-26).

The handgrips are positioned so that body weight is not supported by the axillae. Pressure on the axil-

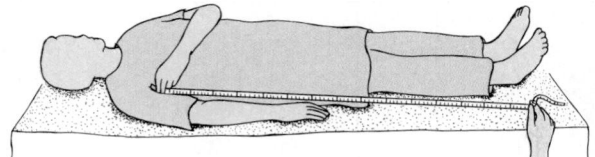

Fig. 43-26   Measuring crutch length.

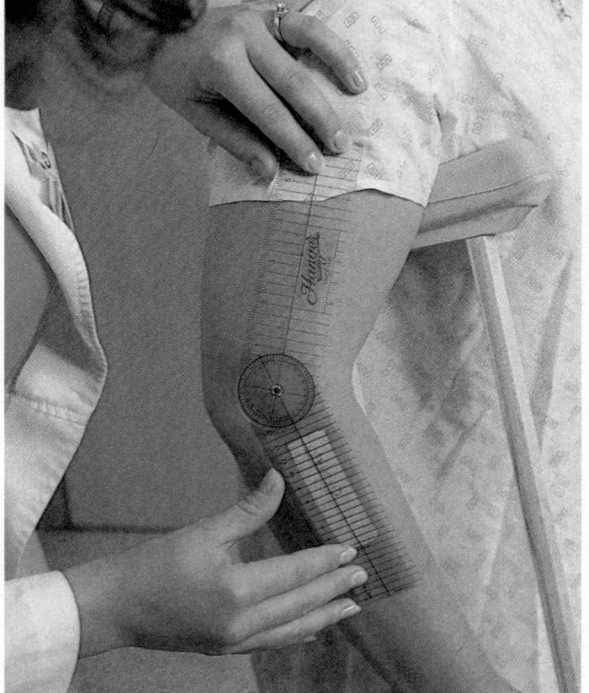

Fig. 43-27   Verifying correct elbow flexion with crutches. Measurement is obtained with a goniometer.

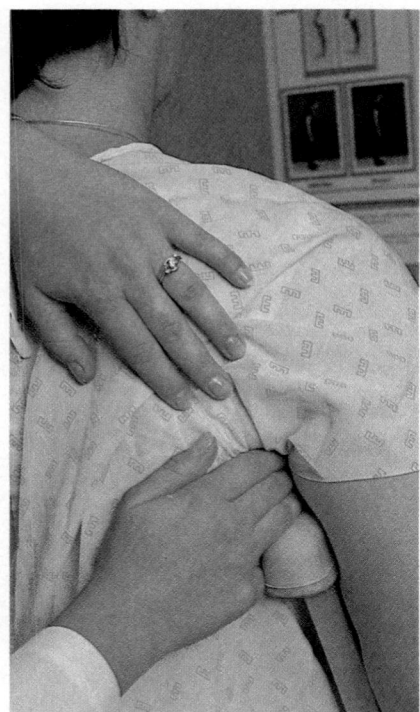

Fig. 43-28   Verifying correct distance between crutch pads and axilla.

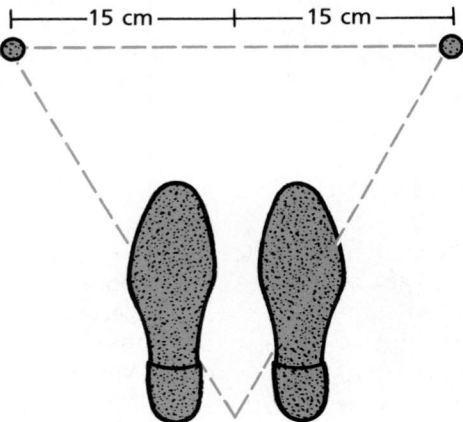

Fig. 43-29   Tripod position, the basic crutch stance.

lae increases risk to underlying nerves, which may cause partial paralysis of the arm. Correct position of the handgrips is determined with the client upright, supporting weight by the handgrips with elbows slightly flexed (20 to 25 degrees). The degree of elbow flexion is verified with a goniometer (Fig. 43-27). After the height and placement of the handgrips have been determined, the nurse verifies that the distance between the crutch pad and axilla is 3 to 4 finger widths (Fig. 43-28).

Teaching Crutch Gait. A **crutch gait** is assumed by alternately bearing weight on one or both legs and on the crutches. The gait used by the client is determined by the nurse's assessment of the client's physical and functional abilities and the disease or injury.

The basic crutch stance is the tripod position, formed when the crutches are placed 15 cm (6 in) in front of and 15 cm to the side of each foot (Fig. 43-29). This position improves balance by providing a wider base of support. Body alignment in the tripod position includes erect head and neck, straight vertebrae, and extended hips and knees. No weight should be borne by the axillae. The tripod position is used before crutch walking.

Four-point alternating or four-point gait gives stability but requires weight bearing on both legs. Three points of support are on the floor at all times (Fig. 43-

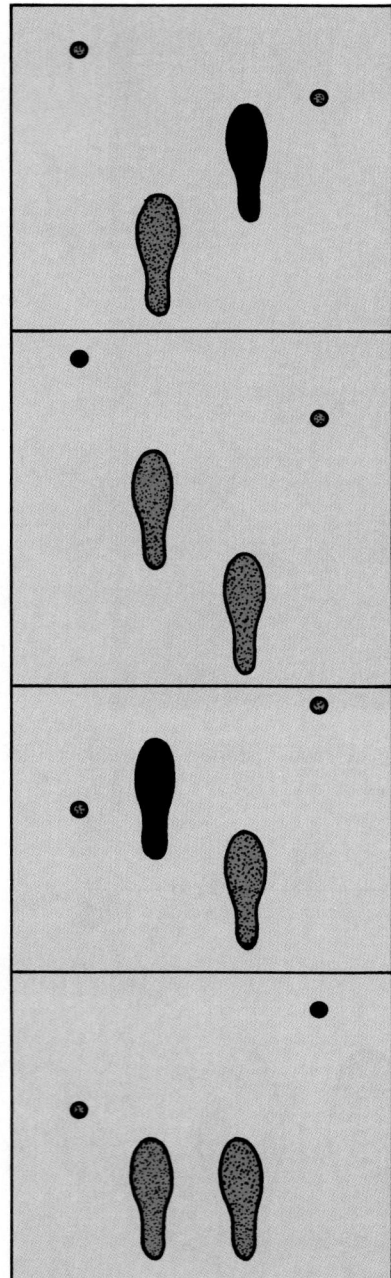

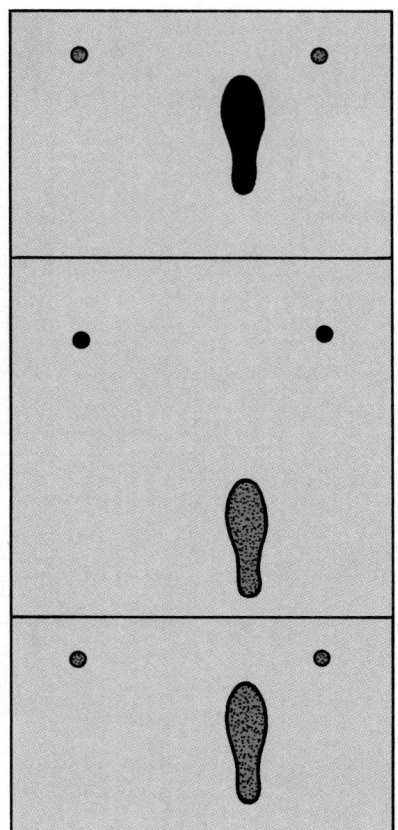

Fig. 43-31 Three-point alternating gait, with weight borne on the uninvolved leg. Black foot and crutch tips show weight bearing in each phase of the gait.

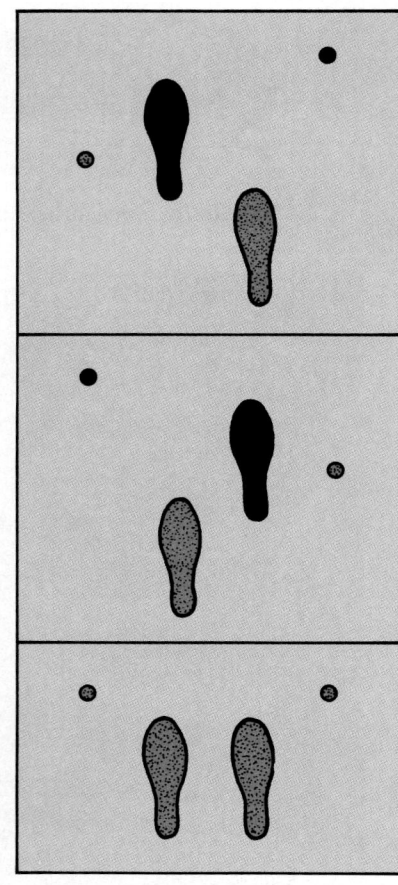

Fig. 43-32 Two-point alternating gait, with weight borne partially on each foot and crutch advancing with the opposing leg. Black areas indicate leg and crutch tips bearing weight.

Fig. 43-30 Four-point alternating gait. Black foot and crutch tips show weight bearing in each phase of the gait.

30). The client first positions a crutch and then positions the opposite foot (for example, right crutch and left foot). The client then repeats this sequence with the other crutch and foot, alternating this pattern (Lane, LeBlanc, 1990).

Three-point alternating or three-point gait requires the client to bear all of the weight on one foot. In a three-point gait, weight is borne on the uninvolved leg (Fig. 43-31) and then on both crutches, and the sequence is repeated. The affected leg does not touch the ground during the early phase of the three-point gait. Gradually the client progresses to touchdown and full weight bearing on the affected leg (Lane, LeBlanc, 1990).

The two-point gait requires at least partial weight bearing on each foot (Fig. 43-32). Each crutch is moved at the same time as the opposing leg so that crutch movements are similar to arm motion during normal walking (Lane, LeBlanc, 1990).

The swing-through or swing-to gait is frequently used by paraplegic clients who wear weight-supporting braces. With weight placed on the supported legs, the client places the crutches one stride in front and then swings to or through the crutches while supporting their weight (Lane, LeBlanc, 1990).

Teaching Crutch Walking on Stairs. When ascending stairs on crutches, the client usually uses a modified three-point gait (Fig. 43-33). First the client stands at the bottom of the stairs and transfers the

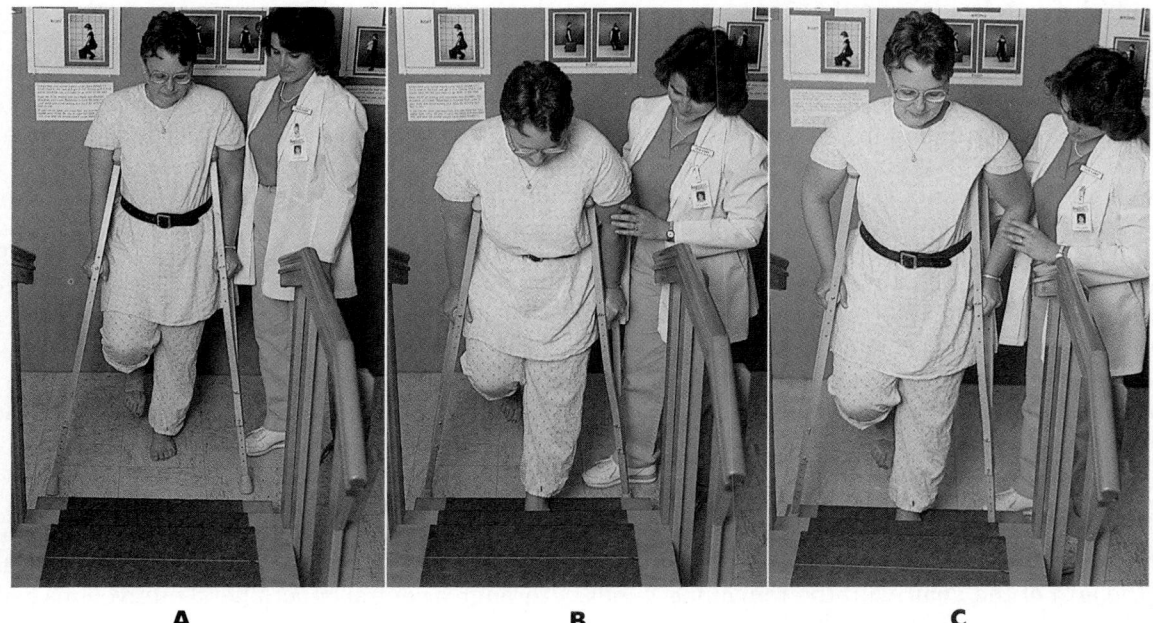

A   **B**   **C**

Fig. 43-33   Ascending stairs. **A,** Weight is placed on crutches. **B,** Weight is transferred from crutches to unaffected leg on the stairs. **C,** Crutches are aligned with unaffected leg on the stairs.

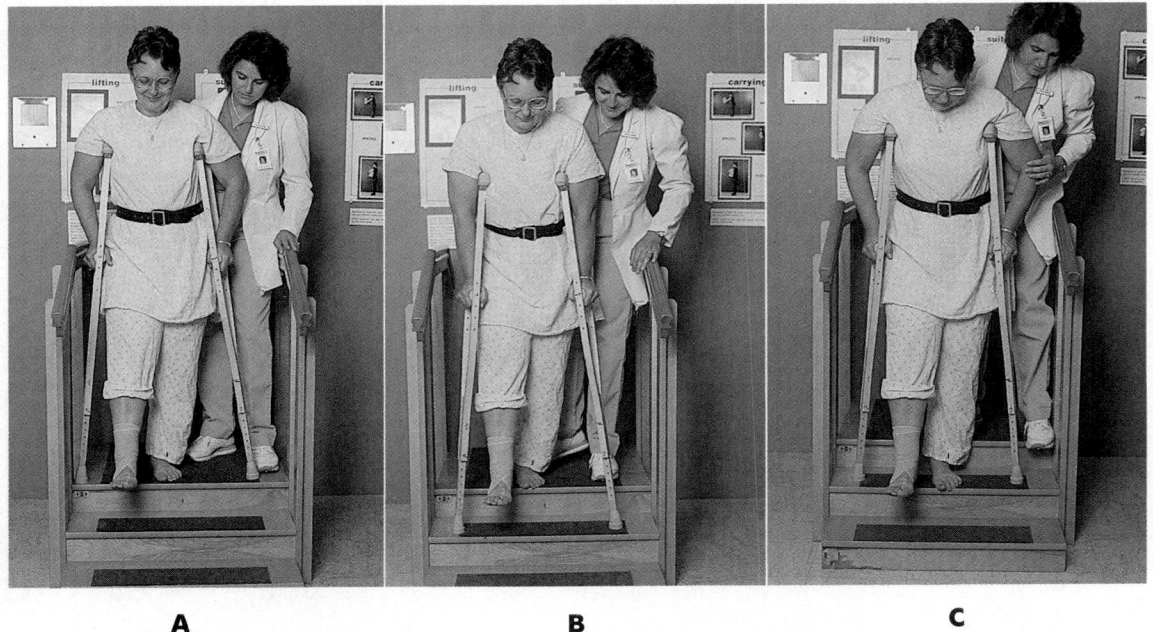

A   **B**   **C**

Fig. 43-34   Descending stairs. **A,** Body weight on unaffected leg. **B,** Body weight transferred to crutches. **C,** Unaffected leg aligned on stairs with crutches.

body weight to the crutches. Second, the unaffected leg is advanced between the crutches to the stairs. Then weight is shifted from the crutches to the unaffected leg. Last, the client aligns both crutches on the stairs. This sequence is repeated until the person reaches the top.

To descend the stairs (Fig. 43-34), a three-phase sequence is also used. First, the client transfers body weight to the unaffected leg. Second, the crutches are placed on the stair and the client begins to transfer body weight to the crutches, moving the affected leg forward. Last, the unaffected leg is moved to the stairs with the crutches. Again, the client repeats the sequence until reaching the bottom.

Clients usually need to use crutches for some time, so they should be taught to use them on stairs before discharge. Instruction in stair climbing applies to all crutch-dependent clients, not only those who have stairs in their homes.

Teaching Sitting With Crutches. The procedure for sitting in a chair requires the client to transfer weight. First, the client should be positioned at the center front of the chair with the posterior aspect of the legs touching the chair. Second, the client holds both crutches in the hand opposite the affected leg. If both legs are affected, as with a paraplegic client who wears weight-supporting braces, the crutches are held on the client's stronger side. With both crutches in one hand the client supports the body's weight on the unaffected leg and crutches (Fig. 43-35). While still holding the crutches, the client grasps the arm of the chair with the remaining hand and lowers the body. To stand, the procedure is reversed, and the client when fully erect should assume the tripod position before walking.

Reduction of Hazards of Immobility

Nursing interventions for an immobilized client should focus on preventing or minimizing the hazards of immobility. Interventions should therefore be directed at maintaining optimal function of all body systems.

METABOLIC SYSTEM. The immobilized client requires a high-protein, high-calorie diet with vitamin B and C supplements. Protein is needed to repair injured tissue and rebuild depleted protein stores. A high-calorie intake provides sufficient fuel to meet metabolic needs and to replace subcutaneous tissue. Supplementation with vitamin C is necessary to replace protein stores. Vitamin B complex is needed for skin integrity and wound healing.

If the client is unable to eat, nutrition must be provided parenterally or enterally. Enteral feedings include delivery through a nasogastric, gastrostomy, or jejunostomy tube of high-protein, high-calorie solutions with complete requirements of vitamins, minerals, and electrolytes (see Chapter 35). Total parenteral nutrition is delivery of nutritional supplements through a central or peripheral intravenous catheter.

RESPIRATORY SYSTEM. Nursing interventions for the respiratory system are aimed at promoting expansion of the chest and lungs, preventing stasis of pulmonary secretions, maintaining a patent airway, and promoting adequate exchange of respiratory gases.

Promoting Expansion of Chest and Lungs. The nurse promotes chest expansion with several inter-

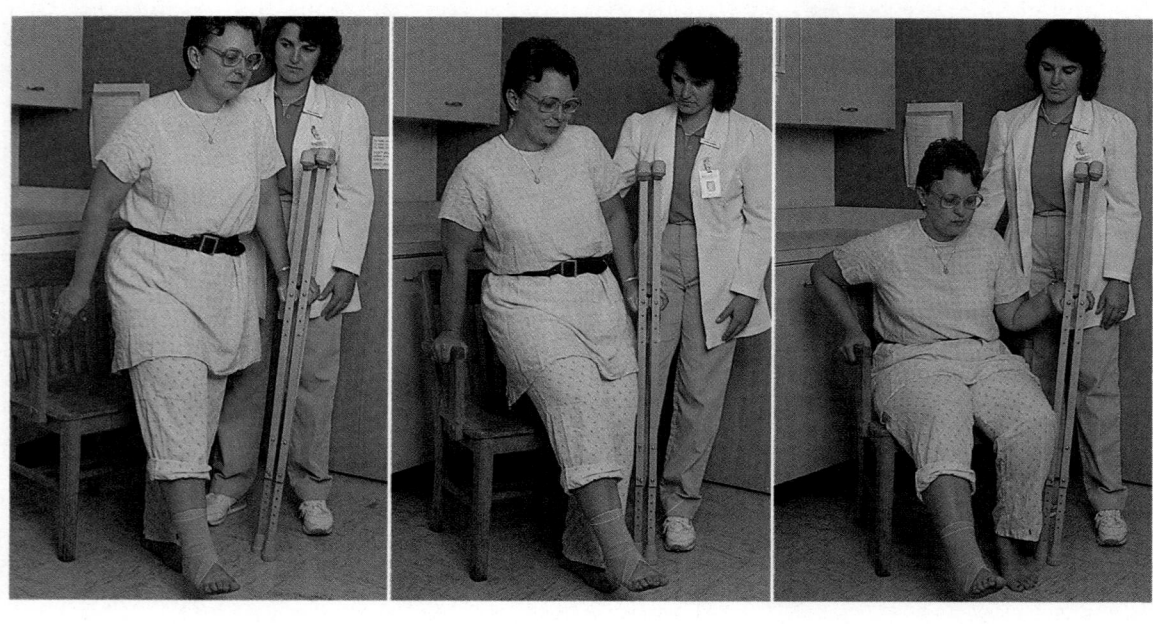

A   **B**   **C**

Fig. 43-35 Sitting in a chair. **A,** Both crutches are held by one hand. Client transfers weight to the crutches and the unaffected leg. **B,** Client grasps arm of the chair with the free hand and begins to lower herself into the chair. **C,** Client completely lowers herself into the chair.

ventions. Changing the position of the client at least every 2 hours allows the dependent lung regions to re-expand. Re-expansion maintains the elastic recoil property of the lungs and clears the dependent lung regions of pulmonary secretions.

The nurse should encourage the client to deep breathe and cough every 1 to 2 hours. Alert clients can be taught to deep breathe or yawn every hour. This action expands all lobes of the lungs and prevents atelectasis. Coughing reduces the stasis of pulmonary secretions. For unconscious clients with an artificial airway, the nurse can expand the chest and lungs by using an Ambu bag (see Chapter 38).

The nurse uses caution when administering postoperative pain medication. These medications can depress the respiratory center, so the rate of respiration or expansion of the lungs is decreased. The nurse should ask a postoperative client who has received pain medication to deep breathe and cough at the peak effect of the analgesic, which is 20 to 30 minutes after administration. This reduces the respiratory-depressant action of the drug.

If abdominal binders and rib supports are required, they should be removed every 2 hours to allow the client to breathe deeply. Removal may be contraindicated, however, for the client who has just had surgery or has just suffered trauma.

Preventing Stasis of Pulmonary Secretions.
Stagnant secretions accumulating in the bronchi and lungs may lead to growth of bacteria and subsequent development of pneumonia. Pulmonary infections still develop despite interventions to prevent them.

Stagnation of secretions can be reduced by changing the client's position every 2 hours. This change repositions the dependent lung and mobilizes secretions.

Chest physiotherapy is an effective method of preventing pulmonary secretions. It uses positioning techniques to drain secretions from specific segments of the bronchi and lungs into the trachea. The client then expels secretions by coughing. Respiratory assessment findings help to identify areas of the lungs that require chest physiotherapy (see Chapter 38).

Maintaining a Patent Airway.
Immobilized clients and those on bed rest are generally weakened. If weakness progresses, the cough reflex gradually becomes inefficient. If the client is too weak or unable to cough up secretions, the nurse must maintain a patent airway using suctioning techniques. The stasis of secretions in the lungs may be life threatening for an immobilized client because hypostatic bronchopneumonia can easily develop. Assessment findings that indicate this condition include productive cough with greenish yellow sputum, fever, pain on breathing, and crackles, wheezes, and dyspnea. Dislodging and mobilizing the stagnant secretions reduce the risk of pneumonia.

In the immobilized client an obstructed airway is usually the result of a mucous plug. The nurse can implement several therapies to reduce the risk of mucous plugs and to maintain the patent airway.

First, the nurse can ask the client to deep breathe and cough every 1 to 2 hr. The nurse instructs the client to take in three deep breaths and cough with the third exhalation. This technique produces a more forceful, productive cough without excessive fatigue.

Second, the nurse may use nasotracheal or orotracheal suction to remove secretions in the upper airways of a client unable to cough productively. This procedure must be performed aseptically. The nurse places a suction catheter in the client's nose or through the mouth and applies suction.

Last, the nurse can suction secretions from an artificial airway such as an endotracheal or tracheal tube. The nurse inserts a catheter into the artificial airway in a sterile procedure. This removes pulmonary secretions from the upper and lower airways (see Chapter 38).

CARDIOVASCULAR SYSTEM. The effects of bed rest or immobilization on the cardiovascular system include orthostatic hypotension, increased cardiac workload, and thrombus formation. Nursing therapies are designed to minimize or prevent these alterations.

Reducing Orthostatic Hypotension.
After a period of bed rest, clients usually have an increased pulse rate, a decreased pulse pressure, and an increase in fainting in response to tilting or erect posture (Winslow, 1985). Interventions should be directed at reducing or eliminating the effects of orthostatic hypotension. The nurse should attempt to get the client out of bed as soon as possible, even if the move is only to a chair. This activity maintains muscle tone and increases venous return. Isometric exercises used during bed rest do not have any beneficial effect on orthostatic hypotension but improve activity tolerance (Winslow, 1985).

When being moved from a supine position into a chair, the client should change positions gradually. When doing this procedure, the nurse should document any orthostatic changes. The nurse obtains baseline vital signs with the client in the supine position. The nurse then raises the client to a high Fowler's position and measures the vital signs again to evaluate decreases in blood pressure or elevations in pulse. The nurse remains with the client and leaves the client in the high Fowler's position for a few moments to allow the body to adapt to any changes in vital signs. The nurse continually monitors the client

Applying Elastic Stockings

STEPS	RATIONALE
1. Identify need for elastic stockings: immobility, lower extremity edema, and varicose veins.	These conditions increase the risk of thrombus formation.
2. Prepare following equipment: a. Tape measure b. Stockings in proper size c. Talcum powder	Stockings must be measured according to directions of specific manufacturer. Measure client's calf circumference length from foot to knee. For thigh-high elastic stockings, measure calf circumference, thigh circumference, and length from foot to thigh.
3. Explain procedure to client.	Relieves anxiety and increases cooperation.
4. Wash hands.	Reduces transmission of microorganisms.
5. Elevate bed to comfortable position, and assist patient to supine position.	Promotes good body mechanics for nurse. Position eases stocking application.
6. After legs have been cleansed, apply small amount of talcum powder to each leg and foot.	Reduces friction and allows for easier application of stocking.
7. Turn elastic stocking inside out by placing one hand into sock, holding toe with other hand, and pulling (see illustration).	Prepares stocking for application.
8. Place client's toe into foot of elastic stocking, making sure that sock is smooth (see illustration).	Wrinkles in sock can impede circulation to lower region of extremity.
9. Slide remaining portion of sock over client's foot, being sure that toes are covered. Sock will now be right side out (see illustration).	If toes remain uncovered, they will become constricted by elastic and their circulation can be reduced.
10. Slide sock over client's calf until it is completely extended. Be sure that sock is smooth and no ridges are present (see illustration).	Ridges impede venous return and can counteract purpose of elastic stocking.
11. Instruct client not to roll socks partially down.	Rolling the sock partially down will have constricting effect and impede venous return.
12. Reposition client for comfort.	Maintains body alignment and promotes comfort.
13. Wash hands.	Reduces transmission of microorganisms.
14. After 1 hr, observe stockings for wrinkles in binding and assess capillary refill in toes and palpate pulses in feet.	Wrinkles increase pressure to skin and impair circulation. Assessment ensures that circulatory status in lower extremities has not been compromised.

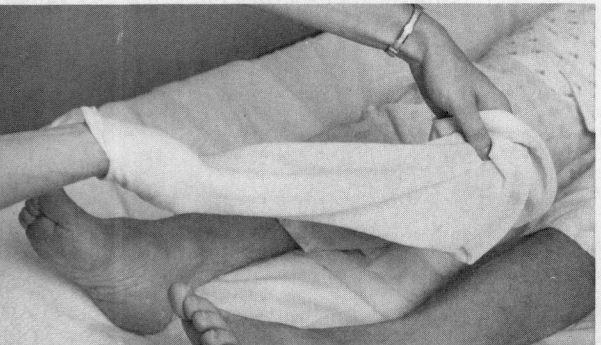

Step 7

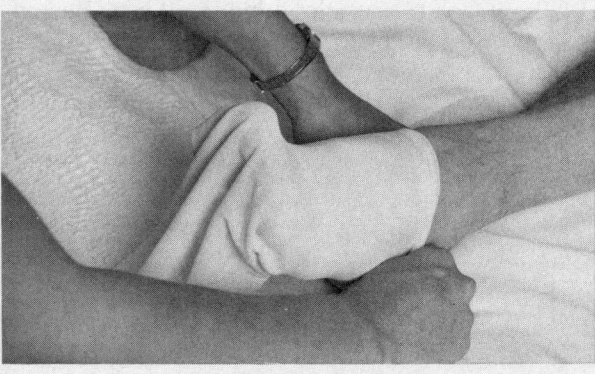

Step 8

STEPS	RATIONALE
15. Remove stockings at least once a shift.	Provides for assessment of skin and circulatory status.
16. Record in nurses' notes date and time of stocking application and condition of skin before application, circulatory status of lower extremities, and stocking length and size.	Documents condition of lower extremities and performance of procedure.

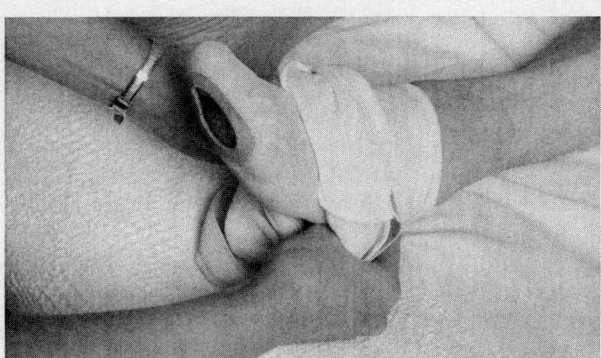

Step 9

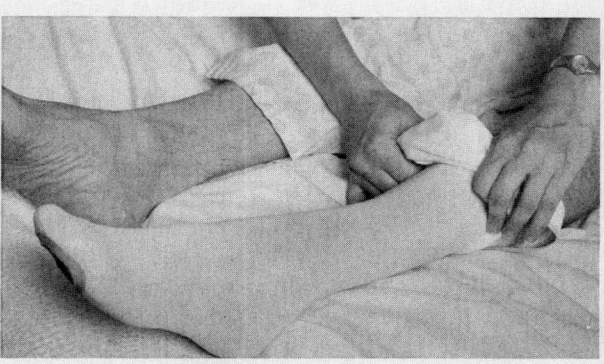

Step 10

for dizziness and light-headedness. The nurse also asks whether the client sees spots.

Then the nurse has the client sit at the side of the bed with the feet on the floor. The client is instructed to lie down and tell the nurse if dizziness or faintness is felt. If there is no dizziness, the nurse assists the client to the chair.

Frequent sitting or standing minimize the orthostatic effect of bed rest. These interventions counteract the headward fluid shift that occurs with bed rest and redistributes venous volume (Winslow, 1985).

Reducing Cardiac Workload. The nurse designs interventions to reduce cardiac workload, which is increased by immobility. The nurses' primary intervention is to discourage the client from using the Valsalva maneuver. When using this maneuver, the client holds the breath, which increases intrathoracic pressure. This decreases venous return and cardiac output. Therefore cardiac workload increases.

Preventing Thrombus Formation. There are multiple interventions designed to reduce the risk for thrombus formation in the immobilized client. Some of these interventions require a physician's order. Others require that clients have certain risk factors before the intervention can be implemented.

Immobilized clients are frequently placed on low-dose heparin therapy to minimize the risk of venous

thromboembolism. Heparin therapy requires a physician's order. The medication is usually administered every 12 hours (5000 units/dose). The usual route of administration is subcutaneous injection, although some clients may receive this therapy through a heparin-lock (Hep-Lock) catheter (Clagett, Reisch, 1988). Heparin is an anticoagulant. Therefore it suppresses clot formation. Because of the action of this medication, the nurse must continually assess the client for signs of bleeding, such as increased bruising, guaiac positive stools, and bleeding gums. Although the majority of clients receiving low-dose heparin do not experience side effects, the risk remains present.

Intermittent pneumatic compression (IPC) devices are designed to provide rhythmic external extremity compression through inflatable "stockings." IPC has proven effective in reducing deep vein thrombosis in general surgical, high-risk oncology, orthopedic, and neurological clients (Clagett, Reisch, 1988).

Therapeutic elastic stockings with graded compressions reduce the risk of thrombus formation (Clagett, Reisch, 1988). Elastic stockings aid in maintaining external pressure on the muscles of the lower extremities and thus may promote venous return. The stockings must be applied properly and removed and reapplied (Procedure 43-5 at least twice a day). In addition, the stockings should always be clean and dry, and it may be useful for the client to have two pair.

Positioning techniques aid in reducing pressure to the skin. Proper positioning used with other therapies (for example, heparin or elastic stockings) aid in reducing the client's risk of thrombus formation. When positioning clients, the nurse uses caution to prevent pressure on the posterior knee and deep veins in the lower extremities.

ROM exercises are designed to reduce the risk of contractures, but these exercises also have beneficial effects in preventing thrombi. The exercise activity causes contraction of the skeletal muscles, which in turn exerts pressure on the veins and promotes venous return. Venous stasis is reduced.

When deep vein thrombosis is suspected, the nurse should report it immediately. The leg should be elevated with no pressure on the thrombus. The family, client, and all health care personnel should be instructed not to massage the area because of the danger of dislodging the thrombus.

MUSCULOSKELETAL SYSTEM. The immobilized client must receive some exercise to prevent excessive muscle wasting, atrophy, and joint contractures. If the client is unable to move part or all of the body, the nurse must perform passive ROM exercises for all immobilized joints while bathing the client and at least 2 or 3 more times a day. If one extremity is paralyzed, the client can be taught to put each joint independently through its ROM.

Some orthopedic conditions require more frequent passive ROM exercises to restore the injured joint's function after surgery. Clients with such conditions may use automatic equipment for passive ROM exercises (Fig. 43-36). The equipment extends an extremity to a prescribed angle for a prescribed period. This is beneficial when the client must gradually increase the degree and duration of extension.

Clients on bed rest should have active ROM exercises incorporated into their daily schedules. They can perform these exercises during activities of daily living. The box describes joint movements that occur with daily activities.

Active ROM exercises maintain functioning of the musculoskeletal system. The nurse should also plan interventions for the gradual return of mobility in clients who will be able to resume normal activity.

The best nursing intervention is a progressive exercise program individualized to the client's health, age, weight, illness, and motivation. A progressive exercise program gradually increases activity to reverse the deconditioning associated with bed rest (Winslow, Weber, 1980).

Progressive exercise programs are used for clients with musculoskeletal, neurological, cardiopulmonary, renal, and other chronic diseases. Before beginning the program, warm-up exercises should be performed, unless they are contraindicated.

INTEGUMENTARY SYSTEM. As discussed previously, the major risk to skin from restricted mobility is pressure ulcers. Nursing interventions therefore focus on prevention and treatment (see Chapter 44).

ELIMINATION SYSTEM. The nursing interventions for maintaining optimal urinary functioning are directed

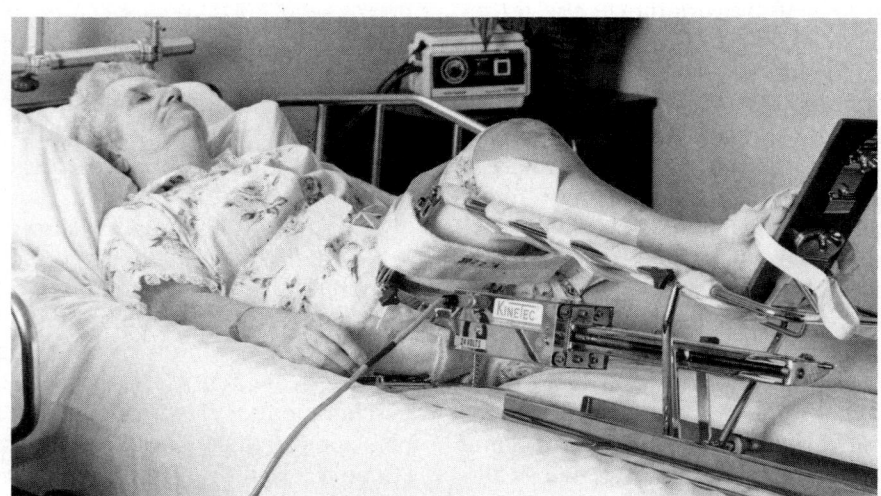

Fig. 43-36   Continuous passive range of motion machine.

at keeping the client well hydrated without causing bladder distention and preventing urinary stasis, calculi, and infections.

Adequate hydration (for example, 2000 to 3000 ml of fluids per day) helps prevent renal calculi and urinary tract infections. The well-hydrated client should void large amounts of dilute urine. If the client is also incontinent, the nurse should modify the care plan to meet the increased urinary elimination needs.

To prevent bladder distention, the nurse assesses the frequency and amount of urinary output. A client who continually dribbles urine and whose bladder is distended has overflow incontinence. If the immobilized client does not have voluntary control of urinary elimination, the nurse may have to insert a straight or indwelling catheter to prevent distention (see Chapter 40).

The nurse must also record the frequency and consistency of bowel movements. A diet rich in fruits, vegetables, and bulk can facilitate normal peristalsis. If a client is unable to maintain regular bowel patterns, the physician may order stool softeners, cathartics, or enemas (see Chapter 41).

PSYCHOSOCIAL CHANGES. Assessment can identify effects of prolonged immobilization on the client's psychosocial dimension. People who have a tendency toward depression or mood swings are at greater risk for developing psychosocial effects during bed rest or immobilization. There are many nursing interventions to meet the client's psychosocial needs.

The nurse should anticipate changes in the client's psychosocial status. The nurse can provide routine and informal socialization. Nursing activities can be planned so that the client can talk and interact with staff. If possible the client should be placed in a room with others who are mobile and interactive. If a private room is required, staff members should be asked to visit at least once a shift.

The nurse also provides stimuli to maintain orientation. A daily newspaper helps the client keep track of events and time. Bedside chats at appropriate moments orient the client to nursing activities, meals, and visiting hours. Books help occupy the client when alone. The client can participate in craft activities. Radio and television provide stimulation and help pass the time.

Clients should be encouraged to wear their glasses or artificial teeth and to shave or apply makeup. These are activities through which people maintain their body images. Maintenance of body image can alleviate depression resulting from immobilization.

Clients should also be involved in their care whenever possible. For example, the nurse should encour-

age the client to determine when the bed should be made. Some clients rest better during the night when fresh sheets are put on in the evening rather than in the morning. The client should provide as much self-care as possible. Hygiene and grooming articles should be kept within easy reach.

Nursing care given between 10 PM and 7 AM should be scheduled to minimize interruptions of sleep. For example, the nurse may administer medi-

---

Incorporating Active Exercises into Activities of Daily Living

- Nodding head "yes" exercises *neck* (flexion and extension).
- Shaking head "no" exercises *neck* (rotation).
- Moving right ear to right shoulder exercises *neck* (lateral flexion).
- Moving left ear to left shoulder exercises *neck* (lateral flexion),
- Reaching to turn on overhead light exercises *shoulder* (flexion).
- Reaching to bedside stand for book exercises *shoulder* (abduction).
- Scratching back exercises *shoulder* (hyperextension and inward rotation).
- Rotating shoulders toward chest exercises *shoulder*.
- Rotating shoulders toward back exercises *shoulder*.
- Eating, bathing, shaving, and grooming exercise *elbow* (flexion, extension).
- All activities requiring fine motor coordination, such as writing and eating, exercise *fingers* and *thumb* (flexion, extension, abduction, adduction, opposition).
- Walking exercises *hip* (flexion, extension, hyperextension).
- Rolling toes inward exercises *hip* (internal rotation).
- Rolling toes outward exercises *hip* (external rotation).
- Walking exercises *knee* (flexion, extension).
- Walking exercises *ankle* (dorsiflexion, plantar flexion).
- Pointing toe toward head of bed exercises *ankle* (dorsiflexion).
- Pointing toe toward foot of bed exercises *ankle* (plantar flexion).
- Walking exercises *toes* (extension, hyperextension).
- Wiggling toes exercises *toes* (abduction, adduction)

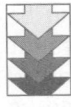

Sample Evaluation of Interventions for Impaired Physical Mobility

Goals	Evaluative Measures	Expected Outcomes
Client will regain normal ROM (180-degree flexion and extension) of left shoulder within 4 months.	Observe client perform ROM to both extremities and compare with initial assessment findings. Ask client about muscle strength to affected extremity.	Client will maintain present ROM in upper extremity joints. Client will perform self-care activities using left arm within 2 days. Client will follow regular exercise program 3-4 times a day by discharge.
Optimal joint motion will be achieved	Observe joint through ROM. Palpate joint during ROM exercises.	Client will have full ROM in affected joint.
Joint contractures will be prevented.	Measure ROM.	Joint contractures will be absent.

cations and assess vital signs at the time when the client is turned or receives special skin care.

The nurse should also observe for failure of the client to cope with restricted mobility. If the nursing care plan is not improving coping patterns, a clinical nurse specialist, counselor, social worker, spiritual adviser, or other consultant may be needed. Their recommendations should be incorporated into the care plan.

DEVELOPMENTAL CHANGES. Ideally, immobilized clients continue normal development. However, this is unrealistic for the very young or very old. Nursing interventions can help.

Nursing care should provide mental and physical stimulation, particularly for a young child. Play activities can be incorporated into the care plan. Completing puzzles, for example, helps a child to develop fine motor skills, and reading helps the child develop cog-

nitively. An immobilized child should be placed with children of the same age who are not immobilized unless a contagious disease is present. Nursing activities, such as dressing changes, cast care, and care of traction, can be designed to require participation of the child. The nurse must recognize significant changes from normal behavioral patterns. If these continue, the nurse should consult with a clinical nurse, counselor, or other health care professional whose specialty is children.

Restricted mobility of older clients presents unique nursing problems. Older clients may have chronic illnesses that place them at increased risk for the hazards of immobility.

Inactive older clients are at greater risk for confusion, depression, and disorientation, which result from immobilization, chronic illness, medications, and aging. To assist in maintaining orientation to time, a calendar and a clock with a large dial should be in the client's room (see Chapter 45). The calendar should be marked so that the client can immediately identify the correct day and date. Chapter 27 describes other measures to assist older clients in meeting developmental needs.

Nursing care should encourage older immobilized clients to perform as many activities of daily living as independently as possible. Clients should continue to perform personal grooming if they did so before their mobility was restricted.

The nurse must remember that older clients are extremely susceptible to the hazards of immobility. A care plan should be designed to prevent or minimize these hazards. Frail older clients may need position changes every hour instead of every 2 hours, and may need more frequent ROM exercises. Not only are older clients more susceptible to the hazards of immobility, but the consequences and severity of immobility are more rapid.

Evaluation

To evaluate outcomes and response to nursing care, the nurse measures the effectiveness of all interventions. The optimal outcomes are the client's ability to maintain or improve body alignment and joint mobility.

The nurse evaluates specific interventions designed to promote body alignment, improve mobility, and protect the client from the hazards of immobility. Client and family teaching to prevent future risks to body alignment and hazards of immobility is also evaluated. Last, the nurse investigates the client's and family's need for additional support services (for example, home health care, physical therapy, and counseling) and initiates the referral process.

Evaluation of nursing care for clients with altered body alignment and mobility is based on objective criteria for each nursing goal (see evaluation box).

Maintaining good body alignment and mobility and preventing the hazards of immobility increase independence and overall mobility. A client with inadequate joint mobility must receive assistance to carry out activities of daily living. The best approach to problems with body alignment and joint mobility is prevention, which begins early in the care plan.

 SUMMARY

The nurse incorporates knowledge of the physiological factors of movement and principles of body mechanics to transfer and position clients safely and to assist clients in using walkers and crutches safely. Through the nursing process, the nurse develops a care plan for clients with potential or actual alterations in body alignment and mobility. The alterations may be temporary or permanent.

Correct body mechanics protects the nurse and client from injuries to the musculoskeletal system. Occasionally, clients with impaired body alignment have restricted mobility or are totally immobilized. Immobilization affects all aspects of the client's life.

CHAPTER 43 REVIEW

Key Concepts

- Body mechanics is the coordinated efforts of the musculoskeletal and nervous systems as the person moves, lifts, bends, stands, sits, lies down, and completes daily activities.
- Coordinated body movement requires integrated functioning of the skeletal system, skeletal muscles, and nervous system.
- The skeleton provides bony support structure for movement, attachment of ligaments and muscles, protection of vital organs, some of the regulation of calcium, and red blood cell production.
- The nervous system provides initiation and voluntary control of movement.
- Muscles primarily associated with movement are located near the skeletal region, where movement results from leverage, which is characteristic of movements of the upper extremities.
- Coordination and regulation of muscle groups depend on muscle tone and activity of antagonistic, synergistic, and antigravity muscles.
- Balance is assisted through nervous system control by the cerebellum and inner ear.
- Body alignment is the condition of joints, tendons, ligaments, and muscles in various body positions.
- Body balance is achieved when there is a wide base of support, the center of gravity falls within the base of support, and a vertical line falls from the center of gravity through the base of support.
- Developmental stages influence body alignment and mobility; the greatest impact of physiological changes on the musculoskeletal system is observed in children and older adults.
- Normal physical mobility depends on intact and functioning nervous and musculoskeletal systems.
- The risk of disabilities related to immobilization depends on the extent and duration of immobilization.
- Immobility may result from illness or trauma or may be prescribed for therapeutic reasons. Immobility presents hazards in the physiological, psychological, and developmental dimensions.
- The nurse uses the nursing process to provide care for clients experiencing or at risk for the adverse effects of impaired body alignment and immobility.
- After identifying nursing diagnoses, the nurse plans and implements interventions to prevent or minimize the hazards and complications of impaired body alignment and immobilization.
- Clients with impaired body alignment require nursing interventions to maintain them in the supported Fowler's, supine, prone, side-lying, and Sims' positions.
- Range of motion exercises include one or all of the body joints.
- Mechanical devices to promote walking include canes, walkers, and crutches.

KEY TERMS

Critical Thinking Exercises

1. You are caring for a client who is in bilateral leg traction. How do you determine what type of mobility this client can safely perform and how this mobility can be incorporated into the care plan?

2. When caring for a client with a spinal cord injury, you note that the client's extremity "stiffens" and resists motion occasionally when the client performs passive range of motion exercises. What do you do so that further injury does not occur to the musculoskeletal system?

3. Mrs. Miller's mobility is limited after a stroke that left her with hemiplegia. She has a history of chronic constipation. What measures can the nurse independently implement to reduce the hazards of immobility to the gastrointestinal system? What evaluative criteria determine that these nursing measures were effective?

4. You're caring for a 27-year-old mother who is immobilized after spinal cord trauma. You note that she is becoming increasingly depressed and withdrawn. What actions are important at this point in the client's care?

REFERENCES

Beckett WS et al: Effect of prolonged bedrest on lung volume in normal individuals, *J Appl Physiol* 61(3):.919, 1986.

Blackburn GL et al: Nutritional and metabolic assessment of the hospitalized patient, *J Parental Nutr* 1:11, 1977.

Booth FW: Effect of limb immobilization on skeletal muscle, *J Appl Physiol* 52:1113, 1982.

Clagett GP, Reisch JS: Prevention of venous thromboembolism in general surgical patients, *Ann Surg* 208(2):227, 1988.

Convertino GP, Goldwater DJ, Sandler H: Bedrest-induced peak VO2 reduction associated with age, gender, and aerobic capacity, *Anat Space Environ Med* 57:17, 1986.

Daniels L, Worthingham C: *Therapeutic exercise for body alignment and function*, ed 2, Philadelphia, 1977, Saunders.

Deitrick JE et al: Effects of immobilization upon various metabolic and physiologic functions of normal men, *Am J Med* 4:3, 1948.

Gordon M: Assessing activity tolerance, *Am J Nurs* 76:72, 1976.

Greenleaf JE: Physiological responses to prolonged bedrest and fluid immersion in humans, *J Appl Physiol* 57(3):619, 1984.

Greenleaf JE, Kozlowski S: Physiological consequences of reduced physical activity during bed rest, *Exerc Sport Sci Rev* 10:84, 1982.

Gröer MW, Shekleton ME: *Basic pathophysiology: a conceptual approach*, ed 3, St Louis, 1989, Mosby–Year Book.

Heebink DM: Effects of bedrest on physical condition, *Resp Care* 26:1278, 1981.

Holm K: Immobility and bone loss in the aging adult, *Crit Care Nurs Q* 12(1):46, 1989.

Hudson MF: Safeguard your elderly patient's health through accurate physical assessment, *Nurs 83 (Can)* 13(11):58, 1983.

Kim MH, McFarland GK, McLane AM: *Pocket guide to nursing diagnoses*, ed 4, St Louis, 1991, Mosby–Year Book.

Knight AL: Medical management of pressure sores, *J Fam Prac* 27 (1):95, 1988.

Lane PL, LeBlanc R: Crutch walking, *Orthop Nurs* 9(5):31, 1990.

Lehmkuhl LD et al: Multidimensional treatment of joint contractures in patients with severe brain injury, *J Head Trauma Rehabil* 5(4):23, 1990.

McCance KL, Huether SE: *Pathophysiology: the biologic basis for disease in adults and children*, St Louis, 1990, Mosby–Year Book.

National Pressure Ulcer Advisory Panel (NPUAP): Pressure ulcer incidence, economics, risk assessment: Consensus Development Conference Statement, *Decubitis* 2(2):24, 2989.

Natlow AB: Nutrition in prevention and treatment of decubitus ulcers, *Top Clin Nurs* 5(2):39, 1983.

Norton D, McLaren R, Exon-Smith A: Pressure sores. In Horsley JA, editor: *Preventing decubitus ulcers: CURN project*, New York, 1981, Grune & Stratton.

Owen BD: How to avoid that aching back, *Am J Nurs* 80:984, 1980.

Owen BD, Garg A: Reducing risk for back pain in nursing personnel, *AAOHN J* 39(1):24, 1991.

Pajk M et al: Investigating the problem of pressure sores, *J Gerontol Nurs* 12(7):11, 1986.

Reddy MP: A guide to early mobilization of bedridden elderly, *Geriatrics* 41(9):59, 1986.

Rubin M: How bedrest changes perception, *Am J Nurs* 88:55, 1988a.

Rubin M: The physiology of bedrest, *Am J Nurs* 88:50, 1988b.

Sine RD et al: *Basic rehabilitation techniques: a self-instructional guide*, ed 2, Rockville, Md, 1981, Aspen.

Stamps JL: "Back" to basics, *Emerg Med Services* 18(2):38, 1989.

Strand FL: *Physiology: a regulatory systems approach*, New York, 1978, Macmillan.

Tompkins ES: Effect of restricted mobility and dominance on perceived duration. *Nurs Res* 29:333, 1980.

Tyler ML: The respiratory effects of body positioning and immobilization, *Resp Care* 29:472, 1984.

West JB: *Respiratory physiology: the essentials*, ed 3, Baltimore, 1985, Williams & Wilkins.

Winslow EH: Cardiovascular consequences of bedrest, *Heart Lung* 14(3):236, 1985.

Winslow EH, Weber TM: Progressive exercises to combat hazards of bedrest, *Am J Nurs* 80:440, 1980.

ADDITIONAL READINGS

Bergstrom N et al: The Braden scale for predicting pressure sore risk, *Nurs Res* 36:205, 1987.

Goldberg WG, Fitzpatrick JJ: Movement with the aged, *Nurs Res* 29:339, 1980.

Marchette L, Marchette R: Back injury: a preventable occupational hazard, *Orthop Nurs* 4(6):25, 1985.

McAbee RR: Nurses and back injury, *AAOHN J* 36(5):221, 1988.

McCauley M: The effect of body mechanics instruction on work performance among young workers, *AM J Occup Ther* 44(4):402, 1990.

Neilson DH et al: Energy, cost, exercise intensity, and gait efficiency of standard versus rocker-bottom axillary crutch walking, *Phys Ther* 70(8):47, 1990.

Owen BD: The magnitude of low-back problems in nursing, *West J Nurs Res* 11(2):234, 1989.

Viellion G: Assessment: examining joints of the upper and lower extremities, *Am J Nurs* 81:763, 1981.

Winters M: *Protective body mechanics in daily life and nursing*, Philadelphia, 1952, Saunders.

CHAPTER 44

Skin Integrity

OBJECTIVES

Mastery of content in this chapter will enable the student to:
- Define the key terms listed.
- Describe the economic consequences of pressure ulcers.
- Describe four risk factors for pressure ulcer development.
- Discuss 10 contributing factors to pressure ulcer formation.
- Discuss the pathogenesis of pressure ulcers.
- List the four stages of pressure ulcer development.
- Complete an assessment for a client with impaired skin integrity.
- List nursing diagnoses associated with impaired skin integrity.
- Develop a nursing care plan for a client with impaired skin integrity.
- List appropriate nursing interventions for a client with impaired skin integrity.
- State evaluation criteria for a client with impaired skin integrity.

CHAPTER OUTLINE

A major aspect of nursing care is the maintenance of skin integrity. Consistent, planned skin-care interventions are critical to ensuring quality in care (Hoff, 1989). Nurses are able to constantly observe their clients' skin for breaks or impairment in skin integrity. Impaired skin integrity can result from a wound, which can result from trauma or surgery (see Chapter 47). Impaired skin integrity also occurs from prolonged pressure, irritation of the skin, or immobility, leading to the development of pressure ulcers. A **pressure ulcer** is a localized area of tissue necrosis (death) that tends to develop when soft tissue is compressed between a bony prominence and an external surface for a prolonged period (National Pressure Ulcer Advisory Panel [NPUAP], 1989).

ECONOMIC CONSEQUENCES OF PRESSURE ULCERS

Pressure ulcers are a continual problem in acute and chronic care settings. The frequency of pressure ulcers ranges from 3% to 14% (NPUAP, 1989). Occurrence among clients admitted to nursing homes is between 15% and 20% (Bryant et al, 1992). A more recent study identified that 58% of clients with pressure ulcers were older adults (Meehan, 1990).

When a pressure ulcer occurs, the length of stay in a hospital and the overall cost of health care increase. The actual cost of treatment is difficult to approximate. Ranges are between $5000 and $27,000, depending on the number and severity of ulcers (Maklebust, 1987; Stotts, 1988; Hoff, 1989; Bryant et al, 1992). Although treatment of pressure ulcers is more costly than prevention, the preventive measures themselves are expensive. Extra equipment such as special beds and mattresses and increased nursing time are needed to administer these mea-

sures. When an ulcer develops, the cost of increased nursing care alone is estimated at 50% (Maklebust, 1987). Prescribed preventive interventions are often uncomfortable for the client and risk complications.

In 1989, the Agency for Health Care and Policy Research (AHCPR) developed guidelines for care of adult clients at risk for pressure ulcers. The AHCPR convened a panel of experts to explore the prevalence, cost, and risk of pressure ulcers. The subsequent research and treatment guidelines are the result of the National Pressure Ulcer Advisory Panel (NPUAP).

Prediction and Prevention of Pressure Ulcers

Prediction

Predictive instruments for pressure ulcer development can readily identify clients at the highest risk for pressure ulcers. Therefore the preventive measures need only be targeted to these high-risk clients. Clients with little risk for pressure ulcer development are spared the unnecessary preventive treatments and the risk of complications (Stotts, 1988). Prevention and treatment of pressure ulcers are major nursing priorities. The ability to identify clients at risk helps maintain health care costs (Gosnell, 1973; Norton, McLaren, Exton-Smith, 1962). The Norton Scale (Table 44-1) is designed to score five risk factors—physical condition, mental condition, activity, mobility, and continence. The range is 5 to 20, with a higher score indicating a higher risk for pressure ulcer development. This tool also offers descriptive information regarding potential risk factors (Hoff, 1989).

In 1987, results of the initial research on the Braden Scale for predicting pressure ulcer risk were published. The Braden Scale is a 23-point instrument composed of six subscales: sensory perception, moisture, activity, mobility, nutrition, friction, and shear. A hos-

---

TABLE 44-1 Norton Scale									
Physical Condition		**Mental Condition**		**Activity**		**Mobility**		**Incontinence (Bowel and/or Bladder)**	
Good	4	Alert	4	Ambulant	4	Full	4	Never	4
Fair	3	Apathetic	3	Walk/help	3	Slightly limited	3	Occasional	3
Poor	2	Confused	2	Chairbound	2	Very limited	2	(<2 per 24 hr)	
Very bad	1	Stuporous	1	Bed	1	Immobile	1	Usually	2
								(>2 per 24 hr)	
								Always	1

Maximum score = 20 (good physical condition); minimum score = 5; high risk for pressure ulcers = 12 or below

From Trelease CC: *Ostomy/Wound Manage* 20:46, 1988.

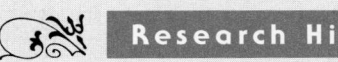

Research Highlight

Bergstrom et al developed a scale for predicting pressure sore risk to identify clients at risk. Research was conducted to determine the Braden Scale's reliability and validity. The tool was found to be highly reliable. It can identify clients who are at greater risk for pressure ulcer development. Subsequently, appropriate nursing interventions can be used to reduce or eliminate the risks.

Bergstrom N et al: The Braden Scale for predicting pressure sore risk, *Nurs Res* 36:205, 1987.

pitalized adult with a score of 16 or below is considered at risk. In older clients, a score of 17 or 18 may be a more efficient prediction of risk (Bryant et al, 1992). This instrument is highly reliable in the identification of clients at greatest risk for pressure ulcers (Bergstrom et al, 1987) (see research highlight).

Prevention

The prevention of pressure ulcers is a priority in caring for clients and is not limited to clients with restrictions in mobility. Impaired skin integrity is not a problem in healthy, immobilized individuals but is a serious and potentially devastating problem in the ill or debilitated client (USDHHS, 1992; Gröer, Shekleton, 1989; Shekleton, Litwack, 1991).

 ## PRESSURE ULCERS

Pressure sore, pressure ulcer, decubitus ulcer, and *bedsore* are terms used to describe impaired skin integrity. The most current terminology is *pressure ulcer,* which is consistent with the NPUAP and the AHCPR's Pressure Ulcer Guidelines Panel (Maklebust, 1991a, 1991b; Lucas, 1991; Green, Katz, 1991; Hastings, 1991; USDHHS, 1992). An ill client experiencing decreased mobility, impaired neurological functioning, decreased sensory perception, or decreased circulation is at risk for pressure ulcer development (Fig. 44-1).

Tissues receive oxygen and nutrients and eliminate metabolic wastes via the blood. Any factor that interferes with this affects cellular metabolism and the function or life of the cell. Pressure affects cellular metabolism by decreasing or obliterating tissue circulation, resulting in tissue ischemia.

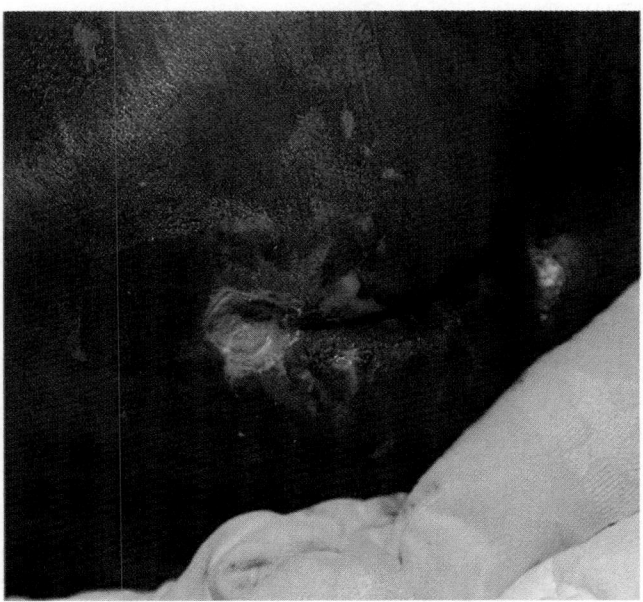

Fig. 44-1   Pressure ulcer with tissue necrosis.

Tissue ischemia is the localized absence of blood or a major reduction of blood flow resulting from mechanical obstruction (Pires, Muller, 1991). The reduction in blood flow causes blanching. **Blanching** is seen when the normal red tones of the skin are absent. Tissue damage occurs when the capillary closing pressure exceeds the normal range of 16 to 32 mm Hg (Gröer, Shekleton, 1989; Maklebust, 1987).

After a period of ischemia the skin can undergo one of two hyperemic changes. **Normal reactive hyperemia** (redness) is the visible effect of localized vasodilation, the body's normal response to lack of blood flow to the underlying tissue (Fig. 44-2, *A* on p. 1520). The area blanches with fingertip pressure (Fig. 44-2, *B*), and reactive hyperemia lasts less than 1 hour. **Abnormal reactive hyperemia** is an excessive vasodilation and induration in response to pressure. The skin appears bright pink to red. The **induration** is an area of localized edema under the skin. Abnormal reactive hyperemia (Fig. 44-3 on p. 1520) can last more than 1 hour up to 2 weeks after the removal of pressure (Pires, Muller, 1991).

When a client is lying or sitting, the weight of the body is heavily placed on bony prominences. The longer the pressure is applied, the greater the risk of skin breakdown. Pressure causes a decrease in blood supply to the tissues, and ischemia occurs. When the pressure is removed, there is a period of reactive hyperemia, or a sudden increase in blood flow to the region. Reactive hyperemia is a compensatory response and is only effective if the pressure on the skin is removed before necrosis or damage occurs.

Risk Factors for Pressure Ulcer Development

A client who is ill with impaired physical mobility is at risk for developing a pressure ulcer. However, a client whose physical mobility is impaired due to a

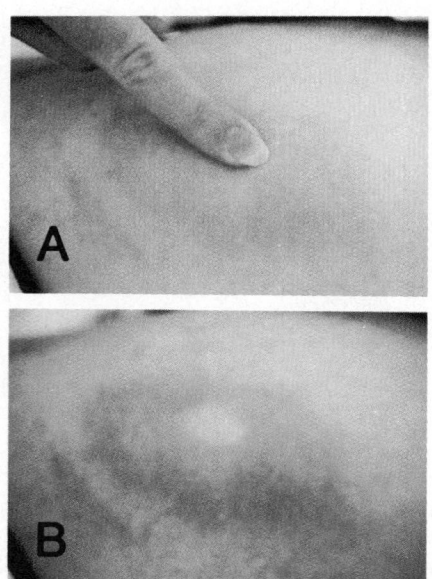

Fig. 44-2 A, Reactive hyperemia. **B,** Blanches with fingertip pressure.
From Pires M, Muller A: *Progressions* 3(3):3, 1991.

number of factors is also at an increased risk for a pressure ulcer.

Impaired Sensory Input

Clients with altered sensory perception for pain and pressure are at greater risk for impaired skin integrity than clients with normal sensation. Clients whose sensory perception of pain and pressure are intact can feel when a portion of their body senses too much pressure or pain. In turn, when clients are alert and oriented, they can change positions or request assistance in changing positions.

Impaired Motor Function

Clients unable to independently change positions are at greater risk for pressure ulcers. These clients can perceive the pressure but are unable to independently change positions and relieve the pressure. Thus the chance of pressure ulcer development increases. In clients with spinal cord injuries, there is motor and sensory impairment. The incidence of pressure ulcers in clients with spinal cord injuries is estimated to be as high as 85%, and ulcers or ulcer-related complications are the cause of death in 8% of this population (Reuler, Cooney, 1981).

Alterations in Level of Consciousness

Clients who are confused or disoriented or have changing levels of consciousness are unable to protect themselves from pressure ulcers. Clients who are confused or disoriented may be able to feel the

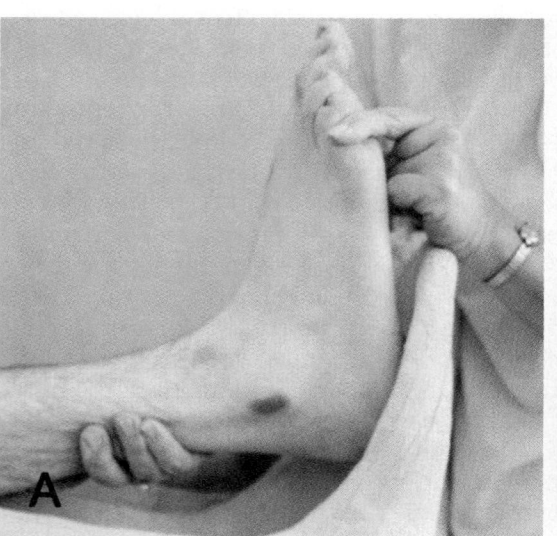
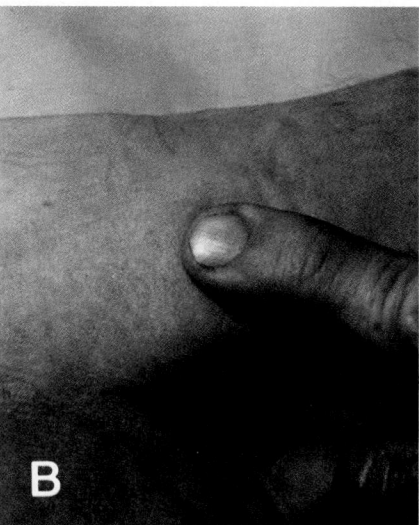
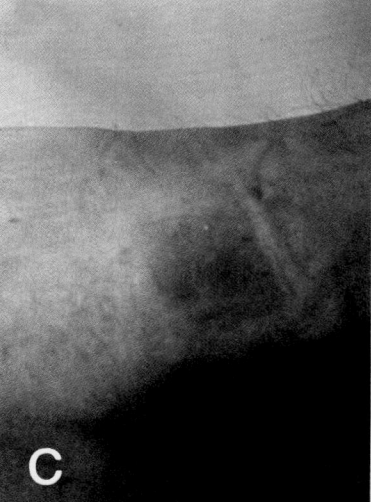

Fig. 44-3 A, Abnormal reactive hyperemia. **B and C,** In abnormal reactive hyperemia the area is much darker than the surrounding skin and does not blanch with fingertip pressure.
From Pires M, Muller A: *Progressions* 3(3):3, 1991.

pressure, but they may not be able to understand how to relieve it. Clients who are in a coma may not perceive pressure and are unable to voluntarily move into a more protective position. In addition, clients whose levels of consciousness change may easily become confused. Thus they are unable to seek out more protective positions.

Casts and Traction

Casts and traction reduce mobility of the client or an extremity. A client with a cast has an increased risk of pressure ulcer development because of the mechanical external force of friction from the surface of the cast rubbing against the skin. A second mechanical force is the pressure exerted by the cast on the skin if the cast dries too tightly or if the extremity swells.

Contributing Factors to Pressure Ulcer Formation

Impaired skin integrity resulting in pressure ulcers is primarily the result of pressure. However, additional factors can further increase the client's risk for pressure ulcer development. These include shearing force, moisture, poor nutrition, anemia, infection, fever, impaired peripheral circulation, obesity, cachexia, and age.

Shearing force is the pressure exerted against the skin when a client is moved or repositioned in bed by being pulled or being allowed to slide down in bed (Fig 44-4). Shearing force is the third major factor contributing to the development of pressure ulcers. When a shearing force is present, the skin and subcutaneous layers adhere to the surface of the bed, and the layers of muscle and even the bones slide in the direction of body movement. The underlying tissue capillaries are compressed and severed by the pressure (Knight, 1988; Bennett, Lee, 1988). As a result, minute layers of bleeding and necrosis occur deep within the tissue layers. In addition, there is a decrease in capillary blood flow from the external pressure against the skin. Subcutaneous fat is more vulnerable to the effects of shearing and the resultant pressure from the underlying bony structure. Eventually a tract opens to the skin to allow drainage from the necrotic area.

The presence of *moisture* on the skin increases the risk of ulcer formation. Moisture reduces the skin's resistance to other physical factors such as pressure or shearing force. The susceptibility to pressure ulcer formation increases with the duration of the exposure to moisture. The presence of moisture increases the risk of pressure ulcer formation fivefold (Reuler, Cooney, 1981).

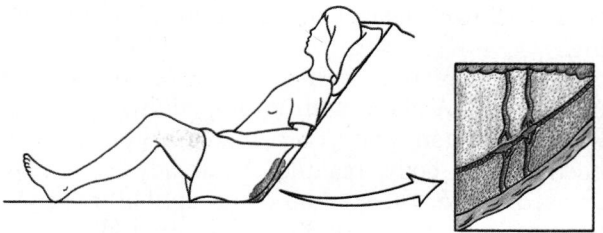

Fig. 44-4   Diagrammatic sketch of shearing force exerted against sacral area.

The immobilized client, who is unable to meet hygiene needs, depends on the nurse to keep the skin dry and intact. The nurse must therefore incorporate hygiene into the care plan. Moisture on the skin can originate from wound drainage, perspiration, condensation from humidified oxygen-delivery systems, vomitus, and incontinence. Certain body fluids (for example, urine, diarrhea, and wound drainage) cause skin erosion, and with pressure the client's risk increases.

Clients with *poor nutrition* often experience serious muscle atrophy and decreases in subcutaneous tissue (see Chapter 35). Because of these changes, less tissue is present to serve as padding between the skin and underlying bone. Therefore the effects of pressure are increased on remaining tissue. The client can have protein deficiency and negative nitrogen balance (see Chapters 35 and 43) and have an inadequate intake of vitamin C (Shekleton, Litwack, 1991). Poor nutritional status may be overlooked if the client has a weight equal to or above the ideal body weight (IBW). Malnutrition is second only to excessive pressure in the etiology, pathogenesis, and nonhealing of pressure ulcers (Hanan, Scheele, 1991; NPUAP, 1989). The client with poor nutritional status frequently has hypoalbuminemia (serum albumin levels below 3.0 g/100 ml) and anemia (Natlow, 1983; Steinberg, 1990).

Poor nutrition can also alter fluid and electrolyte balance. In clients with severe protein loss, hypoalbuminemia leads to a shift of fluid from the extracellular fluid volume to the tissues, resulting in edema. **Edema** increases the affected tissue's risk for pressure ulcers. The blood supply to the edematous tissue is decreased, and waste products remain because of the changing pressures in the capillary circulation and capillary bed (Shekleton, Litwack, 1991; Gröer, Shekleton, 1989).

Clients with **anemia** are at risk for pressure ulcer formation. Decreased levels of hemoglobin reduce the oxygen-carrying capacity of the blood and the amount of oxygen available to tissues. Anemia also alters cellular metabolism and impairs healing.

Infection results from the presence of pathogens in the body. A client with an infection usually has a fever. Infection and *fever* increase the metabolic needs of the body, making an already hypoxic (decreased oxygen) tissue more susceptible to ischemic injury (Shekleton, Litwack, 1991). In addition, fever results in diaphoresis (sweating) and increased skin moisture, which further predispose the client to skin breakdown.

Impaired peripheral circulation is also related to pressure ulcer development. With decreased circulation the tissue becomes hypoxic and more susceptible to ischemic damage. Impaired circulation occurs in clients who have peripheral vascular diseases, who are in shock, or who are receiving vasopressor-type medications.

Obesity can speed pressure ulcer development. Adipose tissue in small quantities protects the skin by cushioning bony prominences against pressure. However, in moderate-to-severe obesity, adipose tissue is poorly vascularized, and the adipose and underlying tissues are more susceptible to ischemic damage.

Cachexia is generalized ill health and malnutrition, marked by weakness and emaciation. It is usually associated with severe diseases such as cancer and end-stage cardiopulmonary diseases. This condition increases the client's risk for pressure ulcers. Basically the cachexic client has lost the adipose tissue necessary to protect bony prominences from pressure.

Pressure ulcer development occurs more frequently in *older adults*. Studies by Stotts (1988) and Kane, Ouslander, and Abrass (1989) note a greater incidence of ulcer development in people over 75 years of age.

Pathogenesis of Pressure Ulcers

A client with impaired physical mobility is at risk of developing a pressure ulcer. A pressure ulcer occurs as a result of a time-pressure relationship (Stotts, 1988). The greater the pressure and the duration of the pressure, the greater the incidence of ulcer formation. The skin and subcutaneous tissue can tolerate some pressure. However, externally applied pressure greater than the pressure in the capillary bed decreases or obliterates blood flow to adjacent tissues. These tissues become hypoxic, and ischemic injury results. If this pressure is greater than 32 mm Hg and remains unrelieved to the point of hypoxia, the vessels collapse and thrombose (develop a clot) (Maklebust, 1987). If the pressure is relieved before the critical point, circulation to the affected tissues is restored through the physiological mechanism of reactive hyperemia.

Pressure ulcers also form as a result of a shearing force when moving the client up in bed. The sacral

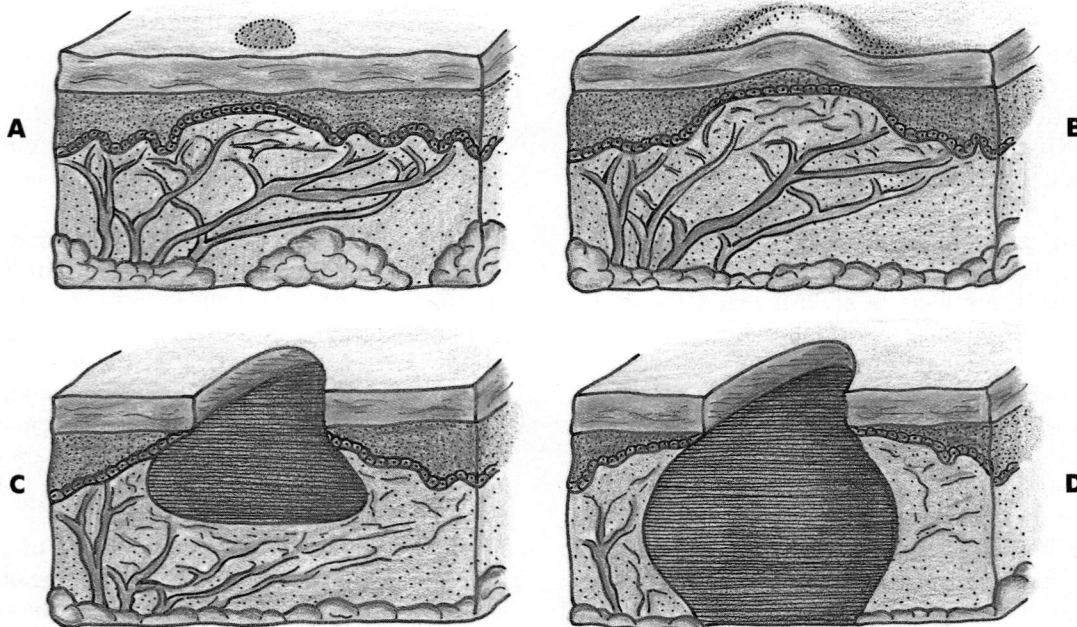

Fig. 44-5   A, Stage I pressure ulcer. B, Stage II pressure ulcer. C, Stage III pressure ulcer. D, Stage IV pressure ulcer.

areas and heels are the most susceptible (Maklebust, 1987). The effect of pressure can be increased by unequal distribution of body weight. Because of gravity, a person is subjected to constant pressures of the body against any surface on which it rests (Berecek, 1975). If the pressure is unevenly distributed on the body, a pressure gradient is increased on tissues receiving the pressure. The cellular metabolism of the skin is altered at the point of pressure.

The compensatory response of the tissues to ischemia, reactive hyperemia, permits ischemic tissue to be flooded with blood when pressure is removed. Increased blood flow increases delivery of oxygen and nutrients to tissue. The metabolic debt resulting from pressure can then be met. Healthy equilibrium is restored, and necrosis of the compressed tissue is avoided (Berecek, 1975; Maklebust, 1991a, 1991b; Pires, Muller, 1991). Reactive hyperemia is effective only if pressure is removed before damage occurs. Some researchers feel that the interval before damage occurs can be between 1 and 2 hours. However, this is a subjective time interval, and it is not based on client assessment data.

Stages of Pressure Ulcers

Pressure ulcers may occur initially in the superficial layers of the skin. Guttman's (1955) criteria, which were modified by Shea (1975), are the most widely used classifications for staging the severity of pressure ulcer formation. The stages below are from the Agency for Health Care Policy and Research's Pressure Ulcer Guideline Panel (USDHHS, 1992).

I   Nonblanchable erythema of the intact skin, the heralding lesion of skin ulceration, occurs (Fig. 44-5, *A*).

II   Partial-thickness skin loss involves epidermis and/or dermis. Ulcer is superficial and presents clinically as an abrasion, blister, or shallow crater (Fig. 44-5, *B*).

III   Full-thickness skin loss involves damage or necrosis of subcutaneous tissue that may extend to the fascia. Ulcer presents clinically as a deep crater with or without undermining of adjacent tissue (Fig. 44-5, *C*).

IV   Full-thickness skin loss occurs with extensive destruction, tissue necrosis, or damage to muscle, bone, or supporting structures (Fig. 44-5, *D*).

NURSING PROCESS AND PRESSURE ULCERS

Assessment

Baseline and continual assessment data provide critical information about the client's skin integrity and the increased risk for pressure ulcer develop-

ment. Assessment for pressure ulcers (Procedure 44-1) is not limited to the skin. Pressure ulcers have multiple etiological factors.

Predictive Measures

A benefit of the predictive instruments is to increase the nurses' early detection of clients at greatest risk for ulcer development. Once these clients are identified, appropriate interventions are instituted to maintain skin integrity.

Two predictive instruments, the Norton Scale (see Table 4-1) and the Braden Scale, are useful in identifying clients at greatest risk. Both instruments have been tested in clinical trials. They are valid and reliable. Of the two instruments, the Braden Scale is more sensitive. Tests have shown that the Norton Scale overpredicts by 64% and the Braden scale overpredicts by 36% (Bergstrom, Demuth, Braden, 1987). It is important to correctly identify clients at risk without overprediction because a majority of the preventive measures are costly and can cause the cost of care to rise unnecessarily.

Skin

The nurse must continually assess the skin for signs of ulcer development. The neurologically impaired client (Sklar, 1985), the chronically ill client in long-term care, the client with diminished mental status (Gosnell, 1987), and the orthopedic client have increased potential for developing pressure ulcers.

Assessment for tissue pressure indicators includes visual and tactile inspection of the skin (Pires, Muller, 1991). Baseline assessment is performed to determine the client's normal skin characteristics and any actual or potential areas of breakdown. The nurse pays particular attention to areas exposed to casts, traction, or splints. The frequency of pressure checks depends on the schedule of appliance application and the skin's response to the external pressure (Figs. 44-6 and 44-7 on p. 1531).

When hyperemia is noted, the nurse documents location, size, and color and reassesses the area after 1 hour (Fig. 44-8, *A* on p.1552). If the nurse suspects abnormal reactive hyperemia, outlining the affected area with a marker makes reassessment easier. Another early warning sign of pressure damage is a blister or pimple over the weight-bearing area with possible hyperemia. Pires and Muller (1991) report that a frequently overlooked sign of early pressure is a scabbing over of the weight-bearing areas in the absence of trauma (Fig. 44-8, *B*). All of these signs are very early indicators of impaired skin integrity, but damage to the underlying tissue may be more progressive. Tactile assessment enables the nurse to use palpation to acquire further data about induration and the damage to the skin and underlying tissues.

Assessment for Risk of Pressure Ulcer Development

STEPS	RATIONALE
1. Identify client's risk for pressure ulcer formation:	Determines need to administer preventive care and use topical agents for existing ulcers.
a. Paralysis or immobilization caused by restrictive devices	Client is unable to turn or reposition independently.
b. Sensory loss	Client feels no discomfort from pressure.
c. Circulatory disorders	Reduce perfusion of skin's tissue layers.
d. Decreased level of consciousness, sedation, or anesthesia	Client is unable to perceive pressure to turn or reposition independently.
e. Shearing force	Causes skin and underlying subcutaneous layers to adhere to surface of bed. Trauma occurs to underlying tissues.
f. Moisture: incontinence, perspiration, wound drainage, or vomitus	Reduces skin's resistance to pressure from shearing force.
g. Malnutrition	Can lead to weight loss, muscle atrophy, and reduced tissue mass. Less tissue is available to pad between skin and underlying bone. Poor protein, vitamin, and caloric intake limit wound-healing capabilities.
h. Anemia	Decreased hemoglobin level reduces oxygen-carrying capacity of blood and amount of oxygen available to tissues.
i. Infection	Causes increase in metabolic demands of tissues. Accompanying diaphoresis leaves skin moist.
j. Obesity	Poorly vascularized excess adipose tissue is more susceptible to pressure.
k. Cachexia	Causes loss of adipose tissue that protects bony prominences from pressure.
l. Hydration: edema or dehydration	Edematous tissue has decreased blood supply and thereby is less tolerant of pressure, friction, and shearing force. Dehydrated skin is less elastic, and skin turgor is poor.
m. Older adulthood	Skin is less elastic and drier; tissue mass is reduced.
n. Existing pressure ulcers	Limits surfaces available for position changes, placing available tissues at increased risk.
2. Assess condition of skin over regions of pressure (see Fig. 44-9). Look for the following areas:	Body weight against bony prominences places underlying skin at risk for breakdown.
a. Normal reactive hyperemia	May indicate that tissue was under pressure. Normal reactive hyperemia is normal physiological response to hypoxemia. In dark-skinned persons, skin that was under pressure will appear darker than surrounding skin and may even take on purplish hue (Pires, Muller, 1991). Normal reactive hyperemia over pressure area lasts less than 1 hr. Affected area blanches at fingertip pressure (Pires, Muller, 1991). Abnormal reactive hyperemia lasts longer than 1 hr. Surrounding tissue does not blanch (Pires, Muller, 1991).
b. Blanching	Blanching is normal, expected response.
c. Induration	Localized edema beneath the skin surface, induration commonly occurs with abnormal reactive hyperemia (Pires, Muller, 1991).
d. Pallor and mottling	Persistent hypoxia in tissues that were under pressure is abnormal physiological response.
e. Absence of superficial skin layers	Represents early pressure ulcer formation.
f. Scabs, blisters, or pimples (see Fig. 44-6, B)	Early signs of skin damage, but damage to underlying tissue may be more progressive (Pires, Muller, 1991).
3. Assess client for additional areas of potential pressure:	Clients at high risk have multiple sites of pressure necrosis.
a. Nares	Site is nasogastric tube.

STEPS	RATIONALE
b. Tongue, lips	Oral airway and endotracheal tube are high-risk locations.
c. Intravenous sites (especially long-term access sites)	Stress occurs at catheter exit sites.
d. Drainage tubes	There is stress against tissue at exit site.
e. Foley catheter	There is pressure against labia, especially with edema.
4. Observe client for preferred positions when in bed or chair.	Weight of body will be placed on bony prominences. Contractures (flexion and fixation of joint) may result in pressure exerted in unexpected places. Phenomenon is best assessed through observation.
5. Observe client's mobility and ability to initiate and assist with position changes.	Potential for friction and shear increases when client is completely dependent for position changes.
6. Obtain risk score: a. Norton Scale b. Braden Scale	Risk score depends on instrument used and predicts client's need for preventive care (USDHHS, 1992).
7. Monitor length of time any area of redness persists:	Redness usually persists for half of time hypoxia occurred. For example, redness lasts 15 min, so hypoxia lasted approximately 30 min.
a. Determine appropriate turning interval, which should be turning interval − hypoxia time = suggested interval.	For example, turning interval is 2 hr, hypoxia time is 30 min. 2 hr − 30 min = 1½ hr suggested turning interval.
b. Use pressure-relief device, if indicated.	Short turning intervals (e.g., 1-2 hr) may not be realistic. Therefore use of device is recommended.
8. Obtain nutritional assessment data, including serum albumin level, total protein level, hemoglobin level, and IBW percentage (see Chapter 35).	Poor nutritional status decreases skin's and underlying tissue's tolerance to pressure, friction, and shearing force (Hanan, Scheele 1991).
9. Assess client's and family's understanding of risks for pressure ulcers.	Provides opportunity to begin prevention education.
10. Document assessment findings.	Provides baseline data for skin integrity and risk of pressure ulcer development.

CONTINUED

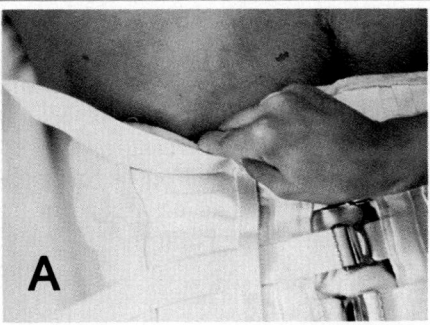

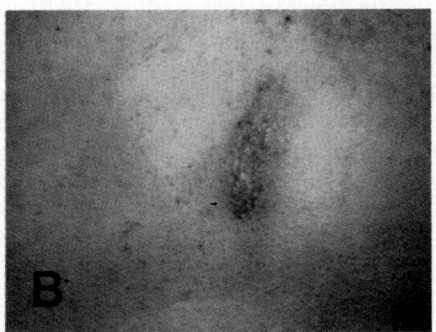

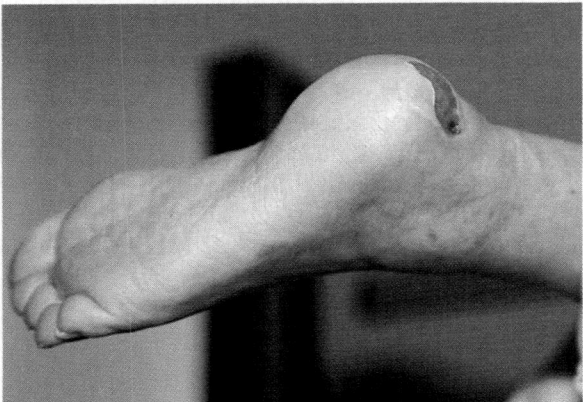

Fig. 44-7 Formation of pressure ulcer on heel resulting from external pressure from mattress of bed.

Fig. 44-6 Benign devices such as this corset (**A**) may result in scabbing or blistering (**B**) resulting from external pressure.
From Pires M, Muller A: *Progressions* 3(3):3, 1991.

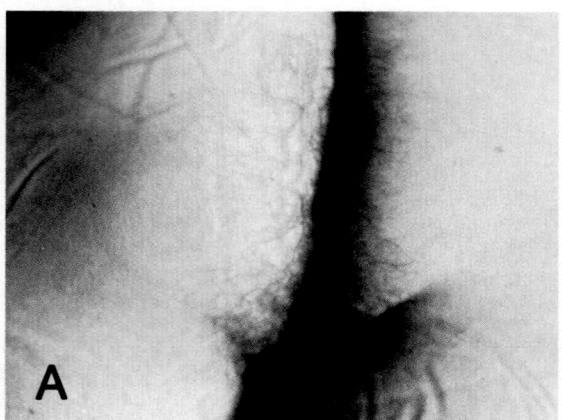

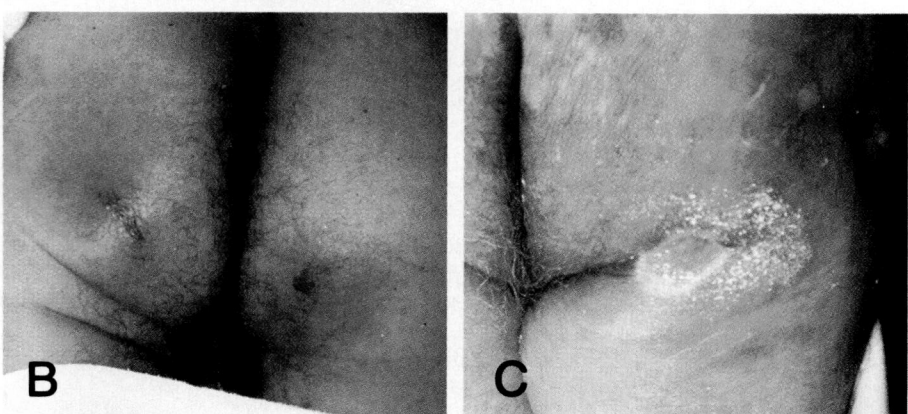

Fig. 44-8 A, Hyperemia on ischial tuberosities. B, Scabbing over bony prominences is a sign of excessive pressure. C, Deeper stages of ulceration.
From Pires M, Muller M: *Progressions* 3(3):3, 1991.

The nurse palpates the tissue adjacent to the observed area of hyperemia. The nurse assesses for blanching with return to normal skin tones. In addition, the nurse palpates for induration, noting the size in millimeters or centimeters of the induration around the injured area. The nurse also notes changes in color, temperature, and hardness of the surrounding skin and tissues (Pires, Muller, 1991).

The nurse includes visual and tactile inspection over the body areas most frequently at risk for pressure ulcer development (Fig. 44-9). When a client lays in bed or sits in a chair, body weight is heavily placed on certain bony prominences. Body surfaces subjected to the greatest weight or pressure are at greatest risk for decubitus ulcer formation.

Mobility

Assessment includes documenting level of mobility and the potential effects of impaired mobility on skin integrity. Assessment of mobility should also include obtaining data regarding the quality of muscle tone and strength. For example, the nurse determines whether the client can lift the weight off the ischial tuberosities and can roll the body to a side-lying position. The client may have adequate range of motion (ROM) to independently move into a more protective position. Finally the nurse notes the client's activity tolerance (see Chapter 43).

Mobility must be assessed as part of baseline data. If the client has some degree of independence in mobility the nurse reinforces the frequency of position changes and measures to relieve pressure. The frequency of position changes is based on ongoing skin assessment and is revised as data change. The following case study illustrates this point:

A nurse is caring for Calvin Jones, a 40-year-old completely rehabilitated paraplegic who is hospitalized for a cholecystectomy. The nurse obtains baseline assessment data regarding skin integrity and mobility status and notes that the client has intact skin, has never had a pressure ulcer, and is able to lift his body weight off his ischial tuberosities. The nurse also notes that the client routinely performs pressure-relieving exercises every 30 minutes for 15 seconds when sitting in his wheelchair at work and home.

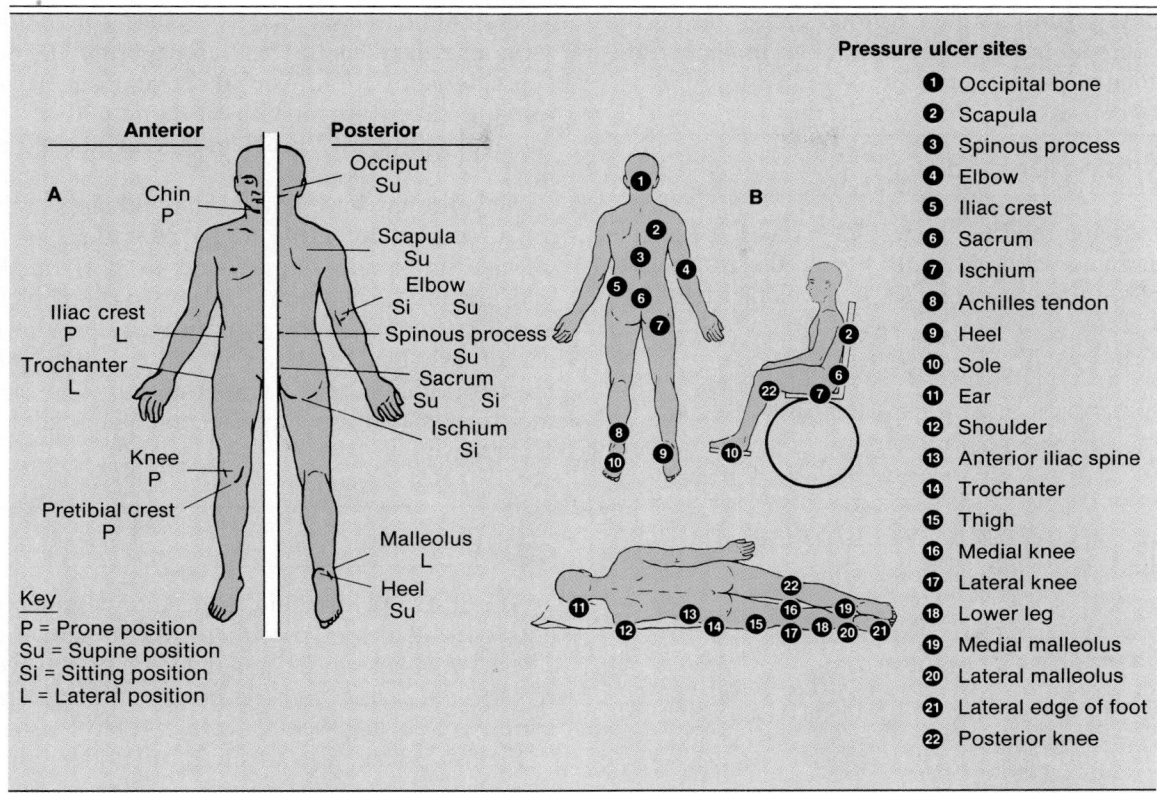

Fig. 44-9 A, Bony prominence most frequently underlying pressure ulcer. B, Pressure ulcer sites.
From Trelease CC: *Ostomy/Wound Manage* 20:46, 1988.

Because Mr. Jones will have general anesthesia, his ability to perform pressure-relieving exercises will change, and the nursing care plan must include nursing measures designed to maintain skin integrity for this client. The nurse must be meticulous in assessing Mr. Jones' pressure sites. Normal reactive hyperemia must be present because once abnormal reactive hyperemia occurs it may take as long as 2 weeks of non-weight-bearing or total pressure relief to heal completely (Pires, Muller, 1991). As a result, if attention is not paid to skin integrity for this client, his lost worktime can increase by an additional 2 weeks beyond the normal postoperative course of treatment.

Nutritional Status

An assessment of the client's nutritional status should be an integral part of the initial assessment data for clients at risk for impaired skin integrity. Albumin is a frequently measured variable used to evaluate the client's protein status. A client with a serum albumin level below 3 g/100 ml is at greater risk for pressure ulcers than a client with a higher albumin level. In addition, low albumin levels are associated with poor wound healing (Hanan, Scheele, 1991; Pinchcofsky-Devin, Kaminski, 1989; Natlow, 1983). Although serum albumin levels are slow to reflect changes in visceral proteins, they are the best predictors of malnutrition in all age groups (Hanan, Scheele, 1991).

Total protein levels are also correlated with pressure ulcer development. Total protein levels below 5.4 g/100 ml decrease colloid osmotic pressure, which leads to interstitial edema and decreased oxygen to the tissues (Hanan, Scheele, 1991). Edema decreases the skin and underlying tissue's tolerance to pressure, friction, and shearing force. In addition, the decreased oxygen levels increase the speed of ischemic injury to the tissue.

The client's percentage of IBW is also obtained. A client who is malnourished or cachexic and whose body weight is less than 90% of IBW or a client whose body weight is greater than 110% of IBW has an increased risk for the development of pressure ulcers (Hanan, Scheele 1991). Percentage of IBW alone is not a good predictor. However, when used with a low serum albumin or total protein level, the client's percentage of IBW can have an impact on the occurrence of pressure ulcers.

Nursing Diagnosis

Assessment reveals clusters of data that indicate whether an actual or a risk for impaired skin integrity exists. The nursing diagnosis is developed based on assessment data (see diagnoses box). In addition, assessment data should contain appropriate defining characteristics to support the diagnostic label. The nursing diagnoses should also include a probable cause of the client's problem (see diagnostic process box).

A client may have one or more problems related to impaired skin integrity. Many alterations in physiological functioning are related to skin breakdown, and impaired functioning in one system may affect another. For example, urinary stasis in the kidney can quickly lead to kidney infection, which produces fever and diaphoresis. The resulting increased skin moisture may then increase the potential for skin breakdown.

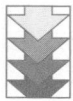

Examples of Nursing Diagnoses Related to Impaired Skin Integrity

---

NANDA-APPROVED NURSING DIAGNOSES

Impaired physical mobility related to:
- Bed Rest
- Decreased strength
- Musculoskeletal impairment

Actual or *high risk for impaired skin integrity* related to:
- Restricted mobility
- Pressure on skin's surface
- Shearing force
- Friction
- Moisture

High risk infection related to:
- Open wound

Planning

The nurse plans therapeutic interventions for clients with actual or potential risks to skin integrity. These therapies are designed according to severity of risks to the client, and the plan is individualized according to developmental stage and level of health.

Planning care also involves an understanding of the client's need to maintain independence. The nurse and client work together to establish ways of maintaining skin integrity. Clients at risk for hazards of pressure ulcers require a nursing care plan directed at meeting their actual or potential positioning, nutritional, and mobility needs (see care plan).

Sample Nursing Diagnostic Process for Impaired Skin Integrity

Assessment Activities	Defining Characteristics	Nursing Diagnosis
Observe skin over bony prominences or area under external pressure (e.g. casts, splints).	Blanching hyperemia Nonblanching hyperemia Scab formation Blister formation Drainage	*Actual* or *high risk for impaired skin integrity* related to pressure on bony prominences
Palpate skin over bony prominences or areas under external pressure (e.g., casts, splints).	Induration Edema Tenderness Moisture Heat	
Observe skin for moisture.	Wound drainage Diaphoresis Vomitus Moisture from oxygen therapy equipment Incontinence	
Observe mobility and activity status.	Fatigue Immobility Restricted mobility	

The plan is based on one or more of the following client goals:

1. Maintaining vitality of the skin through hygiene and topical care
2. Reducing and preventing injuries to the skin and musculoskeletal system from pressure, friction, and shearing force
3. Improving nutritional intake
4. Improving mobility and activity
5. Improving or maintaining body alignment

These goals and the organization of the nursing intervention content are based on the AHCPR Pressure Ulcer Guidelines (Maklebust, 1991a, 1991b).

Implementation

When the client is immobile, the major risk to the skin is the formation of pressure sores. Nursing interventions focus on prevention or treatment of pressure ulcers.

Prevention

The first step in preventing pressure ulcers is to assess the client's risk factors. The nurse then reduces environmental factors that accelerate pressure ulcer formation, such as high room temperature (causing diaphoresis), moisture, or wrinkled bed linen.

Early identification of high-risk clients and their risk factors aids the nurse in preventing pressure sores. Procedure 44-1 identifies frequent pressure ulcer sites. Prevention minimizes the impact that risk factors or contributing factors may have on pressure ulcer development. Table 44-2 on p. 1536 outlines some universal nursing interventions for the prevention of pressure ulcers. Three major areas of nursing interventions for prevention of pressure sores are hy-

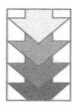

Sample Nursing Care Plan for Impaired Skin Integrity

Nursing diagnosis: *Actual* or *high risk for impaired skin integrity* related to pressure on bony prominences
Definition: Impaired skin integrity is the state in which an individual's skin is at risk of being adversely altered (Kim, McFarland, McLane, 1991).

Goal	Expected Outcomes	Interventions	Rationale
Injury to skin and underlying tissue resulting from pressure on bony prominences will be prevented.	Skin will remain intact (6/1). Normal reactive hyperemia will occur (6/1). Blanching will occur (6/1).	Instruct client to shift body weight every 15 min when sitting.	Redistribution of body weight every 15 min when sitting relieves the downward pressure on the ischial tuberosities (Pires, Muller, 1991).
		Reposition client every 90 min.	Repositioning removes pressure and allows normal hyperemic response. Frequency of turning is based on initial assessment (Maklebust, 1991b).
		Obtain oscillating air mattress for client's bed.	Distributes pressure over a greater area and away from bony pressure points.
Injury to skin and underlying tissue resulting from pressure on bony prominences will be reduced by 6/20.	Wound size will decrease (6/10). Wound drainage will decrease (6/20). Skin will remain intact in unaffected areas (6/1). Normal reactive hyperemia will be observed in unaffected areas (6/1). Decreased hyperemia will be observed in affected areas (6/15).	Apply dressing to wound.	Dressings protect underlying skin and remove drainage from surface of wound (Maklebust, 1991b).
		Implement above measures to reduce risk of other pressure ulcer development.	Clients with pressure ulcer development are at greater risk for new ulcers and need meticulous preventive nursing measures to prevent more ulcers (NPUAP, 1989).

TABLE 44-2 A Quick Guide to Prevention

Risk Factor	Nursing Interventions
Immobility	Establish individualized turning schedule.
	Reduce shear and friction.
	Provide pressure-relief surface.
Inactivity	Provide assistive devices to increase activity.
Incontinence	Assess need for incontinence management.
	Clean and dry skin after soiling.
Malnutrition	Provide adequate nutritional and fluid intake.
	Consult dietitian for nutritional evaluation.
Diminished sensation, decreased mental status	Assess client's and family's ability to provide care.
	Educate care giver regarding pressure ulcer prevention.
Impaired skin integrity	Avoid pressure.
	Do not use donut-shaped cushions.
	Lubricate skin.
	Do not massage red areas.
	Do not use heat lamps.

Adapted from Maklebust J, Sieggreen M: *Pressure ulcers: guidelines for prevention and nursing management*, West Dundee, Ill, 1991, S-N Publications.

giene and topical skin care, positioning, and the use of therapeutic beds and mattresses.

HYGIENE AND SKIN CARE. The nurse must keep the client's skin clean and dry. In this initial line of defense for preventing skin breakdown, the client's skin is continually assessed by nurses, rather than delegated to other personnel. In addition, the types of products available for skin care are numerous, and their uses need to be matched to the specific needs of the client (Maklebust, 1991a, 1991b).

When the skin is cleaned, soaps are avoided. Soaps and alcohol-based lotions cause drying and leave an alkaline residue. The alkaline residue discourages the growth of normal skin bacteria, thus promoting an overgrowth of opportunistic bacteria, which can then enter an open wound (Barnes, 1987).

After the skin is cleansed and completely dried, protective moisturizer should be applied to keep the epidermis well lubricated but not oversaturated. Cornstarch is a dry lubricant and helps to reduce friction (Maklebust, 1991b). A & D, Unicare, and Pericare are bland, water-repellent ointments that protect the skin from moisture (USDHHS, 1992). In addition, these ointments are easily cleansed from the skin (Barnes, 1987). When the nurse uses any water-repellent ointment, the nurse must completely clean the area on a routine basis. Ointment, when left in place too long, can be a medium for bacteria and can cause further skin problems such as maceration and infection.

When clients are incontinent, the area should be cleansed, and a skin barrier containing petrolatum (for example, Vaseline) or zinc oxide is applied. These barriers protect the skin from excessive moisture and toxins from urine or stool (Maklebust, 1991b).

When clients are incontinent, absorptive underpads such as adult diapers or incontinence briefs can be used. The nurse must use those products that drain moisture away from the client's skin (USDHHS, 1992). The absorptive garments have a quilted lining and contain a polymer filling. Disposable, plastic-lined underpads should not be placed directly under the client's skin because they do not drain moisture away from the client's skin. These products protect the bed, not the client. The plastic also causes diaphoresis, which can lead to skin maceration. Moist, macerated skin is more susceptible to pressure, friction, and the shearing force, so tissue breakdown occurs more rapidly. If these pads are necessary to absorb body fluids, they should be placed in pillowcases under a draw sheet (Pajk et al, 1986).

POSITIONING. Positioning interventions are designed to reduce pressure and shearing force to the skin. The immobilized client's position should be changed according to activity level, perceptual ability, and daily routines (Pajk et al, 1986; Bergstrom et al, 1987). Therefore a standard turning interval of 1½ to 2 hours may not prevent pressure sore development in some clients.

When the client can sit in a chair, the time should be limited to 2 hours or less. Again, the exact time interval is individualized (see Procedure 44-1). However, the nurse should not allow the client to sit for a period longer than the recommended time interval that was calculated during assessment. Thus if the timing interval is every 1½ hours, the client should remain in a sitting position less than 1½ hours. In the sitting position, the pressure on the ischial tuberosities is greater than when in the supine position (Pajk et al, 1986). In addition, a high-risk client sitting in a chair should be taught or assisted to shift weight every 15 minutes. Shifting weight provides short-term relief on the ischial tuberosities. A client should also sit on foam, gel, or an air cushion to redistribute weight so that it is not all on the ischium.

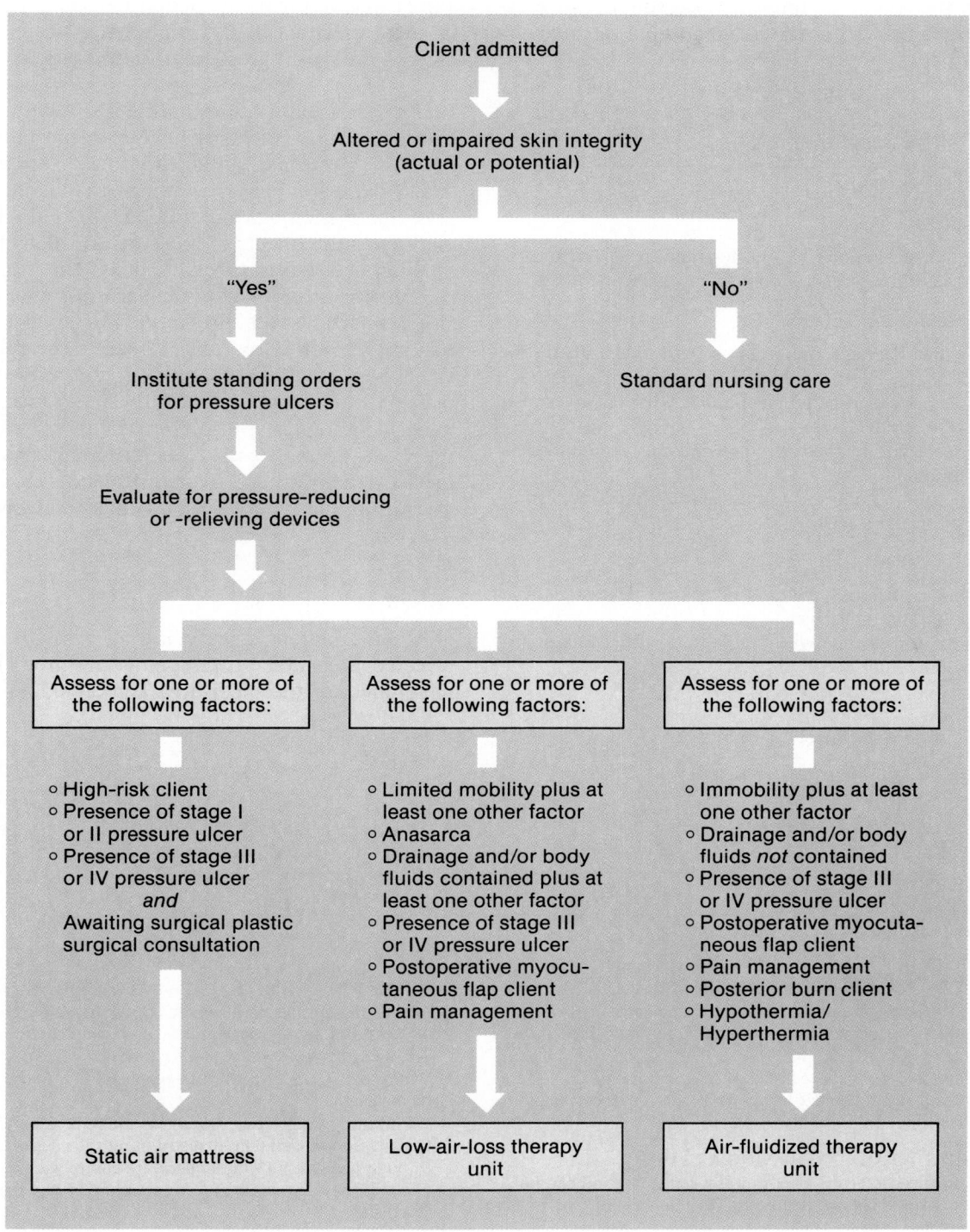

Fig. 44-10   Flow diagram for ordering specialty beds.
From Thomas C: *Ostomy/Wound Manage* 23:51, 1989.

Rigid and donut-shaped cushions are contraindicated because they reduce blood supply to the area, resulting in wider areas of ischemia (Maklebust, 1991a).

After the client is repositioned, the nurse reassesses the skin and observes for normal reactive hyperemia and blanching. The reddened areas should *never* be massaged. This change in practice is a result of nursing research (Maklebust, 1991a; USDHHS, 1992). Massaging the reddened areas increases breaks in the capillaries in the underlying tissues and increases the risk of pressure ulcer formation.

THERAPEUTIC BEDS AND MATTRESSES. A variety of special beds and mattresses have been designed to reduce the hazards of immobility to the skin and musculoskeletal system. However, none eliminates the need for meticulous nursing care. No single device eliminates the effects of pressure on the skin.

When selecting specialty beds, the nurse must thoroughly assess clients' needs. A flow diagram (Fig. 44-10) assists the nurse in clinical decision making. In addition, Table 44-3 lists the specific device, client assessment, and pertinent nurse alerts for using the equipment safely. Clients and families need to be taught the reason for and proper use of the beds or mattresses (see teaching box). When used correctly, these mattresses and specialty beds assist in reducing pressure ulcers in high-risk clients (see box).

Treating Pressure Ulcers

SKIN. In addition to removing all pressure from the affected area and keeping pressure from the area, cleanliness of the ulcer area and all skin surfaces is

---

Client Teaching for Therapeutic Beds and Mattresses

OBJECTIVE
- Client will demonstrate understanding of the purposes and basic operations of the therapeutic bed.

TEACHING STRATEGIES
- Explain to client the reasons for the therapeutic bed.
- Explain proper body mechanics while using the therapeutic bed.
- Educate family about the use and care of the therapeutic bed.
- Explain to client and family about additional pressure-relief measures.

EVALUATION
- Client and family will state basic purposes for the therapeutic mattresses.
- Client and family will be able to describe function of therapeutic bed.

Devices Used to Prevent or Treat Pressure Ulcers

DEVICES TO SUPPORT PRESSURE AREAS
- Flotation pads are pliable pads with a consistency like body fat, which disperse pressure over a larger area (Procedure 44-2).
- Pillows and bridging techniques lift the pressure site off the mattress and separate two points of pressure (see Chapter 43).

DEVICES TO AID IN TURNING A CLIENT
- A CircOlectric bed is electronically controlled and can be rotated vertically 210 degrees to rotate client from prone to supine position.
- A Guttman bed rotates the client from prone to supine positions and from side to side.
- A Rotokinetic treatment table continuously rotates the client 270 degrees every 3 min.
- A Stryker wedge turning frame rotates the client horizontally from the prone to the supine position.

DEVICES TO MINIMIZE OR EQUALIZE PRESSURE
- Alternating air mattresses made of polyvinyl air cells are attached to a pump that inflates and deflates them every 3-7 sec, alternating pressure points (Procedure 42-2).
- Water mattresses disperse and evenly distribute the client's body weight.
- A Clinitron bed decreases pressure and reduces shearing, friction, and maceration by distributing the client's weight through a gentle flow of temperature-controlled air forced upward through a mass of fine ceramic microspheres (Procedure 44-3).
- An egg crate mattress is a foam rubber pad that rests on the bed mattress and disperses the client's body weight evenly over the mattress (Procedure 44-2).

TABLE 44-3 Pressure-Relieving Beds and Mattresses

Brand Names	Manufacturer	Indications	Comments
LOW-AIR-LOSS			
Flexicair	Support Systems International	Pressure relief in clients in whom repositioning is difficult or contraindicated	Nurse must consider need for built-in or underbed scales (may cost extra and be optional feature).
KinAir	Kinetic Concepts		Nurse should use only incontinence pads recommended by manufacturer.
Mediscus	Mediscus Group		Nurse cannot adjust temperature to cool feverish client.
OSCILLATING LOW-AIR-LOSS			
BioDyne	Kinetic Concepts	Hemodynamically unstable clients who cannot tolerate sudden changes in position	If client has small frame, it is difficult to prevent sliding, and there is higher risk of falls.
Pulmonair-40	Mediscus Group	Clients with documented pneumonia and unmanageable secretions requiring frequent position changes to mobilize secretions	Movement of bed may contribute to agitation or cause motion sickness in some clients.
Rescue	Support Systems International		Nurse cannot adjust temperature to cool feverish client. Nurse should use only incontinence pads recommended by manufacturer.
OSCILLATING SUPPORT SURFACE			
Keane Mobility System	Medicus Group	Clients who require frequent turning but have unstable spines	Movement of bed raises risk of skin shearing on support surface.
RotoRest	Kinetic Concepts		Movement of bed may contribute to agitation or cause motion sickness in some clients.
Tilt and Turn Paragon 9000	Egerton Hospital Equipment, UK		Bed does not have built-in scales.
AIR-FLUIDIZED			
Air Plus Therapy System	Air Plus	Clients who require minimal movement to prevent skin damage by shearing forces (e.g., posterior grafts, flaps)	Several people or lift are required to transfer client to and from bed.
Clinitron	Support Systems International		Air flow increases evaporative water loss and can contribute to dehydration. Foam wedge is needed for head elevation.
FluidAir	Kinetic Concepts		Bed requires routine cleaning of beads (check with manufacturer for frequency).
Skytron	Skytron		Nurse should use only incontinence pads recommended by manufacturer

Adapted from Willey T: *Am J Nurs* 89:1142, 1989.

Continued.

TABLE 44-3   Pressure-Relieving Beds and Mattresses—cont'd

Brand Names	Manufacturer	Indications	Comments
OBESE			
Burke Bariatric Treatment System	Kinetic Concepts	Patients over 300 lb	Pressure relief capabilities may vary from client to client.
MegaBed Paragon 8000/ 8500	Egerton Hospital Equipment, UK		
SPECIAL FUNCTION			
TheraPulse	Kinetic Concepts	Same as low-air-loss beds, plus pulsation	No evidence yet exists to support therapeutic effect of pulsation.
Rescue	Support Systems International	Clients needing low-air-loss therapy, oscillating therapy, or pulsation therapy	
FOAM			
Bio Gard	Bio Clinic	Reduction of pressure in clients at risk	Nurse should check with manufacturer regarding flammability of product and to determine whether flame retardation is removed with washing or sterilization.
Geo-Matt	Span-America	Adjunct to care of clients with established ulcer if client can be turned frequently and positioned off ulcer	
High Float	Pre-Foam		
STATIC AIR MATTRESS			
Clini-Care	Gaymar Industries		Nurse should avoid puncturing it (requires mattess replacement with some models).
Sof-Care	Gaymar Industries		Nurse follows manufacturer's instructions for checking inflation level (every 8 hr and as needed).
Roho (see figure)	Roho		
First Step	Kinetic Concepts		Nurse checks for increased perspiration because of plastic surface.
KoalaKair	Pharmaseal		
ALTERNATING AIR MATTRESS			
Bio Flote	Bio Clinic		Nurse should follow manufacturer's instructions for proper functioning of equipment; it may require some assembly.
Grant PCA Systems	Grant		
WATER MATTRESS			
Lotus Water Flotation Mattress	Lotus		Nurse should avoid puncturing it (check every shift and as needed for water leakage).

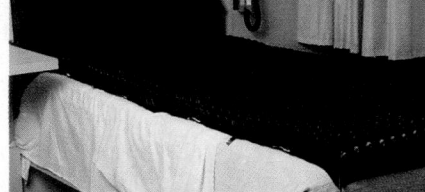

Placing a Client on Support Surface Mattress

STEPS	RATIONALE
1. Assess condition of skin, expecially over dependent sites and bony prominences.	Provides baseline to determine change in skin integrity or change in existing pressure ulcers.
2. Prepare necessary equipment and supplies: a. Flotation pad, foam mattress, air mattress, or sheepskin b. Two bed sheets	Used to cover certain types of support surfaces and bed mattresses.
c. Pillowcases (optional)	Used to cover flotation pads only.
d. Air flow pumping unit	Used only with alternating air-flow mattresses.
3. Explain purpose and application of mattress or pad.	Reduces client anxiety.
4. Wash hands.	Reduces transmission of microorganisms.
5. Close room door or bedside curtain.	Provides client privacy.
6. Apply support surface to bed (bed may be occupied or unoccupied).	Pressure-reducing devices can decrease the incidence of pressure ulcers but must be used with other prevention measures (USDHHS, 1992).
a. *Flotation pad:* (1) Apply foam pad over bed mattress by unrolling it fully.	Pad should lie flat to ensure smooth surface.
(2) Apply sheet over foam pad.	Minimizes soiling.
(3) Place flotation pad in center cut-out portion of foam pad.	Pad is designed to distribute pressure along greater trochanters of hip and sacrum.
b. *Foam mattress:* (1) Apply foam mattress over bed. (With egg crate variety, foam peaks should point up.)	Pad should lie flat to ensure smooth surface. Peaks distribute weight to more effectively relieve pressure.
(2) Apply bed sheet over mattress, being careful to avoid wrinkles.	Prevents soiling.
c. *Air mattress:* (1) Apply deflated mattress flat over bed mattress.	Provides smooth, even surface.
(2) Bring plastic strips or flaps around corners of bed mattress.	Secures air mattress in place.
(3) Attach connector on air mattress to inflation device.	Mattresses vary as to requiring one-time or continuous inflation cycle.
(4) Inflate mattress to proper air pressure determined by air pump or blower.	Manufacturer's directions indicate air pressure to distribute weight evenly.
(5) Place sheet over air mattress, being sure to eliminate all wrinkles.	Prevents soiling of mattress and reduces direct contact of skin against plastic surface.
(6) Check air pumps to be sure pressure cycle alternates.	Produces intermittent cycling, inflating only parts of mattress at any time. Intermittent cycle continually alternates pressure against skin and soft tissue.
7. Position client comfortably as desired over support surface. Reposition routinely.	Location of existing pressure ulcers might influence type of positioning. Regular turning is still required.
8. Wash hands.	Reduces transmission of microorganisms.
9. Inspect skin and bony prominences routinely.	Determines whether pressure sores develop or whether condition of existing sores changes.
10. Record transfer of client to support surface and related information in nurse's notes.	Documents safe completion of the procedure and records initial baseline data.

Placing a Client on a Clinitron Bed

STEPS	RATIONALE
1. Assess condition of client's skin, paying particular attention to potential pressure sites and skin lesions.	Data provide baseline to determine change in client's condition while on bed.
2. For client with severe to moderate pain, premedicate approximately 30 min before transfer.	Promotes client comfort and ability to cooperate.
3. Prepare necessary equipment and supplies: a. Clinitron bed b. Filter sheet	Is permeable to rising airflow from mattress and downward flow of fluids (e.g., sweat, urine, or wound drainage).
4. Explain procedure and purpose of bed to client and family.	Reduces anxiety and promotes cooperation.
5. Obtain additional personnel needed to transfer client to bed.	Ensures client's safety.
6. Wash hands.	Reduces transmission of microorganisms.
7. Close client's room door or bedside curtain.	Maintains client privacy during transfer.
8. Transfer client to bed using appropriate transfer techniques (see Chapter 43).	Appropriate transfer techniques maintain alignment and reduce risk of injury during procedure.
9. Turn fluidization cycle on by depressing continuous or intermittent-mode switch. Regulate temperature in continuous mode.	Fluidization minimizes pressure against skin's surface and reduces friction and shearing force when client moves.
10. Position client and perform ROM exercises as appropriate.	Promotes comfort and reduces contracture formation. Bed reduces pressure on skin, but client must be turned and exercised to avoid joint deformity or contractures.
a. To turn clients, position bed pans, or perform other therapies, set intermittent-fluidization mode. After procedure is completed, set mode to continuous fluidization.	Intermittent fluidization provides firm, molded support that facilitates turning and handling client. Continuous fluidization provides permanent fluid support.
b. In emergencies when cardiopulmonary resuscitation is required, touch button to defluidize bed immediately.	Creates firm surface against which cardiopulmonary resuscitation can be performed.
11. Wash hands.	Reduces transmission of microorganisms.
12. Inspect condition of client's skin periodically.	Evaluates healing progress of existing lesions. Determines whether new pressure areas are forming.
13. Assess client for nausea.	Flotation effects of bed can cause sensation of nausea.
14. Measure client's level of consciousness.	Determines onset of perceptual changes.
15. Record transfer of client to bed, tolerance to procedure, and condition of skin in nurses' notes.	Documents safe completion of procedure and records initial baseline data.

essential (Procedure 44-4). Maintaining cleanliness may be extremely difficult with incontinent, feverish, or confused clients.

Moisture in and around an area of skin breakdown can cause further ulceration and infection. Many products are available for the care of pressure ulcers (Tables 44-4 and 44-5). Before instituting treatment measures, the nurse must thoroughly assess the client's pressure ulcer and determine the correct dressing based on the stage of ulcer development.

The nurse cleans the affected area with an antiseptic solution every 2 hours or as necessary. Caution is needed because antiseptics can damage tissues unprotected by the dermis and may inactivate some drugs. The ulcer should be rinsed with normal saline to minimize the effect of antiseptic (Fowler, 1982).

STEPS	RATIONALE
1. Wash hands; apply disposable gloves.	Reduces transmission of blood-borne pathogens. Gloves should be worn when handling items soiled by body fluids (CDC, 1988).
2. Close door or bedside curtains.	Maintains privacy.
3. Position client comfortably with area of pressure ulcer and surrounding skin easily accessible.	Area should be accessible for cleansing of ulcer and surrounding skin.
4. Assemble supplies at bedside. Open sterile packages and topical solution containers.	Sterile supplies should be ready for easy application so that nurse can use them without contaminating them.
a. Wash basin, warm water, washcloth, and towel	Used to bathe surrounding skin.
b. Cleansing agent (see Table 44-4)	
c. Prescribed topical agent:	
(1) Enzymes: collagenase, fibrinolysin, deoxyribonuclease, or sutilains	Debride dead tissue to allow for granulation.
(2) Antiseptics: providone-iodine (ointment or solution), merbromin (5% or 10% solution), or sodium hypochlorite (1:12 or 1:20 solution)	Reduce bacterial growth in the presence of necrotic tissue, pus, serum, or blood. Reduce infection in weeping ulcer.
(3) Oxydizing agents: benzoyl peroxide (20%) or hydrogen peroxide (half-strength)	Clean wounds, especially with anerobic bacteria. Decreases oxygen supply to devitalized tissues.
(4) Dextranomer beads: Debrisan	Clean wounds with heavy exudate. Absorb fluid, protein, fibrin, fibrinogen, and all products of tissue breakdown and bacterial infection.
d. Sterile dressing (see Table 44-5).	
e. Hypoallergenic tape or adhesive dressing sheet (Hypotix)	Used to apply gauze dressing. Prevents skin irritation and tearing.
f. Sterile gloves	Reduces transmission of microorganisms.
g. Protective paste (e.g., zinc oxide [optional])	Protects nonaffected skin from irritating solutions.
h. Tools to measure wound size:	Used to provide objective measure to evaluate healing.
(1) Transparency film and marker	
(2) Metric ruler	
(3) Camera in some circumstances	Photography provides objective method to assess wound progression.
5. Remove bed linen and client's gown to expose ulcer and surrounding skin. Keep remaining body parts draped.	Prevents unnecessary exposure of body parts.
6. Apply sterile gloves.	Aseptic technique must be maintained during cleansing, measuring, and application of dressings.
7. Assess pressure ulcer and surrounding skin:	
a. Note and document color and appearance of skin around ulcer.	Skin condition may indicate progressive tissue damage.
b. Measure diameter of pressure ulcer with ruler or transparency film.	Provides objective measure of wound size. May determine type of dressing chosen.
c. Measure depth of ulcer using sterile, cotton-tipped applicator or other device that will allow measurement of wound depth.	Depth measure is important for staging ulcer. Kundin scale is a three-dimensional (length, width, and depth) tool for wound volume calculations (Cooper, 1992).
d. Measure depth of undermining skin by lateral tissue necrosis. Use cotton-tipped applicator and gently probe under skin edges.	Undermining may indicate progressive tissue necrosis.
8. Wash skin around ulcer gently with warm water.	Reduces number of resident bacteria.
9. Rinse area thoroughly with water.	

Treating Pressure Ulcers

STEPS	RATIONALE
10. Gently dry skin thoroughly by patting lightly with towel.	Retained moisture causes maceration of skin layers.
11. Cleanse ulcer thoroughly with normal saline or cleansing agent: a. Use irrigating syringe for deep ulcers. b. Use shower with hand-held shower head. c. Use whirlpool treatments to assist with wound cleansing and debridement.	Removes debris from wound from digested material. Previously applied enzymes may require soaking for removal.
12. Apply topical agents, if prescribed: a. Enzymes:	
(1) Keeping gloves sterile, place small amount of enzyme ointment in palm of hand.	Thin layer absorbs and acts more effectively. Excess medication can irritate surrounding skin.
(2) Soften medication by rubbing briskly in palm of hand.	Makes ointment easier to apply to ulcer.
(3) Apply thin, even layer of ointment over necrotic areas. Do not apply enzyme to surrounding skin.	Proper distribution ensures effective action. Enzyme can cause burning, paresthesia, and dermatitis to surrounding skin.
(4) Moisten gauze dressing with saline and apply directly over ulcer.	Protects wound. Keeping ulcer surface moist reduces time needed for healing. Skin cells normally live in moist environment.
(5) Cover moistened gauze with single, dry gauze and tape securely in place.	Prevents bacteria from entering moist dressing.
b. Antiseptics: *Superficial ulcers*	
(1) Moisten sterile gauze with antiseptic solution and paint surface of ulcer.	Distributes antiseptic over entire area to effectively reduce bacterial growth.
(2) Leave ulcer open to air.	If superficial epidermal skin layer is only layer affected, keeping wound dry promotes healing.
Deep ulcers	
(3) Apply antiseptic ointment to dominant gloved hand and spread ointment in and around ulcer.	Antiseptic ointment causes minimal tissue irritation. All surfaces of wound must be covered to effectively control bacterial growth.
(4) Apply sterile gauze pad over ulcer and tape securely in place.	Protects ulcer and prevents removal of ointment during turning or repositioning.
c. Oxidizing agents:	
(1) Spread zinc oxide paste over skin surface around ulcer.	Oxidizing agents can be caustic to healthy tissues.
(2) Apply single layer of gauze dressing moistened in oxidizing solution over ulcer. (Do not apply full-strength peroxide.)	Coats wound surface and retains exposure to tissue surface.
(3) Apply dry gauze dressing over ulcer.	Protects ulcer and prevents loosening or pulling away of moist dressing.
d. Dextranomer beads:	
(1) Hold container of beads approximately 2.5 cm (1 in) above site and lightly sprinkle 5 mm diameter layer over wound.	Absorbs wound exudate.
(2) Apply gauze dressing over ulcer.	Holds beads in place and protects wound.
e. Hydrocolloid beads/paste:	
(1) Fill wound to approximately half of total depth with hydrocolloid beads or paste.	Assists in absorbing wound drainage. Highly draining wounds are best treated with hydrocolloid beads or granules.
(2) Cover with hydrocolloid dressing; extend dressing 1-1½ in beyond edges of wound.	Dressing maintains wound humidity. May be left in place up to 7 days.

CONTINUED

STEPS	RATIONALE
f. Hydrogel agents:	
(1) Cover surface of ulcer with hydrogel using sterile applicator or gloved hand.	Provides maintenance of wound humidity while absorbing excess drainage. May be used as carrier for topical agents.
(2) Apply dry, fluffy gauze over gel to completely cover ulcer.	Holds hydrogel against wound surface. Used as absorbent.
13. Reposition client comfortably off ulcer.	Avoids accidental removal of dressings. Pressure on existing ulcers must be avoided.
14. Remove gloves and dispose of soiled supplies. Wash hands.	Prevents transmission of microorganisms.
15. Report worsening in ulcer's appearance to nurse in charge or physician.	Worsening of condition may indicate need for additional therapy.
16. Record appearance of ulcer in nurses' notes. Describe type of topical agent used, dressing applied, and response.	Documents status of ulcer and specific treatment. Response documents evaluation of treatment.

TABLE 44-4 Topical Cleansing Agents

Name	Type	Comments
Acetic acid	Antimicrobial	Agent is effective against *Pseudomonas aeruginosa*. Use of agent is discontinued when infected organisms are gone.
Biolex	Detergent	Agent is nonionic surfactant for wound cleansing.
Cara-Klenz	Detergent	Agent is wound cleanser.
Hydrogen peroxide	Oxidizing agent	Agent facilitates removal of necrotic debris and crusting. Agent will oxidize healthy tissue. It is *not* used in clean, healing ulcers. Use is discouraged in deep ulcers because gas emboli may result.
Povidone iodine	Antimicrobial	Agent can be irritating to intact skin. If used undiluted, agent may cause toxicity to granulating tissues.
Sodium hypochlorite (Dakin's)	Antimicrobial	Agent is effective for odor control. Nurse should protect intact skin with zinc oxide. Nurse should discontinue use when necrotic tissue is gone.

An ulcer that has necrotic tissue or eschar or shows signs of sloughing must be debrided. **Eschar** is the scab or dry crust that results from excoriation of the skin. **Sloughing** is the shedding of dead tissue as the result of skin ulceration. **Debridement** is the removal of necrotic tissue so that healthy tissue can regenerate.

For reddened areas or areas of broken skin integrity, skin care products that lubricate and protect, stimulate circulation, and promote wound healing are recommended. When the ulcer is pink with granulation tissue throughout, a dressing is indicated to promote healing. A clean, moist environment promotes migration of epithelial cells across the ulcer surface (Fowler, 1982).

NUTRITIONAL STATUS. Maintaining adequate protein intake and hemoglobin levels are important in treatment of pressure ulcers.

Protein Status. Clients with a potential for or decreased serum albumin levels or poor protein intake need a nutritional evaluation to ensure proper caloric intake (Maklebust, 1991a). A client can lose as much as 50 g of protein per day from an open, weeping

TABLE 44-5 Dressing by Ulcer Stage	
Dressing	Comments*

STAGE I

Film dressing (Tegaderm, Bioclusive, Op-site, Uniflex)	Protects from shearing force May be left in place up to 7 days, if occlusive seal remains Will facilitate softening of eschar on deeper ulcers Traps serous exudate and provides moist wound environment
Hydrocolloid dressing (Duoderm, Comfeel, IntraSite)	Is absorbent May be left in place up to 7 days, if occlusive seal remains (Nurse is unable to assess wound with dressing in place.) Reacts with wound fluid to create a soft gel that promotes granulation and epithelialization

STAGE II

Hydrocolloid dressing	See stage I
Composite dressing (Viasorb, film dressing over Telfa)	Provides absorbent, nonadherent layer over wound with occlusive cover
Hydrogel dressing (Vigilon, Geliperm, J&J Gel)	Is absorbent for draining ulcers Usually requires gauze dressing cover
Absorptive dressing (Exu-dry, Bard absorption dressing, Sorbsan)	Is absorbent and nonadherent Protects from shearing force May be used with topical agents Is not occlusive dressing Absorbs exudate and debris while maintaining moist environment*

STAGE III

Polyurethane foam (Lyofoam, Allevyn)	Absorbs exudate Maintains moist wound environment*
Hydrocolloid dressing (see stage I)	Increases absorbency and wear time when hydrocolloid granules or paste is used Can cause damage because of frequent removal (every day or more often) (Recommend other dressing.)
Hydrogel dressing (see stage II)	May be used as carrier for topical agents, including topically applied growth factors
Absorptive dressing	See stage II

STAGE IV

Hydrocolloid dressing (see stages I to III)	May be contraindicated because of location of ulcer, exposed bone, and amount of drainage
Hydrogel dressing	See stages II to III
Gauze dressing	*Kerlix type:* Is absorbent but not occlusive Generally requires dressing changes every 8 to 12 hr *Dry gauze:* Removes drainage away from wound surface† *Moist gauze:* Maintains moist wound environment while removing drainage away from surface† *Moist-to-dry:* Debrides necrotic and healthy tissue nonselectively

*As with *all* occlusive dressing, wounds should *not* be clinically infected.
†Data from Maklebust J: *RN* 41(12):56, 1991.

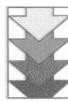

Sample Evaluation of Interventions for Impaired Skin Integrity

Goals	Evaluation Measures	Expected Outcomes
Injury to skin and underlying tissue resulting from pressure on bony prominences will be prevented.	Observe skin over bony prominences.	Skin will remain intact (6/1). Normal reactive hyperemia will occur (6/1). Blanching will occur (6/1).
	Palpate skin and underlying tissue over bony prominence.	
Injury to skin and underlying tissue resulting from pressure on bony prominences will be reduced by 6/20.	Measure perimeter and diameter of wound.	Wound size will decrease (6/10).
	Observe drainage.	There will be decrease in wound drainage (6/20).
	Observe nonaffected areas.	Skin will remain intact in unaffected areas (6/1).
		Normal reactive hyperemia will occur in unaffected areas (6/1).
	Observe and time reactive hyperemic response in affected area.	There will be decreased hyperemia in affected areas (6/15).

pressure ulcer. This is a sizable amount of the daily recommended requirement of 60 g for women and 70 g for men (Kavchak-Keyes, 1977).

Increased protein intake, 2 to 4 times above the daily recommended requirement, helps rebuild epidermal tissue. Increased caloric intake, at least 1½ times the recommended amount, helps replace subcutaneous tissue. Increased intake of vitamin C promotes protein synthesis and tissue repair (Shekleton, Litwack, 1991; Kavchak-Keyes, 1977).

Hemoglobin. A low hemoglobin level decreases delivery of oxygen to the tissues and leads to further ischemia. When possible, hemoglobin should be maintained at 12 g/100 ml.

Evaluation

Because each client has different risk factors for impaired skin integrity, nursing interventions must be individualized. Clients with minimal mobility impairments or relatively stable health status may need only a few measures. Nursing interventions for reducing and treating pressure ulcers are evaluated by determining the client's response to nursing therapies and by determining whether each goal was achieved (see evaluation box).

To evaluate outcomes and responses to care, the nurse measures the effectiveness of interventions. The optimal outcomes are to prevent injury to the skin and tissues, reduce injury to the skin and underlying tissues, and restore skin integrity.

The nurse also evaluates specific interventions designed to promote skin integrity and to teach the client and family to reduce future threats to skin integrity. Using the nursing process, the nurse collects data related to the client's skin integrity, exposure to risks, and physical condition. Nursing interventions are developed to promote skin integrity in the hospital and home or extended care facility after discharge. The nurse also evaluates the client's and family's need for additional support services (for example, home health care, physical therapy, and counseling) and initiates the referral process.

 ## SUMMARY

Pressure ulcers adversely affect the client in all dimensions. Although in some cases immobilization is necessary to promote wound healing, proper skeletal alignment, or rest after an illness, it involves risks. Nursing care prevents the adverse effects of reduced mobility on skin integrity. Using the nursing process, the nurse assesses the risk for pressure ulcers, diagnoses actual or potential problems related to impaired skin integrity, and plans and delivers nursing care to meet the client's needs. Because of the cost, increased nursing time, and prolonged hospital stay to treat pressure ulcers, nursing care aims first to prevent pressure ulcers and then to minimize the effects of pressure ulcers after they develop.

CHAPTER 44 REVIEW

Key Concepts

- Pressure ulcers remain a potential problem in acute and chronic care settings.
- Pressure ulcers increase length of stay in hospitals and extended care settings, as well as the overall cost of nursing care needed to manage the wound.
- The Agency for Health and Policy Research developed guidelines for future research directions and for the prevention and treatment of pressure ulcers.
- Prediction for development of pressure ulcers must focus on clients having the greatest risk for developing impaired skin integrity.
- Alterations in mobility, sensory perception, level of consciousness, and nutrition; the use of casts; and the presence of severe infection or other debilitating diseases increase the risk for pressure ulcer development.
- External pressure, shearing force, moisture, impaired peripheral circulation, edema, and obesity are also contributing factors to the development of pressure ulcers.
- When the external pressure against the skin is greater than the pressure in the capillary bed, blood flow decreases to the adjacent tissues.
- Decreased circulation to the tissues results in tissue hypoxia; if untreated, tissue necrosis results.
- There are four stages of pressure ulcer development.
- Meticulous assessment of the skin and underlying tissue and identification of risk factors are important in decreasing the opportunity for pressure ulcer development.
- In addition to assessing the reactive hyperemia, the nurse must also palpate adjacent tissue for signs of induration.
- Preventive skin care is aimed at controlling external pressure on bony prominences and keeping the skin clean, well lubricated and hydrated, and free of excess moisture.
- Plastic-lined pads protect the bed, not the client's skin, because they do not remove moisture away from the client's skin.
- Proper positioning should reduce the effects of pressure and guard against the shearing force.
- Therapeutic beds and mattresses reduce the effects of pressure; however, selection is based on assessment data to identify the best bed for individual needs.
- Cleansing and topical agents used to treat pressure ulcers vary according to the stage of the pressure ulcer. Assessment of the ulcer enables the nurse to select proper skin care agents.
- Nutritional interventions are directed at improving wound healing through increasing protein and hemoglobin levels.
- The risk of impaired skin integrity related to immobilization depends on the extent and duration of immobilization.

Key Terms

Abnormal reactive hyperemia, p. 1525

Anemia, p. 1527

Blanching, p. 1528

Cachexia, p. 1528

Debridement, p. 1527

Edema, p. 1527

Eschar, p. 1547

Induration, p. 1525

Normal reactive hyperemia, p. 1525

Pressure ulcer, p. 1524

Shearing force, p. 1527

Sloughing, p. 1545

Tissue ischemia, p. 1525

Critical Thinking Exercises

1. You are caring for a client with a spinal cord injury. What are your priorities for reducing the risk for pressure ulcers?

2. Your client's mobility is severely restricted, and he is receiving a medication that causes peripheral vasoconstriction. What interventions are essential in reducing pressure ulcer formation?

3. After changing a client's position, you observe redness over the bony prominences. What type of assessment must you perform to obtain correct information regarding pressure ulcer risk?

4. You have just admitted a client from a nursing home to your division. On initial assessment, you assess a stage III pressure ulcer. How do you determine the type of care and dressing to use with this particular pressure ulcer?

5. You are assigned to care for an older adult with two stage III pressure ulcers. One of your interventions is to place this client on a therapeutic bed. What information do you need to obtain to order the proper therapeutic bed?

REFERENCES

Barnes SH: Patient/family education for the patient with a pressure necrosis, *Nurs Clin North Am* 22:463, 1987.

Bennett L, Lee BY: Vertical shear existence in animal pressure threshold experiments, *Decubitus* 1(1):18, 1988.

Berecek KH: Etiology of decubitus ulcers, *Nurs Clin North Am* 10:157, 1975.

Bergstrom N, Demuth PJ, Braden, B: A clinical trial of the Braden Scale for predicting pressure sore risk, *Nurs Clin North Am* 22(2):417, 1987.

Bergstrom N et al: The Braden Scale for predicting pressure sore risk, *Nur Res* 36:205, 1987.

Bryant RA et al: Pressure ulcer. In Bryant RA, editor: *Acute and chronic wounds: nursing management*, St Louis, 1992, Mosby–Year Book.

Centers for Disease Control: Update: universal precautions for prevention of transmission of human immunodeficiency virus, hepatitis B virus, and other blood-borne pathogens in health care settings, *MMWR* 37:377, 1988.

Cooper DM: Wound assessment and evaluation of healing. In Bryant RA, editor: *Acute and chronic wounds: nursing management,* St Louis, 1992, Mosby–Year Book.

Fowler E: Pressure sores: a deadly nuisance, *J Gerontol Nurs* 12:6809, 1982.

Gosnell DJ: An assessment tool to identify pressure sores, *Nurs Res* 22(1):55 1973.

Gosnell DJ: Assessment and evaluation of pressure sores, *Nurs Clin North Am* 22(2):399, 1987.

Green E, Katz J: Practice guidelines for management of pressure ulcers, *Decubitus* 4(1):36, 1991.

Gröer MW, Shekleton ME: *Basic pathophysiology: a conceptual approach*, ed 3, St Louis, 1989, Mosby–Year Book.

Guttman L: The problem of treatment of pressure sores in patients with spinal paraplegia, *Br J Plast Surg* 8:196, 1955.

Hanan K, Scheele L: Albumin vs. weight as a predictor of nutritional status and pressure ulcer development, *Ostomy/Wound Manage* 33:22-27, 1991.

Hastings KE: Legal aspects of the AHCPR pressure ulcer guidelines, *Decubitus* 4(2):36, 1991.

Hoff J: Effecting a change in nursing practice: pressure ulcer prevention, *J Nurs Qual Assur* 3(4):56, 1989.

Kane RL, Ouslander JG, Abrass IB: *Essentials of clinical geriatrics*, ed 2, New York, 1989, McGraw-Hill.

Kavchak-Keyes MA: Four proven steps tor preventing decubitus ulcers, *Nurs 77* 7:58, 1977.

Kim MJ, McFarland GK, McLane AM: *Pocket guide to nursing diagnoses,* ed 4, St Louis, 1991, Mosby–Year Book.

Knight AL: Medical management of pressure sores, *J Fam Prac* 27(1):95, 1988.

Lucas MD: Research implications of the pressure ulcer guideline, *Decubitus* 4(2):52, 1991.

Maklebust J: Pressure ulcers: etiology and intervention, *Nurs Clin North Am* 22(2):359, 1987.

Maklebust J: Impact of AHCPR pressure ulcer guidelines on nursing practice, *Decubitus* 4(2):46, 1991a.

Maklebust J: Pressure ulcer update, *RN* 41(12):56, 1991b.

Meehan M: Multi-site pressure ulcer prevalence survey, *Decubitus* 3(4):14, 1990.

National Pressure Ulcer Advisory Panel (NPUAP): Pressure ulcers incidence, economics, risk assessment, Consensus Development Conference Statement, *Decubitus* 2(2):24, 1989.

Natlow AB: Nutrition in prevention and treatment of decubitus ulcers, *Top Clin Nurs* 5(2):39, 1983.

Norton D, McLaren R, Exton-Smith AN: An investigation of geriatric nursing problems in a hospital, London, 1962, National Corporation for the Care of Old People.

Pajk M et al: Investigating the problem of pressure sores, *J Gerontol Nurs* 12(7):11, 1986.

Pinchcofsky-Devin GD, Kaminski MV: Correlation of pressure sores and nutritional status, *J Am Geriatr Soc* 34:435, 1989.

Pires M, Muller A: Detection and management of early tissue pressure indicators: a pictorial essay, *Progressions* 3(3):3, 1991.

Reuler JB, Cooney TG: The pressure sore: pathophysiology and principles of management, *Ann Int Med* 94(5):661, 1981.

Shea JD: Pressure sores: classification and management, *Clin Orthop* 112:89, 1975.

Shekleton ME, Litwack K: *Critical care nursing of the surgical patient,* Philadelphia, 1991, Saunders.

Sklar CG: Pressure ulcer management in the neurologically impaired patient, *J Neurosurg Nurs* 17(1):30, 1985.

Steinberg J: Prevalence of decubitus ulcers: issues of concern, *Decubitus* 2(2):50, 1990.

Stotts NA: Predicting pressure ulcer development in surgical patients, *Heart Lung* 17(6):641, 1988.

United States Department of Health and Human Services: *Pressure ulcers in adults: prediction and prevention*, Pub No 92-0047, 92-0050, Rockville, Md, 1992, Public Health Service, Agency for Health Care Policy and Research.

ADDITIONAL READINGS

Barnes S, Rutland BS: Air-fluidized therapy as a cost-effective treatment for a "worst case" pressure necrosis, *J Enterostom Ther* 13(1):27, 1986.

Beckett WS et al: Effect of prolonged bedrest on lung volume in normal individuals, *J Appl Physiol* 61(3):919, 1986.

Booth FW: Effect of limb immobilization on skeletal muscle, *J Appl Physiol* 52:1113, 1982.

Byrne N, Feld M: Overcoming the red menace: preventing and treating decubitus ulcers, *Nurs 84* 14:55, 1984.

Cassell BL: Treating pressure sores stage by stage, *RN* 36:41, 1986.

David JA: Pressure sore treatment: a literature review, *Int J Nurs Stud* 19:183, 1982.

DiMascio S: Debrisan for decubitus ulcers, *Am J Nurs* 79:684, 1979.

Ek A, Boman G: A descriptive study of pressure sores: the prevalence of pressure sore and the characteristics of patient, *J Adv Nurs* 7:51, 1982.

Feustel DE: Pressure sore prevention: age, there is the rub, *Nurs 82* 12:78, 1982.

Jones PL, Millman A: A three-part system to combat pressure sores, *Geriatr Nurs* 7(2):78, 1986.

Kosiak M: Etiology of decubitus ulcers, *Arch Phys Med Rehabil* 42:19, 1961.

Linden O et al: Pressure distribution on the surface of the human body, *Arch Phys Med Rehabil* 46:378, 1965.

McCance KL, Huether SE: *Pathophysiology: the biologic basis for disease in adults and children,* St Louis, 1990, Mosby–Year Book.

Norton D, McLaren R, Exon-Smith A: Pressure sores. In Horsley JA, editor: *Preventing decubitus ulcers: CURN project,* New York, 1981, Grune & Stratton.

Rubin M: How bedrest changes perception, *Am J Nurs* 88:55, 1988.

Rubin M: The physiology of bedrest, *Am J Nurs* 88:50, 1988.

Shannon ML: Five famous fallacies about pressure sores, *Nurs 84* 13:34, 1984.

Steffel PE et al: Reducing devices for pressure sores with respect to nursing care procedures, *Nurs Res* 29:228, 1980.

Thomas C: Specialty beds: decision-making made easy, *Ostomy/ Wound Manage* 23:51, 1989.

Tompkins ES: Effect of restricted mobility and dominance on perceived duration, *Nurs Res* 29:333, 1980.

Tooman T, Patterson J: Decubitus ulcer warfare: product versus process, *Geriatric Nurs* 5:166, 1984.

Trelease CC: Developing standards for wound care, *Ostomy/ Wound Manage* 20:46, 1988.

Willey T: High tech beds and mattress overlays: a decision guide, *Am J Nurs* 89:1142, 1989

CHAPTER 45

Sensory Alterations

OBJECTIVES

Mastery of content in this chapter will enable the student to:
- Define the key terms listed.
- Differentiate among the processes of reception, perception, and reaction to sensory stimuli.
- Discuss common causes and effects of sensory alterations.
- Discuss common sensory changes that normally occur with aging.
- Identify factors to assess in determining sensory status.
- Describe behaviors indicating sensory alterations.
- Identify nursing diagnoses relevant to clients with sensory alterations.
- Develop a plan of care for clients with visual, auditory, tactile, speech, and olfactory deficits.
- Describe how a client's sensory alteration influences the nursing care approaches selected to improve sensory function.
- List interventions for preventing sensory deprivation and controlling sensory overload.
- Describe conditions in the health care agency or client's home that can be adjusted to promote meaningful sensory stimulation.
- Discuss ways to maintain a safe environment for clients with sensory deficits.

CHAPTER OUTLINE

Normal Sensation

Types of Sensory Alterations
Sensory deficits
Sensory deprivation
Sensory overload

Nursing Process and Sensory Alterations
Assessment
Nursing diagnosis
Planning
Implementation
Evaluation

art of the uniqueness of human beings is the ability to sense a variety of stimuli within the environment, perceive and organize those stimuli, and respond appropriately. Stimulation comes from many sources in and outside the body, particularly through the senses of sight (visual), hearing (**auditory**), touch (**tactile**), smell (**olfactory**), and taste (**gustatory**). The body also has a **kinesthetic** sense that enables a person to be aware of the position and movement of body parts without seeing them. **Stereognosis** is a sense that allows a person to recognize an object's size, shape, and texture. The ability to speak is not considered a sense, but it is similar in that the client may lose the ability to interact meaningfully with other human beings. Meaningful stimuli allow a person to learn about the environment and are necessary for healthy functioning and the normal development of the sensory organs. When sensory function is altered, the client's ability to relate to and function within the environment changes drastically.

Many clients enter the health care system with preexisting sensory alterations, or they may develop sensory alterations as a result of surgical intervention (for example, a cataract extraction). Clients who have partial or complete loss of a major sensory modality need to find alternative ways to function safely within the environment. If sensory alterations occur early in life, clients often have developmental and socialization problems because of the difficulty in responding to people and the environment. Clients may also enter health care settings with normal sensory function. However, a health care setting is often a place of unfamiliar sights, sounds, and smells and minimal contact with family and friends. If clients feel depersonalized and are unable to receive meaningful stimuli, serious sensory alterations can develop.

The nurse must understand and help meet the needs of clients with sensory alterations as well as recognize clients most at risk for developing sensory problems. The nurse helps clients who have sensory alterations learn to interact and react safely and effectively in the environment.

NORMAL SENSATION

Normally, the nervous system continually receives thousands of bits of information from sensory nerve organs, relays the information through appropriate channels, and integrates the information into a meaningful response. Sensory stimuli reach the sensory organs and can elicit an immediate reaction or present information to the brain to be stored for future use. The nervous system must be intact for sensory stimuli to reach appropriate brain centers and for the individual to perceive the sensation. After interpreting the significance of a sensation, the person can then react to the stimulus.

Reception, perception, and reaction are the three components of any sensory experience (see Chapter 37). Reception begins with stimulation of a nerve cell called a *receptor*, which is usually designed for only one type of stimulus, such as light or sound. Nerve impulses then travel along pathways from the receptor to the spinal cord or directly to the brain. For example, the retina of the eye receives light, with impulses traveling along the optic nerve to the occipital lobe of the brain.

Only pain receptors receive several forms of stimuli, such as pressure, chemicals, and heat. The movement of a body part stimulates **proprioceptors** to send impulses along peripheral spinal nerves to the spinal cord. From the spinal cord a second set of nerve fibers conducts the sensation of position, travels up the cord, crosses over at the medulla, and travels to the thalamus. At the thalamus, impulses synapse with a third pathway to eventually be sent to the cerebral cortex. Sensory nerve pathways usually cross over to send stimuli to opposite sides of the brain. For example, if a person touches an object with the right hand, the left side of the brain receives the stimulus.

The actual perception or awareness of unique sensations depends on the receiving region of the cerebral cortex, where specialized brain cells interpret the quality and nature of the sensory stimuli. A person's level of consciousness influences how well stimuli are perceived and interpreted. Any factors lowering consciousness impair sensory perception. Perception includes an integration and interpretation of the stimuli based on the person's experiences. If sensation is incomplete or if past experience is inadequate for understanding the stimuli, the person may react inappropriately.

It is impossible to react to each of the multiple stimuli constantly entering the nervous system. The brain is normally capable of discarding and storing sensory information to prevent sensory bombardment. A person will usually react to stimuli that are most meaningful or significant at the time. After continued reception of the same stimulus, however, a person stops responding and the sensory experience goes unnoticed. For example, a person reading a good book is not aware of the pressure of resting the body against the back of a chair. This adaptability phenomenon occurs with most sensory stimuli except for those of pain.

The balance between sensory stimuli entering the brain and those actually reaching the conscious awareness maintains a person's well-being. If an individual attempts to react to every stimulus within the environment or if a variety and quality of stimuli are lacking, sensory alterations will occur.

 ## TYPES OF SENSORY ALTERATIONS

Many factors alter the capacity to receive or perceive sensations (see box). The types of sensory alterations commonly seen by the nurse are sensory deficits, sensory deprivation, and sensory overload. When a client suffers from more than one sensory alteration, the ability to function and relate effectively within the environment is seriously impaired.

Sensory Deficits

A defect in the normal function of sensory reception and perception is a **sensory deficit**. A client may not be able to receive certain stimuli (for example, the client may be blind or deaf), or stimuli become distorted (for example, the client may have cataracts

---

Factors that Influence Sensory Function

AGE

- Infants are unable to discriminate sensory stimuli. Nerve pathways are immature.
- Visual changes during adulthood include presbyopia (inability to focus on near objects) and the need for glasses for reading (usually occurring from ages 40 to 50).
- Hearing changes, which begin at age 30, include decreased hearing acuity, speech intelligibility, pitch discrimination, and hearing threshold. Tinnitus often accompanies a hearing loss as a side effect of drugs. Older adults hear low-pitched sounds the best but have difficulty hearing conversation over background noise.
- Older adults have reduced visual fields, increased glare sensitivity, impaired night vision, reduced accommodation and depth perception, and reduced color discrimination.
- Older adults have difficulty discriminating the consonants (*f, s, th, ch*). Speech sounds are garbled, and there is a delayed reception and reaction to speech.
- Gustatory and olfactory changes include a decrease in the number of taste buds in later years and reduction of olfactory nerve fibers by age 50. Reduced taste discrimination and sensitivity to odors are common.
- Proprioceptive changes after age 60 include increased difficulty with balance, spatial orientation, and coordination.
- Older adults will experience tactile changes, including declining sensitivity to pain, pressure, and temperature.

MEDICATIONS

- Some antibiotics (e.g., streptomycin, gentamicin, aspirin) are ototoxic and can permanently damage the auditory nerve; chloramphenicol can irritate the optic nerve. Narcotic analgesics, sedatives, and antidepressant medications can alter the perception of stimuli.

ENVIRONMENT

- Excessive environmental stimuli (for example, equipment noise and staff conversation in an intensive care unit) can result in sensory overload, marked by confusion, disorientation, and the inability to make decisions. Restricted environmental stimulation (e.g., with isolation) can lead to sensory deprivation. Poor quality of environment (e.g., reduced lighting, narrow walkways, background noise) can worsen sensory impairment.

COMFORT LEVEL

- Pain and fatigue alter the way a person perceives and reacts to stimuli.

PREEXISTING ILLNESSES

- Peripheral vascular disease can cause reduced sensation in the extremities and impaired cognition. Chronic diabetes can lead to reduced vision, blindness, or peripheral neuropathy. Strokes often produce loss of speech. Some neurological disorders impair motor function and sensory reception.

SMOKING

- Chronic tobacco use can atrophy the taste buds, lessening the perception of flavors.

NOISE LEVELS

- Constant exposure to high noise levels (e.g., on a construction job site) can cause hearing loss.

ENDOTRACHEAL INTUBATION

- Temporary loss of speech results from insertion of an endotracheal tube through the mouth or nose into the trachea.

or be confused). A sudden sensory loss can cause fear, anger, and feelings of helplessness in an individual. Initially, a person may withdraw by avoiding communication or socialization with others in an attempt to cope with the sensory loss. It becomes difficult for the person to interact safely with the environment until new skills relying on existing functions are learned. When a deficit develops gradually or when considerable time has passed since the onset of an acute sensory loss, the person learns to rely on unaffected senses. Some senses may even become more acute to compensate for an alteration. For example, a client who is blind often develops an acute sense of hearing.

Clients with sensory deficits may change behaviors in adaptive or maladaptive ways. For example, one client with a hearing impairment may turn the unaffected ear toward a speaker to hear better, whereas another client may shun other people to avoid the embarrassment of not being able to understand their speech.

Sensory Deprivation

Sensory stimulation must be of sufficient quality and quantity to maintain a person's awareness. When a person experiences an inadequate quality or quantity of stimulation such as monotonous or meaningless stimuli, **sensory deprivation** occurs. Three types of sensory deprivation are reduced sensory input (sensory deficit from visual or hearing loss), elimination of order or meaning from input (for example,

clients exposed to strange environments), and restriction of the environment (for example, bed rest) that produces monotony and boredom (Ebersole, Hess, 1990).

There are many effects of sensory deprivation (see box). The symptoms can easily cause nurses and physicians to believe a client is psychologically ill and confused, is suffering from severe electrolyte imbalance, or is under the influence of psychotropic drugs. Therefore the nurse must always be aware of the client's existing sensory function and the quality of stimuli within the environment.

Sensory Overload

When a person receives multiple sensory stimuli and cannot perceptually disregard or selectively ignore some stimuli, **sensory overload** occurs. Excessive sensory stimulation prevents the brain from appropriately responding to or ignoring certain stimuli. Because of the multitude of stimuli leading to overload, the person no longer perceives the environment in a way that makes sense. Overload prevents meaningful response by the brain; the person's thoughts race, attention moves in many directions, and restlessness occurs. As a result, overload causes a state similar to that produced by sensory deprivation.

The acutely ill client may fall victim to sensory overload. The constant pain from the disease process, the nurse's frequent monitoring of vital signs, and the irritation from drainage tubes protruding from the body combine to cause overload. Even if the nurse offers a comforting word or provides a gentle back rub, clients may not benefit because their attention and energy are focused on more stressful stimuli.

Sensory overload differs from deprivation in that the level of stimuli that can cause the condition depends more on individual factors. The point at which stimuli become enough to tax endurance changes according to a person's level of fatigue, attitude, and emotional and physical well-being. Continued overload causes a person to eventually develop many of the same symptoms as are found with sensory deprivation.

 ## NURSING PROCESS AND SENSORY ALTERATIONS

 ### Assessment

When assessing clients with or at risk for sensory alterations, the nurse considers all the factors influ-

---

Effects of Sensory Deprivation

COGNITIVE

Reduced capacity to learn, inability to solve problems, poor task performance, disorientation, bizarre thinking

AFFECTIVE

Boredom, restlessness, increased anxiety, emotional lability, increased need for physical stimulation and socialization

PERCEPTUAL

Reduced attention span, disorganized visual and motor coordination, temporary loss of color perception, disorientation, confusion of sleeping and waking states

encing sensory function (see box on p. 1555), particularly age. The nurse collects a history that also assesses the degree to which a sensory deficit affects the client's lifestyle, psychosocial adjustment, and ability to relate to the environment. The assessment must also focus on the quality and quantity of environmental stimuli.

Persons at Risk

A nurse can quickly assess sensory function for clients most at risk. Older adults are a high risk group because of normal physiological changes involving sensory organs. Clients who are immobilized due to bed rest or physical encumbrances (for example, casts or traction) are unable to experience all the normal sensory sensations of free movement. Another group at risk includes clients isolated in a health care setting or at home. For example, the client placed in isolation because of an infection (see Chapter 18) is often restricted to a hospital room and is unable to enjoy normal interactions with visitors.

A client with a known sensory deficit is obviously at risk for sensory alterations. The length of time a client has had a sensory deficit may not affect the client's response to the environment. Magilvy (1985) found that women with a later onset of hearing loss considered themselves to have a lowered quality of life compared with women who experienced hearing loss at a younger age. Walsh and Eldredge (1989) warn that people who lose their hearing at an early age experience cumulative developmental effects and socialization problems that are compounded with aging.

A hospital environment is full of sensory stimuli, including conversation between staff members, the sounds of electrical monitors and equipment, bright lighting, and the odors of body fluids. A person accustomed to living alone and in a quiet environment may have difficulty coping with the hospital environment and therefore be at risk for sensory alterations.

Physical Assessment

To identify sensory deficits, the nurse should assess vision, hearing, olfaction, taste, and the ability to discriminate light touch, temperature, pain, and position (see Chapter 20). Table 45-1 on p. 1558 summarizes assessment techniques for identifying sensory deficits. The nurse also notes whether the client uses sensory aids (for example, glasses or hearing aids) and whether they are in proper working order. While performing care measures, the nurse may observe the client exhibiting behaviors indicating specific sensory alterations.

A neurological assessment of a client's level of consciousness, orientation, and cognitive thought processes reveals any symptoms of sensory deprivation or overload. This procedure also assesses a client's level of perception. The nurse should remember that factors other than sensory deprivation or overload may cause impaired perception (for example, medications, pain, and reduced oxygenation).

Ability to Perform Self-Care

Clients with sensory or perceptual alterations are often unable to perform activities of daily living. The nurse assesses clients' functional abilities in their home environments and health care settings, including feeding, dressing, grooming, and toileting activities. For example, the nurse assesses whether a client with altered vision can find items on a meal tray and can read directions on a prescription. The nurse also determines a visually impaired client's ability to perform daily routines such as reading bills and writing checks, differentiating money denominations, and driving a vehicle at night. If there is any alteration in the client's ability to perform self-care, the nurse may need to assess resources within the home before the client's discharge from the acute care setting.

Environment

The environment can either minimize or heighten sensory alterations. In some cases the environment is the cause of the problem. The nurse assesses the quality and quantity of stimuli within the health care environment and the home environment.

HAZARDS. A client with sensory alterations may be at risk for injury if the environment is unsafe. Cluttered furniture, dimly lit corridors and stair steps, and torn carpets are dangers for clients with visual impairments (see Chapter 42). In addition, because an older adult client experiences more glare in light, shiny objects such as metal furniture, highly waxed floors, and bright direct lighting can pose problems. An additional problem faced by the visually impaired is the inability to read medication labels and syringe gauges. If a client has a hearing impairment, the nurse checks to see whether the sounds of a doorbell, telephone, smoke alarm, and alarm clock are easy to discriminate.

MEANINGFUL STIMULI. Meaningful stimuli reduce the incidence of sensory deprivation. The nurse observes the environment for stimuli such as pets, a record player or television, pictures of family members, and a calendar and clock. In a health care setting the nurse notes whether clients have roommates or visitors. The presence of others can offer positive stimulation. However, a roommate who constantly watches

TABLE 45-1 Assessment of Sensory Function

Assessment	Behavior Indicating Deficit (Children)	Behavior Indicating Deficit (Adult)
VISION		
Ask client to read newspaper, magazine, or lettering on menu. Measure visual acuity with Snellen chart (see Chapter 20). Assess visual fields and depth perception. Assess pupil size and accommodation to light. Ask client to identify colors on color chart or crayons.	Self-stimulation, including eye rubbing, body rocking, sniffing or smelling, arm twirling; hitching (using legs to propel while in sitting position) instead of crawling	Poor coordination, squinting, underreaching or overreaching for objects, persistent repositioning of objects, impaired night vision, accidental falls
HEARING		
Perform conventional assessment, including ticking watch, whisper, and tuning fork, (see Chapter 20). Perform audiometry. Observe client conversing with others. Compare client's ability to recognize consonants with ability to distinguish vowels. Assess client's perception of hearing ability and history of tinnitus. Inspect ear canal for hardened cerumen.	Frightened when unfamiliar people approach, no reflex or purposeful response to sounds, failure to be awakened by loud noise, slow or absent development of speech, greater response to movement than to sound, avoidance of social interaction with other children	Blank looks, decreased attention span, lack of reaction to loud noises, increased volume of speech, positioning of head toward sound, smiling and nodding of head in approval when someone speaks, use of other means of communication such as lip reading or writing, complaints of ringing in ears
TOUCH		
Assess client for sensitivity to light touch and temperature (see Chapter 20). Check client's ability to discriminate between sharp and full stimuli. Assess whether client can distinguish objects (coin or safety pin) in the hand with eyes closed. Ask whether client feels unusual sensations.	Inability to perform developmental tasks related to grasping objects or drawing, repeated injury from handling of harmful objects (e.g., hot stove, sharp knife)	Clumsiness, overreaction or underreaction to painful stimulus, failure to respond when touched, avoidance of touch, sensation of pins and needles, numbness
SMELL		
Have client close eyes and identify several nonirritating odors (e.g., coffee, vanilla).	Difficult to assess until child is 6 or 7 years old, difficulty discriminating noxious odors	Failure to react to noxious or strong odor, increased body odor, increased sensitivity to odors
TASTE		
Ask client to sample and distinguish different tastes (e.g., lemon, sugar, salt). (Have client drink sip or water and wait 1 min between each taste.) Ask client if recent weight change has occurred.	Inability to tell whether food is salty or sweet, possible ingestion of strange-tasting things	Change in appetite, excessive use of seasoning and sugar, complaints about taste of food, weight change
POSITION SENSE		
Perform conventional tests for balance and position sense (see Chapter 20).	Clumsiness, extraneous movement, excessive arm swinging in those with hyperactivity or learning difficulty	Poor balance and spatial orientation, shuffling gait, reduced response to brace self when falling, more precise and deliberate movements

television, persistently tries to talk, or continuously keeps lights on can contribute to sensory overload. A client can become disoriented in a barren environment that gives few signals for normal sensory perception. The presence or absence of meaningful stimuli influences alertness and the ability to participate in care. In a home or health care setting the nurse checks the environment for bright colors, comfortable furnishings, adequate lighting, good ventilation, and clean surroundings.

With infants and young children, the nurse assesses the toys available. The play area should have developmentally apropriate toys of different sizes, shapes, and colors and should be clean, pleasantly lit, and decorated attractively.

AMOUNT OF STIMULI. Excessive stimuli in an environment can cause sensory overload. In an acute care setting the nurse assesses the level of care required. The frequency of observations and procedures performed may be stressful. If the client is in pain, has many tubes and dressings, or is restricted by casts or traction, overstimulation can be a problem. If the client's room is near the nurses' station, an elevator, or the door leading to the stairs, the noise may be excessive.

Social Development and Support

The amount of contact with supportive family members and significant others can influence the degree of isolation the client feels. The nurse assesses whether a client lives alone and whether family and friends frequently visit. A pattern of social isolation can contribute to sensory changes. The ability to discuss fears or concerns with loved ones is an important coping mechanism for most people. The absence of meaningful conversation can cause a person to become sensorially deprived, and the nurse may not be alerted until behavioral changes occur.

Sensory losses can impair a person's socialization with others. For example, hearing-impaired children do not successfully initiate interactions with others and thus do not learn to relate with those in their environments. Another example is older adult clients who frequently are aware of developing sensory problems. When older adults suspect that sensory functions are deteriorating, they often avoid social interactions to avoid embarrassment.

When clients have socialization problems resulting from sensory deficits, it can become difficult for care givers to adequately plan care. In the case of the severely hearing impaired, nursing staff members may have difficulty planning routine care, providing self-care instructions, and involving the client directly in nursing therapies. The box cites characteristics com-

---

Personality Traits of Deaf Adults

- Withdraw from communication with adults who can hear.
- Are less flexible in their daily routines.
- Demonstrate a negative self-image.
- Possess a narrow range of interests.
- Show a lack of social judgment.
- Show more dependency than hearing adults.

---

monly found among the hearing impaired that can interfere with the way nursing care is delivered (Jackson, 1982; Levine, 1976; Walsh, Eldredge, 1989).

Communication Methods

Clients with existing sensory deficits often develop alternative ways of communicating. The nurse must understand the client's method of communication to interact with the client and to promote interaction with others. A deaf or hearing-impaired client may read lips, use sign language, listen with the help of a hearing aid, or read and write notes. Vision is constantly used in communication as an accompaniment to hearing.

Visually impaired clients are unable to observe facial expressions and other nonverbal behaviors that clarify the content of spoken communication. Instead, they rely on voice tones and inflections to detect the emotional tone of communication. Clients with visual deficits often learn to read Braille.

Clients with **aphasia** may be unable to produce or understand language. **Expressive aphasia,** a motor type of aphasia, is the inability to name common objects or to express simple ideas in words or writing. For example, a client may understand a question but be unable to express an answer. Sensory or receptive aphasia is an inability to understand written or spoken language. The client may be able to express words but is unable to understand inquiries or comments of others. Global aphasia is the inability to understand language or communicate orally.

The temporary or permanent loss of the ability to speak is extremely traumatic to an individual. The nurse quickly assesses a client's alternative communication method to minimize anxiety in the client. Clients who have undergone laryngectomies often write notes, use communication boards, speak with mechanical vibrators, or use esophageal speech. Clients with endotracheal or tracheostomy tubes have a temporary loss of speech. Most use a notepad to write their questions and requests. However, the client may become incapacitated and unable to write messages. The nurse needs to determine whether the client has developed a sign language or system of symbols to communicate needs.

To understand the nature of a communication problem, the nurse must know whether a client has trouble speaking, understanding, naming, reading, or writing. Depending on the nature of the communication problem, the nurse selects the best way to interact with the client.

Mental Status

Mental status assessment is an important component of any evaluation of sensory function (see box). Observation of the client during history taking, the physical examination, and care giving provides valuable data that can serve as the basis for evaluation of mental status.

Self-Perception of Sensory Loss

The nurse should understand the way sensory losses are perceived by clients. Many clients believe that the quality of their lives has been lowered be-

cause of sensory alterations. Of all the disadvantages of aging, sensory deficits are the most likely to cause social isolation (Bernardini, 1985). Simply observing a client interact with others may reveal the person's sense of confidence. The nurse may also ask clients questions such as, "Tell me how have you adjusted to your (hearing, visual, speech) loss?" or "What has changed because of your (hearing, visual, speech) loss?" The nurse then identifies individualized measures that help clients adjust and assesses family members' perceptions of the loss.

Nursing Diagnosis

After gathering data about the client's sensory status, the nurse organizes defining characteristics and

Examples of Nursing Diagnoses for Sensory Alterations

Assessment of Mental Status

PHYSICAL APPEARANCE AND BEHAVIOR

- Motor activity
- Posture
- Facial expression
- Hygiene

COGNITIVE ABILITY

- Level of consciousness
- Abstract reasoning
- Calculation
- Attention
- Judgment
- Ability to carry on conversation
- Ability to read, write, and copy figures
- Recent and remote memory

EMOTIONAL STABILITY

- Agitation, euphoria, irritability, hopelessness, or wide mood swings
- Auditory, visual, or tactile hallucinations
- Illusions
- Delusions

NANDA-APPROVED NURSING DIAGNOSES

Sensory/perceptual alterations: visual related to:
- Aging
- Temporary surgical eye patch

Sensory/perceptual alterations: auditory related to:
- Drug side effects
- Hospitalization in intensive care unit

Sensory/perceptual alterations: kinesthetic related to:
- Bed rest

Sensory/perceptual alterations: gustatory related to:
- Aging
- Side effects of chemotherapy

Bathing/hygiene, dressing/grooming, or *toileting self-care deficit* related to:
- Visual loss
- Reduced tactile sensation

High risk for injury related to:
- Decreased depth perception
- Reduced sense of smell

Impaired verbal communication related to:
- Endotracheal tube
- Motor aphasia

Impaired adjustment related to:
- Sensory overload
- Sensory deficit

Impaired physical mobility related to:
- Altered balance

Social isolation related to:
- Expressive aphasia
- Isolation for infection

Self-esteem disturbance related to:
- Hearing loss

decides on appropriate nursing diagnoses (see diagnostic process box). If a client has sensory alterations that can be treated independently by nursing therapies, the diagnosis is sensory/perceptual alteration. The client may also have health care problems created by a sensory alteration, such as high risk for injury. The nurse may also select nursing diagnoses by predicting the way sensory alterations will affect a client's ability to function (for example, self-care deficit).

The sample nursing diagnoses box lists examples of nursing diagnoses for clients with sensory alterations.

 ## Planning

The plan of care (see care plan) depends on the nurse's assessment of the client's perception and acceptance of the sensory alteration. It also depends on the extent to which the client has adjusted to sensory loss. The nurse should make every effort to provide care that will enable the client to adapt to the health care setting and to the home. The client must actively participate in selecting therapies for the plan of care. Clients who have sensory alterations at the time of entering a health care setting are usually most informed about how to adapt interventions to their lifestyles.

Some sensory alterations are short term, for example, a client suffering sensory/perceptual alterations as a result of sensory overload in an intensive care unit. Appropriate interventions are thus likely to be only temporary. Sensory alterations such as permanent visual loss require long-term goals of care. Sometimes it becomes necessary for the client to make major changes in the way self-care activities, communication, and socialization are performed.

When developing a plan of care, the nurse considers all resources available to clients. The family can play a key role in providing meaningful stimulation and learning ways to help the client adjust to any limitations. The nurse may also refer the client to other health care professionals. Early referrals to occupational or speech therapists, for example, can speed a client's recovery. There are also numerous community-based resources (such as the local chapter of the Society for the Blind and Visually Impaired and the National Federation of the Blind) and organizations whose volunteers assist the deaf. The nurse may be able to arrange a volunteer to visit a client or have printed materials made available that describe ways to cope with sensory problems.

The goals of care for a client with actual or potential sensory alterations may include the following:

1. Maintaining optimal functioning of existing senses
2. Controlling the environment to create meaningful sensory stimuli
3. Establishing a safe environment
4. Preventing additional sensory loss
5. Communicating effectively with existing sensory alterations
6. Understanding the nature and implications of sensory loss
7. Achieving self-care

The nurse establishes priorities among the goals of care. For example, a client who temporarily loses vi-

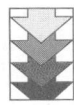 ## Sample Nursing Diagnostic Process for Sensory Alterations

Assessment Activities	Defining Characteristics	Nursing Diagnoses
Observe client converse with others.	Avoidance of conversation with others	*Sensory/perceptual alteration: auditory* related to physiological changes of aging
Ask client to repeat words whispered in each ear.	Inability to hear words, garbled sound	
Ask if client perceives change in hearing.	Inability to hear clearly in group with presence of background noise	
Review history: Note that client has been on bed rest in intensive care unit for 7 days.	Therapeutically restricted environment	*Sensory/perceptual alteration: sensory deprivation* related to bed rest
Assess client's level of orientation.	Confusion as to date and place	
Observe client's behavior.	Restlessness in bed, sudden frantic movement when nurse approaches bedside	

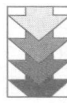

Sample Nursing Care Plan for Sensory/Perceptual Alterations

Nursing diagnosis: *Sensory/perceptual alterations: auditory* related to physiological changes of aging
Definition: Sensory/perceptual alterations is the state in which an individual experiences a change in the amount or patterning of incoming stimuli accompanied by a diminished, exaggerated, distorted, or impaired response to such stimuli (Kim, McFarland, McLane, 1991).

Goal	Expected Outcomes	Interventions	Rationale
Client will communicate successfully with care givers and family members on day of discharge.	Client will describe or demonstrate strategies to optimize ability to hear conversation 2 days before discharge. Client will use communication techniques to converse with family 1 day before discharge.	Instruct client to turn off radio or television or move away from noise source (e.g., fan or running machinery) when conversing with others. Instruct client to maintain eye contact with person speaking. Instruct client and family members to take time to communicate and to look at person and establish eye contact before speaking. Family should keep their mouths clearly visible to hearing impaired (e.g., do not turn head to side, chew gum, or place hands over face).	Presbycusis, a progressive sensorineural hearing loss common in older adults, causes reduction in speech discrimination and speech comprehension, which is complicated by background noise (Kee, 1990). With a hearing deficit, basic communication techniques foster comprehension.

sion following eye surgery will require more assistance in establishing a safe environment than receiving interventions that prevent additional sensory loss. Many clients receive treatment for sensory problems either on an outpatient basis or only after a short stay in a hospital. For this reason, the nurse must be sure to plan therapies that can continue in the home.

Implementation

Nursing interventions involve the client and family so that a safe, pleasant, and stimulating sensory environment can be maintained. The most effective interventions enable the client with sensory alterations to function safely with existing deficits. The client generally is able to continue a normal lifestyle. Nursing interventions are chosen depending on the nursing diagnosis identified and the related factors contributing to the client's problem.

Promoting Function of Existing Senses

The nurse's assessment reveals the functional level of a client's senses. Nursing measures are then implemented that enhance a client's remaining sensory function or maximize other senses. Sensory testing detects sensory problems early so that corrective devices can be made available.

VISION. The most common visual problem during childhood is a **refractive error** such as nearsightedness. Vision screening of school-age children and adolescents can detect visual impairment early. Parents may need encouragement to pursue eye testing by an ophthalmologist.

Because an adult develops visual changes with aging, the nurse uses several strategies to help clients adapt to these changes. A client who wears corrective contact lenses or eyeglasses should make sure they are kept clean, accessible, and functional. Regular ophthalmologic examinations ensure that a client wears the proper lenses. There are many ways the nurse can help the client to maintain existing visual function (see box). The client can be taught to strengthen visual stimuli, use other senses, use sharp visual contrasts, and minimize the effects from glare.

HEARING. Children with chronic middle ear infections—a common cause of impaired hearing—

Client Teaching for Visual Function

OBJECTIVES

- Client will demonstrate use of strategies that enhance visual function.
- Client will report improved vision when using strategies.

TEACHING STRATEGIES
Strengthening Visual Stimuli

- Keep eye glasses and contact lenses clean and functional.
- Use assistive devices (e.g., pocket magnifiers, near-vision microscopic glasses, and large-print wristwatch, telephone dialers, and books).
- Install two side mirrors on cars for enhancing visual field.
- Ask pharmacist to print directions on medication labels in large print.
- Be sure teaching pamphlets have the proper contrast of colors clients are able to see.

Using Other Senses

- Provide books on taped cassettes.
- Install textual cues on walkways or ramps to alert person to intersections.
- Pour salt and pepper into hand before adding to food.
- Fold money according to value and place in different wallet compartments.

Using Sharp Visual Contrasts

- Use warm colors to highlight visual targets. Orange, red, and yellow can be used on hand rails and light switches.
- Color-code the control dials of irons, stoves, dryers, washers, and thermostats. Mark a reference point on dials and on their desired settings. Use colored rims around dishes and cups to reduce spills.
- Have rooms decorated in a visual contrast (e.g., red and yellow, bright blue and light rose) to help distinguish objects.

Minimizing Glare

- Decrease light contrasts by using diffuse, soft lighting.
- Avoid waxed floors and exposure to bright sunlight.
- Install tinted glass windows with adjustable shades or sheer curtains in large windows.
- Shield eyes with sunglasses, visors, or hats with brims.
- Avoid driving at dusk or night when lights from cars are brightest.
- Use dull finish plastic and wood materials, satin finishes, and nongloss paper.

EVALUATION

- Observe client's environment at home.
- Reassess client's visual acuity while selected strategies are used.

---

should undergo auditory testing. Parents must be warned of the risks and should seek medical care when the child has symptoms of earache or respiratory infection. Children should also be immunized against childhood diseases (for example, measles, rubella, and mumps) that can cause hearing loss and should not be treated with **ototoxic** medications.

Older adults frequently experience hearing impairment as a result of impacted cerumen. With aging, cerumen thickens and builds up in the ear canal. Excessive cerumen occluding the ear canal can cause a **conductive hearing loss.** Irrigation of the canal with tepid water in a 60-ml syringe (see Chapter 34) will remove cerumen. Removal of cerumen can improve the client's hearing ability (Lewis-Cullinan, Janken, 1990) (see research highlight on p. 1564).

To maximize residual hearing function, the nurse suggests ways to modify the environment. Telephone rings can be amplified. Special handsets are available

if incoming voices cannot be heard. Important environmental sounds (for example, smoke alarms, doorbells, and alarm clocks) may best be heard if amplified or changed to a more low-pitched, buzzerlike sound. Older adults may not be able to hear with background noise. The nurse can suggest that clients turn off radios, televisions, and appliances during conversations. It is also helpful to have conversations in settings where floor coverings and drapes muffle extraneous background noises (Bernardini, 1985). If a hearing aid is worn, the client should make sure that it is properly cleaned and adjusted and that it contains functioning batteries. The client should wear it at all times. The nurse should also make sure the client knows how and when to change the batteries.

TASTE. The nurse can easily promote the sense of taste by using measures to enhance remaining taste

Research Highlight

The purpose of this experimental study was to estimate the prevalence of impacted cerumen in a population of hospitalized older adults and to evaluate the effect of cerumen removal in reversing hearing impairment. A random sample ($N = 226$) was selected of subjects aged 65 years or older admitted to nonintensive care units of a large teaching hospital. Subjects were placed in one of three study groups: subjects with impacted cerumen in one ear canal who received irrigation in the occluded ear, subjects with both ears occluded who had both ears irrigated, and the control group with unoccluded ear canals. During their hospital stay, subjects received a hearing test and had their ear canals examined for impacted cerumen. Ear canal irrigations were performed on subjects with one or both ears impacted. Repeat hearing tests were then performed on all subjects. Results showed impacted cerumen to be a common condition in hospitalized older adults. In addition, removal of impacted cerumen significantly improved the subjects' hearing ability. Improved hearing scores were obtained in 75% of the ears after impacted cerumen was removed.

Lewis-Cullinan C, Janken JK: Effect of cerumen removal on the hearing ability of geriatric patients, *J Adv Nurs* 15:594, 1990.

Meaningful Environmental Stimuli

VISUAL
- Open the drapes to the client's room so that outside sights can be seen.
- Raise the head of bed and draw back any dividing curtains or partitions so that the client can see a roommate or movement in the hallway.
- Provide attractive decorations on tables or cabinets, such as flowers, plants, a picture, or a greeting card.
- Encourage family to enrich the client's home environment with clean curtains, familiar objects and keepsakes, and perhaps a fresh coat of paint on bedroom walls.

AUDITORY
- Sit down and speak with the client. Listen to the client's thoughts and experiences. Make the conversation meaningful.
- Turn on a radio with the type of music the client enjoys. A favorite radio or television program can also be stimulating.
- Encourage visitors.

TASTE AND SMELL
- Provide attractive, taste-appealing meals. Be sure tableware and glasses are clean. Foods meant to be served warm should be warm, and cold foods should be cold.
- Provide a variety of textures, aromas, and flavors to enhance appetite.

TOUCH
- Therapeutic touch creates meaningful stimuli.

---

perception. Good oral hygiene keeps the taste buds well hydrated. Taste perception will be heightened if foods are well seasoned, differently textured, and eaten separately. The use of vinegar or lemon juice can add tartness to food. The nurse should always ask the client what foods are the most taste appealing. If taste perception is improved, food intake and appetite will also improve.

Stimulation of the sense of smell with aromas such as brewed coffee and baked bread can heighten taste sensation. The client should avoid blending or mixing foods because these actions make it difficult to identify tastes. Older persons should chew food thoroughly to allow more food to contact remaining taste buds.

TOUCH. Clients with reduced tactile sensation usually have the impairment over a limited portion of their bodies. The nurse can stimulate existing function by providing touch therapy. If the client is willing to be touched, hair brushing and combing, a back rub, and touching of the arms or shoulders are ways of increasing tactile contact. When sensation is reduced, a firm pressure may be necessary for the client to feel the nurse's hand. Turning and repositioning can also improve the quality of tactile sensation.

If a client is overly sensitive to tactile stimuli (hyperesthesia), the nurse must minimize irritating stimuli. Keeping bed linens loose to minimize direct contact with the client and protecting the skin from exposure to irritants are other helpful measures.

SMELL. Smell can be improved by strengthening pleasant olfactory stimulation. A client's environment can be made more pleasant with smells such as cologne, mild room deodorizers, fragrant flowers, and sachets. The nurse also encourages clients to sniff food before eating. When the nurse assists clients with eating or sets up a meal tray, naming the foods may help clients imagine the aromas. The client is again an important resource. Certain aromas may actually cause clients to lose their appetites.

Removal of unpleasant odors improves the quality of a person's environment. The nurse should keep a client's room clean, empty bedpans or urinals, and keep bathroom doors closed.

Maintaining Meaningful Stimulation

When a client's environment presents risks of understimulation or overstimulation of the senses, the nurse should provide meaningful stimuli or eliminate confusing or irritating stimuli. With sensory deprivation, the nurse should introduce meaningful stimuli for all senses based on client preferences (see box). The nurse does not force stimulation if the client is more concerned with basic functions such as comfort and nutrition.

A bedridden client has a limited view of the environment. Long intervals of staring at ceilings and walls can heighten sensory problems. Comfort measures such as frequent positioning, washing the face and hands, and providing back rubs can help to improve the quality of stimulation and lessen the chance of sensory deprivation. Planning time to talk with clients is also essential. The client who is well enough to read benefits from a variety of reading materials.

The nurse controls excessive stimuli for clients at risk for sensory overload. Clients need time for rest and freedom from stresses caused by frequent monitoring and repeated tests. The nurse may sit quietly with a client or involve the client in an undemanding repetitive activity such as combing hair or brushing teeth. A client experiencing stress in the home can find relief in simple activities such as meal planning and household chores.

Reorientation to the environment may be provided by wearing name tags on uniforms, addressing the client by name, and using conversational cues as to time or location. The tendency for clients to become confused can be reduced by offering short and simple repeated explanations and reassurance. Helping clients to become as mobile and independent as possible within prescribed limits also provides meaningful stimulation. The nurse encourages the family not to argue with or contradict the confused client but to calmly explain location, identity, and time of day.

The nurse can reduce sensory overload by organizing the care plan. Combining activities such as dressing changes, bathing, and vital sign measurement in one visit prevents the client from becoming overly fatigued. The client also needs scheduled time for rest and quiet. Planning for rest periods often requires cooperation from family and visitors. Coordination with laboratory and radiology departments reduces the amount of time needed for tests and examinations.

Anticipating client needs such as voiding helps reduce uncomfortable stimuli.

The nurse can also try to control extraneous noise in and around the client's room. It may be necessary to ask a roommate to lower the volume on a television or to move the client to a quieter room. Equipment noise should be kept to a minimum. Bedside equipment not in use, such as suction and oxygen equipment, should be turned off. The nurse also avoids abrupt loud noises such as clattering or rinsing bed pans. Nursing staff should also try to control laughter or conversation at the nurses' station. Nurses should allow clients to close room doors.

Providing a Safe Environment

Clients with existing sensory loss must be protected from injury, whereas clients at risk for sensory loss must learn to avoid injury. The nature of the actual or potential sensory loss determines the safety precautions taken.

VISUAL LOSS. The client with recent visual impairment often requires assistance with ambulation. The nurse should stand at the client's nondominant side approximately one step in front of the client (Fig. 45-1). The client can use the nondominant hand to grasp the nurse's arm and reach forward with the dominant hand to feel for any barriers and land-

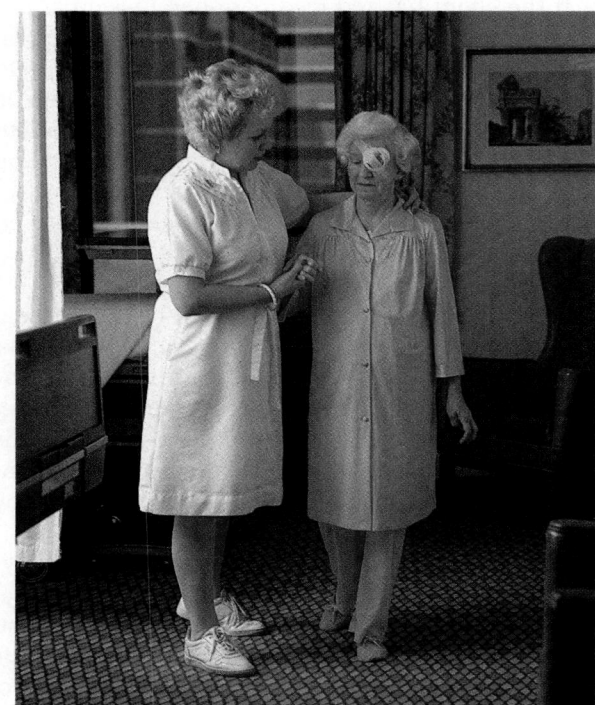

Fig. 45-1 A nurse assists in the ambulation of a client wearing an eye patch.

marks. The nurse should describe the course of movement and ensure that obstacles have been removed. A client with visual impairment should never be left standing alone in an unfamiliar area. For clients who undergo eye surgery, it is important to teach family members ambulation assist techniques.

A visually impaired client who spends considerable time in bed should have a call light nearby. Necessary objects should be placed in front of the client to prevent falls caused by reaching over the bedside. Side rails are also important in this regard. At night a nightlight with a red bulb can help to reduce falls. The red light reduces the time required for the eyes to adapt to the dark and allows the client to see well enough to function without keeping the regular bathroom light on (Matteson, McConnell, 1988).

The nurse removes potential hazards such as furniture that clutters the environment. Adequate lighting should be provided in work areas, corridors, and near steps. More illumination is needed in potentially hazardous areas such as stairs and exits. When possible, steps inside and outside the home should be replaced with ramps.

If a client is partially or totally blind, fire hazards should be removed from the home. Flammable items such as paper and cloth should be kept away from the stove. A client who smokes must learn to discard ashes frequently into an ashtray. Water placed in the bottom of an ashtray helps to ensure that cigarette butts are extinguished.

If the client has reduced peripheral vision and difficulty driving in darkness, the nurse should emphasize precautions such as looking to both sides before passing cars or turning a corner and driving only during the day. When a client's depth perception is poor, the edges of steps and driveway curbs should be painted a bright color (for example, orange) to prevent falls. Rugs should be a bright color to contrast with woodwork and walls.

HEARING LOSS. Nurses may rely on clients in health care settings to report unusual sounds, such as a suction apparatus running improperly or an intravenous pump alarm. However, the client with a hearing loss may not hear such sounds and thus requires more frequent visits by the nurse. The client can also benefit from learning to use vision to discover sources of danger.

In the home, light-signaling devices for burglar alarms, doorbells, alarm clocks, smoke detectors, and telephones are available with red or green flashing lights. Signaling devices allow the deaf person to feel greater independence. Family members or anyone who calls the client regularly should learn to let the phone ring for a longer period. A telecommunications device for the deaf (TDD) is a computer and printer that transfers written words over the telephone to the hearing impaired. Both a sender and receiver must have a TDD to complete a call (Walsh, Eldredge, 1989).

REDUCED OLFACTION. A reduced sensitivity to odors means the client may be unable to smell leaking gas, a smoldering cigarette or fire, and tainted food. The client should use smoke detectors and other alternative precautions such as checking ashtrays or placing cigarette butts in water. A client can learn to check dates on food packages and the color and texture of food. Pilot gas flames should be checked visually.

REDUCED TACTILE SENSATION. Clients with reduced tactile sensation risk injury when their conditions confine them to bed because they are unable to sense pressure on bony prominences or the need to change position. These clients rely on nurses for timely repositioning, moving tubes or devices the client may lie on, and turning to avoid skin breakdown.

When the ability to sense temperature variations is reduced, the nurse should use extra caution in applying heat and cold therapies (see Chapter 48) and preparing bath water. The nurse must frequently check the condition of the client's skin.

SPEECH ALTERATIONS. A client lacking the ability to speak cannot call out for assistance. Clients with aphasia, a laryngectomy, or an artificial airway (see Chapter 38) need alternative means of communication such as message boards and note pads. In the hospital a call light should always be near the client. For the client at home a small bell or alarm at the bedside is helpful.

Preventing Sensory Loss

Occupation or lifestyle may place a person at risk for sensory loss. Persons working around loud noises need to learn potential dangers to hearing function. Protective ear covers are essential if exposure to loud sound is continuous. Ringing of the ears is an early sign of hearing impairment.

Clients exposed to dangerous chemicals or small flying objects should wear eye goggles for protection. A chemical burn to the cornea or a penetrating eye injury can cause permanent blindness. Children should be discouraged from playing with any kind of sharp object because they can be accidentally blinded by a playmate. Care must also be taken to prevent children from placing sharp objects in their ears.

Promoting Communication

A sensory deficit can cause a person to feel isolated because of an inability to communicate with others. This problem can complicate a nurse's effectiveness in teaching clients information and skills. The nature of the sensory loss influences the methods and styles of communication that nurses can use. The methods described in the box can also be taught to family members and significant others.

The client with a hearing impairment may be able to speak normally. However, the deaf client's inability to hear self-spoken words may cause serious speech alterations. A child born deaf is not able to speak at all. Clients may use sign language or lip reading, write with a pad and pencil, rely on a hearing aid, or learn to use a computer for communication. Special communication boards contain common terms used in nursing care and help clients express their needs. If a client has a hearing aid, there are guidelines that can help to ensure the aid works properly (see box).

Depending on the type of aphasia, the inability to communicate can be frustrating and frightening. The nurse should initially establish very basic communication and recognize that aphasia does not indicate intellectual impairment or degeneration of personality.

Understanding Sensory Loss

Clients must understand all implications of sensory loss. The client with a hearing impairment must learn that excessive background noise interferes with the ability to hear conversation. Similarly, an older client with visual loss must know to install proper lighting in hazardous areas to reduce risk of injury. Clients can learn to adapt to sensory alterations so that living environments can be safe and appropriately stimulating. All family members should under-

---

Communication Methods

CLIENTS WITH APHASIA

- Listen to the client and wait for the client to communicate.
- Do not shout or speak loudly (hearing loss is not the problem).
- If the client has problems with comprehension, use simple, short questions and facial gestures to give additional clues.
- If the client has problems speaking, ask questions that require simple yes or no answers or blinking of the eyes. Offer pictures or a communication board so that the client can point.
- Give the client time to understand.
- Do not pressure or tire the client.

CLIENTS WITH AN ARTIFICIAL AIRWAY

- Use pictures, objects, or word cards so that the client can point.
- Offer a pad and pencil or magic slate for the client to write messages.
- Do not shout or speak loudly.
- Provide an artificial voice box (vibrator) for the client with a laryngectomy to use to speak words and phrases.

CLIENTS WITH HEARING IMPAIRMENT

- Get the client's attention. Do not startle the client when entering the room. Do not approach a client from behind. Be sure the client knows you wish to speak.
- Face the client. Be sure your face and lips are illuminated to promote lip reading.
- If the client wears glasses, be sure they are clean so that your gestures and face can be seen. If the client wears a hearing aid, make sure it is in place and working.
- Speak slowly and articulate clearly. Older adults may take longer to process verbal messages.* Use a normal tone of voice and inflections of speech. Refrain from speaking with something in your mouth.
- When you are not understood, rephrase rather than repeat the conversation.
- Use visible aids. Speak with your hands, your face, and your eyes.
- Do not shout. Loud sounds are usually higher pitched and may impede hearing by accentuating vowel sounds and concealing consonants.* If it is necessary to raise your voice, speak in lower tones.
- Talk toward the client's best or normal ear.
- Use gestures or written information to enhance the spoken word.
- Do not restrict a deaf client's hands. Never have intravenous lines in both of the client's hands if the preferred method of communication is sign language.†

*Data from Bernardini L: *Top Clin Nurs* Jan 1985, p 72.
†Data from Chovaz C: *Can Nurs* 85(3):34, 1989.

Guidelines for Checking Hearing Aid Function

- Check the battery. Turn off the aid and remove from client's ear. Cup the aid between your hands and turn the volume up full. A whistle should be heard, otherwise the battery is low.
- The hearing aid should not produce feedback (whistling sound heard when the client talks with others). If it does, check the position of the aid in the ear; note whether a hole is in the tubing or whether hair or cloth interferes with the microphone.
- The hearing aid should not emit scratchy sounds or work intermittently. Assess for any dirt or dust blocking battery contact in the case. Also note whether dirt or dust is present around the volume control.
- The hearing aid should be intact. Check for cracks or separation of the case or receiver and cracks or fraying of the cord or tubing.

---

stand the way a client's sensory loss affects normal daily activities. Family and friends can be more supportive when they understand sensory deficits and the types of elements that worsen or lessen sensory problems. If clients feel socially unaccepted, they will perceive sensory losses as seriously impairing the quality of life.

Promoting Self-Care

The ability to perform self-care is essential for self-esteem. Frequently, family members and nurses believe sensorially impaired persons require assistance, when in fact they can help themselves. Useful guidelines assist clients with visual or tactile impairment when help is required with activities of daily living.

A meal tray can be set up as though food on the tray and condiments and drinks around the tray are numbers on the face of a clock. The visually impaired client can easily become oriented to the items after the nurse explains each item's location.

If tactile sense is diminished, the client can dress more easily with zippers or velcro strips, pullover sweaters or blouses, and elasticized waists. If a client has partial paralysis and reduced sensation, the affected side should be dressed first.

Family members responsible for selecting clothing for visually impaired clients should be encouraged to follow the client's preferences. Any sensory impairment has a significant influence on body image, and it is important for the client to feel well groomed and attractive. The nurse should offer assistance if needed in brushing, combing, and shampooing hair.

The client with visual problems needs assistance in reaching toilet facilities safely. Safety bars should be installed near the toilet. Toilet paper and the call light cord should be within easy reach. Clients with proprioceptive problems may lose their balance when attempting to use the toilet. The nurse must supervise ambulation and sitting, make frequent checks to prevent falls, and caution the client against leaning forward.

 ### Evaluation

When caring for a client with a sensory alteration, the nurse evaluates whether care measures improve or at least maintain a client's ability to interact and function within the environment (see evaluation box). The nature of a client's sensory alteration influences the way the nurse evaluates care. The nurse adapts evaluation measures to the client's sensory deficit to determine whether actual outcomes are the same as expected outcomes. For example, the nurse uses proper communication techniques to evaluate whether a client with a hearing deficit has gained the ability to hear more effectively. Similarly the nurse will use large printed materials to test a visually impaired client's ability to read a prescription. When expected outcomes have not been achieved, there may be a need to change interventions or alter the client's environment. Family members may need to become more involved in support of the client.

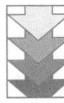

Sample Evaluation of Interventions for Sensory/Perceptual Alterations

Goals	Evaluative Measures	Expected Outcomes
Client will communicate successfully with care givers and family members on discharge.	Ask client about ways to improve ability to hear conversation.	Client will describe ways to optimize hearing (e.g., reducing background noise, watching lips of person speaking through eye contact) 2 days before discharge.
	Observe client interact with family and staff.	Client will use communication techniques to converse with family 1 day before discharge.
Family members will use communication techniques that promote clear comprehension of words by discharge.	Have family and client discuss techniques (e.g., eye contact, speaking in normal voice tones) that help client hear more clearly.	Client and family will identify effective communication techniques 1 day before discharge.
	Observe family members converse with client.	Family members will converse actively with client while using effective communication techniques on day of discharge.

If nursing care has been directed at improving sensory acuity, the nurse evaluates the integrity of the sensory organs and the client's ability to perceive stimuli. Any interventions designed to relieve problems associated with sensory alterations are evaluated on the basis of the client's ability to function normally without injury. When the nurse attempts to directly or indirectly (through education) alter the client's environment, evaluation is directed at observing whether the client makes environmental changes. When client teaching is designed to improve a client's sensory function, it is important to determine whether the client is following recommended therapies. Asking the client to explain or demonstrate self-care skills evaluates the level of learning that has occurred. It may be necessary to reinforce previous instruction if learning has not taken place. The evaluation box demonstrates how the nurse evaluates success at meeting client goals.

When the client leaves an acute care setting for the home environment, nurses should communicate with colleagues in the home care setting about the interventions that helped the client adapt to sensory problems. Similarly, information describing the client's existing sensory deficits should be reported. Continuity of care is achieved when the client is required to make only minimal changes in the home setting.

SUMMARY

The client with sensory alterations often faces a lonely and frightening world. The inability to interact effectively with the environment leads to a loss of security and self-esteem. A healthy balance between incoming sensory stimuli and stimuli to which the person is able to respond is necessary for the person's well-being.

Nurses work with a variety of clients who have actual or potential sensory alterations. Specific physiological changes can create sensory deficits. Exposure to excessive environmental stimulation causes sensory overload. Isolation in an environment without meaningful stimulation causes sensory deprivation. Clients most at risk for sensory problems include older adults, immobilized individuals, and socially isolated persons.

The nature of any sensory alteration influences the choice of nursing interventions. The nurse promotes the ability of the sensorially deprived client to maintain normal functioning with existing sensory deficits. Likewise, the nurse attempts to make changes within the environment to provide safe and meaningful stimulation for clients. Sensory changes can affect various aspects of a client's lifestyle. The nurse uses creative interventions to help clients interact effectively with their environments.

Key Concepts

- Sensory reception involves the stimulation of sensory nerve fibers and the transmission of impulses to higher centers within the brain.

- Sensory perception involves the organization and integration of sensory information into meaningful and conscious awareness.

- Because a person learns to rely on unaffected senses after experiencing a sensory loss, the nurse designs interventions to preserve function of these senses.

- Sensory deprivation results from an inadequate quality or quantity of sensory stimuli.

- Aging results in a gradual decline of acuity in all senses.

- Environmental stimuli within an intensive care unit place a client at risk for sensory overload.

- Clients who are older, immobilized, or confined in isolated environments are at risk for sensory alterations.

- The extent of support from family members and significant others can influence the quality of sensory experiences.

- Assessment of sensory function includes a physical examination and measurement of functional abilities.

- Sensory losses can impair a person's ability to socialize.

- An assessment of environment includes identifying hazards, sources of meaningful stimuli, and the amount of stimuli.

- The plan of care for clients with sensory alterations should include participation by family members.

- Nursing care for clients with sensory alterations includes using stronger sensory stimuli, compensating with other senses, and modifying the environment to maximize remaining sensory function.

- Clients with existing sensory deficits can learn alternative ways to communicate.

- Care of clients at risk for sensory deprivation includes introducing meaningful and pleasant stimuli for all senses.

- To prevent sensory overload, the nurse controls stimuli, orients the client to the environment, and promotes rest by minimizing interruptions.

- To improve communication with the hearing impaired, the nurse speaks clearly, avoids shouting, and makes sure the client can see facial and lip movements.

- Clients with artificial airways can communicate effectively with communication boards and written messages.

Key Terms

Aphasia, p. 1559

Auditory, p. 1554

Conductive hearing loss, p. 1563

Expressive aphasia, p. 1559

Gustatory, p. 1554

Kinesthesic, p. 1554

Olfactory, p. 1554

Ototoxic, p. 1563

Proprioceptors, p. 1554

Refractive error, p. 1562

Sensory deficit, p. 1555

Sensory deprivation, p. 1556

Sensory overload, p. 1556

Stereognosis, p. 1554

Tactile, p. 1554

Critical Thinking Exercises

1. Describe features that you would incorporte into the design of a nursing home for older adult clients with visual deficits.

2. When entering Mrs. James' room, you discover her to be disoriented to name and place. She appears restless and has a reduced attention span. How would you determine whether Mrs. James suffers sensory deprivation or electrolyte imbalance?

3. How would you communicate with a visually impaired client with an artificial airway.

4. Mr. Peters was just transferred to a medical nursing unit after spending 6 days in intensive care. As the nurse caring for Mr. Peters, what interventions would you use to create a meaningful sensory environment?

REFERENCES

Bernardini L: Effective communication as an intervention for sensory deprivation in the elderly client, *Top Clin Nurs* 6(4):72, 1985.

Ebersole P, Hess P: *Toward healthy aging,* ed 3, St Louis, 1990, Mosby–Year Book.

Jackson DL: A psychosocial and economic profile of hearing impaired adult clients. In Hull RH, editor: *Rehabilitative audiology,* Orlando, Fla, 1982, Grune & Stratton.

Kee CC: Sensory impairment: factor X in providing nursing care to the older adult, *J Community Health Nurs* 7(1):45, 1990.

Kim MJ, McFarland GK, McLane AM: *Pocket guide to nursing diagnoses,* ed 4, St Louis, 1991, Mosby–Year Book.

Levine ES: Psychocultural determinants in personality development, *Volta Rev* 78:258, 1976.

Lewis-Cullinan C, Janken JK: Effect of cerumen removal on the hearing ability of geriatric patients, *J Adv Nurs* 15:594, 1990.

Magilvy JK: Quality of life of hearing-impaired older women, *Nurs Res* 34:140, 1985.

Matteson MA, McConnell ES: *Gerontological nursing: concepts and practice,* Philadelphia, 1988, Saunders.

Walsh C, Eldredge N: When deaf people become elderly, *J Gerontol Nurs* 15(12):27, 1989.

ADDITIONAL READINGS

Brinkman K: Why can't your patient hear you? *RN* 54:46, 1991.

Chovaz C: Nursing the hearing impaired patient, *Can Nurse* 85(3):34, 1989.

Christian E et al: Sounds of silence: coping with hearing loss and loneliness, *J Gerontol Nurs* 15(11):4, 1989.

Foreman MJ: Acute confessional states in hospitalized elderly: a research dilemma, *Nurs Res* 35:3, 1986.

Kopac CA: Sensory loss in the aged: the role of the nurse and the family, *Nurs Clin North Am* 18:373, 1983.

Kruczek TM: How hospitals hurt old people, *RN* 49(2):17, 1986.

Palumbo MV: Hearing access 2000: increasing awareness of the hearing impaired, *J Gerontol Nurs* 16(9):26, 1990.

Primental PA: Alteration in communication. In Dudas S, Bukowski L, editors: Nursing care of the stroke patient, *Nurs Clin North Am* 21:321, 1986.

Walsh C: Common sense nursing care for the patient with poor vision, *RN* 49(10):24, 1986.

Whaley LF, Wong DL: *Nursing care of infants and children,* ed 4, St Louis, 1991, Mosby–Year Book.

Zegeer LJ: The effects of sensory changes in older persons, *J Neurosci Nurs* 18:325, 1986.

CHAPTER 46

Substance Abuse

OBJECTIVES

Mastery of content in this chapter will enable the student to:

- Discuss the general health risks related to the abuse of any substance.
- Compare and contrast physiological and psychological dependence.
- List nine major groups of drugs and substances and their signs and symptoms of intoxication.
- Describe several psychosocial causative variables in substance abuse.
- Describe the disease of chemical dependency and its progression.
- Discuss signs and symptoms of chemical dependency and physical, psychological, and social outcomes to the disease.
- Describe the typical course of substance abuse.
- State at least three special groups particularly at risk for substance abuse.
- Describe the nurse's responsibility if a colleague may be abusing a substance.
- Describe special assessment approaches for clients with substance abuse problems.
- List examples of nursing diagnoses related to substance abuse.
- List and discuss seven general types of interventions appropriate for substance abusers.
- Describe major characteristics of the evaluation process for nursing care of substance abusers.

CHAPTER OUTLINE

Substance abuse, or chemical dependency, is one of the major problems faced by every society in the world. If it were possible to add up all the direct and indirect results of substance abuse, including automobile accidents, violent crime and behavior, and the full range of health problems associated with the abuse of alcohol and other drugs, it might be the major health problem in most industrialized countries today. If the economic and social effects of substance abuse are totaled, including the economic costs of health care, job absenteeism, and reduced functioning and effects on the family and other social units, substance abuse can be considered one of the most serious social problems.

A **substance** is any drug, chemical, or biological entity that can be self-administered. Substance abuse occurs because of the substance's real or perceived effects or benefits. Even substances that the general public may consider harmless, such as vitamins, aspirin, and laxatives, can cause health problems if used improperly. The nurse needs to be aware of problems involved in substance abuse because of the wide range of effects on physiological and psychosocial health.

Chemical dependency can affect anyone. Social class, income, education, race, ethnic origin, sex, or occupation does not protect a person from the disease. There is one requirement, however, for developing it. A person must use mood-altering chemicals in sufficient quantity for a sufficient length of time for **chemical dependency** to occur. The person could consume alcohol or drugs in differing patterns, however, and still become chemically dependent. For example, a person could drink daily, never becoming drunk, but still consumes regular and increasing amounts. Eventually, this person could not do without the chemical. Another person could be a "binge" drinker, consuming large quantities on occasion to the point of drunkenness and then not drink at all for a long time. However, after beginning drinking, the binge drinker is unable to control the amount of consumption.

Another characteristic associated with the occurrence of chemical dependency is family history. Children of alcoholics often become alcoholics or drug abusers themselves, even when they have been raised apart from their biological parents. In addition, men have almost double the chance of acquiring the disease, especially when their fathers suffered from alcoholism or drug abuse (Goodwin et al, 1981). Recent research also supports the hereditary nature of chemical dependency (Begleiter et al, 1984).

 ## SUBSTANCE MISUSE, ABUSE, AND DEPENDENCE

Drugs and other substances can be used, misused, or abused, and the nurse must be able to distinguish among these different behaviors when providing care to clients with actual or potential drug or substance problems. These terms are defined in varying ways in different contexts, but the following meanings are generally accepted by health care professionals. Drug or substance *use* occurs if a drug is appropriately taken only as prescribed or generally recommended for its intended physiological or psychological effects. **Misuse** of drug or substance occurs if it is taken indiscriminately, whether as prescribed or self-administered as an over-the-counter (OTC) medication, or if it is taken improperly by a client who does not clearly understand the correct uses and dosage. **Substance abuse** occurs if a drug is regularly taken indiscriminately in excessive quantities to the extent that physiological, psychological, or social functioning is impaired.

The meanings given these terms are related to societal attitudes and values. The ingestion of alcohol to the point of intoxication may be accepted in some groups as social use but viewed as misuse or abuse by other groups. In addition, these behaviors exist on a continuum from cautious and appropriate use at one extreme to self-destructive, violent, chronic abuse at the other. Generally the more extreme cases can be categorized as clear use or abuse, but it is often more difficult to discriminate between use and misuse or misuse and abuse. For example, it is impossible to draw a line between how many alcoholic drinks a month are acceptable and how many constitute abuse.

Many variables are involved in whether the use of any drug or substance becomes misuse, including personality factors, cultural background, social context, and the person's motivations, values, attitudes, and related behavioral patterns. Although misuse of a drug or substance may not immediately compromise functioning, misuse can become abuse and therefore can be viewed as a major risk factor. The concept of the health-illness continuum (see Chapter 2) is useful in assessing the client's health status and risk factors related to abuse patterns if physiological changes have not yet begun to occur.

The nurse may encounter substance abuse in two ways. A person may enter the health care system with a complaint directly or indirectly related to substance abuse, such as a teenager seen in the emergency room with PCP-induced seizures or an alcoholic client being treated for liver disease. The nurse may also discover substance abuse while providing care for other conditions, such as learning in a routine nursing history that the client has been using laxatives daily for several months or in a family counseling situation that a father suspects his son frequently smokes marijuana. Because any type of drug or substance abuse threatens health, the nurse who discovers abuse can provide care directed at resolving the abuse problem.

The nurse must understand the concepts of substance abuse to understand and treat the disease. These include primary and secondary effects, physiological and psychological dependence, tolerance, cross-tolerance, and "remembering."

Alcohol and drugs have dual effects on the client. The **primary effect** of these substances is the self-medicating effect that the individual is seeking by using the drug. For example, the client who uses barbiturates, alcohol, benzodiazepines, marijuana, nonbarbiturate sedative-hypnotics, or inhalants is seeking a depressant effect. The person who uses cocaine, "crack," "ice," amphetamines, or caffeine desires the stimulant effect of the drug. Use of the opiates, such as heroin, methadone, or morphine, is preferred for their pain-killing effects (physical or emotional).

Each substance also possesses secondary effects that occur during **withdrawal**. These **secondary effects** are the opposite of the primary effect. That is, the client who has been using alcohol or barbiturates for the depressant effects experiences a central nervous system (CNS) hyperexcitability on abrupt cessation of the substance. Withdrawal can be extremely uncomfortable and can be fatal if untreated. The cocaine addict who uses cocaine for the euphoric and elated properties will experience profound depression and fatigue during withdrawal. The opiate abuser becomes hypersensitive to pain and emotional discomfort with discontinuation of the drug.

In the eyes of the substance abuser, the only way to avoid the discomfort and obtain relief from the secondary effects of the drug is to use the drug again. Hence the secondary effects of the drug reinforce its use and establish a cycle in which the user is more comfortable with the drug than without. The user's sense of "feeling normal" is associated with the use of the drug. These secondary effects lead to physiological and psychological dependence.

Physiological dependence is a condition in which the body has become so accustomed to the drug or substance that functioning is significantly impaired without it. Physiological dependence is present if a **withdrawal syndrome** occurs when administration of the drug is abruptly stopped. Use of alcohol, opiates, barbiturates, antianxiety drugs, and other agents can lead to physiological dependence.

Psychological dependence is an emotional or psychological reliance on a drug or substance, usually because of its psychological effects. The person prefers the drugged state to a nondrugged state and experiences a desire, craving, or compulsion for the drug or substance. Most physiologically dependent persons are also psychologically dependent on the drug, but psychological dependence can occur alone, as with cocaine, amphetamines, marijuana, and even caffeine.

Dependency occurs when a person experiences actual or potential impairments to functioning related to the chronic use of any drug or substance. In some cases a person may believe that drugs that do not lead to physiological dependence are safer. For example, teenagers may be aware that marijuana is not "addictive" and believe that they can stop using it whenever they want. However, psychological dependence is often as powerful a habit. Chronic abuse of "nonaddictive" drugs can also lead to impaired functioning and physiological damage.

Tolerance is the adaptation in the brain to the chemical. It begins with initial exposure to the substance and results in the need for an increasing dose or increased dose frequency to maintain the original pharmacological and primary effect of the substance. While assessing the extent of the use of the chemically dependent client, the nurse should anticipate the use of large amounts of alcohol or other chemicals.

Cross-tolerance means that the client who is tolerant to a certain substance is tolerant to all substances in the same category. For example, the client who is tolerant to alcohol will also have a tolerance to all CNS depressants, including benzodiazepines and barbiturates. When anesthesia that has CNS depressant properties is administered to an alcoholic surgical client, the nurse must observe for tolerance. In addiction treatment, the cross-tolerance properties permit safe detoxification and medical management of the addicted client. Rather than using alcohol to safely detoxify the alcohol-addicted client or heroin to detoxify the heroin-dependent client, other same-category drugs, such as chlordiazepoxide (Librium) or methadone, provide a safer means to clinically manage the withdrawal process.

"Remembering" is also a concept related to tolerance. It means that after the brain has been programmed for adaptation (tolerance), this tolerance will be remembered for the rest of the addict's life. In other words, once an alcoholic or addict, always an alcoholic or addict.

The client can never return to casual or social use but will always progress quickly, even after years of abstinence, to abuse. This has implications for the substance abuser who assumes that alcohol or drug use can be controlled after prolonged abstinence. In this person, rapid progression to excessive, out-of-control consumption occurs. This is true also for babies born to alcohol-, heroin-, and crack-addicted mothers who are at high risk throughout their lives to the development of a substance abuse problem.

Many clients who are chemically dependent may be receiving nursing care as a result of their physical problems related to alcohol or drug abuse. For example, the nurse working in obstetrics may care for a mother who is a chronic alcoholic and whose infant is born with **fetal alcohol syndrome (FAS)**. FAS is a permanent disorder that may be characterized by retardation and physical abnormalities. A nurse working in a neighborhood clinic may be a primary care provider for an intravenous (IV) substance abuser.

In any clinical setting, the nurse may suspect a drug or alcohol problem when the client has repeated pneumonia, ulcers, pancreatitis, cirrhosis, peripheral neuritis, fractures and other signs of trauma, malnutrition (including weight loss), history of seizures, complaints about impotence, infections or abscesses, hypertension, tuberculosis, or cancer of the mouth or esophagus.

Impaired Health Care Professionals

Nurses are at risk for developing a substance abuse problem. In fact, nurses' problems with chemical dependency have been brought to the attention of the profession (Bissell, Haberman, 1984; Sullivan, 1987) with efforts to assist nurses with recovery (American Nurses Association, 1984; Sullivan, Bissell, Williams, 1988). In fact, one in five nurses may have a substance abuse problem. Risk factors include easy access to abusable substances and the stress of work. Nurses administer medications that can be abused. Fisk and Devoto (1991) assert that meperidine is most often the drug of choice for the nurse with a substance abuse problem. Nurses face life-and-death situations, heavy workload demands, complex technology, and increasingly critical consumers that can appear overwhelming and provoke the desire to obtain immediate tension reduction through the use of drugs and alcohol.

The nurse with an alcohol or drug problem eventually exhibits behaviors that arouse the suspicions of supervisors and peers. These include overuse of sick time, particularly after a few days off; rapid mood changes; use of mints, mouthwash, or perfume to cover the alcohol odor; frequent trips to the bathroom

with a purse; insistence on administering medications or counting narcotics; reduced performance; sleeping at work; sloppy charting; isolation from the work group; or increasing forgetfulness (Fisk, Devoto, 1991).

The co-workers of the addicted nurse are often reluctant to confront their peer and thus participate in a conspiracy of silence. They assume detection of the problem will mean that the addict will be subjected to professional humiliation and the loss of livelihood as a result of license suspension. However, without intervention, chemical dependency is a fatal disease for the addicted nurse. Reporting requirements and professional rehabilitation programs established by state boards of nursing vary from state to state. Inpatient treatment and subsequent back-to-work stipulations permit the addicted nurse to resume nursing practice, determine the employer's expectations regarding aftercare, and avoid high-risk situations that would contribute to a relapse. Many state nurses' associations have developed peer assistance programs that allow the addicted nurse to meet with other ad-

---

Myths and Facts Related to Substance Abuse

Myth: Alcoholics are skid-row bums.
Fact: Only 5% of all alcoholics fit this stereotype. The majority (95%) represent a cross section of people from all walks of life, all professions and occupations, and all socioeconomic levels.
Myth: Providing information on the dangers of alcohol and drugs will prevent addiction.
Fact: Although information is essential, it will not prevent addiction from occurring by itself. Nurses, physicians, and pharmacists, who are all informed about drugs, become addicted at least as often (if not more) than others.
Myth: People just *think* they're addicted to alcohol or other drugs. They could quit if they had more will-power.
Fact: Although initial use is under voluntary control, after a person is physically or psychologically addicted, it becomes nearly impossible to control use.
Myth: Alcoholics (or addicts) must *want* to quit before anything can be done to help them.
Fact: Early treatment is just as beneficial as treating any other disease. By obtaining intervention early in an addiction, an abuser can avoid long-term complications and consequences that come with extensive use.

dicted nurses to address professional and personal issues concerning the chemical dependency. Because nurses care for clients with substance abuse, they may be considered as speakers for schools and community programs, they are at risk themselves for substance abuse, and they must sort fact from myth (see box).

Patterns of Use

Woody (1990) has identified four behavioral patterns of alcohol and drug use. The first pattern is **recreational use** that occurs in social settings for the purpose of experiencing the effects of the substance. Alcohol and drugs play a major role in the social gathering. Although recreational use may be initially infrequent, it can signal the beginning of a substance abuse problem.

Circumstantial use, the second pattern of drug and alcohol use, is inspired by the intent to obtain a specific effect within the context of a certain situation. An example of this would be the use of alcohol at business luncheons.

The third pattern is **intensified use.** With intensified use, alcohol or drugs are taken daily but usually in small-to-moderate amounts. This pattern of use is motivated by the desire for relief from a problem, such as anxiety or depression, or to improve or maintain a level of performance. The car salesman who uses cocaine to work more aggressively and for longer hours would be an example of intensified use.

The last pattern of use is a **compulsive use** of high doses of drugs or alcohol to the exclusion of other meaningful life activities. Unfortunately, compulsive, daily use most often is the only pattern that draws the attention of the medical community. However, recreational, circumstantial, and intensified use are often involved in vehicular accidents, falls, chokings on food, and drownings.

The nurse should not assume that recreational alcohol or drug use is *not* a problem for the client. Considering the prevalence of alcohol and drug use in society, substance abuse assessment on every client regardless of the presenting complaint would provide an opportunity for early intervention.

 DRUGS AND SUBSTANCES

The general public often considers only medically prescribed substances and highly publicized illegal substances to be drugs. Chemically active substances, such as caffeine, nicotine, and alcohol, and nonprescription substances, such as aspirin, laxatives, and antacids, are also drugs and are commonly abused.

Alcohol

Estimates of the prevalence of alcoholism have been made by the National Institute of Alcohol Abuse and Alcoholism (NIAAA). A 1990 national survey revealed that there are 15 million alcohol abusers in the adult population of the United States. The survey showed that approximately 8.6% of the population met the criteria for alcoholism. A higher number of men (13.35%) than women (4.635%) reported alcoholism symptoms (NIAAA, 1991a).

Although considered a stimulant, **alcohol** is actually a CNS depressant that causes a pseudostimulant effect as parts of the brain are released from inhibitory control of the cortex. Alcohol is absorbed rapidly from the stomach and the small intestine over 2 to 6 hours. However, milk or food delays this process. Alcohol is metabolized in the liver with the assistance of the enzyme alcohol dehydrogenase, which oxidizes it to acetaldehyde. Acetaldehyde is further oxidized to acetate and then eliminated through the kidneys and a small amount through the lungs.

Many alcoholics take disulfiram (Antabuse) to deter their impulsive craving for alcohol. Disulfiram inhibits the action of the enzyme alcohol dehydrogenase. If the client drinks while taking disulfiram, the result is toxic accumulation of acetaldehyde. The disulfiram-alcohol interaction consists of nausea, vomiting, flushing, tachycardia, high blood pressure, possible cardiac collapse, or death. The levels of liver enzymes are often elevated due to chronic drinking, but they must return to normal before this medication is prescribed because disulfiram is metabolized in the liver.

The desired effects of alcohol are euphoria and lessened social inhibitions. The person's gait is ataxic, and speech is slurred. In many cases, a personality change occurs during intoxication in which hostile and aggressive impulses are released.

Alcohol withdrawal without medical management can be fatal. Signs and symptoms of withdrawal can occur in the heavy drinker who reduces the daily amount from a quart to a pint a day. The intensity of the withdrawal process is determined by the length of time the person has been drinking and the amount of alcohol consumed. Signs and symptoms occur within 6 to 12 hours after drinking has ceased. The client appears restless and irritable, may exhibit tremors, or report feeling "shaky inside."

Behavioral manifestations of withdrawal may progress to nausea and vomiting, pulse rate greater than 100/minutes, respirations greater than 20/min, and blood pressure greater than 140/90. A critical time during withdrawal is the first and second days, when seizures may develop. Some clients may develop alcohol **hallucinosis,** during which the person may hear persecutory voices while the sensorium remains intact. **Delirium tremens (DTs),** the most severe state of alcohol withdrawal, occurs during the second to fourth day after drinking has stopped and is characterized by visual or tactile hallucinations, disorientation and delirium, fever, diaphoresis, vomiting, tachycardia leading to cardiac collapse, and death. A history of DTs should alert the nurse to monitor the client closely during withdrawal to prevent development because it is difficult to interrupt the process after DTs has begun.

Clinical management of alcohol withdrawal reduces the mortality of DTs significantly. During detoxification, the client's vital signs are monitored, vitamin supplements (thiamine and folic acid) are administered, hydration is encouraged, adequate caloric intake is provided, and medications that are cross-tolerant to alcohol are administered to reduce the anxiety-tremor state and CNS hyperexcitability. Benzodiazepines, such as diazepam (Valium) or chlordiazepoxide (Librium), are frequently used because of their long half-lives. However, with the debilitated client with severely compromised liver disease or the older alcoholic client, vital signs may elevate despite medical management. In fact, the client may appear inebriated from the medication as withdrawal symptoms progress. In these rare cases, it is best to administer oxazepam (Serax) for withdrawal management. The psychological effects of chronic alcohol use include heightened defense mechanisms such as denial and rationalization, a tendency to manipulate others, depression and suicidal tendencies (which must be taken seriously by the clinician), social isolation related to decreased social skills, dependent behaviors, impulsiveness, and a low tolerance for frustration.

Narcotics and Related Drugs

In addition to alcoholism, drug abuse accounts for serious health and economic problems in this country. Determining the prevalence of drug abuse is even more difficult than identifying alcoholics. A survey conducted by the National Institute of Drug Abuse estimated that 3 million people are addicted to heroin and cocaine (National Institute of Drug Abuse, 1991).

The opiates and opiate derivatives, including heroin, morphine, and codeine, are the most commonly used narcotic drugs. The opiate derivatives are generally administered by sniffing (absorption through the mucous membranes) or subcutaneous ("skin popping") or IV injection. **Opiate derivates** are CNS depressants that produce euphoria, analgesia, feelings of well-being, apathy about concerns or the surroundings, giddiness, and lethargy. Psychomotor performance is not impaired. Physical responses to opiate derivatives include nausea and vomiting as chemoreceptors are triggered; generalized itching as histamine is released on injection, which leads to feelings of being flushed; orthostatic hypotension as the vasodilation occurs in response to histamine; constricted pupils; and decreased gastrointestinal motility leading to constipation. Depressed respiration is a major side effect, and respiratory arrest, coma, and pulmonary edema can occur with overdose.

The stages of effects on administration of heroin include the "rush," the "nod," and the emergence of signs and symptoms of withdrawal. The rush lasts several minutes after heroin is taken. The user feels euphoric, flushed (histamine release), and warm, and sensations like sexual orgasm occur. The nod lasts about 4 to 6 hours and is characterized by drowsiness and feelings of well-being. Withdrawal signs and symptoms begin to develop within 5 to 6 hours after use.

Withdrawal symptoms include craving, yawning, and irritability within 6 to 8 hr, followed by influenza-like symptoms within 8 to 12 hours. Rhinorrhea (runny nose); lacrimation; diaphoresis; piloerection; gastrointestinal symptoms such as abdominal cramping, nausea and vomiting, and diarrhea; and musculoskeletal aches are common. Late-stage withdrawal signs, which peak within 36 to 72 hours, include elevated blood pressure, pulse, and respirations; pupil dilation; and muscle spasms. Because of the low purity of street heroin, the addict in withdrawal rarely progresses to exhibit late-stage signs. Detoxification is managed in one of the following ways:

1. The client's tolerance level is determined by monitoring withdrawal. Medicating with methadone (a long half-life opioid) is administered when observable signs appear. The amount of methadone is tapered off over the course of several days.

2. Clonidine (Catapres) and alpha-2 adrenergic antagonists are used to suppress symptoms of withdrawal. Blood pressure is monitored. Some clients attempt to manipulate others and thus seek drugs while being detoxified because they are uncomfortable. This often makes the addict an unpopular client in the health care setting. Firm limits and consistency in carrying out the detoxification protocol prevent this behavior from escalating.

Sedative-Hypnotics

Sedative-hypnotic drugs include barbiturates such as secobarbital (Reds, Redbirds), amobarbital (Blues, Blue Devils), pentobarbital (Yellow Jackets), phenobarbital (the only barbiturate with a low-abuse potential because of its long half-life), and nonbarbiturates such as ethchlorvynol, glutethimide, and methaqualone (Ludes, Sopors). Sedative-hypnotics produce CNS depression and are cross-tolerant with alcohol. Acute intoxication mimics alcohol intoxication. Slowing of mental functions and psychomotor activity, slurred speech, ataxia, emotional lability, delayed reaction time, poor concentration and judgment, drowsiness, and irritation occur. With chronic abuse, paranoia and suicidal behaviors may be demonstrated. Large doses cause respiratory depression, and overdose can cause hypoxia, coma, cardiac depression or arrest, and respiratory failure.

Psychological effects include relaxation or sedation, drowsiness, or a sense of euphoria often followed by depression. Like alcohol withdrawal, withdrawal from sedative-hynotics is life threatening if not medically managed. Seizures can occur between the second and fourth days after the last dose. Hallucinosis and delirium develop within 36 to 72 hours. Often, the temperature of a client in severe withdrawal spikes to more than 106° F. After delirium has developed, it is difficult to interrupt withdrawal, even with medication. Detoxification is accomplished by determining the client's tolerance level, substituting phenobarbital for the shorter half-life sedative-hypnotics, and then tapering the dosage slowly over several weeks if necessary.

Benzodiazepines (Tranquilizers)

The **benzodiazepines** are widely prescribed for antianxiety, management of anxiety and depression, panic disorders, sleep disorders, and musculoskeletal problems, including muscle spasm and low back pain and for medical management of alcohol withdrawal. Diazepam (Valium) follows alcohol as the most commonly abused drug because it is often viewed as harmless by clinicians who prescribe it. Alprozalom (Xanax) is quickly becoming another widely prescribed and abused benzodiazepine. The benzodiazepines possess a greater margin of safety than the barbiturates because they do not depress respirations. Overdose rarely occurs with any benzodiazepine alone, although when the drugs are combined with alcohol, the potentiating effect can be deadly.

The physical effects of the benzodiazepines in large doses include hypotension, tachycardia, and reduced coordination such as slurred speech and ataxia. Psychological effects include fatigue, decreased attentiveness or confusion, emotional bluntness, lethargy, somnolence, and a feeling of tranquility and increased self-confidence.

Early signs and symptoms of withdrawal include anxiety, nausea, vomiting, diarrhea, severe agitation, and emotional lability. This can progress to depression, paranoia, disorientation, hallucinations, twitching, tremors, hypertension, tachypnea, and tachycardia. Seizures and delirium can occur as late as 8 days after the last dose. Safe detoxification includes determining the client's tolerance level and then tapering the dose of the addicting drug slowly to prevent the emergence of withdrawal signs and symptoms.

CNS Sympathomimetics

CNS sympathomimetics include cocaine and amphetamines, which are pharmacologically related to epinephrine and norepinephrine. Both drugs stimulate the CNS and produce physical tolerance. Cocaine and amphetamines produce a strong psychological dependence, and many researchers are questioning the assumption that cocaine does not lead to a physical dependence.

For many substance abusers, cocaine is undeniably the drug of choice. Because it has a very short half-life, to maintain the stimulating effects, it must be taken every 15 to 30 minutes. Physical effects resemble the body's response to stress and include increased pulse, blood pressure, respirations, and temperature; dilated pupils; vasoconstriction with redistribution of blood flow to the brain and skeletal muscles; and elevated serum glucose levels as stored glycogen is converted to glucose, which eventually leads to weight loss. Severe effects include hyperthermia, cerebral hemorrhage, seizures, and status epilepticus.

Cocaine intoxication produces euphoria, a feeling of elation, initially increased intellectual functioning, grandiosity (pomposity or showiness) and feeling of power, hyperalertness, anorexia, insomnia, and hypomanic behaviors (including pressured speech, hyperverbal and hypersexual behavior, and flight of ideas). With progressive abuse, the client may experience a cocaine dysphoria (feelings of anxiety and discontent) with psychomotor agitation, sadness, depression, apathy, and seclusiveness. With continued and high-dose abuse, cocaine hallucinosis may occur in which the abuser begins to experience psychotic symptoms, but sufficient reality testing is present to not act on them. However, growing paranoid delusions can prompt repetitive behavior, such as staring out the window watching for the police. Eventually, the abuser may develop a cocaine psychosis in which reality testing is absent and paranoid delusions can result in harm to self or others. Hallucinations are also common.

Cocaine can be sniffed, injected, or smoked in a converted base form, which is known as "crack." Crack is a beige rock that has undergone the process of combining cocaine with baking soda and water and heating it until the water evaporates. Crack is a serious health threat because it is now cheaper than marijuana, is extremely potent, does not require needles, and is very addicting.

With cocaine, the user experiences a euphoric rush not obtainable in any other illicit drug, so the crash or withdrawal symptoms can be devastating to the user. To avoid these secondary effects, the user compulsively engages in a cycle of "runs" and crashes to escape the agitation and paranoia of abuse and the depression of withdrawal. The cocaine abuser often uses alcohol, heroin, or the benzodiazepines to relieve the anxiety, irritability, and hyperstimulation from the run, leading to polysubstance dependence. Other symptoms of withdrawal from chronic abuse include irritability, anxiety, fatigue and prolonged sleeping, hyperphagia, dysphoria, suicidal tendencies, and violence.

The amphetamines have traditionally been sniffed or injected. Their physical and psychological effects are similar to those of cocaine, with eventual progression to psychosis with chronic high-dose use. However, the amphetamine abuser may develop delusions that last for months after the drug is discontinued. Also, the abuser may engage in compulsive psychomotor behaviors, such as pacing, facial grimacing, or teeth grinding.

Recently, a new drug has emerged to compete with crack. "Ice" is a smokable methamphetamine that possesses the euphoria and rush of cocaine but has a longer half-life than cocaine. Severe depression, often of suicidal proportions, may follow any CNS sympathomimetic high.

Hallucinogens

Hallucinogens include lysergic acid diethylamide (LSD), mescaline, psilocybin, and phencyclidine (PCP). These drugs generally do not lead to physical or psychological dependence, but unpredictable, often violent behavior is associated with their use. PCP use has become more widespread in recent years, and it is sometimes smoked with marijuana.

The effects of PCP include the inability to process incoming sensory stimuli; dreamlike estrangement from reality; feelings of power, strength, and invulnerability; disorientation with the classic "bland stare"; euphoria; and disordered thought processes.

With high-dose levels, the user may develop intensified feelings of depersonalization; auditory and visual hallucinations; grandiose, paranoid, or somatic delusions; psychosis; delirium; seizures; opisthotonos; anesthesia; and the potential for self-harm and violence, which constitutes a psychiatric emergency.

PCP is a long-acting drug with a short half-life because of its high lipid solubility. As a result, the chronic abuser may experience alternating periods of agitation, paranoia, and aggressiveness with calm, "spacy" periods as late as the tenth day after the last use. There is no withdrawal syndrome, but the client should be kept in an area of minimal external stimulation, such as a quiet room to prevent harm to the self or others. In addition, cranberry juice is used to acidify the urine, which hastens the elimination of PCP from the body.

LSD produces relatively mild autonomic nervous system changes, such as tachycardia, hypertension, nausea, and vertigo. The physiological effects of LSD include flushing, sweating, diplopia, nystagmus, analgesia, sedation, ataxia, seizures, hypertension, numbness of extremities, impaired motor skills, respiratory depression, and coma.

LSD causes perceptual changes or hallucinations, impaired judgment, and toxic psychosis characterized by panic, paranoia, and unpredictable behavior. The psychological effects include perceptual distortions, apathy, disorganized thought processes, impaired attention span, hallucinations that can recur unpredictably for days or weeks after use, paranoid behavior, and self-destructive acts.

Marijuana

Marijuana and hashish (a powdered form of the plant's resin) are the most common forms of the cannabis drugs and are derived from a species of hemp. The plant is usually dried and smoked but is sometimes ingested. The pharmacological classification of marijuana is not definite, but the drug seems to act as a CNS depressant.

The physiological effects of marijuana are less dramatic than those of other drugs affecting the CNS. Effects include immediate tachycardia, delayed bradycardia, delayed hypotension, and enhanced appetite. The psychological effects have been the subject of many studies and are still being debated. The drug produces a state of relaxation, distorted perceptions of time and space, moments of excitement or hilarity, impaired decision making, and sometimes fear, panic, or paranoia. Hallucinations occur only with very high doses. Long-term use may cause apathy, memory problems, and some loss of mental acuity. The withdrawal symptoms for high-dose chronic marijuana abuse are mild and include irritability, restlessness, anorexia, and insomnia.

Inhalants

Inhalants are substances, such as volatile hydrocarbons and aerosols, that are abused for their CNS depressant effect. Inhalants include toluene, xylene, benzene, gasoline, paint thinner, lighter fluid, and airplane glue. Inhalant abuse is often the first substance of abuse because it is easily accessible to the young adolescent. Methods of inhalant abuse include "sniffing," "huffing," and "bagging," which lead to a rapid onset of psychoactive effects. Sniffing is direct inhalation from the container. Spraying or pouring the inhalant onto a cloth and then holding this to the nose or mouth is huffing. The huffer can often be identified by redness, tenderness, and skin excoriation around the nose and mouth. Bagging consists of pouring the inhalant into a bag and inflating it by exhaling, waiting several seconds and then inhaling the vapors. The use of plastic bags risks the possibility of suffocation if the abuser loses consciousness from the effects of the inhalant.

The physiological effects of inhalants include ataxia, muscular incoordination, headache, vertigo, slurred speech, bronchial and laryngeal irritation, depressed respirations and reflexes, cardiac dysrythmias, seizures, and death. Coma can result from large doses.

The psychological effects consist of an excitatory phase followed by CNS depression. During the excitatory phase, the user experiences euphoria, excitation, exhilaration, "drunkenness," feelings of omnipotence, distortions of visual and spatial perceptions, and dizziness. CNS depression is characterized by glazed eyes and a vacant stare, ataxia, loss of self-control, and somnolence.

Tolerance develops to inhalant use, and the chronic abuser may use as many as eight tubes of airplane glue a day. Physical dependence and a withdrawal syndrome are not clearly established for inhalants, but reports of tremulousness, irritability, loss of appetite, and insomnia occur with abrupt cessation. Psychological dependence develops because of the state of intoxication rather than the specific chemical.

Nonprescription Substances

Any drug or substance that alters consciousness or physiological functioning can be misused or abused. For example, nicotine in cigarettes causes CNS changes and can be abused for these effects. Similarly, coffee and soft drinks containing caffeine can be misused. Society is generally becoming more aware of the effects and risks of these substances. Many OTC products, however, hold the same potential for misuse and abuse when individuals diagnose their own needs and turn habitually to a commercial product that they can easily buy and self-administer.

Substance abuse does not depend on the presence of psychoactive effects. Often, abuse of OTC products is unintentional and derives from the expected benefit from the drug rather than its consequences. The individual lacks information regarding the limits of the medication's purpose or dosage. "More is better" is the operating principle applied to the self-administration of OTC preparations. Psychologically dependence occurs if the user feels that the medication is necessary for continued good health.

Commonly abused OTC preparations include the following:

1. Sedatives that contain antihistamines, used to treat insomnia (Major side effect is sedation.)
2. Appetite suppressants that contain CNS stimulants, caffeine, or phenylpropanolamine abused by overweight and anorexic individuals
3. Laxatives used by bulimic and anorexic clients to control weight gain
4. Cough and cold preparations that contain alcohol and antihistamines
5. Analgesics used to alleviate aches and pains

Older adults are particularly at risk for abuse of OTC medications because they experience more sickness and physical pain than any other group. Osgood (1990) reports that 25% of all OTC preparations are consumed by older adults.

 ## SUBSTANCE ABUSE AND PSYCHOSOCIAL HEALTH

Because of their mind- and behavior-altering effects, most abused substances can also have serious effects on psychosocial well-being and family functioning. To understand the relationship between abuse and the psychosocial dimension and provide nursing care for a client with substance abuse, the nurse needs to understand the variables that cause substance abuse, the addiction process, attitudes toward abuse, and the psychosocial effects on the abuser's family and other social interactions.

Etiology

Physiological and psychological dependence has a major role in the abuser's pattern of continued use, but the reasons for the initial misuse are more varied. Generally, two kinds of conscious or unconscious motivations may explain the first misuses of a substance (Hahn, Barkin, Oestreich, 1986). The person using mind-altering drugs may be seeking pleasure, euphoria, a new or unusual experience, or self-discovery and may be motivated by factors such as curiosity, boredom, peer pressure, or media attention. The person may be consciously or unconsciously seeking to solve or avoid a problem or cope with stress or other problems. This motivation may apply to a chronic abuser of self-prescribed laxatives and to a businessman who habitually has three martinis at lunch to relieve tension at the office. Many psychologists have examined substance abuse as an **escape mechanism** by which the person attempts to reduce inner tensions, depression, self-concept problems, or problems in social interaction with a spouse, family, or peers.

Theories of Substance Abuse

PRIMARY DISEASE. The success of Alcoholics Anonymous (AA) and Narcotics Anonymous (NA) has forced a recognition of the simple fact that many recover from their dependency and their other problems diminish or disappear when alcoholics stop drinking and adopt abstinence as a goal. This realization has resulted in alcoholism being considered a primary disease (for example, one in which the alcohol problem is seen as primary with other problems [psychological or physical] as secondary to the alcoholism).

In AA and NA, recovery begins with the desire to quit drinking or using drugs, believing that one is powerless over the addiction, and participating in the fellowship of the group. The power of the group and the recognition of a supreme being serves to replace drug or alcohol use. Spirituality is seen as essential to the addict's recovery.

With the development of Adult Children of Alcoholics and Codependents Anonymous, alcohol and drug use are being viewed as only part of a larger problem. These 12-step groups also incorporate a higher power into their structure and identify the user as suffering from many feelings resulting from growing up in a dysfunctional family. These feelings include shame, fear, and confusion.

GENETIC THEORIES. Research has been struggling with the issue of whether chemical dependency is the product of nature or nurture (that is, genetic or environmental factors). One study examined the incidence of alcoholism in children of alcoholics who were raised away from their parents as compared with adoptees without alcoholic biological parents. In this classic study, both groups were adopted into nonalcoholic homes. The men were between 25 and

29 years old at the time of the study. About 20% of those with biological alcoholic parents were alcoholic, whereas only 5% of the men without alcoholic parents had developed alcoholism (Goodwin et al, 1973).

Body-functioning abnormalities has been another area of investigation in which children of alcoholics are viewed as handling alcohol and drugs differently from others. The hypothesis is that the child of an alcoholic lacks acetaldehyde to break alcohol down and instead it accumulates when the individual drinks. The result is immediate intoxication and a compulsion to continue drinking. Many clients are aware of the different effects when they first begin to drink.

PSYCHOLOGICAL THEORIES. Various theories compare psychological factors and substance abuse. One theory suggests that substance abusers possess personality traits that predispose them to seek immediate gratification and pleasure at the expense of other needs. According to the self-medication hypothesis, clients use drugs or alcohol to cope with stress and painful emotional states. This model further suggests that the substance abusers drug of choice is determined by the predominant state that the individual is attempting to manage (Khantzian, 1985).

Behavioral psychological theories are based on the reinforcement principle or learning theory. That is, people begin substance abuse and continue because they have received some reward or reinforcement such as feeling good, having fun, or being accepted. Seeking relief from the discomfort of anxiety or depression serves as a reward for substance abuse behavior. This may be further reinforced by growing up in a family that resorts to alcohol or drugs to manage negative feelings or problems.

SOCIOCULTURAL THEORIES. Sociocultural theories of alcoholism differ from other theories. Instead of examining individuals, these theories focus on group differences. Such theories are based on observation and study of different cultures or groups of people and their drinking practices and the occurrence of chemical dependency. Socialization theorists believe that values, perceptions, norms, and beliefs are passed on from one generation to another and that the way alcohol is used is part of socialization.

Sociological determinants of substance abuse behavior also include the recent trends in social attitudes, such as Mothers Against Drunk Driving (MADD) and Students Against Drunk Driving (SADD). These groups are responsible for societal awareness of the dangers of combining substance abuse and driving.

Obviously, no one cause of chemical dependency has been clearly and consistently identified, but many possible factors exist. A person can be born with a predisposition to a chemical dependency problem, but no one understands the "triggers" that facilitate this process. Although the precise mechanism of the cause of chemical dependency is unknown, the course of substance abuse can be progressive. Compulsive use is the end state.

Addiction Process

Alcohol and other drugs of addiction are mood altering, that is, they change the way a person feels, usually for the better. Mood-altering chemicals affect the CNS and alter its functioning. They help people relax, feel mellow, and enjoy activities. In addition, drugs mediate pain perception, induce sleep, and reduce physical and emotional reactions to stress. Approximately 10% of the population perceive the use of chemicals as necessary for normal daily functioning. These people have become addicted to mood-altering chemicals.

A person rarely sets out to become an alcoholic or addict. Practically all users think that they are in control and can stop using the drug whenever they wish. They do not realize that physical and psychological dependence make stopping impossible.

Addiction is characterized by preoccupation with the acquisition of the chemical, compulsive use in the presence of untoward consequences, and relapse or voluntary return to the substance (Miller, Dackis, Gold, 1987). A definitive indicator of addiction is the loss of control over the chemical. This includes the binge user, as well as the daily user.

As chemical dependency progresses, the user employs a variety of defense mechanisms to cope with the problems that the behaviors cause. Defense mechanisms are unconscious ways people deal with painful events.

The primary defense mechanism used by chemical dependents is denial. The person does not really believe what appears obvious to others. Even with overwhelming evidence that chemical use is impairing life (for example, driving while intoxicated [DWI] arrests, losing jobs and family, or criminal convictions), an addicted person continues to deny that the chemical use is anything but normal and claims, "I can quit anytime I want."

To try to understand the substance abuser, the nurse should try to remember when a shock was felt (for example, a death of someone close or a pet). The nurse probably thought, "this can't be true," and even kept forgetting that it had happened. For example, after waking in the morning, the nurse may have initially thought that the person or pet was still alive. This is denial. Things that appear to be true are not.

Thus abusers really believe that they can quit at any time. Denial helps people deal with difficult and painful events until they are able to assimilate them.

Another example of denial is when chemically dependent individuals assume, after prolonged abstinence, that they can use again but without the loss of control. Many addicts enter treatment programs after acting on such assumptions. They expect to be able to control their use, which quickly gets out of hand. They report that they lose control so fast that it was as if they never stopped using in the first place.

Rationalization is used to explain why they continue to use chemicals. Many users justify their addiction with statements such as "Everyone uses something to relax," "It's just marijuana, what's wrong with that?" or "I don't drink that much." They use any reason to take drugs. Projection is another defense mechanism that allows addicts to continue use in spite of the adverse consequences. Projecting unacceptable behaviors onto another occurs when the substance abuser blames the spouse, children, parents, boss, or any other person for substance abuse. Abusers focus on the faults of others to avoid examining their own.

Attitudes Toward Substance Abuse

To be objective in understanding the problem and to facilitate a therapeutic nurse-client relationship, the nurse should be aware of personal attitudes and values related to use of the substance. The values clarification process is useful in this respect (see Chapter 12). The nurse who adopts a moralistic, judgmental attitude toward drinking has difficulty understanding the contribution of individual factors to the client's behavior. Good listening, communication skills, and the ability to calmly confront the abuser's denial may lead the nurse to realize that the client is not morally weak or bad but rather that chemicals are used as ineffective ways to manage sadness, anger, disappointment, and fear.

Impact on Socialization

Regardless of the pattern of substance use (recreational, circumstantial, intensified, or compulsive), the impact on the user may be financial, legal, emotional, or any combination thereof. Often, jobs are lost (or not done well). Legal problems, such as driving while intoxicated or possession of an illicit substance, may occur and thus require the payment of fines or lawyer fees and may even lead to jail time. Because of impaired judgment, the chemical user may be at risk for victimization from robbery, rape, or assault.

The client's social functioning may deteriorate because the use of alcohol or drugs promotes emotional withdrawal from interpersonal relationships during the intoxication state and because behaviors related to use occur. Such behaviors include missing social engagements, doing embarrassing things, and covering up mistakes. As abuse progresses, the user may become alienated from the nonusing world. Substance abuse also has an impact on the client's family.

Effects on the Family

The magnitude of the effect on the user's family is severe. The spouse's response is often anger and resentment. As the consequences of substance abuse increase, the spouse may try to cover up to prevent embarrassment or to save the addict's job. The effects on the spouse involve all aspects of their relationship and life together. During a nursing history, the spouse may mention matters such as sexual maladjustment, thoughts of separation or divorce, quarreling, economic difficulties, loneliness, confusion, domestic violence, or resentment about increased responsibilities in childrearing and other family roles. All these may be direct or indirect effects of substance abuse because usual roles and coping mechanisms break down with increasing psychological dependence.

Children who have grown up in alcoholic homes often have severe problems with trust, lack of self-esteem, and dependency. So many people have been affected that several self-help groups have formed to assist members in dealing with these issues. These groups are generally associated with Al-Anon and are specified as meetings for adult children of alcoholics.

The effects of substance abuse by either or both parents on their children are often of particular importance to the nurse. The stresses of having an alcoholic parent in the home can have wide-range effects on the child and lead to physical and emotional problems in the early developmental stages. Self-concept may be seriously damaged because most children and adolescents do not understand the complex abuse problem but tend to blame themselves for the parent's emotional neglect. Family conflicts are more likely, and violence often erupts in the presence of children. Children in such families are also at a high risk for child abuse. In addition, children of substance abusers, particularly alcoholics, are at greater risk for later becoming substance abusers themselves.

 ## SUBSTANCE ABUSE IN SPECIAL GROUPS

Developmental Stages

Because substance abuse involves many physiological and psychosocial effects and causative variables, people in different developmental stages have different susceptibilities and are affected in different ways. For example, a 40-year-old businessman may increase alcohol consumption in response to an awareness that physical energy is diminishing with age, or an adolescent may experiment with drugs because of pressures from the peer group. Each developmental stage presents certain kinds of stresses and the potential for maturational crises. These may influence the individual's behavior related to abuse patterns. In addition, the physiological and psychological effects of substance abuse vary according to the person's developmental stage. Unit 5 discusses the developmental stages in detail and the developmental changes that influence the individual's susceptibilities. The nurse should always be alert to the possibility of chemical dependency in any client regardless of age. Risk factors related to developmental phases and maturational and situational crisis should be assessed to detect the presence of a substance abuse problem.

Special attention should be given to the effects of substance abuse in the fetal stage of development. Chapter 22 describes different kinds of teratogens, drugs that cross the placenta into the circulation of the embryo or fetus, with a potential effect on normal growth.

Childhood is a vulnerable time for the start of a substance abuse problem. The age of initiation of smoking, drinking, glue sniffing, and other drug use has steadily dropped from adolescence to that of 8, 9 and 10 year olds within the past decade (Kaplan, Saddock, 1985).

Adolescence is the next phase of development that can be high risk for the establishment of a substance abuse problem. The adolescent faces the major task of separation and individualization from the family of origin. Behavior patterns that seem to be consistent with the adolescent user include the fear of failure, an underlying agitated depression, aggresssive and hopeless feelings, a low frustration tolerance, and limited coping skills (Kaplan, Saddock, 1985).

Early adulthood is the stage in which the individual attempts to establish the roles of spouse, parent, and employee and can be another susceptible stage of development. Particularly at high risk is the individual who is limited to a boring job and who uses drugs and alcohol to escape from the responsibilities of life. Because the person lacks future goals, substance abuse and television become the major activities for retreat.

Middle adulthood is another developmental stage during which addiction may surface. The individual at risk is sometimes the high achiever hiding an unwarranted low self-esteem. While successful in the professional or business world, the person is emotionally isolated by a sense of shame. A major clue to identifying this client is the lack of satisfaction derived from accomplishments. Instead, success brings about feelings of emptiness and the compulsive need to do more. As the work frenzy builds, heavy social drinking or recreational drug use progresses to manage the stress and emotional pain (Bohan, 1990).

Finally, older adults are at high risk for the development of a substance abuse problem. There are two types of older substance abusers: the "survivors" of an early onset of a chemical dependency and those who increase their use after the age of 60 in response to the crises related to aging (for example, retirement, loss of spouse and peers, physical health deterioration and pain, and emotional problems such as depression). Older adults have the highest rate of suicide of all age groups (Osgood, 1990). Although alcohol, tranquilizers, and OTC medications are the major substances of abuse for this population, the nurse should not assume that age precludes the use of illicit drugs.

Substance abuse in older adults is often undetected by health care providers. The client may have aches and pains but deny an underlying problem with drugs or alcohol. Many health care providers are reluctant to assess older adults for substance abuse problems.

NURSING PROCESS FOR THE CHEMICALLY DEPENDENT CLIENT

Assessment

Nurses care for clients who have episodic and chronic use of alcohol or other addictive substances. Episodic care is usually acute, short-term interventions to manage a medical emergency, such as a car accident or drug overdose, whereas chronic abuse problems can result in any number of physical and psychological consequences.

The nurse assists clients and their families in primary, secondary, and tertiary care. Primary prevention includes providing accurate information to the health care system and communities regarding chemical dependency. Secondary care is provided when the nurse serves as a case finder in assisting parents, educators, and other health care professionals in identifying persons with actual or potential chemical abuse problems. Finally, the nurse provides tertiary care to clients in chemical dependency treatment centers, acute care hospitals, home care settings, clinics, and long-term care facilities.

Screening for Chemical Dependency

Identifying the chemically dependent client is the most important step in the nursing process. The nurse must consider the question of substance abuse in any client encountered in the clinical setting, particularly a client who has health conditions related to substance abuse (for example, pancreatitis and pneumonia). The nursing assessment includes a health history and the use of observation skills to determine a client's substance abuse profile. The nurse should ask questions about the individual's and family's substance abuse patterns.

Physical and Behavioral Assessment

Because of the variety of physiological and psychological effects of chronic substance abuse and the often subtle factors that create the potential for an abuse problem, assessment should be thorough and explore the client's health status in all dimensions. The goals of the assessment are to determine whether a substance abuse problem exists; to explore causative factors and effects in all areas of the client's life; to assess the psychological, behavioral, and physiological impact of the abused substance; and to assess the extent of physiological or psychological dependence. Assessment includes observing a client's behaviors that may indicate substance abuse, the interview and nursing history, and the physical examination. A person under the influence of a drug generally manifests a set of behaviors as a result of the drug's psychological and physiological effects (Table 46-1 on p. 1586). Observation of such behaviors in a client, even when the nurse does not otherwise suspect an abuse problem, should prompt further assessment using interview techniques.

The nurse begins a substance abuse history by a physical assessment of the client. The nurse determines whether vital signs are elevated, particularly the pulse and blood pressure, which can indicate a CNS depressant withdrawal syndrome. The client may be fidgety, anxious, easily irritated, or tremulous.

The nurse notes whether the client's arm and legs are edematous, reddened, and warm to the touch,

TABLE 46-1 Summary of Behaviors Associated with Substance Abuse

Substance	Route*	Dependence		Expected Behaviors
		Physical	Psychological	
Alcohol	Ingestion	Yes	Yes	Euphoria followed by depression and sometimes hostility, decreased inhibitions, impaired judgment, incoordination, slurred speech
Opiates				
Heroin	Injection, ingestion, inhalation	Yes	Yes	Euphoria, relaxation, relief from pain, lack of concern, detachment from reality, drowsiness, constricted pupils, nausea, constipation, slurred speech, impaired judgment
Morphine	Injection, ingestion	Yes	Yes	
Meperidine	Ingestion			
Codeine	Ingestion, injection	Yes	Yes	
Opium	Smoking, ingestion	Yes	Yes	
Methadone	Ingestion	Yes	Yes	Relief of craving for drugs without causing impaired functioning
Barbiturates	Ingestion, injection	Yes	Yes	Euphoria followed by depression and sometimes hostility, decreased inhibitions, impaired judgment, slurred speech, incoordination, drowsiness
Amphetamines	Ingestion, injection	No	Yes	Euphoria, hyperactivity, irritability, hyperalertness, insomnia, anorexia, weight loss, tachycardia, hypertension
Cocaine	Inhalation, smoking, injection	No	Yes	Euphoria, elation, agitation, hyperactivity, irritability, grandiosity, presssured speech, tachycardia, hypertension, diaphoresis, anorexia, weight loss, insomnia, glassy eyes
Hallucinogens (psychedelics)	Ingestion, smoking	No	No	Distorted perception, heightened sense of awareness, grandiosity, hallucinations, illusions, distortions of time and space, depersonalization, mystical experiences, dilated pupils, increased blood pressure, increased salivation
Phencyclidine (PCP)	Smoking, ingestion	No	No	Euphoria, perceptual distortion, agitation, violence, delusions, antisocial behavior, elevated blood pressure, increased salivation, diaphoresis, ataxia, nystagmus, decreased pain response
Marijuana	Smoking, ingestion	No	Yes	Relaxation, mild euphoria, loss of inhibition, decreased motivation, red eyes, dry mouth
Antianxiety drugs (benzodiazepines)	Ingestion, injection	Yes	Yes	Relaxation, increased self-confidence, relief of anxiety, drowsiness, ataxia, slurred speech, hypotension

From Stuart GW, Sundeen SJ: *Principles and practice of psychiatric nursing,* ed 4, St Louis, 1991, Mosby–Year Book.

Behaviors Related to Overdose	Withdrawal Syndrome	Special Considerations
Unconsciousness, coma, respiratory depression, death	Tremors, hallucinosis, seizure disorder, DTs (alcohol withdrawal DTs)	Chronic use leads to serious disruptions in most organ systems. Malnutrition and dehydration are common. Vitamin deficiency may lead to Wernick's encephalopathy and alcoholic amnesic syndrome. Alcohol-dependent people are susceptible to other dependencies.
Unconsciousness, coma, respiratory depression, circulatory depression, respiratory arrest, cardiac arrest, death	Watery eyes, dilated pupils, anxiety, abdominal cramps, piloerection, yawning, diaphoresis, rhinorrhea, achiness, anorexia, insomnia, fever, nausea, vomiting, diarrhea	Chronic use leads to lack of concern about physical well-being, resulting in malnutrition and dehydration. Criminal behavior may take place to acquire money for drugs. Injection sites may become infected. Multiple drug use is common.
Same	Same	
Respiratory depression, coma, death	Postural hypotension, tachycardia, fever, insomnia, tremors, agitation, anxiety; *rapid withdrawal*: apprehension, weakness, tremors, postural hypotension, anorexia, grand mal seizures	It is frequently used alternately with stimulants. Combination with alcohol enhances effects and may lead to overdose. Paradoxical responses of hyperactivity may occur in children and older adults.
Restlessness, tremor, rapid respiration, confusion, assaultiveness, hallucinations, pain	Depression, fatigue	Prolonged use can result in psychotic behavior. Paradoxical depressant reaction occurs in children. It is frequently used with depressant substances.
Restlessness, tremor, rapid respiration, confusion, assaultiveness, hallucinations, panic	Depression, fatigue, anxiety	Psychotic behavior may occur after large doses. Prolonged use by inhalation may result in destruction of nasal mucous membranes and deterioration of nasal septum. Use with other substances is dangerous.
Panic, psychosis	None	"Bad trip" may result in panic, unpredictable behavior, and psychotic behaviors. "Flashbacks" may occur for several months after use. Self-destructive behavior may occur while under effect of drug.
Drowsiness, stupor, coma, grand mal seizures, death	None	Use may lead to psychotic behavior, irritationality, and panic.
Psychosis	None	Physiological effects of use are under investigation.
Drowsiness, confusion, hypotension, coma, death	Tremors, agitation, anxiety, grand mal seizures, abdominal cramps, vomiting, diaphoresis	Dependence may occur insidiously. Users may underreport amount taken because of guilt about multiple prescriptions and abuse.

suggesting recent injections. There may be evidence of old injection sites that appear hyperpigmented and shiny or scarred. The palms may be reddened, or the client may have bright spots (petechiae) on the skin, especially the face. These are characteristic of advanced alcoholism. The nurse observes the client for evidence of poor hygiene habits, weight loss, malnourishment, and poor dentition. Physical assessment may alert the nurse to the existence of a substance abuse problem, even if the client initially denies it during the health history. A toxicological blood screening and urinalysis will ascertain the type of drug that the client has used within the past several days.

Interviewing the Chemically Dependent Client

Because of the shame and embarrassment regarding chemical use, clients are often reluctant to reveal the extent of their use or the consequences of it. A man who lost his job because of substance use at work may tell the nurse that he got laid off because of lack of business. It takes a great deal of skill for the nurse to be able to empathize enough with the client so that accurate information can be obtained without encouraging self-pity. It is very difficult to get completely accurate information from the client because the information is often distorted. Even skillful nurses sometimes have difficulty getting accurate data.

The health history, or client interview, begins with less-threatening questions and progresses to the topics of illicit drug and alcohol use. The nurse asks questions about cigarettes; caffeinated beverages; OTC medications, including cold medications containing alcohol and diphenhydramine (Benadryl) that have a particularly high potential for abuse; prescription medications, including the frequently abused benzodiazepines; and alcohol and drugs including opiates, stimulants, hallucinogens, barbiturates, and inhalants.

Questions should be stated in a matter-of-fact manner to imply expectation (for example, "What drugs do you use? Heroin? Cocaine? PCP? Inhalants, such as paint or glue?"). The nurse inquires about individual drugs as the client may not volunteer specific information. The nurse also asks about the amount of alcohol the client consumes on a daily or weekly basis. The nurse does not simply ask, "Do you drink?" Vague answers from the client should alert the nurse to clarify estimates of use in a calm, concerned tone of voice. The nurse should pay attention to the client's nonverbal behavior during the interview, which may reveal whether the client feels threatened, defensive, or angry.

The nurse wants to assess amount, pattern, date, and time of last use. Although alcohol abusers may admit to using half of the actual amount consumed on a daily basis, drug abusers report twice the amount taken. Thus drug abusers may be attempting to convince the health care professional that their tolerance is greater than it really is so that they will receive enough medication during detoxification to get high. The pattern can be daily use of binging episodes in which the client uses for a continuous period of time (hours or days) until forced to stop by illness, accident, or unconsciousness and then goes for extended periods without using. Date and time of last use are important to know when to expect the emergence of signs and symptoms of withdrawal.

The client may be resistant to accepting that substance abuse is a problem. The task of the nurse at this point is to draw a relationship between observable indications of substance abuse and areas of concern, particularly health. Confrontation must be firm but gentle and address the consequences that the client is experiencing secondary to the substance abuse. The nurse cannot force the client to admit to being an alcoholic or drug addict.

The family should be included in the nursing assessment to substantiate the extent of the substance abuse and the effects on the client and family such as emotional, financial, social, or structural problems (for example, who makes the decisions in place of the substance abuser?) (Chychula, 1984). Family members may experience relief that their family problem has been identified or become defensive and guarded about substance abuse in the family or the client. The nurse can provide education regarding self-help groups available to the family and encourage the family's active involvement in treatment.

During the interview and nursing history, the nurse should also listen for any misconceptions the client may have about the substance itself or the nature of substance abuse. Later, interventions may need to include teaching to provide accurate information so that the client can participate more effectively in care.

Nursing Diagnosis

The assessment of chemically dependent clients and their families reveals clusters of data that indicate a variety of problems affecting all dimensions. Many of the nursing diagnoses are closely related to medical diagnoses. The medical diagnoses of chemical dependency are listed and explained in the *Diagnostic and Statistical Manual of Mental Disorders (DSM III-R)* (APA, 1987).

Because chemically dependent people have so many associated physical, psychological, and social problems, multiple nursing diagnostic categories are

Examples of Nursing Diagnoses for Substance Abuse

NANDA-APPROVED NURSING DIAGNOSES

Altered thought processes (disorientation) related to:
- Drug use
- Alcohol ingestion
- Polysubstance use
- Untreated withdrawal

Altered nutrition: less than body requirements related to:
- Drinking patterns
- Use of financial resources to purchase alcohol or drugs
- Effects of drugs

Bathing/hygiene self-care deficit related to:
- Intoxication
- Decreased level of consciousness
- Decreased level of awareness
- Decreased self-image

Sleep pattern disturbance related to:
- Substance withdrawal
- Alcohol use
- Drug use
- Anxiety

Ineffective individual coping related to:
- Denial of substance of use or abuse
- Lack of support system
- Fear and anxiety
- Chronic unexpressed feelings of guilt, shame, hostility, and despair

Ineffective family coping: compromised or *disabled* related to:
- Isolation from others
- Inadequate finances
- Hostility and anger
- Lack of trust
- Denial and distortion of reality

Spiritual distress related to:
- Value conflict
- Guilt and shame from pain inflicted on others
- Isolation from others
- Sense of hopelessness and meaninglessness
- Feelings of emptiness
- Past unresolved trauma and emotional pain

Sample Nursing Diagnostic Process for Substance

Assessment Activities	Defining Characteristics	Nursing Diagnosis
Ask client about daily meal pattern and types of food consumed while using alcohol. Obtain weight measurement and compare it with normal weight for age and height. Observe food choices client makes every meal.	Client verbalizes eating unbalanced diet (e.g., eats sandwich at home or in fast-food restaurant daily with high-sugar snacks throughout day). Client reports loss of 20 lb in past 5 mo. Client should weigh 151-166 lb but weighs 132 lb. Client selects foods high in fat and sugar and does not select fresh fruits and vegetables. Client is often seen eating candy and chips between meals. Client consumes 6 cups of coffee a day.	*Altered nutrition: less than body requirements* related to alcohol abuse

appropriate (see diagnoses box). When developing the nursing diagnostic label, the nurse must be sure that the necessary defining characteristics are present in the client's data base. This ensures an accurate diagnosis suited to the client's needs. The diagnostic process box demonstrates how to derive a nursing diagnosis for clients with substance abuse.

Planning

After identifying each nursing diagnosis, the nurse develops a care plan for the chemically dependent client. The care plan is based on the client's identified needs and problems. Goals are established by the

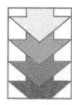 Sample Nursing Care Plan for Substance Abuse

Nursing diagnosis: *altered nutrition: less than body requirements* related to alcohol abuse
Definition: Altered nutrition: less than body requirements is the state in which an individual experiences an intake of nutrients insufficient to meet metabolic needs (Kim, McFarland, McLane, 1991).

Goals	Expected Outcomes	Interventions	Rationale
Client will regain or return to ideal body weight by 30 days.	Client will have weekly weight gain of 3-5 lbs (5/15).	Offer six small, balanced meals a day inclusive of client food preferences.	Small and frequent meals replace high-sugar snacks and one-meal habit.
		Ensure that client eats meals in friendly, relaxed atmosphere.	Relaxed environment aids in mealtime pleasure and digestion.
		Administer vitamins as ordered, and explain rationale for use.	Client is vitamin deficient from prolonged alcohol use.
Client will achieve balanced nutritional status every day.	Client's 24-hr diet history will show improving intake and nutritional status (4/10).	Educate client about rationale and importance of high-protein, high-carbohydrate, low-caffeine diet (see teaching box).	Client lacks knowledge of basic food groups, healthy foods for weight gain, and effects of caffeine as appetite suppressant.
		Teach client to select proper and economical foods.	Actions will reinforce new knowledge and application to everyday meals.
		Have client record everything eaten.	

nurse and client and involve caring for the client's physical health problems, supporting the client and family, and providing education for the client and family (see care plan).

The nurse must first consider providing comfort and safety for the client. For the chemically dependent client, the management of detoxification is the initial goal and first priority. The nurse must determine the client's detoxification needs based on the substance abused, signs and symptoms of withdrawal, and the last use. The client who has an extensive history of alcohol abuse, used several hours before the assessment, and reports a history of DT will have greater safety needs than the client who smokes five marijuana cigarettes a day. The client in cocaine withdrawal who has a complaint of depression and intermittent suicide ideation is at greater risk than the irritable heroin abuser in early withdrawal. The nurse must know about the withdrawal process of every substance to provide individualized care for varying patterns of substance abuse, as well as the client's unique data base. Outcome goals for the client who is in withdrawal include the following:

1. The client will remain free from injury within the first 7 days of hospitalization (as a result of intoxication or detoxification from alcohol or other substances).

2. The client will experience increasing comfort and safety from opiate withdrawal with decreasing complaints of nausea, vomiting, diarrhea, lacrimation, rhinorrhea, chills, and abdominal and muscle cramps within 3 days of hospitalization.

While obtaining the health history, the nurse may discover that the client has numerous physical complaints related to the long-term use of drugs or alcohol. The client may complain of weight loss from inadequate caloric intake, peripheral neuritis from vitamin deficiencies, infections from nonsterile injections, and loss of sexual functioning related to chronic substance abuse. The nurse may also discover that prior health problems have been exacerbated as a result of noncompliance with treatment regimens while using drugs and alcohol (for example, the client who discontinues blood pressure medication or an HIV-positive client who seldom eats, avoids exercise, and expends all energy procuring drugs and alcohol). Outcome goals for the client to maintain or promote physiological integrity may include the following:

1. The client will gradually gain weight (6 to 10 lb) during the 21-day rehabilitation.

2. The client's complaints of stomach pains and requests for antacids will decrease within the first 7 days of hospitalization.

The nurse will also identify client needs and problems related to the promotion and maintenance of psychosocial integrity. The client may deny a substance abuse problem to the nurse by minimizing the effects of the substance abuse with statements such as "I drink as much as the next guy," "My boss has just been waiting to fire me. It doesn't have anything to do with my cocaine use," or "I'm here so that my wife will come back."

The client may admit to a substance abuse problem but lack the knowledge to adequately cope and maintain abstinence. The nurse must plan to educate the client on the availability and importance of compliance with AA or NA as a way to develop a support system and decrease isolation. Also, the client in treatment has a family that is experiencing crisis. Family involvement is essential and may be the only goal if the client's relationships are strained. Family members are often in emotional pain as a result of the consequences of addiction on the functioning of family process. They, too, lack information about the substance abuse and may attempt to deny it, blame others, or resort to violence. The nurse may decide that a referral to Al-Anon will address their needs for knowledge and support, or the threat of family violence may mandate a referral to the local Protective Services Agency to manage the explosive situation. The nurse must be able to establish priorities based on the data. Outcome goals for the client and family to promote and maintain psychosocial integrity may include the following:

1. The client will identify three or more examples of how the substance abuse problem has affected functioning within the first week of hospitalization.
2. The client's spouse will attend two Al-Anon meetings while the client is hospitalized, and the children will attend two Alateen meetings.

Finally, the nurse is concerned with the client's health promotion and maintenance. For the chemically dependent client, the planning stage should include the prevention and management of relapse. The client is vulnerable to relapse for life. Chemical dependency does not go away or get better. The client must find other ways to manage stress. After discontinuing the abuse of alcohol or drugs, the client may be more aware of uncomfortable feelings suppressed by alcohol or drugs. Because these feelings may surface without adequate planning for such stresses, the client will eventually resume substance abuse. Outcome goals related to health promotion and maintenance follow:

1. The client will identify one Alcoholics Anonymous or Adult Children of Alcoholics meeting location and time in the neighborhood to attend after discharge.

2. The client will practice deep breathing as a stress-management technique twice a day while hospitalized.

Modification of goals is an ongoing process when providing care. The nurse must anticipate the long-term needs of the client and family after the immediate care issues have been addressed.

Implementation

Treatment for chemical dependency usually takes place in a unit or treatment center. Based on the principles of AA, treatment helps clients recognize their problems with alcohol or drugs and the effects on their lives, teaches them about chemical dependency, and gives them tools for changing their behavior. Treatment is only the beginning of a continuous, life-long recovery.

An initial intensive phase (inpatient or outpatient) is usually followed by a long-term, outpatient follow-up (from 1 to 2 years). Attendance at self-help groups such as AA or NA is expected. This approach is supported by those who believe that chemical dependency is a primary disease, that genetics and environment play a role in causing it, and that persons can recover by changing their behavior, including abstaining from all mood-altering chemicals.

Detoxification

Alcohol or drug withdrawal is a serious and potentially fatal complication of acute intoxication. **Detoxification** is the process of the removal of mood-altering chemicals from the person's body. Too-rapid removal can result in extreme discomfort, seizures, DT, and sometimes death. Thus most clients are gradually withdrawn from chemicals using long-acting substance medications in place of the short-acting substance. The client is kept quiet, stimuli are reduced, and medications, including vitamins, are given as needed. Good nutrition and fluid balance are also important aspects of treatment.

Detoxification is the first step in treating the chemically dependent client. The client must be free of the immediate effects of chemicals to begin the treatment process. After initial detoxification, which usually lasts a few days unless serious withdrawal symptoms are expected, other health care professionals become involved in the assessment of the client and family and begin to plan and implement care. The nurse continues to manage the client's physical health and participates in other therapeutic activities.

Teaching and Counseling

Often a primary nursing role is to provide information about the potential physiological and psychological effects of substance abuse and the effects of withdrawal for the substance-dependent client. Such information should stress positive aspects rather than attempt to frighten the client into changing abuse habits. Portraying in grisly terms the physiological condition of lung cancer, for example, may cause stress for the chronic cigarette smoker that may increase rather than decrease the desire to smoke. Instead, the nurse can provide information about the success rate of an available treatment program. Other teaching activities include stress-management techniques and self-care activities for hygiene, nutrition, and other areas affected by abuse (see teaching box).

Acute Care Interventions

Acute care interventions, which depend on the client's health status and the body systems affected by the substance, often involve medical interventions, physiological supportive measures, and a variety of nursing interventions. Emergency therapies may be required in cases of alcoholic coma caused by acute intoxication, hepatic coma related to liver malfunctioning, or trauma caused by falls or accidents while under a drug's influence. Emergency treatments may include the administration of narcotic antagonists for opiate overdose, safety measures in cases of acute toxic psychosis, treatment for respiratory or cardiac depression, and treatment for withdrawal syndromes. In most cases the specific substance that resulted in the acute condition must first be identified, followed by a physical assessment and appropriate diagnostic tests.

Interventions for Abusive Behaviors

Nurses may be the recipients of clients' verbal abuse and attempts at manipulation. Chemical effects often lead to anxiety, anger, or paranoia. The verbal attacks on nurses may be clients' expressions of self-hatred related to the substance abuse. In such circumstances, nurses keep themselves and their clients in an emotional balance. Often, nurses react to such abuse and become angry and resentful.

When a client makes critical remarks, the nurse should not become upset. The client may needle or insult the nurse in an attempt to arouse anger, pity, or fear. If the nurse reacts emotionally, verbal attacks are likely to continue. A calm but firm response discourages the client from continuing such manipulative efforts. If the client makes a sexual advance toward the nurse, the nurse confronts the behavior as inappropriate and redirects the client's attention to the present situation, including the reason for being in the nursing unit or the type of care received. The nurse must have a high level of self-esteem to be able to manage the client's physical, mental, or emotional harassment and help the client move beyond these destructive behaviors.

The nurse also takes time out from caring for abusive or manipulative clients. A coffee or lunch break helps relieve emotional tension. The nurse must remember that the client's hostility is the result of intoxication, withdrawal, and illness and that the client will respond to firm limits about behavioral expectations stated in a calm manner.

Community Programs

In many communities, there are a range of substance abuse programs to which the nurse can refer the client. Most notably, AA and NA are self-help groups that assist substance abusers through mutual support to acknowledge the problem and work toward solving it. These groups address the daily issues of recovery and provide an opportunity for the addict to decrease the sense of social isolation. AA and NA resources are listed in the telephone book to provide

---

Client Teaching on Nutrition for a Client with Substance Abuse

OBJECTIVE

- Client will plan a menu for three meals a day for the first week after discharge.

TEACHING STRATEGIES

- Educate client about the basic food groups.
- Discuss how cocaine and alcohol are appetite suppressants and interfere with nutritional status (e.g., elevated liver enzyme and serum cholesterol levels).
- Provide numerous examples of high-protein, high-carbohydrate foods.
- Discuss effective and healthy foods to increase weight.
- Discuss diseases related to a sustained high-fat, high-sugar diet.
- Discuss how a balanced diet contains all the necessary vitamins and minerals.
- Discuss other caffeine-free beverages to replace coffee.
- Suggest quick but healthy recipes.
- Discuss the importance of breakfast.
- Discuss how exercise can stimulate the appetite and desire to eat healthy foods.
- Assist client in developing menu for first day.

EVALUATION

- Observe client plan 1-week menu.

Sample Evaluation of Interventions For Substance Abuse

Goals	Evaluative Measures	Expected Outcomes
Client will regain or return to ideal body weight in 3 days.	Weigh client every Monday, Wednesday, and Friday before breakfast on same scale.	Client will gain 3-5 lb weekly.
Client will achieve balanced nutritional status every day.	Monitor calorie count each day.	Client's 24-hr diet history will show improved intake.
	Monitor liver function tests and serum cholesterol levels every Monday.	Client's liver function tests and serum cholesterol levels will show progressive decreases.
	Observe client's food intake patterns every day.	Client will improve type and quality of food (e.g., food groups, caffeine-free beverage and avoidance of high-sugar, high-fat snacks).
	Test client's knowledge about nutritional value of selected foods.	Client will correctly state nutritional value of selected food.
		Client's 1-week menu will contain foods with high nutritional value.

assistance in locating meetings in the community. Similar support groups exist. These include Al-Anon and Naranon for spouses and relatives of addicts and Alateen for children and adolescents of alcoholics and drug abusers. These self-help groups attempt to understand the addiction as an illness, address how loved ones may enable the disease, and encourage and support family members in helping themselves live fuller lives.

Many inpatient and outpatient substance abuse clinics offer treatment programs independently or in association with hospitals or community mental health centers. These programs may provide counseling, health education, and medical services such as Antabuse clinics or methadone maintenance or withdrawal services.

Detoxification inpatient units generally include a 4- to 7-day stay, whereas rehabilitation programs provide in-depth education and counseling for 2 to 4 weeks. Other types of community resources include employee assistance programs within businesses and industries and student health clinics in high schools and colleges.

Prevention programs are becoming more prominent in community health settings such as schools and mental health clinics. The primary focus of preventive programs is provision of drug education, strengthening family functioning, improving social conditions, and assisting individuals in interpersonal skills and self-esteem. Such a focus helps minimize or eliminate factors that may lead to the abuse of substances as coping or escape mechanisms. The

nurse can initiate preventive interventions of such as educating the client about drugs, promoting effective coping mechanisms, and providing support.

Evaluation

Evaluation of nursing care for clients with substance abuse problems is based on goals of care and expected outcomes (see evaluation box). Evaluation consists of a review of the established goals by examining the outcomes of nursing care with the expected outcomes. The client's progress in meeting the established goals and response to identified nursing interventions are the critical components of this process.

Unfortunately, the client and nurse often choose long-term abstinence as the expected outcome. The client sincerely makes statements never to return to alcohol or drug use again. However, the client may relapse at some point. **Relapse** occurs when the client, who has been abstinent anywhere from several months or years, uses again. The nurse may use the evaluation process to teach the client that "normal" or infrequent substance abuse cannot be resumed for life and that the client must guard against relapse occurrence.

Long-term abstinence is an unrealistic goal and will result in frustration. A more important criteria is that the client make significant progress toward long-term goals. Progress toward long-term goals can be evaluated by the client's involvement in a thorough recovery plan.

Denial of the problem and its severity interferes with the client's understanding that aftercare is essential to maintaining abstinence. The nurse must determine whether the client has identified local self-help groups to attend while in the health care setting or whether this is left to spontaneity after discharge. The nurse asks about the client's intended frequency for attending meetings and an NA or AA group where a "sponsor" could be found for guidance and support when urges and cravings occur. The nurse determines whether the client will be returning for outpatient counseling and whether the client is aware of the need for ongoing treatment. Most clients assume that once the drinking or drugging is stopped, outpatient treatment is not important. However, long-term goals, such as gaining increased self-esteem, learning to use more effective coping mechanisms and internal resources when confronted by stress, and forming behavioral patterns and activities that replace substance-related behaviors, are goals to establish and work toward in outpatient counseling.

Progress toward long-term goals can be evaluated with the family. The nurse asks how family members are planning to take care of themselves and whether they would consider family or couple counseling. They may become involved with Al-Anon to obtain support, examine enabling behaviors, and develop their own personal goals. Often families suffer in isolation with a chemically dependent member because they are not aware of how they can help themselves.

During the evaluation process, the nurse and client also review reasonable and objective short-term goals that were addressed. The nurse evaluates the client's compliance with treatment, including attendance at all group meetings, observance of rules, and active participation in the program. The client may make statements indicating introspection or make comments "romanticizing" the substance of abuse or comparing amounts of consumption. Lack of involvement, limit testing, or "drug/alcohol talk" often indicates whether a client is struggling with denial and whether treatment is really necessary. The nurse modifies the care plan to focus on examination of the aspects affected by the use of drugs or alcohol.

The nurse evaluates whether the client has been unable to refrain from substance abuse while in the treatment program. The nurse and client cannot project the length of time that the client will remain substance free but can establish the treatment period as a short-term goal for abstinence.

The nurse also evaluates short-term goals of weight gain, sleep, stress management, and coping techniques the client has identified and agreed to practice. The client's response to teaching is evaluated by the client's verbalization of understanding and incorporation of these concepts into behavior and daily activities.

Short-term goal evaluation with the family includes their understanding of the information regarding the disease concept of addiction, available family resources in the community, and relapse anticipation and management. The nurse and family may have devised the short-term goal that all family members attend two self-help group meetings before the client's discharge. If the expected and actual outcome is incongruent, the nurse needs to re-evaluate the family's attitude about addiction and the problem. Many family members will state the client, not the family, is the one with the problem. In this case, the family members are struggling with their own denial about the impact of addiction and ineffective family coping.

 ## SUMMARY

Substance abuse takes a variety of forms and may be encountered in any setting. Because substance abuse affects the client in all dimensions, the nurse should be alert to actual and potential health problems associated with abuse patterns. Although any person at any age and in any life situation may become physiologically or psychologically dependent on a drug or substance, including nurses and other health professionals, certain groups may be more susceptible to the problem of abuse at certain developmental stages. The client's family will also be affected in a variety of ways, and the nurse should include the family in the care plan.

The nurse's choice of the appropriate interventions for the client with a substance abuse problem depends on the cause of the abuse and the client's health status. Because society is increasingly aware of substance abuse as a health problem, it carries less stigma than in the past, and individuals with abuse problems are now more likely to seek help before physiological problems bring them to the attention of health care professionals. The increasing societal recognition of the problem has brought a wider variety of support and treatment services, including prevention programs. Substance abuse remains a sensitive area for many clients, however, and the nurse must be particularly aware of communication skills and other aspects of the nurse-client relationship when providing care to clients who are experiencing psychosocial stresses commonly associated with substance abuse.

REFERENCES

American Nurses Association: *Addictions and psychological dysfunctions in nursing: the profession's response to the problem,* Kansas City, Mo, 1984, The Association.

American Psychiatric Association: *Diagnostic and statistical manual of mental disorders (DSM III-R),* Washington, DC, 1987, The Association.

Begleiter H et al: Event-related brain potentials in boys at risk for alcoholism, *Science* 225:1493, 1984.

Bissell L, Haberman PW: *Alcoholism in the professions,* New York, 1984, Oxford University Press.

Bohan M: *Overview of addictions.* Presented at Drugs: the new war, Hampton, Va, Sept 20, 1990.

Chychula N: Screening for substance abuse in a primary care setting, *Nurse Pract* July 1984, p 15.

Fisk N, Devoto D: The nurse employee who uses alcohol/other drugs. In Reed S, editor: *Problem employee behaviors,* Baltimore, 1991, Williams & Wilkins.

Goodwin DW et al: Alcohol problems in adoptees raised apart from alcoholic biological parents, *Arch Gen Psy* 31:238, 1973.

Goodwin DW et al: Genetic component of alcholism, *Ann Rev Med* 32:93, 1981.

Hahn AB, Barkin RL, Oestreich SJK: *Pharmacology in nursing,* ed 16, St Louis, 1986, Mosby–Year Book.

Kaplan H, Saddock B: *Modern synopsis of comprehensve textbook of psychiatry,* ed 4, Baltimore, 1985, Williams & Wilkins.

Khantzian E: The self-medication hypothesis of addictive disorders, *Am J Psych* 142:11, 1985.

Kim MJ, McFarland GK, McLane AM: *Picket guide to nursing diagnoses,* ed 4, St Louis, 1991, Mosby–Year Book.

Miller W, Dackis C, Gold M: The relationship of addiction, tolerance and dependence to alcohol and drugs: a neurochemical approach, *J Sub Abuse Treat* 4:73, 1987.

National Institute of Drug Abuse: *Personal communication,* Nov 13, 1991.

Osgood N: *Alcohol and the elderly.* Presented at Drugs: the new war, Hampton, Va, Sept 20, 1990.

Sullivan EJ: Cost savings of retaining chemically dependent nurses, *Nurs Econ* 4(4):179, 1987.

Sullivan EJ, Bissell L, Williams E: *Chemical dependency in nursing: the deadly diversion,* Menlo Park, Calif, 1988, Addison-Wesley.

Woody G: *Pharmacology of abused drugs.* Presented at Substance abuse treatment in the 90s, St Louis, June 4, 1990.

ADDITIONAL READINGS

Cody B: Alcohol and other drug abuse among adolescents, *Stat Bull Metropol Life Insur Co* 65(1):4, 1984.

Dusek D, Girdano DA: *Drugs: a factual account,* Reading, Mass, 1980, Addison-Wesley.

Estes NJ, Heinemann ME: *Alcoholism: development, consequences, and interventions,* ed 3, St Louis, 1986, Mosby–Year Book.

Estes NJ, Smith-DiJulio K, Heinemann ME, editors: *Nursing diagnosis of the alcoholic person,* St Louis, 1980, Mosby–Year Book.

Freedman AM: Opiate dependence. In Kaplan HI, Freedman AM, Sadock BJ: *Comprehensive textbook of psychiatry,* ed 3, Baltimore, 1980, Williams & Wilkins.

Greene MH et al: Evolving patterns of drug abuse, *Ann Intern Med* 83:402, 1975.

Hughes R, Brewin R: *The tranquilizing of America: pill popping and the American way of life,* New York, 1979, Harcourt Brace Jovanovich.

Isler C: The alcoholic nurse: what we try to deny, *RN* 41:48, 1978.

Lawrence F et al: Admitting an intoxicated patient, *Am J Nurs* 84(5):617, 1984.

Ray O, Ksir C: *Drugs, society, and human behavior,* ed 5, St Louis, 1990, Mosby–Year Book.

Sullivan EJ: A descriptive study of 139 recovering chemically dependent nurses, *Arch Psy Nurs* 1(3):1984, 1987.

Sullivan EJ: Comparison of chemically dependent and nondependent nurses on familial, personal, and professional characteristics, *J Stud Alcohol* 48(6):563, 1987.

Yowell S, Brose C: Working with drug abuse patients in the ER, *Am J Nurs* 77:82, 1977.

CHAPTER 46 REVIEW

Key Concepts

- Chemical dependency is a major health care problem.

- There are many myths surrounding chemical dependency.

- Any substance that produces physiological or psychological effects can be misused or abused.

- Each major group of abused drugs produces distinct psychological and physiological effects.

- The cause of chemical dependency is not known but heredity is a predisposing factor.

- Many psychosocial variables have a causative role in substance abuse, including pleasure-seeking, problem-solving, or avoidance behaviors; personality factors; sociocultural factors; and stressors.

- No one cause or set of causes affects all or most persons who abuse a substance.

- To facilitate the therapeutic relationship and to work toward solving the problems of substance abuse, the client and nurse should be aware of their attitudes toward the abused substance and the causes of the abuse.

- The course of substance abuse varies but typically progresses from social misuse or experimentation through a gradually increasing pattern of abuse to a state of dependence in which all aspects of life are affected.

- Substance abuse affects family functioning, roles, and responsibilities, often with seriously detrimental psychosocial effects on spouse and children.

- Causes and effects of substance abuse vary among developmental stages, and therefore a developmental perspective should be included when a abuse problem is assessed.

- The fetus is susceptible to the effects of substance abuse by the mother.

- Nurses and other health professionals are highly susceptible to abuse problems and need to be aware of how such problems can develop and what interventions may be necessary.

- The assessment of a client with a substance abuse problem may include a tactfully obtained history, observation of behaviors linked to substance abuse, and a complete psychosocial and physical assessment.

- Nursing diagnoses for clients with abuse problems identify needs for physiological support and problems involving stress, interpersonal conflicts, altered work or family roles, and self-concept deficits.

- Intervention and treatment provide an opportunity for the chemically dependent person to alter behavior regarding use of chemicals, as well as begin lifestyle changes.

- Interventions may address the client's needs in all dimensions and may include acute care, teaching and counseling, support systems, family interventions, and the use of community resources.

- Evaluation of the care of substance abusers should be based on realistic goals and focuses on day-to-day progress toward long-term goals.

Key Terms

Addiction, p. 1583

Alcohol, p. 1577

Benzodiazepines, p. 1579

Chemical dependency, p. 1574

Circumstantial use, p. 1577

CNS sympathomimetics, p. 1579

Compulsive use, p. 1577

Cross-tolerance, p. 1575

Delirium tremens (DTs), p. 1578

Detoxification, p. 1591

Escape mechanism, p. 1582

Fetal alcohol syndrome (FAS), p. 1576

Hallucinogens, p. 1580

Hallucinosis, p. 1578

Inhalants, p. 1581

Intensified use, p. 1577

Marijuana, p. 1580

Misuse, p. 1574

Opiate derivatives, p. 1578

Physiological dependence, p. 1575

Primary effect, p. 1574

Psychological dependence, p. 1575

Recreational use, p. 1577

Relapse, p. 1593

"Remembering," p. 1575

Secondary effects, p. 1575

Sedative-hypnotic drugs, p. 1579

Substance, p. 1574

Substance abuse, p. 1574

Tolerance, p. 1575

Withdrawal, p. 1575

Withdrawal syndrome, p. 1575

Critical Thinking Exercises

1. Mr. T. is a 41-year-old client who has been admitted for pneumonia. During the nursing assessment, the client reveals a problem with alcohol and cocaine abuse. What other assessment data do you need to provide for the client's safety needs?

2. Mr. G. has been admitted for gastritis and other gastrointestinal complaints. He makes frequent references to the amount of alcohol he drinks and how alcohol is a major part of his social group. He is beginning to show signs of physical consequences of drinking, such as elevated liver enzyme levels, memory lapses while drinking, and hypertension. His wife tells you that she thinks he drinks too much but that he does not listen to her concerns. Identify four interventions to assist the client and his wife in addressing his problem with alcohol.

3. Ms. A. is a 22-year-old client who was admitted for complaints of chest pain after ingesting large doses of cocaine during a crack "run." She was very frightened about the chest pain and has begun to address her cocaine abuse. What referral resources could you share with her?

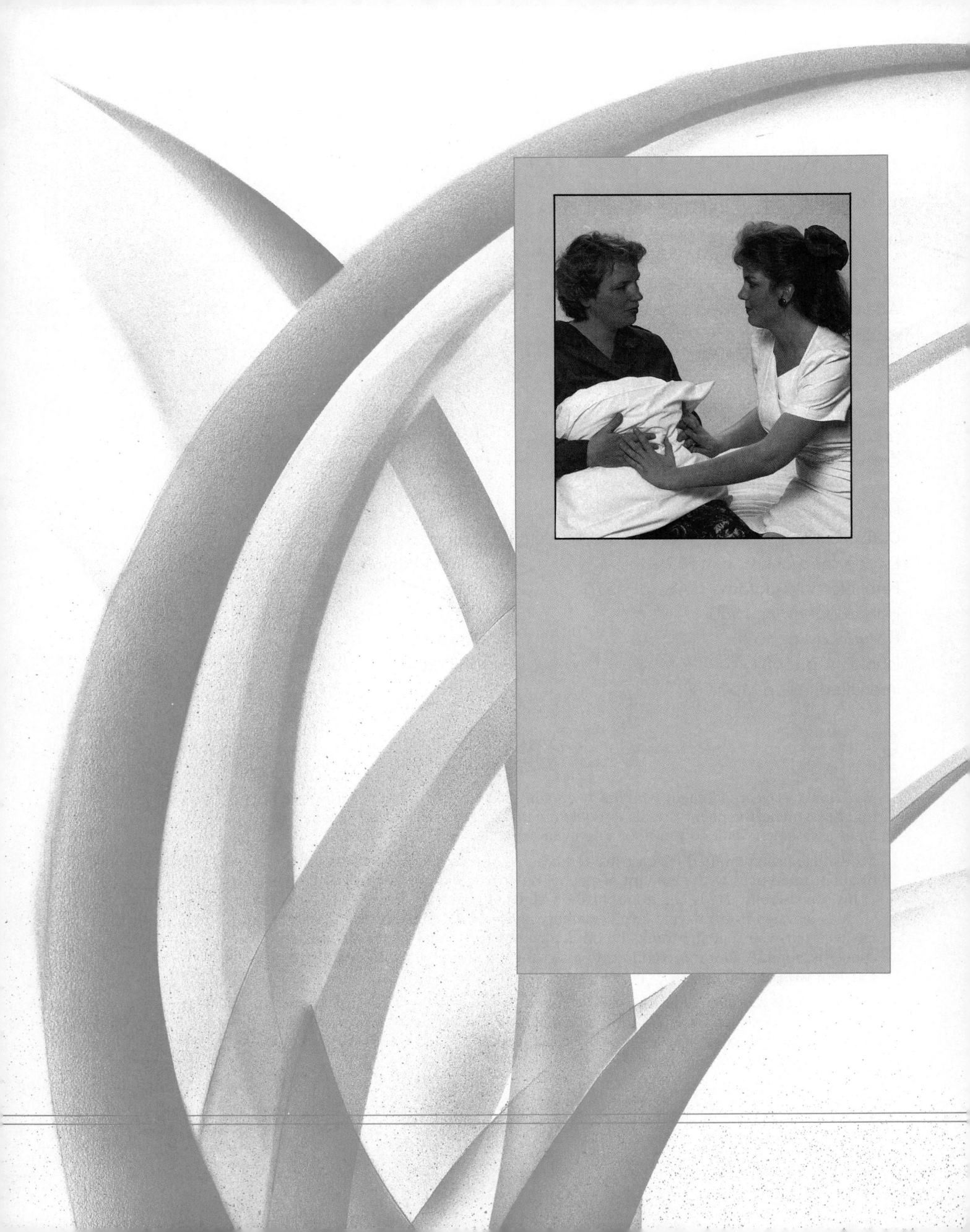

UNIT 9

Caring for the Perioperative Client

CHAPTER 47

Surgical Client

OBJECTIVES

Mastery of content in this chapter will enable the student to:

- Define the key terms listed.
- Explain the concept of perioperative nursing care.
- Differentiate between classifications of surgery.
- List factors to include in the preoperative assessment of a surgical client.
- Describe how to correctly witness a client's informed consent for surgery.
- Demonstrate postoperative exercises: diaphragmatic breathing, coughing, turning, and leg exercises.
- Design a preoperative teaching program.
- Prepare a client for surgery on the morning of a scheduled operation.
- Compare and contrast the actions and side effects of general, regional, and local anesthesia.
- Explain the nurse's role in the operating room.
- Describe the nurse's role in phase I and II recovery.
- Identify factors to include in the postoperative assessment of a client in recovery.
- Describe the rationale for nursing interventions designed to prevent postoperative complications.
- Explain the difference and similarities in caring for outpatient versus inpatient surgical clients.

CHAPTER OUTLINE

client faces a variety of stressors when confronting surgery. Anticipating surgery leads to fear and anxiety for clients who associate surgery with pain, possible disfigurement, dependence, and perhaps even loss of life. Family members often fear a disruption in lifestyle and experience a sense of powerlessness as the surgery approaches. The trauma sustained during surgery creates physical needs requiring close supervision and skilled intervention by the nurse and physician. The client is better able to cooperate and participate in the care plan if the nurse has provided information about events occurring before and after surgery.

Most surgery is performed in hospitals. However, ambulatory outpatient surgical units are increasingly common. A client enters the unit, undergoes surgery, and returns home the same day. Nurses working in both settings must understand the principles of caring for surgical clients.

HISTORY OF SURGICAL NURSING

Surgery became a medical specialty in the mid-nineteenth century. Surgery gave physicians the means to treat conditions that were difficult or impossible to manage only by pure medicine. However, early surgeons had little knowledge of the principles of asepsis, and anesthesia techniques were primitive and unsafe. Nurses working in the first operating rooms cleaned the rooms and equipment, performed technical tasks such as obtaining supplies, and occasionally accompanied the client to the surgical ward to deliver nursing care.

With the advent of antiseptic and later aseptic practices, surgery became a treatment of choice for many conditions. The development of safer anesthetic gases allowed surgeons to conduct longer operative procedures. All surgery was conducted in hospital settings. Operating room nurses required special training for new responsibilities (such as assisting the surgeon during surgery, preparing sterile equipment, and caring for the surgical client). Massachusetts General Hospital provided the first operating room education for nurses in 1876 (Metzger, 1976). This trend continued into the 1900s as nursing schools included operating room experience in each nurse's clinical instruction.

In 1956 the Association of Operating Room Nurses (AORN) was formed to gain knowledge of surgical principles and explore methods to improve nursing care of surgical clients. The association met many challenges, including overcoming the idea that operating room nurses were only technically skilled practitioners. The organization developed standards

of nursing practice to establish the need for registered nurses in the operating room.

During the 1970s a change occurred in nursing education. A focus on the importance of nurses' acquiring a broad knowledge resulted in less emphasis on operating room techniques. Many schools eliminated operating room experience from curriculums. As a result, nurses missed practicing strict aseptic techniques and observing the delicate anatomy of the human body. Today, many nursing schools have reinstituted clinical operating room experience.

There has also been a new development in the setting for operative procedures. Ambulatory surgery, sometimes referred to as *outpatient* or *one-day surgery,* is a health care service that is growing rapidly in numbers and types of procedures performed. **Ambulatory surgery** is a scheduled surgical procedure provided for a client who does not remain overnight in a hospital. Small biopsies, cosmetic surgery, and cataract extractions are just a few examples of ambulatory procedures.

There are distinct benefits for the client undergoing ambulatory surgery. Discovery of anesthetic drugs that metabolize rapidly with few aftereffects allows shorter operative times. Surgeons recognize the benefit of early postoperative ambulation and encourage clients to assume a more active role in recovery. Ambulatory surgery also offers cost savings by eliminating the need for hospital stays. A variety of ambulatory surgical settings have emerged over the past 10 years, but these are the following four basic types:
1. Hospital based. Outpatient and inpatient procedures are done in main operating room suites.
2. Hospital affiliated. A separate, self-contained area is in or next to an inpatient facility.
3. Hospital satellite. A unit is owned by a hospital but is physically separated from it.
4. Private or free-standing. A unit is owned and operated by surgeons or private investors.

In addition to traditional inpatient surgical stays that may last several days and outpatient ambulatory surgery, most hospitals have same-day surgical programs. In a same-day surgical program a client is admitted early on the morning of surgery and stays one night during recovery.

Procedures, such as tumor biopsies and gallbladder removal (**cholecystectomy**) can now be done using laser procedures. For example, a laser cholecystectomy can now be done and involves only a 24- to 48-hour hospital stay and a recovery period of 7 to 10 days (Jackson et al, 1990). By contrast, a traditional cholecystectomy usually involves at least a 4-week recovery period. Thus many surgeons have recently begun using laser procedures instead of traditional surgical procedures, thereby decreasing the length of surgery and hospitalization (Gallagher, Kahn, 1990).

Ambulatory and same-day surgical programs provide challenges for surgical nurses. Before surgery, nurses must find creative ways to educate clients and family members. The preparation time before surgery is shortened, so nurses must perform complete assessments efficiently. The surgical procedures performed in ambulatory surgery also require special considerations by the nurse. Changing trends in care of surgical clients has changed the nurse's role.

PERIOPERATIVE NURSING CARE

Perioperative nursing refers to the role of the nurse during the preoperative, intraoperative, and postoperative phases of a client's surgical experience. The concept of perioperative nursing stresses the importance of providing continuity of care. In many hospitals, operating room nurses assess a client's health status preoperatively, identify specific needs, teach and counsel, attend to the client's needs in the operating room, and then follow recovery. However, in other institutions, different nurses care for the surgical client during each phase of the surgical experience. Involving the operating room nurse in each phase of the client's care provides a smooth course for therapy. The nurse's major responsibility is to provide safe, consistent, and effective nursing care during each phase of surgery.

CLASSIFICATION OF SURGERY

The types of surgical procedures are classified according to the seriousness, urgency, or purpose of surgery (Table 47-1). A procedure may fall into more-

TABLE 47-1	Classification for Surgical Procedures	
Type	Description	Example
SERIOUSNESS		
Major	Involves extensive reconstruction or alteration in body parts; poses great risks to well-being	Coronary artery bypass, colon resection, removal of larynx, resection of lung lobe
Minor	Involves minimal alteration in body parts; often designed to correct deformities; involves minimal risks compared with major procdures	Cataract extraction, facial plastic surgery, skin graft, tooth extraction
URGENCY		
Elective	Is performed on basis of client's choice; is not essential and may not be necessary for health	Bunionectomy, facial plastic surgery, hernia repair, breast reconstruction
Urgent	Is necessary for client's health, may prevent additional problems from developing (e.g., tissue destruction or impaired organ function); not necessarily emergency	Excision of cancerous tumor, removal of gallbladder for stones, vascular repair for obstructed artery (e.g., coronary artery bypass)
Emergency	Must be done immediately to save life or preserve function of body part	Repair of perforated appendix, repair of traumatic amputation, control of internal hemorrhaging
PURPOSE		
Diagnostic	Is surgical exploration that allows physician to confirm diagnosis; may involve removal of tissue for further diagnostic testing	Exploratory laparotomy (incision into peritoneal cavity to inspect abdominal organs), breast mass biopsy
Ablative	Is excision or removal of diseased body part	Amputation, removal of appendix, cholecystectomy
Palliative	Relieves or reduces intensity of disease symptoms; will not produce cure	Colostomy, debridement of necrotic tissue, resection of nerve roots
Reconstructive	Restores function or appearance to traumatized or malfunctioning tissues	Internal fixation of fractures, scar revision
Transplant	Is performed to replace malfunctioning organs or structures	Kidney, cornea, or liver transplant; total hip replacement
Constructive	Restores function lost or reduced as result of congenital anomalies	Repair of cleft palate, closure of atrial septal defect in heart

than one classification. For example, surgical removal of a disfiguring scar is minor in seriousness, elective in urgency, and reconstructive in purpose. Frequently, the classes overlap. An urgent procedure is also considered major in seriousness. The same operation may be performed for different reasons on different clients. For example, a gastrectomy may be performed as an emergency procedure to resect a bleeding ulcer or as an urgent procedure to remove a cancerous growth. The classification indicates to the nurse the level of care a client might require.

 PREOPERATIVE SURGICAL PHASE

Surgical clients enter the health care setting in different stages of health. A client may enter the hospital or ambulatory satellite unit on a predetermined day feeling relatively healthy and prepared to face elective surgery. In contrast, a victim of a vehicle accident may face emergency surgery with no time to prepare.

The surgical client undergoes tests and procedures to confirm or rule out alterations requiring surgery. Many tests can be performed in the physician's office or an outpatient laboratory, preventing the need for hospitalization before surgery. Usually, clients scheduled for ambulatory surgery have tests done several days before surgery. However, the tests can also be done the morning of surgery.

The client meets many health care personnel, including surgeons, nurse anesthetists or anesthesiologists, therapists, and nurses. All play a role in the client's care and recovery. Family members attempt to provide support through their presence but face many of the same stressors as the client. The nurse assesses the client's physical and emotional well-being, recognizes the degree of surgical risk, coordinates diagnostic tests, identifies nursing diagnoses reflecting the client's and family members' needs, prepares the client physically and mentally for surgery, and communicates pertinent information to the surgical team.

 Assessment

Assessment of the surgical client involves collecting a nursing history, performing a physical examination, reviewing the client's and family members' emotional health, and analyzing risk factors and diagnostic data. The length of the preoperative period determines the thoroughness of assessment.

For example, if a client is a same-day admission, it may be difficult to do a comprehensive physical ex-

amination. In this case, the nurse focuses on key measurements for all body systems to ensure that no obvious problems are overlooked. Even though the physician will screen the client before scheduling surgery, preoperative assessment occasionally reveals an abnormality that delays or cancels surgery. Usually, however, the assessment establishes normal values for the client and alerts the nurse to possible postoperative complications.

Nursing History

The nurse conducts an initial interview to collect a history similar to that described in Chapter 6. In the ambulatory surgical setting, the history may be shorter than that collected when the client is hospitalized the evening before surgery. If a client is unable to relate all necessary information, the nurse may ask family members.

MEDICAL HISTORY. A review of the client's medical history should include past illnesses and the primary reason for seeking medical care. The physician's history is an excellent source. Another valuable source of data is medical records from past hospitalizations.

When the nurse first assesses the client, the reasons for surgery may be unclear, or the client may not yet know whether surgery will be required. Preexisting illnesses can influence the ability to tolerate surgery and reach full recovery (Table 47-2). Candidates for ambulatory surgery must be carefully screened for medical conditions that may increase the risk for complications during or after surgery.

PREVIOUS SURGERIES. A client's past experience with surgery can influence physical and psychological responses to a procedure. The type of previous surgery, level of discomfort, extent of disability, and overall level of care provided are some factors the client may recall. The nurse determines any unpleasant factors and complications that the client experienced. This information helps the nurse anticipate the client's preoperative and postoperative needs.

Previous surgery may also influence the level of physical care required after a surgical procedure. For example, a client who has had a previous thoracotomy for resection of a lung lobe has a greater risk for postoperative pulmonary complications than a client with intact normal lungs.

CLIENTS' AND FAMILY MEMBERS' PERCEPTIONS AND UNDERSTANDING OF SURGERY. The nurse must prepare clients and their families for the surgical experience. Identification of clients' knowledge, expectations, and perceptions allows the nurse to plan teaching and emotional preparation measures. If clients are scheduled for ambulatory surgery, assessment

TABLE 47-2   Medical Conditions That Increase the Risks of Surgery

Type of Condition	Reason for Risk
Bleeding disorders (thrombocytopenia, hemophilia)	Disorders increase risk of hemorrhaging during and after surgery.
Diabetes mellitus	Diabetes increases susceptibility to infection and may impair wound healing from altered glucose metabolism and associated circulatory impairment. Fluctuating blood levels may cause central nervous system (CNS) malfunction during anesthesia. Stress of surgery may cause decreased glucose tolerance.
Heart disease (recent myocardial infarction, dysrhythmias, congestive heart failure)	Stress of surgery causes increased demands on myocardium to maintain cardiac output. General anesthetic agents depress cardiac function.
Upper respiratory infection	Infection increases risk of respiratory complications during anesthesia (e.g., pneumonia and spasm of laryngeal muscles).
Liver disease	Liver disease alters metabolism and elimination of drugs administered during surgery and impairs wound healing because of alterations in protein metabolism.
Fever	Fever predisposes client to fluid and electrolyte imbalances and may indicate underlying infection.
Chronic respiratory disease (emphysema, bronchitis, asthma)	Respiratory disease reduces client's means to compensate for acid-base alterations (see Chapter 38). Anesthetic agents reduce respiratory function, increasing risk for severe hypoventilation.
Immunological disorders (leukemia, acquired immunodeficiency syndrome [AIDS], bone marrow depression after use of chemotherapeutic drugs)	Immunological disorders increase risk of infection and delay wound healing after surgery.

may be performed in the physician's office or clients' homes.

Each client brings fears to the surgical setting. Some are due to past hospital experiences, warnings from friends and family, or lack of knowledge. If a client has had previous surgery, the nurse assesses what the experience was like. The course of recovery, occurrence of complications, or perception of the quality of care given by nurses can influence a client's feelings about upcoming surgery. The nurse faces an ethical dilemma when a client is misinformed or unaware of the reason for surgery. The nurse asks for a description of the client's understanding of the surgery planned and its implications. The nurse might ask questions such as "Tell me about what you think will happen before and after surgery" or "Explain to me what you know about surgery." The nurse should confer with the physician before revealing specific information related to the medical diagnosis. The nurse should also determine whether the physician explained routine preoperative and postoperative procedures. When a client is well prepared and knows what to expect, the nurse reinforces the client's knowledge and maintains accuracy and consistency.

MEDICATION HISTORY. If a client regularly uses prescription or over-the-counter drugs, the physician may temporarily discontinue the drugs before surgery or adjust the dosages (Table 47-3 on p. 1606). Certain drugs have special implications for the surgical client. Prescription drugs taken preoperatively are automatically discontinued postoperatively unless a physician reorders them.

ALLERGIES. The nurse is particulary alert for allergies to drugs that may be given during a phase of the surgical experience. If one or more allergies exist, the client receives an allergy identification band to be worn on the wrist before going to surgery. The nurse also makes sure that the front of the client's chart contains a list of allergies.

SMOKING HABITS. The client who smokes is at a greater risk for postoperative pulmonary complications than a client who does not. The chronic smoker already has an increased amount and thickness of mucous secretions in the lungs. General anesthetics increase airway irritation and stimulate pulmonary secretions, which are retained as a result of reduction in ciliary activity during anesthesia. After surgery the

TABLE 47-3 Drugs with Special Implications for the Surgical Client	
Drug Class	**Effects During Surgery**
Antibiotics	Antibiotics potentiate action of anesthetic agents. If taken within 2 wk before surgery, aminoglycosides (gentamicin, tobramycin, neomycin) may cause mild respiratory depression from depressed neuromuscular transmission.
Antidysrhythmics	Antidysrhythmics can reduce cardiac contractility and impair conduction during anesthesia.
Anticoagulants	Anticoagulants alter normal clotting factors and thus increase risk of hemorrhaging. They should be discontinued at least 48 hr before surgery. Aspirin and ibuprofen are commonly used medications that can alter clotting mechanisms.
Anticonvulsants	Long-term use of certain anticonvulsants (e.g., phenytoin [Dilantin] and phenobarbital) can alter metabolism of anesthetic agents.
Antihypertensives	Antihypertensives interact with anesthetic agents to cause bradycardia, hypotension, and impaired circulation. They inhibit synthesis and storage of norepinephrine in sympathetic nerve endings.
Corticosteroids	With prolonged use, corticosteroids cause adrenal atrophy, which reduces body's ability to withstand stress. Before and during surgery, dosages may be temporarily increased.
Insulin	Diabetic client's need for insulin after surgery is reduced because client fasts. Stress response and intravenous (IV) administration of glucose solutions can increase dosage requirements after surgery.
Diuretics	Diuretics potentiate electrolyte imbalances (particularly potassium) after surgery.

client who smokes has greater difficulty clearing the airways of mucous secretions (see Chapter 38).

ALCOHOL INGESTION. Habitual use of alcohol predisposes the client to adverse reactions to anesthetic drugs. The client also experiences a cross-tolerance to anesthetic drugs, necessitating higher-than-normal doses (see Chapter 46). In addition, the physician may need to increase postoperative dosages of analgesics. Excessive alcohol ingestion can also lead to malnutrition, which may contribute to delayed wound healing.

FAMILY SUPPORT. It is important for the nurse to determine the extent of the client's support from family members or friends. Surgery often results in temporary or permanent disability that requires added assistance during recovery. The client cannot always immediately assume the same level of physical activity enjoyed before an illness. Often a client returns home with dressings to change or exercises to perform. With ambulatory surgery, clients and families assume responsibility for postoperative care. The family is an important resource for the client with physical limitations and provides the emotional support needed to motivate the client to return to a previous state of health.

OCCUPATION. Surgery may result in physical alterations that hinder or prevent a person from returning

to work. The nurse assesses the client's occupational history to anticipate the possible effects of surgery on convalescence and eventual work performance. This prepares the nurse to explain any restrictions before a client returns to work. When a client is unable to return to a job, the nurse confers with a social worker to refer the client to job-training programs or to help the client seek economic assistance.

Review of Emotional Health

Surgery is psychologically stressful. The client is anxious about the surgery and its implications. Clients often feel that they have little control over their situations. Family members perceive the client's surgery as a disruption of their lifestyle. Hospitalization and the recovery period at home may be lengthy. The family is usually concerned about the client returning to a normal, productive life. When the client has chronic illness, the family becomes fearful that surgery may result in further disability. To understand the impact of surgery on a client's and family's emotional health, the nurse assesses the client's feelings about surgery, self-concept, coping resources, and body image.

FEELINGS. The nurse may be able to detect the client's feelings about surgery from mannerisms or behaviors. A fearful client often asks many questions, seems uneasy when strangers enter the room, or actively seeks the company of friends and relatives.

It is often difficult to assess feelings thoroughly when ambulatory surgery is scheduled. The nurse usually has limited time for establishing a relationship with the client. In some outpatient surgical programs the nurse may visit with a client in the home or on the phone before surgery. In a hospital room the nurse should choose a time for discussion after admitting procedures or diagnostic tests are completed. The nurse should explain that it is normal to have fears and concerns. The client's ability to share feelings depends on the nurse's willingness to listen, be supportive, and clarify misconceptions.

If the client feels powerless, the nurse determines the reason. The medical diagnosis may generate apprehension of increased dependence and loss of physical or mental function. The thought of being "put to sleep" under anesthesia creates concern about loss of control. Many clients feel the need to retain the power to make decisions about treatment. The nurse must assure clients of their right to ask questions and seek information.

A client may be angry about the need for surgery. A young person may feel that it is unfair to have a disorder that typically affects older people. Surgery may occur at a time when it is inconvenient or potentially disruptive. The client may occasionally express anger by verbally attacking the nurse or physician. Being argumentative or overly demanding, refusing to cooperate, and criticizing the nurse's efforts to provide care are manifestations of anger and anxiety.

SELF-CONCEPT. Clients with a positive self-concept are more likely to approach surgical experiences appropriately. The nurse assesses self-concept by asking clients to identify personal strengths and weaknesses. Clients who are quick to criticize or scorn personal characteristics may have little self-regard or may be testing the nurse's opinion of their characters. Poor self-concept hinders the ability to adapt to the stress of surgery and aggravates feelings of guilt or inadequacy (see Chapter 31).

COPING RESOURCES. Assessment of feelings and self-concept helps reveal whether the client can cope with the stress of surgery. The nurse also asks the client about past stress management. If the client has had previous surgery, the nurse determines behaviors that helped resolve any tension or nervousness. The nurse may instruct the client on relaxation exercises that can help control anxiety (see Chapter 36).

The nurse should ask if family members or friends can provide support. The client may want someone else present when the nurse provides instructions or explanations. Often a family member can become the client's coach, offering valuable support during the postoperative period when the client's participation in care is vital.

BODY IMAGE. Surgical removal of a diseased body part often leaves permanent disfigurement or alteration in body function. Concern over mutilation or loss of a body part compounds a client's fears.

The nurse assesses for the body image alterations that clients perceive will result from surgery. Individuals will react differently, depending on occupation, self-image, and degree of self-esteem (see Chapter 31).

Often, surgery changes the physical or psychological aspects of clients' sexuality. Excision of breast tissue, colostomies or ureterostomies, or removal of prostate glands may affect sexuality. Surgery such as hernia repair or cataract extraction forces clients to refrain from sexual intercourse until they return to normal physical activity.

The nurse should encourage clients to express concerns about sexuality. The client facing even temporary sexual dysfunction requires understanding and support. Discussions about the client's sexuality should be held with the client's sexual partner so that they can gain a shared understanding of how to cope with limitations in sexual function.

Physical Examination

The nurse conducts a partial or complete physical examination, depending on the amount of time available and the client's preoperative condition. Chapter 20 describes techniques used in physical assessment. Assessment focuses on findings related to the client's medical history and on body systems that will be affected by the surgery.

GENERAL SURVEY. The nurse observes the client's general appearance. Gestures and body movements may reflect weakness caused by illness. The client may appear malnourished. Height and body weight are important indicators of nutritional status.

Preoperative assessment of vital signs, including blood pressure while sitting and standing, provides important baseline data with which to compare alterations that occur during and after surgery. Anxiety and fear commonly cause elevations in heart rate and blood pressure. Anesthetic agents typically depress all vital functions. However, adverse drug reactions may include elevations in heart rate and blood pressure. As the effects of the anesthesia diminish after surgery, the nurse closely monitors vital signs and compares findings with preoperative baselines.

Preoperative assessment of vital signs is also important to rule out fluid and electrolyte abnormalities (see Chapter 39). An elevated heart rate may result from a plasma fluid volume deficit, potassium deficit, or sodium excess. If the pulse is full and bounding, a fluid volume excess may be the cause. Cardiac dysrhythmias are commonly caused by electrolyte imbalances.

An elevated temperature before surgery is a cause for concern. If the client has an underlying infection, the surgeon may choose to postpone surgery until the infection has been treated. An elevated body temperature increases the risk of fluid and electrolyte imbalance after surgery.

HEAD AND NECK. The condition of oral mucous membranes reveals the level of hydration. A dehydrated client is at risk for developing serious fluid and electrolyte imbalances during surgery.

Inspection of the soft palate and nasal sinuses can reveal sinus drainage indicative of respiratory or sinus infection. To rule out the possiblity of local or systemic infection, the nurse palpates for cervical lymph node enlargement.

The nurse inspects the jugular veins for distention. Excess fluid within the circulatory system or failure of the heart to contract efficiently may lead to jugular vein distention. A client with heart disease is at risk for cardiovascular complications during surgery.

INTEGUMENT. The nurse carefully inspects the skin overlying all body parts. Particular attention is paid to bony prominences, such as the elbows, sacrum, and scapula. During surgery, a client must lie in a fixed position, often for several hours. Thus a client is susceptible to pressure ulcers (see Chapter 44) if the skin is thin and dry and has poor turgor. The overall condition of the skin also reveals the client's level of hydration.

THORAX AND LUNGS. Assessment of the client's breathing pattern and chest excursion will aid the nurse in determining ventilatory capacity. Clients are encouraged to deep breathe and cough postoperatively (see section on preoperative teaching). A decline in ventilatory function may place the client at risk for respiratory complications. For example, a client who has high abdominal surgery will have difficulty breathing deeply because of a painful abdominal incision. Auscultation of breath sounds will indicate whether the client has pulmonary congestion or narrowing of airways. Crackles or rales signify moisture in the airways, which will be aggravated during surgery. Serious pulmonary congestion may cause postponement. Certain anesthetics can cause laryngeal muscle spasm. If the nurse auscultates wheezing in the airways preoperatively, the client is at risk for further airway narrowing during surgery.

HEART AND VASCULAR SYSTEM. If the client has cardiac disease, the nurse must assess the character of the apical pulse. After surgery, the nurse compares the rate and rhythm of the pulse with preoperative baselines. Anesthetic agents, alterations in fluid balance, and stimulation from the surgical stress response can cause cardiac dysrhythmias.

The nurse assesses peripheral pulses, capillary refill time, and the color and temperature of extremities to determine a client's circulatory status. Capillary refill time is assessed by depressing the client's finger or toe nail bed until the skin blanches, releasing the pressure, and then noting the amount of time that it takes for the color to return to the original appearance. Acceptable capillary refill occurs in less than 3 seconds. Sluggish capillary refill occurs in more than 3 seconds.

This is particularly important for the client having vascular surgery or for a client who may have casts or constricting bandages applied to the extremities after surgery. Postoperative development of a weak or absent pulse in a client who had adequate circulation before surgery indicates impaired circulation.

ABDOMEN. The nurse assesses the abdomen for size, shape, symmetry, and distention. If the client has abdominal surgery, the nurse makes frequent postoperative assessments of the abdominal incision and compares findings with preoperative data. Distention may indicate postoperative alterations in gastrointestinal function. The nurse should know whether the client is simply obese or whether the abdomen has become distended after surgery.

Assessment of preoperative bowel sounds is useful as a baseline. The nurse also determines whether the client has regular bowel movements. If the surgery requires manipulation of the gastrointestinal tract or if a general anesthetic is used, normal peristalsis will not return, and bowel sounds will be absent or diminished for several days after surgery.

NEUROLOGICAL STATUS. During the health history and physical assessment, the nurse observes the client's level of orientation, alertness, and mood, noting whether the client answers questions appropriately and can recall recent and past events. A client who will have surgery for neurological disease (for example, brain tumor or aneurysm) is likely to demonstrate an impaired level of consciousness or altered behavior. Level of consciousness changes as a result of general anesthesia. However, after the effects of anesthesia disappear, the client should return to the preoperative level of responsiveness.

If the client will have spinal anesthesia, preoperative assessment of gross motor function and strength is important. Spinal anesthesia causes temporary paralysis of the lower extremities. The nurse should be aware of a client entering surgery with weakness or impaired mobility of the lower extremities to avoid becoming alarmed when full motor function does not return immediately.

Risk Factors

Various conditions and factors increase a person's risk in surgery. Knowledge of risk factors enables the nurse to take necessary precautions in planning care.

AGE. Very young and old clients are at risk during surgery because of immature or declining physiological status. During surgery, nurses and physicians are especially concerned with maintaining an infant's normal body temperature. The infant's shivering reflex is underdeveloped, and often wide temperature variations occur. Anesthesia adds to the risk because anesthetics can cause vasodilation and heat loss.

During surgery, an infant has difficulty maintaining a normal circulatory blood volume. The total blood volume of an infant is considerably less than that of an older child or an adult. Even a small amount of blood loss can be serious. A reduced circulatory volume makes it difficult for the infant to respond to the need for increased oxygen during surgery. Thus the infant is highly susceptible to dehydration. However, if blood or fluids are replaced too quickly, overhydration may occur.

With advancing age, a client's physical capacity to adapt to the stress of surgery is hampered because of deterioration in certain body functions. Despite the risk, the majority of clients undergoing surgery are older adults. Table 47-4 on p. 1610 summarizes physiological factors that place older clients at risk for surgery.

NUTRITION. Normal tissue repair and resistance to infection depend on adequate nutrients. Surgery intensifies this need. After surgery, a client requires at least 1500 kcal/day to maintain energy reserves (Keithley, 1982). A malnourished client is prone to improper wound healing, reduced energy stores, and infection after surgery. If a client has elective surgery, nutrient imbalances can be corrected before surgery (see Chapter 35). However, if a malnourished client must undergo an emergency procedure, efforts to restore nutrients occur after surgery.

Obesity increases surgical risk. The obese client usually has reduced ventilatory and cardiac function and has difficulty resuming normal physical activity after surgery. The obese client is susceptible to poor wound healing and wound infection because of the structure of fatty tissue, which contains a poor blood supply. This slows delivery of essential nutrients, antibodies, and enzymes needed for wound healing (see Chapter 48). It is often difficult to close the surgical wound of an obese client because of the thick adipose layer. An obese cleint is also at risk for **dehiscence** (opening of the suture line).

RADIOTHERAPY. For the client with cancer, radiotherapy is often given to reduce the size of the cancerous tumor so that it can be removed surgically. Radiation has some unavoidable effects on normal tissue, such as excess thinning of skin layers, destruction of collagen, and impaired vascularization of tissue. Ideally the surgeon waits to perform surgery 4 to 6 weeks after completion of radiation treatments. Otherwise, the client may face serious wound-healing problems.

FLUID AND ELECTROLYTE BALANCE. The body responds to surgery as a form of trauma. As a result of the adrenocortical stress response, hormonal reactions cause sodium and water retention and potassium loss within the first 2 to 5 days after surgery. Severe protein breakdown causes a negative nitrogen balance. The severity of the stress response influences the degree of fluid and electrolyte imbalance. The more extensive the surgery, the more severe the stress. A client who is hypovolemic or who has serious preoperative electrolyte alterations is at significant risk during and after surgery. For example, an excess or depletion of potassium increases the chance of dysrhythmias during or after surgery. If the client has preexisting renal, gastrointestinal, or cardiovascular abnormalities, the risk of fluid and electrolyte alterations is even greater.

Diagnostic Screening

Before a client has surgery, the surgeon orders diagnostic tests to screen for preexisting abnormalities. Many clients are tested on an outpatient basis before surgery or on the morning of surgery. However, a client may also enter the hospital several days in advance to complete all tests. If diagnostic tests reveal severe problems, the surgeon may cancel surgery until the condition stabilizes.

The nurse is responsible for the preparation of clients for diagnostic studies and for coordinating completion of the tests. The nurse also reviews diagnostic results as they become available to alert physicians to findings and to assist with planning appropriate therapy.

Routine screening tests include a complete blood count (CBC), serum electrolyte analysis, coagulation studies, serum creatinine tests, urinalysis, and a chest x-ray study.

TABLE 47-4	Physiological Factors that Place an Older Adult at Risk for Surgery	
Alterations	Risks	Nursing Implications
CARDIOVASCULAR SYSTEM		
Degenerative change in myocardium and valves	Change reduces cardiac reserve.	Assess baseline vital signs.
Rigidity of arterial walls and reduction in sympathetic and parasympathetic innervation to heart	Alterations predispose client to postoperative hemorrhage and rise in systolic and diastolic blood pressure.	
Increase in calcium and cholesterol deposits within small arteries; thickened arterial walls	Problems predispose client to clot formation in lower extremities.	Instruct client on techniques for performing leg exercises and proper turning.
PULMONARY SYSTEM		
Rib cage stiffened and reduced in size	Complication reduces vital capacity.	Instruct client on proper technique for coughing and deep-breathing exercises.
Reduced range of movement in diaphragm	Greater residual capacity of volume of air is left in lung after normal breath increases, reducing amount of new air brought into lungs with each inspiration.	
Stiffened lung tissue and enlarged airspaces	Alteration reduces blood oxygenation.	
RENAL SYSTEM		
Reduced blood flow to kidneys	Reduced flow increases danger of shock when blood loss occurs.	For clients hospitalized before surgery, determine baseline urinary output for 24 hr.
Reduced glomerular filtration rate and excretory times	Problem limits ability to remove drugs or toxic substances.	
Reduced bladder capacity	Voiding frequency increases, and larger amount of urine stays in bladder after voiding.	Instruct client to notify nurse immediately when sensation of bladder fullness develops.
	Sensation of need to void may not occur until bladder is filled.	Keep call light and bedpan within easy reach.
NEUROLOGICAL SYSTEM		
Sensory losses, including reduced tactile sense and increased pain tolerance	Client is less able to respond to early warning signs of surgical complications.	Orient client to surrounding environment. Observe for nonverbal signs of pain.
Decreased reaction time	Client becomes easily confused after anesthesia.	
METABOLIC SYSTEM		
Lower basal metabolic rate	Lower rate reduces total oxygen consumption.	
Reduced number of red blood cells and hemoglobin levels	Ability to carry adequate oxygen to tissues is reduced.	Administer necessary blood products.
Change in total amounts of body potassium and water volume	Greater risk for fluid or electrolyte imbalance occurs.	Monitor electrolyte levels.

COMPLETE BLOOD COUNT. A CBC is the analysis of a peripheral venous blood specimen that measures red blood cell count, white blood cell count, hemoglobin concentration, and hematocrit (packed red cell volume). Each laboratory has a standard for normal laboratory values. An abnormal CBC may indicate a number of alterations (for example, dietary deficiency and chronic blood loss), placing the client at risk for cardiovascular and pulmonary complications. In such a case the surgeon may choose to administer blood products before surgery.

SERUM ELECTROLYTE ANALYSIS. Analysis of serum electrolyte levels also requires a peripheral venous blood sample. Several tests are available to reveal a client's electrolyte balance (Table 47-5). Because of the potential for fluid and electrolyte imbalances after surgery, the surgeon screens preoperative electrolyte levels to determine whether electrolyte replacement is necessary before surgery.

COAGULATION STUDIES. The ability of blood to clot or coagulate is essential for minimizing the risk of hemorrhaging. The prothrombin time (PT), partial thromboplastin time (PTT), and platelet count are routine tests for the clotting ability of blood (Table 47-5). Coagulation studies allow identification of clients at risk for bleeding tendencies and thrombus formation.

SERUM CREATININE TEST. A serum creatinine test assesses renal function. Creatinine is the by-product of muscle metabolism. The body excretes a constant amount through the kidneys, which serves as an excellent measure of the glomerular filtration rate. The creatinine level can be an indicator of renal failure when the value rises (Table 47-5). In the past, many physicians used the serum blood urea nitrogen (BUN) test to assesss renal function. Unlike creatinine, the BUN is affected by a variety of conditions unrelated to kidney function, such as diet, infection, or fluid intake.

URINALYSIS. Analysis of a urine specimen consists of screening for urinary infection, renal disease, and diabetes mellitus. The nurse collects a clean-voided specimen. The urinalysis measures urine color, pH, and specific gravity. It also determines the presence of protein, glucose, ketones, and blood. Chapter 40 discusses normal values in a urinalysis.

CHEST X-RAY STUDY. A chest x-ray examination allows the physician to examine the condition of the heart and lungs before surgery. Although the x-ray study does not always detect subtle pathological changes, it can reveal the overall size and shape of

TABLE 47-5 Common Laboratory Test Values	
Test	Values
Sodium level (Na$^+$)	135-145 mEq/L
Potassium level (K$^+$)	3.5-5.0 mEq/L
Chloride level (Cl$^-$)	100-106 mEq/l
Bicarbonate level (HCO$_3^-$)	24-32 mEq/L
Serum creatinine level	0.6-1.5 mg/100 ml
Prothrombin time (PT)	Less than 2-sec deviation from control
Partial thromboplastin time (PTT)	25-27 sec
Platelet count	150,000-350,000/mm^3

the heart, lung lesions and chest wall abnormalities, and position of the diaphragm and aorta. If the physician detects lung abnormalities, a different type and dosage of sedatives or anesthetic agents may be used. Before sending a female client for an x-ray examination, the nurse should be sure she is not pregnant. Exposure of the fetus to radiation may cause injury.

ADDITIONAL SCREENING TESTS. If a client is over the age of 40 or has heart disease, the physician orders an electrocardiogram (ECG). The test involves painless application of electrodes to the chest and extremities. An ECG measures the heart's electrical activity to determine whether the heart rate, rhythm, and other factors are normal. The procedure takes less than 5 minutes and requires the client simply to lie flat and relax.

Depending on the type of surgery, the client will undergo, there are several diagnostic tests for specific anatomical structures and physiological functions. If the client is likely to lose a large amount of blood during surgery, the physician orders a blood specimen for type and crossmatching. This enables the laboratory to determine the proper blood type and Rh factor. The surgeon usually designates the number of blood units to have available during surgery. **Autotransfusion** is an option for some clients who choose to donate their own blood before surgery to reduce the risk of transfusion-related infections. The donation usually must be made several weeks before the scheduled surgery.

Nursing Diagnosis

The nurse clusters defining characteristics gathered during assessment to identify nursing diagnoses

Examples of Nursing Diagnoses for Preoperative Client

NANDA-APPROVED NURSING DIAGNOSES

Ineffective airway clearance related to:
■ Diminished cough
■ Increased pulmonary congestion
Anxiety related to:
■ Knowledge deficit of impending surgery
■ Threat of loss of body part
Ineffective family coping: compromised related to:
■ Temporary role change of client
■ Impending severity of surgery
Fear related to:
■ Impending surgery
■ Anticipation of postoperative pain
Knowledge deficit regarding implications of surgery related to:
■ Lack of experience with surgery
■ Information misinterpretation
Altered nutrition: less than body requirements related to:
■ Preoperative malnourishment
Altered nutrition: more than body requirements related to:
■ Excess intake of food
Powerlessness related to:
■ Emergency nature of surgery
High risk for impaired skin integrity related to:
■ Preoperative radiation
■ Immobilization during surgery
Sleep pattern disturbance related to:
■ Fear of surgery
■ Preoperative hospital routines

for the surgical client (see diagnoses box). The diagnoses establish direction for care that will be provided during one or all surgical phases. Preoperative nursing diagnoses allow the nurse to take precautions and actions so that care provided during the intraoperative and postoperative phases is consistent with the client's needs.

Nursing diagnoses made preoperatively may also focus on the potential risks a client may face after surgery. Preventive care is essential so that the surgical client can be managed effectively. The nature and type of surgery, as well as the client's health status, provide defining characteristics for a number of nursing diagnoses (see diagnostic process box).

Planning

It is essential to include any client, especially the surgical client, in health care planning. Involving the client early when developing the surgical care plan minimizes surgical risks and postoperative complications. For example, nursing research has shown that structured preoperative teaching can reduce the length of the client's hospital stay (Lindeman, Van Aernam, 1971). A client informed about the surgical experience is less likely to be fearful and can prepare for expected outcomes. The box provides a sample care plan for a preoperative surgical client.

For the ambulatory surgical client, the preoperative planning phase occurs in the home or in the outpatient surgery unit on the morning of surgery. Ideally, it is done in the home. This gives the client time to think about the surgical experience, make neces-

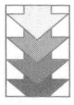

Sample Nursing Diagnostic Process for Knowledge Deficit

Assessment Activities	Defining Characteristics	Nursing Diagnoses
Ask client about previous surgical experiences.	Client reports no previous surgical experience either personally or involving family Client asks questions about what to expect	*Knowledge deficit regarding implications of surgery* related to first surgical experience
Ask client about preoperative preparation from physician.	Has received minimal preparation by physician	
Observe client's nonverbal behavior.	Alert and responsive to discussion	
Ask client about previous smoking history.	History of smoking	*High risk for ineffective airway clearance* related to diminished cough and increased pulmonary congestion
Auscultate client's breath sounds.	Abnormal breath sounds	
Assess for presence of a cough, noting character and productivity.	Chronic, nonproductive cough present	
Note client's surgical procedure and type of anesthesia.	Scheduled for anesthesia Scheduled for abdominal surgery	

sary physical preparations (for example, altering diet or discontinuing medication use), and ask questions about postoperative procedures. The ambulatory surgical client returns home on the day of surgery. Thus well-planned, preoperative care ensures that the client is well informed and able to be an active participant during recovery. The family or spouse can also play an active supportive role for the client.

The preoperative care plan is based on nursing diagnoses and is thus individualized. However, each client must undergo basic preparations. Goals of care for the preoperative client include the following:
1. Understanding physiological and psychological responses to surgery
2. Understanding intraoperative and postoperative events
3. Acquiring emotional comfort
4. Gaining a return of normal physiological function after surgery
5. Maintaining a normal fluid and electrolyte balance during and after surgery
6. Achieving comfort and rest
7. Remaining free of postoperative surgical wound infection
8. Remaining safe from harm during surgery

 ## Implementation

Preoperative nursing interventions provide the client with a complete understanding of the surgery and prepare the client physically for surgical intervention.

Informed Consent

A surgeon cannot legally perform surgery until a client understands the need for a procedure, the steps involved, risks, expected results, and alternative treatments. The primary responsibility for informing the client rests with the surgeon. Consent is not informed if the client is confused, unconscious, mentally incompetent, or under the influence of sedatives. All consent forms must be signed by the client before the nurse administers preoperative medications. Ideally a surgeon obtains consent before a client is admitted to the hospital or satellite surgical setting.

The surgeon's explanation should be witnessed by a qualified member of the health care team. The form's structure allows the physician to write information related to the surgery. A client's signature on a consent form implies that the client has been thoroughly informed about the procedure. The nurse frequently witnesses signing of the form and examines the document for the correct date, time, and signature, which must be in ink. A client who is illiterate can sign by making a mark as long as it is properly witnessed. As a witness the nurse is able to attest that the client's signature is on the form but not that the client was properly informed. In many institutions, a time limit is placed on consent forms (for example, 30 days).

 ### Sample Nursing Care Plan for Knowledge Deficit

Nursing diagnosis: *Knowledge deficit regarding implications of surgery* related to first surgical experience
Definition: Knowledge deficit is the state in which specific information is lacking (Kim, McFarland, McLane, 1991).

Goal	Expected Outcomes	Interventions	Rationale
Client will understand intra-operative and postoperative events.	Client and family will describe routine procedures that nurses perform after surgery.	Offer teaching booklet *Your Surgical Experience*.	Structured preoperative teaching has positive influence on recovery.
	Client will describe ways to participate in care after surgery.	Provide planned teaching session to explain common events that occur after surgery (e.g., monitoring, IV care, exercise).	
	Client and family will describe events that commonly occur in holding area and operating room.	Explain events that will occur in holding area (e.g., IV insertion, vital sign check) and in operating room (e.g., positioning, anesthesia).	Preparatory information helps clients form realistic image of surgical experience and be better able to cope and attend to it when it occurs.

Individuals must personally sign the consent form if they are of legal age (varies among states and provinces), under legal age but have valid marriage certificates, designated as emancipated minors (certain states), and not at present under legal guardianship. In some provinces a teenager may sign a consent form under certain conditions. If the client is a minor or legally considered to be incompetent and is not included in these categories, a parent or legal guardian signs the consent form. A spouse or next of kin signs for an adult who is unconscious or mentally incompetent.

In emergencies, the client may be unable to sign, and family members may be unavailable. The surgeon is legally permitted to perform surgery without consent in such a case. However, every effort must be made to obtain permission from a responsible family member by telephone, telegram, or in some states by court order. A telephone consent must be witnessed by two persons who hear the family member's oral consent. The two witnesses sign the consent with the name of the family member, noting that an oral consent was obtained. Informed consent is critical to protect not only the client but also health personnel so that the surgical team can practice without fear of legal reprisal.

After the client's consent form has been completed, the nurse makes sure that the form is placed in the medical client's record. The record goes to the operating room with the client. Chapter 14 discusses in detail the nurse's responsibilities for informed consent.

Preoperative Teaching

Structured preoperative teaching has proven benefits. Preoperative teaching concerning a client's expected postoperative behaviors, provided in a systematic and structured format with teaching and learning principles, has a positive influence on the client's recovery. Structured preoperative teaching can influence postoperative factors such as the following:

1. Ventilatory function. Teaching improves the ability to cough and deep breathe effectively.
2. Physical functional capacity. Teaching improves the ability to ambulate and resume activities of daily living early.
3. Sense of well-being. Clients who are prepared for surgery experience less anxiety and report a greater sense of psychological well-being.
4. Length of hospital stay. Structured preoperative teaching can reduce the length of stay.

The most effective teaching program for surgical clients is planned so that all clients receive the same information. Detailed discussion and demonstration of postoperative exercises are vital. If the client understands why these exercises are important to post-

operative recovery and knows how to perform them correctly, the recovery period will be less complicated. Today, because many clients come to the hospital on the day of surgery, preoperative teaching may occur in the home. Printed literature, instructions, and videotapes are made available to clients (Fig. 47-1). Preadmission nurses may call clients the evening before surgery to clarify questions and reinforce explanations. One study (Lepczyk et al, 1990) demonstrated that it made little difference in knowledge or anxiety measures if clients received preoperative education up to a week before surgery or immediately before. Another study found that clients preferred receiving preoperation information between admission to the hospital and the time of surgery, even if the time span was only a few hours or less (Schoessler, 1989). Therefore it seemed ideal to attempt outpatient preoperative education before admission and then to reinforce the information before surgery.

Including family members in preoperative preparation is advised. Often a family member is the coach for postoperative exercises when the client returns from surgery. If anxious relatives do not understand routine postoperative events, it is likely their anxiety will heighten the client's fears or concerns. Preoperative preparation of family members minimizes anxiety and misunderstanding.

The nurse should provide clients with information about sensations typically experienced after surgery. Preparatory information helps clients anticipate the steps of a procedure and thus helps them form realistic images of the surgical experience. When events occur as predicted, clients are better able to cope and attend to the experiences. For example, in the operating room the anesthesiologist may apply petrolatum ointment to clients' eyes to prevent corneal damage. Warning clients about sensations of blurred vision will reduce their anxiety on awakening from surgery. Sensations that the nurse may describe include the expected pain at the surgical site, the tightness of dressings, dryness of the mouth, or the sensation of a sore throat resulting from an endotracheal tube.

It is best to begin preoperative teaching well in advance of scheduled surgery. If the nurse can teach a client 1 or 2 days before surgery, the client will be better able to learn. Anxiety and fear are barriers to learning, and both emotions are heightened as surgery approaches. The nurse assesses the surgical client's readiness and ability to learn. If the client is capable of and receptive to learning, the nurse presents information in a logical sequence, beginning with preoperative events and advancing to intraoperative and postoperative routines. Preoperative teaching checklists give nurses useful guidelines for presenting comprehensive instructions.

INSTRUCTIONS FOR OUTPATIENT SURGERY

Your surgery will take place at:

DATE: _____ SURGERY TIME: _____ ARRIVE: _____

Anesthesia: Local _____ General _____ Block _____

1. Please be at the facility one to one and a half hours prior to scheduled time of operation.
2. You should have nothing to eat or drink for eight to twelve hours before surgery.
3. Register at the Reception Desk when you arrive.
4. It is best to leave valuables at home. However, any valuables you do have will be checked with the receptionist for safe keeping. You will then change into a hospital gown. Your clothing will be placed in a locker until after surgery.
5. After the operation, you will recover in the Recovery Room, if necessary, and then be discharged to your home.
6. Someone must accompany you. They should wait for you in the Outpatient Waiting Room until you come out of the OR.
7. When riding home in your car or a taxi, use shoulder belts, seat straps, or ride in the rear seat.
8. Routine laboratory tests, cardiogram and/or x-rays will be ordered as needed. The patient will be asked for a urine specimen the morning of surgery.
9. We request that you take *no aspirin* for two weeks before surgery. You may take aspirin substitute (non-aspirin compound).
10. If facial surgery is indicated, *DO NOT WEAR cosmetics to surgery.* Wash your face the night before and the morning of surgery. Cosmetics in the area of surgery could cause infection.
11. If surgery of the hand is indicated, the hand should be clean and the nails trimmed. *DO NOT wear nail polish.*
12. Hand surgery patients should wear clothing with large sleeves that will fit over a bulky dressing.
13. It is imperative that your insurance forms be in order for surgery. If forms are requested, be sure to have them with you the day of surgery.
14. You will be called the night before surgery. The main purpose of this call is to confirm your time on the schedule. If you cannot be reached, your surgery may be cancelled. If you have any questions, please call our office.
15. You will also be called the evening after your surgery. If you are not going to be home, leave the number where you can be reached with the nurse.

Fig. 47-1 Instructions for outpatient surgery.
From Kasdan AS et al: *Todays OR Nurse* 6(12):19, 1984.

The American Nurses Association and the Association of Operating Room Nurses (AORN) (1972) established the following criteria by which the client demonstrates understanding of the surgical experience. Extensive preoperative teaching not only improves the client's understanding, but also promotes return of normal physiological function.

CLIENT CITING REASONS FOR EACH PREOPERATIVE INSTRUCTION AND EXERCISES. Given a rationale for preoperative and postoperative procedures, the client is better prepared to participate in care. Every preoperative teaching program includes explanation and demonstration of the five postoperative exercises: diaphragmatic breathing, incentive spirometry, coughing, turning, and leg exercises. These exercises are designed to prevent postoperative complications (Procedure 47-1).

When a client is under general anesthesia, the lungs do not ventilate fully. After surgery the client has a reduced lung volume and needs greater effort to breathe. During surgery, venous blood flow to the

Demonstrating Postoperative Exercises

STEPS	RATIONALE
1. Assess client's risk for postoperative respiratory complications. Review medical history to identify presence of chronic pulmonary conditions (e.g., emphysema, asthma), any condition that affects chest wall movement, history of smoking, and presence of reduced hemoglobin.	General anesthesia predisposes client to respiratory problems because lungs are not fully inflated during surgery; cough reflex is suppressed, so mucous collects within airway passages. After surgery, client may have reduced lung volume and require greater efforts to cough and deep breathe; inadequate lung expansion can lead to atelectasis and pneumonia. Client is at greater risk to develop respiratory complications if other chronic lung conditions are present. Smoking damages ciliary clearance and increases mucous secretion. Reduced hemoglobin level can lead to inadequate oxygenation.
2. Assess ability to cough and deep breathe by having client take deep breath and observing movement of shoulders and chest wall. Measure chest excursion during deep breath. Ask client to cough after taking deep breath.	Reveals maximum potential for chest expansion and ability to cough forcefully; serves as baseline to measure ability to perform exercises after surgery.
3. Assess risk for postoperative thrombus formation. (Older, immobilized clients are most at risk.) Observe for positive Homan's sign by monitoring calf pain when dorsiflexing client's foot with knee flexed. Observe for calf pain, redness, warmth, swelling, or vein distention.	After general anesthesia, circulation is slowed, and when rate of blood flow is slowed, there is greater tendency for clot formation. Immobilization results in decreased muscular contraction in lower extremities, which promotes venous stasis.
4. Prepare necessary supplies: a. Pillow (optional)	Client may prefer to use pillow to splint incision when coughing to reduce discomfort.
5. Explain postoperative exercises to client, including importance to recovery and physiological benefits.	Information allows client to attend and can motivate learning. Persons tend to learn new skills when benefits can be gained.

DIAPHRAGMATIC BREATHING

STEPS	RATIONALE
6. Assist client to comfortable sitting or standing position. If client chooses to sit, assist to side of bed or to upright position in chair.	Upright position facilitates diaphragmatic excursion.
7. Stand or sit facing client.	Allows client to observe breathing exercise.

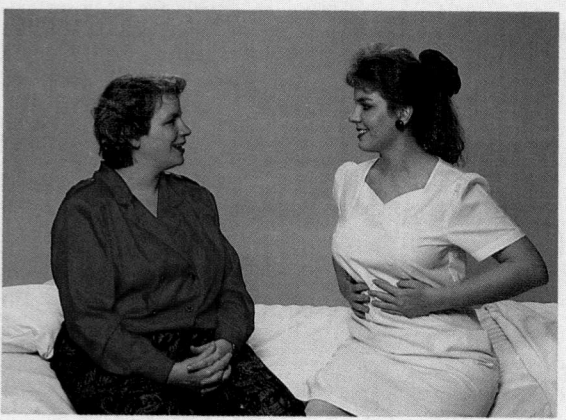

Step 8

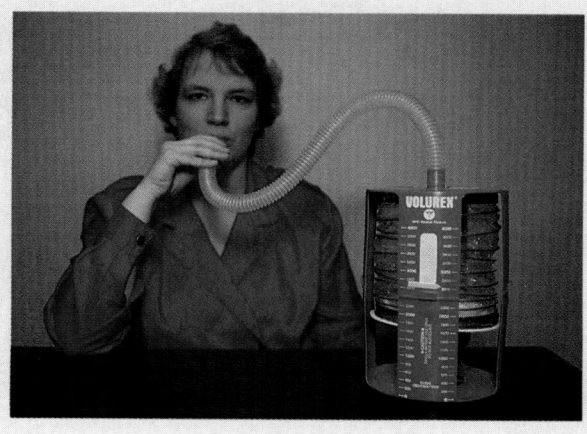

Step 17

STEPS	RATIONALE
8. Instruct client to place palms of hands across from each other, down and along lower borders of anterior rib cage. Place tips of third fingers lightly together (see illustration). Demonstrate for client.	Position of hands allows client to feel movement of chest and abdomen as diaphragm descends and lungs expand.
9. Have client take slow, deep breaths, inhaling through nose. Tell client to feel middle fingers separate during inhalation. Demonstrate.	Slow, deep breath prevents panting or hyperventilation. Inhaling through nose warms, humidifies, and filters air.
10. Explain that client will feel normal downward movement of diaphragm during inspiration. Explain that abdominal organs descend and chest wall expands.	Explanation and demonstration focus on normal ventilatory movement of chest wall. Client develops understanding of how diaphragmatic breathing feels.
11. Avoid using chest and shoulders while inhaling and instruct client in same manner.	Using auxiliary chest and shoulder muscles increases useless energy expenditures.
12. Have client hold slow, deep breath for count of three and then slowly exhale through mouth. Tell client middle fingertips will touch as chest wall contracts.	Allows for gradual expulsion of all air.
13. Repeat breathing exercise 3 to 5 times.	Allows client to observe slow, rhythmic breathing pattern.
14. Have client practice exercise. Instruct client to take 10 slow, deep breaths every 2 hr while awake during postoperative period until mobile.	Repetition of exercise reinforces learning. Regular deep breathing prevents postoperative complications.

INCENTIVE SPIROMETRY

STEPS	RATIONALE
15. Wash hands.	Reduces transmission of microorganisms.
16. Instruct client to assume semi-Fowler's or high Fowler's position.	Promotes optimal lung expansion during respiratory maneuver.
17. Demonstrate to client how to place mouthpiece so that lips completely cover mouthpiece (see illustration).	Demonstration is reliable technique for teaching psychomotor skill and enables client to ask questions.
18. Instruct client to inhale slowly and maintain constant flow through unit. When maximal inspiration is reached, client should hold breath for 2-3 sec and then exhale slowly. Number of breaths should not exceed 10-12 per min (Dettenmeier, 1992).	Maintains maximal inspiration and reduces risk of progressive collapse of individual alveoli. Slow breath prevents or minimizes pain from sudden pressure changes in chest (Dettenmeier, 1992).
19. Instruct client to breathe normally for short period.	Prevents hyperventilation and fatigue.
20. Have client repeat maneuver until goals are achieved.	Ensures correct use of spirometer.
21. Wash hands.	Reduces transmission of microorganisms.

CONTROLLED COUGHING

STEPS	RATIONALE
22. Explain importance of maintaining upright position.	Position facilitates diaphragm excursion and enhances thorax expansion.
23. Demonstrate coughing. Take two slow, deep breaths, inhaling through nose and exhaling through mouth.	Deep breaths expand lungs fully so that air moves behind mucus and facilitates effects of coughing.
24. Inhale deeply third time and hold breath to count of 3. Cough fully for two or three consecutive coughs without inhaling between coughs. (Tell client to push all air out of lungs.)	Consecutive coughs help remove mucus more effectively and completely than one forceful cough.
25. Caution client against just clearing throat instead of coughing.	Clearing throat does not remove mucus from deep in airways.

Demonstrating Postoperative Exercises

STEPS	RATIONALE
26. If surgical incision will be abdominal or thoracic, teach client to place one hand over incisional area and other hand on top of first. During breathing and coughing exercises, client presses gently against incisional area to splint or support it. Pillow over incision is optional (see illustration).	Surgical incision cuts through muscles, tissues, and nerve endings. Deep breathing and coughing exercises place additional stress on suture line and cause discomfort. Splinting incision with hands provides firm support and reduces incisional pulling. (Some clients prefer to have pilow to place over incision.)
27. Client continues to practice coughing exercises, splinting imaginary incision. Instruct client to cough 2 to 3 times every 2 hr while awake.	Value of deep coughing with splinting is stressed to effectively expectorate mucus with minimal discomfort.
28. Instruct client to examine sputum for consistency, amount, and color changes.	Sputum consistency, amount, and color changes may indicate presence of pulmonary complication, such as pneumonia.

TURNING

STEPS	RATIONALE
29. Instruct client to assume supine position to right side of bed. Side rails on both sides of bed should be in up position.	Positioning begins on right side of bed so that turning to left side will not cause client to roll toward bed's edge.
30. Instruct client to place left hand over incisional area to splint it.	Supports and minimizes pulling on suture line during turning.
31. Instruct client to keep left leg straight and flex right knee up and over left leg.	Straight leg stabilizes client's position. Flexed right leg shifts weight for easier turning.
32. Have client grab left side rail with right hand, pull toward left, and roll onto left side.	Pulling toward side rail reduces effort needed for turning.
33. Instruct client to turn every 2 hr while awake.	Reduces risk of vascular and pulmonary complications.

LEG EXERCISES

STEPS	RATIONALE
34. Have client assume supine position in bed. Demonstrate leg exercises by performing passive range of motion exercises and simultaneously explaining exercise.	Provides normal anatomical position of lower extremities.
35. Rotate each ankle in complete circle. Instruct client to draw imaginary circles with big toe. Repeat 5 times.	Leg exercises maintain joint mobility and promote venous return.

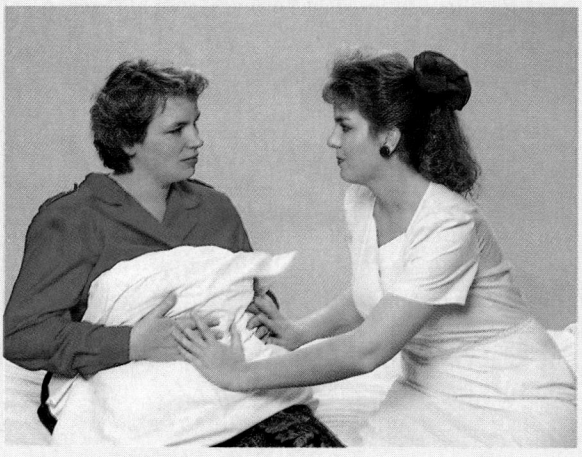

Step 26

STEPS	RATIONALE
36. Alternate dorsiflexion and plantar flexion of both feet. Direct client to feel calf muscles contract and relax alternately (see illustration). Repeat 5 times.	Stretches and contracts gastrocnemius muscles.
37. Have client continue leg exercises by alternately flexing and extending knees. Repeat 5 times (see illustration).	Contracts muscles of upper legs and maintains knee mobility.
38. Have client alternately raise each leg straight up from bed surface, keeping legs straight. Repeat 5 times.	Promotes contraction and relaxation of quadriceps muscles.
39. Have client practice exercises at least every 2 hr while awake. Instruct client to coordinate turning and leg exercises with diaphragmatic breathing, incentive spirometry, and coughing exercises.	Repetition of sequence reinforces learning. Establishes routine for exercises that develops habit for performance. Sequence of exercises should be leg exercises, turning, breathing, incentive spirometry, and coughing.
40. Observe client's ability to perform all five exercises independently.	Ensures that client has learned correct technique.
41. Record exercises demonstrated and client's ability to perform them independently.	Documents client's education and provides data for instructional follow-up.

CONTINUED

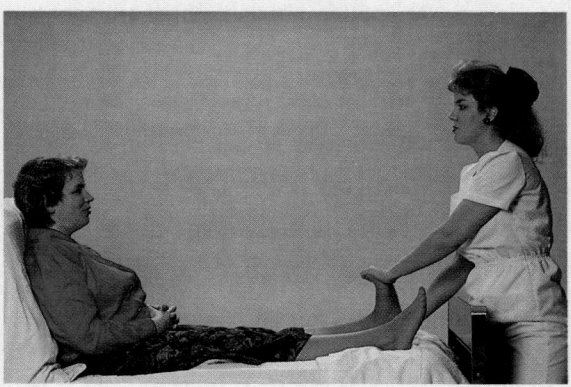

Step 36

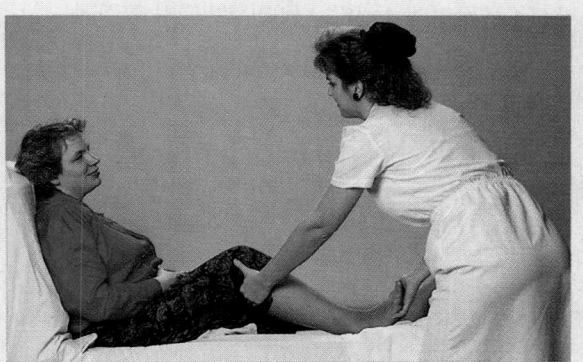

Step 37

legs slows. Stasis of circulation may lead to thrombi or clots. A clot can break off and travel to the brain, heart, or lungs to cause potentially fatal complications.

Diaphragmatic breathing improves lung expansion and oxygen delivery without using excess energy. The client learns to use the diaphragm during deep breathing to take slow, deep, and relaxed breaths. Eventually the client's lung volume improves. Deep breathing also helps clear out anesthetic gases remaining in the airways. To facilitate deep breathing the physician may order an incentive spirometer for the client, which encourages effective deep breathing through sustained maximal inspiration (see Chapter 38).

Coughing assists in removing retained mucus in the airways. A deep, productive cough is more beneficial than merely clearing the throat. Postoperative incisional pain makes coughing difficult. The client must anticipate the pain and understand the importance of coughing. The nurse also teaches the client to splint an incision to minimize pain during coughing. Nurses direct clients to cough and deep breathe at least every 2 hours while awake.

Leg exercises and turning improve blood flow to the extremities and thus reduce stasis. Contraction of lower leg muscles promotes venous return, making it difficult for clots to form. The nurse encourages the client to perform exercises at least every 2 hours while awake.

After explaining each exercise, the nurse demonstrates it. The nurse acts as a coach, guiding the client through each exercise. For example, the nurse says whether the client is sitting properly and helps the client place the hands in the proper position during breathing. The nurse then allows the client time (at least 15 minutes) for independent practice. The nurse can attend to other duties before returning to watch each exercise independently. The nurse gives feedback, telling the client what aspect of each exercise is done correctly and what needs improvement.

CLIENT STATING TIME OF SURGERY. The client and family should be told the approximate time that surgery will begin. If the hospital has a busy operating room schedule, it is best to let them know how many procedures are scheduled before the client's. It is unwise to tell the client and family the anticipated length of surgery. Unanticipated delays may occur for many reasons. If the client fails to return at the time expected, the family will be highly anxious. Family members should be told that nurses in the postoperative surgical division will inform them of the client's arrival in the recovery room.

CLIENT STATING POSTOPERATIVE UNIT AND LOCATION OF FAMILY DURING SURGERY AND RECOVERY. The unit to which the client is admitted before surgery may be different from the postoperative unit. The family needs to know where the client will be taken after surgery. The nurse also explains where the family can wait and where the surgeon will attempt to find family members after surgery. If the client will be taken to a special unit, it helps to orient the client and family members to the unit's environment before surgery.

CLIENT DISCUSSING ANTICIPATED POSTOPERATIVE MONITORING AND THERAPIES. The client and family want to know about postoperative events. If they understand routine postoperative vital sign monitoring before surgery, they will be less apprehensive when nurses make these checks. The nurse can also explain whether the client is likely to have IV lines, dressings, or drainage tubes. The nurse should neither overprepare nor underprepare the client and family. The nurse cannot predict all of the client's postoperative therapies because each surgeon follows different practices for each type of surgery. Although the nurse becomes familiar with each surgeon's preferences, it is easy to misinform a client about a ther-

apy that may not be initiated. Contradictions between the nurse's explanations and postoperative reality can cause great anxiety.

CLIENT DESCRIBING SURGICAL PROCEDURES AND POSTOPERATIVE TREATMENT. After the surgeon has explained the basic purpose of a surgical procedure, the client may ask the nurse additional questions to clarify misunderstandings. The nurse is careful to avoid saying anything that contradicts the surgeon's explanation. One way to avoid problems is to first ask what the client has been told. When the client has little or no understanding about the surgery, the nurse first checks with the physician to determine what explanation can be given. Before surgery, certain predictable aspects of the client's treatment plan (for example, dressing changes and respiratory therapy) and level of supportive nursing care are explained. The nurse can also describe plans for postoperative rehabilitation and drug therapy.

CLIENT DESCRIBING POSTOPERATIVE ACTIVITY RESUMPTION. The type of surgery a client undergoes affects the speed with which normal physical activity and regular eating habits can be resumed. The nurse explains that it is normal to progress gradually in activity and eating. If the client tolerates activity and diet well, activity levels will progress more quickly.

CLIENT VERBALIZING PAIN-RELIEF MEASURES. One of the surgical client's greatest fears is pain. The family is also concerned for the client's comfort. Pain after surgery is normal. The nurse informs the client and family of therapies available for pain relief (for example, analgesics, positioning, splinting, and relaxation exercises) (see Chapter 37). The client needs to know the schedule for analgesic drugs, the route of administration, and their effects.

The client should be encouraged to inform the nurses as soon as pain becomes a constant discomfort. If a client waits until pain becomes excruciating, an analgesic will not provide relief. The client should also know the length of time that it takes for a drug to act and that all discomfort is rarely eliminated.

Surgical clients often avoid taking pain-relief drugs for fear of becoming dependent. But most drug doses and the required intervals between administration are not sufficient to cause dependence. During assessment, the nurse should asscertain the client's drug history and the use of recreational drugs, prescribed analgesics, and any history of abuse or dependence. The nurse should encourage the client to use analgesics as needed. Unless the pain is controlled, it will be difficult for the client to participate in postoperative therapy. Hospitalized clients initially receive parenteral injections, depending on the nature of surgery. As they become able to tolerate food, the physician replaces parenteral analgesics with oral forms.

CLIENT EXPRESSING FEELINGS REGARDING SURGERY. The client may feel like part of an assembly line during the preoperative surgical phase. Frequent visits by staff, diagnostic testing, and physical preparation for surgery consume a lot of time, and the client has few opportunities to reflect on the surgical experience. The nurse makes sure that the client feels like an individual. The client and family need time to express feelings about surgery. The client's level of anxiety influences the frequency of discussions. While delivering routine care, the nurse can encourage expression of concerns. The family may wish to discuss concerns without the client so that their fears will not frighten the client.

Physical Preparation

The degree of preoperative physical preparation depends on the client's health status, the surgery to be performed, and the surgeon's preferences. A seriously ill client receives more supportive care in the form of medications, IV fluid therapy, and monitoring than the client facing a minor elective procedure. The nurse explains the purpose of all procedures.

MAINTENANCE OF NORMAL FLUID AND ELECTROLYTE BALANCE. The surgical client is vulnerable to fluid and electrolyte imbalances as a result of inadequate preoperative intake or excessive fluid losses during surgery (see Chapter 39). A client takes nothing by mouth (NPO) after midnight on the morning of surgery. The nurse removes fluids and solid foods from the client's bedside and posts a sign over the bed to alert hospital personnel and family members about fasting restrictions. After 6 to 8 hours of fasting, the client's gastrointestinal tract will be relatively empty, so the risks of vomiting or aspirating emesis during surgery are minimal. General anesthetics typically cause slowing of gastrointestinal peristalsis.

A client who is at home the evening before surgery must understand the importance of not taking food or fluids and be willing to follow restrictions. The nurse can allow the client to rinse the mouth with water or mouthwash and brush the teeth as long as the client does not swallow water. In the hospital the nurse notifies the surgeon if the client eats or drinks during the fasting period.

During surgery, normal mechanisms for controlling fluid and electrolyte balance, including respiration, digestion, circulation, and elimination, are disturbed. The surgical procedure may cause extensive losses of blood and other body fluids. The surgical stress response aggravates any fluid and electrolyte imbalance. The nurse determines whether the client eats and drinks sufficient amounts before fasting to ensure adequate fluid and nutrition intake. This prevents fluid and electrolyte imbalances and reduces the risk of infection. The client's diet should include foods high in protein, with sufficient carbohydrates, fat, and vitamins. If a client cannot eat because of gastrointestinal alterations or impairments in consciousness, an IV route for fluid replacement is started. The physician relies on serum electrolyte levels to determine the type of IV fluids and electrolyte additives to administer. Clients with severe nutritional imbalances may require supplements with concentrated protein and glucose (see Chapter 35).

REDUCTION OF RISK OF SURGICAL WOUND INFECTION. The risk of developing a surgical wound infection is determined by the amount and type of microorganisms contaminating a wound, susceptibility of the host, and condition of the wound at the end of the operation (largely determined by the surgeon's operative technique). All three factors may interact to cause infection.

The skin is a favorite site for microorganisms to grow and multiply. Without proper skin preparation (Procedure 47-2), the risk of postoperative wound infection is high. Bathing the evening before surgery with an antimicrobial soap (for example, Triclosan or Chlorhexidine) is believed to effectively reduce the incidence of postoperative wound infections (Ayliffe et al, 1983). Many surgeons have clients bathe or shower the evening before surgery. Some physicians may order clients to bathe or shower more than once, whereas others may have clients give special attention to cleansing the proposed operative site. Depending on the surgical procedure, a client may repeat a shower the morning of surgery.

If the surgical procedure involves the head, neck, or upper chest area, the client may also be required to shampoo the hair. Cleansing and trimming of fingernails and toenails are necessary when the surgeon desires strict asepsis, as in the case of certain transplant procedures.

In the past a surgical client's skin was thoroughly shaved to remove hair around the incision site. The rationale for the procedure was to remove microorganisms residing in body hair. However, studies have shown that shaving the surgical site increases the incidence of postoperative wound infection (Cruse, Foord, 1980). Shaving with a razor can cause superficial cuts and nicks in the skin that allow microorganisms to grow. The CDC recommends avoiding hair removal or, if necessary, shaving only immedi-

Skin Preparation For Surgery

STEPS	RATIONALE
1. Inspect general condition of skin.	If lesions, irritations, or signs of skin infection are present, shaving should not be done. These conditions increase chances for postoperative wound infections.
2. Review physician's order for area to be clipped. (Review institution's operating room manual as needed.)	Extent of area for hair removal depends on site of incision, nature of surgery, and physician's preference. Area is always larger than actual incision to ensure wide perimeter with minimal bacteria.
3. Prepare necessary equipment and supplies:	Ensures smooth procedure.
a. Portable lamp	Needed if room light is insufficient. Good lighting is important to inspect skin condition.
b. Bath blanket	Used to drape client to provide privacy.
c. Towel or waterproof pad	
d. Electric clippers	Used to remove short hair.
e. Scissors	Used to cut long body hair.
f. Towel	
g. Cotton balls, applicators, and antiseptic solution (optional)	
4. Explain procedure and rationale for removal of hair over large surface area.	Promotes cooperation and minimizes anxiety because client may think incision will be as large as clipped site.
5. Wash hands.	Reduces transmission of infection.
6. Close room doors or bedside curtains.	Provides privacy.
7. Raise bed to high position. Position client comfortably with surgical site accessible.	Avoids need to bend over for long periods of time. Hair removal and skin preparation can take several minutes. Nurse should have easy access to hard-to-reach areas.
8. Clip hair:	
a. Lightly dry area to be clipped with towel.	Removes moisture, which interferes with clean cut of clippers.
b. Hold clippers in dominant hand, about 1 cm above skin, and cut hair in direction it grows. Clip small area at time.	Prevents pulling on hair and abrasion of skin.
c. Arrange drapes as necessary.	Prevents unnecessary exposure of body parts.
d. Lightly brush off cut hair with towel.	Removes contaminated hair and promotes comfort. Improves visibility of area being clipped.
e. When clipped area is over body crevices, (e.g., umbilicus or groin), clean crevices with cotton-tipped applicators or cotton ball dipped in antiseptic solution, then dry.	Removes secretions, dirt, and hair clippings, which harbor microorganisms.
9. Tell client that procedure is completed.	Relieves anxiety.
10. Clean and dispose of equipment according to policy and dispose of gloves.	Prevents spread of infection.
11. Inspect condition of skin after completion of hair removal.	Determines whether there is remaining hair.
12. Record procedure, area clipped, and condition of skin before and after clip in nurses' notes.	Documents procedure performed and condition of skin before surgery.

ately before the operation (Garner, 1985). **Depilatories** and clipping are preferred over shaving. However, there are hospitals and surgical clinics that still perform shaving. The nurse should consult an institution's policy and procedure manual.

Another way to reduce the risk of a postoperative wound infection is to keep a client's preoperative hospital stay short. A number of researchers have shown that a short stay is associated with low wound infection rates (Cruse, Foord, 1980; Halsey et al, 1981). Thus clients have less opportunity to acquire pathogens from the hospital.

PREVENTION OF BOWEL AND BLADDER INCONTINENCE. The client may not receive a bowel preparation (for example, a cathartic or enema) unless surgery involves the gastrointestinal system. Manipulation of portions of the gastrointestinal tract during surgery results in absence of peristalsis for 24 hours and sometimes longer. Enemas and cathartics cleanse the gastrointestinal tract to prevent intraoperative incontinence and postoperative constipation. An empty bowel reduces risk of injury to the intestines and prevents contamination of the operative wound in case a portion of the bowel is incised or opened. The surgeon's order may read "Give enemas until clear." This means that the nurse is to administer enemas until the enema return contains no fecal material (see Chapter 41). Too many enemas given over a short time, however, can cause serious fluid and electrolyte imbalances. Most agencies recommend a limit to the number of enemas a nurse may administer successively.

The bladder is not prepared until the morning of surgery. The nurse instructs the client to void just before leaving for the operating room. An empty bladder prevents a client from being incontinent during surgery. This is important during abdominal surgery, when it may become necessary for the surgeon to manipulate the bladder. An empty bladder also makes abdominal organs more accessible during surgery. The nurse in the operating room often inserts a Foley catheter to maintain an empty bladder.

PROMOTION OF REST AND COMFORT. Rest is essential for normal healing. Anxiety about surgery can easily interfere with the ability to relax or sleep. The underlying condition requiring surgery may be painful, further impairing rest.

The nurse should attempt to make the client's environment quiet and comfortable. Frequently, the physician orders a sedative-hypnotic or antianxiety agent for the night before surgery. Sedative-hypnotics (for example, flurazepam [Dalmane]) affect and promote sleep. Antianxiety agents (for example, al-

prazolam [Xanax] and diazepam [Valium]) act on the cerebral cortex and limbic system to relieve anxiety.

An advantage to ambulatory surgery or same-day surgical admissions is that the client is able to sleep at home the night before surgery. The client is likely to get more rest in a familiar environment.

Day of Surgery

On the morning before surgery the nurse completes a number of routine procedures before releasing the client for surgery.

CHECKING MEDICAL RECORD CONTENTS AND COMPLETING RECORDING. Before the client goes to the operating room, the nurse checks the contents of the medical record to be sure that pertinent laboratory results are present. The nurse checks consent forms for accuracy of information. A preoperative checklist (Fig. 47-2) provides the nurse with guidelines for en-

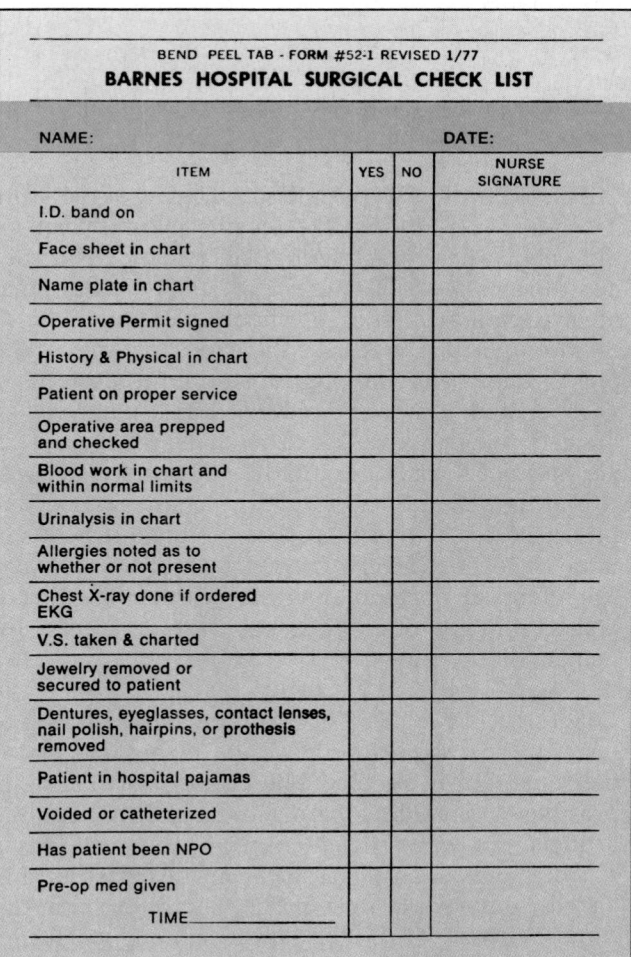

BEND PEEL TAB - FORM #52-1 REVISED 1/77
BARNES HOSPITAL SURGICAL CHECK LIST

NAME:			DATE:
ITEM	YES	NO	NURSE SIGNATURE
I.D. band on			
Face sheet in chart			
Name plate in chart			
Operative Permit signed			
History & Physical in chart			
Patient on proper service			
Operative area prepped and checked			
Blood work in chart and within normal limits			
Urinalysis in chart			
Allergies noted as to whether or not present			
Chest X-ray done if ordered EKG			
V.S. taken & charted			
Jewelry removed or secured to patient			
Dentures, eyeglasses, contact lenses, nail polish, hairpins, or prothesis removed			
Patient in hospital pajamas			
Voided or catheterized			
Has patient been NPO			
Pre-op med given			
TIME_____			

Fig. 47-2 Preoperative checklist.
Courtesy Barnes Hospital, St Louis.

suring completion of nursing interventions. The nurse also checks the nurses' notes to be sure that documentation of care is current. This is especially important if the hospitalized client experienced unpredicted problems the night before surgery.

CHECKING VITAL SIGNS. The nurse makes a final preoperative assessment of vital signs. The anesthesiologist uses these values as baselines for intraoperative vital signs. If preoperative vital signs are abnormal, surgery may need to be postponed. For example, an elevated temperature increases the client's surgical risk. The nurse notifies the physician of abnormalities before sending the client to surgery.

PROVIDING HYGIENE. Basic hygiene measures provide an additional level of comfort before surgery. If the hospitalized client is unwilling to take a complete bath, a partial bath is refreshing and removes irritating secretions or drainage from the skin. Because the client cannot wear personal nightwear to the operating room, the nurse provides a clean hospital gown. After being NPO throughout the night, the client usually has a very dry mouth. The nurse may offer mouthwash and toothpaste, again cautioning the client not to swallow water.

CHECKING HAIR AND COSMETICS. During surgery under general anesthesia, the anesthesiologist positions the client's head to introduce an endotracheal tube into the airway (see Chapter 38). This procedure may involve manipulation of the client's hair and scalp. To avoid injury the nurse asks the client to remove hairpins or clips before leaving for surgery. Hairpieces or wigs should also be removed. Long hair can be braided to keep it in place. The client will wear a paper hair net before entering the operating room.

During and after surgery, the anesthesiologist and nurses assess skin and mucous membranes to determine the client's level of oxygenation and circulation. Therefore all makeup (lipstick, powder, blush, nail polish) must be removed to expose normal skin and nail coloring.

CHECKING FOR REMOVAL OF PROSTHESES. It is easy for any type of prosthetic device to become lost or damaged during surgery. The client must remove all prostheses, including partial or complete dentures, artificial limbs, artificial eyes, and contact lenses. Hearing aids, false eyelashes, and eyeglasses must also be removed. If a client has a brace or splint, the nurse checks with the physician to determine whether it should remain with the client.

For many clients, it is embarrassing to remove dentures or other devices that enhance appearance.

Thus privacy should be offered as the dentures are removed. Dentures must be placed in special containers for safekeeping to prevent loss or breakage, and the client is assessed for any loose teeth. A broken tooth can become dislodged during insertion of an endotracheal tube and obstruct the airway.

In many agencies, nurses must inventory all prosthetic devices and have them locked away for safekeeping. It is also common practice for nurses to give prostheses to family members or to keep the devices at the client's bedside.

PREPARING BOWEL AND BLADDER. The client may require an enema or cathartic the morning of surgery. If so, it should be given at least an hour before the client is scheduled to leave, allowing time for the client to defecate without rushing. The client should void before surgery. If the client is unable to void, it should be noted on the preoperative checklist.

APPLYING ANTIEMBOLISM STOCKINGS. Many physicians prefer clients to wear **antiembolism stockings** during surgery. These are designed to support the lower extremities and maintain compression of small veins and capillaries. The constant compression forces blood into larger vessels, thus promoting venous return and preventing circulatory stasis. When correctly sized and properly applied, antiembolism stockings can reduce the risk of thrombi. Chapter 43 reviews the procedure for sizing and application.

PROMOTING CLIENT DIGNITY. During preoperative preparations, care can become depersonalized unless the nurse maintains the client's privacy and reduces sources of anxiety. Ambulatory and same-day surgical admission clients often must sit in a waiting room before surgery. To protect client modesty the nurse allows them to wear underclothes when possible and provides cover robes. Hospitalized clients should be ensured privacy by closing room curtains or doors during preoperative preparation. Family may be allowed to stay until it is time for transport to the operating room.

PERFORMING SPECIAL PROCEDURES. A client's condition may warrant special interventions before surgery. The surgeon's orders inform nurses of the need to start IV infusions, insert Foley catheters, or administer medications.

One special procedure involves insertion of a nasogastric (NG) tube, a pliable plastic tube, through the client's nasopharynx into the stomach (Procedure 47-3). The tube has a hollow lumen that allows removal of gastric secretions and introduction of solutions into the stomach. NG intubation has several pur-

Text continued on p. 1629.

STEPS	RATIONALE
1. Inspect condition of client's oral cavity. (Use of gloves is recommended.)	Baseline condition determines need for special nursing measures for oral hygiene after tube placement.
2. Palpate client's abdomen.	Baseline determination will later serve as comparison after tube is inserted.
3. Check medical record for surgeon's order, type of NG tube to be placed, and whether tube is to be attached to suction or drainage bag.	Procedure requires physician's order. Adequate decompression depends on suction.
4. Prepare equipment and supplies:	
a. 14 or 16 Fr NG tube (smaller lumen for child)	For decompression, smaller lumen catheters are not used because they must be used to remove thick secretions.
b. Water-soluble lubricating jelly	Used to lubricate tube for insertion.
c. pH test strips	Used to measure gastric aspirate acidity.
d. Tongue blade	
e. Flashlight	
f. Asepto bulb or cone-tip syringe	Used to irrigate or instill fluid into tube.
g. 2.5-cm (1-in) wide hypoallergenic tape	Prevents loss of skin on nose.
h. Safety pin and rubber band	
i. Clamp, drainage bag, or suction machine	Tube may be open or closed to drainage.
j. Bath towel	
k. Glass of water with straw	
l. Facial tissues	
m. Normal saline	Used for irrigation of tube.
n. Tincture of benzoin (optional)	
o. Nonsterile gloves	Increases adhesion of tape to nose.
5. Identify client and explain procedure.	Prevents error and gains client's cooperation to facilitate passage of tube and lessen possibility that client will remove tube.
6. Wash hands and don gloves.	Reduces transmission of microorganisms.
7. Position client in high Fowler's position with pillows behind head and shoulders. Raise bed to its highest horizontal level.	Promotes client's ability to swallow during procedure. Good body mechanics prevents injury to nurse or client.
8. Assemble all equipment at bedside and place on your side of bed. Pull curtain around bed or close room door.	Procedure should be organized to limit discomfort. Provides privacy.
9. Stand at right side of bed if right-handed and left side if left-handed.	Allows easiest manipulation of tubing.
10. Place bath towel over chest; give tissues to client.	Prevents soiling of gown. Tube insertion through nasal passages may cause tearing.
11. Instruct client to relax and breathe normally while occluding one naris. Then repeat this action for other naris. Select nostril with greater air flow.	Tube passes more easily through naris that is more patent.
12. Measure distance to insert tube:	Tube should extend from nares to stomach; distance varies with each client. Length provides distance from nose to stomach in 98% of clients (Grant, Kennedy-Caldwell, 1988).
a. Traditional method: measure distance from tip of nose to earlobe to xiphoid process to sterum (see illustration on p. 1626).	
b. Hanson method: first mark 50-cm (20-in) point on tube and then do traditional measurement. Tube insertion should be to midway point between 50 cm and traditional mark.	

Inserting and Maintaining an NG Tube

STEPS	RATIONALE
13. Mark length of tube to be inserted with piece of tape or note distance from next tube marking.	Marks amount of tube to be inserted from nares to stomach.
14. Cut 10-cm (4-in) long piece of tape. Split one end lengthwise 5 cm (2 in).	Tape will be used after tube insertion to anchor tube securely.
15. Curve 10-15 cm (4-6 in) of end of tube tightly around index finger; release.	Curving tube tip aids insertion.
16. Lubricate 7.5-10 cm (3-4 in) of end of tube with water-soluble lubricating jelly.	Minimizes friction against nasal mucosa.
17. Initially instruct client to extend neck back against pillow; insert tube slowly through naris with curved end pointing downward (see illustration).	Facilitates initial passage of tube through naris and maintains clear airway for open naris.
18. Continue to pass tube along floor of nasal passage, aiming down toward ear. When resistance is felt, apply gentle downward pressure to advance tube (do not force past resistance).	Minimizes discomfort of tube rubbing against upper nasal turbinates. Resistance is caused by posterior nasopharynx. Downward pressure helps tube to curl around corner of nasopharynx.
19. If resistance is met, withdraw tube, allow client to rest, relubricate tube, and insert into other naris.	Forcing against resistance can cause trauma to mucosa. Helps relieve anxiety.

20. Continue insertion of tube until just past nasopharynx by gently rotating tube toward opposite naris:
  a. Stop tube advancement, allow client to relax, and provide tissues.
  b. Explain that next step requires swallowing.
	Relieves anxiety; tearing is natural response to mucosal irritation.
	Tube is about to enter esophagus.

21. With tube just above oropharynx, instruct client to flex head forward and dry swallow or suck in air through straw. Advance tube 2.5-5 cm (1-2 in) with each swallow. If client has trouble swallowing and is allowed fluids, offer glass of water. Advance tube with each swallow of water.	Flexed position closes off upper airway to trachea and opens esophagus. Swallowing closes epiglottis over trachea and helps to move tube into esophagus. Swallowing water reduces gagging or choking.
22. If client begins to cough, gag, or choke, stop tube advancement. Instruct client to breathe easily and take sips of water.	Tubing may accidentally enter larynx and initiate cough reflex. Gagging is eased by swallowing water.

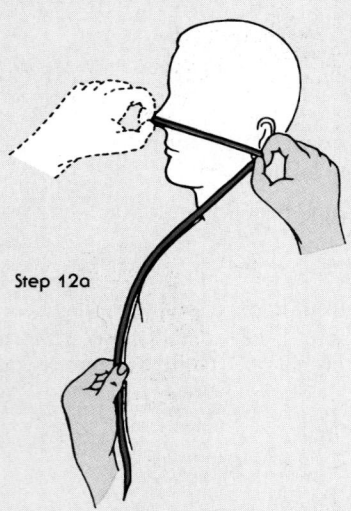

Step 12a

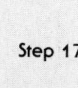

Step 17

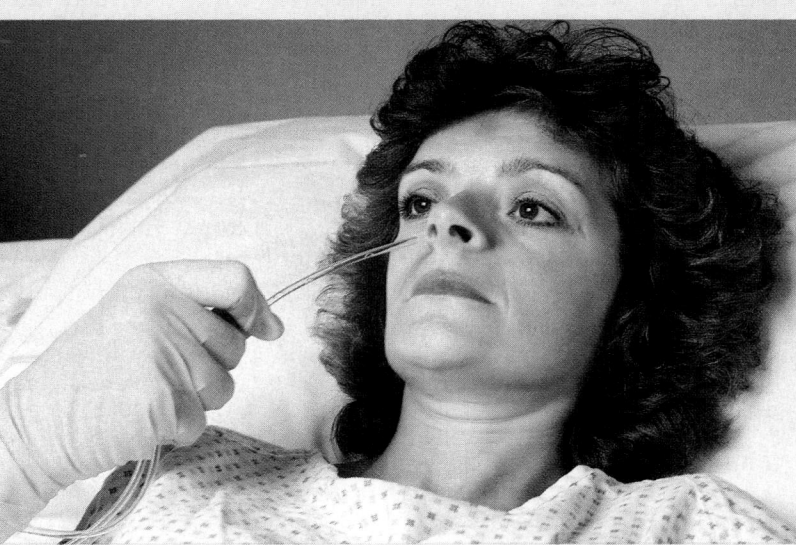

STEPS	RATIONALE
23. If client continues to cough, pull tube back slightly.	Tube may enter larynx and obstruct airway.
24. If client continues to gag, check back of pharynx using flashlight and tongue blade.	Tube may coil around itself in back of throat.
25. After client relaxes, continue to advance tube desired distance.	Tip of tube should be within stomach to decompress properly.

CHECKING TUBE PLACEMENT

26. Ask client to talk.	Client would be unable to talk if tube passed through vocal cords.
27. Check posterior pharynx for presence of coiled tube.	Tube is pliable and can coil up in back of pharynx instead of advancing into esophagus.
28. Attach cone-tipped syringe to end of tube. Aspirate gently back on syringe to obtain gastric contents. (Insufflation of air into tube followed by auscultation of sounds is no longer considered most effective in determining tube placement.) Check institutional policy for preferred method.	Aspiration of contents provides means to measure fluid pH and thus determine tube tip placement in gastrointestinal tract. (Sounds transmitted by insufflation of air may be transmitted from pleural space to upper abdomen, giving false impression of placement [Metheny, 1988; Metheny et al, 1989b]).
29. Measure pH of aspirate with color-coded pH paper with range of whole numbers from 1-11 (see research highlight on p. 1629).	Gastric aspirates have decidedly acidic pH values, preferably 4 or less (Metheny et al, 1989a).
30. If tube is not in stomach, advance another 2.5-5 cm (1-2 in) and repeat Steps 29 and 30 to check tube position.	Tube must be in stomach to provide decompression.

ANCHORING TUBE

31. After tube is properly inserted, clamp end or connect it to drainage bag or suction machine.	Drainage bag is used for gravity drainage. Intermittent suction is most effective for decompression. Tube is often clamped in client going to operating room.
32. Tape tube to nose; avoid putting pressure on nares.	Prevents tissue necrosis. Tape anchors tube securely. Benzoin prevents loosening of tape if client perspires.

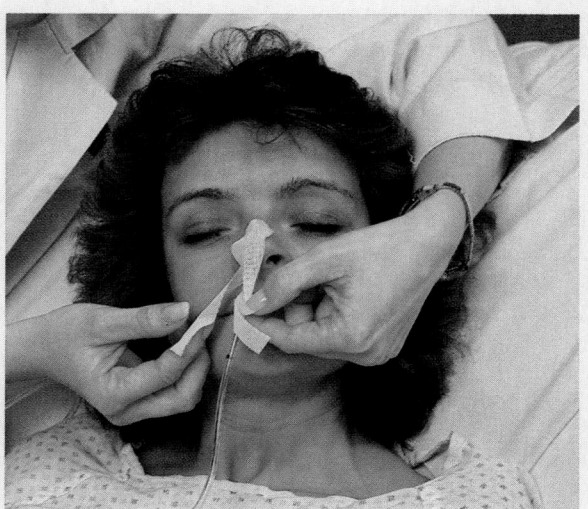 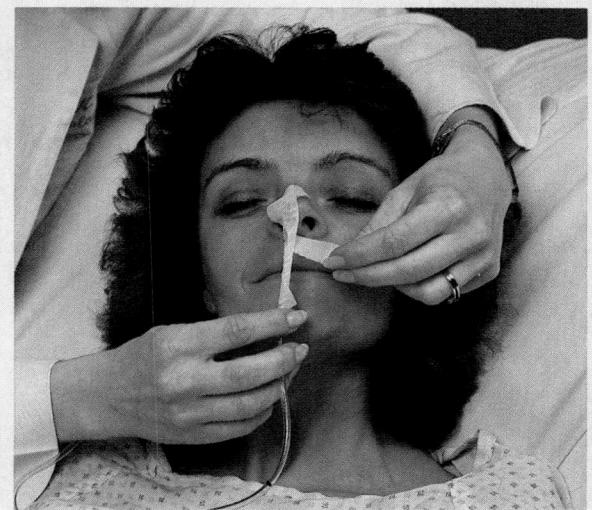

Step 32b

Inserting and Maintaining
an NG Tube

STEPS	RATIONALE
a. OPTIONAL: Apply small amount of tincture of benzoin to lower end of nose and allow to dry. Place top end of tape over nose.	
b. Carefully wrap two split ends around tube (see illustrations).	
33. Fasten end of tube to gown by looping rubber band around tube in slip knot. Pin rubber band to gown.	Reduces pressure on nares if tube moves. Pinning provides slack for movement.
34. Unless physician orders otherwise, head of bed should be elevated 30 degrees.	Helps prevent esophageal reflux and minimizes irritation of tube against posterior pharynx.
35. Explain that sensation of tube will decrease somewhat.	Helps adaptation to continued sensory stimulus.
36. Wash hands.	Reduces transmission of microorganisms.
37. Record in nurses' notes time and type of tube inserted, tolerance to procedure, confirmation of placement, character of gastric contents, and whether tube is changed or connected to drainage device.	Documents that procedure was performed correctly. Description of gastric contents provides baseline to determine change.

TUBE IRRIGATION

38. Check tube placement if it remains patent.	Prevents accidental entrance of irrigating solution into lungs.
39. Draw up 30 ml of normal saline into Asepto or cone-tipped syringe.	Minimizes loss of electrolytes from stomach fluids.
40. Clamp connection tubing proximal to connection site for drainage or suction apparatus. Disconnect tubing and lay end on towel.	Reduces backflow of secretions and soiling of gown and bed linen.
41. Insert tip of irrigating syringe into end of tube. Hold syringe with tip pointed at floor and inject saline slowly and evenly. (Do not force solution.)	Position prevents introduction of air into vent tubing, which could cause gastric distention. Solution introduced under pressure can cause trauma.
42. If resistance occurs, check for kinks in tubing. Turn client onto left side. Repeated resistance should be reported to surgeon.	Tip of tube may lie against stomach lining. Buildup of secretions causes distention.
43. After instilling saline, immediately aspirate or pull back slowly on syringe to withdraw fluid. Measure volume returned as output.	Irrigation clears tubing, so stomach should remain empty. Fluid remaining in stomach is measured as intake.
44. Reconnect tube to drainage or suction. (If solution does not return, repeat irrigation.)	Reestablishes drainage collection; may repeat irrigation or repositioning of tube until tube drains properly.
45. Wash hands.	Reduces transmission of microorganisms.
46. Record each irrigation: type and amount of solution used and character and volume of aspirate.	Documents procedure and results.

DISCONTINUATION OF TUBE

47. Apply nonsterile gloves.	Reduces transmission of microorganisms.
48. Turn off suction and disconnect tube from drainage bag or suction. Remove tape from bridge of nose and unpin tube from gown.	Tube is free of connections before removal.
49. Explain procedure to client and reassure that removal is less distressing than insertion.	Minimizes anxiety and increases cooperation. Tube passes out smoothly.

STEPS	RATIONALE
50. Hand client facial tissue; place clean towel across chest. Instruct client to take and hold deep breath.	Airway will be temporarily obstructed during removal. Client may wish to blow nose after removal.
51. Clamp or kink tubing securely and pull tube out steadily and smoothly while client holds breath.	Clamping prevents tube contents from draining into oropharynx.
52. Measure unit of drainage and note character of content. Dispose of tube and drainage equipment.	Provides accurate measure of fluid output. Reduces transfer of microorganisms.
53. Wash hands.	Reduces transmission of microorganisms.
54. Clean nares and provide mouth care.	Promotes comfort.
55. Position client comfortably and explain procedure for drinking fluid, if not contraindicated.	Depends on physician's order; usually begins with small amount of ice chips each hour and increases as client is able to tolerate more.
56. Clean equipment and return to proper place. Place soiled linen in "dirty" utility room or proper receptacle.	Proper disposal of equipment prevents spread of microorganisms and ensures proper exchange procedures.
57. Remove gloves and wash hands.	Reduces transmission of microorganisms.
58. Palpate abdomen periodically, noting distention.	Determines success of abdominal decompression.
59. Inspect condition of nares and nose.	Evaluates onset of skin and tissue irritation.
60. Record removal of NG tube, client's tolerance of procedure, presence of bowel sounds, and abdominal assessment.	Documents procedure and provides baseline information regarding abdominal assessment and bowel sounds.

 Research Highlight

The purpose of this clinical study by Metheny et al was to investigate whether pH values of aspirates could be used to differentiate between gastric and intestinal placement and gastric and respiratory placement. The sample consisted of 181 adults ($N = 181$), 94 with NG tubes and 87 with nasointestinal tubes. Tube placement was confirmed by x-ray determination made with the pH aspirate readings. The researchers found, after making a total of 247 pH aspirate readings, that pH readings were effective in differentiating between gastric and intestinal placement. The majority of pH aspirates from NG tubes had values that ranged from 1 to 4, whereas the pH aspirates from nasointestinal tubes had values of 6 or greater.

Metheny N et al: Effectiveness of pH measurements in predicting feeding tube placement, *Nurs Res* 38(5):280, 1989.

poses (Table 47-6 on p. 1630). For a surgical client the main purpose is stomach decompression to prevent abdominal distention. The physician often waits to order NG tube insertion until the client is in the operating room.

The Levin and Salem sump tubes are the most common for stomach decompression. The Levin tube is a single-lumen tube with holes near the tip. It may be connected to a drainage bag or an intermittent suction device to drain stomach secretions.

The Salem sump tube is preferable for stomach decompression. The tube has two lumina: one for removal of gastric contents and one to provide an air vent. A blue "pigtail" is the air vent that connects with the second lumen. When the sump tube's main lumen is connected to suction, the air vent permits free, continuous drainage of secretions. The air vent should never be clamped off, connected to suction, or used for irrigation.

The procedure for tube insertion (Procedure 47-3) does not require sterile technique. The nurse simply uses clean technique. The procedure is uncomfortable. The client experiences a burning sensation as

TABLE 47-6	Purposes of NG Intubation	
Purpose	Description	Type of Tube
Decompression	Removal of secretions and gaseous substances from gastrointestinal tract; prevention or relief of abdominal distention	Salem sump, Levin, Miller-Abbott
Feeding (gavage) (see Chapter 35)	Instillation of liquid nutritional supplements or feedings into stomach for clients unable to swallow fluid	Duo, Dobhoff, Levin
Compression	Internal application of pressure by means of inflated balloon to prevent internal gastrointestinal hemorrhage	Sengstaken-Blakemore
Lavage	Irrigation of stomach in cases of active bleeding, poisoning, or gastric dilation	Levin, Ewald, Salem sump

the tube passes through the sensitive nasal mucosa. When the tube reaches the back of the pharynx, the client may begin to gag. The nurse must help the client relax to make tube insertion easier.

One of the greatest problems in caring for a client with an NG tube is maintaining comfort. The tube is a constant irritation to nasal mucosa. The nurse must assess the condition of the nares and mucosa for inflammation and excoriation. The tape used to anchor the tube becomes soiled. The nurse changes it every day to lessen irritation. Frequent lubrication of the nares also minimizes excoriation. With one naris occluded, the client may breathe through the mouth. Frequent mouth care (at least every 2 hours) helps minimize dehydration. A glass of cool water for rinsing is useful, but the client who is NPO should not swallow the water. The client will frequently complain of a sore throat. An ice bag applied externally to the throat sometimes helps.

After the tube is introduced, the nurse must maintain its patency. If the tip of the tubing rests against the stomach wall or if the tube becomes blocked with thick secretions, regular irrigation is necessary. Flushing the tube with normal saline by way of a cone-tipped syringe clears blockage within the tube (Procedure 47-3). If an NG tube continues to drain improperly after irrigation, the nurse must reposition it by advancing or withdrawing it slightly. Any change in position requires reassessment of tube placement.

The NG tube can cause distention. The presence of the tube causes many clients to swallow large volumes of air. Channels of gastric secretions also form along the walls of the stomach and bypass the suction holes. Turning the client regularly helps to collapse the channels and promote emptying of stomach contents.

SAFEGUARDING VALUABLES. If a client has any valuables, the nurse should turn them over to family members or secure them for safekeeping. Many hospitals require clients to sign a release to free the institution of responsibility for lost valuables. Valuables can usually be stored and locked in a designated location. Often, clients are reluctant to remove wedding rings or religious medals. A wedding band can be taped in place. However, if there is a risk that the client will experience swelling of the hand or fingers, the band should be removed. Many hospitals allow clients to pin religious medals to their gowns, although the risk of loss increases.

ADMINISTERING PREOPERATIVE MEDICATIONS. The anesthesiologist or surgeon orders preanesthetic drugs that reduce the client's anxiety, the amount of general anesthesia required, and respiratory tract secretions. Tranquilizers, such as chlorpromazine (Thorazine) or diazepam (Valium), reduce anxiety and relax skeletal muscles. Narcotic analgesics, such as meperidine (Demerol) or morphine, provide sedation, reduce pain and anxiety, and reduce the amount of anesthetic required during surgery. Drugs, such as glycopyrrolate (Robinul) or atropine, create anticholinergic effects to inhibit mucous secretions in the oral and respiratory passages and prevent spasm of laryngeal muscles.

Typically the physician orders preoperative medications to be administered when the client leaves for the operating room or at an earlier prescribed time. The nurse provides all nursing care measures before giving the client preoperative medications. Because the drugs cause sedation, the client should not be allowed to leave the bed or stretcher until surgical orderlies and nurses arrive to transport the client to the operating room. The client should be warned to an-

Sample Evaluation of Interventions for Knowledge Deficit

Goals	Evaluative Measures	Expected Outcomes
Client will understand intraoperative and postoperative events.	Ask client and family to identify appropriate times of surgery and routine postoperative monitoring and treatment procedures.	Client and family will describe routine procedures that nurses perform after surgery.
Client will understand physiological and psychological responses to surgery.	Ask client and family to identify basic purpose of surgery and changes to expect after surgery.	Client will describe purpose of surgery and physical or psychological changes to expect.
Client will achieve return of normal physiological function after surgery.	Have client demonstrate deep breathing, coughing, splinting, foot and leg exercises, and turning.	Client will be able to ventilate to maximum ability, cough forcibly, perform exercises, and turn correctly after surgery.
Client will achieve rest and comfort.	Observe time client falls asleep after bedtime. Ask if client feels rested on awakening in morning.	Client will fall asleep within 30 min after bedtime. Client will report feeling rested and at ease.

ticipate drowsiness and dry mouth. The side rails should be raised and the bed or stretcher kept in the low position for client safety.

Evaluation

Often, there is limited time to evaluate the outcomes of the preoperative care plan. The client's surgery may be an emergency, or performance of various procedures may make it difficult for the nurse to find time for evaluation. The nurse's interventions may continue during and after surgery so that evaluation does not occur until after surgery. For example, the nurse will not be able to evaluate the success of reducing postoperative wound infection or promoting return of normal physiological function until a few days after surgery.

The nurse evaluates success at preoperative teaching and promotes the client's physiological function and achievement of rest and physical comfort (see evaluation box). However, evaluation of these interventions must also continue after surgery.

Transport to the Operating Room

Personnel in the operating room notify the nursing division or ambulatory surgical waiting area when it is time for surgery. In many hospitals a nursing orderly or transporter brings a stretcher for transporting the client. The transporter checks the client's identification bracelet against the client's chart to be sure that the right person is going to surgery. Because the client has already received preoperative

drugs, the nurses and transporter assist the client in transferring from bed to stretcher to prevent falls.

The family gets one last opportunity to visit before the client is transported to the operating room. Nurses then direct the family to a waiting area.

After the client leaves the nursing division, the nurse prepares the bed and room for the client's return if the client is returning to the same nursing division. A postoperative bedside unit should include the following:

1. Sphygmomanometer, stethoscope, and thermometer
2. Emesis basin
3. Clean gown
4. Washcloth, towel, and facial tissues
5. IV pole
6. Suction equipment
7. Oxygen equipment
8. Extra pillows for positioning the client comfortably
9. Bed pads to protect bed linen from drainage
10. Bed raised to stretcher height with bed linens pulled back

The nurse will be better prepared to care for the client after surgery if the room is readied before the client's return.

INTRAOPERATIVE SURGICAL PHASE

Care of the client during surgery requires careful preparation and knowledge of the events that occur during the surgical procedure.

Holding Area

In most hospitals the client enters a holding area outside the operating room. There, the nurse explains the steps to be taken in preparing the client for surgery. Nurses in the holding area are usually part of the operating room staff and wear surgical scrub suits, hats, and footwear in accordance with infection-control policies. In some ambulatory surgical settings a perioperative primary nurse admits the client, circulates for the operative procedure, and recovers and discharges the client.

In the holding area the nurse or anesthesiologist inserts an IV catheter into the arm to establish a route for fluid replacement and IV drugs. A large-bore IV catheter is used for easy infusion of fluids. The nurse also applies a blood pressure cuff. The cuff will remain in place throughout surgery so that the anesthesiologist can assess blood pressure readings.

By this time the client begins to feel drowsy. Because the temperature in the holding area and adjacent operating room suites is usually cool, the client should be offered an extra blanket. The client's stay in the holding area should be brief.

Admission to the Operating Room

Nurses transfer the client to the operating room via stretcher. The client is usually still awake and will notice nurses and physicians wearing complete surgical masks and gowns. The staff carefully transfers the client to the operating table, being sure that the stretcher and table are locked in place. After the client is on the table, the nurse fastens a safety strap around the client.

The operating room nurse checks the client's identification and chart; reviews consent forms, medical history, physical assessment findings, and test results; makes sure that prosthetic devices and valuables have been removed; and reviews the care plan to establish an intraoperative care plan.

The nurse may apply monitoring devices to the client before surgery. Clients receiving general and regional anesthesia undergo continuous ECG monitoring during surgery. Small, plastic electrodes are placed on the chest and extremities to record electrical activity of the heart. A monitor in the operating room displays the heart's electrical activity.

Many ambulatory surgical clients remain awake during the procedure because only local anesthetic is used. The nurse supports the client by explaining procedures and encouraging the client to ask questions. Sights and sounds in the surgical suite can frighten clients.

Introduction of Anesthesia

Clients undergoing surgical procedures receive anesthesia in one of three ways: general, regional, or local.

General Anesthesia

Under **general anesthesia,** a client loses all sensation and consciousness. Muscles relax to ease manipulation of body parts. The client also experiences amnesia of all surgical events. Surgery using general anesthesia involves major procedures requiring extensive tissue manipulation.

An anesthesiologist gives general anesthetics by IV and inhalation routes through the four stages of anesthesia. Stage 1 begins with the client awake. The client gradually becomes drowsy and loses consciousness, and a state of analgesia begins. Stage 2 is the stage of excitement. The client's muscles are often tense and almost spasmodic. Swallowing and vomiting reflexes remain intact, and the client may have an irregular breathing pattern. Stage 3 begins with the onset of regular rhythmical breathing. Vital functions are depressed, reflexes are depressed or temporarily lost, and the surgeon begins the operation during this phase. Stage 4 is the stage of complete respiratory depression, which can be fatal.

To move the client quickly to stage 3 of general anesthesia, the anesthesiologist usually gives an IV dose of a barbiturate. To prevent possible aspiration and other respiratory complications, the anesthesiologist puts an endotracheal tube into the client's airway. Succinylcholine causes temporary paralysis of vocal cords and respiratory muscles while the tube is in place. The anesthesiologist then provides artificial ventilation until succinylcholine's effects wear off and the client again breathes spontaneously. From that point, anesthetic gases or vapors are usually delivered by inhalation through the endotracheal tube. The client also receives a continuous supply of oxygen.

The duration of anesthesia depends on the length of surgery. Surgical risks influence the duration of surgery. The greatest risks from general anesthesia are the side effects of anesthetic agents, including cardiovascular depression or irritability, respiratory depression, and liver and kidney damage.

Regional Anesthesia

Induction of **regional anesthesia** results in loss of sensation in an area of the body. The method of induction influences the portion of sensory pathways that is anesthetized. The anesthesiologist gives regional anesthetics by infiltration and local application (see Chapter 37). In major surgery, such as a hernia repair, vaginal hysterectomy, or vascular repair of leg blood vessels, only infiltrative induction is used. Infiltration of anesthetic agents may involve one of the following induction methods:

1. Nerve block. Local anesthetic is injected into a nerve (for example, brachial plexus in the arm), blocking the nerve supply to the operative site.
2. Spinal anesthesia. The anesthesiologist performs a lumbar puncture and introduces local anesthetic into the cerebrospinal fluid in the spinal subarachnoid space. Anesthesia can extend from the tip of the xiphoid process down to the feet. Positioning of the client influences movement of the anesthetic agent up or down the spinal cord.
3. Epidural anesthesia. This is a safer procedure than spinal anesthesia because the anesthetic agent is injected into the epidural space outside the dura mater and the level of anesthesia is not as great as spinal anesthesia. Because epidural anesthesia provides an effective loss of sensation in the vaginal and perineal areas, it is the best anesthetic for obstetrical procedures.
4. Caudal anesthesia. This is a form of epidural anesthesia achieved by giving the local anesthetic at the base of the spine. The extent of anesthesia affects only the pelvic region and legs.

There are risks involved with infiltrative anesthetics, particularly in the case of spinal anesthesia, because the level of anesthesia may rise. The client may have a sudden fall in blood pressure, which results from extensive vasodilation caused by the anesthetic block to sympathetic vasomotor nerves, pain, and motor fibers. If the level of anesthesia rises, respiratory paralysis may develop, requiring resuscitation by the anesthesiologist. The client requires careful monitoring during and immediately after surgery.

The client under regional anesthesia is awake throughout the surgery unless the physician orders a tranquilizer that promotes sleep. Because the client is responsive and capable of breathing voluntarily, it is unnecessary for the anesthesiologist to use an endotracheal tube. Operating room personnel often gain a false sense of security because of the client's relative alertness. Nurses must remember that burns and other trauma can occur on the anesthetized part of the body without the client being aware of the injury. It is therefore necessary to frequently observe the position of extremities and the condition of the skin.

Local Anesthesia

Local anesthesia involves loss of sensation at the desired site (for example, a growth on the skin or the cornea of the eye). The anesthetic agent (for example, lidocaine) inhibits nerve conduction until the drug diffuses into the circulation. The client experiences a loss in pain sensation and touch, motor, and autonomic activities (for example, bladder emptying). Local anesthesia is commonly used for minor procedures performed in ambulatory surgery.

Positioning the Client for Surgery

During general anesthesia, the nursing personnel and surgeon often do not position the client until the stage of complete relaxation. The choice of position is usually determined by the surgical approach. Ideally the client's position provides good access to the operative site and sustains adequate circulatory and respiratory function. It should not impair neuromuscular structures. The client's comfort and safety must be considered.

It is sometimes difficult for nurses in postoperative divisions to appreciate the discomfort a client may feel after surgery (for example, discomfort of the left arm or side of a client whose right kidney was removed) (Fig. 47-3). Normal range of joint motion is maintained in an alert person by pain and pressure receptors. If a joint is extended too far, pain stimuli provide a warning that muscle and joint strain are too great. In a client who is anesthetized, normal defense mechanisms cannot guard against joint damage, muscle stretch, and strain. The mucles are so relaxed that it is relatively easy to place the client in a position the individual normally could not assume while awake. The client often remains in a given position for several hours. Although it may be necessary to place a client in an unusual position, the nurse should attempt to maintain correct alignment and protect the client from pressure, abrasion, and other injuries. Attachments to the operating table allow protection and padding of extremities and bony prominences. Positioning should not impede normal movement of the diaphragm or interfere with circulation to body parts. If restraints are necessary, the nurse pads the area to be restrained to prevent skin trauma.

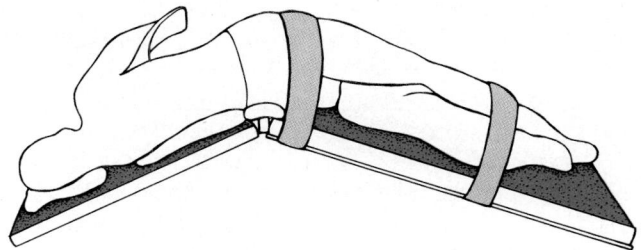

Fig 47-3 Client's position on operating room table for a nephrectomy.

BARNES

OPERATIVE NURSES NOTES AND OR RECORD

DATE / /	OR RM NO.	SER	☐ SCHEDULED ☐ EMERGENCY	RECORD NO.

PREOPERATIVE ASSESSMENT

PATIENT IDENTIFICATION VERIFIED BY: ☐ PATIENT   ☐ OTHER _____

☐ ARMBAND   ☐ STAMP PLATE   ☐ FACE SHEET   ☐ CHART REVIEWED

☐ OPERATIVE PERMIT VERIFIED

NPO: ☐ YES ☐ NO   SINCE _____

☐ **ALLERGIES TO:** _____

_____ ☐ NKA

VERIFICATION OF PROCEDURE/LOCATION: ☐ VERBAL   ☐ CONSENT FORM

☐ SPECIAL PROCEDURE PERMIT (SPECIFY) _____ ☐ NA

MENTAL/EMOTIONAL STATUS: ☐ ALERT/ORIENTED ☐ DROWSY/SEDATED ☐ CONFUSED/DISORIENTED

☐ UNCONSCIOUS/UNRESPONSIVE ☐ INTUBATED/TRACH   ☐ NERVOUS/ANXIOUS

PHYSICAL ABNORMALITIES/LIMITATIONS: ☐ NONE   ☐ AUDITORY   ☐ VISUAL

☐ LANGUAGE ☐ MOBILITY   ☐ OTHER _____

PERSONAL ITEMS: ☐ YES   ☐ NO   LIST: _____

_____ DISPOSITION _____

SKIN CONDITION: ☐ INTACT   ☐ OTHER _____

COMFORT MEASURES IMPLEMENTED: ☐ WARM BLANKET ☐ OTHER _____

IV   ☐ NA

☐ SITE _____ FLUID _____ ☐ SITE _____ FLUID _____

☐ ARTERIAL LINE   ☐ NA   LOCATION _____   ☐ O2 ☐ NA   ☐ NG TUBE ☐ NA

☐ SWAN GANZ ☐ NA   LOCATION _____   ☐ FOLEY CATHETER ☐ NA

☐ CVP LINE ☐ NA   LOCATION _____   ☐ OTHER _____ ☐ NA

TIME _____ RN

PATIENT ESCORTED TO OR ROOM BY: ☐ MD   ☐ ANESTH   ☐ RN

NAME: _____

NURSING DIAGNOSIS: Potential For Anxiety Related To Knowledge Deficit.

PLAN & IMPLEMENTATION-GOAL: Demonstrates Decreased Anxiety.

☐ GIVE CLEAR CONCISE EXPLANATIONS   ☐ CONVEY CARING, SUPPORTIVE ATTITUDE

☐ COMMUNICATE PATIENT CONCERNS TO OTHER HEALTHCARE MEMBERS   ☐ REMAIN WITH PATIENT DURING INDUCTION   ☐ OTHER _____

EVALUATION: Demonstrated Understanding Of Explanations.   ☐ YES   ☐ NO

INITIALS _____   IF NO, EXPLAIN _____

NURSES NOTES: _____

_____

_____

_____

_____

_____

_____

_____

_____

_____

_____

_____

_____

_____

_____

_____

_____

_____

ROOM READY	LC	PT IN OR	LC	INCISION	DRESSING	TIME OUT

PRE-OP DIAGNOSIS

PROCEDURE

☐ X-RAY PROCEDURE ☐ NA   ☐ LASER TYPE _____   ☐ NA

POST-OP DIAGNOSIS

ANESTHETIC ROUTE ☐ GEN ☐ SPINAL/EPID   ☐ LOCAL ☐ REGIONAL   ☐ MAC ☐ BLOCK TYPE _____   ☐ NONE   FACTOR

	FIRST PROCEDURE	SECOND PROCEDURE/RELIEF
SURGEON		
1ST ASSISTANT		
2ND ASSISTANT		
3RD ASSISTANT		
OTHER		
ATTENDING ANESTHESIOLOGIST	RELIEF	
RESIDENT ANESTHESIOLOGIST	RELIEF	
ANESTHETIST	RELIEF	

SCRUB NURSES/TITLE/INITIAL/ID# ☐ NA	TIME IN/OUT	TIME IN/OUT	TIME IN/OUT
CIRCULATING NURSES/TITLE/INITIAL/ID#			
CELL SAVER/TITLE/INITIAL/ID# ☐ NA			
PERFUSIONIST/TITLE/INITIAL/ID# ☐ NA			
OBSERVERS ☐ NA			

Fig. 47-4 Operative nursing note.
Courtesy Barnes Hospital, St Louis.

Nurse's Role During Surgery

The nurse assumes one of two roles during the surgical procedure: scrub nurse or circulating nurse. The **scrub nurse** provides the surgeon with instruments and supplies, which requires strict surgical asepsis (see Chapter 48) and familiarity with surgical instruments. Each instrument is designed for a specific purpose during a phase or step in surgery. It takes knowledge and skill to anticipate which instrument the surgeon requires and to pass it quickly and smoothly. The scrub nurse also disposes of soiled gauze sponges and accounts for sponges, needles, and instruments on the surgical field and in body cavities.

The **circulating nurse** is an assistant to the scrub nurse and surgeon. When the client first enters the operating room, the circulator helps position the client and applies necessary equipment and surgical drapes. During surgery, the circulator provides the scrub nurse with supplies, disposes of soiled equipment and sponges, and keeps a count of instruments, needles, and sponges used. If there is a need to help reposition the client or move the operating room lights, the circulating nurse is available to assist. Like all members of the surgical team the circulator follows surgical aseptic technique. If a break in asepsis occurs, the circulator assists team members with regowning and regloving.

At the end of each surgical procedure, the scrub and circulating nurses count the number of used instruments, needles, and gauze sponges. This procedure prevents the accidental loss of such items within the client's surgical wound. It is not difficult for a sponge saturated with blood to be overlooked within a wound. Careful monitoring of items is essential for the client's safety. The nurse who fails to make accurate counts can be held legally accountable. If a client is injured by a misplaced needle or instrument the nurse may be judged negligent (see Chapter 14).

Documentation of Intraoperative Care

During the intraoperative phase, the nursing staff continues the preoperative care plan. For example, strict asepsis must be followed to minimize the risk of surgical wound infection (see Chapter 48). IV fluid infusion and monitoring of urinary and NG output are actions the nurse takes to maintain fluid balance. Throughout the surgical procedure, the nurse keeps an accurate record of client care activities and procedures performed by operating room personnel (Fig. 47-4). Documentation of intraoperative care provides useful data for the nurse who cares for the client postoperatively.

 ## POSTOPERATIVE SURGICAL PHASE

After surgery, a client's care can become complex as a result of physiological changes that may occur. Clients who have undergone general anesthesia are more likely to face complications than those who have only had local anesthesia. The client who requires general anesthesia usually has undergone extensive surgery as well. In contrast an ambulatory surgical client who had local anesthesia with no sedation and has stable vital signs may be discharged immediately.

To assess a client's postoperative condition the nurse relies on information from the preoperative nursing assessment and on knowledge regarding the surgical procedure performed and events occurring during surgery. The nurse must be able to detect change. A variation from the norm may indicate onset of surgically related complications.

A client's postoperative course involves two phases: the immediate recovery period and postoperative convalescence. For an ambulatory surgical client, **recovery** normally lasts only 1 to 2 hours, and **convalescence** takes place at home. For a hospitalized client, recovery may last a few hours, and convalescence takes 1 or more days, depending on the extent of surgery and the client's response.

Immediate Postoperative Recovery

Before the arrival of the client in the recovery room or postanesthesia room, the recovery room nurse obtains data from the surgical team in the operating room regarding the client's general status and need for special equipment and nursing care. Careful planning allows the nursing staff to consider placement of clients in the recovery room. For example, clients who undergo spinal anesthesia are aware of their surroundings and may benefit from being in a quieter part of the recovery room, away from clients needing frequent monitoring. The client with a serious infection should be isolated from other clients.

When the client enters the recovery room, the nurse and members of the surgical team confer about the client's status. The surgical team's report includes a review of anesthetic agents administered so that the recovery room nurse can anticipate the ease with which a client should regain consciousness. A report on IV fluids or blood products administered during surgery alerts the nurse to the fluid and electrolyte balance. The surgeon often reports special concerns (for example, whether the client is at risk for hemorrhaging or infection). The operating room nurse discusses whether there were complications during surgery, such as excessive blood loss or cardiac irregularities.

After reviewing events in the operating room, the recovery room nurse makes a complete assessment of the client's status. Until stabilized, the client remains in the recovery room.

The recovery room personnel notify the nursing division of the client's arrival. This allows the nursing staff to inform family members of the client's operative course. The nurse usually advises family members to remain in the designated waiting area so that they can be found when the surgeon arrives to explain the client's condition. The surgeon describes the client's status, the results of surgery, and the occurrence of any complications.

Anxiety can arise if the surgeon has informed the family of the anticipated length of surgery and if the client remains in the operating room past this time. Nurses can help relieve concerns by explaining normal delays, such as room preparation or delay in the previous surgery. If the client's stay in recovery is extended, the nurses can explain to the family that the client is being held longer for observation. If the client has complications, it is the surgeon's responsibility to explain what occurred during surgery.

If the client's surgery was unsuccessful or the surgeon discovered an inoperable condition (for example, a malignant tumor), the nurse provides support to the family. Directing the family to the location of public telephones, providing a cup of coffee, and encouraging expression of fears in a private location are a few ways to help the family cope with the waiting period. The family's initial shock requires the nurse to be available and serve as a resource for the family. After the initial assessment on the client's arrival to recovery, the nurse repeats evaluation of vital signs and other key observations at least every 15 minutes.

Respiration

Certain anesthetic agents may cause respiratory depression. Thus the nurse is especially alert for shallow, slow breathing and a weak cough. The nurse assesses respiratory rate, rhythm, depth of ventilation, symmetry of chest wall movement, breath sounds, and color of mucous membranes. If breathing is unusually shallow, placement of the hand over the client's face or mouth allows the nurse to feel exhaled air.

The client often has an oral or nasal airway (see Chapter 38) inserted to maintain a patent airway until comfortable breathing at a normal rate resumes.

As respiratory function returns, the nurse asks the client to spit out the airway. The ability to do so signifies the return of a normal gag reflex.

One of the nurse's greatest concerns is airway obstruction resulting from aspiration of emesis, accumulation of mucous secretions in the pharynx, or swelling or spasm of the larynx. The following measures maintain airway patency:

1. The nurse positions the client on one side with the face down and the neck slightly extended. A small, folded towel supports the head. Neck extension prevents occlusion of the airway at the pharynx. When the face is kept turned downward, the tongue moves forward and mucous secretions flow out of the mouth instead of accumulating in the pharynx. If the nature of the surgery prevents turning the client on one side, the head of the bed is slightly elevated and the client's neck slightly extended, with the head turned to the side. The client should never be positioned with arms over or across the chest because this position reduces maximal chest expansion.
2. The nurse begins coughing and deep breathing exercises as soon as the client is responsive.
3. The nurse suctions artificial airways and the oral cavity for mucous secretions. Care must be taken to avoid continually eliciting the gag reflex, which might cause vomiting. Before the nurse or client removes an airway, the back of the airway should be suctioned so that mucous plugs and secretions are not retained.
4. The nurse administers oxygen as ordered.

Circulation

The client is at risk for cardiovascular complications resulting from actual or potential blood loss from the surgical site, side effects of anesthesia, electrolyte imbalances, and depression of normal circulatory regulating mechanisms. Careful assessment of heart rate and rhythm along with blood pressure reveals the client's cardiovascular status. The values are monitored at least every 15 minutes throughout the recovery phase. The nurse compares preoperative vital signs with postoperative values. The surgeon's postoperative orders may specify when vital sign changes should be reported. For example, a heart rate above 110 beats/min or below 60 beats/min should be reported immediately. However, the nurse must use judgment in reporting vital sign changes. If the client's blood pressure drops progressively after each check or if the heart rate becomes more irregular, the physician should be notified.

The nurse assesses circulatory perfusion by noting the color of nail beds and skin. If the client has had vascular surgery or has casts or constricting devices that may impair circulation, the nurse assesses peripheral pulses distal to the site of surgery. For example, after surgery to the femoral artery, the nurse assesses popliteal and dorsalis pedis pulses. The nurse also compares pulses in the affected extremity with those in the nonaffected extremity.

A common circulatory problem is hemorrhage. Blood loss may occur externally through a drain or incision or internally within the surgical wound. Either type of hemorrhage may manifest itself by a fall in blood pressure; elevated heart and respiratory rate; thready pulse; cool, clammy, pale skin; and restlessness. If hemorrhage is external, the nurse notes increased bloody drainage on dressings or through drains. If a dressing becomes saturated, the blood oozes down the client's sides and collect in a pool under bedclothes. An alert nurse always checks under the client for drainage. When hemorrhage is internal, the operative site becomes swollen and tight. For example, if a client bleeds within the abdomen, the abdomen becomes tight and distended. The first signs of suspected hemorrhaging should be reported to the physician immediately. The nurse maintains IV fluid infusion and monitors the client's vital signs every 15 minutes or more frequently until the client's condition stabilizes.

Temperature Control

The operating room and recovery room environments are extremely cool. The client's depressed level of body function results in a lowering of metabolism and fall in body temperature. When clients begin to awaken, they complain of feeling cold and uncomfortable.

The nurse measures the client's body temperature and provides warmed blankets. Increasing body warmth causes the client's metabolism to rise and circulatory and respiratory functions to improve.

Shivering may not be a sign of hypothermia but rather a side effect of certain anesthetic agents. Deep breathing and coughing help expel retained anesthetic gases. In rare instances, **malignant hyperpyrexia,** a life-threatening complication of anesthesia, develops. Malignant hyperpyrexia causes a high fever, tachycardia, metabolic changes, and even convulsions. Without proper treatment, it can be fatal.

Neurological Functions

On arrival in the recovery room, the client is usually asleep or reacting to verbal commands. However, medications, electrolyte and metabolic changes, pain, and emotional factors can influence the level of consciousness. The nurse rouses the client by calling the name in a moderate tone of voice. The nurse notes whether the client responds appropriately or seems confused and disoriented. If the client remains asleep or unresponsive, the nurse attempts arousal through touch or by gently moving a body part. If a painful stimulus is needed to arouse the client, the nurse should notify the anesthesiologist.

As the effects of anesthesia wear off, the client's reflexes return, muscle strength is regained, and a normal level of orientation returns. The nurse can easily check for pupillary and gag reflexes (see Chapter 20). If a client has had surgery involving a portion of the neurological system, the nurse conducts a more thorough neurological assessment. For example, if the client had low back surgery, the nurse assesses leg movement, sensation, and strength. Clients with regional anesthesia begin to experience a return in motor function before tactile sensation returns.

Orientation to the recovery room environment is important in maintaining the client's alertness. The nurse explains that surgery is completed and describes procedures and nursing measures within the recovery area. The client who was properly prepared before surgery is less likely to be as anxious when recovery nurses begin their care.

Skin Integrity and Condition of Wound

In the recovery room, the nurse assesses the condition of the client's skin, noting rashes, petechiae, abrasions, or burns. A rash may indicate a drug sensitivity or allergy. Abrasions or petechiae may result from inappropriate positioning or restraining that injures skin layers. Burns may indicate that an electrical cautery grounding pad was incorrectly placed on the client's skin. Burns or serious injury to the skin should be documented by an incident report (see Chapter 14).

After surgery, most surgical wounds are covered with a dressing that protects the wound site and collects drainage. The nurse observes the amount, color, odor, and consistency of drainage on dressings. The nurse estimates the amount of drainage by noting the number of saturated gauze sponges. If drainage appears on the outer surface of a dressing, another way of assessing drainage is by drawing a circle around the outer perimeter of the drainage and dating it with the time noted. If the perimeter expands, drainage is increasing (see Chapter 48). However, this is not the most accurate measure of volume of fluid lost.

Many physicians prefer to change dressings the first time so that they can inspect the incisional area. Therefore the recovery room nurse may simply add an extra layer of gauze on top of the original dressing, thereby reinforcing the dressing.

Genitourinary Function

A client may not regain voluntary control over urinary function for 6 to 8 hours after anesthesia. An epidural or spinal anesthetic may prevent the client from feeling bladder fullness or distention. The nurse palpates the lower abdomen just above the symphysis pubis for bladder distention. Because a full bladder can be painful and often cause restlessness in recovery, it may become necessary to insert a catheter. If the client has a Foley catheter, there should be a continuous flow of urine of at least 2 ml/kg/hr in adults. The nurse observes the color and odor of urine. Surgery involving portions of the urinary tract normally causes bloody urine for at least 12 to 24 hours, depending on the type of surgery.

Gastrointestinal Function

Anesthetics slow gastrointestinal motility and cause nausea. Normally, during the immediate recovery phase, a nurse hears faint or absent bowel sounds in all four quadrants. Inspection of the abdomen rules out distention that may be caused by accumulation of gas. In a client who has had abdominal surgery, distention will develop if internal bleeding occurs.

To minimize nausea the nurse avoids sudden movement of the client. If the client has an NG tube, the nurse keeps it patent by regular irrigations. Occlusion of NG tubes results in accumulation of gastric contents within the stomach. Because stomach emptying slows under anesthesia, the accumulated contents cannot escape, and nausea and vomiting develop. Normally a client does not receive fluids to drink in the recovery room because of the risk of vomiting.

Fluid and Electrolyte Balance

Because of the surgical client's risk for fluid and electrolyte abnormalities, the nurse assesses the hydration status and monitors cardiac and neurological function for signs of electrolyte alterations (see Chapter 39). The nurse also has an important responsibility for maintaining patency of IV infusions. The client's only source of fluid intake immediately after surgery is through IV catheters. The nurse inspects a catheter insertion site to be sure that it is properly positioned within a vein so that fluid flows freely. The physician orders a prescribed rate for each infusion. To ensure adequate fluid intake the nurse should not allow infusion of fluids to fall behind. The client may also receive blood products after surgery, depending on the blood loss during surgery.

Accurate recording of intake and output helps assess renal and circulatory function. The nurse measures all sources of output, including urine, gastric drainage, drainage from wounds, and any insensible loss from diaphoresis. Mucus suctioned from airways is not included in output measurements.

Comfort

As clients awaken from general anesthesia, the sensation of pain becomes prominent. Pain can be perceived before full consciousness is regained. Acute incisional pain causes clients to become restless and may be responsible for changes in vital signs. It is difficult for clients to begin coughing and deep breathing exercises when they experience pain. The client who had regional or local anesthesia usually does not experience pain initially because the incisional area is still anesthetized.

It is common to administer narcotic analgesics immediately after surgery to expedite pain relief and minimize respiratory depression. After a hospitalized client is transferred to a hospital room, patient-controlled analgesia (PCA) given intravenously or epidural analgesia may be continued (see Chapter 37). Intramuscular injections may initially be given in divided doses, but this is not the preferred route of administration immediately after surgery.

Recovery in Ambulatory Surgery

The thoroughness and extent of postoperative assessment depend on the ambulatory client's condition, type of surgery, and anesthesia. In many cases the assessment is identical to that conducted for hospitalized clients. However, if the client has undergone minor surgery (for example, cosmetic removal of a mole), the postoperative recovery phase requires minimal assessment.

If an ambulatory client has received general or regional anesthesia or intensive IV sedation, the client will be transferred to the recovery room. In phase I recovery, clients in need of close monitoring are frequently assessed for vital sign changes, respiratory and circulatory status, level of consciousness, condition of the surgical wound, and pain level.

The time that a client spends in phase I recovery depends on several factors. Outpatient anesthesia is gauged to provide a quick recovery time, few aftereffects, and a speedy return to daily routines. The average time spent in phase I is 1 hour, without complications. Clients are encouraged to gradually sit up on the stretcher or bed and begin to take ice chips or sips of water while regaining full alertness. After clients become stable and no longer require close monitoring, the nurse transfers them to phase II recovery. Clients who have undergone minor surgery may be transferred directly to phase II recovery.

Phase II recovery consists of a room equipped with medical recliner chairs, side tables, and foot rests. Kitchen facilities for preparing light snacks and beverages are usually located in the area, along with bathrooms. The phase II environment is designed to promote the client's and families' comfort and well-being until discharge. The nurse monitors clients but not at the same intensity as phase I. In phase II recovery, nurses initiate postoperative teaching with clients and family members (see box).

Postoperative Convalescence

After the client's condition stabilizes, the client is returned to the postoperative nursing division. Ambulatory surgical clients will, in contrast, be discharged. Nursing care focuses on returning the client to a relatively functional level of wellness as soon as possible. The speed of convalescence depends on the type or extent of surgery, risk factors, postoperative complications, and the nurse's care plan.

Discharge from the Recovery Room

The nurse evaluates readiness for discharge from recovery on the basis of vital sign stability, body temperature control, good ventilatory function, orientation to surroundings, absence of complications, minimal pain and nausea, controlled wound drainage, adequate urine output, and fluid and electrolyte balance. If the client's condition is still poor after 2 to 3 hours, the stay will lengthen or the surgeon may transfer the client to an intensive care unit (ICU).

When the client is discharged from recovery, the nurse calls the nursing division to report vital signs, the type of surgery and anesthesia performed, blood loss, level of consciousness, general physical condition, and presence of IV lines or drainage tubes. The nurse's report helps the nurse on the division anticipate special client needs and obtain necessary equipment.

A nurse and transporter return the client on a stretcher. Staff members assist in safely transferring

the client to a bed (see Chapter 43). The recovery room nurse shows the division nurse the recovery room record and reviews the client's condition and course of care. The recovery room nurse also points out physician orders that require attention. Before the recovery nurse leaves, the division nurse takes a complete set of vital signs to compare with recovery room findings. Minor vital sign variations normally occur after transporting the client.

Assessment

The nurse's assessment includes an initial check of the client's general condition, including vital signs, level of consciousness, condition of dressings and drains, IV fluid status, comfort level, and skin integrity.

The same physical measurements and observations performed in the recovery room are also carried out on the postoperative division. The nurse routinely assesses the client at least every 15 minutes the first hour, every 30 minutes for 1 to 2 hours, every hour for 4 hr, and then every 4 hours. Frequency of assessment depends on the client's condition. A nurse should not assume that further monitoring is unnecessary if the client appears normal during the initial assessment. A client's postoperative condition can change rapidly. A nurse is guilty of neglect when failing to follow the assessment schedule.

The nurse thoroughly documents the initial assessment and makes entries in the nurses' notes. Vital signs, IV fluid intake, and urinary output measurements can be entered on flowsheets. The initial findings are a baseline for comparing postoperative changes.

After the nurse completes the first assessment and has attended to immediate needs, the family is allowed to visit. The nurse can explain the purpose of postoperative procedures or equipment. The family wants to know how the client is doing. The nurse explains whether vital signs are stable and whether the client seems to be awakening without difficulty. The family should know that the client will fall in and out of sleep for most of the rest of the day from the effects of general anesthesia. The family should also be reminded that frequent assessments are to be expected and that loss of sensation and movement in the extremities remains for several hours if the client had spinal anesthesia.

Nursing Diagnosis

The nurse determines the status of problems identified from preoperative nursing diagnoses and clus-

---

Postoperative Instructions for Ambulatory Surgical Clients

- Physician's office phone number
- Surgery center's phone number
- Follow-up appointment, date, and time
- Review of prescribed medications
- Guidelines related to specific surgery (for example, dressing and wound care, activity restrictions, and warning signs of complications)

ters new relevant data to identify new diagnoses (see diagnoses box). Previously defined diagnoses, such as *impaired skin integrity,* may continue as a postoperative problem. The nurse may also identify risk factors leading to identification of potential nursing diagnoses (see diagnostic process box). For example, an older client who has undergone major abdominal surgery and who has a preexisting problem of reduced hip mobility resulting from arthritis will be at risk for the diagnosis of *high risk of impaired physical mobility.* The nurse also considers needs of a client's family when making diagnoses. For example, the inability of the family to cope with the client's condition requires the nurse's intervention.

 Examples of Nursing Diagnoses for Postoperative Client

NANDA-APPROVED NURSING DIAGNOSES

Ineffective airway clearance related to:
- Diminished cough
- Retained secretions
- Prolonged sedation

Ineffective breathing pattern related to:
- Incisional pain
- Analgesia effects on ventilation

Pain related to:
- Surgical incision
- NG tube placement

Ineffective individual coping related to:
- Constraints imposed by surgery
- Postoperative therapies

High risk for fluid volume deficit related to:
- Wound drainage
- Inadequate fluid intake

High risk for or *actual impaired skin integrity* related to:
- Wound drainage
- Impaired mobility

Anticipatory grieving related to:
- Client's critical condition

Impaired physical mobility related to:
- Pain
- Postoperative activity restrictions
- Casts or dressings

Altered oral mucous membranes related to:
- Irritation of nasogastric or endotracheal tube
- NPO status

Feeding, bathing/hygiene, dressing/grooming, toileting self-care deficit related to:
- Postoperative activity restrictions

High risk for altered body temperature related to:
- Lowered metabolism

High risk for infection related to:
- Surgical wound incision

Impaired verbal communication related to:
- Endotracheal or airway tube placement

 Sample Nursing Diagnostic Process for Postoperative Client

Assessment Activities	Defining Characteristics	Nursing Diagnoses
Monitor the rate and depth of client's respirations.	Elevated respiratory rate Shallow respirations	*Ineffective airway clearance* related to incisional pain.
Auscultate lungs. Observe client's postoperative coughing technique.	Abnormal breath sounds Dyspnea Ineffective cough with splinting	
Ask client if discomfort is noted in area of abdominal incision; have client describe nature and character of pain. Observe client's nonverbal behavior while moving and when coughing or deep breathing.	Right upper quadrant incision of 6 in Verbalizes sharp pain present in abdomen, increased with breathing Grimaces when coughs or breathes deeply Attempts to splint abdomen during moving	*Pain* related to trauma of surgical incision.

Planning

At the convalescent phase the nurse has much information to plan the client's care. Current physical assessment data and analysis of the preoperative nursing history allow the nurse to plan specific nursing interventions. The surgeon's postoperative orders also offer guidelines. Typical postoperative orders include the following:

1. Frequency of vital signs and special assessments
2. Types of IV fluids and rate of infusion
3. Postoperative medications (especially those for pain and nausea)
4. Fluids and food allowed by mouth
5. Level of activity that the client is allowed to resume
6. Position that the client is to maintain while in bed
7. Intake and output
8. Laboratory tests and x-ray studies
9. Special directions

The nurse considers the effects of the stress of surgery and limitations it produces when establishing goals of care for the client. Likewise, the nurse considers goals of care established during the preoperative surgical phase. Typical goals of care postoperatively include the following:

1. Gaining a return of normal physiological function

2. Remaining free of postoperative surgical wound infection
3. Achieving rest and comfort
4. Maintaining self-concept
5. Returning to a functional state of health within limitations posed by surgery

The box outlines a typical sample care plan for a postoperative surgical client.

Implementation

Regaining Normal Physioloigcal Function

A surgical wound, the effects of prolonged immobilization during surgery and convalescence, and the influence of anesthesia and analgesics are the principal causes for postoperative complications. Nursing interventions are directed at preventing complications so that the client returns to the highest level of functioning possible. Failure of the client to become actively involved in recovery adds to the risk of complications (Table 47-7 on p. 1642). Virtually any body system can be affected. The nurse must consider the interrelationship of all systems and therapies provided.

MAINTAINING RESPIRATORY FUNCTION. To prevent respiratory complications the nurse begins aggressive pulmonary hygiene measures early. The benefits of thorough preoperative teaching are realized when cli-

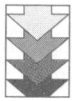
Sample Nursing Care Plan for Ineffective Airway Clearance

Nursing diagnosis: *Ineffective airway clearance* related to incisional pain
Definition: Ineffective airway clearance is the state in which an individual is unable to clear secretions or obstructions from the respiratory tract to maintain airway patency (Kim, McFarland, McLane, 1991).

Goal	Expected Outcomes	Interventions	Rationale
Client will achieve normal ventilatory function with patent airway by second postoperative day.	Client will be able to breathe deeply.	Have client perform diaphragmatic breathing using incentive spirometer every 2 hr while awake.	Adequate lung expansion can prevent atelectasis.
	Cough will be clear and nonproductive.	Have client splint abdominal incision while performing coughing exercises.	Splinting incision helps prevent discomfort while performing coughing exercises.
		Offer preferred fluids (iced tea and cranberry juice), 1500 ml/day minimum.	Increased fluid intake helps prevent thickening of mucus.
	Lung sounds will be clear.	Turn client side to side every 1-2 hr while awake.	Turning permits lung expansion.

TABLE 47-7 Postoperative Complications

Complication	Cause

RESPIRATORY SYSTEM

Atelectasis is collapse of alveoli with retained mucous secretions. Signs and symptoms include elevated respiratory rate, dyspnea, fever, crackles auscultated over involved lobes of lungs, and productive cough.

Atelectasis is caused by inadequate lung expansion. Anesthesia, analgesia, analgesics, and immobilized position prevent full lung expansion. There is greater risk in clients with upper abdominal surgery who have pain during inspiration and repress deep breathing.

Pneumonia is inflammation of alveoli caused by infectious process. It may involve one or several lobes of lung. Development of pneumonia in lower dependent lobes of lung is common in immobilized surgical client. Signs and symptoms include fever, chills, productive cough, chest pain, purulent mucus, and dyspnea.

Pneumonia is caused by poor lung expansion with retained secretions. Common resident bacteria in respiratory tract is *Diplococcus pneumoniae*, which causes most cases of pneumonia.

Hypoxia is inadequate concentration of oxygen in arterial blood. Signs and symptoms include restlessness, dyspnea, high blood pressure, tachycardia, diaphoresis, and cyanosis.

Respirations are depressed by anesthetics or analgesics. Increased retention of mucus with impaired ventilation occurs because of pain or poor positioning.

Pulmonary embolism is embolus blocking pulmonary artery and disrupting blood flow to one or more lobes of lung. Signs and symptoms include dyspnea, sudden chest pain, cyanosis, tachycardia, and drop in blood pressure.

Same factors lead to formation of thrombus or embolus. Immobilized surgical client with preexisting circulatory or coagulation disorders is at high risk.

CIRCULATORY SYSTEM

Hemorrhage is loss of large amount of blood externally or internally in short period of time. Signs and symptoms same as hypovolemic shock.

Hemorrhage is caused by slipping of suture or dislodged clot at incisional site. Clients with coagulation disorders are at greater risk.

Hypovolemic shock is perfusion of tissues and cells from loss of circulatory fluid volume. Signs and symptoms include hypotension, weak and rapid pulse, cool and clammy skin, rapid breathing, restlessness, and reduced urine output.

In surgical client, hypovolemic shock is usually caused by hemorrhage.

Thrombophlebitis is inflammation of vein often accompanied by clot formation. Veins in legs are most commonly affected. Signs and symptoms include swelling and inflammation of involved site and aching or cramping pain. Vein feels hard, cordlike, and sensitive to touch. Pain in calf occurs when client walks or dorsiflexes foot (Homans' sign).

Venous stasis is aggravated by prolonged sitting or immobilization. Trauma to vessel wall and hypercoagulability of blood increase risk of vessel inflammation.

Thrombus is formation of clot attached to interior wall of a vein or artery, which can occlude the vessel lumen.

Thrombus is caused by venous stasis (see thrombophlebitis) and vessel trauma. Venous injury is common after surgery of legs, abdomen, pelvis, and major vessels. Thrombi also form from increased coagulability of blood (e.g., polycythemia and use of birth control pills containing estrogen).

Embolus is piece of thrombus that has dislodged and circulates in bloodstream until it lodges in another vessel, commonly lungs, heart, or brain.

GASTROINTESTINAL SYSTEM

Abdominal distention is retention of air within intestines. Signs and symptoms include increased abdominal girth and tympanic percussion over abdominal quadrants. Client complains of fullness and "gas pains."

Distention is caused by slowed peristalsis from anesthesia, bowel manipulation, or immobilization.

Constipation is infrequent passage of stools. It should not be immediate concern after surgery, especially if client has preoperative bowel preparation. After client resumes solid diet, failure to pass stool within 48 hr is cause for concern.

Slowed peristalsis (see causes of distention) and delay in resuming normal diet cause constipation.

TABLE 47-7	Postoperative Complications—cont'd	
Complication		Cause

GASTROINTESTINAL SYSTEM—CONT'D

Nausea and vomiting are symptoms of improper gastric emptying or chemical stimulation of vomiting center. Client complains of gagging or feeling full or sick to stomach.

Nausea and vomiting are caused by severe pain, abdominal distention, fear, medications, eating or drinking before peristalsis returns, and initiation of gag reflex.

GENITOURINARY SYSTEM

Urinary retention is involuntary accumulation of urine in bladder as result of loss of muscle tone. Signs and symptoms include inability to void, restlessness, and bladder distention. It appears 6-8 hr after surgery.

Retention is caused by effects of anesthesia and narcotic analgesics. Local manipulation of tissues surrounding bladder and edema interferes with bladder tone. Poor positioning of client impairs voiding reflexes.

INTEGUMENTARY SYSTEM

Wound infection is an invasion of deep or superficial wound tissues by pathogenic microorganisms; signs and symptoms include warm, red, and tender skin around incision. Client may have fever and chills. Purulent material may exit from drains or from separated wound edges. It appears 3-6 days after surgery.

Infection is caused by poor aseptic technique and contaminated wound before surgical exploration.

Wound dehiscence is separation of wound edges at suture line. Signs and symptoms include increased drainage and appearance of underlying tissues. It usualy occurs 6-8 days after surgery.

Malnutrition, obesity, preoperative radiation to surgical site, old age, poor circulation to tissues, and unusual strain on suture line from coughing cause dehiscence.

Wound evisceration is protrusion of internal organs and tissues through incision. It usually occurs 6-8 days after surgery.

See dehiscence. Client with dehiscence is at risk for developing evisceration.

---

ents are able to participate actively. The following measures promote expansion of the lungs:

1. The nurse encourages diaphragmatic breathing exercises at least every 2 hours while clients are awake. Maximal inspirations lasting 3 to 5 seconds open up alveoli.
2. The nurse instructs clients to use incentive spirometers for maximum inspiration (see Chapter 38).
3. The nurse encourages early ambulation. Walking causes clients to assume a position that does not restrict chest wall expansion and stimulates an increased respiratory rate.
4. The nurse assists clients who are restricted to bed to turn on their sides every 1 to 2 hours while awake and to sit when possible. Turning permits expansion of the lungs. Sitting causes lowering of abdominal organs, thus facilitating diaphragmatic movement and lung expansion.

The following measures promote removal of pulmonary secretions:

1. The nurse encourages coughing exercises every 2 hours while clients are awake and maintains pain control to promote a full productive cough.
2. The nurse provides oral hygiene to expectorate mucus. Oral mucosa becomes dry when clients are NPO or are placed on limited fluid intake.
3. The nurse initiates orotracheal or nasotracheal suction for clients who are too weak or unable to cough (see Chapter 38).

PREVENTING CIRCULATORY STASIS. Early measures directed at preventing circulatory complications prevent circulatory stasis. Some clients are at greater risk of venous stasis because of the nature of their surgery. The following measures promote normal venous return and circulatory blood flow:

1. The nurse encourages clients to perform leg exercises at least every hour while awake. Exercise may be contraindicated in an affected extremity involving vascular repair or realignment of fractured bones and torn cartilage.
2. The nurse applies elastic antiembolism stockings as ordered by the physician. The stockings should be removed every 8 hours and left off for 1 hours (see Chapter 43).
3. The nurse applies pneumatic antiembolism stockings. Each stocking wraps around a cli-

ent's leg and is kept in place with a velcro attachment. Compressed air inflates the padded plastic stocking systematically from ankle to calf to thigh and then deflates. The stocking reduces venous stasis.

4. The nurse encourages early ambulation. Most clients are ordered to ambulate the evening of surgery, depending on the severity of surgery and their condition. The degree of activity allowed progresses as the condition improves. Before ambulation the nurse assesses vital signs. Abnormalities may contraindicate ambulation. If vital signs are normal, the nurse first assists the client to sit on the side of the bed. Clients' complaints of dizziness are a sign of postural hypotension. A recheck of blood pressure determines whether ambulation is safe. The nurse assists with ambulation by standing at the client's side, making sure that the client can walk steadily. In the first few times out of bed, clients may be able to walk only a few feet. This improves each time. The nurse evaluates tolerance to activity by periodically assessing the pulse rate.

5. The nurse avoids positioning clients in a manner that interrupts blood flow to extremities. While in bed, clients should not have pillows or rolled blankets placed under the knees. Compression of the popliteal vessels can cause thrombi. When clients sit in chairs, their legs should be elevated on footstools. A client should never be allowed to sit with one leg crossed over the other.

6. The nurse administers anticoagulant drugs as ordered. Physicians often order small doses of anticoagulants, such as heparin, for clients at greatest risk for thrombus formation. Orthopedic clients often receive aspirin for anticoagulation.

7. The nurse promotes adequate fluid intake orally or intravenously. Adequate hydration prevents concentrated buildup of formed blood elements, such as platelets and red blood cells. When the plasma volume is low, these elements may gather to form small clots within blood vessels.

PROMOTING NORMAL ELIMINATION AND ADEQUATE NUTRITION. Interventions for preventing gastrointestinal complications promote return of normal elimination and faster resumption of normal nutritional intake. It takes several days for a client who has had surgery on gastrointestinal structures (for example, a colon resection) to resume a normal dietary intake. Normal peristalsis may not return for 2 to 3 days. In contrast, the client whose gastrointestinal tract is un-

affected directly by surgery must simply endure the effects of anesthesia before resuming dietary intake. The following measures promote return of normal elimination:

1. The nurse assesses for return of peristalsis. The nurse routinely auscultates the abdomen to detect return of normal bowel sounds; 5 to 30 loud gurgles per minute over each quadrant indicates that peristalsis has returned. High-pitched tinkling sounds accompanied by abdominal distention suggest the bowel is not functioning properly. The nurse asks if the client is passing flatus. This is an important sign indicating normal bowel function.

2. The nurse maintains a gradual progression in dietary intake. For the first few hours after surgery a client receives only IV fluids. If the physician orders a normal diet the first evening after surgery, the nurse first provides clear liquids, such as water, apple juice, or tea, after nausea subsides. Overloading with large amounts of fluids may lead to distention and vomiting. If the client tolerates liquids without nausea, the diet is advanced as ordered. Clients who have had abdominal surgery are usually NPO the first 24 to 48 hours. As peristalsis returns, the nurse provides clear liquids, followed by full liquids, a light diet of solid foods, and finally a regular diet.

3. The nurse promotes ambulation and exercise. Physical activity stimulates a return of peristalsis. The client who suffers abdominal distention and "gas pain" will obtain relief while walking.

4. The nurse maintains an adequate fluid intake. Fluids keep fecal material soft for easy passage. Fruit juices and warm liquids are especially effective.

5. The nurse administers enemas, rectal suppositories, and rectal tubes as ordered. If constipation or distention develops, the physician attempts to stimulate peristalsis with cathartics or enemas. A rectal tube or return-flow enema promotes passage of flatus (see Chapter 41).

The following measures maintain an adequate dietary intake:

1. The nurse removes sources of noxious odors.

2. The nurse assists the client to a comfortable position during mealtime. The client should sit if possible to minimize pressure on the abdomen.

3. The nurse provides small servings of food. A client is more willing to face the first meal when servings are not large.

4. The nurse provides frequent oral hygiene. Adequate hydration and cleansing of the oral cavity eliminate dryness and bad tastes.

5. The nurse provides meals when the client is rested and free from pain. Often a client loses in-

terest in eating if mealtime has been preceded by exhausting activities, such as ambulation, coughing and deep breathing exercises, or extensive dressing changes. When a client has pain, the associated nausea often causes a loss of appetite.

PROMOTING URINARY ELIMINATION. The depressant effects of anesthetics and analgesics impair the sensation of bladder fullness. If bladder tone is reduced, the client has difficulty starting urination. Clients who undergo surgery of the urinary system frequently have Foley catheters inserted to maintain free urinary flow until voluntary control of urination returns. The following measures promote normal urinary elimination (see Chapter 40):

1. The nurse assists the client to assume normal positions during voiding. The male client may need assistance to stand to void. Bedpans make voiding difficult. A female client will have better results if she is able to use a toilet.
2. The nurse checks the client frequently for the need to void. A surgical client restricted to bed needs assistance in handling and using bedpans or urinals. Often the client acquires a sudden feeling of bladder fullness and urgency to void, and the nurse must respond quickly when the client calls for help.
3. The nurse assesses for bladder distention. If a client does not void within 8 hours of surgery, it may be necessary to insert a urinary catheter. A physician's order is needed.
4. The nurse monitors intake and output. An accepted level of urine output is at least 2 ml/kg/hr for adults. If the urine is dark, concentrated, and low in volume, a physician should be notified. A client can easily become dehydrated as a result of fluid loss from the surgical wound. The nurse measures intake and output for several days after surgery until normal fluid intake and urinary output are achieved.

Promoting Wound Healing

A surgical wound undergoes considerable stress during convalescence. The stress of inadequate nutrition, impaired circulation, and metabolic alterations increases the risk for delayed healing (see Chapter 48). A wound may also undergo considerable physical stress. Strain on sutures from coughing, vomiting, distention, and movement of body parts can disrupt the wound layers. The nurse protects the wound and promotes healing. A critical time for wound healing is 24 to 72 hours after surgery. If a wound becomes infected, it usually occurs 3 to 6 days after surgery. A clean surgical wound usually does not regain strength against normal stress for 15

to 20 days after surgery. The nurse uses aseptic technique during dressing changes and wound care (see Chapter 18). Surgical drains must remain patent so that accumulated secretions can escape from the wound bed. Ongoing observation of the wound identifies early signs and symptoms of infection.

Achieving Rest and Comfort

A surgical client's pain increases as the effects of anesthesia wear off. The client becomes more aware of the surroundings and more perceptive of discomfort. The incisional area may be only one source of pain. Irritation from drainage tubes, tight dressings, or casts and the muscular strains caused from positioning on the operating room table can make the client feel miserable.

Pain can significantly slow recovery. The client becomes reluctant to cough, breathe deeply, turn, ambulate, or perform necessary exercises. The nurse assesses the client's pain thoroughly (see Chapter 37). It should not be assumed that the pain is incisional. When the client calls for a pain medication, the nurse determines the nature and character of the pain. The nurse should provide analgesics as often as allowed the first 24 to 48 hours after surgery to improve pain control. The PCA system allows clients to administer their own IV analgesics from a specially prepared IV pump (Bast, Hayes, 1986). If clients gain a sense of control over their pain, they usually have fewer postoperative problems.

Epidural infusion of narcotics, such as morphine, fentanyl, and meperidine, is also a popular method of postoperative analgesia for many surgical clients (Powell, Bora, 1989). Epidural narcotics relieve severe pain, often without the central nervous system depression that often occurs with systemic narcotics.

Maintaining Self-Concept

The appearance of wounds, bulky dressings, and extruding drains and tubes threatens a client's self-concept. The effects of surgery, such as disfiguring scars, may create permanent changes in the client's body image. If surgery leads to impairment in body function, the client's role within the family can change significantly.

The nurse observes clients for alterations in self-concept. Clients may show a revulsion toward their appearance by refusing to look at incisions, carefully covering dressings with bedclothes, or refusing to get out of bed because of tubes and devices. The fear of not being able to return to a functional role in their families may even cause clients to avoid participating in the nurse's care plan.

The family becomes an important part of the nurse's efforts to improve the client's self-concept.

The nurse explains the client's appearance and ways to avoid nonverbal expressions of revulsion or surprise to the family. The family needs to be accepting of the client's needs and still encourage the client's independence. If the condition is terminal, the family learns to assist the client through the grieving process so that they can reach a stage of acceptance. The following measures maintain the client's self-concept:

1. The nurse provides privacy during dressing changes or inspection of the wound. Room curtains are kept closed around the bed, and the client is draped so that only the dressing or incisional area is exposed.

2. The nurse maintains the client's hygiene. Wound drainage and antiseptic solutions from the surgical skin preparation dry on the skin's surface and act as sources of irritation. A complete bath the first day after surgery can make the client feel renewed. When the gown becomes soiled by wound drainage, the nurse offers a clean gown and washcloth. The nurse keeps the client's hair neatly combed and offers frequent oral hygiene, especially for the client who is NPO.

3. The nurse prevents drainage sets from overflowing. Typically the physician orders contents of drainage sets to be measured every 8 hours for output recording. The client sometimes becomes preoccupied with observing the gradual collection of drainage, and some drainage sets can leak contents if they become too full. The nurse should empty the sets periodically to prevent accidental spills and hampering of the client's movement.

4. The nurse maintains a pleasant environment. Self-concept is heightened by being in pleasant, comfortable surroundings. Frequently the room of a surgical client becomes cluttered with extra dressings, rolls of tape, and bottles of antiseptic solution. If the client requires frequent dressing changes, the room may take on the appearance of a supply room. The nurse should store or remove unused supplies and keep the client's bedside orderly and clean.

5. The nurse offers opportunities for the client to discuss feelings about appearance. If the nurse notices that the client avoids looking at an incision, the client may need to discuss any fears or concerns. A client having surgery for the first time is often more anxious than one who has had multiple surgeries. Both male and female clients may worry about permanent scarring. A client is more apt to look at an incision several days after surgery when healing is occurring and energy and well-being are increased. If the client chooses to look at an incision for the first time, the area should be clean. Eventually the client should be able to care for the incision site by applying simple dressings or bathing the affected area.

6. The nurse provides the family with opportunities to discuss ways to promote the client's self-concept. Encouraging independence can be difficult for a family member who has a strong desire to assist the client in any way. By knowing about the appearance of a wound or incision, family members can be supportive during dressing changes. The topic or tone of a conversation can also help family members distract a client from dwelling on fears and concerns. Family members should not avoid discussing the future. However, the nurse must help them to know when it is appropriate to discuss future plans. Then the client and family can work together to discuss realistic plans for the client's return home.

PROMOTING RETURN TO A FUNCTIONAL STATE OF HEALTH. Throughout the postoperative convalescent period the nurse promotes the client's independence and active participation in care. When a client is in pain or suffers from complications, there is little motive for self-care. The nurse must maintain a balance of providing for clients' needs when they are physically dependent and promoting more involvement when their conditions allow.

The goals a nurse sets for a client's involvement in care must be realistic. Surgery may limit the ability to participate effectively. It is unrealistic for the nurse to involve the client if movement is highly restricted or if participation increases discomfort.

The nurse should keep the client and family informed of recovery progress. Many clients become depressed if they think recovery is slow. The nurse explains that it normally takes many days to reach a level of maximal recovery. Surgery may also cause permanent physical limitations that require time for acceptance.

The nurse plans care daily, keeping in mind the ultimate goals for recovery. From the moment that the client enters the hospital, through surgery, and during the postoperative phase, the nurse anticipates the client's return home.

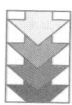

Sample Evaluation of Interventions for Ineffective Airway Clearance for Postoperative Client

Goals	Evaluation Measures	Expected Outcomes
Client will remain free of surgical wound infection.	Inspect condition of wound edges and character of drainage.	Wound edges will be approximated and slightly reddened and drainage will be minimal and clear.
	Assess body temperature.	Client will remain afebrile.
Client will achieve rest and comfort by discharge.	Evaluate client for verbal and nonverbal behaviors indicative of pain.	Client will report less discomfort compared with baseline.
		Client will be able to perform activities of daily living without signs of discomfort.
Client will maintain self-concept.	Observe client inspecting and caring for wound or dressing.	Client will observe and care for wound openly and freely.
	Observe client discussing changes experienced as a result of surgery.	Client will talk about physical changes with others.
	Note client's personal apperance.	Client will maintain personal grooming.
Client will return to functional state of health by discharge.	Observe client participate in self-care activities.	Client will initiate self-care independently.
	Observe client's level of ambulation.	Client will exercise progressively.

Involvement of family members in the client's care plan can facilitate recovery. If the client requires additional care at home, such as dressing changes, assistance with ambulation, or drug administration, the nurse instructs family members on proper care techniques. If family members are unable to assist the client, the nurse works with the physician and social worker in making plans for home care. The client will be more able to assume a functional state of health when family members understand the limitations a client faces.

Evaluation

The nurse evaluates the effectiveness of care provided to the surgical client on the basis of expected outcomes of nursing interventions. In all surgical settings the nurse consults with the client and family to gather evaluation data. The nurse can evaluate the ambulatory surgical client's outcomes by making a telephone call to the client's home. The call is usually placed 24 hours after surgery and reassures the client that the nurse is concerned and allows the nurse to evaluate the progress of recovery.

In an acute care setting the evaluation of a surgical client is ongoing. If a client fails to progress as expected, the nurse revises the care plan based on the priorities of the client's needs. Every effort is made to assist the client to return to as healthy and functional a state as possible.

Part of the nurse's evaluation is determining the extent to which the client and family have learned self-care measures. A client often has to continue dressing care, follow activity restrictions, continue medication therapy, and observe for signs and symptoms of complications on returning home. A referral to home health care assists clients unable to perform self-care activities. It is useful to have a home health nurse in attendance at discharge to know what a client can effectively perform. The evaluation box outlines criteria used for postoperative clients.

SUMMARY

Care for the client during all phases of the surgical experience needs to be continuous and integrated. Before surgery the nurse prepares the client and family for the surgery, performs diagnostic tests, and assesses the client in preparation for the operation. During surgery the nurse assists surgeons and other operating room nurses to ensure that the client receives optimal care. After surgery, the nurse assists the client to physical stability and wakefulness and institutes measures to help the client achieve maximal recovery. Through all phases of care, the nurse involves the client and family as much as possible in the care plan and helps maintain the client's dignity.

CHAPTER 47 REVIEW

Key Concepts

- Perioperative nursing is professional nursing care afforded the surgical client before, during, and after surgery.
- Surgery is classified by level of severity, urgency, and purpose.
- In addition to the nature of nursing care provided, previous illnesses and past surgeries influence the client's ability to tolerate surgery.
- The duration of the preoperative period may be several days or only a few hours.
- All medications taken before surgery are automatically discontinued after surgery unless a physician reorders the drugs.
- Family members are important in assisting clients with any physical limitations and in providing emotional support during postoperative recovery.
- Preoperative assessment of vital signs and physical findings provides an important baseline with which to compare postoperative assessment data.
- A client's feelings about surgery can have a significant impact on relationships with the nursing staff and the client's ability to participate in care.
- Surgical removal of a body part may permanently alter a person's body image, as well as the individual's sexuality.
- Nursing diagnoses of the surgical client may pose implications for nursing care during one or all phases of surgery.
- Primary responsibility for informed consent rests with the client's surgeon.
- Informed consent should not be obtained if a client is confused, unconscious, mentally incompetent, or under the influence of sedatives.
- Structured preoperative teaching has a positive influence on postoperative recovery.
- Basic to preoperative teaching is explanation of all preoperative and postoperative routines and demonstration of postoperative exercises.
- Clipping of a surgical site should be done as close as possible to the time of surgery to minimize infection.
- In ambulatory surgery, nurses must use the limited time available to educate clients, assess their health status, and prepare them for surgery.
- A routine preoperative checklist is a guide for final preparation of the client before surgery.
- Many responsibilities of nurses within the operating room focus on protecting the client from potential harm.
- Assessment of the postoperative client centers on the body systems most likely to be affected by anesthesia, immobilization, and surgical trauma.
- The recovery room nurse reports to the nurse on the postoperative division information pertaining to the client's current physical status and risk for postoperative complications.
- From the time of admission the nurse plans for the surgical client's discharge.

Key Terms

Ambulatory surgery, p. 1602

Antiembolism stockings, p. 1624

Cholecystectomy, p. 1602

Circulating nurse, p. 1635

Convalescence, p. 1635

Dehiscence, p. 1609

Depilatories, p. 1623

General anesthesia, p. 1632

Local anesthesia, p. 1633

Malignant hyperpyrexia, p. 1637

Perioperative nursing, p. 1603

Recovery, p. 1635

Regional anesthesia, p. 1632

Scrub nurse, p. 1635

Critical Thinking Exercises

1. Your 76-year-old client is being admitted for a cataract extraction. Name three of the physiological changes occurring in older adults that would place your client at risk for surgery.

2. Mrs. B. is a 52-year-old client who will have abdominal surgery in the morning. She has a history of smoking one pack of cigarettes per day for 30 years. What areas would you concentrate on during Mrs. B.'s preoperative teaching?

3. Your client has undergone abdominal surgery to remove a cancerous growth. Describe postoperative measures you would use to promote rest and comfort.

4. Mrs. R. is a 39-year-old client who has undergone a right modified mastectomy. You notice that she refuses to look at her incision and has been remaining in bed even though she has been instructed to increase her activity as tolerated. How can you encourage Mrs. R.'s independence and maintain her self-concept?

REFERENCES

American Nurses Association and Association of Operating Room Nurses: *Standards of perioperative nursing care,* Kansas City, Mo, 1972, The Associations.

Ayliffe GAJ et al: A comparison of preoperative bathing with chlorhexidine detergent and non-medicated soap in the prevention of wound infection, *J Hosp Infect*4(3):237, 1983.

Bast C, Hayes P: Patient-controlled analgesia, *Nurs 86* 16:25, 1986.

Cruse PJE, Foord R: The epidemiology of wound infection: a ten-year prospective study of 62,939 wounds, *Surg Clin North Am* 60:1, 1980.

Dettenmeier PA: *Pulmonary nursing care,* St Louis, 1992, Mosby-Year Book.

Gallagher MT, Kahn C: Lasers: scalpels of light, *RN* 53:46, 1990.

Garner JS: *Guidelines for prevention of surgical wound infections,* 1985, Hospital Infections Program, CDC, PHS, US Department of Health and Human Services.

Grant JA, Kennedy-Caldwell C: *Nutritional support in nursing,* New York, 1988, Grune & Stratton.

Halsey RW et al: Nosocomial infections in U.S. hospitals, 1975-1976: estimated frequency by selected characteristics of patients, *Am J Med* 70:947, 1981.

Jackson DC et al: Endoscopic laser cholecystectomy: a new approach to gallbladder removal, *AORN J* 51:1546, 1990.

Keithley JK: Wound healing in malnourished patients, *AORN J* 35:1094, 1982.

Kim MJ, McFarland GK, McLane AM: *Pocket guide to nursing diagnosis,* ed 4, St Louis, 1991, Mosby–Year Book.

Lepczyk M et al: Timing of preoperative patient teaching, *J Adv Nurs* 15:300, 1990.

Lindeman C, VanAernam B: Nursing intervention with the presurgical patient—the effects of structured and unstructured preoperative teaching, *Nurs Res* 20:319, 1971.

Metheny N: Measures to test placement of nasogastric and nasointestinal feeding tubes: a review, *Nurs Res* 37:324, 1988.

Metheny N et al: Effectiveness of pH measurements in predicting feeding tube placement, *Nurs Res* 38:280, 1989a.

Metheny N et al: Effectiveness of the ausculatory method in predicting feeding tube location, *Nurs Res* 39:262:1990.

Metzger RS: The beginning of OR nursing education, *AORN J* 24:73, 1976.

Powell AN, Bora MB: How do you give continuous epidural fentanyl? *Am J Nurs* 89:1197, 1989.

Schoessler M: Perceptions of preoperative education in patients admitted the morning of surgery, *Patient Educ Couns* 14:127, 1989.

ADDITIONAL READINGS

Andrews DR, Taylor C: Documenting post-anesthesia recovery, *Am J Nurs* 85:290, 1985.

Bean M: Preparation for surgery in an ambulatory surgery unit, *J Post Anesesth Nurs* 5:42, 1990.

Blackwood S: Back to basics, the preop exam, *Am J Nurs* 86:39, 1986.

Breslin EF: Prevention and treatment of pulmonary complications in patients after surgery of the upper abdomen, *Heart Lung* 10:511, 1981.

Burtman F, Salminer CA: Back to basics: controlling postoperative infection, *Nurs 84* 14:43, 1984.

Cummings C: Taking the fear out of surgery, *Nurs 87* 17:64b, 1987.

Faherty BS, Grien MR: Analgesic medication for elderly people post-surgery, *Nurs Res* 33:369, 1984.

Frogge MH: Promoting wound healing in the irradiated patient, *J Am Assoc OR Nurs* 35:1088, 1982.

Hathaway A: Effect of preoperative instruction on postoperative outcomes: a meta-analysis, *Nurs Res* 35:269, 1986.

Hogan P, Bell S: How to handle postanesthetic hypertension, *Nurs 86* 16:58, 1986.

Kneedler J, Dodge G: *Perioperative patient care*, Boston, 1987, Blackwell.

Lynch S: Ambulatory surgery: families can watch surgery while they wait, *AORN J* 46:522, 1987.

Meeker MH, Rothrock JC: *Alexander's care of the patient in surgery*, St Louis, 1991, Mosby–Year Book.

Metheny N et al: Effect of feeding tube properties and three irrigants on clogging rates, *Nurs Res* 37:165, 1988.

Pagana KD, Pagana TJ: *Diagnostic testing and nursing implications*, ed 3, St Louis, 1990, Mosby–Year Book.

Ross R: Overcoming fear: a review on research on patient, family instruction, *AORN J* 43:1107, 1986.

Seneca CM: How we streamlined preop paperwork, *RN* 49:42, 1986.

Ziemer MM: Effects of information on postsurgical coping, *Nurs Res* 32:232, 1983.

CHAPTER 48

Clients with Wounds

OBJECTIVES

Mastery of content in this chapter will enable the student to:

- Define the key terms listed.
- Discuss normal stages of wound healing by primary intention.
- Describe complications of wound healing and their usual time of occurrence.
- Explain the factors that impair or promote wound healing.
- Describe differences in assessing a wound in a stable versus emergency setting.
- Conduct an assessment of a closed and open wound.
- Identify nursing diagnoses related to clients with wounds.
- Discuss principles of first aid in wound care.
- Explain nursing care implications in the use of dressings.
- Apply a sterile dry or wet-to-dry dressing.
- Discuss the purpose of bandages and binders.
- Describe the effects of heat and cold on wound healing.
- Apply warm and cold applications safely to an injured body part.

CHAPTER OUTLINE

Normal Integument

Wound Classifications

Wound Healing Process

Healing by primary intention

Healing by secondary intention

Complications of Wound Healing

Hemorrhage

Infection

Dehiscence

Evisceration

Fistulas

Delayed wound closure

Factors Influencing Wound Healing

Nutrition

Aging

Psychosocial Impact of Wounds

Nursing Process and Wound Healing

Assessment

Nursing diagnosis

Planning

Implementation

Evaluation

The body's integument is a protective barrier against disease-causing organisms and a sensory organ for pain, temperature, and touch. Injury to the integument poses risks to safety and triggers a complex healing response. Knowing the normal healing pattern helps the nurse recognize alterations that require intervention. The nurse's main responsibilities are to prevent invasion of microorganisms into wounds and to support the body's defenses in achieving wound repair. When choosing interventions, the nurse considers the type of wound, the pain associated with it, conditions that affect healing, and the client's psychological well-being.

NORMAL INTEGUMENT

In relation to wound healing the integument has two principal layers: the epidermis and the dermis (Fig. 48-1). The **epidermis,** or outer layer, has two layers. The stratum corneum is the thin, outermost layer of the epidermis. It consists of flattened, dead cells. The cells originate from the second epidermal layer, the stratum malpighii. Cells in the stratum malpighii divide, proliferate, and migrate toward the epidermal surface. After cells reach the stratum corneum, they flatten and die. This constant movement ensures replacement of surface cells sloughed off during normal **desquamation.** The thin stratum corneum protects underlying cells and tissues from dehydration and prevents entrance of certain chemical agents. However, the stratum corneum does allow evaporation of water from the skin and permits absorption of certain topically applied medications.

The **dermis** differs from the epidermis in that it contains no skin cells. **Collagen** (a tough, fibrous protein), blood vessels, and nerves compose it. Fibroblasts, which are responsible for collagen formation, are the only distinctive cell type within the dermis.

Understanding the integument's layers helps the nurse promote wound healing. The epidermis functions to resurface wounds and restore the barrier against invading organisms. The dermis responds to restore the structural integrity and the physical properties of the skin. Even though a wound may close in the upper epidermal layer, the client is at risk for infection, circulatory impairment, and tissue breakdown if the underlying dermis fails to heal.

WOUND CLASSIFICATIONS

There are many ways to classify wounds. Wound classification systems describe the status of skin in-

tegrity, cause of the wound, severity of tissue injury, cleanliness of the wound, or descriptive qualities of the wound (Table 48-1). These classifications overlap. For example, a penetrating knife wound is also an open wound, and a contused wound is a closed wound. Wound classifications enable the nurse to understand the risks associated with a wound and implications for its care. An open wound, for example, presents a greater risk of infection than a closed wound, whereas an abrasion requires less extensive dressings than a deep-penetrating wound.

WOUND HEALING PROCESS

Wound healing involves integrated physiological processes. The nature of healing is the same for all wounds with variations, depending on the location, severity, and extent of injury. The ability of cells and tissues to regenerate or return to normal structure by cell growth also affects healing. Cells of the liver, renal tubules, and neurons of the central nervous system typically regenerate slowly or not at all.

There are two types of wounds: those with loss with tissue and those without. A clean surgical incision is an example of a wound with little tissue loss. The surgical wound heals by **primary intention.** The skin edges **approximate,** or close together, and the risk of infection is lower. In contrast a wound involving loss of tissue, such as a burn, pressure ulcer, or severe laceration, heals by **secondary intention.** The wound edges do not approximate. The wound is left open until it becomes filled by scar tissue. It takes longer for a wound to heal by secondary intention, and thus the chance of infection is greater. If scarring from secondary intention is severe, there may be permanent loss of tissue function.

Healing by Primary Intention

An example of the normal healing process is repair of a clean surgical wound. Healing occurs in four

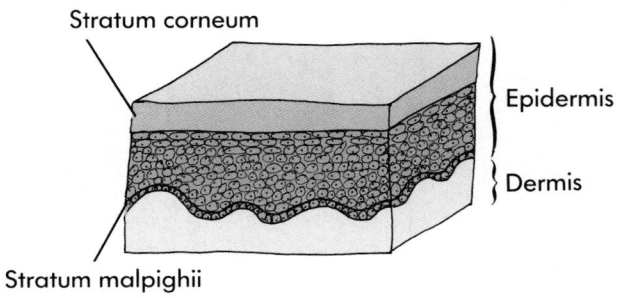

Fig. 48-1 Layers of the integument.

TABLE 48-1   Wound Classification

Description	Causes	Implications for Healing
STATUS OF SKIN INTEGRITY **Open**		
Wound involving a break in skin or mucous membranes	Trauma by sharp object or blow (surgical incision, venipuncture, gunshot wound)	Break in skin exposes body to invasion by microorganisms. Loss of blood and body fluids through wound occurs. Function of body part is reduced.
Closed		
Wound involving no break in skin integrity	Part of body being stuck by blunt object; twisting, straining, or deceleration force against body (bone fracture, tear of visceral organ)	Wound may predispose person to internal hemorrhage. Function of affected body part is reduced.
CAUSE **Intentional**		
Wound resulting from therapy	Surgical incision; introduction of needle into body part	Incision is usually performed under aseptic technique to minimize chance of infection. Wound edges are usually smooth and clean.
Unintentional		
Wound that occurs unexpectedly	Traumatic injury (knife wound, burn)	Wound occurs under unsterile conditions. Wound edges are often jagged.
SEVERITY OF INJURY **Superficial**		
Wound that involves only epidermal layer of skin	Result of friction applied to skin surface (abrasion, first-degree burn, shearing)	Break creates risk of infection. Wound does not involve underlying injury to tissues or organs. Blood supply to area is intact.
Penetrating		
Wound involving break in epidermal skin layer, as well as dermis and deeper tissues or organs	Foreign object or instrument entering deep into body tissues; usually unintentional (gunshot wound, stab wound)	There is high risk of infection because foreign object is contaminated. Wound may cause internal and external hemorrhage; damage to organs causes temporary or permanent loss of function.
Perforating		
Penetrating wound in which foreign object enters and exits an internal organ	(See above entry)	There is high risk of infection. Nature of injury depends on organ perforated (lung, compromised oxygenation; major vessel, hemorrhage; intestine, contamination of abdominal cavity by feces).
CLEANLINESS **Clean**		
Wound containing no pathogenic organisms.	Closed surgical wound not entering gastrointestinal, respiratory, genital, or uninfected urinary tract or oropharyngeal cavity	There is low risk of infection.

Continued.

TABLE 48-1 Wound Classification—cont'd		
Description	Causes	Implications for Healing
CLEANLINESS—cont'd		
Clean-contaminated		
Wound made under aseptic conditions but involving body cavity that normally harbors microorganisms	Surgical wound entering gastrointestinal, respiratory, genital, or urinary tract or oropharyngeal cavity under controlled conditions	There is greater risk of infection than with clean wound.
Contaminated		
Wound existing under conditions in which presence of microorganisms is likely	Open, traumatic, accidental wounds; surgical wound in which break in asepsis occurred	Tissues are often not healthy and show inflammation. There is high risk of infection.
Infected		
Bacterial organisms present in wound site usually above 10^5 organisms per gram of tissue	Any wound that does not properly heal and grows organisms, old traumatic wound, surgical incision into area infected (e.g., ruptured bowel)	Wound presents signs of infection (inflammation, purulent drainage, skin separation).
Colonized		
Wound containing microorganisms (usually multiple)	Chronic wound (vascular stasis ulcer, pressure ulcer)	Wound healing is slow, and high risk of infection exists.
DESCRIPTIVE QUALITIES **Laceration**		
Tearing of tissues with irregular wound edges	Severe traumatic injury (knife wound, industrial accident involving machinery, tissues cut by broken glass)	Wound is usually created by contaminated object. Depth of wound determines other complications.
Abrasion		
Superficial wound involving scraping or rubbing of skin's surface by friction	Wound often resulting from fall (skinned knee or elbow); wound also resulting from dermatological procedure for removing scar tissue	Wound is painful resulting from exposure of superficial nerves; deeper tissues are not involved. There is risk of infection from exposure to contaminated surface.
Contusion		
Closed wound caused by a blow to body by blunt object; contusion or bruise characterized by swelling, discoloration, and pain	Bleeding in underlying tissues caused by blunt force against body part	Wound is more severe if internal organ is contused. Wound may cause temporary loss of function of body part. Localized bleeding into tissues may form hematoma (collection of blood).

stages as described by Westaby (1986): inflammatory, destructive, proliferative, and maturation.

Inflammatory Phase

The stage of inflammation begins within minutes of injury and lasts about 3 days. Reparative processes control bleeding (**hemostasis**), deliver blood and cells to the injured area (inflammation), and form epithelial cells at the injury site (**epithelization**). During hemostasis, injured blood vessels constrict and platelets gather to stop bleeding. Clots form a **fibrin** matrix that later provides a framework for cellular repair. Damaged tissue and mast cells secrete histamine, resulting in vasodilation of surrounding capillaries and exudation of serum and white blood cells into damaged tissues. This results in localized redness, edema, warmth, and throbbing. The inflammatory response is beneficial, and there is no value in attempting to cool the area or reduce the swelling unless the swelling occurs within a closed compartment (for example, fascial compartment or neck).

Leukocytes reach the wound within a few hours. The primary acting white blood cell is the neutrophil, which begins to ingest bacteria and small debris. The neutrophils die in a few days and leave behind an enzyme **exudate** that attacks bacteria or interferes with tissue repair. In chronic inflammation the dying neutrophils create pus. The second important leukocyte is the monocyte, which transforms into macrophages. The macrophages are "garbage cells" that clean a wound of bacteria, dead cells, and debris by phagocytosis. The macrophages also digest and recycle substances, such as amino acids and sugars, that aid in wound repair.

After the macrophages clean the wound and make it ready for tissue repair, epithelial cells move from the wound margins under the base of the clot or scab. Epithelial cells continue to gather under the wound space for about 48 hours. Eventually a thin layer of epithelial tissue forms over the wound as a barrier against infectious organisms and toxic materials.

Growth hormones are released by platelets and macrophages. There is increasing evidence that these factors promote wound healing.

The inflammatory phase is prolonged and repair processes are slowed if too little inflammation occurs, as in debilitating disease or after administration of steroids. Too much inflammation also prolongs healing because arriving cells compete for available nutrients.

Destructive Phase

The destructive phase (2 to 5 days) begins before inflammation ends. Macrophages continue the process of clearing the wound of debris, attracting further macrophages, and stimulating formation of **fibroblasts,** the cells that synthesize collagen. Collagen can be found as early as the second day and is the main component of scar tissue. Fibroblasts require vitamins B and C, oxygen, and amino acids to function properly. Collagen provides strength and structural integrity to a wound.

Proliferative Phase

With the appearance of new blood vessels as reconstruction progresses, the proliferative phase begins and lasts from 3 to 24 days. During this period, the wound begins to close with new tissue. As reconstruction progresses, the tensile strength of the wound increases, and the risk of wound separation or rupture is less likely. The degree of stress on a wound influences the amount of scar tissue formed. For example, more scar tissue forms in an extremity wound than in a less mobile area such as the scalp or chest. Impairment of healing during this stage usually results from systemic factors such as age, anemia, hypoproteinemia, and zinc deficiency.

Maturation

Maturation, the final stage of healing, may take more than a year, depending on the depth and extent of the wound. The collagen scar continues to gain strength for several months. However, a healed wound usually does not have the strength of the tissue it replaces. Collagen fibers undergo remodeling or organization before assuming their normal appearance. Usually, scar tissue contains fewer pigmented cells (melanocytes) and has a lighter color than normal skin.

Healing by Secondary Intention

When tissue loss in a wound is extensive, wound healing takes longer. A large open wound typically drains more fluid than a closed wound. Inflammation is often chronic, and tissue defects become filled with fragile granulation tissue rather than collagen. **Granulation tissue** is a form of connective tissue that has a more abundant blood supply than collagen. Because the wound is larger, the amount of connective tissue scarring is larger.

When epithelial and connective tissue cells are unable to close a wound defect, contraction may occur. **Wound contraction** involves movement of the dermis and epidermis on each side of the wound. The mechanism of contracture is not completely understood. It is known, however, that collagen is not essential and any event that interferes with cell viability at the wound margin inhibits contraction. Wound contraction begins on about the fourth day and occurs simultaneously with epithelization. The cell that provides the motive force is the myofibroblast. Wound contraction results in thinning of surrounding tissues, and the size and shape of the final scar corresponds to tension lines in the damaged area. For example, a square wound in the abdomen assumes the shape of two Ys, end to end. There are areas of the body where contraction gives poor results, such as wounds on the face, sternum, and anterior lower leg. Wound contraction is not the same as a contracture or deformity resulting from muscle shortening and joint fixation.

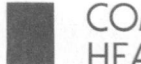

COMPLICATIONS OF WOUND HEALING

Hemorrhage

Hemorrhage, or bleeding from a wound site, is normal during and immediately after the initial trauma. Hemostasis occurs within several minutes unless large blood vessels are involved or the client has poor clotting function. Hemorrhage occurring after hemostasis indicates a slipped surgical suture, a dislodged clot, infection, or erosion of a blood vessel by a foreign object (for example, a drain). Hemorrhage may occur externally or internally. For example, if a surgical suture slips off a blood vessel, bleeding occurs within the tissues, and there are no visible signs of blood unless a surgical drain is present. (The surgeon often inserts a drain into tissues beneath a wound to remove fluid that collects in underlying tissues.) The nurse can detect internal bleeding by looking for distention or swelling of the affected body part, a change in the type and amount of drainage from a surgical drain, or signs of **hypovolemic shock** (for example, fall in blood pressure, increased thready pulse, increased respirations, restlessness, and diaphoresis). A **hematoma** is a localized collection of blood underneath the tissues. It appears as a swelling or mass that often takes on a bluish discoloration. A hematoma near a major artery or vein is dangerous because pressure from the expanding hematoma may obstruct blood flow.

External hemorrhaging is more obvious. The nurse observes dressings covering the wound for bloody drainage. If bleeding is extensive, the dressing soon becomes saturated, and frequently blood escapes along the sides of the dressing and pools beneath the client. The nurse observes all wounds closely, particularly surgical wounds in which the risk of hemorrhage is great during the first 24 to 48 hours after surgery.

Infection

Wound infection is the second most common **nosocomial** (hospital-related) **infection** (see Chapter 18). According to the Centers for Disease Control (CDC) (Garner, 1985), a wound is infected if purulent material drains from it, even if a culture is not taken or has negative results. A sample of drainage from an infected wound may not reveal bacteria in a culture because of poor culture technique or because the client has already received antibiotics. Positive culture findings do not always indicate an infection because many wounds contain colonies of noninfective resident bacteria. The chances of wound infection are greater when the wound contains dead or necrotic tissue, when there are foreign bodies in or near the wound, and when blood supply and local tissue defenses are reduced. Bacterial wound infection inhibits wound healing.

A contaminated or traumatic wound may show signs of infection early, within 2 to 3 days. A surgical wound infection usually does not develop until the fourth or fifth day. The client has a fever, tenderness and pain at the wound site, and an elevated white blood cell count. The edges of the wound may appear inflamed. If drainage is present, it is purulent, odorous, and has a yellow, green, or brown color, depending on the causative organism.

Dehiscence

When a wound fails to heal properly, the layers of skin and tissue may separate. This most commonly occurs before collagen formation (3 to 11 days after injury). **Dehiscence** is the partial or total separation of wound layers. A client with poor wound healing is at risk for dehiscence. However, obese clients have a high risk because of the constant strain placed on their wounds and the poor healing qualities of fatty tissue. Dehiscence often involves abdominal surgical wounds and occurs after a sudden strain, such as coughing, vomiting, or sitting up in bed. Clients often report feeling as though something has given way. When there is an increase in serosanguineous drainage from a wound, the nurse should be alert for dehiscence.

Evisceration

With total separation of wound layers, **evisceration** (protrusion of visceral organs through a wound opening) may occur. The condition is a medical emergency that requires surgical repair. When evisceration occurs, the nurse places sterile towels soaked in sterile saline over the extruding tissues to reduce chances of bacterial invasion and drying. If the organs protrude through the wound, blood supply to the tissues is compromised.

Fistulas

A **fistula** is an abnormal passage between two organs or between an organ and the outside of the body. A surgeon may create a fistula for therapeutic purposes (for example, making an opening between the stomach and the outer abdominal wall to insert a gastrostomy tube for feeding). Most fistulas, however, form as a result of poor wound healing. Trauma, infection, radiation exposure, and diseases such as cancer prevent tissue layers from closing

Risks for Skin Breakdown from Body Fluids

LOW RISK
- Saliva
- Serosanguineous drainage

HIGH RISK
- Gastric drainage
- Pancreatic drainage

MODERATE RISK
- Bile
- Stool
- Urine
- Ascitic fluid
- Purulent exudate

properly and allow the fistula tract to form. Fistulas increase the risk of infection and fluid and electrolyte imbalances from fluid loss. Chronic drainage of fluids through a fistula can also predispose a person to skin breakdown (see box).

Delayed Wound Closure

Sometimes referred to as *third-intention wound healing,* delayed wound closure is a deliberate attempt by the surgeon to allow effective drainage of a clean-contaminated or contaminated wound. The wound is not closed until all evidence of edema and wound debris has been removed, usually several days, occasionally weeks. An occlusive dressing is used to prevent bacterial contamination of the wound. Then the wound is closed as in primary closure, or first intention. Experimentally, it has been demonstrated that scarring or delayed healing does not significantly increase when this technique is used (Cooper, 1992b).

 ## FACTORS INFLUENCING WOUND HEALING

A number of factors influence the rate of wound healing. A client with any factors listed in Table 48-2 on p. 1660 is at risk for wound complications. The nurse's knowledge of factors influencing healing helps in providing preventive care and selecting appropriate wound care therapies.

Nutrition

Normal wound healing requires proper nutrition. Physiological processes of wound healing depend on the ready availability of protein, vitamins (especially A and C), and the trace minerals zinc and copper.

Collagen is a protein formed from amino acids acquired by fibroblasts from protein ingested in food. Vitamin C is needed for synthesis of collagen. Vitamin A reduces the negative effects of steroids on wound healing (see Table 48-2). Trace elements are needed for epithelization (zinc), collagen synthesis (zinc), and collagen fiber linking (copper).

For clients weakened or debilitated by illness, nutritional therapy is especially important. A client who has undergone surgery (see Chapter 47) and is well nourished still requires at least 1500 kcal/day for nutritional maintenance. Alternatives such as enteral feedings (see Chapter 35) and parenteral nutrition (see Chapter 39) are made available for clients unable to maintain normal food intake.

Aging

Although the rates for the stages of healing among older clients may be slowed, the physiological aspects of healing are unchanged from the younger adult. Problems that arise during healing are difficult to assign to the aging process or to other possible causes, such as poor nutrition, environment, or individual response to stress. Before surgery, the nurse assesses any factors that may influence or alter the wound healing in older clients. (see Table 48-2).

 ## PSYCHOSOCIAL IMPACT OF WOUNDS

Although not directly involved in the physiological process of healing, the client's psychological response to any wound is part of the nurse's assessment. Body-image changes may impose a great stress on the client's adaptive mechanisms. In addition, body-image changes influence self-concept (see Chapter 31) and sexuality (see Chapter 32). The client's personal and social resources for adaptation should also be a part of the assessment. Factors that may affect the client's perception of the wound include the presence of scars, drains (drains may be necessary for weeks or even months after certain procedures), odor from drainage, and temporary or permanent prosthetic devices.

 ## NURSING PROCESS AND WOUND HEALING

 ### Assessment

The nurse often assesses wounds under two conditions: at the time of injury before treatment and after therapy when the wound is relatively stable. Each

TABLE 48-2 Factors that Impair Wound Healing

Physiological Effects	Nursing Implications
AGE Aging alters all phases of wound healing. Vascular changes impair circulation to wound site. Reduced liver function alters synthesis of clotting factors. Inflammatory response is slowed. Reduced formation of antibodies and lymphocytes occurs. Collagen tissue is less pliable. Scar tissue is less elastic.	Instruct client on safety precautions to avoid injuries. Be prepare to provide wound care for longer time period. Teach support persons in home wound care techniques.
MALNUTRITION All phases of wound healing are impaired. Stress from burns or severe trauma increases nutritional requirements.	Provide balanced diet rich in protein, carbohydrates, lipids, vitamins A and C, and minerals (e.g., zinc, copper).
OBESITY Fatty tissue lacks adequate blood supply to resist bacterial infection and deliver nutrients and cellular elements for healing.	Observe obese client for signs of wound infection and evisceration.
IMPAIRED OXYGENATION Low arterial oxygen tension alters synthesis of collagen and formation of epithelial cells. If local circulating blood flow is poor, tissues fail to receive needed oxygen. Decreased hemoglobin in blood (anemia) reduces arterial oxygen levels in capillaries and interferes with tissue repair.	Provide diet adequate in iron. Monitor hematocrit and hemoglobin levels of clients with wounds.
SMOKING Smoking reduces amount of functional hemoglobin in blood, thus decreasing tissue oxygenation. Smoking may increase platelet aggregation and cause hypercoagulability. Smoking interferes with normal cellular mechanisms that promote release of oxygen to tissues.	Discourage client from smoking by explaining its effects on wound healing.
DRUGS Steroids reduce inflammatory response and slow collagen synthesis. Antiinflammatory drugs suppress protein synthesis, wound contraction, epithelialization, and inflammation. Prolonged antibiotic use may increase risk of superinfection. Chemotherapeutic drugs can depress bone marrow function, lower number of leukocytes, and impair inflammatory response.	Carefully observe clients receiving these drugs because signs of inflammation may not be obvious.
DIABETES Chronic disease causes small blood vessel disease that impairs tissue perfusion. Diabetes causes hemoglobin to have greater affinity for oxygen, so it fails to release oxygen to tissues. Hyperglycemia alters ability of leukocytes to perform phagocytosis and also supports overgrowth of fungal and yeast infection.	Instruct diabetic clients to take preventive measures to avoid cuts or breaks in skin. Provide preventive foot care. Control blood sugar to reduce the physiological changes associated with diabetes.

TABLE 48-2 Factors that Impair Wound Healing—cont'd	
Physiological Effects	Nursing Implications
RADIATION	
Fibrosis and vascular scarring eventually develop in irradiated skin layers. Tissues become fragile and poorly oxygenated.	Closely observe clients who have surgery after radiation for wound complications.
WOUND STRESS	
Vomiting, abdominal distention, and respiratory effort may stress suture line and disrupt wound layer. Sudden, unexpected tension on incision inhibits formation of endothelial cell and collagen networks.	Control nausea with ordered antiemetics. Keep nasogastric tubes patent and draining to avoid accumulation of secretions. Instruct and assist cient to splint abdominal wound during coughing.

condition requires the nurse to make different observations and to take different actions.

Emergency Setting

The nurse may see wounds in any setting, including a clinic, emergency room, rural youth camp, or the nurse's own backyard. The type of wound determines the criteria for inspection. For example, the nurse need not inspect for signs of internal bleeding after an abrasion but should do so in the event of a puncture wound.

When a client's condition is judged to be stable because of the presence of spontaneous breathing, a clear airway, and a strong carotid pulse (see Chapter 38), the nurse inspects the wound for bleeding. An **abrasion** is usually superficial with little bleeding. The wound may appear "weepy" because of plasma leakage from damaged capillaries. A **laceration** may bleed more profusely, depending on the wound's depth and location. For example, minor scalp lacerations tend to bleed profusely because of the rich blood supply to the scalp. Lacerations greater than 5 cm (2 in) long or 2.5 cm (1 in) deep can cause serious bleeding. **Puncture** wounds bleed in relation to the depth and size of the wound: for example, a nail puncture does not cause as much bleeding as a knife wound. The primary dangers of puncture wounds are internal bleeding and infection.

The nurse next inspects the wound for foreign bodies or contaminant material. Most traumatic wounds are dirty. Soil, broken glass, shreds of cloth, and foreign substances clinging to penetrating objects can become embedded in the wound.

The size of the wound is the next criterion for inspection. A deep laceration requires suturing by a physician. A large open wound may expose bone or tissue that should be protected.

When the injury is the result of trauma from a dirty penetrating object, the nurse determines when the client last received a tetanus toxoid injection. Tetanus bacteria reside in soil and in the gut of humans and animals. A tetanus antitoxin injection is necessary if the client has not had one within 5 years.

Stable Setting

When the client's condition is stabilized (for example, after surgery or treatment) the nurse assesses the wound to determine its progress toward healing. If the wound is covered by a dressing and the physician has not ordered it changed, the nurse should not directly inspect the wound unless serious complications are suspected. In such a situation the nurse should inspect only the dressing and any external drains. If the physician prefers to change the dressing, the physician will assess the wound at least daily. When the nurse removes dressings, care is taken to avoid accidental removal or displacement of underlying drains. Because removal of dressings can be painful, it may help to give an analgesic at least 30 minutes before exposing a wound.

WOUND APPEARANCE. The nurse notes whether wound edges are closed. A surgical incision should have clean, well-approximated edges. Crusts often form along the wound edges from exudate. A puncture wound is usually a small, circular wound with the edges coming together toward the center. If a wound is open, the wound edges are separated, and the nurse inspects the condition of underlying tissue such as adipose and connective tissue. The nurse also looks for complications such as dehiscence and evisceration. The outer edges of a wound normally appear inflamed for the first 2 to 3 days, but this slowly disappears. Within 7 to 10 days a normally healing wound fills with epithelial cells, and edges close. If infection develops, the wound edges become brightly inflamed and swollen.

Skin discoloration usually results from bruising of interstitial tissues or possibly hematoma formation. Blood collecting beneath the skin first takes on a bluish or purplish appearance. Gradually, as the clotted blood is broken down, shades of brown and yellow appear.

Character of Wound Drainage

The nurse notes the amount, color, odor, and consistency of drainage. The amount of drainage depends on the location and extent of the wound. For example, drainage is minimal after a simple appendectomy. In contrast, wound drainage is moderate for 1 to 2 days after resection of a portion of the small bowel. If the nurse needs an accurate measurement of the amount of drainage within a dressing, the dressing can be weighed and compared with the weight of the same dressing when clean and dry. A rule of thumb is 1 g of drainage equals 1 ml. The color and consistency of drainage vary depending on the components. Types of drainage include the following:

1. **Serous,** which is a clear, watery plasma
2. **Sanguineous,** which indicates fresh bleeding
3. **Serosanguineous,** which is a pale, more watery drainage than sanguineous drainage
4. **Purulent,** which is a thick, yellow, green, or brown drainage

If the drainage has a pungent or strong odor, an infection should be suspected.

The nurse objectively records the wound integrity and drainage character. Phrases such as "appears to be healing well" or "minimal drainage" do not give a clear picture of the wound's condition. The nurse should describe the wound's appearance according to characteristics observed. An example of accurate recording follows:

> Abdominal incision is approximately 5 cm long across RLQ (right lower quadrant); edges well approximated without inflammation or exudate. 1.2-cm diameter circle of serous drainage present on one 4 × 4 gauze.

DRAINS. The physician inserts a drain into or close to a surgical wound if a large amount of drainage is expected and if keeping wound layers closed is especially important. If fluid is allowed to accumulate under tissues, the inner wound edges may never close.

A drain such as a penrose may lie under a dressing, extend through a dressing, or be connected to a drainage bag or a suction apparatus. The physician often places a pin or clip through the drain to prevent it from slipping farther into a wound (Fig. 48-2). It is usually the physician's responsibility to pull or advance the drain as drainage decreases to permit healing deep within the drain site.

The nurse assesses drain placement, character of drainage, and condition of collecting apparatus. First, the nurse observes the security of the drain and its location with respect to the wound. Next the nurse notes the character of drainage. If there is a collecting device, the nurse measures the drainage volume. Because a drainage system must be patent, the nurse looks for drainage flow through the tubing. A sudden decrease may indicate a blocked drain, and the physician should be notified. When a drain is connected to suction, the nurse assesses the system to be sure that the pressure ordered is being exerted. Evacuator units, such as a Hemovac or Jackson-Pratt (Fig. 48-3), exert a constant low pressure as long as the suction bladder or bag is fully compressed. When the evacuator device is unable to maintain a vacuum on its own, the nurse notifies the surgeon, who will then order a secondary vacuum system. If fluid is allowed to accumulate within the tissues, wound healing will not progress at an optimal rate, and the risk of infection is increased.

WOUND CLOSURES. Surgical wounds are closed with staples, sutures, or wound closures. A popular skin closure is the stainless-steel staple. The staple provides more strength than nylon or silk sutures and tends to cause less irritation to the skin. The nurse looks for irritation around staple or suture sites and notes whether closures are intact. The nurse may choose to count sutures when the physician has removed a portion of them. Normally for the first 2 to 3 days after surgery the skin around sutures or staples is swollen. Continued swelling may indicate that the closures are too tight. The skin can be cut by overly tight suture material, leading to wound separation. Sutures that are too tight are a common cause of wound dehiscence. Early suture removal reduces formation of defects along the suture line and minimizes chances of unattractive scar formation.

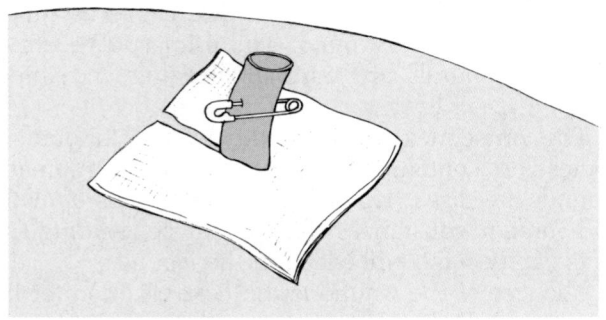

Fig. 48-2 Penrose drain.

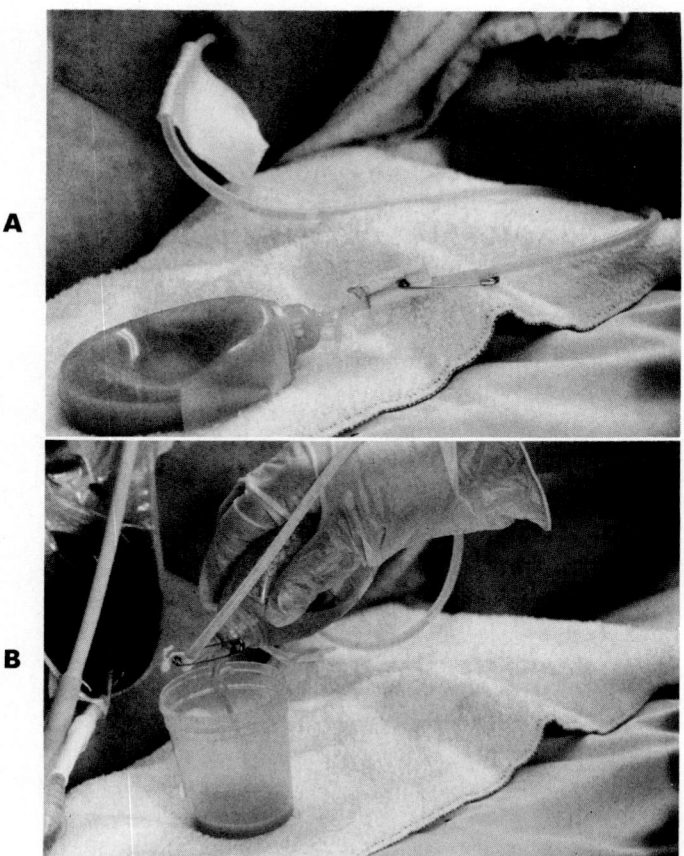

Fig. 48-3 Jackson-Pratt drainage device. **A,** Drainage tubes and reservoir. **B,** Emptying drainage reservoir.

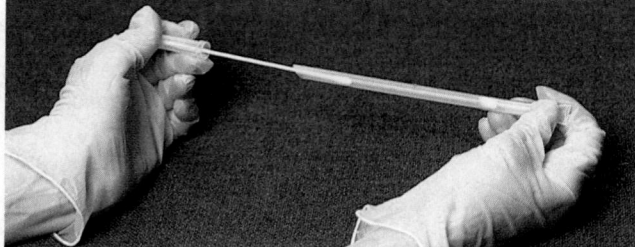

Fig. 48-4 Wound culturette tube.

lated to tape removal, use of an adhesive removal may make it painless.

Wound Cultures

If the nurse detects purulent or suspicious-looking drainage, collecting a specimen for culture may be necessary (see Chapter 44). The nurse never collects a wound culture sample from old drainage. Resident colonies of bacteria from the skin grow within exudate and may not be the true causative organisms of a wound infection. The nurse cleans a wound first to remove skin flora. Aerobic organisms grow in superficial wounds exposed to the air, and anaerobic organisms tend to grow within body cavities. The nurse uses a different method of specimen collection for each type of organism.

To collect an aerobic specimen the nurse uses a sterile swab from a culturette tube (Fig. 48-4). If wound edges are separated, the nurse slowly and gently inserts the tip of the swab into the wound to collect deeper secretions. After collecting the specimen the nurse returns the swab to the culturette tube, caps the tube, and crushes the inner ampule containing the medium for organism growth. The medium must moisten and coat the swab tip. The nurse immediately sends the labeled specimen to the laboratory.

If drainage from a deep body cavity has a foul odor, there is a chance of anaerobic organism growth. The nurse uses a sterile syringe tip to aspirate drainage from the inner wound. Afterward the nurse applies a sterile needle to the syringe, expels air from the syringe and needle, and places a cork over the needle to prevent entrance of air. In some institutions the nurse may inject the specimen into a special vacuum container with a culture medium.

Gram's stains are often performed, as well. This test often allows the physician to order appropriate treatment earlier than when only cultures are done. No additional specimens are usually required. The microbiology laboratory needs only to be notified to perform the additional test.

PALPATION OF WOUND. When inspecting a wound, the nurse may observe swelling or separation of wound edges. Using light palpation on wound edges, the nurse can detect localized areas of tenderness or drainage collection. The nurse should apply sterile gloves before palpating any wound. The nurse gently applies the fingertips along the wound edges. If pressure causes fluid to be expressed, the nurse notes the character of the drainage. It may be necessary to collect the drainage for culture. The client is normally sensitive to palpation of wound edges. Extreme tenderness may indicate infection.

PAIN. Pain assessment is an important part of wound assessment in terms of detecting complications and planning for future wound care. If the client experiences serious discomfort while the nurse inspects or palpates the wound, the nurse should look for underlying problems. If the wound is extensive and discomfort seems to be related to dressing removal or application, the nurse plans to administer analgesics before future dressing changes. If discomfort is re-

Nursing Diagnosis

After completing an assessment of the client's wound, the nurse identifies nursing diagnoses that

Examples of Nursing Diagnoses Related to Wound Healing

NANDA-APPROVED NURSING DIAGNOSES

Impaired skin integrity related to:
- Surgical incision
- Pressure
- Chemical injury
- Secretions and excretions

High risk for impaired skin integrity related to:
- Physical immobilization
- Exposure to secretions

High risk for infection related to:
- Malnutrition
- Tissue loss and increased environmental exposure

Acute pain related to:
- Abdominal incision

Impaired physical mobility related to:
- Pain of surgical wound

Altered nutrition: less than body requirements related to:
- Inability to ingest food

Ineffective breathing pattern related to:
- Pain of abdominal incision

Altered tissue perfusion related to:
- Interruption of arterial flow
- Interruption of venous flow

Self-esteem disturbance related to:
- Perception of scars
- Perception of surgical drains
- Reaction to surgically removed body part

---

will direct supportive and preventive care (see diagnoses box). Existence of a wound clearly indicates a diagnosis for actual impaired skin integrity. This diagnosis directs the nurse to initiate interventions that promote the healing process.

The client may be at risk for poor wound healing because of previously defined factors that impair healing. Thus even though the client's wound may appear normal, the nurse identifies nursing diagnoses such as *altered nutrition* or *altered tissue perfusion* that direct nursing care toward support of wound repair.

The nature of a wound can cause problems unrelated to wound healing. Alteration in comfort and impaired mobility are problems that have implications for the client's eventual recovery. For example, a large abdominal incision can cause enough pain to interfere with the client's ability to turn in bed effectively. The diagnostic process box lists nursing diagnoses related to problems of wound healing.

Planning

After identifying nursing diagnosises, the nurse develops a care plan for the client needing wound management. The plan is based on the client's identified needs and priorities. Goals are established, and from the goals the nurse plans therapies according to severity and type of wound and the presence of any complicating conditions (for example, infection, poor nutrition, immunosupression, and diabetes) that may affect wound healing.

Because of earlier discharges, it is important to consider the client's home when planning therapies to promote wound healing. Clients and their families may need to continue the objectives of wound management after discharge. The nurse and client work together to establish ways of maintaining client in-

---

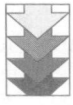

Sample Nursing Diagnostic Process for Wound Healing

Assessment Activities	Defining Characteristics	Nursing Diagnoses
Inspect surface of skin.	Presence of wound Edges of wound not approximated Sutures remain in place	*Impaired skin integrity* related to contaminated wound
Inspect wound for signs of healing.	Tan-red drainage 5 days after surgery Edges of wound not approximated	*High risk for infection* related to traumatic, contaminated wound
Obtain client's temperature, heart rate, and white blood cell count.	Client is febrile, heart rate is 125 beats/min, leukocyte (white blood cell) count is 12,000/mm^3	

volvement in nursing care and to promote wound healing whether the client is in the hospital or home.

The nurse's priorities in wound care depend on whether the client's condition is stable or emergent. The type of wound care administered depends on the type of wound, its size and location, and complications. Nursing interventions will be both dependent and independent (see care plan). Goals of care for clients with wounds include the following:

1. Promoting wound hemostasis
2. Preventing infection
3. Preventing further tissue injury
4. Promoting wound healing
5. Maintaining skin integrity
6. Regaining normal function
7. Gaining comfort

Implementation

In an emergency setting the nurse uses first aid measures for wound care. Under more stable conditions the nurse uses a variety of interventions to ensure wound healing.

First Aid for Wounds

When a client suffers a traumatic wound, first aid interventions include stabilizing cardiopulmonary function (see Chapter 38), promoting hemostasis, cleansing the wound, and protecting the wound from further injury.

HEMOSTASIS. After assessing the type and extent of the wound the nurse controls bleeding of a laceration by applying direct pressure on the wound with a sterile or clean dressing, such as a washcloth. After bleeding subsides, an adhesive bandage strip or gauze dressing taped over the laceration allows skin edges to close and a blood clot to form. If a dressing becomes saturated with blood, the nurse adds another layer of dressing, continues to apply pressure, and elevates the affected part. Further disruption of skin layers should be avoided. More serious lacerations should be sutured by a physician. Pressure dressings used the first 24 to 48 hours after trauma help maintain hemostasis.

A puncture wound is allowed to bleed to remove dirt and other contaminants, such as saliva from a dog bite. If a penetrating object, such as a knife blade, is in a client's body, removal could cause massive, uncontrolled bleeding. Therefore the penetrating object should not be removed. The nurse may apply pressure around the object but not on it, and the client should be transported to an emergency clinic or hospital.

GROWTH FACTORS. Topical and parenteral growth factors have been used to treat nonhealing wounds and fistula formation (see research highlight on p. 1666). The nurse is responsible for the use of this treatment modality after the physician determines that it may provide a benefit for the client's wound care. Teaching the client or significant other about the use of growth factors is also the nurse's responsibility. Including the use of the medication, the nurse

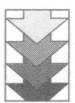

Sample Nursing Care Plan for Impaired Skin Integrity

Nursing diagnosis: Impaired skin integrity related to contaminated wound
Definition: Impaired skin integrity is the state in which an individual's skin is adversely altered (Kim, McFarland, McLane, 1991).

Goals	Expected Outcomes	Interventions	Rationale
Skin integrity wil be improved in area of surgical wound (3/20).	Wound will be clean and intact without inflammation, drainage, or maceration (3/18). Wound edges will be approximated.	Keep wound clean and dry. Perform prescribed dressing changes, including debridement and application of treatments. Instruct client or significant other to perform wound assessment and care. Include return demonstration.	Wound healing depends on clean, moist environment for epithelization and deposition of granulation tissue (Atwater, 1989; Cooper, 1990). Accurate and regular assessment of wound and surrounding skin are critical to nursing care plan for wound management (Cooper, 1992a).

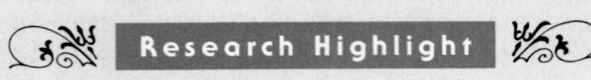

Research Highlight

The purpose of Fylling's study was to determine the effectiveness of topical growth factors in promoting the healing process in nonhealing wounds. In this prospective study, wounds were treated in a double-blind, randomized crossover trial. A solution of five different growth factors (GF) were applied to 21 wounds, and a collagen solution (CS) was applied to the control group of 13 wounds. The wounds and etiologies were similar in each group. All wounds were treated identically, other than the treatment variable, as part of a comprehensive wound-care program. By the 8-week crossover time, 81% of the wounds in the GF group had achieved 100% epithelization, whereas only 15% of the wounds in the control group had achieved that level of healing. About 54% of the wounds in the control group actually increased in size during that time. After the 85% unhealed wounds in the control group were crossed over to the GF group, all achieved 100% epithelization. The average time to 100% epithelization from the start of the study was 8.6 weeks in the GF group and 15 weeks in the CS group ($p = 0.0002$).

Fylling CP: Comprehensive wound management with topical growth factors, *Ostomy/Wound Manage* 22:62, 1989.

also teaches wound care and the prevention of wound breakdown and recurrence.

CLEANSING. Gentle cleansing of a wound removes contaminants that might serve as sources of infection. However, vigorous cleaning can cause bleeding or further injury. For abrasions, minor lacerations, and small puncture wounds the nurse first rinses the wound in running water, cleans it with mild soap and water, and may apply an over-the-counter antiseptic. Topical antibiotics applied to wound edges may slow microorganism growth. However, prolonged application of topical antibiotics can foster growth of nonsusceptible organisms. When a laceration is bleeding profusely, the nurse should only brush away surface contaminants and concentrate on hemostasis until the client can be cared for in a clinic or hospital.

Topical Agents for Cleansing Wounds. Topical agents used to clean wounds include povidone-iodine solutions, Dakin's solution, acetic acid solution, hydrogen peroxide, and saline.

Povidone-Iodine Solutions (Iodophor). When diluted to a 1:1000 solution, iodophor is bacteriocidal for *Staphylococcus aureus* and not cytotoxic to hu-

man fibroblasts. The nurse should know that iodine may be absorbed systemically during prolonged use. In addition, the use of iodophor in exudative wounds weakens and inactivates the antiseptic effect as the iodine is bound to the serum proteins of the drainage.

Dakin's Solution. Dakin's solution is a combination of 0.45% to 0.5% sodium hypochlorite and 0.4% boric acid. It is bacteriocidal against staphylococcal and streptococcal organisms. When applied as a full-strength solution, Dakin's solution can be very irritating to skin around the wound. Consequently, Dakin's solution is most often used in a 0.25% to 0.5% dilution.

Acetic Acid Solution. Although a solution of 0.5% acetic acid is effective against gram-positive and gram-negative bacteria, there is no evidence that progress of tissue healing is enhanced.

Hydrogen Peroxide. The primary function of hydrogen peroxide is its action as a **debriding** agent. When this solution is applied to a wound, it combines with catalase (a common enzyme found in most tissues) and decomposes to oxygen and water, thus forming its familiar effervescence. There is no antimicrobial action with hydrogen peroxide. The nurse does not apply hydrogen peroxide to granulation tissue because it is likely to destroy healthy new growth. The nurse also does not irrigate deep closed wounds with hydrogen peroxide. In the confined space the resultant gas may be absorbed into the vascular system as an embolism.

Saline. Gentle cleansing with normal saline and the application of saline dressings (wet-to-wet, wet-to-damp, damp-to-dry) are most often used to debride wounds. The nurse uses saline to maintain the moist surface needed to promote the development and migration of epithelial tissue.

PROTECTION. Regardless of whether bleeding has stopped, the nurse protects the wound from further injury by applying sterile or clean dressings and immobilizing the body part. A light dressing applied over minor wounds prevents entrance of microorganisms. In the case of small abrasions, it is acceptable to leave the wound open to air so that a scab can form.

The more extensive the wound, the larger the bandage required. In the home a clean towel or diaper may be the best dressing. A bulky dressing applied with pressure minimizes movement of underlying tissues and helps immobilize the entire body part. A bandage or cloth wrapped around a penetrating object should immobilize it adequately.

Dressings

The use of dressings requires an understanding of wound healing. A variety of dressing materials is commercially available. Unless a dressing is suited to the characteristics of a wound, the dressing can hinder wound repair.

The choice of dressings and the method of dressing a wound influence the progress of wound healing. The proper dressing should not allow a draining wound to become overly dry with extensive scab formation. When this occurs, the dermis dehydrates and crusts. As a result, a barrier forms against normal epidermal cell growth, leaving a depression or defect in the new epidermal surface. Furthermore, dryness of the wound may increase the client's discomfort. Ideally a dressing leaves a wound slightly moist to promote epithelial cell migration. The dressing should also absorb drainage to prevent pooling of exudate that may promote bacterial growth.

For surgical wounds that heal by primary intention, it is common to remove dressings as soon as drainage stops. In contrast, when the nurse dresses an open wound healing by secondary intention, the dressing material becomes a means for mechanically removing exudate and necrotic tissue.

PURPOSES OF DRESSINGS. A dressing may serve several purposes:

1. Protecting a wound from microorganism contamination
2. Aiding hemostasis
3. Promoting healing by absorbing drainage and debriding a wound
4. Supporting or splinting the wound site
5. Protecting the client from seeing the wound (if perceived as unpleasant)
6. Promoting thermal insulation to the wound surface
7. Providing maintenance of high humidity between the wound and dressing

When the skin becomes broken, a dressing helps reduce exposure to microorganisms. However, when wound drainage is minimal, the healing process forms a natural fibrin seal that can eliminate the need for a dressing. A dressing is always needed for extensive wounds.

Pressure dressings promote hemostasis. Applied with elastic bandages, a pressure dressing exerts localized downward pressure over an actual or potential bleeding site. A pressure dressing eliminates dead space in underlying tissues so that wound healing progresses normally. The nurse checks pressure dressings to be sure that they do not interfere with circulation of a body part. The nurse assesses skin color, pulses in distal extremities, the client's comfort, and changes in sensation. Pressure dressings are not routinely removed.

A primary function of a dressing is to absorb drainage. Most surgical dressings have three layers: a contact or primary layer, an absorbent layer, and an outer protective layer. The contact dressing covers the incision and part of the adjacent skin. Fibrin, blood products, and debris adhere to the contact dressing's surface. A problem occurs if the wound drainage dries, causing the dressing to stick to the suture line. Early or improper removal of the dressing can cause tearing of the healing epidermal surface. The nurse must either remove the dressing gently and moisten the attached area with sterile normal saline before removal or leave the dressing unchanged for several days. When wounds require debriding, such as infected or necrotic wounds, the contact dressing debrides necrotic tissue and debris. In this case the contact dressing sticks to underlying tissue, and debridement occurs during removal. Dressings applied to a draining wound require frequent changing to prevent microorganism growth and skin breakdown. Bacteria grow readily in the dark, warm, moist environment under a dressing. Skin surfaces become macerated and irritated. Skin breakdown can be minimized by keeping the skin clean and dry and reducing the use of tape.

The absorbent dressing layer serves as a reservoir for additional secretions. The wicking action of gauze dressings pulls excess drainage into the dressing and away from the wound.

The final outer layer of a dressing helps prevent bacteria and other external contaminants from reaching the wound surface. Usually the outer dressing is made of a thicker dressing material.

A firmly taped or wrapped dressing supports or immobilizes a body part, minimizing movement of the underlying incision and injured tissues. Finally, a dressing insulates and keeps a wound's surface well hydrated. The humidity between a dressing and the client's skin surface promotes normal epithelial cell growth.

TYPES OF DRESSINGS. Dressings vary by type of material and mode of application (wet or dry). They should be easy to apply, comfortable, and made of materials that promote wound healing.

Gauze dressings are the most common. They do not interact with wound tissues and thus cause little wound irritation. Gauze is available in different textures and in squares of 10 × 10 cm (4 × 4 in) or 5 × 5 cm (2 × 2 in), rectangles of 10 × 20 cm (4 × 8 in), and rolls of various lengths.

Wet dressings are preferred in treating wounds that require debridement. The nurse moistens the contact dressing layer, increasing the gauze's ability to collect exudate and wound debris, and then applies a dry second layer of absorbent dressing. This wet-to-dry dressing effectively cleanses infected and necrotic wounds.

Nonadherent gauze dressings such as Telfa are used over clean wounds. Telfa gauze has a shiny, nonadherent surface that does not stick to incisions or wound openings but allows drainage to pass through to the softened gauze above.

Another type of dressing is a self-adhesive, transparent film that acts as a temporary second skin (Fig. 48-5). The transparent dressing is ideal for small, superficial wounds or those that do not require debridement. It has the following advantages:

1. It adheres to undamaged skin.
2. It serves as a barrier to external fluids and bacteria but still allows the wound surface to "breathe."
3. It promotes a moist environment that speeds epithelial cell growth.
4. It can be removed without damaging underlying tissues.
5. It permits viewing the wound.

Hydrocolloid (HCD) and hydrogel dressings (Comfeel Ulcus, Duoderm, Vigilon) are occlusive. This type of dressing has the following functions:

1. It absorbs drainage through the use of exudate absorbers (Duoderm granules, Bard absorption dressing, Comfeel Ulcus powder) beneath the dressing.
2. It maintains wound humidity.
3. It slowly liquefies necrotic debris.
4. It provides protective cushioning.

This type of dressing is most useful on shallow to moderately deep dermal ulcers.

CHANGING DRESSINGS. To prepare for changing a dressing, the nurse must know the type of dressing, the presence of underlying drains or tubing, and the type of supplies needed for wound care. Poor preparation may cause a break in aseptic technique (see

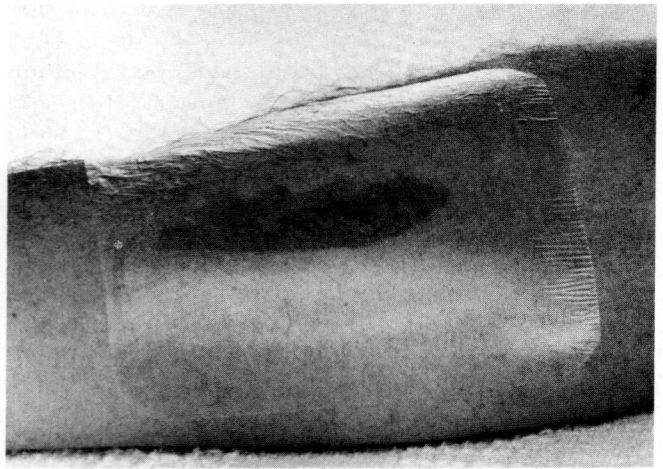

Fig. 48-5 Transparent film dressing.

Chapter 18) or an accidental dislodging of a drain. The nurse's judgment in modifying a dressing change procedure is important during wound care, particularly if the character of a wound changes. Notifying the physician of any change is essential.

The physician's order for changing a dressing should indicate the dressing type, the frequency of changing and any solutions or ointments to be applied to the wound. An order to "reinforce dressing prn" (add dressings without removing original one) is common right after surgery when the physician does not want accidental disruption of the suture line or bleeding. The medical or operating room record usually tells whether drains are present and from what body cavity they drain. After the first dressing change, the nurse describes the location of drains and the type of dressing materials and solutions to use in the client's care plan. The CDC (Garner, 1985) recommends the following guidelines during dressing change procedure:

1. The nurse should perform thorough handwashing before and after wound care.
2. Personnel should not touch an open or fresh wound directly without wearing sterile gloves (see Chapter 18).
3. If a wound is sealed, dressings may be changed without gloves.
4. Dressings over closed wounds should be removed or changed when they become wet or if the client has signs or symptoms of infection.

To prepare a client for a dressing change the nurse does the following:

1. Administers required analgesics so that peak effects occur during the dressing change
2. Describes steps of the procedure to lessen anxiety
3. Describes normal signs of healing
4. Answers questions about the procedure or the wound

Often the physician orders clients to learn how to change dressings so that they will be prepared for home care. In this situation the nurse must demonstrate dressing change to the client and family and then provide an opportunity for the client or family member to practice (see teaching box). Usually, in this situation wound healing has progressed to the point that risks of complications such as dehiscence or evisceration are minimal. The client should be able to change a dressing independently or with assistance from a family member before discharge. Procedure 48-1 on p. 1670 outlines the steps for changing dry and wet-to-dry dressings.

SECURING DRESSINGS. The nurse may use tape, ties, or bandages and cloth binders to secure a dressing over a wound site. The choice of anchoring depends

Client Teaching for Dressing Application	

OBJECTIVE

- Client (or family member) will demonstrate the correct technique for the application of dressing.

TEACHING STRATEGIES

- Discuss with client and significant other the importance of infection control.
- Demonstrate the correct technique for the dressing change for the client and the family member.
- Discuss signs and symptoms of wound infection.

EVALUATION

- Observe client and family member perform the dressing change.
- Client and family state symptoms of wound infection.

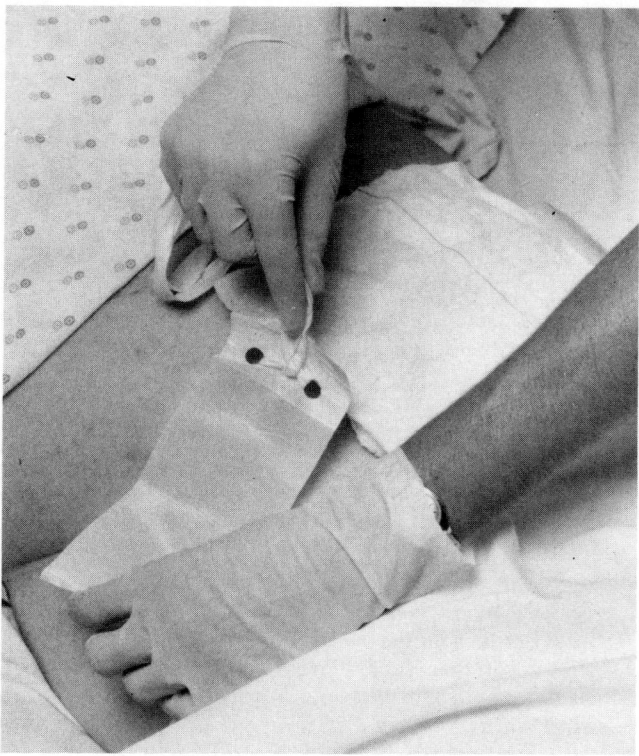

Fig. 48-6   Montgomery ties.

on the wound size, location, presence of drainage, frequency of dressing changes, and client's level of activity.

The nurse most often uses strips of tape to secure dressings if the client is not allergic to tape. Nonallergenic paper and plastic tapes minimize skin reactions. Common adhesive tape adheres well to the skin's surface, whereas elastic adhesive tape compresses closely around pressure bandages and permits more movement of a body part. Skin sensitive to adhesive tape can become severely inflamed and excoriated and may even slough when the tape is removed.

Tape is available in various widths such as 1.2, 2.5, 5, and 7.5 cm (½, 1, 2, and 3 in). The nurse chooses the size that sufficiently secures the dressing. For example, a large abdominal wound dressing must remain secure over a large area despite frequent stress from movement, respiratory effort, and possibly abdominal distention. Strips of 7.5-cm (3-in) adhesive better stabilize such a large dressing so that it does not continually slip off. When applying tape, a nurse ensures that it adheres to several inches of skin on both sides of the dressing and that it is placed across the middle of the dressing. When securing the dressing, the nurse presses the tape gently, exerting pressure away from the wound. This way tension occurs in both directions away from the wound, minimizing skin distortion and irritation. Tape is never applied over irritated or broken skin.

To remove tape safely the nurse loosens the tape ends and gently pulls the outer end parallel with the skin surface toward the wound. The nurse applies

light traction to the skin away from the wound as the tape is loosened and removed. The traction minimizes pulling of the skin. If tape covers an area of hair growth, the client experiences less discomfort if the nurse pulls the tape in the direction of hair growth.

To avoid repeated removal of tape from sensitive skin, the nurse can secure dressings with pairs of reusable Montgomery ties (Fig. 48-6). Each tie consists of a long strip; half contains an adhesive backing to apply to the skin and the other half folds back and contains a cloth tie or a safety pin and rubber band combination to be fastened across a dressing and untied at dressing changes. A large, bulky dressing may require two or more sets of Montgomery ties. To provide even support to a wound and immobilize a body part the nurse may apply elastic gauze or cloth bandages and binders over a dressing.

COMFORT MEASURES. A wound can be painful, depending on the extent of tissue injury. The nurse uses several techniques to minimize discomfort during wound care. Careful removal of tape, gentle cleansing of wound edges, and careful manipulation of dressings and drains minimize stress on sensitive tissues. Careful turning and positioning also reduce strain on a wound. Administration of analgesic medi-

Applying Dry and Wet-to-Dry Dressings

STEPS	RATIONALE
1. Assess size and location of wound to be dressed.	Assists nurse to plan for proper type and amount of supplies needed. Alerts nurse when assistance is needed to hold dressings in place.
2. Assess client's level of comfort.	Removal of dry dressing can be painful; client may require pain medication.
3. Review medical orders for dressing change procedure.	Indicates type of dressing or applictions to use.
4. Prepare necessary equipment and supplies: a. Sterile gloves b. Dressing set (sterile), scissors, forceps c. Sterile drape (optional) d. Gauze dressings and pads e. Fine-mesh gauze (wet-to-dry only) f. Sterile basin g. Antiseptic ointment (optional for dry dressing) h. Cleansing solution i. Sterile solution (wet-to-dry only) j. Clean disposable gloves k. Tape, ties, or bandage as needed l. Waterproof bag m. Extra gauze dressings, Surgi-Pads, or ABD pads n. Bath blanket o. Adhesive remover (optional) p. Disposable mask (optional)	Used to apply dressing and cut gauze to size. For antiseptic or cleansing solution. Used to moisten dressing. For disposal of old dressing and supplies.
5. Explain procedure to client and instruct client not to touch wound area or sterile supplies.	Decreases anxiety. Sudden, unexpected movement by client could result in contamination of wound and supplies.
6. Close room or cubicle curtains; close open windows.	Provides privacy and reduces airborne microorganisms.
7. Position client comfortably and drape with bath blanket to expose only wound site.	Draping provides access to wound and minimizes unnecessary exposure.
8. Place disposable bag within reach of work area. Fold top of bag to make cuff.	Ensures easy disposal of soiled dressings. Prevents soiling of bag's outer surface.
9. Apply face mask (usually required when wound has drainage that may splash into eyes of nurse) and wash hands thoroughly.	Reduces transmission of pathogens to exposed tissues.
10. Put on clean disposable gloves and remove tape, bandage, or ties.	Prevents transmission of infectious organisms from soiled dressings to nurse's hands.
11. Remove tape, pulling parallel to skin and toward dressing. Remove remaining adhesive from skin.	Pulling tape toward dressing reduces stress on suture line or wound edges.
12. With gloved hand, carefully remove gauze dressings, taking care not to dislodge drains or tubes. Keep soiled undersurface away from client's sight. (If dressing sticks on wet-to-dry dressing, do not moisten it; instead gently free dressing and warn client of discomfort.)	Appearance of drainage may be upsetting to client. (Wet-to-dry dressing should debride wound.)
13. Observe character and amount of drainage on dressing and appearance of wound.	Provides estimate of drainage amount and assessment of wound's condition.
14. Dispose of soiled dressings in disposable bag.	Reduces transmission of microorganisms.
15. Remove gloves by pulling them inside out. Dispose in bag.	Prevents contact of your hands with material on gloves.

STEPS	RATIONALE
16. Open sterile dressing tray or individually wrapped sterile supplies. Place on bedside table (see illustration).	Sterile dressings remain sterile while on or within sterile surface. Preparation of supplies prevents break in technique during dressing change.
17. Apply dry dressing:	
a. Open bottle of antiseptic solution and pour into sterile basin.	Keeps supplies sterile.
b. Apply sterile gloves.	Allows handling of sterile supplies without contamination.
c. Inspect wound for appearance, drainage, and integrity (see illustration). Avoid contact with contaminated material.	Indicates status of healing.
d. Cleanse wound with antiseptic solution:	
(1) Use separate swab for each cleansing stroke.	Prevents contaminating previously cleaned area.
(2) Clean from least contaminated area to most contaminated (Fig. 48-7).	Prevents introduction of organisms into wound.
e. Use dry gauze to swab in same manner as Step 17d to dry wound.	Reduces excess moisture, which could eventually harbor microorganisms.
f. Apply antiseptic ointment if ordered, using same technique as for cleansing.	Reduces growth of microorganisms. Ointment may be applied to dressing if direct application causes discomfort.
g. Apply dry sterile dressings to incision or wound site:	
(1) Apply loose woven gauze as contact layer.	Promotes proper absorption of drainage.
(2) Cut 4 × 4 gauze flat to fit around drain, if present. Precut gauze is also available.	Secures drain and promotes drainage absorption at site.
(3) Apply second layer of gauze.	Ensures proper coverage and optimal absorption.
(4) Apply thicker woven pad (Surgi-Pad).	Protects wound from external environment.
18. Apply wet-to-dry dressing:	
a. Pour prescribed solution into sterile basin and add fine-mesh gauze.	Contact layer must be totally moistened to increase dressing's absorptive abilities.
b. Apply sterile gloves.	Allows handling of sterile supplies without contamination.
c. Inspect wound for color, character of drainage, type of sutures, and drains.	Provides assessment of wound healing.
d. Cleanse wound with prescribed antiseptic solution or normal saline. Clean from least to most contaminated area.	Assists in debridement and cleanses wound of debris.

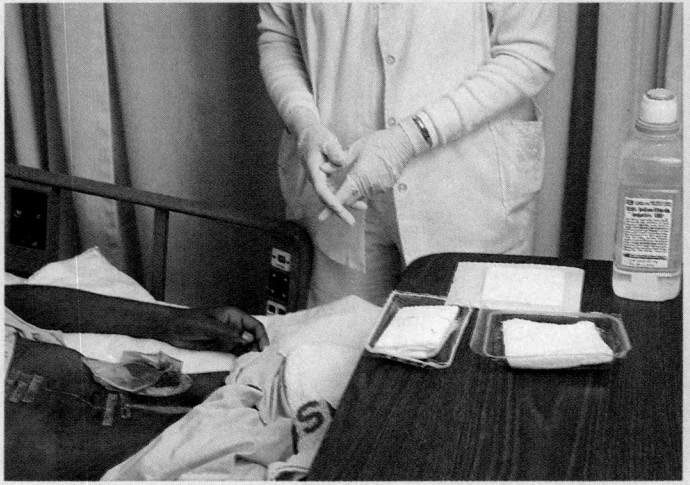
Step 16

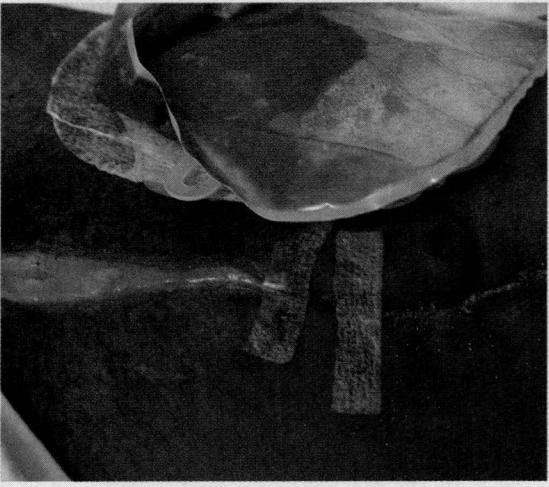
Step 17c

Applying Dry and Wet-to-Dry Dressings

STEPS	RATIONALE
e. Apply moist, fine-mesh gauze directly onto wound surface. If wound is deep, gently pack gauze into wound with forceps until all wound surfaces are in contact with moist gauze (see illustrations).	Moist gauze absorbs drainage and adheres to debris. Wound should be loosely packed to facilitate wicking of drainage into absorbent outer layer of dressing.
f. Apply dry sterile 4 × 4 gauze over wet gauze.	Pulls moisture from wound.
g. Cover with ABD pad, Surgi-Pad, or gauze.	Protects wound from entrance of microorganisms.
19. Apply tape over dressing, Kling roll (for circumferential dressings), or Montgomery ties. For application of Montgomery ties:	
a. Expose adhesive surface of tape on end of each tie.	Allows frequent dressing changes without removal of adhesive tape.
b. Place ties on opposite side of dressing.	
c. Place adhesive directly on client's skin or use skin barrier.	
d. Secure dressing by lacing ties across it or using safety pins and rubber bands.	Ensures dressing remains intact and covers wound.
20. Remove gloves and dispose in bag.	Reduces transmission of infection.
21. Assist client to comfortable position.	Promotes well-being.
22. Dispose of all supplies and wash hands.	Clean environment enhances comfort. Reduces transmission of infection.
23. Reassess client to determine response to dressing change.	Determines client's comfort level.
24. Monitor status of dressing at least every shift.	Evaluates extent of drainage and integrity of dressing.
25. Record appearance of wound and drainage, client's tolerance, and type of dressing applied in nurses' notes.	Documents progress of wound healing and promotes continuity in dressing change techniques.
26. Record frequency of dressing change and supplies needed on Kardex.	Alerts staff members to dressing change times and supplies needed.

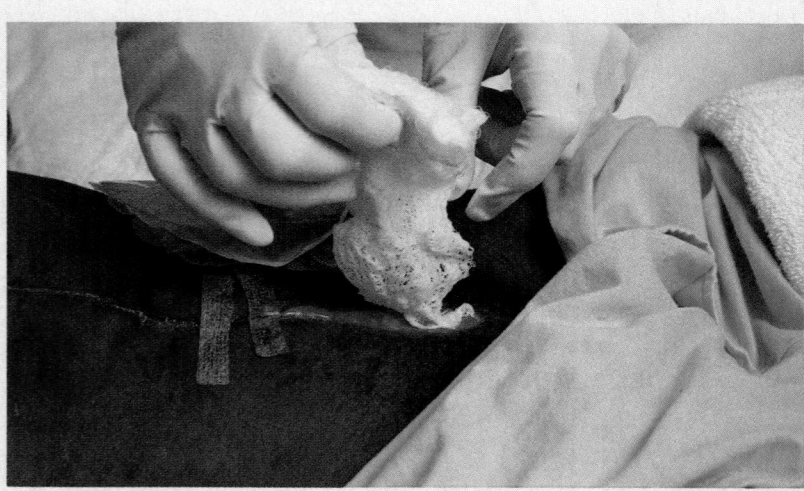

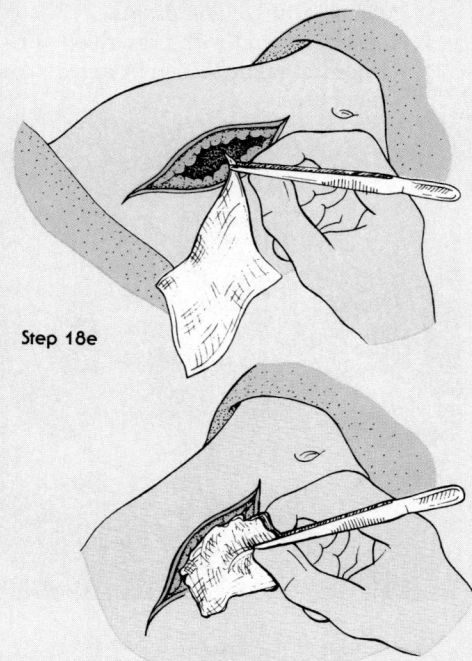

Step 18e

cations 30 to 60 minutes before dressing changes (depending on a drug's time of peak action) also reduces discomfort.

Cleansing Skin and Drain Sites

Although a moderate amount of wound exudate promotes epithelial cell growth, the physician may order cleansing of a wound or drain site if a dressing does not properly absorb drainage or if an open drain deposits drainage onto the skin. Wound cleansing requires good handwashing and aseptic techniques (see Chapter 18). The nurse may apply antiseptics locally (Table 48-3) to remove pathogens or may use irrigation to remove debris. The most effective antiseptic solutions for skin cleansing are tincture of chlorhexidine (Hibiclens) and the iodophors (such as Betadine), which persist in acting against bacteria as they remain on the skin. Alcohol (70%) acts rapidly on bacteria but has no persistent effect because it evaporates. Hydrogen peroxide is useful when cleaning open wounds containing necrotic debris.

BASIC SKIN CLEANSING. The nurse cleanses surgical or traumatic wounds by applying antiseptic solutions with sterile gauze or by irrigation. The following three principles are important when cleaning an incision or the area surrounding a drain:

1. Cleanse in a direction from the least contaminated area, such as from the wound or incision to the surrounding skin (Fig. 48-7) or from an isolated drain site to the surrounding skin (Fig. 48-8).

TABLE 48-3 Cleansing Agents		
Solution	Indications	Effects
Acetic acid (bactericidal)	Effective against *Pseudomonas aeruginosa*, some gram-positive and gram-negative organisms	May change color of wound exudate, does not significantly aid healing
Povidone-iodine (antibacterial)	Reported to be active against bacteria, spores, fungi, and viruses	Liberates 10% free iodine
Sodium hypochloride (antimicrobial)	Effective against staphylococci, streptococci	Releases elemental chlorine, which is tissue irritant
Chlorhexidine (bactericidal)	Effective against gram-negative and gram-positive organisms and some fungi	
Hydrogen peroxide (oxidizing agent)	Useful for softening and removing crusted exudate and debris	Should not be used in presence of granulation tissue
Normal saline (irrigant)	Useful for irrigation of clean or noninfected wounds	May be used under gentle pressure (35-ml syringe with 19-gauge needle) to assist in wound debridement
Cara-Klenz (cleanser) PharmaClens (cleanser)	Useful for cleaning dead tissue and secretions	Does not delay wound healing

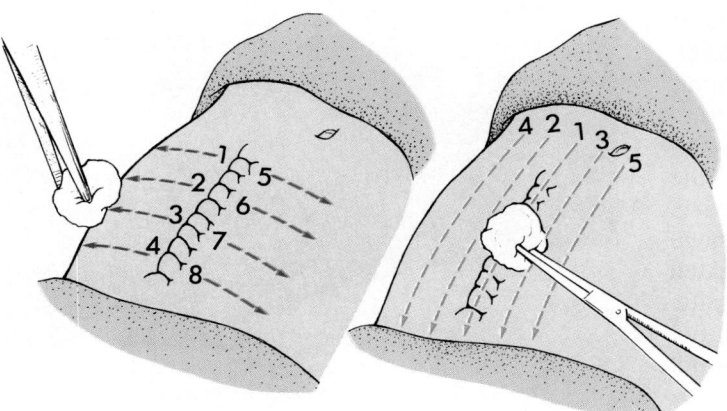

Fig. 48-7 Methods for cleansing a wound site.

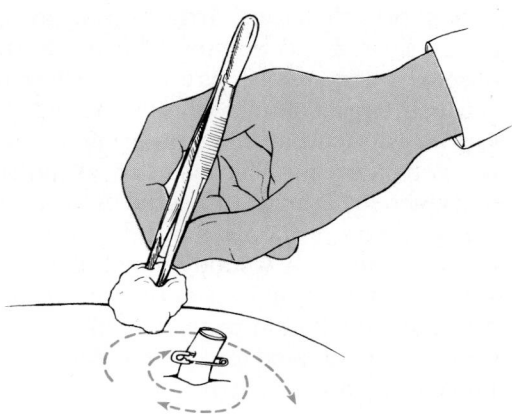

Fig. 48-8 Cleansing a drain site.

2. Use gentle friction when applying antiseptics locally to the skin.
3. When irrigating, allow the solution to flow from the least to most contaminated area.

A wound is thought to be less contaminated than the surrounding skin. After applying an antiseptic solution to sterile gauze the nurse cleans away from the wound. The nurse never uses the same piece of gauze to cleanse across an incision or wound twice.

A drain site is highly contaminated because the moist drainage harbors microorganisms. If a wound has a dry incisional area and a moist drain site, cleansing moves from the incisional area toward the drain. The nurse uses two separate swabs, one to clean from the top of the incision toward the drain and one to clean from the bottom of the incision toward the drain. To cleanse the area of an isolated drain site the nurse swabs around the drain, moving in circular rotations outward from a point closest to the drain. In this situation the skin near the site is more contaminated than the site itself. To cleanse circular wounds the nurse uses the same technique as cleansing around a drain.

IRRIGATIONS. Irrigations are a special way of cleansing wounds. The nurse uses an irrigating syringe to flush the area with a constant flow of solution. The gentle washing action of the irrigation cleans a wound of exudate and debris. Irrigations are particularly useful for open deep wounds involving an inaccessible body part, such as the ear canal, or when cleansing sensitive body parts, such as the conjunctival lining of the eye.

In addition to wound cleansing, irrigations serve to apply heat to an affected area and apply locally acting medications in the form of sterile solutions. The prescribed solution is usually sterile water, saline, or antiseptic solution. Administration of irrigating solutions at body temperature enhances comfort and provides the added benefit of local heat application.

Wound Irrigations. Irrigation of an open wound requires sterile technique. The nurse uses a large Asepto or cone-tipped syringe to deliver the solution because large volumes of solution are often necessary. It is important never to occlude a wound opening with a syringe because this would result in the introduction of irrigating fluid into a closed space. The pressure of the fluid could cause tissue damage and discomfort. A wound should always be irrigated with the syringe tip over but not in the drainage site. Fluid should flow directly into the wound and not over a contaminated area before entering the wound. Procedure 48-2 lists steps for wound irrigation.

Suture Care

A surgeon closes a wound by bringing the wound edges as close together as possible to reduce scar formation. Proper wound closure involves minimal trauma and tension to tissues with control of bleeding.

Sutures are threads or wire used to sew body tissues together. The client's history of wound healing, site of surgery, tissues involved, and purpose of the sutures determine the suture material to be used. For example, if the client has had repeated surgery for an abdominal hernia, the physician might choose wire sutures to provide greater strength for wound closure. In contrast a small laceration of the face calls for the use of very fine Dacron (polyester) sutures to minimize scar formation.

Sutures are available in a variety of materials, including silk, steel, cotton, linen, wire, nylon, and Dacron. Sutures come with or without sharp surgical needles attached. Commonly seen are steel staples (Fig. 48-9), a type of outer skin closure that causes less trauma to tissues than sutures, yet provides extra strength. It is also common to see wounds closed with Steri-Strips. A **Steri-Strip** is a sterile butterfly tape, applied along both sides of a wound to keep the edges closed.

Sutures are placed within tissue layers in deep wounds and superficially as the final means for wound closure. The deeper sutures are usually an absorbable material that disappears in several days. Sutures are foreign bodies and thus are capable of causing local inflammation. The surgeon can minimize tissue injury by using the finest suture possible and the smallest number necessary.

Policies vary within institutions as to who may remove sutures. If the nurse is allowed to remove them, a physician's order is required. An order for su-

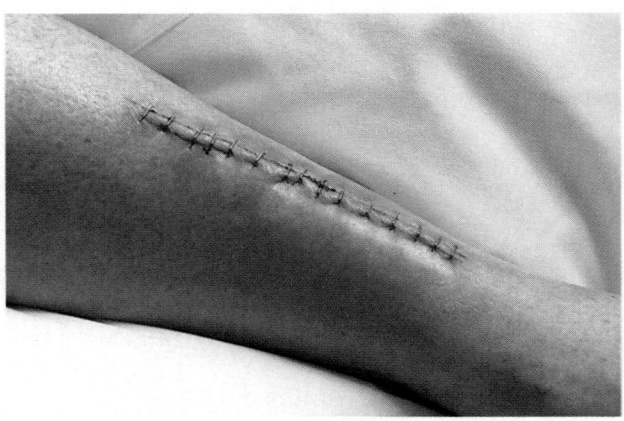

Fig. 48-9 Incision closed with wire staples.

STEPS	RATIONALE
1. Assess client's level of pain.	Discomfort may be related directly to wound or i... muscle tension or immobility.
2. Review medical record for physician's prescription for irrigation of open wound and type of solution to be used.	Open wound irrigation requires medical order including type of solutions to use.
3. Identify recent recording of signs and symptoms related to client's open wound: a. Extent of impairment of skin integrity b. Elevation of body temperature c. Drainage from wound (amount, color)	Data are used as baseline to indicate change in condition of wound. May indicate response to infection. Amount will decrease as healing takes place; serous drainage is clear; bright red drainage indicates fresh bleeding; purulent drainage is thick and yellow, pale green, or white.
d. Odor e. Consistency of drainage f. Size of wounds, including depth, length, and width	Strong odor indicates infectious process. Leukocytes produce thick drainage. Determines stage of healing.
4. Administer prescribed analgesic 30-45 min before starting wound irrigation procedure.	Increased comfort level will permit client to move more easily and be positioned to facilitate infection control during irrigation.
5. Gather equipment at bedside: a. Sterile basin	Increases efficiency. Used to hold sterile irrigation solution in preparation for irrigation.
b. 150- to 500-ml prescribed sterile irrigating solution warmed to body temperature	Warming adds to comfort level.
c. Sterile irrigation syringe, sterile soft catheter, if needed	Used to prevent introduction of additional pathogens during procedure; soft catheter is used to irrigate deep wounds with small openings.
d. Clean basin e. Clean gloves (check policy of institution)	Used to collect contaminated irrigating solution. Protect nurse from infection while removing wound dressing.
f. Sterile gloves	Used to maintain asepsis during irrigation and redressing procedures.
g. Waterproof underpad h. Sterile dressing tray and supplies for dressing change, including packing, if ordered	Prevents soiling of bed linen; is cost and time effective. Prevents infection and promotes wound healing.
i. Leakproof refuse bag	Used to gather soiled and contaminated dressings and prevent cross-infection.
j. Gown	Gown may or may not be indicated to protect uniform from contamination. Mask and goggles may be indicated if spraying of drainage is possible.
6. Explain procedure.	Reduces anxiety.
7. Position client comfortably to permit gravitational flow of irrigating solution through wound and into collection basin. Position client so that wound is vertical to collection basin.	Directing solution from top to bottom of wound and from clean area to contaminated area prevents further infection. Positioning client during planning stage provides bed surfaces for later preparation.
8. Warm sterile irrigating solution to approximate body temperature.	Increases comfort and reduces vascular constriction response in tissues.
9. Form cuff on leakproof refuse bag and place it near bed.	Helps maintain large opening, thereby permitting placement of contaminated dressing without soiling bag's outer surface.
10. Close room door or bed curtains.	Maintains privacy.

STEPS	RATIONALE
11. Place waterproof underpad on bed surface in front of wound.	Protection of bedding eliminates need to change linens.
12. Place clean basin directly under wound.	Collects contaminated irrigating solution.
13. Wash hands	Reduces transmission of infection.
14. If gown is needed, apply it now.	Protects your clothing and prevents cross-infection.
15. Prepare sterile field using sterile dressing set and supplies.	Reduces risk of introducing microorganisms into wound.
16. Add sterile basin and pour in estimated volume of warm sterile irrigating solution and set irrigating syringe in basin with solution.	Prepares solution for wound irrigation.
17. Place several strips of adhesive tape within reach and *not* on sterile field.	Provides easy access to tape for securing dressing.
18. Put on clean gloves and remove soiled dressing and discard in leakproof refuse bag.	Reduces transmission of microorganisms.
19. Remove and discard gloves.	
20. Inspect wound and make mental note of healing process, inflammation, drainage, or purulent matter.	Facilitates accurate description later.
21. Apply sterile gloves.	Reduces transmission of microorganisms.
22. Irrigate wound with wide opening: a. Fill syringe with irrigating solution. b. Hold syringe tip 2.5 cm (1 in) above upper end of wound. c. Using slow, continuous pressure, flush wound. d. Repeat Steps 22a–22c until solution draining into basin is clear.	Aids in removal of debris and facilitates healing by secondary intention. Prevents trauma to granulation tissue from syringe. Ensures removal of all debris.
23. Irrigate deep wound with very small opening: a. Attach soft catheter to filled irrigating syringe. b. Lubricate tip of catheter with irrigating solution. Gently insert tip of catheter until resistance is felt, and then pull out about 1.2 cm (½ in) to remove tip from fragile inner wall of wound. c. Using slow, continuous pressure, flush wound. d. Pinch off catheter just below syringe. e. Remove syringe, fill, and reattach to catheter. Repeat until return is clear.	Permits direct flow of irrigant into wound. Ensures removal of debris without traumatizing new granulation tissue. Avoids contamination of sterile solution or basin.
24. Dry wound edges with sterile gauze.	Prevents maceration of surrounding tissue from excess moisture.
25. Apply sterile dressing.	Maintains sterile protective barrier over wound.
26. Remove and dispose of gloves.	Facilitates placement of adhesive tape.
27. Secure dressing with adhesive tape.	
28. Assist client to comfortable position.	Relieves tension on wound site.
29. Dispose of equipment; retain remaining bottle of sterile solution.	Sterile solution can be used for subsequent irrigations.
30. Wash hands.	Reduces transmission of infection.

CONTINUED

STEPS	RATIONALE
31. Inspect dressing periodically.	Determines response to wound irrigation and need to modify care plan.
32. Evaluate skin integrity.	Determines whether extension of wound has occurred.
33. Record wound appearance, irrigation, and client response in nurses' notes.	Fulfills legal responsibility and provides information needed to ensure continuity of care.

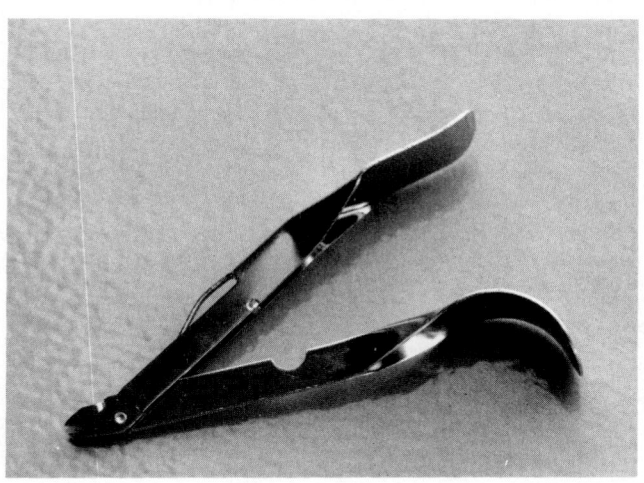

Fig. 48-10   Staple remover.

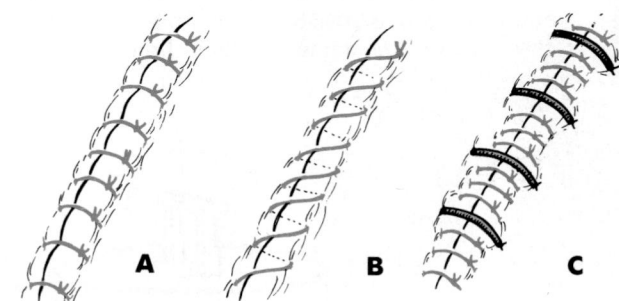

Fig. 48-11   Examples of suturing methods. A, Intermittent. B, Continuous. C, Retention.

ture removal is not written until the physician believes that the wound has closed (usually 7 to 10 days). Special scissors with curved cutting tips or special staple removers slide under the skin closures for suture removal (Fig. 48-10). The physician usually signifies the number of sutures or staples to remove. If the suture line appears to be healing in certain locations better than in others, the physician may choose to have only some sutures removed (for example, every other one).

To remove staples, the nurse simply inserts the tips of the staple remover under each wire staple. While slowly closing the ends of the staple remover together, the nurse squeezes the center of the staple with the tips, freeing the staple from the skin.

To remove sutures the nurse first checks the type of suturing used (Fig. 48-11). With interrupted suturing the surgeon ties each individual suture made in the skin. Continuous suturing, as the name implies, is a series of sutures with only two knots, one

at the beginning and one at the end of the suture line. Retention sutures are placed more deeply than skin sutures and may or may not be removed by the nurse, depending on agency policy. The manner in which the suture crosses and penetrates the skin determines the method for removal. The most important principle in suture removal is to *never* pull the visible portion of a suture through underlying tissue. Sutures on the skin's surface harbor microorganisms and debris. The portion of the suture beneath the skin is sterile. Pulling the contaminated portion of the suture through tissues may lead to infection. The nurse clips suture materials as close to the skin edge on one side as possible and then pulls the suture through from the other side (Fig. 48-12 on p. 1678).

Drainage Evacuation

When drainage interferes with healing, drainage evacuation can be achieved by using either a drain alone or a drainage tube with continuous suction. The nurse may apply special skin barriers, similar to those used with ostomies (see Chapter 41), around drain sites. The **skin barriers** are soft, waferlike, plastic materials that are applied to the skin with ad-

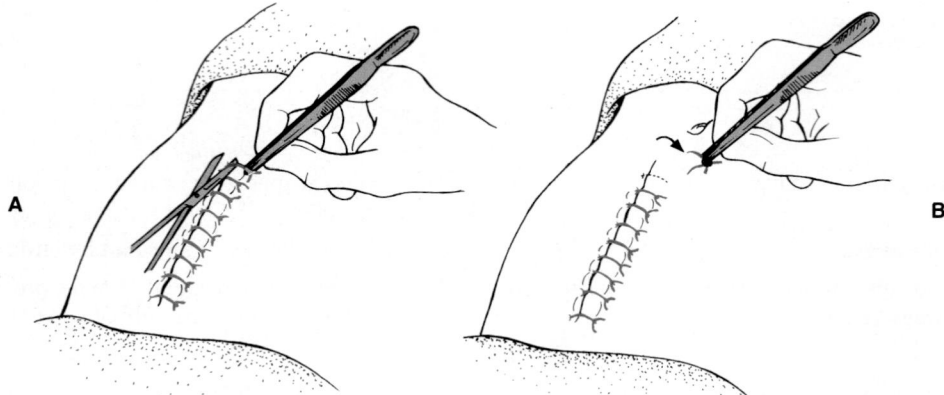

Fig. 48-12   Removal of intermittent suture. **A,** The nurse cuts the suture as close to the skin as possible, away from the knot. **B,** The nurse removes the suture and never pulls the contaminated stitch through tissues.

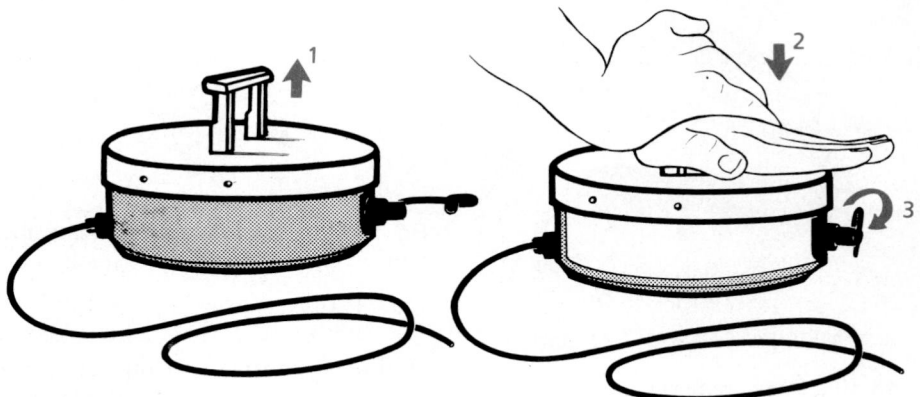

Fig. 48-13   Setting the suction on a drainage evacuator. **1,** With drainage port open, the lever to the vacuum diaphragm is raised. **2,** The nurse pushes straight down on the lever to lower the diaphragm. **3,** Closure of the port prevents escape of air and creates vacuum pressure.

hesive. Drainage flows on the barrier but not directly on the skin. **Drainage evacuators** (Fig. 48-13) are convenient, portable units that connect to tubular drains lying within a wound bed and exert a safe, constant, low-pressure vacuum to remove and collect drainage. The nurse ensures that suction is exerted and that connection points between the evacuator and tubing are intact. The evacuator collects drainage that the nurse assesses for volume and character every shift and as needed. When the evacuator fills, the nurse measures output by emptying the contents into a graduated cylinder and immediately resets the evacuator to apply suction.

Bandages and Binders

A simple gauze dressing is often not enough to immobilize or provide support to a wound. **Binders** and bandages applied over or around dressings can provide extra protection and therapeutic benefits by:

1. Creating pressure over a body part (for example, an elastic pressure bandage applied over an arterial puncture site)
2. Immobilizing a body part (for example, an elastic bandage applied around a sprained ankle)
3. Supporting a wound (for example, an abdominal binder applied over a large abdominal incision and dressing)
4. Reducing or preventing edema (for example, a breast binder used to minimize swelling between skin and tissue layers after a mastectomy)
5. Securing a splint (for example, a bandage applied around hand splints for correction of deformities)

TABLE 48-4   Principles for Bandage and Binder Application

Principle	Rationale
Position body part to be bandaged in comfortable position of normal anatomical alignment.	Bandages cause restriction in movement. Immobilization in normal functioning position reduces risks of deformity or injury.
Prevent friction between and against skin surfaces by applying gauze or cotton padding.	Skin surfaces in contact with each other (e.g., between toes, under breasts) can rub against each other to cause abrasion or chafing. Bandages over bony prominences may rub against skin to cause breakdown.
Apply bandages securely to prevent slippage during movement.	Friction between bandage and skin can cause skin breakdown.
When bandaging extremities, apply bandage first at distal end and progress toward trunk.	Gradual application of pressure from distal toward proximal portion of extremity promotes venous return and minimizes risk of edema or circulatory impairment.
Apply bandages firmly with equal tension exerted over each turn or layer. Avoid excess overlapping of bandage layers.	Application prevents unequal pressure distribution over bandaged body part. Localized pressure causes circulatory impairment.
Position pins, knots, or ties away from wound or sensitive skin areas.	Materials can exert localized pressure and irritation.

6. Securing dressings (for example, elastic webbing applied around leg dressings after a vein stripping)

Bandages are available in rolls of various widths and materials, including gauze, elasticized knit, elastic webbing, flannel, and muslin. Gauze bandages are lightweight and inexpensive, mold easily around contours of the body, and permit air circulation to prevent skin maceration. Elastic bandages conform well to body parts but can also be used to exert pressure over a body part. Flannel and muslin bandages are thicker than gauze and thus stronger for supporting or applying pressure. A flannel bandage also insulates to provide warmth.

Binders are bandages that are made of large pieces of material to fit a specific body part. Most binders are made of elastic, cotton, muslin, or flannel. An abdominal binder and a breast binder are examples.

PRINCIPLES FOR APPLYING BANDAGES AND BINDERS.
Correctly applied bandages and binders do not cause injury to underlying and nearby body parts or create discomfort for the client. For example, a chest binder must not be so tight as to restrict chest wall expansion. Before a bandage or binder is applied, the nurse's responsibilities include the following:

1. Inspecting the skin for abrasions, edema, discoloration, or exposed wound edges
2. Covering exposed wounds or open abrasions with a sterile dressing

3. Assessing the condition of underlying dressings and changing them if soiled
4. Assessing the skin of underlying body parts and parts that will be distal to the bandage for signs of circulatory impairment (coolness, pallor or cyanosis, diminished or absent pulses, swelling, numbness, and tingling) to provide a means for comparing changes in circulation after bandage application

Table 48-4 outlines the principles of bandage and binder application. After a bandage is applied, the nurse assesses, documents, and immediately reports changes in circulation, skin integrity, comfort level, and body function such as ventilation or movement. The nurse who applies a bandage can loosen or readjust it as necessary. The nurse should have a physician's order before loosening or removing a bandage applied by a physician. The nurse explains to the client that any bandage or binder feels relatively firm or tight. A bandage should be carefully assessed to be sure that it is properly applied and is providing therapeutic benefit, and soiled bandages should be replaced. Like a damp dressing, a bandage or binder can harbor microorganisms.

BINDER APPLICATION. Binders are especially designed for the body part to be supported. The most common types of binders are the breast binder, abdominal binder, and **T** binder (Procedure 48-3).

Breast Binder. A breast binder looks like a tight-fitting sleeveless vest. It conforms to the shape of the

Applying an Abdominal Binder, T Binder, or Breast Binder

STEPS	RATIONALE
1. Observe client with need for support of thorax or abdomen. Observe ability to breathe deeply and cough effectively.	Baseline assessment determines client's ability to breathe and cough. Impaired ventilation of lung can lead to alveolar atelectasis and inadequate arterial oxygenation.
2. Inspect skin for actual or potential alterations in integrity. Observe for irritation, abrasions; skin surfaces that rub against each other; allergic response to adhesive tape used to secure dressing.	Actual impairments in skin integrity can be worsened with application of binder. Binder can cause pressure and excoriation.
3. Review medical record if medical prescription for particular binder is required and reasons for application.	Application of supportive binders may be based on nursing judgment. In some situations, physician input is required.
4. Gather necessary data regarding size of client and appropriate binder.	Ensures proper fit of binder.

5. Prepare necessray equipment and supplies:
  a. Abdominal binder:
    (1) Correct size cloth or elastic straight binder
    (2) Safety pins (unless Velcro closure is attached)
  b. T and double-T binder:
    (1) Correct size binder
    (2) Safety pins: 2 pins for T binders; 3 pins for double-T binder
  c. Breast binders:
    (1) Correct size binder
	Binder must be large enough to surround abdomen and overlap to secure closure.
	One pin secures horizontal waistband. Second pin secures each tail, placing pin through all thicknesses at horizontal level.
	
	Binder must be large enough to overlap to secure Velcro closure.

6. Explain procedure to client and close curtains or room door.	Promotes understanding. Provides privacy.
7. Wash hands	Maintains medical asepsis and infection control.

8. Apply abdominal binder:
  a. Position client in supine position with head slightly elevated and knees slightly flexed.
  b. Fanfold far side of binder toward midline of binder.
  c. Instruct and assist client to roll away from you toward raised side rail while firmly supporting abdominal incision and dressing with hands.
  d. Place fanfolded ends of binder under client.
 	
  e. Instruct and assist client to roll over folded ends.
  f. Unfold and stretch ends out smoothly on far side of bed. (Binder should extend from just above symphysis pubis to just below costal margin.)
  g. Instruct client to roll back into supine position.
 	
  h. Adjust binder so that supine client is centered over binder using symphysis pubis and costal margins as lower and upper landmarks.
  i. Straight binder: Pull distal end of binder over center of client's abdomen. While maintaining tension on that end of binder, pull opposite end of binder over center and secure with Velcro closure tabs or safety pins.
	Minimizes muscular tension on abdominal organs.
	
	Reduces time client remains in uncomfortable position. Reduces pain and discomfort.
	
	Permits placement and centering of binder with minimal discomfort.
	
	Maintains skin integrity and comfort.
	
	Facilitates chest expansion and adequate wound support when binder is closed.
	Centers support from binder over abdominal structures.
	
	Provides continuous wound support and comfort.

CONTINUED

STEPS	RATIONALE
j. Assess client's ability to breathe deeply and cough effectively.	Determines ventilation and clears airways of pulmonary secretions.
k. Ask client about comfort level.	Excess discomfort may inhibit expirations.
l. Adjust binder as necessary.	
9. Apply T and double-T binders:	
a. Assist client to dorsal recumbent position.	
b. Have client raise hips and place horizontal band around waist (or above iliac crests) with vertical tails extending past buttocks. Overlap waist-band in front and secure with safety pins.	Minimizes muscular tension on perineal organs. Secures binder around client.
c. Complete binder application:	Single-T and double-T binders provide support to perineal muscles and organs.
(1) *T binder:* Bring remaining vertical strip over perineal dressing and continue up and under center front of horizontal band. Bring ends over waistband and secure all thicknesses with safety pin.	
(2) *Double-T binder:* Bring remaining vertical strips over perineal or suprapubic dressing with each tail supporting one side of scrotum and proceeding upward on either side of penis. Continue upward on either side of penis. Continue drawing ends behind and then downward in front of horizontal band. Secure all thicknesses with one safety pin.	
d. Assess comfort level with client in lying, sitting, and standing positions. Readjust front pins as necessary. Increase padding if any area rubs against surrounding tissues.	Determines efficacy of binder to maintain dressings and support perineal structures.
e. Instruct client regarding removal of binder before defecating or urinating and need to replace binder after these bodily functions.	Cleanliness of binder reduces infection risk.
10. Apply breast binder:	
a. Assist client in placing arms through binder's armholes.	Binder placement process.
b. Assist client to supine position in bed.	Facilitates normal anatomical situation of breasts. Maintains normal anatomical alignment of breasts. Facilitates healing and comfort.
c. Pad area under breasts if necessary.	Prevents skin contact with undersurface.
d. Using Velcro closure tabs, secure binder at nipple level first. Continue closure process above and then below nipple line until entire binder is closed.	Reduces risk of uneven pressure or localized irritation.
e. Make appropriate adjustments including individualizing fit of shoulder straps.	Maintains support to client's breasts.
f. Instruct and observe skill development in self-care related to reapplying breast binder.	Self-care is an integral aspect of discharge planning. Skin integrity and comfort level goals are ensured.
11. Wash hands.	Prevents cross-infections.
12. Observe site for skin integrity, circulation, and characteristics of the wound. Note comfort level of client	Determines that binder has not resulted in irritation to skin or underlying organs. Binders should not impede breathing or increase discomfort.
13. Record application of binder, condition of skin and circulation, integrity of dressings, and comfort level.	Documents procedure. Baseline data ensure continuity of care.

chest wall and is available in different sizes. Breast binders can provide support after breast surgery or exert pressure to reduce lactation in a woman after childbirth. It is essential that excess pressure be avoided when clients or family members are learning how to apply binders. Chest expansion should remain unimpaired.

Abdominal Binders. An abdominal binder supports large abdominal incisions that are vulnerable to tension or stress as the client moves or coughs (Fig. 48-14). The nurse secures an abdominal binder with safety pins, Velcro strips, or metal stays. Procedure 48-3 describes steps for an abdominal binder application.

T Binders. As the name implies, the T binder looks like the letter T (Fig. 48-15) and is used to secure rectal or perineal dressings. The single T is for female clients, and the double T fits male clients.

The belt of the binder fits securely around the client's waist with the tail passing between the client's legs from back to front and attaching to the belt's front. The nurse must be sure that the tail fits smoothly and against the dressing. T binders become soiled easily and often require frequent changing. Irritation to the urethra or scrotum must be avoided.

SLINGS. Slings support arms with muscular sprains or fractures. A commercially made sling consists of a long sleeve that extends above the elbow, with a strap that fits around the neck. In the home a large triangular piece of cloth can be used. The client may sit or lie supine during sling application (Fig. 48-16). The nurse instructs the client to bend the affected arm, bringing the forearm straight across the chest. The open sling fits under the client's arm and over the chest, with the base of the triangle under the wrist and the triangle's point at the client's elbow. One end of the sling fits around the back of the client's neck. The nurse brings the other end up and over the affected arm while supporting the extremity. The nurse ties the two ends at the side of the neck so that the knot does not press against the cervical spine. The loose material at the elbow can be folded evenly around the elbow and pinned. The lower arm and hand should always be supported at a level above the elbow to prevent formation of dependent edema.

BANDAGE APPLICATION. Rolls of bandage can secure or support dressings over irregularly shaped body parts. Each roll has a free outer end and a terminal end at the center of the roll. The rolled portion of the bandage is its body, and its outer surface is placed against the client's skin or dressing. Procedure 48-4 describes the steps for applying an elastic bandage. The nurse may use a variety of bandage turns depending on the body part to be bandaged (Table 48-5). Care must be taken to prevent the applied bandage from exerting a tourniquet effect.

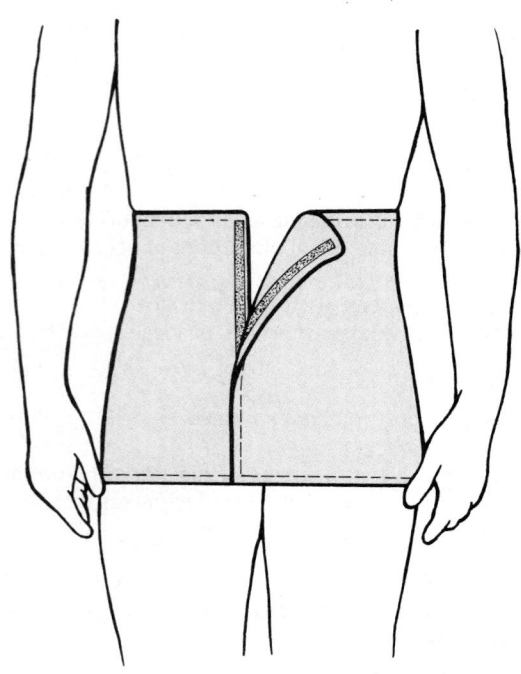

Fig. 48-14 An abdominal binder secures with velcro.

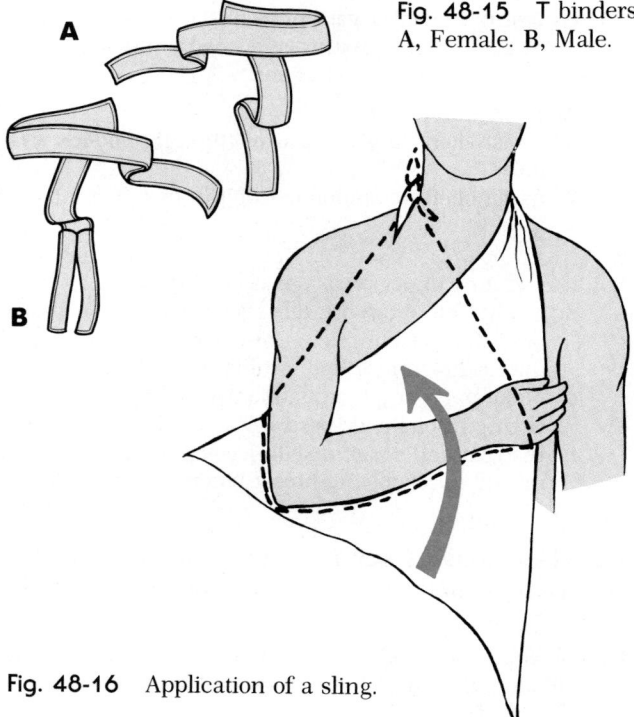

Fig. 48-15 T binders. A, Female. B, Male.

Fig. 48-16 Application of a sling.

Applying an Elastic Bandage

STEPS	RATIONALE
1. Inspect skin for alterations in integrity as indicated by abrasions, discoloration, chafing, or edema. (Look carefully at bony prominences.)	Altered skin integrity contraindicates the use of elastic bandage.
2. Observe adequacy of circulation by noting surface temperature, skin color, and sensation of body parts to be wrapped.	Comparison of area before and after application of bandage is necessary to ensure continued adequate circulation. Impairment of circulation may result in coolness to touch when compared with opposite side of body, cyanosis or pallor of skin, diminished or absent pulses, edema or localized pooling, and numbness or tingling of part.
3. Review medical record for specific orders related to application of elastic bandage. Note area to be covered, type of bandage required, frequency of change, and previous response to treatment.	Specific prescription may direct procedure, including factors such as extent of application (e.g., toe to knee, toe to groin) and duration of treatment.
4. Obtain necessary equipment and supplies (determine if present bandage will be reused or replacement be obtained):	
a. Correct widths and number of bandages (Elastic bandages are available in 2, 2½, 3, 4, 6, and 8 in and 1½ and 3 yd [5, 6.25, 7.5, 10, 15, and 20 cm and 135 and 270 cm]; 7.5- and 10-cm bandages are most often appropriate.)	Increasingly wider bandages are used as size of body part increases (e.g., 7.5-, 10-, and 15-cm bandages may be used to cover foot, calf, thigh).
b. Safety pins, tape	Secures bandage in place.
5. Explain procedure. Reinforce teaching that smooth, even, light pressure will be applied to improve venous circulation, prevent clot formation, reduce or prevent swelling, immobilize arms, secure surgical dressings, and provide pressure.	Promotes cooperation and reduces anxiety. Improves knowledge level regarding need for elastic bandages.
6. Wash hands.	Reduces transmission of infection.
7. Close room door or curtains. Assist client to assume comfortable, anatomically correct position	Maintains comfort and dignity. Maintains alignment. Prevents musculoskeletal deformity.
8. Hold roll of elastic bandage in dominant hand and use other hand to lightly hold beginning of bandage at distal body part. Continue transferring roll to dominant hand as bandage is wrapped.	Maintains appropriate and consistent bandage tension.
9. Apply bandage from distal point toward proximal boundary using variety of turns to cover various shapes of body parts (Table 48-5).	Bandage is applied in manner that conforms evenly to body part and promotes venous return.
10. Unroll and very slightly stretch bandage. Overlap turns	Maintains uniform bandage tension. Prevents uneven bandage tension and circulatory impairment.
11. Secure first bandage before applying additional rolls.	Prevents wrinkling or loose ends.
12. Wash hands.	Reduces transmission of microorganisms.
13. Evaluate distal circulation as application is completed and at least twice during 8-hr period (note color, warmth, pulses, and numbness).	Early detection of circulatory difficulties ensures healthy neuromuscular status.
14. Record bandage application and client's response in nurses' notes.	Documents procedures and ensures continuity of care.

TABLE 48-5 Types of Bandage Turns

Type	Description	Purpose or Use
Circular	Bandage turn overlapping previous turn completely	Anchors bandage at the first and final turn; covers small part (finger, toe)
Spiral	Bandage ascending body part with each turn overlapping previous one by one-half or two-thirds width of bandage	Covers cylindrical body parts such as wrist or upper arm
Spiral—reverse	Turn requiring twist (reversal) of bandage halfway through each turn	Covers cone-shaped body parts such as the forearm, thigh, or calf; useful with nonstretching bandages such as gauze or flannel
Figure eight	Oblique overlapping turns alternately ascending and descending over bandaged part; each turn crossing previous one to form figure eight	Covers joints; snug fit provides excellent immobilization
Recurrent	Bandage first secured with two circular turns around proximal end of body part; half turn made perpendicular up from bandage edge; body of bandage brought over distal end of body part to be covered with each turn folded back over on itself	Covers uneven body parts such as head or stump

Heat and Cold Therapy

Local application of heat and cold to an injured body part can be therapeutic. Before using these therapies, however, the nurse must understand normal body responses to local temperature variations, assess the integrity of the body part, determine the client's ability to sense temperature variations, and ensure proper operation of equipment. The nurse is legally responsible for safe administration of heat and cold applications.

BODILY RESPONSES TO HEAT AND COLD. Exposure to heat and cold can cause systemic and local responses. Systemic responses occur through heat-loss mechanisms (sweating and vasodilation) or mechanisms promoting heat conservation (vasoconstriction and piloerection) and heat production (shivering) (see Chapter 19). Local responses to heat and cold occur through stimulation of temperature-sensitive nerve endings within the skin. This stimulation sends impulses from the periphery to the hypothalamus, which becomes aware of local temperature sensations and triggers adaptive responses for maintenance of normal body temperature. If alterations occur along temperature sensation pathways, the reception and eventual perception of stimuli will be altered.

The body also possesses a protective reflex response so that, when a person touches an extremely hot or cold stimulus, impulses travel to the spinal cord, synapse within the cord, and return by way of a motor nerve to cause withdrawal from the stimulus. The person simultaneously becomes aware of the discomfort.

The body can tolerate wide variations in temperature. The normal temperature of the skin's surface is 34° C (93.2° F), but temperature receptors usually adapt quickly to local temperatures between 45° and 15° C (113° and 59° F). Pain develops when local temperatures exceed this range. Excessive heat causes a burning sensation. Cold produces a numbing sensation before pain.

The body's adaptive ability creates the major problem in protecting clients from injury resulting from temperature extremes. A person initially feels an extreme change in temperature but within a short time hardly notices it. This can be dangerous because a person insensitive to heat and cold extremes can suffer serious tissue injury. The nurse must recognize clients most at risk for injuries from heat and cold applications (Table 48-6).

LOCAL EFFECTS OF HEAT AND COLD. Heat and cold stimuli create different physiological responses. The choice of heat or cold therapy depends on local responses desired for wound healing.

Effects of Heat Application. Table 48-7 summarizes the benefits of heat application. Heat generally is quite therapeutic, improving blood flow to an injured part. If heat is applied for 1 hour or more, however, blood flow is reduced by a reflex vasoconstriction as the body attempts to control heat loss from the area. Periodic removal and reapplication of local heat restores vasodilation. Continuous exposure to heat damages epithelial cells, causing redness, localized tenderness, and even blistering.

Effects of Cold Application. Table 48-7 on p. 1186 also summarizes the benefits of cold application. Prolonged exposure of the skin to cold results in a reflex vasodilation. The cell's inability to receive adequate blood flow and nutrients results in tissue ischemia. The skin initially takes on a reddened appear-

---

TABLE 48-6   Conditions That Increase Risk of Injury from Heat and Cold Application

Condition	Risk Factors
Very young clients or older clients	Thinner skin layers in children increase risk of burns. Older clients have reduced sensitivity to pain.
Open wounds, broken skin, stomas	Subcutaneous and visceral tissues are more sensitive to temperature variations. They also contain no temperature and fewer pain receptors.
Areas of edema or scar formation	Reduced sensation to temperature stimuli occurs because of thickening of skin layers from fluid buildup or scar formation.
Peripheral vascular disease (e.g., diabetes, arteriosclerosis)	Body's extremities are less sensitive to temperature and pain stimuli because of circulatory impairment and local tissue injury. Cold application would further compromise blood flow.
Confusion or unconsciousness	Reduced perception of sensory or painful stimuli occurs.
Spinal cord injury	Alterations in nerve pathways prevent reception of sensory or painful stimuli.
Abscessed tooth or appendix	Infection is highly localized. Application of heat may cause rupture with spread of microorganisms systemically.

TABLE 48-7	Therapeutic Effects of Heat and Cold Applications	
Physiological Response	Therapeutic Benefit	Examples of Conditions Treated

HEAT

Vasodilation	Improves blood flow to injured body part; promotes delivery of nutrients and removal of wastes; lessens venous congestion in injured tissues	Inflamed or edematous body part; new surgical wound; infected wound; arthritis, degenerative joint disease; localized joint pain, muscle strains; low back pain; menstrual cramping, hemorrhoidal, perianal, and vaginal inflammation; local abscesses
Reduced blood viscosity	Improves delivery of leukocytes and antibiotics to wound site	
Reduced muscle tension	Promotes muscle relaxation and reduces pain from spasm or stiffness	
Increased tissue metabolism	Increases blood flow; provides local warmth	
Increased capillary permeability	Promotes movement of waste products and nutrients	

COLD

Vasoconstriction	Reduces blood flow to injured body part, preventing edema formation; reduces inflammation	Direct trauma (sprains, strains, fractures, muscle spasms); superficial laceration or puncture wound; minor burn; suspected malignancy in area of injury or pain; injections; arthritis and joint trauma
Local anesthesia	Reduces localized pain	
Reduced cell metabolism	Reduces oxygen needs of tissues	
Increased blood viscosity	Promotes blood coagulation at injury site	
Decreased muscle tension	Relieves pain	

ance, followed by a bluish purple mottling with numbness and a burning type of pain. The skin's tissues can freeze from exposure to extreme cold.

FACTORS INFLUENCING HEAT AND COLD TOLERANCE. The body's response to heat and cold therapies depends on the following factors:

1. Duration of application. A person is better able to tolerate short exposure to temperature extremes.
2. Body part. Certain areas of the skin are more sensitive to temperature variations. These include the neck, inner aspect of the wrist and forearm, and perineal region. The foot and palm of the hand are less sensitive.
3. Damage to body surface. Exposed skin layers are more sensitive to temperature variations.
4. Prior skin temperature. The body responds best to minor temperature adjustments. If a body part is cool and a hot stimulus touches the skin, the response is greater than if the stimulus were only warm.

5. Body surface area. A person has less tolerance to temperature changes when a large area of the body is exposed to heat or cold.
6. Age and physical condition. Tolerance to temperature variations changes with age. Clients who are very young and old are most sensitive to the heat and cold. If a client's physical condition reduces the reception or perception of sensory stimuli, tolerance to temperature extremes is high, but the risk of injury is also high.

ASSESSMENT FOR TEMPERATURE TOLERANCE. Before applying heat or cold therapies, the nurse assesses the client's physical condition for signs of potential intolerance to heat and cold. The nurse first observes the area to be treated. Alterations in skin integrity, such as abrasions, open wounds, edema, bruising, bleeding, or localized areas of inflammation, increase the client's risk of injury. Because the physician commonly orders heat and cold applications to be placed on traumatized areas, the baseline assessment provides a guide for evaluating skin changes that might occur during therapy.

Assessment includes identification of conditions that contraindicate heat or cold therapy. An active area of bleeding should not be covered by a warm application because bleeding will continue. Warm applications are contraindicated when the client has an acute, localized inflammation such as appendicitis because the heat could cause the appendix to rupture. If a client has cardiovascular problems, it is unwise to apply heat to large portions of the body because the resulting massive vasodilation may disrupt blood supply to vital organs.

Cold is contraindicated if the site of injury is already edematous. Cold further retards circulation to the area and prevents absorption of the interstitial fluid. If the client has impairment in circulation (for example, arteriosclerosis), cold further reduces blood supply to the affected area. One other contraindication for cold therapy is shivering. Cold applications may intensify shivering and dangerously increase body temperature. The nurse also assesses the client's response to stimuli. Sensation to light touch, pinprick, and mild temperature variations (see Chapter 20) reveals the ability of the client to recognize when heat or cold becomes excessive. If a client has peripheral vascular disease, the nurse pays particular attention to the integrity of extremities. For example, if the physician's order is to apply a cold compress to a lower extremity, the nurse should assess circulation to the leg by observing skin color and palpating skin temperatures, distal pulses, and edematous areas. If signs of circulatory inadequacy are present, the nurse should question the order.

Level of consciousness influences the ability to perceive heat, cold, and pain. If a client is confused or unresponsive, the nurse must make frequent observations of skin integrity after therapy begins.

The nurse must also assess the condition of equipment being used. Electrical equipment should be checked for cracked cords, frayed wires, damaged insulation, and exposed heating components. Equipment containing circulating fluids should not have leaks. The nurse also checks equipment for evenness of temperature distribution. Uneven temperature distribution suggests that the equipment is functioning improperly.

CLIENT EDUCATION AND SAFETY. Before application of heat or cold therapy the client should understand its purpose, the symptoms of temperature exposure, and precautions taken to prevent injury. The box provides hints for safely applying heat and cold therapy.

Safety Suggestions for Applying Heat or Cold Therapy

- *Do* explain to the client sensations to be felt during the procedure.
- Do instruct the client to report changes in sensation or discomfort immediately.
- *Do* provide a timer, clock, or watch so that the client can help the nurse time the application.
- *Do* keep the call light within the client's reach.
- *Do* refer to the institution's policy and procedure manual for safe temperatures.
- *Do not* allow the client to adjust temperature settings.
- *Do not* allow the client to move an application or place hands on the wound site.
- *Do not* place the client in a position that prevents movement away from the temperature source.
- *Do not* leave unattended a client who is unable to sense temperature changes or move from the temperature source.

APPLYING HEAT AND COLD. A prerequisite to using any heat or cold application is a physician's order, which should include the body site to be treated and the type, frequency, and duration of application. The nurse should consult the agency's procedure manual for correct temperatures to use.

Choice of Moist or Dry. Heat and cold applications can be administered in dry or moist forms. The type of wound or injury, the location of the body part, and the presence of drainage or inflammation are factors considered in selecting dry or moist applications. Table 48-8 on p. 1188 summarizes advantages and disadvantages of both.

Hot, Moist Compresses. For open wounds, sterile, hot, moist compresses improve circulation, relieve edema, and promote consolidation of pus and drainage. A **compress** is a piece of gauze dressing moistened in a prescribed warmed solution. A **pack** is a larger cloth or dressing applied to a larger body area.

Heat from hot compresses dissipates quickly. To maintain a constant temperature the nurse must change the compress often or apply a warm aquathermic pad or waterproof heating pad over the compress. Because moisture conducts heat, any device's temperature setting should be lower for a moist compress than for a dry application. A layer of plastic wrap or a dry towel can also be used to insulate the

TABLE 48-8 Choice of Dry or Moist Applications	
Advantages	Disadvantages

MOIST APPLICATIONS

Moist application reduces drying of skin and softens wound exudate.	Prolonged exposure can cause maceration of skin.
Moist compresses conform well to body area being treated.	Moist heat will cool rapidly because of moisture evaporation.
Moist heat penetrates deeply into tissue layers.	Moist heat creates greater risk for burns to skin because moisture conducts heat.
Warm moist heat does not promote sweating and insensible fluid loss.	

DRY APPLICATIONS

Dry heat has less risk of burns to skin than moist applications.	Dry heat increases body fluid loss through sweating.
Dry application does not cause skin maceration.	Dry applications do not penetrate deep into tissues.
Dry heat retains temperature longer because it is not influenced by evaporation.	Dry heat causes increased drying of skin.

compress and retain heat. Moist heat promotes vasodilation and evaporation of heat from the skin's surface. For this reason a client may feel chilly. The nurse controls drafts within the room and keeps the client covered with a blanket or robe. Procedure 48-5 describes the steps for applying a hot, moist compress.

Warm Soaks. Immersion of a body part in a warmed solution promotes circulation, lessens edema, increases muscle relaxation, and can provide a means to debride wounds and apply medicated solution. A soak can also be accompanied by wrapping the body part in dressings and saturating them with the warmed solution.

The nurse positions the client comfortably, places waterproof pads under the area to be treated, and heats the solution to about 40.5° to 43° C (105° to 110° F). After immersing the body part, the nurse covers the container and extremity with a towel to reduce heat loss. It is usually necessary to remove the cooled solution and add heated solution after about 10 minutes. The problem is to keep the solution at a constant temperature. The nurse never adds a hotter solution while the body part remains immersed. After any soak the nurse dries the body part thoroughly to prevent maceration.

Sitz Baths. The client who has had rectal surgery, an episiotomy during childbirth, painful hemorrhoids, or vaginal inflammation may benefit from a **sitz bath,** a bath in which only the pelvic area is immersed in warm fluid. The client sits in a special tub or chair or in a basin that fits on the toilet seat so that the legs and feet remain out of the water. Immersing the entire body causes widespread vasodilation and nullifies the effect of local heat application to the pelvic area.

The desired temperature for a sitz bath depends on whether the purpose is to promote relaxation or to clean a wound. It may be necessary to add warm water during the procedure, which normally lasts 20 minutes, to maintain a constant temperature. Agency procedure manuals recommend safe water temperatures. A disposable sitz basin contains an attachment resembling an enema bag that allows gradual introduction of warmer water (Fig. 48-17 on p. 1691).

The nurse prevents overexposure of the client by draping bath blankets around the client's shoulders and thighs and controlling drafts. The client should be able to sit in the basin or tub with feet flat on the floor and without pressure on the sacrum or thighs. Because exposure of a large portion of the body to heat can cause extensive vasodilation, the nurse should assess the pulse and facial color and ask whether the client feels light-headed or nauseated.

Paraffin Baths. A paraffin bath consists of a mixture of heated paraffin wax and mineral oil (1 part oil to 5 parts paraffin). Clients with painful arthritis or other joint discomforts of the hands and feet benefit most from the baths. In many institutions, only physical therapists administer the applications. Clients often heat paraffin baths at home in double boilers (53.3° to 54.4° C [128° to 130° F]).

Aquathermia (Water-Flow) Pads. A popular device in health-care institutions is the **aquathermia**

STEPS	RATIONALE
1. Inspect condition of exposed skin and wound on which compress is to be applied (see illustration).	Provides baseline to determine changes in skin during heat application. Very thin or damaged skin is more susceptible to injury from heat.
2. Assess client's extremities for sensitivity to temperature and pain by measuring light touch, pinprick, and temperature sensation tests.	Determines whether client is insensitive to heat and cold extremes.
3. Refer to physician's order for type of compress, location and duration of application, and desired temperature.	Ensures likelihood of safe application.
4. Prepare necessary equipment and supplies:	
a. Prescribed solution warmed to proper temperature, approximately 43°-46° C (110°-115° F)	Correct temperature prevents accidental burns.
b. Sterile gauze dressings	
c. Sterile container for solution	
d. Commercially prepared compresses (optional)	Premoistened compress reduces preparation.
e. Sterile gloves	
f. Petrolatum jelly, if desired	Protects untreated skin surface.
g. Sterile cotton swabs	
h. Waterproof pad	Prevents soiling of bed linen.
i. Tape or ties	
j. Dry bath towel	
k. Aquathermic or heating pad (optional)	Provides continuous source of heat.
l. Disposable gloves	
m. Bath thermometer	Measures solution temperature.
n. Bath blanket	
5. Explain steps of procedure and purpose. Describe sensation to be felt (e.g., feeling of warmth and wetness). Explain precautions to prevent burning.	Minimizes anxiety and promotes cooperation.
6. Assist client in assuming comfortable position in proper body alignment.	Compress remains in place for several minutes. Limited mobility in uncomfortable position causes muscular stress.
7. Place waterproof pad under area to be treated.	Prevents soiling of bed linen.
8. Expose body part to be covered with compress and drape client with bath blanket. Close bedside curtains.	Prevents unnecessary cooling and exposure of body part. Provides privacy.

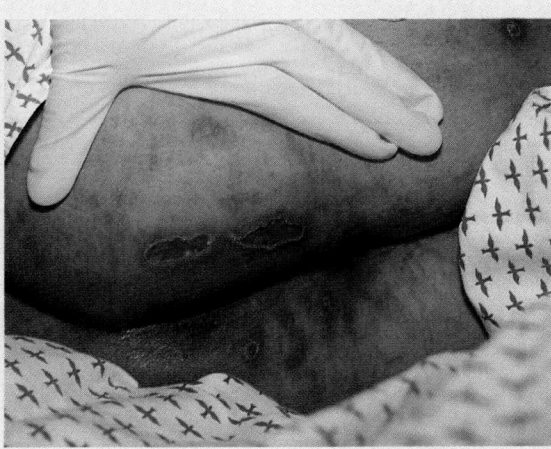

Step 1

Applying a Hot, Moist Compress to an Open Wound

STEPS	RATIONALE
9. Wash hands.	Reduces transmission of infection.
10. Assemble equipment. Pour warmed solution into sterile container. (If using portable heating source, keep solution warm. Commercially prepared compresses may remain under infrared lamp until just before use.) Open sterile packages and drop gauze into container to become immersed in solution. Turn aquathermia pad (if desired) to correct temperature.	Compresses must retain warmth for therapeutic benefit.
11. Apply disposable gloves. Remove any existing dressing covering wound. Dispose of gloves and dressing in proper receptacle.	Reduces transmission of microorganisms.
12. If wound was covered, assess condition of it and surrounding skin.	Provides baseline to determine skin changes after compress application.
13. Apply sterile gloves.	Allows nurse to manipulate sterile dressing and touch open wound.
14. Apply sterile petrolatum jelly, if desired, with cotton swab to skin surrounding wound. Do not apply jelly on broken areas of skin.	Protects skin from possible burns and maceration.
15. Pick up one layer of immersed gauze and wring out excess water.	Excess moisture macerates skin and increases risk of burns and infection.
16. Apply gauze lightly to open wound. Watch response and ask whether cient feels discomfort. In a few seconds, lift edge of gauze to assess for redness.	Skin is sensitive to sudden change in temperature. Redness indicates burn.
17. If client tolerates compress, pack gauze snugly against wound. Be sure all wound surfaces are covered by hot compress.	Prevents rapid cooling from underlying air currents.
18. Wrap or cover moist compress with dry bath towel. If necessary, pin or tie in place.	Insulates compress to prevent heat loss.
19. Change hot compress every 5 min or as ordered.	Prevents cooling and maintains therapeutic benefit of compress.
20. Apply aquathermic or waterproof heating pad over towel (optional). Keep it in place for desired duration of application (about 20-30 min).	Provides constant temperature to compress. Local application of heat for more than 60 min often results in reflex vasoconstriction. Removing hot compress after 30 min and then reapplying in 15 min, if desired, maintains vasodilation and positive therapeutic effects.
21. Ask client periodically whether there is discomfort or burning sensation. Observe area of skin not covered by compress.	Continued exposure to heat can cause burning of skin.
22. Remove pad, towel, and compress in 30 min. Again assess wound and condition of skin.	Continued exposure to moisture will macerate skin.
23. Replace dry sterile dressing as ordered.	Prevents entrance of microorganisms into wound site.
24. Assist client to preferred comfortable position.	Maintains comfort.
25. Dispose of equipment and soiled compress. Wash hands.	Reduces transmission of infection.
26. Inspect affected area covered by compress and heating pad.	Assists in determining effects of application.

CONTINUED

STEPS	RATIONALE
27. Ask client whether an unusual burning sensation is noticed that was not felt before.	It may be difficult to assess burn merely by color changes if wound is inflamed or drainage is present
28. Record type, location, and duration of application. Note temperature used in nurses' notes.	Documents therapy administered.
29. Describe condition of wound, skin, and response.	Documents response to therapy.

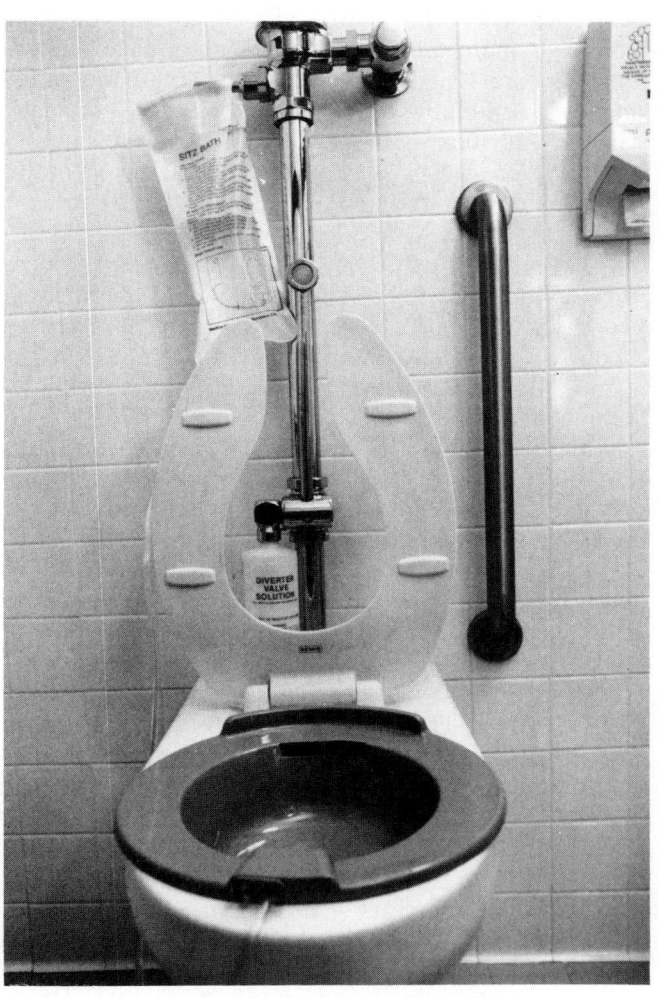

Fig. 48-17   Disposable sitz bath.

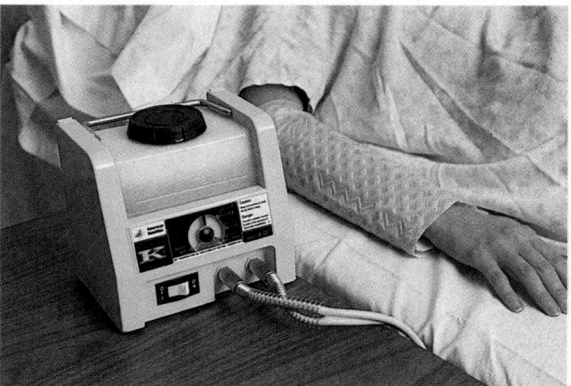

Fig. 48-18   Aquathermia pad.

pad or water-flow pad (Fig. 48-18), used for treating muscle sprains and areas of mild inflammation or edema. The aquathermia unit consists of a water-proof plastic or rubber pad connected by two hoses to an electrical control unit that has a heating element and motor. Distilled water circulates through hollowed channels within the pad to the control unit where water is heated or cooled (depending on temperature setting). Some pads have an absorbent surface to apply moist heat. The units are safer than conventional heating pads. However, the nurse should still check for equipment malfunctions. The temperature setting is fixed by inserting a plastic key into the temperature regulator. In many institutions the central supply room sets the regulators to the recommended temperature (40.5° to 43° C [105° to 110° F]). If the distilled water in the unit runs low, the nurse simply fills the reservoir two-thirds full. Plain tap water is never added because it might leave mineral deposits in the unit.

To avoid burning the client's skin the nurse does not place the pad directly on it. A thin towel or pillow case fits easily over the heating pad. Tape, ties, or a gauze roll holds the pad in place. Pins are never used because they might cause a leak. The nurse checks the client's skin often for signs of burning. An application should last only 20 to 30 minutes. The nurse does not allow a client to lie on a pad. Pressure against a mattress prevents normal heat dissipation. If the pad is to be applied to a region of the back, the client should lie prone or on one side.

Warm Air Blower. When wounds require drying (such as the donor site in split-thickness skin grafting), the nurse may use a hair-dryer. The hair-dryer is set on medium warm setting and then held about 8 to 10 inches from the wound. The nurse then gently waves the device over the site for about 5 minutes or the time prescribed by the surgeon. This procedure is repeated 3 or 4 times a day until the wound is completely dry.

Heat Lamps. Heat lamps use infrared or regular (40 to 75 watt) light bulbs to expose superficial layers of the skin to heat. Because nothing touches the skin surface, this therapy is valuable for clients with sensitive or painful skin lesions or wounds. The lamp is used mainly to increase circulation to a wound.

After explaining the procedure, the nurse provides the client privacy, covers any scars or stomas, cleans and dries the area to be heated, positions the lamp a safe distance from the exposed body surface, and instructs the client not to touch the lamp's hot surface. A 60-watt bulb should be placed at least 50 cm (24 in) away. A larger watt bulb should be about 75 cm (30 in) away. Treatments last about 20 minutes. The nurse checks the condition of the client's skin at least every 5 minutes.

The nurse takes precautions to protect the client's skin, but these low-watt bulbs can be positioned closer to the skin and left on longer than heat lamps. The bulb should be at least 40 to 45 cm (16 to 18 in) away from the client's skin. The nurse checks the client for discomfort or redness of the skin every 5 to 10 min.

Commercial Hot Packs. Commercially prepared, disposable hot packs apply warm, dry heat to an injured area. By striking, kneading, or squeezing the pack, chemicals are mixed and release heat. Package directions recommend the time for heat application.

Hot Water Bottles. Hot water bottles are rarely used in hospitals or other health care settings because of the risk of causing serious burns. In the home the hot water bottle is still economical to use. Nurses must give clients and family members the following instructions on the safe use of water bottles:

1. First ensure that there are no leaks. Fill the bottle with tap water, secure the cap, and turn the bottle upside down.

2. Use tap water at a temperature of 40.5° to 46° C (105° to 115° F).

3. Fill the bag only two-thirds full, expel any air at the top, and secure the cap. The bag is then easier to mold over a body part.

4. Wipe off any moisture on the outside of the bag.

5. Never apply a water bottle directly to the skin surface. Cover it with a towel or pillow case.

6. Keep the bottle in place for 20 to 30 minutes.

7. Never apply a water bottle if the client has sensorineural deficits.

Electric Heating Pads. Another conventional form of heat therapy is the heating pad, an electric coil enclosed within a waterproof pad covered with cotton or flannel cloth. The pad is connected to an electric cord that has a temperature-regulating unit for a high, medium, or low setting. Nurses should advise clients to avoid using the high setting and to never lie on the pad. Another precaution to note is that a safety pin inserted through a pad can result in an electrical shock.

Cold, Moist and Dry Compresses. The procedure for applying cold, moist compresses is the same as that for warm compresses. Cold compresses should be applied for 20 minutes at a temperature of 15° C (59° F) to relieve inflammation and swelling. They may be clean or sterile.

There are commercially prepared cold packs similar to the disposable hot packs for dry applications. They come in various shapes and sizes to fit different body parts. When using cold compresses, the nurse observes for adverse reactions such as burning or numbness, mottling of the skin, redness, extreme paleness, and a bluish skin discoloration.

Cold Soaks. The procedure for preparing cold soaks and immersing a body part is the same as for warm soaks. The desired temperature for a 20-minute cold soak is 15° C (59° F). The nurse controls drafts and uses outer coverings to protect the client from chilling. It may be necessary to add cold water during the procedure to maintain a constant temperature.

Ice Bags or Collars. For a client who has a muscle sprain, localized hemorrhage, or hematoma or has undergone dental surgery, an ice bag is ideal to prevent edema formation, control bleeding, and anesthetize the body part. Proper use of the bag requires the following steps:

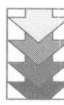

Sample Evaluation of Interventions for Impaired Skin Integrity

Goals	Evaluative Measures	Expected Outcomes
Skin integrity will be improved in area of surgical wound.	Inspect skin surfaces next to wound and around drain sites.	Skin surrounding wound will be clean and intact without maceration or inflammation.
Wound healing will be promoted. Infection will be prevented.	Observe condition of wound and character of drainage.	Incision line will be clean and approximated, without drainage and tenderness.
		Client wil be afebrile.
		Inflammation will diminish progressively.
Client will be comfortable.	Observe nonverbal responses as client moves or places stress on wound. Ask client if discomfort is experienced at wound site.	Client will deny discomfort around wound site.

1. Fill the bag with water, secure the cap, invert to check for leaks, and pour out the water.
2. Fill the bag two-thirds full with crushed ice so that the bag can mold easily over a body part.
3. Release any air from the bag by squeezing its sides before securing the cap because excess air interferes with conduction of cold.
4. Wipe off excess moisture.
5. Cover the bag with a flannel cover, towel, or pillow case.
6. Apply the bag to the injury site for 30 minutes; the bag can be reapplied in an hour.

Evaluation

The nurse evaluates wound healing on an ongoing basis (see evaluation box). This occurs during dressing changes, when therapies are administered, and as a client attempts to perform self-care in the presence of a wound. The nurse instructs clients and family members about how to evaluate wound healing after discharge from a health care setting. For example, clients should be warned to notify a physician if signs of infection develop.

The nurse evaluates each intervention designed to promote wound healing and compares the status of the wound with the assessment data. Together the nurse and the client review any teaching plans de-

signed to enable the client and family to care for the wound. The nursing care and teaching plans are modified based on evaluation data. Last, the nurse investigates the client's and family's need for additional support services (for example, home health care, physical therapy, and counseling) and initiates the referral process.

 SUMMARY

The nurse delivers various forms of therapy to clients with surgical or traumatic wounds. The type of wound determines the types of dressing used, their methods of application, the manner of caring for drains and sutures, and observations to make for monitoring wound repair. Clients most at risk for impaired wound healing require close observation and may benefit from the use of bandages and binders to support and protect wounds or the use of heat and cold therapies.

Principles the nurse follows to promote wound healing include use of aseptic technique, protection of the wound from further injury, and promotion of the stages of healing. These principles are also used in the application of hot and cold therapies. In addition, the nurse uses knowledge of the effects of heat and cold to recognize wounds that will benefit from heat or cold applications.

Key Concepts

- In normal wound healing the epidermal skin layer resurfaces wounds, and the dermis restores the structural integrity and physical properties of the skin.

- A clean surgical incision with little tissue loss heals by primary intention.

- Healing by primary intention proceeds through four stages: inflammation, destruction, proliferation, and maturation.

- When there is extensive tissue loss, a wound heals by secondary intention.

- Hemorrhaging often occurs during the destructive stage of wound healing.

- The chances of wound infection are greater when the wound contains dead or necrotic tissue, when foreign bodies lie on or near the wound, and when blood supply and tissue defenses are reduced.

- Any factor that lowers a client's immune response impairs wound healing.

- Physical stress from vomiting, coughing, or sudden muscular contraction can cause separation of wound edges.

- Wound assessment requires a description of the appearance of the wound, palpation of the area, and information regarding character of drainage, drains and wound closures, and pain.

- Wound drains remove secretions within tissue layers to promote wound closure.

- The nurse never collects a wound culture from old drainage.

- Principles of wound first aid include control of bleeding, cleansing, and protection.

- The layers of a dry dressing protect the wound edges, absorb drainage, and prevent entrance of bacteria.

- The wet-to-dry dressing mechanically removes dead tissue and wound exudate to debride the wound.

- When cleaning wounds or drain sites, the nurse cleans from the least to most contaminated area, away from wound edges.

- The type of suture securing a wound influences the method of suture removal.

- A bandage or binder should be applied in a manner that does not impair circulation or irritate the skin.

- The safe use of heat or cold therapy requires an assessment of the client's sensory function, identification of risk factors, and understanding of the physiological effects of heat and cold.

- An acute sprain, fracture, or bruise responds best to cold applications.

- Warm applications are effective for improving circulation to wound sites and promoting muscle relaxation.

- The choice of moist or dry applications depends on the type of wound, location of body part, and presence of drainage or inflammation.

Key Terms

Critical Thinking Exercises

1. On the second day after surgery, you observe an increased amount of dark-red drainage in the client's Jackson-Pratt device. What type of action is required?

2. When changing your client's dressing, you note that the Penrose drain is no longer in place. What do you do?

3. While changing your client's dressing, you note a foul odor and observe serous yellow drainage from the suture line. What physician's order would you anticipate?

4. When removing a wet-to-dry dressing, you note that the underlying gauze is wet with saline. The skin surrounding the wound is macerated. What conclusions can you make about the previous dressing? What would you do to avoid recurrence of this type of wet-to-dry application?

REFERENCES

Atwater EE: Care of the surgically created granulating wound, *Dermatol Nurs* 1:43, 1989.

Cooper DM: Optimizing wound healing: a practice within nursing domain, *Nurs Clin North Am* 25:165, 1990.

Cooper DM: Wound assessment and evaluation of healing. In Bryant RA: *Acute and chronic wounds: nursing management*, St Louis, 1992a, Mosby–Year Book.

Cooper DM: Acute surgical wounds. In Bryant RA: , *Acute and chronic wounds: nursing management*, St Louis, 1992b, Mosby–Year Book.

Garner JS: Guidelines for prevention of surgical wound infections, Atlanta, 1985, Centers for Disease Control.

Kim MJ, McFarland GK, McLane AM: *Pocket guide to nursing diagnosis*, ed 4, St Louis, 1991, Mosby–Year Book.

Westaby S: *Wound care*, St Louis, 1986, Mosby–Year Book.

ADDITIONAL READINGS

AACN: Clinical issues in critical care nursing, 1:553-601, 1990.

Alsbjorn BF, Oversen H, Walther-Larsen B: Occlusive dressing versus petroleum gauze on drainage wounds, *Acta Chir Scand* 156:211, 1990.

Bale S, Harding KG: Using modern dressings to effect debridement, *Prof Nurs* 5:244, 1990.

Bauer MS, Aiken S: The healing of open wounds, *Semin Vet Med Surg* 4:268, 1989.

Carrieri VK, Lindsey AM, West CM, editors: *Pathophysiological phenomena in nursing: human responses to illness*, Philadelphia, 1986, Saunders.

Cuzzell JZ: The new RYB color code: next time you assess an open wound, remember to protect red, cleanse yellow, and debride black, *Am J Nurs* 88:1342, 1988.

Cuzzell JZ, Stotts NA: Wound care: trial and error yields to knowledge, *Am J Nurs* 90:53, 1990.

Dimick AR: Delayed wound closure: indications and techniques, *Ann Emerg* 17:1303, 1988.

Esclamado RM, Damiano GA, Cummings CW: Effect of local hypothermia on early wound repair, *Arch Otolaryngol—Head Neck Surg* 116:803, 1990.

Fay MF: Drainage systems: their role in wound healing, *CONA-J* 10:12, 1988.

Fowler E, Cuzzell JZ, Papen JC: Healing with thin-film dressing, *Am J Nurs* 91:36, 1991.

Fylling CP: Comprehensive wound management with topical growth factors, *Ostomy/Wound Manage* 22:62, 1989.

Gallo JA, Todd BA: Mediastinitis after cardiac surgery, *Crit Care Nurs* 10:64, 1990.

Hess CT, Miller P: The management of open wounds: acute and chronic, *Ostomy/Wound Manage* 31:58, 1990.

Hill PD: Effects of heat and cold on the perineum after episiotomy/laceration, *JOGNN* 18:124, 1989.

Hotter AN: Wound healing and immunocompromise, *Nurs Clin North Am* 25:193, 1990.

Hudson-Goodman P, Girard N, Jones MB: Wound repair and the potential use of growth factors, *Heart Lung* 19:379, 1990.

Hunt TK: Basic principles of wound healing, *J Trauma* 30:S122, 1990.

Hutchinson JJ, McGuckin M: Occlusive dressing: a microbiologic and clinical review, *Am J Infect Control* 18:257, 1990.

Jones PL, Millman A: Wound healing and the aged patient, *Nurs Clin North Am*, 25:263, 1990.

Kloth LC, McCulloch JM, Feedar JA, editors: *Wound healing: alternatives in management*, Philadelphia, 1990, Davis.

Lange MP et al: Management of multiple enterocutaneous fistulas, *Heart Lung* 18:386, 1989.

LaVan FB, Hunt TK: Oxygen and wound healing, *Clin Plast Surg* 17:463, 1990.

Lee KA, Stotts NA: Support of the growth hormone-somatomedin system to facilitate healing, *Heart Lung* 19:157, 1990.

Mash N: Protocols for wound management: standards of care as a systematic approach, *Ostomy/Wound Manage* 22:23, 1989.

Meehan PA, Mayz EJ: Nursing management of an open abdominal wound, *Crit Care Nurs* 8:29, 1988.

Messer MS: Wound care, *Crit Care Nurs Q* 11:17, 1989.

Nightengale K: Making sense of . . . wound closure, *Nurs Times* 86:35, 1990.

Norris SD, Provo B, Stotts NA: Physiology of wound healing and risk factors that impede the healing process, *AACN Clin Iss Crit Care Nurs* 1:545, 1990.

North A: The effect of sleep on wound healing, *Ostomy/Wound Manage* 27:56, 1990.

Pinchcofsky DG: Why won't this wound heal? *Ostomy/Wound Manage* 27:56, 1990.

Reese JL: Nursing interventions for wound healing in plastic and reconstructive surgery, *Nurs Clin North Am* 25:223.

Robson MC: Disturbances of wound healing, *Ann Emerg Med* 17:1274, 1988.

Rosenberg CS: Wound healing in the patient with diabetes mellitus, *Nurs Clin North Am* 25:247, 1990.

Ross MC: Healing under pressure, *Amer J Nurs*, 86:1118, 1988.

Schmidt JM, Schimpeler SM: Obstetric and gynecologic abdominal wound infections: a comprehensive nurse-managed program, *J Perinat Neonat Nurs* 4:25, 1990.

Shira L: Seeking an optimum dressing: a nursing intervention implemented and evaluated, *Ostomy/Wound Manage* 15:72, 1987.

Smith TM: Management of difficult or chronic wounds, *Top Emerg Med* 11:45, 1989.

Swaim SF: The effects of dressing and bandages on wound healing, *Sem Vet Med Surg* 4:274, 1989.

Thomas AC, Wysocki AB: The healing wound: a comparison of three clinically useful methods of measurement, *Decubitus* 3:18, 1990.

Turner V: Standardization of wound care, *Nurs Stand* 5:25, 1991.

Wallace DM et al: Use of directional flow irrigation (ingress-egress tubes) for complex wound care management, *Ostomy/Wound Manage* 22:34, 1989.

Whitney JD: Physiologic effects of tissue oxygenation on wound healing, *Heart Lung* 18:466, 1989.

Wroblewski JR: Ointments, creams, gels: working with topical skin care preparation, *Ostomy/Wound Manage* 15:46, 1987.

Young ME: Malnutrition and wound healing, *Heart Lung* 17:60, 1988.

Zitelli J: Wound healing for the clinician, *Adv Derm* 2:243, 1987.

APPENDIX

Normal Reference Laboratory Values

Blood, Plasma, or Serum Values

Determination	Reference Range	
	Conventional	SI
Acetoacetate plus acetone	0.3-2.0 mg/100 ml	3-20 mg/L
Aldolase	1.3-8.2 mU/ml	12-75 nmol $\cdot$ s^{-1}/L
Alpha amino nitrogen	3.0-5.5 mg/100 ml	2.1-3.9 mmol/L
Ammonia	80-110 µg/100 ml	47-65 µmol/L
Ascorbic acid	0.4-1.5 mg/100 ml	23-85 µmol/L
Barbiturate	0; coma level: phenobarbital, approximately 10 mg/100 ml; most other drugs, 1-3 mg/100 ml	0 µmol/L
Bilirubin (van den Bergh test)	1 minute: 0.4 mg/100 ml	Up to 7 µmol/L
	Direct: 0.4 mg/100 ml	Up to 17 µmol/L
	Total: 1.0 mg/100 ml	
	Indirect is total minus direct	
Blood volume	8.5%-9.0% of body weight in kg	80-85 ml/kg
Bromide	0; toxic level: 17 mEq/L	0 mmol/L
Bromsulfalein (BSP)	Less than 5% retention 45 min after 5 mg/kg IV	<0.051
Calcium	8.5-10.5 mg/100 ml (slightly higher in children)	2.1-2.6 mmol/L
Carbon dioxide content	24-30 mEq/L; 20-26 mEq/L in infants (as HCO$_3^-$)	24-30 mmol/L
Carbon monoxide	Symptoms with over 20% saturation	0(1)
Carotenoids	0.8-4.0 µg/ml	1.5-7.4 µmol/L
Ceruloplasmin	27-37 mg/100 ml	1.8-2.5 µmol/L
Chloride	100-106 mEq/L	100-106 mmol/L
Cholinesterase (pseudocholinesterase)	0.5 pH U or more/hr; 0.7 pH U or more/hr for packed cells	0.5 or more arb. unit
Copper	Total: 100-200 µg/100 ml	16-31 µmol/L
Creatine phosphokinase (CPK)	Female 5-35 mU/ml	0.08-0.58 µmol $\cdot$ s^{-1}/L
	Male 5-55 mU/ml	
Creatinine	0.6-1.5 mg/100 ml	60-130 µmol/L
Ethanol	0.3%-0.4%, marked intoxication; 0.4%-0.5%, alcoholic stupor; 0.5% or over, alcoholic coma	65-87 mmol/L
		87-109 mmol/L
		>109 mmol/L

Modified from Kaye DA, Rose LF: *Fundamentals of internal medicine*, St Louis, 1983, Mosby Year Book. Adapted by from *New Engl J Med* 302:37, 1980.

Abbreviations used: *SI*, Système international d'Unités (The SI for the Health Professions. World Health Organization, Office of Publications, Geneva, Switzerland, 1977); *d*, 24 hours; *P*, plasma; *S*, serum; *B*, blood; *U*, urine; *L*, liter; *hr*, hour; and *sec*, second.

Continued.

Determination	Reference Range Conventional	SI
Glucose	Fasting: 70-110 mg/100 ml	3.9-5.6 mmol/L
Iron	50-150 μg/100 ml (higher in males)	9.0-26.9 μmol/L
Iron-binding capacity	250-410 μg/100 ml	44.8-73.4 μmol/L
Lactic acid	0.6-1.8 mEq/l	0.6-1.8 mmol/L
Lactic dehydrogenase	60-120 U/ml	1.00-2.00 μmol •$^{-1}$/L
Lead	50 μg/100 ml or less	Up to 2.4 μmol/L
Lipase	2 U/ml or less	Up to 2 arb. unit
Lipids		
Cholesterol	120-220 mg/100 ml	3.10-5.69 mmol/L
Cholesterol esters	60-75% of cholesterol	
Phospholipids	9-16 mg/100 ml as lipid phosphorus	2.9-5.2 mmol/L
Total fatty acids	190-420 mg/100 ml	1.9-4.2 g/L
Total lipids	450-1000 mg/100 ml	4.5-10.0 g/L
Triglycerides	40-150 mg/100 ml	0.4-1.5 g/l
Lithium	Toxic level 2 mEq/L	2 mmol/L
Magnesium	1.5-2.0 mEq/L	0.8-1.3 mmol/L
5'Nucleotidase	0.3-3.2 Bodansky U	30-290 nmol • s^{-1}/L
Osmolality	285-295 mOsm/kg water	285-295 mmol/kg
Oxygen saturation (arterial)	96%-100%	0.96-1.00 L
Pco_2	35-43 mm Hg	4.7-6.0 kPa
pH	7.35-7.45	Same
Po_2	75-100 mm Hg (dependent on age) while breathing room air; above 500 mm Hg while on 100% O_2 10.0-13.3 kPa	
Phenylalanine	0-2 mg/100 ml	0-120 μmol/L
Phenytoin (Dilantin)	Therapeutic level: 5-20 μg/ml	19.8-79.5 μmol/L
Phosphorus (inorganic)	3.0-4.5 mg/100 ml (infants in 1st yr up to 6.0 mg/100 ml)	1.0-1.5 mmol/L
Potassium	3.5-5.0 mEq/L	3.5-5.0 mmol/L
Primidone (Mysoline)	Therapeutic level: 4-12 μg/ml	18-55 μmol/L
Protein: Total	6.0-8.4 g/100 ml	60-84 g/L
Albumin	3.5-5.0 g/100 ml	35-50 g/L
Globulin	2.3-3.5 g/100 ml	23-35 g/L
Electrophoresis	% of total protein	Of total protein
Albumin	52-68	0.52-0.68
Globulin:		
$Alpha_1$	4.2-7.2	0.042-0.072
$Alpha_2$	6.8-12	0.068-0.12
Beta	9.3-15	0.093-0.15
Gamma	13-23	0.13-0.23
Pyruvic acid	0-0.11 mEq/L	0-0.11 mmol/L
Quinidine	Therapeutic: 1.5-3 μg/ml	4.6-9.2 μmol/L
	Toxic: 5-6 μg/ml	15.4-18.5 μmol/L
Salicylate:	0	
Therapeutic	20-25 mg/100 ml; 25-30 mg/100 ml to age 10 yr 3 hr postdose	1.4-1.8 mmol/L 1.8-2.2 mmol/L
Toxic	Over 30 mg/100 ml	>2.2 mmol/L
	Over 20 mg/100 ml after age 60	>1.4 mmol/L
Sodium	135-145 mEq/l	135-145 mmol/L
Sulfate	0.5-1.5 mg/100 ml	0.05-1.2 mmol/L
Sulfonamide	0 mg/100 ml; therapeutic: 5-15 mg/100 ml	0 mmol/L
Transaminase (SGOT) (aspartate amino-transferase)	10-40 U/ml	0.08-0.32 μmol · s^{-1}/L
Urea nitrogen (BUN)	8-25 mg/100 ml	2.9-8.9 mmol/L
Uric acid	3.0-7.0 mg/100 ml	0.18-0.42 mmol/L
Vitamin A	0.15-0.6 μg/ml	0.5-2.1 μmol/L
Vitamin A tolerance test	Rise to twice fasting level in 3 to 5 hr	

Urine Values

Determination	Reference Range Conventional	Reference Range SI
Acetone plus acetoacetate (quantitative)	0	0 mg/L
Alpha amino nitrogen	64-199 mg/d; not over 1.5% of total nitrogen	4.6-14.2 mmol/d
Amylase	24-76 U/ml	24-76 arb. unit
Calcium	150 mg/d or less	3.8 ≤ mmol/d
Catecholamines	Epinephrine: under 20 μg/d	<55 nmol/d
	Norepinephrine: under 100 μg/d	<590 nmol/d
Copper	0-100 μg/d	0-1.6 μmol/d
Coproporphyrin	50-250 μg/d	80-380 nmol/d
	Children under 80 lb 0-75 μg/d	0-115 nmol/d
Creatine	Under 100 mg/d or less than 6% of creatinine. In pregnancy: up to 12%. In children under 1 yr: may equal creatinine. In older children: up to 30% of creatinine	<0.75 mmol/d
Cystine or cysteine	0	0
Follicle-stimulating hormone:		
Follicular phase	5-20 IU/d	Same
Midcycle	15-60 IU/d	
Luteal phase	5-15 IU/d	
Menopausal	50-100 IU/d	
Men	5-25 IU/d	
Hemoglobin and myoglobin	0	
5-Hydroxyindole acetic acid	2-9 mg/d (women lower than men)	10-45 μmol/d
Lead	0.08 μg/ml or 120 μg or less/d	≤0.39 μmol/L
Phenolsulfonphthalein (PSP)	At least 25% excreted by 15 min; 40% by 30 min; 60% by 120 min	0.25 l
Phosphorus (inorganic)	Varies with intake; average 1 g/d	32 mmol/d
Porphobilinogen	0	0
Protein:		
Quantitative	<150 mg/d	<0.15 g/d

Steroids

17-Ketosteroids (per day)

Age	Male (mg)	Female (mg)	Male (μmol/d)	Female (μmol/d)
10	1-4	1-4	3-14	3-14
20	6-21	4-16	21-73	14-56
30	8-26	4-14	28-90	14-49
50	5-18	3-9	17-62	10-31
70	2-10	1-7	7-35	3-24

Determination	Reference Range Conventional	Reference Range SI
17-Hydroxysteroids	3-8 mg/d (women lower than men)	8-22 μmol/d as hydrocortisone
Sugar		
Quantitative glucose	0	0 mmol/L
Identification of reducing substances		
Fructose	0	0 mmol/L
Pentose	0	0 mmol/L
Titratable acidity	24-40 mEq/d	20-40 mmol/d
Urobilinogen	Up to 1.0 Ehrlich U	To 1.0 arb. unit
Uroporphyrin	0	0 nmol/d
Vanillylmandelic acid (VMA)	Up to 9 mg/d	Up to 45 μmol/d

Special Endocrine Tests

Determination	Reference Range	
	Conventional	SI
STEROID HORMONES		
Aldosterone	Excretion: 5-19 μg/d	14-53 nmol/d
Fasting, at rest, 210 mEq sodium diet	Supine: 48 ± 29 pg/ml Upright: (2 hr) 65 ± 23 pg/ml	180 ± 64 pmol/L
Fasting, at rest, 110 mEq sodium diet	Supine: 107 ± 45 pg/ml Upright: (2 hr) 239 ± 123 pg/ml	279 ± 125 pmol/L 663 ± 341 pmol/L
Fasting at rest, 10 mEq sodium diet	Supine: 175 ± 75 pg/ml Upright: (2 hr) 532 ± 228 pg/ml	485 ± 208 pmol/L 1476 ± 632 pmol/L
Cortisol		
Fasting	8 AM: 5-25 μg/100 ml	0.14-0.69 μmol/L
At rest	8 PM: Below 10 μg/100 ml	0-0.28 μmol/L
20 U ACTH	4 hr ACTH test: 30-45 μg/100 ml	0.83-1.24 μmol/L
Dexamethasone at midnight	Overnight suppression test: Below 5 μg/100 ml Excretion: 20-70 μg/d	<0.14 nmol/L 55-193 nmol/d
11-Deoxycortisol	Responsive: over 7.5 μg/100 ml (after metyrapone)	>0.22 μmol/L
Testosterone	Adult male: 300-1100 ng/100 ml Adolescent male: over 100 ng/100 ml Female: 25-90 ng/100 ml	10.4-38.1 nmol/L >3.5 nmol/L 0.87-3.12 nmol/L
Unbound testosterone	Adult male: 3.06-24.0 ng/100 ml Adult female: 0.09-1.28 ng/100 ml	106-832 pmol/L 3.1-44.4 pmol/L
POLYPEPTIDE HORMONES		
Adrenocorticotropin (ACTH)	15-70 pg/ml	3.3-15.4 pmol/L
Calcitonin	Undetectable in normals >100 pg/ml in medullary carcinoma	0 >29.3 pmol/L
Growth hormone		
Fasting, at rest	Below 5 ng/ml	<233 pmol/L
After exercise	Child: Over 10 ng/ml Male: Below 5 ng/ml Female: Up to 30 ng/ml	>465 pmol/L <233 pmol/L 0-1395 pmol/L
After glucose	Male: Below 5 ng/ml Female: Below 10 ng/ml	<233 pmol/L 0-465 pmol/L
Insulin		
Fasting	6-26 μU/ml	43-187 pmol/L
During hypoglycemia	Below 20 μU/ml	<144 pmol/L
After glucose	Up to 150 μU/ml	0-1078 pmol/L
Leuteinizing hormone	Male: 6-18 mU/ml	6-18 u/L
Pre- or postovulatory	Female: 5-22 mU/ml	5-22 u/L
Midcycle peak	30-250 mU/ml	30-250 u/L
Parathyroid hormone	<10 μl equiv/ml	<10 mEq/L
Prolactin	2-15 ng/ml	0.08-6.0 nmol/L
Renin activity		
Normal diet	Supine: 1.1 ± 0.8 ng/ml/hr Upright: 1.9 ± 1.7 ng/ml/hr	0.9 ± 0.6 (nmol/L)hr 1.5 ± 1.3 (nmol/L)hr
Low-sodium diet	Supine: 2.7 ± 1.8 ng/ml/hr Upright: 6.6 ± 2.5 ng/ml/hr	2.1 ± 1.4 (nmol/L)hr 5.1 ± 1.9 (nmol/L)hr
Low-sodium diet	Diuretics: 10.0 ± 3.7 ng/ml/hr	7.7 ± 2.9 (nmol/L)hr

Special Endocrine Tests—cont'd

Determination	Reference Range	
	Conventional	SI
THYROID HORMONES		
Thyroid-stimulating hormone (TSH)	0.5-3.5 μU/ml	0.5-3.5 mU/L
Thyroxine-binding globulin capacity	15-25 μg T_4/100 ml	193-322 nmol/L
Total triiodothyronine by radioimmunoassay (T_3)	70-190 ng/100 ml	1.08-2.92 nmol/L
Total thyroxine by RIA (T_4)	4-12 μg/100 ml	52-154 nmol/L
T_3 resin uptake	25%-35%	0.25-0.35
Free thyroxine index (FT_4I)	1-4 ng/100 ml	12.8-51.2 pmol/L

Hematologic Values

Determination	Reference Range	
	Conventional	SI
Coagulation factors		
Factor I (fibrinogen)	0.15-0.35 g/100 ml	4.0-10.0 μmol/L
Factor II (prothrombin)	60%-140%	0.60-1.40
Factor V (accelerator globulin)	60%-140%	0.60-1.40
Factor VII-X (proconvertin-Stuart)	70%-130%	0.70-1.30
Factor X (Stuart factor)	70%-130%	0.70-1.30
Factor VIII (antihemophilic globulin)	50%-200%	0.50-2.0
Factor IX (plasma thromboplastic cofactor)	60%-140%	0.60-1.40
Factor XI (plasma thromboplastic-antecedent)	60%-140%	0.60-1.40
Factor XII (Hageman factor)	60%-140%	0.60-1.40
Coagulation screening tests		
Bleeding time (Simplate)	3-9 min	180-540 sec
Prothrombin time	Less than 2-sec deviation from control	Less than 2-sec deviation from control
Partial thromboplastin time (activated)	25-37 sec	25-37 sec
Whole-blood clot lysis	No clot lysis in 24 hr	0/d
Fibrinolytic studies		
Euglobin lysis	No lysis in 2 hr	0 (in 2 hr)
Fibrinogen split products	Negative reaction at greater than 1:4 dilution	0 (at > 1:4 dilution)
Thrombin time	Control ± 5 sec	Control ± 5 sec
Complete blood count		
Hematocrit	Male: 45%-52%	Male: 0.42-0.52
	Female: 37%-48%	Female: 0.37-0.48
Hemoglobin	Male: 13-18 g/100 ml	Male 8.1-11.2 mmol/L
	Female: 12-16 g/100 ml	Female: 7.4-9.9 mmol/L

Continued.

Hematologic Values—cont'd

Determination	Reference Range	
	Conventional	SI
Leukocyte count	4300-10,800/mm^3	4.3-10.8 × 10^9/L
Erythrocyte count	4.2-5.9 10^6/mm^3	4.2-5.9 × 10^{12}/L
Mean corpuscular volume (MCV)	80-94 μm^3	80-94 fl
Mean corpuscular hemoglobin (MCH)	27-32 pg	1.7-2.0 fmol
Mean corpuscular hemoglobin concentration (MCHC)	32%-36%	19-22.8 mmol/L
Erythrocyte sedimentation rate (Westergren method)	Male: 1-13 mm/hr Female: 1-20 mm/hr	Male: 1-13 mm/hr Female: 1-20 mm/hr
Erythrocyte enzymes		
Glucose-6-phosphate dehydrogenase	5-15 U/gHb	5-15 U/g
Pyruvate kinase	13-17 U/gHb	13-17 U/g
Ferritin (serum)		
Iron deficiency	0-20 ng/ml	0-20 μg/L
Iron excess	Greater than 400 ng/L	>400 μg/L
Folic acid		
Normal	Greater than 1.9 ng/ml	>4.3 mmol/L
Borderline	1.0-1.9 ng/ml	2.3-4.3 mmol/L
Haptoglobin	100-300 mg/100 ml	1.0-3.0 g/L
Hemoglobin studies		
Electrophoresis for A$_2$ hemoglobin	1.5%-3.5%	0.015-0.035
Hemoglobin F (fetal hemoglobin)	Less than 2%	<0.02
Hemoglobin, met- and sulf-	0	0
Serum hemoglobin	2-3 mg/100 ml	1.2-1.9 μmol/L
Thermolabile hemoglobin	0	0
LE (lupus erythematosus) preparation		
Heparin as anticoagulant	0	0
Defibrinated blood	0	0
Leukocyte alkaline phosphatase		
Quantitative method	15-40 mg of phosphorus liberated/hr 10^{10} cells	15-40 mg/hr
Qualitative method	Males: 33-188 U	33-188 U
	Females (off contraceptive pill): 30-160 U	30-160 U
Muramidase	Serum, 3-7 μg/ml	3-7 mg/L
	Urine, 0-2 μg/ml	0-2 mg/L
Osmotic fragility of erythrocytes	Increased if hemolysis occurs in over 0.5% NaCl; decreased if hemolysis is incomplete in 0.3% of NaCl	
Peroxide hemolysis	Less than 10%	<0.10
Platelet count	150,000-350,000/mm^3	150-350 × 10^9/L
Clot retraction	50%-100%/2 hr	0.50-1.00/2 hr
Platelet aggregation	Full response to ADP, epinephrine, and collagen	1.0
Platelet factor 3	33-57 sec	33-57 sec
Reticulocyte count	0.5%-1.5% red cells	0.005-0.015
Vitamin B$_{12}$	90-280 pg/ml (borderline: 70-90)	66-207 pmol/L (borderline: 52-66)

Cerebrospinal Fluid Values

Determination	Reference Range		Determination	Reference Range	
	Conventional	SI		Conventional	SI
Bilirubin	0	0 μmol/L	Glucose	50-75 mg/100 ml	2.8-4.2 mmol/L
Chloride	120-130 mEq/L (20 mEq/L higher than serum)			(30-50% less than blood)	
Albumin	Mean: 29.5 mg/100 ml	0.295 g/L	Pressure (initial)	70-180 mm of water	70-80 arb. units
	±2 SD: 11-48 mg/100 ml	±2 SD: 0.11-0.48	Protein		
			Lumbar	15-45 mg/100 ml	0.15-0.45 g/L
IgG	Mean: 4.3 mg/100 ml	0.043 g/L	Cisternal	15-25 mg/100 ml	0.15-0.25 g/L
	±2 SD: 0-8.6 mg/100 ml	± 2 SD: 0-0.086	Ventricular	5-15 mg/100 ml	0.05-0.15 g/L

Miscellaneous Values

Determination	Reference Range	
	Conventional	SI
Autoantibodies in serum		
Thyroid colloid and microsomal antigens	Absent	
Stomach parietal cells	Absent	
Smooth muscle	Absent	
Kidney mitochondria	Absent	
Rabbit renal collecting ducts	Absent	
Cytoplasm of ova, theca cells, testicular interstitial cells	Absent	
Skeletal muscle	Absent	
Adrenal gland	Absent	
Carcinoembryonic antigen (CEA) in blood	0-2.5 ng/ml, 97% healthy non-smokers	0-2.5 μg/L, 97% healthy nonsmokers
Cryoprecipitable proteins in blood	0	0 arb. unit
Digitoxin in serum	17 ± 6 ng/ml	22 ± 7.8 nmol/L
Digoxin in serum		
0.25 mg/d	1.2 ± 0.4 ng/ml	1.54 ± 0.5 nmol/L
0.5 mg/d	1.5 ± 0.4 ng/ml	1.92 ± 0.5 nmol/L
Duodenal drainage:		
pH	5.5-7.5	5.5-7.5
Amylase	Over 1200 U/total sample	>1.2 arb. unit
Trypsin	Values from 35%-160% "normal"	0.35-1.60
Viscosity	3 min or less	180 sec or less
Gastric analysis	Basal	0.6 ± 0.5
	Females 2.0 ± 1.8 mEq/hr	0.8 ± 0.6 μmol/sec
	Males 3.0 ± 2.0 mEq/hr	
	Maximal (after histalog or gastrin)	4.4 ± 1.4 μmol/sec
	Females 16 ± 5 mEq/hr	6.4 ± 1.4 μmol/sec
	Males 23 ± 5 mEq/hr	
Gastrin-1 in blood	0-200 pg/ml	0-95 pmol/L

Continued.

Miscellaneous Values—cont'd

Determination	Reference Range Conventional	SI
Immunological tests		
Alpha-feto-globulin	Abnormal if present	
Alpha 1-antitrypsin	200-400 mg/100 ml	2.0-4.0 g/L
Antinuclear antibodies	Positive if detected with serum diluted 1:10	
Anti-DNA antibodies	Less than 15 units/ml	
Complement, total hemolytic	150-250 U/ml	
C3	Range 55-120 mg/100 ml	0.55-1.2 g/L
C4	Range 20-50 mg/100 ml	0.2-0.5 g/L
Immunoglobulins in blood:		
IgG	1140 mg/100 ml	11.4 g/L
	Range 540-1663	5.5-16.6 g/L
IgA	214 mg/100 ml	2.14 g/L
	Range 66-344	0.66-3.44 g/L
IgM	168 mg/100 ml	1.68 g/L
	Range 39-290	0.39-2.9 g/L
Viscosity	1.4-1.8 expressed as relative viscosity of serum compared to water	
Iontophoresis	Children: 0-40 mEq sodium/L	0-40 mmol/L
	Adults: 0-60 mEq sodium/L	0-60 mmol/L
Propranolol (includes bioactive 4-OH metabolite) in serum 4 hr after last dose	100-300 ng/ml	386-1158 nmol/L
Stool fat	Less than 5 g in 24 hr or less than 4% of measured fat intake in 3-day period	<5 g/day
Stool nitrogen	Less than 2 g/day or 10% of urinary nitrogen	<2 g/day
Synovial fluid		
Glucose	Not less than 20 mg/100 ml lower than simultaneously drawn blood sugar	See blood glucose mmol/L
Mucin	Type 1 or 2	1-2 arb. unit
	Grades as:	
	Type 1-tight clump	
	Type 2-soft clump	
	Type 3-soft clump that breaks up	
	Type 4-cloudy, no clump	
D-Xylose absorption	5-8 g/5 hr in urine	33-53 mmol
	40 mg/100 ml in blood 2 hr after ingestion of 25 g of D-Xylose	2.7 mmol/L

Glossary

abdominal-diaphragmatic breathing Respiration in which the abdomen moves out while the diaphragm descends on inspiration.

ablate (ablation) An amputation, an excision of any body part, or removal of a growth or harmful substance.

abortion Spontaneous or induced termination of pregnancy before the fetus has developed enough to be expected to live if born.

absorption The passage of substances across and into tissues (for example, intestinal and parenteral absorption).

abstract thought Final stage in the development of the cognitive thought processes that occurs between the ages of 12 and 15 years; it is characterized by adaptability, flexibility, the use of abstractions and generalizations, and logical problem solving based on observations.

abuse Indiscriminate chronic or acute use of a drug or other substance such that physiological or psychosocial functioning is impaired.

accessory muscles Muscles in the anterior thorax that increase or decrease chest expansion (e.g., sternocleidomastoid, trapezius).

accommodation Process of responding to the environment through new activity and thinking.

accommodation reflex Adjustment of the eyes for near vision, composed of pupillary constriction, convergence of the visual axes, and increased convexity of the lens.

accountability State of being answerable for one's actions—the professional nurse answers to the self, the client, the profession, the employing institution, and society for the effectiveness of nursing care performed.

accrediting (accreditation) A process whereby a professional association or nongovernmental body grants recognition to a school or institution for demonstrated ability in a special area of practice or training, as the accreditation of hospitals by the Joint Commission of Accreditation for Hospitals or of nursing schools by the National League for Nursing.

Achilles tendon Thickest and strongest tendon in the body, beginning near the middle of the posterior part of the calf and ending at the calcaneus.

acidemia Increased concentration of hydrogen ions in the blood, causing a reduced pH of less than 7.3%.

acne Inflammatory, papulopustular skin eruption, usually occurring on the face, neck, shoulders, and upper back.

acromegaly Chronic metabolic condition caused by overproduction of growth hormone and characterized by gradual, marked enlargement and elongation of bones of the face, jaw, and extremities.

active strategies of health promotion Activities that depend on the client being motivated to adopt a specific health program.

active transport Movement of materials across the cell membrane by means of chemical activity that allows the cell to admit larger molecules than would otherwise be possible.

activities of daily living Activities usually performed in the course of a normal day in the client's life, such as eating, dressing, bathing, brushing the teeth, and grooming.

activity tolerance Kind and amount of exercise or work that a person is able to perform.

actual health care problem Health problem currently being perceived or experienced by the client.

acuity Intensity of nursing care required to meet the needs of a client; higher acuity usually requires longer and more frequent visits and more supplies and equipment.

acute illness Illness characterized by symptoms that are of relatively short duration, are usually severe, and affect the functioning of the client in all dimensions.

adaptation Process by which changes occur in any of a person's dimensions in response to stress.

addiction Compulsive, uncontrollable, physical and psychological dependence on a substance or habit, for example, a narcotic, to the point that withdrawal causes severe emotional, mental, and physiological reactions.

ADH Hormone affecting fluid and electrolyte balance; decreases the production of urine by increasing reabsorption of water by the kidney tubules.

adherence Process in which a client follows the prescriptions and recommendations of a regimen of care.

advance directives A written agreement established between a client and physician to withhold heroic measures or life-sustaining treatment if the patient's condition becomes irreversible. Advance directives are usually written at a time when clients are healthy or able to make conscious decisions regarding their welfare.

adverse reaction Harmful or unintended effect of a medication, diagnostic test, or therapeutic intervention.

advocacy Process whereby a nurse objectively provides clients with the information they need to make decisions and supports clients in whatever decisions they make.

aerobic *1.* Of or pertaining to the presence of air or oxygen. 2. Requiring oxygen for the maintenance of life.

aerobic metabolism Production of energy and body fuels by the tissues in the presence of oxygen.

afebrile Without fever.

affective learning   Acquisition of behaviors involved in expressing feelings in attitudes, appreciations, and values.

afferent   Proceeding to a center, as with nerves, arteries, and veins (e.g., afferent nerves lead to the spinal cord).

ageism   Attitude that disadvantages, separates, and stigmatizes older adults on the basis of age-related characteristics.

agent   Element of the agent-host-environment model of health and illness; any biological, chemical, physical or mechanical, or psychosocial factor whose presence or absence can lead to disease or illness.

air pollution   Contamination of the environmental atmosphere with substances known as pollutants that are not normally found in the air.

Alcoholics Anonymous   International, nonprofit organization of recovering alcoholics whose purpose is to help alcoholics stop drinking and maintain sobriety through group support, shared experiences, and a faith in a power greater than themselves.

aldosterone   Minerocorticoid, produced by the adrenal cortex, that regulates sodium and potassium balance.

algor mortis   Reduction in body temperature after death accompanied by loss of skin elasticity.

alkalemia   Decreased concentration of hydrogen ions in the blood, causing an elevated pH greater than 7.44.

alopecia   Partial or complete loss of hair; baldness.

alveolar hyperventilation   Respiratory rate in excess of that required to maintain normal carbon dioxide levels in the body tissues.

alveolar hypoventilation   Respiratory rate insufficient to prevent carbon dioxide retention.

Alzheimer's disease   A brain disorder that causes gradual and progressive decline in cognitive functioning. The most frequent cause of irreversible dementia; also known as senile dementia of the Alzheimer type, or SDAT.

ambiguous genitalia   Newborn genitalia that are not clearly identifiable as female or male; external genitalia may appear male in an infant with female internal sex organs or vice versa.

ambulatory surgery   Scheduled outpatient procedures provided for clients who do not remain overnight in a hospital.

American Nurses' Association (ANA)   Organization of professional nurses in the United States that focuses on standards of health care, nurses' professional development, and economic and general welfare of nurses.

ampule   Small, sterile, glass or plastic container that usually contains a single dose of solution to be administered parenterally.

amylase   Enzyme secreted in saliva and pancreatic juice to digest starch.

anabolism   Constructive metabolism characterized by conversion of simple substances into more complex compounds of living matter.

anaerobic   The absence of oxygen.

anaerobic metabolism   Production of energy and body fuels by the tissues without oxygen.

analgesic   Relieving pain; a drug that relieves pain.

analogy   Resemblance made between things otherwise unlike.

anemia   Disorder characterized by a decrease in hemoglobin in the blood.

anesthesia   Absence of normal sensation, especially sensitivity to pain.

aneurysm   Localized dilatation of the wall of a blood vessel, usually caused by atherosclerosis, hypertension, or a congenital weakness in the vessel wall.

angina   Episodic chest pain caused most often by myocardial anoxia, resulting from atherosclerosis of the coronary arteries. Pain radiates down inner aspect of left arm and is often accompanied by feeling of suffocation and impending death.

animism   The attribution of life to inanimate objects (Piagetian term).

anions   Negatively charged electrolytes.

anlingus   Sexual stimulation by licking the anus. Anal-oral sexual activity.

anonymity   Nondisclosure of a client's or other person's name or identification, such as is used in research to ensure the privacy of research subjects.

anorexia   Lack or loss of appetite resulting in the inability to eat.

anoxia   Condition characterized by a relative or total lack of oxygen; may be local or systemic.

antagonistic muscles   Group of muscles that works together to bring about movement at the joint.

antibody   Immunoglobulin, essential to the immune system, which is produced by lymphoid tissue in response to bacteria, viruses, or other antigens.

anticipatory grief   Grief response in which the person begins the grieving process before an actual loss.

anticipatory guidance   Psychological and physical preparation of a client to help relieve fear and anxiety of an event or outcome that is expected to be stressful.

antidiuretic hormone (ADH)   Hormone that decreases the production of urine by increasing reabsorption of water by the kidney tubules.

antiemetic   Medication that prevents or alleviates nausea and vomiting.

antigen   Substance, usually a protein, that causes the formation of an antibody and reacts specifically with that antibody.

antigravity muscles   Muscles involved with stabilization of joints by opposing the effect of gravity on the body.

antipyretic   Of or pertaining to a substance or procedure that reduces fever.

antiseptic   Tending to inhibit the growth and reproduction of microorganisms.

anuria   Cessation of urine production.

anxiety   Feeling of apprehension, uneasiness, agitation, uncertainty, and fear resulting from the anticipation of something perceived as negative.

Apgar scale   Assessment tool that rates the newborn's physiological status 1 to 5 minutes after birth. Includes assessment of respiratory effort, heart rate, muscle tone, reflex irritability, and color.

Apgar score   Rating describing a newborn's physiological status at birth and thereafter. Assists in determining the newborn's ability to adjust to extrauterine life.

aphasia   Neurological disorder influencing the production and understanding of language.

apical pulse   The heartbeat taken with the bell or diaphragm of a stethoscope placed on the apex, or pointed extremity of the heart.

apical-radial pulse deficit Comparison of apical and radial pulses measured at the same time. If a deficit exists, the radial pulse is usually slower, indicating ineffective heart contractions.

apnea Cessation of airflow through the nose and mouth.

apocrine gland One of the large, deep exocrine glands located in the axillary, anal, genital, and mammary areas of the body; secretes sweat having a strong odor.

apothecary system A system of graduated liquid volumes based on the minim and on a system of graduated amounts arranged in order of heaviness and based on the grain.

approximate To come close together, as in the edges of a wound.

arcus senilis An opaque ring, gray to white in color, that surrounds the periphery of the cornea. Caused by deposits of fat granules in the cornea.

ariboflavinosis Condition caused by dietary deficiency of vitamin B_2.

arterial blood gases Oxygen (PO_2) and carbon dioxide (Pco_2) concentrations, hydrogen ion concentration (pH), and oxygen saturation (O_2 sat) of the hemoglobin in arterial blood; also refers to the laboratory tests that measure these levels.

artificialism The belief that all things in the universe have been created by man (Piagetian term).

ascites Abnormal accumulation of fluid in the intraperitoneal space.

asepsis Absence of germs or microorganisms.

assault Unlawful threatening or inflicting of harm on another.

assertiveness (training) A technique focusing on the direct, honest statement of feelings and beliefs, both positive and negative, helping individuals become more self-assertive and self-confident.

assimilation To become absorbed into another culture and to adopt its characteristics.

asymptomatic Without symptoms.

atelectasis Collapse of alveoli, preventing the normal respiratory exchange of oxygen and carbon dioxide.

atherosclerosis Common arterial disorder characterized by yellowish plaques of cholesterol, lipids, and cellular debris in the inner layers of the walls of the large- and medium-sized arteries.

atrophy Wasting or diminution of size or physiological activity of a part of the body caused by disease or other influences.

attachment The deep emotional tie between parents and child that is reciprocal and becomes progressively stronger during the first year.

attitudinal isolation Social isolation that occurs because of the older adult's personal or cultural values.

attribute (physical, cognitive, or psychosocial) An inherent characteristic or a quality of an individual.

audit Methodical examination or review of written records with the intent to verify or deny the accuracy of information based on established standards.

auditory Related to, or experienced through, hearing.

auscultation Act of listening for sounds within the body to evaluate the condition of body organs; usually performed with a stethoscope.

authoritarian style Leadership style in which the leader retains all authority and responsibility and is concerned primarily with tasks and goal achievement.

autonomy Ability or tendency to function independently.

autopsy Examination performed after a person's death to confirm or determine the cause of death.

autotransfusion The collection, anticoagulation, filtration, and reinfusion of blood from an active bleeding site.

bactericidal Destructive to bacteria.

bacteriuria Presence of bacteria in the urine.

basal metabolism rate (BMR) Amount of energy used in a unit of time by a fasting, resting subject to maintain vital functions.

basic human needs Needs for things, such as food, water, safety, and love, that people require to maintain vital functions.

battery Legal term for touching of another's body without consent.

bed rest Placement of the client in bed for therapeutic reasons for a prescribed period.

behavioral isolation Social isolation that occurs because of the older adult's socially unacceptable behaviors.

beneficence The doing or active promotion of doing good. One of the four principles of the ethical theory of deontology.

bereavement Response to loss through death; a subjective experience that a person suffers after losing a person with whom there has been a significant relationship.

beriberi Disease of the peripheral nerves caused by a deficiency of or an inability to assimilate thiamine.

bias Prejudice or mental inclination to collect or interpret data according to a person's opinions or beliefs.

bilirubin Orange-yellow pigment of bile formed principally by the breakdown of hemoglobin in red blood cells.

binder Bandage made of a large piece of material to fit a specific body part.

binocular vision Vision involving the use of both eyes.

bioethics Study of the ethical problems in health care delivery and the obligations of health professionals.

biological clock Cyclical nature of body functions; functions controlled from within the body as synchronized with environmental factors; same meaning as biorhythm.

biological identity (sex) Chromosomal masculinity or femininity (XY or XX).

biopsy Removal of a small piece of living tissue from an organ or other part of the body for microscopic examination.

bisexual Sexual orientation involving erotic preferences for members of either sex.

blastocyst Embryonic form that arises as a cavity within the morula, where cellular differentiation begins.

blended family Family formed when parents bring together unrelated children from previous marriages.

blood pressure (BP) The pressure exerted by the circulating volume of blood on the walls of the arteries, veins, and chambers of the heart. The pressure in the aorta and the large arteries of a healthy young adult is approximately 120 mm Hg during systole and 70 mm Hg during diastole.

body image Mental picture of one's body internally and externally.

body mechanics Coordinated efforts of the musculoskeletal and nervous systems to maintain proper balance, posture, and body alignment.

body substance isolation (BSI) Isolation system that uses generic infection precautions all clients, emphasizing the potential infectiousness of all moist body substances.

bolus Round mass of chewed food ready to be swallowed.

bonding The parent's emotional tie to their child that usually develops soon after birth as a result of their interaction.

bone resorption Destruction of bone cells and release of calcium into the blood.

borborygmus Audible abdominal sound produced by hyperactive intestinal peristalsis.

bradycardia Slower than normal heart rate; heart contracts fewer than 60 times per minute.

bradypnea An abnormally slow rate of breathing. Also called oligopnea.

brain death Irreversible, complete loss of brain function while the heart continues to beat.

bronchoscopy Visual examination of the tracheal and bronchial tree using a flexible fiberoptic bronchoscope.

bruit Abnormal sound or murmur heard while auscultating an organ, gland, or artery.

buccal Of or pertaining to the inside of the cheek or the gum next to the cheek.

buffer Substance or group of substances that can absorb or release hydrogen ions to correct an acid-base imbalance.

cachexia General ill health and malnutrition marked by weakness and emaciation.

calorie Amount of heat required to raise 1 gram of water 1° centigrade at atmospheric pressure; a kilocalorie or large calorie, used to represent energy values of food, is 1000 times as large as the small calorie, the unit used in physics to describe energy exchange in the body.

Canadian Nurses Association (CNA) Organization of professional nurses in Canada that focuses on standards of health care, nurses' professional development, and economic and general welfare of nurses.

cannulation Insertion of a flexible tube (cannula) into a body duct or cavity, such as the bladder or a blood vessel.

carbon dioxide (CO$_2$) Respiratory gas formed in the body as an end product of tissue metabolism.

carbon monoxide (CO) Colorless, odorless, poisonous gas produced by the combustion of carbon or organic fuels.

carbon monoxide poisoning Toxic condition in which carbon monoxide gas has been inhaled and absorbed in the lungs, displacing oxygen from hemoglobin and decreasing the capacity of the blood to carry oxygen.

carcinoma Malignant epithelial neoplasm that tends to invade surrounding tissue and spread to distant regions of the body.

cardiac arrest Sudden cessation of cardiac output and effective circulation.

cardiac output The volume of blood expelled by the ventricles of the heart, equal to the amount of blood ejected at each beat (the stroke output), multiplied by the number of beats in the period of time used in the computation.

cardiac telemetry Transmission of a client's ECG signals by way of a small, battery-powered unit connected to the client. Signals travel to a receiving location near a nurses' station where the ECG is displayed on a monitor.

cardiopulmonary rehabilitation Process of actively assisting the cardiopulmonary client to achieve and maintain an optimal level of health through controlled physical exercise, nutritional counseling, relaxation and stress management techniques, prescribed medication, oxygen therapy, and adherence to the rehabilitation program.

cardiopulmonary resuscitation (CPR) Basic emergency procedures for life support consisting of artificial respiration and manual external cardiac massage.

caring The sense of dedication to another person.

carrier Animal or person who harbors and spreads a disease-causing organism but who does not become ill.

cartilage Nonvascular, supporting connective tissue located mainly in the joints and in the thorax, trachea, larynx, nose, and ear.

cartilaginous joint Slightly movable, highly elastic cartilage that unites bony surfaces.

case management Organized system for delivering health care to an individual client or group of clients; includes assessment and development of a plan of care, coordination of all services, referral, and follow-up; usually assigned to one professional.

catabolism Complex metabolic process in which energy is liberated for use in work, energy, storage, or heat production by oxidation of carbohydrates, lipids, and proteins; carbon dioxide and water, as well as energy, are produced.

catalyst Substance that influences the rate of a chemical reaction without being permanently altered by the process.

catalytic Pertaining to a chemical reaction caused by an agent unchanged by the reaction.

cataplexy Condition characterized by sudden muscular weakness and loss of muscle tone.

cataract Abnormal opacity of the lens of the eye causing interference with light reaching the retina.

cathartic Drug that acts to promote bowel evacuation.

cations Positively charged electrolytes.

Centers for Disease Control (CDC) Agency of the U.S. government that provides facilities and services for the investigation, identification, prevention, and control of disease.

centigrade Denotes a temperature scale in which 0° is the freezing point of water and 100° is the boiling point of water at sea level; also called Celsius.

central line An intravenous line inserted through the skin and into a vein entering the vena cava. Central lines are used to infuse substances that are irritating to smaller peripheral veins.

central nervous system sympathomimetic A pharmacological agent that mimics the effects of stimulations of organs and structures by the sympathetic nervous system by occupying adrenergic receptor sites and acting as an agonist or by increasing the release of the neurotransmitter norepinephrine at postganglionic nerve endings.

central sleep apnea Sleep disorder characterized by the absence of attempts to breathe; the person is momentarily unable to move respiratory muscles or maintain airflow through the nose and mouth.

cerebellum Portion of the brain located in the posterior cranial fossa behind the brainstem.

certified nurse-midwife (CNM) Nurse who is educated in midwifery and possesses certification in accordance with criteria of the American College of Midwives.

cerumen Waxy substance secreted in the ear.

change Dynamic process by which alterations occur within the behavior and function of a person, family, group, or community.

change agent A person or group who identifies need, initiates strategies, and implements alterations.

change process (*See* change.)

channel A passageway or groove that conveys fluid, as the central channels that connect the arterioles with the venules.

chart *n.,* Informal term for the client's record; *v.,* to enter data into a client's record.

charting by exception A charting methodology in which data is entered only when there is an exception from what is normal or expected. Reduces time spent documenting.

chemical dependency Continued use of mood-altering chemicals despite the emotional, physical, social, and legal problems created.

chemicals Substances that alter senses, emotions, physical condition, or mood when ingested by mouth, injected, or inhaled; includes both legal and illegal drugs: alcohol, narcotics, tranquilizers, barbiturates, amphetamines, cocaine, marijuana, and others.

chemotherapy Medication used for the treatment of cancer. The actions and side effects of these drugs can lead to serious physical problems. The knowledge required to safely administer these medications is quite specialized. Nurses may be required to have special training and certification before giving these drugs.

chest percussion Striking the chest wall with a cupped hand to promote mobilization and drainage of pulmonary secretions.

chest physiotherapy Group of therapies used to mobilize pulmonary secretions.

cholecystectomy Surgical removal of the gallbladder.

chordotomy Surgical resection of the anterolateral nerve tracts in the spinal cord for pain relief.

chromosomes Strands of DNA from the ovum and sperm that carry genes and thus determine genetic inheritance.

chronic illness Illness that persists over a long period of time and affects physical, emotional, intellectual, social, and spiritual functioning.

chyme Viscous, semifluid contents of the stomach present during digestion of a meal, which eventually pass into the intestines.

circadian rhythm Repetition of certain physiological phenomena within a 24-hour cycle.

cirrhosis Chronic degenerative disease of the liver.

citation Reference notation to the source of an idea or quotation.

civil law The law established by a nation or state for its own jurisdiction.

client-centered goal Specific measurable objective designed to reflect the client's highest level of wellness and independence in function.

climacteric Physiological, developmental change that occurs in the male reproductive system between the ages of 45 and 60.

clinical nurse specialist (CNS) Nurse with a master's degree in nursing and expertise in a specific area of practice.

clinical reasoning Cognitive skills by which the nurse gathers relevant data about the client, analyzes the client's response to the health care problem, organizes the data, and formulates the nursing diagnosis.

CNS sympathomimetic Drug, such as cocaine and amphetamines, whose effects mimic the effects of sympathetic nervous system stimulation.

coccidioidomycosis Infectious fungal disease caused by the inhalation of windborne spores of the bacterium *Coccidiodes immits,* also called valley fever.

code of ethics Formal statement that delineates a profession's guidelines for ethical behavior; a code of ethics sets standards or expectations for the professional to achieve.

coercive change Alterations in behavior or lifestyle that are forced on the person, family, or group.

cognitive learning Acquisition of intellectual skills that encompass behaviors such as thinking, understanding, and evaluating.

coitus interruptus Withdrawal of the penis from the vagina during intercourse before ejaculation. While ineffective, it is often practiced by adolescents as a method of contraception.

colic Sharp visceral pain resulting from obstruction or smooth muscle spasm of a hollow organ, such as the ureter or the intestines.

colitis Inflammatory condition of the large intestine.

collagen Substance that combines to form the white, glistening, inelastic fibers of tendons, ligaments, and fasciae.

colon Portion of the large intestine from the cecum to the rectum.

colonized Referring to the establishment of a mass of microorganisms, often nonpathogenic, in or on the body.

communal family Form of family composed of unrelated adults rearing their children together in a communal living arrangement.

communicable disease Any disease that can be transmitted from one person or animal to another by direct or indirect contact, or by vectors.

communication Ongoing, dynamic series of events that involves the transmission of information or feelings from sender to receiver.

comorbidity An accompanying illness or disease that coexists with an already established medical diagnosis.

comparison group Group of subjects in a study who are equivalent to the subjects in the experimental group but do not receive the treatment or intervention the study is examining; also known as a control group.

compensation *1.* Action by the body's chemical, biological, or physiological buffering system to correct an acid-base imbalance. *2.* An adaptive ego-defense mechanism in which a person avoids feelings of inferiority or inadequacy in one area through achievement in another area.

compliance Person's fulfillment of the prescribed course of treatment.

compress Soft pad of gauze or cloth used to apply heat, cold, or medications to the surface of a body part.

computer-assisted instruction (CAI) Self-instructed teaching method utilizing computers.

concentration (concentrate) A substance, particularly a liquid, that has been strengthened and reduced in volume though evaporation or other means.

concept Abstract idea summarized in a word or phrase.

concomitant symptoms Symptoms that accompany a primary symptom.

concrete thought Stage in the development of cognitive thought processes that occurs at ages 7 to 11 years; it is characterized by increasingly logical and coherent thought, the ability to classify, sort, order, and organize facts, and an inability to generalize or think in abstractions.

concurrent nursing audit Evaluation of nursing care while the client is receiving the care.

conductive hearing loss A form of hearing loss in which sound is inadequately conducted through the external or middle ear to the sensorineural apparatus of the inner ear.

confabulation Defense mechanism in which the person fabricates experiences or situations and often recounts them in a detailed and plausible way in order to fill in and cover up gaps in memory.

confidentiality Privacy; a nurse must maintain the confidentiality of information related to a client's health care.

Congress for Nursing Practice Unit of the ANA whose activities concern the scope of nursing practice, legal aspects of nursing practice, public recognition of the significance of nursing in health care, and implications of health care trends for nursing practice.

connotative Tending to suggest meaning by a word apart from the thing it explicitly describes.

consensual light reflex Constriction of the pupil of one eye when the other eye is illuminated.

constipation Condition characterized by difficulty in passing stool or an infrequent passage of hard stool.

consultation Process in which the help of a specialist is sought to identify ways to handle problems in client management or in the planning and implementation of programs.

contagious Communicable, as a disease.

continuing education Formal educational programs designed to further the knowledge, skills, and professional attitudes of practicing nurses.

contraception Prevention of pregnancy by means of a medication, device, or method that blocks or alters one or more of the processes of reproduction in such a way that sexual union can occur without impregnation.

contrast medium Radiopaque substance injected into the body to improve visualization of internal structures that are otherwise difficult to see on x-ray examination.

control To regulate or limit error or distortion of information.

controlled substance A drug whose distribution is controlled by federal and/or state government regulation. An example is narcotics.

contusion An injury that does not break the skin, characterized by swelling, discoloration, and pain.

convalescence Period of recovery after an illness, injury, or surgery.

coping mechanism Any effort directed toward stress management, including task-oriented and ego-defense mechanisms.

corpus luteum Ovarian site of ruptured graafian follicle after ovulation. The corpus luteum is maintained through the secretory phase of the menstrual cycle and produces progesterone.

costal Of or referring to the ribs.

cough Sudden, audible expulsion of air from the lungs.

counseling Implementation method that helps the client use a problem-solving process to recognize and manage stress and that facilitates interpersonal relationships between the client and the family, significant others, or the health care team.

crackle Fine bubbling sound heard on auscultation of the lung; produced by air entering distal airways and alveoli containing serous secretions.

cretinism Condition characterized by severe congenital hypothyroidism.

crime Act that violates a law and that may include criminal intent.

criminal law The law of crimes and their punishment.

crisis Stressful encounter with a change or obstacle to life goals that is perceived as insurmountable.

crisis intervention Use of therapeutic techniques directed toward helping a client resolve a particular and immediate problem.

crisis intervention centers Agencies providing emergency psychiatric and counseling assistance to clients experiencing extreme stress or conflict, often involving attempted suicide, drug or alcohol abuse, or other crisis behaviors.

critical pathway Tool used in managed care. A critical pathway incorporates the treatment interventions of care givers from all disciplines who normally care for a client. Designed for a specific case type, a pathway is used to manage the care of a client throughout a projected length of stay.

critical period The time when development of a specific attribute (physical, cognitive, or psychosocial) is most vulnerable to both advantageous and harmful agents.

critical period of development Time span during which the environment has its greatest impact on an individual's development.

Crohn's disease Disease involving inflammation of the small intestine.

cross tolerance Adaptation to substance in one group (narcotics, central nervous system depressants, or stimulants) results in adaptation to all other substances in that group.

crutch gait Gait assumed by a person on crutches by alternately bearing weight on one or both legs and on the crutches.

culture Nonphysical traits such as values, beliefs, attitudes, and customs shared by a group and passed from one generation to the next.

culture shock Disorder that occurs in response to transition from one setting to another; former behavior patterns are ineffective in such an unfamiliar situation, and basic cues for social behavior are absent.

cunnilingus Oral stimulation of the female external genitalia; oral-genital sex.

curing Traditionally, a two-dimensional phenomena that results in ridding disease from the body or mind.

cutaneous stimulation Stimulation of a person's skin to prevent or reduce pain perception. A massage, warm bath, application of liniment, hot and cold therapies, and transcutaneous electric nerve stimulation are some ways to reduce pain perception.

cyanosis Bluish discoloration of the skin and mucous membranes caused by deoxygenated hemoglobin in the blood or a structural defect in hemoglobin.

cystitis Inflammation of the urinary bladder, characterized by pain, urgency, and frequency of urination.

cytotoxic Pharmacological compound that inhibits the proliferation of cells within the body.

data clustering Grouping of related information from the nursing health history, physical examination, and laboratory results as part of the process of determining the nursing diagnosis.

data source Origin of information relevant to the client's level of wellness and health patterns.

data validation Process of determining if information gathered during assessment is complete and accurate.

day-care centers Agencies that provide health care during the day to children or adults with special needs.

debridement Removal of dead tissue from a wound.

decibel Unit of measure of the intensity of sound.

defamation of character To harm the reputation of a person by libel or slander.

defecation Passage of feces from the digestive tract through the rectum.

defining characteristic Cluster of signs and symptoms that are observed in the client having a specific nursing diagnosis.

dehiscence Separation of a wound's edges, revealing underlying tissues.

dehydration Excessive loss of water from the body tissues, accompanied by a disturbance of body electrolytes.

delirium Syndrome involving impairment of memory and other cognitive abilities and characterized by clouding of consciousness.

delusion Presistent belief or perception held by a person even though it is illogical and probably wrong.

dementia Irreversible mental state characterized by decreased impairment of memory, intellectual function, and other cognitive abilities that can have a variety of causes.

democratic style People-centered leadership style in which the group participates openly in decision making for group goals.

denial Defense mechanism by which a person avoids emotional conflicts and anxiety by refusing to acknowledge thoughts, feelings, desires, impulses, and other factors that would cause intolerable pain.

denotative Denoting or tending to denote.

dependent intervention Action completed with a physician's order but requiring nursing judgment or decision making.

depersonalization Extreme form of identity confusion in which a person is unable to distinguish between inner and outer realities or between the self and others.

depilatory Substance that removes hair.

depression Abnormal emotional state characterized by exaggerated or inappropriate feelings of sadness, melancholy, dejection, worthlessness, emptiness, and hopelessness.

dermatitis Inflammation of skin characterized by itching, redness, and skin lesions.

dermis Layer of skin just below the epidermis, containing blood and lymphatic vessels, nerves and nerve endings, glands, and hair follicles.

desquamation Normal process in which the dead cells of the epidermal skin layer slough off.

development Qualitative or observable aspects of the progressive changes an individual makes in adapting to the environment.

developmental change Biopsychosocial alterations that occur normally within the life cycle of the person or family.

diagnosis Identification of a health problem by analyzing the assessment data about a client's health status.

diagnostic process Process of determining a client's health status and evaluating the factors influencing that status.

diagnostic related groups (DRGs) Group of patients classified for measuring a hospital's delivery of care; classification is based on the following variables: primary and secondary diagnosis, primary and secondary procedures, age, and length of stay.

dialysis A medical procedure for the removal of certain elements from the blood or lymph.

diaphoresis Secretion of sweat, especially profuse secretion associated with an elevated body temperature, physical exertion, or emotional stress.

diarrhea Increase in the number of stools and the passage of liquid, unformed feces.

diastolic pressure The minimum level of blood pressure measured between contractions of the heart.

diffusion Movement of molecules from an area of higher concentration to an area of lower concentration.

direct-question interview Type of inquiry that requires one- or two-word answers.

discharge planning Set of decisions and activities involved in providing continuity and coordination of nursing care when a client is discharged from a health care agency.

disinfection The process of killing pathogenic organisms.

diuresis Increased formation and excretion of urine.

diurnal Daily.

diverticula Pouchlike herniations through the muscular wall of a tubular organ; may be present in the stomach, small intestine, or most commonly the colon.

documentation Act of authenticating events or activities by keeping written records.

domains of learning Areas in which learning occurs: cognitive, affective, and psychomotor.

dorsal Pertaining to the back or posterior.

drainage tube Hollow tube used for evacuation of air or fluid from a cavity or wound in the body.

driving forces for change Motivating or facilitating factors in the change process.

drug allergy Hypersensitivity to a pharmacological agent, manifested by reactions ranging from a mild rash to anaphylactic shock.

drug dependence   Psychological or physiological reliance on a chemical agent.

drug interaction   A modification of the effect of a drug when administered with food or another drug. The effect may increase or decrease the action of the drug or other substance.

drug rehabilitation centers   Agencies providing long-term care for a gradual return to the community of a person with chemical or drug dependency.

durable medical equipment (DME)   Equipment leased or sold to clients for use in their homes, for example, wheelchairs, hospital beds, walkers, canes, and so on.

dysarthria   Difficulty in articulating speech.

dysfunctional grief   Actual or perceived object loss; objects may include people, possessions, a job, status, home, and parts of the body.

dyspareunia   Painful intercourse in a woman.

dysphagia   Difficulty in swallowing.

dyspnea   A shortness of breath or difficulty in breathing that may be caused by certain heart or lung conditions or strenuous exercise.

dysrhythmia   Deviation from the normal pattern of the heart beat.

dysuria   Painful urination resulting from bacterial infection of the bladder and obstructive conditions of the urethra.

ear oximeter   Continuous measurement of capillary oxygen saturation through the use of a cutaneous monitoring system attached to a client's ear lobe.

ecchymosis   Discoloration of skin or bruise caused by leakage of blood into subcutaneous tissues as a result of trauma to underlying vessels.

edema   Abnormal accumulation of fluid in interstitial spaces of tissues.

efferent   Direct away from a center, as with nerves, arteries, and veins.

ego-defense mechanism   Unconscious behavior that protects a person from an emotional stress.

electrolyte   Element or compound that, when melted or dissolved in water or other solvent, dissociates into ions and can carry an electrical current.

emaciation   Excessive leanness caused by disease or malnutrition.

embolus   Small amount of air, fat, or other substance that circulates in the blood until becoming lodged in a blood vessel.

embryo   Stage of human development from implantation of the fertilized ovum to the eighth week of intrauterine life.

emphysematous   Of or pertaining to emphysema, an abnormal condition of the lungs, characterized by overinflation and destructive changes of alveolar walls.

empirical data   Information that has been collected through the human senses and can be verified through research.

endocrine   Pertaining to one of the ductless glands in the endocrine system.

endogenous   Produced within a cell or organism.

endorphin   Naturally occurring neuropeptide with morphine like properties secreted within the CNS to inhibit pain-impulse transmission.

endoscopy   Visualization of the interior of body organs and cavities with an endoscope.

enema   Procedure involving introduction of a solution into the rectum for cleansing or therapeutic purposes.

enteral nutrition   Provision of nutrients through the gastrointestinal tract when the client cannot ingest, chew, or swallow food but can digest and absorb nutrients.

enterostomal therapist   Specially trained nurse for care of patients with ostomies.

enucleation   Removal of the eyeball; a procedure used in corneal tissue recovery.

enuresis   Involuntary passage of urine; incontinence.

enzyme   Protein produced by living cells that catalyzes chemical reactions in organic matter.

epidemiology   Study of the occurrence, distribution, and causes of disease.

epidermis   Superficial, avascular layers of the skin, made up of an outer, dead, cornified portion of cells and a deeper, living cellular portion.

epidural   Type of nerve block local anesthesia, in which an anesthetic is injected in the lumbosacral region of the spinal cord to prevent or eliminate pain in the lower trunk and extremities.

epitheliazation   Refers to the stage of wound-healing that is characterized by growth of epithelial tissue.

erectile dysfunction   Inability of a male to attain or maintain an erection sufficient to achieve penetration during sexual contact; the dysfunction may be primary or secondary.

error of commission   Mistake resulting from overdiagnosis or diagnosing a nonexistent health problem.

error of omission   Mistake resulting from failure of the nurse to diagnose a health problem.

erythema   Redness or inflammation of the skin or mucous membranes that is a result of dilation and congestion of superficial capillaries; sunburn is an example.

erythrocyte   Red blood cell.

erythropoietin (EPO)   A glycoprotein hormone synthesized mainly in the kidneys and released into the bloodstream in response to anoxia.

escape mechanism   Behavioral response by which a person consciously or unconsciously attempts to avoid a problem or stressor.

estrogen   Hormonal steroid compound that promotes the development of female secondary sex characteristics.

ethics   Principles or standards that govern proper conduct as they apply to professional issues or problems.

ethnicity   Cultural group's sense of identification associated with the group's common social and cultural heritage.

ethnocentrism   Tendency of members of one cultural group to view the members of other cultural groups in terms of the standards of behavior, attitudes, and values of their own group.

etiological factor   Probable cause contributing to or maintaining the nursing diagnosis.

eupnea   Normal respiration that is quiet, effortless, and rhythmical.

euthanasia   Deliberately bringing about the death of a person who is suffering from an incurable disease or condition; actively, as by administering a lethal drug, or passively, as by allowing the person to die without medical treatment.

evaluation   Category of nursing behavior in which a determination is made and recorded regarding the extent to which the client's goals have been met.

evisceration   Protrusion of visceral organs through a surgical wound.

exacerbation   Increase in the seriousness of a disease or disorder as marked by greater intensity in signs or symptoms.

excise   To remove completely, as in the surgical excision of the appendix.

excoriation   Injury to the skin's surface caused by abrasion.

exercise   Performance of any physical activity for the purpose of conditioning the body, improving health, maintaining fitness, or as a therapeutic measure.

exogenous   Originating outside an organ or part.

exophthalmos   Abnormal protrusion of one or both eyeballs.

expected outcome   Expected condition of a client at the end of therapy or of a disease process, including the degree of wellness and the need for continuing care, medications, support, counseling, or education.

expectorate   Ejection of mucus, sputum, or fluids from the trachea and lungs by coughing or spitting.

experiment   Research study designed to examine a cause-and-effect relationship.

expressive aphasia   Inability to name common objects or to express simple ideas in words or writing.

extended care facility   Institution providing medical, nursing, or custodial care for clients over a prolonged period.

extended family   Form of family composed of the nuclear family and all other relatives in both of the couple's families.

external environment   Set of factors outside and distinct from a person that may influence health, including the physical environment, social relationships, economic variables, and so on.

external stressor   Stressor originating outside a person.

extracellular fluid   Portion of the body fluid composed of the interstitial fluid and blood plasma.

exudate   Fluid, cells, or other substances that have been slowly discharged from cells or blood vessels through small pores or breaks in cell membranes.

family   *1.* A group of people related by heredity, as parents, children, and siblings. 2. Group of interacting individuals composing a basic unit of society. Although concepts of what constitutes a family vary, the family usually has some degree of permanence, commitment, and attachment.

family as client   Nursing perspective in which the family is viewed as a unit of interacting members having attributes, functions, and goals separate from those of the individual family members; the nurse provides care to the family as a whole.

family as environment   Nursing perspective in which the family is viewed as the significant provider of physical, psychosocial, and emotional support to individual family members; the nurse provides care primarily to one of the family members.

family functions   Processes by which the family operates as a whole, including communication and manipulation of the environment for problem solving.

family health   Phenomenon that is more than the sum of the health of individual family members, including the achievement of satisfying family functioning and the attainment of family goals.

family of origin   Family into which a person is born, as distinct from the person's family of procreation.

family of procreation   Family a person forms through marriage and/or having children, as distinct from the person's family of origin.

family stress   Stress related to the individual's roles, relationships, or functions within the family.

family structure   Composition of the family organization of relationships among family members.

fatigue   State of exhaustion or loss of strength or endurance.

febrile   Pertaining to or characterized by an elevated body temperature.

feces   Waste or excrement from the gastrointestinal tract.

feedback   In communication theory, information produced by a receiver and perceived by a sender that informs the sender about the receiver's reaction to the message. Feedback is a cyclical part of the process of communication that regulates and modifies the content of messages.

fellatio   Sexual stimulation by licking, sucking, or placing the penis in the mouth; oral-genital sex.

felony   Crime of serious nature that carries a penalty of imprisonment or death.

female genitalia   Female's external sex organs (vulva, mons veneris, labia majora, labia minora, clitoris, and vaginal opening or introitus) and internal sex organs (vagina, uterus, fallopian tubes, and ovaries).

fetal alcohol syndrome   Fetal abnormalities associated with heavy alcohol consumption by the pregnant woman.

fetus   Stage of human development from the end of the embryonic period until birth.

fever   Elevation in the hypothalamic set-point so that body temperature is regulated at a higher level.

fibrin   Protein product formed from the action of thrombin on fibrinogen in the clotting process.

fibrous joint   Tough layer of fibrous connective tissue that binds bones firmly together.

fidelity   The quality or state of being faithful.

fistula   Abnormal passage from an internal organ to the body surface or between two internal organs.

flail chest   Condition caused by multiple rib fractures, resulting in instability in part of the chest wall and paradoxical breathing. The chest wall underlying the injured area contracts on inspiration and expands on expiration.

flat bones   Bones providing for structural contours of the skeleton.

flatulence   Condition characterized by the accumulation of gas within the lumen of the intestines.

"flight-or-fight" syndrome   Set of sympathetic physiological responses to a stressor that prepares a person to attempt to overcome or avoid stress.

fluid volume deficit   An alteration characterized by the loss of fluids and electrolytes in an isotonic fashion.

fluid volume excess   An alteration characterized by the abnormal retention of fluids and electrolytes in an isotonic fashion.

focus charting A charting methodology for structuring progress notes according to the focus of the note, for example, symptoms and nursing diagnosis. Each note includes data, actions, and client response.

follicular phase First part of the menstrual cycle, in which ovarian follicles grow to prepare for ovulation and the menstrual flow signifies that the uterus has shed its lining from the preceding cycle.

fomites Inanimate substances or objects, such as clothing and paper, that absorb and transmit infectious material.

Food and Drug Administration (FDA) Federal agency responsible for the enforcement of federal regulations regarding the manufacture and distribution of food, drugs, and cosmetics to ensure protection against the sale of impure or dangerous substances.

food poisoning Toxic processes resulting from the ingestion of a food contaminated by toxic substances or by bacteria containing toxins.

footboard Board placed perpendicular to the mattress, parallel to and touching the plantar surface of the client's foot, and used to maintain dorsiflexion of the feet.

forceps Pair of any of a large variety and number of surgical instruments, with two handles or sides each attached to a blade.

formulary Listing of drugs and information about them used by health practitioners to prescribe therapy.

fracture Breakage of bone caused by violence to the body; disruption of bone tissue continuity.

friction Effect of rubbing or the resistance that a moving body meets from the surface on which it moves; a force that occurs in a direction to oppose movement.

friction rub Dry, grating sound heard during auscultation, caused by rubbing of tissue surfaces.

frostbite Traumatic effect of extreme cold on the skin and subcutaneous tissues, first manifested by distinct pallor.

fungus Simple parasitic plant dependent on other life forms for food.

gait Manner or style of walking, including rhythm, cadence, and speed.

gangrene Necrosis or death of tissue, usually the result of loss of blood supply.

gastrocolic reflex Mass peristaltic activity in the colon in response to food entering the stomach.

gender identity Awareness of being male or female that develops from infancy.

gender role (sex role) Expression of one's maleness or femaleness to both oneself and others.

general adaptation syndrome (GAS) Generalized defense response of the body to stress, consisting of three stages: alarm, resistance, and exhaustion.

generalization Application of findings from a research study in a broader situation.

geographic isolation Social isolation of the older adult resulting from urban crime, institutional barriers, and distance from family.

geriatrics Branch of health care dealing with the physiology and psychology of aging and with the diagnosis and treatment of illnesses affecting the older adult.

gerontology Study of all aspects of the aging processes and their consequences.

gingiva Gum of the mouth; a mucous membrane with supporting fibrous tissue that overlies the crowns of unerupted teeth and encircles the necks of those that have erupted.

glaucoma Abnormal condition of elevated pressure within the anterior chamber of the eye caused by obstructed outflow of aqueous humor.

glomerulus Cluster or collection of capillary vessels within the kidney involved in the initial formation of urine.

gluconeogenesis Formation of glucose or glycogen from substances that are not carbohydrates, such as protein or lipid.

glycerol Alcohol that is a component of lipids and that is soluble in ethyl alcohol and water.

glycogen Polysaccharide that is the major carbohydrate stored in animal cells.

glycolysis Series of enzymatically catalyzed reactions within cells by which glucose and other sugars are broken down to yield lactic acid or pyruvic acid, releasing energy in the form of adenosine triphosphate.

glycosuria Abnormal presence of glucose in the urine.

gonadotropic hormones Substances that are produced and secreted by the anterior pituitary gland and stimulate the function of the testes and ovaries.

governmental agencies Clinics, hospitals, and health services that are supported by local, state or provincial, or national taxes.

graafian follicle Ovarian follicle that continues to mature through a given menstrual cycle and ruptures to release an ova at the time of ovulation.

granulation tissue Soft, pink, fleshy projections of tissue that form during the healing process in a wound not healing by primary intention.

gravity Heaviness of an object resulting from the universal effect of the attraction of a planetary body.

grief Form of sorrow involving the person's thoughts, feelings, and behaviors, occurring as a response to an actual or perceived loss.

grieving process Sequence of affective, cognitive, and physiological states through which the person responds to and finally accepts an irretrievable loss.

growth Quantitative or measurable aspect of an individual's increase in physical measurements.

guaiac test Test of feces for the presence of occult (hidden) blood.

gurgle Abnormal coarse sound heard during auscultation of the lung; produced by air entering large, mucus-containing airways.

gustatory Pertaining to the sense of taste.

half-life Time required for elimination processes to reduce the blood concentration of a drug by half.

halitosis Offensive breath resulting from poor oral hygiene, dental or oral infection, ingestion of certain foods, or systemic disease.

hallucinogens Drugs such as LSD or PCP that cause excitation of the central nervous system, including hallucinations, sensory distortions, and other effects.

hand rolls A roll of cloth that keeps the thumb slightly adducted and in opposition to the fingers.

hand-wrist splints Splints individually molded for the client to maintain proper alignment of the thumb, slight adduction of the wrist, and slight dorsiflexion.

haustral contraction Type of peristaltic contraction that occurs in the large intestine; produces a large sac in the colon's wall to increase surface area for nutrient absorption.

healing Traditionally, a holistic or three-dimensional phenomena that results in the restoration of balance or harmony to the body, mind, and spirit.

health Dynamic state in which an individual adapts to internal and external environments so that there is a state of physical, emotional, intellectual, social, and spiritual well-being.

health behavior Activities through which a person maintains, attains, or regains good health and prevents illness.

health belief model Conceptual framework that predicts a person's health behavior as an expression of personal health beliefs.

health care delivery system Total complex of preventive, remedial, and therapeutic services provided by hospitals and other institutions, governmental and voluntary agencies, health care professionals, pharmaceutical and medical equipment manufacturers, and governmental and private insurance agencies.

health care need Condition or problem that results when clients are unable to meet their physiological, psychological, sociocultural, developmental, and spiritual needs within the context of daily living.

health-illness continuum Scale by means of which a person's level of health can be described, ranging from high-level wellness to severe illness. The scale takes into account the presence of risk factors.

health maintenance organization (HMO) Group health care agency that provides basic and supplemental health maintenance and treatment services to voluntary enrollees who prepay a fixed periodic fee that is set without regard to the amount or kind of services received.

health promotion Activities directed toward maintaining or enhancing the health and well-being of clients.

heat exhaustion An abnormal condition characterized by weakness, vertigo, nausea, muscle cramps, and loss of consciousness, caused by depletion of body fluid and electrolytes resulting from exposure to intense heat or the inability to acclimatize to heat.

heat stroke A severe and sometimes fatal condition resulting from the failure of the temperature-regulating capacity of the body, caused by prolonged exposure to the sun or to high temperatures.

hematemesis Vomiting of blood indicating upper gastrointestinal bleeding.

hematocrit Measure of the packed cell volume of red cells, expressed as a percentage of the total blood volume.

hematoma Collection of blood trapped in the tissues of the skin or an organ.

hematuria Abnormal presence of blood in the urine.

hemodynamics Study of the circulation of the blood.

hemolysis Breakdown of red blood cells and release of hemoglobin as may result by administration of hypotonic intravenous solutions that cause progressive swelling and rupture of the erythrocytes.

hemoptysis Coughing of blood from the respiratory tract.

hemorrhage External or internal loss of a large amount of blood in a short period of time.

hemorrhoids Permanent dilation and engorgement of veins within the lining of the rectum.

hemosiderin Iron-rich pigment that is the product of red blood cell hemolysis.

hemosiderosis Abnormal deposition of iron in a variety of tissues.

hemostasis Termination of bleeding by mechanical or chemical means or by the coagulation process of the body.

hemothorax Accumulation of blood and fluid in the pleural cavity between the parietal and visceral pleurae.

heredity Primary natural force influencing an individual's genetic development.

heterosexual Sexual orientation involving erotic preference for members of the opposite sex.

hierarchy of basic human needs Categorization of human needs from the most basic to those at a higher level.

hirsutism Excessive body hair in a masculine distribution caused by heredity, hormonal dysfunction, or medication.

Holter monitor Portable ECG device, similar to the size of a miniature tape recorder; records a continuous ECG over 24 hours or longer.

home health agency Public or private organization that complies with all conditions for participation in government insurance programs. Services provided may include nursing, rehabilitation, social work, home health aides, and homemakers.

home health care Professional and paraprofessional services and equipment provided to clients and families in their place of residence for purposes of health promotion and maintenance, client and family education, illness prevention, diagnosis and treatment of disease, and palliation and rehabilitation.

home health care agencies Organizations providing skilled, intermittent health care services usually in the form of nursing, home care aides, or rehabilitative therapies.

homosexual Sexual orientation involving erotic preference for members of one's own sex.

hope Confident, yet uncertain, expectation of achieving a future goal.

hospice Philosophy of client care that advocates physical and psychosocial support for palliative care of persons in the last months of an incurable illness so that life can be lived as fully and comfortably as possible.

host Element of the agent-host-environment model of health and illness. A host is a person or group who, because of risk factors, may be susceptible to disease or illness.

human relations movement Leadership theory that emphasizes the role of interpersonal relationships and human needs for improving productivity in the workplace.

hydrostatic pressure Pressure exerted by a liquid.

hygiene Science of health.

hypercarbia Greater than normal amounts of carbon dioxide in the blood; also called hypercapnia.

hypercoagulability Increased tendency for blood to clot.

hypermetabolism Increased metabolism, producing above-normal body heat.

hyperpigmentation Unusual darkening of the skin.

hypertension Disorder characterized by an elevated blood pressure persistently exceeding 140/90 mm Hg.

hyperthermia Situation in which body temperature exceeds the set-point.

hypertonic The situation where one solution has a smaller concentration of solute than another solution; therefore the first solution exerts less osmotic pressure.

hypervolemia Increase in the amount of fluid in the circulating blood volume.

hypnotic Class of drug that causes insensibility to pain and induces sleep.

hypotension Abnormal lowering of blood pressure, which is inadequate for normal perfusion and oxygenation of tissues.

hypothermia Abnormal lowering of body temperature below 93° F or 35° C, usually caused by prolonged exposure to cold.

hypoventilation Reduction in the volume of air that enters the lung for gas exchange; oxygen exchange is insufficient to meet metabolic demands of the body.

hypovolemia Decreased circulatory blood volume resulting from extracellular fluid losses.

hypoxia Inadequate cellular oxygenation that may result from a deficiency in the delivery or use of oxygen at the cellular level.

iatrogenic disease Disease caused by a treatment or diagnostic procedure.

identification Internalizing beliefs, values, and behavior of another through imitation and introjection with a unique individual expression.

identity Component of self-concept; sense of continuity and sameness; one's persisting consciousness of being oneself, separate, unique, and distinct from others.

identity confusion Form of self-concept disturbance in which a person does not maintain a clear consciousness of a consistent and continuous self; sense of fragmentation or distortion.

illegal chemicals Mood-altering substances not available on the open market, including cocaine, marijuana, heroin, and prescription drugs sold without a prescription.

illiterate Having little education, especially in relation to the ability to read or write.

illness Abnormal process in which any aspect of a person's functioning is diminished or impaired as compared with the previous condition.

illness behavior Ways in which people monitor their bodies, define and interpret their symptoms, take remedial actions, and use the health care system.

illness prevention Health education programs or activities directed toward protecting clients from threats or potential threats to health and toward minimizing risk factors.

immobility Inability to move about freely, caused by any condition in which movement is impaired or therapeutically restricted.

immunocompromised Abnormal condition of the immune system in which cellular or humoral immunity is inadequate.

immunoglobulin Humoral antibody produced by the body and present in serum and external secretions; formed in response to specific antigens.

impairment A reduction in a person's physical and/or mental functioning as a result of chemical dependency.

implementation Category of nursing behavior in which the action necessary for achieving the projected outcomes of the health care plan are initiated and completed.

incentive spirometry Method of encouraging voluntary deep breathing by providing visual feedback to clients of the inspiratory volume they have achieved.

incident report Confidential document that describes any client accident while the person is on the premises of a health care agency.

independent intervention Nursing action that can solve the client's problems without consultation or collaboration with physicians or other nonnursing health professionals.

individual practice association Prospective payment plans requiring the client to pay a fixed annual payment; the plan pays the provider when the services are used.

induction of anesthesia All portions of the anesthetic process that occur before attaining the desired stage of anesthesia, including premedication, intubation, and administration of oxygen.

indurated Hardened tissue, particularly the skin, due to edema, inflammation, or infiltration by a tumor.

induration Hardening of a tissue, particularly the skin, because of edema or inflammation.

industry Diligence in the pursuit of a goal.

infancy Stage of life from 1 month to 1 year of age.

infertility Man's, woman's, or couple's involuntary inability to conceive.

infestation Presence of animal parasites on the skin or in the hair of a host (person or animal).

inflammation Protective responses of body tissues to irritation or injury.

informed consent Process of obtaining permission from a client to perform a specific test or procedure, after describing all risks, side effects, and benefits.

infradian rhythm Repetition of certain physiological phenomena within a cycle exceeding 24 hours.

infusion Introduction of a substance, such as a fluid, drug, electrolyte, or nutrient, directly into a vein by means of gravity flow.

inhalants Medications administered via the nasal passage.

inhibition Process of socialization in which one learns to refrain from a behavior even when motivated to engage in that behavior.

initiative Energy displayed in starting an action.

injection Act of introducing a liquid into the body by means of a syringe.

inpatient Client admitted for treatment within a hospital over the course of more than 1 day.

insensible water loss Loss of fluid from the body by evaporation, as normally occurs during respiration.

in-service education Instruction or training provided by an agency or institution to nurses practicing within the agency or institution.

insomnia Condition characterized by chronic inability to sleep or remain asleep through the night.

inspection Assessment process during which the nurse observes the client.

instillation Procedure in which a fluid is slowly introduced into a cavity or passage of the body (for example, rectum) and allowed to remain for a specific length of time before being withdrawn or drained.

integument Skin and its appendages: hair, nails, and sweat and sebaceous glands.

intercostal muscles Muscles inserted between the ribs, responsible for expansion and contraction of the rib cage during inspiration and expiration.

interdependent intervention Action with or without physician's order or written at a nurse's suggestion that can provide the solution to the client's problem in a collaborative manner with judgment and recommendations of the interdisciplinary health team.

interference Behavior(s) that deliberately delays or impedes the change process.

internal environment Set of factors inside people that may influence their health, including genetic factors, physiological processes, psychological variables, and intellectual and spiritual dimensions.

internal stressor Stress-causing stimulus that arises within a person.

International Council of Nurses (ICN) International organization for professional nurses; the ANA and CNA are members.

interpersonal communication Exchange of information between two persons or among persons in a small group.

interstitial fluid Fluid that fills the spaces between most of the cells of the body and provides a substantial portion of the liquid environment of the body.

interview Type of communication with a client initiated for a specific purpose and focused on a specific content area.

intonation Rise and fall in pitch of the voice in speech.

intraarterial Within an artery.

intraarticular Within a joint.

intracardiac Within the myocardium.

intracellular fluid Liquid within the cell membrane.

intractable pain Pain not easily relieved, as may occur with some types of cancer.

intradermal injection Form of injection in which the solution is introduced into the dermis of the skin.

intramuscular (IM) injection Form of injection in which the solution is introduced into the body of a muscle.

intraoperative Pertaining to the period of time during a surgical procedure.

intrapersonal communication Communication that occurs within an individual, for example, a person who "talks with the self" silently or forms an idea in the mind.

intrathecal Within the sheath surrounding the spinal cord.

intravenous (IV) injection Form of injection in which the solution is introduced into a vein.

intravenous piggyback (IVPB) A special coupling for the primary IV tubing that allows a supplementary or piggyback solution to run into the IV system.

intravenous therapy Delivery of fluids, medications, and nutrients through a small catheter placed in a vein. Home IV therapy usually involves electronic control devices (infusion pumps) to regulate the rate of infusion of the fluids and medications.

intrinsic factor Substance that is secreted by the gastric mucosa and is essential for the intestinal absorption of vitamin B_{12}.

intubation Passage of a tube into a body opening, for example, insertion of a breathing tube through the mouth or nose into the trachea.

invasion of privacy Release of personal information, for example, health records, financial statements, or employment history, without the person's permission.

invasive Referring to procedures that involve puncture, incision, or insertion of a foreign object, such as a needle or catheter, into the body.

irregular bones Bones of the vertebral column and some bones of the skull.

irrigation Process of washing out a body cavity or wounded area with a stream of fluid.

ischemia Decreased blood supply to a body part such as skin tissue or to an organ such as the heart.

isometric contraction Increased muscle tension without muscle shortening.

isotonic The situation where two solutions have the same concentration of solute; therefore both solutions exert the same osmotic pressure.

isotonic contraction Increased muscle tension resulting in muscle contraction and muscle shortening.

jaundice Yellow discoloration of the skin, mucous membranes, and sclera, caused by greater than normal amounts of bilirubin in the blood.

job stress Condition in which some factor or combination of factors at work disrupts the worker's psychological or physiological balance.

Joint Commission on Accreditation of Healthcare Organizations (JCAHO) A private, nongovernmental agency that establishes guidelines for the operation of hospitals and other health care facilities.

joints Connections between bones; classified according to structure and degree of mobility.

justice Fairness or equity in the manner decisions are made. One of the principles of the ethical theory of deontology.

Kardex Trade name for card-filing system that allows quick reference to the particular need of the client for certain aspects of nursing care.

keratosis Any skin condition in which there is overgrowth and thickening of the cornified epithelium; types are actinic and seborrheic.

ketoacidosis Acidosis accompanied by an accumulation of ketones in the body, resulting from faulty carbohydrate metabolism.

ketonuria Presence in the urine of excessive amounts of ketone bodies (products of fat metabolism), such as occurs in diabetes mellitus.

kinesthesia Perception of position of body parts, weight, and movement.

Korsakoff's syndrome Psychosis characterized by disorientation of time, place, and person by amnesia for recent events and by confabulation.

laceration Torn, jagged wound.

lactation Process and period in which the mother produces milk for the infant.

laissez-faire Philosophy characterized by an individual freedom of choice and action.

laissez-faire style Leadership style in which the leader denies responsibility, abdicates authority, and allows the group to direct themselves.

lanugo Fine hair that normally covers the fetus after the fifth month of intrauterine life and is mostly shed by birth.

laxative   Drug that acts to promote bowel evacuation.

leader   Person with the ability to influence the behavior of others toward the accomplishment of common goals; not necessarily a manager.

leadership style   Specific means by which a leader influences a group to accomplish goals.

learning   Acquisition of new knowledge and skills as a result of reinforcement, practice, and experience.

learning objectives   Written statement that describes the behavior a teacher expects from an individual following a learning activity.

legal chemicals   Mood-altering substances that may be purchased legally, including alcohol, prescription drugs, and over-the-counter medications.

legal right   Claim that is due according to legal guarantees.

legume   Fruit or pod of beans, peas, and lentils.

lesbian   Female with homosexual partner preference.

leukocytosis   Abnormal increase in the number of circulating white blood cells.

leukoplakia   Thick, raised, pearly-white patch of precancerous tissue found on the lips, buccal mucosa, penis, or vulva.

libel   Written false statement about a person that may injure reputation.

libido   Psychological term for sexual desire.

licensed practical or vocational nurse   Person trained in basic nursing techniques and direct client care who practices under the supervision of a registered nurse.

lifesaving measure   Independent, dependent, or interdependent nursing intervention that is implemented when a client's physiological or psychological status is threatened.

ligaments   White, shiny, flexible bands of fibrous tissues binding joints together and connecting various bones and cartilage.

litigation   Practice of taking legal action.

living will   Instrument by which a dying person makes wishes known to those care givers; a living will has no legal validity in most states.

livor mortis   Purple discoloration of the skin in dependent body parts after death; results from red blood cell destruction.

local adaptation syndrome (LAS)   Localized response of tissue, an organ, or a system that occurs as a direct reaction to stress.

local anesthesia   Loss of sensation at the desired site of action.

localized pain   Pain caused by injury in a specific location and perceived in that location, in contrast to diffuse, radiating, or referred pain.

long bones   Bones that contribute to height of the person, to the length of an extremity such as the arm, or to the length of a portion of an extremity such as the hand.

luteal phase   Third and final phase of the menstrual cycle, in which the corpus luteum develops, preparing for implantation of the egg, and deteriorates if an egg is not implanted.

lymphocyte   One type of leukocyte developing in the bone marrow; responsible for synthesizing antibodies and T cells that attack antigens.

maceration   Softening something solid, such as the skin, by soaking.

macrophage   Large phagocytic cell of the reticuloendothelial system.

malabsorption syndrome   Set of symptoms resulting from disorders in the intestinal absorption of nutrients, characterized by anorexia, weight loss, bloating of the abdomen, and muscle cramps.

male genitalia   Male external sex organs (penis and scrotum) and internal sex organs (testicles, epididymis, vas deferens, prostate gland, seminal vesicles, and Cowper's gland).

malignant tumor   Neoplasm that is anaplastic and invasive and that spreads to other body tissues.

malnutrition   Any nutritional disorder such as unbalanced, insufficient, or excessive diet or impaired absorption, assimilation, or utilization of food.

malpractice   Injurious or unprofessional actions that harm another.

management process   (as described by Fayol) Involves planning, organizing, directing, and controlling activities so that what is planned actually happens.

manager   Person with an official organizational position to guide and direct the work of subordinate employees.

mastication   Chewing, tearing, or grinding food with the teeth while it becomes mixed with saliva.

masturbation   Erotic self-stimulation by touching the genitals.

maturation   Process of becoming fully developed and grown, involving the individual's biological ability and environmental opportunities to alter functions and learning.

maturational loss   Loss, usually of an aspect of self, resulting from the normal changes of growth and development.

maturity   State of adulthood in which the person has attained independence with a balanced development in physiological, psychosocial, and cognitive dimensions.

meatus   Opening through any part of the body, for example, the urethral meatus.

Medicaid   State medical assistance based on Title XIX of the Social Security Act. States receive 50% in matching federal funds to provide medical care and services to people meeting categorical and income requirements. Covers home health services based on Medicare guidelines. Many innovative home health programs can be covered by Medicaid as long as they meet the recipient's needs and cost less than institutionalization.

medical diagnosis   Identification of a specific disease or pathological process.

Medicare   Federal government insurance coverage for persons over 65 years of age (or disabled and under 65) who have paid into the Social Security or Railroad Retirement system. Covers inpatient hospital charges and some home health services.

medulla oblongata   Portion of the brain that controls vital functions necessary for homeostasis and survival.

megadose   Dose greatly in excess of that usually prescribed.

melanin   Black or dark brown pigment that occurs naturally in the skin, hair, and iris.

melena   Abnormal black, tarry stool containing digested blood; indicative of gastrointestinal bleeding.

menarche Onset of a girl's first menstruation, usually occurring between 9 and 16 years of age.

meniscus Interface between a liquid (for example, mercury and air) that causes a convex shape to the liquid.

menopause Natural cessation of menses by the ovaries; normally occurs in women between ages 45 and 60.

menses Normal flow of blood, secretions, and tissue debris that occurs during menstruation, beginning on the first day of the menstrual cycle.

menstrual cycle Recurring cycle of changes in the ovaries, uterus, and hormone levels, involving the development of an egg, ovulation, and implantation of the egg or sloughing of the corpus luteum and lining. The cycle can be divided into proliferative and secretory phases by uterine changes or follicular, ovulation, and luteal phases based on ovarian activity.

menstruation Time of menstrual flow during the menstrual cycle.

message Information sent or expressed by sender in the communication process.

metabolism Aggregate of all chemical processes that take place in living organisms, resulting in growth, generation of energy, elimination of wastes, and other functions concerned with the distribution of nutrients in the blood after digestion.

metacognition Act of reflecting on one's own thought processes.

metacommunication Dependent not only on what is said but also on the relationship to the other person involved in the interaction. It is a message that conveys the sender's attitude toward the self and the message and the attitudes, feelings, and intentions toward the listener.

metric system A decimal system of measurement based on the meter (39.37 inches) as the unit of length, on the gram (15.432 grains) as the unit of weight or mass, and as a derived unit, on the liter (0.908 U.S. dry quart or 1.0567 U.S. liquid quart) as the unit of volume.

microorganism Any microscopic entity capable of carrying on living processes, such as bacteria, viruses, and fungi.

micturition Urination; act of passing or expelling urine voluntarily through the urethra.

mild stress situation Type of stress situation that is encountered by most people on a daily or weekly basis.

milliequivalent Number of grams of a specific electrolyte dissolved in 1 liter of plasma.

misdemeanor Lesser crime; the penalty is usually a fine or imprisonment for less than 1 year.

misuse Indiscriminate use of a drug or substance but to a lesser extent than with chronic abuse and dependence.

modeling Technique in which a person learns a desired response by observing it performed.

moderate stress situation Stress situation that lasts from several hours to a number of days.

modern Present-day beliefs and practices of the providers within the American, or western, health care delivery system.

molding Overlapping and shaping of the soft skull bones during birth, usually resolved during the first few days of life.

monocular Relating to vision through only one eye.

morality Behavior involving judgment, attitudes, and actions based on nationally conceived norms.

moralize Explain or interpret behavior on the basis of rigid principles of right or wrong.

morals Personal conviction that something is absolutely right or wrong in all situations.

morbidity *1.* An illness or abnormal condition. 2. The rate at which an illness occurs in a particular area or population.

morning sickness Pregnant woman's symptoms of nausea and vomiting related to changes in serum hormone levels.

mortician Person trained in the care of the dead.

morula Early stage of human development in which a solid mass of cells form from the zygote approximately 3 days after fertilization.

motivation Internal impulse that causes a person to take action.

mourning A psychological process of reaction activated by an individual to assist in overcoming a great personal loss. The process is finally resolved when a new object relationship is established.

muscle tone Normal state of balanced muscle tension.

myalgia Diffuse muscle pain.

mydriatic An ophthalmic preparation that dilates the pupil and paralyzes the ocular muscles of accomodation.

myoneural junction Point at which impulses traveling along motor nerves are transferred to muscle fibers.

narcolepsy Syndrome involving sudden sleep attacks that a person cannot inhibit; uncontrollable desire to sleep may occur several times during a day.

narcotic Drug substance, derived from opium or produced synthetically, that alters perception of pain and that with repeated use may result in physical and psychological dependence.

nasal Of or pertaining to the nose and the nasal cavity.

National League for Nursing (NLN) Organization of nurses and lay people concerned with improving nursing education, nursing service, and the delivery of health care in the United States. The NLN is the official accrediting agency for nursing schools.

nebulization Process of adding moisture to inspired air by the addition of water droplets.

necrotic Of or pertaining to the death of tissue in response to disease or injury.

negative nitrogen balance Condition occurring when the body excretes more nitrogen than it takes in.

negligence Careless act of omission or commission that results in injury to another.

neonate Stage of life from birth to 1 month of age.

nephron Structural and functional unit of the kidney containing a renal glomerulus and tubule.

neurogenic bladder Dysfunctional urinary bladder resulting from impaired neurological innervation.

neurolinguistic programming A communication model derived from the fields of linguistics, psychology, neurophysiology, kinetics, and cybernetics. When effectively used, this programming communicate trust and safety to another person.

neuropathy Abnormal condition characterized by inflammation and degeneration of peripheral nerves that alter sensory or motor function.

neurotransmitter Chemical that transfers the electrical impulse from the nerve fiber to the muscle fiber.

nocturia Urination at night; can be a symptom of renal disease or may occur in persons who drink excessive amounts of fluids before bedtime.

nocturnal enuresis Incontinence of urine during the night.

noise pollution Noise level in an environment when it becomes uncomfortable to its inhabitants.

nonmaleficence The duty to do no harm to another person. One of the principles of the ethical theory of deontology.

nonREM or NREM sleep Abbreviation for nonrapid eye movement, which occurs during the first four stages of normal sleep.

nonverbal communication Communication using expressions, gestures, body posture, and positioning rather than words.

norm Measure of a phenomenon generally accepted as the ideal standard performance against which other measures of the phenomenon may be measured.

nosocomial infection Infection acquired during hospitalization or stay in a health care facility.

noxious Painful or harmful to health.

nuclear family Form of family consisting of husband and wife and their children.

nurse administrator Nurse in management position with an agency who focuses on the delivery of nursing services.

nurse anesthetist Nurse with advanced training and accreditation in the speciality of nurse anesthesia; manages the anesthetic care of clients in certain surgical situations.

nurse-client relationship Association between the nurse and the client that has as a mutual concern the well-being of the client.

nurse educator Nurse with a background in clinical nursing who works in a school of nursing as a faculty member, in a staff development department of a health care agency, or in an inpatient education department.

nurse practice acts Statutes enacted by the legislature of any state delineating the legal scope of the practice of nursing within the geographical boundaries of the jurisdiction.

nurse practitioner Nurse with advanced training or education who provides primary care for nonemergency clients, usually in an outpatient or community setting.

nurse researcher Nurse with graduate nursing education who investigates problems related to nursing practice.

nursing Profession concerned with the diagnosis and treatment of human responses to actual and potential health problems.

nursing audit Thorough investigation designed to identify, examine, or verify the performance of certain specified aspects of nursing care using established professional standards.

nursing care plan Written guidelines of nursing care, documenting specific nursing diagnoses for the client and goals, interventions, and projected outcomes.

nursing care strategy Detailed nursing care plans that include direct and indirect care for the client.

nursing diagnosis A statement that describes the client's actual or potential response to a health problem that the nurse is licensed and competent to treat.

nursing health history Data collected about a client's present level of wellness, changes in the life patterns, sociocultural role, and mental and emotional reactions to illness.

nursing intervention Any action by a nurse that implements the nursing care plan or any specific objective of the plan.

nursing research A detailed process in which a systematic study of a problem in the field of nursing is performed.

nursing theory Organized framework of concepts and purposes designed to guide the practice of nursing.

object permanence The Piagetian term for the understanding that a person or object out of sight still exists.

objective data Data relating to a client's health problem that are obtained through observation or diagnostic measurements.

observation Report of what is seen or noticed about the client.

obstructive sleep apnea Temporary cessation of airflow (apnea) but with continuation of chest and abdominal movements; occurs while a person is sleeping.

occupational therapist Health care professional certified to develop and use adaptive devices that help the chronically ill or handicapped carry out activities of daily living.

olfactory Pertaining to the sense of smell.

oliguria Diminished capacity to form and pass urine.

oncotic pressure The total influence of the protein on the osmotic activity of plasma water.

open-ended question interview Inquiry aimed at obtaining a full client response and discussion between the client and the nurse.

ophthalmic Of or pertaining to the eye.

oral hygiene Condition or practice of maintaining the tissues and structures of the mouth.

oral report Verbal exchange of information from one nurse to another.

organic foods Foods grown in soils that have been treated only with organic matter (manure or compost).

orgasm Climax phase of sexual response, in which reflex muscular contractions, genital vasocongestion, and increased heart and respiratory rates occur.

orgasmic maturity Physiological maturity of the reproductive system enabling completion of the adult sexual response cycle.

orthopnea Abnormal condition in which a person must sit or stand to breathe deeply or comfortably.

orthostatic hypotension A drop in systolic blood pressure of 15mm Hg when a person rises from a recumbent position to a sitting or standing position.

osmolality The concentration or osmotic pressure of a solution expressed in osmols or milliosmols per kilogram of water (normal = 280-295 mOsm/kg).

osmosis Movement of a pure solvent through a semipermeable membrane from a solution with a lower solute concentration to one with a higher solute concentration.

osmotic pressure Drawing power for water, which depends on the number of molecules in the solution.

ostomate Person with an ostomy.

ostomy Surgical procedure in which an opening is made into the abdominal wall to allow the passage of intestinal contents from the bowel (colostomy) or urine from the bladder (urostomy).

ototoxic Having a harmful effect on the eighth cranial (auditory) nerve or the organs of hearing and balance.

ototoxicity Referring to any drug or substance that has a harmful effect on the eighth cranial nerve or the organs of hearing and balance.

outcome Condition of a client at the end of therapy, including the degree of wellness and the need for continuing care, medication, support, counseling, or education.

outpatient Client who has not been admitted to a hospital but receives treatment in a clinic or facility associated with the hospital.

outpatient setting Physician's office, clinic, or other ambulatory care facility for the provision of health care services.

overhydration Excess of water in the extracellular fluid.

over-the-counter drug Drug available to a consumer without a prescription.

ovulation Second phase of the menstrual cycle, in which a mature egg is released from the ovary and moves down the fallopian tubes.

oxidation Any process in which the oxygen content of a compound is increased.

oxygen therapy Administration of oxygen to a client by any route to prevent or relieve hypoxia.

pain Subjective, unpleasant sensation caused by noxious stimulation of sensory nerve endings.

pain perception Threshold or point at which a person experiences pain.

palliative therapy Treatment designed to relieve or reduce intensity of uncomfortable symptoms but not to produce a cure.

pallor Unnatural paleness or absence of color in the skin.

palpation Use of the hands and the sense of tough to gather data.

palpebra Portion of the conjunctiva that lines the inner surface of the eyelids; it is thick, opaque, and highly vascular.

paralytic ileus Usually temporary paralysis of intestinal wall that may occur after abdominal surgery or peritoneal injury and that causes cessation of peristalis. Leads to abdominal distention and symptoms of obstruction.

paranoia Disorder characterized by a system of thinking with delusions of persecution and grandeur, usually centered on one major theme.

paraphrasing Restating a passage or phrase to give the same meaning in another form.

parasite Organism living in or on another organism and obtaining nourishment from it.

parenteral Not in or through the digestive system; typically refers to administering medications by injection.

paronychia Infection of the fold of skin at the margin of a nail.

partial bed bath Bath in which body parts that might cause the client discomfort if left unbathed, that is, face, hands, axillary areas, back, and perineum, are washed in bed.

passive smoking Smoke and toxic fumes inhaled by a nonsmoker from a smoker's cigarette, cigar, or pipe.

passive strategies of health promotion Activities that involve the client as the recipient of actions by health care professionals.

pathogen Any microorganism capable of producing disease.

pathological fractures Fractures resulting from weakened bone tissue; frequently caused by osteoporosis or neoplasms.

patient-controlled analgesia (PCA) Drug delivery system that allows patients to self-administer analgesic medications when they want.

peer review Appraisal, by professional co-workers of equal status, of the way a nurse conducts practice, education, or research.

pellagra Disorder resulting from a deficiency of niacin or tryptophan.

perception Person's mental image or concept of elements in the environment, including information gained through the senses.

percussion Tapping of various body organs and structures to produce vibration and sound.

perineal care Cleansing procedure prescribed for cleansing the genital and anal areas as part of the daily bath or after various obstetrical and gynecological procedures.

periodontal disease (pyorrhea) Disease of the tissues around the tooth, such as inflammation of the periodontal membrane or ligament.

perioperative nursing Refers to the role of the operating room nurse during the preoperative, intraoperative, and postoperative phases of surgery.

peristalsis Coordinated, rhythmical, serial contractions of smooth muscle that force food through the digestive tract.

peritoneal dialysis A dialysis procedure performed to correct an imbalance of fluids or electrolytes in the blood or to remove toxins, drugs, or other wastes normally excreted by the kidney.

peritonitis Inflammation of the peritoneum produced by bacteria or irritating substances introduced into the abdominal cavity by a penetrating wound or perforation of an organ in the GI tract or the reproductive tract.

PERRLA Acronym for "pupils equal, round, reactive to light, accommodative"; the acronym is recorded in the physical examination if eye and pupil assessments are normal.

petechiae Tiny purple or red spots that appear on skin as minute hemorrhages within dermal layers.

phagocytosis Process by which certain cells, such as macrophages, engulf and dispose of microorganisms.

pharmacist Licensed professional who formulates and dispenses medications.

pharmacokinetics Study of how drugs enter the body, reach their site of action, are metabolized, and exit from the body.

phenomena Data that can be observed in reality.

phlebitis Inflammation of a vein.

physical examination Scrutinization of all body parts through the use of inspection, palpation, percussion, and auscultation.

physical therapist Health care professional licensed to assist in the management of physically disabled or handicapped clients through techniques such as special exercise, application of heat and cold, and sonar wave methods.

physician Health care professional who has the degree of Doctor of Medicine (MD) or Doctor of Osteopath (DO) and is licensed to provide medical, surgical, and other treatment.

physician assistant Health care professional trained in aspects of the practice of medicine to provide support to physicians.

physiological anorexia A decrease in appetite that occurs with slower growth rates, decreased caloric need, and smaller food intake during toddlerhood.

physiological dependence Condition in which the body is so accustomed to a drug or substance that functioning is impaired without it.

physiological needs Needs necessary for human survival, including those for oxygen, fluid, nutrition, temperature, elimination, and shelter.

PIE (Problem-Intervention-Evaluation) A format for documenting client care that unifies the care plan and progress notes into a complete record.

pigmentation Organic coloring material, such as melanin, that gives color to the skin.

pituitary gland Small gland attached to the hypothalamus that supplies numerous hormones for the control of vital functions and the maintenance of homeostasis.

placebo Dosage form that contains no pharmacologically active ingredients but may relieve pain through psychological effects.

placenta Organ surrounding the embryo and fetus through which nutrients and other substances from the mother and waste products from the fetus pass.

planned change Goal-directed, collaborated efforts to alter a situation or environment.

plantar wart Painful lesion on the sole of the foot, primarily at pressure points, caused by the common wart virus.

plasma Watery, colorless, fluid portion of the lymph and blood.

plasma proteins Albumin, fibrinogen, prothrombin, and the gamma globulins, which constitute about 6% to 7% of the blood plasma in the body.

pleura Delicate serous membrane enclosing the lung.

pleural cavity Cavity within the thorax that contains the lungs.

pneumothorax Collection of air or gas in the pleural space.

podiatrist Practitioner trained to diagnose and treat diseases and other disorders of the feet.

point of maximal impulse (PMI) Anatomic point along the fourth to fifth intercostal space at the midclavicular line where the heart beat can most easily be palpated through the chest wall.

poison Any substance that impairs health or destroys life when ingested, inhaled, or absorbed by the body in relatively small amounts.

poison control center One of a network of facilities that provides information regarding all aspects of poisoning or intoxication, maintains records of their occurrence, and refers clients to treatment centers.

pollutant A harmful chemical or waste material discharged into the water or atmosphere.

polycythemia Abnormal increase in the number of erythrocytes in the blood.

polysomnogram Monitoring device that involves placement of electrodes on the scalp, face, chin, and legs to measure brain waves, eye movements, and muscle activity; used to diagnose sleep disorders.

polyuria Excretion of an abnormally large volume of urine.

postoperative Pertaining to the period of time after surgery.

postural drainage Use of positioning along with percussion and vibration to drain secretions from specific segments of the lungs and bronchi into the trachea.

posture Position of the body in relation to the surrounding space.

potential health care problem Health problem for which the client is at risk.

potentiation Synergistic action in which the effect of two drugs given simultaneously is greater than the effect of the drugs given separately.

power Ability to influence, direct, produce, or control; to exert authority, force, or strength.

precipitating force Element that causes or contributes to the occurrence of a symptom.

Preferred Provider Organization (PPO) Group of physicians or hospital that provides company employees and their dependents with comprehensive health services at a discount.

premenstrual syndrome (PMS) Complex of physical and psychological symptoms experienced by some women just before menstruation.

prenatal Stage of life from conception to birth.

preoperational thought Children can think about things not physically present by using mental representations but are limited by their inability to use logic.

preoperative Pertaining to the period before surgery.

presbycusis Condition that affects the client's ability to hear high-pitched sounds and sibilant consonants such as "s," "sh," and "ch" because of the aging process.

presbyopia Farsightedness with inability to focus on near objects, resulting from loss of elasticity of the lens; occurs with age.

preschooler Stage of life from 3 to 5 years of age.

prescription Authorized order for medication, therapy, or a therapeutic device.

presentational isolation Social isolation that occurs because of the older adult's socially unacceptable appearance or presentation of self to others.

pressure ulcer Inflammation, sore, or ulcer in the skin over a bony prominence.

preventive nursing action Interventions directed toward preventing illness and promoting health to avoid the need for secondary or tertiary health care.

primary care The first contact in a given episode of illness that leads to a decision regarding a course of action to resolve the health problem.

primary intention Primary union of the edges of a wound, progressing to complete scar formation without granulation.

primary nursing System of nursing care in which the care of a client is managed for the hospital stay by one nurse, who directs and coordinates other nurses and other personnel in the care of the client. When on duty, the primary nurse cares for the client personally.

primary prevention Activities directed toward decreasing the probability of specific illnesses or dysfunctions.

primary source Research report written by an investigator in an original study.

private duty agencies Organizations that provide professional and paraprofessional home health care services on a continuous basis.

private insurance   Health insurance other than government coverage. Insurance provided for profit by citizen-owned companies.

proactive decision   Decision made by an individual directed at attaining a goal.

problem-oriented medical record (POMR or POR)   Method of recording data about the health status of a client that fosters a collaborative problem-solving approach by all members of the health care team.

problem-seeking interview   Type of inquiry that focuses on gathering data to identify problems the client needs to resolve.

problem-solving interview   Type of inquiry that focuses on specific problems that have been identified by the client or nurse.

profession   Vocation requiring specialized knowledge and intensive academic preparation.

professional organization   Association of professionals created to deal with issues of concern to the profession as a whole.

prophylactic   Preventing the spread of infection.

proposition   Statement that defines or explains a relationship between two or more concepts.

proprioception   Sensation achieved through stimuli from within the body regarding spatial position and muscular activity.

proprioceptors   Nerve endings located in muscles, tendons, and joints that respond to stimuli originating from within the body regarding spatial position or movement.

prospective payment   Procedure by which the federal government sets rates for hospitals in advance for treatment of specific illnesses; this replaces the previous policy of reimbursing each hospital based on actual cost.

prospective reimbursement   Predetermined amount of payment before delivery of services.

protocol   Written and approved plan specifying the procedures to be followed during an assessment or in providing treatment.

proxemics   The study of spatial distances between people and its effect on interpersonal behavior.

pruritus   Symptom of itching, an uncomfortable sensation leading to the urge to scratch, which may result in secondary infections.

psychiatric hospital   Institution providing inpatient and outpatient counseling services to clients with behavioral or emotional illnesses.

psychological dependence   Chronic emotional or psychological reliance on a drug or substance such that the person feels unable to handle stress without it.

psychomotor learning   Acquisition of ability to perform motor skills.

psychosurgery   Surgical interruption of certain nerve pathways in the brain; performed in selected cases of agitation, unremitting anxiety, and other forms of abnormal behavior.

psychotherapy   Treatment of mental and emotional disorders by any of a large number of psychological techniques rather than by physical means.

psychotomimetic   Drug or substance whose effects mimic the symptoms of psychosis, such as hallucinations.

ptosis   Abnormal condition of one or both upper eyelids in which the eyelid droops; caused by weakness of the levator muscle or paralysis of the third cranial nerve.

ptyalin   Salivary amylase that breaks starch down to maltose.

puberty   Developmental period of emotional and physical changes, including the development of secondary sex characteristics and the onset of menstruation and ejaculation.

public communication   Interaction between one person and a large group of people.

puerperium   Period of approximately 6 weeks after childbirth during which the woman's reproductive system is in transition to the nonpregnant state.

pulmonary function tests   Procedures for determining the capacity of the lungs to exchange oxygen and carbon dioxide efficiently.

pulse   The regular, recurrent expansion and contraction of an artery produced by waves of pressure caused by the ejection of blood from the left ventricle of the heart as it contracts.

pulse deficit   Condition that exists when the radial pulse is less than the ventricular rate as auscultated at the apex or seen on an electrocardiogram. The conditions indicate a lack of peripheral perfusion for some of the heart contractions.

pulse pressure   The difference between the systolic and diastolic pressures, normally 30 to 40 mm Hg.

pursed-lip breathing   Deep inspiration through the nose and mouth, not using pursed lips, followed by prolonged expiration through pursed lips.

purulent   Producing or containing pus.

pyrogen   Any substance that causes a rise in body temperature, as in the case of bacterial toxins.

qualitative research   Research that is descriptive in nature and studies the quality, value, or nature of variables measured.

quality assurance   Evaluation of the quality and appropriateness of nursing care provided and the results achieved as compared with accepted standards.

quality improvement   The monitoring and evaluation of processes and outcomes in health care or any other business to identify opportunities for improvement.

radial pulse   Pulse of the radial artery palpated at the wrist over the radius. The radial pulse is the one most often taken.

radiating pain   A sensation of pain extending from the initial site of injury to another body part.

random selection   Method of choosing subjects for a research study in which all members of a particular group are equally likely to be included.

reaction   Component of the pain experience that may include both physiological responses such as in the general adaptation syndrome and behavioral responses.

reactive decision   Decision made by an individual in response to the influence of others.

reality orientation   Therapeutic modality for restoring an individual's sense of the present.

receiver   Person to whom message is sent during the communication process.

reception   Neurophysiological components of the pain experience, in which nervous system receptors receive painful stimuli and transmit them through peripheral nerves to the spinal cord and brain.

receptor   A sensory nerve ending that responds to various kinds of stimulation.

recommended daily allowances (RDAs) Suggested or recommended amounts of various nutrients used in planning diets.

record Written form of communication that permanently documents information relevant to health care management.

recovery room Area adjoining the operating room to which surgical clients are taken while still under anesthesia.

recumbent Lying down or leaning backward.

referent Factor that motivates a person to communicate with another individual.

referred pain Pain perceived in an area separate from and unaffected by the source of pain, as sensory neurons from the affected organ meet neurons in the spinal cord from organs where the pain is perceived.

reflux Abnormal backward flow or return of fluid, as in the case of gastric contents reentering the esophagus.

refractive error Defect in the ability of the lens of the eye to focus light, such as occurs in nearsightedness and farsightedness.

refractory period Postejaculation recovery time during which further ejaculation is physiologically impossible.

refreezing stage of change Incorporation of change or modifications as standard procedure or function.

regional anesthesia Loss of sensation in an area of the body supplied by sensory nerve pathways.

registered nurse Health care professional who has completed a course of study at an accredited school of professional nursing and has passed an examination administered by a state board of nursing or the Canadian Nurses Association Testing Service.

regurgitation Return of swallowed food into the mouth.

rehabilitation Restoration of an individual to normal or near-normal function following a physical or mental illness, injury, or chemical addiction.

rehabilitation center Facility that provides therapy and training to restore a client to an optimal level of functioning and independence.

reinforcement Provision of a contingent response to a learner's behavior that increases the probability of the behavior recurring.

reinforcement-extinction Process of socialization in which one learns to engage in certain behaviors (reinforcement) or to avoid certain behaviors (extinction).

relative humidity Amount of moisture in the air as compared with the maximum amount that the air could contain at the same temperature.

relieving factor Element that alleviates a symptom.

religion Belief in a divine or superhuman power or powers to be obeyed and worshipped as the creator(s) and ruler(s) of the universe.

religious Relating to specific practices, rites, and rituals of one's professed religion.

REM sleep Abbreviation for rapid eye movement, occurring during stage of sleep in which dreaming and rapid eye movements are prominent; important for mental restoration.

remembering Lifelong tolerance to chemicals established by earlier abuse or exposure and situations.

reminiscence Recalling the past for the purpose of assigning new meaning to past experiences.

remission Partial or complete disappearance of the clinical and subjective characteristics of a chronic or malignant disease; remission may be spontaneous or the result of therapy.

renal Of or pertaining to the kidney.

renal calculus Calcium stone in the renal pelvis.

renal replacement therapy Treatments designed to carry out kidney function. Currently two methods of renal replacement exist: dialysis, peritoneal and hemodialysis and organ transplantation.

renin A proteolytic enzyme, produced by and stored in the juxtaglomerular apparatus that surrounds each arteriole as it enters a glomerulus. The enzyme affects the blood pressure by catalyzing the change of angiotensinogen to angiotensin, a strong repressor.

research process Systematic collection and analysis of data to obtain new knowledge, add to existing knowledge, or find solutions to problems.

research utilization Systematic process for determining the scientific worth of a group of conceptually related nursing research studies and whether or not the findings can be used to solve a nursing care problem with a particular group of clients in a setting other than the one in which the studies were conducted.

residual urine Volume of urine remaining in the bladder after a normal voiding; the bladder normally is almost completely empty after micturition.

resistance An overtly active or covertly passive set of behaviors, whether conscious or unconscious in motivation, to avoid or to prevent the change process.

resocialization Technique that assists older adults to expand their social networks within their community.

respiratory therapist Health care professional licensed to deliver treatment to improve ventilatory function or oxygenation.

respite Temporary relief services for the primary care giver of a dependent older adult in the home or institutional setting.

responsibility Carrying out duties associated with a particular role.

restraining forces against change Factors that resist, slow, or interfere with the occurrence of the change process.

restraint Device to aid in the immobilization of a client or client's extremity.

resuscitation Process of sustaining the vital functions of persons in respiratory or cardiac arrest while reviving them.

reticular activating system Group of specialized nerve cells located in the brainstem, upper spinal cord, and cerebral cortex.

reticular formation Small cluster of neurons in the brainstem and spinal cord that continuously monitor and control vital functions to maintain homeostasis.

retinopathy A noninflammatory eye disorder resulting from changes in the retinal blood vessels.

retroperitoneal Of or pertaining to organs closely attached to the posterior abdominal wall and partly covered by peritoneum.

***Rickettsia* organisms** Group of microorganisms that occupies an intermediate position between viruses and bacteria.

rigidity Condition of stiffness or inflexibility, as in muscle rigidity.

rigor mortis Stiffening of the body shortly after death because of the contraction of skeletal and smooth muscle.

Rinne test Method of assessing auditory acuity useful in distinguishing conductive from sensorineural hearing loss.

role A person's pattern of behavior in a particular social group or situation.

role ambiguity State in which a person has unclear role expectations and feels unable to predict the outcomes of behavior.

role conflict State in which a person experiences incongruent or incompatible expectations within one role or between two or more simultaneously held roles.

role overload State in which a person experiences conflicting role priorities and must decide with which pressures to comply.

role strain Generalized state of frustration or anxiety produced by the stress of role conflict and ambiguity.

safety and security needs Needs for freedom from threats to one's physical and psychological well-being.

sample Portion of a larger group of subjects.

satiety Satisfied feeling of being full.

scientific management theory Leadership theory that emphasizes technology and task analysis, rather than human factors, as a means of improving productivity.

scientific rationale Reason, based on supporting literature, why a specific nursing action was chosen.

sebaceous gland One of the small organs in the dermis that secretes an oily substance (sebum) on the skin's surface and in the hair.

sebum Normal secretion of the sebaceous glands of the skin; when combined with sweat, forms a moist, oily, acidic film that protects the skin from drying.

secondary intention Wound closure in which the edges are separated, granulation tissue develops to fill the gap, and finally, epithelium grows in over the granulation, producing a larger scar than results with healing by primary intention.

secondary prevention Activities directed toward early diagnosis and prompt intervention, thereby shortening severity and enabling the client to return to the highest level of health at the earliest possible point.

secondary sex characteristics Physical characteristics other than genitals that distinguish females from males, for example, the breasts.

secondary source Report that interprets research data written by someone not involved in the original research.

sedative Medication that produces a calming effect by decreasing functional activity, diminishing irritability, and allaying excitement.

sedative-hypnotics Drugs, such as barbiturates, that depress the central nervous system and produce a sense of euphoria or relaxation.

self-actualization State of being in which one is fully achieving one's potential and is able to cope realistically with problems.

self-concept 1. Complex, dynamic integration of conscious and unconscious feelings, attitudes, and perceptions about one's identity, physical being, worth, and roles. 2. How people perceive and define themselves.

self-esteem Feeling of self-worth characterized by feelings of achievement, adequacy, self-confidence, and usefulness.

self-ideal Aspirations, goals, values, and standards of behavior that a person considers ideal and strives to attain.

sender Person who initiates interpersonal communication by conveying a message.

senile keratosis A slowly developing, localized thickening of the outer layers of the skin as a result of chronic, excessive exposure to the sun. Commonly develops in older adults.

sensate exercises Series of pleasurable touching exercises that focus on sensual (not sexual) activities.

sensory deficit Defect in the function of one or more of the senses, resulting in visual, auditory, or olfactory impairments.

sensory deprivation State in which stimulation to one or more of the senses is lacking, resulting in impaired sensory perception.

sensory overload State in which stimulation to one or more of the senses is so excessive that the brain disregards or does not meaningfully respond to stimuli.

separation anxiety Behavioral manifestation created by fear of being apart from primary caretaker.

serosanguineous Thin red drainage composed of serum and blood.

serous fluid Clear fluid that reduces friction between structures covered by serous membranes, such as the lung.

severe stress situation Chronic stress situation that may last from several weeks to years.

severe stress syndrome The stage of illness development in stress-related diseases that occurs just prior to appearance of early clinical signs.

sex 1. Classification of male or female based on many criteria, among them anatomical and chromosomal characteristics. 2. Refers also to biological aspects of sexuality and genital sexual activity.

sex skin Term used for the labia minora because of the distinctive color changes that occur during sexual arousal.

sexual dysfunction Inability or difficulty in sexual function caused by physiological or psychological factors or both.

sexuality Dynamic and diverse facet of the personality involving the biological, psychological, sociological, spiritual, and cultural dimensions, depending in part on the person's sense of sexual identity and affecting the person's values, attitudes, behaviors, and relationships with others.

sexual orientation Clear, persistent desire of a person for one sex rather than the other.

sexual response cycle Four phases of biological sexual response: excitement, plateau, orgasm, and resolution as defined by Masters and Johnson.

sexually transmitted diseases (STDs) Infectious diseases transmitted to any part of the body through contact with body fluids during sexual activities.

sign Objective finding perceived by an examiner, such as a fever, rash, abnormal reflex, or abnormal breath sound.

single-parent family A form of family composed of single, divorced, or widowed parents and their children.

situational change Unplanned events that alter behavior of a person, family, group, or community.

situational crisis Crisis occurring suddenly in response to a specific external event or conflict.

situational leadership A leadership theory developed by Hersey and Blanchard that is concerned with the extent of structure and socioemotional support provided by a leader on the basis of subordinates' maturity.

situational loss Loss of a person, thing, or quality resulting from a change in a life situation, including changes related to illness, body image, environment, and death.

situational theory Leadership theory in which the manager chooses a leadership style to match the particular situation.

sitz bath Bath in which only the hips or buttocks are immersed in fluid.

slander Utterance of a false statement about another that harms that person's reputation.

sleep deprivation Condition resulting from a decrease in the amount, quality, and consistency of sleep.

SOAP Acronym for subjective, objective, assessment, and plan, the four parts of the written account of a client's health problem in a problem-oriented record.

social worker Professional trained to counsel clients and families to help them seek community and financial resources and to assist them in selecting long-term and extended care facilities.

socialization Process that begins in infancy by which a person acquires values, behavior, skills, and roles from social norms and significant others.

sodium pump Physiological mechanism that transports sodium ions across cellular membranes against an opposing concentration gradient.

solution Mixture of one or more substances dissolved in another substance. The molecules of each of the substances disperse homogeneously and do not change chemically. A solution may be a liquid, gas, or solid.

somnolence Condition characterized by constant sleepiness or drowsiness.

spasm Involuntary muscle contraction of sudden onset.

specific gravity Measurement of the degree of concentration of a liquid.

spiritual distress State of being out of harmony with a system of beliefs, a supreme being, or god.

spiritual health Awareness and openness to a system of beliefs, a supreme being, or god; a presence with or in each person and in the world.

spirituality Spiritual dimension of a person, including the relationship with humanity, nature, and a system of beliefs, a supreme being, or god.

spirometer Instrument that measures and records the volume of inhaled and exhaled air; used to assess pulmonary function.

standard Measure or guide that serves as a basis for comparison when evaluating similar phenomena or substances.

standardized care plan (SCP) Written care plan used for clients who have similar health care problems.

standards of care The minimum level of care accepted to ensure high quality of care to clients. Standards of care define the types of therapies typically administered to clients with defined problems or needs.

standards of practice The minimum required level of performance expected of care givers to ensure quality care is delivered to clients. Standards of practice are reflected in procedures and job descriptions. They define nurses' responsibilities to clients.

standing order Written and approved document containing rules, policies, procedures, regulations, and orders for the conduct of client care in various stipulated clinical settings.

statistics Mathematical science concerned with measuring, classifying, and analyzing objective information.

statutory law Of or related to laws enacted by a legislative branch of the government.

stereognosis Ability to recognize objects by the sense of touch.

stereotype A generalization about a form of behavior, an individual, or a group.

sterile Aseptic, without germs.

sterile field Specified area, such as within a tray or on a sterile towel, that is considered free of microorganisms.

sterilization Rendering a person unable to produce children; accomplished by surgical, chemical, or other means.

Steri-strip Trade name for butterfly tape used as a wound closure.

stoma Artificially created opening between a body cavity and the body's surface—for example, a colostomy, formed from a portion of the colon pulled through the abdominal wall.

stomatitis Any inflammatory condition of the mouth.

stress Physiological or psychological tension that threatens homeostasis or a person's psychological equilibrium.

stress behaviors Changes from a person's normal behaviors in response to a stressor.

stressor Any event, situation, or other stimulus encountered in a person's external or internal environment that necessitates change or adaptation by the person.

stridor An abnormal, high-pitched, musical respiratory sound, caused by an obstruction in the trachea or larynx.

stroke volume The amount of blood ejected by the ventricle during a ventricular contraction.

subcutaneous injection Form of injection in which the solution is introduced into subcutaneous tissues.

subjective data Data relating to a client's health problem described in the client's own words.

subjects People or events selected for a study in order to examine a particular variable or condition.

substance Any drug, chemical, or biological entity; specifically, any material capable of being self-administered or abused because of its physiological or psychological effects.

substance abuse Commonly used as synonymous for chemical dependency; a less precise term that only indicates abuse of a substance, not dependence on it.

sundown syndrome Nocturnal confusion in clients who are usually not confused at other times during the day. Institutional tempo changes, sensory deficit, and environmental change are major contributors to this confusion.

superinfection Infection occurring during antimicrobial treatment for another infection; usually caused by a change in normal tissue flora.

suppurative Producing or associated with formation of pus.

sustained maximal inspiration Alveolar inflation to total lung capacity produced by high negative transpulmonary pressures.

suture Surgical stitch taken to repair an incision or wound.

symptom Subjective indication of a disease or a change in condition as perceived by a client; some symptoms, such as numbness of a body part, may be objectively confirmed.

synapse Region surrounding the point of contact between two neurons or between a neuron and an effector organ.

syncope A brief lapse in consciousness caused by transient cerebral hypoxia.

synergistic agent Substance that augments or adds to the activity of another substance or agent.

syntax Arrangement of words as elements in a phrase, clause, or sentence.

system Unit made up of separate parts or elements; the parts rely on each other, are interrelated, have a common purpose, and together form a collective whole.

systemic Of or pertaining to the whole body rather than to a localized area.

systolic pressure The pressure exerted in the aorta and large arteries of a human during systolic contraction of the left ventricle. Indicated during blood pressure measurement as the point when sound can first be heard during deflation of the pressure cuff.

tachycardia Rapid, regular heart rate ranging between 100 and 150 beats per minute.

tachypnea An abnormally rapid rate of breathing, as seen with hyperpyrexia.

tactile Relating to the sense of touch.

tarry Sticky quality of feces containing blood.

teaching Interaction between a teacher and a student that promotes learning.

teaching-learning process Interaction between the teacher and learner in which specific learning objectives are presented and met.

technique Method followed in performing a specific procedure such as administering medication, changing a client's dressing, or inserting a Foley catheter.

temperament The child's characteristic style of approaching and reacting to people and situations.

temperature A measure of sensible heat associated with the metabolism of the human body, normally maintained at a constant level of 98.6° F (37° C).

teratogen Chemical or physiological agents that may produce adverse effects in the embryo or fetus.

teratogenic Any chemical or physiological agent that may produce adverse effects in the embryo or fetus.

terminal illness Condition of a client for whom medical technology cannot offer curative treatment.

territoriality Persistent attachment of a person to a specific area or space.

tertiary prevention Activities directed toward rehabilitation rather than diagnosis and treatment.

testosterone Naturally occurring male sex hormone.

theory General statement about relationships among concepts or facts, based on existing information.

theory X and theory Y Developed by McGregor to differentiate the attitudes about human nature often reflected in a managing behavior.

theory Z Japanese adaptation of the human relations theory. The focus is participative management involving employees in decisions that affect them.

therapeutic Of or pertaining to a treatment or beneficial act.

thermoregulation Internal control of body temperature.

third space syndrome A shift of body fluid into a space from which it is not easily exchanged with the extracellular fluid.

thoracentesis Surgical perforation of the chest wall and pleural space with a needle for the aspiration of fluid or to obtain a specimen for diagnostic or therapeutic purposes.

threshold Point at which a person first perceives a painful stimulus as being painful.

thrombus Accumulation of platelets, fibrin, clotting factors, and the cellular elements of the blood attached to the interior wall of a vein or artery, sometimes occluding the lumen of the vessel.

tidal breath Volume of air. The mechanical activity of the lungs and thoracic cage that occurs during normal relaxed breathing. The volume inhaled during tidal breath is approximately 500 cc of air.

tidal volume Amount of air inhaled and exhaled during normal ventilation.

tinnitus Ringing heard in one or both ears.

toddlerhood Stage of life from 1 to 3 years of age.

tolerance The ability to endure hardship, pain, or ordinarily injurious substances, such as drugs, without apparent physiological or psychological injury.

tolerance (chemical substance) Need for increasingly larger amounts of a drug (alcohol or other) to achieve the same physical and/or psychological effect.

tolerance (pain) Point at which a person is not willing to accept pain of greater severity or duration.

topical Pertaining to a drug or treatment applied to the surface of a part of the body.

tort Act that causes injury for which the injured party can bring civil action.

total parenteral nutrition (TPN) The administration of a nutritionally adequate hypertonic solution consisting of glucose, protein hydrolysates, minerals, and vitamins through an indwelling catheter into the superior vena cava.

tracheostomy Opening through the neck into the trachea with an indwelling tube inserted, which is created surgically to produce an airway.

traditional Ancient ethnocultural-religious beliefs and practices handed down through the generations.

trait development theory Leadership theory that analyzes successful leadership in terms of the leader's personal qualities, including intelligence, energy level, aggressiveness, and friendliness.

tranquilizer Medication that calms agitated or anxious persons without causing loss of consciousness.

transcutaneous electrical nerve stimulation (TENS) Technique in which a battery-powered device blocks pain impulses from reaching the spinal cord by delivering weak electrical pulses directly to the skin's surface.

transit time Time required to propel a bolus of intestinal contents from one location in the gastrointestinal tract to another.

transplantation Transfer of an organ or tissue from one person to another or from one part of the body to another in order to replace a diseased structure or to restore function.

transsexual People whose gender identities are opposite their biological sex identities.

transvestism Tendency to achieve psychic and sexual relief by dressing in clothing of the opposite sex.

Trendelenburg position Position in which the body and legs are on an inclined plane with the head lowermost.

triage A process in which a group of clients is sorted according to their needs for care. The kind of illness or injury, the severity of the problem, and the facilities available govern the process.

tryptophan Essential amino acid, precursor of serotonin and niacin.

tumescence To become swollen, as with genital vasocongestion during sexual arousal.

turgor Normal resiliency of the skin caused by the outward pressure of the cells and interstitial fluid.

ultradian rhythm Repetition of certain physiological phenomena within a cycle lasting less than 24 hours.

unfreezing stage of change Identifying the problem and need for alterations.

unresolved grief Severe chronic grief reaction in which the person does not complete the resolution stage of the grieving process within a reasonable time.

uremia Presence of excessive amounts of urea and other nitrogenous wastes in the blood; occurs in renal failure.

uremic syndrome Symptoms characterized by the presence of urinary constituents in the blood and altered regulatory functions, causing marked fluid and electrolyte abnormalities, nausea, vomiting, headache, coma, or convulsions.

ureterostomy Diversion of urine away from a diseased or defective bladder through an artificial opening in the skin.

urgency Sensation of the need to void soon.

urinary diversion A surgically created diversion of the ureter to the abdominal wall for the drainage of urine following removal of a diseased bladder.

urinary frequency Symptom involving increased voiding.

urinary incontinence Inability to control urination.

urinometer Device for determining the specific gravity of urine.

utilization review (UR) An assessment of the appropriateness and economy of an admission to a health care facility or continued hospitalization.

validation therapy Technique used with severely confused and disoriented older adults to provide a sense of dignity and self-worth and validate their feelings.

value Personal belief about the worth of a given idea or behavior.

values clarification Technique for clarifying values, developed by Louis Raths; process designed to give an individual the opportunity to find meaning and significance in personal values.

values clarification strategy An exercise that assists the participants in clarifying values toward a specific concept or issue.

varicosity Abnormal condition of a vein, characterized by swelling and irregular shape or course.

vascular access devices Catheters, cannulas, or infusion ports designed for long-term, repeated access to the vascular system.

vascularization Process by which body tissue becomes vascular and develops proliferating capillaries.

venipuncture Technique in which a vein is punctured transcutaneously by a sharp, rigid stylet or by a needle attached to a syringe.

venous stasis Disorder in which the normal flow of blood through a vein is slowed or halted.

ventilation Respiratory process by which gases are moved into and out of the lungs.

ventilators Mechanical devices used to artificially support breathing in clients with ventilatory failure. Small electronic ventilators with battery back-up have been specifically designed for home use.

ventral Of or pertaining to anterior position, toward the abdomen.

veracity The ability to tell the truth.

verbal communication The sending of messages from one individual to another or to a group of individuals through the spoken word.

verbal report *See* oral report.

vernix caseosa A grayish-white cheeselike substance consisting of sebaceous gland secretions, lanugo, and epithelial cells that coats the skin of the fetus and newborn.

vial Glass container with a metal-enclosed rubber seal.

vibration Fine, shaking pressure applied by hands to the chest wall only during exhalation.

virulent Of or pertaining to a very pathogenic or rapidly progressive condition.

virus Minute microorganism (smaller than a bacterium) having no independent metabolic activity, which may only replicate within a cell of a living animal or plant host.

viscera Internal organs of the abdominal cavity.

visual Of or pertaining to the sense of sight.

vital signs Temperature, pulse, respirations, and blood pressure.

vitiligo Benign acquired skin disease consisting of irregular patches of various sizes totally lacking in pigment; exposed areas of skin are most affected.

volunteer agencies Not-for-profit health care agencies established within a community to meet specific needs.

water deficit An alteration characterized by the loss of fluid in greater proportion than electrolytes.

water excess An alteration characterized by the retention of fluid in greater proportion than electrolytes.

water pollution Contamination of lakes, rivers, and streams by industrial pollutants.

Wernicke's syndrome Illness occurring with advanced stages of vitamin B_1 depletion and accompanied by nystagmus, papillary abnormalities, ataxia, tremor, and stupor.

withdrawal syndrome Physiological and psychological responses that occur when a person physiologically dependent on a substance abruptly withdraws from its use.

witness Person who is present and can testify that he has observed something (such as the signing of a will or consent form).

xenophobia Morbid fear of strangers.

xerostomia Dryness of the mouth caused by cessation of normal salivary secretion caused by various diseases (for example, diabetes) facial nerve paralysis, or may be an adverse reaction to drugs.

zygote Fertilized ovum created by the joining of the mother's ovum and father's sperm.

Index

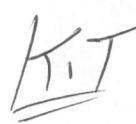

Common Abbreviations

NOTE: Abbreviations in common use can vary widely from place to place. Each institution's list of acceptable abbreviations is the best authority for its records.

°C	degrees Centigrade		EBV	Epstein-Barr virus
°F	degrees Farenheit		ECF	extracellular fluid
µg	microgram		ECG	electrocardiogram
µm	micrometer		ECT	electroconvulsive therapy
ʒ	dram		EDC	estimated date of confinement
@	at		EDD	estimated date of delivery
aa	of each		EEG	electroencephalogram
ABG	arterial blood gas		EKG	electrocardiogram
ac	before meals		elix	elixer
ad lib	freely as desired		EMG	electromyogram
ADL	activities of daily living		ENG	electronystagmography
Ag	silver, antigen		ER	emergency room
AIDS	acquired immunodeficiency syndrome		ERG	electroretinogram
			ESR	erythrocyte sedimentation rate
ALS	amyotrophic lateral sclerosis		ESRD	end-stage renal disease
AM	morning		EST	electroshock therapy
a.m.a.	against medical advice		f ʒ	fluid ounce
AMI	acute myocardial infarction		FANA	fluorescent antinuclear antibody test
amp	ampule		Fe	iron
ARC	AIDS-related complex		FEV	forced expiratory volume
ARDs	adult respiratory distress syndrome		FHR	fetal heart rate
AS	aortic stenosis		FRC	functional residual capacity
ASD	atrial septal defect		FUO	fever of unknown origin
Ba	barium		Fx, fx	fracture, fractional urine test
BE	barium enema		g, gm, Gm	gram
bid	two times a day		Gc, GC	gonococcus
BM, bm	bowel movement		GI	gastrointestinal
BMR	basal metabolic rate		gr	grain
BP	blood pressure		grav, I, II, III, etc	pregnancy one, two, three, etc
BPH	benign prostatic hypertrophy		gtt, gt	drop, drops
BRP	bathroom privileges		GTT	glucose tolerance test
BSA	body surface area		GU	genitourinary
BUN	blood urea nitrogen		GYN, Gyn	gynecological
c̄	with		H_2O	water
c/o	complains of		h	hour
Ca	calcium, cancer, carcinoma		H^+	hydrogen ion
CAD	coronary artery disease		h/o	history of
cap	capsule		H&P	history and physical examination
CAT	computed axial tomography		HAV	hepatitis A virus
cath.	catheter, catheterize		Hb	hemoglobin
CBC	complete blood count		HBAg	hepatitis B antigen
CBR	complete bed rest		HBV	hepatitis B virus
CC	chief complaint		Hct, HCT	hematocrit
cc	cubic centimeter		Hg	mercury
CCU	coronary care unit, critical care unit		Hgb	hemoglobin
CDC	Centers for Disease Control		HIV	human immunodeficiency (AIDS) virus
CEA	carcinoembryonic antigen			
CFT	complement-fixation test		HLA	human lymphocyte antigen
cg	centigram		hs	at bedtime
CHF	congestive heart failure		HSV	herpes simplex virus
CHO	carbohydrate		I&O	intake and output
Cl	chlorine		IC	inspiratory capacity
cm	centimeter		ICP	intracranial pressure
cm^3	cubic centimeter		ICU	intensive care unit
CNS	central nervous system		IDDM	insulin-dependent diabetes mellitus
CO	carbon monoxide		IE	immunoelectrophoresis
CO_2	carbon dioxide		Ig	immunoglobulin
COPD	chronic obstructive pulmonary disease		IgA, etc	immunoglobulin A, etc
			IM	intramuscular
CPK	creatine phosphokinase		IOP	intraocular pressure
CPR	cardiopulmonary resuscitation		IPPB	intermittent positive pressure breathing
CSF	cerebrospinal fluid			
CT	computed tomography		IV	intravenous
CVA	cerebrovascular accident, costovertebral angle		IVP	intravenous push; intravenous pyelogram
CVP	central venous pressure		IVU	intravenous urogram
D&C	dilation and curettage		JRA	juvenile rheumatoid arthritis
D5W	5% dextrose in water		K	potassium
db, dB	decibles		kg	kilogram
dc	discontinue		KUB	kidney, ureters, and bladder (radiograph)
DIC	disseminated intravascular coagulation			
			KVO	keep vein open
diff	differential blood count		L	liter
dil	dilute		L&A	light and accommodation
DJD	degenerative joint disease		LBBB	left bundle branch block
dl	deciliter		LE	lupus erythematosus
DM	diastolic mumur		LGV	lymphogranuloma venereum
DNR	do not resuscitate		LLL	left lower lobe
DOE	dyspnea on exertion		LLQ	left lower quadrant
dx, DX	diagnosis		LMP	last menstrual period